PEDIATRIC SURGERY

PEDIATRIC SURGERY

THIRD EDITION

Keith W. Ashcraft, MD

Emeritus Professor of Surgery
University of Missouri—Kansas City
School of Medicine
Former Surgeon-in-Chief
The Children's Mercy Hospital
Kansas City, Missouri

Associate Editors

J. Patrick Murphy, MD
The Children's Mercy Hospital
Kansas City, Missouri

Ronald J. Sharp, MD
The Children's Mercy Hospital
Kansas City, Missouri

David L. Sigalet, MD, PhD, FRCSC, MSc
Alberta Children's Hospital
Calgary, Alberta, Canada

Charles L. Snyder, MD
The Children's Mercy Hospital
Kansas City, Missouri

W.B. SAUNDERS COMPANY

A Harcourt Health Sciences Company
Philadelphia London New York St. Louis Sydney Toronto

161322

W.B. SAUNDERS COMPANY
A Harcourt Health Sciences Company

The Curtis Center
Independence Square West
Philadelphia, Pennsylvania 19106

Library of Congress Cataloging-in-Publication Data

Pediatric surgery / editor, Keith W. Ashcraft; associate editors, J. Patrick Murphy, Ronald J. Sharp, David L. Sigalet, Charles L. Snyder.—3rd ed.

p.   cm.

Includes bibliographical references and index.

ISBN 0–7216–7312–0

1. Children—Surgery.   I. Ashcraft, Keith W. [DNLM: 1. Surgical Procedures, Operative—in infancy & childhood. WO 925 P3715 2000]

RD137.P43 2000   617.9′8—dc21

DNLM/DLC   98–31214

Editor: Richard H. Lampert
Editorial Assistant: Beth LoGiudice
Senior Production Manager: Frank Polizzano
Copy Editor: Amy L. Cannon
Illustration Specialist: Lisa Lambert
Indexer: Angela Holt

PEDIATRIC SURGERY   ISBN 0–7216–7312–0

Printed in the United States of America.

Last digit is the print number: 9   8   7   6   5   4   3   2   1

CONTRIBUTORS

Elaine J. Abrams, MD
Associate Professor of Clinical Pediatrics, College of Physicians and Surgeons of Columbia University; Director, Family Care Center, Harlem Hospital Center, New York, New York
HUMAN IMMUNODEFICIENCY VIRUS

Craig T. Albanese, MD
Assistant Professor of Surgery and Pediatrics, University of California, San Francisco, Fetal Treatment Center, San Francisco, California
PRENATAL DIAGNOSIS AND SURGICAL INTERVENTION

Uri S. Alon, MD
Professor of Pediatrics, University of Missouri—Kansas City School of Medicine; Pediatric Nephrologist, The Children's Mercy Hospital, Kansas City, Missouri
RENAL IMPAIRMENT

Maria H. Alonso, MD
Assistant Professor of Surgery, Division of Pediatric Surgery, Department of Surgery; Surgical Director, Kidney Transplantation, Children's Hospital Medical Center, Cincinnati, Ohio
SOLID ORGAN TRANSPLANTATION IN CHILDREN

Robert M. Arensman, MD
Lydia J. Fredrickson Professor of Pediatric Surgery, Northwestern University School of Medicine; Surgeon-in-Chief, Children's Memorial Hospital, Chicago, Illinois
CONGENITAL DIAPHRAGMATIC HERNIA AND EVENTRATION

Keith W. Ashcraft, MD
Emeritus Professor of Surgery, University of Missouri—Kansas City School of Medicine; Former Surgeon-in-Chief, The Children's Mercy Hospital, Kansas City, Missouri
THE ESOPHAGUS; ACQUIRED ANORECTAL DISORDERS

Richard G. Azizkhan, MD
Chief of The Division of Pediatric Surgery, Department of Surgery, Director of Pediatric Surgery Training Program, and Professor of Surgery and Pediatrics, University of Cincinnati School of Medicine; Surgeon-in-Chief, Children's Hospital Medical Center, Cincinnati, Ohio
NECROTIZING ENTEROCOLITIS

Daniel A. Bambini, MD
Fellow in Pediatric Surgery, Children's Memorial Hospital, Chicago, Illinois
CONGENITAL DIAPHRAGMATIC HERNIA AND EVENTRATION

Gillian Barker, FRCS
Senior Registrar, Pediatric Surgery, The Hospital for Sick Children, London, England
NEUROBLASTOMA

Edward M. Barksdale, Jr., MD
University of Pittsburgh School of Medicine; Assistant Professor of Pediatric Surgery, Children's Hospital of Pittsburgh, Pittsburgh, Pennsylvania
RHABDOMYOSARCOMA

Robert E. Binda, Jr., MD
Associate Professor of Pediatrics/Anesthesiology, University of Missouri—Kansas City School of Medicine, Kansas City, Missouri
ANESTHETIC CONSIDERATIONS

Jose Boix-Ochoa, MD
Professor of Pediatric Surgery; Chair and Chief of Division of Pediatric Surgery, Department of Pediatric Surgery, Children's Hospital "Vall d'Hebron," Universidad Autônoma de Barcelona, Barcelona, Spain
GASTROESOPHAGEAL REFLUX

Scott J. Boley, MD
Professor of Surgery and Pediatrics, Albert Einstein College of Medicine; Chief of Pediatric Surgical Services, Montefiore Medical Center, Bronx, New York
ANORECTAL CONTINENCE AND MANAGEMENT OF CONSTIPATION

Douglas L. Brockmeyer, MD
Assistant Professor of Neurosurgery, Assistant Professor of Pediatrics, University of Utah Medical Center; Attending Neurosurgeon, Primary Children's Medical Center, Salt Lake City, Utah
HEAD INJURIES IN CHILDREN

Patrick C. Cartwright, MD
Associate Professor of Surgery and Pediatrics, University of Utah; Primary Children's Medical Center, Salt Lake City, Utah
BLADDER AND URETHRA

Michael G. Caty, MD
Assistant Professor of Surgery and Pediatrics, School of Biomedical Sciences, State University of New York at Buffalo; Attending Surgeon, Children's Hospital of Buffalo, Buffalo, New York
NECROTIZING ENTEROCOLITIS

Clinton Cavett, MD
Assistant Professor of Clinical Surgery, University of Virginia School of Medicine, Charlottesville; Director, Pediatric Surgery, Carilion Medical Center for Children, Roanoke, Virginia
MEDIASTINAL TUMORS

Robert E. Cilley, MD
Associate Professor of Surgery and Pediatrics, Pennsylvania State University College of Medicine; Pennsylvania State University Children's Hospital, The Milton S. Hershey Medical Center, Hershey, Pennsylvania
LESIONS OF THE STOMACH

Lisa A. Clark, MD
General Surgery Resident, Duke University, Durham, North Carolina
MALROTATION

Arthur Cooper, MD, MS
Associate Professor of Clinical Surgery, College of Physicians and Surgeons of Columbia University; Chief of Pediatric Surgery, Harlem Hospital Center, New York, New York
HUMAN IMMUNODEFICIENCY VIRUS

Douglas E. Coplen, MD
Assistant Professor, Division of Urology, Washington University School of Medicine; Director of Pediatric Urology, St. Louis Children's Hospital, St. Louis, Missouri
DEVELOPMENTAL AND POSITIONAL ANOMALIES OF THE KIDNEY; URETERAL OBSTRUCTION AND MALFORMATIONS

Arnold G. Coran, MD
Professor of Surgery and Head, Section of Pediatric Surgery, University of Michigan, Pediatric Surgery Associates, Mott Children's Hospital, Ann Arbor, Michigan
NUTRITIONAL SUPPORT OF THE PEDIATRIC SURGICAL PATIENT

Robin T. Cotton, MD
University of Cincinnati Medical Center; Professor, Otolaryngology—Head and Neck Surgery and Director, Pediatric Otolaryngology—Head and Neck Surgery, Children's Hospital Medical Center, Cincinnati, Ohio
AIRWAY MALFORMATIONS AND RECONSTRUCTION

Sidney Cywes, MMed (Surg), FRCS, FRCS(Edin)
Emeritus Professor of Pediatric Surgery, University of Cape Town and Red Cross War Memorial Children's Hospital, Cape Town, South Africa
INTESTINAL ATRESIA AND STENOSIS

Peter W. Dillon, MD
Associate Professor of Surgery and Pediatrics, Pennsylvania State University College of Medicine; Chief, Section of Pediatric Surgery, Pennsylvania State University Children's Hospital, The Milton S. Hershey Medical Center, Hershey, Pennsylvania
LESIONS OF THE STOMACH

Sigmund H. Ein, FRCSC
Associate Professor, Department of Surgery, Faculty of Medicine, University of Toronto; Staff Surgeon, Division of General Surgery, The Hospital for Sick Children; Consultant Staff, Department of Newborn and Developmental Paediatrics, Women's College Campus, Sunnybrook and Women's College, Health Sciences Centre; Associate Staff, Department of Surgery, Mount Sinai Hospital; Provisional Staff, Department of Obstetrics, Gynecology and Pediatrics, Wellesley Hospital, Toronto, Ontario, Canada
APPENDICITIS

Mary E. Fallat, MD
Associate Professor of Surgery, Division of Pediatric Surgery, University of Louisville, Louisville, Kentucky
INTUSSUSCEPTION

Howard C. Filston, MD
Professor of Pediatric Surgery and Pediatrics, University of Tennessee Graduate Medical Center; Chief of Pediatric Surgery and Vice Chair, Department of Surgery, University of Tennessee Memorial Hospital, Knoxville, Tennessee
ESOPHAGEAL ATRESIA AND TRACHEOESOPHAGEAL MALFORMATIONS

Eric W. Fonkalsrud, MD
Professor and Chief of Pediatric Surgery, University of California, Los Angeles, School of Medicine, Los Angeles, California
INFLAMMATORY BOWEL DISEASE AND GASTROINTESTINAL NEOPLASMS

Barbara A. Gaines, MD
Chief Resident, Surgery, Children's Hospital of Pittsburgh, University of Pittsburgh, Pittsburgh, Pennsylvania
GASTROSCHISIS AND OMPHALOCELE

Alan S. Gamis, MD, MPH
Assistant Professor of Pediatrics, University of Missouri—Kansas City; Pediatric Hematologist/Oncologist, The Children's Mercy Hospital, Kansas City, Missouri
LYMPHOMAS

Victor F. Garcia, MD
Pediatric and General Surgeon and Director, Trauma Services, Children's Hospital Medical Center, Cincinnati, Ohio
UMBILICAL AND OTHER ABDOMINAL WALL HERNIAS

Brian F. Gilchrist, MD
Assistant Professor, Surgery and Pediatrics, State University of New York, College of Medicine; Assistant Professor, Pediatric Surgery, University Hospital, Brooklyn, New York
INITIAL HOSPITAL ASSESSMENT AND MANAGEMENT OF THE TRAUMA PATIENT

George K. Gittes, MD
Associate Professor of Surgery, University of Missouri—Kansas City School of Medicine; Director of Surgical Research, The Children's Mercy Hospital, Kansas City, Missouri
LESIONS OF THE PANCREAS AND SPLEEN

Diller B. Groff, MD
Professor of Surgery and Director, Division of Pediatric Surgery, University of Louisville; Chief of Surgery, Kosair Children's Hospital, Louisville, Kentucky
MECONIUM DISEASE

Jonathan I. Groner, MD
Assistant Professor of Surgery, College of Medicine, Ohio State University; Director of Trauma Services, The Children's Hospital, Columbus, Ohio
RENAL NEOPLASMS

David P. Gruber, MD
Fellow, Division of Pediatric Neurosurgery, University of Utah School of Medicine, Primary Children's Medical Center, Salt Lake City, Utah
HEAD INJURIES IN CHILDREN

Gerald M. Haase, MD
Clinical Professor of Surgery, University of Colorado School of Medicine; Attending Staff Surgeon and Former Chair, Department of Surgery, The Children's Hospital, Denver, Colorado
ADJUVANT THERAPY IN CHILDHOOD CANCER

Michael R. Harrison, MD
Professor of Surgery and Pediatrics, Department of Surgery, Chief, Division of Pediatric Surgery, and Director, Fetal Treatment Center, University of California, San Francisco; Surgeon-in-Chief, Packard Children's Health Services, Lucile Packard Children's Hospital, Palo Alto, California
PRENATAL DIAGNOSIS AND SURGICAL INTERVENTION

André Hebra, MD
Assistant Professor of Surgery and Pediatrics, Division of Pediatric Surgery, Medical University of South Carolina, Charleston, South Carolina
BRONCHOPULMONARY MALFORMATIONS

Stanley Hellerstein, MD
Professor of Pediatrics, Pediatric Nephrologist, and Ernest L. Glasscock, MD, Chair in Pediatric Research, The Children's Mercy Hospital, University of Missouri—Kansas City School of Medicine, Kansas City, Missouri
RENAL IMPAIRMENT

W. Hardy Hendren, MD
Robert Gross Professor of Surgery, Harvard Medical School; Chief of Surgery Emeritus, Children's Hospital; Visiting Surgeon, Massachusetts General Hospital, Boston, Massachusetts
URETHRAL VALVES

M. John Hicks, MD, DDS, PhD
Associate Professor of Pathology, Baylor College of Medicine; Director of Surgical Pathology, Texas Children's Hospital, Houston, Texas
NEVUS AND MELANOMA

J. Laurance Hill, MD
Professor of Surgery, University of Maryland, Baltimore, Maryland
FOREIGN BODIES

Ronald B. Hirschl, MD, MS
Associate Professor of Surgery, University of Michigan, Ann Arbor, Michigan
MECHANICAL VENTILATION IN PEDIATRIC SURGICAL DISEASE

George W. Holcomb III, MD
Katharine B. Richardson Professor of Pediatric Surgery, University of Missouri—Kansas City School of Medicine; Surgeon-in-Chief, The Children's Mercy Hospital, Kansas City, Missouri
GASTROSCHISIS AND OMPHALOCELE

Robert S. Hollabaugh, MD
Clinical Associate Professor of Surgery and Pediatrics, University of Tennessee Center for Health Sciences; Active Staff, Le Bonheur Children's Medical Center, Memphis, Tennessee
ALIMENTARY TRACT DUPLICATIONS

Alexander Holschneider, MD, PhD
Professor, University of Cologne; Chief of The Hospital for Sick Children, Department of Pediatric Surgery, Cologne, Germany
HIRSCHSPRUNG'S DISEASE

Joseph A. Iocono, MD
Senior Resident, General Surgery, Pennsylvania State University College of Medicine, The Milton S. Hershey Medical Center, Hershey, Pennsylvania
SURGICAL INFECTIOUS DISEASE

Tom Jaksic, MD, PhD
Associate Professor of Surgery, Baylor College of Medicine; Staff Surgeon, Texas Children's Hospital, Houston, Texas
NEVUS AND MELANOMA

Douglas A. Katz, MD
Fellow in Pediatric Surgery, Arkansas Children's Hospital, University of Arkansas, Little Rock, Arkansas
PHYSIOLOGY OF THE NEWBORN

Michael A. Keating, MD
Division of Pediatric Urology, Nemours Children's Clinic; Chair, Department of Children's Surgery, Arnold Palmer Hospital for Children and Women, Orlando, Florida
PRUNE-BELLY SYNDROME

Edward M. Kiely, FRCSI, FRCS, FRCPCH
Consultant Paediatric Surgeon, The Hospital for Sick Children, London, England
NEUROBLASTOMA

Denis R. King, MD
Clinical Associate Professor of Surgery, The Ohio State University College of Medicine; Staff Surgeon and Director of the Nutrition Support Service, The Children's Hospital, Columbus, Ohio
RENAL NEOPLASMS

Susan G. Kreissman, MD
Associate Professor of Pediatrics, Indiana University School of Medicine; Member, Medical Staff, Department of Pediatrics, Section of Pediatric Hematology/Oncology, James Whitcomb Riley Hospital for Children, Indianapolis, Indiana
ADJUVANT THERAPY IN CHILDHOOD CANCER

Thomas M. Krummel, MD
John A. and Marian T. Waldhausen Professor and Chair, Department of Surgery, Pennsylvania State University College of Medicine, The Milton S. Hershey Medical Center, Hershey, Pennsylvania
SURGICAL INFECTIOUS DISEASE

Jean-Martin Laberge, MD, FRCSC
Associate Professor, Department of Surgery and Program Director, Pediatric General Surgery, McGill University; Director, Pediatric General Surgery, Montreal Children's Hospital, Montreal, Quebec, Canada
TERATOMAS, DERMOIDS AND OTHER SOFT TISSUE TUMORS

Michael P. La Quaglia, MD
Associate Professor of Surgery, Cornell University Medical College; Chief, Pediatric Surgical Service, Memorial Sloan-Kettering Cancer Center, New York, New York
LESIONS OF THE LIVER

Gary K. Lofland, MD
Clinical Professor of Surgery, University of Missouri—Kansas City School of Medicine; Joseph Boon Gregg Chair, Section of Cardiac Surgery, The Children's Mercy Hospital, Kansas City, Missouri
THORACIC TRAUMA IN CHILDREN

Valerie K. Logsdon-Pokorny, MD
Assistant Professor, University of Utah School of Medicine, Salt Lake City, Utah
PEDIATRIC GYNECOLOGY

Claudia Marhuenda, MD
Attending Pediatric Surgeon, Department of Pediatric Surgery, Children's Hospital "Vall d'Hebron," Universidad Autôuoma de Barcelona, Barcelona, Spain
GASTROESOPHAGEAL REFLUX

Ruth D. Mayforth, MD, PhD
Chief Resident, Pediatric Surgery, Washington University; St. Louis Children's Hospital, St. Louis, Missouri
ENDOCRINE DISORDERS AND TUMORS

Charles W. McGill, MD
Pediatric Surgeon, Marshfield Clinic, Marshfield, Wisconsin
BITES

Peter H. Mestad, MD
Associate Professor, Pediatric Anesthesiology, University of Missouri—Kansas City School of Medicine; Chief, Department of Anesthesiology, The Children's Mercy Hospital, Kansas City, Missouri
ANESTHETIC CONSIDERATIONS

Alastair J. W. Millar, MBChB, FRCS, FRCS(Edin)
Associate Professor and Principal Pediatric Surgeon, University of Cape Town and Red Cross War Memorial Children's Hospital, Cape Town, South Africa
INTESTINAL ATRESIA AND STENOSIS

Eugene Minevich, MD
Clinical Instructor, University of Cincinnati Medical Center; Attending Urologist, Children's Hospital Medical Center, Cincinnati, Ohio
URINARY TRACT INFECTION AND VESICOURETERAL REFLUX

J. Patrick Murphy, MD
Associate Professor of Surgery, University of Missouri—Kansas City; Chief of Section of Urology, The Children's Mercy Hospital, Kansas City, Missouri
EXSTROPHY OF THE BLADDER; HYPOSPADIAS

Don K. Nakayama, MD
Colin G. Thomas, Jr, Distinguished Professor of Surgery and Pediatrics, University of North Carolina at Chapel Hill; Surgeon-in-Chief, North Carolina Children's Hospital, Chapel Hill, North Carolina
BREAST DISEASES IN CHILDREN

Wallace W. Neblett III, MD
Professor of Surgery and Pediatrics, Vanderbilt
University School of Medicine; Chair, Department
of Pediatric Surgery, Vanderbilt University Medical
Center, Nashville, Tennessee
GASTROSCHISIS AND OMPHALOCELE

Kurt D. Newman, MD
Professor of Surgery and Pediatrics, George
Washington University School of Medicine; Senior
Attending Surgeon and Vice-Chair, Department of
Surgery, Children's Hospital, Washington, D.C.
EXTRACORPOREAL MEMBRANE OXYGENATION

Luong T. Nguyen, MD, FRCSC
Associate Professor, Department of Surgery, McGill
University; Attending Surgeon, Pediatric General
Surgery, Montreal Children's Hospital, Montreal,
Quebec, Canada
TERATOMAS, DERMOIDS, AND OTHER SOFT TISSUE TUMORS

Stephen W. Nicholas, MD
Associate Professor of Clinical Pediatrics, College
of Physicians and Surgeons of Columbia
University; Director, Incarnation Children's Center,
New York, New York
HUMAN IMMUNODEFICIENCY VIRUS

James F. Nigro, MD
Assistant Professor of Pediatrics and Dermatology,
Baylor College of Medicine, Houston, Texas
NEVUS AND MELANOMA

John Noseworthy, MD
Professor of Surgery, Jefferson Medical College,
Philadelphia, Pennsylvania; Associate Professor of
Surgery, Mayo Medical School, Rochester,
Minnesota; Chair, Department of Surgery and
Associate Medical Director, Nemours Children's
Clinic, Jacksonville, Florida
TESTICULAR TORSION

Keith T. Oldham, MD
Professor and Chief, Division of Pediatric Surgery,
Vice-Chair, Department of Surgery, Medical College
of Wisconsin; Surgeon-in-Chief, Children's Hospital
of Wisconsin, Milwaukee, Wisconsin
MALROTATION

H. Biemann Othersen, Jr., MD
Professor of Surgery and Pediatrics, Chief, Division
of Pediatric Surgery, Medical University of South
Carolina, Charleston, South Carolina
BRONCHOPULMONARY MALFORMATIONS

Alberto Peña, MD
Professor of Surgery, Albert Einstein College of
Medicine, Bronx; Chief of Surgery, Schneider
Children's Hospital, Long Island Jewish Medical
Center, New Hyde Park, New York
IMPERFORATE ANUS AND CLOACAL MALFORMATIONS

Susan Pokorny, MD
Chair, Department of Obstetrics/Gynecology, Kelsey
Seybold Clinics, Houston, Texas
PEDIATRIC GYNECOLOGY

Nigel J. Price, MD, FRCSC
Assistant Professor of Orthopaedic Surgery,
University of Missouri—Kansas City; Director,
Spinal Deformities, The Children's Mercy Hospital,
Kansas City, Missouri
PEDIATRIC ORTHOPEDIC TRAUMA

Max L. Ramenofsky, MD
Professor of Surgery and Chief, Pediatric Surgery,
State University of New York, College of Medicine;
Professor and Chief, Pediatric Surgery, University
Hospital—Brooklyn, New York
INITIAL HOSPITAL ASSESSMENT AND MANAGEMENT OF THE
TRAUMA PATIENT

Stephen C. Raynor, MD
Assistant Clinical Professor of Surgery, University
of Nebraska Medical Center, Omaha, Nebraska
CIRCUMCISION

Mark A. Rich, MD
Director, Division of Pediatric Urology, Nemours
Children's Clinic; Staff Urologist, Arnold Palmer
Hospital for Children and Women, Orlando,
Florida
PRUNE-BELLY SYNDROME

Heinz Rode, MBChB, MMed(Surg), FRCS(Edin)
Professor, University of Cape Town; Chief Pediatric
Surgeon, Red Cross War Memorial Children's
Hospital, Cape Town, South Africa
INTESTINAL ATRESIA AND STENOSIS

Frederick C. Ryckman, MD
Associate Professor of Surgery, Division of
Pediatric Surgery, Department of Surgery; Surgical
Director, Liver Transplantation, Children's Hospital
Medical Center, Cincinnati, Ohio
SOLID ORGAN TRANSPLANTATION IN CHILDREN

Thomas T. Sato, MD
Assistant Professor of Surgery, Medical College of
Wisconsin; Attending Pediatric Surgeon, Children's
Hospital of Wisconsin, Milwaukee, Wisconsin
EXTRACORPOREAL MEMBRANE OXYGENATION

Robert C. Shamberger, MD
Associate Professor of Surgery, Harvard Medical
School; Senior Associate in Surgery, Children's
Hospital, Boston, Massachusetts
CHEST WALL DEFORMITIES

Ronald J. Sharp, MD
Associate Professor of Surgery, University of
Missouri—Kansas City School of Medicine;
Director, Burn Unit and Trauma Service, The
Children's Mercy Hospital, Kansas City, Missouri
BURNS; INTERSEX

Kenneth S. Shaw, MD, FRCSC
Assistant Professor, Department of Surgery, McGill
University; Attending Surgeon, Pediatric General
Surgery, Montreal Children's Hospital, Montreal,
Quebec, Canada
TERATOMAS, DERMOIDS, AND OTHER SOFT TISSUE TUMORS

Curtis A. Sheldon, MD
Professor of Surgery, University of Cincinnati
Medical Center; Director, Division of Pediatric
Urology, Children's Hospital Medical Center,
Cincinnati, Ohio
URINARY TRACT INFECTION AND VESICOURETERAL REFLUX

Nicholas A. Shorter, MD
Associate Professor of Surgery and Pediatrics,
Dartmouth Medical School, Hanover; Attending
Surgeon, Children's Hospital at Dartmouth,
Dartmouth-Hitchcock Medical Center, Lebanon,
New Hampshire
ESOPHAGEAL ATRESIA AND TRACHEOESOPHAGEAL
MALFORMATIONS

Linda M. D. Shortliffe, MD
Professor and Chair, Department of Urology,
Stanford University School of Medicine; Chief of
Urology, Stanford University Medical Center; Chief
of Pediatric Urology, Lucile Salter Packard
Children's Hospital at Stanford, Stanford,
California
UNDESCENDED TESTIS AND TESTICULAR TUMORS

David L. Sigalet, MD, PhD, FRCSC, MSc
Associate Professor, University of Calgary;
Pediatric Surgeon, Alberta Children's Hospital,
Calgary, Alberta, Canada
BILIARY TRACT DISORDERS AND PORTAL HYPERTENSION

Michael A. Skinner, MD
Associate Professor of Surgery, Duke University
Medical Center, Durham, North Carolina
ENDOCRINE DISORDERS AND TUMORS

Samuel D. Smith, MD
Professor of Surgery, University of Arkansas for
Medical Sciences; Chief of Pediatric Surgery,
Arkansas Children's Hospital, Little Rock, Arkansas
PHYSIOLOGY OF THE NEWBORN

Brent W. Snow, MD
Professor of Surgery and Pediatrics, University of
Utah; Primary Children's Medical Center, Salt Lake
City, Utah
BLADDER AND URETHRA

Charles L. Snyder, MD
Assistant Professor of Surgery, University of
Missouri—Kansas City School of Medicine; Staff
Surgeon, The Children's Mercy Hospital, Kansas
City, Missouri
ABDOMINAL AND GENITOURINARY TRAUMA; MECKEL'S
DIVERTICULUM

Howard M. Snyder III, MD
Professor of Surgery in Urology, University of
Pennsylvania School of Medicine; Academic
Director, Pediatric Urology, Children's Hospital of
Philadelphia, Philadelphia, Pennsylvania
URETERAL OBSTRUCTION AND MALFORMATIONS

Rowena Spencer, MD
Former Associate Professor of Surgery, Louisiana
State University School of Medicine; Former
Clinical Associate Professor of Surgery, Tulane
University School of Medicine, New Orleans,
Louisiana
CONJOINED TWINS

James C. Stanley, MD
Professor of Surgery, University of Michigan; Head,
Section of Vascular Surgery, University Hospital,
Ann Arbor, Michigan
RENOVASCULAR HYPERTENSION

Gustavo Stringel, MD
Professor of Surgery and Pediatrics, New York
Medical College; Attending Surgeon, Westchester
Medical Center, Valhalla, New York
HEMANGIOMAS AND LYMPHANGIOMAS

Edward P. Tagge, MD
Associate Professor of Surgery and Pediatrics,
Division of Pediatric Surgery, Medical University
of South Carolina, Charleston, South Carolina
BRONCHOPULMONARY MALFORMATIONS

David Tapper, MD
Professor of Surgery and Vice-Chair, Department of
Surgery, University of Washington School of
Medicine; Surgeon-in-Chief and Director,
Department of Surgery, Children's Hospital and
Regional Medical Center, Seattle, Washington
HEAD AND NECK SINUSES AND MASSES

Daniel H. Teitelbaum, MD
Assistant Professor of Surgery, Section of Pediatric
Surgery, University of Michigan, Pediatric Surgery
Associates, Mott Children's Hospital, Ann Arbor,
Michigan
NUTRITIONAL SUPPORT OF THE PEDIATRIC SURGICAL
PATIENT

Thomas F. Tracy, Jr., MD
Professor of Surgery and Pediatrics, Brown
University School of Medicine; Chief, Division of
Pediatric Surgery and Pediatric Surgeon-in-Chief,
Rhode Island Hospital/Hasbro Children's Hospital,
Providence, Rhode Island
GROIN HERNIAS AND HYDROCELES

David W. Tuggle, MD
Associate Professor of Surgery, University of Oklahoma College of Medicine; Chief, Section of Pediatric Surgery, Children's Hospital of Oklahoma, University of Oklahoma College of Medicine, Oklahoma City, Oklahoma
ACQUIRED PULMONARY AND PLEURAL DISORDERS

Charles S. Turner, MD
Associate Professor of Surgery and Pediatrics, Wake Forest University School of Medicine, Winston-Salem, North Carolina
VASCULAR ACCESS

Benno M. Ure, MD, PhD
Consultant Pediatric Surgeon, Wilhelmina Children's Hospital, University Medical Center Utrecht, Utrecht, The Netherlands
HIRSCHSPRUNG'S DISEASE

Roger W. Voigt, MB, ChB
Assistant Professor of Surgery, University of Maryland, Baltimore, Maryland
FOREIGN BODIES

Jeffrey Wacksman, MD
Associate Professor of Clinical Surgery, University of Cincinnati Medical Center; Associate Director, Division of Pediatric Urology, Children's Hospital Medical Center, Cincinnati, Ohio
URINARY TRACT INFECTION AND VESICOURETERAL REFLUX

John H. T. Waldhausen, MD
Assistant Professor of Surgery, University of Washington School of Medicine; Attending Surgeon, Children's Hospital and Regional Medical Center, Seattle, Washington
HEAD AND NECK SINUSES AND MASSES

Marion L. Walker, MD
Professor of Neurosurgery and Division of Pediatric Neurosurgery, University of Utah, Primary Children's Medical Center, Salt Lake City, Utah
HEAD INJURIES IN CHILDREN

Eric M. Wallen, MD
Senior Resident, Department of Urology, Stanford University Medical Center, Stanford, California
UNDESCENDED TESTIS AND TESTICULAR TUMORS

Bradley A. Warady, MD
Professor of Pediatrics, University of Missouri—Kansas City School of Medicine; Chief, Section of Pediatric Nephrology and Director, Dialysis and Transplantation, The Children's Mercy Hospital, Kansas City, Missouri
RENAL IMPAIRMENT

Brad W. Warner, MD
Associate Professor of Surgery, Division of Pediatric Surgery, University of Cincinnati College of Medicine; Attending Surgeon, Division of

Pediatric Surgery, Children's Hospital Medical Center, Cincinnati, Ohio
EXSTROPHY OF THE CLOACA

Thomas R. Weber, MD
Professor of Surgery and Pediatrics, St. Louis University School of Medicine; Director of Pediatric Surgery, Cardinal Glennon Children's Hospital, St. Louis, Missouri
GROIN HERNIAS AND HYDROCELES

Gerard Weinberg, MD
Associate Professor of Surgery and Pediatrics, Albert Einstein College of Medicine; Director of Pediatric Surgery, Weiler Hospital/Montefiore Medical Center, Bronx, New York
ANORECTAL CONTINENCE AND MANAGEMENT OF CONSTIPATION

Brian M. Wicklund, MD, CM, MPh
Assistant Professor, Department of Pediatrics, University of Missouri—Kansas City School of Medicine; Director, Pediatric Hemophilia Center, Kansas City Regional Hemophilia Treatment Center; Pediatric Hematologist/Oncologist, The Children's Mercy Hospital, Kansas City, Missouri
COAGULOPATHIES AND SICKLE CELL DISEASE

Eugene S. Wiener, MD
Professor of Surgery, University of Pittsburgh School of Medicine; Surgeon-in-Chief, Chief of General Pediatric Surgery, Children's Hospital of Pittsburgh, Pittsburgh, Pennsylvania
RHABDOMYOSARCOMA

J. Paul Willging, MD
University of Cincinnati Medical Center; Associate Professor, Otolaryngology—Head and Neck Surgery, Cincinnati Children's Hospital, Cincinnati, Ohio
AIRWAY MALFORMATIONS AND RECONSTRUCTION

Gerald M. Woods, MD
Professor of Pediatrics, University of Missouri—Kansas City School of Medicine; Chief, Section of Hematology-Oncology, Director, Sickle Cell Program, and Pediatric Hematologist/Oncologist, The Children's Mercy Hospital, Kansas City, Missouri
COAGULOPATHIES AND SICKLE CELL DISEASE

Earle L. Wrenn, Jr., MD
Le Bonheur Children's Medical Center; Clinical Professor of Surgery, University of Tennessee School of Medicine, Memphis, Tennessee
ALIMENTARY TRACT DUPLICATIONS

Moritz M. Ziegler, MD
Professor of Surgery, Harvard Medical School; Chair, Department of Surgery and Surgeon-in-Chief, Children's Hospital, Boston, Massachusetts
EXSTROPHY OF THE CLOACA

PREFACE

The preparation of a textbook on the subject of pediatric surgery becomes more difficult with the passage of time. The first edition of this book, which Tom Holder and I put together 20 years ago, contained as many pages as does this third edition. The amount of knowledge, however, has grown exponentially in some areas and arithmetically in others, but it has grown in all. The attempt to summarize this information while keeping to one volume and to a size that is portable requires compression, which will not bother the experienced reader but may confuse the student. The study of the history of pediatric surgery has been of great value in the development of almost all of the advances in the surgical practice of pediatrics. It is helpful to return, on occasion, to the older books in order to both appreciate the state of the art at present and to consider avenues to be taken for further progress.

This book intentionally contains little in the way of surgical technique. The technical changes in both general and pediatric surgery are progressing at such a rate that many of the procedures done at the time a chapter was written are being superseded by more popular, less invasive methods today. There are a great number of surgical technical books being published for those whose questions center on the cur-

rent techniques. That is not to say all of the newer methods are necessarily better than the old. There is an aspect of art to the practice of a surgical procedure that, in my opinion, requires the handling of tissues with tenderness and skill not yet seen using elongated instruments thrust through small ports with organs visualized on a large screen rather than up close and personal. Perhaps it is that loss of the personal touch that bothers me so much. I have often told pediatric surgical resident candidates that if they can learn to successfully correct hypospadias, they will have mastered surgical technique. I don't think that the construction of a urethra for correction of hypospadias will ever be done using gadgets much more sophisticated than delicate tissue forceps and fine instruments with which precise sutures may be placed in tissue that is handled with great respect. So we forego surgical techniques and allot more space than ever before to the basics of surgical information that will be useful to all types of surgeons.

I have just retired from the practice of pediatric surgery. I leave the future of this book in the capable hands of my associate editors. We all hope that this edition will be a source of solid information and great help in the treatment of your patients.

Keith W. Ashcraft, MD
January 2000

CONTENTS

1

PHYSIOLOGY OF THE NEWBORN

Douglas A. Katz, MD • Samuel D. Smith, MD

Of all pediatric patients, the neonate possesses the most distinctive and rapidly changing physiologic characteristics. These changes are due to the newborn's adaptation from placental support to the extrauterine environment, early organ maturation, and the demands of rapid growth and development. Due to these dynamic physiologic alterations, this chapter emphasizes the neonate.

Newborns may be classified based on gestational age and weight. Preterm babies are those born before 38 weeks of gestation. Term babies are those born between 38 and 42 weeks of gestation. Postterm babies have a gestation that exceeds 42 weeks. Babies whose weight is below the 10th percentile for age are small-for-gestational-age (SGA), whereas those whose weight is at or above the 98th percentile are large-for-gestational-age (LGA). The babies whose weight falls between these extremes are appropriate-for-gestational-age (AGA).

SGA newborns are thought to suffer intrauterine growth retardation as a result of placental, maternal, or fetal abnormalities. Conditions associated with deviation in intrauterine growth are shown in Figure 1–1. SGA infants have a body weight below what is appropriate for their age, yet their body length and head circumference are age appropriate. To classify an infant as SGA, the gestational age must be estimated by the physical findings summarized in Table 1–1.

Although SGA infants may weigh the same as premature infants, they have different physiologic characteristics. Due to intrauterine malnutrition, body fat levels are frequently below 1% of the total body weight. This lack of insulation increases the risk of cold stress with SGA infants. Hypoglycemia develops earlier in SGA infants due to higher metabolic activity, and SGA infants have reduced liver glycogen levels due to intrauterine malnutrition. The red blood cell (RBC) volume and the total blood volume are much higher in the SGA infant compared with the preterm average for gestational age or the non-SGA full-term infant. This rise in RBC volume frequently leads to polycythemia, with an associated rise in blood viscosity. Due to the ade-

quate length of gestation, the SGA infant has pulmonary function approaching that of an average-for-gestational-age or a full-term infant.

Infants born before 38 weeks of gestation, regardless of birth weight, are considered premature. The premature infant's skin is thin and transparent with an absence of plantar creases. Fingers are soft and malleable; ears have poorly developed cartilage. In females, the labia minora appear enlarged, but the labia majora are small. In males, the testicles are usually undescended, and the scrotum is undevel-

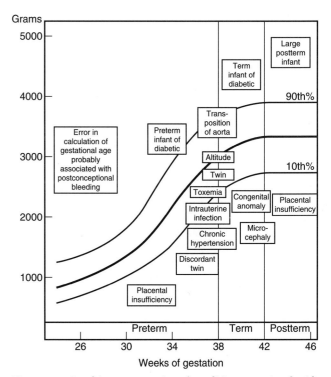

Figure 1–1. Graphic representation of conditions associated with deviations in intrauterine growth. The boxes symbolize the approximate birth weight and gestational age at which the condition is likely to occur. (Adapted from Avery ME, Villee D, Baker S, et al: Neonatology. In Avery ME, First LR [eds]: Pediatric Medicine. Baltimore, Williams & Wilkins, 1989, p 148.)

TABLE 1-1. Clinical Criteria for Classification of Low-Birth-Weight Infants

Criteria	36 wk (Premature)	37–38 wk (Borderline Premature)	39 wk (Full Term)
Plantar creases	Rare, shallow	Heel remains smooth	Creases throughout sole
Size of breast nodule	Not palpable to <3 mm	4 mm	Visible (7 mm)
Head hair	Cotton-wool quality		Silky; each strand can be distinguished
Earlobe	Shapeless, pliable with little cartilage		Rigid with cartilage
Testicular descent and scrotal changes	Small scrotum with rugal patch; testes not completely descended	Gradual descent	Enlarged scrotum creased with rugae; fully descended testes

Adapted from Avery ME, Villee D, Baker S, et al: Neonatology. In Avery ME, First LR (eds): Pediatric Medicine. Baltimore, Williams & Wilkins, 1989, p 148.

oped. Special problems with the preterm infant include the following:

1. Weak suck reflex
2. Inadequate gastrointestinal absorption
3. Hyaline membrane disease (HMD)
4. Intraventricular hemorrhage
5. Hypothermia
6. Patent ductus arteriosus
7. Apnea
8. Hyperbilirubinemia

□ Specific Physiologic Problems of the Newborn

Fetal levels of glucose, calcium, and magnesium are carefully maintained by maternal regulation. The transition to extrauterine life can have profound effects on the physiologic well-being of the newborn.

GLUCOSE METABOLISM

The fetus maintains a blood glucose value 70 to 80% of maternal value by facilitated diffusion across the placenta. There is a buildup of glycogen stores in the liver, skeleton, and cardiac muscles during the later stages of fetal development but little gluconeogenesis. The newborn must depend on glycolysis until exogenous glucose is supplied. Following delivery, the baby depletes its hepatic glycogen stores within 2 to 3 hours. Glycogen stores are more rapidly reduced in premature and SGA babies. The newborn is severely limited in his or her ability to use fat and protein as substrates to synthesize glucose.

Hypoglycemia

Clinical signs of hypoglycemia are nonspecific and may include a weak or high-pitched cry, cyanosis, apnea, jitteriness, apathy, seizures, abnormal eye movements, temperature instability, hypotonia, and weak suck. Some infants, however, exhibit no signs, despite extremely low blood glucose levels.

Neonatal hypoglycemia is generally defined as a glucose level lower than 40 mg/dl. After 72 hours of age, plasma glucose levels should be 40 mg/dl or more.[1] Infants who are at high risk for developing hypoglycemia require frequent glucose monitoring. Because most newborns who require surgical procedures are at risk to develop hypoglycemia, a 10% glucose infusion is usually started on admission to the hospital, and blood glucose levels are measured at the bedside and confirmed by periodic laboratory determinations. If the blood glucose level falls below 40 mg/dl or if any signs of hypoglycemia are present, an hourly bolus infusion of 1 to 2 ml/kg (4 to 8 mg/kg/min) of 10% glucose is given intravenously (IV). If a central venous line is present, concentrations of up to 50% glucose may be used. During the first 36 to 48 hours after a major surgical procedure, because fluid and electrolyte adjustments are necessary, the dextrose concentration in the maintenance IV solution may need to be varied from 5 to 15%, depending on the blood and urine glucose determinations. Rarely, hydrocortisone, glucagon, or somatostatin is used to treat persistent hypoglycemia.

Hyperglycemia

Hyperglycemia is a common problem with the use of total parenteral nutrition (TPN) in very immature infants who are less than 30 weeks' gestation and less than 1.1 kg birth weight. These infants are usually fewer than 3 days of age and are frequently septic.[2] The cause of hyperglycemia appears to be an inadequate insulin response to glucose. Hyperglycemia may cause intraventricular hemorrhage and water and electrolyte losses from glucosuria. The glucose concentration and infusion rate of the TPN must be adjusted based on serum glucose levels. Full parenteral caloric support is achieved with incremental increases in glucose, usually over several days. Occasionally, IV insulin at 0.001 to 0.01 U/kg/min is needed to maintain normoglycemia.

CALCIUM

Calcium is continuously delivered to the fetus by active transport across the placenta. Of the total amount of calcium transferred across the placenta,

75% occurs after 28 weeks' gestation.[3] This observation partially accounts for the high incidence of hypocalcemia in extremely preterm infants. Any neonate has a tendency for hypocalcemia due to limited calcium stores, renal immaturity, and relative hypoparathyroidism secondary to suppression by high fetal calcium levels. Newborn calcium levels usually reach their nadir 24 to 48 hours after delivery, when parathormone responses become effective. Hypocalcemia is defined as an ionized calcium level of less than 1 mg/dl. At greatest risk for hypocalcemia are preterm infants, newborn surgical patients, and infants of complicated pregnancies, such as those of diabetic mothers or those receiving bicarbonate infusions. Calcitonin, which inhibits calcium mobilization from the bone, is increased in premature and asphyxiated infants.

Exchange transfusions or massive transfusions of citrated blood can result in the formation of calcium citrate complexes, reducing the ionized serum calcium levels to dangerous or even fatal levels. Late-onset (>48 hours of age) hypocalcemia is less frequent now that most formulas are low in phosphate.

Signs of hypocalcemia may include jitteriness, seizures, cyanosis, vomiting, and myocardial depression, some of which are similar to the signs of hypoglycemia. Hypocalcemic infants have increased muscle tone, which helps differentiate infants with hypocalcemia from those with hypoglycemia. Ionized calcium levels are easily determined in most intensive care settings. Symptomatic hypocalcemia is treated with 10% calcium gluconate administered IV at a dosage of 1 to 2 ml/kg over 10 minutes while monitoring the electrocardiogram. Asymptomatic hypocalcemia is best treated with calcium gluconate in a dose of 50 mg of elemental calcium/kg/day added to the maintenance fluid: 1 ml of 10% calcium gluconate contains 9 mg of elemental calcium. Calcium mixed with sodium bicarbonate forms an insoluble precipitate. If possible, parenteral calcium should be given through a central venous line.

MAGNESIUM

Magnesium is actively transported across the placenta. Half of total body magnesium is in the plasma and soft tissues. Hypomagnesemia occurs with growth retardation, with maternal diabetes, after exchange transfusions, and with hypoparathyroidism. Magnesium and calcium metabolism are interrelated. The same infants at risk for hypocalcemia are also at risk for hypomagnesemia. Whenever an infant who has seizures that are believed to be associated with hypocalcemia does not respond to calcium therapy, magnesium deficiency should be suspected and confirmed by obtaining a serum magnesium level. Emergent treatment consists of magnesium sulfate solution, 25 to 50 mg/kg IV every 6 hours until normal levels are obtained.

BLOOD VOLUME

Total RBC volume is at its highest point at delivery. Estimation of blood volume for premature in-

TABLE 1-2. Estimation of Blood Volume

Group	Blood Volume (ml/kg)
Premature infants	85–100
Term newborns	85
>1 mo	75
3 mo–adult	70

Adapted from Rowe PC (ed): The Harriet Lane Handbook (11th ed). Chicago, Year Book Medical, 1987, p 25.

fants, term neonates, and infants are summarized in Table 1–2. By about 3 months of age, total blood volume per kilogram is nearly equal to adult levels. The newborn blood volume is affected by shifts of blood between the placenta and the baby prior to clamping the cord. Infants with delayed cord clamping have higher hemoglobin levels.[4] A hematocrit greater than 50% suggests placental transfusion has occurred.

Polycythemia

A central venous hemoglobin level greater than 22 g/dl or a hematocrit value greater than 65% during the 1st week of life is defined as polycythemia. After the central venous hematocrit value reaches 65%, further increases result in rapid exponential increases in blood viscosity. Neonatal polycythemia occurs in infants of diabetic mothers, infants of mothers with toxemia of pregnancy, or SGA infants. Polycythemia is treated using a partial exchange of the infant's blood with fresh whole blood or 5% albumin. This is frequently done for hematocrit greater than 65%. Capillary hematocrits are poor predictors of viscosity; therefore, decisions to perform exchange transfusions should be based on central hematocrits only.

Anemia

Anemia present at birth is due to hemolysis, blood loss, or decreased erythrocyte production.

Hemolytic Anemia

Hemolytic anemia is most often a result of placental transfer of maternal antibodies that are destroying the infant's erythrocytes. This can be determined by the direct Coombs' test. The most common severe anemia is Rh incompatibility. Hemolytic disease in the newborn produces jaundice, pallor, and hepatosplenomegaly. The most severely affected infants manifest hydrops. This massive edema is not strictly related to the hemoglobin level of this infant. ABO incompatibility frequently results in hyperbilirubinemia but rarely causes anemia.

Congenital infections, hemoglobinopathies (sickle cell disease), and thalassemias produce hemolytic anemia. In a severely affected infant with a positive-reacting direct Coombs' test result, a cord hemoglobin level of less than 10.5 g/dl, or a cord bilirubin level of greater than 4.5 mg/dl, immediate exchange transfusion is indicated. For less severely affected infants, exchange transfusion is indicated when total indirect bilirubin level is greater than 20 mg/dl.

Hemorrhagic Anemia

Significant anemia can develop from hemorrhage that occurs during placental abruption. Internal bleeding (intraventricular, subgaleal, mediastinal, intraabdominal) in infants can also often lead to severe anemia. Usually, hemorrhage occurs acutely during delivery, and the baby occasionally requires transfusion. Twin-twin transfusion reactions can produce polycythemia in one baby and profound anemia in the other. Severe cases can lead to death in the donor and hydrops in the recipient.

Anemia of Prematurity

Decreased RBC production frequently contributes to anemia of prematurity. Erythropoietin is not released until a gestational age of 30 to 34 weeks has been reached. These infants, however, have large numbers of erythropoietin-sensitive RBC progenitors. Research has focused on the role of recombinant erythropoietin (Epogen) in treating anemia in preterm infants.[5-7] Successful increases in hematocrit levels using Epogen may obviate the need for blood transfusions and reduce the risk of blood-borne infections and reactions. Studies suggest that routine use of Epogen is probably helpful for the very-low-birth-weight infant (<750 g), but its regular use for other preterm infants is not likely to significantly reduce the transfusion rate.

Hemoglobin

At birth, nearly 80% of circulating hemoglobin is fetal ($a_2{}^A\gamma_2{}^F$). When infant erythropoiesis resumes at about 2 to 3 months of age, most new hemoglobin is adult. When the oxygen level is 27 mm Hg, 50% of the bound oxygen is released from adult hemoglobin (P-50). Therefore, the P-50 of adult hemoglobin is 27 mm Hg. Reduction of hemoglobin's affinity for oxygen allows more oxygen to be released into the tissues at a given oxygen level.

Fetal hemoglobin has a P-50 value 6- to 8-mm Hg higher than that of adult hemoglobin. This higher P-50 value allows more efficient oxygen delivery from the placenta to the fetal tissues. In this situation, the hemoglobin equilibrium curve is considered to be shifted to the left of normal. This increase in P-50 is thought to be due to the failure of fetal hemoglobin to bind 2,3-diphosphoglycerate to the same degree as does adult hemoglobin.[8] This is somewhat of a disadvantage to the newborn because lower peripheral oxygen levels are needed before oxygen is released from fetal hemoglobin. By 4 to 6 months of age in a term infant, the hemoglobin equilibrium curve gradually shifts to the right and the P-50 value approximates that of a normal adult.

JAUNDICE

In the hepatocyte, bilirubin created by hemolysis is conjugated to glucuronic acid and rendered water soluble. This conjugated or direct bilirubin is excreted in bile. Without this mechanism of conjugation, unconjugated bilirubin acts as a neural cell poison, interfering with cellular respiration. This neural damage is termed *kernicterus* and produces athetoid cerebral palsy, seizures, sensorineural hearing loss, and, rarely, death.

The newborn's liver has a metabolic excretory capacity for bilirubin that is not equal to its task. Even healthy full-term infants usually have an elevated unconjugated bilirubin level. This peaks about the 3rd day of life at approximately 6.5 to 7.0 mg/dl and does not return to normal until the 10th day of life. A total bilirubin level greater than 7 mg/dl in the first 24 hours or greater than 13 mg/dl at any time in full-term newborns often prompts an investigation for the cause. Breast-fed infants usually have serum bilirubin levels 1 to 2 mg/dl greater than formula-fed babies. The common causes of prolonged indirect hyperbilirubinemia are listed in Table 1–3.

Pathologic jaundice within the first 36 hours of life is usually due to excessive production of bilirubin. Hyperbilirubinemia is managed based on the infant's weight. Phototherapy is initiated for newborns (1) less than 1500 g, when the serum bilirubin level reaches 5 mg/dl; (2) 1500 to 2000 g, when the serum bilirubin level reaches 8 mg/dl; or (3) 2000 to 2500 g, when the serum bilirubin level reaches 10 mg/dl. Formula-fed term infants without hemolytic disease are treated by phototherapy when levels reach 13 mg/dl. For hemolytic-related hyperbilirubinemia, phototherapy is recommended when the serum bilirubin level exceeds 10 mg/dl by 12 hours of life, 12 mg/dl by 18 hours, 14 mg/dl by 24 hours, or 15 mg/dl by 36 hours.[9] An absolute bilirubin level that triggers exchange transfusion is still not established, but most exchange transfusion decisions are based on the serum bilirubin level and its rate of rise.

RETINOPATHY OF PREMATURITY

Retinopathy of prematurity (ROP) develops during the active phases of retinal vascular development in the first 3 or 4 months of life. The exact causes are unknown, but oxygen exposure and extreme prematurity are the only risk factors that have

TABLE 1–3. Causes of Prolonged Indirect Hyperbilirubinemia

Breast milk jaundice	Pyloric stenosis
Hemolytic disease	Crigler-Najjar syndrome
Hypothyroidism	Extravascular blood

Data from Maisels MJ: Neonatal jaundice. In Avery GB (ed): Neonatology. Pathophysiology and Management of the Newborn. Philadelphia, JB Lippincott, 1987, p 566.

been repeatedly and convincingly demonstrated. The risk of ROP is probably related to the degree of immaturity, length of exposure, and oxygen concentration. ROP is found in 1.9% of premature infants in large neonatal units.[10] Retrolental fibroplasia (RLF) is the pathologic change observed in the retina and overlying vitreous after the acute phases of ROP subside. A study conducted by the National Institutes of Health found that cryotherapy was effective in preventing retinal detachment, macular fold, and RLF.[11]

American Academy of Pediatrics' guidelines recommend that all infants who received oxygen therapy who weigh less than 1800 g and are fewer than 35 weeks' gestation and any infants who weigh less than 1300 g and are fewer than 30 weeks' gestation should undergo an ophthalmologic examination to rule out ROP.[12] Babies younger than 4 to 6 weeks of age often have a vitreous haze that may obscure the view of the retina. An examination at 7 to 9 weeks of age is more likely to be reliable.

Thermoregulation

A homeotherm is a mammal that can maintain a constant deep body temperature. Although human beings are homeothermic, newborns have difficulty maintaining constant deep body temperature due to their relatively large surface area, poor thermal regulation, and small mass to act as a heat sink. Heat loss may occur owing to (1) evaporation (a wet baby or a baby in contact with a wet surface), (2) conduction (direct skin contact with a cool surface), (3) convection (air currents blowing over the baby), and (4) radiation (the baby radiates heat to a cooler surface not in contact with him or her).

Of these, radiation is the most difficult to control. Infants produce heat by increasing metabolic activ-

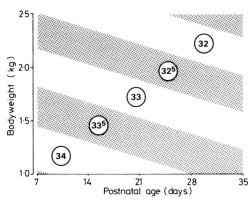

Figure 1–3. Neutral thermal environment (°C) from day 7 to 35. Dew point of air 18°C, flow 10 l/min. Body weight is current weight. Values for body weight more than 2.0 kg are calculated by extrapolation. (From Sauer PJJ, Dane HJ, Visser HKA: New standards for neutral thermal environment of healthy very low birthweight infants in week one of life. Arch Dis Child 59:18–22, 1984.)

ity either by shivering like an adult or by nonshivering thermogenesis, using brown fat. Brown-fat thermogenesis may be rendered inactive by vasopressors,[13] by anesthetic agents,[14] and through nutritional depletion.[15] *Thermoneutrality* (the optimal thermal environment for the newborn) is the range of ambient temperatures in which the newborn with a normal body temperature and a minimal metabolic rate can maintain a constant body temperature by vasomotor control. The *critical temperature* is the temperature below which a metabolic response to cold is necessary to replace lost heat. The appropriate incubator temperature is determined by the patient's weight and postnatal age (Figs. 1–2 and 1–3). For low-birth-weight infants, thermoneutrality is approximately 34 to 35°C up to 6 weeks of age and 31 to 32°C until 12 weeks of age. Infants who weigh 2 to 3 kg have a thermoneutrality zone of 31° to 34°C on the 1st day of life and 29° to 31°C until 12 days. Double-walled incubators offer the best thermoneutral environment. Radiant warmers cannot prevent convection heat loss and lead to higher insensible water loss.

Failure to maintain thermoneutrality leads to serious metabolic and physiologic consequences. Special care must be exercised to maintain the body temperature within normal limits in the operating room.

Fluids and Electrolytes

At 12 weeks of gestation, the fetus has a total body water content that is 94% of body weight. This amount decreases to 80% by 32 weeks' gestation and 78% by term (Fig. 1–4). A further 3 to 5% reduction in total body water content occurs in the first 3 to 5 days of life. Body water continues to decline and reaches adult levels (approximately 60% of body weight) by 1½ years of age. Extracellular water also declines by 1 to 3 years of age. These water composition changes progress in an orderly

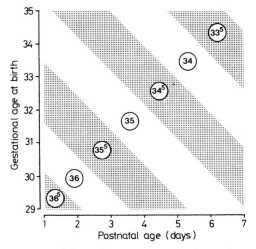

Figure 1–2. Neutral thermal environment (°C) during the 1st week of life calculated from these measurements: dew point of the air 18°C, flow 10 l/min. (From Sauer PJJ, Dane HJ, Visser HKA: New standards for neutral thermal environment of healthy very low birthweight infants in week one of life. Arch Dis Child 59:18–22, 1984.)

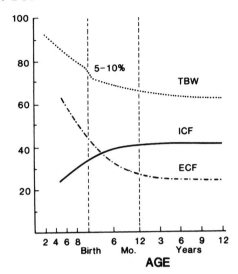

% BODY WEIGHT

Figure 1–4. Friss-Hansen's classic chart relating total body weight (TBW) and extracellular (ECF) and intracellular fluid (ICF) to percentage of body weight, from early gestation to adolescence. (Adapted from Welch KJ, Randolph JG, Ravitch MM, et al [eds]: Pediatric Surgery [4th ed]. Chicago, Year Book Medical, 1986, p 24.)

fashion in utero. Premature delivery requires the newborn to complete both fetal and term water unloading tasks. Surprisingly, the premature infant can complete fetal water unloading by 1 week following birth. Postnatal reduction in extracellular fluid volume has such a high physiologic priority that it occurs even in the presence of relatively large variations of fluid intake.[16]

Glomerular Filtration Rate

The glomerular filtration rate (GFR) of newborns is slower than that of adults.[17] From 21 ml/min/1.73 m² at birth in the term infant, GFR quickly increases to 60 ml/min/1.73 m² by 2 weeks of age. GFR reaches adult levels by 1½ to 2 years of age. A preterm infant has a GFR that is only slightly slower than that of a full-term infant. In addition to this difference in GFR, the concentrating capacity of the preterm and the full-term infant is well below that of the adult. An infant responding to water deprivation increases urine osmolarity to a maximum of only 600 mOsm/kg. This is in contrast to the adult, whose urine concentration can reach 1200 mOsm/kg. It appears that the difference in concentrating capacity is due to the insensitivity of the collecting tubules of the newborn to antidiuretic hormone. Although the newborn cannot concentrate urine as efficiently as the adult, the newborn can excrete very dilute urine at 30 to 50 mOsm/kg. Newborns are unable to excrete excess sodium, an inability thought to be due to a tubular defect. Term babies are able to conserve sodium, but premature infants are considered "salt wasters" because they have an inappropriate urinary sodium excretion, even with restricted sodium intake.

Insensible Water Loss

Insensible water loss from the lungs can be essentially eliminated by humidification of inspired air. Transepithelial water loss occurs by the diffusion of water molecules through the stratum corneum of the skin. Due to the immature skin, preterm infants of 25 to 27 weeks' gestation can lose more than 120 ml H_2O/kg/day by this mechanism. Transepithelial water loss decreases as age increases.

Neonatal Fluid Requirements

To estimate fluid requirements in the newborn requires an understanding of (1) preexisting fluid deficit or excess, (2) metabolic demands, and (3) losses.

Because these factors change quickly in the critically ill newborn, frequent adjustments in fluid management are necessary. Hourly monitoring of intake and output allows early recognition of fluid balance that will affect treatment decisions. This dynamic approach requires two components: an initial hourly fluid intake that is safe and a monitoring system to detect the patient's response to the treatment program selected. A table of initial volumes expressed in rates of milliliters per kilogram per 24 hours for various surgical conditions has been developed as a result of a study of a large group of infants followed during their first 3 postoperative days (Table 1–4). The patients were divided into three groups, according to conditions: moderate surgical conditions, such as colostomies, laparotomies, and intestinal atresia; severe surgical conditions, such as midgut volvulus or gastroschisis; and necrotizing enterocolitis with perforation of the bowel or bowel necrosis requiring exploration.

No "normal" urine output exists for a given neonate. Ideal urine output can be estimated by measuring the osmolar load presented to the kidney for excretion and calculating the amount of urine necessary to clear this load, if the urine is maintained at an isotonic level of 280 mOsm/dl (Table 1–5).

After administering the initial hourly volume for 4 to 8 hours, depending on the patient's condition, the newborn is reassessed by observing urine output and concentration. With these two factors, it is pos-

TABLE 1–4. Newborn Fluid Volume Requirements (ml/kg/24 h) for Various Surgical Conditions

Group	Day 1	Day 2	Day 3
Moderate surgical conditions (e.g., colostomies, laparotomies for intestinal atresia, Hirschsprung's disease)	80 ± 25	80 ± 30	80 ± 30
Severe surgical conditions (e.g., gastroschisis, midgut volvulus, meconium peritonitis)	140 ± 45	90 ± 20	80 ± 15
Necrotizing enterocolitis with perforation	145 ± 70	135 ± 50	130 ± 40

TABLE 1-5. Minimum Newborn Ideal Urine Output (ml/kg/h) for Various Surgical Conditions

Group	Day 1	Day 2	Day 3
Moderate surgical conditions (e.g., colostomies, laparotomies for intestinal atresia, Hirschsprung's disease)	2 ± 0.96	2.63 ± 1.71	2.38 ± 0.92
Severe surgical conditions (e.g., gastroschisis, midgut volvulus, meconium peritonitis)	2.67 ± 0.92	2.96 ± 0.54	2.96 ± 1.0
Necrotizing enterocolitis with perforation	2.58 ± 1.04	3.17 ± 1.67	3.46 ± 1.46

sible to determine the state of hydration of most neonates and their responses to the initial volume. In more difficult cases, changes in serial serum sodium (Na), blood urea nitrogen (BUN), creatinine, and osmolarity along with urine Na, creatinine, and osmolarity make it possible to assess the infant's response to the initial volume and to use fluid status to guide the next 4 to 8 hours' fluid intake.

Illustrative Examples

INSUFFICIENT FLUID. A 1-kg premature infant, during the first 8 hours postoperatively, has 0.3 ml/kg/hour of urine output. Specific gravity is 1.025. Previous initial volume was 5 ml/kg/hour. Serum BUN has increased from 4 mg/dl to 8 mg/dl; hematocrit value has increased from 35 to 37%, without transfusion. This child is dry. The treatment is to increase the hourly volume to 7 ml/kg/hour for the next 4 hours and to monitor the subsequent urine output and concentration to reassess fluid status.

INAPPROPRIATE ANTIDIURETIC HORMONE RESPONSE. A 3-kg newborn with congenital diaphragmatic hernia during the first 8 hours postoperatively has a 0.2 ml/kg/hour of urine output, with a urine osmolarity of 360 mOsm/l. The previous initial volume was 120 ml/kg/day (15 ml/h). The serum osmolarity value has decreased from 300 mOsm preoperatively to 278 mOsm/l; BUN, from 12 mg/dl to 8 mg/dl. The inappropriate antidiuretic hormone response requires reduction in fluid volume from 120 ml/kg/day to 90 ml/kg/day for the next 4 to 8 hours. Repeat urine and serum measurements will allow the further adjustment of fluid administration.

OVERHYDRATION. A 3-kg baby, 24 hours following operative closure of gastroschisis, had an average urine output of 3 ml/kg/hour for the past 4 hours. During that time period, the infant received fluids at a rate of 180 ml/kg/day. The specific gravity of the urine has decreased to 1.006; serum BUN is 4 mg/dl; hematocrit value is 30%, down from 35% preoperatively. The total serum protein concentration is 4.0 mg/dl, down from 4.5 mg/dl. This child is being overhydrated. The treatment is to decrease the fluids to 3 ml/kg/hour for the next 4 hours and then to reassess urine output and concentration.

RENAL FAILURE. A 5-kg infant with severe sepsis secondary to Hirschsprung's enterocolitis has had a urine output of 0.1 ml/kg/hour for the past 8 hours. The specific gravity is 1.012; serum sodium, 150; BUN, 25 mg/dl; creatinine, 1.5 mg/dl; urine sodium, 130; and urine creatinine, 20 mg/dl.

Fractional Na Excretion (FE Na)

$$\frac{Ur\,Na \times Pl\,Cr}{Pl\,Na \times Ur\,Cr} = \frac{130 \times 1.5}{150 \times 20}$$

FE Na = 193/3000 × 100
FE Na = 6.5% (normal = 2 to 3%)

FE Na less than 2% usually indicates a prerenal cause of oliguria, whereas greater than 3% usually implies a renal cause (ATN). This patient is in acute renal failure. The plan is to restrict fluids to insensible losses plus measured losses for the next 4 hours and to then reassess the plan using both urine and serum studies.

□ Pulmonary System of the Newborn

The dichotomous branching of the bronchial tree is usually completed by 16 weeks' gestation. No actual alveoli are seen until 24 to 26 weeks' gestation. Therefore, the air-blood surface area for gas diffusion is limited should the fetus be delivered at this age. Between 24 and 28 weeks, the cuboidal and columnar cells become flatter and start differentiating into type I (lining cells) and/or type II (granular) pneumocytes. Between 26 and 32 weeks of gestation, terminal air sacs begin to give way to air spaces. From 32 to 36 weeks, further budding of these air spaces occurs and alveoli become numerous. At the same time, the phospholipids that constitute pulmonary surfactant begin to line the terminal lung air spaces. Surfactant is produced by type II pneumocytes and is extremely important in maintaining alveolar stability.

The change in the ratio of the amniotic phospholipids, lecithin and sphingomyelin, is used to assess fetal lung maturity. A ratio greater than 2 is considered compatible with mature lung function. Absence of adequate surfactant leads to HMD or respiratory distress syndrome. HMD is present in nearly 10% of all premature infants and is the leading cause of morbidity and mortality (30%) among premature infants in the United States. Other conditions associated with pulmonary distress in the newborn include delayed fetal lung absorption, (wet lung syndrome), intrauterine aspiration pneumonia (meconium aspiration), and intrapartum pneumonia. In all of these conditions, endotracheal intubation and mechanical ventilation may be required for hypoxia, CO_2 retention, or apnea. Ventilator options and management are discussed in Chapter 6.

SURFACTANT

Surfactant deficiency is believed to be the major cause of HMD. Surfactant replacement therapy improves effective oxygenation. Three surfactant preparations have been under investigation: (1) surfactant derived from bovine or porcine lung, (2) human surfactant extracted from amniotic fluid, and (3) artificial surfactant. Multicenter-based, randomized trials for modified bovine surfactant (Survanta)[18] and artificial surfactant (Exosurf Neonatal)[19] have been published.

In one study in 1990, Survanta was given as a single dose via an endotracheal tube an average of 12 minutes after birth. The patients who received this bovine surfactant demonstrated less severe radiographic changes at 24 hours of age compared with infants who received placebo. No difference occurred in clinical status 7 and 28 days after treatment compared with placebo.

In the Exosurf Neonatal study done in 1991, the premature infants were randomized to receive one dose of the artificial surfactant or air placebo. In this study, a significant reduction was noted in the surfactant-treated infants compared with the control group in all of the following: number of deaths attributed to HMD, incidence of pulmonary air leaks, oxygen requirements, and mean airway pressure.

An uncontrolled case series has also been reported in which surfactant was given to full-term newborns with pneumonia and meconium aspiration, with a significant improvement in oxygenation after treatment.[20] Although these and other reports are promising, more studies are needed to determine the most effective dose, the number of doses, and the best timing for surfactant treatment. Surfactant therapy is an important addition to the pulmonary care of the preterm newborn.

One recent multicenter study reported that surfactant therapy early in the course of full-term newborn respiratory failure resulted in a significantly lower requirement for extracorporeal membrane oxygenation and produced no additional morbidity. Several recent multicenter studies compared the efficacy and complication rates of synthetic versus calf-lung cannula surfactant therapies for neonatal respiratory failure.[21–24]

Results from one study suggest that a calf lung surfactant preparation (Infasurf) is preferred over synthetic owing to reduced incidence of RDS, severity of early pulmonary disease, development of air leaks, and overall mortality from RDS. However, calf-lung surfactant was associated with a greater risk of developing an intraventricular hemorrhage. Other studies reported that calf-lung surfactants produce more rapid onset of effects but noted no significant difference in the rate of complications compared with synthetic surfactants. However, support exists for the synthetic surfactant preparations. This support is based on the theoretical advantage of a possibly reduced risk of intraventricular hemorrhage, less exposure to animal antigen with subsequent reactions, and lower overall cost. Future studies will hopefully provide additional insight into the appropriate applications of the available agents.

MONITORING

Continuous monitoring of physiologic indices provides data that assist in assessing response to therapy and trends that may be used to predict catastrophe. Many episodes of "sudden deterioration" in critically ill patients are viewed, in retrospect, as changes in clinical condition that had been occurring for some time.

Arterial Blood Gases and Derived Indices

Arterial oxygen tension (PaO_2) is measured, most commonly, by obtaining an arterial blood sample and by measuring the partial pressure of oxygen with a polarographic electrode. Defining normal parameters for PaO_2 depends on the maturation and age of the patient. In the term newborn, the general definition for hypoxia is a PaO_2 less than 55 mm Hg, whereas hyperoxia is greater than 80 mm Hg.

Capillary blood samples are "arterialized" by topical vasodilators or heat to increase blood flow to a peripheral site. Blood must be freely flowing and collected quickly to prevent exposure to the atmosphere. Blood flowing sluggishly and exposed to atmospheric oxygen falsely raises the PaO_2 from a capillary sample, especially in the 40 to 60 mm Hg range.[25] Capillary blood pH and carbon dioxide tension (PCO_2) correlate well with arterial samples, except when perfusion is poor. PaO_2 is the least reliable of all capillary blood gas determinations. In patients receiving oxygen therapy in whom arterial PaO_2 exceeds 60 mm Hg, the capillary PaO_2 correlates poorly with the arterial measurement.[26, 27]

In newborns, umbilical artery catheterization provides arterial access. The catheter tip should rest at the level of the diaphragm or below L3. The second frequently used arterial site is the radial artery. Complications of arterial blood sampling include repeated blood loss and anemia. Changes in oxygenation are such that intermittent blood gas sampling may miss critical episodes of hypoxia or hyperoxia. Due to the drawbacks of ex vivo monitoring, several in vivo monitoring systems have been used.

Pulse Oximetry

The noninvasive determination of oxygen saturation (SaO_2) gives moment-to-moment information regarding the availability of O_2 to the tissues. If the PaO_2 is plotted against the oxygen saturation of hemoglobin, the S-shaped hemoglobin dissociation curve is obtained (Fig. 1–5). Referring to this curve,

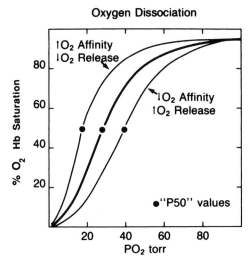

Figure 1–5. The oxygen dissociation curve of normal adult blood. The P-50, the oxygen tension at 50% oxygen saturation, is approximately 27 mm Hg (torr). As the curve shifts to the right, the oxygen affinity of hemoglobin decreases and more oxygen is released at a given oxygen tension. With a shift to the left, the opposite effects are observed. A decrease in pH or an increase in temperature reduces the affinity of hemoglobin for oxygen. (From Blancette V, Zipursky A: Neonatal hematology. In Avery GB [ed]: Neonatology. Philadelphia, JB Lippincott, 1987, p 663.)

hemoglobin is 50% saturated at 25 mm Hg PaO_2 and 90% saturated at 50 mm Hg. Pulse oximetry has a rapid (5- to 7-second) response time, requires no calibration, and may be left in place continuously.

Pulse oximetry is not possible if the patient is in shock, has peripheral vasospasm, or has vascular constriction due to hypothermia. Inaccurate readings may occur in the presence of jaundice, direct high-intensity light, dark skin pigmentation, and greater than 80% fetal hemoglobin. Oximetry is not a sensitive guide to gas exchange in patients with high PaO_2 due to the shape of the oxygen dissociation curve. On the upper horizontal portion of the curve, large changes in PaO_2 may occur with little change in SaO_2. An oximeter reading of 95% could represent a PaO_2 between 60 and 160 mm Hg.

A study to compare pulse oximetry with PaO_2 determined from indwelling arterial catheters has shown that SaO_2 greater than or equal to 85% corresponds to a PaO_2 greater than 55 mm Hg and saturations less than or equal to 90% correspond with a PaO_2 less than 80 mm Hg.[28] Guidelines for monitoring infants using pulse oximetry have been suggested for the following three conditions:

1. In the infant with acute respiratory distress without direct arterial access, saturation limits of 85% (lower) and 92% (upper) should be set.
2. In the older infant with chronic respiratory distress who is at low risk for ROP, the upper saturation limit may be set at 95%; the lower limit should be set at 87% to avoid pulmonary vasoconstriction and pulmonary hypertension.
3. Because the concentration of fetal hemoglobin in newborns affects the accuracy of pulse oximetry, infants with arterial access should have

both PaO_2 and SaO_2 monitored closely. A graph should be kept at the bedside documenting the SaO_2 each time the PaO_2 is measured. Limits for the SaO_2 alarm can be changed because the characteristics of this relationship change.

Carbon Dioxide Tension

Arterial carbon dioxide tension ($PaCO_2$) is a direct reflection of gas exchange in the lungs and of the metabolic rate. In most clinical situations, changes in $PaCO_2$ are due to changes in ventilation. For this reason, serial measurement of $PaCO_2$ is a practical method to assess the adequacy of ventilation. The discrepancy among venous, capillary, and arterial carbon dioxide tensions is not great under most conditions, although one study noted a significant increase in $PaCO_2$ in venous samples compared with simultaneous arterial samples.[29]

Because it is possible to monitor $PaCO_2$ and pH satisfactorily with venous or capillary blood samples and because pulse oximetry is now commonly used to assess oxygenation, many infants with respiratory insufficiency no longer require arterial catheters for monitoring.

End-Tidal Carbon Dioxide

Measuring expired CO_2 by capnography provides a noninvasive means of continuously monitoring alveolar PCO_2. Capnometry measures CO_2 by an infrared sensor either placed in line between the ventilator circuit and the endotracheal tube, or off to the side of the air flow, both of which are applicable only to the intubated patient. A comparative study of end-tidal carbon dioxide in critically ill neonates demonstrated that both sidestream and mainstream end-tidal carbon dioxide measurements approximated $PaCO_2$.[30] When the mainstream sensor was inserted into the breathing circuit, the $PaCO_2$ increased an average of 2 mm Hg. Although this is not likely to significantly affect infants who are ventilated, it might create fatigue in weaning infants from mechanical ventilation. The accuracy of the end-tidal carbon dioxide is diminished with small endotracheal tubes.

Central Venous Catheter

Indications for central venous catheter placement include (1) hemodynamic monitoring, (2) inability to establish other venous access, (3) TPN, and (4) infusion of inotropic drugs or other medications that cannot be given peripherally. Measuring central venous pressure (CVP) to monitor volume status is frequently used in the resuscitation of a critically ill patient. A catheter placed in the superior vena cava or right atrium measures the filling pressure of the right side of the heart, which usually reflects left atrial and filling pressure of the left ventricle. Often, a wide discrepancy exists between left and right atrial pressure when pulmonary disease, overwhelming sepsis, or cardiac lesions are present. To employ the monitor effectively, continuous measurements must be taken with a pressure transducer connected to a catheter accurately placed in the central venous system. Positive-pressure ventilation, pneumothorax, abdominal distention, or pericardial tamponade all elevate CVP.

Pulmonary Artery

The pulmonary artery pressure catheter has altered the care of the child with severe cardiopulmonary derangement by allowing direct measurement of cardiovascular variables at the bedside. The indications for pulmonary catheter placement are listed in Table 1–6. With this catheter, it is possible to monitor CVP, pulmonary artery pressure, pulmonary wedge pressure, and cardiac output. A 4-French, double-lumen catheter and a 5- to 8-French, triple-lumen catheter are available. The catheter is usually placed by percutaneous methods (as in the adult) except in the smallest pediatric patient, in whom a cutdown is sometimes required.

When the tip of the catheter is in a distal pulmonary artery and the balloon is inflated, the resulting pressure is generally an accurate reflection of left atrial pressure because the pulmonary veins have no valves. This pulmonary "wedge" pressure represents left ventricular filling pressure, which is used as a reflection of preload. The monitors display phasic pressures, but treatment decisions are made based on the electronically derived mean CVP. A low pulmonary wedge pressure suggests that blood volume must be expanded. A high or normal pulmonary wedge pressure in the presence of continued signs of shock suggests left ventricular dysfunction.

Cardiac output is usually measured in liters per minute. When related to body surface area, the output is represented as the *cardiac index*, which is simply the cardiac output divided by the body surface area. The normalized cardiac index allows the evaluation of cardiac performance without regard to body size. The usual resting value for cardiac index is between 3.5 and 4.5 l/min/m². The determination of cardiac output by the thermodilution technique, which is possible with a Swan-Ganz pulmonary artery catheter, is widely used and has a good correlation with other methods. Accurate cardiac output determination depends on rapid injection, accurate measurement of the injectant temperatures and volume, and absence of shunting. Because ventilation affects the flow into and out of the right ventricle, three injections should be made at a consistent point in the ventilatory cycle, typically at end-expiration.

Doppler measurement of aortic flow velocity allows measurement of cardiac output by the following formula:

$$\text{Cardiac Output (ml/min)} = \\ \text{Mean Aortic Blood Flow Velocity (cm/sec)} \times \\ \text{Aortic Cross-Sectional Area (cm}^2) \times 60$$

Aortic cross-sectional area is determined by standard ultrasonographic techniques. Using this cross-sectional measurement, pulsed Doppler aortic flow velocity is measured by a transducer placed at the suprasternal notch, in the esophagus, or in the trachea, with a specially modified endotracheal tube, to derive cardiac output. Studies are underway to determine if cardiac output measured by this technique correlates well with thermodilution or the Fick method in critically ill pediatric patients. Previous studies have shown that cardiac output measured by intermittent Doppler measurement at the suprasternal notch was not of sufficient reliability to be employed for hemodynamic monitoring in critically ill children.[31]

Impedance cardiography (bioimpedance) is another noninvasive technique that measures stroke volume on a beat-by-beat basis.[32] Bioimpedance employs a low-level current applied to the thorax, where changes in the volume and velocity of blood flow in the thoracic aorta result in detectable changes in thoracic conductivity. Previous application of this technique in critically ill patients met with only limited success.[33] Late refinements in electrode configuration, algorithms, and microprocessors have produced more acceptable results. A 1990 study in pigs demonstrated a good correlation of bioimpedance-derived cardiac output with thermodilutional cardiac output over a wide hemodynamic range.[34] These techniques have yet to be proved effective in children.

Another study concluded that using right heart catheters in treating critically ill adult patients resulted in an increased mortality.[35] However, a consensus committee report documents the continued safety and efficacy of right heart catheters in the care of critically ill children.[36]

Venous Oximetry

Mixed venous oxygen saturation (SvO_2) is an indicator of the adequacy of oxygen supply and of the demand in perfused tissues. Oxygen consumption is defined as the amount of oxygen consumed by the tissue as calculated by the Fick equation:

TABLE 1-6. Indications for Pulmonary Artery Catheter Placement

---

Inadequate systemic perfusion in the presence of elevated central venous pressure
Fluid management in noncardiogenic pulmonary edema
Evaluation of therapeutic interventions, such as changes in positive end-expiratory pressure, use of vasoactive drugs, or assisted circulation
Hemodynamic evaluation in children with pulmonary hypertension
Severe pulmonary disease with profound hypoxemia

Adapted from Perkin RM: Invasive monitoring in the pediatric intensive care unit. In Nussbaum E (ed): Pediatric Intensive Care (2nd ed). Mt. Kisco, NY, Futura Publishing Co, 1989, p 259.

$$O_2 \text{ Consumption} = \text{Cardiac Output} \times \text{Arterial-Venous Oxygen Content Difference}$$

Reflectance spectrophotometry is currently used for continuous venous oximetry. Multiple wavelengths of light are transmitted at a known intensity by means of fiberoptic bundles in a special pulmonary artery or right atrial catheter. The light is reflected by RBCs flowing past the tip of the catheter. The wavelengths of light are chosen so that both oxyhemoglobin and deoxyhemoglobin are measured to determine the fraction of hemoglobin saturated with oxygen. The system requires either in vitro calibration by reflecting light from a standardized target that represents a known oxygen saturation or in vivo calibration by withdrawing blood from the pulmonary artery catheter and measuring the saturation by laboratory cooximetry.

Mixed venous oxygen saturation values within the normal range (68 to 77%) indicate a normal balance between oxygen supply and demand, provided that vasoregulation is intact and distribution of peripheral blood flow is normal. Values greater than 77% are most commonly associated with syndromes of vasoderegulation, such as sepsis. Uncompensated changes in O_2 saturation, hemoglobin level, or cardiac output lead to a decrease in SvO_2. A sustained decrease in SvO_2 greater than 10% should lead to measuring SaO_2, hemoglobin level, and cardiac output to determine the cause of the decline.[37] The most common sources of error in measuring SvO_2 are calibration and catheter malposition. The most important concept in SvO_2 monitoring is the advantage of continuous monitoring, which allows early warning of a developing problem.[38]

Although most clinical experience has been with pulmonary artery catheters, right atrial catheters are more easily placed and may thus provide better information to detect hemodynamic deterioration earlier and permit more rapid treatment of physiologic derangements.[39] A study has shown that, when oxygen consumption was monitored and maintained at a consistent level, the right atrial venous saturation was thought to be an excellent monitoring device.[40]

□ Shock

Shock is a state in which the cardiac output is insufficient to deliver adequate oxygen to meet metabolic demands of the tissues. Cardiovascular function is determined by preload, cardiac contractility, heart rate, and afterload. Shock may be classified broadly as hypovolemic, cardiogenic, or septic.

HYPOVOLEMIC SHOCK

Preload represents the volume of blood presented to the ventricles. Preload is a function of blood volume. Due to the impracticality of measuring volume, preload is commonly monitored by atrial pressure measurements. In most clinical situations, right atrial pressure or CVP is the index of cardiac preload. In situations in which left ventricular or right ventricular compliance is abnormal or in certain forms of congenital heart disease, right atrial pressure may not correlate well with left atrial pressure. In infants and children, most shock situations are the result of reduced preload secondary to fluid loss, such as from diarrhea or vomiting.

Virtually all forms of pediatric shock have significant intravascular and functional interstitial fluid deficits. Hypovolemia results in decreased venous return to the heart. Preload is reduced, cardiac output falls, and the overall result is a decrease in tissue perfusion. Invasive infection and hypovolemia are the most common causes of shock in both children and adults. The first step in treating all forms of shock is to correct existing fluid deficits. Inotropic drugs should not be initiated until adequate intravascular fluid volume has been established. The speed and volume of the infusate are determined by the patient's responses, particularly changes in blood pressure, pulse rate, urine output, and CVP. Shock resulting from acute hemorrhage is treated with the administration of 10 to 20 ml/kg of Ringer's lactate solution or normal saline as a fluid bolus. If the patient does not respond, a second bolus of crystalloid is given. Type-specific or cross-matched blood is given, when available.

The choice of resuscitation fluid in shock that results from sepsis or from loss of extracellular fluid (conditions such as peritonitis, intestinal obstruction, and pancreatitis) is less clear. Our initial resuscitation fluids include Ringer's lactate, half-normal saline, or normal saline in older infants and children and half-strength Ringer's or half normal saline in the newborn. In spite of our reluctance to use colloid-containing solutions for shock, we make an exception in the desperately ill newborn or premature infant with septicemia. To replace the reduced serum factors, such as fibronectin and complement, we provide fresh frozen plasma as the resuscitation fluid.

The rate and volume of resuscitation fluid given is adjusted based on feedback data obtained from monitoring the effects of the initial resuscitation. After the initial volume is given, the adequacy of replacement is assessed by monitoring urine output, urine concentration, plasma acidosis, oxygenation, arterial pressure, CVP, and pulmonary wedge pressure, if indicated. When cardiac failure is present, continued vigorous delivery of large volumes of fluid may cause further increases in preload to the failing myocardium and accelerates the downhill course. In this setting, inotropic agents are given while monitoring cardiac and pulmonary function, as outlined previously.

CARDIOGENIC SHOCK

Myocardial contractility is usually expressed in terms of the proportion of ventricular volume pumped, <u>the</u> ejection fraction. Myocardial contractility is reduced with hypoxemia and acidosis. Inotropic drugs increase cardiac contractility but have their best effect when hypoxemia and acidosis are corrected.

Adrenergic receptors are important in regulating calcium flux, which, in turn, is important in controlling myocardial contractility. α and β receptors are proteins present in the sarcolemma of myocardial and vascular smooth muscle cells. β_1 receptors are predominantly in the heart and, when stimulated, result in increased contractility of myocardium. β_2 receptors are predominately in respiratory and vascular smooth muscle. When stimulated, these receptors result in bronchodilation and vasodilation. α_1-adrenergic receptors are located on vascular smooth muscle and result in vascular constriction when stimulated. α_2 receptors are found mainly on prejunctional sympathetic nerve terminals. The concept of dopaminergic receptors has also been used to account for the cardiovascular effects of dopamine not mediated through α or β receptors. Activation of dopaminergic receptors results in decreased renal and mesenteric vascular resistance and, usually, increased blood flow. The most commonly used inotrophic drugs are listed in Table 1–7.

Epinephrine

Epinephrine is an endogenous catecholamine with α- and β-adrenergic effects. At low doses, the β-adrenergic effect predominates. These effects include an increase in heart rate, cardiac contractility, cardiac output, and bronchiolar dilation. Blood pressure rises, in part, not only due to increased cardiac output but also due to increased peripheral vascular resistance, which is noted with higher doses in which α-adrenergic effects become predominant. Renal blood flow may increase slightly, remain unchanged, or decrease depending on the bal-

TABLE 1–7. Vasoactive Medications Commonly Used in the Newborn

Vasoactive Agent	Principal Modes of Action	Major Hemodynamic Effects	Administration and Dosage	Indications
Epinephrine	A- and B-agonist	Increases heart rate and myocardial contractility by activating B_1 receptors	0.1 ml/kg of 1:10,000 solution given IV intracardial; *OR* endotracheal 0.05–1.0 μg/kg/min IV	Cardiac resuscitation; short-term use when severe heart failure resistant to other drugs
Dopamine low dose	Stimulates dopamine receptors	Decrease in vascular resistance in splanchnic, renal, and cerebral vessels	<2 μg/kg/min IV	Useful in managing cardiogenic or hypovolemic shock or following cardiac surgery
Dopamine intermediate dose	Stimulates B_1 receptors; myocardial norepinephrine release	Inotropic response	2–10 μg/kg/min IV	Blood pressure unresponsive to low dose
Dopamine high dose	Stimulates A receptors	Increased peripheral and renal vascular resistance	>10 μg/kg/min IV	Septic shock with low systemic vascular resistance
Dobutamine	Synthetic B_1-agonist in low doses; A and B_2 effects in higher doses	Increased cardiac output, increased arterial pressure; less increase in heart rate than dopamine	1–15 μg/kg/min IV	Useful alternative to dopamine if increase in heart rate undesirable
Isoproterenol	B_1- and B_2-agonist	Increased cardiac output by positive inotropic and chronotropic action and increase in venous return; systemic vascular resistance generally reduced; pulmonary vascular resistance generally reduced	0.05–2.0 μg/kg/min IV	Useful in low output situations, especially when heart rate is slow
Sodium nitroprusside	Direct-acting vasodilator that relaxes arteriolar and venous smooth muscle	Afterload reduction; reduced arterial pressure	1–10 μg/kg/min IV (for up to 10 min); 0.5–2 μg/kg/min IV	Hypertensive crisis; vasodilator therapy
Milrinone	Phosphodiesterase inhibitor relaxes arteriolar and venous smooth muscle via calcium/cyclic AMP	Increased cardiac output, slight decreased blood pressure, increased oxygen delivery	75 μg/kg bolus IV, then 0.75–1.0 mg/kg IV	Useful as an alternative or in addition to dopamine (may act synergistically) if increased HR undesirable

IV, intravenous.
Adapted from Lees MH, King DH: Cardiogenic shock in the neonate. Pediatr Rev 9:263, 1988.

ance between greater cardiac output and changes in peripheral vascular resistance, which lead to regional redistribution of blood flow. Cardiac arrhythmias can be seen with epinephrine, especially with higher doses. Dosages for treating compromised cardiovascular function range from 0.05 to 1.0 μg/kg/min. Excessive doses of epinephrine can cause worsening cardiac ischemia and dysfunction from increased myocardial oxygen demand.

Isoproterenol

Isoproterenol is a β-adrenergic agonist. It increases cardiac contractility and heart rate, with little change in systemic vascular resistance (SVR). The peripheral vascular β-adrenergic effect and lack of a peripheral vascular α-adrenergic effect may allow reduction of left ventricular afterload. Isoproterenol's intense chronotropic effect produces tachycardia, which can limit its usefulness. Isoproterenol is administered IV at a dosage of 0.05 to 2.0 μg/kg/min.

Dopamine

Dopamine is an endogenous catecholamine with β-adrenergic, α-adrenergic, and dopaminergic effects. It is both a direct and an indirect β-adrenergic agonist. Dopamine elicits positive inotropic and chronotropic responses by direct interaction with the β receptor (direct effect) and by stimulating the release of norepinephrine from the sympathetic nerve endings, which interacts with the β receptor (indirect effect). At low dosages (<3 μg/kg/min), the dopaminergic effect of the drug predominates, resulting in reduced renal and mesenteric vascular resistance and further blood flow to these organs. The β-adrenergic effects become more prominent at intermediate dosages (3 to 10 μg/kg/min), producing a higher cardiac output. At relatively high dosages (>15 to 20 μg/kg/min), the α-adrenergic effects become prominent with peripheral vasoconstriction.

Experience with the use of dopamine in pediatric patients suggests that it is effective in increasing blood pressure in neonates, infants, and children. The precise dosages at which the desired hemodynamic effects are maximized are not known. The effects of low dosages of dopamine on blood pressure, heart rate, and renal function were studied in 18 hypotensive, preterm infants.[41] The blood pressure and diuretic effects were observed at 2, 4, and 8 μg/kg/min. Elevations in heart rate were seen only at 8 μg/kg/min. Further work is needed to better characterize the pharmacokinetics and pharmacodynamics of dopamine in children, especially in newborns.

Recent clinical evidence has demonstrated some beneficial effects from orally administered levodopa for treating cardiac failure in pediatric patients. Because enteral medications for heart failure are currently limited to digoxin and diuretics, using levodopa may improve our ability to treat heart failure without using parenteral ionotropes.[42]

Dobutamine

Dobutamine, a synthetic catecholamine, has predominantly β-adrenergic effects with minimal α-adrenergic effects. The hemodynamic effect of dobutamine in infants and children with shock has been studied.[43] Dobutamine infusion significantly increased cardiac index, stroke index, and pulmonary capillary wedge pressure, and it decreased SVR. The drug appears more efficacious in treating cardiogenic shock than septic shock. The advantage of dobutamine over isoproterenol is its lesser chronotrophic effect and its tendency to maintain systemic pressure. The advantage over dopamine is dobutamine's lesser peripheral vasoconstrictor effect. The usual range of dosages for dobutamine is 2 to 15 μg/kg/min. The combination of dopamine and dobutamine has been increasingly used. Little information regarding their combined advantages or effectiveness in pediatric patients has been published.

Milrinone

Milrinone, a phosphodiesterase inhibitor, is a potent positive inotrope and vasodilator that has been shown to improve cardiac function in infants and children.[44–46] The proposed action is due, in part, to an increase in intracellular cyclic adenosine monophosphate and calcium transport secondary to inhibition of cardiac phosphodiesterase. This effect is independent of β-agonist stimulation and, in fact, may act synergistically with β agonist to improve cardiac performance. Milrinone increases cardiac index and oxygen delivery without affecting heart rate, blood pressure, or pulmonary wedge pressure. Milrinone is administered as a 75-μg/kg bolus followed by infusion of 0.75 to 1.0 μg/kg/min.

SEPTIC SHOCK

Afterload represents the force against which the left ventricle must contract to eject blood. It is related to SVR and myocardial wall stress. SVR is defined as the systemic mean arterial blood pressure minus right arterial pressure divided by cardiac output. Cardiac contractility is affected by SVR and afterload. In general, increases in afterload reduce cardiac contractility, and decreases in afterload increase cardiac contractility.

Septic shock is a distributive form of shock that differs from other forms of shock. Cardiogenic and hypovolemic shock lead to increased SVR and decreased cardiac output. Septic shock results from a severe decrease in SVR and a generalized maldistribution of blood and leads to a hyperdynamic state.[47] The pathophysiology of septic shock begins with a nidus of infection. Organisms may invade the blood stream, or they may proliferate at the infected site and release various mediators into the blood stream.

Evidence now supports the finding that substances produced by the microorganism, such as lipopolysaccharide, endotoxin, exotoxin, lipid moieties, and other products can induce septic shock by stimulating host cells to release cytokines, leukotrienes, and endorphins.

Endotoxin is a lipopolysaccharide found in the outer membrane of gram-negative bacteria. Functionally, the molecule is divided into three parts: (1) the highly variable O-specific polysaccharide side chain (conveys serotypic specificity to bacteria and can activate the alternate pathway of complement); (2) the R-core region (less variable among different gram-negative bacteria; antibodies to this region could be cross protective); and (3) lipid-A (responsible for most of the toxicity of endotoxin). Endotoxin stimulates tumor necrosis factor (TNF) and can directly activate the classic complement pathway in the absence of antibody. Endotoxin has been implicated as an important factor in the pathogenesis of human septic shock and gram-negative sepsis.[48] Therapy has focused on developing antibodies to endotoxin to treat septic shock. Antibodies to endotoxin have been used in clinical trials of sepsis with variable results.[49–51]

Cytokines, especially TNF, play a dominant role in the host's response. Endotoxin and exotoxin both induce TNF release in vivo and produce many other toxic effects via this endogenous mediator.[52–54] TNF is released primarily from monocytes and macrophages; however, it is also released from natural killer cells, mast cells, and some activated T-lymphocytes. Antibodies against TNF protect animals from exotoxin and bacterial challenge.[55, 56] Other stimuli for its release include viruses, fungi, parasites, and interleukin-1 (IL-1). In sepsis, the effects of TNF release may include cardiac dysfunction, disseminated intravascular coagulation, and cardiovascular collapse. TNF release also causes the release of granulocyte-macrophage colony-stimulating factor (GM-CSF), interferon-α, and IL-1.

IL-1 is produced primarily by macrophages and monocytes. IL-1, previously known as the endogenous pyrogen, plays a central role in stimulating a variety of host responses, including fever production, lymphocyte activation, and endothelial cell stimulation, to produce procoagulant activity and to increase adhesiveness. IL-1 also causes the induction of the inhibitor of tissue plasminogen activator and the production of GM-CSF. These effects are balanced by the release of platelet-activating factor and arachidonic metabolites.

IL-2, also known as *T-cell growth factor,* is produced by activated T lymphocytes and strengthens the immune response by stimulating cell proliferation. Its clinically apparent side effects include capillary leak syndrome, tachycardia, hypotension, increased cardiac index, decreased SVR, and decreased left ventricular ejection fraction.[57, 58]

Studies done on dogs have suggested that in immature animals, septic shock is more lethal and has different mechanisms of tissue injury.[59] These include more dramatic aberrations in blood pressure (more constant decline), heart rate (progressive, persistent tachycardia), blood sugar level (severe, progressive hypoglycemia), acid base status (severe acidosis), and oxygenation (severe hypoxemia). These changes are significantly different from those seen in the adult animals that also experience improved survival of almost 600% (18.5 vs. 3.1 hours) compared with the immature animal.

The neonate's host defense can usually respond successfully to ordinary microbial challenge. However, defense against major challenges appears limited, which provides an explanation for the high mortality rate with major neonatal sepsis. As in adults, the immune system consists of four major components: cell-mediated immunity (T cells), complement system, antibody-mediated immunity (B cells), and macrophage-neutrophil phagocytic system. The two most important deficits in newborn host defenses that seem to increase the risk of bacterial sepsis are the quantitative and qualitative changes in the phagocytic system and the defects in antibody-mediated immunity.

The proliferative rate of the granulocyte-macrophage precursor has been reported to be at near-maximal capacity in the neonate. However, the neutrophil storage pool is markedly reduced in the newborn compared with the adult. After bacterial challenge, newborns fail to increase stem cell proliferation and deplete their already reduced neutrophil storage pool. Numerous in vitro abnormalities have been demonstrated in neonatal polymorphonuclear neutrophils, especially in times of stress or infection.[60] These abnormalities include decreased deformability, chemotaxis, phagocytosis, C3b receptor expression, adherence, bacterial killing, and depressed oxidative metabolism. Chemotaxis is impaired in neonatal neutrophils in response to various bacterial organisms and antigen-antibody complexes.[61] Although phagocytosis has additionally been demonstrated to be abnormal in neonatal phagocytes, it appears that this phenomenon is most likely secondary to decreased opsonic activity rather than an intrinsic defect of the neonatal polymorphonuclear neutrophils.[62, 63]

Preterm and term newborns have poor responses to various antigenic stimuli, reduced gamma globulin levels at birth, and reduced maternal immunoglobulin supply from placental transport. Almost 33% of infants with a birth weight less than 1500 g develop substantial hypogammaglobulinemia.[64] IgA and IgM are also low due to the inability of these two immunoglobulins to cross the placenta. Neonates, therefore, are usually more susceptible to pyogenic bacterial infections because most of the antibodies that opsonize pyrogenic bacterial capsular antigens are IgG and IgM. In addition, neonates do not produce type-specific antibodies, which appears to be secondary to a defect in the differentiation of B lymphocytes into immunoglobulin-secreting plasma cells and T-lymphocyte-mediated facilitation of antibody synthesis. In the term infant, total hemolytic complement activity, which measures the classic complement pathway, constitutes approximately 50% of adult activity.[65] The activity of the alternative complement pathway, secondary to lowered levels of factor B, is also decreased in the neonate.[66] Fibronectin, a plasma protein that promotes reticuloendothelial clearance of invading microorganisms, is deficient in neonatal cord plasma.[67]

Using IV immunoglobulins (IVIGs) for the prophylaxis and treatment of sepsis in the newborn, especially the preterm, low-birth-weight infant, has been studied in numerous trials with varied outcomes. In one study, a group of infants weighing 1500 g was treated with 500 mg/kg of IVIG each week for 4 weeks and compared with infants who were not treated with immunoglobulin.[68] The death rate was 16% in IVIG-treated group compared with 32% in the untreated controlled group. Another recent analysis examined the role of IVIG to prevent and treat neonatal sepsis.[69] A significant, but only marginal, benefit was noted from prophylactic use of IVIG to prevent sepsis in low-birth-weight premature infants. However, using IVIG to treat neonatal sepsis produced a greater than 6% decrease in the mortality rate.

There are no prospective trials examining the routine use of IVIG to prevent neonatal sepsis. Until data are available, its prophylactic use cannot be recommended.

CSFs are a family of glycoproteins that stimulate proliferation and differentiation of hematopoietic cells of various lineages. GM-CSF and CSF have similar physiologic actions. Both stimulate the proliferation of bone marrow myeloid progenitor cells, induce the release of bone marrow neutrophil storage pools, and enhance mature neutrophil effect or function.[69, 70] Preliminary studies of GM-CSF in neonatal animals demonstrate enhancement of neutrophil oxidative metabolism, as well as priming of neonatal neutrophils for enhanced chemotaxis and bacterial killing. Both GM-CSF and granulocyte colony-stimulating factor (G-CSF) induce peripheral neutrophilia within 2 to 6 hours of intraperitoneal administration. This enhanced affinity for neutrophils returns to normal baseline level by 24 hours.[71] Recent studies confirm the efficacy and safety of G-CSF therapy for neonatal sepsis and neutropenia.[72] Other studies have demonstrated no long-term adverse hematologic, immunologic, or developmental effects from G-CSF therapy in the septic neonate. The current recommended daily pediatric dose is 5 μg/kg/dose given subcutaneously.

REFERENCES

1. Cornblath M, Schwartz R: Disorders of Carbohydrate Metabolism in Infancy (2nd ed). Philadelphia, WB Saunders, 1976.
2. Dweck HS, Cassady G: Glucose intolerance in infants of very low birth weight, I: Incidence of hyperglycemia in infants of birth weights 1,110 grams or less. Pediatrics 53:189–195, 1974.
3. Ziegler EE, O'Donnell AM, Nelson SE, et al: Body composition of reference fetus. Growth 40:329, 1976.
4. Colozzi AE: Clamping of the umbilical cord. Its effect on the placental transfusion. N Engl J Med 250:629, 1954.
5. Asch J, Wedgwood JF: Optimizing the approach to anemia in the preterm infant: Is there a role for erythropoietin therapy? J Perinatol 17:276–282, 1997.
6. Doyle JJ: The role of erythropoietin in the anemia of prematurity. Semin Perinatol 21:20–27, 1997.
7. King PJ, Sullivan TM, Leftwich ME, et al: Score for neonatal acute physiology and phlebotomy blood loss predict erythrocyte transfusions in premature infants. Arch Pediatr Adolesc Med 151:27–31, 1997.
8. Bauer C, Ludwig I, Ludwig M: Different effects of 2,3-diphosphoglycerate and adenosine triphosphate on the oxygen affinity of adult and fetal human hemoglobin. Life Sci 7:1339, 1968.
9. Osborn LM, Lenarsky C, Oakes RC, et al: Phototherapy in full-term infants with hemolytic disease secondary to ABO incompatibility. Pediatrics 73:520–526, 1984.
10. Biglan AW, Cheng KP, Brown DR: Update on retinopathy of prematurity. Intern Ophthalmol Clin 29:2–4, 1989.
11. National Institutes of Health: Cryotherapy for retinopathy of prematurity cooperative group. Multicenter trial of cryotherapy for retinopathy of prematurity. Arch Ophthalmol 106:471–479, 1988.
12. Ferson WM, et al: Retinopathy of prematurity guidelines [letter]. Pediatrics 101:1093, 1998.
13. Karlberg P, Moore RE, Oliver TK: The thermogenic response of the newborn infant to noradrenaline. Acta Paediatr Scand 51:284, 1962.
14. Stein J, Cheu H, Lee M, et al: Effects of muscle relaxants, sedatives, narcotics and anesthetics on neonatal thermogenesis. In Pannell M (ed): Surgical Forum. Vol. 38. Chicago, American College of Surgeons, 1987, p 76.
15. Landsberg L, Young JB: Fasting, feeding and regulation of the sympathetic nervous system. N Engl J Med 198:1295, 1978.
16. Lorenz JM, Kleinman LI, Kotagal UR, et al: Water balance in very low birth weight infants: Relationship to water and sodium intake and effect on outcome. J Pediatr 101:423–432, 1982.
17. Aperia A, Broberger O, Herin P, et al: Postnatal control of water and electrolyte homeostatis in pre-term and full-term infants. Acta Paediatr Scand 305:61–65, 1983.
18. Soll RF, Holkstra RE, Fangman JJ, et al: Multicenter trial of single-dose modified bovine surfactant extract (Survanta) for prevention of respiratory distress syndrome. Pediatrics 85:1092–1102, 1990.
19. Corbet A, Bucciarelli R, Goldman S, et al: Decreased mortality rate among small premature infants treated at birth with a single dose of synthetic surfactant: A multicenter controlled trial. J Pediatr 118:277–284, 1991.
20. Auten RL, Notter RH, Kendig JW, et al: Surfactant treatment of full-term newborns with respiratory failure. Pediatrics 87:101–107, 1991.
21. Hudak ML, Martin DJ, Egan EA, et al: A multicenter randomized masked comparison trial of synthetic surfactant versus calf lung surfactant extract in the prevention of neonatal respiratory distress syndrome. Pediatrics 100:39–50, 1997.
22. Bloom BT, Kattwinkel J, Hall RT, et al: Comparison of Infasurf (calf lung surfactant extract) to Survanta (Beractant) in the treatment and prevention of respiratory distress syndrome. Pediatrics 100:31–38, 1997.
23. Halliday HL: Controversies: Synthetic or natural surfactant. The case for natural surfactant. J Perinat Med 24:417–426, 1996.
24. Whitelaw A: Controversies: Synthetic or natural surfactant treatment for respiratory distress syndrome? The case for synthetic surfactant. J Perinat Med 24:427–435, 1996.
25. Garg AK: "Arterialized" capillary blood [letter]. CMAJ 107:16, 1972.
26. Glasgow JF, Flynn DM, Swyer PR: A comparison of descending aortic and "arterialized" capillary blood in the sick newborn. CMAJ 106:660, 1972.
27. Siggaard-Andersen O: Acid-base and blood gas parameters—arterial or capillary blood? Scand J Clin Lab Invest 21:289, 1968.

28. Reynolds GJ, Yu VYH: Guidelines for the use of pulse oximetry in the non-invasive estimation of oxygen saturation in oxygen-dependent newborn infants. Aust Paediatr J 24:346–350, 1988.

29. Weil MH, Rackow EC, Trevino R, et al: Difference in acid-base state between venous and arterial blood during cardiopulmonary resuscitation. N Engl J Med 315:153–156, 1986.

30. McEvedy BAB, McLeod ME, Kirpalani H, et al: End-tidal carbon dioxide measurements in critically ill neonates: A comparison of sidestream capnometers. Can J Anaesth 37:322–326, 1990.

31. Notterman DA, Castello FV, Steinberg C, et al: A comparison of thermodilution and pulsed Doppler cardiac output measurement in critically ill children. J Pediatr 115:554–560, 1989.

32. Pianesi P: Comparison of impedance cardiopathy with indirect FiO_2 (CO_2) method of measuring cardiac output in healthy children during exercise. Am J Cardiol 77:745–749, 1996.

33. Van de Water JM, Phillips PA, Thouin LG, et al: Bioelectric impedance: New developments and clinical application. Arch Surg 102:541, 1971.

34. Spinale FG: Relationship of bioimpedance to thermodilution and electrocardiographic measurements of cardiac function. Crit Care Med 18:414–418, 1990.

35. Connors A: The effectiveness of right heart catheterization in the initial care of critically ill patients. JAMA 276:889–897, 1996.

36. Thompson AE: Pulmonary artery catheterization in children. New Horiz 5:244–250, 1997.

37. Nelson LD: Application of venous saturation monitoring. In Civetta JM, Taylor RW, Kirby RR (eds): Critical Care. Philadelphia, JB Lippincott, 1988, pp 327–334.

38. Norfleet EA, Watson CB: Continuous mixed venous oxygen saturation measurement: A significant advance in hemodynamic monitoring? J Clin Monit Comput 1:245–258, 1985.

39. Ko WJ, Chang CI, Chiu IS: Continuous monitoring of venous oxygen saturation in critically-ill infants. J Formos Med Assoc 95:258–262, 1996.

40. Hirschl RB, Palmer P, Heiss KF, et al: Evaluation of the right atrial venous oxygen saturation as a physiologic monitor in a neonatal model. J Pediatr Surg 28:901–905, 1993.

41. DiSessa TG, Leitner M, Ti CC, et al: The cardiovascular effects of dopamine in the severely asphyxiated neonate. J Pediatr 99:772–776, 1981.

42. Mendelson AM, Johnson CE, Brown CE, et al: Hemodynamic and clinical effects of oral levodopa in children with congestive heart failure. J Am Coll Cardiol 30:237–242, 1997.

43. Perkin RM, Levin DL, Webb R, et al: Dobutamine: A hemodynamic evaluation in children with shock. J Pediatr 100:977–983, 1982.

44. Ramamoorthy C, Anderson GD, Williams GD, et al: Pharmacokinetics and side effects of milrinone in infants and children after open heart surgery. Anesth Analg 86:283–289, 1998.

45. Barton P, Garcia JK, Kitchen A, et al: Hemodynamic effects of i.v. milrinone lactate in pediatric patients with septic shock. A prospective double-blinded, randomized, placebo-controlled interventional study. Chest 109:1302–1312, 1996.

46. Chang AC, Am A, Wernovsky G, et al: Milrinone: Systemic and pulmonary hemodynamic effects in neonates after cardiac surgery. Crit Care Med 23:1907–1914, 1995.

47. Parrillo JE: Septic shock in humans. Advances in the understanding of pathogenesis, cardiovascular dysfunction, and therapy. Ann Intern Med 113:227–242, 1990.

48. Danner R, Elin RJ, Hosline KM, et al: Endotoxin determinations in 100 patients with septic shock. Clinical Research 36:453A, 1988.

49. McCloskey RV, Straube KC, Sanders C, et al: Treatment of septic shock with human monoclonal antibody HA-1A. A randomized, double-blind, placebo-contolled trial. CHESS Trial Study Group. Ann Intern Med 121:1–5, 1994.

50. Rogy MA, Moldawer LL, Oldenburg HS, et al: Anti-endotoxin therapy in primate bacteremia with HA-1A and BPI. Ann Surg 220:77–85, 1994.

51. Ziegler EJ, Fisher CJ Jr, Sprung CL, et al: Treatment of gram-negative bacteremia and septic shock with HA-1A human monoclonal antibody against endotoxin. A randomized, double-blind, placebo-controlled trial. The HA-1A Sepsis Study Group. N Engl J Med 324:429–436, 1991.

52. Tracey KJ, Lowry SF, Cerami A: Chachectin: A hormone that triggers acute shock and chronic cachexia. J Infect Dis 157:413–420, 1988.

53. Nedwin GE, Svedersky LP, Bringman TS: Effect of interleukin-2, interferon-gamma and mitogens on the production of tumor necrosis factors alpha and beta. J Immunol 135:2492–2497, 1985.

54. Jupin C, Anderson S, Damais C, et al: Toxic shock syndrome toxin 1 as an inducer of human tumor necrosis factors and gamma interferon. J Exp Med 167:752–761, 1988.

55. Tracey KJ, Fong Y, Hesse DG, et al: Anti-cachectin/TNF monoclonal antibodies prevent septic shock during lethal bacteraemia. Nature 330:662–664, 1987.

56. Beutler B, Milsaark IW, Cerami AC: Passive immunization against cachectin/tumor necrosis factor protects mice from the lethal effects of endotoxin. Science 229:869–871, 1981.

57. Rosenstein M, Ettinghausen SE, Rosenberg SA: Extravasation of intravascular fluid mediated by the systemic administration of recombinant interleukin-2. Immunology 137:1735, 1986.

58. Ognibene FP, Rosenberg SA, Lotze M, et al: Interleukin-2 administration causes reversible hemodynamic changes and left ventricular dysfunction similar to those seen in septic shock. Chest 94:750, 1988.

59. Pryor RW, Hinshaw LB: Sepsis/septic shock in adults and children. Pathol Immunopathol Res 8:222–230, 1989.

60. Hill HR: Biochemical, structural and functional abnormalities of polymorphonuclear leukocytes in the neonate. Pediatr Res 22:375–382, 1987.

61. Miller M: Chemotactic function in the human neonate: Humoral and cellular aspects. Pediatr Res 5:487–492, 1971.

62. Miller ME: Phagocytosis in the newborn: Humoral and cellular factors. J Pediatr 75:255–259, 1969.

63. Forman ML, Stiehm ER: Impaired opsonic activity but normal phagocytosis in low-birth-weight infants. N Engl J Med 281:926–931, 1969.

64. Cates KL, Rowe JC, Ballow M: The premature infant as a compromised host. Curr Probl Pediatr 13:1–63, 1983.

65. Anderson DC, Hughes J, Edwards MS, et al: Impaired chemotaxigenesis by type III group B streptococci in neonatal sera: Relationship to diminished concentration of specific anticapsular antibody and abnormalities of serum complement. Pediatr Res 17:496–502, 1983.

66. Stossel TP, Alper CH, Rosen F: Opsonic activity in the newborn: Role of properidin. Pediatrics 52:134–137, 1973.

67. Gerdes JS, Yoder MC, Douglas SD, et al: Decreased plasma fibronectin in neonatal sepsis. Pediatrics 72:877–881, 1983.

68. Chirico G, Rondini G, Plebani A, et al: Intravenous gamma globulin therapy for prophylaxis of infection in high-risk neonates. J Pediatr 110:437–442, 1987.

69. Clark SC, Kamen R: The human hematopoietic colony-stimulating factors. Science 236:1229–1237, 1987.

70. Sieff CA: Hematopoietic growth factors. J Clin Invest 79:1549, 1987.

71. Barak Y, Leibovitz E, Mogilner B, et al: The in vivo effect of recombinant human granulocyte-colony stimulating factor in neutropenic neonates with sepsis. Eur J Pediatr 156:643–646, 1997.

72. Wolach B: Neonatal sepsis: Pathogenesis and supportive therapy [Review]. Semin Perinatol 21:28–38, 1997.

2

NUTRITIONAL SUPPORT OF THE PEDIATRIC SURGICAL PATIENT

Daniel H. Teitelbaum, MD •
Arnold G. Coran, MD

Nutritional support in the pediatric surgical patient must take into account that the patient is growing and developing while he or she is recovering from an injury or operation. The full-term newborn infant grows at a rate of 25 to 30 g/day, leading to a doubling of the birth weight by about 4 months of age.[1] The average infant triples his or her birth weight by 12 months of age. By 3 years of age, the weight is four times the birth weight, and by completion of the first decade, the weight has increased nearly 20-fold. Body length increases 50% by the end of the first year of life and increases three-fold at the end of the first decade of life.

The preterm infant's growth pattern is quite distinct from that of a term infant, since most nutrients are accumulated by the fetus in the third trimester of pregnancy. For instance, fat accounts for only 1 to 2% of body weight in a 1-kg infant compared with 16% in a 3.5-kg infant. An anticipated loss of 15% of a preterm infant's birth weight is usual in the first 7 to 10 days of life, compared with a 10% weight loss for a term infant. After this initial period of weight loss, an infant younger than 27 weeks' gestation gains approximately 10 to 20 g/day because he or she has not yet entered the accelerated weight gain of the third trimester. A 27- to 40-week gestational age infant may gain as many as 35 grams per day.[2]

□ Assessment of Nutritional Status

The pediatric surgeon faces unique nutritional challenges because many infants and children suffer from malnutrition owing to either prematurity or the underlying disease process for which they require surgical therapy. Nutritional assessment is a critical aspect of the initial evaluation of all surgical patients. Malnutrition in pediatric patients has been demonstrated to be quite high.[3] Although a signifi-

cantly malnourished patient can be easily identified, identification of those patients with mild to moderate malnutrition is frequently difficult. A baseline assessment begins with a subjective global assessment, which consists of a history and a physical examination, including an evaluation of weight loss, anorexia, or vomiting and physical evidence of muscle wasting.[4] Beyond this initial subjective assessment, a variety of indexes can be used to measure the child's nutritional status.

Objective nutritional assessment begins with the basic anthropomorphic measurements of height, weight, and head circumference to be plotted on a standardized growth curve. Using these growth charts, the expected weight-for-height index can be calculated. As length and head circumference are less affected by excess fat or fluid fluctuations, length is a better indicator of body growth. Acute changes in nutritional status have an immediate effect on body weight rather than length and decrease the child's weight-for-height index. Chronic undernutrition, however, will show a lag in body weight as well as linear growth.

For a child whose nutritional status requires further evaluation, the measurement of mid-upper-arm circumference and triceps skinfold thickness can be helpful. Mid-arm circumference is a good indicator of the body's somatic muscle mass size. Triceps skinfold thickness best reflects the degree of subcutaneous fat reserves. Both these measurements are good indicators of a patient's calorie and protein reserves, but there may be variations in measurements between observers, and measurements can change dramatically with alternations in the child's fluid status.

DIRECT MEASUREMENT OF BODY COMPOSITION

A variety of methods have been created since the mid-1970s to measure body composition more directly. Body water has been measured using isotope dilution techniques, which are based on the principle that because fat is anhydrous, the majority of the isotope is directed into the water compartments of the body.[5] Although this assumption is not always correct, an excellent approximation of body fat and water may be obtained.[6, 7] Bioelectrical impedance to the flow of electrical current is another method used to measure total body water. Extrapolation of these measurements can allow for the determination of other body compartments, including total body adipose tissue. More recently, dual-photon absorptiometry and dual-energy x-ray absorptiometry have been used to measure bone mineral content as well as amounts of fat and body water.[8, 9] The accuracy of the instruments is excellent, but they require special adaptation for the young infant. Because of the low amounts of x-ray exposure, dual energy x-ray absorptiometry may become the eventual method of choice for measuring pediatric body composition.

BIOCHEMICAL MEASUREMENTS OF NUTRITIONAL STATUS

Albumin is the classic biochemical marker used to assess the malnourished state.[10] Albumin levels can be altered by a variety of factors, including disturbances of hepatic synthesis, distribution of the plasma space, protein loss from the vascular compartment, and alterations in the child's hydration state.[11] The biologic half-life of albumin is 20 days, making it difficult to determine acute changes in nutritional status. Hypoalbuminemia has been associated with increased morbidity and mortality rates in hospitalized children.[12]

Transferrin is a transport glycoprotein that is synthesized in the liver and binds and transports ferric iron. Its biologic half-life is 8.8 days, and the body pool of transferrin is smaller than that of albumin, which makes transferrin levels a better indicator of protein status than are serum albumin levels.[13] Infants with iron deficiency anemia may have abnormal transferrin levels unrelated to their nutritional status. Transferrin levels may also be abnormal in patients with liver failure, patients receiving large doses of antibiotics, and surgical patients with large fluid shifts.[14]

Prealbumin binding protein, or *transthyretin*, is a transport protein for thyroxine. Transthyretin has a half-life of 2 days and a relatively small distribution pool, making it a good marker of nutritional status. Further, because prealbumin is comprised of a large amount of the amino acid tryptophan, it reflects visceral protein status better than either albumin or transferrin. Levels of prealbumin correlate nicely with nitrogen balance studies.[15] Prealbumin levels have also been used to monitor nutritional therapy during the transition from total parenteral nutrition (TPN) to enteral feedings.[13]

Retinol-binding protein is a useful marker of nutritional status because of its extremely short bio-

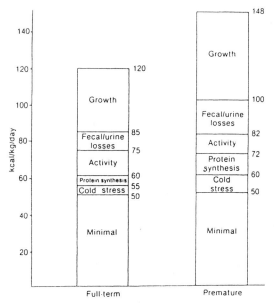

Figure 2–1. Energy requirements for full-term and premature infants broken down into the actual distribution of energy usage.

logic half-life of 12 hours as well as its small body pool size. It is excreted in the urine and thus is not useful in patients with renal failure.[16]

☐ Nutritional Requirements

The energy needs and reserves of infants and children are unique (Fig. 2–1). A 1-kg infant has only a 4-day nutritional reserve, and a full-term infant may live for no more than a month without nutrition.[17] Energy in a child is required for the maintenance of body metabolism as well as for growth. The estimated energy needs of an infant and an older child are shown in Table 2–1. In general, infants require more calories enterally than parenterally.[18] Most simply, energy needs can be viewed as being nearly equivalent to the child's daily water requirements. Energy requirements for most pediatric patients can be calculated based on standard nomograms such as Recommended Daily Allowance tables. Nomograms usually provide an estimated basal energy expenditure based on age, height, and weight and allow the computation of additional energy needs related to such conditions as postoperative stress, multiple

TABLE 2-1. Kilocalorie and Protein Requirements

Age (y)	Kilocalories (kcal/kg Body Weight)	Protein (g/kg Body Weight)
0–1	90–120	2.0–3.5
1–7	75–90	2.0–2.5
7–12	60–75	2.0
12–18	30–60	1.5
>18	25–30	1.0

trauma, fever, and severe infection. Actual measurement or estimation of metabolic rate is the best method of following nutritional status.[19]

The most common method of measuring energy expenditure is *indirect calorimetry*. In this method, the amount of oxygen absorbed across the lung is assumed to be exactly equal to the amount of oxygen consumed in metabolic processes. Commonly used nomograms may significantly underestimate or often overestimate energy expenditure determined by calorimetry.[20–22]

Advances and miniaturization of equipment have allowed the measurement of indirect calorimetry in children during and immediately after major abdominal operations to establish the resting energy expenditure (REE).[23, 24] Initial investigations of REE in the postoperative infant did not detect the increases that had been demonstrated using hormonal and metabolic substrates in postoperative neonates. An explanation for this discrepancy may lie in the timing of these measurements. A more recent study in infants demonstrated a rise in REE, peaking 4 hours after the start of an operation, with a return to baseline by 24 hours.[25] Timing of this increase closely corresponded to increases in postoperative catecholamine levels[26] and interleukin-6 levels.[27] After this increase in energy expenditure, REE has been shown to decline significantly, thus potentially leading to a state of overfeeding if such changes are not anticipated.[28]

WATER AND ELECTROLYTE REQUIREMENTS

Water requirements depend on the patient's age, size, and environment. Table 2–2 shows the normal water requirements based on the age of the patient. The water content of infants is higher than that of adults (75% of body weight vs. 60%).[6] In addition to the water provided by fluid intake, the oxidation of food provides small amounts of water. Despite the large fluid intake of most infants and children, only 0.5 to 3% is retained; the rest is excreted by the kidney (50%) and is lost through the gastrointestinal tract (3 to 10%) and through insensible losses (40 to 50%). Electrolyte requirements are also unique in the pediatric patient.

PROTEIN REQUIREMENTS

The average intake of protein should comprise approximately 15% of the total calories adminis-

TABLE 2-2. Daily Fluid Requirements

Category	Volume Administered/Day
Premature (<2 kg)	150 ml/kg
Neonates and infants (2–10 kg)	100 ml/kg for the first 10 kg
Infants and children (10/20 kg)	1000 ml + 50 ml/kg over 10 kg
Children (>20 kg)	1500 ml + 20 ml/kg over 20 kg

tered. Two percent of the infant's body weight, compared with 3% of the adult's body weight, consists of nitrogen, and the majority of the increase in body nitrogen occurs during the first year of life. Protein needs are thus markedly higher in the neonate and infant. Protein requirements in the neonate range from 2 to 3 g/kg/day and up to 3.5 g/kg/day in the premature infant. Extrapolation of fetal absorption across the placenta during the last trimester indicates that protein needs to be 2.2 g/kg/day.[29, 30] Delivery of excessive amounts of protein to neonates has generally been associated with elevated blood urea nitrogen levels, but amounts in excess of 6 g/kg/day may produce central nervous system injury and impair neurologic development.[31] Estimates of protein needs based on the amount of protein in human milk suggests that 1.9 g/kg/day of protein should suffice. There is a fairly rapid decline in protein needs over the first 6 months of life. In general, the provision of 2.5 g/kg/day to the non-stressed term neonate and 1.5 g/kg/day to older infants may be adequate for normal growth.[31, 32]

The protein requirements in the premature infant are greater than those of the term infant. The American Academy of Pediatrics currently recommends 3.5 to 4.0 g/kg/day of protein for infants weighing less than 1800 g if given by the enteral route and approximately 3 g/kg/day or more if given parenterally.[30]

Protein requirments in the postoperative patient are increased because of the breakdown of visceral protein and decreased extrahepatic protein synthesis. Protein is used for gluconeogenesis and for hepatic synthesis of acute phase reactants. Urinary nitrogen losses of 200 to 300 mg/kg/24 hours in the postoperative patient compare with 80 mg/kg/24 hours in neonates who have not had surgery.[33] Such losses may rapidly lead to protein-calorie malnutrition.[34] Protein breakdown, as measured by an elevation in 3-methylhistidine–creatinine ratios, has been seen in clinically ill premature infants[35] and in postoperative neonates.[26]

Protein breakdown is enhanced by catecholamine release and is reduced by the administration of fentanyl during the postoperative period, which presumably blocks catecholamine release.[26] A study of preterm surgical neonates demonstrated protein sparing with the addition of 3.9 g/kg/day of amino acids, compared with 2.3 g/kg/day.[36] Because of the risk of azotemia, hyperammonemia, and metabolic acidosis, protein sparing effects can probably more safely be achieved by the administration of a balanced prescription of parenteral nutrition (PN).[37] Experimental work with the administration of insulin-like growth factor in highly catabolic patients suggests that this may be another way to reduce somatic muscle breakdown.

Essential Amino Acids In Neonates

Of the 20 standard amino acids, 8 are classically essential, in that no enzymatic pathways are avail-

TABLE 2-3. Essential Amino Acids

Threonine	Methionine	Cystine†
Leucine	Phenylalanine	Proline†
Isoleucine	Tryptophan	Glutamine‡
Valine	Histidine*	Arginine‡
Lysine	Tyrosine†	

*Essential only in infancy.
†May be essential in the premature baby.
‡May be essential in times of excess stress and energy demands.

able in humans to synthesize them (Table 2–3). Unique to the neonate are three or possibly four additional essential amino acids which, because of immature amino acid synthetic mechanisms, are not formed in sufficient amounts. This has become apparent by the development of deficiencies in cysteine, taurine, and tyrosine after chronic administration of adult parenteral formulations to neonates.[38, 39] The deficiencies are most likely due to low levels of phenylalanine, hydroxylase, and cystathionase activity (Fig. 2–2).[40] It has more recently been suggested that proline is an essential amino acid in preterm infants, although this has yet to be confirmed by others.[41] The administration of a

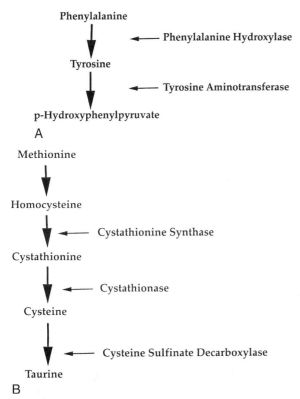

Figure 2–2. Metabolic pathways demonstrating two enzymes that are deficient in neonates. *A,* Metabolic pathway for the formation of tyrosine and p-hydroxyphenylpyruvate. Neonates appear to lack sufficient phenylalanine hydroxylase, thus making tyrosine a relatively essential amino acid in this age group. *B,* Metabolic pathway for the formation of cysteine and taurine. Neonates appear to lack sufficient cystathionase activity, thus making both cysteine and taurine relatively essential amino acids in this age group.

specially designed pediatric formulation leads to a normalization of the neonate's plasma aminogram levels.[42, 43] Despite claims that such formulas can lead to improved weight gain, nitrogen balance, and a decreased incidence of PN-associated jaundice, no controlled study has effectively proved these claims.[44] One substantial benefit of a specialized formula with taurine supplementation is the prevention of retinal degenerative changes.[45]

Two additional amino acids, glutamine and arginine, although not defined as essential, appear to have special functions relevant to metabolism and may be classified as relatively essential.

Glutamine is a vital source of protein and energy for several organs.[46] It is the most abundant amino acid in whole tissues and in blood, and is the most important vehicle for the transfer of nitrogen for renal ammoniagenesis and hepatic ureagenesis. Glutamine is an essential percursor for nucleic acid biosynthesis and is therefore essential for the proliferation of cells that are rapidly turning over, such as the intestinal mucosa and lymphocytes. The gastrointestinal tract is the principal organ of glutamine utilization.[46–48] Glutamine plays multiple roles in intestinal metabolism, structure, and function. Gut mucosal cells have high glutaminase activity, and the human gastrointestinal tract extracts 12 to 13% of circulating glutamine.[49] Glutamine is a major energy source and appears to be more important than glucose for enterocytes and colonocytes. Although glutamine is readily available in healthy individuals, in pathophysiologic states this carefully balanced homeostasis may be lost. Such conditions as sepsis, trauma, surgery, or shock may cause blood glutamine levels to fall, possibly indicating an increased level of glutamine consumption in some tissues despite accelerated skeletal muscle release (Fig. 2–3).

A significant degree of intestinal mucosal atrophy has been demonstrated in rats maintained on standard TPN as compared with TPN supplemented with glutamine.[50, 51] Another group of investigators failed to show that glutamine can prevent TPN-induced mucosal atrophy.[52] In addition, nitrogen retention was also higher in the rats receiving the 2% glutamine solution.[47] Animal studies have shown the potential benefits of glutamine in reducing radiation toxicity as well as intestinal injury from chemotherapy.[46] In a well-controlled human study on bone marrow transplant patients, the high-dose glutamine group showed improved nitrogen balance.[53] The incidence of infection, microbial colonization, and length of hospital stay were also decreased in the high-dose glutamine group. However, a more recent study of transplant patients failed to demonstrate many of these benefits.[54] Although quite appealing, it remains to be proved whether glutamine will have a true impact on the clinical course of patients.[55]

Glutamine is not currently added to PN solutions because the enzyme necessary for its synthesis—glutamine synthetase—is present in humans. This

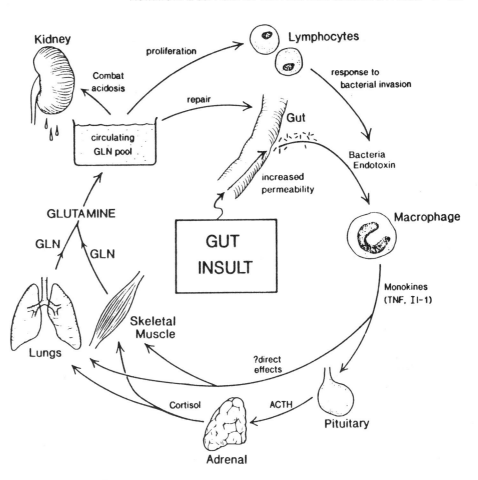

Figure 2–3. Metabolic routes in which glutamine is utilized during a septic event. A primary insult to the gut causes increased gastrointestinal permeability, which results in the passage of bacterial endotoxin into the portal venous system, causing macrophages to release the cytokines tumor necrosis factor and interleukin-1. These cytokines act on multiple end organs to stimulate the production of glutamine, with a resultant replenishment of the glutamine pool. This increase in glutamine is needed for the removal of acid through the kidney and for the generation of new lymphocytes and enterocytes. During periods of increased stress, the circulating pool of glutamine may drop, despite this mechanism, causing a relative dependency on exogenous sources. ACTH, adrenocorticotropic hormone; GLN, glutamine; TNF, tumor necrosis factor. (From Souba WW, Herskowitz K, Austgen TR, et al: Glutamine nutrition: Theoretical considerations and therapeutic impact. JPEN J Parenter Enteral Nutr 14[5 suppl]: 237S–243S, 1990.)

enzyme catalyzes the synthesis of glutamine from glutamate and ammonia. An additional reason that glutamine is not currently added to amino acid formulations is that its solubility has been a problem. Glutamine dipeptides, including l-ananyl, l-glutamine and l-glycyl, l-glutamine have prolonged stability and improved solubility, which makes them more practical.[50] Hopefully the availability of these newer products will allow a greater evaluation and use of glutamine in PN.

Arginine is a dibasic amino acid that has also been considered essential during times of metabolic stress.[2, 56] Studies have demonstrated that arginine supplementation improves nitrogen retention and wound healing in postoperative and malnourished states.[57, 58] Improvement has been demonstrated in the immunologic status of patients maintained on arginine supplemental diets.[59] The mechanism for arginine's actions has not been fully demonstrated, although its function appears to require an intact hepothalamic-pituitary axis. Further, arginine infusion induces the secretion of growth hormone, insulin, prolactin, and somatostatin.[59] Over the past few years, the association between arginine metabolism and the formation of nitric oxide has been examined extensively.[60] Arginine serves as the substrate for nitric oxide synthesis. The production of nitric oxide requires the cellular incorporation of arginine and the enzyme nitric oxide synthase, which medi-

ates its formation. A complex, interdependent control mechanism for the formation of arginine and nitric oxide exists, whereby the formation of argininosuccinate synthetase, the rate-limiting enzyme for arginine formation, is dependent on lipopolysaccharide and interferon-γ, both of which also induce the formation of nitric oxide synthetase.[61] Arginine is present in all commercially available amino acid mixtures, with higher concentrations found in pediatric formulations (approximately 123 mg/g of amino acid) compared with adult formulations (95 to 99 mg/g).

CARBOHYDRATE REQUIREMENTS

Carbohydrates provide a major source of nutrition through both parenteral and enteral routes. Because the body is capable of forming sugars from lipids as well as amino acids, there is no essential amount of carbohydrate needed. However, the addition of small amounts of carbohydrates reduces the breakdown of somatic protein sources and thus acts as a protein-sparing substrate.[62]

The body has a limited ability to store glucose despite an almost essential and continuous need for this substrate by the central nervous system. Immediately after a meal, glucose absorption contributes to the bulk of circulating glucose. As soon as 4 hours after the meal, these sources are rapidly depleted, and glycogen from the liver becomes a major source of energy for the next 8 to 12 hours. The newborn has relatively limited (34 g) glycogen reserves, most of which reside in the liver. Thus, relatively short periods of fasting can lead to a hypoglycemic state.[63]

The primary enteral carbohydrate delivered to neonates and young infants is lactose. In the intestine, lactose is broken down into glucose and galactose by disaccharidases (e.g., lactase) located along the intestinal epithelial border. Because the lactose is the predominant carbohydrate of small children, lactase levels remain sufficiently high in most infants to at least 2 to 3 years of age. Nonlactose formulas may provide adequate amounts of carbohydrates through formulas that are soy based and contain sucrose or corn syrup. Preterm infants may be unable to digest certain carbohydrates, particularly lactose, because of inadequate intestinal lactase activity. Thus, in a small preterm infant, formulas that have a 50:50 mixture of lactose and glucose polymers are ideal. Stable infants should receive approximately 40 to 45% of their total caloric intake as carbohydrate.

Overfeeding of glucose, or the rapid administration of glucose, may lead to an osmotic diuresis and dehydration as a result of exceeding the renal tubular glucose reabsorption threshold. Immunologic suppression has also been associated with overfeeding and is believed to be caused by inactivation of the complement system.[64] Excessive glucose may lead to excessive triglyceride levels and hepatic steatosis.

Carbohydrate requirements in the postoperative patient are sometimes difficult to ascertain. Hyperglycemia may result from a decrease in insulin concentration and may in part be due to an increase in gluconeogenesis.[65, 66] Hyperglycemia resolves quickly in neonates; glucose levels twice the preoperative values returned to baseline levels after 12 hours.[67] Stimulated by catecholamines, postoperative hyperglycemia also appears to be associated with an increased production of lactate and pyruvate.[68] Substrate use has not been shown to increase substantially in neonates after surgery. In fact, previous estimates of early postoperative energy requirements may be significantly higher than suggested by a more recent study.[28] This study showed that the administration of calories at 50% above REE levels led to a significant state of overfeeding.

PN for the neonate should begin at approximately 6 to 8 mg/kg/min of dextrose to prevent hypoglycemia in a young neonate. Older neonates tolerate twice as much glucose, provided it is administered through a central venous catheter. Because of significant hypersomality, central venous administration is essential.

Finally, overfeeding, with the development of lipogenesis, has the potential to exacerbate ventilatory impairment in a critically ill child owing to the increased CO_2 production. Overfeeding these critically ill patients can also lead to fluid retention, which may compromise respiratory function. As indirect calorimetry devices become more readily available in smaller patients, their use will help guide nutritional therapy in these infants.

FAT REQUIREMENTS

The child's diet usually contains sufficient quantities of fat to provide calories and supply essential fatty acids. Fat requirements in the postoperative patient have been determined largely by the experience derived from TPN. Intravenous fats have the highest caloric density of the three major nutrients (9 kcal/g) and are an excellent source of energy. In general, intravenous fats should comprise 30 to 50% of all nonnitrogen calories. Linoleic acid is essential for neonates as well as older children; in general, 2 to 4% of dietary energy should come from this essential fatty acid. Deficiencies of linoleic acid may occur rapidly in neonates. Withholding of lipids from a neonate's parenteral nutrition for as little as 2 days may lead to fatty acid deficiency.[69] Manifestations of fatty acid deficiency include scaly skin, hair loss, diarrhea, and impaired wound healing.[70] Absence of trace amounts of linolenic acid may also be the cause of visual and behavioral disorders.

There are essentially two types of fatty acids: saturated and unsaturated. The two major polyunsaturated fatty acids are linoleic acid, which is an ω-6 fatty acid, and α-linolenic acid, which is an ω-3 fatty acid. Both these polyunsaturated fats are essential for the development of cell membranes and the central nervous system as well as for the synthesis of arachidonic acid and related prostaglandins. Thromboxanes derived from ω-6 fatty acids are potential mediators of platelet aggregation, whereas prostaglandins derived from ω-3 fatty acids are potent anticoagulants. ω-6 fatty acids, which form arachidonic acid, also contribute to the formation of prostaglandin E_2, a known immunosuppressant, whereas ω-3 fatty acids contribute to the formation of prostaglandin E_1 and prostaglandin E_3, which do not have an immunosuppressive effect (Fig. 2–4). A ratio of 50:50 (ω-6:ω-3) appears to be the most ideal,

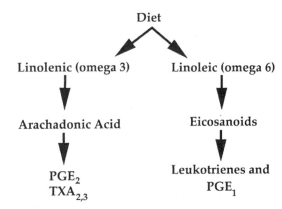

Figure 2–4. Formation of prostaglandins and thromboxanes derived from ω-3 and ω-6 fatty acids. See text for explanation. PGE, prostaglandin E; TXA, thromboxane.

based on burn survival data from experimental animals.[5] No data are available on an ideal ratio in neonates or children.

Patients who have steatorrhea need the provision of fatty acids either in the form of intravenous lipids or with the addition of enteral medium-chain triglycerides, which are absorbed directly across the intestinal epithelium. Medium-chain triglycerides, however, do not contain essential fatty acids. Thus, infants who malabsorb fat are at risk for developing essential fatty acid deficiency.

For PN, the choice of 10% versus 20% lipids has been examined extensively. Both are safe and effective formulas for lipid administration.[71] Each of these lipid emulsions contain similar amounts of egg yolk and phospholipids (1 to 2g/dl), but they differ in the amount of triglycerides. Therefore, formula with 20% lipids contains a similar amount of phospholipid but twice the triglyceride content as formula with 10% lipids.[72] Higher amounts of phospholipids have been associated with higher plasma triclyceride levels and the accumulation of cholesterol and low-density lipoproteins, thus making 20% lipids the preferred source of parenteral fat. The additional advantage of 20% lipids is the delivery of the same amount of calories in a smaller volume of fluid.

ADDITIONAL GROWTH FACTORS AND NUTRIENTS

Carnitine is required for the transport of long-chain fatty acids into mitochrondria. Although the liver is able to synthesize this factor, carnitine is present in human milk and cow milk formulas. It is felt that the newborn, and particularly the preterm infant, may not be able to manufacture sufficient amounts of carnitine.[73] At present, it is difficult to determine whether carnitine supplementation should be given. In general, 5 to 10 mg/kg/day should suffice in neonates and older patients on chronic TPN as a maintenance dose.[74]

Nucleotides, which are based on the parent compounds of purines and pyrimidines, are structural units required for the production of DNA and RNA. Laboratory findings suggest that nucleotides are required for normal T-cell maturation and function. It has been hypothesized that supplementing these may enhance immune function and maintain gastrointestinal barrier function. The clinical use of formulas that contain nucleotides appears to result in the reduction of operative infectious complications.[75–77] However, because the formulas used in these studies also contained arginine and ω-3 fatty acids, the relative contribution of the nucleotides is unclear.

A variety of growth factors have a beneficial effect on intestinal growth, and their absence prevents normal growth of an organism. Many of these factors are not produced in sufficient amounts during the administration of parenteral nutrition and may, therefore, need to be given to patients on TPN. Some of these factors are found in breast milk and appear to play a major role in the transition of a neonate's intestine from one that is maternally supported to one that must actively absorb nutrients. In addition, malnutrition is associated with decreased levels of insulin-like growth factor 1. A potential use of this growth factor has been in the prevention of protein losses during a severe catabolic state such as sepsis or burn injury, in which large losses of protein cannot be compensated for by the administration of amino acids. Insulin-like growth factor 1, however, can inhibit protein breakdown during such injuries and may have great clinical applicability.[78–79]

☐ Enteral Nutrition

The most ideal route of feeding is enteral. Even small amounts of enteral feedings allow for the preservation of normal intestinal villus and microvillus structure, which helps maintain epithelial barrier function.[80] Such preservation also helps maintain normal absorptive processes and prevents injurious luminal factors, such as endotoxins, from entering the host. It appears that the loss of enteral feedings, with TPN administration, leads to an increased expression of interferon-γ in the mucosal epithelium, which may mediate the observed loss of epithelial barrier function.[81] Septic complications are far more common in patients on PN than in patients on enteral nutrition.[82, 83] It is possible that the loss of epithelial barrier function may allow for the development of bacterial translocation from the intestinal lumen and contribute to septicemia.[84, 85] The administration of enteral feeds is associated with a much lower rate of iatrogenic complications. Enteral nutrition obviates the need for intravenous access and has a lower rate of metabolic complications. Enteral feedings are also a more economical route, costing less than one tenth the daily cost of PN.

Early oral intake is critical in preventing the occurrence of feeding aversion. Because suck and swallow reflexes are not developed until the 34th week of gestation, a feeding tube should initially be used in the premature infant.[86] In general, most healthy term infants tolerate oral feeds without difficulty. For infants who have an abnormal suck or swallow or who are not alert enough to swallow, consideration should be given to feeding tube placement. Gastric feedings are preferred because they allow for a normal digestive process. Children receiving gastric feeds tolerate a higher osmolarity and volume than those being fed into the small bowel. Furthermore, gastric acid may benefit digestion and has a bactericidal effect with less frequent gastrointestinal complications.[1] Transpyloric tube placement may be considered for those infants who are at a high risk for aspiration, and a gastrostomy tube should be placed for those infants that will require enteral nutritional support for more than 6 to 8 weeks. The decision to place a gastrostomy tube generally requires an evaluation of the patient for associated gastroesophageal reflux. It has been shown that patients without a strong clinical history of reflux rarely develop clinical reflux after the placement of a percutaneous gastrostomy, suggesting that an extensive preoperative evaluation may not be necessary.[87]

Formula selection depends on the age of the patient and the condition of their gastrointestinal tract. In general, term infants should be maintained on human milk or standard 20 kcal/oz formula (0.67 kcal/ml). The composition of various formulas is given in Table 2–4. A lactose-based formula is generally the first choice, as it is the most like human milk and the least expensive. Lactose-free, soy protein–based formula may be used for those infants who are intolerant of lactose. Calories can be provided by increasing the volume delivered, increasing the concentration of the formula, or supplementing the feedings. As many as 2 g of Polycose or 1 g of oil per oz of feedings can be added quite safely.

Human milk has a variety of advantages over commercial formulas. Breast-feeding provides nutrition as well as passive immunologic protection to the neonate. Breast milk contains 87% water and provides 0.64 to 0.67 kcal per ml. The fat content of breast milk is fairly high at 3.4 g/dl. The protein content of human milk (0.9%) is lower than that of bovine milk or commercial formulas but appears to be much better absorbed because of the higher amounts of whey content. Casein, which predominates in bovine milk, is a complex of protein and calcium. The whey fraction contains primarily lactalbumin and lactoferrin, an iron binding protein that is bacteriostatic to *Staphylococcus aureus* and *Escherichia coli* by restricting iron availability.[88] Breast milk contains elevated levels of cysteine, which is probably essential for a neonate, and taurine, which is needed for bile salt excretion and neurologic and retinal development. Despite similar amounts of trace elements, human milk allows for more efficient absorption of these elements compared with commercial formulas.

The immunologic advantages of breast milk include the transmission of humoral as well as cellular factors to the neonate. Passive immunity is conferred by the passage of secretory immunoglobulin A. Human milk also contains bifidus factor, which supports the growth of *Lactobacillus bifidus* and inhibits the growth of potential pathogens, lysozyme, lactoferrin, and interferon.[89] The highest concentration of immunoglobulin A occurs in colostrum during the first week of life. Levels peak on the first postpartum day at approximately 160 μ/g of protein and decline by the fifth day of life to 20 to 30 μ/g of protein and remain at this level for the first half year.[90] Cellular factors include macrophages and lymphocytes that the infant ingests. The number of cells is approximately 3×10^6 cells/ml on the first postpartum day and declines to one tenth that over the next several days. The lymphocytes are derived from the mother's gut-associated lymphoid tissue and specifically home to the breast for excretion during milk production.[91]

The composition of human milk changes with the gestational and postpartum age of the infant. Milk from mothers of preterm infants contains higher amounts of energy, fat, protein, immunoglobulin A, and sodium.[92] This may offer an advantage to a preterm infant; however, consumption of 180 to more than 200 ml/kg/day may be needed to provide adequate nutritional supplementation. Further, the demands for calcium, phosphorus, electrolytes, and trace elements cannot be achieved with human milk alone. Because of this, human milk fortifiers should be added to breast milk that is fed to preterm infants. Supplementation should continue until the child achieves the weight of a term infant.

Postoperative enteral feeding is well tolerated once the postoperative ileus has resolved. The critically ill child may sustain a loss of a significant portion of intestinal absorptive function. Symptoms are generally manifested by cramping, diarrhea, or emesis. Not uncommonly, the intolerance is due to a lactase deficiency that often improves with the initiation of a lactose-free diet. Other alterations in the diet can also improve feeding tolerance. First, the gastrointestinal tract generally tolerates increased volume more readily than increased osmolarity. Therefore, such adverse symptoms can be avoided by initiating feedings of ⅛- or ¼-strength formula and slowly advancing the formula concentration. Second, the administration of formula by continuous drip may be better tolerated than bolus feedings. The threat of gastroesophageal reflux, vomiting, and subsequent aspiration is thereby reduced. Third, care must be taken to ensure that the enteral formula does not become contaminated, either during preparation or at the bedside. Expiration times should be observed. Finally, pectin, psyllium (Metamucil), diphenoxylate (Lomotil), paregoric, or loperamide (Imodium) are required for those who have lost a significant amount of their bowel length. Assessment of adequate absorption can be carried out most readily by testing the stool for pH and reducing substances. A stool pH below 5.5 or a reducing substance of greater than 0.5% indicates unabsorbed carbohydrates in the stool and should lead to a dilution of the formula. Alternatively, a change in the type of formula may be helpful, such as changing from a formula predominating in lactose to a sucrose-based or glucose polymer–based formula (see Table 2–4). Detection of fat malabsorption using a qualitative or quantitative fecal fat test may be helpful; in general, however, isolated fat malabsorption is unusual unless due to pancreatic insufficiency (e.g., cystic fibrosis).

☐ Parenteral Nutrition

The decision to institute PN to reduce morbidity and mortality must be weighed against the risk of serious complications of the technique, especially

TABLE 2-4. Formulas for Infant Feeding

	Mature Human Milk	Enfamil with Iron*	Pregestimil	RCF†	Nursoy	Enfamil Premature	Whole Cow Milk‡	Peptamen Junior
Protein§	1.1	1.4	1.9	1.8	2.1	2.0	3.6	3.0
Casein	40%	40%				40%	82%	
Whey	60%	60%				60%	18%	
Soy				100%	100%			
Hydrolyzed casein			100%					100%
Osmolarity (mOsm/kg H$_2$O)	300	270	320	70	296	260	290	260
Fat§	3.9	3.5	2.7	3.7	3.6	3.4	3.7	3.9
LCT	100%	100%	60%	100%	100%	60%	100%	40%
MCT	—	—	40%	—	—	40%	—	60%
Carbohydrate§	7.2	7.3	9.0	0	6.9	7.4	4.8	13.8
Formula type	Lactose	Lactose	Partially hydrolyzed starch		Sucrose	Lactose, glucose polymer	Lactose	Maltodextrin, starch
Selected mineral (mg/l)								
Sodium¶	150	180	315	320	200	260	520	460
Potassium**	550	720	730	950	700	690	1480	1320
Calcium	340	520	630	710	600	400	1220	1080
Phosphorus	140	350	415	510	420	550	960	800
Iron	0.5	12	12.5	12	12	12	0.6	14
Energy (kcal/30 ml)	20	20	20		20	20		30
Indication			Malabsorption, hypoallergenic; also for short bowel syndrome and biliary atresia	CHO intolerance (CHO added as tolerated)	Lactose intolerance	For premature, up to full-term birth weight infants		For children with impaired GI function, ages 1–6 y
Similar formulas		Similac with iron Carnation	Nutramigen* Portagen Alimentum	3232A	Isomil Prosobee 1-Soyalac	Similac Special Care		

*Lacks medium-chain triglycerides (MCTs).
†Ross Carbohydrate Free formula. This is not a complete formula as provided by the manufacturer and contains no carbohydrates. Ideal for carbohydrate intolerance, particularly in infants with malabsorption or severe enteritis. Carbohydrate can be reintroduced as dextrose; up to 7 g/dl, and slowly changed from dextrose to sucrose.
‡For comparison only. Whole cow milk should not be fed to infants until they are at least 6 months of age and have developed renal maturity.
§Values stated are percentages of weight per volume. Percentages are the relative percentages of long-chain triglycerides (LCTs) versus MCTs.
¶To determine mEq/l, divide by 23.
**To determine mEq/l, divide by 39.1.
CHO, carbohydrate; GI, gastrointestinal.

sepsis. Two general approaches can be taken to intravenous feeding in infants and children. These are a central venous infusion of a hypertonic glucose solution and peripheral infusion of a moderately hypertonic glucose solution.

PN is an ideal way to maintain nutrition in those infants and children who are unable to tolerate enteral feedings. In the newborn period, extremely premature infants should be started on PN after the first 24 to 48 hours of life. The term infant will require PN support if periods of starvation last more than 4 to 5 days. Other infants who may require PN are those who will be in an anticipated state of prolonged starvation. Older children and adults generally do not require PN unless periods of starvation go beyond 7 to 10 days. Those with inadequate intestinal length require long-term PN. Other indications for PN include chronic malabsorption or diarrhea, inflammatory bowel disease, and receiving either radiotherapy or chemotherapy with resultant gastrointestinal dysfunction.

The type of venous access varies depending on the nutritional needs of the patient. For fewer than 10 to 14 days, peripheral TPN is an ideal route. Peripheral PN has the advantage of relatively few serious complications, with each intravenous catheter lasting approximately 2 to 3 days. The amount of calories that can be delivered with peripheral PN is limited because glucose solutions greater than 12.5% are associated with a high degree of venous sclerosis. Lipid solutions are well tolerated and act to protect the venous endothelium.

Central venous PN may be administered through a tunneled silastic catheter. More recently, the percutaneous intravenous central catheter line has been used in a large portion of patients on TPN. Maintenance of all these catheters requires that the skin site be cleansed with an antiseptic solution and dressed in a dry fashion every other day.[93] Tubing and infusion bags are changed every 72 hours along with a new Millipore filter (0.22-μm) which is placed in line to remove particulate matter such as calcium salts or microorganisms that may contaminate the solution; a 1.2-μm filter is used when infusing lipids in a 3:1 mixture. The lipid tubing must be changed every 24 hours. Adequate maintenance of these lines and prevention of an infection demand meticulous care, because these catheters are a common source of sepsis in the very small neonate.[94]

COMPOSITION OF PARENTERAL SOLUTIONS

Neonates are generally kept on a dextrose and electrolyte solution (e.g., D_{10} 0.2 NS w/20 MEq KCl/l) at maintenance rates (120 ml/kg/day for the first day of life, 100 ml/kg/day for the second day) and are then begun on PN 48 hours after birth. Typically the small neonate is somewhat intolerant of large amounts of dextrose or amino acids for the first 2 or 3 days of life. Dextrose concentrations are generally initiated at 10 to 12.5% and are slowly advanced on

a daily basis to between 20 and 25%. In general, the small neonate has limited glycogen reserves and thus needs to be maintained at approximately 8 mg/kg/min of dextrose. Dextrose administration in the neonate should generally not exceed 12 to 15 mg/kg/min. Amino acid administration should begin at 0.5 to 1.0 g/kg/day. Amino acids are advanced approximately 0.5 to 1 g/kg/day to a maximal goal of 2.5 to 3.0 g/kg/day, which appears to be the ideal range for most neonates. Markedly higher levels result in an elevated blood urea nitrogen level and aminoaciduria. Lipid administration begins at 0.5 to 1 g/kg/day and is similarly advanced to a total of 3.0 g/kg/day. This amount of lipid is generally well tolerated in children. Standard amounts of electrolytes, trace elements, and vitamins are added to this PN solution (Table 2–5). In addition, heparin, at a concentration of 0.5 U/ml may also be added to the solution. The addition of heparin may have the beneficial effect of decreasing thrombotic events, although heparin may interfere with drug absorption.[95, 96] Neonates may not be able to metabolize lipids fully if large amounts of heparin have been added to the PN solution, although heparin in general allows for an improved utilization of lipids.[97] Further, the use of lipids in infants with an indirect hyperbilirubinemia is no longer considered a con-

TABLE 2–5. Central Parenteral Nutrition in Infants*

Constituent	Amount (g/kg/24 h)
Glucose	150–30 g
Protein	2.0–3.5 g
Sodium	2.4 mEq
Potassium	2.4 mEq
Chloride	3–6 mEq
Magnesium	0.5–1.0 mEq
Calcium	0.5–3.0 mEq
Phosphate	0.5–1.0 mM
Trace elements†	0.2 ml
Multivitamin infusion (MVI)‡	
<1750 g body weight	2 ml
>1750 g body weight	3 ml
Heparin	1.0 IU/ml
Glucose-protein volume	60–114 ml
Fat	1–4
10% fat emulsion volume	10–40 ml
Total volume	70–154 ml
Total kilocalories	70–154 kcal

*Each 1000 ml of a standard solution is prepared by mixing 500 ml of 50% dextrose and water with 500 ml of 7% amino acids to give a final concentration of 25% dextrose and 3.5% amino acids. The appropriate amounts of electrolytes, vitamins, and trace elements are added according to the patient's weight.

†Each 0.1 ml of trace element solution (American Regent Laboratories) contains 100 μg of zinc, 20 μg of copper, 10 μg of manganese, 0.2 μg of chromium, and 1.2 μg of selenium. A special neonatal trace element solution contains 300 μg of zinc in 0.3 ml and the same amounts of the other elements.

‡Each vial (diluted to 3 ml) of pediatric MVI (Astra, Merck Corporation) contains vitamin A, 2300 IU; vitamin D, 400 IU; ascorbic acid, 80 IU; thiamine (vitamin B_1), 1.2 mg; riboflavin (vitamin B_2), 1.4 mg; niacinamide, 17 mg; pyridoxine (vitamin B_6), 1 mg; dexpanthenol, 5 mg; vitamin E, 7 IU; folic acid, 140 μg; cyanocobalamin (vitamin B_{12}), 1 μg; phytonadione (vitamin K_1), 200 μg; and biotin, 200 μg.

traindication.[97] In addition, medications such as H2 blockers may be added to the PN solution. Nutritional goals for total energy delivery are shown in Table 2–1.

MONITORING OF LABORATORY VALUES

Monitoring of laboratory values is essential, as aberrations in these values are common in small infants and children, particularly at the onset of PN. A complete blood count should be obtained at the initiation of TPN. Glucose, blood urea nitrogen, creatinine, and electrolytes (Na^+, K^+, Cl^-, HCO_3^-) should be obtained at initiation and biweekly thereafter. Liver function tests (alkaline phosphatase, alanine transaminase, aspartate transaminase, and lactate dehydrogenase, alkaline phosphatase and total/direct bilirubin) and levels of magnesium, albumin, calcium, and phosphorus should be obtained at initiation and weekly until stable. Triglyceride levels should be assessed until the child reaches his or her goal of fat intake.

COMPLICATIONS OF PARENTERAL NUTRITION

Sepsis is one of the most frequent and serious complications of TPN. Long-term central venous catheters are sources of bacteremia and septicemia. Microorganisms usually infect the catheter by entrance at the connections or migration along the subcutaneous tract.[98, 99] Alternatively, the organism may travel through the bloodstream from a distant septic site. The most important factors in reducing the incidence of septic complications are the placement of catheters under strict aseptic conditions and the use of meticulous care when the catheters are "entered." A standardized, dry dressing change every 48 hours should be employed. In addition, the use of the catheter for PN alone, with strict avoidance of drawing blood, giving blood products, or administering medications through the same catheter, minimizes the risk of contamination and mechanical failure. The establishment of PN teams and the use of standardized protocols have resulted in a marked decrease in sepsis rates. Most series report an incidence of 0.5 to 2.0 infections per 1000 catheter days for an nonimmunosuppressed patient with a central venous catheter.[100, 101] For those patients who are immunosuppressed (e.g., hematology or oncology patients), a rate of 2 to 3 infections per 1000 catheter days is generally reported.[102, 103] A considerably higher rate of infections is found in children with the short bowel syndrome, ranging from 7 to 9 infections per 1000 catheter days.[94, 104]

Catheter sepsis in a patient receiving PN is suggested primarily by the development of a fever. Leukocytosis and an unexplained glucosuria may also be seen.[100] Infection is confirmed by culturing microorganisms from blood drawn through the central venous line or from another venous site. Multiple organisms, although previously thought to be due to

contamination, have been found in as many as 25% of catheter infections.[105] If the patient is not toxic, the catheter should remain in place during the initial 48 hours of evaluation, because approximately 50% of febrile patients with central catheters have another source of fever. In general, if no other site of sepsis is found, the catheter should be presumed to be the source. Intravenous antibiotics should be initiated via the catheter after the appropriate cultures have been drawn. If the patient is stable and is improving on appropriate antibiotics, an attempt should be made to salvage the line. In the majority (80 to 90%) of cases, the central venous catheter may be salvaged by 7 to 10 days of intravenous antibiotics. Initial antibiotics should be vancomycin and gentamicin. After 48 hours of treatment, sensitivity results will be available and the antibiotics changed accordingly. Prolonged or inappropriate use of vancomycin can lead to vancomycin-resistant enterococci, and this practice should therefore be avoided.[106] Although initially thought to be useful, the addition of urokinase flushes has shown no benefit in the treatment of infected catheters.[107] Another technique to treat central venous catheter infections is the antibiotic lock technique. This technique allows one to place markedly higher doses of antibiotic within the catheter itself and to leave them there while not in use.[108, 109] It allows antibiotics to be used that normally would be ineffective if given systemically because of such high minimum inhibitory concentrations (e.g., nafcillin for a staphylococcal line infection). Antibiotic lock methods are used routinely in some centers but probably have their greatest utility in those patients who may not tolerate aminoglycoside or vancomycin administration.

Because febrile patients are frequently the most in need of nutritional support, it is important to have a protocol for managing central catheters in these high-risk patients. Parenteral nutrition is never an emergency procedure, and a febrile patient should undergo a thorough investigation of the source of the fever before being started on central PN. If PN begins while a patient is febrile, periodic blood cultures should be drawn until the patient becomes afebrile.

In most series, fungal sepsis comprises 3 to 15% of all catheter infections and is increasing. The most common organism is *Candida* sp., which is associated with considerable morbidity and mortality. Most *Candida* infections require removal of the silastic catheter because of the high risk (25%) of mortality and low chance of attaining clearance of the infection with the line in place (13%).[110] Only a relatively short course (7 to 14 days) of antifungal agents needs to be given after the catheter is removed, and blood cultures must be confirmed as negative.[111] In the unusual case of the loss of central venous access due to the previous placement of multiple catheters, a trial of antifungal agents with the line in place may be attempted. A more uncommon fungal organism associated with TPN is *Malassezia furfur*. This organism thrives in a lipid-rich environment and generally responds to antifungal treatment without catheter removal as long as lipids are withheld.

Catheter Failure

Catheter occlusion or fracture is the second most common reason for catheter removal. Although external fractures of silastic catheters can be repaired, internal breaks can result in embolization of the catheter or extravasation. Therefore, if a kinking of the catheter is detected on plain radiograph, removal is generally indicated.[112] Silastic catheters may become occluded by thrombus, calcium precipitates, or lipid deposition. An initial trial of two flushes of urokinase (5000 U/ml), each with a 20-minute dwell time, should be attempted. Should this fail, a trial of two flushes of 0.1 N hydrochloric acid (HCl), with a similar dwell time, should be tried. If the HCl is unsuccessful, 70% ethanol should be tried. The HCl dissolves calcium precipitates and is most effective in long-term nutrition patients. The ethanol dissolves lipid deposits as well as most drug precipitates.[113] The volume of most Silastic catheters is small, and very small volumes of these potentially harmful agents can be infused. A pediatric size 4 French-Broviac catheter has a volume of 0.004 ml/cm length and a 2.7 French-Broviac catheter has a volume of 0.002 ml/cm length.

Metabolic Complications

Although almost every conceivable metabolic abnormality has been reported during TPN, the more common ones are discussed below. Serious consequences may ensue if these complications go undetected for any length of time. However, careful monitoring with appropriate adjustment of the PN solution allows most patients to tolerate TPN quite well.

Hyperglycemia does not require treatment unless the glucose level exceeds 300 mg/dl or there is a significant osmotic diuresis. Insulin production normally compensates as the glucose load is increased over a 48- to 72-hour period, returning the blood glucose to normal. If hyperglycemia does not autoregulate, regular human insulin may be added to the infusate. Nondiabetic infants and children rarely require insulin. Patients who are stable on PN and suddenly develop a blood glucose level greater than 200 mg/dl or who require increasing doses of insulin should be evaluated for sepsis. Marked hyperglycemia is quite deleterious to the infant. Aside from causing an osmotic diuresis, hyperglycemia can predispose to an increased risk of infection rates owing to the blood becoming a rich environment for bacterial growth as well as impairment of the complement system.[64] Hyperglycemia causes a dissociation of the insulin effect on glucose and potassium transport. Thus, although insulin can assist in transporting glucose into the cell, potassium does not enter the cell and no actual anabolic benefit may occur.[114] Finally, marked hyperglycemia can result in significant fluid shifts in the central nervous system, which can cause intracranial bleeding, especially in the premature infant. These fluid shifts can also occur in the kidney and can cause renal cortical bleeding. One group at particular risk for hyperglycemia is the infant with a very low birth weight who has a low renal threshold for glucose.[115–117] Careful use of an insulin drip (beginning at 0.01 U/kg/hour) in this particular population has been shown to be quite effective, with improvement in glucose utilization and weight gain.[118, 119]

Although symptoms of hypoglycemia, such as diaphoresis, confusion, or agitation, have been reported when PN is abruptly terminated, we have rarely observed this complication in children even with many accidental interruptions of infusions. Nevertheless, 10% dextrose should always be administered when the TPN solution is interrupted for any reason. PN should be tapered gradually when nutrition by vein is no longer required, ideally by decreasing the rate to half the original dosage during the last hour before termination. Such a routine should be standard for patients on cycled PN.

Patients undergoing major surgical procedures frequently become glucose intolerant because of endogenous hormone secretion or insulin resistance. Therefore, we recommend that the PN infusion rate be routinely decreased by half, or stopped altogether, when the patient is taken to the operating room. The infusion can usually be returned to the preoperative rate within 24 to 48 hours after the surgical procedure, provided that the blood glucose concentration has returned to an acceptable range after the first phase of surgical convalescence. For minor procedures, PN need not be interrupted.

Hypokalemia may develop when a patient on PN becomes anabolic and begins to synthesize new protein. Intravenous potassium is administered at a level of 2 to 4 mEq/kg/day in infants and small children, or at a concentration of 40 mEq/l in older children and adolescents. Higher dosages may be required in the early phase of refeeding, which will become evident by monitoring the patient's serum potassium concentration.

Hyperkalemia may develop in patients receiving PN if they are not significantly anabolic. Other causes of hyperkalemia include decreased renal function, metabolic acidosis, tissue necrosis, and systemic sepsis. Potassium should be reduced or withheld from the PN solution until the underlying problem is resolved.

Calcium and phosphorus disturbances have been reported in patients who receive TPN because of inappropriate amounts of calcium and phosphorus being added to the TPN solution. These extremes can be avoided by careful monitoring of serum calcium and phosphorus levels. Because of growth requirements, infants and children need relatively more calcium and phosphorus than do adolescents or adults.

Hypomagnesemia results in hallucinations, vertigo, ileus, and hyperreflexia. The addition of appropriate amounts of magnesium to the infusate completely eliminates this complication.

Essential fatty acid deficiency may be detectable by laboratory assessment after as little as 2 to 3 weeks of fat-free TPN and consists of a raised serum level of 5,8,11 eicosatrienoic acid, low levels of linoleic and arachidonic acids, and an eicosatrienoic:arachidonic (triene:tetranene) ratio greater than 0.4.[120] Clinical signs of fatty acid deficiency usually do not appear until after 2 to 3 months of fat-free therapy except in the small neonate. Typically, a flaking erythematous, papular rash develops, which is generally limited to the legs, chest, and face. This rash can be corrected by administering at least 3% of the child's daily caloric requirements in the form of linoleic acid. Because most pediatric patients who receive PN also routinely receive intravenous fat as part of their daily caloric budget, the complication of fatty acid deficiency has largely been eliminated.

Triglyceride and cholesterol levels are normal in most patients receiving a fat emulsion. A few who receive PN for longer than 1 month have serum triglyceride levels in the range of 300 to 350 mg/dl (normal levels are 50 to 150 mg/dl) and serum cholesterol values of 150 to 250 mg/dl (normal, 100 to 150 mg/dl). These elevations appear to be of little consequence and return to normal once the fat infusion is discontinued.[121] In general, high triglyceride levels are most consistent with excessive carbohydrates and are not due to excessive lipid administration. Another important cause of high triglyceride levels is carnitine deficiency. This is particularly common in premature infants, those on long courses of TPN, and those with renal failure. In general, total plasma carnitine levels are the most accurate way to determine a deficiency. Supplementation of carnitine in neonates should be given if they are on TPN for more than 10 to 14 days.

Metabolic acidosis usually develops because the added chloride exceeds 6 mEq/kg/day. The problem is most commonly seen in premature infants who are not able to excrete a sufficient amount of acid load through their kidneys. Balancing the chloride:acetate ratio with the TPN solution is a useful method to correct or control the metabolic state of an infant. In addition, the administration of cysteine may lead to acidosis.

Fluid overload in the form of pulmonary edema, peripheral edema, or congestive heart failure is rare in patients treated according to the techniques previously outlined, provided that proper patient selection and monitoring are carried out. Studies at our institution that have employed the tracers deuterium oxide and sodium bromide have shown that total body water and extracellular fluid volumes during PN do not increase, but rather decrease, concomitant with an increase in body weight.[17] The results strongly support the hypothesis that weight gain during PN is due to tissue accretion rather than water retention.

Respiratory failure, in patients with compromised pulmonary function, may be due to the large dextrose loads associated with PN. If these patients are already receiving ventilatory assistance, weaning from the ventilator may be difficult. This complication can be resolved by decreasing the total caloric load for the patient.

☐ Home Parenteral Nutrition

Home parenteral nutrition (HPN) is a rapidly developing area of nutritional support. Approximately 40,000 patients per year receive this therapy in the United States, and its usage in this country is 4 to 10 times that of other developed countries.[122] The cost of HPN exceeds $800 million per year in the United States excluding the added costs of hospitalizations. The average cost of maintaining a pediatric patient on HPN ranges from $100,000 to 150,000 per year. The most common diagnosis among HPN patients is cancer, followed by inflammatory bowel disease and the short bowel syndrome.

HPN for infants and children provides well-documented psychological, social, and economic advantages over continued hospitalization, provided that patients and parents have been selected carefully and continued support is available. The major indications for HPN are (1) that the primary diagnosis precludes normal growth and development without supplemental parenteral nutrition and (2) the potential need for 14 to 30 days or more of conventional PN. Although many third-party payers are unwilling to pay for patients on short-term (i.e., <90 days) HPN, many patients can derive a significant benefit from this form of treatment, and therapy at home both reduces cost and improves patient well-being. Once a Silastic central venous catheter has been placed, a detailed protocol for HPN is adapted to each patient and family, and the method of infusion and catheter care is described stepwise. Once the patient is stable, with optimal PN volume and concentration given over 24 hours, an adaptive phase is begun. This consists of decreasing the duration of infusion by 2 hours each day while holding the total daily volume constant via an appropriate increase in the infusion rate. An electric volumetric infusion pump that can be programmed to increase and decrease rates of infusion at the initiation and termination of TPN is ideally suited for this. Eventually, the patient can tolerate infusion of his or her 24-hour nutritional needs over 10 to 12 hours at night. Irrigating the catheter with a heparinized saline solution and capping it off during the day permits both the parents and child a more normal lifestyle. The nutrient solution may be prepared by the hospital pharmacy or supplied to the patient at home by one of several commercial vendors.

An HPN program is one half to one third the cost of in-hospital PN support and is ideally carried out by the pharmacists, dietitians, and nurses on the parenteral and enteral nutrition team. Complications, unfortunately, have not been well documented, but HPN appears to be relatively safe. Based on the largest analysis of HPN patients, the Oley Foundation documented a survival in children of approximately 92%.[122] Rehabilitation to normal activity occurred in the majority of children, and a mean of 1.8 complications/year of HPN therapy was seen.

□ Special Problems in Nutritional Support of the Pediatric Surgical Patient

BILIARY ATRESIA

The infant with biliary atresia, even after a clinically successful hepatic portoenterostomy, generally has lower than normal amounts of bile flow into the intestine. This subsequently leads to a profound defect in fat digestion and absorption.[123] Such a deficit may leave the infant with an essential fatty acid deficiency and inadequate absorption of fat soluble vitamins, leading to a lack of bone mineralization as well as failure to thrive. The essential goals for such an infant are to provide adequate calories using a formula that maximizes fat intake. Portagen (Mead Johnson & Company) has been used for a variety of causes of liver failure in infancy because of its high content of medium-chain triglycerides. Medium-chain triglycerides, which undergo intestinal luminal triglyceride hydrolysis, are less dependent on bile acids for absorption than are long-chain fatty acids. Portagen, however, contains a limited amount of linoleic acid. A more ideal formula is Pregestimil (Mead Johnson & Company). Although Pregestimil contains fewer medium-chain triglycerides than does Portagen (60% vs. 80%), the former contains approximately 11% of its calories as linoleic acid. Thus, provision of essential fatty acid is better. When PN is needed, a standard crystalline amino acid solution appears to be best. Although there are claims that branch chain amino acid formulas are better, no proven benefit has been shown in pediatric patients. Breast-feeding, although generally ideal in infancy, may actually be detrimental in patients with biliary atresia because breast milk has a much higher fat content than commercially available formulas. Vitamin supplementation is critical in patients with biliary atresia. Table 2–6 gives the current recommendations for fat-soluble vitamin administration in patients with this condition. Frequent monitoring of vitamin levels is essential to ensure that sufficient supplementation is being achieved. Water-soluble vitamins in addition to those provided in standard infant formulas should be administered in a multivitamin preparation. There should be careful screening for iron, zinc, and calcium deficiencies.

SHORT BOWEL SYNDROME

Nutritional support of a child with the short bowel syndrome is complex and requires a multidis-

TABLE 2-6. Vitamins and Supplements for Children with Liver Disease*

Medications to be Given at Diagnosis	
Vitamin	Amount
A†	10,000–25,000 IU/day Aquasol A (Astra, Inc.)
D	0.05–0.2 µg/kg/day Rocaltrol (1.25-dihydroxycholecalciferol) (Roche Laboratories)
E	20 IU/kg/day Aquasol E (Astra, Inc.)
K	2.5 mg biweekly to 5 mg/day AquaMEPHYTON (Merck)

Additional Potential Deficiencies in Patients with Biliary Atresia

Iron: Iron deficiency is common. Supplementation: 2 mg/kg of Fer-in-Sol (Mead Johnson) should be given one to three times daily depending on the level of deficiency.
Calcium and zinc: Both can be decreased in cases of fat malabsorption, and levels should be monitored.
Additional supplements: Multivitamins for infants once daily.

*Vitamin levels should initially be measured every 3 months then yearly, and adjusted appropriately.
†If levels remain low, suspect additional zinc deficiency.

ciplinary approach involving the pediatric surgeon, pediatric gastroenterologist, pharmacist, and dietitian. The care of such an infant can be divided into three stages.[124] The first stage of care begins after resuscitation of the patient during the postoperative period or when the diagnosis of short bowel syndrome is made. The syndrome is associated with increased gastric output, owing to a loss of intrinsic intestinal negative feedback, and increased stool output, which often leads to fluid and electrolyte shifts and losses of nutrients and trace elements. During this time a permanent Silastic central venous catheter (e.g., Broviac) needs to be inserted. Because the child will need long-term venous access, each access site must be carefully cared for and protected. The child's main or sole caloric source will be via the parenteral route for a considerable period. Nevertheless, enteral feedings should be initiated within 1 to 2 weeks after the onset of the short bowel syndrome. Enteral feedings stimulate small bowel adaptation and prevent the development of PN-associated cholestasis. The ideal enteral solution is isotonic, or nearly isotonic, as this is better tolerated by the gastrointestinal tract. The protein source should be predominately dipeptides and tripeptides, since this source of protein is absorbed most easily and efficiently.[125] The solution should have a fair amount of medium-chain triglycerides, as this source of fat is well absorbed through the basolateral wall of the intestinal enterocytes. However, medium-chain triglycerides contain no essential fatty acids, thus these fats cannot be the sole source of lipids in these patients. Table 2–4 lists recommended formulas for children of different ages. In infants, we prefer to initiate feedings with Pregestimil, and in children older than 1 year, we generally use Petamen Junior (Clintec), which can be given to children as old as 10 years). High stool output is associated with excessive losses of zinc; thus, levels of zinc above those normally required should be provided in the PN solution. Finally, the loss of sodium and bicarbonate in such patients can be dramatic, and a total body sodium depletion has been shown to be associated with failure to thrive, despite the administration of adequate amounts of calories.[126, 127] A simple way to detect such a deficit is to measure a spot urine sodium. A urine sodium of less than 10 mEq/l may well indicate total body sodium depletion, and supplementation via the oral route should be given on a daily basis.

During the second phase of support, a more stabilized state has been reached, at which point careful monitoring of the patient's nutritional status is very important. Electrolytes, liver function, and protein status (total protein albumin and total iron binding capacity) should be assessed initially and on a weekly basis thereafter. Fat-soluble vitamin levels should be assessed approximately every 6 months to assure that adequate amounts are being absorbed. Serum levels of vitamins A, D, and E can be assayed. A prothrombin time is indicative of vitamin K levels. Patients with a significant loss of the terminal ileum should have their vitamin B_{12} level assessed on a yearly basis. The supplementation of fat-soluble vitamins, if depleted, should follow the recommendation outlined in the previous section on biliary atresia. The child's stool should intermittently be assessed for pH, reducing substances and qualitative fecal fats. A stool pH of 5.5 or less or a reducing substance level greater than 0.5% indicates the malabsorption of carbohydrates. Elevation in fecal fats suggests fat malabsorption, which may require modification of the child's enteral diet (i.e., increase the percentage of medium-chain triglycerides). Formulas with sucrose as the carbohydrate do not yield a positive reducing substance test despite carbohydrate malabsorption.

The final phase of nutritional support consists of weaning the patient off of PN. During this stage, which may last from months to years, a variety of factors must be monitored. These include an assurance that the child will develop normal suck and swallow reflexes and not develop an aversion to oral feedings. Also, the child should be monitored for normal length and weight gain. Patients with an intact colon should be evaluated for the development of renal oxalate stones, and thus should avoid a diet high in oxalates.

Recently, an interest in "rehabilitating" the intestinal remnant in these in patients has surfaced. The use of enteral glutamine, a high-fiber diet, and systemic growth hormone has been tried in patients on long-term TPN. A 3-week course of this therapy apparently resulted in improved caloric absorption from the intestine and decreased stool output.[128] Experience in children, however, is lacking, and further work in this age group is needed to confirm these findings. More recent work in this area has actually demonstrated no improvements in small bowel morphology, stool losses, or macronutrient absorption.[129]

FAILURE TO THRIVE

Malnutrition in childhood is associated with poor growth and development. The diagnosis of failure to thrive is based on a weight more than 2½ SD below the mean weight percentile of both parents. Failure to thrive is either symmetric, in which case height, length, and the development of other body organs all are below the fifth percentile, or asymmetric, in which case weight is lower than the fifth percentile but length and head circumference are within normal limits. In general, those patients with symmetrical failure to thrive have more profound malnutrition and suffer from greater neurologic maldevelopment than those with asymmetric failure to thrive, who have reasonably normal cognitive development. More recent investigations have shown that abnormal cognitive development in patients with failure to thrive may well be due to a poor social environment and is often reversible.[130, 131]

The approach to feeding a patient with failure to thrive should include a multidisciplinary assessment of medical, social, and psychological factors. A systematic evaluation should be carried out to rule out neurologic pathology, swallowing disorders, feeding aversion, malabsorption, and metabolic disorders. A trial of feeding the child in a hospital setting can often identify a problem with the child's home and social environment. Nutritional support for an infant should begin at approximately 50 kcal/kg/day and advance by 20 to 25 kcal/kg/day, as long as there is adequate gastrointestinal tolerance to the feedings. Stool weight should be less than 150 g/day in young infants. Feedings may increase to 150 to 240 kcal/kg/day to achieve adequate catch-up growth.[132] Additional potassium up to 5 mEq/kg/day may also be required during the first week of nutritional rehabilitation. Levels of potassium, magnesium, and phosphate need to be closely monitored, as they often drop rapidly during the initiation of feedings. The following is a commonly used formula for estimating catch-up growth[133]:

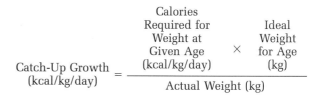

$$\text{Catch-Up Growth (kcal/kg/day)} = \frac{\substack{\text{Calories Required for Weight at Given Age (kcal/kg/day)}} \times \substack{\text{Ideal Weight for Age (kg)}}}{\text{Actual Weight (kg)}}$$

Estimated protein requirements can similarly be estimated using a similar formula by substituting protein required (g/kg) for calories required. However, this formula not infrequently overestimates nutritional needs. Another simple formula is to provide five additional calories for each gram of tissue weight gain per day that is desired.

THE CHILD WITH DISABILITIES

Between 10 and 20% of children in the United States have special healthcare needs because of chronic illness and developmental disorders.[134] Among these disorders are several in which pediatric surgeons take an active part in nutritional care, including neurologic impairment; developmental delay; cerebral palsy; and a variety of genetic syndromes such as trisomies 13, 18, and 21 and de Lange's and Rett syndromes. The pediatric surgeon is often responsible for providing nutritional access in many of these patients as well as for maintaining nutritional care before and after surgery. Potential factors that may contribute to poor nutrition in these patients include feeding disorders, uncoordinated tongue movements, poorly coordinated swallowing reflexes, gastroesophageal reflux with associated nutrient loss, and increased energy expenditure due to muscle spasticity or athetosis. Because measuring energy expenditure in these children may be impractical, estimates of energy needs can be based on previous studies of resting energy expenditure. Children with spastic type (hypertonia) cerebral palsy may have lower energy needs than normal. These children with cerebral palsy have approximately 1200 to 1300 kcal/day in total energy needs for an adolescent.[135, 136] Children with athetosis (consisting of a mixed pattern of too much and too little muscle tone) may require a higher than normal calorie intake, sometimes more than double the recommended daily allowance. Children with myelomeningocele are quite inactive compared with their peers and may therefore need only 50 to 60% of estimated energy needs of normal children (Table 2–7).

Often the child's body habitus is markedly abnormal; in this instance, a more appropriate estimate of energy needs is based on surface area rather than weight. Repeated assessments of the child's growth during nutritional supplementation are essential, since the development of obesity in these impaired children is common and can cause a considerable burden on the family and caregivers because of the increased difficulty in moving an overweight child.

METABOLIC BONE DISEASE IN THE PREMATURE INFANT

With improved medical and surgical care, pediatric surgeons are caring for a larger number of preterm infants. The incidence of metabolic bone disease in these infants is as high as 30% in infants weighing less than 1500 g and is 70% in infants weighing less than 800 g at birth.[137] Factors that tend to exacerbate the development of rickets in preterm infants include the prolonged use of PN as well as the use of thiazide diuretics. It is essential to detect this disorder, using biochemical tests and radiologic assessment. Biochemical tests include measurements of calcium phosphate, vitamin D, and serum alkaline phosphatase levels. Calcium levels

TABLE 2-7. Guidelines for Estimating Caloric Requirements Based on Height in Children with Developmental Disabilities

Condition	Caloric Recommendation
Ambulatory, ages 5–12 y	13.9 kcal/cm height
Nonambulatory, ages 5–12 y	11.1 kcal/cm height
Cerebral palsy with severely restricted activity	10 kcal/cm height
Cerebral palsy with mild to moderate activity	15 kcal/cm height
Athetoid cerebral palsy, adolescence	Up to 6000 kcal/day
Down's syndrome, boys, ages 1–14 y	16.1 kcal/cm height
Down's syndrome, girls, ages 1–14 y	14.3 kcal/cm height
Myelomeningocele	Approximately 50% of recommended daily allowance for age after infancy. May need as little as 7 kcal/cm height to maintain normal weight.
Prader-Willi syndrome	10–11 kcal/cm height (maintenance) 8–9 kcal/cm height (weight loss)

Adapted from DeYoung L (ed): Mayo Clinic Diet Manual: A Handbook of Nutrition Practices (7th ed). St. Louis, Mosby–Year Book, 1994.

are often normal in patients with rickets; however, phosphate levels are characteristically low in these patients. Alkaline phosphatase levels are elevated in many infants with rickets.[138] Because elevated levels of alkaline phosphates may also be due to PN-associated cholestasis, interpretation may be somewhat difficult. Alkaline phosphatase levels are characteristically five times higher than normal adult levels. Fractionation of the alkaline phosphates may help determine the etiology of its elevation (i.e., bone vs. liver). Unfortunately, standard chest and extremity radiographs detect only advanced cases of rickets, well after the full clinical development of the process. A more precise assessment of rickets can be done using x-ray or photon absorptiometry.[8]

Treatment of neonatal rickets ideally begins with prevention. Neonates receiving long-term PN should receive maximal amounts of calcium and phosphate, at a calcium:phosphate ratio of 1.3:1 to 1.7:1, which provides good retention rates with little or no disturbance to mineral homeostasis.[137] Further increases in calcium concentration run the risk of the development of calcium phosphate salt precipitation and occlusion of the intravenous catheter or ectopic calcium deposition.[139] The administration of cysteine HCl has been used to improve calcium and phosphate solubility by decreasing the pH of the PN solution. The risks of adding such a solution include the development of a metabolic acidosis as well as a potential leaching of calcium salts from bone. Probably no more than 4 mg/dl of cysteine should be added to the PN formula. For neonates receiving enteral feedings, liquid or powdered human milk fortifiers or a preterm infant formula should be used (see Table 2–4). If commercial fortifiers are not available, calcium disodium phosphate should be added to breast milk or standard formula. Both the level and activity of vitamin D are quite adequate in most preterm infants, and thus, no additional vitamin D is needed. Supplementation should continue until the infant obtains a weight of 3 to 3.5 kg (term weight).

PARENTERAL NUTRITION–ASSOCIATED CHOLESTASIS

The initial association between cholestasis and PN was made 4 years after this therapy was first used in neonates.[140] Histologically, the liver shows bile duct proliferation in the portal triad region, with the subsequent formation of large tracts of fibrosis between normal-appearing hepatocytes.

Several factors have been found to be associated with parenteral nutrition-associated cholestasis (PNAC). The most prominent risk factors are low birth weight and prematurity.[141–143] The duration of TPN administration has also been shown to increase the risk of cholestasis. PNAC leads to cirrhosis, sepsis, and increased mortality rates. Although reversible in its early stage, cirrhosis eventually becomes irreversible; clearly, liver failure is the ultimate complication. The group at greatest risk of PNAC are those infants on long-term TPN for the short bowel syndrome. In one series, the incidence of sepsis was 56% in PNAC babies, compared with 13% in those babies on TPN with normal bilirubin levels.[144] The higher infection rates in these patients can most likely be explained by a number of immunologic deficiencies that develop as shown in animal models of bile duct ligation and that include decreased T-lymphocyte function and lymphocytic proliferation.[145, 146] Infants with PNAC have a 31% mortality compared with a 3% mortality for those on TPN without cholestasis.[144] In our group of patients with the short bowel syndrome, the majority of those who died developed a significant rise in direct bilirubin level within 4 months of their development of short bowel syndrome. Those patients given sustained direct bilirubin at a level of more than 4 mg/dl for more than 6 months had an 80% mortality.

The etiology of cholestasis is unknown. The PN solution may contain something toxic to the liver, or it may be missing one or more critical nutritional factors that are needed to prevent liver injury. Virtually every possible factor included in the TPN formula has been implicated as the causative agent at one time or another. Among the more likely factors is a lack of taurine. A lack of taurine prevents the conjugation of bile salts, which are needed for their excretion. Taurine-supplemented TPN has been compared with the standard PN in a limited number of studies. Although some of these studies have

suggested a decreased incidence of cholestasis in those neonates receiving taurine, no adequate study has been performed.[43] Phytosterols found in intravenous lipid compounds and derived from plant products have been suspected to have a role in the development of PNAC. Patients with PNAC have been shown to have elevated plasma levels of phytosterols,[147] and these levels may accumulate in other types of patients with cholestasis.[148] More recently, phytosterols have been implicated in the pathogenesis of PNAC itself, using a rabbit model.[149] Methionine, although needed in premature infants, has been suggested as a cause of PNAC.[150]

One clear cause of liver injury is overfeeding, most commonly with excessive carbohydrates. The liver pathology in this condition, however, is different in that the only finding is hepatic steatosis, without bile duct proliferation. Clearly, by limiting the amount and type of delivered calories, this problem can be avoided.

A more recently proposed cause is bacterial translocation, which has a higher incidence in fasting animals. During the process of bacterial translocation, a release of endotoxins can lead to the secretion of various cytokines, including TNF and α-interferon, by either peritoneal or hepatic macrophages. These cytokines could then potentially cause liver injury. The administration of antimicrobial agents such as metronidazole has been hypothesized to reduce the incidence of cholestasis by decreasing the colonization of the gastrointestinal tract and subsequently the incidence of bacterial translocation. In one study on rats receiving TPN, the degree of hepatic steatosis was reduced with oral antibiotic treatment; however, bilirubin levels remained unchanged, suggesting that the cause of hepatic steatosis most likely differs from that of cholestasis.[151]

The last area that has been considered in the etiology of PNAC is the lack of enteral stimulation. During prolonged periods of fasting, the gastrointestinal tract lacks sufficient enteral stimulation for the release of a variety of hormones that promote bile flow. Such hormones may be critical in preventing biliary stasis. The use of cholecystokinin to relieve this problem has been attempted in experimental animals and in clinical trials with moderate success.[152, 153] Cholecystokinin given near the beginning of the TPN administration appeared to have an even greater benefit in preventing the development and severity of PNAC.[154]

An associated problem related to the prolonged use of TPN is the development of cholelithiasis. Approximately 10% of patients with the short bowel syndrome develop gallstones.[155] Because many of these infants were not specifically studied for the presence of gallstones, the incidence of cholelithiasis may in fact be much higher. In general, many of these stones regress over time. The majority are asymptomatic and thus do not require cholecystectomy.

REFERENCES

1. Marian M: Pediatric nutrition support. Nutr Clin Pract 8:199–209, 1993.
2. Rose J, Gibbons K, Carlson SE, Koo WWK: Nutrient needs of the preterm infant. Nutr Clin Pract 8:226–232, 1993.
3. Wright JA, Ashenburg CA, Whitaker RC. Comparison of methods to categorize undernutrition in children. J Pediatr 124:944–946, 1994.
4. Detsky AS, McLaughlin JR, Baker JP, et al: What is subjective global assessment of nutritional status? JPEN J Parenter Enteral Nutr 11:8–13, 1987.
5. Coran AG, Drongowski RA, Wesley JR: Changes in total body water and extracellular fluid volume in infants receiving total parenteral nutrition. J Pediatr Surg 19:771–776, 1984.
6. Coran AG, Drongowski RA: Body fluid compartment changes following neonatal surgery. J Pediatr Surg 24:829–832, 1989.
7. Jensen MD: Research techniques for body composition assessment. J Am Diet Assoc 92:454–460, 1992.
8. Braillon PM, Salle BL, Brunet J, et al: Dual energy X-ray absorptiometry measurement of bone mineral content in newborns: Validation of the technique. Pediatr Res 12:77–80, 1992.
9. Rico HM, Revilla LF, Villa ER, et al: Body composition in children and Tanner's stages: A study with dual-energy X-ray absorptiometry. Metabolism 42:967–970, 1993.
10. Bistrian BR: Interaction of nutrition and infection in the hospital setting. Am J Clin Nutr 30:1228–1235, 1977.
11. Merritt RJ, Kalsch M, Roux LD: Significance of hypoalbuminemia in pediatric oncology patients—malnutrition or infection? JPEN J Parenter Enteral Nutr 9:303–306, 1985.
12. Kenny SE, Pierro A, Isherwood D, et al: Hypoalbuminaemia in surgical neonates receiving parenteral nutrition. J Pediatr Surg 30:454–457, 1995.
13. Katz MD, Lor E, Norris K: Comparison of serum prealbumin and transferrin for nutritional assessment of TPN patients: A preliminary study. Nutr Support Serv 6:22–24, 1986.
14. Roza AM, Tuitt D, Shizgal HM: Transferrin—a poor measure of nutritional status. JPEN J Parenter Enteral Nutr 8:523–528, 1984.
15. Bernstein LH, Leukhardt-Fairfield CJ, Pleban W: Usefulness of data on albumin and prealbumin concentrations in determining effectiveness of nutritional support. Clin Chem 35:271–274, 1989.
16. Spiekerman M: Proteins used in nutritional assessment. Clin Lab Med 13:353–369, 1993.
17. Heird W, Driscoll J, Schullinger J: Intravenous alimentation in pediatric patients. J Pediatr 80:351–355, 1972.
18. Reichman B, Chessex P, Putet G, et al: Diet, fat accretion, and growth in premature infants. N Engl J Med 305:1495–1500, 1981.
19. Baker J, Detsky A, Wesson D: Nutritional assessment: A comparison of clinical judgment and objective measurements. N Engl J Med 306:969–972, 1982.
20. Kaplan AS, Zemel BS, Neiswender KM, Stallings VA: Resting energy expenditure in clinical pediatrics: Measured versus prediction equations. J Pediatr 127:200–205, 1995.
21. Mendeloff E, Wesley J, Deckert R: Comparison of measured resting energy expenditure (REE) versus estimated energy expenditure (EEE) in infants. JEPN J Parenter Enteral Nutr 10(suppl):65–69, 1986.
22. Mitchell IM, Davies PSW, Day JME, et al: Energy expenditure in children with congenital heart disease, before and after cardiac surgery. J Thorac Cardiovasc Surg 107:374–380, 1994.
23. Chwals WJ, Lally KP, Woolley MM: Indirect calorimetry in mechanically ventilated infants and children: Measurement accuracy with absence of audible airleak. Crit Care Med 20:768–770, 1992.
24. Groner JI, Brown MF, Stallings VA, et al: Resting energy expenditure in children following major operative procedures. J Pediatr Surg 24:825–828, 1989.
25. Jones M, Pierro A, Hammond P, Lloyd D: The metabolic response to operative stress in infants. J Pediatr Surg 28:1258–1263, 1993.
26. Anand K, Sippell M, Aynsley-Green A: Randomised trial of fentanyl anaesthesia in preterm babies undergoing surgery: Effects on the stress response. Lancet 1:243–248, 1987.
27. Jones MO, Pierro A, Hashim IA, et al: Postoperative changes in resting energy expenditure and interleukin 6 level in infants. Br J Surg 81:536–538, 1994.
28. Letton RW, Chwals WJ, Jamie A, Charles B: Early postoperative alterations in infant energy use increase the risk of overfeeding. J Pediatr Surg 30:988–993, 1995.
29. Lemons JA: Fetal-placental nitrogen metabolism. Semin Perinatol 3:177–190, 1979.
30. Zlotkin SH, Bryan MH, Anderson GH: Intravenous nitrogen and energy intakes required to duplicate in utero nitrogen accretion in prematurely born human infants. J Pediatr 99:115–120, 1981.
31. Goldman HI, Goldman JS, Kaufman I, Liebman OB: Late effects of early dietary protein intake on low-birth-weight infants. J Pediatr 85:764–769, 1974.
32. Fomon S: Requirements and recommended dietary intakes of protein during infancy. Pediatr Res 30:391–395, 1991.
33. Colle E, Paulsen E: Response of the newborn infant to major surgery. I. Effects on water, electrolyte, and nitrogen balance. Pediatrics 23:1063–1084, 1959.
34. Coran A: Nutrition of the surgical patient. In Welch K (ed): Pediatric Surgery. Chicago, Year Book Medical, 1986, pp 96–108.
35. Seashore J, Huszar G, Davis E: 1981. Urinary 3-methylhistidine/creatinine ratio as a clinical tool: Correlation between 3-methylhistidine excretion and metabolic clinical states in healthy and stressed premature infants. Metabolism 30:959–969, 1981.
36. Duffy B, Pencharz P: The effects of surgery on the nitrogen metabolism of parenterally fed human neonates. Pediatr Res 20:32–35, 1986.
37. Pierro A, Carnielli V, Filler R, et al: Characteristics of protein sparing effect of total parenteral nutrition in the surgical infant. J Pediatr Surg 23:538–542, 1988.
38. Dahlstrom KA, Ament ME, Laidlaw SA, Kopple JD: Plasma amino acid concentrations in children receiving long-term parenteral nutrition. J Pediatr Gastroenterol Nutr 7:748–754, 1988.
39. Das JB, Filler PM: Amino acid utilization during total parenteral nutrition in the surgical neonate. J Pediatr Surg 8:793–799, 1973.
40. Zlotkin SH, Anderson SH: The development of cystathionase activity during the first year of life. Pediatr Res 16:65–68, 1982.
41. Miller R, Jahoor F, Jaksic T: Decreased cysteine and proline synthesis in parenterally fed, premature infants. J Pediatr Surg 30:953–958, 1995.
42. Heird WC, Dell RB, Helms RA, et al: Amino acid mixture designed to maintain normal plasma amino acid patterns in infants and children requiring parenteral nutrition. Pediatrics 80:401–408, 1987.
43. Heird WC, Hay W, Helms RA, et al: Pediatric parenteral amino acid mixture in low birth weight infants. Pediatrics 81:41–50, 1988.
44. Okamoto E, Rassin DK, Zucker CL, et al: Role of taurine in feeding the low-birth-weight infant. J Pediatr 104:936–940, 1984.
45. Tyson JE, Lasky R, Flood D, et al: Randomized trial of taurine supplementation for infants less than or equal to 1,300-gram birth weight: Effect on auditory brainstem-evoked responses. Pediatrics 83:406–415, 1989.
46. Souba WW, Herskowitz K, Austgen TR, et al: Glutamine nutrition: Theoretical considerations and therapeutic impact. JPEN J Parenter Enteral Nutr 14:237S–243S, 1990.
47. O'Dwyer S, Smith R, Hwang T, Wilmore D: Maintenance of small bowel mucosa with glutamine-enriched parenteral nutrition. JPEN J Parenter Enteral Nutr 13:579–585, 1989.
48. Alverdy JC: Effects of glutamine-supplemented diets on immunology of the gut. JPEN J Parenter Enteral Nutr 14:109S–113S, 1990.

49. Loch H, Hubl W: Metabolic basis for selecting glutamine-containing substrates for parenteral nutrition. JPEN J Parenter Enteral Nutr 14:114S–117S, 1990.

50. Tremel H, Kienle B, Weilemann LS, et al: Glutamine dipeptide-supplemented parenteral nutrition maintains intestinal function in the critically ill. Gastroenterology 107:1595–1601, 1994.

51. Tamada H, Nezu R, Imamura I, et al: The dipeptide alanyl-glutamine prevents intestinal mucosal atrophy in parenterally fed rats. JPEN J Parenter Enteral Nutr 16:110–116, 1992.

52. Spaeth G, Gottwald T, Haas W, Holmer M: Glutamine peptide does not improve gut barrier function and mucosal immunity in total parenteral nutrition. JPEN J Parenter Enteral Nutr 17:317–323, 1993.

53. Ziegler TR, Young LS, Benfell K, et al: Clinical and metabolic efficacy of glutamine-supplemented parenteral nutrition after bone marrow transplantation. A randomized, double-blind, controlled study. Ann Intern Med 116:821–828, 1992.

54. Schloerb PR, Amare M: Total parenteral nutrition with glutamine in bone marrow transplantation and other clinical applications (a randomized, double-blind study). JPEN J Parenter Enteral Nutr 17:407–413, 1993.

55. Buchman AL: Glutamine: Is it a conditionally required nutrient for the human gastrointestinal system? J Am Coll Nutr 15:199–205, 1996.

56. Scull CW, Rose WC: Arginine metabolism. I. The relation of the arginine content of the diet to the increments in tissue arginine during growth. J Biol Chem 89:109–121, 1930.

57. Barbul A: Arginine: Biochemistry, physiology and therapeutic implications. J Parenter Enteral Nutr JPEN 10:227–238, 1986.

58. Hibbs JB, Vavrin Z, Taintor RR: L-arginine is required for expression of the activated macrophage effector mechanism causing selective metabolic inhibition in target cells. J Immunol 138:550–565, 1987.

59. Daly JM, Reynolds J, Thom A, et al: Immune and metabolic effects of arginine in the surgical patient. Ann Surg 208:512–528, 1988.

60. Kelly E, Morris S, Billiar T: Nitric oxide, sepsis and arginine metabolism. JPEN J Parenter Enteral Nutr 19:234–238, 1995.

61. Nussler AK, Billiar TR, Liu ZZ, Morris SM Jr: Coinduction of nitric oxide synthase and argininosuccinate synthetase in a murine macrophage cell line: Implications for regulation of nitric oxide production. J Biol Chem 269:1257–1269, 1994.

62. Kien L: 1993. Carbohydrates. In Tsang RC, Lucas A, Vauy R (eds): Nutritional Needs of the Preterm Infant, Scientific Basis and Practical Guidelines. Baltimore, Williams & Wilkins, 1993, pp 47–63.

63. American Academy of Pediatrics Committee on Nutrition: Practical significance of lactose intolerance in children. Pediatrics 86(suppl):643–644, 1990.

64. Hennessey PJ, Black CT, Andrassy RJ: Nonenzymatic glycosylation of immunoglobulin G impairs complement fixation. JPEN J Parenter Enteral Nutr 15:60–64, 1991.

65. Wilmore D: Glucose metabolism following severe injury. J Trauma 21:705–707, 1981.

66. Watters J, Bessey P, Dinarello C: Both inflammatory and endocrine mediators stimulate host response to sepsis. Arch Surg 121:179–190, 1986.

67. Elphick M, Wilkinson A: The effects of starvation and surgical injury on the plasma levels of glucose, free fatty acids, and neutral lipids in newborn babies suffering from various congenital anomalies. Pediatr Res 15:313–318, 1981.

68. Anand K, Sippell W, Schofield N: Does halothane anaesthesia decrease the metabolic and endocrine stress response of newborn infants undergoing operation? Br Med J 296:668–672, 1988.

69. Friedman Z, Danon A, Stahlman MT, Oates JA: Rapid onset of essential fatty acid deficiency in the newborn. Pediatrics 58:640–649, 1976.

70. Feuerstein G, Hallenbeck JM: Leukotrienes in health and disease. FASEB J 1:186–192, 1987.

71. Coran AG, Drongowski R, Sarahan TM, Wesley JR: Comparison of a new 10% and 20% safflower oil fat emulsion in pediatric parenteral nutrition. JPEN J Parenter Enteral Nutr 5:236–239, 1981.

72. Haumont D, Deckelbaum RJ, Richelle M, et al: Plasma lipid and plasma lipoprotein concentration in low birth weight infants given parenteral nutrition with twenty or ten percent lipid emulsion. J Pediatr 115:787–793, 1989.

73. Penn D, Ludwigs B, Schmidt-Sommerfeld E: Effect of nutrition on tissue carnitine concentrations in infants of different gestational ages. Biol Neonate 47:130–135, 1985.

74. Roe C: Clinical experience with carnitine deficiency. J Rare Dis 111:5–11, 1997.

75. Senkal M, Mumme A, Eickhoff U, et al: Early postoperative enteral immunonutrition: Clinical outcome and cost-comparison analysis in surgical patients. Crit Care Med 25:1489–1496, 1997.

76. Schilling J, Vranjes N, Fierz W, et al: Clinical outcome and immunology of postoperative arginine, omega-3 fatty acids, and nucleotide-enriched enteral feeding: A randomized prospective comparison with standard enteral and low calorie/low fat i.v. solutions. Nutrition 12:423–429, 1996.

77. Bower RH, Cerra FB, Bershadsky B, et al: Early enteral administration of a formula (Impact) supplemented with arginine, nucleotides, and fish oil in intensive care unit patients: results of a multicenter, prospective, randomized, clinical trial. Crit Care Med 23:436–449, 1995.

78. Cioffi W, Gore D, Rue L: Insulin-like growth factor-1 lowers protein oxidation in thermally injured patients. Ann Surg 220:310–316, 1994.

79. Fang C, Li B, Wand J, et al: Insulin-like growth factor 1 stimulates protein synthesis and inhibits protein breakdown in muscle from burned rats. JPEN J Parenter Enteral Nutr 21:245–251, 1997.

80. Pang KY, Bresson JL, Walker WA: Development of the gastrointestinal mucosal barrier. Evidence for structural differences in microvillus membranes from newborn and adult rabbits. Biochim Biophys Acta 727:201–208, 1983.

81. Kiristioglu I, Teitelbaum DH: Alteration of intestinal intraepithelial lymphocytes during total parenteral nutrition. J Surg Res 79:91–96, 1998.

82. Kudsk K, Croce M, Favian T, et al: Enteral versus parenteral feeding. Effects on septic morbidity after blunt and penetrating abdominal trauma. Ann Surg 215:503–511, 1992.

83. Moore FA, Moore EE, Kudsk KA, et al: Clinical benefits of an immune-enhancing diet for early postinjury enteral feeding. J Trauma 37:607–615, 1994.

84. Alverdy J, Aoys E, Moss G: Total parenteral nutrition promotes bacterial translocation from the gut. Surgery 104:185–190, 1988.

85. Cummins A, Chu G, Faust L, et al: Malabsorption and villous atrophy in patients receiving enteral feeding. JPEN J Parenter Enteral Nutr 19:193–198, 1995.

86. Groh-Wargo S: Prematurity and low birth weight. In Lang C (ed): Nutrition Support in Critical Care. Rockville, MD, Aspen Publishers, 1987, pp 287–313.

87. Isch JA, Rescorla FJ, Scherer LR III, et al: The development of gastroesophageal reflux after percutaneous endoscopic gastrostomy. J Pediatr Surg 32:321–323, 1997.

88. Motil KJ: 1987. Breast-feeding: Public health and clinical overview. In Grand RJ, Sutphen JL, Dietz WH Jr (eds): Pediatric Nutrition Theory and Practice. Stoneham, MA, Butterworth, 1987, pp 251–263.

89. Wright JA, Walker WA: Breast milk and host defense of the infant. In Grand RJ, Sutphen JL, Dietz WH Jr (eds): Pediatric Nutrition Theory and Practice. Stoneham, MA, Butterworth, 1987, pp 293–303.

90. Ogra SS, Ogra PL: Immunological aspects of human colostrum and milk. J Pediatr 92:550, 1978.

91. Kleinman RE, Walker WA: The enteromammary immune system. Dig Dis Sci 24:876–878, 1979.

92. Gross S, David R, Bauman L, Tomarelli R: Nutritional composition of milk produced by mothers delivering preterm. J Pediatr 96:641–644, 1980.

93. Reed CR, Sessler CN, Glauser FL, Phelan BA: Central ve-

nous catheter infections: Concepts and controversies. Intensive Care Med 21:177–183, 1995.

94. Kurkchubasche AG, Smith SD, Rowe MI: Catheter sepsis in short-bowel syndrome. Arch Surg 127:21–25, 1992.

95. Fabri PJ, Mirtallo JM, Ebbert ML, et al: Clinical effect of nonthrombotic total parenteral nutrition catheters. JPEN J Parenter Enteral Nutr 8:705–707, 1984.

96. Yao JD, Arkin CF, Karchmer AW: Vancomycin stability in heparin and total parenteral nutrition solutions: Novel approach to therapy of central venous catheter-related infections. JPEN J Parenter Enteral Nutr 16:268–274, 1992.

97. Spear ML, Stahl GE, Hamosh M, et al: Effect of heparin dose and infusion rate on lipid clearance and bilirubin binding in premature infants receiving intravenous fat emulsions. J Pediatr 112:94–98, 1988.

98. Sitges-Serra A, Puig P, Linares J, et al: Hub colonization as the initial step in an outbreak of catheter-related sepsis due to coagulase-negative staphylococci during parenteral nutrition. JPEN J Parenter Enteral Nutr 8:668–672, 1984.

99. Cercenado E, Ena J, Rodriguez-Creixems M, et al: A conservative procedure for the diagnosis of catheter-related infections. Arch Intern Med 150:1417–1420, 1990.

100. King DR, Komer M, Hoffman J, et al: Broviac catheter sepsis: The natural history of an iatrogenic infection. J Pediatr Surg 20:728–733, 1985.

101. Wurzel CL, Halom K, Feldman JG, Rubin LG: Infection rates of Broviac-Hickman catheters and implantable venous devices. Am J Dis Child 142:536–540, 1988.

102. Dawson S, Pai MKR, Smith S, et al: Right atrial catheters in children with cancer: A decade of experience in the use of tunnelled, exteriorized devices at a single institution. Am J Pediatr Hematol Oncol 13:126–129, 1991.

103. Johnson PR, Decker MD, Edwards KM, et al: Frequency of broviac catheter infections in pediatric oncology patients. J Infect Dis 154:570–578, 1986.

104. Caniano DA, Starr J, Ginn-Pease ME: Extensive short-bowel syndrome in neonates: Outcome in the 1980s. Surgery 105:119–124, 1989.

105. Wang E, Prober C, Ford-Jones L, Gold R: The management of central intravenous catheter infections. Ped Infect Dis 3:110–113, 1984.

106. Goldstein E, Bartholomew W, Parr T, Vickers J: Monitoring vancomycin blood levels: When to start? [letter]. JAMA 270:1426, 1993.

107. La Quaglia MP, Caldwell C, Lucas A, Corbally M: A prospective randomized double-blind trial of bolus urokinase in the treatment of established Hickman catheter sepsis in children. J Pediatr Surg 29:742–745, 1994.

108. Cowan CE: Antibiotic lock technique. J Intraven Nurs 15:283–287, 1992.

109. Messing B, Peitra-Cohen S, Debure A, et al: Antibiotic-lock technique: A new approach to optimal therapy for catheter-related sepsis in home-parenteral nutrition patients. JPEN J Parenter Enteral Nutr 12:185–189, 1988.

110. Eppes SC, Troutman JL, Gutman LT: Outcome of treatment of candidemia in children whose central catheters were removed or retained. Pediatr Infect Dis J 8:99–104, 1989.

111. Donowitz LG, Hendley JO: Short-course amphotericin B therapy for candidemia in pediatric patients. Pediatrics 95:888–891, 1995.

112. Hinke DH, Zandt-Stastny DA, Goodman LR, et al: Pinch-off syndrome: A complication of implantable subclavian venous access devices. Radiology 177:353–356, 1990.

113. Werlin SL, Lausten T, Jessen S, et al: Treatment of central venous catheter occlusions with ethanol and hydrochloric acid. JPEN J Parenter Enteral Nutr 19:416–418, 1995.

114. Shangraw RE, Jahoor F, Miyoshi H, et al: Differentiation between septic and postburn insulin resistance. Metabolism 38:983–989, 1989.

115. Hay WW, Sparks JW: Placental, fetal and neonatal carbohydrate metabolism. Clin Obstet Gynecol 28:473–485, 1985.

116. Lilien DP, Rosenfeld RL, Baccaro MM: Hyperglycemia in stressed, small premature infants. J Pediatr 94:454–459, 1979.

117. Varma S: Homeostatic response to glucose loading in newborn and young dogs. Metabolism 22:1367–1375, 1973.

118. Collins JWJ, Hoppe M, Brown K: A controlled trial of insulin infusion and parenteral nutrition in extremely low birth weight infants with glucose intolerance. J Pediatr 118:921–927, 1991.

119. Ostertag SG, Jovanovic L, Lewis B: Insulin pump therapy in the very low birth weight infant. Pediatrics 78:625–630, 1986.

120. Wesley J, Coran A: Intravenous nutrition for the pediatric patient. Semin Ped Surg 1:212–230, 1992.

121. Coran A, Edwards B, Zaleska R: The value of heparin in the hyperalimentation of infants and children with a fat emulsion. J Pediatr Surg 9:725–732, 1974.

122. Howard L, Ament M, Fleming CR, et al: Current use and clinical outcome of home parenteral and enteral nutrition therapies in the United States. Gastroenterology 109:355–365, 1995.

123. Kaufman SS, Murray ND, Wood P, et al: Nutritional support for the infant with extrahepatic biliary atresia. J Pediatr 110:679–686, 1987.

124. Farrell MM: Nutrition in gastrointestinal disorders of infancy and childhood. In Walberg-Ekvall S (ed): Pediatric Nutrition and Chronic Diseases in Developmental Disorders. New York, Oxford University Press, 1993, pp 293–300.

125. Schmitz J: Malabsorption. In Walker W, Durie P, Hamilton J, et al (eds): Pediatric Gastrointestinal Disease. Vol. 1. Philadelphia, BC Decker, 1991, pp 79–89.

126. Bower TR, Pringle KC, Soper RT: Sodium deficit causing decreased weight gain and metabolic acidosis in infants with ileostomy. J Pediatr Surg 23:567–572, 1988.

127. Sacher P, Hirsig J, Gresser J, Spitz L: The importance of oral sodium replacement in ileostomy patients. Prog Pediatr Surg 24:226–231, 1989.

128. Byrne TA, Morrissey TB, Nattakom TV, et al: Growth hormone, glutamine, and a modified diet enhance nutrient absorption in patients with severe short bowel syndrome. JPEN J Parenter Enteral Nutr 19:296–302, 1995.

129. Scolapio JS, Camilleri M, Fleming CR, et al: Effect of growth hormone, glutamine, and diet on adaptation in short-bowel syndrome: A randomized, controlled study. Gastroenterology 113:1074–1081, 1997.

130. Levitsky DA, Strupp BJ: Malnutrition and the brain: Changing concepts, changing concerns. J Nutr 125:2212S–2220S, 1995.

131. Strupp BJ, Levitsky DA: Enduring cognitive effects of early malnutrition: A theoretical reappraisal. J Nutr 125:2221S–2232S, 1995.

132. Peterson KE, Washington J, Rathbun JM: Team management of failure to thrive. J Am Diet Assoc 84:810–815, 1984.

133. Rathbun J, Peterson K: Nutrition in Failure to Thrive. In Grand R, Sutphen J, Dietz W (eds): Pediatric Nutrition, Theory and Practice. Stoneham, MA, Butterworth, 1987, pp 627–643.

134. Roche A: Growth and assessment of handicapped children. Diet Curr 6:25, 1970.

135. Eddy T, Nicholson A, Wheeler E: Energy expenditures and dietary intakes in cerebral palsy. Dev Med Child Neurol 7:377–380, 1965.

136. Krick J, Murphy P, Markham J, Shapiro B: A proposed formula for calculating energy needs of children with cerebral palsy. Devel Med Child Neurol 34:481–487, 1992.

137. Greene HL, Hambidge KM, Schanler R, Tsang RC: Guidelines for the use of vitamins, trace elements, calcium, magnesium, and phosphorus in infants and children receiving total parenteral nutrition: Report of the Subcommittee on Pediatric Parenteral Nutrient Requirements from the Committee on Clinical Practice Issues of The American Society for Clinical Nutrition. Am J Clin Nutr 48:1324–1342, 1988.

138. Lipkin E, Ott S, Klein G: Serum markers of bone formation in parenteral nutrition patients. Calcif Tissue Int 47:75–81, 1990.

139. Hamoudi AC, Singley CT, Teitelbaum DH, et al: Intravascular calcium deposits in a critically ill patient. Light- and electron-microscopic findings. Arch Pathol Lab Med 117:1257–1260, 1993.

140. Peden V, Witzleben C, Skelton M: Total parenteral nutrition [letter]. J Pediatr 78:180–181, 1971.

141. Drongowski RA, Coran AG: An analysis of factors contributing to the development of total parenteral nutrition-induced cholestasis. JPEN J Parenter Enteral Nutr 13:586–589, 1989.
142. Merritt R: Cholestasis associated with total parenteral nutrition. J Pediatr Gastroenterol Nutr 5:9–22, 1986.
143. Sax HC, Bower RH: Hepatic complications of total parenteral nutrition. JPEN J Parenter Enteral Nutr 12:615–618, 1988.
144. Ginn-Pease M, Pantalos D, King D: TPN-associated hyperbilirubinemia: A common problem in newborn surgical patients. J Pediatr Surg 20:436–439, 1985.
145. Feduccia TD, Scott-Conner CE, Grogan JB: Profound suppression of lymphocyte function in early biliary obstruction. Am J Med Sci 296:39–44, 1988.
146. Maggiore G, De Giacomo C, Scotta MS, et al: Cell-mediated immunity in children with chronic cholestasis. J Pediatr Gastroenterol Nutr 1:385–388, 1982.
147. Clayton PT, Bowron A, Mills KA, et al: Phytosterolemia in children with parenteral nutrition–associated cholestatic liver disease. Gastroenterology 105:1806–1813, 1993.
148. Gylling H, Vuoristo M, Farkkila M, Miettinen TA: The metabolism of cholestanol in primary biliary cirrhosis. J Hepatol 24:444–451, 1996.
149. Iyer K, Spitz L, Clayton P: New insight into mechanisms of parenteral nutrition–associated cholestasis: Role of plant sterols. J Pediatr Surg 33:1–6, 1998.
150. Moss R, Haynes A, Enomoto M, Glew R: Methionine infusion reproduces liver injury of parenteral nutrition cholestasis. Surg Forum 48:642–644, 1997.
151. Pappo I, Bercovier H, Berry EM, et al: Polymyxin B reduces total parenteral nutrition–associated hepatic steatosis by its antibacterial activity and by blocking deleterious effects of lipopolysaccharide. JPEN J Parenter Enteral Nutr 16:529–532, 1992.
152. Rintala RJ, Lindahl H, Pohjavuori M: Total parenteral nutrition-associated cholestasis in surgical neonates may be reversed by intravenous cholecystokinin: A preliminary report. J Pediatr Surg 30:827–830, 1995.
153. Teitelbaum DH, Han-Markey T, Schumacher RE: Treatment of parenteral nutrition–associated cholestasis with cholecystokinin-octapeptide. J Pediatr Surg 30:1082–1085, 1995.
154. Teitelbaum D, Han-Markey T, Drongowski R, et al: Use of cholelcystokinin to prevent the development of parenteral nutrition–associated cholestasis. JPEN J Parenter Enteral Nutr 20:100–103, 1997.
155. Manji N, Bistrian B, Mascioli E, et al: Gallstone disease in patients with severe short bowel syndrome dependent on parenteral nutrition. JPEN J Parenter Enteral Nutr 13:461–464, 1989.

3

ANESTHETIC CONSIDERATIONS

Robert E. Binda, Jr., MD • Peter H. Mestad, MD

☐ Preanesthetic Evaluation

Pediatric surgical procedures are frequently performed on an outpatient basis, or the patients are admitted from the postanesthetic care unit (PACU). As a consequence, information that can be used in evaluating the patient's readiness for surgery is often limited to that obtained in a telephone interview or on the day of surgery. This amount of information is generally adequate, but at times clarification of complicating factors may necessitate postponement or delay of the procedure. Some centers are developing the preoperative evaluation center, in which patients can be evaluated more thoroughly prior to the day of surgery. Exposure that pediatric patients and parents have to the healthcare facility can be abrupt and intimidating. "Preop parties" acquaint the children and parents to the surgical environment prior to the day of surgery and often alleviate many of these concerns.

A focused history provides valuable information. A history of pseudocholinesterase deficiency, malignant hyperthermia, or porphyria in family members or the patient is important, although the absence of these complications does not exclude them from consideration. Approximately 33% of patients who develop malignant hyperthermia, for example, have had a previous uneventful anesthetia. Drug allergies and adverse reactions are common. Focused questions often reveal an allergy that was previously denied or has been forgotten. Allergy to latex is an increasing problem that can result in life-threatening complications during a surgical procedure. Extensive exposure to latex is usually related in the history. Institutional protocols that deal with the prevention and treatment of latex allergy and latex susceptibility can be helpful in minimizing confusion and optimizing the care of this problem. The preanesthetic interview should include a short review of major organ systems and recent illnesses.

The preanesthetic physical examination should be appropriate for the surgical procedure and the patient's physical status. Frequently, children have evidence of upper respiratory infection. Common sense should dictate whether these patients should undergo an anesthetic. If the rhinorrhea and cough are chronic problems and no other signs of acute illness are present, it is appropriate to proceed with the operation. However, if onset of the "runny nose" is recent or if the child has other signs of illness, such as decreased activity or appetite or an elevated temperature, it is best to postpone the procedure until the illness has run its course. Fever cannot be ignored, and unless a satisfactory alternative explanation for the temperature elevation is present, the operation should be postponed. Children who have an acute upper respiratory infection have a two- to sevenfold greater risk of having an adverse respiratory event during the anesthetic and recovery period.[1]

Routine laboratory testing is not indicated. Little new or useful information is gained from routine testing, and in most cases management decisions are not changed as a result of the testing.[2, 3] In 1987, the American Society of Anesthesiologists' House of Delegates stated that routine laboratory or diagnostic screening test is not necessary for the preanesthetic evaluation of patients. Decisions regarding the need for laboratory tests should be based on the individual patient and the proposed operative procedure. Trauma to the pediatric patients and indirectly to their parents is lessened, and healthcare costs are decreased by eliminating venipuncture.

Many children being operated on have preexisting illnesses for which they are taking medication. In general, medications, including oral as well as aerosolized medications, should be continued up to the time of operation. By doing this, it is hoped that exacerbations of illness will be avoided, making the anesthetic course smoother and safer. The possible exception is digoxin (Lanoxin) for cardiac surgery patients.

Frequently, children who have cardiac anomalies must undergo extracardiac operations. Some of these patients are at risk for subacute bacterial endocarditis. Recommendations for prophylaxis of this disease have been clarified and simplified.[4] Only one preoperative antibiotic dose is now recommended. Young children often have a heart murmur that can be heard during a physical examination. It may be difficult to differentiate significant from innocent murmurs. The type of surgery that is planned as well as the physical status of the child dictates whether a more thorough evaluation is necessary prior to performing the surgical procedure.

Aspiration pneumonitis can be a serious complication to any anesthetic. However, the incidence and morbidity of aspiration may be decreasing.[5–7] Prolonged preoperative fasting may result in dehydration and hypoglycemia and thereby add to parental and patient stress.[8] Policies that allow ingestion of clear liquids up to 2 or 3 hours before surgery and solids up to 6 or 8 hours before surgery are now common in many pediatric facilities. Milk and formula are considered solids.[9] The incidence of aspiration has not increased following the adoption of these policies, and the patients and parents have been more satisfied. Because of the low incidence of significant aspiration, the routine use of gastric antisecretory medications is not justified. The use of these agents in emergency procedures may be warranted, however.

Preoperative medication is another controversial issue. Preoperative medications were initially intended to make a safer anesthetic by shortening the excitation period of anesthetic induction. Anesthetics that are used today have a short induction time and therefore have a short excitation period. Preoperative medication may also be used to lessen the psychological trauma that children may experience prior to their operation. Although a calm environment and a well-presented preanesthetic visit decrease anxiety in many cases, many medications have been administered by various routes. One technique that should be abandoned in most instances is the intramuscular injection, since oral medication has the same effect with less trauma to the patient.[10] Midazolam 0.3 to 0.5 mg/kg given orally is effective in decreasing patient anxiety without demonstrable delay in awakening time or the time to discharge from the facility.[11] Fentanyl given in lozenge form is similarly effective but may be associated with undesirable side effects such as preoperative and postoperative vomiting and facial itching.[12] Regardless of the medication used, 30 to 45 minutes are required for peak effectiveness. In addition, it is prudent to monitor the oxygen saturation after administration and before the induction of anesthesia. Induction rooms, which allow the parents to be present during the induction, may be as effective as pharmacologic agents and are so utilized in some institutions.

☐ Management of Outpatient Surgery

Ambulatory surgery comprises 70% or more of the case load in most pediatric centers. Multiple factors need to be considered when evaluating whether a child is suitable for outpatient surgery. Communication between surgeons and anesthesiologists is essential in this evaluation. Individual circumstances vary, and no set of rules can be applied to all situations. In most cases, the child should be free of severe systemic disease. However, a well-controlled systemic illness should not adversely affect the postoperative course. Operative procedures in which major organ systems are significantly affected may not be suitable in an outpatient facility. Other factors that may determine the suitability of a child for outpatient surgery are family and social dynamics. For instance, will this child be cared for by a responsible and capable adult? Is the child to be cared for by a single parent who must work? How far must the child travel to receive appropriate medical attention, if needed? These and other individual factors should be considered when evaluating a pediatric patient for outpatient surgery.

Today's ideal anesthetic should have a rapid onset of action, allow for a rapid recovery with minimal or no side effects, and be maximally effective at reasonable cost. The emphasis is on minimizing anesthetic time and hospital exposure. These demands present challenges to the anesthesiologist and have required reevaluation of the type of care given to patients during the perioperative period as well as the way effectiveness is evaluated.[13] Routine admission to the PACU, for example, may no longer be required using newer anesthetics. Indeed, controlling admissions to the PACU may be the only way to decrease anesthetic costs significantly.[14] This issue is being actively investigated.

Anesthesiologists have at their disposal a wide choice of anesthetics that are suitable for outpatient use. Children are frightened of needles, and the use of inhalation anesthetics still predominates in most pediatric centers. Halothane is the most frequently used volatile agent. However, two new agents, sevoflurane and desflurane, are both reported to have shorter induction and recovery times.[15] An added advantage of sevoflurane is that it has an odor that is usually acceptable to most children. Desflurane, on the other hand, has a pungent odor that limits its use as an induction agent. In addition, recovery from desflurane may be associated with an increase in agitation and delirium.[16] Regardless of the reported advantages that these newer agents have over halothane, clear benefits will need to be demonstrated prior to replacing an agent that has a 40-year record of safety and low cost.

Newer drugs have made intravenous anesthesia more attractive in pediatrics. Opioids such as fentanyl and alfentanil are frequently used as adjuncts to inhalation anesthetics. Remifentanil, an ultra–short acting opioid with a half-life of 11 minutes, is being used more frequently because of its rapid emergence time. Propofol has become very popular, again due to its short half-life and apparent lack of significant side effects. This lipid emulsion agent has been used as an induction and maintenance agent for operative and diagnostic procedures that require deep sedation. As an added benefit, it appears to act as an antiemetic.[17]

Fear of needles has limited the use of intravenous agents. Preoperative medication may mitigate this fear to some extent. In addition, the use of local anesthetics such as Emla cream has been effective in reducing the pain of needle insertions. Intravenous agents will certainly continue to play a role in pediatric anesthesia, and techniques are constantly being developed that will ensure their use to the greatest advantage.

Regional anesthetics, in particular spinal or caudal blocks, are used in some institutions for outpatient surgical procedures.[18] The regional technique may be used alone with sedation or in association with a general anesthetic. Personal preference will control how the procedure is performed.

To maximize safety, outpatients should be given the same consideration as inpatients when deciding on monitoring and postoperative care. It is often helpful to establish venous access after induction to partially rehydrate the patient, provide an avenue for intraoperative drug administration, and provide an avenue for postoperative pain relief in the recovery room. We try to administer at least 30 ml/kg of crystalloid while the intravenous line is in place. This amount provides adequate hydration if oral intake be diminished postoperatively and may help decrease nausea after surgery.

□ Recovery of Outpatients

The recovery period for pediatric patients may be more crucial than that for adult patients. Although the risks of intraoperative problems are similar in adults and children, 3 to 4% of infants and children experience major complications in the recovery period, whereas only 0.5% of adults experience these complications.[19, 20]

Because of the increased use of same-day surgery and because of the frequency of postoperative complications in children, clinicians must readdress some of the problems common in children who are recovering from surgery.

The outpatient who is experiencing pain can be managed in much the same manner as the inpatient. Local anesthetic blocks have proved to be extremely valuable in managing the postoperative pain of pediatric outpatients.[21] Bupivacaine may give a patient 12 to 24 hours of reasonable pain relief, thereby reducing the need for narcotics during the postoperative period.

Vomiting occurs in about 2 to 5% of all pediatric surgical patients.[20] Its incidence is much higher in adolescent patients, in whom it may be twice as high without regard to the procedure[20]; in patients with a history of motion sickness; and in patients undergoing certain procedures, such as eye muscle surgery, in whom it may occur with a frequency of 80%.[22] We no longer require that children be free from vomiting and be able to tolerate liquids before

discharge from the hospital, since it is now recognized that oral intake before discharge may cause vomiting.[23] We make certain that the patients are well hydrated before discharge, typically by providing intravenous fluids intraoperatively. We also provide antiemetic therapy to children who have had a prior history of postoperative vomiting and to those who are undergoing a procedure that is associated with a high incidence of nausea and vomiting (e.g., strabismus surgery, dental rehabilitation, tonsillectomy, and middle ear surgery). Antiemetic medications include ondansetron, droperidol, and metoclopramide. Ondansetron appears to be the treatment of choice in many centers, but expense limits its use.[24–26]

Airway problems are common in the pediatric age group, and they account for many of the problems in the recovery room. In a large study of pediatric perioperative problems, airway obstructions occurred in 3% of cases overall.[11] Our incidence is similar, occurring in 2% of all our patients. This problem usually occurs in patients who arrive in the recovery room still deeply anesthetized, without mechanical airway support.

Another common airway problem in children is postintubation croup. When outpatient surgery was first offered for pediatric patients, many centers went to great lengths to avoid intubating outpatients because of the concern for this complication. If intubation was necessary, it often precluded that patient from being treated as an outpatient. With experience, it was noted that this type of croup, unlike viral croup, had a somewhat defined time course and was not associated with rebound edema when treated with racemic epinephrine.[27] It gradually became routine to provide endotracheal intubations wherever indicated and to exclude the need for intubation from the criteria for admission to the hospital after surgery.

Postintubation croup occurs in about 1 to 6% of all pediatric patients and is most common after surgery involving the head and neck region, in children between the ages of 1 and 4 years, in traumatic or repeated attempts at intubation, and after excessive coughing or straining on the endotracheal tube.[28] Treatment is usually limited to nebulized racemic epinephrine (0.5 ml in 2.5 ml of saline), although some investigators have recommended steroids.[29] Currently, our practice is to observe patients who require racemic epinephrine for 2 hours and then allow them to leave the hospital. The parents are instructed about signs and symptoms of increasing stridor or respiratory distress and whom to contact in the event that either occurs.

The final complication we have noted in the recovery room is oxygen desaturation. Reduction in oxygen saturation occurs in approximately 3% of patients. The most common cause for this complication is the admission to the PACU with a marginal airway because of still being deeply anesthetized. However, some patients have difficulty in maintaining adequate (95%) oxygen saturations on room air for no discernible reason. These patients are observed on oxygen, with the saturation monitored in the hospital for several hours postoperatively. If they improve, they are discharged; if not, they are admitted to the hospital overnight for oxygen therapy.

☐ Care of the Former Preterm Infant

The potential dangers in performing outpatient surgery on former premature infants were first published in 1982.[30] The most life-threatening hazard is apnea following the surgical procedure, normally within the first 12 to 18 hours. Factors that contribute to the increased risk are not completely understood but may include immature neurologic development, particularly in the brain stem's respiratory center, and less developed diaphragmatic musculature that leads to easier fatigability.[31] The age after birth at which this increased risk of apnea disappears is still being debated despite numerous studies of this issue. A metaanalysis of pertinent studies was reported in 1995.[32] The results of this analysis indicated that there was a significant reduction in the incidence of apnea at 52 to 54 weeks postconceptional age, depending on the gestational age. A hematocrit below 30% was identified as a risk factor, and it was recommended that infants with this degree of anemia be hospitalized postoperatively for observation no matter what the age. However, conclusions drawn using metaanalysis have been challenged for their validity, and the sample size of this study may not have been large enough to draw valid conclusions.[33]

No anesthetic technique appears to be clearly superior to other techniques, although some evidence has suggested an advantage to spinal anesthesia.[34] General anesthesia is still the preferred anesthetic in most institutions.[35] Likewise, no medications can predictably prevent apnea, although caffeine may hold some promise.[36] Until more patients are systematically studied, the choice of when former preterm infants can be operated on as outpatients is up to the discretion and personal bias of the anesthesiologist and surgeon. Institutional policies most commonly mention ages of 44 to 46 weeks, 50 weeks, or 60 weeks postconceptual age. Indeed, a recent survey of surgical practices showed that approximately one third of the surgeons chose to wait until 50 weeks and that one third waited until 60 weeks postconceptual age.[35] Legal issues direct such practices in some institutions. More important, regardless of the postconceptual age at time of surgery, an infant should be hospitalized if any safety concerns arise during the operative or PACU period.

☐ Monitoring

In 1954, Beecher and Todd were the first to analyze factors leading to anesthetic mortality.[37] They assumed that the major risk of anesthetic mishaps was the use of dangerous and potent drugs, in this case the muscle relaxant curare. Although their conclusions have subsequently been proved to be wrong, their methodology was sound and continues as the basis for most medical outcome studies. For instance, they were the first investigators to use a denominator when expressing mortality statistics.

Little change occurred in the thinking about anesthetic mishaps until the 1970s. It was then that experts began to attribute the majority of anesthetic mishaps to human error[38–43] and not to the anesthetic drugs or the equipment used to deliver them. These findings led to a precedent that all individuals administering anesthetics maintain a heightened awareness and vigilance. One study reported that 50% of the errors were the result of inexperience, haste, inattention, or fatigue on the part of the anesthetist.[42] It was a logical conclusion that increasing the monitoring of the patient might prevent many of these mishaps by alerting the anesthesia provider(s) to changes in the patient's condition.

It soon became evident that the major problems, although human in origin, most often resulted in events that were respiratory in nature. Hypoventilation and hypoxemia were the most frequently noted complications. A landmark study of the Harvard hospitals, which looked at their malpractice losses, reported that 82% of all alleged anesthesia claims were respiratory in origin and that 90% of these were thought to be preventable.[44] These findings therefore began two decades of technological advances directed at providing more intraoperative information to the anesthetist in the hopes of reducing adverse outcomes.

Prior to 1970, intraoperative monitoring consisted mainly of noninvasive blood pressure and heart rate measurements. Invasive monitoring of arterial, central venous, pulmonary arterial, and intracranial pressures began to be employed during prolonged anesthetics or when the patient's medical condition(s) dictated that more careful monitoring would be beneficial. The noninvasive monitors that were heralded as providing the most valuable information (with the least risk) were oxygen saturation and exhaled carbon dioxide (capnography).

What is often overlooked in reviews of anesthetic safety is that the anesthetic experience was actually becoming safer before the introduction of hi-tech monitoring.[45] The improvement in anesthesia safety has not been critically evaluated and instead is offered simply as evidence that increased monitoring was responsible. Thus, the anesthetic experience was not only becoming safer but much more expensive because of increased monitoring.

In 1985 and 1986, standards for monitoring (which attempted to codify monitoring usage in the United States) were proposed by Harvard University and the American Society of Anesthesiologists. Insurance carriers assumed, as did the majority of physicians, that increased monitoring would produce increased safety. As anesthetic outcomes subsequently improved, malpractice premiums dropped dramatically for anesthesiologists. Once again, this was taken as evidence that the anesthetic experience had become safer solely because of increased monitoring. No critical scientific studies were undertaken to test the relationship between improved outcome and monitoring.

Several recent studies, however, have examined the impact that monitors have had on the safety of anesthesia. One of the first was a retrospective study claiming that the major difference in outcomes between cases performed at Harvard University hospitals before and after 1985 must have resulted from the impact of monitoring introduced in 1985.[46] As with most retrospective studies, many variables such as newer anesthetics, new anesthetic techniques, better preoperative and postoperative care, and different surgical techniques were not considered in this study. A recent prospective study of 20,000 anesthetics concluded that although the detection of hypoxia increased 19-fold in the group whose oxygen saturation was monitored, the overall incidence of complications was no different in the nonmonitored control group.[47] The relatively small numbers involved in this study may compromise its value.

Although no one would advocate the return to premonitoring days, we must guard against assuming that the more technological information we have, the better the care will be for the patient. There is also the risk that false information or false interpretation of correct information can lead to bad decisions and bad patient consequences.[48]

Having offered this long disclaimer, we have to accept the fact that monitoring of infants and children during surgery is here to stay. Those monitors and their basis for use are now briefly summarized.

The electrocardiogram (ECG) monitor has been used primarily to determine abnormal cardiac rhythms and the presence or absence of myocardial ischemia. Significant arrhythmias are usually bradyarrhythmias and extrasystoles that may portend a serious cardiac event. It is not uncommon to have healthy children become bradycardic during various procedures. On rare occasions, healthy children have developed complete heart block on being anesthetized. In these children, subsequent cardiology evaluations often reveal previously undetected conduction defects. The other common use for ECG monitoring is the detection of myocardial ischemia. This condition is not often an important consideration in the pediatric population, and even in the adult age group it is estimated that standard ECG monitors detect only 30% of ischemic events.

Because most (90%) pediatric anesthetic mishaps[49] are the result of respiratory events, the detection of hypoxemia and its correction have become the basis for most quality improvement efforts of anesthesia departments. The advent of reliable practical oxygen saturation technology has been hailed as a major advance in pediatric anesthesia. When anesthetists were allowed to view the saturation

monitor only 14% of cases were associated with hypoxemia at any time during the anesthsia.[50] The control group, in which the anesthetist was blinded to the oxygen monitor, experienced saturations below 90% in 42% of the cases.

The other part of respiratory monitoring is capnography or mass spectrometry. The purported advantages of capnography include its ability to confirm endotracheal intubation, to measure $PaCO_2$ indirectly, and, when minute ventilation is controlled, to indicate changes in pulmonary blood flow (i.e., cardiac output).

Automated noninvasive blood pressure monitors have improved anesthetic care mainly by freeing the anesthetist from manual measurements of blood pressure, especially in critical situations.

The final part of monitoring is the use of multiple alarms to alert the anesthetist to changes in the patient's condition that exceed predetermined limits. All vital sign monitors, along with most aspects of the anesthesia machine (including ventilators), are now equipped with alarms. Again, in theory these should increase the safety of anesthesia functioning as an early warning system. Unfortunately, as with the rest of the monitors discussed, the benefits of alarms are largely unproved. One study reported that these alarms sounded an average of 10 times per case.[51] In addition, 75% were false and only 3% indicated a possible risk to the patient. Most of the time, they served as distractions to the anesthetists and other members of the surgical team. Alarms were often ignored and many times were turned off.

If monitors are to warrant their added expense, their reliability and true benefit to the care of the patient must be critically proved. Unfortunately, however, in our litigious society the use of expensive monitoring, no matter how unproved, is here to stay.

☐ Pain

The incidence of postoperative pain in the pediatric population, although difficult to evaluate objectively, is probably similar to that in the adult population. It is reasonable, therefore, to assume that about 75% of children will report significant pain on the first postoperative day.[52]

Ineffective treatment of postoperative discomfort in children is most often the result of four factors:

1. Individuals involved in the care of children are working with an evolving knowledge of the mechanisms of pain and its transmission in children. Attitudes toward the management of pain in children have often been biased by several observations made on newborns. It has been known for many years that newborns may cry for relatively short periods after experiencing noxious stimuli and then settle down and sleep without the use of analgesics.[53] In addition, microscopic examination of thalamocorti-

cal tracts in the newborn has shown a lack of myelin, leading investigators and clinicians to postulate that the pain perception of neonates is immature and rudimentary.[54] Finally, higher concentrations of endogenous opioids are present in the plasma and cerebrospinal fluid of neonates when compared with those of older children.[55] This type of information has led to the erronious conclusion that babies do not have a normal sensation of pain and therefore do not require postoperative pain therapy. Evidence now indicates that neonates do experience pain in a manner similar to that of adults. Sophisticated observations of cry patterns, facial expressions, movements, and cardiovascular variables allow for reproducible documentation of painful experiences in these smallest of patients.

2. There remain misperceptions regarding the pharmacokinetics of pain medications in children. Clearly, the neonate presents differences from older children and adults that must be taken into account. For instance, neonates appear to have a greater sensitivity to the respiratory depressant effects of narcotics. This may be explained by the fact that there are relatively fewer Mu-1 narcotic receptors (mediating analgesia) relative to the Mu-2 receptors (mediating respiratory depression) in neonates when compared with older individuals.[56] Evidence also suggests that for some narcotics the volume of distribution is larger and the elimination half-life prolonged in premature infants. The elimination half-life of fentanyl is 129 minutes in the adult and 230 minutes in the neonate. As a result of these two differences, higher levels of narcotics persist in the cerebrospinal fluid for longer periods. Many experts feel that narcotics should be used in neonates to 6-month-olds only in patients for whom observation in an intensive care setting is possible or postoperative ventilation is planned.[57]

3. The management of pain in the pediatric population is hampered by the difficulty that exists assessing pain. Many children may respond to pain by emotionally withdrawing from their surroundings, and this may be misinterpreted by the medical and nursing staffs as evidence that they have no pain. In addition, when questioned as to their degree of pain, children may not volunteer useful information for fear of painful interventions. To circumvent these difficulties, several visual and verbal scales have been developed for quantifying painful sensations or describing typical painful behaviors. These have met with varying degrees of success because they are difficult to implement, time consuming to employ, and still rely on patient comprehension and cooperation.

4. There are individual biases that exist in medical professionals caring for children. These biases run from the belief that pain is a natural consequence of surgery to the beliefs that the risks of respiratory depression and narcotic addiction outweigh the benefits that are associated with aggressive pain management.

Given these difficulties in managing the child who is in pain, what options are available to the clinician? The mainstay in pain control remains the use of narcotics. Not only is there a bewildering array of narcotics available, but the methods of their administration are also changing.

Dose-dependent respiratory depression is common to the use of all narcotics and goes hand in hand with their analgesic properties. Other side effects that vary from drug to drug and patient to patient are somnolence, nausea and vomiting, pruritus, constipation, and urinary retention. Given time, patients develop tolerance to most, if not all, of these side effects while they continue to experience their analgesic properties. The side effects may be treated symptomatically while tolerance is developing, thereby making the patient much more comfortable and manageable. Often changing the narcotics reduces or eliminates the side effects.

Morphine remains the standard by which most pain therapy is measured. Some pharmacologic differences between morphine and other analgesics need to be appreciated to best utilize this narcotic. Although morphine has roughly the same plasma elimination half-life as other narcotics, its effect and duration of action may have considerable variability because of the dmg's low lipid solubility. A fourfold variation has been measured in the plasma concentration of morphine at which patients medicate themselves for pain.

Because there is a poor correlation between the plasma concentration of morphine and its desired analgesic effect, many clinicians feel that morphine is best administered in a patient-controlled device—patient-controlled analgesia (PCA). As the patient experiences changes in the level of morphine in the central nervous system, he or she is able to administer supplemental doses.

PCA dosing recommendations for morphine include a loading dose ranging from 0.04 to 0.06 mg/kg followed by use of intermittent PCA doses of 0.01 to 0.03 mg/kg. A lockout interval of 6 to 15 minutes and 0.2 to 0.4 mg/kg every 4 hours is the limit generally employed with morphine.

When PCA devices are not used, the intermittent administration of morphine to opioid-naive children should be started at 0.05 to 0.1 mg/kg every 2 to 4 hours. If the treatment of pain is undertaken in a recovery room or intensive care setting, similar doses may be administered every 5 to 10 minutes until the child is comfortable.

The efficacy of a continuous background infusion of narcotics along with PCA would theoretically make sense by maintaining a consistent blood level of drug especially during sleep. However, studies of continuous infusions in both children[58] and adults[59] have failed to show any documented improvement in pain scores. If any benefit is seen in sleep patterns it might occur only on the first night postoperatively.[58] Therefore, although in theory continuous infusions in addition to PCA would seem beneficial, in reality they serve only to increase the complications and dosages of narcotics used.[60]

It appears that the only indication for continuous infusion of narcotics may be for pain control in children who are unable to manage the PCA techniques because of age or mental capacity. The recommended dose for continuous infusion of morphine is 0.015 to 0.03 mg/kg/hour. Because feedback controls are not present with continuous infusions of narcotics, close observation and careful respiratory monitoring are mandatory.

Fentanyl is a synthetic narcotic that usually has a relatively short duration of action as a result of rapid distribution into fat and muscle because of its high lipid solubility. With repeat dosing, the duration of action appears to increase.[61] When compared with morphine, fentanyl is about 100 times more potent. (Fentanyl dosages are calculated in μg rather than mg.) In controlled comparisons using equipotent dosages, morphine is generally found to provide better analgesia than fentanyl but with more side effects, such as pruritus, hypotension, nausea, and vomiting.[62–64]

When using fentanyl for procedures, incremental dosing of 0.25 to 0.5 μg/kg every 5 minutes is safe. All of the respiratory depression from a single dose of fentanyl is evident within 5 minutes because of its rapid equilibration across the blood-brain barrier. The elimination rate of a single dose of fentanyl is reported to be about 1 μg/kg/hour.[65] A safe cumulative dose for procedures is 4 to 5 μg/kg.[66]

Other formulations of fentanyl are available that have clinical applications in pain management. Although not approved for pediatrics at present, transdermal fentanyl in doses of 25 to 100 μg/hour, has proved more efficacious in the treatment of chronic pain than some of the more traditional modalities.[67] Fentanyl has more recently been released in a transmucosal oralet formulation that can be used for sedation and analgesia in pain of short duration. Dosage recommended is 10 to 15 μg/kg.[66]

Hydromorphone is a well-tolerated alternative to morphine and fentanyl and is associated with less pruritis and sedation than morphine and a longer duration of action than fentanyl. It is five to seven times more potent than morphine. The dosing schedule for PCA hydromorphone uses a loading dose of 0.005 to 0.015 mg/kg, a lockout of 6 to 15 minutes, supplemental PCA doses of 0.003 to 0.005 mg/kg, and a 4-hour limit of 0.1 mg/kg.

As more and more of pediatric surgery is being performed on an outpatient basis, there has been significant interest in the role of nonnarcotic analgesics for the management of postoperative pain.

Many physicians have questioned the efficacy of acetaminophen for significant pain relief, although this may be more a question of the dosage employed. Recent investigators have challenged established dosing recommendations for rectal aceta-

minophen.[68, 69] Dosages for analgesia were based on recommendations for fever control (10 to 20 mg/kg), but these doses failed to produce serum levels shown to be effective even in reducing temperature. To achieve adequate serum levels for analgesia, doses of 30 to 40 mg/kg rectally are required. A dose of 30 mg/kg of acetaminophen rectally has proved to have similar analgesic properties as 1 mg/kg of ketorolac.[70] Further controlled studies are needed to delineate the benefits and doses of acetaminophen in the management of postoperative analgesia.

Ketorolac is an oral and parenteral nonsteroidal antiinflammatory drug shown to have excellent pain control characteristics with few side effects. Dosage recommendations are 0.5 mg/kg intravenously every 6 to 8 hours for 48 hours. One of the drawbacks associated with ketorolac is its inhibition of platelet aggregation, which has been associated with increased bleeding after a tonsillectomy.[71]

Regional anesthetic techniques used concomitantly with general anesthesia have had a resurgence in both adult and pediatric patients. These techniques include local infiltration of the wound, peripheral nerve blocks (i.e., ilioinguinal blocks), and epidural or spinal blocks. The intent of these techniques is to prevent sensitization of the peripheral and central nervous systems, which could result in prolonged or excessive postoperative pain. This approach is often referred to as preemptive analgesia. Whether preemptive analgesia exists in children is still unresolved.[72] Anecdotal reports of improved, prolonged analgesia during the postoperative period when regional anesthetic techniques are employed preemptively still await scientific validation.

Pediatric patients, whether undergoing an operation on an inpatient or outpatient basis, should be afforded maximal pain relief. Recent developments in and understanding of pain-relieving techniques place this goal within the reach of all clinicians caring for children during the postoperative period.

Acknowledgment

We gratefully acknowledge the assistance of Denise Gardonia in the preparation of this manuscript.

REFERENCES

1. Cohen M, Cameron C: Should you cancel the operation when a child has an upper respiratory tract infection? Anesth Analg 72:282–288, 1991.
2. Roizen MF: Preoperative laboratory testing—what is necessary? International Anesthesia Research Society Review Course Lectures, 1989, pp 29–35.
3. Leonard JV, Clayton BE, Colley JRT: Use of biochemical profile in children's hospital: Results of two controlled trials. Br Med J 21:662–665, 1975.
4. Dajan A, Taubert K, Wilson W, Bolger A, et al: Prevention of bacterial endocarditis—recommendations of the American Heart Association. Circulation 96:358–366, 1997.
5. Olson GL, Hallen B, Hambraeus-Jonzon K: Aspiration during anesthesia: A computer-aided study of 185,358 anaesthetics. Acta Anaesthesiol Scand 30:84–92, 1986.
6. Tiret L, Hivoche Y, Halton F, et al: Complications related to

anesthesia in infants and children. A prospective survey of 40,240 anaesthetics. Br J Anaesth 61:263–269, 1988.

7. Borland L, Woelfel S, Saitz M, et al: Pulmonary aspiration in pediatric patients under general anesthesia: Frequency and outcome [abstract]. Anesthesiology 83:A1150, 1995.

8. Welborn LG, McCail WA, Hannallah RS, et al: Perioperative blood glucose concentrations in pediatric outpatients. Anesthesiology 65:543–547, 1986.

9. Schreiner M, Nicholson S: Pediatric Ambulatory Anesthesia: NPO—before or after surgery? J Clin Anesth 7:589–596, 1995.

10. Nicholson S, Betts E, Jobes D, et al: Comparison of oral and intramuscular preanesthetic medication for pediatric inpatient surgery. Anesthesiology 71:8–10, 1989.

11. Weldon B, Watcha M, White P: Oral midazolam in children: Effect of time and adjunctive therapy. Anesthesia and Analgesia: 75, 51–55, 1992.

12. Epstein R, Mendel H, Witwaski T, et al. The safety and efficacy of oral transmucosal fentanyl citrate for preoperative sedation in young children. Anesth Analg 83:1200–1205, 1996.

13. Fisher D: Surrogate end points—are they meaningful? Anesthesiology 81:795–796, 1994.

14. Dexter F, Tinker J: Analysis of strategies to decrease postanesthesia care unit costs. Anesthesiology 82:94–101, 1995.

15. Welborn L, Hannallah R, Norden J, et al: Comparison of emergence and recovery characteristics of sevoflurane, desflurone and halothane in pediatric ambulatory patients. Anesth Analg 83:917–920, 1996.

16. Davis P, Cohen I, McGowan F, Letta K: Recovery characteristics of desflurane versus halothane for maintenance in pediatric ambulatory patients. Anesthesiology 80:298–302, 1994.

17. Hanannallah R, Bulton J, Schaefer P, et al: Propofol anesthesia in pediatric ambulatory patients: A comparison with thiopental and halothane. Can J Anaesth 41:12–18, 1994.

18. Broadman LM: Regional anesthesia for the pediatric outpatient. Anesth Clin North Am 5:53–72, 1987.

19. Cohen MM, Duncan P, Pope W, Wolkenstein C: A survey of 112,000 anesthetics at one teaching hospital (1975–1983). Can Anaesth Soc J 33:22–31, 1986.

20. Cohen MM, Cameron C, Duncan P: Pediatric morbidity and mortality in the perioperative period. Anesth Analg 70:160–167, 1990.

21. Shandling B, Steward DJ: Regional analgesia for postoperative pain in pediatric outpatient surgery. J Pediatr Surg 15:477, 1980.

22. Abramowitz MD, Elder P, Friendly D, et al: Antiemetic effectiveness of intraoperatively administered droperidol in pediatric strabismus outpatient surgery. Anesthesiology 53:5323, 1980.

23. Schreiner M, Nicholsen S, Martin T, Whitney L: Should children drink before discharge from day surgery? Anesthesiology 76:528–533, 1992.

24. Davis P, McGowen F, Landsman I, et al: Effect of antiemetic therapy on recovery and hospital discharge time: A double blind assessment of ondansetron, droperidol and placebo in pediatric patients undergoing ambulatory surgery. Anesthesiology 83:956–960, 1995.

25. Watcha M, Smith I: Cost effectiveness analysis of antiemetic therapy for ambulatory surgery. J Clin Anesth 6:370–377, 1994.

26. Ummenhofer W, Frie F, Urwyler A, et al: Effects of ondansetron in the prevention of post operative nausea and vomiting in children. Anesthesiology 81:804–810, 1994.

27. Koka BY, Jean I, Andre J, et al: Postintubation croup in children. Anesth Analg 56:501, 1977.

28. Gregory G (ed): Pediatric Anesthesia (2nd ed). New York, Churchill Livingstone, 1989, p 635.

29. Goddard JE: Betamethasone for prophylaxis of postintubation inflammation. Anesth Analg 46:348, 1967.

30. Steward DJ: Preterm infants are more prone to complications following minor surgery than are term infants. Anesthesiology 56:304–306, 1982.

31. Rigatto H, Brady JP: Periodic breathing and apnea in preterm infants. Evidence for hypoventilation possibly due to central respiratory depression. Pediatrics 50:202–218, 1972.

32. Cote C, Zaslavsky A, Downe J, et al: Postoperative apnea in former preterm infants after inguinal herniorraphy: A combined analysis. Anesthesiology 82:809–822, 1995.

33. Fisher D: When Is the ex-premature infant no longer at risk for apnea? Anesthesiology 82:807–808, 1995.

34. Welborn L, Rice L, Hannallah R, et al: Postoperative apnea in former preterm infants: Prospective comparison of spinal and general anesthesia. Anesthesiology 72:838–842, 1990.

35. Wiener E, Touloukian R, Rodgers B, et al: Hernia survey of the section on surgery of the American Academy of Pediatrics. J Pediatr Surg 31:1166–1169, 1996.

36. Welborn LG, Hannallah RS, Fiwle R, et al: High-dose caffeine suppresses postoperative apnea in former premature infants. Anesthesiology 71:347–349, 1989.

37. Beecher HK, Todd DP: A study of the deaths associated with anesthesia and surgery based on a study of 599,458 anesthesias in ten institutions, 1948–1952, inclusive. Ann Surg 140:2–35, 1954.

38. Dripps RD, Lamont A, Eckenhoff J: The role of anesthesia in surgical mortality. JAMA 178:261–266, 1961.

39. Macintosh RR: Deaths under anesthetics. Br J Anaesth 21:107–136, 1948.

40. Wylie WD: "There, but for the grace of God . . ." Ann R Coll Surg Engl 56:171–180, 1975.

41. Marx G, Mateo C, Orkin L: Computer analysis of postanesthetic deaths. Anesthesiology 39:54–58, 1973.

42. Cooper JB, et al: Preventable anesthesia mishaps. Anesthesiology 49:399–406, 1978.

43. Green WA, Taylor TH: An analysis of anesthesia medical liability claims in the United Kingdom 1977–1982. Int Anesthiol Clin 22:73–90, 1984.

44. Eichhorn JH: Standards for patient monitoring during anesthesia at Harvard Medical School. JAMA 256:1017–1020, 1986.

45. Orkin FK: Practice standards. The Midas touch or the emperor's new clothes? Anesthesiology 70:567–571, 1989.

46. Eichhorn JH: Prevention of intraoperative anesthesia accidents and related severe injury through safety monitoring. Anesthesiology 70:572–577, 1989.

47. Moller JT, Johannessen NW, Espersen K, et al: Randomized evaluation of pulse oximetry in 20,802 patients: Perioperative events and postoperative complications clinical investigation. Anesthesiology 78:445–453, 1993.

48. Keats A: What do we know about anesthetic mortality? Anesthesiology 50:387–392, 1979.

49. Morray JP, Geiduschek JM, Caplan RA: A comparison of pediatric and adult anesthesia closed malpractice claims. Anesthesiology 78:461–467, 1993.

50. Cote CJ, Goldstein EA, Cote MA, et al: A single-blind study of pulse oximetry in children. Anesthesiology 68:184–188, 1988.

51. Kestin IG, Miller BR, Lockhart CH: Auditory alarms during anesthesia monitoring. Anesthesiology 69:106–109, 1988.

52. Mather L, Mackie J: The incidence of postoperative pain in children. Pain 15:271–282, 1983.

53. Hatch DJ: Analgesia in the neonate [editorial] Br Med J 294:920, 1987.

54. Tilney F, Rossett J: The value of brain lipoids in an index of brain development. Bull Neurol Inst N Y 1:28–71, 1931.

55. Orlowski JP: Cerebrospinal fluid endorphines and the infant apnea syndrome. Pediatrics 78:233–237, 1986.

56. Pasternak GW, Zhang A, Tecott L: Developmental differences between high and low affinity opiate binding sites: Their relationship to analgesia and respiratory depression. Life Sci 27:1185–1190, 1980.

57. Lloyd-Thomas AR: Pain management in paediatric patients. Br J Anaesth 64:85–104, 1990.

58. Doyle E, Harper I, Morton NS: Comparison of patient-controlled analgesia with and without a background infusion after lower abdominal surgery in children. Br J Anesth 71:670–673, 1993.

59. Parker RK, Holtmann B, White PF: Patient-controlled analgesia. Does a concurrent opioid improve pain management after surgery? JAMA 266:1947–1952, 1991.

60. McNeely JK, Trentadue NC: Comparison of patient-controlled

analgesia with and without nighttime morphine infusion following lower extremity surgery in children. J Pain Symptom Manage 13:268–273, 1997.

61. Kay B, Rolly G: Duration of action of analgesia supplement of anesthesia. A double-blind comparison between morphine, fentanyl, and sufentanil. Acta Anaesthesiol Belg 28:25–32, 1977.
62. Claxton AR, McGuire G, Chung F, Cruise C: Evaluation of morphine versus fentanyl for postoperative analgesia after ambulatory surgical procedures. Anesth Analg 84:509–514, 1997.
63. Sanford TJ Jr, Smith NT, Dec-Silver H, Harrison WK: A comparison of morphine, fentanyl, and sufentanil anesthesia for cardiac surgery: induction, emergence, and extubation. Anesth Analg 65:259–266, 1986.
64. Lejus C, Roussiere G, Testa S, et al: Postoperative extradural analgesia in children: Comparison of morphine with fentanyl. Br J Anesth 72:156–159, 1994.
65. Kastrup EK, Hebel SK, Rivard R, et al: Narcotic agonist analgesics. Facts and Comparisons, 1997 Edition. St. Louis, 1997, pp 1316–1318.

66. Hill K, Anderson C: Pediatric pain management: Clinical aspects for the nineties. Semin Anesth 16:136–151, 1997.
67. Ahmedzai S, Brooks D: Transdermal fentanyl versus sustained release morphine in cancer pain: preference, efficacy, and quality of life. The TTS-Fentanyl Compatative Trial Group. J Pain Symptom Manage 13:254–261, 1997.
68. Birmingham PK, Tobin MJ, Henthom TK, Fisher DM, et al: Twenty-four hour pharmacokinetics of rectal acetaminophen in children. Anesthesiology 87:244–252, 1997.
69. Montgomery CJ, McCormack JP, Reichert CC, Marsland CP: Plasma concentrations after high-dose (45 mg·kg-1) rectal acetaminophen in children. Can J Anaesth 42:982–986, 1995.
70. Rusy LM, Houck CS, Sullivan LJ, et al: A double-blind evaluation of ketorolac tromethamine versus acetaminophen in pediatric tonsillectomy: Analgesia and bleeding. Anesth Analg 80:226–229, 1995.
71. Gunter JB, Varughese AM, Harrington JF, et al: Recovery and complications after tonsillectomy in children: A comparison of ketorolac and morphine. Anesth Analg 81:1136–1141, 1995.
72. Ho JW, Khambatta HJ, Pang LM, et al: Preemptive analgesia in children—does it exist? Reg Anesth 22:12–130, 1997.

4

RENAL IMPAIRMENT

Stanley Hellerstein, MD • Uri S. Alon, MD •
Bradley A. Warady, MD

□ Body Fluid Regulation

Effective kidney function maintains the normal volume and composition of body fluids even though there is wide variation in dietary intake and nonrenal expenditures of water and solute. Water and electrolyte balance is maintained by the excretion of urine, with the volume and composition defined by physiologic needs. Fluid balance is accomplished by glomerular ultrafiltration of plasma coupled with modification of the ultrafiltrate by tubular reabsorption and secretion.[1, 2] The excreted urine, or modified glomerular filtrate, is the small residuum of the large volume of nonselective ultrafiltrate modified by transport processes operating along the nephron. The glomerular capillaries permit free passage of water and solutes of low molecular weight while restraining formed elements and macromolecules. The glomerular capillary wall functions as a barrier to the filtration of macromolecules based on their size, shape, and charge characteristics. The glomerular filtrate is modified during passage through the tubules via the active and passive transport of certain solutes into and out of the luminal fluid and the permeability characteristics of specific nephron segments. The ionic transport systems in renal epithelial cells serve to maintain global water, salt, and acid-base homeostasis rather than to regulate local cellular processes, such as volume and metabolic substrate uptake, as do nonrenal epithelial cells.

An adequate volume of glomerular filtrate is essential for the kidney to regulate water and solute balance effectively. Blood flow to the kidneys accounts for 20 to 30% of cardiac output. Of the total renal plasma flow, 92% passes through the functioning excretory tissue and is known as the *effective renal plasma flow* (ERPF). Glomerular filtration rate (GFR) is usually about one fifth of ERPF, giving a filtration fraction of about 0.2.

The rate of ultrafiltration across the glomerular capillaries is determined by the same forces that allow the transmural movement of fluid in other capillary networks.[3] These forces are the transcapillary hydraulic and osmotic pressure gradients and the characteristics of capillary wall permeability. A renal autoregulatory mechanism enables the kidney to maintain relative constancy of blood flow in the presence of changing systemic arterial and renal perfusion pressures.[1] This intrinsic renal autoregulatory mechanism appears to be mediated in individual nephrons by tubuloglomerular feedback involving the macula densa (a region in the early distal tubule that juxtaposes the glomerulus) and the afferent and efferent arterioles. A decrease in arteriolar resistance in the afferent arteriole, with maintenance of the resistance in the efferent arteriole, sustains glomerular hydraulic pressure despite a fall in systemic and renal arterial pressures.

Under normal conditions, the reabsorption of water and the reabsorption and secretion of solute during passage of the filtrate through the nephron are subservient to the maintenance of body fluid homeostasis. In the healthy, nongrowing individual, the intake and the expenditure of water and solute are equal, and the hydrogen-ion balance is zero. Renal function may be impaired by systemic or renal disease and by medications such as vasoactive drugs, nonsteroidal antiinflammatory drugs, diuretics, and antibiotics. Hypoxia and renal hypoperfusion appear to be the events most commonly associated with postoperative renal dysfunction.

□ Renal Function Evaluation

The evaluation of kidney function begins with a thorough history and physical examination and is followed by laboratory studies to estimate GFR and renal tubular function. An abnormal voiding pattern or significant impairment in renal concentrating capacity should be evident from the patient's history. Examination of the urinary sediment may provide direct evidence of renal glomerular or interstitial disease. Levels of serum electrolytes, calcium, and phosphorus are useful in screening for renal tubular disorders. In a clinical setting, serum creatinine concentration is the usual laboratory test used to estimate GFR, although creatinine is not only filtered by the glomerular capillaries but also secreted by the renal tubules. Serum creatinine concentration is also affected by diet.

URINE VOLUME

The appropriate urine volume for a patient depends on the status of body fluids, fluid intake and extrarenal losses, and obligatory renal solute load. Patients with defects in renal concentrating capacity require a larger minimum urinary volume for excretion of the obligatory renal solute load than patients with normal renal concentrating capacity.

Although the estimation of an appropriate urinary volume in most clinical settings involves many caveats, the determination is based on an estimate of the minimum urinary volume needed to excrete the obligatory renal solute load. The calculations should be made per 100 ml of maintenance water to obtain an estimate applicable to patients of all sizes. Usual maintenance water requirements for this purpose are conveniently calculated using the method of Holliday and Segar (Table 4–1).[4] A maintenance water allowance of 100 ml/kg/24 h applies only to 10 kg of body weight. The 15-kg child has a maintenance water requirement of 1250 ml/24 h, and the 30-kg child has a maintenance water requirement of 1700 ml/24 h.

The minimum urinary volume for excretion of the obligatory renal solute load is derived using the following assumptions:

1. The obligatory renal solute load in the patient being evaluated for ischemic acute renal failure (ARF) is more than the minimum endogenous renal solute load of 10 to 15 mOsm/100 ml of maintenance water and is probably less than 40 mOsm/100 ml of maintenance water generated by the usual diet.[4] Approximately 30 mOsm of obligatory renal solute/100 ml of usual maintenance water is taken as the obligatory renal solute load in children 2 months of age and older.

2. Urinary concentrating capacity increases rapidly during the 1st year of life and reaches the adult level of 1200 to 1400 mOsm/kg at about the 2nd year.[5, 6] The maximum urinary concentrating capacity of the term infant, aged 1 week to 2 months, ranges from 600 to 1100 mOsm/kg. By age 10 to 12 months, a patient's average maximum urinary osmolality is slightly greater than 1000 mOsm/kg. Table 4–2 provides an estimate of the minimum urinary volumes that permit excretion of the obligatory renal solute load, assuming an appropriate physiologic response to renal hypoperfusion. Significantly lower urinary volumes are usually present with ischemic ARF. Urinary volumes have been calculated according to the following relationship:

$$\text{Urinary Volume} = \frac{\text{Solute Load (mOsm)}}{\text{Solute Concentration (mOsm/kg)}}$$

The presence of oliguric renal failure, based on urine volume, can be diagnosed only in the hydrated patient who has adequate blood pressure for renal perfusion and has no urinary tract obstruction. Ischemic ARF is probably not present in an infant as old as 2 months with a urinary volume equal to or greater than 1.25 ml/h/100 ml maintenance water or in an older patient with a urinary volume equal to or greater than 1.0 ml/h/100 ml of maintenance water. Urine output less than this requires further evaluation for oliguric renal failure. Nonoliguric renal failure occurs about as frequently as does oliguric renal failure. It is diagnosed when a patient with a normal urinary volume exhibits other evidence of decreased GFR, such as an elevated serum creatinine concentration or a decreased creatinine clearance.

GLOMERULAR FILTRATION RATE

GFR is the most useful index of renal function because it reflects the volume of plasma ultrafiltrate presented to the tubules.[7] Decline in GFR is the principal functional abnormality in both acute and chronic renal failure. Assessment of GFR is important not only for evaluating the patient with respect to renal function but also for guiding the administration of antibiotics and other drugs.

Inulin clearance, which is the accepted standard for measurement of GFR, is too time consuming and inconvenient to be used in the clinical evaluation of most patients. Serum urea nitrogen concentration shows so much variation with dietary intake of nitrogen that it is not a satisfactory index of GFR. Almost by default, serum creatinine concentration and creatinine clearance have become the usual clinical measures for estimation of GFR. A number of precautions should be taken when using creatinine to estimate GFR. Ingestion of a meal containing a large quantity of animal protein for example, increases serum creatinine levels about 0.25 mg/dl in 2 hours and increases creatinine excretion rate about 75% over the next 3 to 4 hours.[8] It follows that serum creatinine concentration should be measured

TABLE 4-1. Usual Maintenance Water Requirements

Weight Range (kg)	Maintenance Water
2.5–10	100 ml/kg
10–20	1000 ml + 50 ml/kg > 10 kg
20	1500 ml + 20 ml/kg > 20 kg

TABLE 4-2. Minimum Urinary Volumes for Excretion of Obligatory Renal Solute

| Age | Assumptions | | Urinary Volume | |
	Renal Solute Load (mOsm/100 cal)	Maximum Urine Concentration (mOsm/kg)	ml of Urine per 100 ml Maintenance Water (Per 24 h)	(Per h)
1 wk to 2 mo	25 (?)	800	31.3	1.3
2 mo to 2 y	30 (?)	1000	25.0	1.0
2 y	30	1200	20.8	1.0

while the patient is fasting. A diet with a high intake of meat, fowl, or fish should be avoided when urine is being collected for measurement of creatinine clearance. Serum creatinine levels are sometimes increased by medication, such as trimethoprim, which competes with creatinine for tubular secretion through a base-secreting pathway. Trimethoprim does not alter GFR, only the serum creatinine level. Trimethoprim-induced elevation of serum creatinine concentration may cause concern in the evaluation of an individual with impaired renal function because the fraction of urinary creatinine derived from tubular secretion rises as the GFR falls.

Serum creatinine concentration in the neonate reflects the maternal level for approximately the 1st week of life. After this time, serum creatinine concentration should decrease. If it does not, a more indepth evaluation of kidney function is warranted. From 2 weeks to 2 years of age, serum creatinine concentration averages about 0.4 ± .04 mg/dl (35 ± 3.5 μmol/l).[9] The serum creatinine concentration is relatively constant because the increase in endogenous creatinine production, which is directly correlated with muscle mass, is matched by the increase in GFR. During the first 2 years, GFR rises from 35 to 45 ml/min/1.73 m² to the normal adult range of 80 to 170 ml/min/1.73 m². The normal

range for serum creatinine concentration increases from 2 years through puberty, although GFR remains essentially constant when expressed per unit of surface area. This occurs because growth during childhood is associated with increased muscle mass and, therefore, increased creatinine production, which is greater than the increased GFR per unit of body weight. Table 4–3 shows the mean values and ranges for plasma or serum creatinine levels at different ages.

FRACTIONAL EXCRETION OF SODIUM (FE_{Na}) AND BICARBONATE (FE_{HCO_3})

Fractional excretions are indexes of renal function that are helpful in evaluating specific clinical conditions. Conceptually, a fractional excretion is the fraction of the filtered substance that is excreted in the urine. Fractional excretions are calculated by using creatinine clearance to estimate GFR and the serum and urine concentrations of the substance studied. The quantity of the substance filtered is taken as the GFR multiplied by the serum concentration of the substance being evaluated, and the quantity excreted is taken as the concentration in the urine multiplied by the urine volume. The fractional excretion of sodium is derived as follows:

TABLE 4-3. Plasma Creatinine Levels at Different Ages

| Age | Height (cm) | True Plasma Creatinine* (mg/dl) | |
		Mean	Range (± 2 SD)
Fetal cord blood		0.75	0.51–0.99
0–2 wk	50	0.50	0.34–0.66
2–26 wk	60	0.39	0.23–0.55
26 wk–1 y	70	0.32	0.18–0.46
2 y	87	0.32	0.20–0.44
4 y	101	0.37	0.25–0.49
6 y	114	0.43	0.27–0.59
8 y	126	0.48	0.31–0.65
10 y	137	0.52	0.34–0.70
12 y	147	0.59	0.41–0.78
Adult male	174	0.97	0.72–1.22
Adult female	163	0.77	0.53–1.01

*Conversion factor μmol/l = mg/dl × 88.4.

Adapted from Chantler C, Barratt TM: Laboratory evaluation. In Holliday MA (ed): Pediatric Nephrology (2nd ed). Baltimore, Williams & Wilkins, 1987, pp 282–299.

$$\begin{aligned}
\%\mathrm{FE_{Na}} &= \frac{\mathrm{Na\ Excreted}}{\mathrm{Na\ Filtered}} \times (100) \\[4pt]
&= \frac{(\mathrm{U_{Na}} \times \mathrm{V})\,(100)}{(\mathrm{P_{Na}})\,\dfrac{(\mathrm{U_{Cr}} \times \mathrm{V})}{(\mathrm{P_{Cr}})}} \\[4pt]
&= \frac{\mathrm{U_{Na}}}{\mathrm{P_{Na}}} \times \frac{\mathrm{P_{Cr}}}{\mathrm{U_{Cr}}} \times 100
\end{aligned}$$

where $\mathrm{U_{Na}}$ and $\mathrm{U_{Cr}}$ = urine sodium and creatinine, respectively, and $\mathrm{P_{Na}}$ and $\mathrm{P_{Cr}}$ = plasma sodium and creatinine, respectively.

Volumes cancel out; the fractional excretion is calculated from the determination of sodium and creatinine concentrations in samples of blood and urine obtained at approximately the same time.

Fractional Excretion of Sodium

FE_{Na} is usually less than 1% but may be elevated with greater salt intake, adaptation to chronic renal failure, and diuretic administration.[10] With a decrease in renal perfusion pressure, which is common in extracellular volume depletion or congestive heart failure, the normal renal response results in a marked increase in the tubular resorption of sodium and water and in the excretion of a small volume of concentrated urine. The physiologic response to decreased renal perfusion is an FE_{Na} below 1%. FE_{Na} is usually greater than 2% in ischemic ARF.

When using FE_{Na} to aid in differentiating prerenal azotemia from ARF, it is essential that there has been no recent diuretic therapy. Prerenal azotemia may occur in patients with preexisting chronic renal disease who have FE_{Na} levels above 1% as a consequence of the adaptation to chronic renal failure. When these patients are volume deficient, the elevated serum levels of urea nitrogen and creatinine and the high FE_{Na} may be partially volume responsive. FE_{Na} as well as the other diagnostic indices employed to help differentiate prerenal azotemia from ischemic ARF are not pathognomonic for either disorder. However, FE_{Na} provides helpful information when integrated into the overall clinical evaluation.

Fractional Excretion of Bicarbonate

Renal tubular acidosis (RTA) describes a group of disorders in which metabolic acidosis occurs as a result of an impairment in the reclamation of filtered HCO_3^- or as a result of a defect in the renal hydrogen ion excretion, in the absence of significant reduction in GFR.[11] Typically, RTA is considered in the differential diagnosis of the patient with metabolic acidosis, a normal serum anion gap (hyperchloremic metabolic acidosis), and a urinary pH above 6.0. In the patient with proximal RTA, due to the decreased reclamation of filtered HCO_3^-, urinary pH may be below 6.0 when the plasma HCO_3^- concentration is below the decreased renal threshold for HCO_3^- resorption. Another exception with respect to urinary pH occurs in type IV RTA, a form of distal RTA in which the normal serum anion gap metabolic acidosis is associated with hyperkalemia and acid urine (see later). In patients with proximal RTA, when the plasma HCO_3^- concentration is normalized by administering sufficient alkali, the distal nephron is flooded with HCO_3^-, and the urine becomes highly alkaline. The diagnosis of a defect in proximal tubular reabsorption of HCO_3^- is made by showing that FE_{HCO_3} is greater than 15% when the serum HCO_3^- concentration is increased to the normal range. FE_{HCO_3} is calculated just as FE_{Na} but with serum and urine HCO_3^- substituted for Na. A normal individual ingesting a usual diet resorbs all the filtered HCO_3^-, and the FE_{HCO_3} is zero. A urinary pH of 6.2 or less indicates that urinary HCO_3^- is negligible.

URINARY P_{CO_2} OR URINE MINUS BLOOD P_{CO_2} (U-B P_{CO_2})

Classic distal RTA is caused by a defect in the secretion of H^+ by the cells of the distal nephron. It is characterized by hyperchloremic metabolic acidosis, urine with a pH greater than 6.0 at normal as well as at low serum HCO_3^- concentrations, and an FE_{HCO_3} below 5% when serum HCO_3^- is normal.[11, 12] Normally, the cells of the distal nephron secrete H^+ into the lumen where, in the presence of filtered HCO_3^-, carbonic acid (H_2CO_3) is formed. Slow dehydration of the H_2CO_3 into $CO_2 + H_2O$ in the medullary collecting ducts, renal pelvis, and urinary bladder results in urinary P_{CO_2} greater than 80 mm Hg or (U-B P_{CO_2}) greater than 30 mm Hg. Urinary P_{CO_2} is evaluated after administering a single dose of $NaHCO_3$ (2 to 3 mEq/kg) or acetazolamide (17 ± 2 mg/kg) to flood the distal nephron with HCO_3^-. Sodium bicarbonate, rather than acetazolamide, should be used in a patient with significantly reduced serum HCO_3^- levels at the time of the test. Urinary P_{CO_2} should be measured only after urinary pH exceeds 7.4 or urinary HCO_3^- concentration exceeds 40 mEq/l or both. A defect in distal nephron secretion of H^+ is diagnosed if U-B P_{CO_2} is greater than 20 mm Hg or urine P_{CO_2} is below 60 mm Hg.

Type IV RTA, a form of distal RTA associated with low urinary pH (<6.0) and hyperkalemia,[11, 12] involves both H^+ and K^+ secretion in the distal tubule and is related to a failure to reabsorb sodium. This fosters development of a negative potential in the tubular lumen (i.e., a voltage-dependent defect). Type IV RTA is probably the most commonly recognized type in both adults and children. The hyperkalemia inhibits ammonia synthesis, resulting in decreased ammonia to serve as a urinary buffer. Therefore, a low urinary pH occurs despite decreased H^+ secretion ($NH_3 + H^+ = NH_4^+$). Type IV RTA is physiologically equivalent to aldosterone deficiency, which is one cause of the disorder. In children, it may reflect true hypoaldosteronism, but it is much more common as a consequence of renal parenchymal damage, especially that due to obstructive uropathy. In pediatric patients, the physiologic impairment of type IV RTA resolves in a few weeks to months after relief of an obstructive disorder.

☐ Medical Aspects of Managing the Patient with Postoperative Impairment of Renal Function

PATHOPHYSIOLOGY OF ACUTE RENAL FAILURE

ARF is characterized by an abrupt decrease in renal function. Because ARF is caused by a fall in GFR, the initial clinical manifestations are elevations in serum urea nitrogen and creatinine concentrations and, frequently, reduction in urine output. With improved standards of neonatal and pediatric care, the incidence of ARF associated with medical diseases and with surgery has reduced. Among pediatric surgical patients, an impairment in renal function is most common in those who are undergoing cardiopulmonary procedures.[13, 14]

The most important factor in the pathogenesis of postoperative renal failure is decreased renal perfusion. In the early phase, the reduction in renal blood flow results in a decline in GFR. Intact tubular function results in enhanced resorption of sodium and water. This clinical condition is recognized as prerenal azotemia. Analysis of the patient's urine reveals a high urinary osmolality of greater than 300 mOsm/kg H_2O, a urine-to-plasma urea concentration ratio greater than 5, and a urine sodium concentration greater than 20 mEq/l. The most useful index of the tubular response to renal hypoperfusion with intact renal function is FE_{Na}. The FE_{Na} test is invalid if the patient received diuretics before giving the urine sample. When kidney function is intact in the hypoperfused state, FE_{Na} is below 1% in term infants and children and below 2.5% in premature infants.[15] In most patients with prerenal azotemia, intravascular volume depletion is clinically evident. However, in patients with diminished cardiac output (pump failure), clinical appreciation of reduced renal perfusion can be obscured because body weight and central venous pressure may suggest fluid overload. The reduced effective intraarterial volume is usually evident from the reduced systemic blood pressure, tachycardia, and prolonged capillary refill time.

Prerenal azotemia can be alleviated by improving renal perfusion via either repleting the intravascular fluid volume or improving the cardiac output. The improved kidney function is recognized by increased urine output and normalization of serum urea nitrogen and creatinine concentrations. However, if renal hypoperfusion persists for a significant period or if other nephrotoxic factors are present, parenchymal renal failure can ensue. Factors that may predispose the patient to ARF include preexisting congenital urinary anomalies, septicemia, hypoxemia, hemolysis, rhabdomyolysis, hyperuricemia, drug toxicity, and use of radiocontrast agents.

MEDICAL MANAGEMENT

The child with postoperative oliguria and elevated serum creatinine concentration should be assessed for possible prerenal azotemia. If the child is found to be hypovolemic, an intravenous (IV) fluid challenge of 20 ml/kg of isotonic saline or plasma is commonly infused. In most instances, however, it may be physiologically advantageous to provide a solution in which bicarbonate accounts for 25 to 40 mEq/l of the anions in the fluid bolus (½ isotonic NaCl in 5% glucose to which is added 25 to 40 mEq/l of 1 M of $NaHCO_3$). If no response is observed and the child is still dehydrated, the dose can be repeated. When the urine output is satisfactory after fluid replenishment, the child should receive appropriate maintenance and replacement fluids and should be monitored. Body weight, urinary volume, and serum concentrations of urea nitrogen, creatinine, and electrolytes also should be monitored.

If urinary output is inadequate after the fluid challenge, an IV infusion of furosemide of 1 mg/kg may be given in a bolus. Patients with renal failure may require higher doses, up to 5 mg/kg. If no response occurs after the initial infusion of furosemide, a second, higher dose can be repeated after 1 hour. Some patients may require furosemide every 4 to 8 hours to maintain satisfactory urinary volume. A protocol with constant furosemide infusion has been successfully employed in oliguric children after cardiac surgery.[16] Furosemide is infused at 0.1 mg/kg/h, with the dose increased by 0.1 mg after 2 hours if the urinary volume remains less than 1 ml/kg/h. The maximum dose is 0.4 mg/kg/h. Urine output can at times be increased by the use of vasoactive agents such as dopamine; however, their efficacy in otherwise altering the course of ARF is not well established.[17]

Careful monitoring of the patient's fluid and electrolyte status is essential. Those children who fail to respond to furosemide are at risk for fluid overload. Overzealous fluid administration during anesthesia and surgery and for the management of persistent hypoperfusion along with decreased urinary output can result in hypervolemia, hypertension, heart failure, and pulmonary edema. In extreme cases, fluid administration must be decreased to the minimum necessary to deliver essential medications. In less severe instances, and in euvolemic patients with impaired kidney function, total fluid intake should equal insensible water loss, urine volume, and any significant extrarenal fluid losses. Urine output must be monitored hourly, and fluid management must be reevaluated every 4 to 12 hours, as clinically indicated. Valuable information about the patient's overall fluid status can be obtained by carefully monitoring blood pressure, pulse, and body weight. The preoperative values of these parameters help serve as a baseline for postoperative evaluation. Ideally, the patient's hemodynamic status should be assessed continuously using central venous pressure monitoring. In patients with complicated cardiac problems, a Swan-Ganz catheter that monitors pulmonary wedge pressure should be used.

Fluid overload can lead to hyponatremia. Because, in most cases, total body sodium remains normal or high, the best way to normalize serum sodium concentration is by restriction of fluid intake and enhancement of urinary volume.[18] In patients with acute symptomatic hyponatremia, careful infusion of NaCl 3% solution (512 mEq Na/l or 0.5 mEq/ml) may be given to correct hyponatremia. Rapid correction at a rate of 1 to 2 mEq/h over 2 to 3 hours, with an increase of serum sodium level by 4 to 6 mEq/l, is usually well tolerated and adequate. Infusion of 6 ml/kg of 3% NaCl increases serum sodium concentration by about 5 mEq/l. Hyponatremia that is present more than 24 to 48 hours should not be corrected at a rate more rapid than 0.5 mEq/l/h.

Children with ARF often develop hyperkalemia. The early sign of potassium cardiotoxicity is peaked T waves on the electrocardiogram. Higher levels of serum potassium can cause ventricular fibrillation and cardiac asystole. The treatment for hyperkalemia is shown in Table 4–4. Emergent treatment of hyperkalemia is indicated when serum potassium concentration reaches 7.0 mEq/l or when electrocardiographic changes are noted.

Children with ARF rapidly develop metabolic acidosis. Owing to decreased kidney function, fewer hydrogen ions are excreted. Organic acids then accumulate in the body, causing a reduction in the serum bicarbonate concentration. Although a child with uncompromised ventilatory capacity is able to hyperventilate and achieve partial compensation, a child with compromised pulmonary function or a hypercatabolic state is at risk for profound acidosis. Metabolic acidosis is usually treated by administering sodium bicarbonate. However, attention should be directed toward the excess sodium load associated with this mode of therapy. Because many patients with ARF also develop hypocalcemia, treatment with alkali should be done with care to protect them from hypocalcemic tetany. It is not necessary to completely correct the metabolic acidosis to prevent the untoward effects of acidemia. Increasing the serum bicarbonate concentration to 15 mEq/l is usually satisfactory.[19]

DIALYSIS

The inability to medically control the fluid-and-electrolyte or acid-base disorders caused by renal failure necessitates the initiation of dialysis therapy.

Indications for Acute Dialysis

The indications for acute dialysis follow:
Prolonged oligoanuria
Hyperkalemia
Metabolic acidosis
Fluid overload
Severe electrolyte and mineral disturbances
Uremic syndrome
The most common indication for postoperative dialysis in a child is the hypervolemia caused by repeated attempts at fluid resuscitation, administration of medications, and total parenteral nutrition. Repeated catheter flushes and endotracheal tube lavages can add a significant amount of water and solute to the total intake.[20] Fluid overload in the postoperative patient can cause pulmonary edema and, less commonly, hypertension.

Dialysis Therapy

The three modes of therapy include hemodialysis, hemofiltration, and peritoneal dialysis. The last of these is employed most commonly in children. The intrinsic factors that affect the efficacy of peritoneal dialysis include peritoneal blood flow, peritoneal vascular permeability, and peritoneal surface area.[21] Although removal of up to 50% of the peritoneal surface area does not seem to interfere with dialysis efficacy,[22] hypoperfusion of the peritoneal membrane vasculature renders dialysis ineffective.[23] Dialysis in the postoperative patient is feasible even in the presence of peritonitis or immediately after major abdominal surgery.[24, 25] Increased intraabdominal pressure caused by the administration of peritoneal fluid can cause respiratory embarrassment and contribute to fluid leakage from the sites of the surgical incisions and the entrance of the peritoneal catheter. Under such circumstances, the smallest effective dialysis fluid volume is used. It can be gradually increased with time after surgery. Common complications associated with peritoneal dialysis are peritonitis, exit site infection, leaking dialysate, catheter obstruction, and abdominal wall hernia. A rare complication is abdominal organ perforation.[26]

Dialysate solution with a 1.5% glucose concentration has an osmolality of 350 mOsm/kg H_2O, which is moderately hypertonic to normal plasma (280 to

---

TABLE 4-4. Treatment of Hyperkalemia

Cardiac Protection

Calcium gluconate 10%, 0.5–1.0 ml/kg body weight injected intravenously and slowly over 5–10 min, with continuous monitoring of heart rate

Shift of Potassium into the Intracellular Compartment

Sodium bicarbonate, 1–2 mEq/kg body weight intravenously over 10–20 min, provided that salt and water overload is not a problem

Glucose, 1 g/kg body weight, and insulin, 1 unit per every 4 g of glucose, intravenously over 20–30 min

Stimulants of β_2-adrenergic receptors, such as salbutamol, intravenously or by inhalation

Elimination of Excess Potassium

Cation exchange resin, sodium polystyrene sulfonate, 1 g/kg body weight, administered orally or rectally in 20–30% sorbitol or 10% glucose, 1 g resin/4 ml

Additional 70% sorbitol syrup may be given if constipation occurs

Dialysis, peritoneal or hemodialysis

295 mOsm/kg H_2O). With increased glucose concentration in the dialysate solution, the tonicity of the solution increases, reaching 490 mOsm/kg H_2O with 4.25% glucose, the highest concentration commercially available. Other factors being equal, the higher the tonicity of the dialysate, the greater the ultrafiltrate (fluid removed from the body). Owing to the rapid movement of water and glucose across the peritoneal membrane, the effect of peritoneal dialysis on fluid removal is maximum when short dialysis cycles of 20 to 30 minutes are used. When solutions containing glucose concentrations higher than 1.5% are given, close monitoring of the serum glucose concentration is necessary. If hyperglycemia above 200 mg/dl develops, it can be controlled by the addition of insulin to the dialysate solution or by IV insulin drip. The volume of fluid removed by dialysis in a 24-hour period should be limited to 500 ml in the neonate, range from 500 to 1000 ml in infants and 1000 to 1500 ml in young children, and be limited to 3000 ml in children weighing more than 30 kg.[27] The effect of dialysis on the removal of solutes depends mainly on the length of the dwell time in the peritoneal cavity and the molecular weight of the solute. The following are the relative rates of diffusion of common substances[28]:

Urea > Potassium > Sodium > Creatinine > Phosphate > Uric Acid > Calcium > Magnesium

Standard dialysate solutions do not contain potassium. Hyperkalemia, therefore may be controlled with a few hours of effective peritoneal dialysis.

In children in whom peritoneal dialysis is not feasible, hemodialysis and hemofiltration are options. The latter may be preferred, especially in those patients who are hemodynamically unstable.[29] The most common mode of hemofiltration is the pump-assisted continuous venovenous hemofiltration. When indicated it can be combined with dialysis.

☐ Acute Renal Failure in the Neonate

ARF occurs in as many as 23% of all patients admitted to the neonatal intensive care unit.[30] The definition of ARF in a neonate is most often considered to be a serum creatinine level above 1.5 mg/dl for more than 24 hours in the setting of normal maternal renal function.[31] ARF is of the oliguric variety when the elevated serum creatinine is accompanied by a urine output below 1 ml/kg/h after the initial 24 hours of life and when urine output fails to improve in response to a fluid challenge. In contrast, some patients develop solute retention; as evidenced by an elevated serum creatinine level, with a normal (>1.0 ml/kg/h) urine flow rate: they are diagnosed as having nonoliguric ARF.[32] The nonoliguric form is particularly common in neonates with ARF secondary to perinatal asphyxia and appears to be associated with a better prognosis than the oliguric form.[32] The diagnosis of nonoliguric ARF can be overlooked if patients at risk for developing renal insufficiency are monitored solely by the evaluation of urine output without repeated assessments of the serum creatinine.

The causes of ARF traditionally have been divided into three categories: prerenal, intrinsic, and postrenal (Table 4–5). This division, based on the site of the lesion, has important implications because the evaluation, treatment, and prognosis of the three groups can be quite different.

PRERENAL ACUTE RENAL FAILURE

Impairment of renal perfusion is the cause of 70% of ARF in the neonatal period.[30, 31] Prerenal ARF may occur in any patient with hypoperfusion of an otherwise normal kidney. Although prompt correction of the low perfusion state usually reverses kidney function impairment, delay in fluid resuscitation may result in renal parenchymal damage.

INTRINSIC ACUTE RENAL FAILURE

Intrinsic ARF occurs in 6 to 8% of admissions to the neonatal intensive care unit and implies the presence of renal cellular damage associated with impaired kidney function.[31] Intrinsic ARF usually falls into one of the following categories: ischemic (acute tubular necrosis), nephrotoxic (aminoglyco-

TABLE 4-5. Major Causes of Acute Renal Failure in the Newborn

Prerenal Failure

Systemic hypovolemia: fetal hemorrhage, neonatal hemorrhage, septic shock, necrotizing enterocolitis, dehydration
Renal hypoperfusion: perinatal asphyxia, congestive heart failure, cardiac surgery, respiratory distress syndrome, pharmacologic (tolazoline, captopril, indomethacin)

Intrinsic Renal Failure

Acute tubular necrosis
Congenital malformations: bilateral agenesis, renal dysplasia, polycystic kidney disease, glomerular maturational arrest
Infection: congenital (syphilis, toxoplasmosis), pyelonephritis
Renal vascular: renal artery thrombosis, renal venous thrombosis, disseminated intravascular coagulation
Nephrotoxins: aminoglycosides, indomethacin, amphotericin B, contrast media
Intrarenal obstruction: uric acid nephropathy, myoglobinuria, hemoglobinuria

Postrenal (Obstructive) Renal Failure

Congenital malformations: imperforate prepuce, urethral stricture, posterior urethral valves, urethral diverticulum, primary vesicoureteral reflux, ureterocele, megacystis megaureter, Eagle-Barrett syndrome, ureteropelvic junction obstruction
Extrinsic compression: sacrococcygeal teratoma, hematocolpos
Intrinsic obstruction: renal calculi, fungus balls
Neurogenic bladder

Adapted from Karlowicz MG, Adelman RD. Acute renal failure in the neonate. Clin Perinatol 19:139–158, 1992.

side antibiotics, indomethacin), congenital renal anomalies (infantile [autosomal recessive] polycystic kidney disease), and vascular lesions (renal artery or vein thrombosis, especially with a solitary kidney).[33]

POSTRENAL ACUTE RENAL FAILURE

Postrenal ARF results from urine flow obstruction from both kidneys or from a solitary kidney. The most common causes of postrenal ARF in neonates are posterior urethral valves and bilateral ureteropelvic junction obstructions.[34] Although this type of obstruction is usually reversible, neonates with long-standing intrauterine obstruction have varying degrees of permanent impairment of renal function. This impairment may be due to not only the presence of renal dysplasia but also cellular damage secondary to ARF.

CLINICAL PRESENTATION

Clinical presentation of the neonate with ARF often reflects the condition that has precipitated development of the renal insufficiency. Accordingly, sepsis, shock, dehydration, severe respiratory distress syndrome, and other related conditions may be present. Nonspecific symptoms related to uremia, such as poor feeding, lethargy, emesis, seizures, hypertension, and anemia, also are frequently present.

DIAGNOSTIC EVALUATION

Evaluation of the neonate with ARF should include a thorough patient and family history and a physical examination. Suspected prerenal causes of acute oliguria are usually addressed diagnostically and therapeutically by volume expansion, with or without furosemide. If this approach does not result in increased urine output, a more extensive evaluation of renal function is indicated.

Laboratory studies are an important component of the evaluation and should include the following measures: complete blood count, serum concentrations of urea nitrogen, creatinine, electrolytes, uric acid, calcium, glucose, and phosphorus. The serum creatinine value during the first several days of life is a reflection of the maternal value. In full-term infants, a value of 0.4 to 0.5 mg/dl is expected after the first week of life.[35] A urinalysis should be obtained to check for the presence of red blood cells, protein, and casts suggestive of intrinsic renal disease.

Urine indexes can help distinguish intrinsic renal failure from prerenal azotemia in the oliguric patient. The index usually found to be the most useful is FE_{Na}. This factor is based on the assumption that the renal tubules of the poorly perfused kidney reabsorb sodium avidly, whereas the kidney with intrinsic renal disease and tubular damage is unable to do so. Accordingly, in most cases of neonatal oliguric renal failure secondary to intrinsic disease,

FE_{Na} is greater than 2.5%.[36] FE_{Na} should be measured prior to administering furosemide. In addition, the results should be interpreted with caution in a very premature infant who normally has a high (e.g., >5%) FE_{Na}.[37]

Ultrasonography is commonly the initial imaging study performed. The urinary tract should be evaluated for the presence of one or two kidneys and for their size, shape, and location. Dilation of the collecting system and the size and appearance of the urinary bladder should be evident. A voiding cystourethrogram may also be necessary, specifically when the diagnosis of posterior urethral valves or vesicoureteral reflux is entertained. Antegrade pyelography may be needed to evaluate for ureterovesicular junction obstruction. The limited GFR and renal tubular function of the neonate result in poor visualization of the kidneys and urinary tract by IV pyelography during the first several weeks of life. Radiocontrast agents may be nephrotoxic.[38] Radiologic assessment of the renal function should be performed with radioisotope scanning, using agents such as technetium[99m]-dimercaptosuccinic acid or technetium[99m]-MAG-3.

MANAGEMENT

The treatment of neonatal ARF should proceed simultaneously with the diagnostic workup. A fluid challenge, with or without subsequent furosemide therapy, usually enhances urine flow and fosters improved renal function in an infant with prerenal oliguria. Bladder catheter placement is good immediate therapy for posterior urethral valves, whereas high surgical drainage may be needed for other obstructive lesions in the neonate. The fluid challenge should consist of 20 ml/kg of an isotonic solution containing 25 mEq/l of sodium bicarbonate infused over 1 to 2 hours. In the absence of a prompt diuresis of 2 ml or more of urine/kg over 1 to 2 hours, intravenous furosemide at 2 to 5 mg/kg may be helpful. The role of dopamine as therapy for neonatal oliguric ARF, owing to its ability to cause renal vasodilation, remains unclear.[39] If used, the initial dose should be 1 µg/kg/min and should not exceed 5 µg/kg/min owing to its potential to induce vasoconstriction at the higher doses.[40] The failure to achieve increased urinary output after volume expansion in the neonate with an adequate cardiac output (i.e., renal perfusion) and an unobstructed urinary tract indicates the presence of intrinsic renal disease and the need to appropriately manage oliguric or anuric renal failure.

Maintenance of normal fluid balance is of primary concern in the management of the patient with ARF. Daily fluid intake should equal insensible water loss, urine output, and fluid losses from nonrenal sources. In full-term infants, insensible water losses amount to 30 to 40 ml/kg/day, whereas premature infants may require as much as 50 to 100 ml/kg/day.[37, 41] A frequent assessment of the neonate's body weight is essential for fluid management. The electrolyte content of the fluids administered should be guided by frequent laboratory studies. Insensible water losses are electrolyte free and should be replaced using glucose in water.

Important systemic disturbances that may arise secondary to ARF include hyperkalemia, hyponatremia, hypertension, hypocalcemia, hyperphosphatemia, and metabolic acidosis. All exogenous sources of potassium should be discontinued in patients with ARF. Despite this restriction, many develop elevated serum potassium levels, which must be treated aggressively owing to the potential for cardiac toxicity.[42] Treatment should be initiated with a sodium-potassium exchange resin (sodium polystyrene sulfonate in sorbitol, 1 g/kg by enema) if a progressive rise in the serum potassium level is noted (see Table 4–4). More rapid management intended to prevent or treat a cardiac arrhythmia consists of IV sodium bicarbonate (1 to 2 mEq/kg), 10% calcium gluconate solution (0.5 ml/kg), and glucose (0.5 to 1.0 g/kg) followed by insulin (0.1 to 0.2 U/kg).

Hyponatremia and systemic hypertension are most often related to overhydration in the infant with oliguria and initially should be treated with fluid restriction. The addition of high-dose IV furosemide (5 mg/kg) may be beneficial. The approximate amount of sodium needed to correct symptomatic hyponatremia in neonates is calculated as follows:

$$Na^+ (mEq) = ([Na^+] \text{ Desired} - [Na^+] \text{ Actual}) \times \text{Weight (kg)} \times 0.8$$

The treatment of persistent hypertension may include parenterally administered hydralazine (0.2 to 0.4 mg/kg/dose), labetalol (0.25 to 2 mg/kg/h as bolus or steady infusion) or enalaprilat (0.005 to 0.05 mg/kg/dose) for the patient without symptoms. Treatment for the patient with marked or refractory hypertension can include IV diazoxide (5 mg/kg), sodium nitroprusside (0.5 to 8 mg/kg/min), and labetalol or oral nifedipine (0.25 to 0.5 mg/kg/dose). Caution should be exercised when initiating therapy with captopril (initial oral dose, 0.03 to 0.15 mg/kg) owing to the profound hypotension that can occur in neonates in association with higher doses.[43]

Hyperphosphatemia (serum phosphorus level >7 mg/dl), which is often the cause of associated hypocalcemia, necessitates the use of a low-phosphorus infant formula (Similac PM 60/40) and calcium carbonate, as a phosphate binder (50–100 mg/kg/day).[44] Aluminum hydroxide as a binder is contraindicated, owing to its association with aluminum toxicity in infants and children with renal insufficiency.[45]

Hypocalcemia, as reflected by a low total serum calcium level, often occurs in ARF in association with hypoalbuminemia. Less commonly, the ionized calcium level is low and the patient is symptomatic. In these cases, IV 10% calcium gluconate should be given until the ionized calcium level is restored to the normal range.

Metabolic acidosis may arise as a result of retention of hydrogen ions and may require sodium bicarbonate for correction. The dose of sodium bicarbonate to be given can be calculated as follows:

$$(\text{Desired Bicarbonate} - \text{Observed Bicarbonate}) \times \text{Weight (kg)} \times 0.5 = \text{mEq of Sodium Bicarbonate to Be Given}$$

This dose may be given orally or added to parenteral fluids and infused over several hours.

Adequate nutrition should be provided with the goal of 100 to 120 calories and 1 to 2 g of protein/kg/day, provided via IV or orally. For neonates who can tolerate oral fluids, a formula containing low levels of phosphorus and aluminum, such as Similac PM 60/40, is recommended. An aggressive approach to nutrition may well contribute to renal recovery by providing necessary energy at the cellular level.[42]

Although most neonates with ARF can be managed conservatively, occasional patients require peritoneal dialysis, continuous arteriovenous hemofiltration, or continuous venovenous hemofiltration for the treatment of the metabolic complications of fluid overload.[24, 27] The mortality rate in this group of patients commonly exceeds 60%. Twenty-three patients who received peritoneal dialysis at Children's Mercy Hospital during the neonatal period had a 35% mortality at 1 year.[46] The somewhat lower mortality rate in our center probably reflects the improved outcome of neonates with renal structural abnormalities leading to renal failure (17% mortality rate) compared to those infants with multisystem disease. In a recent report of 12 neonates who developed ARF following cardiac surgery and received continuous venovenous hemofiltration, 7 (59%) of the infants survived and no complications were noted related to the hemofiltration procedure.[47]

☐ Obstructive Uropathy

Obstructive uropathy in the neonate is most often the result of posterior urethral valves or ureteropelvic junction obstruction.[34] Obstruction also represents a significant cause of end-stage renal disease (ESRD) in children and is the underlying cause of ESRD in nearly 90% of affected boys younger than 4 years.[48] Accordingly, early recognition and treatment of these lesions are desirable, due to the adverse effects obstruction can have on renal function. Regardless, following surgical intervention and relief of obstruction, there may be alterations of GFR, renal blood flow, and renal tubular function.[49] Specifically, injury to the renal tubule may result in an impaired capacity to reabsorb sodium, to concentrate urine, and to secrete potassium and hydrogen, all of which may have profound clinical implications. The resorption of other solutes, such as magnesium, calcium, and phosphorus, may also be affected.[49]

The ability of the renal tubule to reabsorb salt and water after relief of obstruction depends on whether the obstruction was unilateral or bilateral. In unilateral obstruction, the proximal tubules of the juxtamedullary nephrons are unable to maximally reabsorb salt and water, whereas the fractional reabsorption of salt and water is increased in the superficial nephrons.[49] However, the amount of sodium excreted by the previously obstructed kidney is not different from that of the contralateral kidney, because tubuloglomerular balance is maintained. In contrast, relief of bilateral obstruction results in a marked elevation in the absolute amount of sodium and water lost. In part, these changes are a result of an osmotic diuresis secondary to retained solutes, such as urea.[50] Some contribution may also occur from atrial natriuretic factor, the plasma level of which is elevated during obstruction, as well as from enhanced synthesis of prostaglandins.[49, 51] Decreased renal medullary tonicity and decreased hydraulic water permeability of the collecting duct in response to antidiuretic hormone both contribute to the kidney's impaired concentrating ability.[52]

The clinical conditions associated with the concentrating abnormalities are secondary nephrogenic diabetes insipidus and hypernatremic dehydration. Accordingly, management must ensure the provision of adequate amounts of fluid and salt. Fluid intake should equal insensible losses, urine output, and nonrenal losses and should be guided by frequent assessments of body weight. Sodium intake should be monitored by serum and urine electrolyte determinations.

Ureteral obstruction can result in the impairment of hydrogen and potassium secretion and the syndrome of hyperkalemic hyperchloremic metabolic acidosis, or type IV renal tubular acidosis.[53, 54] This clinical situation appears to be the result of the impaired turnover of the sodium-potassium pump or a decreased responsiveness of the distal renal tubule to the actions of aldosterone. In a portion of the patients with this presentation, FE_{Na} is normal and FE_K is inappropriately low, relative to the elevated serum level. Treatment is directed toward correcting the underlying obstructive abnormality with surgery as well as providing sodium bicarbonate to alleviate the metabolic acidosis and hyperkalemia.

In older children and adults, release of bilateral ureteral obstruction results in a nonspecific increase in potassium excretion. In part, this effect is related to an increased delivery of sodium to the distal tubule, which results in an accelerated sodium-potassium exchange.[41] Close monitoring of the serum potassium level to detect the need for potassium replacement therapy is necessary to avoid development of hypokalemia.

REFERENCES

1. Brenner BM, Dworkin LD, Kchikawa L: Glomerular ultrafiltration. In Brenner BM, Rector FC Jr (eds): The Kidney. Vol. 1 (3rd ed). Philadelphia, WB Saunders, 1986, pp 124–144.
2. Hogg RJ, Stapleton FB: Renal tubular function. In Holliday MA, Barratt TM, Vernier RL (eds): Pediatric Nephrology (2nd ed). Baltimore, Williams & Wilkins, 1987, pp 59–77.
3. Yared A, Ichikawa I: Renal blood flow and glomerular filtration rate. In Holliday MA, Barratt TM, Vernier RL (eds): Pediatric Nephrology (2nd ed). Baltimore, Williams & Wilkins, 1987, pp 45–58.
4. Holliday MA, Segar WE: The maintenance need for water in parenteral fluid therapy. Pediatrics 19:823–832, 1957.
5. Edelmann CM Jr, Barnett HL: Role of the kidney in water metabolism in young infants. J Pediatr 56:154–179, 1960.
6. Polacek B, Vocel J, Neugebauerova L, et al: The osmotic concentrating ability in healthy infants and children. Arch Dis Child 40:291–295, 1965.
7. Chantler C, Barratt TM: Laboratory evaluation. In Holliday MA, Barratt RM, Vernier RL (eds): Pediatric Nephrology (2nd ed). Baltimore, Williams & Wilkins, 1987, pp 282–299.
8. Hellerstein S, Hunter JL, Warady BA: Creatinine excretion rates for evaluation of kidney function in children. Pediatr Nephrol 2:419–424, 1988.
9. Hellerstein S, Holliday MA, Grupe WE, et al: Nutritional management of children with chronic renal failure. Pediatr Nephrol 1:195–211, 1987.
10. Steiner RW: Interpreting the fractional excretion of sodium. Am J Med 77:699–702, 1984.
11. Halperin ML, Goldstein MB, Stinebaugh BJ, Richardson RMA: Renal tubular acidosis. In Maxwell MH, Kleeman CR, Narins RG (eds): Clinical Disorders of Fluid and Electrolyte Metabolism (4th ed). New York, McGraw-Hill, 1987, pp 675–689.
12. Rodriguez-Soriana J, Vallo A: Renal tubular acidosis. Pediatr Nephrol 4:268–275, 1990.
13. Rigden SPA, Barratt TM, Dillon MJ, et al: Acute renal failure complicating cardiopulmonary bypass surgery. Arch Dis Child 57:425–430, 1982.
14. Gomez-Campadra FJ, Maroto-Alvaro E, Galinanes M, et al: Acute renal failure with cardiac surgery. Child Nephrol Urol 9:138–143, 1989.
15. Siegel NJ, Gaudio KM: Pathogenesis and treatment of acute renal failure. Pediatr Clin North Am 34:771–787, 1971.
16. Singh N, Kissoon N, Al-Mofada S, et al: Furosemide infusion versus furosemide bolus in the postoperative pediatric cardiac patient. Pediatr Res 27:35A, 1990.
17. Alkhunaaizi AM, Schrier RW: Management of acute renal failure: New perspectives. Am J Kidney Dis 28:315–328, 1996.
18. Trachtman H: Sodium and water homeostasis. Pediatr Clin North Am 42:1343–1363, 1995.
19. Feld LG, Cachero S, Springate JE: Fluid needs in acute renal failure. Pediatr Clin North Am 37:337–350, 1990.
20. Noble-Jamieson CM, Kuzim P, Airede KI: Hidden sources of fluid and sodium intake in ill newborns. Arch Dis Child 61:645–696, 1986.
21. Gruskin AB, Morgenstern BZ, Perlman S: Kinetics of peritoneal dialysis in children. In Fine RN, Grustin AB (eds): End Stage Renal Disease in Children. Philadelphia, WB Saunders, 1984, pp 95–117.
22. Alon U, Bar-Maor JA, Bar-Joseph G: Effective peritoneal dialysis in an infant with extensive resection of the small intestine. Am J Nephrol 8:65–67, 1988.
23. Erbe RW, Greene JA Jr, Weller JM: Peritoneal dialysis during hemorrhagic shock. J Appl Physiol 22:131–135, 1967.
24. Fine RN: Peritoneal dialysis update. J Pediatr 100:1–7, 1982.
25. Tzamaloukas AH, Garella S, Chazan JA: Peritoneal dialysis for acute renal failure after major abdominal surgery. Arch Surg 106:639–643, 1973.
26. Matthews DE, West KW, Rescoria FJ, et al: Peritoneal dialysis in the first 60 days of life. J Pediatr Surg 25:111–116, 1990.
27. Chan JCM: Peritoneal dialysis for renal failure in childhood: Clinical aspects and electrolyte changes as observed in 20 cases. Clin Pediatr 17:349–354, 1978.
28. Miller RB, Tassistro CR: Peritoneal dialysis. N Engl J Med 17:945–948, 1969.
29. Evans ED, Greenbaum LA, Ettenger RB: Principles of renal replacement therapy in children. Pediatr Clin North Am 42:1579–1602, 1995.

30. Norman ME, Asadi FK: A prospective study of acute renal failure in the newborn infant. Pediatrics 63:475–479, 1979.
31. Stapleton FB, Jones DP, Green RS: Acute renal failure in neonates: Incidence, etiology and outcome. Pediatr Nephrol 1:314–320, 1987.
32. Karlowicz MG, Adelman RD: Nonoliguric and oliguric acute renal failure in asphyxiated term neonates. Pediatr Nephrol 9:718–722, 1995.
33. Blowey DL, Ben-David S, Koren G: Interactions of drugs with the developing kidney. Pediatr Clin North Am 42:1415–1431, 1995.
34. Elder JS, Duckett JW: Management of the fetus and neonate with hydronephrosis detected by prenatal ultrasonography. Pediatr Ann 17:19–28, 1988.
35. Feldman H, Guignard J-P: Plasma creatinine in the first month of life. Arch Dis Child 57:123–126, 1982.
36. Karlowicz MG, Adelman RD: Acute renal failure in the neonate. Clin Perinatol 19:139–158, 1992.
37. Anand SK: Acute renal failure. In Taeusch HW, Ballard RA, Avery ME (eds): Diseases of the Newborn. Philadelphia, WB Saunders, 1991, pp 894–895.
38. Gruskin AB, Oetliker O, Wolfish NM, et al: Effects of angiography on renal function and histology in infants and piglets. J Pediatr 76:41–50, 1970.
39. Tulassay T, Seri I, Machay T, et al: Effects of dopamine on renal functions in premature infants with respiratory distress syndrome. Int J Pediatr Nephrol 4:19–23, 1983.
40. Roberts RJ: Drug Therapy in Infants: Pharmacologic Principles and Clinical Experience. Philadelphia, WB Saunders, 1984, pp 165–166.
41. Roy NR, Sinclair JC: Hydration of the low birth weight infant. Clin Perinatol 2:393–410, 1975.
42. Gaudio KM, Siegel NJ: Pathogenesis and treatment of acute renal failure. Pediatr Clin North Am 34:771–787, 1987.
43. Tack ED, Periman JM: Renal failure in sick hypertensive premature infants receiving captopril therapy. J Pediatr 112:805–810, 1988.
44. Alon U, Davidai G, Bentur L, et al: Oral calcium carbonate as phosphate binder in infants and children with chronic renal failure. Miner Electrolyte Metab 12:320–325, 1986.
45. American Academy of Pediatrics, Committee on Nutrition. Aluminum toxicity in infants and children. Pediatrics 97:412–416, 1996.
46. Blowey DL, McFarland K, Alon U, et al: Peritoneal dialysis in the neonatal period: Outcome data. J Perinatol 13:59–64, 1993.
47. Leyh RG, Nötzold A, Kraatz EG, et al: Continuous venovenous haemofiltration in neonates with renal insufficiency resulting from low cardiac output syndrome after cardiac surgery. Cardiovasc Surg 4:520–525, 1996.
48. Minoja M, Hirschman G, Jones C, et al: Incidence and causes of ESRD in children in the USA [abstract]. J Am Soc Nephrol 6:396, 1995.
49. Klahr S, Harris K, Purkerson ML: Effects of obstruction on renal functions. Pediatr Nephrol 2:34–42, 1988.
50. Harris RH, Yarger WE: The pathogenesis of postobstructive diuresis: The role of circulating natriuretic and diuretic factors, including urea. J Clin Invest 56:880–887, 1975.
51. Peters CA: Obstruction of the fetal urinary tract. J Am Soc Nephrol 653–663, 1997.
52. Hanley MJ, Davidson K: Isolated nephron segments from rabbit models of obstructive nephropathy. J Clin Invest 69:165–174, 1982.
53. Rodriguez-Soriano J, Vallo A, Oliveros R, et al: Transient pseudohypoaldosteronism secondary to obstructive uropathy in infancy. J Pediatr 103:375–380, 1983.
54. Yarger WE, Buerkert J: Effect of urinary tract obstruction on renal tublar function. Semin Nephrol 2:17–30, 1982.

5

COAGULOPATHIES AND SICKLE CELL DISEASE

Brian M. Wicklund, MD, CM, MPh •
Gerald M. Woods, MD

The pediatric surgeon encounters patients with various hematologic disorders, including hemophilia, immune thrombocytopenia purpura, sickle cell disease, and spherocytosis. Children with hemophilia and sickle cell disease represent the largest populations that have been followed by the hematologist over an extended period. Although there is no association between hemophilia and sickle cell disease from a pathophysiologic standpoint, we discuss these two conditions because of the unique surgical challenges that these patients provide the pediatric surgeon, pediatric hematologist, and other physicians involved.

☐ Coagulopathies

The hemostatic system arrests bleeding from injured blood vessels and prevents the loss of blood from intact vessels. It keeps unwanted clots from forming and resolves blood clots that have served their purpose. A complex, three-part system of proteins, platelets, and vessels containing them has evolved to maintain hemostasis. Pathologic defects in this regulatory system result in either bleeding or thrombosis when too little or too much clot is formed or when the dissolution of a clot is not properly controlled.

Obtaining a complete history about the patient and his or her family is essential to anticipating hemostatic disorders. Laboratory studies help identify and characterize the problems that are uncovered by the history. The pediatric surgeon who takes no history may eventually have a patient on the operating table who will not stop bleeding.

BIOCHEMISTRY AND PHYSIOLOGY OF HEMOSTASIS

Three distinct structures are involved in the process of hemostasis: blood vessels, platelets, and circulating hemostatic proteins. These parts together form the coagulation system, the naturally occurring anticoagulation system, and the fibrinolytic system. These systems serve to amplify the stimulus that activated the coagulation system and to control the amount of response to that initial stimulus. Coagulation must act rapidly to stop the loss of blood from an injured vessel, but the blood clot formed must remain localized so that it does not interfere with the passage of blood in the intact circulation. The anticoagulation system prevents the extension of the forming clot beyond the site of injury. The fibrinolytic system removes excess hemostatic material that has been released into the circulation and slowly lyses the clot once it is no longer needed.

The initial stimulus to the formation of a clot comes from the disruption of endothelial cells, exposing collagen, and subendothelial tissues. The hemostatic response to tissue injury consists of four stages. First, vasoconstriction by the contraction of smooth muscle in the injured vessel wall reduces blood flow and promotes more effective activation of platelets and other coagulation sequences. Second, platelets adhere to the exposed endothelium, aggregate, and release their granular contents. This activity stimulates further vasoconstriction and recruits more platelets. Primary hemostasis results from platelets occluding the hole in the blood vessel and halting the escape of blood. Third, the intrinsic and extrinsic coagulation systems are activated to form fibrin, which stabilizes the platelets and prevents disaggregation. Fourth, fibrinolysis results from the release of plasminogen activators from the injured vessel wall. These activators limit the coagulation process and, once healing has taken place, begin the resolution of formed clot so that vascular patency can be restored.[1]

Endothelial Cells

Endothelial cells line the lumen of all blood vessels, maintain the integrity of the blood vessel, and prevent the egression of blood into the surrounding tissue.[1] When the vessel is intact, they provide a thromboresistant surface that prevents the activation of the coagulation system. Passive thromboresistance is provided by endothelial proteoglycans, primarily heparin sulfate. Heparin is an anticoagulant compound that acts as a cofactor in converting antithrombin III to a potent inhibitor of activated clotting factors. Active thromboresistance is achieved through several mechanisms, including the synthesis and release of prostacyclin (PGI₂).[1, 2]

Prostacyclin is a potent vasodilator and an inhibitor of platelet adhesion and aggregation. It opposes the vasoconstriction caused by thromboxane A₂ and triggers adenyl cyclase in the platelet membrane to increase the production of cyclic adenosine monophosphate (cAMP). cAMP inhibits the expression of fibrinogen receptors and factor VIII:von Willebrand's factor receptors on the platelet membrane, thereby decreasing platelet adhesion and aggregation. The two actions of prostacyclin serve to prevent the excess accumulation of platelets and to limit the duration of vasoconstriction. Prostacyclin is synthesized and released in response to thrombin and other substances produced at the site of tissue injury.[2]

Intact endothelium inactivates or clears adenosine diphosphate (ADP), several proaggregatory vasoactive amines, and thrombin.[3] The endothelium produces thrombomodulin, a cofactor in the thrombin-dependent activation of protein C. The activation of protein C results in the destruction of factors Va and VIIIa and thereby decreases the formation of fibrin through the intrinsic and common pathways. Endothelial cells synthesize and release both tissue plasminogen activator (t-PA) and tissue plasminogen activator inhibitor (t-PAI), which control the activation of the fibrinolytic system.[4] The release of t-PA and t-PAI serves to control the degree of response of the coagulation system and to limit the propagation of clot.

When endothelium is injured, tissue factor (thromboplastin) is produced and rapidly promotes local thrombin formation.[5] Tissue factor binds factor VII and converts it to factor VIIa. The production of factor VIIa is the first step in activation of the extrinsic coagulation pathway, which, when activated, then activates the common pathway, leading to the formation of fibrin.[6] The contribution these processes make to the control of bleeding depends on the size of the interrupted vessel. Capillaries seal with little dependence on the hemostatic system, but arterioles and venules require the presence of platelets to form an occluding plug. In arteries and veins, hemostasis depends on both vascular contraction and clot formation around an occluding primary hemostatic plug.[7]

Platelets

In the resting state, platelets circulate as disk-shaped, anuclear cells that have been released from megakaryocytes in the bone marrow. They are 2 to 3 μm in size, have a volume of 10 fl, and remain in circulation for as many as 8 days unless they participate in coagulation reactions, bind to formed clot, or are removed by the spleen.[8] Platelets have a circumferential cytoskeleton of microtubules and actin filaments that provides a contractile system and, through the actin, participates in clot retraction. The surface membrane of the platelet is contiguous with a sponge-like, open canalicular membrane system that comes into close proximity with a dense tubular system that is not surface connected. In the resting state, platelets do not bind to intact endothelium. Platelets release growth factors to facilitate the proliferation of vascular endothelial and smooth muscle cells. These cells play a significant role in restoring the structure of injured blood vessels.[8]

Platelet Adhesion

Once platelets bind to injured tissue and activate, their diskoid shape changes; they spread on the subendothelial connective tissue and degranulate. Degranulation occurs when platelets internally contract and extrude storage granule contents into the open canalicular system. Dense granules release serotonin, ADP, calcium, and adenosine triphosphate (ATP). Alpha granules release factor V, fibrinogen, factor VIII:von Willebrand's factor, fibronectin, platelet factor IV, β-thromboglobulin, and platelet-derived growth factor.[8, 9] Lysosomal vesicles are also present within platelets. The material released from the granules recruits and aggregates more platelets from the circulation onto the already adherent platelets.

When a vessel is disrupted, platelet adhesion occurs via the binding of collagen and von Willebrand's factor found in the subendothelium to the platelet membrane. For platelet adhesion to occur, platelets must express specific glycoprotein Ib receptors on their surface to bind the von Willebrand factor complex. If this specific glycoprotein is missing, platelets are unable to adhere to areas of injury.[10] Platelets in Bernard-Soulier syndrome lack glycoprotein Ib and are unable to adhere and form the initial hemostatic plug.[11] If the von Willebrand factor is defective or deficient in amount, platelets do not adhere to sites of vascular injury. The result is von Willebrand's disease, for which several specific types and subtypes have been defined.[12, 13] In either Bernard-Soulier syndrome or von Willebrand's disease, if an operation is performed without the replacement of normal amounts and types of platelets or von Willebrand's factor, respectively, serious bleeding can result from the inability to form an initial hemostatic platelet plug. Very high concentrations of PGI₂ can also inhibit platelet adhesion to exposed subendothelium.[7]

After platelet adhesion has occurred, in addition to degranulation and an increased local concentration of ADP, small amounts of thrombin are formed and platelet membrane phospholipase is activated to generate thromboxane A$_2$. Thromboxane A$_2$ and serotonin released from the dense granules stimulate vasoconstriction and induce the exposure of membrane receptors for fibrinogen (glycoproteins IIb/IIIa). Fibrinogen binding to stimulated platelets then induces aggregation by linking platelets together.[8]

Platelet Aggregation

Aggregation is a complex reaction that involves platelet granule release, cleavage of membrane phospholipids, by phospholipases A$_2$ and C, alterations in intracellular cAMP levels, mobilization of intracellular calcium, and the expression of fibrinogen receptors on the platelet surface. If fibrinogen receptors (glycoproteins IIb and IIIa) or fibrinogen are missing, platelets do not aggregate.[14] Glanzmann's thrombasthenia is a deficiency of glycoproteins IIb and IIIa in which platelets adhere normally but do not aggregate. These patients have a serious, lifelong bleeding disorder.[9]

After aggregation, platelets function to enhance thrombin formation. Platelet membrane provides specific binding sites for factors Xa and V. The result is an efficient site for the assembly of the prothrombinase complex, which converts prothrombin into thrombin.[8] Thrombin formation results in the formation of a stable hemostatic plug of adherent platelets surrounded by a network of fibrin strands.

Generation of Thrombin

Tissue injury induces activation of the plasma-based coagulation system, resulting in the generation of thrombin from prothrombin. Thrombin is the enzyme responsible for transforming liquid blood into a fibrin gel. The initial activation of factor VII by tissue factor (thromboplastin) results in the production of thrombin by the extrinsic system. Tissue factor is released after injury to the endothelial cells but is not expressed on the surface of the cells.[3]

The majority of thrombin production results from the activation of the intrinsic coagulation system, not the extrinsic system. Exposed subendothelium converts factor XII to factor XIIa and thereby activates the intrinsic pathway. Activation of factors XI and IX follows, and activated factor IX in combination with factor VIII, calcium, and platelet phospholipid activates factor X. Factor Xa with factor V then cleaves prothrombin into the active molecule thrombin. When thrombin is free of the platelet membrane, it can convert fibrinogen into fibrin.[3, 6]

Formation of Fibrin

When thrombin acts on fibrinogen, fibrin monomers result after the proteolytic release of fibrinopeptides A and B. The monomeric fibrin then polymerizes into a gel.[3, 6] With additional stabilization of the fibrin gel provided by factor XIII, fibrin surrounds and stabilizes the platelet plug. This process makes the multimeric fibrin more resistant to plasmin digestion and completes the formation and stabilization of the blood clot.[15]

Several regulatory proteins serve to localize thrombin formation to the surface of the blood vessel. Endothelial cells have receptors for protein C, an anticoagulant protein. Protein C from the plasma binds to these receptors. Thrombomodulin is an endothelial surface protein that acts in combination with thrombin to activate the bound protein C. Activated protein C then degrades factors Va and VIIIa, which inhibit thrombin formation.[16]

Heparin-like anticoagulant molecules are present on endothelial cells. They act in combination with antithrombin III to inhibit factors XIIa, XIa, IXa, and Xa and thrombin. Inhibition of these factors prevents the spread of clot to uninjured adjacent vessels and the blockage of large vessels by excessive clot formation.[3, 16] Endothelial cells, as mentioned previously, produce PGI$_2$, a potent vasodilator and inhibitor of platelet aggregation and adhesion.

Fibrinolysis

The regulatory system that dissolves fibrin and preserves vessel patency is called *fibrinolysis*. Circulating plasminogen is converted into plasmin by tissue plasminogen activators. These activators are released from the vessel walls at the site of blood clotting. They bind to the fibrin clot and convert plasminogen to plasmin. Plasmin enzymatically degrades fibrin, fibrinogen, and other plasma proteins, and this process results in the dissolution of formed clot.[3, 16]

CLINICAL EVALUATION

Currently, there is no screening test of hemostasis that is completely reliable for the preoperative evaluation of patients.[17] A careful history, including a full family history, is still the best means of uncovering mild bleeding problems, such as von Willebrand's disease or qualitative platelet abnormalities. These disorders may easily escape standard laboratory screening procedures, such as prothrombin time (PT), activated partial thromboplastin time (aPTT), platelet count, and bleeding time. However, patients with mild hemophilia who have not previously undergone surgical procedures may have absolutely no history of bleeding problems and might be identified preoperatively only if an aPTT is done. Any of the preceding clinical situations is associated with a risk of excessive bleeding in surgery that is great enough to recommend the completion of a reasonable combination of history, physical examination, and clinically indicated laboratory tests.[18, 19] It is important to consider the history as the most sensitive of the three testing procedures and to thoroughly investigate any story of unusual bleeding, even if the screening tests are normal. Conversely, preoperative coagulation testing done in the absence of a suggestive history can result in false-positive results.[20] Several studies have examined the utility of the preoperative PT and PTT in patients undergoing tonsillectomy and adenoidectomy and have concluded that routine screening with a PT and PTT of all patients cannot be recommended.[21, 22]

In obtaining a history from a patient and parents,[17, 23] positive answers to any of the following questions should indicate the need for further evaluation:

- Is there any history of easy bruising, bleeding problems, or an established bleeding disorder in the patient or any family members?
- Has there been excessive bleeding after any previous surgery or dental work? Have the parents or any siblings had excessive bleeding after any surgical or dental procedures, specifically tonsillectomy or adenoidectomy?
- Have frequent nosebleeds occurred, and has nasal packing or cautery been needed? Has bleeding without trauma occurred into any joint or muscle?
- Does excessive bleeding or bruising occur after aspirin ingestion?
- Does significant gingival bleeding occur after tooth brushing?
- Has the patient been on any medication that might affect platelets or the coagulation system?
- If the patient is male and was circumcised, were there any problems with prolonged oozing after the circumcision?
- If the patient is a child, do the parents remember any bleeding problems when the umbilical cord separated?
- If the patient is menstruating, does she have profuse menstruation?
- Has the patient ever received any transfusions of blood or blood products? If so, what was the reason for the transfusion?

If there is a history of abnormal bleeding, the following points need to be established. The type of bleeding (i.e., petechiae, purpura, ecchymosis, and single or generalized bleeding sites) can give an indication of the underlying defect. Petechiae and purpura are most frequently associated with platelet abnormalities, either of function or numbers. von Willebrand's disease is most frequently associated with mucosal bleeding, including epistaxis, whereas hemophilia is most often associated with bleeding into joints and or soft tissue ecchymosis. Bleeding when the umbilical cord separates is most often associated with a deficiency in factor XIII.[15] A single bleeding site is frequently indicative of a localized mechanical problem and not a system-wide coagulation defect.

The course or pattern of the bleeding (i.e., spontaneous or posttrauma) and its frequency, duration of problems, and severity can provide clues to the cause of the problem. A family history of bleeding is important to define, and the pattern of inheritance (i.e., X-linked or autosomal; recessive or dominant) can help narrow the differential diagnosis. Hemophilia A and B are X-linked recessive diseases, whereas von Willebrand's disease is an autosomal dominant trait.[24]

Any previous or current drug therapy must be fully documented, and a search is made for any over-the-counter medications that the patient might be taking but does not consider "medicine" and has therefore not mentioned. Ibuprofen, cough medications containing guaifenesin, and antihistamines can uncover a preexisting bleeding disorder such as von Willebrand's disease when they would not alone cause sufficient platelet dysfunction to result in clinically apparent bleeding.[25] The presence of other medical problems is important to establish, because renal failure with uremia, hepatic failure, malignancies, or collagen vascular diseases may have associated coagulopathies.

The physical examination is used to help narrow the differential diagnosis and guide the laboratory investigation of hemostatic disorders. Certain physical findings may be associated with a specific coagulation abnormality, whereas others may be indicative of an underlying systemic disease with an associated coagulopathy. Petechiae and purpuric bleeding occur with platelet and vascular abnormalities. If the petechiae are raised, a vasculitis is likely, whereas petechiae due to thrombocytopenia are not elevated and initially occur on ankles or mucosa. Acquired coagulation defects usually result in widespread ecchymotic bleeding with or without gastrointestinal or urinary tract bleeding. Bleeding into joints and bleeding that stops and restarts are characteristic of congenital coagulation factor deficiencies. Hemophilia patients often have bruises with a raised central nodule, called *palpable purpura*. Findings compatible with a collagen vascular disorder include the body habitus of Marfan's syndrome; blue sclera; skeletal deformities; hyperextensible joints and skin; and nodular, spider-like, or pinpoint telangiectasias. Hepatosplenomegaly and lymphadenopathy may suggest an underlying malignancy, and jaundice plus hepatomegaly may indicate hepatic dysfunction.

LABORATORY EVALUATION

At present, the usual tests for screening the hemostatic system are the platelet count, PT, and aPTT.[24, 26] Additional tests can be done to measure fibrinogen levels, assess the thrombin time, screen for inhibitors of specific coagulation factors, measure specific factor levels, and test for platelet function. Patients can also be evaluated for evidence of disseminated intravascular coagulation (DIC) using multiple assays to test for the presence of various fibrinopeptides and products from the breakdown of fibrin or fibrinogen.

PLATELET COUNT. The platelet count measures the adequacy of platelet numbers to provide initial hemostasis. Platelet counts are usually performed using an automated hematology counter. The normal range is 150,000 to 400,000 platelets/mm³, and excess bleeding with surgical procedures usually does not occur until the count is below 50,000 platelets/mm³.[8, 20] At counts between 50,000 and 20,000 platelets/mm³, increased bruising and petechiae are expected, and when the platelet count is below 20,000/mm³, spontaneous bleeding may occur. It is the usual practice to transfuse the patient with platelet concentrates to raise the platelet count above 100,000/mm³ prior to any major operation.[18, 26]

BLEEDING TIME. The bleeding time is defined as the length of time a standardized incision takes to stop oozing blood that can be absorbed onto filter paper. A variety of procedures have been used, including the Duke method with a stab incision of the earlobe and the Ivy method with a standardized cut on the forearm, but both have been difficult to reproduce accurately. At present, the *simplate* test using a spring-load blade to make a controlled cut of a specific length and depth on the volar surface of the forearm is the most frequently used procedure and provides a reasonable reproducibility. The normal values vary, depending on the procedure used and the individual laboratory, but are usually less than 10 min.[1, 7]

The bleeding time is dependent on platelet count and function, vascular function, and von Willebrand's factor. It is the best in vivo test of platelet function involved in producing the primary hemostatic plug. Patients with coagulopathies such as hemophilia have a normal bleeding time, as their platelet function is normal.[24] When the platelet count is below 100,000/mm³, the bleeding time prolongs in a linear fashion until the count is below 10,000/mm³, at which point it then prolongs asymptomatically.[27] Other reasons for a prolonged bleeding time include an inherited defect in platelet function, a defect or deficiency in the patient's von Willebrand factor, and an acquired defect in platelet function, such as that caused by aspirin ingestion or uremia. Patients with an immune destruction of platelets (e.g., immune thrombocytopenic purpura) may have normal hemostasis and a normal bleeding time with platelet counts of 50,000/mm³ or less, owing to the production of young, hemostatically competent platelets.[27]

PROTHROMBIN TIME. The PT screens the function of the extrinsic and common coagulation pathways. It is the time required to clot platelet-poor plasma after the addition of tissue factor, calcium, and phospholipid, the tissue factor being the material that is "extrinsic" to the plasma-based coagulation system.[1] Isolated prolongations of the PT are seen in factor VII deficiency and in patients on warfarin sodium anticoagulation. It is also considered the most sensitive screening test for liver dysfunction coagulopathies.[1]

PARTIAL THROMBOPLASTIN TIME. The aPTT screens the function of the intrinsic and common coagulation pathways. Platelet-poor plasma is incubated with kaolin, Celite, or ellagic acid to form activated factor

XII (factor XIIa). Calcium and phospholipid are then added, and the time to formation of clot is measured.[1] Factor levels below 30 to 50% of normal levels are needed to produce an abnormal test result; the level at which the test becomes abnormal depends on the reagents and testing equipment used. The aPTT detects deficiencies in factors XII, XI, IX, and VIII and in the common pathway, but mild factor deficiencies may be missed. The aPTT is also used to monitor anticoagulation with heparin.[1]

Several inherited disorders of coagulation are not detected by the preceding tests. Factor XIII deficiency is detected by a urea clot solubility test.[1] von Willebrand's disease patients may have normal or prolonged aPTTs, and patients with a deficiency in α-2-plasmin inhibitor have a normal aPTT. Both the PT and aPTT are prolonged in patients with deficiencies of factors X and V, prothrombin, and fibrinogen and in patients with DIC or severe liver disease.[1, 24]

THROMBIN TIME. The thrombin time is a measure of fibrin formation, the final reaction of the clotting cascade. The test is performed by adding thrombin to platelet-poor plasma and measuring the time required for the formation of a fibrin gel.[1] The thrombin time is normal in patients with defects in the intrinsic or extrinsic pathway but is abnormal with low levels of fibrinogen or a dysfunctional fibrinogen or in the presence of thrombin inhibitors such as heparin or fibrin-split products. This test is extremely sensitive to the presence of heparin.[1]

FIBRINOGEN. The standard method for fibrinogen determination measures clottable fibrinogen using a kinetic assay. Normal levels of fibrinogen are 150 to 350 mg/dl. Because fibrinogen is the substrate for the final reaction in the formation of a clot and all plasma-based screening tests depend on the formation of a clot as the endpoint of the reaction, fibrinogen levels below 80 mg/dl prolong the PT, aPTT, and thrombin time and therefore make the results uninterpretable.[1, 2] Large amounts of fibrin degradation products interfere with the formation of fibrin and cause an artificially low level of fibrinogen to be measured. Partially clotted samples also cause a low level of fibrinogen to be assayed. An immunologic-based assay for fibrinogen is available and is used to measure both clottable and nonclottable fibrinogen. This test is most often used in identifying patients with a dysfibrinogenemia, in whom the functional level of fibrinogen is low and the immunologic level is normal.[1, 24]

INHIBITOR SCREENING TESTS. Repeating the PT or aPTT using a 1:1 mix of patient plasma with normal plasma is a useful procedure for investigating a prolonged PT or aPTT. Normal plasma has, by definition, 100% levels of all factors. When mixed with an equal volume of patient plasma, a minimum of 50% of any given factor is present, which should normalize the PT or aPTT. If the test normalizes, it suggests the presence of a factor deficiency, whereas lack of normalization suggests the presence of an inhibitor that interferes with either thrombin or fibrin formation.[1]

Two types of acquired inhibitors prolong the aPTT. One blocks or inactivates one of the intrinsic factors, whereas the other is a lupus-like inhibitor that interferes with phospholipid-based clotting reactions. The first type of inhibitor occurs in 5 to 15% of hemophiliacs and can occur spontaneously, but it is extremely rare in nonhemophiliac children.[24] The lupus-like inhibitor is not associated with bleeding problems but rather with an increased risk of thrombotic problems in adults. Lupus-like inhibitors are mentioned because they commonly cause prolongations of the aPTT.[28] Specific investigation of either of these situations should be referred to a skilled coagulation reference laboratory.

PLATELET FUNCTION STUDIES. Platelet function studies measure in vitro platelet aggregation. In this procedure, platelet-rich plasma is incubated with an agonist, and changes in the amount of light transmitted through the platelet suspension are recorded. Agonists used to induce platelet aggregation include collagen, epinephrine, ADP, thrombin, and ristocetin. Three distinct phases are seen in the reaction. The first is an initial change in the shape of the platelets, leading to a temporary decrease in light transmission. Next is the first wave of aggregation, which is a reversible platelet-platelet interaction. With additional stimulation, the final phase—the second wave of aggregation—occurs and produces irreversible platelet aggregation. The second wave of aggregation is due to the release reaction of the platelet granules and thromboxane A_2 synthesis. The release reaction is extinguished by aspirin and is absent in patients with an inherited storage pool defect, congenital deficiency in thromboxane A_2 synthesis, or cyclooxygenase deficiency.[8]

SPECIFIC FACTOR ASSAYS. Specific factor assays are available for all known coagulation, fibrinolysis, and anticoagulation factors to quantify their levels in plasma. These tests are not indicated unless a screening test result is abnormal. The only exception involves the patient with a history that is suspicious for von Willebrand's disease and in whom the aPTT may therefore not be sensitive enough to detect the decreased level or activity of von Willebrand's factor. Further testing may be justified by clinical suspicion based on the patient's history and would consist of measuring factor VIII levels, factor VIII–related antigen levels, ristocetin cofactor activity, and ristocetin-induced platelet aggregation. Analysis of the distribution of von Willebrand's factor multimers can be useful to the hematologist in identifying the specific type of von Willebrand's disease.[12, 13]

TESTS FOR DISSEMINATED INTRAVASCULAR COAGULATION. The usually available tests in most hospital laboratories for identification of DIC are semiquantitative fibrin or fibrinogen degradation product assays, which involve a slide agglutination procedure. An increased amount of these degradation products suggests that either plasmin has circulated to lyse fibrin and fibrinogen or the patient's hepatic function is insufficient to clear the small amounts of regularly produced degradation products. The D-dimer test is also a slide agglutination procedure that tests for the presence of two D subunits of fibrin that are cross-linked by factor XIII. This test provides specific evidence that plasmin has digested fibrin clot and not fibrinogen. It is positive in patients with DIC, in patients resolving large intravascular clots, and in patients with hepatic insufficiency. Specific assays to demonstrate the presence of soluble fibrin monomer complexes or fibrinopeptides produced by the conversion of prothrombin to thrombin are available in specialized coagulation laboratories.[29]

☐ Surgery in Hemophilia A and B

Hemophilia A and B are X-linked recessive bleeding disorders caused by decreased levels of functional procoagulant factors VIII and IX, respectively. Approximately 80% of all hemophilia patients have factor VIII deficiency, which is *classic hemophilia*. The remaining 20% have factor IX deficiency, which is called *Christmas disease*. Until 1964, the therapy of both types of hemophilia was limited by volume restrictions imposed by the use of whole blood or fresh frozen plasma, at which time the factor VIII–rich fraction of fresh frozen plasma called cryoprecipitate was discovered.[30] Specific lyophilized factor VIII concentrates have since been developed, as have prothrombin-complex concentrates containing factors II, VII, IX, and X and concentrates containing only factor IX for the treatment of hemophilia B patients.[31–33] The lyophilized factor concentrates have allowed storage of the clotting factor using standard refrigeration and have permitted the outpatient treatment of bleeding episodes plus the development of home, self-infusion programs.[34] This treatment, combined with the development of comprehensive hemophilia treatment centers, has produced a remarkable change in the outlook for these patients, who previously began to develop significant joint deformities in their teens to twenties and were frequently wheelchair bound in adult life. Rapid home therapy has decreased the damage caused by hemarthroses, with hemophiliac children born since the mid-1970s having far fewer joint deformities than older hemophiliacs. These factor concentrates have allowed surgical procedures to be performed with much less risk, even to the point that orthopedic procedures can be readily accomplished.[35]

Viral infections transmitted by cryoprecipitate and factor concentrates have become one of the major problems faced by hemophilia patients. Approximately 60 to 70% of all hemophilia patients are positive for HIV, and more than 1200 have died of AIDS.[35, 36] This number is out of a total population of only 20,000 hemophiliacs in the United States.[37] Hepatitis is the other major viral infection transmitted by the factor concentrates used to treat hemophilia. Estimates from the mid-1980s are that more than 90% of multiply transfused hemophiliacs were positive for non-A, non-B hepatitis and that more than 95% had been infected with hepatitis B.[38] A more recent study shows that 75% of hemophiliacs who are HIV negative have evidence of hepatitis C infection.[39] All medical personnel working with hemophiliacs must strictly observe universal blood precautions, and all patients should be assumed to be positive for HIV or hepatitis. Special precautions are warranted in the operating room, such as wearing double gloves as well as a plastic apron under the surgical gown and making special arrangements to deal with aerosolized material during orthopedic procedures.

Hemophilia patients are classified into three categories based on their level of circulating procoagulant. Those with factor levels below 1% are *severe hemophiliacs,* are at a high risk of bleeding, and usually require replacement therapy two to four times per month.[37, 40] Bleeding occurs in areas subject to mechanized stress or minor trauma. Hemarthroses, hematomas, and ecchymoses are common. Recurrent hemarthroses can cause pseudotumors of the bone, and hematomas can cause compression damage to tissue or nerves and even ischemic compartment syndromes. Bleeding episodes in severe hemophiliacs can be irregularly spaced, with periods of recurrent hemarthrosis requiring frequent replacement doses of factor concentrate, interspersed with periods during which little or no concentrate is used.[37] In *moderate hemophiliacs,* who have procoagulant levels of 1 to 5%, spontaneous hemorrhage occurs infrequently, but relatively minor trauma can cause bleeding into joints or soft tissues. *Mild hemophiliacs,* with levels greater than 5%, rarely have bleeding problems and typically have problems only with major trauma or surgery.[24, 37] Some mild hemophiliacs may not be diagnosed until late childhood or adulthood and as children may therefore not give any history to alert the pediatric surgeon to a risk of bleeding. Because one third of all cases of hemophilia are caused by new mutations, there may not be any family history to alert the clinician.[24] Preoperative laboratory testing may provide the only point at which a mild hemophiliac is diagnosed.

The indications for surgery in hemophiliacs are the same as for patients with a normal clotting system, but they most frequently center on areas of damage secondary to bleeding episodes. In 1985, the results of a review of 350 consecutive operations performed at Orthopedic Hospital in Los Angeles were published.[41] The study examined patients with hemophilia A between 1967 and 1983. Because the study group represented patients from before the start of home therapy and comprehensive care, the group was expected to have significant orthopedic problems secondary to multiple hemarthroses. Of the 350 procedures reviewed, 312 were characterized as serious and 38 as of lesser intensity. There

were 318 operations on hemophiliacs with moderate and severe hemophilia and 30 on patients with mild hemophilia. As predicted by the time period, musculoskeletal procedures made up two thirds of all operations on moderate and severe hemophiliacs and half of all operations on mild hemophiliacs. Pseudotumors of the bone were removed in 15 operations, and there was one death, in a child with a massive intracranial hemorrhage who did not survive an emergency craniotomy.[41]

Bleeding problems during operation were not observed, but 23% of all serious operations were complicated by postoperative hemorrhages. Only operations on the knee had significantly more postoperative hemorrhages (40%), with other joints and soft tissue areas having similar rates of complications (15%). Hemophilia management changed during the time of the patient series, causing increased amounts of factor concentrate to be given to maintain higher minimum factor levels yet producing no decrease in the number of postoperative hemorrhages. Most of the postoperative hemorrhages occurred with plasma factor levels greater than 30%, which is the minimum level that is considered hemostatic. During the course of this patient series, intermittent infusions of factor concentrates were used. These infusions are wasteful in that they create unnecessarily high levels of factor immediately after infusion, yet factor levels may fall to less than those required for hemostasis before the next dose. The authors were not sure what role this might have played, but they suggested the use of continuous infusion for factor VIII concentrate to avoid these problems and provide greater physiologic stability of factor levels. The authors also noted that the incidence of postoperative hemorrhages dropped after the 11th postoperative day, although other studies have found that vigorous physical therapy may cause postoperative hemorrhage and have therefore recommended the continuation of factor replacement throughout the period of physical therapy.[41, 42]

The management of the hemophilic patient requires close cooperation among surgeons; hematologists; and personnel of the hemophilia center, the coagulation laboratory, and the pharmacy or blood bank. Careful preoperative planning is essential to the success of the procedure, and an adequate supply of clotting factor concentrate must be available to cover the patient's needs before the patient is admitted. The patient must also be screened for the presence of an inhibitor to either factor VIII or IX during the 2 to 4 weeks before surgery. If an inhibitor is present, management of the patient becomes much more complex and depends on the strength of the inhibitor. A low-titer inhibitor may be overcome with increased doses of human clotting factor, but high-titer inhibitors may require the use of porcine factor VIII, prothrombin complex concentrates, or activated prothrombin complex concentrates such as Feiba or Autoplex. These patients have been desensitized with daily doses of human factor concentrate over several months, and extracorporeal antibody absorption has been used to augment immune-tolerance therapy.[35] Finally, recombinant factor VIIa has been used to provide hemostasis for inhibitor patients on an experimental basis.[43]

We previously admitted the hemophilia patient scheduled for a surgical procedure on the afternoon before the scheduled operation. That evening, after a bolus dose of factor (usually 50 units/kg body weight of factor VIII in patients with hemophilia A), a continuous infusion of 4 to 5 units/kg/hr of factor VIII (for the hemophilia A patient) was started to maintain a factor level greater than 75%.[44] At present, owing to the influence of managed care, the patients are now admitted on the day of surgery, and administration of the initial bolus of factor plus initiation of the continuous factor infusion is done in the hematology clinic. The factor level is checked immediately before the operation and is the final screen for the presence of an inhibitor. The infusion is maintained throughout the procedure and is then lowered on the second or third postoperative day to allow the plasma levels to decrease to 30 to 50% range. Replacement is continued for a full 10 to 14 days after surgery. Daily measurement of factor levels is necessary to ensure maintenance of appropriate levels. For neurosurgical or orthopedic procedures, much longer periods of factor coverage—even 4 to 6 weeks—are needed if significant physical therapy is planned.[35, 37]

Many hemophiliacs now have home factor supply systems, and, with the advent of home nursing services, we are now discharging patients home on prolonged periods of factor coverage. Hemophilia center personnel must be closely involved in the planning of these discharges to ensure that sufficient clotting factor is available at home and that close follow-up is maintained during periods of scheduled home therapy. Hemophilia patients should not receive any compounds that contain aspirin, and their charts should be clearly marked. They should also avoid Darvon Compound and Percodan, as these compounds contain aspirin. Intramuscular injections should be avoided, and any minor procedures that would require factor correction should be combined with the major procedure, if possible, to save on the use of factor concentrate.

☐ Problems in Patients with Hemophilia B

Previously, the hemophilia B patient undergoing surgery had specific problems due to the thrombogenic risk inherent in the use of older factor IX concentrates. Thromboembolic complications were seen postoperatively, particularly in orthopedic surgery patients. The risk was not limited solely to these patients, however, as thrombosis had also been seen in other hemophilia B patients.[35, 40] Heparin in low doses was added to factor IX concentrate to reduce the risk of thrombosis. Since the advent of newer, more purified factor IX concentrates with a decreased risk of thrombosis, surgical procedures in hemophilia B patients have been performed without excess thrombotic problems.[33]

Factor VIII is dosed differently from factor IX based on their half-lives. Factor VIII has an 8- to 12-hour half-life, and the infusion of one unit of factor/kg body weight increases the plasma level by 2%. Thus, if a severe hemophilia A patient weighs 50 kg, an infusion of 25 units/kg × 50 kg, or 1250 units, of factor VIII will raise his factor level to 50%. Factor IX has a half-life of 24 hours and must be infused in larger amounts than factor VIII to raise the plasma level. Infusion of 1 unit/kg of factor IX will raise the plasma level only by 1%. Continuous infusion of highly purified factor IX, as well as factor VIII, has been shown to prevent excessive peaks and troughs of factor levels, is simpler to manage, and decreases the cost by decreasing the overall amount of factor used. It has not shown any problems with excess thrombosis.[45, 46]

NEONATAL HEMOSTASIS

The newborn's coagulation system is not fully mature until 6 months after birth. The lower levels of procoagulant, fibrinolytic, and anticoagulant proteins in neonatal patients complicate both surgical procedures and the care of sick and preterm infants. Platelet counts are within the usual adult normal ranges of 150,000 to 450,000/mm³ in healthy term and preterm infants. These platelets have a lower function than that of adults, but they function properly in hemostasis and produce a normal bleeding time.[47] Circulating coagulation factors do not cross the placenta, and infants with inherited deficiencies of clotting factors, fibrinolytic proteins, or natural anticoagulants may present in the neonatal period. Levels of fibrinogen, factor V, factor VIII, and von Willebrand's factor are within the adult normal range at birth.[48] All other procoagulants are at reduced levels, depending on gestational age. Vitamin K–dependent factors may become further depressed in infants who are breast-fed and not given vitamin K at birth.[47]

Of more concern are the low levels of anticoagulant and fibrinolytic proteins. Very low levels of protein C have been associated with purpura fulminans in newborns. In sick infants, levels of antithrombin III and plasminogen may be inadequate to deal with increased levels of clot-promoting activity in the blood. Sick infants with indwelling catheters are at significant risk of thrombotic complications and may endanger their renal circulation when umbilical venous lines are used.[49]

DISSEMINATED INTRAVASCULAR COAGULATION

Disseminated intravascular coagulation is the inappropriate activation of both thrombin and fibrin. It may follow sepsis, hypotension, hypoxemia, trauma, malignancy, burns, and extracorporeal circulation. Hemorrhage due to the depletion of clotting factors as well as thrombosis due to the excess formation of clot are seen, and it is the end-organ damage caused by ischemia and impairment of blood flow that causes irreversible disease and death.[29]

Acute DIC is associated with the consumption of factors II, V, VIII, X, and XIII as well as fibrinogen, antithrombin III, plasminogen, and platelets. Review of the peripheral smear usually shows a microangiopathic hemolytic anemia. The PT and PTT may both be prolonged, and the fibrinogen level may be initially elevated as an acute phase reactant but ultimately falls as the DIC worsens. In active DIC, the presence of soluble fibrin monomer complexes indicates the ongoing formation of new clot. The presence of D dimers indicates the circulation of plasmin digesting formed fibrin. Antithrombin III levels may be low, and recent work on the use of antithrombin III concentrates in septic shock indicates that they may play an important role in the future treatment of DIC. At present, the major therapy of DIC is correction of the underlying disorder, with fresh frozen plasma and platelet transfusions as indicated to support hemostasis. Low-dose heparin infusions have been used to stop the ongoing consumption of clotting factors prior to starting replacement therapy but have not been shown to appreciably improve the outcome.[29]

☐ Management of Quantitative and Qualitative Platelet Disorders

Thrombocytopenias are caused by either inadequate production of platelets by the bone marrow or increased destruction or sequestration of the platelets in the circulation. The destruction can be immunologic, as in immune thrombocytopenic purpura; mechanical, as in septicemia; or drug-induced, as in patients with sensitivity to heparin or cimetidine. Establishing the cause of the thrombocytopenia determines the therapy needed to restore the platelet count in preparing the patient for operation. The most important test is usually a bone marrow examination to establish the number of megakaryocytes and rule out a malignancy. This test can be followed by a transfusion of platelet concentrate, with 1- and 4-hour postinfusion platelet counts to determine if there is any response to the transfusion and, if there is, the rate of consumption of the platelets. In patients with immune-based platelet consumptions such as immune thrombocytopenic purpura, there is usually no response to platelet transfusion, and there may be only a very short response in patients with other causes of increased consumption. Management of the patient is then aimed at reducing the consumption and should involve consultation with a hematologist about the use of steroids, the use of

intravenous immunoglobulin, the discontinuation of medications, and other treatment modalities.[8, 50]

If the thrombocytopenia is caused by a lack of production of platelets, due to either aplastic anemia, malignancy, or chemotherapy, transfusion with platelet concentrate to raise the platelet count above a minimum of 50,000 cells/mm³ will allow minor surgery to be performed safely. Most surgeons and anesthesiologists prefer for the platelet count to be greater than 100,000 cells/mm³ before undertaking major surgery. Continued monitoring of platelet counts is vital, as further transfusions may be needed to keep the platelet count above 50,000 cells/mm³ for 3 to 5 days after operations.[50]

Qualitative platelet defects can be caused by rare congenital defects, such as Bernard-Soulier syndrome, Glanzmann's thrombasthenia, or platelet storage pool disease. Alternatively, they can be caused by drug ingestions such as an aspirin-induced cyclooxygenase deficiency. In these situations, transfusion of normal donor platelets provides adequate hemostasis for surgery. Discontinuation of all aspirin-containing products 1 week before surgery permits correction of the cyclooxygenase deficiency as new platelets are produced.[9, 25]

DISORDERS OF THROMBIN GENERATION AND FIBRIN FORMATION

Patients with rare deficiencies of other clotting factors, such as factors XI, X, VII, and V and prothrombin and fibrinogen, can have clinical bleeding, depending on the level of deficiency. Most of these disorders are inherited in an autosomal recessive manner and can therefore affect both males and females. Replacement therapy with fresh frozen plasma, or in certain situations with prothrombin complex concentrates, corrects the deficiency[35, 51] and should be conducted under the direction of a hematologist.

Vitamin K deficiency, both in the neonatal period and due to malabsorption, can cause deficiencies of factors II, VIII, IX, and X. Treatment with 1 to 2 mg of intravenous vitamin K may begin to correct the deficiencies within 4 to 6 hours, but if a surgical procedure is contemplated, fresh frozen plasma (15 ml/kg body weight) should be given with the vitamin K, and prothrombin times are monitored for correction of the coagulopathy prior to the operation. Laboratory monitoring should be maintained during the postoperative period to ensure continuation of the appropriate factor levels; repeat doses of fresh frozen plasma and vitamin K may be needed.[7]

Patients with factor XIII deficiency usually present with delayed bleeding from the umbilical cord, rebleeding from wounds that have stopped bleeding, and poor wound healing. These problems may be treated with relatively small amounts of fresh frozen plasma, namely 5 to 10 ml/kg. Because factor XIII has a half-life of 6 days, this treatment is usually needed only once to stop bleeding or at the time of surgery.[15, 35] Patients with dysfibrinogenemia or afibrinogenemia may be treated with fresh frozen plasma or cryoprecipitate. Because fibrinogen has a long half-life, repeated infusions are usually not required.[35]

FIBRINOLYTIC AND THROMBOTIC DISORDERS

Failure to properly control excess fibrinolysis can result in a bleeding disorder, and deficiencies of the naturally occurring anticoagulants may result in excess clot formations. A severe hemorrhagic disorder due to a deficiency of α-2-antiplasmin has responded to treatment with tranexamic acid, an antifibrinolytic agent.[24] Congenital antithrombin III, protein S, and protein C deficiencies are associated with recurrent thrombosis and are usually controlled with oral anticoagulants.[24] Operation requires discontinuation of the anticoagulation, and the patients will require replacement therapy during the procedure and the postoperative healing period until oral anticoagulants can be restarted. Depending on the deficiency, antithrombin III concentrate or fresh frozen plasma can be used for replacement therapy, which should be conducted under the guidance of a hematologist with ready access to a full coagulation laboratory.

□ Sickle Cell Disease

Sickle cell disease (SCD) is caused by a genetic mutation that results in the production of sickle hemoglobin (Hg S) instead of normal hemoglobin (Hg A). Hg S is a β-globin defect. The sickle cell gene in combination with any other abnormal β-globin gene results in SCD. Sickle cell anemia (Hg SS) is the most common and in general the most severe form of SCD. Sickle β⁰-thalassemia patients have clinical manifestations similar to those in patients with Hg SS disease. Sickle-C (Hg SC disease) is the second most common form of SCD and generally has a more benign clinical course than Hg SS disease. Sickle B⁺-thalassemia patients have clinical manifestations similar to those in patients with Hg SC disease. There are many other forms of SCD, among which the sickle–hereditary persistence of fetal hemoglobin (S/H) is the most common. Patients with Hg SS disease and sickle β⁰-thalassemia generally have lower hemoglobin levels and present a greater risk under general anesthesia than do patients with Hg SC disease and sickle β⁺ thalassemia. Patients with sickle–hereditary persistence of fetal hemoglobin may actually have normal hemoglobin levels.

The red cell membrane is abnormal in patients with SCD. The red cell lifespan is shortened by hemolysis. Intermittent episodes of vascular occlusion cause tissue ischemia, which results in acute and chronic organ dysfunction.[52] Patients with SCD require special considerations to prevent perioperative complications due to hemolysis and vasoocclusion.

Children with SCD require surgical evaluation and treatment due to either complications of their SCD or an unrelated process. The differential diagnosis for acute abdominal pain in a patient with SCD includes uncomplicated sickle cell pain episode ("crises"), cholelithiasis, appendicitis, pancreatitis, ulcer, and splenic sequestration. Previous episodes of similar pain point toward a sickle cell crisis. A study that reviewed the presentation and management of acute abdomen in adults with SCD suggested that a surgical condition is more likely if the pain does not resemble previous crises and there is no precipitating event.[53] Sickle crisis pain was relieved within 48 hours with hydration and oxygen in 97% of patients, whereas no patient with a surgical disease achieved pain relief over the same period with these modalities. Leukocyte count and serum bilirubin were not helpful in establishing the correct diagnosis.

Vasoocclusive episodes produce bone pain and fever, symptoms that are difficult to differentiate from osteomyelitis. The majority of bone pain in SCD is due to vasoocclusion, but osteomyelitis secondary to *Salmonella* species or *Staphylococcus aureus* is not infrequent.[54] The presence of an immature white blood cell count, elevation of sedimentation rate, C-reactive protein, or leukocyte alkaline phosphatase points toward a bone infection and may be an indication for aspiration of the bone lesion. Radiographic studies, including simple plain films, bone scan, or magnetic resonance imaging, are generally not helpful unless they are performed within 2 days of the onset of pain.

The patient with SCD may require an operation. The most common procedures according to one recent study were cholecystectomy; ear, nose, and throat procedures; orthopedic procedures; splenectomy; or herniorrhaphy.[55] Cholecystectomy, splenectomy, and orthopedic procedures are often required to treat complications of SCD.

PREOPERATIVE ASSESSMENT AND MANAGEMENT

The outcome of children with SCD requiring surgery is improved by careful attention to the cardiorespiratory, hemodynamic, hydration, infectious, and nutritional status of the child.[56, 57] It may be helpful to consult a pediatric hematologist who has expertise in the preparation of the patient for anesthesia and surgery.

If possible, the operation should be performed when the child is in his or her usual steady state in regard to the SCD. Particular attention should be directed toward any recent history of acute chest syndrome, pneumonia, wheezing, and alloimmunization. Special efforts must be made to avoid perioperative hypoxia, hypothermia, acidosis, and dehydration. Any of these events can result in serious complications.

The use of preoperative blood transfusions is somewhat controversial. Although most centers administer preoperative transfusions for sickle cell patients, there are no controlled trials documenting the benefit of these transfusions.[58] An aggressive transfusion regimen would involve decreasing Hg S to less than 30%, whereas a conservative transfusion regimen would simply increase the Hg level to 10 gm/dl. A national cooperative preoperative sickle cell transfusion study concluded that the conservative transfusion regimen was as effective as the aggressive regimen in preventing preoperative complications. The conservative approach reduced the risk of transfusion-associated complications by 55%.[55] The authors of this study and others have suggested that surgical procedures can be performed more safely in sickle cell patients if a multidisciplinary team is used.[59, 60]

INTRAOPERATIVE MANAGEMENT

Anesthestic considerations are based more on the type of surgical procedure planned than on the presence of SCD. Careful monitoring for hypoxia, hypothermia, acidosis, and dehydration is essential in any case. Monitoring should include arterial blood gases, digital oxygen saturation, end-tidal carbon dioxide, temperature, electrocardiogram, blood pressure, and urine output.[61]

POSTOPERATIVE MANAGEMENT

A critical phase of postoperative management occurs when the patient is moved to the recovery room and from there to the nursing ward. It is important to prevent hypothermia, hypoxia, and hypotension. Before extubation, the patient should be awake and oxygenating well. The extubated patient must be carefully monitored with a digital oxygen saturation monitor and the pulmonary status critically assessed before transfer to the floor. Continuous pulse oximetry should be provided in the early postoperative period. Assessment of fluid status should continue until the patient has resumed adequate oral intake and is able to maintain hydration without intravenous supplementation.

Appropriate levels of analgesic (preferably by a continuous intravenous line and patient-controlled analgesia, if appropriate) should be provided so the patient is comfortable enough to cooperate with ambulation and maintain pulmonary toilet without oversedation. Experienced respiratory therapists should administer a vigorous program for pulmonary toilet. The patient must be monitored closely for the occurrence of pulmonary edema or atelectasis that can progress to acute chest syndrome.[62]

☐ Specific Surgical Conditions

CHOLETHIASIS AND CHOLECYSTECTOMY

At present, there is no clear consensus regarding the appropriate therapy for SCD children who have cholelithiasis. The reported prevalence of cholelithiasis varies from 4 to 55%.[63, 64] The diagnosis is dependent on the age of the patient population and the diagnostic modalities used. The higher prevalence figures were obtained using ultrasonography. We routinely screen symptomatic children with ultrasonography and laboratory studies (e.g., total and direct bilirubin, serum glutamic-oxaloacetic transaminase, serum glutamate-pyruvate transaminase, alk phos and gamma-glutamyl-transpeptidase). It is our practice to screen all SCD children for gallstones no later than 12 years of age.

A child with SCD and cholelithiasis should undergo cholecystectomy after appropriate preoperative preparation to avoid the increased morbidity of an emergent operation on an unprepared patient.[65–68] Intraoperative cholangiography is recommended because of the high prevalence of common duct stones and the low sensitivity of preoperative ultrasonography.[69]

The utility of laparoscopic cholecystectomy in SCD was first reported in 1990.[70] Since that time, laparoscopic cholecystectomy has been performed with increasing frequency in children with SCD.[71, 72] The advantages of laparoscopic cholecystectomy over open cholecystectomy are decreased pain, earlier feeding, earlier discharge, earlier return to school, and improved cosmesis. The presence of common duct stones at times complicates the laparoscopic approach and may require conversion to an open operation for removal. At present, the role of extracorporeal shock wave lithotripsy as a palliative therapeutic modality is uncertain.

SPLENIC SEQUESTRATION AND SPLENECTOMY

Before the advent of routine newborn screening for hemoglobinopathies, acute splenic sequestration was the second-most common cause of mortality in children younger than 5 years with sickle cell anemia.[73] Splenic sequestration classically presented with the acute onset of pallor and listlessness, a precipitous fall in hemoglobin, thrombocytopenia, and massive splenomegaly.[74] It now appears that parental education along with earlier recognition and immediate treatment with volume support (including red blood cell transfusions) has resulted in significantly decreased mortality. It is rare for an uncomplicated patient with Hg SS disease who is older than 6 years to suffer an acute splenic sequestration; however, patients with Hg SC and sickle β+-thalassemia disease can experience splenic sequestration at an older age.[75]

The ultimate management of the sickle cell child with splenic sequestration is a clinical dilemma. Options include immediate splenectomy, observation with splenectomy after two acute episodes, or a prophylactic transfusion protocol to prevent splenic sequestration. The current trend is toward earlier splenectomy.[76, 77] The benefit of splenectomy must be balanced with the increased risk of overwhelming bacterial sepsis in the younger asplenic sickle cell patient.[78] Most recently, partial splenectomy[79, 80] and laparoscopic splenectomy[81] procedures are being explored.

OTHER SURGICAL CONDITIONS

Children with sickle cell disease may require various surgical procedures for which the same principles should be employed. As a consequence of their disease, school-aged and adolescent patients are at higher risk for other medical complications, such as priapism. If a patient with priapism is refractory to medical management, operative treatment may be required.[82]

REFERENCES

1. Thompson AR, Harker LA: Manual of Hemostasis and Thrombosis (3rd ed). Philadelphia, FA Davis, 1983.
2. Moncada S, Gryglewski R, Bunting S, Vane JR: An enzyme isolated from arteries transforms prostaglandin endoperoxides to an unstable substance that inhibits platelet aggregation. Nature 263:663, 1976.
3. Mackie IJ, Bull HA: Normal haemostasis and its regulation. Blood Rev 3:237, 1989.
4. Esmon CT: The regulation of natural anticoagulant pathways. Science 235:1348, 1987.
5. Stern D, Nawroth P, Handley D, et al: An endothelial cell dependent pathway of coagulation. Proc Natl Acad Sci U S A 82:2523, 1985.
6. Esmon CT: Blood coagulation. In Nathan DG, Orkin SA (eds): Nathan and Oski's Hematology of Infancy and Childhood (5th ed). Philadelphia, WB Saunders, 1998, p 1532.
7. Saito H: Normal hemostatic mechanisms. In Ratnoff OD, Forbes CD (eds): Disorders of Hemostasis (2nd ed). Philadelphia, WB Saunders, 1991, p 18.
8. Marcus AJ: Platelets and their disorders. In Ratnoff OD, Forbes CD (eds): Disorders of Hemostasis (2nd ed). Philadelphia, WB Saunders, 1991, p 57.
9. George JN, Nurden AT, Phillips DR: Molecular defects in interactions of platelets with the vessel wall. N Engl J Med 311:1084, 1984.
10. Turitto VT, Baumgartner HR: Platelet-surface interactions. In Coleman RW, Hirsh J, Marder VJ, Salzman EW (eds): Hemostasis and Thrombosis. Basic Principles and Clinical Practice (2nd ed). Philadelphia, JB Lippincott, 1987, p 555.
11. Nurden AT, Didry D, Rosa JP: Molecular defects of platelets in Bernard-Soulier syndrome. Blood Cells 9:333, 1983.
12. Tuddenham EGD: von Willebrand factor and its disorders: An overview of recent molecular studies. Blood Rev 3:251, 1989.
13. Sadler JE. Appendix II: A revised classification of von Willebrand disease. Haemophilia 3(suppl 2):11, 1997.
14. Colman RW, Walsh PN: Mechanisms of platelet aggregation. In Colman RW, Hirsh J, Marder VJ, Salzman EW (eds): Hemostasis and Thrombosis. Basic Principles and Clinical Practice (2nd ed). Philadelphia, JB Lippincott, 1987, p 594.
15. Lorand L, Losowsky MS, Miloszewski KJM: Human factor XIII: Fibrin-stabilizing factor. Prog Hemostasis Thromb 5:245, 1980.
16. Rosenberg RD, Rosenberg JS: Natural anticoagulant mechanisms. J Clin Invest 74:1, 1984.
17. Rappaport SI: Preoperative hemostatic evaluation: Which tests, if any? Blood 61:229, 1983.
18. Stockman JA III: Hematologic evaluations. In Raffensperger JG (ed): Swenson's Pediatric Surgery (5th ed). Norwalk, CT, Appleton & Lange, 1990, p 37.
19. Messmore HL, Godwin J: Medical assessment of bleeding in the surgical patient. Med Clin N Amer 78:627, 1994.
20. Rohrer MJ, Michelotti MC, Nahrwold DL: A prospective eval-

21. uation of the efficacy of preoperative coagulation testing. Ann Surg 208:554, 1988.
21. Zwack GC, Derkay CS: The utility of preoperative hemostatic assessment in adenotonsillectomy. Int J Pediatr Otorhinolaryngol 39:75, 1997.
22. Close HL, Kryzer TC, Nowlin JH, Alving BA: Hemostatic assessment of patients before tonsillectomy: A prospective study. Otolaryngol Head Neck Surg 111:737, 1994.
23. Sramek A, Eikenboom JCJ, Briet E, et al: Usefulness of patient interview in bleeding disorders. Arch Intern Med 155:1413, 1995.
24. Lusher JM: Approach to the bleeding patient. In Nathan DG, Orkin SA (eds): Nathan and Oski's Hematology of Infancy and Childhood (5th ed). Philadelphia, WB Saunders, 1998, p 1574.
25. George JN, Shattil SJ: The clinical importance of acquired abnormalities of platelet function. N Engl J Med 324:27, 1991.
26. Salzman EW: Hemostatic problems in surgical patients. In Coleman RW, Hirsh J, Marder VJ, Salzman EW (eds): Hemostasis and Thrombosis: Basic Principles and Clinical Practice (2nd ed). Philadelphia, JB Lippincott, 1987, p 920.
27. Harker LA, Slichter SJ: The bleeding time as a screening test for evaluation of platelet function. N Engl J Med 287:155, 1972.
28. Thiagarjan P, Shapiro SS: Lupus anticoagulants. Prog Hemost Thromb 5:198, 1982.
29. Bick RL: Disseminated intravascular coagulation and related syndromes: A clinical review. Semin Thromb Hemostasis 14:299, 1988.
30. Pool JG, Hershgold EJ, Pappenhagen AR: High potency antihaemophilic factor concentrate prepared from cryoglobulin precipitate. Nature 203:312, 1964.
31. Tullis JL, Melin M, Jurigian P: Clinical use of prothrombin complexes. N Engl J Med 273:667, 1965.
32. Johnson AJ, Newman J, Howell MB, Puszkin S: Purification of antihemophilic factor (AHF) for clinical and experimental use. Thromb Diath Haemorrh 26(suppl):377, 1967.
33. Scharrer I: The need for highly purified products to treat hemophilia B. Acta Haematol 94(suppl 1):2, 1995.
34. Levine PH: Delivery of health care in hemophilia. Ann N Y Acad Sci 240:201, 1975.
35. Hilgartner MW: Factor replacement therapy. In Hilgartner MW, Pochedly C (eds): Hemophilia in the Child and Adult (3rd ed). New York, Raven Press, 1989, p 1.
36. Centers for Disease Control: HIV/AIDS Surveillance Report. Atlanta, GA, May 8, 1991, p 1.
37. Levine PH: Clinical manifestations and therapy of hemophilias A and B. In Colman RW, Hirsh J, Marder VJ, Salzman EW (eds): Hemostasis and Thrombosis: Basic Principles and Clinical Practice (2nd ed). Philadelphia, JB Lippincott, 1987, p 97.
38. Kernoff PB, Lee CA, Karayiannis P, Thomas HC: High risk of non-A non-B hepatitis after a first exposure to volunteer or commercial clotting factor concentrates: Effects of prophylactic immune serum globulin. Br J Haematol 60:469, 1985.
39. Troisi CL, Hollinger FB, Hoots WK, et al: A multicenter study of viral hepatitis in a United States hemophilic population. Blood 81:412, 1993.
40. Lusher JM, Warrier I: Hemophilia. Pediatr Rev 12:275, 1991.
41. Kasper CK, Boylen AL, Ewing NP, et al: Hematologic management of hemophilia A for surgery. JAMA 253:1279, 1985.
42. Nilsson IM, Hedner U, Ahlberg A, et al: Surgery of hemophiliacs: 20 years' experience. World J Surg 1:55, 1977.
43. Hedner U, Bjoern S, Bernvil SS, et al: Clinical experience with human plasma-derived factor VIIa in patients with hemophilia A and higher titer inhibitors. Haemostasis 19:335, 1989.
44. Hathaway WE, Christian MJ, Clarke SL, Hasiba U: Comparison of continuous and intermittent factor VIII concentrate therapy in hemophilia A. Am J Hematol 17:85, 1984.
45. Kobrinsky NL, Stegman DA: Management of hemophilia during surgery. In Forbes CD, Aledort LM, Madhok R (eds): Hemophilia. Oxford, Chapman & Hall, 1997, p 242.
46. Shapiro AD, White GC II, Kim HC, et al: Efficacy and safety

of monoclonal antibody purified factor IX concentrate in haemophilia B patients undergoing surgical procedures. Haemophilia 3:248, 1997.

47. Andrew M: Developmental hemostasis: Relevance to newborns and infants. In Nathan DG, Orkin SA (eds): Nathan and Oski's Hematology of Infancy and Childhood (5th ed). Philadelphia, WB Saunders, 1998, p 115.

48. Andrew M, Paes B, Milner R, et al: Development of the human coagulation system in the full-term infant. Blood 70:165, 1987.

49. Gibson BES: Normal and disordered coagulation. In Hann IM, Gibson BES, Letsky EA (eds): Fetal and Neonatal Hematology. London, Baillière Tindall, 1991, p 123.

50. Jackson DP: Management of thrombocytopenia. In Colman RW, Hirsh J, Marder VJ, Salzman EW (eds): Hemostasis and Thrombosis. Basic Principles and Clinical Practice (2nd ed). Philadelphia, JB Lippincott, 1987, p 530.

51. Greenberg CS: Hemostasis: Pathophysiology and management of clinical disorders. In Sabiston DC Jr (ed): Sabiston's Essentials of Surgery. Philadelphia, WB Saunders, 1987, p 79.

52. Lane PA: Sickle cell disease. Pediatr Clin North Am 43:639, 1996.

53. Baumgartner F, Klein S: The presentation and management of the acute abdomen in the patient with sickle cell anemia. Amer Surgeon 55:660, 1989.

54. Epps CH, Bryant DD, Coles MJ, et al: Osteomyelitis in patients who have sickle cell disease. Diagnosis and management. J Bone Joint Surg 73:1281, 1991.

55. Vichinsky EP, Haberkern CM, Neumayr L, et al: A comparison of conservative and aggressive transfusion regimens in the perioperative management of sickle cell disease. N Engl J Med 333:206, 1995.

56. Ware RE, Filston HC: Surgical management of children with hemoglobinopathies. Surg Clin North Am 72:1223, 1992.

57. Sutton JP, Farrer JJ, Rodning CB: Surgical management of patients with sickle cell syndromes. In Mankad VN, Moore RB (eds): Sickle Cell Disease—Pathophysiology, Diagnosis, and Management. Westport, CT, Praeger Publishers, 1992, pp 364–386.

58. Griffin TC, Buchanan GR: Elective surgery in children with sickle cell disease without preoperative blood transfusion. J Pediatr Surg 28:681, 1993.

59. Wayne AS, Kevy SV, Nathan DG: Transfusion management of sickle cell disease. Blood 81:1109, 1993.

60. Koshy M, Weiner SJ, Miller ST, et al: Surgery and anesthesia in sickle cell disease. Blood 86:3676, 1995.

61. Mankad AV: Anesthetic management of patients with sickle cell disease. In Mankad VN, Moore RB (eds): Sickle Cell Disease—Pathophysiology, Diagnosis, and Management. Westport, CT, Praeger Publishers, 1992, pp 351–363.

62. Castro O, Brambilla DJ, Thorington B, et al: The acute chest syndrome in sickle cell disease: Incidence and risk factors. Blood 84:643, 1994.

63. Lachman BS, Lazerson J, Starshak RJ, et al: The prevalence of cholelithiasis in sickle cell disease as diagnosed by ultrasound and cholecystography. Pediatrics 64:601, 1979.

64. Sarnaik S, Slovis TL, Corbett DP, et al: Incidence of cholelithiasis in sickle cell anemia using the ultrasonic gray-scale technique. J Pediatr 96:1005, 1980.

65. Pappis CH, Galanakis S, Moussatos G, et al: Experience of splenectomy and cholecystectomy in children with chronic hemolytic anemia. J Pediatr Surg 24:543, 1989.

66. Stephens CG, Scott RB: Cholelithiasis in sickle cell anemia: Surgical or medical management. Arch Intern Med 140:648, 1980.

67. Ware R, Filston HC, Schultz WH, et al: Elective cholecystectomy in children with sickle hemoglobinopathies. Ann Surg 208:17, 1988.

68. Haberkern CM, Neumayr LD, et al: Cholecystectomy in sickle cell anemia patients: Perioperative outcome of 364 cases from the National Preoperative Transfusion Study. Blood 89:1533, 1997.

69. Ware RE, Schultz WH, Filston HC, et al: Diagnosis and management of common bile duct stones in patients with sickle hemoglobinopathies. J Pediatr Surg 27:572, 1992.

70. Dubois F, Icard P, Berthelot G, et al: Coelioscopic cholecystectomy: Preliminary report of 36 cases. Ann Surg 211:60, 1990.

71. Gadacz TR, Talamini MA, Lillemoe KD, et al: Laparoscopic cholecystectomy. Surg Clin North Am 70:1249, 1990.

72. Tagge EP, Othersen HB Jr, Jackson SM, et al: Impact of laparoscopic cholecystectomy on the management of cholelithiasis in children with sickle cell disease. J Pediatr Surg 29:209, 1994.

73. Gill FM, Sleeper LA, Weiner SJ, et al: Clinical events in the first decade in a cohort of infants with sickle cell disease. Blood 86:776, 1995.

74. Emond AM, Collis R, Darvill D, et al: Acute splenic sequestration in homozygous sickle cell disease: Natural history and management. J Pediatr 107:201, 1985.

75. Aquino VM, Norvell JM, Buchanan GR: Acute splenic complications in children with sickle cell–hemoglobin C disease. J Pediatr 130:961, 1997.

76. Al-Salem AH, Qaisaruddin S, Nasserallah Z, et al: Splenectomy in patients with sickle cell disease. Am J Surg 172:254, 1996.

77. Kinney TR, Ware RE, Schultz WH, et al: Long-term management of splenic sequestration in children with sickle cell disease. J Pediatr 117:194, 1990.

78. Pegelow CH, Wilson B, Overturf GD, et al: Infection in splenectomized sickle cell patients. Clin Pediatr 19:102, 1980.

79. Svarch E, Vilorio P, Nordet I, et al: Partial splenectomy in children with sickle cell disease and repeated episodes of splenic sequestration. Hemoglobin 20:393, 1996.

80. Nouri A, de Montalembert M, Revillon Y, et al: Partial splenectomy in sickle cell syndromes. Arch Dis Child 66:1070, 1991.

81. Hicks BA, Thompson WE, Rogers ZR, et al: Laparoscopic splenectomy in childhood hematologic disorders. J Laparoendosc Surg 6:531, 1996.

82. Miller ST, Rao SP, Dunn EK, et al: Priapism in children with sickle cell disease. J Urol 154:844, 1995.

6

MECHANICAL VENTILATION IN PEDIATRIC SURGICAL DISEASE

Ronald B. Hirschl, MD

□ History

Amazingly, ventilation via tracheal cannulation was performed as early as 1543 when Vesalius demonstrated the ability to maintain the beating heart in animals with open chests.[1] Such techniques were first applied to human beings in 1780, but little progress in the development of positive pressure ventilation was achieved until the Fell-O'Dwyer apparatus, which provided translaryngeal ventilation via a bellows, was used in 1887 in both adults and children.[2, 3] The Drinker-Shaw iron lung, which allowed piston pump cyclic ventilation of a metal cylinder and associated negative pressure ventilation, became available in 1928 and was followed by a simplified design built by Emerson in 1931.[4] Such ventilators were the mainstays in the ventilation of victims of polio epidemics that occurred in the 1930s through 1950s.

In 1928, the technique of tracheal intubation was refined by Magill and Rowbotham, and in World War II, the Bennett valve, which allowed cyclic application of high pressure, was devised to allow pilots to tolerate high altitude bombing missions.[5–7] Subsequently, the use of translaryngeal intubation and mechanical ventilation became commonplace both in the operating room as well as in the treatment of respiratory insufficiency. However, application of mechanical ventilation to newborns both in the operating room as well as in the intensive care unit lagged behind their pediatric and adult counterparts. Stahlman and colleagues described the use of positive pressure mechanical ventilation in the management of the respiratory distress syndrome (RDS) in 1962.[8] However, it was the death in 1963 of President John F. Kennedy's son, Patrick Bouvier Kennedy, at 32 weeks' gestation that resulted in additional National Institutes of Health (NIH) funding for research in the management of newborns with respiratory failure.[9] The discovery of surfactant deficiency as the etiology of RDS in 1959, documentation of the ability to provide positive pressure ventilation in newborns with respiratory insufficiency in 1965, and demonstration of the effectiveness of continuous positive airway pressure (CPAP) in enhancing lung volume and ventilation in patients with RDS in 1971 set the stage in the 1970s for the development of continuous flow ventilators specifically designed for neonates.[10–12] The development of neonatal intensive care units, hyperalimentation, and neonatal invasive and noninvasive monitoring enhanced the care of newborns with respiratory failure and increased survival in preterm newborns from 50% in the early 1970s to over 90% currently.[13]

□ Gas Exchange During Mechanical Ventilation

The approach to mechanical ventilation is best understood if the two variables—oxygenation and carbon dioxide elimination—are considered separately.[14]

CARBON DIOXIDE ELIMINATION

The primary purpose of ventilation is to eliminate CO_2. This is accomplished by delivering tidal volume (V_T) breaths at a designated rate. The product, $V_T \times$ rate, determines the minute volume ventilation (V_E). Although CO_2 elimination is proportional to V_E, it is, in fact, directly related to the volume of gas ventilating the alveoli. This is because part of the V_E resides in the conducting airways or in nonperfused alveoli (Fig. 6–1). As such, this portion of the ventilation does not participate in CO_2 exchange and is termed the *dead space* (V_{DS}).[15] In the patient with healthy lungs, this dead space is fixed or "anatomic" and consists of about one third of the tidal volume ($V_{DS}/V_R = 0.33$). This fixed anatomic dead space can unwittingly be increased through the presence of extensions of the trachea such as the

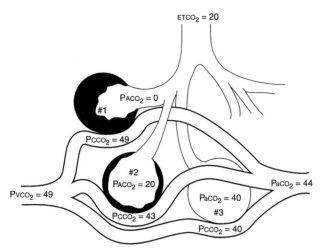

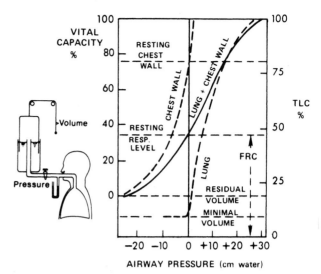

Figure 6–1. Pulmonary deadspace (VD) and ventilation/perfusion matching (V̇/Q̇). VD is a function of the conducting airways, the number of nonperfused alveoli, and the volume of the ventilator tubing beyond the "Y." V̇/Q̇ is demonstrated as regions with normal V̇/Q̇ (#3) and low V̇/Q̇ (minimal/no ventilation, reasonable perfusion, #1). (From Hirschl RB, Heiss K: Cardiopulmonary critical care and shock. In Oldham KT, Colombani PM, Foglia RP [eds]: Surgery of Infants and Children: Scientific Principles and Practice. Philadelphia, Lippincott-Raven, 1997, p 158.)

Figure 6–2. Pulmonary function as a function of chest wall and lung compliance in healthy patients. At functional residual capacity (FRC), the tendency for the chest wall to expand and the lung to collapse balance. (From West JB: Respiratory Physiology—The Essentials [4th ed]. Baltimore, Williams & Wilkins, 1985, p 100.) (Modified from Rahn H, et al: Am J Physiol 146:161, 1946.)

endotracheal tube, a pneumotachometer to measure tidal volume, an end tidal carbon dioxide monitor, or an extension of the ventilator tubing beyond the "Y." It is critical, therefore, that endotracheal tubes be shortened as much as is reasonable and that other safeguards be applied to ensure that the anatomic VDS is minimized in the mechanically ventilated patient. In the setting of respiratory insufficiency, the proportion of dead space (VDS/VT) may be augmented by the presence of nonperfused alveoli and a reduction in tidal volume.

The tidal volume is a function of the applied ventilator pressure and the volume-pressure relationship (compliance) that describes the distensibility of the lung and chest. At the functional residual capacity (FRC), which is the static point of end-

expiration, the tendency for the lung to collapse (elastic recoil) is in balance with the forces that promote chest wall expansion[15] (Fig. 6–2). As each breath develops, however, the elastic recoil of both the lung and chest wall work in concert to oppose lung inflation. Pulmonary compliance, then, is a function of both the lung elastic recoil (lung compliance) and the distensibility of the rib cage and diaphragm (chest wall compliance).

The compliance can be determined in a dynamic or static mode. The lung, at an inflating pressure of 30 cm H_2O when compared to ambient (transpulmonary) pressure, is considered to be at total lung capacity (TLC) (Fig. 6–3) (Table 6–1). Note that the loop observed during both inspiration and expiration is curvilinear (Fig. 6–4). This is due to the

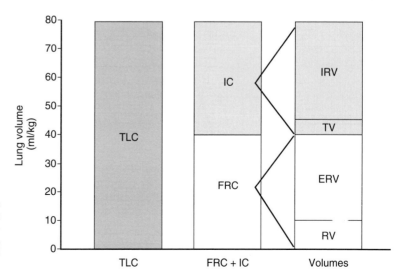

Figure 6–3. Demonstration of the various volumes and capacities of the lung. ERV, expiratory reserve volume; FRC, functional residual capacity; IC, inspiratory capacity; IRV, inspiratory reserve volume; RV, residual volume; TLC, total lung capacity; TV, tidal volume.

TABLE 6-1. Definitions and Normal Values
for Respiratory Physiologic Parameters

Variable	Definition	Normal Value
TLC	Total lung capacity	80 ml/kg
FRC	Functional residual capacity	40 ml/kg
IC	Inspiratory capacity	40 ml/kg
ERV	Expiratory reserve volume	30 ml/kg
RV	Residual volume	10 ml/kg
Tv	Tidal volume	5 ml/kg
V_E	Minute volume ventilation	100 ml/kg/min
V_A	Alveolar ventilation	60 ml/kg/h
V_D	Deadspace	ml = wt in lbs
V_{DS}/V_T	Percentage deadspace	0.33
C_{ST}	Static compliance	2 ml/cm H_2O/kg
C_{EFF}	Effective compliance	1 ml/cm H_2O/kg

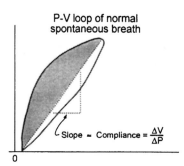

Figure 6–4. Dynamic pressure/volume relationship and effective pulmonary compliance (C_{eff}) in the normal lung. The volume at 30 cm H_2O is considered total lung capacity (TLC). C_{eff} is calculated by V/P. (From Bhutani VK, Sivieri EM: Physiological principles for bedside assessment of pulmonary graphics. In Donn SM [ed]: Neonatal and Pediatric Pulmonary Graphics: Principles and Applications. Futura Publishing, Armonk, NY, 1998, p 70.)

resistance that is present in the airways and describes the work required to overcome airflow resistance. As a result, at any given point of active flow, the measured pressure in the airways is higher during inspiration and lower during expiration than at the same volume under zero flow conditions. Therefore, pulmonary compliance measurements, as well as alveolar pressure measurements, can be effectively performed only when there is no flow in the airways (zero flow) (i.e., at FRC and TLC). A line drawn between the two points describes the "effective" compliance. It is termed *effective compliance* because this analysis only provides assessment of compliance between the two arbitrary points of end-inspiration and end-expiration. The volume-pressure relationship is not linear over the range of most inflating pressures when a static compliance curve is developed. Such static compliance assessments are most commonly performed via a large syringe in which aliquots of 1 to 2 ml/kg of oxygen, up to a total of 15 to 20 ml/kg, are instilled sequentially with 3 to 5 second pauses between each. At the end of each pause, zero flow pressures

are measured. By graphing the data, a static compliance curve may be generated, which demonstrates how the calculated compliance can change depending on the arbitrary points used for assessment of the effective compliance[16] (Fig. 6–5). The compliance changes as the FRC or end-expiratory lung volume (EELV) increases or decreases. For instance, at low FRC, atelectasis is present and a given ΔP will not optimally inflate alveoli. Likewise, at a high FRC, due to air trapping or application of high PEEP, the lung is already distended and application of the same ΔP will only result in overdistention and potential lung injury with little benefit in terms of added tidal volume. Optimal compliance is provided, then, when the pressure-volume range is on the linear portion of the static compliance curve. Clinically, the compliance at a variety of FRC or PEEP values can be monitored to establish optimal FRC.[17]

Typical ventilator rate requirements in patients with healthy lungs range from 10 breaths per minute in an adult to 30 breaths per minute in a newborn.

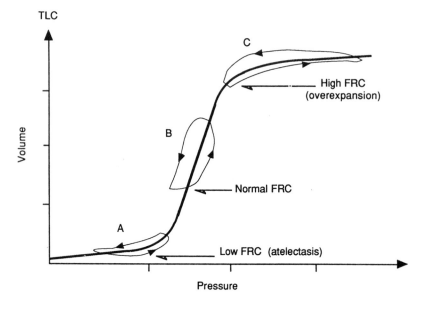

Figure 6–5. Static lung compliance curve in a normal lung. Effective compliance would be altered depending on whether FRC were to be at a level resulting in lung atelectasis (A) or overdistention (C). Optimal lung mechanics are observed when FRC is set on the steepest portion of the curve (B). FRC, functional residual capacity; TLC, total lung capacity. (From Harris TR: Physiological principles. In Goldsmith JP, Karotkin EH [eds]: Assisted Ventilation of the Newborn. WB Saunders, Philadelphia, 1998, p 34.)

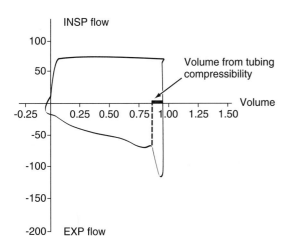

Figure 6–6. Flow-volume loops demonstrating the effect of ventilator tubing gas compression volume in the ventilator tubing of a patient with respiratory insufficiency. The high flow during expiration results from gas decompressing from the ventilator tubing. (Adapted from Pilbeam SP: Mechanical Ventilation: Physiological and Clinical Applications [3rd ed.]. St. Louis, MO, CV Mosby, 1998, p 50.)

Tidal volume is maintained at 5 to 10 ml/kg. This affords a minute volume ventilation of up to 100 ml/kg/min in adolescents and 150 ml/kg/min in newborns. These settings should provide sufficient ventilation to maintain normal $PaCO_2$ levels of approximately 40 mm Hg and should generate peak inspiratory pressures (PIPs) of between 15 and 20 cm H_2O above an applied PEEP of 5 cm H_2O. Clinical assessment by observing chest wall movement, auscultation, and evaluation of gas exchange determine the appropriate tidal volume.

It is important to recognize that a portion of the tidal volume generated by the ventilator is actually compression of gas within both the ventilator tubing and the airways (Fig. 6–6). The ratio of gas compressed in the ventilator tubing to that entering the lungs is a function of the compliance of the ventilator tubing and the lung. The compliance of the ventilator tubing is 0.3 to 4.5 ml/cm H_2O.[18] A ΔP of 15 cm H_2O in a 3 kg newborn with respiratory insufficiency and a pulmonary compliance of 0.4 ml/cm H_2O/kg would result in a lung tidal volume of 18 ml and an impressive ventilator tubing gas compression volume of 15 ml if the tubing compliance equals 1.0 ml/cm H_2O. The relative ventilator tubing gas compression volume would not be as striking in an adult. The ventilator tubing compliance is characterized for all current ventilators and should be accounted for when considering tidal volume data. The software in many ventilators now corrects for ventilator tubing compliance when displaying tidal volume values.

OXYGENATION

In contrast to CO_2, oxygenation is determined by the fraction of inspired oxygen (FiO_2) and the degree of lung distention or alveolar recruitment, which is determined by the level of PEEP and the mean airway pressure (Paw) during each ventilator cycle. In fact, were CO_2 not to be a competing gas at the alveolar level, oxygen absorbed by pulmonary capillary blood would simply be replaced by that provided at the airway as long as alveolar distention were maintained. Such apneic oxygenation has been used in conjunction with extracorporeal carbon dioxide removal ($ECCO_2R$), in which oxygen is delivered at the carina while lung distention is maintained via application of PEEP.[19] Under normal circumstances, however, alveolar ventilation serves to remove CO_2 from the alveolus and to replenish the partial pressure of oxygen, thereby maintaining the alveolar–pulmonary capillary blood oxygen gradient.

Rather than depending on the degree of alveolar ventilation, oxygenation predominantly is a function of the appropriate matching of pulmonary blood flow to inflated alveoli (ventilation/perfusion matching, $\dot{V}/\dot{Q}$).[15] Areas of ventilation but no perfusion (high $\dot{V}/\dot{Q}$), such as in the setting of pulmonary embolus, do not contribute to oxygenation. Hypoxemia supervenes in this situation once the average residence time of blood in the remaining perfused pulmonary capillaries exceeds that necessary for complete oxygenation: normal residence time is threefold that required for full oxygenation of pulmonary capillary blood. The common pathophysiology observed in the setting of respiratory insufficiency is that of minimal or no ventilation with persistent perfusion (low $\dot{V}/\dot{Q}$) resulting in right-to-left shunt and hypoxemia. Patients with the acute respiratory distress syndrome (ARDS) have collapse of the posterior, or dependent, regions of the lungs when supine (Fig. 6–7).[20, 21] As the majority of blood flow is distributed to these dependent regions, one can easily imagine the limited oxygen transfer, large shunt, ventilation/perfusion mismatch, and resulting hypoxemia that occurs in patients with ARDS. Attempts to inflate the alveoli in these regions, with interventions such as application of PEEP, can reduce $\dot{V}/\dot{Q}$ mismatch and enhance oxygenation.

In normal lungs, the PEEP should be maintained at 5 cm H_2O, an expiratory pressure that allows maintenance of alveolar inflation at end-expiration. An FiO_2 equal to 0.50 should be administered initially. However, one should be able to wean the FiO_2 rapidly in the patient with healthy lungs and normal $\dot{V}/\dot{Q}$ matching. The arterial oxygen (PaO_2) and arterial oxygen saturation (SaO_2) levels are measured most frequently to evaluate oxygenation. Lung oxygenation capabilities are frequently assessed as a function of the difference between the ideal alveolar and the measured systemic arterial oxygen levels $[(A - a)DO_2 = (FiO_2 \times (P_B - P_{H_2O}) - PaCO_2 \times RQ) - PaO_2]$, the ratio of the PaO_2 to the FiO_2 (P/F ratio), the physiologic shunt ($Qps/Qt = \dfrac{CiO_2 - CaO_2}{CiO_2 - CvO_2}$), and the oxygen index ($OI = \dfrac{Paw \times FiO_2 \times 100}{PaO_2}$) where

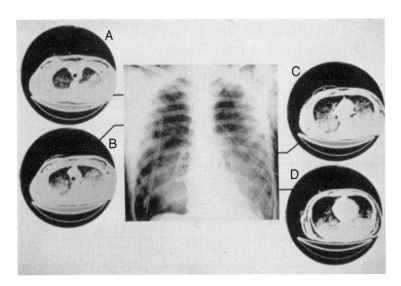

Figure 6–7. Cross-sectional image of the lungs at various levels in a patient with acute respiratory distress syndrome. Note the diffuse infiltrates on chest radiograph but the regional posterior, dependent atelectasis on computed tomography. The anterior, or nondependent, regions are well inflated. (From Maunder RJ, Shuman WP, McHugh JW, et al: Preservation of normal lung regions in the adult respiratory distress syndrome. Analysis by computed tomography. JAMA 255:2463–2465, 1986.)

P_B is barometric pressure, P_{H_2O} is partial pressure of water, RQ is the respiratory quotient or the ratio of the oxygen consumption ($\dot{V}O_2$) and the CO_2 production ($\dot{V}CO_2$), and $CvO_2/CaO_2/CiO_2$ are the oxygen content of venous, arterial, and expected pulmonary capillary blood, respectively.[15]

The overall therapeutic goal of optimizing parameters of oxygenation is to maintain oxygen delivery (DO_2) to the tissues. Three variables ascertain oxygen delivery: cardiac output (Q), hemoglobin concentration (Hgb), and arterial blood oxygen saturation (SaO_2). The product of these three variables determines oxygen delivery by the relationship:

$$DO_2 = Q \times CaO_2 \text{ where } CaO_2 = \\ [(1.36 \times Hgb \times SaO_2) + (0.003 \times PaO_2)]$$

Note that the contribution of the PaO_2 to oxygen delivery is minimal and, therefore, may be disregarded in most circumstances. If the hemoglobin concentration of the blood is normal (15 g/dl) and the hemoglobin is fully saturated with oxygen, the amount of oxygen bound to hemoglobin is 20.4 ml/dl (Fig. 6–8). In addition, approximately 0.3 ml of oxygen is physically dissolved in each deciliter of plasma, which makes the oxygen content of normal arterial blood equal to approximately 20.7 ml O_2/dl. Similar calculations reveal that the normal venous blood oxygen content is approximately 15 mlO_2/dl.

Typically oxygen delivery is four to five times greater than oxygen consumption. As DO_2 increases or oxygen consumption ($\dot{V}O_2$) decreases, more oxygen remains in the venous blood. The result is an increase in the oxygen hemoglobin saturation in the mixed venous pulmonary artery blood (SvO_2). In contrast, if the DO_2 decreases or $\dot{V}O_2$ increases, relatively more oxygen is extracted from the blood and, therefore, less oxygen remains in the venous blood. A decrease in SvO_2 is the result. In general, the SvO_2 serves as an excellent monitor of oxygen kinetics because it specifically assesses the adequacy of oxygen delivery in relation to oxygen consumption

($DO_2/\dot{V}O_2$ ratio) (Fig. 6–9).[22] Many pulmonary arterial catheters now contain fiberoptic bundles, which provide continuous mixed venous oximetry data. Such monitoring provides a means for assessing the adequacy of oxygen delivery, rapid assessment of the response to interventions such as mechanical ventilation, and cost savings due to a diminished need for sequential blood gas monitoring.[22, 23]

Four factors are manipulated in an attempt to improve the $DO_2/\dot{V}O_2$ ratio: cardiac output, hemoglobin concentration, SaO_2, and $\dot{V}O_2$. The result of various interventions designed to increase cardiac output such as volume administration, infusion of inotropic agents, administration of afterload-reducing drugs, and correction of acid-base abnormalities may be assessed by the effect on the SvO_2 (Fig. 6–10). One of the most efficient ways to enhance oxygen delivery is to increase the oxygen carrying capacity of the blood. For instance, an increase in hemoglobin from 7.5 to 15 g/dl will be associated with a twofold increase in oxygen delivery at constant cardiac output. However, blood viscosity is

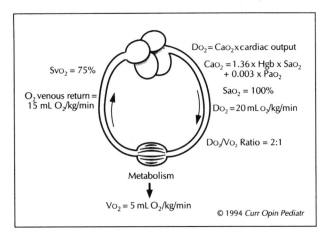

Figure 6–8. Oxygen consumption ($\dot{V}O_2$) and delivery (DO_2) relationships. (Adapted from Hirschl RB: Oxygen delivery in the pediatric surgical patient. Curr Opin Pediatr 6:341–347, 1994.)

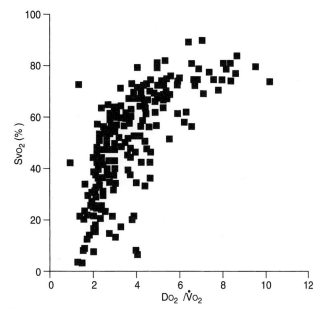

Figure 6–9. The relationship of the mixed venous oxygen saturation (SvO_2) and the ratio of oxygen delivery to oxygen consumption (DO_2/VO_2) in normal eumetabolic, hypermetabolic septic, and hypermetabolic exercising canines. (From Hirschl RB, Heiss K: Cardiopulmonary critical care and shock. In Oldham KT, Colombani PM, Foglia RP [eds]: Surgery of Infants and Children: Scientific Principles and Practice. Philadelphia, Lippincott-Raven, 1997, p 154.)

increased with blood transfusion, which may result in a reduction in cardiac output.[24]

The SaO_2 can often be enhanced through application of supplemental oxygen and mechanical ventilation. The use of PEEP and mechanical ventilation are, however, limited by the adverse effects observed on cardiac output, the incidence of barotrauma, and the risk for ventilator-induced lung injury with application of peak inspiratory pressures higher than 30 to 40 cm H_2O.[25, 26] Assessment of the "best PEEP" identifies the level at which oxygen delivery and SvO_2 are optimal.[27] Evaluation of the best PEEP should be performed in any patient requiring an FiO_2 >0.60 and may be determined by

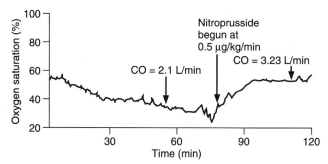

Figure 6–10. Alterations in mixed venous blood oxygen saturation are shown as sodium nitroprusside is administered to reduce left ventricular afterload in the setting of cardiac insufficiency. (From Hirschl RB, Heiss K: Cardiopulmonary critical care and shock. In Oldham KT, Colombani PM, Foglia RP [eds]: Surgery of Infants and Children: Scientific Principles and Practice. Philadelphia, Lippincott-Raven, 1997, p 177.)

continuous monitoring of the SvO_2 as the PEEP is sequentially increased from 5 to 15 cm H_2O over a short period of time. The point at which the SvO_2 is maximal indicates the PEEP at which oxygen delivery is optimal.

Oxygen consumption may be elevated due to sepsis, burns, agitation, seizures, hyperthermia, hyperthyroidism, and increased catecholamine production or infusion. A number of interventions may be applied to reduce oxygen consumption such as sedation and mechanical ventilation. Paralysis may enhance the effectiveness of mechanical ventilation while simultaneously reducing oxygen consumption.[28, 29] In the appropriate setting, hypothermia may be induced with an associated reduction of 7% in VO_2 with each 1°C decrease in core temperature.[30]

☐ The Mechanical Ventilator

The ventilator must overcome the pressure generated by the elastic recoil of the lung at end-inspiration plus the resistance to flow at the airway. To do so, most current ventilators in the intensive care unit are pneumatically powered via gas pressurized at 50 psi. Microprocessor controls allow accurate management of proportional solenoid-driven valves, which carefully control infusion of a blend of air or oxygen into the ventilator circuit while simultaneously opening and closing an expiratory valve.[31] Additional components of a ventilator include a bacterial filter, a pneumotachometer, a humidifier, a heater and thermostat, an oxygen analyzer, and a pressure manometer. A chamber for nebulizing drugs is usually incorporated into the inspiratory circuit. Tidal volume is not usually measured directly. Rather, flow is assessed as a function of time, thereby allowing calculation of tidal volume.

The modes of ventilation are characterized by three variables: the parameter used to initiate or "trigger" a breath, the parameter used to "limit" the size of the breath, and the parameter used to terminate inspiration or "cycle" the breath (Fig. 6–11).[32] Gas flow in most ventilators is triggered either by time (controlled breath) or by patient effort (assisted breath). Controlled ventilation modes are time triggered: the inspiratory phase is concluded once a desired volume, pressure, or flow is attained, and the expiratory time (ET) forms the difference between the inspiratory time (IT) and the preset respiratory cycle time. In the assist mode, the ventilator is pressure- or flow-triggered: with the former, a pressure generated by the patient of approximately −1 cm H_2O triggers the initiation of a breath. The sensitivity of the triggering device can be adjusted so that patient work is minimized. Other ventilators detect the reduction in constant ventilator tubing gas flow that is associated with patient initiation of a breath. Detection of this decrease in flow results in initiation of a positive pressure breath.

The magnitude of the breath is controlled or lim-

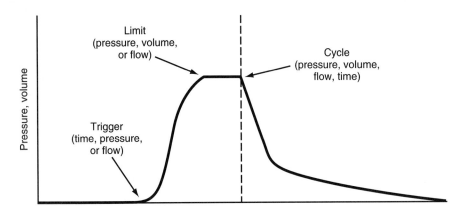

Figure 6–11. Variables that characterize the mode of mechanical ventilation.

ited by one of three variables: volume, pressure, or flow. When a breath is volume, pressure, or flow "controlled," it indicates that inspiration concludes once the limiting variable is reached. In contrast, a factor that "limits" inspiration suggests that the chosen value limits the level of the variable during inspiration, but the inspiratory phase does not conclude once this value is attained. For instance, during pressure-limited ventilation, gas flow continues until a given pressure limit is attained. However, the inspiratory phase does not necessarily conclude at that point. In contrast, during pressure-controlled ventilation both gas flow and the inspiratory phase terminate once the preset pressure is reached.

Pressure-controlled or pressure-limited modes are currently the most popular for all age groups, although volume-controlled ventilation may be of advantage in preterm newborns.[33] In this mode, the respiratory rate, the inspiratory gas flow, the PEEP level, the It:Et ratio, and the peak airway pressure (PIP) are determined. The ventilator infuses gas until the desired PIP is provided. Zero flow conditions are realized at end-inspiration during pressure-limited ventilation. Therefore, in this mode, PIP is frequently equivalent to end-inspiratory pressure (EIP) or plateau pressure. In many ventilators, the gas flow rate is fixed, although newer ventilators allow manipulation of the flow rate and, therefore, the rate of positive pressure development. Those with rapid flow rates provide rapid ascent of pressure to the preset maximum where it remains for the duration of the inspiratory phase. This square wave pressure pattern results in decelerating flow during inspiration. Airway pressure is "front loaded," which increases Paw, alveolar volume, and oxygenation without increasing PIP.[34] However, one of the biggest advantages of pressure-controlled or pressure-limited ventilation is the ability to avoid lung overdistention and barotrauma or volutrauma (discussed later). The disadvantage of pressure-controlled or pressure-limited ventilation is that delivered volume varies with airway resistance and pulmonary compliance and may be reduced when short inspiratory times are applied.[35] For this reason, tidal volume and minute volume ventilation both must be monitored carefully.

Volume-controlled or volume-limited ventilation requires delineation of the tidal volume, respiratory rate, and inspiratory gas flow. Gas is inspired until the preset tidal volume is attained. The volume remains constant despite changes in pulmonary mechanics, although the resulting EIP and PIP may be altered. Flow-controlled or flow-limited ventilation is similar in many respects to volume-controlled or volume-limited ventilation. A flow pattern is predetermined, which effectively results in a fixed volume as the limiting component of inspiration.

The ventilator breath is concluded based on one of four variables: pressure, flow, volume, or time. With volume-cycled ventilation, inspiration is terminated when a prescribed volume is obtained. Likewise, with time-cycled, pressure-cycled, or flow-cycled ventilation, expiration begins once a certain time period has passed, the airway pressure reaches a certain value, or the flow has decreased to a predetermined level respectively.

☐ Modes of Mechanical Ventilation

CONTROLLED MECHANICAL VENTILATION

Controlled mechanical ventilation (CMV) is time triggered, flow limited, and volume or pressure cycled. Spontaneous breaths may be taken between the mandatory breaths. However, there is no additional gas provided during spontaneous breaths. Therefore, the work of breathing is markedly increased in the spontaneously breathing patient. This mode of ventilation is no longer used.

INTERMITTENT MANDATORY VENTILATION

Intermittent mandatory ventilation (IMV) is time triggered; volume or pressure limited; and time, volume, or pressure cycled. A rate is set, as is a volume or pressure parameter. Additional inspired gas is provided by the ventilator to support spontaneous breathing when additional breaths are desired. This constitutes the difference between CMV and IMV: in the latter, inspired gases are provided to the patient during spontaneous breaths.[36] IMV is useful in patients who do not have respiratory drive, for example, those who are neurologically impaired or pharmacologically paralyzed. Work of breathing is still elevated in this mode in the awake and spontaneously breathing patient.

SYNCHRONIZED INTERMITTENT MANDATORY VENTILATION

In the synchronized intermittent mandatory ventilation (SIMV) mode, the ventilator synchronizes IMV breaths with the patient's spontaneous breaths. Small, patient-initiated negative deflections in airway pressure (pressure-triggered) or decreases in the constant ventilator gas flow (bias flow) passing through the exhalation valve (flow-triggered) provide a signal to the ventilator that a patient breath has been initiated. Ventilated breaths are timed with the patient's spontaneous respiration, but the number of supported breaths each minute is predetermined and remains constant. Additional constant inspired gas flow is provided for use during any other spontaneous breaths. Recent advances in neonatal ventilators have provided the means for detecting small alterations in bias flow. As such, flow-triggered SIMV may now be applied to newborns; it appears to enhance ventilatory patterns and allows ventilation with reduced airway pressures and FiO_2.[37, 38] SIMV may be associated with a reduction in duration of ventilation and incidence of bronchopulmonary dysplasia (BPD) and intraventricular hemorrhage in preterm neonates.[39]

ASSIST CONTROL VENTILATION

In the spontaneously breathing patient, brainstem reflexes dependent on cerebral spinal fluid levels of CO_2 and pH can be harnessed to determine the appropriate breathing rate.[15] As in SIMV, the assisted breaths can be either pressure triggered or flow triggered. The triggering mechanism sensitivity can be set in most ventilators. In contrast to SIMV, the ventilator supports all patient-initiated breaths. This mode is similar to IMV but allows the patient to inherently control his or her ventilation needs and minimizes work of breathing in adults and neonates.[40, 41] Occasionally, patients may hyperventilate, such as when they are agitated or have neurologic injury. Heavy sedation may be required if agitation is present. A minimum ventilator rate below the patient's assist rate should be established in case of apnea.

PRESSURE SUPPORT VENTILATION

Pressure support ventilation (PSV) is a pressure- or flow-triggered, pressure-limited, and flow-cycled mode of ventilation. It is similar in concept to assist control in that mechanical support is provided for each spontaneous breath and the patient determines ventilator rate. During each breath, inspiratory flow is applied until a predetermined pressure is attained.[42] As the end of inspiration approaches, flow

decreases to a level below a specified value (2 to 6 l/min) or a percentage of peak inspiratory flow (≤25%). At this point, inspiration terminates. Although it may apply full support, PSV is frequently used to partially support the patient by assigning a pressure limit for each breath that is less than that required for full support.[43] For example, in the spontaneously breathing patient, PSV can be sequentially decreased from full support to a PSV 5 to 10 cm H_2O above PEEP.[44, 45] This allows weaning while providing partial support with each breath. Therefore, during PSV, tidal volume may be dependent on patient effort. PSV provides two advantages during ventilation of spontaneously breathing patients: (1) it provides excellent support and decreases the work of breathing associated with ventilation and (2) lower PIP and Paw and higher VT and cardiac output levels may be observed.[42, 46, 47]

Pressure-triggered SIMV and PSV may now be applied to newborns using the VIP ventilator (VIP Products Corp., Palm Springs, California). Inspiration is terminated when the peak airway flow drops to a set percentage of between 5 and 25%. This flow cutoff for inspiration is known as the *termination sensitivity*, which may be adjusted: the higher the termination sensitivity value, the shorter the inspiratory time. The termination sensitivity function may also be disabled, at which point ventilation is time-cycled instead of flow-cycled. Studies have demonstrated a reduction in work of breathing and sedation requirements when SIMV with pressure support is applied to newborns.

VOLUME ASSURED PRESSURE SUPPORT VENTILATION

Volume assured pressure support ventilation (VAPSV) modes attempt to combine volume- and pressure-controlled ventilation in order to ensure a desired tidal volume within the constraints of the pressure limit set. This mode has the advantage of maintaining inflation to a point below an injurious PIP level while maintaining tidal volume constant in the face of changing pulmonary mechanics. Work of breathing may be markedly decreased and effective compliance increased during VAPSV.[48]

PROPORTIONAL ASSIST VENTILATION

Proportional assist ventilation (PAV) is an intriguing approach to the support of the spontaneously breathing patient. It relies on the concept that the combined pressure generated by the ventilator (Paw) and respiratory muscles (Pmus) is equivalent to that required to overcome the resistance to flow of the endotracheal tube or airways (Pres) and the tendency for the inflated lungs to collapse (elastic recoil or elastance $= \dfrac{1}{\text{compliance}}$, Pel):

$$Paw + Pmus = Pel + Pres$$

Elastance and resistance can be assessed in patients during periods of mechanical ventilation in which there are no spontaneous breaths via the following equations:

$$\text{Elastance} = \frac{\text{Plateau Pressure} - \text{PEEP}}{V_T} \text{ and}$$

$$\text{Airway Resistance} = \frac{\text{PIP} - \text{PEEP}}{\text{Flow}}$$

The pressure required to overcome lung elastic recoil is equivalent to the product of the current lung volume and the elastance (Pel = volume × elastance), and the pressure required to overcome airway resistance is equivalent to the product of the current flow and the resistance (Pres = flow × resistance). At any point during inspiration, therefore, instantaneous patient pressure generation (Pmus) may be assessed if elastance and resistance have already been calculated and volume, flow, and Paw are instantaneously measured:

$$\text{Pmus} = (V \times E + \text{flow} \times R) - \text{Paw}.[49]$$

With PAV, airway pressure generation by the ventilator is proportional at any instant to the respiratory effort (Pmus) generated by the patient. Small efforts, therefore, result in small breaths, whereas greater patient effort results in development of a greater tidal volume. Inspiration is patient triggered and terminates with discontinuation of patient effort. Rate, V_T, and T_I are entirely patient controlled. In fact, the predominant variable to be set on the ventilator is the proportional response between Pmus and the applied ventilator pressure. This proportional assist (Paw/Pmus) can be increased until nearly all patient effort is provided by the ventilator.[50] Patient work of breathing, dyspnea, and PIP are reduced.[51, 52] Elastance and resistance are set as is applied PEEP. V_T is variable and risk of atelectasis may be present. Overall, the adult clinical experience is limited and its use has not been reported in pediatric and newborn patients. However, this is an exciting first step in servoregulating ventilators to patient requirements.

CONTINUOUS POSITIVE AIRWAY PRESSURE

During CPAP, pressures above those of ambient are continuously applied to the airways in order to enhance alveolar distention and oxygenation.[53] Both airway resistance and work of breathing may be substantially reduced. However, there is no support of ventilation. This mode requires, therefore, that the patient provide all of the work of breathing. It is to be avoided in patients with hypovolemia, untreated pneumothorax, lung hyperinflation, or elevated intracranial pressure and in infants with nasal obstruction, cleft palate, tracheoesophageal fistula, or untreated congenital diaphragmatic hernia. CPAP is frequently applied via nasal prongs, although it can be delivered in adult patients with a nasal mask.

INVERSE RATIO VENTILATION

In the setting of respiratory failure, one would wish to enhance alveolar distention in order to reduce hypoxemia and shunt. One means to accomplish this is to maintain the inspiratory plateau pressure for a longer proportion of the breath.[54] Although some studies have failed to demonstrate enhanced gas exchange with this mode of ventilation, others have revealed an increase in Paw and oxygenation while protecting the lungs with a reduction in PIP.[55–58] The I_T may be prolonged to the point at which the ratio of I_T to E_T may be as high as 4:1.[59] In most circumstances, however, the I_T:E_T ratio is maintained at approximately 2:1. Inverse ratio ventilation (IRV) is usually performed during pressure-controlled ventilation (PC-IRV), although a prolonged I_T can be applied during volume-controlled ventilation by adding a decelerating flow pattern or an end-inspiratory pause to the volume-controlled ventilator breath.[60] One advantage of IRV is the ability to recruit alveoli that are associated with high-resistance airways, and, therefore, inflate only with prolonged application of positive pressure.[61]

Unfortunately, IRV is associated with a profound sense of dyspnea in patients who are awake and spontaneously breathing. Therefore, heavy sedation and pharmacologic paralysis is required during this ventilator mode. One must also be cognizant of the risk for incomplete expiration as the E_T is reduced. This may be identified by the failure to achieve zero flow conditions at end-expiration. The result is "auto-PEEP" or a total PEEP greater than that of the preset or applied PEEP. Care should be taken to recognize the presence of auto-PEEP and to incorporate it into the ventilation strategy. IRV may also affect cardiac output and, therefore, oxygen delivery.[62] Continuous monitoring of the SvO_2 may aid in determining whether the addition of IRV has enhanced Do_2 in addition to PaO_2 and SaO_2.

AIRWAY PRESSURE RELEASE VENTILATION

Airway pressure release ventilation (APRV) is a unique approach to ventilation in which CPAP at high levels is used to enhance mean alveolar volume while intermittent reductions in pressure to a "release" level provide a period of expiration (Fig. 6–12). Reestablishment of CPAP results in inspiration and return of lung volume back to the baseline level. The advantage of APRV is a reduction in PIP of approximately 50% in adult patients with ARDS supported with this technique when compared to other more conventional modes of mechanical ventilation.[63, 64] There are also data to suggest that $\dot{V}/\dot{Q}$ matching may be improved and dead space reduced.[65, 66] In performing APRV, tidal volume is altered by adjusting the release pressure. Conceptually, ventilator management during APRV is the inverse of other modes of positive pressure ventilation in that the peak inspiratory pressure, or CPAP, deter-

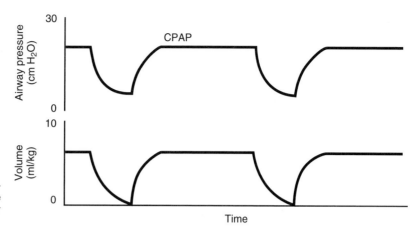

Figure 6–12. Typical pressure and volume waveforms observed during airway pressure release ventilation. CPAP, continuous positive airway pressure.

mines oxygenation while the expiratory pressure (release pressure) is used to adjust tidal volume and CO_2 elimination. APRV is very similar to modes of ventilation which use prolonged $I_T:E_T$ ratios such as low frequency positive pressure–inverse ratio ventilation (LFPP-IRV). In some studies, the physiologic shunt decreased during APRV, whereas in others, PaO_2 was decreased due to the development of atelectasis.[67] The clinical experience with APRV is limited and the newborn and infant experience is only in animal models.[68]

BILEVEL CONTROL OF POSITIVE AIRWAY PRESSURE

Although sometimes used in the acute lung setting, the bilevel control of positive airway pressure (BIPAP) simple ventilator system is frequently used for home respiratory support by varying airway pressure between one of two settings: the inspiratory positive airway pressure (IPAP) and the expiratory positive airway pressure (EPAP).[69, 70] With patient effort, a change in flow is detected and the IPAP pressure level is developed. With reduced flow at end-expiration, EPAP is reestablished. This device, therefore, provides both ventilatory support as well as airway distention during the expiratory phase. However, BIPAP ventilators should be used only to support the patient who is spontaneously breathing.

□ Monitoring During Mechanical Ventilation

Current mechanical ventilators incorporate highly accurate solid-state pressure transducers that provide data on a variety of pressures and gas flows. Volume is not measured directly; rather, flow is integrated over time in the determination of volume. Low-pressure alarms are present to detect disconnection and leaks and are set at approximately 10 cm H_2O below the anticipated PIP, whereas high-pressure alarms are set at approximately 10 cm H_2O above PIP to avoid incidental application of excessive pressure to the lungs. Apnea alarms typically are triggered if tidal volume is not delivered for more than 10 seconds. Alarms for numerous other parameters such as PEEP, low tidal volume, low and high rate, and low and high FiO_2 may be adjusted on various ventilators. Most ventilators also have an indicator that notifies the operator if the ventilator settings result in an $I_T:E_T$ ratio that is greater than 1:1. Current ventilators can calculate and display a variety of pressure-volume, flow-volume, or volume-pressure waveforms as well as demonstrate volume, flow, and pressure over time. In the setting of respiratory insufficiency, mechanical ventilation should be used in conjunction with invasive monitoring, such as systemic arterial and pulmonary arterial (PA) catheters, as well as pulse oximetry and end-tidal CO_2 monitoring. Technology that allows frequent blood gas sampling without blood loss is now available for newborns and infants. It is likely that ventilators in the future will incorporate PA catheter-derived SvO_2, pulse oximeter–derived SaO_2, and oxygen consumption data in determining online cardiac output and oxygen delivery values (Fig. 6–13).[71] As online blood gas monitoring becomes more accurate, FiO_2, rate, PIP, and PEEP will be servoregulated on the basis of SaO_2, SvO_2, and $PaCO_2$.

□ Management of the Mechanical Ventilator

IMV and SIMV may suffice for patients with normal lungs such as those who are postoperation.[72] If a patient is spontaneously breathing and is to be ventilated for more than a brief period, a flow- or pressure-triggered assist mode, pressure support, or proportional assist ventilation will result in maximal support and minimal work of breathing.[40, 41] Ventilator modes that allow adjustment of specific details of pressure, flow, and volume are required in the patient with severe respiratory failure. With all these modes, the ventilator rate; tidal volume or PIP; PEEP; and either I_T alone or $I_T:E_T$, if ventilation is pressure limited, must be assigned. Other secondary controls such as the flow rate, the flow pattern,

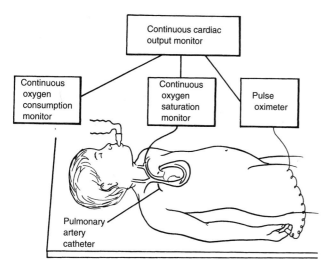

Figure 6–13. Continuous Fick cardiac output monitoring is illustrated schematically. (From Hirschl RB, Heiss K: Cardiopulmonary critical care and shock. In Oldham KT, Colombani PM, Foglia RP [eds]: Surgery of Infants and Children: Scientific Principles and Practice. Philadelphia, Lippincott-Raven, 1997, p 168.)

the trigger sensitivity for assisted breaths, the inspiratory hold, the termination sensitivity, and the safety pressure limit are also set on individual ventilators. The normal minute volume ventilation is 100 to 150 ml/kg/min. The FiO_2 is usually initiated at 0.50 and decreased based on pulse oximetry. All efforts should be made to maintain the FiO_2 less than 0.60 in order to avoid alveolar nitrogen depletion and the development of atelectasis.[73, 74] Oxygen toxicity likely is a result of this phenomenon, although free oxygen radical formation may play a role when an FiO_2 greater than 0.40 is applied for prolonged periods.[75] A short inspiratory phase with a low IT:ET ratio favors the expiratory phase and CO_2 elimination whereas longer IT:ET ratios enhance oxygenation. In the normal lung, IT:ET ratios of 1:3 and IT equal to 0.5 to 1 second are typical.

☐ Mechanical Ventilation in the Patient with Respiratory Failure

VENTILATOR-INDUCED LUNG INJURY

One typically observes both a decrease in pulmonary compliance as well as functional residual capacity in the patient with acute lung injury (ALI, PaO_2/FiO_2 ratio = 200 to 300) or ARDS (PaO_2/FiO_2 ratio <200). These two parameters are related as the loss of FRC associated with alveolar collapse results in a decrease in the volume of lung available for ventilation and, therefore, a decrease in pulmonary compliance. As a result, higher ventilator pressures are necessary to maintain tidal volume and minute volume ventilation.

However, the adverse effects of prolonged lung exposure to high ventilating pressures (plateau pressures >35 cm H_2O) were elucidated in the 1980s

and 1990s.[76] Electron microscopy reveals an increased incidence of alveolar stress fractures in ex vivo, perfused rabbit lungs exposed to transalveolar pressures greater than 30 cm H_2O (Fig. 6–14).[77] Other investigators have demonstrated increases in albumin leak, elevation of the capillary leak coefficient, enhanced wet-to-dry lung weight, deterioration in gas exchange, and augmented diffuse alveolar damage on histology with application of increased airway pressure (45 to 50 cm H_2O) in otherwise normal rats and sheep over 1 to 24 hours.[26, 78, 79] Pulmonary exposure to high pressures may worsen nascent respiratory insufficiency and, ultimately, lead to the development of pulmonary fibrosis. Such injury may be prevented during application of high peak inspiratory pressures by strapping the chest, thereby preventing lung overdistention, suggesting that alveolar distention or "volutrauma" is the injurious element rather than application of high pressures or "barotrauma."[80]

These data suggest that avoidance of high peak inspiratory pressures should be a primary goal of any mechanical ventilatory approach to the lung. However, two multicenter studies have attempted to randomize patients with ARDS to high and low peak pressure or volume strategies. The first failed to demonstrate a difference in mortality or duration of mechanical ventilation in patients randomized to either the low (7.2 ± 0.8 ml/kg) or the high (10.8 ± 1.0 ml) volume strategy, although the applied PIP was not elevated to injurious levels in either group (low = 23.6 ± 5.8 cm H_2O; high = 34.0 ± 11.0 cm H_2O).[81] Another study revealed similar results but had similar limitations.[82] One recent randomized, controlled study revealed a significant increase in survival from 38 to 71% among patients with respiratory failure who were approached with a lung protective ventilation strategy (see Permissive Hypercapnia).[83] The NIH ARDS consortium is now in-

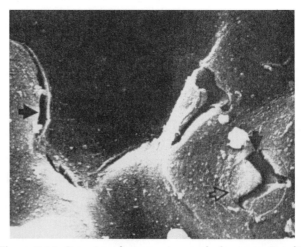

Figure 6–14. Scanning electron micrograph demonstrating disruptions in the blood-gas barriers (arrows) in rabbit lungs subjected to 20 cm H_2O airway pressure and 75 cm H_2O pulmonary arterial pressure. (From Fu Z, Costello ML, Tsukimoto K, et al: High lung volume increases stress failure in pulmonary capillaries. J Appl Physiol 73:123–133, 1992.)

vestigating the efficacy of low volume (6 ml/kg) compared with high volume (12 ml/kg) ventilation in adult patients with ARDS, with preliminary results suggesting a lower mortality in the low when compared to the high volume ventilation group.[84]

PERMISSIVE HYPERCAPNIA

The use of high ventilator pressures in an attempt to hyperventilate the newborn with pulmonary hypertension can actually result in compromise of cardiopulmonary physiology and the development of ventilator-induced lung injury (VILI) or BPD.[85] To avoid VILI, practitioners have applied the concept of permissive hypercapnia, in which arterial CO_2 is allowed to rise to levels as high as 120 mm Hg as long as the blood pH is maintained in the 7.1 to 7.2 range by administration of buffers.[86] Mortality was reduced to 26% when compared with that expected (53%, P <.004) based on Acute Physiology and Chronic Health Evaluation (APACHE) II scores when low-volume, pressure-limited ventilation with permissive hypercapnia was applied in the setting of ARDS in adults.[87]

PROTECTIVE EFFECTS OF POSITIVE END-EXPIRATORY PRESSURE

Although application of high, overdistending airway pressures appears to be associated with the development of lung injury, a number of studies have demonstrated that application of PEEP or high-frequency oscillatory ventilation (HFOV) may allow avoidance of lung injury by the following mechanisms[88, 89]:

1. Recruitment of collapsed alveoli, which reduces the risk for overdistention of healthy units
2. Resolution of alveolar collapse, which in and of itself, is injurious
3. Avoidance of the shear forces associated with the opening and closing of alveoli

In the older child with injured lungs, a pressure of 8 to 12 cm H_2O is required to open alveoli and to begin tidal volume generation.[83, 90, 91] Alveoli will subsequently close unless the end-expiratory pressure is maintained at such pressures. This cyclic opening and closing is thought to be particularly injurious due to application of large shear forces.[90] One way to avoid this process is through the application of PEEP to a point above the inflection pressure (Pflex) such that alveolar distention is maintained throughout the ventilatory cycle.[92, 93] In addition, the distribution of infiltrates and atelectasis in the supine patient with ARDS is predominantly in the dependent regions of the lung (Fig. 6–15).[94] This is likely the result of compression due to the increased weight of the overlying edematous lung. The application of PEEP results in recruitment of these atelectatic lung regions, simultaneously enhancing pulmonary compliance and oxygenation.[20]

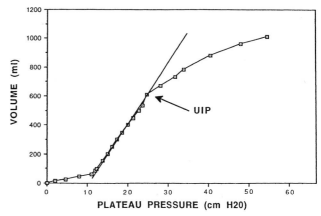

Figure 6–15. Static pressure/volume curve demonstrating the Pflex point (the lower inflection point) at approximately 12 cm H_2O in a patient with acute respiratory distress syndrome. Peak end-expiratory pressure should be maintained approximately 2 cm H_2O above that point. The upper inflection point (UIP) indicates the point at which lung overdistention is beginning to occur. Ventilation to points above the UIP should be avoided in most circumstances. (From Roupie E, Dambrosio M, Servillo G, et al, 1995, Titration of tidal volume and induced hypercapnia in acute respiratory distress syndrome. *American Journal of Respiratory and Critical Care Medicine,* 152:121–128. Official Journal of the American Thoracic Society © American Lung Association.

APPROACH TO THE PATIENT WITH RESPIRATORY FAILURE

As a result of these new data and concepts, the approach to mechanical ventilation in the patient with respiratory failure changed drastically in the 1990s (Table 6–2). Time-cycled, pressure-controlled ventilation has become favored because of the ability to limit EIP to noninjurious levels at a maximum of 35 cm H_2O.[91] In infants and newborns, this EIP limit is set lower at 30 cm H_2O. A lung-protective approach also incorporates lung distention and prevention of alveolar closure. Static pressure/volume (PV) curves should be developed on each individual patient at least daily so that the Pflex can be identified and the PEEP maintained at least 2 cm H_2O above Pflex. If a static PV curve cannot be determined, then a PEEP of at least 8 to 12 cm H_2O, and perhaps even >15 cm H_2O, should be empirically applied in older patients.[91, 95] As both PIP and PEEP are increased, enhancements in compliance and reductions in V_D/V_T and shunt are to be expected. If they are not observed, then one should suspect the presence of overdistention of currently inflated alveoli instead of the desired recruitment of collapsed

TABLE 6-2. Current Favored Approaches to the Treatment of Acute Respiratory Distress Syndrome

Pressure-limited ventilation	SvO_2 ≥65%
Inverse ratio ventilation	SaO_2 ≥80–85%
EIP ≤35 cm H_2O	Transfusion to Hgb >13 g/dl
PEEP >Pflex or 12 cm H_2O	Diuresis to dry weight
Permissive hypercapnia	Prone positioning
FiO_2 ≤0.06	Extracorporeal support

EIP, end-inspiratory pressure; PEEP, positive end-expiratory pressure.

lung units. Application of increased levels of PEEP may also result in a decrease in venous return and cardiac output. In addition, West's zone I physiology, which predicts diminished or absent pulmonary capillary flow in the nondependent regions of the lungs at end-inspiration, may be exacerbated with application of higher airway pressures. This may be especially detrimental because it is the nondependent regions that are best inflated and to which one would wish to direct as much pulmonary blood flow as possible.[15]

As a result, parameters of oxygen delivery should be carefully monitored during application of increased PEEP.[96] One means for doing so is via attention to the SvO_2 whenever the PEEP is raised above 5 cm H_2O. As mentioned, one approach is to gradually increase the PEEP in increments of 2.5 cm H_2O until the desired level of oxygenation or lung protection is achieved or a decrease in SvO_2 to below the maximum is observed. Effective lung compliance also should be monitored to ensure that alveolar recruitment is being achieved.

If oxygenation remains inadequate with application of higher levels of PEEP, FiO_2 should be increased to maintain an SaO_2 greater than 90%, although levels as low as 80% may be acceptable in patients with adequate oxygen delivery. One of the most effective ways to enhance oxygen delivery is via transfusion. All attempts should be made to avoid the atelectasis and oxygen toxicity associated with FiO_2 levels >0.60.[73] Extending FiO_2 to levels greater than 0.60 often has little effect on oxygenation because severe respiratory failure is frequently associated with a large transpulmonary shunt. If inadequate oxygen delivery persists, a trial increase in PEEP level should be performed or institution of extracorporeal support considered.[97, 98]

Inflation of the lungs can also be enhanced by prolonging the inspiratory time via PC-IRV. Pharmacologic paralysis and sedation are required during performance of PC-IRV, although paralysis may have the additional benefit of decreasing oxygen consumption and enhancing ventilator efficiency.[29] PaO_2 may improve with application of PC-IRV.[99, 100] However, again, monitoring of the effect on oxygen delivery and the SvO_2 is critical to ensure the benefit of this intervention. The advantages of the alveolar inflation associated with a decelerating flow waveform during pressure-limited modes of ventilation also should be employed.[34]

Altering the patient from the supine to the prone position appears to enhance gas exchange (Fig. 6–16).[101, 102] This improvement was initially thought to be secondary to redistribution of pulmonary blood flow toward the better inflated anterior lung regions (previously nondependent, now dependent).[103] However, data in lung-injured sheep suggest that the enhancement in gas exchange may be predominantly due to more homogenous distribution of ventilation.[104] This effect may be reversed after a number of hours. However, enhanced posterior region lung inflation frequently accounts for persistent increases in oxygenation when the patient

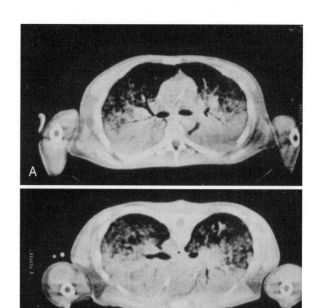

Figure 6–16. Cross-sectional images at the level of the carina in a patient with ARDS who is in the supine (A) followed by the prone (B) position. Note the redistribution of densities from the posterior to the anterior region with prone positioning. (From Langer M, Mascheroni D, Marcolin R, et al: The prone position in ARDS patients. A clinical study. Chest 94:103–107, 1988.)

is re-placed into the supine position.[105] Therefore, benefit may be seen when the prone and supine positions are alternated, usually every 4 to 6 hours. Some patients may not respond to altered positioning, in which case the intervention should be discontinued. Attention to careful patient padding and avoidance of dislodgment of tubes and catheters are critical to successful implementation of this approach.

Another means for enhancing oxygenation may be through administration of diuretics and the associated reduction of left atrial and pulmonary capillary hydrostatic pressure.[106] Diuresis results in a decrease in lung interstitial edema. In addition, reduction of lung edema decreases compression of the underlying dependent lung.[107] Collapsed dependent lung regions are thereby recruited. Although this treatment approach has not been proved in clinical trials, reduction in total body fluid in adult patients with ARDS is associated with an increase in survival.[108]

One protects the lung by applying noninjurious PIPs and enhancing PEEP levels, which limits the ΔP and V_T. This results in compromise of CO_2 elimination. Therefore, the concept of permissive hypercapnia, which was discussed previously, is integral to the successful application of lung protective strategies. $PaCO_2$ levels greater than 100 mm Hg have been allowed with this approach, although most practitioners prefer to maintain the $PaCO_2$ less than 60 to 70 mm Hg.[87] Bicarbonate or trishydroxymethylaminomethane (THAM) may be used to induce a metabolic alkalosis to maintain the pH greater than 7.20. Few significant physiologic effects are observed with elevated $PaCO_2$ levels, as long as the pH is maintained at reasonable levels.[109] If adequate CO_2 elimination cannot be achieved while limiting EIP to noninjurious levels, then initiation of ECLS should be considered.

The one situation in which it may be acceptable to increase EIP to levels greater than 35 cm H_2O (30 cm H_2O in the infant and newborn) is in the patient with reduced chest wall compliance and relatively normal pulmonary compliance. Because pulmonary compliance is composed of a combination of lung compliance and chest wall compliance, a decrease in chest wall compliance, such as due to abdominal distention or chest wall edema, can markedly reduce pulmonary compliance despite reasonable lung compliance. This situation is analogous to studies in which lungs remain uninjured despite application of high airway pressures because the chest is strapped to prevent lung overdistention.[80] This is a frequent problem in secondary respiratory failure due to trauma, sepsis, and other frequent disease processes observed among surgical patients. Cautious increase in EIP in such patients may be warranted. A simple intervention such as raising the head of the bed may have marked effects on FRC and gas exchange in such patients.

WEANING FROM MECHANICAL VENTILATION

Once a patient is spontaneously breathing and able to protect the airway, consideration should be given to weaning from ventilator support. The FiO_2 should be decreased to ≤0.40 before extubation. Simultaneously, PEEP should be weaned down to 5 cm H_2O. The pressure support mode of ventilation is an efficient means for weaning because the preset inspiratory pressure can be gradually decreased while partial support is provided for each breath.[110] Adequate gas exchange during a pressure support of 7 to 10 cm H_2O above PEEP in adults and newborns is predictive of successful extubation.[111] However, another study in adults demonstrated that simple transition from full ventilator support to a "T-piece," in which oxygen flowby is provided, is as effective at weaning as is gradual reduction in rate during IMV or pressure during PSV.[112] In all circumstances, brief trials of spontaneous breathing before extubation should be performed with flowby oxygen and CPAP. Prophylactic dexamethasone administration does not appear to increase the odds of a successful trial in infants.[113] Parameters during a T-piece trial that indicate readiness for extubation include the following:

1. Maintenance of the pretrial respiratory and heart rate
2. Inspiratory force greater than 20 cm H_2O
3. Minute volume ventilation less than 100 cc/kg/min
4. SaO_2 greater than 95%

If the patient's status is in question, transcutaneous CO_2 monitoring, along with arterial blood gas analysis ($PaCO_2$ ≤40 mm Hg, PaO_2 ≥60 mm Hg), may

TABLE 6-3. Management of the Patient Who Has Failed Extubation Attempts

Frequent spontaneous breathing trials
Pressure support ventilation
Caloric intake ≤10% above expenditure
Minimize carbohydrate calories
Diuresis to dry weight
Treat infection
Tracheostomy

help to ascertain whether extubation is appropriate. The weaning trial should be brief and under no circumstances longer than 1 hour because the narrow endotracheal tube provides substantial resistance to spontaneous ventilation. In most cases, the patient who tolerates spontaneous breathing through an endotracheal tube for only a few minutes will demonstrate enhanced capabilities once the airway access device is removed.

Frequent causes of failed extubation include persistent pulmonary parenchymal disease, interstitial fibrosis, and reduced breathing endurance. Pressure support ventilation is ideal for use in the difficult-to-wean patient because it allows gradual application of spontaneous support to enhance respiratory strength and conditioning (Table 6–3).[110] Enteral and parenteral nutrition should be adjusted to maintain the total caloric intake no more than 10% above the estimated caloric needs of the patient. Excess calories will be converted to fat with a high respiratory quotient and increased CO_2 production. Nutritional support high in glucose has a similar effect.[114] Manipulation of feedings along with treatment of sepsis may reduce VCO_2 and enhance weaning. Pulmonary edema should be treated with diuretics. Some patients benefit from a tracheostomy to avoid ongoing upper airway contamination, to decrease dead space and airway resistance, and to provide airway access for evacuation of secretions during the weaning process. In addition, the issue of extubating the patient is removed by tracheostomy tube placement. Spontaneous breathing trials, therefore, are easy to perform and the transition to liberation from the mechanical ventilator is a much more smooth and efficient process. Tracheostomy tube placement in older patients can be performed by percutaneous means at the bedside.[115] Long-term complications of a tracheostomy tube are fairly minimal in older patients, but in newborns and infants, the rate of development of stenoses and granulation tissue may be significant.[116, 117]

☐ Nonconventional Modes and Adjuncts to Mechanical Ventilation

HIGH FREQUENCY VENTILATION

The concept of high frequency jet ventilation (HFJV) was developed in the early 1970s to provide

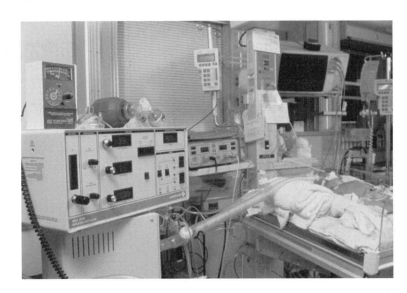

Figure 6–17. The SensorMedics 3100 (Yorba Linda, California) high frequency oscillatory ventilation (HFOV) device. The amplitude, Paw, Hz, and IT are set by the operator.

gas exchange during procedures performed on the trachea. HFJV employs small bursts of gas through a small "jet port" in the endotracheal tube typically at a rate of 420/min, with the range being 240 to 660 breaths per minute.[118] The expiratory phase is passive.[119] Tidal volume is adjusted by controlling the PIP, which is usually initiated at 90% of conventional PIP. CO_2 removal is most affected by the ΔP, or amplitude between the PIP and the PEEP. Therefore, an increase in the PIP or decrease in the PEEP will result in enhanced CO_2 elimination. Adjusting the Paw, PEEP, and FiO_2 alters oxygenation. HFJV is typically superimposed on background conventional tidal volume mechanical ventilation.

High frequency oscillatory ventilation (HFOV) employs a piston pump–driven diaphragm, which delivers small volumes at frequencies between 3 and 15 Hz (Fig. 6–17).[118] Both inspiration and expiration are active. Oxygenation is manipulated by adjusting Paw, which controls lung inflation similar to the role of PEEP in conventional mechanical ventilation. CO_2 elimination is controlled by manipulating the tidal volume, also known as the *amplitude* or *power*. In short, only four variables are adjusted during HFOV:

1. Mean airway pressure (Paw) is typically initiated at a level 1 to 2 cm H_2O higher in premature newborns and 2 to 4 cm H_2O higher in full-term newborns and children than that used during conventional mechanical ventilation.[120] For most disease processes, Paw is adjusted thereafter to maintain the right hemidiaphragm at the 8 to 9 rib level on the anteroposterior chest film.
2. Frequency (Hz) is usually set at 12 Hz in premature newborns and 10 Hz in full-term patients. Lowering the frequency tends to result in an increase in tidal volume and a decrease in $PaCO_2$.
3. Inspiratory time (IT), which may be increased to enhance tidal volume, is usually set at 33%.
4. Amplitude or power (ΔP) is set to achieve good chest wall movement and adequate CO_2 elimination.

Gas exchange during high frequency ventilation is thought to occur by convection in those alveoli located close to airways and for others by streaming, a phenomenon by which inspiratory gas, which has a parabolic profile, tends to flow down the center of the airways while the expiratory flow, which has a square profile, takes place at the periphery (Fig. 6–18).[121] Other effects may play a role:

1. Pendelluft, in which gas exchange takes place between lung units with different time constants as some are filling while others are emptying
2. The movement of the heart itself, which may enhance mixing of gases in distal airways
3. Taylor dispersion, in which convective flow and diffusion together function to enhance distribution of gas
4. Local diffusion

High frequency ventilation should be applied to the newborn and pediatric patient who is failing conventional ventilation either due to parameters of

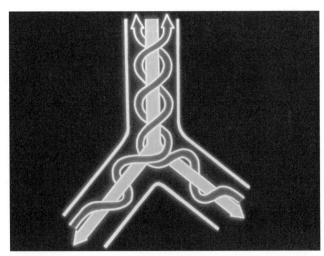

Figure 6–18. Streaming as a mechanism of gas exchange during high frequency ventilation. Note that the parabolic wavefront of the inspiratory gas induces central flow in the airways while expiratory gas flows at the periphery.

oxygenation or CO_2 elimination. The advantage of high-frequency ventilation lies in the alveolar distention and recruitment that is provided while limiting exposure to potentially injurious high ventilator pressures.[122] Thus, the approach during high-frequency ventilation should be to apply a mean airway pressure that will effectively recruit alveoli and maintain oxygenation while limiting the ΔP to that which will provide chest wall movement and adequate CO_2 elimination. Carbon dioxide elimination at lower PIPs may be a specific advantage in patients with air leak, especially those with bronchopleural fistulas.[123] Once again, the effect on oxygen delivery, rather than simply PaO_2, should be considered.

Although initial studies with HFOV in preterm newborns suggested that the incidence of BPD was similar to the conventional ventilation group and that there were adverse effects on intraventricular hemorrhage and periventricular leukomalacia, other trials have noted an increase in the rescue rate and a reduction in BPD.[124–126] Still other studies have suggested that the rescue rate or survival of full-term newborns and pediatric patients with respiratory insufficiency treated with HFOV was significantly increased when compared to conventional mechanical ventilation.[127–129] Reductions in oxygenation index and FiO_2 were observed during HFOV in 17 adult patients with ARDS.[130] Some reports suggest that mean airway pressure during HFJV in adults is reduced as is the incidence of barotrauma.[131, 132]

Intratracheal Pulmonary Ventilation

Intratracheal pulmonary ventilation (ITPV) involves infusion of fresh gas (oxygen) into the trachea via a cannula placed at the tip of the endotracheal tube. This gas flow effectively replaces the central airway deadspace with fresh oxygen during the expiratory phase of the ventilatory cycle and functions to reduce deadspace, which augments CO_2 elimination. For this purpose, a special reverse thruster catheter (RTC) is used for gas insufflation that reverses the flow of gas at the tip such that it follows a retrograde path up the endotracheal tube (Fig. 6–19).[133] This provides a Venturi effect that entrains gas, providing for more effective deadspace reduction during expiration. ITPV has been demonstrated to maintain reasonable levels of ventilation in normal animals at PIPs one half to one third those required during conventional mechanical ventilation. Using ITPV, it is possible to maintain adequate levels of CO_2 in lambs in whom only 12.5% of the lung parenchyma remained available for gas exchange.[134] This same concept has been applied with use of a simple catheter, rather than the RTC, in adults with respiratory insufficiency and has been termed *tracheal gas insufflation* (TGI).[35, 135] Studies have demonstrated the ability of ITPV to reduce airway deadspace and, therefore, the ventilator pressures required to achieve equivalent rates of CO_2 elimination when compared with those observed during conventional mechanical ventilation in pedi-

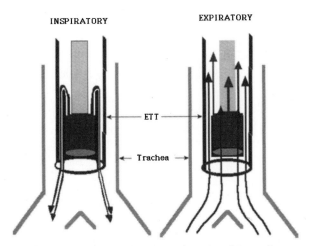

Figure 6–19. The reverse thruster catheter used in performance of intratracheal pulmonary ventilation (ITPV). During inspiration, the exhalation valve on the ventilator closes and gas flows prograde, filling the lung with a tidal volume of oxygen gas. During expiration, the gas flows retrograde, entraining and replacing the gas in the airways, thereby reducing deadspace and $PaCO_2$. (From Wilson JM, Thompson JR, Schnitzer JJ, et al: Intratracheal pulmonary ventilation and congenital diaphragmatic hernia. J Pediatr Surg 28:484–487, 1993.)

atric patients on venoarterial extracorporeal life support (ECLS) and in newborns with congenital diaphragmatic hernia (CDH) following ECLS.[136, 137]

Inhaled Nitric Oxide Administration

Nitric oxide (NO) is an endogenous mediator that serves to stimulate guanylate cyclase in the endothelial cell to produce cyclic guanosine monophosphate (cGMP), which results in relaxation of vascular smooth muscle (Fig. 6–20).[138] NO is rapidly

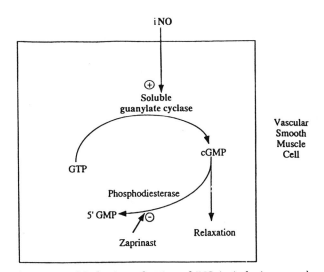

Figure 6–20. Mechanism of action of iNO in inducing vascular smooth muscle relaxation. Zaprinast is a phosphodiesterase inhibitor that may increase the potency and duration of the effect of iNO. cGMP, 5′GMP, cyclic guanosine monophosphate; GTP, guanosine triphosphate; iNO, inhaled nitric oxide. (From Hirschl RB: Innovative therapies in the management of newborns with congenital diaphragmatic hernia. Semin Pediatr Surg 5:256–265, 1996.)

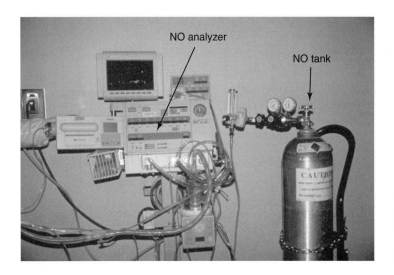

Figure 6–21. Apparatus for administering iNO to the neonate. The tank of 800 ppm NO is blended with the flow by gas to form a dose between 1 and 80 ppm. The NO analyzer allows accurate assessment of the concentration administered. iNO, inhaled nitric oxide; NO, nitric oxide.

scavenged by heme moieties. As such, inhaled nitric oxide (iNO) serves as a selective vasodilator of the pulmonary circulation because it is inactivated before reaching the systemic circulation. It is typically diluted in nitrogen and then mixed with blended oxygen and air to administer it in doses of from 1 to 80 parts per million (ppm) (Fig. 6–21).

Although initial studies demonstrated a decrease in pulmonary vascular resistance and an increase in PaO₂ without change in systemic arterial pressure, in adults with ARDS who were treated with iNO, a randomized, controlled study recently failed to demonstrate a difference in parameters of oxygenation or survival between the iNO and the control groups.[139–141] However, a subgroup analysis revealed an increase in survival in those patients treated with 5 ppm iNO. Further trials evaluating this dosing strategy are underway. Pediatric patients with ARDS demonstrated improvement in oxygenation in 15 of 17 patients after 30 minutes of iNO at 20 ppm, although other investigators have demonstrated that the improvement was not sustained beyond 24 hours.[142, 143]

Multiple studies have confirmed the utility of iNO in increasing oxygenation in newborns with pulmonary hypertension associated with various diagnoses.[144, 145] The Neonatal Inhaled Nitric Oxide Study (NINOS) demonstrated a reduction in oxygen index (NO = −14.1 ± 21.1 versus control = 0.8 ± 21.1, P <.001) and use of ECLS (NO = 39%, control = 55%, P = .014) among non-CDH newborns with pulmonary hypertension who were treated with either 20 or 80 ppm iNO when compared with control patients in a randomized, controlled, blinded trial.[146] In contrast, those patients with CDH demonstrated no effectiveness from iNO administration in a similar study.[147] It should be noted, however, that some investigators have suggested that the efficacy of iNO in patients with CDH may be more substantial following surfactant administration or at the point at which recurrent pulmonary hypertension occurs.[148] iNO administration may also be indicated

in the moribund CDH patient until ECLS can be initiated.

It should be recognized that iNO is still an experimental drug that is associated with the production of potentially toxic metabolites. When combined with O₂, iNO produces peroxynitrates, which can be damaging to epithelial cells and can also inhibit surfactant function.[149, 150] Nitrogen dioxide, which is toxic, can also be produced and hemoglobin may be oxidized to methemoglobin. There are additional concerns about the carcinogenicity of iNO, the immunosuppressive effects, and the potential for platelet dysfunction and intracranial hemorrhage in premature patients. In view of these concerns, iNO should only be used in situations in which efficacy has been demonstrated.

Surfactant Replacement Therapy

The use of exogenous surfactant has been responsible for a 30 to 40% reduction in the odds of death among very low birth weight newborns with RDS.[151, 152] In addition, in those premature neonates with birth weight greater than 1250 g, mortality in a controlled, randomized, blinded study decreased from 7% to 4%.[153] There are, in general, two forms of surfactant: synthetic surfactant (e.g., colfosceril palmitate [Exosurf, Neonatal]), which are made of dipalmitoylphosphatidylcholine and are protein free, and bovine surfactant extracts (e.g., beractant [Survanta]), which contain natural surfactants and associated proteins. Although it has been thought that there is a substantial difference in effect between the natural and synthetic surfactants, studies reveal no difference between colfosceril palmitate and beractant in terms of outcome, but a significantly lower risk of chronic lung disease or death at 28 days in the beractant (27%) when compared to the colfosceril palmitate (34%) infants with birth weights of 1001 to 1500 g.[154]

A randomized, prospective, controlled study in full-term newborns with respiratory insufficiency demonstrated an increased failure rate as defined by OI greater than 40 in the control group when compared with the group in whom surfactant was administered.[155] Another controlled, randomized study demonstrated the utility of surfactant in full-term newborns with the meconium aspiration syndrome.[156] The OI minimally decreased with the initial dose but markedly decreased with the second and third doses of surfactant from a baseline of 23.7 to 5.9. After three doses of surfactant, persistent pulmonary hypertension had resolved in all but one of the infants in the study group compared with none of the infants in the control group. The incidence of air leaks and need for ECLS were markedly reduced in the surfactant group when compared with the control patients.

It appears that patients with CDH are surfactant deficient.[157] Animal and human studies have suggested that surfactant administration before the first breath is associated with enhancement in PaO$_2$ and pulmonary mechanics.[158, 159] However, among CDH patients on ECLS, no difference between those randomized to receive surfactant (n = 9) and those control patients receiving air (n = 8) was noted in terms of lung compliance, time to extubation, period of oxygen requirement, and total number of hospital days.[157]

Liquid Ventilation with Perfluorocarbon

Perfluorocarbons are clear, colorless, odorless fluids that carry large amounts of oxygen (50 ml O$_2$/dl) and CO$_2$ (210 ml CO$_2$/dl).[160] They are relatively dense fluids (1.9 g/ml) and have low surface tension (19 dyne/cm). Liquid ventilation has been performed by one of two methods.[161] The first is *total liquid ventilation* (TLV), in which the lungs are filled with perfluorocarbon to a volume equivalent to FRC on which a device is used to generate tidal volumes of perfluorocarbon in the perfluorocarbon-filled lung.[162] The second technique of liquid ventilation involves administration of intratracheal perfluorocarbon to a volume equivalent to functional residual capacity followed by standard gas mechanical ventilation of the perfluorocarbon-filled lung, otherwise known as *partial liquid ventilation* (PLV).[163] TLV appears to be somewhat more effective at enhancing gas exchange, whereas PLV is a technique that is more easily generalized to critical care physicians managing patients with severe respiratory insufficiency.

Studies have demonstrated the efficacy of PLV in enhancing gas exchange in animal models of respiratory insufficiency.[164–167] It appears that intratracheal administration of perfluorocarbon acts as a surrogate surfactant, recruits atelectatic lung regions, and redistributes pulmonary blood flow toward the better-ventilated, nondependent regions of the lungs in the patient with ARDS.[19, 168] Phase I and II clinical studies have demonstrated the efficacy of partial liquid ventilation in enhancing oxygenation and pulmonary mechanics in adults, children, and

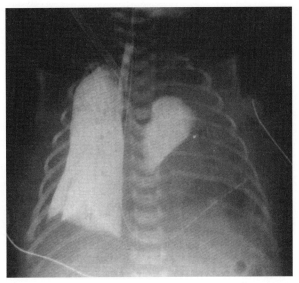

Figure 6–22. Chest radiograph of a newborn with congenital diaphragmatic hernia after initiation of partial liquid ventilation. Note the radiopaque perflubron filling the lungs, including the hypoplastic lung on the left. (From Pranikoff T, Gauger PG, Hirschl RB: Partial liquid ventilation in newborn patients with congenital diaphragmatic hernia. J Pediatr Surg 31:613–618, 1996.)

newborns with respiratory insufficiency, including those with CDH and those who are premature (Fig. 6–22).[169–172] Studies in pediatric and adult patients have demonstrated decreases in the (A − a)DO$_2$ from approximately 450 to 250 mm Hg within the first 48 hours after initiation of PLV.[173] In addition, in a separate uncontrolled study in premature newborns who had an a/A less than 0.2 following two doses of surfactant, the OI decreased from approximately 50 to 10 over the first 4 hours after initiation of PLV. Studies evaluating the safety and efficacy of PLV in adult and pediatric patients with respiratory insufficiency in a prospective, controlled, randomized fashion have been completed. No differences between PLV and conventional groups were observed.[174] A surprisingly low mortality in pediatric patients with isolated respiratory failure of 15 to 20% made successful completion of the study impossible. Subgroup analysis of adult patients younger than 55 years of age with ALI and ARDS demonstrated trends toward an increase in survival and the number of days free from the ventilator in the PLV when compared to the conventional gas ventilated group. Randomized, controlled trials in adult patients with respiratory insufficiency are now underway.

Studies have demonstrated the ability of in utero tracheal ligation to correct the structural and physiologic effects of pulmonary hypoplasia in the sheep fetus with CDH.[175, 176] It is also possible to induce lung growth via distention of the isolated right upper lobe in newborn sheep with perflubron (Liqui-Vent) to a pressure of 7 to 10 mm Hg (Fig. 6–23).[177] This study demonstrated an increase in size and alveolar number in the right upper lobe while main-

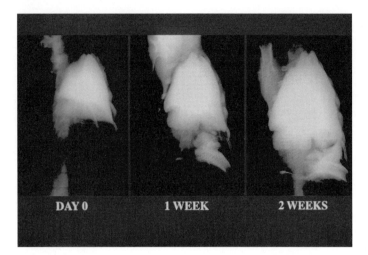

Figure 6–23. Enhancement in growth of the right upper lobe of the sheep after 2 weeks of distention with perflubron to a continuous pressure of 7–10 mm Hg. (From Fauza DO, DiFiore JW, Hines MH, et al: Continuous intrapulmonary distention with perfluorocarbon accelerates postnatal lung growth: Possible application for congenital diaphragmatic hernia. Surg Forum 46:666–669, 1995.)

taining the air space fraction, the protein-DNA ratio, and the alveolar-arterial ratio unchanged when compared with nondistended control animals. This technique would apply to patients with CDH who required ECLS.

REFERENCES

1. Baker AB: Artificial respiration, the history of an idea. Med Hist 15:336–351, 1971.
2. Matas R: Intralaryngeal insufflation. JAMA 34:1468–1473, 1900.
3. Daily WJR, Smith PC: Mechanical ventilation of the newborn infant. Curr Probl Pediatr 1:3–37, 1971.
4. Emerson JH: The Evolution of Iron Lungs. Cambridge, MA: JH Emerson, 1978.
5. Magill IW: Endotracheal anesthesia. Proc R Soc Med 22:83–88, 1928.
6. Rowbotham S: Intratracheal anesthesia by the nasal route for operation on the mouth and lips. BMJ 1:590–591, 1920.
7. Eckman M, Barach B, Fox C, et al: An appraisal of intermittent pressure breathing as a method of increasing altitude tolerance. J Aviat Med 18:565–574, 1947.
8. Stahlman MT, Young WC, Payne G: Studies of ventilatory aids in hyaline membrane disease. Am J Dis Child 104:526, 1962.
9. Cassani VL: We've come a long way baby! Mechanical ventilation of the newborn. Neonatal Net 13:63–68, 1994.
10. Avery ME, Mead J: Surface properties in relation to atelectasis and hyaline membrane disease. Am J Dis Child 17:517–523, 1959.
11. Thomas DV, et al: Prolonged respiratory use in pulmonary insufficiency of the newborn. JAMA 193:183, 1965.
12. Gregory GA, Kitterman JA, Phibbs RH, et al: Treatment of the idiopathic respiratory-distress syndrome with continuous positive airway pressure. N Engl J Med 284:1333–1340, 1971.
13. Kossel H, Versmold H: 25 years of respiratory support of newborn infants. J Perinat Med 25:421–432, 1997.
14. Bartlett RH: Use of the mechanical ventilator. In Douglas W, Wilmore MD, Laurence Y, et al (eds): Surgery. Vol. 1. New York, Scientific American, 1988.
15. Satterfield TS (ed): Respiratory Physiology—The Essentials. Baltimore, Williams & Wilkins, 1990, pp 1–185.
16. Gattinoni L, Mascheroni D, Basilico E, et al: Volume/pressure curve of total respiratory system in paralysed patients: Artefacts and correction factors. Intensive Care Med 13:19–25, 1987.
17. Putensen C, Baum M, Hormann C: Selecting ventilator settings according to variables derived from the quasi-static pressure/volume relationship in patients with acute lung injury. Anesth Analg 77:436–447, 1993.
18. Bartel LP, Bazik JR, Powner DJ: Compression volume during mechanical ventilation: Comparison of ventilators and tubing circuits. Crit Care Med 13:851–854, 1985.
19. Gattinoni L, Pesenti A, Mascheroni D, et al: Low-frequency positive-pressure ventilation with extracorporeal CO_2 removal in severe acute respiratory failure. JAMA 256:881–886, 1986.
20. Gattinoni L, D'Andrea L, Pelosi P, et al: Regional effects and mechanism of positive end-expiratory pressure in early adult respiratory distress syndrome. JAMA 269:2122–2127, 1993.
21. Maunder RJ, Shuman WP, McHugh JW, et al: Preservation of normal lung regions in the adult respiratory distress syndrome: Analysis by computed tomography. JAMA 255:2463–2465, 1986.
22. White KM: Completing the hemodynamic picture: SvO_2. Heart Lung 14:272–280, 1985.
23. Nelson L: Continuous venous oximetry in surgical patients. Ann Surg 203:329–333, 1986.
24. Jan K, Usami S, Smith JA: Effects of transfusion on rheological properties of blood in sickle cell anemia. Transfusion 22:17–20, 1982.
25. Marini JJ: Pressure-targeted, lung-protective ventilatory support in acute lung injury. Chest 105(suppl):109S–116S, 1994.
26. Parker JC, Townsley MI, Rippe B, et al: Increased microvascular permeability in dog lungs due to high peak airway pressures. J Appl Physiol 57:1809–1816, 1984.
27. Ranieri VM, Mascia L, Fiore T, et al: Cardiorespiratory effects of positive end-expiratory pressure during progressive tidal volume reduction (permissive hypercapnia) in patients with acute respiratory distress syndrome. Anesthesiology 83:710–720, 1995.
28. Palmisano BW, Fisher DM, Willis M, et al: The effect of paralysis on oxygen consumption in normoxic children after cardiac surgery. Anesthesiology 61:518, 1984.
29. Coggeshall JW, Marini JJ, Newman JH: Improved oxygenation after muscle relaxation in adult respiratory distress syndrome. Arch Intern Med 145:1718–1720, 1985.
30. Ganong WF: Energy Balance, Metabolism, and Nutrition: Review of Medical Physiology. Los Altos, CA, Lange Medical Publications, 1979.
31. Kacmarek RM, Hess D: Basic principles of ventilator machinery. In Tobin MJ (ed). Principles and Practice of Mechanical Ventilation. New York, McGraw-Hill, 1994, pp 65–110.
32. Pilbeam SP: Physical aspects of mechanical ventilators. In Russell J (ed). Mechanical Ventilation: Physiological and Clinical Applications. St. Louis, MO, CV Mosby, 1998, pp 62–91.
33. Piotrowski A, Sobala W, Kawczynski P: Patient-initiated, pressure-regulated, volume-controlled ventilation compared with intermittent mandatory ventilation in neonates:

A prospective, randomised study. Intensive Care Med 23:975–981, 1997.
34. Abraham E, Yoshihara G: Cardiorespiratory effects of pressure controlled ventilation in severe respiratory failure. Chest 98:1445–1449, 1990.
35. Nahum A, Burke WC, Ravenscraft SA, et al: Lung mechanics and gas exchange during pressure-control ventilation in dogs: Augmentation of CO_2 elimination by an intratracheal catheter. Am Rev Respir Dis 146:965–973, 1992.
36. Kirby RR: Intermittent mandatory ventilation in the neonate. Crit Care Med 5:18–22, 1977.
37. Bernstein G, Mannino FL, Heldt GP, et al: Randomized multicenter trial comparing synchronized and conventional intermittent mandatory ventilation in neonates. J Pediatr 129:948–950, 1996.
38. Cleary JP, Bernstein G, Mannino FL, et al: Improved oxygenation during synchronized intermittent mandatory ventilation in neonates with respiratory distress syndrome: A randomized, crossover study. J Pediatr 126:407–411, 1995.
39. Chen JY, Ling UP, Chen JH: Comparison of synchronized and conventional intermittent mandatory ventilation in neonates. Acta Paediatr Jpn 39:578–583, 1997.
40. Leung P, Jubran A, Tobin MJ: Comparison of assisted ventilator modes on triggering, patient effort, and dyspnea. Am J Respir Crit Care Med 155:1940–1948, 1997.
41. Jarreau PH, Moriette G, Mussat P, et al: Patient-triggered ventilation decreases the work of breathing in neonates. Am J Respir Crit Care Med 153:1176–1181, 1996.
42. Dekel B, Segal E, Perel A: Pressure support ventilation. Arch Intern Med 156:369–373, 1996.
43. Banner MJ, Kirby RR, Blanch PB, et al: Decreasing imposed work of the breathing apparatus to zero using pressure-support ventilation. Crit Care Med 21:1333–1338, 1993.
44. Kacmarek RM: The role of pressure support ventilation in reducing the work of breathing. Respir Care 33:99–120, 1988.
45. Brochard L, Pluskwa F, Lemaire F: Improved efficacy of spontaneous breathing with inspiratory pressure support. Crit Care Med 136:411–415, 1987.
46. Gullberg N, Winberg P, Sellden H: Pressure support ventilation increases cardiac output in neonates and infants. Paediatr Anaesth 6:311–315, 1996.
47. Tokioka H, Kinjo M, Hirakawa M: The effectiveness of pressure support ventilation for mechanical ventilatory support in children. Anesthesiology 78:880–884, 1993.
48. Amato MB, Barbas CS, Bonassa J, et al: Volume-assured pressure support ventilation (VAPSV): A new approach for reducing muscle workload during acute respiratory failure. Chest 102:1225–1234, 1992.
49. Younes M: Proportional assist ventilation: A new approach to ventilatory support. Crit Care Med 149:268, 1994.
50. Younes M: Proportional assist ventilation and pressure support ventilation: Similarities and differences. Intensive Care Emerg Med 15:361–380, 1991.
51. Bigatello LM, Nishimura M, Imanaka H, et al: Unloading of the work of breathing by proportional assist ventilation in a lung model. Crit Care Med 25:267–272, 1997.
52. Younes M, Puddy A, Roberts D, et al: Proportional assist ventilation. Results of an initial clinical trial. Am Rev Respir Dis 145:121–129, 1992.
53. Gittermann MK, Fusch C, Gittermann AR, et al: Early nasal continuous positive airway pressure treatment reduces the need for intubation in very low birth weight infants. Eur J Pediatr 156:384–388, 1997.
54. Lain DC, DiBenedetto R, Morris SL, et al: Pressure control inverse ratio ventilation as a method to reduce peak inspiratory pressure and provide adequate ventilation and oxygenation. Chest 95:1081–1088, 1989.
55. Armstrong BWJ, MacIntyre NR: Pressure-controlled, inverse ratio ventilation that avoids air trapping in the adult respiratory distress syndrome. Crit Care Med 23:279–285, 1995.
56. Mancebo J, Vallverdu I, Bak E, et al: Volume-controlled ventilation and pressure-controlled inverse ratio ventilation: A comparison of their effects in ARDS patients. Monaldi Arch Chest Dis 49:201–207, 1994.
57. Lessard MR, Guerot E, Lorino H, et al: Effects of pressure-controlled with different I:E ratios versus volume-controlled ventilation on respiratory mechanics, gas exchange, and hemodynamics in patients with adult respiratory distress syndrome. Anesthesiology 80:983–991, 1994.
58. Goldstein B, Papadokos PJ: Pressure-controlled inverse-ratio ventilation in children with acute respiratory failure. Am J Crit Care 3:11–15, 1994.
59. Tharratt RS, Allen RP, Albertson TE: Pressure controlled inverse ratio ventilation in severe adult respiratory failure. Chest 94:755–762, 1988.
60. Marcy TW, Marini JJ: Inverse ratio ventilation in ARDS: Rationale and implementation. Chest 100:494–504, 1991.
61. Porembka DT: Inverse ratio ventilation. Probl Respir Care 2:69–76, 1989.
62. Mercat A, Titiriga M, Anguel N, et al: Inverse ratio ventilation (I/E = 2/1) in acute respiratory distress syndrome: A six-hour controlled study. Am J Respir Crit Care Med 155:1637–1642, 1997.
63. Chiang AA, Steinfeld A, Cooper C, et al: Demand-flow airway pressure release ventilation as a partial ventilatory support mode: Comparison with synchronized intermittent mandatory ventilation and pressure support ventilation. Crit Care Med 22:1431–1437, 1994.
64. Rasanen J, Cane RD, Downs JV, et al: Airway pressure release ventilation during acute lung injury: A prospective multicenter trial. Crit Care Med 19:1234–1241, 1991.
65. Cane RD, Peruzzi WT, Shapiro BA: Airway pressure release ventilation in severe acute respiratory failure. Chest 100:460–463, 1991.
66. Valentine DD, Hammond MD, Downs JB, et al: Distribution of ventilation perfusion with different modes of mechanical ventilation. Am Rev Respir Dis 143:1262–1266, 1991.
67. Sydow M, Burchardi H, Ephraim E, et al: Long-term effects of two different ventilatory modes on oxygenation in acute lung injury: Comparison of airway pressure release ventilation and volume-controlled inverse ratio ventilation. Am J Respir Crit Care Med 149:1550–1556, 1994.
68. Martin LD, Wetzel RC, Bilenki AL: Airway pressure release ventilation in a neonatal lamb model of acute lung injury. Crit Care Med 19:373–378, 1991.
69. Padman R, Lawless ST, Kettrick RG: Noninvasive ventilation via bilevel positive airway pressure support in pediatric practice. Crit Care Med 26:169–173, 1998.
70. Lofaso F, Brochard L, Hang T, et al: Home versus intensive care pressure support devices: Experimental and clinical comparison. Am J Respir Crit Care Med 153:1591–1599, 1996.
71. Baxley WA, Cavender JB, Knoblock J: Continuous cardiac output monitoring by the Fick method. Cathet Cardiovasc Diagn 28:89–92, 1993.
72. Hollinger IB: Postoperative management: Ventilation. International Anesthesiol Clin 18:205–216, 1980.
73. Jenkinson SG: Oxygen toxicity. New Horiz 1:504–511, 1993.
74. Wolfe WG, DeVries WC: Oxygen toxicity. Annu Rev Med 26:203–217, 1975.
75. Gladstone IM Jr, Levine RL: Oxidation of proteins in neonatal lungs. Pediatrics 93:764–768, 1994.
76. Dreyfuss D, Saumon G: Ventilator-induced lung injury: Lessons from experimental studies. Am J Respir Crit Care Med 157:294–323, 1998.
77. Fu Z, Costello ML, Tsukimoto K, et al: High lung volume increases stress failure in pulmonary capillaries. J Appl Physiol 73:123–133, 1992.
78. Kolobow T, Moretti MP, Fumagalli R, et al: Severe impairment in lung function induced by high peak airway pressure during mechanical ventilation. Am Rev Respir Dis 135:312–315, 1987.
79. Dreyfuss D, Basset G, Soler P, et al: Intermittent positive-pressure hyperventilation with high inflation pressures produces pulmonary microvascular injury in rats. Am Rev Respir Dis 132:880–884, 1985.
80. Hernandez LA, Peevy K, Moise AA, et al: Chest wall restriction limits high airway pressure-induced lung injury in young rabbits. J Appl Physiol 66:2364–2368, 1989.

81. Stewart TE, Meade M, Cook DJ, et al: Evaluation of a ventilation strategy to prevent barotrauma in patients at high risk for acute respiratory distress syndrome. N Engl J Med 338:355–361, 1998.

82. Brochard L: Low versus high tidal volumes. In Vincent JL (ed). Acute Lung Injury. Vol. 30. Brussels, Belgium, Springer-Verlag, 1998, pp 276–281.

83. Amato MB, Barbas CS, Mederios DM, et al: Effect of a protective-ventilation strategy on mortality in the acute respiratory distress syndrome. N Engl J Med 338:347–354, 1998.

84. Bernard GR, Brown RG: NIH ARDS Network report of ongoing and proposed clinical trials. Presented at the Meeting of the American Thoracic Society; San Diego, CA; April 26, 1999.

85. Wung JT, James LS, Kilchevsky E, et al: Management of infants with severe respiratory failure and persistence of the fetal circulation without hyperventilation. Pediatrics 76:488, 1985.

86. Hickling KG: Low volume ventilation with permissive hypercapnea in the adult respiratory distress syndrome. Clin Intensive Care 3:67–78, 1992.

87. Hickling KG, Walsh J, Henderson S, et al: Low mortality rate in adult respiratory distress syndrome using low-volume, pressure-limited ventilation with permissive hypercapnia: A prospective study. Crit Care Med 22:1568–1578, 1994.

88. McCulloch PR, Forkert PG, Forese AB: Lung volume maintenance prevents lung injury during high frequency oscillatory ventilation in surfactant-deficient rabbits. Am Rev Respir Dis 137:1185–1192, 1988.

89. Dreyfuss D, Sjoer P, Basset G, et al: High inflation pressure pulmonary edema: Respective effects of high airway pressure, high tidal volume, and positive end-expiratory pressure. Am Rev Respir Dis 137:1159–1164, 1988.

90. Lachmann B: Open up the lung and keep the lung open. Intensive Care Med 18:319–321, 1992.

91. Mancebo J: PEEP, ARDS, and alveolar recruitment. Intensive Care Med 18:383–385, 1992.

92. Gattinoni L, Pesenti A, Avalli L, et al: Pressure-volume curve of total respiratory system in acute respiratory failure. Am Rev Respir Dis 136:730–736, 1987.

93. Roupie E, Dambrosio M, Servillo G, et al: Titration of tidal volume and induced hypercapnia in acute respiratory distress syndrome. Am J Respir Crit Care Med 152:121–128, 1995.

94. Gattinoni L, Presenti A, Torresin A, et al: Adult respiratory distress syndrome profiles by computed tomography. J Thorac Imag 1:25–30, 1986.

95. DiRusso SM, Nelson LD, Safcsak K, et al: Survival in patients with severe adult respiratory distress syndrome treated with high-level positive end-expiratory pressure. Crit Care Med 23:1485–1496, 1995.

96. Witte MK, Galli SA, Ghatburn RL, et al: Optimal positive end-expiratory pressure therapy in infants and children with acute respiratory failure. Pediatr Res 24:217–221, 1988.

97. Pranikoff T, Hirschl R, Steimle C, et al: Efficacy of extracorporeal life support in the setting of adult cardiorespiratory failure. ASAIO J 40:M339–M343, 1994.

98. Moler FW, Palmisano J, Custer JR: Extracorporeal life support for pediatric respiratory failure: Predictors of survival from 220 patients. Crit Care Med 21:1604–1611, 1993.

99. Sjostrand UH, Lichtwarch-Aschoff M, Nielsen JB, et al: Different ventilatory approaches to keep the lung open. Intensive Care Med 21:310–318, 1995.

100. Papadakos PJ, Halloran W, Hessney JI, et al: The use of pressure-controlled inverse ratio ventilation in the surgical intensive care unit. J Trauma 31:1211–1214, 1991.

101. Pappert D, Rossaint R, Slama K, et al: Influence of positioning on ventilation-perfusion relationships in severe adult respiratory distress syndrome. Chest 106:1511–1516, 1994.

102. Fridrich P, Krafft P, Hochleuthner H, et al: Anesth Analg 83:1206–1211, 1996.

103. Wiener CM, Kirk W, Albert RK: Prone position reverses gravitational distribution of perfusion in dog lungs with oleic acid-induced injury. J Appl Physiol 68:1386–1392, 1990.

104. Mutoh T, Guest RJ, Lamm WJE, et al: Prone position alters the effect of volume overload on regional pleural pressures and improves hypoxemia in pigs in vivo. Am Rev Respir Dis 146:300–306, 1992.

105. Gattinoni L, Presenti A: Adult respiratory distress syndrome: Computed tomography scanning in acute respiratory failure. In Zapol WM, Lemaire S (eds): Adult Respiratory Distress Syndrome. New York: Marcel Dekker, 1991, p 199.

106. Baltopoulos G, Zakynthinos S, Dimpoulos A, et al: Effects of furosemide on pulmonary shunts. Chest 96:494–498, 1989.

107. Gattinoni L: Decreasing edema results in improved pulmonary function and survival in patients with ARDS. Intensive Care Med 12:137, 1986.

108. Simmons RS, Berdine GG, Seidenfeld JJ, et al: Fluid balance in the respiratory distress syndrome. Am Rev Respir Dis 135:924, 1987.

109. McIntyre RC Jr, Haenel JB, Moore FA, et al: Cardiopulmonary effects of permissive hypercapnia in the management of adult respiratory distress syndrome. J Trauma 37:433–438, 1994.

110. Brochard L, Rauss A, Benito S, et al: Comparison of three methods of gradual withdrawal from ventilation support during weaning from mechanical ventilation. Am J Respir Crit Care Med 150:896–903, 1995.

111. Leitch EA, Moran JL, Grealy B: Weaning and extubation in the intensive care unit: Clinical or index-driven approach? Intensive Care Med 22:752–759, 1996.

112. Esteban A, Frutos F, Tobin MJ, et al: A comparison of four methods of weaning patients from mechanical ventilation. N Engl J Med 332:345–350, 1995.

113. Ferrara TB, Georgieff MK, Ebert J, et al: Routine use of dexamethasone for the prevention of postextubation respiratory distress. J Perinatol 9:287–290, 1989.

114. Dries DJ: Weaning from mechanical ventilation. J Trauma 43:372–384, 1997.

115. Holdgaard HO, Pedersen J, Jensen RH, et al: Percutaneous dilatational tracheostomy versus conventional surgical tracheostomy: A clinical randomised study. Acta Anaesthesiol Scand 42:545–550, 1998.

116. Rosenbower TJ, Morris JA Jr, Eddy VA, et al: The long-term complications of percutaneous dilatational tracheostomy. Am Surg 64:82–87, 1998.

117. Citta-Pietrolungo TJ, Alexander MA, Cook SP, et al: Complications of tracheostomy and decannulation in pediatric and young patients with traumatic brain injury. Arch Phys Med Rehabil 74:905–909, 1993.

118. Nicks JJ, Becker MA: High-frequency ventilation of the newborn: Past, present, and future. J Respir Care Pract 16–21.

119. Clark RH: High-frequency ventilation. J Pediatr 124:661–670, 1994.

120. Minton SD, Gerstmann DR, Stoddard RA: High-frequency oscillation: Ventilator strategies to interrupt pulmonary injury sequence. J Respir Care Pract 1992, Oct/Nov: 15–31.

121. Froese AB, Bryan AC: High frequency ventilation. Am Rev Respir Dis 135:1363–1374, 1987.

122. Rouby JJ, Simonneau G, Benhamou D, et al: Factors influencing pulmonary volumes and CO_2 elimination during high-frequency jet ventilation. Anesthesiology 63:473–482, 1985.

123. Baumann MH, Sahn SA: Medical management and therapy of bronchopleural fistulas in the mechanically ventilated patient. Chest 97:721–728, 1991.

124. The HIFI Study Group: High-frequency oscillatory ventilation compared with conventional mechanical ventilation in the treatment of respiratory failure in preterm infants. N Engl J Med 320:88–93, 1989.

125. Clark RH, Gerstmann DR, Null DMJ, et al: Prospective randomized comparison of high-frequency oscillatory and conventional ventilation in respiratory distress syndrome. Pediatrics 89:5–12, 1992.

126. Keszler M, Donn SM, Bucciarelli RL, et al: Multicenter control trial comparing high frequency jet ventilation and conventional ventilation in newborn patients with pulmonary interstitial emphysema. J Pediatr 119:85–93, 1991.

127. Clark RH, Yoder BA, Sell MS: Prospective, randomized comparison of high-frequency oscillation and conventional ventilation in candidates for extracorporeal membrane oxygenation. J Pediatr 124:447–454, 1994.

128. Arnold JH, Hanson JH, Toro-Figuero LO, et al: Prospective, randomized comparison of high-frequency oscillatory ventilation and conventional mechanical ventilation in pediatric respiratory failure. Crit Care Med 22:1530–1539, 1994.

129. Rosenberg RB, Broner CW, Peters KJ, et al: High-frequency ventilation for acute pediatric respiratory failure. Chest 104:1216–1221, 1994.

130. Fort P, Farmer C, Westerman J, et al: High-frequency oscillatory ventilation for adult respiratory distress syndrome—a pilot study. Crit Care Med 25:937–947, 1997.

131. Carlon GC, Gu Y, Groeger JS, et al: Early prediction of outcome of respiratory failure: Comparison of high-frequency jet ventilation and volume-cycled ventilation. Chest 86:194–197, 1984.

132. Borg UR, Stoklosa JC, Siegel JH, et al: Prospective evaluation of combined high-frequency ventilation in post-traumatic patients with adult respiratory distress syndrome refractory to optimized conventional ventilatory management. Crit Care Med 17:1129–1142, 1990.

133. Kolobow T, Powers T, Mandava S, et al: Intratracheal pulmonary ventilation (ITPV): Control of positive end-expiratory pressure at the level of the carina through the use of a novel ITPV catheter design. Anesth Analg 78:455–461, 1994.

134. Muller EE, Kolobow T, Mandava S, et al: How to ventilate lungs as small as 12.5% of normal: The new technique of intratracheal pulmonary ventilation. Pediatr Res 34:606–610, 1993.

135. Ravenscraft SA, Burke WC, Nahum A, et al: Tracheal gas insufflation augments CO_2 clearance during mechanical ventilation. Am Rev Respir Dis 148:345–351, 1993.

136. Raszynski A, Hultquist KA, Latif H, et al: Rescue from pediatric ECMO with prolonged hybrid intratracheal pulmonary ventilation: A technique for reducing dead space ventilation and preventing ventilator induced lung injury. ASAIO J 39:M681–M685, 1993.

137. Wilson JM, Thompson JR, Schnitzer JJ, et al: Intratracheal pulmonary ventilation and congenital diaphragmatic hernia: A report of two cases. J Pediatr Surg 28:484–487, 1993.

138. Murad F: Cyclic guanosine monophosphate as a mediator of vasodilation. J Clin Invest 78:1–5, 1986.

139. Rossaint R, Falke KJ, Lopez F, et al: Inhaled nitric oxide for the adult respiratory distress syndrome. N Engl J Med 328:399–405, 1993.

140. Rossaint R, Slama K, Steudel W, et al: Effects of inhaled nitric oxide on right ventricular function in severe acute respiratory distress syndrome [see comments]. Intensive Care Med 21:197–203, 1995.

141. Dellinger RP, Zimmerman JL, Taylor RW, et al: Effects of inhaled nitric oxide in patients with acute respiratory distress syndrome: Results of a randomized phase II trial. Crit Care Med 26:15–23, 1998.

142. Day RW, Allen EM, Witte MK: A randomized, controlled study of the 1-hour and 24-hour effects of inhaled nitric oxide therapy in children with acute hypoxemic respiratory failure. Chest 112:1324–1331, 1997.

143. Abman SH, Griebel JL, Parker DK, et al: Acute effects of inhaled nitric oxide in children with severe hypoxemic respiratory failure. J Pediatr 124:881–888, 1994.

144. Kinsella JP, Neish SR, Ivy DD, et al: Clinical responses to prolonged treatment of persistent pulmonary hypertension of the newborn with low doses of inhaled nitric oxide. J Pediatr 123:103–108, 1993.

145. Finer NN, Etches PC, Kamstra B, et al: Inhaled nitric oxide in infants referred for extracorporeal membrane oxygenation: Dose response. J Pediatr 124:302–308, 1994.

146. Inhaled nitric oxide in full-term and nearly full-term infants with hypoxic respiratory failure. The Neonatal Inhaled Nitric Oxide Study Group. N Engl J Med 336:597–604, 1997.

147. Inhaled nitric oxide and hypoxic respiratory failure in infants with congenital diaphragmatic hernia. NINOS. Pediatrics 99:838–845, 1997.

148. Karamanoukian HL, Glick PL, Wilcox DT, et al: Pathophysiology of congenital diaphragmatic hernia, VIII: Inhaled nitric oxide requires exogenous surfactant therapy in the lamb model of congenital diaphragmatic hernia. J Pediatr Surg 30:1–4, 1995.

149. Haddad IY, Ischiropoulos H, Holm BA, et al: Mechanisms of peroxynitrite-induced injury to pulmonary surfactants. Am J Physiol 265:L555–L564, 1993.

150. Beckman JS, Beckman TW, Chen J, et al: Apparent hydroxyl radical production by peroxynitrite: Implications for endothelial injury from nitric oxide and superoxide. Proc Natl Acad Sci U S A 87:1620–1624, 1990.

151. Jobe AH: Pulmonary surfactant therapy. N Engl J Med 328:861–868, 1993.

152. Hallman M, Merritt TA, Jarvenpaa AL, et al: Exogenous human surfactant for treatment of severe respiratory distress syndrome: A randomized prospective clinical trial. J Pediatr 106:963–969, 1985.

153. Long W, Corbet A, Cotton R, et al: A controlled trial of synthetic surfactant in infants weighing 1250 g or more with respiratory distress syndrome. The American Exosurf Neonatal Study Group I, and the Canadian Exosurf Neonatal Study Group. N Engl J Med 325:1696–1703, 1991.

154. Vermont-Oxford NN: A multicenter, randomized trial comparing synthetic surfactant with modified bovine surfactant extract in the treatment of neonatal respiratory distress syndrome. Vermont-Oxford Neonatal Network. Pediatrics 97:1–6, 1996.

155. Lotze A, Mitchell BR, Bulas DI, et al: Multicenter study of surfactant (beractant) use in the treatment of term infants with severe respiratory failure. Survanta in Term Infants Study Group. J Pediatr 132:40–47, 1998.

156. Findlay RD, Taeusch HW, Walther FJ: Surfactant replacement therapy for meconium aspiration syndrome. Pediatrics 97:48–52, 1996.

157. Lotze A, Knight GR, Anderson KD, et al: Surfactant (beractant) therapy for infants with congenital diaphragmatic hernia on ECMO: Evidence of persistent surfactant deficiency [see comments]. J Pediatr Surg 29:407–412, 1994.

158. Wilcox DT, Glick PL, Karamanoukian H, et al: Pathophysiology of congenital diaphragmatic hernia, V: Effect of exogenous surfactant therapy on gas exchange and lung mechanics in the lamb congenital diaphragmatic hernia model. J Pediatr 124:289–293, 1994.

159. Glick PL, Leach CL, Besner GE, et al: Pathophysiology of congenital diaphragmatic hernia, III: Exogenous surfactant therapy for the high-risk neonate with CDH. J Pediatr Surg 27:866–869, 1992.

160. Shaffer TH: A brief review: Liquid ventilation. Undersea Biomed Res 14:169–179, 1987.

161. Shaffer TH, Wolfson MR, Clark L Jr: State of the art review: Liquid ventilation. Pediatr Pulmonol 14:102–109, 1992.

162. Hirschl RB, Merz S, Montoya P, et al: Development of a simplified liquid ventilator. Crit Care Med 23:157–163, 1995.

163. Fuhrman BP, Paczan PR, DeFrancisis M: Perfluorocarbon-associated gas exchange. Crit Care Med 19:712–722, 1991.

164. Hirschl RB, Tooley R, Parent AC, et al: Improvement of gas exchange, pulmonary function, and lung injury with partial liquid ventilation: A study model in a setting of severe respiratory failure. Chest 108:500–508, 1995.

165. Leach CL, Fuhrman BP, Morin FD, et al: Perfluorocarbon-associated gas exchange (partial liquid ventilation) in respiratory distress syndrome: A prospective, randomized, controlled study. Crit Care Med 21:1270–1278, 1993.

166. Major D, Cadenas M, Cloutier R, et al: Combined gas ventilation and perfluorochemical tracheal instillation as an alternative treatment for lethal congenital diaphragmatic hernia in lambs. J Pediatr Surg 30:1178–1182, 1995.

167. Wilcox DT, Glick PL, Karamanoukian HL, et al: Perfluorocarbon-associated gas exchange improves pulmonary mechanics, oxygenation, ventilation, and allows nitric oxide delivery in the hypoplastic lung congenital diaphragmatic hernia lamb model. Crit Care Med 23:1858–1863, 1995.

168. Hirschl RB, Overbeck MC, Parent A, et al: Liquid ventilation

provides uniform distribution of perfluorocarbon in the setting of respiratory failure. Surgery 116:159–167, 1994.

169. Greenspan JS, Wolfson MR, Rubenstein SD, et al: Liquid ventilation of human preterm neonates. J Pediatr 117:106–111, 1990.

170. Gauger PG, Pranikoff T, Schreiner RJ, et al: Initial experience with partial liquid ventilation in pediatric patients with the acute respiratory distress syndrome. Crit Care Med 24:16–22, 1996.

171. Hirschl RB, Pranikoff P, Wise C, et al: Initial experience with partial liquid ventilation in adult patients with the acute respiratory distress syndrome. JAMA 275:383–389, 1996.

172. Pranikoff T, Gauger P, Hirschl RB: Partial liquid ventilation in newborn patients with congenital diaphragmatic hernia. J Pediatr Surg 31:613–618, 1996.

173. Toro-Figueroa LO, Melinoes JN, Curtis SE, et al: Perflubron partial liquid ventilation (PLV) in children with ARDS: A safety and efficacy pilot study. Crit Care Med 24:A150, 1996.

174. Bartlett R, Croce M, Hirschl R, et al: Phase II randomized, controlled trial of partial liquid ventilation (PLV) in adult patients with acute hypoxemic respiratory failure (AHRF). Crit Care Med 25:A35, 1997.

175. DiFiore JW, Fauza DO, Slavin R, et al: Experimental fetal tracheal ligation reverses the structural and physiological effects of pulmonary hypoplasia in congenital diaphragmatic hernia. J Pediatr Surg 29:248–256, 1994.

176. Hedrick MH, Estes JM, Sullivan KM, et al: Plug the lung until it grows (PLUG): A new method to treat congenital diaphragmatic hernia in utero. J Pediatr Surg 29:612–617, 1994.

177. Fauza D, Hines M, Fackler J, et al: Continuous positive airway pressure with perfluorocarbon accelerates postnatal lung growth. Surg Forum 46:666–669, 1995.

7

EXTRACORPOREAL MEMBRANE OXYGENATION

Thomas T. Sato, MD • Kurt D. Newman, MD

A major, contemporary advancement in neonatal and pediatric critical care is treating respiratory failure by using extracorporeal devices capable of providing effective gas exchange and, when necessary, cardiopulmonary life support. The clinical success that extracorporeal membrane oxygenation (ECMO) has achieved reflects the effective fusion of biomedical technology, the improved understanding of the pathophysiology of respiratory failure, and the dedication of clinicians devoted to this field.

Developing and refining mechanical ventilation for infants and children since the 1970s led to an increasing number of children surviving following respiratory failure. However, a subset of infants with respiratory failure died with conventional ventilation. The clinical course of these infants was characterized by progressive respiratory failure with inadequate ventilation, ineffective gas exchange, and persistent pulmonary hypertension despite more aggressive use of conventional ventilator techniques. Ultimately, the vast majority of these critically ill newborns died from respiratory failure.

The scientific foundation for developing ECMO was laid by cardiac surgeons. The initial desire to repair congenital heart lesions under direct, intracardiac viewing led to developing techniques that diverted the circulation to an extracorporeal oxygenator. The first cardiopulmonary bypass circuits used for surgical procedures involved direct cross-circulation between the patient and another subject (usually the patient's mother or father) acting as both the pump and the oxygenator.[1] Attempts at establishing cardiopulmonary bypass using "artificial" admixture bubble oxygenators were limited by troublesome hemolysis encountered from the direct mixing of blood and oxygen.

The subsequent emergence of successful extracorporeal devices capable of supporting long-term cardiac and pulmonary function relied on the discovery of heparin use for anticoagulation and the development of semipermeable membranes capable of supporting gas exchange by diffusion.[2] Bartlett and colleagues reported the first successful application of ECMO for neonatal respiratory failure in 1976, involving a newborn with severe meconium aspiration syndrome.[3] Since that time, improvements in technology, as well as a better understanding of both the pathophysiology of diseases causing respiratory failure and the effects of extracorporeal support, have contributed to ECMO being used in more than 14,000 critically ill patients of all ages. Given the fact that most of these patients meet criteria that predict an 80% risk of death from respiratory failure, the clinical effectiveness of ECMO is demonstrated by an approximate overall survival of 80% for neonates, 53% for pediatric patients, and 41% survival for adults.[4]

The Extracorporeal Life Support Organization (ELSO) was formed in 1989. It represents the collaboration of investigators with a clinical and scientific interest in ECMO. ELSO members provide the medical community with standards, training manuals, and guidelines for the effective use of ECMO. In addition, the ELSO Registry provides investigators with a means of accruing an ECMO patient database for analysis and evaluation of this technique.

☐ Clinical Applications of ECMO

The application of extracorporeal life support has emerged since the late 1980s to include both common and uncommon newborn and pediatric conditions. The most common use of ECMO is for cardiopulmonary support of the term or near-term neonate with failure to oxygenate secondary to meconium aspiration syndrome, persistent pulmonary hypertension of the newborn (PPHN), sepsis, pneumonia, hyaline membrane disease, and congenital diaphragmatic hernia. Experience with pediatric ECMO has increased significantly since the late 1980s, particularly with respiratory failure secondary to pneumonia and for babies unweanable from bypass following cardiac surgery. Continued success with temporary extracorporeal life support has helped many institutions establish ECMO as an effective means of saving patients with an otherwise high-predicted mortality from respiratory failure.

Uncommon uses of ECMO include support of the child with respiratory failure secondary to smoke inhalation[5] and with severe asthma.[6] ECMO has also been reported to be a potentially useful strategy in complex tracheal surgery[7] and during planned hypothermic hypoperfusion for resection of large tumors such as massive sacrococcygeal teratoma.[8] ECMO, in conjunction with hemodialysis, has been used successfully for acebutolol overdose.[9] The use of ECMO to maintain a "brain-dead" organ donor before successful liver allograft harvest and transplantation was reported in 1997.[10]

☐ Pathophysiology of PPHN

Normal fetal circulation is characterized by pulmonary vascular resistance that exceeds systemic vascular resistance, resulting in higher right-sided heart pressures and preferential right-to-left blood flow. Placental blood oxygenated in the chorionic villi travels through the fetal umbilical vein to the inferior vena cava via the ductus venosus. Owing to the relatively high pulmonary vascular resistance, the vast majority of the blood that reaches the right atrium via the inferior vena cava empties directly into the left atrium through the foramen ovale. Deoxygenated venous blood returning through the superior vena cava preferentially flows into the right ventricle and pulmonary artery. Again, owing to the high pulmonary vascular resistance, the majority of this blood shunts through the ductus arteriosus into the aorta. Therefore, the upper body and head of the fetus are perfused with relatively more well-oxygenated blood than the lower body. Approximately 7 to 10% of the deoxygenated blood that enters the pulmonary artery with a Po_2 less than 20 mm Hg perfuses the pulmonary vascular bed and returns to the left atrium. As a consequence of these anatomic right-to-left shunts, most of the fetal circulating blood volume bypasses the lungs completely.

Immediately following birth, the newborn's initial breath distends the fluid-filled alveoli with air. The mechanical distention of the lungs is paralleled by expansion of the pulmonary vascular bed, causing a rapid drop in pulmonary vascular resistance to below systemic vascular resistance. The decrease in right atrial pressure to below left atrial pressure leads to closure of the foramen ovale; consequently, right atrial blood flow is redirected to the pulmonary vascular bed. Closure of the ductus arteriosus also occurs during this time, thereby closing the fetal right-to-left circulation and effectively isolating perfusion of the pulmonary vascular bed for gas exchange. This initial transition of fetal to newborn circulation is dependent on the establishment and maintenance of pressure gradients in the pulmonary and systemic circulations. Anatomic closure of the foramen ovale and ductus arteriosus occurs days to weeks following birth.

PPHN is characterized by failure of the transition from fetal circulation with high pulmonary vascular resistance to newborn circulation with low pulmonary vascular resistance and high blood flow. This condition is also known as *persistent fetal circulation*,[11] emphasizing the persistence of high pulmonary resistance and consequent right-to-left shunting through a patent foramen ovale and patent ductus arteriosus. Clinically, PPHN presents as hypoxemia that is out of proportion to the degree of pulmonary parenchymal disease.

Normally, in fetal and term infant lungs, fully muscularized, preacinar arteries extend to the terminal bronchioles. In the first few days following birth, the muscularized arteries begin to decrease in thickness and undergo structural remodeling.[12] Hypoxia in utero can induce proliferation of smooth muscle cells in the arterial media of intraacinar and alveolar arteries, resulting in abnormally thickened and reactive pulmonary vessels.[13] These vessels undergo significant vasoconstriction in response to hypoxemia, leading to a spiraling course of worsening hypoxemia in the setting of persistent pulmonary hypertension and right-to-left shunting.

Therapy for PPHN is directed at increasing pulmonary blood flow and decreasing the right-to-left shunt. Using mechanical ventilation to provide adequate gas exchange and oxygenation and using supportive management and correction of polycythemia, hypothermia, and acidosis are useful therapeutic interventions. Establishing and maintaining respiratory or metabolic alkalosis (pH 7.50) is a reasonable clinical treatment goal. Hypotension may need to be treated with volume expansion and with the judicious use of inotropic agents such as dopamine. Intravenous (IV) pharmacologic agents used to induce pulmonary vasodilation, such as tolazoline hydrochloride and nitroprusside, are relatively nonspecific, and the effects of systemic vasodilation are unpredictable. Recently, using inhaled nitric oxide to treat pulmonary hypertension in the infant with respiratory failure by transiently improving oxygenation has shown some promise; however, no improvement in overall mortality rates in these critically ill infants has been demonstrated.[14, 15]

☐ Patient Selection Criteria

Selecting patients for ECMO based on clinical criteria remains controversial. The risks of placing a critically ill newborn on an invasive and heparinized extracorporeal bypass circuit must be weighed against the estimated mortality of the infant with conventional therapy alone. Most institutions follow clinical criteria designed to select those infants who have a predicted mortality rate of 80% or greater with "optimal" conventional therapy. The definition of optimal conventional therapy remains inexact because it is largely institution specific, depending, in part, on the experience of the clinicians using currently available knowledge and technologies. Therefore, all ECMO centers must develop and continually evaluate their patient selection criteria based on their institutional experience.

Generally accepted selection criteria for using neonatal ECMO follow.

GESTATIONAL AGE >34 WEEKS OR BIRTH WEIGHT >2000 g. The use of systemic heparinization during ECMO in premature infants younger than 34 weeks' gestational age or infants weighing less than 2000 g is associated with significant morbidity and mortality from intracranial hemorrhage.[16] Data from Children's National Medical Center in Washington, D.C., suggest that the incidence of intracranial hemorrhage and subsequent death during ECMO in infants with birth weights from 2000 g to 2500 g is higher than in infants weighing more than 2500 g, validating the inherent risk of heparinization and ECMO in these children.[17] Additionally, infants weighing less than 2000 g present technical considerations secondary to the small diameter of the carotid artery available for cannulation and the flow restrictions imposed by the size of the cannula. The changes in cerebral perfusion during ECMO and the effects of ipsilateral ligation of the carotid artery and internal jugular vein following decannulation are incompletely understood.

LACK OF ACTIVE BLEEDING OR COAGULOPATHY. Infants with ongoing, uncontrolled bleeding or uncorrectable coagulopathy are at increased risk for bleeding complications during ECMO secondary to the need for systemic heparinization.[18] Infants with respiratory failure secondary to sepsis often have associated coagulopathy and can be successfully treated with ECMO with aggressive, early correction of the coagulopathy using appropriate blood products, along with vigilant attention to anticoagulation with heparin.[19] Infants with grade I intraventricular hemorrhage or small intraparenchymal hemorrhage, if deemed necessary, can be successfully treated with ECMO using lower activated clotting times (ACTs) in the range of 180 to 200 seconds. Patients with more extensive intracranial hemorrhage, infarction, or ischemic injury should be considered at high risk for complications, and care must be individualized.

REVERSIBLE LUNG DYSFUNCTION. Effective use of ECMO relies on the concepts that the cause of the respiratory failure is acute, the underlying pulmonary disease is reversible, and the reversal of pulmonary dysfunction will occur in a relatively short period. Exposure to high-inspired concentrations of oxygen and repetitive, high-positive-pressure mechanical ventilation have been implicated in developing bronchopulmonary dysplasia. The risk of developing this more chronic form of pulmonary dysfunction may occur within the first 4 days of aggressive conventional ventilation.[20]

The pulmonary dysfunction induced by oxygen toxicity or barotrauma typically requires weeks to months for resolution, making it unsuitable for short-term therapy with ECMO. Therefore, a maximum limit of 10 to 14 days of mechanical ventilation prior to ECMO is widely accepted owing to the high probability of developing more chronic pulmonary dysfunction during this interval. Although the maximal duration that a patient can be supported by ECMO is unknown, the risk of complications with ECMO increases directly with the duration of bypass, and, consequently, most centers use 21 days as the upper limit of time on bypass.

ABSENCE OF LETHAL CONGENITAL OR UNCORRECTABLE CARDIAC DISEASE. Every attempt must be made to identify infants with congenital anomalies incompatible with survival before considering ECMO for respiratory failure. Infants with congenital anomalies do not benefit from ECMO.

Additionally, infants with uncorrectable cardiac disease should be identified by echocardiography and, if necessary, angiography, before offering ECMO therapy. Technical considerations may also be influenced by local anatomic findings; for example, venoarterial (VA) ECMO is contraindicated in infants with coarctation of the aorta. Infants with reversible respiratory failure and correctable cardiac disease should be considered for ECMO on an individual basis because a successful ECMO run can provide effective cardiopulmonary support prior to definitive cardiac surgery.

NEONATAL ECMO RISK ASSESSMENT

For the infant with respiratory failure despite aggressive, optimal medical therapy, ECMO may provide an effective means of rescue. In neonates, because of the invasive nature of ECMO and the potentially life-threatening complications, several investigators have tried to characterize factors capable of predicting which infants have 80% mortality without ECMO. Two such measurements are the alveolar-arterial oxygen gradient (PaO_2-PaO_2) and the oxygenation index (OI), calculated as follows:

Alveolar-Arterial Oxygen Gradient

$$AaDO_2 = (P_{atm} - 47)(FiO_2) - \frac{(PaCO_2)}{0.8} - PaO_2$$

where P_{atm} = atmospheric pressure
FiO_2 = inspired concentration of oxygen

Oxygenation Index

$$OI = \frac{MAP \times FiO_2 \times 100}{PaO_2}$$

where MAP = mean airway pressure

Each institution's criteria for ECMO varies according to the cause of respiratory failure and the local clinician's experience. In addition, the definition of optimal medical management for respiratory failure evolves as refinements and improved therapies emerge. However, it is generally accepted that, in the setting of maximal therapy, a PaO_2-PaO_2 greater than 600 to 620 mm Hg for 4 to 12 hours, or an oxygenation index of 25 to 60 for 30 minutes to

6 hours establishes both a relatively sensitive and specific predictor of mortality. Other qualifying criteria to consider for ECMO include a PaO_2 less than 35 to 50 mm Hg for 2 to 12 hours; acute clinical deterioration manifested as a PaO_2 less than 35 to 40 mm Hg; or a pH less than 7.25 for 2 hours with intractable hypotension. These are sustained values as measured over time, reflecting the fact that a single measurement does not accurately predict mortality or outcome. Recommended pre-ECMO studies are listed in Table 7–1.

☐ Venoarterial Versus Venovenous ECMO

There are two major modes of ECMO: VA and venovenous (VV). VA ECMO uses two separate cannulas: one for venous outflow placed in the right atrium and another for arterial return placed at the aortic arch. Typical cannulation sites are the right internal jugular vein and the right common carotid artery via a single cervical incision. Although most infants requiring ECMO have isolated respiratory failure, some infants have significant cardiac dysfunction resulting from hypoxia and right heart failure secondary to pulmonary hypertension. VA ECMO provides both gas exchange and cardiac support for these patients, and is the standard of therapy in many institutions. Some concerns have been raised regarding VA ECMO, however, including ligation of the carotid artery, loss of pulsatile cerebral and systemic blood flow dynamics, and particulate or air emboli reaching the cerebral or coronary vascular beds. Carotid artery ligation alone does not consistently change cerebral arterial blood flow velocity, but the addition of venous occlusion can cause significant reduction of cerebral arterial blood flow velocity during VA ECMO.[21] However, no consistent differences in the incidence of intracranial hemorrhage have been identified in comparing VA and VV ECMO.[22]

In response to the concerns with VA ECMO, VV ECMO has emerged as an alternative therapy option in selected infants. VV ECMO uses a single cannula with two separate lumina placed into the right atrium via the internal jugular vein. Both venous outflow and oxygenated "arterial" return occur in the right atrium. This technique requires intact cardiac function, and, at high flow rates, there can be significant recirculation in the right atrium, leading to limited oxygenation.[23, 24] Reduction of recirculation and improvement of oxygenation has been achieved with improvements in cannula design.[25] The potential problems with ligation of the carotid artery, loss of pulsatile blood flow dynamics, and emboli are reduced or eliminated with VV ECMO.

Retrospective data from the ELSO Registry evaluating complications during ECMO suggest an overall higher survival rate and lower incidence of major neurologic events (seizures, infarction) with VV ECMO.[26] In a matched comparison of infants with respiratory failure from the ELSO Registry treated with either VA or VV ECMO, survival advantage for VV ECMO was observed when matched for respiratory failure alone, but survival was not significantly greater with VV ECMO when matched for degree of respiratory and hemodynamic failure; however, hemolysis and cannula kinking were more common with VV ECMO.[22]

Because blood flow rates are directly proportional to the fourth power of the tubing radius and inversely proportional to the tubing length, the rate of blood flow through the circuit depends on cannula size and length of raceway tubing. To maximize circuit flow and hence, oxygenation, the largest-lumen venous cannula with the shortest circuit length possible should be used. The arterial cannula is typically the smallest diameter element in the circuit and therefore represents the highest resistance to flow. Once again, the largest-diameter arterial cannula that can fit in the infant's carotid artery with the shortest circuit tubing distance is ideal.

CANNULATION AND INITIATION OF BYPASS

Techniques for ECMO cannulation and decannulation vary with institutional and individual preferences. However, we have found it beneficial to use a standardized operative approach for cannulation and decannulation. The vast majority of ECMO procedures are performed in neonatal and pediatric intensive care units. A full operating team should be assembled with adequate equipment, including mobile electrocautery and light sources. All team members—neonatologists, surgeons, critical care nursing staff, perfusionists, and respiratory therapists—should be immediately available. When time permits, cross-matched blood should be available and brought to the intensive care unit; with the emergent need for cannulation, O Rh-negative blood may be used. A syringe of blood (10 ml/kg) should be drawn and available for transfusion and emergencies. All infants requiring ECMO should be considered candidates for surfactant replacement therapy.[27]

The infant is placed on a bed with an overhead warmer, with the infant's head at the foot of the bed. The ventilator and tubing are extended to the

TABLE 7–1. Recommended Pre-ECMO Studies

Head ultrasound
Cardiac echocardiogram
Chest radiograph
Complete blood count, platelets
Type and cross
Electrolytes, calcium
Coagulation studies (PT, PTT, fibrinogen, fibrin degradation
  products)
Serial arterial blood gases

ECMO, extracorporeal membrane oxygenation; PT, prothrombin time; PTT, partial thromboplastin time.

infant's left side, and the primed ECMO circuit is positioned on the infant's right side. Placing a towel roll underneath the shoulders places the infant's neck in slight hyperextension. Adequate analgesia is administered along with a long-acting muscle relaxant. Local infiltrative anesthesia with lidocaine is also used.

A 2-cm incision is made over the right sternocleidomastoid muscle using electrocautery. Meticulous hemostasis is necessary throughout the procedure. Exposure of the internal jugular vein and common carotid artery is achieved by dissecting through the sternocleidomastoid muscle. The carotid artery and internal jugular vein are encircled with 2-0 silk ties, and the infant is systemically anticoagulated with 75 to 150 units/kg of heparin. The dose of heparin can be modulated based on the estimated risk of bleeding and guided by the ACT. Following adequate circulation time, the carotid artery is ligated cephalad, with proximal control obtained with a bulldog clamp. A transverse arteriotomy is made, and two 6-0 polypropylene (Prolene) stay sutures are used to control the arteriotomy and prevent intimal dissection. The artery is dilated if necessary, and an appropriate-size cannula is inserted through the arteriotomy and to the level of the aortic arch. The arterial cannula is secured into place using additional 2-0 silk sutures tied over a small piece of vessel loop. The cephalad tie used to ligate the carotid artery is also secured around the cannula. A blood specimen for an ACT measurement can be obtained from the cannula at this time.

Venous cannulation is performed in identical fashion. Owing to the multiple fenestrations in the venous cannula and the relative fragility of the vein, care must be taken during cannulation. Compressing the liver and momentarily holding ventilation during venous cannulation helps prevent an air embolus. Air bubbles remaining in the cannulas or circuit tubing are removed using heparized saline, and the cannulas are firmly secured to the circuit tubing. Bypass can be initiated either immediately in the unstable patient or following confirmation of cannula position by chest film or sonography[28] in the stable patient. In patients with coagulopathy, using a modified topical fibrin sealant may help improve hemostasis in the cannulation wound.[29] The skin incision is closed with a running suture using an atraumatic needle, and the cannulas are sutured to the infant's skin to prevent dislodgment. A transparent dressing is preferred because it allows monitoring of the wound during systemic anticoagulation.

Bypass flow is initiated and increased as determined by pulse oximetry and an in-line venous saturation monitor. Estimation of neonatal cardiac output at approximately 200 ml/kg/min is used to calculate percent bypass. The goal of ECMO is to perfuse the infant and provide adequate oxygen delivery, allowing the lungs to "rest." This can be achieved with ECMO flow rates of 120 to 150 ml/kg/min, or approximately 60% of total cardiac output. In general, VA ECMO bypass flow rates are

increased 50 ml every 5 minutes. Concomitantly, the ventilator settings are incrementally decreased as long as adequate arterial and venous oxygen saturation are maintained. Typical resting ventilator settings for an infant on full VA ECMO support include a pressure limit at 15 to 18 cm H_2O, intermittent mandatory ventilation rate 15 to 20 breaths per minute, positive end-expiratory pressure 5 cm H_2O, and an FiO_2 of .21. The initiation of VV ECMO bypass must be done more slowly, usually at 30 ml every 5 minutes, and conversion to VA ECMO should be considered if the infant remains persistently hypotensive or hypoxemic or if ventilator settings cannot be decreased in the face of increasing bypass.

Some patients exhibit significant reduction in cardiac output or myocardial "stun" following initiation of bypass, characterized by a narrow pulse pressure and nearly equivalent PaO_2 values between patient and pump.[30] Although this condition is not well understood, infants with more pronounced hypoxia or prebypass ischemia are more likely to develop cardiac stun. Therapy consists of providing enough ECMO flow to supply cardiac output until the myocardium recovers.

Following establishment of bypass, pressors can be weaned and systemic anticoagulation must be maintained with ACT measurements between 200 to 220 seconds. IV antibiotics such as ampicillin and gentamicin are also given for the duration of bypass. Serial blood samples for a complete blood count, platelets, electrolytes, glucose, and calcium are obtained every 8 hours. The hemoglobin is kept at 14 to 18 g/dl, and the platelet count is maintained above 60,000 mm³. Given the relatively high risk of cerebrovascular injury in infants treated with ECMO, daily head ultrasonographic (US) surveillance is extremely useful to help identify major intracranial hemorrhage.[31]

Owing to the need for systemic heparinization while on ECMO, invasive procedures are relatively contraindicated. We discourage nasopharyngeal suctioning, heel sticks, venipunctures, and intramuscular injections during ECMO. Should bedside invasive procedures such as chest tube placement become necessary while on bypass, we use electrocautery and maintain meticulous hemostasis.

Maintenance fluid requirements while on ECMO are 80 to 120 ml/kg/day, with parenteral caloric requirements of approximately 378 kJ (90 kcal)/kg/day. Urinary output of 1 to 2 ml/kg/h is adequate. Maintenance sodium requirements are somewhat lower, about 1 to 2 mEq/kg/day, with potassium requirements as high as 4 to 5 mEq/kg/day. Sedation without neuromuscular blockade is used throughout most of the ECMO run. Virtually all medications, fluids, and parenteral nutrition can be given via the ECMO circuit ports. Should renal failure develop, hemofiltration or ultrafiltration can be accomplished via the ECMO circuit. Care must be exercised during the run to periodically monitor the arterial blood gas values, hemoglobin, platelet count, and coagulation factor studies.

Following initiation of ECMO, the chest radiograph often demonstrates complete opacification of the lung fields ("white-out").[32] This effect is probably multifactorial, including reducing ventilatory peak inspiratory pressure and positive end-expiratory pressure with establishment of cardiopulmonary bypass. The ECMO circuit itself may also contribute to initiating and maintaining a systemic inflammatory response in the neonate, producing diffuse pulmonary infiltrates as a manifestation of this process. Early pulmonary deterioration after neonatal ECMO initiation is associated with the activation of circulating neutrophils and the production of proinflammatory cytokines.[33, 34] In addition, there are measurable, systemic activation and consumption of coagulation factors during ECMO, reflecting a generalized inflammatory process that may, in part, be a host response to the ECMO membrane and circuit.[35]

ECMO CIRCUIT

Blood is removed from the infant by passive gravity drainage through the venous outflow cannula into a venous bladder or reservoir (Fig. 7–1). An in-line circuit venous return monitor (VRM) continuously analyzes the amount of venous blood in the bladder and ensures that the venous outflow from the patient equals the arterial flow from the pump. The VRM alarms and automatically shuts off the pump if venous return to the bladder decreases for any reason. Once the lost volume in the bladder is restored, the VRM stops alarming and the pump continues to run.

One of the most common causes of decreased venous inflow to the ECMO circuit is hypovolemia. The height of the infant's bed can also be raised to improve venous drainage by gravity. Without the VRM, running the pump without adequate venous inflow causes the raceway tubing to collapse; the resultant negative pressure generated pulls air out of solution ("cavitation") and causes air emboli in the circuit. Figure 7–2 outlines a suggested algorithm for managing inadequate venous return during ECMO.

A displacement roller pump directs the blood through the membrane lung, where gas exchange occurs as a consequence of gas pressure gradients. Most ECMO roller pumps currently used are designed with a microprocessor that allows for calculation of blood flow based on the pump head revolutions per minute and the size of tubing in the circuit. Blood is then rewarmed to body temperature in a countercurrent heat exchanger and returned to the infant via the arterial cannula.

Control of the gas mixture in the membrane lung is achieved by a gas delivery system with three major components: (1) oxygen flowmeter assembly (both high and low flow); (2) carbon dioxide flowmeter; and (3) air-oxygen blender. A precise Fio_2

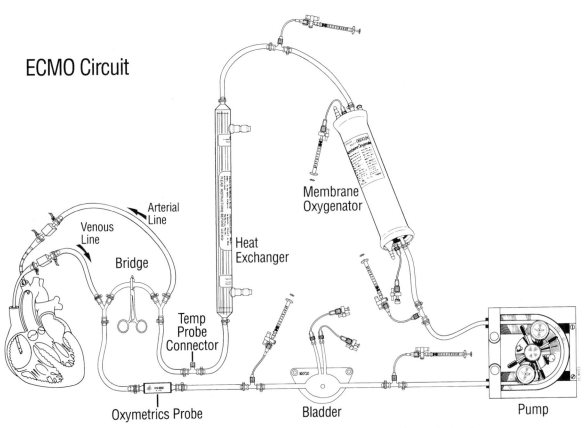

ECMO Circuit

Venous Line

Arterial Line

Bridge

Heat Exchanger

Membrane Oxygenator

Temp Probe Connector

Oxymetrics Probe

Bladder

Pump

Figure 7–1. Diagram of extracorporeal membrane oxygenation (ECMO) circuit.

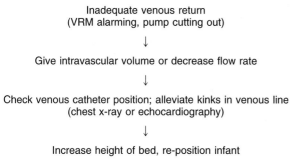

Inadequate venous return
(VRM alarming, pump cutting out)

↓

Give intravascular volume or decrease flow rate

↓

Check venous catheter position; alleviate kinks in venous line
(chest x-ray or echocardiography)

↓

Increase height of bed, re-position infant

↓

Check venous bladder function

↓

Sedate infant; consider trial of neuromuscular blockade

↓

Place additional venous cannula if required

Figure 7–2. Suggested algorithm for the management of inadequate venous return during extracorporeal membrane oxygenation. VRM, venous return monitor. (Adapted from Zwischenberger JB, Upp JR Jr: Emergencies during extracorporeal membrane oxygenation and their management. In Zwischenberger JB, Bartlett RH [eds]: ECMO: Extracorporeal cardiopulmonary support in critical care. Ann Arbor, Extracorporeal Life Support Organization, 1995, pp 221–249.)

can be achieved using the air-oxygen blender at low- or high-flow rates. While the infant is on ECMO, his or her oxygen delivery is determined primarily by the ECMO blood flow rates and the hemoglobin level; this reflects the fact that the functioning membrane oxygen gradient is extremely large (approximately 760 mm Hg in the membrane and 40 mm Hg in the infant's blood). Therefore, with a PO_2 greater than 100 mm Hg, the infant's blood traveling through the ECMO circuit is maximally saturated with oxygen, and raising the infant's PO_2 further does not significantly increase oxygen delivery. To increase the infant's oxygen delivery, either (1) the ECMO flow rates (i.e., the amount of cardiac bypass) must be increased; or (2) the hemoglobin must be increased. The PCO_2 is determined predominantly by the ECMO membrane gas flow. CO_2 elimination is extremely efficient in the membrane lung, and CO_2 must be added to maintain a normal PCO_2 in the range 40 to 45 mm Hg. Because blood returning to the infant is via the aortic arch (during VA ECMO), the pump PCO_2 is more reflective of the blood reaching the brain's respiratory center. During weaning, a low pump PCO_2 inhibits the infant's spontaneous respiratory efforts and causes relative hypoventilation and systemic hypercarbia. Vigilant monitoring allows for the timely adjustments of gas mixture and flow rates during ECMO bypass.

The current membrane oxygenator in use in the United States consists of a reinforced silicone rubber membrane that surrounds a plastic screen. The membrane envelope is wound around a polycarbonate spool and is enclosed by a silicone sleeve. Gas flows into the inside of the membrane envelope and exchanges by diffusion with the blood flowing on the external surface of the membrane. The surface area of the membrane is typically chosen for the weight of the patient; in most newborns, a membrane with surface area of 0.8 m² is used. With this surface area, oxygen transfer can reach approximately 70 ml/min/m². The blood compartment pressure gradient across the membrane oxygenator should be kept around 100 to 200 mm Hg, always exceeding the gas compartment pressure to avoid air embolization.

WEANING AND DECANNULATION

"Typical" neonatal ECMO runs have a duration of approximately 5 days (cardiac and congenital diaphragmatic hernia patients are exceptions). With improvement in the lungs, less blood flow is required to pass through the ECMO circuit, and the flow can be weaned slowly in 10 to 20 ml/min increments. The measurement of mixed venous oxygen saturation from the right atrial venous cannula can be used to effectively wean bypass as long as there is no hemodynamically significant intracardiac shunt and the infant's cardiac output, hemoglobin, and metabolic rate remain stable.

ECMO flow rates are weaned as conventional ventilatory support is increased until successfully achieving 10% bypass. This "idle" flow rate is maintained for 6 to 8 hours to ensure that the infant can be maintained on acceptable settings using conventional ventilation. Measuring lung compliance as an indicator of pulmonary recovery has also been useful; neonatal lung compliance of 0.8 ml/cm H_2O/kg or greater is associated with a level of pulmonary improvement allowing successful ECMO decannulation.[36]

Decannulation is performed in nearly identical fashion to cannulation; when possible, the same ECMO team members perform the procedure. Cross-matched blood should be brought to the patient's bedside, and 10 ml/kg of blood is drawn into a syringe for emergency transfusion. We have routinely used IV sedation, analgesia, and neuromuscular blockade to prevent spontaneous inspiration and possible air embolus caused by negative inspiratory effort during venous cannula removal. The infant's ventilator settings must be increased following paralysis.

Following positioning of the infant, the neck and cannulas are prepped in sterile fashion. Care should be taken to prepare enough of the chest wall in the unlikely event that partial sternotomy is necessary for emergent proximal control of the vessels during decannulation. The neck wound is reopened and explored, and the arterial and venous cannulas are isolated. The infant is taken off bypass and the cannulas are clamped. The venous cannula is typically removed first to allow better exposure. An inspiratory hold must be performed during venous cannula removal to prevent air embolus. The venous cannula is removed and the vessel controlled with a Satinsky clamp. The vessel is ligated. The arterial cannula is removed in similar fashion; however, there is no need for inspiratory hold or liver compression. Following decannulation, the wound is examined for hemostasis, and 1 mg of protamine is often given to reverse the effects of the remaining heparin. The wound is closed according to surgeon preference.

Some patients should be considered "at risk" for requiring a second course of ECMO despite successful weaning to idle flow. This group includes infants with congenital diaphragmatic hernia, patients with a high oxygenation index prior to ECMO, and patients requiring a lengthy initial ECMO run. In a survey of ELSO centers, approximately one third used a technique of retaining the ECMO cannulas in position for high-risk patients.[37] This strategy evolved to avoid the need to reexplore the neck for replacing ECMO cannulas should a second course of ECMO be required. The infant must remain anticoagulated to prevent thromboembolic complications. If retention of ECMO cannulas is considered, a definitive time period should be set, usually less than 24 hours, during which the infant is either placed back on ECMO or decannulated. The risk of retaining, or "hanging," the ECMO cannulas with the potential for lethal thrombotic complications must be carefully weighed against the benefit of being able to immediately place the infant back on ECMO.

Some institutions consider repair of the common carotid artery rather than ligation following decannulation.[38, 39] The infants selected for carotid artery reconstruction should be without major intracranial hemorrhage or cerebral injury, have adequate vessels for reconstruction, and have a favorable prognosis. Short-term follow-up demonstrates acceptable patency rates[39, 40] and an equivalent 1-year neurodevelopmental outcome when compared with infants undergoing carotid artery ligation.[39] Long-term follow-up is necessary to determine whether carotid artery reconstruction is a durable and desirable technical procedure to perform in ECMO survivors.

COMPLICATIONS

Mechanical Complications

Membrane Failure

Membrane failure is characterized by retention of carbon dioxide or a decrease in oxygenation. Both water condensation and fibrin clot formation can obstruct the membrane's ability to perform gas exchange by diffusion. Additionally, the membrane should not be subjected to extremely high outflow pressures as determined by flow rate and arterial cannula size. The formation of water vapor coming from the membrane gas exit port, along with an increase in pump Pco_2, can be the first sign of impending membrane failure secondary to water condensation and should be handled emergently. Similarly, the progressive consumption of coagulation factors, including platelets, indicates that the mem-

brane may need to be changed if ECMO is still required.

Raceway Tubing Rupture

Tubing rupture was more commonly seen with the polyvinyl chloride tubing used in the past. Contemporary circuit tubing is now modified for increased durability and better fatigue characteristics, making raceway tubing rupture infrequent. The circuit tubing can rupture when the roller occlusion pressure is too high; therefore, the circuit must be inspected carefully throughout the bypass run. In addition, the circuit connections must be secured properly and replaced if broken or defective. Should raceway rupture occur, the pump must be turned off immediately and the infant must be emergently taken off bypass until a new raceway and pump roller head are installed.

Accidental Decannulation

Securely fixing the cannulas into position and closely supervising the area around the infant's head can prevent accidental decannulation. Unexpected decannulation is a surgical emergency, and immediate pressure must be placed on the neck wound. The infant must be taken off bypass immediately, and conventional ventilatory settings must be increased. There is significant blood loss, and backup blood should be obtained. The neck incision must be reexplored to prevent further hemorrhage and to replace cannula(s) for reestablishing bypass.

Patient Complications

Air Embolism

Air in the ECMO circuit, with the potential for causing air embolism, is one of the most feared and devastating complications that can occur on bypass. Removal of all visible air bubbles using heparinized saline is essential during cannulation. Care must be exercised when performing venous cannulation and decannulation to prevent the accidental entry of air into the right heart. There are numerous entry points for air in the circuit, including connectors, stopcocks, and the oxygenator, and the circuit must be continually watched by bedside personnel. Air on the arterial side of the circuit demands that the infant be taken immediately off bypass. Air on the venous side of the circuit typically is trapped near the bridge or venous return bladder and can usually be "walked" to a convenient site proximal to the oxygenator and aspirated.

If air enters the patient via the aortic cannula, the infant must be immediately taken off ECMO, hand-bagged, and placed in Trendelenburg's position in an attempt to prevent air from entering the cerebral circulation. Vigorous aspiration of the arterial cannula should be performed to remove any air remaining in the cannula or proximal aorta. Inotropic support may be required if air has entered the coronary circulation. The infant should not be placed back on the ECMO circuit until the cause of the air embolus is identified and corrected.

Intracranial Hemorrhage and Other Bleeding

One of the most frequently observed patient complications in neonatal ECMO is related to intracranial hemorrhage, infarction, or cerebral edema. These central nervous system injuries occur in as many as 35% of infants on ECMO[25] and, in part, may reflect the degree and duration of pre-ECMO hypoxemia or hypotension. The neurologic status of the infant must be constantly evaluated, and a careful search must be performed in the presence of new-onset seizure activity while on ECMO. Daily head US examinations are essential, and in the presence of a new onset moderate (grade II) hemorrhage or expanding intracranial hematoma, discontinuation of ECMO and reversal of anticoagulation are advisable.

Bleeding from the neck cannulation wound is not uncommon, and efforts should be made to ensure that the infant has an appropriate ACT, a platelet count greater than 100,000/mm^3 and adequate coagulation factors. Some data suggest that maintaining a platelet count greater than 200,000/mm^3 may help decrease the overall bleeding complication rate.[42] Persistent bleeding from the wound that exceeds 10 ml/h for longer than 2 hours, despite optimizing coagulation status, necessitates local wound exploration.

One strategy for infants at risk for bleeding while on ECMO (i.e., prebypass coagulopathy, preexisting intraventricular hemorrhage, or recent or planned invasive procedures) is to use high-flow, low-ACT bypass. The high flow (60 to 70% of estimated total cardiac output) allows relatively less anticoagulation, as reflected by lower ACT values (160 to 170 seconds). In this situation, lung compliance measurements can help determine when an infant is capable of coming off bypass. ECMO flow is then weaned relatively rapidly, and as flow is decreased, additional heparin is given to prolong the ACT and prevent thrombosis in the circuit. The use of heparin-bonded tubing with ECMO may also help to prevent circuit thrombosis during bypass.[43]

Infants at risk for bleeding on ECMO can also be treated with agents that inhibit fibrinolysis to help prevent hemorrhagic complications. Administering IV aminocaproic acid at an initial bolus of 100 mg/kg, followed by continuous infusion at 30 mg/kg/h, either just before or after cannulation, has been shown to decrease bleeding and subsequent transfusion requirements, particularly in infants requiring operative procedures; additionally, a significant reduction in the incidence of intracranial hemorrhage was noted in the infants treated with aminocaproic acid.[44] Other antifibrinolytic agents, such as tranexamic acid, have been used during operative diaphragmatic hernia repair during ECMO to significantly decrease bleeding and transfusion requirements; however, thrombotic complications thought to be secondary to the antifibrinolytic therapy have also been observed.[45]

Patent Ductus Arteriosus

With the dramatic decrease in pulmonary artery pressure, most infants develop a left-to-right shunt through the patent ductus arteriosus (PDA) during the first 48 hours on ECMO. The manifestations of a PDA on ECMO include less efficient oxygenation, persistent pulmonary edema, poor urinary output secondary to poor peripheral perfusion, and an ability to obtain unexpectedly high ECMO flow rates without setting off the VRM. In general, the PDA closes spontaneously with medical management, including fluid restriction to 80 to 100 ml/kg/day and diuresis by the administration of furosemide. Owing to the effects on platelet function, we have not advocated using indomethacin during ECMO. Rarely is operative closure of a persistent PDA required while on ECMO.

Miscellaneous Complications

Aortic dissection complicating arterial cannulation can occur with VA ECMO and can manifest as diminished lower extremity pulses following decannulation.[46] Diagnosis is confirmed with either transthoracic or transesophageal echocardiography or aortic arch angiography. We have employed routine transmural vascular stay sutures during arterial cannulation to prevent intimal dissection. We have also used stay sutures during venous cannulation to prevent inadvertent loss of the internal jugular vein deep to the clavicle and into the mediastinum.

An extremely rare form of acquired hypercoagulability associated with the use of heparin (heparin-induced or associated thrombocytopenia and thrombosis) has been reported during ECMO.[47] Induction of this hypercoaguable state is thought to be secondary to antibodies directed against heparin–platelet factor 4 complexes.

Exposure to the plasticizer di(2-ethylhexyl)phthalate (DEHP) during ECMO has also been reported.[48] DEHP leaches from the circuit tubing, with the concentrations related to the total tubing surface area. This exposure appears to be eliminated by using heparin-bonded circuit tubing. Although short-term toxicity has not been observed, the effect of exposure to this plasticizer remains unknown.

The overall incidence of nosocomial infections during ECMO has been reported as high as 30%, with associated risk factors for infection including the duration of ECMO, the length of hospitalization, and surgical procedures prior to or during ECMO.[49] ELSO Registry data from 5001 neonatal VA ECMO patients documented bacterial infection in 2.9% and fungal infection in 0.6% of patients, with fungal infection carrying a significantly higher hospital mortality rate.[50] Overall morbidity and mortality appear to be greater in neonates with the onset of sepsis while on ECMO.[51] Given the need for blood products, infants treated with ECMO are also at risk for developing bloodborne infectious disease. In a recent study, approximately 8% of a group of children who were treated with ECMO as newborns were seropositive for antibodies to hepatitis C virus.[52]

□ Operative Procedures While on ECMO

Although the infant on ECMO is systemically anticoagulated, operative procedures, when deemed necessary, can be performed successfully during extracorporeal bypass. Unlike cardiopulmonary bypass for repair of congenital heart defects, however, immediate reversal of anticoagulation following operation may not be possible in the infant on ECMO owing to the need for continued extracorporeal support. Therefore, surgical approaches to the infant requiring invasive procedures while on ECMO must take into account the need for continued postoperative anticoagulation.

The ECMO team is assembled, and the infant is placed on high-flow, low-ACT bypass settings. Platelets are given to maintain an adequate level, and blood products are made immediately available. The continuous IV infusion of aminocaproic acid should be considered for all major operations. To minimize the risk of transport during ECMO, we have typically performed operations either in the neonatal intensive care unit (NICU) or in the operating room immediately adjacent to the NICU. The basic principles of meticulous surgical technique should be emphasized. The liberal use of electrocautery while minimizing dissection is recommended.

The issues regarding the timing of and techniques for repair of congenital diaphragmatic hernia (CDH) are discussed elsewhere in this text. It should be noted that CDH repair while on ECMO has been associated with a higher occurrence of surgical-site hemorrhage requiring transfusion (38%) when compared with CDH repair either before or after ECMO (18% and 6%, respectively).[53] Large diaphragmatic defects or defects that cannot be closed primarily without significant dissection are closed with a Gore-Tex soft-tissue patch to minimize surgical site bleeding. Temporary abdominal wall reconstruction and closure using a prosthetic patch[54] can effectively manage difficulty or inability replacing the viscera into the infant's abdominal cavity while he or she is on ECMO.

Open lung biopsy during ECMO has also been reported in pediatric patients and may be useful in some instances to provide diagnostic and prognostic data.[55] Bronchoscopy and thoracic and abdominal operations can be performed successfully during ECMO, with the caveats that hemostasis must be exact and vigilance for surgical-site bleeding must be maintained.

□ Results

The contemporary use of ECMO in managing neonatal respiratory failure reflects the evolution and

TABLE 7–2. ECMO Cases by Patient Group (ELSO Registry, 1980–1995)

Indication	No. of Cases	Survival (%)
Neonatal respiratory failure	10,391	80
Pediatric	982	53
Neonatal/pediatric cardiac failure	1,491	43
Adult	197	41

ECMO, extracorporeal membrane oxygenation; ELSO, Extracorporeal Life Support Organization.

refinement of a previously experimental technique that is now accepted therapy. The establishment of an international ECMO Registry by ELSO has allowed patient data accumulation and analysis from 111 active ECMO centers throughout the world. An overall survival of 75% for all ECMO patients was observed in the first 10,000 patients registered, with a higher survival rate in neonates and lower survival rates in children and adults (Table 7–2).

A decline in the overall number of ECMO cases reported to the ELSO Registry has been noted since the mid-1990s. The observed decrease in case volume is thought to reflect improvements in less invasive ventilatory management strategies in selected infants and children, including the use of exogenous surfactant, high-frequency oscillatory ventilation, and inhaled nitric oxide. Review of 1995 ELSO Registry data demonstrates that newborns with meconium aspiration requiring ECMO continue to have the best survival rate (93%), whereas ECMO survival for infants with congenital diaphragmatic hernia is 58% (Table 7–3). Infants with PPHN or respiratory distress syndrome have ECMO survival rates of 83% and 84%, respectively. In patients with cardiac arrest or failure prior to going on ECMO, the survival is 60%, whereas infants placed on ECMO based on measured $AaDO_2$ or oxygenation index criteria predicting 80% mortality have an 86% survival. There have been no significant differences in the ECMO survival rates for any neonatal diagnostic group since 1991.[56]

TABLE 7–3. Neonatal ECMO Cases (ELSO Registry, July 1995)

Indication	No. of Cases	Survival (%)
Meconium aspiration syndrome	3,771	94
Respiratory distress syndrome	1,116	84
PFC/PPHN	1,391	83
Pneumonia/sepsis	1,611	76
Congenital diaphragmatic hernia	2,081	58
Other	379	74
TOTAL	**10,349**	**80**

ECMO, extracorporeal membrane oxygenation; ELSO, Extracorporeal Life Support Organization; PFC, persistent fetal circulation; PPHN, persistent pulmonary hypertension of the newborn.

Neurodevelopmental outcome in ECMO survivors has been generally encouraging. Approximately 60 to 70% of neonatal ECMO survivors are developmentally normal when evaluated at 1 to 2 years of age.[57, 58] In a prospective cohort study of 103 5-year-old children treated with ECMO at Children's National Medical Center in Washington, D.C., major disability was present in 17 (16%), and an increased risk for school-age academic difficulties and behavioral problems was observed.[59] The fact that a percentage of ECMO survivors have developmental delay must be weighed against the almost certain mortality without ECMO.

Baseline neurologic assessment, including diagnostic imaging of the brain with either computed tomography or magnetic resonance imaging, and hearing screening are recommended for all ECMO survivors[60] because some of these patients have neuroimaging abnormalities not detected by cranial US alone. Both intracranial hemorrhage and ischemic lesions can be demonstrated in both cerebral hemispheres, and the extent of these abnormalities has been found to correlate well with the severity of neurologic delay.[61] Extension of a preexisting intracranial hemorrhage secondary to systemic anticoagulation and ischemia or infarction secondary to cerebral emboli are constant risks during ECMO. However, a large proportion of cerebrovascular injury in this high-risk group may occur as a result of hypoxia before ECMO rather than directly relate to the effects of cannulation, carotid artery ligation, and changes in cerebral blood flow. Long-term multidisciplinary follow-up is recommended for all ECMO survivors.

A total of 942 pediatric cases of respiratory failure managed with ECMO were recorded in the ELSO Registry as of July 1995, with an overall survival of 53% (Table 7–4).[62] The pediatric population is represented by a wide age range, as well as by diverse causes of respiratory failure. The delineation of selection criteria in this population remains inexact. The vast majority of pediatric patients are treated with ECMO for respiratory failure unresponsive to conventional medical management. As noted, the mortality is higher, and the duration of

ECMO bypass required tends to be longer. Both VA and VV ECMO have been used, albeit with a higher rate of mechanical complications recorded as compared to the neonatal ECMO data. It is generally felt that the higher complication rate with pediatric ECMO reflects the longer duration of bypass required for reversal of respiratory failure in this group.

ECMO has also been used for isolated cardiac failure in both the neonatal and pediatric population; there were 1491 cases in the ELSO Registry as of July 1995 with an overall survival of 44%.[56] The largest clinical use of ECMO in this category is for postoperative support following cardiac surgery (1164 cases with 42% survival), followed by preoperative or postoperative support for cardiac transplantation (87 cases with 41% survival). In these groups, the vast majority of patients were placed on ECMO for failure to wean off cardiopulmonary bypass. Similar to pediatric ECMO for respiratory failure, the mechanical complication rate in the cardiac ECMO group is higher, and surgical site bleeding is not uncommon.

Increasing experience has accrued with adult ECMO, with an overall survival of 46% recorded by the ELSO Registry.[62] Several individual institutions report similar survival statistics.[63–65] The initial results with adult ECMO were somewhat disappointing, and several modifications were developed to improve overall survival. These technical modifications included using VV ECMO when possible, using large membranes for effective gas exchange, maintaining ACT values between 180 and 200 seconds, and selecting patients with a predicted mortality of 90%.[66] There appears to be an inverse relationship between survival and the duration of mechanical ventilation prior to the institution of ECMO, suggesting that early initiation of ECMO in severe adult respiratory failure may improve outcome.[67]

□ Future Directions

A key trend for the future is the integration of ECMO technology with newer innovative therapies for respiratory failure. The role of ECMO will necessarily evolve as newer strategies emerge. Already, many institutions are experiencing a transition in both the quantity and types of ECMO cases. Despite a significant drop in the number of cases, a trend toward more complex pediatric and cardiac ECMO cases requiring longer runs with a higher patient complication rate has been observed.[68] This tendency will, in all likelihood, create a greater need for regionalization of ECMO centers. As such, the early identification and transfer of ECMO-eligible patients remain helpful, particularly to institutions that can provide alternative therapies as well as ECMO.

The timing of transfer of a critically ill newborn with severe respiratory failure can be aided by tele-

TABLE 7–4. Pediatric ECMO Cases
(ELSO Registry, July 1995)

Indication	No. of Cases	Survival (%)
Pneumonia		
Bacterial	88	45
Viral	304	56
Pneumocystis	13	38
Aspiration	88	65
Adult respiratory distress syndrome	61	51
Other	406	49
TOTAL	**942**	**53**

ECMO, extracorporeal membrane oxygenation; ELSO, Extracorporeal Life Support Organization.

medicine and early communication and, if appropriate, expedient referral to an ECMO center. A "hidden" mortality as high as 39.1% has been observed for ECMO-eligible infants dying before or during transport or immediately after arrival to an ECMO center.[69] A recent report from Germany documented experience with interhospital transfer of eight patients on VV ECMO.[70] This alternative strategy may help to salvage some infants who would otherwise die before or during transport to an ECMO center.

Stratification of children for appropriate therapeutic interventions will become more accurate. Some infants with conditions such as congenital diaphragmatic hernia will remain problematic despite ECMO. A recently conducted multiinstitutional trial of inhaled nitric oxide in neonates with congenital diaphragmatic hernia and hypoxemic respiratory failure was unable to demonstrate a reduced need for ECMO or a lower death rate in this difficult group.[71] Initial experience with partial liquid ventilation using perfluorocarbon in neonates with congenital diaphragmatic hernia and severe respiratory failure has been reported to improve pulmonary compliance and gas exchange.[72] Whether intrapulmonary perfluorocarbon can induce lung growth, improve lung function, and ultimately improve survival in infants with congenital diaphragmatic hernia on ECMO remains to be determined.[73]

The only certainty is that scientific and technologic progress will occur and the goal of clinicians will remain to select and treat the appropriate groups of infants and children with both the new and old therapies. The continuing success of ECMO in treating previously lethal conditions is an important example of multidisciplinary progress in treating infants with respiratory failure.

REFERENCES

1. Lillehei CW, Cohen M, Warden HE, et al: The direct-vision intracardiac correction of congenital anomalies by controlled cross circulation. Surgery 38:11–29, 1955.
2. Clowes GHA Jr, Hopkins AL, Neville WE: An artificial lung dependent upon diffusion of oxygen and carbon dioxide through plastic membranes. J Thorac Surg 32:630–637, 1956.
3. Bartlett RH, Gazzaniga AB, Jefferies MR, et al: Extracorporeal membrane oxygenation (ECMO) cardiopulmonary support in infancy. Trans Am Soc Artif Intern Organs 22:80–93, 1976.
4. Tracy TF Jr, DeLosh T, Stolar CJH: The registry of the extracorporeal life support organization. In Zwischenberger JB, Bartlett RH (eds): ECMO: Extracorporeal Cardiopulmonary Support in Critical Care. Ann Arbor, Extracorporeal Life Support Organization, 1995, pp 251–260.
5. Lessin JS, el-Eid SE, Klein MD, et al: Extracorporeal membrane oxygenation in pediatric respiratory failure secondary to smoke inhalation injury. J Pediatr Surg 31:1285–1287, 1996.
6. Tobias JD, Garrett JS: Therapeutic options for severe, refractory status asthmaticus: Inhalational anesthetic agents, extracorporeal membrane oxygenation and helium/oxygen ventilation. Paediatr Anesth 7:47–57, 1997.
7. Goldman AP, Macrae DJ, Tasker RC, et al: Extracorporeal membrane oxygenation as a bridge to definitive tracheal surgery in children. J Pediatr 128:386–388, 1996.
8. Lund DP, Soriano SG, Fauza D, et al: Resection of a massive sacrococcygeal teratoma using hypothermic hypoperfusion: A novel use of extracorporeal membrane oxygenation. J Pediatr Surg 30:1557–1559, 1995.
9. Rooney M, Massey KL, Jamali F, et al: Acebutolol overdose treated with hemodialysis and extracorporeal membrane oxygenation. J Clin Pharmacol 36:760–763, 1996.
10. Johnson LB, Plotkin JS, Howell CD, et al: Successful emergency transplantation of a liver allograft from a donor maintained on extracorporeal membrane oxygenation. Transplantation 63:910–911, 1997.
11. Gersony WM, Duc GV, Sinclair JC: "PFC" syndrome (persistence of the fetal circulation). Circulation 40(suppl 111):87, 1969.
12. Rabinovitch M: Structure and function of the pulmonary vascular bed: An update. Cardiol Clin 1989;7:895–914.
13. Wohrley JD, Frid MG, Moiseeva EP, et al: Hypoxia selectively induces proliferation in a specific subpopulation of smooth muscle cells in the bovine neonatal pulmonary arterial media. J Clin Invest 96:273–281, 1995.
14. Barefield ES, Karle VA, Phillips JB III, et al: Inhaled nitric oxide in term infants with respiratory failure. J Pediatr 129:279–286, 1996.
15. Anonymous: Inhaled nitric oxide in full-term and nearly full-term infants with hypoxic respiratory failure. N Engl J Med 336:597–604, 1997.
16. Cilley RE, Zwischenberger JB, Andrews AF, et al: Intracranial hemorrhage during extracorporeal membrane oxygenation in neonates. Pediatrics 78:699–704, 1986.
17. Revenis ME, Glass P, Short BL: Mortality and morbidity rates among lower birth weight infants (2000 to 2500 grams) treated with extracorporeal membrane oxygenation. J Pediatr 121:452–458, 1992.
18. Sell LL, Cullen ML, Whittlesey GC, et al: Hemorrhagic complications during extracorporeal membrane oxygenation: Prevention and treatment. J Pediatr Surg 21:1087–1091, 1986.
19. McCune S, Short BL, Miller MK, et al: Extracorporeal membrane oxygenation therapy in neonates with septic shock. J Pediatr Surg 25:479–482, 1990.
20. Kornhauser MS, Cullen JA, Baumgart S, et al: Risk factors for bronchopulmonary dysplasia after extracorporeal membrane oxygenation. Arch Pediatr Adolesc Med 148:820–825, 1994.
21. Weber TR, Kountzman B: The effects of venous occlusion on cerebral blood flow characteristics during ECMO. J Pediatr Surg 31:1124–1127, 1996.
22. Gauger PG, Hirschl RB, Delosh TN, et al: A matched pairs analysis of venoarterial and venovenous extracorporeal life support in neonatal respiratory failure. ASAIO J 41:M573–M579, 1995.
23. Anderson HL III, Otsu T, Chapman RA, et al: Venovenous extracorporeal life support in neonates using a double lumen catheter. ASAIO Trans 35:650–653, 1989.
24. Short BL: Extracorporeal membrane oxygenation. In Avery GB, Fletcher MA, MacDonald MG (eds): Neonatology (4th ed). Philadelphia, JB Lippincott, 1994, pp 504–515.
25. Rais-Bahrami K, Rivera O, Mikesell GT, et al: Improved oxygenation with reduced recirculation during venovenous extracorporeal membrane oxygenation: Evaluation of a test catheter. Crit Care Med 23:1722–1725, 1995.
26. Zwischenberger JB, Nguyen TT, Upp JR Jr, et al: Complications of neonatal extracorporeal membrane oxygenation. Collective experience from the extracorporeal life support organization. J Thorac Cardiovasc Surg 107:838–848, 1994.
27. Lotze A, Knight GR, Martin GR, et al: Improved pulmonary outcome after exogenous surfactant therapy for respiratory failure in term infants requiring extracorporeal membrane oxygenation. J Pediatr 122:261–268, 1993.
28. Riccabona M, Dacar D, Zobel G, et al: Sonographically guided cannula positioning for extracorporeal membrane oxygenation. Pediatr Radiol 25:643–645, 1995.
29. Atkinson JB, Gomperts ED, Kang R, et al: Prospective, randomized evaluation of the efficacy of fibrin sealant at the cannulation site in neonates undergoing extracorporeal membrane oxygenation. Am J Surg 173:479–484, 1997.
30. Martin GR, Short BL, Abbott C, et al: Cardiac stun in infants undergoing extracorporeal membrane oxygenation. J Thorac Cardiovasc Surg 101:607–611, 1991.

31. Bulas DI, Taylor GA, O'Donnell RM, et al: Intracranial abnormalities in infants treated with extracorporeal membrane oxygenation: Update on sonographic and CT findings. Am J Neuroradiol 17:287–294, 1996.
32. Taylor GA, Short BL, Kreismer P: Extracorporeal membrane oxygenation: Radiographic appearance of the neonatal chest. Am J Roentgen 146:1257–1260, 1986.
33. Fortenberry JD, Bhardwaj V, Niemer P, et al: Neutrophil and cytokine activation with neonatal extracorporeal membrane oxygenation. J Pediatr 128(pt 1):670–678, 1996.
34. Underwood MJ, Pearson JA, Waggoner J, et al: Changes in "inflammatory" mediators and total body water during extracorporeal membrane oxygenation (ECMO). A preliminary study. Int J Artif Organs 18:627–632, 1995.
35. Urlesberger B, Zobel G, Zenz W, et al: Activation of the clotting system during extracorporeal membrane oxygenation in term newborn infants. J Pediatr 129:264–268, 1996.
36. Lotze A, Short BL, Taylor GA: Lung compliance as a measure of lung function in newborns with respiratory failure requiring extracorporeal membrane oxygenation. Crit Care Med 15:226–229, 1987.
37. McKay VJ, Stewart DL, Massey MT, et al: Retaining extracorporeal membrane oxygenation cannulae after extracorporeal support in the neonate: Is it safe? J Pediatr Surg 32:703–707, 1997.
38. Crombleholme TM, Adzick NS, deLorimier AA, et al: Carotid artery reconstruction following extracorporeal membrane oxygenation. Am J Dis Child 144:872–874, 1990.
39. Levy MS, Share JC, Fauza DO, et al: Fate of the reconstructed carotid artery after extracorporeal membrane oxygenation. J Pediatr Surg 30:1046–1049, 1995.
40. Cheung PY, Vickar DB, Hallgren RA, et al: Carotid artery reconstruction in neonates receiving extracorporeal membrane oxygenation: A 4-year follow-up study. J Pediatr Surg 32:560–564, 1997.
41. Baumgart S, Streletz LJ, Needleman L, et al: Right common carotid artery reconstruction after extracorporeal membrane oxygenation: Vascular imaging, cerebral circulation, electroencephalographic, and neurodevelopmental correlates to recovery. J Pediatr 125:295–304, 1994.
42. Stallion A, Cofer BR, Rafferty JA, et al: The significant relationship between platelet count and haemorrhagic complications on ECMO. Perfusion 9:265–269, 1994.
43. Rossaint R, Slama K, Lewandowski K, et al: Extracorporeal lung assist with heparin-coated systems. Int J Artif Organs 15:29–34, 1992.
44. Wilson JM, Bower LK, Fackler JC, et al: Aminocaproic acid decreases the incidence of intracranial hemorrhage and other hemorrhagic complications of ECMO. J Pediatr Surg 28:536–540, 1993.
45. Van der Staak FH, de Haan AF, Geven WB, et al: Surgical repair of congenital diaphragmatic hernia during extracorporeal membrane oxygenation: Hemorrhagic complications and the effect of tranexamic acid. J Pediatr Surg 32:594–599, 1997.
46. Paul JJ, Desai H, Baumgart S, et al: Aortic dissection in a neonate associated with arterial cannulation for extracorporeal life support. ASAIO J 43:92–94, 1997.
47. Butler TJ, Sodoma LJ, Doski JJ, et al: Heparin-associated thrombocytopenia and thrombosis as the cause of a fatal thrombus on extracorporeal membrane oxygenation. J Pediatr Surg 32:768–771, 1997.
48. Karle VA, Short BL, Martin GR, et al: Extracorporeal membrane oxygenation exposes infants to the plasticizer, di(2-ethylhexyl)phthalate. Crit Care Med 25:696–703, 1997.
49. Coffin SE, Bell LM, Manning M, et al: Nosocomial infections in neonates receiving extracorporeal membrane oxygenation. Infect Control Hosp Epidemiol 18:93–96, 1997.
50. Douglass BH, Keenan AL, Purohit DM: Bacterial and fungal infection in neonates undergoing venoarterial extracorporeal membrane oxygenation: An analysis of the registry data of the Extracorporeal Life Support Organization. Artif Organs 20:202–208, 1996.
51. Meyer DM, Jessen ME, Eberhart RC: Neonatal extracorporeal membrane oxygenation complicated by sepsis. Extracorporeal Life Support Organization. Ann Thorac Surg 59:975–980, 1995.
52. Nelson SP, Jonas MM: Hepatitis C infection in children who received extracorporeal membrane oxygenation. J Pediatr Surg 31:644–648, 1996.
53. Vazquez WD, Cheu HW: Hemorrhagic complications and repair of congenital diaphragmatic hernias: Does timing of the repair make a difference? Data from the extracorporeal life support organization. J Pediatr Surg 29:1002–1005, 1994.
54. Schnitzer JJ, Kikiros CS, Short BL, et al: Experience with abdominal wall closure for patients with congenital diaphragmatic hernia repaired on ECMO. J Pediatr Surg 30:19–22, 1995.
55. Bond SJ, Lee DJ, Stewart DL, et al: Open lung biopsy in pediatric patients on extracorporeal membrane oxygenation. J Pediatr Surg 31:1376–1378, 1996.
56. Tracy TF Jr, Delosh TN, Stolar CJH: The Registry of the Extracorporeal Life Support Organization. Ann Arbor, ELSO, 1997.
57. Glass P, Miller M, Short BL: Morbidity for survivors of extracorporeal membrane oxygenation: Neurodevelopmental outcome at 1 year of age. Pediatrics 83:72–78, 1989.
58. Schumacher RE, Palmer TW, Roloff DW, et al: Follow-up of infants treated with extracorporeal membrane oxygenation for newborn respiratory failure. Pediatrics 87:451–457, 1991.
59. Glass P, Wagner AE, Papero PH, et al: Neurodevelopmental status at age five years of neonates treated with extracorporeal membrane oxygenation. J Pediatr 127:447–457, 1995.
60. Taylor GA, Short BL, Fitz CR: Imaging of cerebrovascular injury in infants treated with extracorporeal membrane oxygenation. J Pediatr 114(pt 1):635–639, 1989.
61. Taylor GA, Fitz CR, Glass P, et al: CT of cerebrovascular injury after neonatal extracorporeal membrane oxygenation: Implications for neurodevelopmental outcome. Am J Roentgenol 153:121–126, 1989.
62. Bartlett RH: Extracorporeal life support registry report 1995. ASAIO J 43:104–107, 1997.
63. Pranikoff T, Hirschl RB, Steimle CN, et al: Efficacy of extracorporeal life support in the setting of adult cardiorespiratory failure. ASAIO J 40:M339–M343, 1994.
64. Macha M, Griffith BP, Keenan R, et al: ECMO support for adult patients with acute respiratory failure. ASAIO J 42:M841–M844, 1996.
65. Peek GJ, Moore HM, Moore N, et al: Extracorporeal membrane oxygenation for adult respiratory failure. Chest 112:759–764, 1997.
66. Anderson HL III, Delius RE, Sinard JM, et al: Early experience with adult extracorporeal membrane oxygenation in the modern era. Ann Thorac Surg 53:553–563, 1992.
67. Pranikoff T, Hirschl RB, Steimle CN, et al: Mortality is directly related to the duration of mechanical ventilation before the initiation of extracorporeal life support for severe respiratory failure. Crit Care Med 25:28–32, 1997.
68. Wilson JM, Bower LK, Thompson JE, et al: ECMO in evolution: The impact of changing patient demographics and alternative therapies on ECMO. J Pediatr Surg 31:1116–1122, 1996.
69. Boedy RF, Howell CG, Kanto WP Jr: Hidden mortality rate associated with extracorporeal membrane oxygenation. J Pediatr 117:462–464, 1990.
70. Rossaint R, Pappert D, Gerlach H, et al: Extracorporeal membrane oxygenation for transport of hypoxaemic patients with severe ARDS. Br J Anaesth 78:241–246, 1977.
71. Anonymous: Inhaled nitric oxide and hypoxic respiratory failure in infants with congenital diaphragmatic hernia. The Neonatal Inhaled Nitric Oxide Study Group (NINOS). Pediatrics 99:838–845, 1997.
72. Pranikoff T, Gauger PG, Hirschl RB: Partial liquid ventilation in newborn patients with congenital diaphragmatic hernia. J Pediatr Surg 31:613–618, 1996.
73. Hirschl RB: Innovative therapies in the management of newborns with congenital diaphragmatic hernia. Semin Pediatr Surg 5:256–265, 1996.

8

VASCULAR ACCESS

Charles S. Turner, MD

Vascular access in infants and children is one of the most frustrating and exasperating aspects of pediatric surgery. What is delegated to the role of an ancillary surgical procedure in adults may become a major task in children and may, in the operating arena, take as long as the surgical procedure itself. The least experienced physician is often given the task of starting the intravenous (IV) line.

Nowhere is this situation more critical than during attempted resuscitation of a child. In a study of 66 emergency department cardiac arrests in children, IV access required 10 or more minutes in 24% of the cases.[1] Indeed, in 6% of resuscitations, access was never established. When resuscitation was successful, access had been established significantly sooner than when resuscitation failed. Placing an IV catheter took the most time in children younger than 2 years of age.

In 1986, a prospective study was undertaken to determine the effectiveness of a protocol designed to standardize the route and site of pediatric IV access in an emergency situation.[2] This study found that resuscitations using the protocol achieved IV access more rapidly (median, 4.5 minutes) than those deviating from the protocol (median, 10 minutes) (Fig. 8–1). Therefore, surgeons must develop and maintain a high degree of expertise in vascular access in infants and children. Beyond the immediate need for IV access in resuscitative efforts, the surgeon must often establish arterial access lines for monitoring and central venous access lines for hemodialysis, parenteral nutrition, chemotherapy, and critical care monitoring.

This chapter reviews the options available for vascular access so that this aspect of pediatric surgical care can be improved.

□ Peripheral Venous Access

Peripheral venous access in infants and children is usually accomplished employing the veins of the hand and forearm, the distal leg and foot, and the scalp (Table 8–1). A thorough knowledge of anatomy is mandatory for successful access.

In infants, the superficial veins on the dorsum of the hand are most frequently selected. These veins are straight and flat on the metacarpals. They feed the larger dorsal branch of the distal cephalic vein, which is also stabilized for access without difficulty. The lateral branch of the distal cephalic vein is difficult to stabilize and is less accessible for venous puncture and catheter placement.

The median vein tributaries located on the ventral surface of the wrist are accessible, but they are small and acutely angulated. Therefore, they require a small catheter, which is difficult to advance into the vein. These tributaries may be used during an operation, but they become unreliable in the awakened patient. The cephalic and basilic veins in the

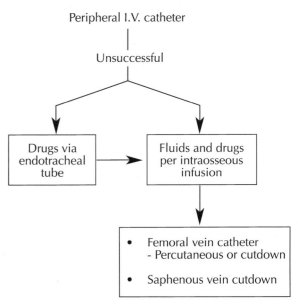

Figure 8–1. Access for emergency resuscitation (protocol example). I.V., intravenous.

TABLE 8-1. Peripheral Vein Access Priority in Infants and Children

1. Dorsal veins of the hands
2. Antecubital veins of the arms
3. Saphenous vein at the ankle
4. Dorsal veins of the foot
5. Median vein tributary at the wrist
6. External jugular veins
7. Scalp

antecubital fossa are accessible, but advancement of the cannula may be difficult owing to the angulation of the veins across the fossa.

In the lower extremity, the tributaries of the dorsal venous arch on the dorsal aspect of the foot are useful. The largest reliable vein is the saphenous vein just anterior and lateral to the medial malleolus. This vein is always palpable, although it is only sometimes visible. A larger catheter can be accommodated.

Although the external jugular vein can be seen, cannulation is difficult. Once the catheter is in place, it serves well during anesthesia. However, the jugular vein infuses poorly when the child awakens because, with motion, the acute angle of the external jugular into the subclavian vein makes the adequacy of infusion "positional." The external jugular vein catheter is also difficult to stabilize and easy to dislodge.

EMERGENCY SITUATION

The next step for venous access, when percutaneous peripheral venous access is unsuccessful, depends on the speed with which access is needed. In an emergency situation, when difficult venous access is secondary to cardiac arrest or hypovolemia, the options are tracheal instillation, intraosseous infusion,[3] venous cutdown,[4–6] and central venous access.[6–8]

The sites for intraosseous infusion in infants and small children are the tibia, iliac crest, and femur. Access can be accomplished with a bone marrow aspiration needle or a 16- or 19-gauge butterfly needle. In the femur, the needle is introduced in a cephalad direction, 3 cm proximal to the condyles. Tibial introduction is 1 to 3 cm distal to the tibial tuberosity; the needle is placed in a distal direction. Most drugs, crystalloid solutions, and blood products can be given by interosseous infusion in an emergency. Infusion is as rapid as through IV routes. Intramedullary vessels do not collapse in the hypovolemic, "shocky" patient.[3]

In the past, the venous cutdown has been the mainstay of difficult venous access by the pediatric surgeon. An American Pediatric Surgical Association survey showed that an average of 56 cutdowns per pediatric surgeon per year were performed.[4] The time required for venous cutdowns in neonates, children younger than 5 years of age, and children older than 5 years was 11, 8, and 6 minutes, respec-

tively. The saphenous vein was preferred (79%) over the brachial and external jugular veins (21%). However, the time required even by the surgeons most experienced in the procedure made the cutdown in an emergency situation supplementary, at best. Alternative routes must be established to give medications (endotracheal instillation) and fluids (interosseous infusion) while cutdowns are being prepared.[3]

NONEMERGENCY SITUATIONS

In nonemergency situations, are peripheral venous cutdowns necessary? The option is central venous catheterization, but two specific contraindications to central venous insertion exist: an uncorrected coagulopathy and an undefined major cardiac anomaly. Otherwise, percutaneous central venous lines are preferred when peripheral lines are unavailable or when long-term access is required.

A comparison study of percutaneous central venous catheterization versus peripheral venous cutdowns in children aged 1 day to 17 years was conducted. Within age groups, the children were similar in weight and size. More successful placements, fewer complications, and longer functional states were found in the patients with central venous catheters versus those with peripheral venous cutdowns.[6] Surgical cutdowns also carry a significantly greater risk of infectious complications than do percutaneous catheterizations.[7] Therefore, percutaneous central venous catheterization is the method of choice when venous access other than routine peripheral IV access is required.

Butterfly needles are used now to introduce small Silastic catheters percutaneously into neonates.[8] This needle enhances the ability to obtain central venous access in very small infants without cutdown. The catheter is Silastic medical grade tubing (0.012 mm inside diameter and 0.025 mm outside diameter)[8] (Fig. 8–2). The catheter is inserted into a peripheral vein (scalp, neck, or arm) through a 19-gauge scalp vein needle or through a 20-gauge angiocatheter.[8, 9] The catheter is threaded centrally.

Owing to the small catheter size, the flow rate is limited to 25 ml/hour. An increased risk of calcium phosphate precipitation may exist if lipid emulsions are given simultaneously with parenteral nutrition.[9, 10] For short-term use in a neonate who weighs less than 6 kg, these small-diameter catheters introduced percutaneously offer a good alternative to the large-diameter lines that require cutdown or subclavian insertion. Certainly, however, the surgeon must perfect the technique of peripheral venous cutdown and employ the newer Silastic catheters, which are less thrombogenic than the older polyethylene catheters.

☐ Central Venous Access

Access to the central veins of the chest has altered the outcome of a multitude of pediatric surgical

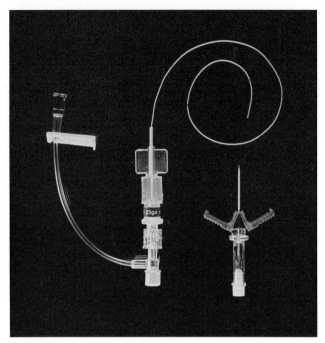

Figure 8–2. Butterfly peel-away angiocatheter with Silastic catheter.

problems. With this access, the hemodynamics in a critically ill child can be monitored precisely. Children with problems such as short-gut syndrome, intestinal pseudoobstruction, and gastroschisis can be kept alive with central parenteral nutrition. Survival among extremely premature babies has increased owing to the ability to provide adequate calories, protein, and fat via central venous catheters (Fig. 8–3).

Pediatric oncology patients require central venous access not only for reliable delivery of chemotherapeutic agents but also for nutritional support. Central venous access has also allowed catheters to be placed for both short-term and long-term hemodialysis and for plasmapheresis in the treatment of certain metabolic disorders.

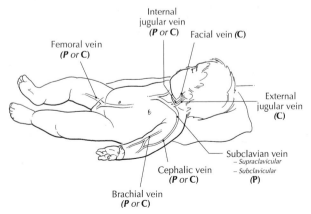

Figure 8–3. Most common sites for central venous access. P, percutaneous; C, cutdown.

CATHETER TYPE

The first consideration is the type of catheter, which is primarily dictated by the intended use and by the size of the patient. Duration, patient compliance, and ability to care for the catheter also enter into the catheter-selection process. For short periods in the critical care or emergency situation, single- to triple-lumen polyethylene catheters are available. These can be inserted percutaneously into the internal jugular, subclavian, or femoral veins by Seldinger's technique.

For long-term application in parenteral nutrition or oncology, the silicone rubber catheters are preferred owing to their pliability and decreased thrombogenicity.[11] Broviac or Hickman catheters are made of silicone rubber with a Dacron cuff around the nonvascular portion of the catheter. These catheters can be placed percutaneously into the subclavian, internal jugular, or femoral veins, using Seldinger's technique and "peel-away" introducers.

The tip is advanced to the caval-atrial junction under fluoroscopy. The extravascular portion with its Dacron cuff is brought out through a long subcutaneous tunnel to the anterior chest wall or to the abdominal wall, if the femoral approach is taken. The Dacron cuff should be midway between the skin and the vein entrance site.[11] Other veins for the cutdown technique include the external jugular, common facial, inferior thyroid, saphenous, and inferior epigastric. When those veins are exhausted, the azygos vein can be cannulated via the intercostal veins on the right, although this requires thoracotomy or thoracoscopy. The inferior vena cava has also been accessed through a percutaneous translumbar approach for central venous catheter placement.[12, 13]

Implantable access devices consist of an injection reservoir connected to a silicone rubber catheter (Fig. 8–4). The port or reservoir is placed in a subcutaneous pocket on the anterior chest. The catheter is tunneled under the skin to the vein entrance site. The vein can be accessed with a percutaneous Seldinger's technique or a cutdown technique. The subcutaneous reservoirs have a Silastic diaphragm, which can be punctured by a side hole (Huber) needle, without a core of Silastic being taken with entrance of the needle.

The back and side walls of the reservoir are metal so that it is known when the needle is completely inserted. This type of device allows access to the central venous system without the need to care for an external catheter. These implantable reservoirs are also available as double- and triple-lumen types and as low-profile types for infants. The ease of care, the absence of protruding tubes, and the compatibility with normal activities are their major advantages.[14] The complication rate of central venous access is not increased with their use[15–17]; in fact, the infection rate is lower.[18, 19] For patients who require intermittent but long-term central venous access (as for managing cancer, cystic fibrosis, and

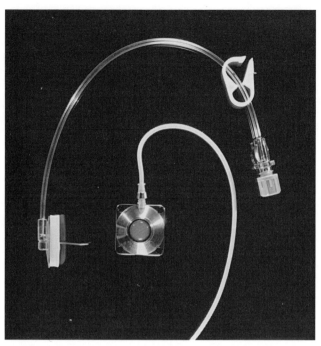

Figure 8–4. Implantable access device with "side-hole" access needle.

hemophilia),[20] an implantable system seems appropriate. Whether a continuous need, such as chronic home parenteral nutrition, is better met with an implantable device or an external catheter is still unanswered.

Special catheters for hemodialysis allow a single-needle dialysis technique to be used. These catheters (Cook, Inc., Bloomington, IN), which have offset inflow and outflow ports, are made of polyurethane[21] (Fig. 8–5). They can be introduced percutaneously using a peel-away catheter technique; they also have Dacron cuffs that are tunneled in, as de-

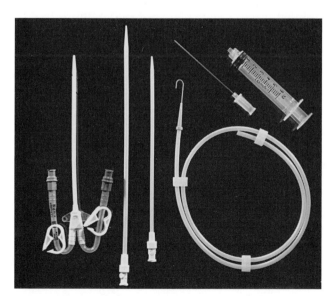

Figure 8–5. Hemodialysis catheter *(right)* with Seldinger introducer kit *(left)*.

scribed for Broviac catheters.[11] They can be employed in children who weigh as little as 7 kg.[21]

Centrally placed Hickman (Evermed) catheters have also been used for hemodialysis with the single-needle dialysis technique. Various sizes, depending on the size of the patient, provide adequate hemodialysis in children as light as 7.7 kg.[22] These catheters are best suited for acute hemodialysis in children with acute renal failure without availability of peritoneal dialysis, in children with peritonitis that requires temporary removal of a peritoneal dialysis catheter, and in children with unsuccessful peritoneal dialysis outcome who are awaiting kidney transplant. These catheters have also been used for long-term dialysis,[21] although the best long-term dialysis for children is believed to be peritoneal.

If long-term hemodialysis is required because of chronic peritonitis and problematic transplant matching, a Brescia-Cimino arteriovenous fistula is possible in children weighing no more than 15 kg.[23]

The site of insertion of a central venous catheter in a child depends greatly on the expertise and training of the surgeon. The percutaneous route to the subclavian vein is feasible even in very small infants.[24, 25] As mentioned before, long lines from the antecubital fossa by a cutdown technique or a percutaneous technique have been placed in neonates weighing as little as 0.5 kg.[9]

COMPLICATIONS

The femoral route for central line placement has been thought to be associated with increased thrombophlebitis of the ipsilateral leg and with wound infection due to proximity of the groin.[26–28] Gangrene of the lower extremity,[29] septic arthritis of the hip[30] and arteriovenous fistula,[31] penetration of a viscus in an unrecognized femoral hernia, and infused fluid into the abdominal wall[32] have also been reported as complications of femoral vein cannulation. However, because the femoral approach has been the route of choice for cardiac catheterization,[27] the femoral approach for central venous catheter placement has been accepted for use in pediatric patients.[26–28, 33, 34] The advantages listed are the anatomy, the attained hemostasis, and the distance from other lifesaving maneuver sites in a multiply injured patient.

Therefore, for rapid central venous access in cases of cardiac arrest, hypotension, respiratory arrest, and multiple trauma, the femoral vein approach, either by percutaneous or cutdown technique, is the route of choice. In neonates, infants, and children who require long-term central venous lines, the femoral approach is acceptable and is available with the exit site or reservoir located on the lower abdominal wall.

Except for the complications listed earlier, those for central venous catheters are primarily associated with percutaneous placement of the catheter in the subclavian or internal jugular veins. Acute complications include aberrant location of the catheter;

perforation of the vein or artery with resultant hemothorax, hydrothorax, or extravasation of fluid into surrounding tissues; perforation of the lung with pneumothorax; and perforation of the heart with resultant pericardial tamponade.[35-39] Misplacing the tip of the catheter into a small tributary can lead to phlebitis when hypertonic solutions are infused. Fluoroscopy and immediate postinsertion radiographs allow accurate placement of the catheter and early detection of these complications.

Long-term complications include tunnel infection, sepsis, venous thrombosis, superior vena caval obstruction, thrombosis of the catheter tip, and septic emboli.[10, 36-40] A review of central venous catheter infections is available.[10] It should be studied by anyone who works with patients who require vascular access.

The overall rate of septic infections in central venous catheters is 1.7 cases per 1000 days of catheter use. This rate varies, depending on whether the patient is on total parenteral nutrition only or is also on chemotherapy, and whether more than one lumen is being employed (not just being in position). The diagnosis of catheter-related sepsis is assumed in any case with fever. Quantitative blood cultures obtained centrally and peripherally that show a 5:1 or greater ratio of colonies per milliliter suggest the catheter as the most likely source.

Initial therapy should be removal of the catheter if the patient can get along without it. If the line is still needed, antibiotics can be given through the catheter. A thrombolytic agent is added if thrombus is seen on echocardiography or if flow is restricted.[40] If no clinical improvement is seen within 48 hours or if the patient's condition deteriorates sooner, the catheter must be removed. Although bacterial infections may be cured without removal of the catheter, *Candida* infections are unlikely to be cured.[10]

TREATMENT OF INFECTION

The best treatment for infection is prevention. Strict aseptic technique at the time of insertion as well as following the protocols of meticulous aseptic care of the catheter site is essential. This care includes the iodoform ointments (most effective against *Candida* and gram-negative bacilli) at the entrance site and gauze and tape dressings[10] or transparent semipermeable adhesive dressings, which should be changed every 48 to 72 hours.[41]

Thrombosis of the Silastic catheter can be suggested before complete occlusion by difficulty in flushing, inability to withdraw blood, and measured increase in resistance to flow.[38] When partial or total occlusion occurs, urokinase, 5000 IU/ml, can be administered.[39, 40] The volume of urokinase depends on the size of the catheter (e.g., 1.8 to 2.0 ml for Hickman catheters and 0.8 ml for Broviac catheters). After 30 to 60 minutes, the catheter is aspirated and then flushed with heparinized saline. Regular administration of dilute heparin decreases thrombus formation and may also lead to a reduction in septic

complications.[10, 41] An intracardiac thrombus at the tip of the catheter can become infected.[40] The presence of such a thrombus usually causes symptoms (septic, respiratory, cardiac insufficiency, or catheter malfunction).[37] Detection is confirmed by echocardiography.

Various modes of treatment include thrombolytic agents (urokinase infusion at 2000 to 10,000 U/kg/hour for 1 to 8 days) and heparin, with or without catheter removal; catheter removal only; observation only[37]; a regimen of aspirin, dipyridamole, and antibiotics[40]; and atriotomy.[37] On the basis of published reports, thrombolytic therapy through the catheter, with the addition of antibiotics in the case of sepsis, would be the first line of treatment. Atriotomy is saved for deteriorating sepsis or cardiac compromise due to the mechanical presence of the thrombus.

☐ Arterial Access

Intraarterial catheters in infants are frequently employed to monitor blood pressure and to provide access to arterial blood for blood gas and other laboratory determinations, thereby eliminating the need for intermittent arterial puncture.[42, 43] The arterial sites of cannulization include the umbilical,[44-46] radial,[47-50] femoral,[26, 51] posterior tibial,[42] and temporal[52-54] arteries (Fig. 8–6).

UMBILICAL ARTERY

The umbilical artery usually constricts minutes after birth, although this constriction is delayed by hypoxia and acidosis. The artery can usually be catheterized within 2 to 4 days of life. The usual approach is at the umbilical stump itself, although the umbilical artery can be cannulated through a minilaparotomy.[45] The advantages of catheterizing the umbilical artery are the ease of access, the longer functional life for umbilical catheters than for peripheral arterial catheters, and the ability to infuse fluids, glucose, electrolytes, and drugs by such a direct route.[55] Its use also allows postductal blood

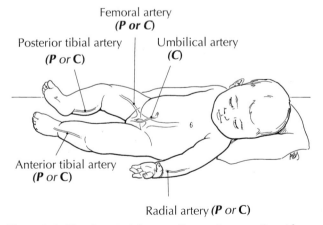

Figure 8–6. Sites for arterial access. P, percutaneous; C, cutdown.

gas evaluations, which are helpful in determining the amount of right-to-left shunting in neonates with persistent fetal circulation. The umbilical artery is also used for access in cardiac catheterization.[46]

Complications from umbilical artery catheters include thrombosis, distal embolism, vasospasm, vascular perforation with hemoperitoneum, hemorrhage from catheter disconnection, and, after catheter removal, visceral infarction, paraplegia, hypertension, and sepsis.[43, 46, 48] All of these situations require immediate removal of the catheter. Additionally, thrombosis of the aorta may require thrombolytic or surgical therapy. Multiple aortic aneurysms in a neonate after umbilical artery catheter insertion have been reported.[56] The umbilical artery cannot be catheterized in 5 to 10% of patients, nor can it be catheterized after the neonatal period. Complications from the umbilical artery catheter may require premature removal. In these instances, 22- to 24-gauge catheters can be placed by percutaneous technique or by cutdown in the peripheral arteries.

RADIAL ARTERY

The most frequently employed peripheral artery is the radial artery. It carries a low risk of infection (12% for catheters in place more than 48 hours) and of thrombosis. The catheter allows preductal gas determinations if in the right radial artery. The overall incidence of complications from peripheral artery catheters is approximately 7% compared with 27% from umbilical artery catheters.[48] The catheters in the artery are of 22- to 24-gauge Teflon. They can be placed either by percutaneous or cutdown technique. If placed by cutdown, the catheter can be inserted through the skin and then, under direct vision, into the artery without ligating the artery.[49] A palpable pulse usually returns within 3 to 5 days after removal of a radial artery catheter.[47]

Complications from radial artery catheters include skin ischemia, radial artery obstruction, and inability to withdraw blood through the catheter. In patients who need insertion via a cutdown technique, the interval to recanalization after catheter removal is longer than that in patients with percutaneously placed catheters.[49] The radial artery catheter must be flushed continuously because catheters infused continuously with heparin, 1 U/ml of saline, last longer than those flushed intermittently[50] and because continuous slow flushing avoids the possible catastrophic complication of retrograde embolization of clot and air to the cerebral circulation.[57] If the patency of the ulnar artery is proved before placement of the radial artery catheter and if continuous flushing is done, few significant complications of radial artery catheterization will occur.[49]

TEMPORAL ARTERY

Temporal artery catheterization has been suggested for infants whose radial arteries are no longer

patent.[54] Although this technique is technically feasible, reports of hemiparesis and cerebral infarcts (confirmed by computed tomography to be on the side of the temporal artery catheter) have decreased the initial enthusiasm for this approach. Although this complication is rare (1 in 600 patients when heparin is infused continuously and the catheter is not flushed[52]), the possibility of such a catastrophic complication contraindicates this approach.

Lastly, the indications for arterial access must constantly be reassessed. With the increasing sophistication of noninvasive monitoring systems, often arterial access is not mandatory.[58] The needs of the patient should determine the use of this approach rather than the convenience of the physician.

REFERENCES

1. Rossetti V, Thompson BM, Aprahamian C, et al: Difficulty and delay in intravascular access in pediatric arrests [abstract]. Ann Emerg Med 13:406, 1984.
2. Kanter RK, Zimmerman JJ, Strauss RH, et al: Pediatric emergency intravenous access: Evaluation of a protocol. Am J Dis Child 140:132–134, 1986.
3. Orlowski JP: My kingdom for an intravenous line [editorial]. Am J Dis Child 138:803, 1984.
4. Iserson KV, Criss EA: Pediatric venous cutdowns: Utility in emergency situations. Pediatr Emerg Care 2:231–234, 1986.
5. Peter G, Lloyd-Still JD, Lovejoy FH Jr: Local infection and bacteremia from scalp vein needles and polyethylene catheters in children. J Pediatr 80:78–83, 1972.
6. Newman BM, Jewett TC Jr, Karp MP, et al: Percutaneous central venous catheterization in children: First-line choice for venous access. J Pediatr Surg 21:685–688, 1986.
7. Meignier M, Heloury Y, Roze J-C, et al: Surgical central venous access in low birth infants [letter]. J Pediatr Surg 23:596, 1988.
8. Durand M, Ramanathan R, Martinelli B, et al: Prospective evaluation of percutaneous central venous Silastic catheters in newborn infants with birth weights of 510 to 3,920 grams. Pediatrics 78:245–250, 1986.
9. Loeff DS, Matlak ME, Black RE, et al: Insertion of a small central venous catheter in neonates and young infants. J Pediatr Surg 17:944–949, 1982.
10. Decker MD, Edwards KM: Central venous catheter infections. Pediatr Clin North Am 35:579–612, 1988.
11. Broviac JW, Cole JJ, Scribner BH: A silicone rubber atrial catheter for prolonged parenteral alimentation. Surg Gynecol Obstet 136:602–606, 1973.
12. Robards JB, Jaques PF, Mauro MA, et al: Percutaneous translumbar inferior vena cava central line placement in a critically ill child. Pediatr Radiol 19:140–141, 1989.
13. Denny DF Jr, Greenwood LH, Morse SS, et al: Inferior vena cava: Translumbar catheterization for central venous access. Radiology 170:1013–1014, 1989.
14. Pegelow CH, Narvaez M, Toledano SR, et al: Experience with a totally implantable venous device in children. Am J Dis Child 140:69–71, 1986.
15. Krul EJ, van Leeuwen EF, Vos A, et al: Continuous venous access in children for long-term chemotherapy by means of an implantable system. J Pediatr Surg 21:689–690, 1986.
16. Kappers-Klunne MC, Degener JE, Stijnen T, et al: Complications from long-term indwelling central venous catheters in hematologic patients with special reference to infection. Cancer 64:1747–1752, 1989.
17. Guenier C, Ferreira J, Pector JC: Prolonged venous access in cancer patients. Eur J Surg Oncol 15:553–555, 1989.
18. Mirro J Jr, Rao BN, Kumar M, et al: A comparison of placement techniques and complications of externalized catheters and implantable port use in children with cancer. J Pediatr Surg 25:120–124, 1990.

19. Ross MN, Haase GM, Poole MA, et al: Comparison of totally implanted reservoirs with external catheters as venous access devices in pediatric oncologic patients. Surg Gynecol Obstet 167:141–144, 1988.
20. Schultz WH, Ware R, Filston HC, et al: Prolonged use of an implantable central venous access system in a child with severe hemophilia. J Pediatr 114:100–101, 1989.
21. Lally KP, Brennan LP, Sherman NJ, et al: Use of a subclavian venous catheter for short- and long-term hemodialysis in children. J Pediatr Surg 22:603–605, 1987.
22. Gibson TC, Dyer DP, Postlethwaite RJ, et al: Vascular access for acute haemodialysis. Arch Dis Child 62:141–145, 1987.
23. Matlak ME: Vascular access in pediatric patients. In Wilson SE, Owens ML (eds): Vascular Access Surgery. Chicago, Year Book Medical, 1980, pp 273–292.
24. Morgan WW Jr, Harkins GA: Percutaneous introduction of long-term indwelling venous catheters in infants. J Pediatr Surg 7:538–541, 1972.
25. Groff DB, Ahmed N: Subclavian vein catheterization in the infant. J Pediatr Surg 9:171–174, 1974.
26. Purdue GF, Hunt JL: Vascular access through the femoral vessels: Indications and complications. J Burn Care Rehabil 7:498–500, 1986.
27. Meland NB, Wilson W, Soontharotoke C-Y, et al: Sapheno-femoral venous cutdowns in the premature infant. J Pediatr Surg 21:341–343, 1986.
28. Stenzel JP, Green TP, Fuhrman BP, et al: Percutaneous femoral venous catheterizations: A prospective study of complications. J Pediatr 114:411–415, 1989.
29. Nabseth DC, Jones JE: Gangrene of the lower extremities of infants after femoral venipuncture: Report of two cases. N Engl J Med 268:1003–1005, 1961.
30. Asnes RS, Arendar GM: Septic arthritis of the hip: A complication of femoral venipuncture. Pediatrics 38:837–841, 1966.
31. Fuller TJ, Mahoney JJ, Juncos LI, et al: Arteriovenous fistula after femoral vein catheterization [letter]. JAMA 236:2943–2944, 1976.
32. Bonadio WA, Losek JD, Melzer-Lange M: An unusual complication from a femoral venous catheter. Pediatr Emerg Care 4:27–29, 1988.
33. Kanter RK, Gorton JM, Palmieri K, et al: Anatomy of femoral vessels in infants and guidelines for venous catheterization. Pediatrics 83:1020–1022, 1989.
34. Kanter RK, Zimmerman JJ, Strauss RH, et al: Central venous catheter insertion by femoral vein: Safety and effectiveness for the pediatric patient. Pediatrics 77:842–847, 1986.
35. Dunbar RD, Mitchell R, Lavine M: Aberrant locations of central venous catheters. Lancet 1:711–715, 1981.
36. Stine KC, Friedman HS, Kurtzberg J, et al: Pulmonary septic emboli mimicking metastatic rhabdomyosarcoma. J Pediatr Surg 24:491–493, 1989.
37. Ross P Jr, Ehrenkranz R, Kleinman CS, et al: Thrombus associated with central venous catheters in infants and children. J Pediatr Surg 24:253–256, 1989.
38. Stokes DC, Rao BN, Mirro J Jr, et al: Early detection and simplified management of obstructed Hickman and Broviac catheters. J Pediatr Surg 24:257–262, 1989.
39. Ross P Jr, Seashore JH: Bilateral hydrothorax complicating central venous catheterization in a child: Case report. J Pediatr Surg 24:263–264, 1989.
40. Teitelbaum DH, Caniano DA, Wheller JK: Resolution of an infected intracardiac thrombus. J Pediatr Surg 24:1118–1120, 1989.
41. Chathas MK: Percutaneous central venous catheters in neonates. J Obstet Gynecol Neonatal Nurs 15:324–332, 1986.
42. Spahr RC, MacDonald HM, Holzman IR: Catheterization of the posterior tibial artery in the neonate. Am J Dis Child 133:945–946, 1979.
43. Randel SN, Tsang BHL, Wung J-T, et al: Experience with percutaneous indwelling peripheral arterial catheterization in neonates. Am J Dis Child 141:848–851, 1987.
44. Pourcyrous M, Korones SB, Bada HS, et al: Indwelling umbilical arterial catheter: A preferred sampling site for blood culture. Pediatrics 81:821–825, 1988.
45. Singer RL, Wolfson PJ: Experience with umbilical artery cut-downs in neonates. Pediatr Surg Int 5:295–297, 1990.
46. Kitterman JA, Phibbs RH, Tooley WH: Catheterization of umbilical vessels in newborn infants. Pediatr Clin North Am 17:895–912, 1970.
47. Adams JM, Rudolph AJ: The use of indwelling radial artery catheters in neonates. Pediatrics 55:261–265, 1975.
48. Barr PA, Sumners J, Wirtschafter D, et al: Percutaneous peripheral arterial cannulation in the neonate. Pediatrics 59(suppl 6, pt 2):1058–1062, 1977.
49. Miyasaka K, Edmonds JF, Conn AW: Complications of radial artery lines in the paediatric patient. Can Anaesth Soc J 23:9–14, 1976.
50. Sellden H, Nilsson K, Larsson LE, et al: Radial arterial catheters in children and neonates: A prospective study. Crit Care Med 15:1106–1109, 1987.
51. Taylor LM Jr, Troutman R, Feliciano P, et al: Late complications after femoral artery catheterization in children less than five years of age. J Vasc Surg 11:297–306, 1990.
52. Prian GW: Complications and sequelae of temporal artery catheterization in the high-risk newborn. J Pediatr Surg 12:829–835, 1977.
53. Bull MJ, Schreiner RL, Garg BP, et al: Neurologic complications following temporal artery catheterization. J Pediatr 96:1071–1073, 1980.
54. Gauderer M, Holgersen LO: Peripheral arterial line insertion in neonates and infants: A simplified method of temporal artery cannulation. J Pediatr Surg 9:875–877, 1974.
55. Goetzman BW: Arterial access in the newborn [editorial]. Am J Dis Child 141:841, 1987.
56. Kirpekar M, Augenstein H, Abiri M: Sequential development of multiple aortic aneurysms in a neonate post umbilical arterial catheter insertion. Pediatr Radiol 19:452–453, 1989.
57. Lowenstein E, Little JW III, Lo HH: Prevention of cerebral embolization from flushing radial-artery cannulas. N Engl J Med 285:1414–1415, 1971.
58. Willard D, Messer J: Arterial access and monitoring in the newborn [letter]. Am J Dis Child 142:480, 1988.

9

SURGICAL INFECTIOUS DISEASE

Joseph A. Iocono, MD •
Thomas M. Krummel, MD

Despite advances in antimicrobial therapy and surgical and aseptic techniques, infection continues to be an enormous problem for the surgeon. Widespread antibiotic use has not significantly decreased the number of infections since the 1950s and has brought with it the deadly complication of resistant organisms.[1] Antibiotic selection has also become increasingly complex as newer antibiotics are continually released.[2]

There are two broad classes of infectious disease processes that affect a surgical practice: those infectious conditions that present to the pediatric surgeon for treatment and cure[3] and those that arise in the postoperative period that are a complication of surgical intervention.

☐ Components of Infection

The pathogenesis of infection involves a complex interaction between host and pathogens. Four components, present in varying degrees, are present in any infection: virulence of organism, size of inoculum, presence of nutrient source for the organism, and breakdown of host defense.

VIRULENCE OF ORGANISM

The virulence of any microorganism depends on its ability to cause damage to the host. Exotoxins, such as Streptococcal hyaluronidase, are digestive enzymes released locally that allow the spread of infection by breaking down host extracellular matrix proteins. Exotoxins may also be absorbed systemically by the host and cause remote damage. Endotoxins, such as lipopolysaccharides, are components of gram-negative cell walls that are released only after bacterial cell death. Endotoxin causes no local injury; rather, once systemically absorbed, endotoxin triggers a severe and rapid systemic inflammatory response.[4]

Infections are often polymicrobial, thus the concept of virulence requires an understanding of the types of interaction among species of microorganisms.[5] Different species may exist together within tissue through three separate mechanisms. *Species indifference* exists when there is a relatively stable balance between colonies of different species within the same environment. The best example of this is the complex flora of the human intestinal tract, which contains more than 100 species of bacteria.[6] *Species antagonism* is common and occurs when one or a few species emerge predominant from an initial large group as a result of external forces. A clinical example occurs when *Clostridium difficile* grows disproportionately owing to antibiotic disruption of the balance of colonic flora. *Species synergism* is seen when two or more species act in concert to allow continued growth of both species. In this mechanism, the observed damage to the host outweighs an additive affect of the individual organisms. The most common example of species synergism is seen in the mixed anaerobic and aerobic infections of an intraabdominal abscess.[7] Anaerobic bacteria have high invasive potential but have difficulty propagating in an aerobic environment. However, when mixed with aerobic species, the oxygen content of the local tissues is consumed, allowing anaerobes to flourish while aerobes benefit from the increased soft tissue invasion.

SIZE OF INOCULUM

The size of inoculum is the second component of an infection. The number of colonies of microorganisms per gram of tissue is a key determinant to infection. A minimum number of colonies is necessary for survival against host defenses. The smallest number of bacteria required to cause clinical infection varies from species to species, and, predictably, any decrease in host resistance decreases the absolute number of colonies necessary to cause clinical disease. In general, if the bacterial population in a wound exceeds 100,000 organisms per gram of tissue, invasive infection is present.[8]

PRESENCE OF NUTRIENT SOURCE

For any inoculum, the ability for the organism(s) to find suitable nutrients is essential for their survival and comprises the third component of any clinical infection. The only other requirement for most microorganisms is water; microorganisms do poorly in dry environments. Accumulation of necrotic tissue, hematoma, or other environmental contamination offers nutrient medium for continued growth and spread. Of special importance to the surgeon is the concept of necrotic tissue and infection. Retained necrotic tissue plays a dual role in the pathogenesis of infection. This tissue is recognized as a nutrient source for invading microorganisms,[9] and recent data have also shown that necrotic tissue accumulates complement proteins.[10] Therefore, necrotic tissue at a wound site attracts neutrophils and diverts them from invading microorganisms.

BREAKDOWN OF HOST DEFENSE

Finally, for a clinical infection to arise, the body's resistance to infection must be broken. Even highly virulent organisms can be eradicated before clinical infection occurs if resistance is intact and nutrients are scarce. Evolution has equipped humans with redundant mechanisms of defense, both anatomic and systemic.

☐ Defense Against Infection

ANATOMIC BARRIERS

Intact skin and mucous membranes provide an effective surface barrier to infection.[11] These tissues are not merely a mechanical obstacle; physiologic aspects of skin and mucous membranes provide additional protection. The constant turnover of keratinocytes leaves the uppermost surface of the skin dry, causing microorganisms to desiccate there. Skin temperature tends to be about 5°C less than physiologic, which inhibits bacterial growth. Acid secretion from sebaceous glands creates an environment on the skin surface with a pH of 5.5, further inhibiting bacterial cell growth. Finally, keratinocytes themselves can express the antigen responsible for recognition of cytotoxic T cell and can excrete proinflammatory cytokines in certain disease states.

Those mucosal surfaces that are exposed to the environment have also developed advanced defense mechanisms to prevent and combat microbial invasion. Specialized epithelial layers provide a defense to prevent bacterial invasion. The respiratory bronchial tree is protected by the mucociliary transport mechanism, which efficiently removes particulate contamination from inspired air. In the gastrointestinal (GI) tract, the harsh acidic environment of the stomach effectively kills most invading bacteria. Distally, the normal colonic flora competes with pathogenic organisms and prevents their emergence.

In the urinary tract, the bladder also possesses an acidic environment and undergoes continuous and near-complete evacuation, diluting and eliminating organisms. In the eye, the surface of the cornea is continually bathed in the bacteriocidal enzyme lysozyme.[12]

Any pathologic situation affecting the normal function of these anatomic barriers increases the host's susceptibility to infection. A skin wound or a burn provides open access to soft tissues, tobacco damages the mucociliary transport system in the respiratory tree,[13] and antibiotic use disrupts normal colonic flora.[14] Such breakdowns in surface barriers are dealt with by the second line of defenses, the immune system.

IMMUNE RESPONSE

The mammalian immune system involves complex pathways and many specialized effector responses.[15] Multiple overlapping mechanisms of intercellular communication (paracrine) act in concert with endocrine mechanisms to constitute this essential protective system.

The immune response is triggered by any infectious, traumatic, or foreign body invasion, resulting in inflammation (calor, rubor, dolor, and tumor). The components of acute inflammation are changes in local blood flow, presence of vascular permeability, and exudation of leukocytes. An initial vasoconstriction response is followed by vasodilation. Injury stimulates macrophages, production of proinflammatory cytokines, and microcirculation with activation of endothelial cells, blood elements, and a capillary leak. These processes are potentiated by ischemia, impaired oxygen delivery, and necrotic tissue, each of which exacerbates the inflammatory response. The classic hypothalamic-pituitary-adrenal axis, activated via neurologic afferent pathways, significantly influences inflammation by producing catecholamines and glucocorticoids.

Once initiated, the immune response operates by releasing cytokines and by receptors interacting on cell membranes.[16] Cytokines are endogenously produced proteins of low molecular weight and multiple biologic effects that are released locally by activated leukocytes. They exert both local and systemic responses. The best understood of these cytokines are tumor necrosis factor (TNF) and interleukin-1 (IL-1), which act to increase local synthesis of nitric oxide, prostaglandins, platelet-activating factor (PAF), and endothelial cell adhesion molecules. Cytokines also have the ability to exert control over the cells that produce them in an autocrine fashion. Sepsis, hemorrhage, ischemia, ischemia-reperfusion, and soft tissue trauma all share an ability to activate macrophages and produce proinflammatory cytokines that may progress to the uncontrolled systemic inflammatory response syndrome (SIRS).[17] Second-message compounds and effector molecules mediate the observed clinical phenomena (Fig. 9–1).

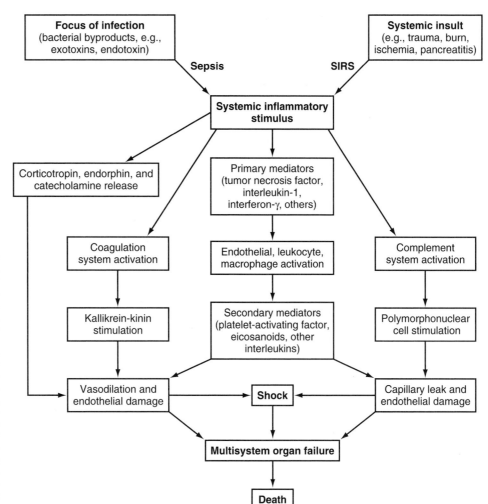

Figure 9–1. The parallel systemic inflammatory response that can result from infection, trauma, or critical illness. All of these types of insult may progress to shock, multisystem organ failure, and death. SIRS, systemic inflammatory response syndrome. (Data from Saez-Llorens X, McCracken GH Jr: Sepsis syndrome and septic shock in pediatrics: Current concepts of terminology, pathophysiology, and management. J Pediatr 123:497–508, 1993; and American College of Chest Physicians/Society of Critical Care Medicine Consensus Conference: Definitions for sepsis and organ failure and guidelines for the use of innovative therapies in sepsis. Crit Care Med 20:864–874, 1992.)

The local effect of these cytokines is chemotaxis, a targeted migration of the phagocyte toward an infectious focus. Most bacteria and fungi are destroyed by phagocytosis, the single most important process in the control of infection.[18] There are three important aspects of microbe recognition prior to phagocytosis: receptor redundancy, receptor cooperation, and transduction of specific cellular signals following receptor binding. Multiple receptors on leukocytes often participate in a given microbial recognition event. This cooperation among multiple receptors often increases the apparent affinity of the receptors for their ligand, thereby increasing the killing power of the leukocyte. Further, the receptor may orchestrate subsequent intracellular events during phagocytosis by transducing specific cellular signals. For example, the mannose and Fc γ-receptors direct particles to lysosomes and trigger a respiratory burst, whereas other receptors may not. Ingesting is an ameboid process in which the microbe is incorporated into the cytoplasm of the cell via endocytosis. Occasionally, however, ingested bacteria or their products are sufficiently potent to destroy the phagocyte before digestion. If this occurs, the release of contained lysozymes can lead to a destructive autodigestion of local host tissues. These defense mechanisms are nonspecific and do not rely on the host's targeted recognition of the invading organism.

Humoral and Cell-Mediated Immunity

Specific immunity has two major components. The *humoral mechanism* (B-cell system) is based on bursal cell lymphocytes and plasma cells and is independent of the thymus. The *cellular mechanism* (T-cell system) consists of the thymic-dependent lymphocytes.[19]

Humoral antibodies may neutralize toxins, tag foreign matter to aid phagocytosis (opsonization), or lyse invading cellular pathogens. Plasma cells and non–thymic-dependent lymphocytes that reside in the bone marrow and in the germinal centers and medullary cords of lymph nodes produce the reactive components of this humoral system. These components account for most of the human immunity against extracellular bacterial species.

Immunity provided by the B-cell system consists both of relatively specific antibodies, which are heat stable, and complement, which is heat labile and relatively nonspecific. Antibody receptor sites combine with antigen to form either soluble macromolecular compounds or insoluble complexes that precipitate or agglutinate. Human antibodies are classified into five basic types of immunoglobulins that vary considerably in concentration, diffusibility, size, and other properties. Complement is consumed whenever the humoral system has been activated, usually as a cascading system of at least nine complement components. Endotoxin and other proteins are also known to activate the sequence in what is called the *alternative pathway.*

The cellular or T-cell component of immunity is based on sensitized lymphocytes, probably of thymic origin, located in the subcortical regions of lymph nodes and in the periarterial spaces of the spleen; these lymphocytes form a part of the recirculating lymphocyte pool. The T cells are specifically responsible for immunity to viruses, most fungi, and intracellular bacteria. They produce a variety of lymphokines, such as transfer factors, that activate further lymphocytes, chemotactic factors, leukotrienes, and interferons.

☐ Immunodeficiencies

Susceptibility to infection is increased when some component of the host defense mechanism is absent, reduced in absolute numbers, or significantly curtailed in function. Such derangements may have a congenital basis, although the majority are acquired as a direct result of drugs, radiation, endocrine disease, surgical ablation, tumors, or bacterial toxins.

Any alteration in the timing, magnitude, or quality of the host inflammatory response may permit the immediate invasion of pathogens. These defects, in local reaction to injury, are observed with extreme degrees of vasoconstriction, as in shock, and under certain other conditions. If the barrier has been injured (e.g., burns), fails to repair, or increases its permeability, microbial invasion can occur. Whenever a normal drainage system becomes obstructed (e.g., nephrolithiasis, cholelithiasis) or fails to function, infection may occur.

In diabetes mellitus, leukocytes often fail to respond normally to chemotaxis. Measurable reductions in the number of mature phagocytes occur in leukemia, agranulocytosis, and marrow dysplasia.[20] Tumors, drugs (e.g., chloramphenicol, steroids), radiation, or other agents that impair hematopoiesis may account for derangements in phagocytosis. Poor nutritional status has adverse effects on immune function. In general, cell-mediated and nonspecific immunity are more sensitive than humoral immunity.[21]

In patients with a primary immune defect, susceptibility to a specific infection is based on whether the defect is humoral, cellular, or a combination. Primary immunodeficiencies are rare but important because prompt recognition can lead to lifesaving treatment or significant improvement in the quality

of life.[22] B-cell deficiencies are associated with sepsis from encapsulated bacteria, especially pneumococcus, *Haemophilus influenzae,* and meningococcus. Often, there is a fulminating course that rapidly ends in death, despite timely therapeutic measures. Although congenital agammaglobulinemia or dysgammaglobulinemia has been widely recognized, other causes of humoral defects include radiation, steroid and antimetabolite therapy, sepsis, splenectomy, and starvation.

T-cell deficiencies are responsible for many viral, fungal, and bacterial infections. Cutaneous candidiasis is a good example of a common infection seen with a T-cell deficiency. DiGeorge syndrome is a developmental anomaly in which both the thymus and the parathyroid glands are deficient, thus increasing the risk for infection and hypocalcemic tetany during infancy. Bacterial toxins, immunosuppressive drugs, malnutrition, and radiation can also produce defects in cellular immunity.[19]

☐ Prevention of Infections

The most effective way to deal with surgical infectious complications is to avoid them. The clinician must recognize the variables that increase the risk of infection and eliminate them.

SURGICAL TECHNIQUE AND SKIN PREPARATION

Preoperative preparation of the operative site and hands of the entire surgical team is of utmost importance in reducing the risk of postoperative infection. Hand scrubbing remains the most important proactive mechanism to reduce infection. Although debated, a 5-minute first scrub followed by subsequent 2- or 3-minute scrubs for secondary cases with one of several different cleansing solutions is adequate.[23, 24] Using either 5% povidone iodine or 4% chlorhexidine gluconate, a consistent 95% decrease in skin flora can be achieved.

Similar reduction in the patient's skin flora can be achieved with aggressive preoperative cleansing and sterile draping. Shaving the operative field, if necessary, should only be done just prior to prepping the skin.[25, 26]

ANTIBIOTIC PROPHYLAXIS

Operative procedures can be classified into one of four types, based on clinical situation and anatomic site, as outlined in Table 9–1. In adults, several well-designed prospective trials document decreased infection rates for all types of operative procedures with established antibiotic recommendations.[27] Timing of the perioperative antibiotic coverage is crucial; the first dose must be given less than 1 hour before the surgical incision to achieve bacteriocidal levels of antibiotic at the site of the incision.

In pediatric surgery, it is clear that antibiotic cov-

TABLE 9-1. Surgical Wound Classification System

Wound Category	Clinical Scenario	Technique Notes
Clean	Elective operation, primarily closed, no drains, no hollow viscus opened	No break in technique
Clean Contaminated	Elective operation; respiratory, GI, or GU tracts entered under controlled conditions	Minor break in technique or entry into a hollow viscus without significant spillage
Contaminated	Open fresh traumatic wounds, from relatively clean source; entrance into respiratory, GI, or GU systems in presence of known infection	Major break in technique resulting in significant spillage from hollow viscus
Dirty	Open, fresh, or late traumatic wounds from dirty source or gross spillage (pus) encountered during operation	Delayed treatment

GI, gastrointestinal; GU, genitourinary.

erage is required during clean-contaminated, contaminated, or dirty cases. However, there is still some disagreement concerning antimicrobial prophylaxis in clean operations. In clean cases in children with no other associated risk factors for infection, some pediatric surgeons still believe that preoperative antibiotics are necessary. Review of the pediatric surgical literature yields studies that advocate the use of antibiotics[28] and those that do not.[29] Currently, antibiotic prophylaxis in a clean case in the pediatric population is at the discretion of the operating surgeon.

BOWEL PREPARATION

The efficacy of bowel preparation before elective colon surgery has been established.[30] There are three components to the technique, although each has its own variations: mechanical irrigation and flushing of the colon to remove stool; oral topical antibiotics against colonic aerobes and anaerobes; and preoperative intravenous (IV) antibiotics that cover both common skin and colonic flora.[31] The preparation can be started on an outpatient basis the day before surgery, and the parenteral drugs are added to the regimen just prior to the procedure. One must be careful in the pediatric population, however, to avoid dehydration associated with bowel preps.

DRAINS AND IRRIGATION

The use of drains varies widely; drains are indicated in those surgical procedures where one expects accumulation of blood, serum, and exudates from wounds, and potential dead space.[32] Drains are also indicated when closure of a hollow viscus is imperfect. In the absence of infection, a closed drainage system is indicated and a drain should be brought out via a separate stab wound away from the operative incision. Drains should be removed as soon as possible because they are foreign bodies that can impede wound closure and because bacteria can colonize the wound via a drain or its exit site.[33]

Irrigating the operative field is an important component in preventing postoperative infectious complications.[34] Irrigation with copious amounts of sterile saline mechanically removes loose debris, necrotic tissue, serum, and excess clot. Usage of antibiotics in the irrigation solution has not been proved to be efficacious,[35] but noxious solutions, such as povidone-iodine or hydrogen peroxide, are deleterious.[36]

SUBACUTE BACTERIAL ENDOCARDITIS PROPHYLAXIS

Prophylaxis for endocarditis is a special situation. Patients with a history of prosthetic valves, congenital cardiac defects, rheumatic fever, or previous endocarditis should receive parenteral coverage with a penicillin and aminoglycoside preparation prior to any intraabdominal procedure. Minor dental procedures, endoscopy, and simple lacerations can be covered effectively simply with oral penicillin.[37]

☐ Treatment of Infection

Despite meticulous technique, perioperative antibiotics, and proper use of drains and irrigation, surgical infectious complications still occur. The fundamental principles of surgical treatment of an infectious process are straightforward: (1) drain pus, (2) débride the wound, (3) reestablish anatomic continuity, and (4) treat with appropriate antibiotic(s).

ANTIBIOTICS

There are several classes of antibiotics, based on their molecular structure and site of action. The varying classes of antibiotics may be divided into bacteriostatic, which inhibit bacterial growth, and bacteriocidal, which destroy bacteria.

PENICILLINS. Penicillins were originally derived from molds and were the first major class of antibiotics developed. Penicillins are bacteriocidal and act by disrupting the cell wall of gram-positive organisms. They have a short half-life and a narrow spectrum, and they carry a significant risk of sensitivity. Penicillins are inactivated by β-lactamase. Synthetic derivatives have somewhat greater activity but are still susceptible to enzyme degradation.

CEPHALOSPORINS. Also bacteriocidal, cephalosporins are subdivided into generations based on increasing gram-negative activity. Adverse reactions include hypersensitivity reactions and alcohol intolerance. On the whole, they are less susceptible to β-lactamases and, like penicillins, act by inhibiting cell wall synthesis. First-generation cephalosporins are effective against most aerobic gram-positive organisms. Second-generation drugs have increased gram-negative and anaerobic coverage. Third-generation cephalosporins have the broadest gram-negative coverage of the family, but they lose most of the gram-positive activity of the first generation. Fourth-generation cephalosporins are projected to have an extended spectrum of activity for gram-negative and gram-positive organisms and minimal β-lactamase susceptibility.

AMINOGLYCOSIDES. Used to treat susceptible aerobic gram-negative bacteria, the aminoglycosides act by inhibiting protein synthesis. Aminoglycosides have a narrow margin of safety within the therapeutic dose range. Aminoglycosides can produce four types of dose-related adverse effects: (1) renal proximal tubular cell damage, (2) destruction of sensory cells in the cochlea, (3) destruction of sensory cells in the vestibular apparatus, and (4) neuromuscular paralysis.

TETRACYCLINES. Tetracyclines inhibit protein synthesis but are only bacteriostatic. They are active against gram-negative and gram-positive bacteria, mycoplasmas, chlamydiae, and protozoans. Tetracyclines remain a good first-line antibiotic in the penicillin-allergic patient.

QUINOLONES. Quinolones are bactericidal. The fluoroquinolones destroy aerobic Enterobacteriaceae, staphylococci, *Pseudomonas aeruginosa,* and some streptococci. The quinolones are excreted in the urine and are useful in treating urinary tract infections.

MACROLIDES. The macrolides erythromycin, azithromycin, and clarithromycin are similar to each other in activity. They are primarily bacteriostatic agents active against aerobic and anaerobic gram-positive cocci and gram-negative anaerobes. Hypersensitivity reactions are rare, but pseudomembranous enterocolitis due to *C. difficile* does occur.

IMIPENEM. Imipenem is an extremely active bacteriocidal antibiotic with a spectrum against almost all gram-positive and gram-negative organisms, both aerobic and anaerobic. Enterococci, *Bacteroides fragilis,* and *P. aeruginosa* are all susceptible.

AZTREONAM. Aztreonam is a parenteral antibiotic with excellent activity against *P. aeruginosa* equivalent to that of imipenem, ceftazidine, piperacillin, and azlocillin. Gram-positive organisms and anaerobes are resistant to aztreonam.

VANCOMYCIN. A bactericidal antibiotic active against all gram-positive cocci and bacilli, including *Staphylococcus aureus* and *Staphylococcus epidermidis* resistant to penicillins and cephalosporins, vancomycin also has bacteriostatic activity against enterococci. Vancomycin is the drug of choice for serious staphylococcal infection and endocarditis caused by *Streptococcus viridans* or enterococci or when penicillins or cephalosporins cannot be used because of drug allergy. Oral vancomycin is the drug of choice in *C. difficile* colitis, when it is resistant to metronidazole (Flagyl). Nephrotoxicity occurs occasionally, and deafness may be associated with very high blood levels, usually in patients with renal insufficiency.

TRIMETHOPRIM AND SULFAMETHOXAZOLE (BACTRIM). This bacteriostatic combination is active against most aerobic gram-positive and gram-negative organisms. Trimethoprim and sulfamethoxazole combined is the drug of choice to treat *Pneumocystis carinii* pneumonia. It is also effective in prophylaxis of this infection in children with AIDS or with malignancies. The side effects are nausea, vomiting, rash, and folate deficiency, resulting in macrocytic anemia.

METRONIDAZOLE. A bacteriocidal agent used primarily to treat protozoal infections and infections caused by anaerobes, particularly *B. fragilis,* metronidazole has also been used successfully in Hirschsprung's enterocolitis and for bowel prep. It is the agent of choice in treatment of *C. difficile* colitis.

ANTIFUNGALS

AMPHOTERICIN B. Amphotericin B is a fungicidal and fungistatic antibiotic useful in any systemic fungal infection. Many attempts at reducing the toxicity of amphotericin have been investigated.[39] New lipid-encapsulated amphotericin formulations are available that allow increased dosing (efficacy) and decreased toxicity.

FLUCONAZOLE. A fungistatic agent useful against oropharyngeal and esophageal candidiasis, fluconazole has been successfully used in systemic fungal infections with *Candida* species not including *Candida glabrata.* Fluconazole has rarely been associated with hepatic toxicity, which is sometimes fatal in patients with serious comorbid conditions.

FLUCYTOSINE. Flucytosine is an antifungal agent active against a number of fungi. Patients with AIDS do not tolerate flucytosine.

NYSTATIN. Both fungistatic and fungicidal against a wide variety of yeast and yeast-like fungi, nystatin is passed unchanged in the stool. It is used to treat intestinal and oral cavity infections caused by *Candida albicans.* Large oral doses occasionally produce diarrhea, gastrointestinal (CGI) distress, nausea, or vomiting.

ANTIVIRALS

ACYCLOVIR. Acyclovir is an antiviral agent effective for preventing and treating viruses in the herpes family. Both IV and oral formulations are approved for use in children. Very little active drug accumulates in uninfected cells, which accounts for the low toxicity of the drug.

GANCICLOVIR. Related to acyclovir but with greater efficacy against cytomegalovirus, ganciclovir inhibits viral replication by interfering with cellular DNA. Adverse reactions include bone marrow suppression, mild nephrotoxicity, and transient hepatic enzyme elevation.

PHARMACOKINETICS AND MONITORING

The efficacy and safety of many drugs have not been established in the pediatric patient, especially in the newborn.[40] Dosages based on pediatric pharmacokinetic data offer the most rational approach. The assumption that a child is a miniature adult as the basis for extrapolation of adult dosages to children is certainly not ideal. Dosage requirements constantly change as a function of age and body weight. Knowledge of a drug's pharmacokinetic profile allows manipulation of the dose to achieve and maintain a given plasma concentration. For example, penicillins and cephalosporins have a distribution in children which prolongs their half-life.[41] Many drugs exhibit a biexponential plasma disappearance curve in neonates and children in that a certain fraction of the drug remaining in the body is eliminated per unit of time. Some drugs (e.g., gentamicin) exhibit saturation kinetics in which a specific amount, not a fraction, of the drug is eliminated per unit of time.[42] The body surface area (BSA) method of calculating drug dosages

$$\text{BSA} = (\text{Weight [kg]} \div 1.73) \times \text{adult dose}$$

approximates the pediatric dose of many drugs but does not always accurately determine dosage requirements in the premature and full-term newborn.

Newborns usually have extremely skewed drug distribution patterns. Thus, the entire body during the newborn period could be considered as if it were a single compartment for purposes of dose calculations. For the majority of drugs, dose adjustments can be based on plasma drug concentration. Administering a loading dose is advisable when rapid onset of drug action is required. For many drugs, loading doses (milligrams per kilogram) are generally greater in neonates and young infants than in older children or adults.[42] However, prolonged elimination of drugs in the neonate requires lower maintenance doses, given at longer intervals, to prevent toxicity. Monitoring serum drug concentrations is useful if the desired effect is not attained or if adverse reactions occur. In the sick premature newborn, almost all medications are administered IV because GI function and drug absorption are unreliable. Intramuscular injection is impractical because these neonates have little muscle mass. In older preterm neonates, full-term newborns, and older pediatric patients who do not have vomiting or diarrhea, oral drugs may be used. Drug absorption

through the skin is enhanced in the neonate and is currently being evaluated.[43]

The neonate undergoing extracorporeal membrane oxygenation (ECMO) presents a special challenge to drug delivery and elimination. Because the ECMO circuit may bind drugs and make them unavailable to the patient, dosing of drugs requires careful attention to drug response and serum levels. In one in vitro study, drug levels of common medications were significantly lowered depending, partially, on the age of the membrane.[44]

☐ Types of Infection

POSTOPERATIVE SOFT TISSUE INFECTIONS

Postoperative soft tissue infections can be divided into confined local lesions and invasive, spreading ones. Early diagnosis and prompt intervention help to avoid morbidity and occasional mortality. Erythema, fever, leukocytosis, tenderness, crepitus, and suppuration in a wound are diagnostic signs that are not always present. When confronted with a suspicious wound, clinical judgments must be made. Treatment should be suited to the extent of the infection and may include oral or IV antibiotics, simple incision and drainage, or extensive surgical débridement. Fortunately, soft tissue infections are uncommon in the pediatric surgical population. The incidence of wound infection varies from 1 to 11% in clean wounds and from 6 to 20.7% in contaminated wounds.[45, 46]

A localized surgical wound infection with seroma or pus requires drainage and packing to allow healing by secondary intention. Antibiotic therapy should be reserved for those infections with associated cellulitis. Localized cellulitis without fluid accumulation sometimes is amenable to antibiotic treatment only.

An abscess is a localized collection of pus in a cavity formed by an expanding infectious process. The pus is a combination of leukocytes, necrotic material, bacteria, and extracellular fluid. The usual cause is staphylococcal species in combination with one or more organisms; treatment is incision and drainage followed by antibiotic therapy. Drainage must be complete or the abscess will reform. A phlegmon is an area of diffuse inflammation with little pus and some necrotic tissue. A phlegmon usually progresses to an abscess if untreated.

Necrotizing fasciitis is a rapidly progressing infection of the fascial tissues and overlying skin. Although it can occur as a postoperative complication or as a primary infection, necrotizing fasciitis is more likely in immunocompromised patients.[47] Because the diagnosis is often not obvious, the clinician must look for clinical clues such as edema beyond the area of erythema, crepitus, skin vesicles, or cellulitis refractory to IV antibiotics. Prompt surgical intervention, including wide excision of all necrotic and infected tissue, along with the institution of antibiotics, is mandatory to avoid progression and mortality. Approximately half of pediatric cases occur in neonates. Combining the 47 patients reported in three series, the most common associated diagnosis was varicella infection (46%).[48–50] The mortality was 25% and was usually associated with delayed diagnosis. All survivors were operated on within 3 hours of diagnosis. Extensive débridement and triple antibiotic therapy were the hallmarks of survival.

DEHISCENCE

Dehiscence is defined as breakdown of the fascial components of a surgically closed wound. In any incision, the long-term tensile strength lies in the healing of the fascial component of the closure. By definition, dehiscence can occur in any surgically closed wound. Poor nutrition, renal failure, corticosteroid use, immune compromise, and poor wound closure technique increase the chance of wound dehiscence.[51]

PERITONITIS

Peritonitis is defined as inflammation of the peritoneum.[52] Peritonitis is divided into primary, secondary, and tertiary, depending on the etiology. Spontaneous primary peritonitis is a bacterial infection without enteric perforation. It is usually caused by a single organism of gut origin; however, if an invasive catheter is present, the most likely organism is gram positive.[53] Susceptible infants are those with ascites, indwelling peritoneal dialysis catheters, ventriculoperitoneal shunts, or compromised immunity. An infant with primary peritonitis usually does not exhibit signs of peritonitis but may have poor feeding, lethargy, distention, vomiting, and mild to severe abdominal tenderness. Definitive treatment may require only a course of broad-spectrum antibiotics. Primary peritonitis in children now represents approximately 1% of all cases of peritonitis.

Secondary peritonitis is associated with GI tract disruption.[54] This can be caused directly by perforation, bowel wall necrosis, or trauma or postoperatively as a result of iatrogenic injury or anastomotic leak. Treatment of secondary peritonitis is a combination of surgery and antibiotics.

Tertiary peritonitis is inflammation without bacteria or fungi.

LYMPHANGITIS

Lymphangitis is often accompanied by a red streak extending up an extremity. The causative organism is usually *Staphylococcus* or *Streptococcus* species. Prompt, aggressive therapy includes immobilization and IV antibiotics. The infection worsens without treatment, and obliteration of the lymphatic channels can result.

SEPSIS

Sepsis, by contemporary definition, distinguishes between the systemic derangements that are caused by the infectious organisms and their byproducts and those that are caused by the host systemic inflammatory response.[55] In 1992, the Society of Critical Care Medicine published the results of a consensus conference to accurately define the terms regarding sepsis and the inflammatory response to injury and infection[56] (Table 9–2). Independent of the original infection, SIRS may progress to multiorgan dysfunction and death. Gram-negative organisms possess a lipopolysaccharide moiety on the cell wall that has been shown to incite most, if not all, of the toxic effects of end-organ failure. In animal models, injection of lipopolysaccharide can induce a septic response by both direct and indirect effects. Directly, it activates macrophages and neutrophils to release the cytokines, TNF, IL-1, and IL-6, which are the primary host mediators of end-organ failure.[57]

The indirect host responses to these cytokines include release of PAF, IL-8, prostaglandins, and nitric oxide. These secondary mediators induce vasodilation, more polymorphonuclear cell stimulation, endothelial cell damage and leak, as well as platelet activation. The systemic response to these derangements is hypotension, fever, hypoxia, and end-organ failure. The process is self-propagating. Figure 9–1 shows a schematic of the current understanding of the pathogenesis of the inflammatory response in sepsis.[58]

Therefore, in addition to conventional surgical débridement and drainage, antibiotic treatment and supportive intensive therapy, modulating the host inflammatory mediators as a therapeutic addition, have been explored since the mid-1980s. Although successful in animal models of sepsis, inhibiting host inflammatory response in human sepsis has not improved survival. New treatment modalities, such as granulocyte-stimulating factor, immunoglobulin infusion, and cytokine antagonists offer theoretical promise but so far have not improved the results of clinical trials.[59]

Neonatal sepsis is defined as a generalized bacterial infection accompanied by a positive blood culture within the first month of life.[60] Neonatal sepsis occuring during the first week of life is caused primarily by maternal organisms transferred during delivery. Maternal contamination of the neonate can be transmitted through the placenta, via the birth canal or by direct contamination of the amniotic fluid. The mortality of this early onset variety approaches 50%. Late-onset neonatal sepsis is primarily nosocomial, most often secondary to indwelling catheters or bacterial translocation from the gut. In the surgical neonate, three factors promote bacterial translocation and sepsis: (1) intestinal bacterial colonization and overgrowth, (2) compromised host defenses, and (3) disruption of the mucosal epithelial barrier.[61] The mortality of late-onset sepsis is

TABLE 9-2. Definitions

Term	Definition
Infection	Microbial phenomenon characterized by an inflammatory response to the presence of microorganisms or to the invasion of normally sterile host tissues by microorganisms
Bacteremia	Presence of viable bacteria in the blood
Systemic inflammatory response syndrome	Systemic inflammatory response to a variety of severe clinical insults (noninfectious); the response is manifested by two or more of the following: Temperature >38°C or <36°C Heart rate >90 beats/min Respiration rate >20 breaths/min or $PaCO_2$ <32 mm Hg × 2 White blood cell count >12,000 cells/mm³, <4000 cells/mm³, or > 10% immature forms
Sepsis	Systemic response to infection manifested by two or more of the following conditions as a result of infection: Temperature >38°C or <36°C Heart rate >90 beats/min Respiration rate >20 breaths/min or $PaCO_2$ <32 mm Hg × 2 White blood cell count >12,000 cells/mm³, <4000 cells/mm³, or > 10% immature forms
Severe sepsis	Sepsis associated with organ dysfunction; hypotension; or hypoperfusion (hypoperfusion abnormalities may include but are not limited to lactic acidosis, oliguria, and acute alteration in mental status)
Septic shock	Sepsis with hypotension, despite adequate fluid resuscitation, along with perfusion abnormalities, which may include but are not limited to lactic acidosis, oliguria, and acute alteration in mental status (patients who are on inotropic or vasopressor agents may not be hypotensive at the time perfusion abnormalities are measured)
Hypotension	Systolic blood pressure of <90 mm Hg or a reduction of >40 mm Hg from baseline in the absence of other causes of hypotension
Multiple organ dysfunction syndrome	Presence of altered organ function in an acutely ill patient such that hemostasis cannot be maintained without any and all interventions

Adapted from American College of Chest Physicians/Society of Critical Care Medicine Consensus Conference: Crit Care Med 20:864–874, 1992.

20%. The clinician must be alert for the subtle signs and symptoms of neonatal sepsis, which include lethargy, irritability, temperature instability, and change in respiratory or feeding pattern. Neonates may not demonstrate leukocytosis. Empirical triple-antibiotic coverage may be started, pending the results of blood and other cultures.

MYCOTIC INFECTION

Mycotic infections are an increasing problem in immunocompromised pediatric patients.[62] Successful management of fungal infections requires recognition of the potential for infection, understanding of the organisms that can cause infection, and identification of the organ system(s) affected. The immature immune system of neonates is partially responsible for some specific diseases and poses unique management problems. Hospitalized infants today are increasingly stressed to degrees not previously seen in intensive care nurseries and may be on long-term antibiotic therapy for other illnesses. Chemotherapy for malignancy, bone marrow transplant,

trauma, and chronic illness increase the risk of immunocompromise and systemic fungal infection.[63] The frequent use of long-term intravascular catheters contributes to fungal infections. Therapy includes administration of topical and parenteral antifungal agents and supportive care.

NOSOCOMIAL INFECTION

Nosocomial infections are hospital acquired.[64] They are a potential threat to all hospitalized patients and increase morbidity and mortality significantly.[65] A recent report described a total of 676 operative procedures performed in 608 pediatric patients. Nosocomial infection occurred in 38 (6.2%). A total of 53 infectious complications were tabulated: wound 17 (2.5%), septicemia 14 (2.1%), pulmonary 10 (1.5%), urinary tract 5 (0.7%), abdominal 5 (0.7%), and diarrhea 2 (0.3%). Broviac catheter sepsis occurred in 7 (11.5%) of 61 lines. The highest overall occurrence of infection was in the infant group (1 month–1 year), (13 [8.1%] of 161). The probability of septicemia was highest in neonates

(4.2%) compared with infants (3.1%) and older children (1.2%) (P < .05). The most common isolates were *Staphylococcus epidermidis* (10 of 17) from septic patients, and gram-negative enteric bacteria (27 of 50) from organ and wound infections. Infection was associated with impaired nutrition, multiple disease processes, and multiple operations. The risk of nosocomial infection in this population was comparable to that reported in adult surgical patients. In one study, ECMO use correlated with increased incidence of nosocomial infection.[66] Two factors that increase the risk of nosocomial infection in surgical wounds as well as other sites are length of the preoperative stay and exposure to invasive medical devices.[67]

Using central venous catheters is essential in managing critically ill pediatric patients. However, the complication of catheter-related infection prevails despite a great deal of effort to reduce its occurrence. It is important to recognize the difference between colonization of the catheter and central venous catheter infection. Colonization is defined as the presence of a positive culture without signs and symptoms of clinical infection. Five major factors are associated with the development of the following catheter-related nosocomial infections:

1. Sterility of the insertion technique
2. Type of solution being administered through the line
3. Care of the catheter once inserted
4. Proximity of the catheter to another wound
5. Presence of another infection elsewhere

Absolute sterile techniques should be maintained in all instances of line insertion except in a trauma or other emergency situation in which the need for expedient line placement may necessitate less-than-sterile technique. Infusion of hyperalimentation has been shown to increase the incidence of infection in central venous catheters.[68] Bacteria from a local or distant source may seed the catheter.[69]

Pneumonitis is the most lethal nosocomial infection, with mortality ranging from 20 to 70% and accounting for 10 to 15% of all pediatric hospital-acquired infections.[70] The mortality rate is dependent on the causative organism. The risk factors for nosocomial pneumonia in the pediatric population include serious underlying illness, immunosuppression, length of time on a ventilator, and nasopharyngeal floral changes with prolonged hospitalization.[6] There may be increased risk in patients with gastric alkalinization because use of antacids in the intensive care unit to prevent stress ulceration increases bacterial counts in the stomach and may predispose the patient to increased bacterial translocation.[71]

REFERENCES

1. Neu HC: The changing ecology of bacterial infections in children. Compr Ther 2:47–52, 1976.
2. Liu HH: Antibiotics and infectious diseases. Prim Care 17:745–774, 1990.
3. Kosloske AM: Surgical infections in children. Curr Opin Pediatr 6:353–359, 1994.
4. DeLa Cadena RA, Majluf-Cruz A, Stadnicki A, et al: Activation of the contact and fibrinolytic systems after intravenous administration of endotoxin to normal human volunteers: Correlation with the cytokine profile. Immunopharmacology 33:231–237, 1996.
5. White RL, Burgess DS, Manduru M, et al: Comparison of three different in vitro methods of detecting synergy: Time-kill, checkerboard, and E test. Antimicrob Agents Chemother 40:1914–1918, 1996.
6. Jarvis WR: The epidemiology of colonization. Infect Control Hosp Epidemiol 17:47–52, 1996.
7. Brook I: Anaerobic infections in childhood. Rev Infect Dis 6(suppl 1):S187–S192, 1984.
8. Robson MC, Stenberg BD, Heggers JP: Wound healing alterations caused by infection. Clin Plast Surg 17:485–492, 1990.
9. Baxter CR: Immunologic reactions in chronic wounds. Am J Surg 167:12S–14S, 1994.
10. Harris BH, Gelfand JA: The immune response to trauma. Semin Pediatr Surg 4:77–82, 1995.
11. Forslind B, Lindberg M, Roomans GM, et al: Aspects on the physiology of human skin: Studies using particle probe analysis. Microsc Res Tech 38:373–386, 1997.
12. Bleacher JC, Krummel TM: Host resistence to infection. In Fonkalsrud EW, Krummel TM (eds): Infections and Immunologic Disorders in Pediatric Surgery. Philadelphia, WB Saunders, 1993, pp 63–75.
13. Brown R, Pinkerton R, Tuttle M: Respiratory infections in smokers. Am Fam Physician 36:133–140, 1987.
14. Godet AS, Williams RD: Postoperative *Clostridium difficile* gastroenteritis. J Urol 149:142–144, 1993.
15. Daynes RA, Araneo BA, Hennebold J, et al: Steroids as regulators of the mammalian immune response. J Invest Dermatol 105(1 suppl):14S–19S, 1995.
16. del Guercio P: The self and the nonself: Immunorecognition and immunologic functions. Immunol Res 12:168–182, 1993.
17. Karzai W, Reinhart K: Immune modulation and sepsis. Int J Clin Pract 51:232–237, 1997.
18. Mosser DM: Receptors on phagocytic cells involved in microbial recognition. Immunol Ser 60:99–114, 1994.
19. Fleisher TA: Immune function. Pediatr Rev 18:351–356, 1997.
20. Bessman AN, Sapico FL: Infections in the diabetic patient: The role of immune dysfunction and pathogen virulence factors. J Diabetes Complications 6:258–262, 1992.
21. Scrimshaw NS, SanGiovanni JP: Synergism of nutrition, infection, and immunity: An overview. Am J Clin Nutr 66:464S–477S, 1997.
22. Puck JM: Primary immunodeficiency diseases. JAMA 278:1835–1841, 1997.
23. Pereira LJ, Lee GM, Wade KJ: The effect of surgical hand-washing routines on the microbial counts of operating room nurses. Am J Infect Control 18:354–364, 1990.
24. Wheelock SM, Lookinland S: Effect of surgical hand scrub time on subsequent bacterial growth. AORN J 65:1087–1092, 1094–1098, 1997.
25. Mishriki SF, Law DJ, Jeffery PJ: Factors affecting the incidence of postoperative wound infection. J Hosp Infect 16:223–230, 1990.
26. Kovach T: Nip it in the bud: Controlling wound infection with preoperative shaving. Todays OR Nurse 12:23–26, 1990.
27. Nichols RL: Surgical antibiotic prophylaxis. Med Clin North Am 79:509–522, 1995.
28. Inserra A, Serventi P, Ciprandi G, et al: Antibioticoprofilassi con ceftazidime in chirurgia pediatrica. Clin Ter 136:393–398, 1996.
29. Kesler RW, Guhlow LJ, Saulsbury FT: Prophylactic antibiotics in pediatric surgery. Pediatrics 69:1–3, 1982.
30. Debo Adeyemi S, Tai da Rocha-Afodu J: Clinical studies of 4 methods of bowel preparation in colorectal surgery. Eur Surg Res 18:331–336, 1986.
31. Le TH, Timmcke AE, Gathright JB Jr, et al: Outpatient bowel preparation for elective colon resection. South Med J 90:526–530, 1997.
32. Samelson SL, Reyes HM: Management of perforated appendicitis in children—revisited. Arch Surg 122:691–699, 1987.

33. Raves JJ, Slifkin M, Diamond DL: A bacteriologic study comparing closed suction and simple conduit drainage. Am J Surg 148:618–620, 1984.
34. Badia JM, Torres JM, Tur C, et al: Saline wound irrigation reduces the postoperative infection rate in guinea pigs. J Surg Res 63:457–459, 1996.
35. Oestreicher M, Tschantz P: Prevention de l'infection de la plaie operatoire: Lavage par dérive iode, ou NaCl. Étude prospective et randomisée en chirurgie generale. Hel Chir Acta 56:133–137, 1989.
36. Kaysinger KK, Nicholson NC, Ramp WK, et al: Toxic effects of wound irrigation solutions on cultured tibiae and osteoblasts. J Orthop Trauma 9:303–311, 1995.
37. Cetta F, Bell TJ, Podlecki DD, et al: Parental knowledge of bacterial endocarditis prophylaxis. Pediatr Cardiol 14:220–222, 1993.
38. MacGowan AP, Bowker KE: Pharmacodynamics of antimicrobial agents and rationale for their dosing. J Chemother 9(suppl 1):64–73, 1997.
39. Leenders AC, de Marie S: The use of lipid formulations of amphotericin B for systemic fungal infections. Leukemia 10:1570–1575, 1996.
40. Musoke RN: Rational use of antibiotics in neonatal infections. East Afr Med J 74:147–150, 1997.
41. Butler DR, Kuhn RJ, Chandler MH: Pharmacokinetics of anti-infective agents in paediatric patients. Clin Pharmacokinet 26:374–395, 1994.
42. Routledge P: Pharmacokinetics in children [review]. J Antimicrob Chemother 34(suppl A):19–24, 1994.
43. Amato M, Huppi P, Isenschmid M, et al: Developmental aspects of percutaneous caffeine absorption in premature infants. Am J Perinatol 9:431–434, 1992.
44. Dagan O, Klein J, Gruenwald C, et al: Preliminary studies of the effects of extracorporeal membrane oxygenator on the disposition of common pediatric drugs. Ther Drug Monit 15:263–266, 1993.
45. Davenport M, Doig CM: Wound infection in pediatric surgery: A study in 1,094 neonates. J Pediatr Surg 28:26–30, 1993.
46. Bhattacharyya N, Kosloske AM: Postoperative wound infection in pediatric surgical patients: A study of 676 infants and children. J Pediatr Surg 25:125–129, 1990.
47. Farrell LD, Karl SR, Davis PK, et al: Postoperative necrotizing fasciitis in children. Pediatrics 82:874–879, 1988.
48. Murphy JJ, Granger R, Blair GK: Necrotizing fasciitis in childhood. J Pediatr Surg 30:1131–1134, 1995.
49. Moss RL, Musemeche CA, Kosloske AM: Necrotizing fasciitis in children: Prompt recognition and aggressive therapy improve survival. J Pediatr Surg 31:1142–1146, 1996.
50. Waldhausen JH, Holterman MJ, Sawin RS: Surgical implications of necrotizing fasciitis in children with chickenpox. J Pediatr Surg 31:1138–1141, 1996.
51. Poon TS, Zhang AL, Cartmill T, et al: Changing patterns of diagnosis and treatment of infantile hypertrophic pyloric stenosis: A clinical audit of 303 patients. J Pediatr Surg 31:1611–1165, 1996.
52. Heemken R, Gandawidjaja L, Hau T: Peritonitis: Pathophysiology and local defense mechanisms. Hepatogastroenterology 44:927–936, 1997.
53. Levy M, Balfe JW, Geary D, et al: Exit-site infection during continuous and cycling peritoneal dialysis in children. Perit Dial Int 10:31–35, 1990.
54. Ohmann C, Hau T: Prognostic indices in peritonitis. Hepatogastroenterology 44:937–946, 1997.
55. Kelly JL, Osullivan C, Oriordain M, et al: Is circulating endotoxin the trigger for the systemic inflammatory response syndrome seen after Injury. Ann Surg 225:530–541, 1997.
56. SCCM Consensus Committee: American College of Chest Physicians/Society of Critical Care Medicine Consensus Conference: Definitions for sepsis and organ failure and guidelines for the use of innovative therapies in sepsis. Crit Care Med 20:864–874, 1992.
57. Horn DL, Opal SM, Lomastro E: Antibiotics, cytokines, and endotoxin: A complex and evolving relationship in gram-negative sepsis. Scand J Infect Dis 101(suppl):9–13, 1996.
58. Shapiro L, Gelfand JA: Cytokines and sepsis: Pathophysiology and therapy. New Horiz 1:13–22, 1993.
59. Wexler LH, Weaver-McClure L, Steinberg SM, et al: Randomized trial of recombinant human granulocyte-macrophage colony-stimulating factor in pediatric patients receiving intensive myelosuppressive chemotherapy. J Clin Oncol 14:901–910, 1996.
60. Wolach B: Neonatal sepsis: Pathogenesis and supportive therapy. Semin Perinatol 21:28–38, 1997.
61. Jackson RJ, Smith SD, Wadowsky RM, et al: The effect of E. coli virulence on bacterial translocation and systemic sepsis in the neonatal rabbit model. J Pediatr Surg 26:483–485; discussion, 485–486, 1991.
62. Hilfiker ML, Azizkhan RG: Mycotic infections in pediatric surgical patients. Semin Pediatr Surg 4:239–244, 1995.
63. Barson WJ, Brady MT: Management of infections in children with cancer. Hematol Oncol Clin North Am 1:801–839, 1987.
64. Allen U, Ford-Jones EL: Nosocomial infections in the pediatric patient: An update. Am J Infect Control 18:176–193, 1990.
65. Bhattacharyya N, Kosloske AM, MacArthur C: Nosocomial infection in pediatric surgical patients: A study of 608 infants and children. J Pediatr Surg 28:338–343; discussion, 343–344, 1993.
66. Coffin SE, Bell LM, Manning M, et al: Nosocomial infections in neonates receiving extracorporeal membrane oxygenation. Infect Control Hosp Epidemiol 18:93–96, 1997.
67. Martin MA: Nosocomial infections in intensive care units: An overview of their epidemiology, outcome, and prevention. New Horiz 1:162–171, 1993.
68. Christensen ML, Hancock ML, Gattuso J, et al: Parenteral nutrition associated with increased infection rate in children with cancer. Cancer 72:2732–2738, 1993.
69. Reed CR, Sessler CN, Glauser FL, et al: Central venous catheter infections: Concepts and controversies. Intensive Care Med 21:177–183, 1995.
70. Stein F, Trevino R: Nosocomial infections in the pediatric intensive care unit. Pediatr Clin North Am 41:1245–1257, 1994.
71. Avanoglu A, Herek O, Ulman I, et al: Effects of H_2 receptor blocking agents on bacterial translocation in burn injury. Eur J Pediatr Surg 7:278–281, 1997.

10

HUMAN IMMUNODEFICIENCY VIRUS

Arthur Cooper, MD, MS • Elaine J. Abrams, MD • Stephen W. Nicholas, MD

Since the beginning of the HIV pandemic in the late 1970s, great strides have been made in reducing the mortality and morbidity rates of HIV infection in children. Widespread availability of laboratory tests that facilitate early diagnosis and aggressive prophylaxis of opportunistic infections have limited the debilitating effects of these conditions and improved the duration and quality of life for HIV-infected children. The two most important recent developments in the management of this illness relate to measures that prevent the development of HIV infection in newborns and delay the onset of AIDS in older children. The vertical transmission of HIV infection can be reduced by two thirds (from 24% to 8%) via maternal ingestion of zidovudine (ZDV, previously known as azidothymidine [AZT]), during the second and third trimesters of pregnancy, followed by neonatal administration of this drug for 6 weeks following delivery.[1] Long-term combination therapy with antiretroviral agents (both reverse transcriptase inhibitors and protease inhibitors) has greatly slowed the progression of illness among infants who are infected.[2] The resultant dramatic increases in overall survival and in life expectancy have changed the outlook for infants and children infected with HIV, from inexorable decline toward early death to chronic disability that can be effectively managed.

Nowhere are these changes more apparent than among children requiring surgical treatment for HIV-related complications. The decreasing incidence of opportunistic infections, particularly those affecting the lungs, has greatly reduced the need for minimally invasive diagnostic procedures, such as bronchoscopy with bronchoalveolar lavage, and virtually eliminated the need for fully invasive diagnostic procedures, such as open lung biopsy. At the same time, as larger numbers of children survive until chronic central nervous system or gastrointestinal infection develops, which may preclude ade-

quate oral alimentation, the need for supplemental nutritional support has resulted in more frequent reliance on artificial feeding via percutaneous endoscopic gastrostomy or central venous catheterization. Finally, as children are exposed to immunocompromised states for ever longer time intervals, the need for surgical assistance with tissue diagnosis of pathologic lesions, both infectious and neoplastic, has assumed an increasingly important role in overall surgical management.

☐ Epidemiology and Transmission

As of 1997, 7902 children younger than 13 years of age met the case surveillance definition developed by the U.S. Centers for Disease Control and Prevention (CDC) for AIDS, the end stage of HIV infection heralded by the presence of certain pathognomic "indicator diseases."[3] The case surveillance definition was revised in 1993 to include additional indicator diseases, but it has come to be applied to adults and adolescents only. The CDC developed a revised classification system for HIV infection in children younger than 13 years of age in 1994 that supersedes the original classification developed in 1987.[4] It incorporates the surveillance definition of AIDS promulgated in 1987. The revised classification permits staging by mild, moderate, and severe categories, based on clinical criteria as well as age-specific definitions of CD4-positive T-lymphocytopenia (Tables 10–1 to 10–4).[5] It is estimated that the number of HIV-infected infants and children outnumber those with documented AIDS by a factor of 3; hence, it is believed that more than 20,000 infants and children are infected in the United States—the majority of whom are of African American (61%) or Hispanic (24%) descent and reside in densely populated urban areas in the Northeast (44%) and South (36%).[3]

126

TABLE 10-1. Diagnosis of HIV Infection in Children

Diagnosis: HIV Infected

a) A child <18 mo of age who is known to be HIV seropositive or born to an HIV-infected mother and
  • has positive results on two separate determinations (excluding cord blood) from one or more of the following HIV detection tests:
     HIV culture
     HIV polymerase chain reaction
     HIV antigen (p24)
                    or
  • meets criteria for AIDS diagnosis based on the 1987 AIDS surveillance case definition
b) A child ≥ 18 mo of age born to an HIV-infected mother or any child infected by blood, blood products, or other known modes of transmission (e.g., sexual contact) who
  • is HIV-antibody positive by repeatedly reactive enzyme immunoassay (EIA) and confirmatory test (e.g., Western blot or immunofluorescence assay [IFA])
                    or
  • meets any of the criteria in a) above

Diagnosis: Perinatally Exposed (Prefix E in Table 10–2)

A child who does not meet the criteria above who
  • is HIV seropositive by EIA and confirmatory test (e.g., Western blot or IFA) and is <18 mo of age at the time of test
                    or
  • has unknown antibody status, but was born to a mother known to be infected with HIV

Diagnosis: Seroreverter (SR)

A child who is born to an HIV-infected mother and who
  • has been documented as HIV-antibody negative (i.e., two or more negative EIA tests performed at 6–18 mo of age or one negative EIA test after 18 mo of age)
                    and
  • has had no other laboratory evidence of infection (has not had two positive viral detection tests, if performed)
                    and
  • has not had an AIDS-defining condition

Adapted from Centers for Disease Control and Prevention: 1994 revised classification system for human immunodeficiency virus infection in children less than 13 years of age. MMWR Morb Mortal Wkly Rep 43:RR-12, 1994.

Vertical transmission is the cause of HIV infection in nearly 100% of infants and children. Routine use of recombinant blood clotting factors has dramatically reduced the risk of contracting HIV disease among hemophiliacs, and routine screening of do-nated blood products has virtually eliminated this risk among transfusion recipients.[6] Infection can be acquired prenatally via the placenta, perinatally during passage through the birth canal, or postnatally via breast milk, but most infants appear to become exposed at or near the time of birth. Although all infants born to HIV-infected women test seropositive at birth as a result of passive transfer of maternal antibody to the fetus during pregnancy, only 15 to 40% are actually infected. Hence, 60 to 85% of HIV-seropositive infants lose their maternal antibodies by 18 months of life, revert to HIV-seronegative status, and remain uninfected.[7, 8]

The number of HIV-infected women giving birth each year in the United States appears to be decreasing, in some areas by as much as one third.[9] Although the annual incidence of perinatally acquired disease appears to be similarly decreasing, an estimated 6000 to 7000 HIV-exposed infants are born each year.[10] Heterosexual contact has become the most common type of HIV exposure in American women, particularly for women younger than 25 years of age, accounting for 40% of recently reported AIDS cases among this population group.[6, 11] By contrast, intravenous drug use is responsible for only 33% of recently reported AIDS cases in American women.

Perinatally acquired HIV infection was initially considered to be a rapidly progressive disease with a short survival time, a median of approximately 38 months from diagnosis to death.[8, 12, 13] However, there appears to be a bimodal pattern of HIV disease.[14] Approximately one third of HIV-infected children suffer an early onset of severe immunodeficiency, opportunistic infection, and encephalopathy. Half of these children die by their third birthday. Approximately two thirds of HIV-infected children exhibit a later onset of advanced symptoms. Nearly all of these children live well beyond their third birthday. Thus, even though clinical evidence of HIV infection develops in most infants by 6 months of age, the mortality rate is less than 10% during the 1st year of life and decreases to less than 5% during years 1 to 7 of life before increasing toward 10% during years 8 to 12 of life, yielding a 5-year survival rate of 75% and a median survival time of 8 years.[15–18] Moreover, these statistics will

TABLE 10-2. Pediatric HIV Classification*

	Clinical Category			
Immunologic Category	N: No Signs/Symptoms	A: Mild Signs/Symptoms	B†: Moderate Signs/Symptoms	C†: Severe Signs/Symptoms
1. No evidence of suppression	N1	A1	B1	C1
2. Evidence of moderate suppression	N2	A2	B2	C2
3. Severe suppression	N3	A3	B3	C3

*Children whose HIV infection status is not confirmed are classified by using the above grid with a letter E (for perinatally exposed) placed before the appropriate classification code (e.g., EN2).
†Both category C and lymphoid interstitial pneumonitis in category B are reportable to state and local health departments as AIDS.
Adapted from Centers for Disease Control and Prevention: 1994 revised classification system for human immunodeficiency virus infection in children less than 13 years of age. MMWR Morb Mortal Wkly Rep 43:RR-12, 1994.

TABLE 10-3. Clinical Categories for Children with HIV Infection

---

Category N: Not Symptomatic

Children who have no signs or symptoms considered to be the result of HIV infection or who have only one of the conditions listed in category A.

Category A: Mildly Symptomatic

Children with two or more of the conditions listed below but none of the conditions listed in categories B and C:
- Lymphadenopathy (≥0.5 cm at more than two sites; bilateral = one site)
- Hepatomegaly
- Splenomegaly
- Dermatitis
- Parotitis
- Recurrent or persistent upper respiratory infection, sinusitis, or otitis media

Category B: Moderately Symptomatic

Children who have symptomatic conditions other than those listed for Category A or C that are attributed to HIV infection. Examples of conditions in clinical category B include but are not limited to
- Anemia (<8 g/dl), neutropenia (<1000/mm³), or thrombocytopenia (<100,000/mm³) persisting ≥30 d
- Bacterial meningitis, pneumonia, or sepsis (single episode)
- Candidiasis, oropharyngeal (thrush), persisting (>2 mo) in children >6 mo of age
- Cardiomyopathy
- Cytomegalovirus infection, with onset before 1 mo of age
- Diarrhea, recurrent or chronic
- Hepatitis
- Herpes simplex virus stomatitis, recurrent (more than two episodes within 1 y)
- HSV bronchitis, pneumonitis, or esophagitis with onset before 1 mo of age
- Herpes zoster (shingles) involving at least two distinct episodes or more than one dermatome
- Leiomyosarcoma
- Lymphoid interstitial pneumonia or pulmonary lymphoid hyperplasia complex
- Nephropathy
- Nocardiosis
- Persistent fever (lasting >1 mo)
- Toxoplasmosis, onset before 1 mo of age
- Varicella, disseminated (complicated chickenpox)

Category C: Severely Symptomatic

Children who have any condition listed in the 1987 surveillance case definition for AIDS, with the exception of lymphocytic interstitial pneumonitis:
- Serious bacterial infections, multiple or recurrent (i.e., any combination of at least two culture-confirmed infections within a 2-y period), of the following types: septicemia, pneumonia, meningitis, bone or joint infection, or abscess of an internal organ or body cavity (excluding otitis media, superficial skin or mucosal abscesses, and indwelling catheter-related infections)
- Candidiasis, esophageal or pulmonary (bronchi, trachea, lungs)
- Coccidioidomycosis, disseminated (at site other than or in addition to lungs or cervical or hilar lymph nodes)
- Cryptococcosis, extrapulmonary
- Cryptosporidiosis or isosporiasis with diarrhea persisting >1 mo
- Cytomegalovirus disease with onset of symptoms at age >1 mo (at a site other than liver, spleen, or lymph nodes)
- Encephalopathy (at least one of the following progressive findings present for at least 2 mo in the absence of a concurrent illness other than HIV infection that could explain the findings: (a) failure to attain or loss of developmental milestones or loss of intellectual ability, verified by standard developmental goals or neuropsychological tests; (b) impaired brain growth or acquired microcephaly demonstrated by head circumference measurements or brain atrophy demonstrated by computerized tomography or magnetic resonance imaging (serial imaging is required for children <2 y of age); (c) acquired symmetric motor deficit manifested by two or more of the following: paresis, pathologic reflexes, ataxis, or gait disturbance
- Herpes simplex virus infection causing a mucocutaneous ulcer that persists for >1 mo; or bronchitis, pneumonitis, or esophagitis for any duration affecting a child >1 mo of age
- Histoplasmosis, disseminated (at a site other than or in addition to lungs or cervical or hilar lymph nodes)
- Kaposi's sarcoma
- Lymphoma, primary, in brain
- Lymphoma, small, noncleaved cell (Burkitt's), or immunoblastic or large cell lymphoma of B-cell or unknown immunologic phenotype
- *Mycobacterium tuberculosis,* disseminated or extrapulmonary
- *Mycobacterium,* other species or unidentified species, disseminated (at a site other than or in addition to lungs, skin, or cervical or hilar lymph nodes)
- *Mycobacterium avium* complex or *Mycobacterium kansasii,* disseminated (at site other than or in addition to lungs, skin, or cervical or hilar lymph nodes)
- *Pneumocystis carinii* pneumonia
- Progressive multifocal leukoencaphalopathy
- *Salmonella* (nontyphoid) septicemia, recurrent
- Toxoplasmosis of the brain with onset at >1 mo of age
- Wasting syndrome in the absence of a concurrent illness other than HIV infection that could explain the following findings: (a) persistent weight loss >10% of baseline, (b) downward crossing of at least two of the following percentile lines on the weight-for-age chart (e.g., 95th, 75th, 50th, 25th, 5th) in a child ≥1 y of age; (c) <5th percentile on weight-for-height chart on two consecutive measurements, ≥30 d apart plus (1) chronic diarrhea (i.e., at least two loose stools/d for ≥30 d); (2) documented fever (for ≥30 d, intermittent or constant)

Adapted from Centers for Disease Control and Prevention: 1994 revised classification system for human immunodeficiency virus infection in children less than 13 years of age. MMWR Morb Mortal Wkly Rep 43:RR-12, 1994; and Centers for Disease Control: Revision of the CDC surveillance case definition for acquired immunodeficiency syndrome. MMWR Morb Mortal Wkly Rep 36:1S, 1987.

TABLE 10-4. Immunologic Categories for Children with HIV Infection Based on Age-Specific CD4+ T-Lymphocyte Counts and Percentage of Total Lymphocytes

	Age of Child					
	<12 mo		1-5 y		6-12 y	
Immunologic Category	μl	(%)	μl	(%)	μl	(%)
1. No evidence of suppression	≥1500	(≥25)	≥1000	(≥25)	≥500	(≥25)
2. Evidence of moderate suppression	750–1499	(15–24)	500–999	(15–24)	200–499	(15–24)
3. Severe suppression	<750	(<15)	<500	(<15)	<200	(<15)

Adapted from Centers for Disease Control and Prevention: 1994 revised classification system for human immunodeficiency virus infection in children less than 13 years of age. MMWR Morb Mortal Wkly Rep 43:RR-12, 1994.

continue to improve because combination antiretroviral therapy is the standard of care.

The long-term prognosis for older vertically infected children is also much improved. Indeed, some authors have described small cohorts of vertically infected children in their teens,[19, 20] whereas other authors have estimated that as many as one third to one half of all such children will survive until adolescence.[21, 22] Moreover, although HIV-related immunologic abnormalities become increasingly common after the first birthday, the proportion of HIV-infected children who show HIV-related clinical manifestations continues to decline steadily. These facts vividly demonstrate both the clinical "plateau" observed in many HIV-infected school-age children and the gradual "aging" of the pediatric HIV population, hence the need to provide routine medical and surgical treatment to all children, regardless of HIV status.

The most commonly reported AIDS indicator diseases among children with perinatally acquired infection continue to be *Pneumocystis carinii* pneumonia (PCP), lymphoid interstitial pneumonitis (LIP), recurrent bacterial infections, HIV wasting syndrome, candidal esophagitis, and HIV encephalopathy.[23] Without medical intervention, PCP, which remains the leading cause of death among children with AIDS, occurs in up to 25% of HIV-infected infants during the 1st year of life, mostly during the first 6 months of life, but universal prophylaxis of HIV-seropositive newborns with trimethoprim/sulfamethoxazole (TMP/SMX), which can prevent PCP, is leading to measurable decreases in the incidence of PCP.[24–26] Similarly, aggressive chemoprophylaxis of severely immunocompromised children against *Mycobacterium avium* complex, coupled with aggressive therapy of advanced disease, appears to be decreasing the incidence of this syndrome as well.[27, 28] Efforts to prevent serious bacterial infections with intravenous immunoglobulin, prophylactic antibiotics, and pneumococcal vaccine also have met with some success.[29, 30]

The key advance in current understanding of HIV disease has resulted from the development of methods to quantify the content of viral RNA in host serum. What initially was believed to be a period of latency following infection is actually a period of vigorous viral replication in the face of diminishing immune function. Viral loads, often undetectable at birth, increase rapidly during the first weeks of life, with higher loads being associated with more rapid disease progression, early development of AIDS and early death.[31, 32] Similar patterns are observed both in very young children (<30 months of age), among whom early death or disease progression is five times more common (52% versus 11%) if viral loads are high (>1,700,000 copies/ml) than if viral loads are low (<150,000 copies/ml), and in older children (>30 months of age), among whom disease progression is evident if viral loads are high (>150,000 copies/ml) but it is not clinically evident if viral loads are low (<15,000 copies/ml).[33, 34]

Detailed knowledge of the viral dynamics of HIV infection has facilitated rapid evolution of antiretroviral therapy. Currently, five nucleoside reverse transcriptase inhibitors (ZDV, didanosine [ddI], zalcitabine [ddC], stavudine, [d4T], lamivudine [3TC]), two nonnucleoside reverse transcriptase inhibitors (nevirapine, delaviridine), and four protease inhibitors (ritonavir, saquanivir, indinavir, nelfinavir) have been approved for use in HIV-infected adults by the U.S. Food and Drug Administration, and aggressive combination therapies designed to decrease viral load have been shown both to restore immunocompetence and reduce mortality and morbidity rates.[35, 36] Even though experience with antiretroviral therapy in children is less than that in adults, children with advanced disease appear to have a similar response to therapy, as demonstrated by improvement in viral load, immunologic function, and weight gain.[37–39] Thus, although age-specific pharmacokinetic data are still limited, antiretroviral therapy has become the standard of care in HIV-infected children as well as adults; CDC guidelines currently recommend treatment for all infants younger than 12 months of age and all children with clinical symptoms or evidence of immunosuppression.[40]

□ Clinical Manifestations

The first case report of pediatric AIDS appeared in 1982.[41] Children are diagnosed earlier in the course of infection than adults, are more likely to have recurrent bacterial infections, and are predisposed to chronic pulmonary diseases. Kaposi's sarcoma is less commonly seen in the pediatric age group, and, except for PCP, opportunistic infections are less frequent in children than in adults. Overall, however, the course of untreated disease in children closely resembles that of untreated disease in adults: A progressively deteriorating immune system leads to increasingly severe clinical abnormalities and ultimately death.

Children with HIV disease are also at high risk for serious bacterial infections, such as meningitis, pneumonia, bacteremia, sepsis, and osteomyelitis, caused by pathogens such as *Streptococcus pneumoniae, Haemophilus influenzae, Staphylococcus aureus,* and *Salmonella typhi.*[42, 43] A number of minor infections can assume much larger proportions in the child with HIV infection; for example, oral candidiasis can interfere with appropriate feeding and may progress to esophageal disease. Treatment with oral nystatin may not be sufficient, and clotrimazole troches or ketoconazole suspension may be required. Otitis media, sinusitis, and subcutaneous abscesses also occur with increased frequency and severity in pediatric HIV patients.

Children with HIV infection are especially susceptible to opportunistic pulmonary diseases. LIP is a chronic, interstitial pneumonitis seen principally in children with HIV disease, although it is recognized occasionally in adults.[44–46] Epstein-Barr virus (EBV) DNA and HIV RNA have been identified in lung tissue of children with this diagnosis, but the precise origin remains unknown.[47]

Whether the result of direct effect, immune deregulation, or secondary infection, HIV can involve nearly every organ system in the body. Cardiac abnormalities include pericardial effusions, dysrhythmias, and cardiomyopathy.[48, 49] Liver disease is manifested chiefly as hepatitis, characterized by moderate elevations of both serum transaminases and total and direct bilirubin levels; renal insufficiency can occur as nephrotic syndrome, associated with focal and segmental glomerulosclerosis, proteinuria, azotemia, and progressive renal failure.[50–52] Hematologic disorders include anemia, leukopenia, and thrombocytopenia.[53, 54] Encephalopathy is debilitating.[55–57]

□ Diagnostic Evaluation

HIV disease is most commonly diagnosed in the pediatric age group by the primary care physician. Initial screening is by enzyme-linked immunosorbent assay (ELISA), an exquisitely sensitive but insufficiently specific test that requires subsequent confirmation by Western blot analysis, an equally sensitive but far more specific paper chromatographic technique. However, neither test is capable of differentiating between passively transferred maternal antibody and actively produced infant anti-

body. Definitive diagnosis therefore is based on polymerase chain reaction, a method that relies on molecular gene amplification and its subsequent detection by a specific synthetic probe, or on viral culture. The early diagnosis of HIV infection by laboratory methods in the infant optimizes medical management of the HIV-exposed infant, guidelines for which have been recently promulgated.[58] It also maximizes the potential for highly active antiretroviral therapy of the HIV-infected infant who can be identified routinely within the first 6 months of life. The goal of this therapy is to decrease viral loads to undetectable levels, stop active viral replication, and delay onset of immune deficiency. However, because these regimens are complex, difficult to tolerate, and have numerous side effects, long-term adherence to multidrug therapy remains a major challenge.

□ Surgical Management

The surgical management of HIV disease in infants and children has changed dramatically since the beginning of the HIV pandemic in the late 1970s. In the early 1980s, HIV infection and its complications were unfamiliar to all but a small number of pediatric surgeons located in the epicenters of the epidemic. Medical management was limited chiefly to the diagnosis and treatment of opportunistic infections associated with HIV disease, and surgical involvement was a frequent occurrence. Currently, HIV disease is encountered in nearly every urban center in the United States, medical management has been fully systemized, and surgically remediable complications of end-stage disease have been sharply reduced, largely obviating the need for operative intervention. This experience is clearly reflected by the relative paucity of HIV disease-related articles in the recent surgical literature: fewer than 2 dozen such articles have been published in major American surgical journals since 1990.[59–76]

Not only has the absolute number of surgical operations required for the care of HIV-infected children decreased but the spectrum of these procedures has also changed. Widespread use of TMP/SMX as prophylaxis against PCP has largely obviated the need for bronchoscopy with bronchoalveolar lavage and essentially eliminated the need for diagnostic open lung biopsy.[25, 26] It has also decreased both the number of serious bacterial infections and their surgical complications, such as subcutaneous abscesses requiring incision and drainage. However, the number of children requiring percutaneous endoscopic gastrostomy for supplemental enteral nutrition and combination antiretroviral therapy has markedly increased. The number of infected children requiring routine surgical treatment has also increased, for example, for repair of inguinal hernias. These procedures can be accomplished with morbidity and mortality rates comparable to those observed in uninfected patients, except in those with advanced stage disease and low serum albumin.[66, 67]

Nevertheless, the pediatric surgeon is occasionally enlisted for assistance with definitive diagnosis of pulmonary infections. Tracheal aspiration consists of controlled bedside intubation and deep tracheal suctioning, with care being taken to provide adequate hyperinflation and preoxygenation before aspiration. Bronchoscopy with bronchoalveolar lavage may be carried out at the bedside or in an endoscopic suite, using intravenous sedation, or in an operating theater, using general anesthesia. Care must be taken (1) to protect the airway from excessive trauma during the procedure, (2) to instill at least 50 ml of bronchial wash fluid in aliquots of no more than approximately 10 ml, (3) to ensure that the lavage fluid reaches the terminal airways before it is retrieved, by hyperinflating between episodes of suctioning, and (4) to allow sufficient time to elapse between episodes of suctioning to maintain adequate oxygenation. Open lung biopsy has been rarely required in our recent experience. When necessary, we continue to favor lingular biopsy via a small left anterior thoracotomy so that adequate tissue can be obtained for pathologic and microbiologic study. Great care is taken during the procedure to minimize tissue trauma and to avoid the possibility of postoperative air leak. The integrity of the suture line—constructed by hand with fine silk, using an overlapping horizontal mattress technique—is tested underwater, with application of 40 cm H_2O mean airway pressure, following completion of biopsy. The chest is closed and underwater seal drainage used for a period of approximately 24 hours to be sure an air leak does not develop in the early postoperative period.

Central venous access remains an important part of the surgical care of children with HIV infections. The chief indication for this procedure is the need for total parenteral nutrition, although permanent venous access occasionally may be required for medication administration. Systemic infections are the the most common complication of this procedure and are due to a variety of pathogens, including *Staphylococcus epidermidis, Candida albicans,* and *Escherichia coli.* Although the overall rate of infection is high, the per diem rate of infection compares favorably with the rate in other children, considering the nature and severity of the underlying illness.

Peripherally inserted central catheters (PIC lines) are our first choice in patients requiring short-term central venous access. If these fail, or if long-term central venous access is required, we continue to prefer indwelling, tunneled Silastic catheters, such as a Broviac catheters, placed via venous cutdown of the external jugular vein and passed to the level of the cavoatrial junction. We take care to close the wounds in two layers with absorbable, interrupted, vertical, subcuticular sutures, and to dress the skin with flexible collodion. We credit these techniques with the absence of local infection and the lack of

wound breakdown in our series. In infants, we use the saphenous vein approach whenever feasible, which allows us to perform most of these procedures using ketamine anesthesia, thus avoiding the use of inhalational agents in these patients, virtually all of whom have some degree of underlying pulmonary interstitial disease. The catheter is tunneled from high on the abdominal wall, well above the diaper to avoid contamination by stool, and is passed to the level of the diaphragm.

We continue to use forced feeding programs when intake of protein and calories is inadequate. When these fail, the diet can be supplemented with gavage feedings via an indwelling, narrow-gauge, Silastic nasogastric feeding tube, which can be replaced when dislodged. Nevertheless, gastrostomy tube placement is a viable solution for HIV-infected patients who cannot or will not eat, particularly those with gastrointestinal complications or HIV encephalopathy. Gastrostomy tube placement should also be considered for patients in whom highly active antiretroviral therapy is used to facilitate administration of medications that are not palatable yet require multiple doses.

Candidates for percutaneous endoscopic gastrostomy in HIV-infected infants and children must have a patent, functioning upper gastrointestinal tract, as demonstrated by contrast fluoroscopy. Careful preparation, including broad-spectrum and long-duration perioperative antibiotic coverage, is warranted, because local infections—frequently caused by *Pseudomonas aeruginosa*—have occurred with some frequency. Finally, meticulous attention to surgical technique is advised, and multiple passes of the introducing needle should be avoided, because they may traumatize or seed the abdominal wall, predisposing to local infection (R. Gandhi, A. Cooper, unpublished data, 1997).

Unusual types of neoplastic conditions continue to constitute a special problem in the pediatric HIV population. Although rare, they continue to appear in far greater numbers among HIV-infected children than among the general population. Non-Hodgkin's lymphomas, for which surgical assistance is occasionally required in establishing the diagnosis, continue to account for the greatest number of tumors encountered (approximately 70%), and thymoma has also been reported in the pediatric population (W. Middlesworth, S.M. Alaish, unpublished data, 1997). Kaposi's sarcoma remains the most common solid tumor encountered in children with AIDS, accounting for approximately 20% of documented malignancies in these children, with a variety of other soft tissue malignancies accounting for the remaining 10%, including both rhabdomyosarcomas in unusual locations and leiomyomas and leiomyosarcomas of the gastrointestinal tract.[77–88]

Certain nonneoplastic conditions, such as benign, typically bilateral, lymphoepithelial cysts, are occasionally observed in older children.[89, 90] Although they can be successfully removed by simple, elective, surgical enucleation, they also may undergo spontaneous resolution as CD4-positive T-lymphpocyte counts decrease below 200 cells/mm (D. Larague, A. Cooper, unpublished data, 1995).[68] Rectal bleeding, which sometimes can be massive and usually is caused by cytomegalovirus infection, continues to remain a major diagnostic and therapeutic challenge. It usually stops spontaneously and therefore infrequently requires surgical intervention.[91, 92]

Somewhat more troublesome is a group of necrotizing soft tissue infections that do not respond well to antibiotics or surgical débridement. Most of these occur late in the course of the illness and should be managed conservatively. The development of soft tissue infections that do not heal appears limited to the preterminal stages of HIV disease; anal fissures are especially problematic, because they are associated with severe pain. The symptoms have been reported to remit following direct intralesional corticosteroid injection, although injection does not produce healing. Finally, acquired rectovaginal fistula has recently been recognized as an unusual but serious complication of the severe anorectal inflammatory disease occasionally encountered in infants.[93] These fistulae are treated conservatively without resort to colostomy, except when necessitated by obstruction or fasciitis. As with anal fissures, none have yet been known to heal; the vaginal discharge has reportedly been well tolerated, except when associated with unremitting diarrhea.

A number of nonoperable lesions that affect the integrity of the gastrointestinal tract may also come to the attention of the pediatric surgeon, chiefly for diagnosis. These lesions include esophagitis and gastritis, and severe chronic diarrhea. In these cases, esophagogastroduodenoscopy or colonoscopy with biopsy usually is performed for the purpose of obtaining tissue for culture. In a few patients with advanced disease, we have recognized a severe form of enteropathy characterized by abdominal distention, small and large bowel diltation, hypoperistalsis, and the need for long-term total parenteral nutrition (E. J. Abrams, A. Cooper, unpublished data, 1989).

Pediatric surgical consultation is also sought for complications of the aggressive medical therapy required to treat advanced disease. Opportunistic pulmonary infections may progress to acute respiratory failure and adult respiratory distress syndrome, for which oxygen delivery at high concentration and pressure is frequently required. This treatment predisposes to barotraumatic complications such as pneumothorax—also a recognized complication of PCP itself—which is often refractory to conservative treatment by means of tube thoracostomy, necessitating operative management in selected cases.[94, 95] Deep venous thrombophlebitis has also been observed in patients requiring central venous catheters for monitoring and administration of vasoactive drugs—even among patients with profound thrombocytopenia—but typically responds to conservative management once the catheter has been removed (W. Moss, A. Cooper, unpublished data, 1993).

Although the surgical management of infants and children with HIV disease constitutes only a small part of total patient management, it is nevertheless essential to optimal medical care. The pediatric surgeon's role should be principally that of a consultant, not merely a technician, in that it cannot be assumed that primary care physicians fully understand the benefits and risks of surgical intervention in these fragile children. Knowledgeable involvement by the surgeon in decisions regarding children with HIV infections, in our experience, facilitates optimal management, minimizing risks to patients and physicians alike. If such conditions are met, surgical interventions can be performed safely and successfully in most patients, providing maximum benefit at minimum risk.

☐ Occupational Considerations for Caregivers

The risk of parenteral exposure of surgical personnel to HIV during operative procedures is approximately 2%, the risk being highest in bloody operations more than 3 hours in length; risk is not altered by preoperative knowledge of patient HIV status.[96] The risk of seroconversion among surgical personnel who sustain deep needlestick injuries or sharp object cuts—particularly those involving needles placed in blood vessels, devices contaminated with visible blood, emergency procedures, and terminal illness—is approximately 0.5%, although postexposure prophylaxis with ZDV may be protective; the risk approaches zero among those exposed via simple contact with mucous membranes, open wounds, or nonintact skin of HIV-infected patients.[97, 98] However, because the surgeon and first assistant are recipients of as many as 80% of all intraoperative needlestick injuries, the risk to the individual surgeon of seroconversion associated with a single operation may be not so small as the 1 in 10,000 chance that simple arithmetic might suggest.[99, 100] Moreover, the overall statistical risk is cumulative, having been estimated in various studies to range from 0.26% to 2.0% for the individual surgeon over an entire career.[101–107] This risk is also dependent on the frequency of contact with HIV-infected patients, which is small; such patients make up less than 0.5% of the elective surgical population and less than 1% of the trauma surgical population, even in urban environments—although the prevalence of HIV seropositivity appears higher, approximately 2.5%, among children seeking urgent medical treatment in pediatric emergency departments in metropolitan areas.[108–110] Although clinical studies do not support the notion that solid-bore suture needles are less dangerous than hollow-bore hypodermic needles, there is a small body of laboratory evidence to suggest that the type of parenteral exposure typically sustained in the operating room may be less hazardous than that sustained elsewhere. Hollow-bore needles—the devices most frequently implicated in parenteral exposures resulting in seroconversion—have been shown, using various laboratory methods, to result in inocula ranging in volume from 34 nl for a 25-gauge phlebotomy needle to 138 nl for a 22-gauge phlebotomy needle.[111–114] However, recent studies conducted using a model designed to simulate living tissue showed that the average inocula were 311 nl for a 22-gauge phlebotomy needle and 196 to 266 nl for suture needles of various sizes.[115] An increase in the depth of penetration of the needle from 2 to 5 mm substantially increased the volume of each inoculum, but this volume was decreased almost to zero for solid-bore suture needles if first passed through a double layer of surgical gloves—a decrease that did not occur for hollow-bore hypodermic needles.

The use of a double layer of surgical gloves also appears to reduce the actual incidence of needlestick injuries in the operating room. A number of recent studies confirm that, whereas the outer of the two gloves may perforate as frequently as a single glove, the inner glove is infrequently perforated.[116–121]

Given that a minimum of four cell culture infectious units are required to produce HIV infection in nonhuman primates and that approximately one cell culture infectious unit is contained in 100 nl of HIV-infected blood, it is highly unlikely that a sufficient quantity of virus could penetrate the skin to cause HIV infection if double gloves are routinely worn.[115, 122–124] Thus, it is recommended that surgeons operating on patients at risk for HIV infection regularly avail themselves of this, and other, simple protections, such as use of blunt suture needles for fascial closure, "hands off" surgical technique for the handling of sharps in the operative field, and, possibly, polymer-iodine coating of surgical instruments, and that such precautions should be routinely used in all operative cases, even when the patient tests negative for HIV, because such a result may lull the surgical team into a false sense of security.[125–128]

The problem of provider-to-patient transmission of HIV, although of great theoretical interest, is of little actual concern. This issue was raised in 1991 following documented reports that a Florida dentist known to be infected with HIV had transmitted the virus to five of his patients via mechanisms, which, to date, remain unknown. It intensified in 1992 following a report suggesting that a European surgeon had infected a patient during an orthopedic procedure, the specifics of which have not as yet been published. No other cases of provider-to-patient transmission are known to have occurred, despite extensive seroprevalence studies of patients whose practitioners—including surgeons—were known to be HIV-infected. Nevertheless, although the risk of provider-to-patient transmission during surgical procedures is currently zero, even among HIV-infected surgeons, those with open lesions on their

hands should refrain from performing operative procedures, particularly those that are classified as "exposure prone" in accordance with universal precautions, which should be followed by all health care providers having direct contact with the blood or body fluids of potentially infected patients.[129, 130]

Universal precautions are not universally followed by surgeons, even though in following such precautions, a greater benefit accrues to the surgeon than to the patient.[131] Unlike the risk of provider-to-patient transmission, the risk of patient-to-provider transmission is *not* zero. Yet, infractions typically occur in up to 60% of cases, regardless of surgeons' participation in educational programs specifically designed to increase compliance with universal precautions.[132] The reasons for such behavior remain unclear, but they seem to be based more on emotion than reason; educational programs aimed solely at increasing cognitive knowledge appear to have little effect on psychomotor routines. Perhaps this is not surprising in view of the documented ambivalence of many surgeons toward HIV disease. As recently as 1990, approximately 6% of surgeons in two high-seroprevalence areas refused to treat HIV-infected patients, whereas fewer than 50% recommended use of barrier precautions for all their patients.[133] Moreover, as recently as 1992, 72% of surgeons favored routine testing of operative candidates despite clear evidence that knowledge of the result does not influence the rate of parenteral exposure, and an identical percentage erroneously believed that HIV-infected surgeons should have operating privileges restricted despite unequivocal proof that the risk of provider-to-patient transmission is nil.[132]

The American College of Surgeons has taken a leadership role in the issue of provider-to-patient transmission and has recently published a revised "Statement on the Surgeon and HIV Infection" outlining its position on this subject.[134] At the heart of these recommendations are the conclusions that enforced limitations on the surgical practices of HIV-infected surgeons are not justified by the scientific evidence and that high standards of infection control are the best means of avoiding the slim possibility of provider-to-patient transmission in the future. This document further calls for dedicated epidemiologic research efforts as the best means of obtaining the knowledge required to define the true extent of the problem as well as the appropriate solution. Most important, it reconfirms the ethical obligations of the surgeon to render care to HIV-infected patients whenever this need may arise.

REFERENCES

1. Connor EM, Sperling RS, Gelber R, et al: Reduction of maternal-infant transmission of human immunodeficiency virus type 1 with zidovudine treatment. *N Engl J Med* 331:1173–1180, 1994.
2. Nielsen K, McSherry G, Petru A, et al: A descriptive survey of pediatric human immunodeficiency virus-infected long-term survivors. *Pediatrics* 99(4):e4. URL:http://www.pediatrics.org/cgi/content/full/99/4/e4.

3. Centers for Disease Control and Prevention: *HIV/AIDS Surveillance Report* [Vol. 9, No. 1]. Atlanta: United States Department of Health and Human Services, 1997.
4. Centers for Disease Control: Revision of CDC surveillance case definition for acquired immunodeficiency syndrome. *MMWR* Morb Mortal Wkly Rep 36(suppl 1S):1S–15S, 1987.
5. Centers for Disease Control and Prevention: 1994 revised classification system for human immunodeficiency virus infection in children less than 13 years of age. *MMWR* Morb Mortal Wkly Rep 43:RR-12, 1994.
6. Centers for Disease Control and Prevention: *HIV/AIDS Surveillance Report* [Vol. 8, No. 2]. Atlanta, United States Department of Health and Human Services, 1996.
7. New York State Department of Health: *AIDS in New York State, 1988–1992*. Albany, New York State Department of Health, 1993.
8. Oxtoby MJ: Vertically acquired HIV infection in the United States. In Pizzo PA, Wilfert CM (eds): Pediatric AIDS: *The Challenge of HIV Infection in Infants, Children, and Adolescents* (2nd ed) Baltimore, Williams & Wilkins, 1994, pp 3–20.
9. New York State Department of Health: *AIDS Surveillance.* Albany, New York State Department of Health, 1997.
10. Davis SF, Byers RH, Lindegren ML, et al: Prevalence of HIV infection in the United States, 1985–1992. *JAMA* 274:952–955, 1995.
11. Centers for Disease Control and Prevention: *Progress in Prevention: HIV and AIDS Trends.* Atlanta, United States Department of Health and Human Services, November 1996.
12. Rogers MF, Thomas PA, Starcher ET, et al: Acquired immunodeficiency syndrome in children: Report of the Centers for Disease Control National Surveillance, 1982 to 1985. *Pediatrics* 79:1008–1014, 1987.
13. Scott GB, Hutto C, Makuch RW, et al: Survival in children with perinatally acquired human immunodeficiency virus type 1 infection. N Engl J Med 321:1791–1796, 1989.
14. Blanche S, Tardieu M, Duliege AM, et al: Longitudinal study of 94 symptomatic infants with perinatally acquired human immunodeficiency virus infection: Evidence for a bimodal expression of clinical and biological symptoms. *Am J Dis Child* 144:1210–1215, 1990.
15. Tovo PA, deMartino M, Gabiano C, et al: Prognostic factors and survival in children with perinatal HIV-1 infection. *Lancet* 339:1249–1253, 1992.
16. Italian Register for HIV Infection in Children: Features of children perinatally infected with HIV-1 surviving longer than 5 years. *Lancet* 343:191–195, 1992.
17. The European Collaborative Study: Natural history of vertically acquired human immunodeficiency virus-1 infection. *Pediatrics* 94:815–823, 1994.
18. Barnhart HX, Caldwell MB, Thomas P, et al: Natural history of human immunodeficiency virus disease in perinatally infected children: An analysis for the pediatric spectrum of disease project. *Pediatrics* 97:710–716, 1996.
19. Persaud D, Chandwani S, Rigaud M, et al: Delayed recognition of human immunodeficiency virus infection in preadolescent children. *Pediatrics* 90:688–691, 1992.
20. Grubman S, Gross E, Lerner-Weiss N, et al: Older children and adolescents living with perinatally acquired human immunodeficiency virus infection. *Pediatrics* 95:657–663, 1995.
21. Pliner V, Weedon J, Thomas PA, et al: Incubation period of HIV-1 perinatally infected children [abstract We. C. 3473]. Presented at the XIth International Congress on AIDS, Vancouver, British Columbia; July 1996.
22. Kuhn L, Thomas PA, Singh T, et al: Long-term survival of children with human immunodeficiency virus infection in New York City: Estimates from population-based surveillance data. *Am J Epidemiol* 147:846–854, 1998.
23. Centers for Disease Control and Prevention: *HIV/AIDS Surveillance Report* [Vol. 5, No. 1]. Atlanta, United States Department of Health and Human Services, 1993.
24. Simonds RJ, Oxtoby MJ, Caldwell B, et al: *Pneumocystis carinii* pneumonia among US children with perinatally acquired HIV infection. JAMA 270:470–473, 1993.
25. Thea DM, Lambert G, Weedon J, et al: Benefit of primary prophylaxis before 18 months of age in reducing the incidence of *Pneumocystis carinii* pneumonia and early death in a cohort of 112 human immunodeficiency virus-infected infants. Pediatrics 97:59–64, 1996.
26. Rigaud M, Pollack H, Leibovitz E, et al: Efficacy of primary prophylaxis against *Pneumocystic carinii* pneumomia during the first year of life in infants infected with human immunodeficiency virus type 1. J Pediatr 125:476–480, 1994.
27. Hoyt L, Oleske J, Holland B, et al: Nontuberculous mycobacteria in children with acquired immunodeficiency syndrome. *Pediatr Infect Dis J* 11:354–360, 1992.
28. Centers for Disease Control: 1997 USPHS/IDSA guidelines for the prevention of opportunistic infections in persons infected with human immunodeficiency virus. *MMWR* Morb Mortal Wkly Rep 46:RR-12, 1997.
29. The National Institute of Child Health and Development Intravenous Immunoglobulin Study Group: Intravenous immune globulin for the prevention of bacterial infections in children with symptomatic human immunodeficiency virus infection. *N Engl J Med* 32:73–80, 1991.
30. Spector SA, Gelber RD, McGrath N, et al: A controlled trial of intravenous immune globulin for the prevention of serious bacterial infections in children receiving zidovudine for advanced human immunodeficiency virus infection. *N Engl J Med* 331:1181–1187, 1994.
31. Abrams EJ, Weedon J, Steketee RW, et al: Association of human immunodeficiency virus (HIV) load early in life with disease progression among HIV-infected infants. New York City Perinatal HIV Transmission Collaborative Study Group. *J Infect Dis* 178:101–108, 1998.
32. Shearer WT, Quinn TC, LaRussa P, et al: Viral load and disease progression in infants infected with human immunodeficiency virus type 1. *N Engl J Med* 336:1337–1342, 1997.
33. Mofenson LM, Korelitz J, Meyer WA, et al: The relationship between serum human immunodeficiency virus type 1 (HIV-1) RNA level, CD4 lymphocyte percent, and long-term mortality risk in HIV-1 infected children. *J Infect Dis* 175:1029–1038, 1997.
34. Palumbo PE, Raskino C, Fiscus S, et al: Predictive value of quantitative plasma HIV RNA and CD4+ lymphocyte count in HIV-infected infants and children. *JAMA* 279:756–761, 1998.
35. Hammer SM, Katzenstein DA, Hughes MD, et al: A trial comparing nucleoside monotherapy with combination therapy in HIV-infected adults with CD4 cell counts from 200 to 500 per cubic millimeter. AIDS Clinical Trials Group Study 175 Study Team. *N Engl J Med* 375:1081–1090, 1996.
36. Katzenstein DA, Hammer SM, Hughes MD, et al: The relation of virologic and immunologic markers to clinical outcomes after nucleoside therapy in HIV-infected adults with 200 to 500 CD4 cells per cubic millimeter. AIDS Clinical Trials Group Study 175 Virology Study Team. *N Engl J Med* 335:1091–1098, 1996.
37. Melvin A, Mohan K, Manns Arcuino LA, et al: Clinical, virologic and immunologic responses of children with advanced human immunodeficiency virus type 1 disease treated with protease inhibitors. *Pediatr Infect Dis J* 16:968–974, 1997.
38. Rutstein RM, Feingold A, Meislich D, et al: Protease inhibitor therapy in children with perinatally acquired HIV infection. *AIDS* 11:F107–F111, 1997.
39. Luzuriaga K, Bryson YJ, Krogstad P, et al: Combination treatment with zidovudine, didanosine, and nevirapine in infants with human immunodeficiency virus type 1 infection. *N Engl J Med* 336:1343–1349, 1997.
40. Centers for Disease Control and Prevention: Guidelines for the use of antiretroviral agents in pediatric HIV infection. *MMWR* Morb Mortal Wkly Rep 47(RR-4):1–43, 1998.
41. Centers for Disease Control: Unexplained immunodeficiency and opportunistic infections in infants—New York, New Jersey, California. *MMWR* Morb Mortal Wkly Rep 31:665–667, 1982.

42. Bernstein LJ, Krieger BZ, Novick B, et al: Bacterial infection in the acquired immunodeficiency syndrome of children. *Pediatr Infect Dis* 4:472–475, 1985.
43. Krasinski K, Borkowsky W, Bonk S, et al: Bacterial infections in human immunodeficiency virus-infected children. *Pediatr Infect Dis* 7:323–328, 1988.
44. Grieco MH, Chinoy-Acharya P: Lymphocytic interstitial pneumonitis associated with the acquired immunodeficiency symndrome. *Am Rev Respir Dis* 131:952–955, 1985.
45. Joshi VV, Oleske JM, Minnefore AB, et al: Pathologic pulmonary findings in children with the acquired immunodeficiency syndrome: A study of ten cases. *Hum Pathol* 16:241–246, 1985.
46. Rubenstein A, Morecki R, Silverman B, et al: Pulmonary disease in children with acquired immunodeficiency syndrome and AIDS-related complex. *J Pediatr* 108:498–503, 1986.
47. Andiman W, Eastman R, Martin K, et al: Opportunistic lymphoproliferations associated with Epstein-Barr viral DNA in infants and children with AIDS. *Lancet* 2:1390–1393, 1985.
48. Stewart JM, Kaul A, Gromish DS, et al: Symptomatic cardiac dysfunction in children with human immunodeficiency virus. *Am Heart J* 117:140–144, 1989.
49. Lipshultz SE, Chanock S, Sanders SP, et al: Cardiovascular manifestations of human immunodeficiency virus infection in infants and children. *Am J Cardiol* 63:1489–1497, 1989.
50. Jonas MM, Roldan EO, Lyons HJ, et al: Histopathologic features of the liver in pediatric acquired immune deficiency syndrome. *J Pediatr Gastroenterol Nutr* 9:73–81, 1989.
51. Connor E, Gupta S, Joshi V, et al: Acquired immunodeficiency syndrome-associated renal disease in children. *J Pediatr* 113:39–44, 1988.
52. Strauss J, Abitbol C, Zilleruelo G, et al: Renal disease in children with the acquired immunodeficiency syndrome. *N Engl J Med* 321:625–630, 1989.
53. Saulsbury FT, Boyle RJ, Wykoff RF, et al: Thrombocytopenia as the presenting manifestation of human T-lymphotropic virus type III infection in infants. *J Pediatr* 109:30–34, 1986.
54. Ellaurie M, Burns ER, Bernstein LJ, et al: Thrombocytopenia and human immunodeficiency virus in children. *Pediatrics* 82:905–908, 1988.
55. Epstein LG, Sharer LR, Oleske JM, et al: Neurologic manifestations of human immunodeficiency virus infection in children. *Pediatrics* 78:678–687, 1986.
56. Belman AL, Diamond G, Dickson D, et al: Pediatric acquired immunodeficiency syndrome: Neurologic syndromes. *Am J Dis Child* 142:29–35, 1988.
57. Ultman MH, Belman AL, Ruff H, et al: Developmental abnormalities in infants and children with acquired immune deficiency syndrome (AIDS) and AIDS-related complex. *Dev Med Child Neurol* 27:56–571, 1985.
58. American Academy of Pediatrics Committee on Pediatric AIDS: Evaluation and medical treatment of the HIV-exposed infant. *Pediatrics* 99:909–917, 1997.
59. Binderow SR, Shaked AA: Acute appendicitis in patients with AIDS/HIV infection. *Am J Surg* 162:9–12, 1991.
60. Terry JH, Loree TR, Thomas MD, et al: Major salivary gland lymphoepithelial lesions and the acquired immunodeficiency syndrome. *Am J Surg* 162:324–329, 1991.
61. Wond R, Rappaport W, Gorman S, et al: Value of lymph node biopsy in the treatment of patients with the human immunodeficiency virus. *Am J Surg* 162:590–593, 1991.
62. Diettrich NA, Cacioppo JC, Kaplan G, et al: A growing spectrum of surgical disease in patients with human immunodeficiency virus/acquired immunodeficiency syndrome: Experience with 120 major cases. *Arch Surg* 126:860–866, 1991.
63. Shaha AR, DiMaio T, Webber C, et al: Benign lymphoepithelial lesions of the parotid. *Am J Surg* 166:403–406, 1993.
64. Heneghen SJ, Li J, Bizer LS: Intestinal perforation from gastrointestinal histoplasmosis in acquired immunodeficiency syndrome. Case report and review of the literature. *Arch Surg* 128:464–466, 1993.
65. Adolph MD, Bass SN, Lee SK, et al: Cytomegaloviral acalculous cholecystitis in acquired immunodeficiency syndrome. *Am Surg* 59:679–684, 1993.
66. Burke EC, Orloff SL, Freise CE, et al: Wound healing after anorectal surgery in human immunodeficiency virus-infected patients. *Arch Surg* 126:1267–1271, 1991.
67. Binderow SR, Cavallo RJ, Freed J: Laboratory parameters as predictors of operative outcome after major abdominal surgery in AIDS- and HIV-infected patients. *Am Surg* 59:754–757, 1993.
68. Ferraro FJ, Rush BF, Ruark D, et al: Enucleation of parotid lymphoepithelial cyst in patients who are human immunodeficiency virus positive. *Surg Gynecol Obstet* 177:524–526, 1993.
69. Carrillo EH, Carrillo LE, Byers PM, et al: Penetrating trauma and emergency surgery in patients with AIDS. *Am J Surg* 170:341–344, 1995.
70. Spivak H, Schlasinger MH, Tabanda-Lichauco R, et al: Small bowel obstruction from gastrointestinal histoplasmosis in acquired immune deficiency syndrome. *Am Surg* 62:369–372, 1996.
71. Wastel C, Corless D, Keeling N: Surgery and human immunodeficiency virus-1 infection. *Am J Surg* 172:89–92, 1996.
72. Spivak H, Keller S: Spontaneous pneumothorax in the AIDS population. *Am Surg* 62:753–756, 1996.
73. Golshan MM, McHenry CR, deVente J, et al: Acute suppurative thyroiditis and necrosis of the thyroid gland: A rare endocrine manifestation of acquired immunodeficiency syndrome. *Surgery* 121:593–596, 1997.
74. Lord RVN: Anorectal surgery in patients infected with human immunodeficiency virus: Factors associated with delayed wound healing. *Ann Surg* 226:92–99, 1997.
75. Leiva JI, Etter EL, Gathe J, et al: Surgical therapy for 101 patients with acquired immunodeficiency syndrome and symptomatic cholecystitis. *Am J Surg* 174:414–416, 1997.
76. Modesto VL, Gottesman L: Surgical debridement and intralesional steroid injection in the treatment of idiopathic AIDS-related anal ulcerations. *Am J Surg* 174:439–441, 1997.
77. Buck BE, Scott GB, Valdes-Dapena M, et al: Kaposi sarcoma in two infants with acquired immunodeficiency syndrome. *J Pediatr* 103:911–913, 1986.
78. Gutierrez-Ortega P, Hierro-Orozco S, Sanchez-Cisneros R, et al: Kaposi's sarcoma in a 6-day-old infant with human immunodeficiency virus. *Arch Dermatol* 125:432–433, 1989.
79. Baum LG, Vinters HV: Lymphoadenopathic Kaposi's sarcoma in a pediatric patient with acquired immunodeficiency syndrome. *Pediatr Pathol* 9:459–465, 1989.
80. Connor E, Boccon-Gibod L, Joshi V, et al: Cutaneous acquired immunodeficiency syndrome-associated Kaposi's sarcoma in pediatric patients. *Arch Dermatol* 126:791–793, 1991.
81. Ravalli S, Chabon AB, Khan AA: Gastrointestinal neoplasia in young HIV antibody-positive patients. *Am J Clin Pathol* 91:458–461, 1989.
82. Scully RE, Mark RE, McNeely BU: Case records of the Massachusetts Hospital: Case 9-1986. *N Engl J Med* 314:629–640, 1986.
83. Martinez S, Young R, Moll B, et al: Simultaneous leiomyosarcoma and leiomyoma in pediatric HIV infection [abstract]. *Ann Allergy* 64:89, 1990.
84. Chadwick EG, Connor EJ, Guerra Hanson IC, et al: Tumors of smooth muscle origin in HIV-infected children. *JAMA* 263:3182–3184, 1990.
85. Sabatino D, Martinez S, Young R, et al: Simultaneous pulmonary leiomyosarcoma and leiomyoma in pediátric HIV infection. *Pediatr Hematol Oncol* 8:355–359, 1991.
86. Orlow SJ, Kamino H, Lawrence RL: Multiple subcutaneous leiomyosarcomas in an adolescent with AIDS. *Am J Pediatr Hematol Oncol* 14:265–268, 1992.
87. Mueller BU, Butler KM, Feuerstein IM, et al: Smooth muscle tumors in children with human immunodeficiency virus infection. *Pediatrics* 90:460–463, 1992.
88. Ninane J, Moulin D, Latinne D, et al: AIDS in two African

children—one with fibrosarcoma of the liver. *Eur J Pediatr* 144:385–390, 1985.

89. Goddart D, Francois A, Ninane NJ, et al: Parotid gland abnormalities found in children seropositive for HIV. *Pediatr Radiol* 20:355–357, 1990.

90. Soberman N, Leonidas JC, Berdon WE, et al: Parotid enlargement in children seropositive for HIV: Imaging findings. *AJR Am J Roentgenol* 157:553–556, 1991.

91. Schwartz DL, So HB, Bungarz WR, et al: A case of life-threatening gastrointestinal hemorrhage in an infant with AIDS. *J Pediatr Surg* 24:313–315, 1989.

92. Dolgin SE, Larsen JG, Shah KD, et al: CMV enteritis causing hemorrhage and obstruction in an infant with AIDS. *J Pediatr Surg* 25:696–698, 1990.

93. Hyde GA, Sarbah S: Acquired rectovaginal fistula in human immunodeficiency virus-positive children. *Pediatrics* 84:940–941, 1994.

94. Gerein AN, Brumwell ML, Lawson LM, et al: Surgical management of pneumothorax in patients with acquired immunodeficiency syndrome. *Arch Surg* 126:1272–1277, 1991.

95. Horowitz MD, Oliva H: Pneumothorax in AIDS patients: Operative management. *Am Surg* 59:200–204, 1993.

96. Geberding JL, Littell C, Tarkington H, et al: Risk of exposure to surgical personnel to patients' blood during surgery at San Francisco General Hospital. *N Engl J Med* 322:1788–1793, 1990.

97. AIDS and HIV update: Acquired immunodeficiency syndrome and human immunodeficiency virus infection among health care workers. *MMWR Morb Mortal Wkly Rep* 37:229–234, 1988.

98. Cardo DM, Culver DH, Ciesielski CA, et al: A case-control study of HIV seroconversion in health care workers after percutaneous exposure. *N Engl J Med* 337:1485–1490, 1997.

99. Popejoy SL, Fry DE: Blood contact and exposure in the operating room. *Surg Gynecol Obstet* 172:480–483, 1991.

100. Quebbeman EJ, Telford GL, Hubbard S, et al: Risk of blood contamination and injury to operating room personnel. *Ann Surg* 214:614–620, 1991.

101. Wormser GP, Rabkin CS, Joline C: Frequency of nosocomial transmission of HIV infection among health care workers. *N Engl J Med* 319:307–308, 1988.

102. Schiff SJ: A surgeon's risk of AIDS. *J Neurosurg* 73:615–660, 1990.

103. Hagen MD, Meyer KB, Pauler SG: Routine preoperative screening for HIV: Does the risk to the surgeon outweigh the risk to the patient? *JAMA* 259:1357–1359, 1988.

104. Wilson SE, Williams RA, Robinson G: Operating on HIV positive patients: What are the risks to health care workers? To patients? *Postgrad Med* 88:193–203, 1990.

105. McKinney WP, Young MJ: The cumulative probability of occupationally acquired HIV infection: The risks of repeated exposures during a surgical career. *Infect Control Hosp Epidemiol* 11:243–247, 1990.

106. Howard RJ: Human immunodeficiency virus testing and the risk to the surgeon of acquiring HIV. *Surg Gynecol Obstet* 171:22–25, 1990.

107. Charache P, Cameron JL, Maters AW, et al: Prevalence of infection with human immunodeficiency virus in elective surgery patients. *Ann Surg* 214:562–568, 1991.

108. Rudolph R, Bowen DG, Boyd CR, et al: Seroprevalence of human immunodeficiency virus in admitted trauma patients at a southeastern metropolitan/rural trauma center. *Am Surg* 59:384–387, 1993.

109. Mullins JR, Harrison PB: The questionable utility of mandatory screening for the human immunodeficiency virus. *Am J Surg* 166:676–679, 1993.

110. Schweich PJ, Fosarelli PD, Duggan AK, et al: Prevalence of human immunodeficiency virus seropositivity in pediatric emergency room patients undergoing phlebotomy. *Pediatrics* 86:660–665, 1990.

111. Napoli VM, McGowan JE: How much blood in a needlestick? *J Infect Dis* 155:828, 1987.

112. Hoffman PN, Larkin DP, Samuel D: Needlestick and needle—share the difference. *J Infect Dis* 160:545, 1989.

113. Mast ST, Geberding JL: Factors predicting infectivity following needlestick exposure to HIV: An in vitro model. *Clin Res* 39:58A, 1991.

114. Shirizian D, Herzlich BC, Mokhtarian F, et al: Detection of HIV antibody and antigen (p24) in residual blood on needles and glass. *Infect Control Hosp Epidemiol* 11:180–184, 1990.

115. Bennett NT, Howard RJ: Quantity of blood inoculated in a needlestick injury from suture needles. *J Am Coll Surg* 2:107–110, 1994.

116. Matta H, Thompson AM, Rainey JB: Does wearing two pairs of gloves protect operating theatre staff from skin contamination? *BMJ* 297:597–598, 1988.

117. Cole RP, Gault DT: Glove perforation during plastic surgery. *Br J Plast Surg* 42:481–483, 1989.

118. Dodds RD, Barker SG, Morgan NH, et al: Self protection in surgery: The use of double gloves. *Br J Surg* 77:219–220, 1990.

119. Gani JS, Anseline PF, Bissett RL: Efficacy of double versus single gloving in protecting the operating team. *Aust N Z J Surg* 60:171–175, 1990.

120. Cohn GM, Seifer DB: Blood exposure in single versus double gloving during pelvic surgery. *Am J Obstet Gynecol* 162:715–717, 1990.

121. Bennett B, Duff. P: The effect of double gloving on the frequency of glove perforations. *Obstet Gynecol* 78:1019–1022, 1991.

122. Arthur LO, Bess JW, Water DJ, et al: Challenge of chimpanzees (*Pan troqdolytes*) immunized with human immunodeficiency virus envelope glycoprotein gp120. *J Virol* 63:5046–5053, 1989.

123. Ho DD, Mougil T, Alam M: Quantitation of human immunodeficiency virus type 1 in the blood of infected persons. *N Engl J Med* 321:1621–1625, 1989.

124. Coombs RW, Collier AC, Allain JP, et al: Plasma viremia in human immunodeficiency virus infection. *N Engl J Med* 321:1626–1631, 1989.

125. Fontz FJ, Fowler JM, Farias-Eisner R, et al: Blunt needles in fascial closure. *Surg Gynecol Obstet* 173:147–148, 1991.

126. Telford GL, Quebbeman EJ, Condon RE: A protocol to reduce risk of contracting AIDS and other blood-borne diseases in the OR. *Surg Rounds* 11:30–37, 1987.

127. Bessinger CD: Preventing transmission of human immunodeficiency virus during operations. *Surg Gynecol Obstet* 167:287–289, 1988.

128. Skikani AH, St. Clair M, Domb A: Polymer-iodine inactivation of the human immunodeficiency virus. *J Am Coll Surg* 183:195–200, 1996.

129. Centers for Disease Control: Recommendations for preventing transmission of human immunodeficiency virus and hepatitis B virus to patients during exposure-prone invasive procedures. *MMWR* Morb Mortal Wkly Rep 40:RR-8, 1991.

130. Centers for Disease Control: Update: Universal precautions for prevention of human immunodeficiency virus, hepatitis B virus, and other blood-borne pathogens in health-care settings. *MMWR* Morb Mortal Wkly Rep 37:377–382, 1988.

131. Courington KR, Patterson SL, Howard RJ: Universal precautions are not universally followed. *Arch Surg* 126:93–96, 1991.

132. Shelley GA, Howard RJ: A national survey of surgeons' attitudes about patients with human immunodeficiency virus infection and acquired immunodeficiency syndrome. *Arch Surg* 127:206–212, 1992.

133. Mandelbrot DA, Smythe WR, Norman SA, et al: A survey of exposures, practices, and recommendations of surgeons in the care of patients with human immunodeficiency virus. *Surg Gynecol Obstet* 171:99–106, 1990.

134. American College of Surgeons: Statement on the Surgeon and HIV Infection. *Bull Am Coll Surg* 83:27–29, 1998.

11

PRENATAL DIAGNOSIS AND SURGICAL INTERVENTION

Craig T. Albanese, MD •
Michael R. Harrison, MD

Since the 1970s, sophisticated ultrasonographic imaging and fetal sampling techniques have had a profound impact on the study of abnormal fetal development.[1] Serial sonographic study of fetuses with anatomic lesions has made it possible to define the natural history of these anomalies, determine the pathophysiologic features that affect clinical outcome, and formulate management plans based on prognosis. Prenatal diagnosis has defined a "hidden mortality rate" for some lesions, such as congenital diaphragmatic hernia (CDH), bilateral hydronephrosis, sacrococcygeal teratoma (SCT), and congenital cystic adenomatoid malformation (CCAM) of the lung. These lesions, when first evaluated and treated postnatally, demonstrate a favorable selection bias because the most severely affected fetuses often die in utero or immediately after birth.[2]

Although most prenatally diagnosed malformations are best managed by medical and surgical therapy after planned delivery near term, an increasing number of simple anatomic abnormalities with predictably devastating developmental consequences have been successfully corrected before birth. However, fetal surgery is justifiable only if all of the following criteria are met:

1. Natural history and pathophysiology of the disease are well understood
2. Prenatal diagnosis is accurate, capable of excluding other anomalies, and able to predict which fetuses have a prognosis poor enough to justify in utero intervention
3. In utero correction is shown to be efficacious in animal models
4. Maternal risk is proved to be acceptably low

In the 1980s, the pathophysiology of several potentially correctable fetal lesions was elucidated using a variety of animal models. Concomitantly, the natural history of these abnormalities was determined by serial observation of human fetuses; selection criteria for prenatal intervention were developed; and anesthetic, tocolytic, and surgical techniques for hysterotomy and fetal surgery were refined.[1, 3, 4] In the 1990s, this investment in basic and clinical research benefitted an increasing number of fetal patients. This chapter reviews the current status of fetal surgery for prenatally diagnosed life-threatening anatomic anomalies.

☐ Risks and Benefits

For the fetus, the risk of the procedure is weighed against the benefit of correcting a lethal or debilitating defect. However, risks and benefits for the mother are more difficult to assess. Maternal safety is paramount; most fetal malformations do not directly threaten the mother's health, but if she chooses fetal surgery, she must bear significant risk and discomfort from the surgical procedure and the postoperative tocolytic therapy.

Because fetal surgery has rarely been attempted elsewhere, the 75 procedures we performed at the Fetal Treatment Center of the University of California, San Francisco, through June 1997 provide the best data about maternal outcome (Table 11–1). Intraoperatively, 11 of the 75 mothers required blood transfusions. In our early experience, 2 patients developed amniotic fluid leaks through the hysterotomy site, which required repair, and 5 patients developed amniotic fluid leaks from the vagina. None of the patients developed a leak from a trocar site following a fetoscopic procedure (see Fetal Surgery Techniques, later). There have been no maternal deaths and no infectious complications. All patients experienced labor after hysterotomy, and treatment of preterm labor accounted for the majority of maternal morbidity.[4, 5] Eleven patients developed pulmonary edema while receiving high doses of tocolytic drugs. Although reversible, this complication em-

TABLE 11-1. Maternal Outcome with
Open and Fetal Endoscopic Surgery*

Variable	Median	Range
Maternal age (y)	27	18–43
Gestational age of fetus (wk)	26.0	17–28
Operative time, total (min)	135.4	69–365
Operative time, fetal repair (min)	32	5–92
Blood loss (ml)	455	150–2500
Interval to delivery (wk)	4.5	1–15

Subsequent Pregnancy History	Number
Term cesarean delivery, healthy	31†
Currently pregnant	1
Pregnancy not attempted, not desired, too early, etc.	29

*University of California, San Francisco, Fetal Treatment Center, 75 cases through June 1997.

†Three women had two subsequent pregnancies each.

Adapted from Harrison MR: Fetal surgery. Am J Obstet Gynecol 174:1255–1264, 1996.

phasized the need for close monitoring in an intensive care setting. This complication has been rarely seen after fetoscopic procedures because they incite less uterine irritability compared to the open hysterotomy procedure. Because the midgestation hysterotomy is not performed in the lower uterine segment, delivery after fetal surgery and all future deliveries require cesarean section.

Early in our series, five uterine dehiscences occurred in subsequent pregnancies allowed to labor; uterine closure and neonatal outcome were excellent in all cases. There were two cases of maternal morbidity directly related to the fetal condition, termed the *maternal mirror syndrome*.[5] Two mothers with hydropic fetuses from an SCT and a CCAM developed high-output cardiac failure and physiologic manifestations that "mirrored" those of the distressed fetus. The maternal condition was not alleviated by correction of the fetal defect. Preterm labor ensued and early cesarean delivery was performed, with resolution of the maternal syndrome. However, both preterm neonates died from respiratory insufficiency.

Finally, the ability to carry and deliver in subsequent pregnancies does not appear to be jeopardized by fetal surgery. The potential for future childbearing after fetal surgery was first evaluated in a large series of nonhuman primates.[6] In this study, the subsequent fertility of animals that had uterine closure with absorbable sutures after fetal surgery was not diminished. However, animals that had metal staple hysterotomy closure had a markedly decreased fertility rate. We now use a stapler with absorbable staples for hysterotomy.[7, 8] Since 1981, we have follow-up data from 35 mothers who have attempted to become pregnant after fetal surgery: 32 conceived and 31 delivered normal babies.[9] One mother has yet to deliver. Of the 3 who could not conceive, 2 had a strong history of infertility before fetal surgery and the 3rd had attempted only for 6 months to become pregnant.

☐ Fetal Surgery Techniques

Numerous technical aspects of fetal surgical procedures have evolved over 15 years of experimental and clinical work.[1, 3–8, 10–17] In the operating room, the mother is positioned with left uterine displacement to avoid inferior vena cava compression by the gravid uterus, and she and her baby are anesthetized with a halogenated agent. Maternal monitoring is accomplished with routine noninvasive monitors plus central venous and arterial catheters. There are two surgical approaches to the fetus: one involves opening the uterus and delivering the fetal part to be repaired, and the other employs minimally invasive fetal endosurgical (FETENDO) techniques.

TECHNIQUES FOR OPEN HYSTEROTOMY

The uterus is exposed through a low, transverse abdominal incision; a large abdominal ring retractor is used to maintain exposure (Fig. 11–1). Ultrasonography (US) is used to localize the placenta and to determine the position of the fetus, in order to inject the fetus with a narcotic and a paralytic agent. Depending on the position of the placenta, the uterus is opened either anteriorly or posteriorly using absorbable staples that provide hemostasis and seal the membranes against the myometrium. Four specially designed, gentle, reverse-biting clamps, along with the staples, provide uterine hemostasis and help expose the pertinent fetal part. A miniaturized pulse oximeter records fetal pulse rate and oxygen saturation intraoperatively. Warm lactated Ringer's solution is continuously infused around the fetus.

After fetal repair, a radiotelemeter is implanted in a submuscular pocket before closing the fetal incision. This provides postoperative monitoring of fetal heart rate, temperature, and amniotic pressure. The uterine incision is closed with two layers of absorbable sutures and fibrin glue. Amniotic fluid is restored with warm lactated Ringer's solution containing 500 mg of nafcillin.

TECHNIQUES FOR MINIMALLY INVASIVE FETAL SURGERY

To date, we have nearly exclusively used Fetendo techniques to perform fetal tracheal occlusion to treat CDH[17] (see Congenital Diaphragmatic Hernia, later). Maternal positioning, monitoring, anesthesia, and abdominal incision to expose the uterus are as described earlier, except the mother is placed in lithotomy position (Fig. 11–2). To date, we have not performed this procedure percutaneously. Intraoperative US maps the placental position and guides trocar placement. An anterior placenta necessitates tipping the uterus forward and placing the trocars superiorly, posteriorly, or both.

Three to four 5- and 10-mm trocars with compressive flanges and balloons are used to perform Fet-

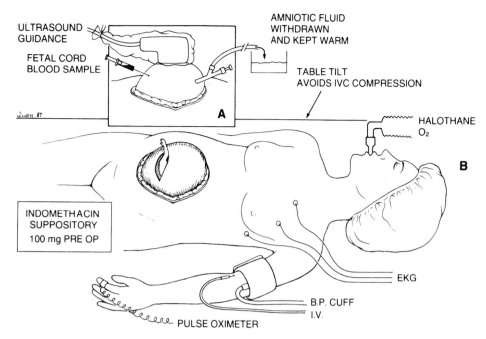

Figure 11–1. Maternal positioning and monitoring for open fetal surgery.

endo procedures. Continuous irrigation to optimize visibility is performed using a high-flow pump irrigation system via the sheath of a 12-degree hysteroscope. This system maintains a constant intrauterine fluid volume, avoids risk of air embolus with gas distention of the uterus, ensures a continuously washed operative field, improves visibility by exchanging the cloudy amniotic fluid with lactated Ringer's solution, and keeps the fetus warm. The fetus is monitored by transuterine US. A miniaturized telemeter that can be placed into the amniotic cavity via a trocar site has been developed and is being tested.

The fetal neck is exposed by placing a transuterine fetal mandibular stitch, which maintains neck extension (Fig. 11–3). The midline of the fetal neck is localized by a T-fastener sonographically placed within the lumen of the trachea. The trachea is occluded with two standard, large titanium hemoclips. The skin incision is left open. Each uterine puncture site is closed with one or two absorbable sutures and fibrin glue after instillation of intraamniotic antibiotic.

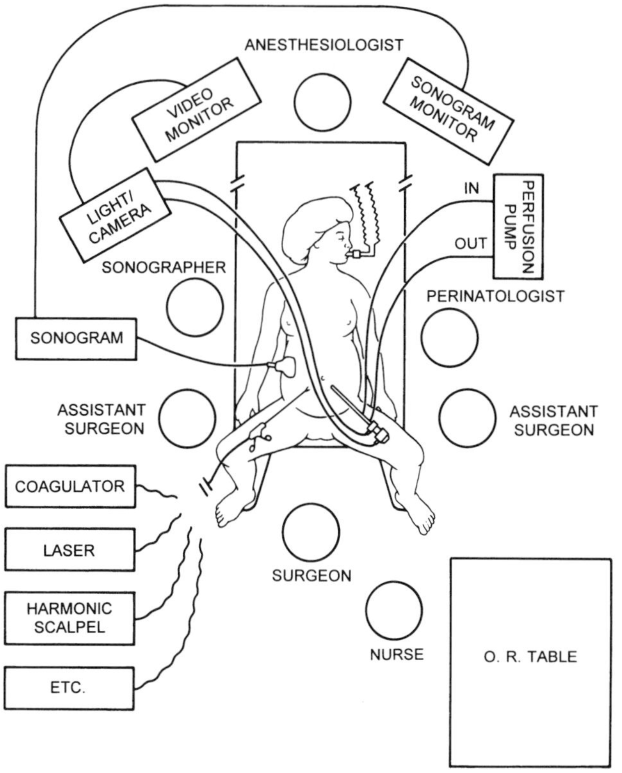

Figure 11–2. Operating room setup and maternal positioning for fetoscopic tracheal occlusion procedure.

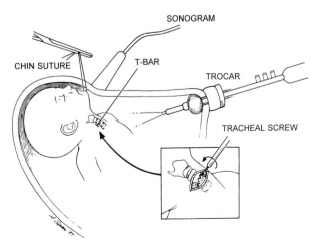

Figure 11–3. Under sonographic guidance, (1) the fetus' neck is exposed and head stabilized by placing a transuterine chin suture, and (2) a T-bar is placed in the fetal trachea to aid in localizing the midline fetal neck. After anterior tracheal dissection, a tracheal "screw" *(inset)* is placed in the tracheal wall and anterior traction applied, allowing safe posterolateral tracheal dissection.

POSTOPERATIVE MANAGEMENT OF MOTHER AND FETUS

Maternal arterial pressure, central venous pressure, urine output, and oxygen saturation are continuously monitored in an intensive care setting. Fetal well-being and uterine activity are recorded externally by a tocodynamometer and a radiotelemeter implanted at surgery, which continuously record the fetal electrocardiogram, fetal temperature, and intraamniotic pressure.[15] Continuous epidural analgesics ease maternal pain and aid tocolysis. The average hospital stay for open and Fetendo procedures is 12 and 6 days, respectively. Outpatient tocolysis is administered with oral or subcutaneous terbutaline or oral nifedipine. Fetal sonograms are performed at least weekly. Cesarean delivery is performed when membranes rupture or labor cannot be controlled, usually before 36 weeks' gestation.

☐ Preterm Labor

Breaching the uterus, whether by puncture or incision, incites uterine contractions. In spite of technical advances, preterm labor remains the Achilles heel of fetal therapy. The regimen—preoperative indomethacin; intraoperative deep halogenated inhalation anesthesia; and postoperative indomethacin, magnesium sulfate, and betamimetics—which was first perfected in sheep and monkeys,[11] has been only marginally successful in extensive procedures in humans.

Additionally, there are many potential side effects of tocolysis. Although halogenated inhalation agents provide satisfactory anesthesia for mother and fetus, the depth of anesthesia necessary to achieve intraoperative uterine relaxation can produce fetal and maternal myocardial depression and affect placental perfusion.[12] Indomethacin can constrict the fetal ductus arteriosus and the combination of magnesium sulfate and β-mimetics can produce maternal pulmonary edema. Fluid restriction to avoid this complication can compromise maternal-placental-fetal circulation and contribute to recalcitrant preterm labor.

The search for a more effective and less toxic tocolytic regimen led to the demonstration in monkeys that exogenous nitric oxide ablates preterm labor induced by hysterotomy.[13] Since 1996, we have used intravenous nitroglycerin (a nitric oxide donor) intraoperatively and postoperatively. It is a potent tocolytic, but it requires careful control to avoid serious complications.

☐ Fetal Problems Amenable to Surgical Correction Before Birth

The only anatomic malformations that warrant consideration are those that interfere with fetal organ development and that, if alleviated, would allow normal development to proceed. At present, only a small number of life-threatening malformations have been successfully corrected. A few others should be considered for treatment as their prenatal pathophysiology (natural history) is unraveled.

As minimally invasive interventional techniques continue to be developed and proved safe and treatment and prevention of preterm labor improve, prenatal treatment of select nonlethal anomalies (e.g., myelomeningocele[18, 19] and cleft lip or palate[20, 21]) may be considered.

CONGENITAL DIAPHRAGMATIC HERNIA

CDH is an anatomically simple defect that is correctable after birth by removing the herniated viscera from the chest and closing the diaphragm. Although less severely affected babies survive with modern postnatal surgical care, including extracorporeal membrane oxygenation (ECMO) support, the majority of babies die despite all intervention because their lungs are underdeveloped (hypoplastic) and there is associated pulmonary hypertension. Because retrospective estimates of mortality for CDH vary widely and are flawed by a hidden mortality of unknown magnitude, we prospectively studied 52 fetuses with potentially correctable, isolated diaphragmatic hernias diagnosed before 24 weeks' gestation.[22] The mortality was 58%, despite the best postnatal care including ECMO. Babies who die in utero and soon after birth contribute to a substantial hidden mortality. Salvage of these severely affected babies remains an unsolved problem.

The pulmonary hypoplasia of CDH is reversible after repair, but weeks or months are required. After birth, pulmonary support with ECMO is limited to 1 or 2 weeks and cannot save severely affected babies. We have shown experimentally that repair before birth, when the lungs can grow while the fetus remains on placental support, is physiologically sound and technically feasible.[23] But repair in utero has proved to be a formidable challenge, particularly when the left lobe of the liver is incarcerated in the chest, because reduction of the liver compromises umbilical blood flow.[24, 25]

Many technical problems associated with this difficult repair led to the development of the "CDH two-step," a carefully orchestrated approach that necessitates both a thoracotomy and a laparotomy, allowing reduction of the herniated viscera, reconstruction of the diaphragm with a Gore-Tex patch, and enlargement of the abdomen to accept the returned viscera.[26] The efficacy, safety, and cost-effectiveness of in utero repair have been prospectively evaluated in a National Institutes of Health–sponsored trial.[27] The results indicate that children in whom the liver is not incarcerated in the left hemithorax can be successfully treated by the in utero repair. However, in utero repair in this group has not led to an increased survival compared to matched controls who received standard postnatal therapy.

When an isolated fetal CDH is diagnosed prior to 24 weeks' gestation, the family has three choices: (1) terminate the pregnancy; (2) carry to term and deliver in a tertiary neonatal center for intensive care with an expected mortality of 58%, and considerable morbidity; or (3) attempt prenatal intervention (Fig. 11–4). The family's dilemma in choosing management is particularly difficult: the natural history of fetal CDH is quite variable because there are no direct biochemical or imaging parameters that reliably predict postnatal lung function.

We established a sonographic prognostic measure of severity, the lung-to-head ratio (LHR).[28] It is determined by measuring right lung volume corrected for gestational age by dividing by the head circumference; the greater the mediastinal shift, the greater the ipsilateral and contralateral lung compression, and the lower the LHR. An LHR less than 1.0 is highly predictive of a poor postnatal outcome. It is known that fetuses that herniate late in gestation (>25 weeks) will do well with modern postnatal surgical and neonatal care after delivery at a tertiary center. Conversely, fetuses with early herniation, severe mediastinal shift, low LHR, dilated intrathoracic stomach (gastric outlet obstruction produces polyhydramnios and gastric dilation), and herniated liver have a poor outlook.

Fetuses with herniated liver have never been successfully repaired using the two-step technique in utero, despite extensive efforts using a variety of techniques. Indeed, it took many years to recognize the significance of liver herniation and to be able to reliably predict it sonographically. For fetuses deemed unfixable by virtue of liver herniation, we have developed experimentally and now tested clinically an approach to improving fetal lung development. We have shown, in lamb fetuses, that impeding the normal egress of fetal lung fluid by controlled tracheal obstruction enlarges the hypoplastic lungs and pushes the viscera back into the abdomen.[29–31] Initial experience with this procedure, which we call PLUG (*P*lug the *L*ung *U*ntil It *G*rows), suggests that temporary occlusion of the fetal trachea accelerates fetal lung growth and ameliorates the often fatal pulmonary hypoplasia associated with severe CDH.

We initially achieved clinical prenatal tracheal occlusion using open fetal surgical techniques. Then we developed a fetoscopic approach, used in 8 "poor prognosis" patients (i.e., the liver was herniated into the hemithorax, the diagnosis was made before 25 weeks' gestation, and the LHR was low) that resulted in a 75% survival rate, compared to a 38% survival in matched controls. This technique has proved safe and efficacious, and it has resulted in less preterm labor and less maternal morbidity.[16, 17] Delivery and reestablishment of the airway are discussed later (see Ex Utero Intrapartum Treatment Procedure).

CONGENITAL CYSTIC ADENOMATOID MALFORMATION

Although CCAM often presents as a benign pulmonary mass in infancy or childhood, some fetuses with large lesions die in utero or at birth from either

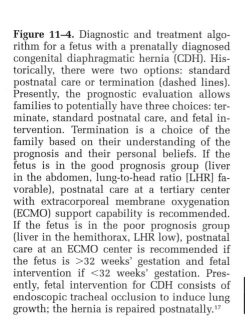

Figure 11–4. Diagnostic and treatment algorithm for a fetus with a prenatally diagnosed congenital diaphragmatic hernia (CDH). Historically, there were two options: standard postnatal care or termination (dashed lines). Presently, the prognostic evaluation allows families to potentially have three choices: terminate, standard postnatal care, and fetal intervention. Termination is a choice of the family based on their understanding of the prognosis and their personal beliefs. If the fetus is in the good prognosis group (liver in the abdomen, lung-to-head ratio [LHR] favorable), postnatal care at a tertiary center with extracorporeal membrane oxygenation (ECMO) support capability is recommended. If the fetus is in the poor prognosis group (liver in the hemithorax, LHR low), postnatal care at an ECMO center is recommended if the fetus is >32 weeks' gestation and fetal intervention if <32 weeks' gestation. Presently, fetal intervention for CDH consists of endoscopic tracheal occlusion to induce lung growth; the hernia is repaired postnatally.[17]

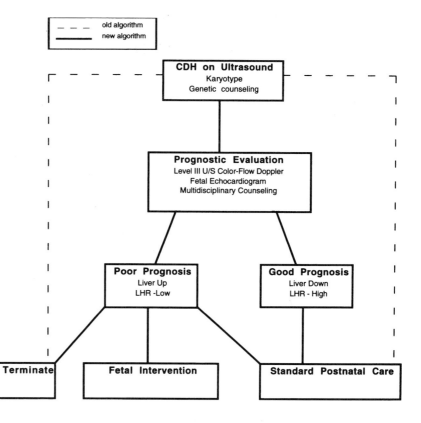

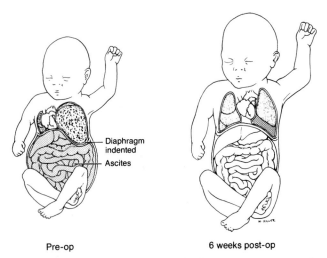

Pre-op   6 weeks post-op

Figure 11–5. Schematic drawing of fetal anatomy preoperatively *(left)* and 6 weeks after fetal surgery for cystic adenomatoid malformation *(right)*. Postoperatively, the fetal ascites resolved, the mediastinum returned to the midline, and the remaining left upper lobe and right lung showed remarkable growth.

hydrops or pulmonary hypoplasia.[32] Differences in the survival rate of patients with CCAM are not related to the histologic type of the lesion but rather to the associated hydrops. Hydrops is probably secondary to vena cava obstruction or cardiac compression caused by the extreme mediastinal shift caused by these lesions.[33] The potentially fatal outcome with large CCAM lesions may also be related to lung hypoplasia secondary to prolonged compression in utero.

Experimentally, fetal pulmonary resection is feasible and compensatory growth of the opposite lung occurs.[34] Experience managing 111 cases suggests that most lesions can be successfully treated after birth, and that some lesions resolve or significantly regress before birth.[35] Although only a few fetuses with very large lesions will develop hydrops before 26 weeks' gestation, almost all of these lesions progress rapidly and lead to in utero death. Careful US surveillance of large lesions is necessary to detect the first signs of hydrops because fetuses that develop hydrops (<10% of all fetuses with CCAMs) can be successfully treated by emergency resection of the cystic lobe in utero. When hydrops is accompanied by placentomegaly and signs of maternal preeclampsia (maternal mirror syndrome), it is too late for fetal intervention. Early in our experience, this clinical scenario was responsible for some of the postoperative deaths.

Twelve fetuses have undergone open surgical resection of the massively enlarged pulmonary lobe (Fig. 11–5) based on well-established selection criteria (Fig. 11–6). Seven had rapid resolution of hydrops, impressive in utero lung growth bilaterally, and normal postnatal growth and development with a follow-up of 52 to 84 months.[36, 37] For lesions with a single large cyst, percutaneous thoracoamniotic shunting with a double-J pigtail catheter has also been successful.[38]

SACROCOCCYGEAL TERATOMA

Most neonates with SCT survive and malignant invasion is unusual. However, the outcome for SCT diagnosed prenatally (by elevated alphafetoprotein or US) is less favorable. The prognostic importance of the gestational age at diagnosis was reported in a series in which six of eight fetuses survived when the diagnosis was made after 30 weeks' gestation, but only 1 of 14 survived when the diagnosis was made earlier.[39] When SCT was diagnosed prior to 30

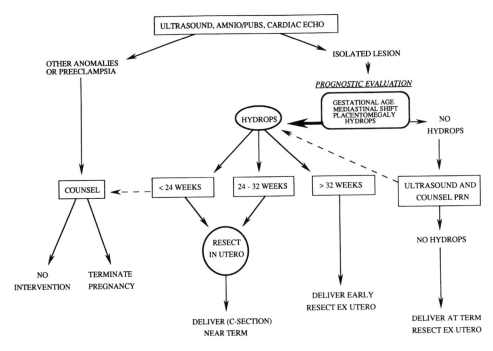

Figure 11–6. Algorithm for management of the fetus with a congenital cystic adenomatoid malformation. amnio, amniocentesis; c-section, cesarean section; echo, echography.

weeks' gestation, invariably, massive tumor enlargement, fetal hydrops, and placentomegaly were present. In all of six cases diagnosed prior to 23 weeks' gestation, the mothers developed the maternal mirror syndrome, with vomiting, hypertension, edema, and proteinuria.

Less than 20% of fetuses with large tumors develop hydrops from high-output failure secondary to high blood flow through the extremely vascular tumor. The tumor behaves as a large arteriovenous fistula with markedly increased distal aortic blood flow and shunting of blood away from the placenta.[40] Because hydrops progresses very rapidly to fetal death, frequent sonographic follow-up is mandatory.

These findings have important implications for management. Fetuses with lesions larger than 5 cm should be delivered by cesarean section to avoid dystocia, tumor rupture, or hemorrhage into the tumor.[39] Fetuses with hydrops diagnosed after 30 weeks' gestation should be delivered when pulmonary maturity is attained. Hydropic fetuses diagnosed prior to 30 weeks' gestation have a poor outcome. In these patients, excision of the tumor reverses the pathophysiology[40] and has been successful in two patients.[41, 42]

URINARY TRACT OBSTRUCTION

Fetal urethral obstruction produces pulmonary hypoplasia and renal dysplasia, and these often fatal consequences can be ameliorated by urinary tract

TABLE 11-2. Prognostic Criteria* for the Fetus with Bilateral Obstructive Uropathy

Predicted Function	Sodium (mEq/l)	Chloride (mEq/l)	Osmolarity (mOsm)	Output (ml/h)
Poor	>100	>90	>210	<2
Good	<100	<90	<210	>2

*Fetal urine composition and volume.

decompression before birth.[43] The natural history of untreated fetal urinary tract obstruction is well documented, and selection criteria based on fetal urine volume and electrolyte levels (Table 11–2) and the sonographic appearance of the fetal kidneys have proved reliable.[44, 45]

Of all fetuses with urinary tract dilation, as many as 90% do not require intervention (Fig. 11–7). The fetus with a dilated low-pressure system that continues to have good urine output and adequate amniotic fluid volume requires no intervention. The fetus with severe renal dysplasia that is not reversible, even with decompression, clearly should not be treated. The fetus with unilateral disease of any type with a normally functioning contralateral kidney can be managed conservatively, because the disease is not life-threatening. However, fetuses with bilateral severe hydronephrosis due to urethral obstruction that have good renal function and develop oligohydramnios require treatment. If the lungs are mature, the fetus can be delivered early for postnatal

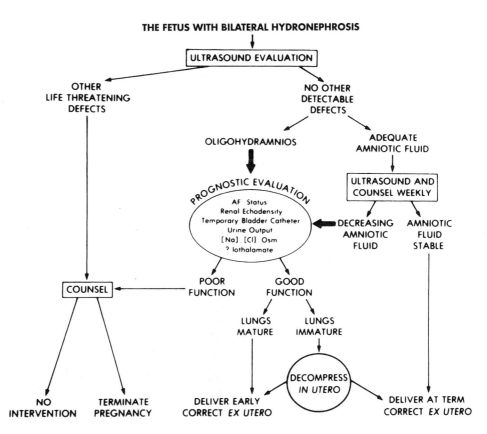

Figure 11–7. Management scheme for the fetus with bilateral hydronephrosis. (From Glick PL, Harrison MR, Golbus MS, et al: Management of the fetus with congenital hydronephrosis, II: Prognostic criteria and selection for treatment. J Pediatr Surg 20:376–387, 1985.)

decompression. If the lungs are immature, the bladder can be decompressed in utero by a catheter shunt placed percutaneously under sonographic guidance,[46] by open fetal vesicostomy,[47] by fetoscopic vesicostomy,[48] or by placement of a wire mesh stent that may solve the technical problems historically encountered with shunts (malfunction, dislodgment, and abdominal wall disruption).[49]

Experience treating several hundred fetuses in many institutions suggests that selection is good enough to avoid inappropriate intervention and that restoration of amniotic fluid can prevent the development of fatal pulmonary hypoplasia. It is still unclear whether in utero intervention can arrest or reverse cystic dysplastic changes caused by obstructive uropathy. It is possible that the dysplastic changes initiated in utero will compromise renal function progressively as demand increases with growth. Relief of obstruction during the most active phase of nephrogenesis, between 20 and 30 weeks' gestation, may obviate further damage and allow nephrogenesis to proceed normally.[23]

□ Ex Utero Intrapartum Treatment Procedure

Tracheal occlusion for the treatment of CDH requires a technique to safely "unobstruct" the trachea at birth and establish a stable airway. The ex utero intrapartum treatment (EXIT) procedure relies on maintaining fetoplacental circulation until the fetal airway is secure. Provided uterine relaxation is maintained (preventing placental separation), fetal manipulations have been performed for up to 60 minutes before dividing the umbilical cord.[50]

For the child with external tracheal clips for the treatment of CDH, clip removal is performed via a "partial" cesarean section. Only the head and shoulders are delivered. One surgeon performs bronchoscopy while another removes the tracheal clips. Lung fluid is suctioned, the child is intubated, and surfactant is administered, allowing delivery of the child with a secure airway.

The EXIT strategy has also been used to manage a variety of prenatally diagnosed conditions that may threaten the airway at birth, such as large airway tumors[51] and congenital high airway obstruction syndrome (CHAOS) due to a laryngeal web. Fetuses with CHAOS have large echogenic lungs due to overdistention by lung fluid, and they uniformly develop hydrops.[51] The EXIT strategy allowed delivery of a hydropic early third-trimester child with creation of a tracheostomy before dividing the umbilical cord. This child is now 14 months old and is thriving, awaiting airway reconstruction.

REFERENCES

 1. Harrison MR, Golbus MS, Filly RA (eds): The Unborn Patient: Prenatal Diagnosis and Treatment (2nd ed). Philadelphia, WB Saunders, 1990.
 2. Harrison MR, Bjordal RI, Landmark F, et al: Congenital diaphragmatic hernia: The hidden mortality. J Pediatr Surg 13:227–231, 1979.
 3. Harrison MR, Adzick NS: The fetus as a patient: Surgical considerations. Ann Surg 213:279–291, 1990.
 4. Harrison MR: Fetal surgery. West J Med 159:341–349, 1993.
 5. Longaker MT, Golbus MS, Filly RA, et al: Maternal outcome after open fetal surgery. JAMA 265:737–741, 1991.
 6. Adzick NS, Harrison MR, Anderson JV, et al: Fetal surgery in the primate, III: Maternal outcome after fetal surgery. J Pediatr Surg 21:477–480, 1986.
 7. Adzick NS, Harrison MR, Flake AW, et al: Automatic uterine stapling device in fetal surgery: Experience in a primate model. Surg Forum 36:476–481, 1985.
 8. Bond SJ, Harrison MR, Slotnick RN, et al: Cesarean delivery and hysterotomy using an absorbable stapling device. Obstet Gynecol 74:25–28, 1989.
 9. Farrell JA, Albanese CT, Jennings RW, et al: Maternal fertility is not affected by fetal surgery. Fetal Diagn Ther: in press.
10. Adzick NS, Harrison MR: Fetal surgical therapy. Lancet 343:897–902, 1994.
11. Harrison MR, Anderson J, Rosen MA, et al: Fetal surgery in the primate, I: Anesthetic, surgical, and tocolytic management to maximize fetal-neonatal survival. J Pediatr Surg 17:115–122, 1982.
12. Sabik JF, Assad RS, Hanley FL: Halothane as an anesthetic for fetal surgery. J Pediatr Surg 28:542–546, 1993.
13. Jennings RW, MacGillivray TE, Harrison MR: Nitric oxide inhibits preterm labor in the rhesus monkey. J Matern Fetal Med 2:170–175, 1993.
14. Harrison MR, Adzick NS: Fetal surgical techniques. Semin Pediatr Surg 2:136–142, 1993.
15. Jennings RW, Adzick NS, Longaker MT, et al: Radiotelemetric fetal monitoring during and after open fetal surgery. Surg Obstet Gynecol 176:59–64, 1993.
16. VanderWall KJ, Bruch SW, Meuli M, et al: Fetal endoscopic (FETENDO) tracheal clip. J Pediatr Surg 31:1101–1104, 1996.
17. Harrison MR, Mychaliska GB, Albanese CT, et al: Correction of congenital diaphragmatic hernia in utero, IX: Fetuses with poor prognosis (liver herniation and low lung-to-head ratio) can be saved by fetoscopic temporary tracheal occlusion. J Pediatr Surg 33:1017–1022, 1998.
18. Meuli M, Meuli-Simmen C, Yingling CD, et al: A new model of myelomeningocele: Studies in the fetal lamb. J Pediatr Surg 30:1034–1037, 1995.
19. Meuli M, Meuli-Simmen C, Hutchins GM, et al: In utero surgery rescues neurologic function at birth in sheep with spina bifida. Nat Med 1:342–347, 1995.
20. Longaker MT, Whitby DJ, Adzick NS, et al: Fetal surgery for cleft lip: A plea for caution. Plast Reconstr Surg 88:1087–1092, 1991.
21. Estes JM, MacGillivray TE, Hedrick MH, et al: Fetoscopic surgery for the treatment of congenital anomalies. J Pediatr Surg 27:950–954, 1992.
22. Harrison MR, Adzick NS, Estes JM, et al: A prospective study of the outcome of fetuses with congenital diaphragmatic hernia. JAMA 271:382–384, 1994.
23. Harrison MR, Ross NA, deLorimier AA: Correction of congenital diaphragmatic hernia in utero, III: Development of a successful surgical technique using abdominoplasty to avoid compromise of umbilical blood flow. J Pediatr Surg 16:934–942, 1981.
24. Harrison MR, Langer JC, Adzick NS, et al: Correction of congenital diaphragmatic hernia in utero, V: Initial clinical experience. J Pediatr Surg 25:47–57, 1990.
25. Harrison MR, Adzick NS, Flake AW, et al: Correction of congenital diaphragmatic hernia in utero, VI: Hard-earned lessons. J Pediatr Surg 28:1411–1418, 1993.
26. Harrison MR, Adzick NS, Flake AW, et al: The CDH two-step: A dance of necessity. J Pediatr Surg 28:813–816, 1993.
27. Harrison MR, Adzick NS, Bullard KM, et al: Correction of congenital diaphragmatic hernia in utero, VII: A prospective trial. J Pediatr Surg 32:1637–1642, 1997.
28. Lipshutz GS, Albanese CT, Feldstein VA, et al: Prospective analysis of lung-to-head ratio predicts survival for patients

with prenatally diagnosed congenital diaphragmatic hernia. J Pediatr Surg 32:1634–1636, 1997.

29. DiFiore JW, Fauza DO, Slavin D, et al: Experimental fetal tracheal ligation reverses the structural and physiologic effects of pulmonary hypoplasia in congenital diaphragmatic hernia. J Pediatr Surg 29:248–257, 1994.

30. Hedrick MH, Estes JM, Sullivan KM, et al: Plug the lung until it grows (PLUG): A new method to treat congenital diaphragmatic hernia in utero. J Pediatr Surg 29:612–617, 1994.

31. Harrison MR, Adzick NS, Flake AW, et al: Correction of congenital diaphragmatic hernia in utero, VIII: Response of the hypoplastic lung to trachea. J Pediatr Surg 31:1339–1348, 1996.

32. Adzick NS, Harrison MR, Glick PL, et al: Fetal cystic adenomatoid malformation: Prenatal diagnosis and natural history. J Pediatr Surg 20:483–488, 1985.

33. Rice HE, Estes JM, Hedrick MH, et al: Congenital cystic adenomatoid malformation: A sheep model of fetal hydrops. J Pediatr Surg 29:692–696, 1994.

34. Adzick NS, Harrison MR, Hu LM, et al: Compensatory lung growth after pneumonectomy in fetal lambs: A morphometric study. Surg Forum 37:309–314, 1986.

35. MacGillivray TE, Harrison MR, Goldstein RB, et al: Disappearing fetal lung lesions. J Pediatr Surg 28:1321–1325, 1993.

36. Harrison MR, Adzick NS, Jennings RW, et al: Antenatal intervention for congenital cystic adenomatoid malformation. Lancet 336:965–967, 1990.

37. Adzick NS, Harrison MR, Flake AW, et al: Fetal surgery for cystic adenomatoid malformation of the lung. J Pediatr Surg 28:806–812, 1993.

38. Blott M, Nicolaides KH, Greenough A: Postnatal respiratory function after chronic drainage of fetal pulmonary cyst. Am J Obstet Gynecol 159:858–859, 1988.

39. Flake AW, Harrison MR, Adzick NS, et al: Fetal sacrococcygeal teratoma. J Pediatr Surg 21:563–566, 1986.

40. Langer JC, Harrison MR, Schmidt KG, et al: Fetal hydrops and demise from sacrococcygeal teratoma: Rationale for fetal surgery. Am J Obstet Gynecol 160:1145–1150, 1989.

41. Graf JL, Beech R, Jennings RW, et al: Successful fetal sacrococcygeal teratoma resection in a hydropic fetus. J Pediatr Surg: in press.

42. Graf JL, Housely HT, Albanese CT, et al: A surprising histologic evolution of preterm sacrococcygeal teratomas. J Pediatr Surg 33:177–179, 1998.

43. Adzick NS, Harrison MR, Flake AW, et al: Fetal urinary tract obstruction: Experimental pathophysiology. Semin Perinatol 9:79–80, 1985.

44. Nicolaides KH, Cheng HH, Snijders RJM, et al: Fetal urine biochemistry in the assessment of obstructive uropathy. Am J Obstet Gynecol 166:932–937, 1992.

45. Johnson MP, Bukowski TP, Reitleman C, et al: In utero surgical treatment of fetal obstructive uropathy: A new comprehensive approach to identify appropriate candidates for vesicoamniotic shunt therapy. Am J Obstet Gynecol 170:1770–1779, 1994.

46. Manning FA, Harrison MR, Rodeck CH, et al: Special report. Catheter shunts for fetal hydronephrosis and hydrocephalus. N Engl J Med 315:336–340, 1986.

47. Crombleholme TM, Harrison MR, Langer JC, et al: Early experience with open fetal surgery for congenital hydronephrosis. J Pediatr Surg 23:1114–1121, 1988.

48. MacMahan RA, Renou PM, Shekelton PA, et al: In utero cystostomy. Lancet 340:1234, 1992.

49. Estes JM, Harrison MR: Fetal obstructive uropathy. Semin Pediatr Surg 2:129–135, 1993.

50. Mychaliska GB, Bealer JF, Graf JL, et al: Operating on placental support: The ex utero intrapartum treatment procedure. J Pediatr Surg 32:227–231, 1997.

51. Martinez-Ferro M, Hedrick MH, Flake AW, et al: Prenatal diagnosis of congenital high airway obstruction (CHAOS): Potential for perinatal intervention. J Pediatr Surg 29:271–274, 1994.

12

FOREIGN BODIES

J. Laurance Hill, MD • Roger W. Voigt, MB, ChB

The proclivity of infants and children to place all manner of foreign bodies into their mouths, noses, and ears frequently results in the need for surgical removal. The complications of foreign bodies in the airway, gut, and soft tissue can be fatal. The frightening and true emergency of an obstructed airway or the serious infection resulting from a perforated viscus or soft tissue foreign body is long remembered. Although many practitioners are interested in the removal of foreign bodies, it is our opinion that the patient is best treated by an experienced surgeon trained in and comfortable with operating on a child's chest or abdomen, when necessary. The benefit of a children's center that has modern equipment and pediatric anesthesia immediately available cannot be overestimated.

The development of small diameter flexible endoscopes has allowed medical specialists access to the esophagus and airway in the conscious, sedated patient. This has, in turn, led to suggestions that foreign bodies in these structures might be removed in an efficacious and cost-effective manner.[1] The complexities of some foreign bodies and the tissue reaction that is generated by their presence often make removal under conscious sedation impossible. The ultimate result of such an undertaking is that what is intended to be a simple procedure becomes a matter of endoscopy by two different specialists. This increases not only the costs but also the risks to the patient. Dislodging a foreign body that is obstructing a bronchus to a position of occluding the glottis may be disastrous.

A history that suggests the possibility of a foreign body should mandate the most effective and safest method for diagnosis *and* removal of the foreign body. Topical anesthetics and sedation do not control the anxieties and defensive hyperreflexes of children undergoing complicated and possibly prolonged endoscopic procedures. In small children, the endoscopes that allow ventilation, suction of secretions, access for extracting forceps, and access for light and vision are rigid. The setting is the operating room; the appropriate team consists of anesthesiologist, surgeon, and nursing staff familiar with the intricacies of the procedure and the equipment. The equipment must be demonstrated to be in good working order and the extraction equipment must fit the sheath. The key principle is to prepare for and to prevent the potential disaster. Rigid endoscopy provides the best airway control and channel for the safe removal of airway and esophageal foreign bodies.

About 2 centuries have passed since Bozzini (1806)[2] used a candle as a light source to remove foreign bodies from the airway. More than 60 years have passed since Chevalier Jackson (1936) would not open his black box of instruments until the room had been darkened enough so that his inventive tools could not be copied (B. Blades, personal communication).

The security of ventilation and especially the visibility of modern instruments were markedly enhanced by the development of an integrated pediatric endoscopy system by Karl Storz.[3] This system brought four major advantages that reduced the risks of pediatric endoscopy. The first and most ingenious of these was the magnification system of Harold Hopkins, which reversed the function of air and glass within the telescope. Convex air spaces between glass rods provided the needed magnification and vastly improved the second improvement, light transmission, to the end of the telescope and back to the viewer. The third improvement was the separate channel for the delivery of oxygen and anesthetic gases to the patient. This safety feature continues to be one of the most important of the modern day endoscopy equipment. The fourth improvement was the development of miniaturized graspers that are built into the telescopic carrier. These four improvements have become features that make present day foreign body removal more controlled than before their institution. Further refinements in cameras and monitors have made teaching foreign body removal more effective than before their use.

Although there are flexible fiberoptic endoscopes as small as 1.7 mm available for passage through an endotracheal tube or for awake diagnostic endoscopy, it is not possible to ventilate or manipulate instruments with these devices. The smallest diameter rigid endoscope that contains a working channel and a ventilation channel is the 3.5 mm sheath, through which a 1.9 mm telescope can be passed while leaving enough room for ventilation.[4] This instrument passes through almost any full-term infant's glottis. In neonates whose airways do not accommodate this sheath, the unprotected rigid telescope may be used to visualize foreign bodies, although the surgeon must be extremely careful to avoid bending the telescope; bending it destroys its optical characteristics forever. Although devices are manufactured to eliminate fogging of the lens by airflow, the simplest way to avoid this problem is to apply an antifogging agent before insertion (Fig. 12–1).

The delicate, intricate instruments that have been developed to grasp foreign bodies or biopsy tissues are an extremely important part of the endoscopist's armamentarium (Fig. 12–2). This array of instruments allows the removal of foreign bodies as hard as glass or as soft and soggy as paper. The optics that go with these instruments allow the surgeon to manipulate the grasping device to contact a foreign body without pushing it distally. The experienced endoscopist occasionally uses vascular balloon catheters, urologic catheters, and devices for the extraction of ureteral stones to remove foreign bodies.

☐ Clinical Problems

EAR AND NOSE FOREIGN BODIES

Although the ears and nose are usually considered the realm of the otolaryngologist and patients are directly referred to this specialist, occasionally the pediatric surgeon or primary care physician is called on to manage foreign bodies in these cavities. Insects may invade the external auditory canal, and small objects such as peas, peanuts, paper, or beans may be inserted by the child. A live insect usually produces a buzzing noise, which the child will describe if he or she is old enough to verbalize, but the child may be more reticent to admit to self-inflicted foreign objects. An inflammatory process may be the first indication of a foreign body in the ear or nose. Drainage, fever, and bleeding may all be seen with a foreign body that has been in place for several days or more. The foreign body may be dislodged by irrigation with tepid water using a Water-Pik, or a cerumen scoop, loop, or bayonet forceps may be used to remove it. If the ear canal is inflamed and tender, sedation or even general anesthesia may be required for safe foreign body removal.

Irrigation is not effective for nasal foreign bodies. A nasal foreign body generates a prompt mucus discharge and may easily be mistaken for a viral illness. Epistaxis may be an early or a late symptom, depending on the nature of the foreign body and its potential to erode the mucosa. Fever and a foul odor sometimes accompany the nasal foreign body. A nasal foreign body often requires manipulation into the pharynx or application of a grasper for removal and thus may well require general anesthesia. Once it is removed, saline or antibiotic nose drops may help promote healing.

LARYNGEAL AND TRACHEAL FOREIGN BODIES

Children from age 9 to 30 months are susceptible to airway foreign bodies due to these children's mo-

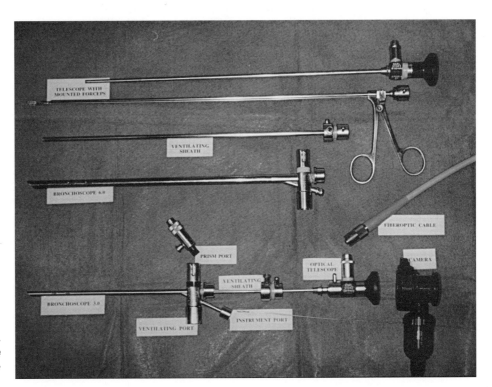

Figure 12–1. Instruments for pediatric bronchoscopy, which come in a series of calibers and lengths, are also used for esophagoscopy.

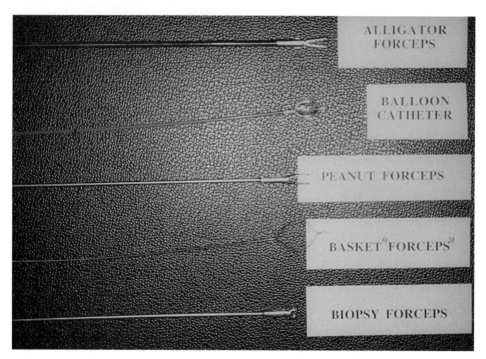

Figure 12–2. Various devices useful in the extraction of foreign bodies.

bility and their oral orientation. Older children and adults add to the problem by giving the toddler inappropriate foods, such as peanuts and popcorn, or small objects, which the child promptly puts into his or her mouth and which can be aspirated. Pointed objects are likely to become fixed and to result in laryngeal obstruction, but flimsy pieces of plastic and rubber balloons are more modern threats. Poorly chewed fruits, vegetables, and meat are frequently aspirated when the child inhales with a full pharynx.

An object touching the glottis provokes immediate coughing, choking, and loss of phonation. The stridor, wheezing, and retractions that follow draw attention immediately to the possibility of aspiration. If the foreign body has lodged within the glottic opening, the child struggles to take in enough air with which to cough. He or she rapidly becomes cyanotic. At this point, the Heimlich maneuver may dislodge the foreign body and restore the airway. Manual dislodgement of larger objects by an adult also may be effective. Inverting the child and pounding on the back may help dislodge the foreign material. Otherwise, the child progresses to hypoxia and cardiac arrest within a few minutes. A small child struggling to breathe represents a true life or death emergency and demands quick action. These lifesaving efforts take place outside the hospital. An emergency tracheotomy or cricothyrotomy is not likely to solve the problem of glottic obstruction under the usual circumstances.

Most aspirated foreign bodies pass through the glottis and lodge in a bronchus or one of its branches. In these cases, the acute, life-threatening phase was not seen, but the child often wheezes and continues coughing. There may be no symptoms. Often, only if the parent or someone else remembers the choking incidence at the initial aspiration is the situation further investigated, unless inflammation has produced illness.

Physical examination often reveals audible wheezes over the ipsilateral chest. Total occlusion of the bronchus results in atelectasis and no breath sounds. Pneumonitis quickly develops in cases in which the bronchus is even partially occluded, leading to findings of a febrile illness. Chronic, less occlusive foreign bodies in a minor airway may lead to bronchiectasis, abscess, hemorrhage, empyema, and systemic sepsis.

Radiographic findings may be minimal in the early stages of foreign body bronchial occlusion, particularly if both inspiration and expiration films are not taken. The radiolucent foreign body often is only evident due to the ball-valve effect, which prevents the egress of air from the involved lung. The ipsilateral diaphragm may be depressed and the intercostal spaces relatively widened by the effects of air trapping. Tracheal deviation toward the normal lung occurs early. Prolonged occlusion or more complete occlusion of the bronchus results in atelectasis, which remains fixed on the inspiratory-expiratory radiographic studies.

☐ Surgical Problems

A brief discussion of the plan for the removal of an airway foreign body is essential between the surgeon and the anesthesiologist. The nature of the foreign body and its suspected location help both parties understand the maneuvers needed to remove it and the problems to be avoided. Such preparation can significantly shorten the duration and enhance both the accuracy and safety of the procedure. Effective positioning of the patient may prevent the "good" lung from being contaminated by pus that is liberated when a long-standing bronchial foreign body obstruction is removed. Mask induction of the anesthetic and spraying of the vocal cords with local anesthetic agents reduce the likelihood of laryngospasm on introduction of the endoscope, but the anesthetic agent may interfere with bacterial cultures if the airway is sprayed. Hypoxia and bradycardia may be prevented by repositioning the bronchoscope into the trachea if the anesthesiologist alerts the surgeon to falling saturation. The vigor with which the child is ventilated may be unintentionally reduced when the surgeon is intently removing a foreign body and has the endoscope lodged distally in one bronchus. The smaller and sicker the patient, the more competition for the airway becomes crucial to the patient's well-being and the more important becomes good communication between the surgeon and the anesthesiologist.

Bronchoscopic removal of a foreign body should be done with as much attention to sterility as possible. The head is wrapped in sterile towels. The lips and teeth must be protected from injury. The endoscope is usually introduced using the laryngoscope to expose the glottis. It may be necessary to rotate the bronchoscope 90 degrees to pass the vocal cords. An endoscope should be sufficiently small to avoid trauma on introduction. The surgeon may observe the passage of the endoscope through the glottis either by looking alongside the endoscope or by looking through the telescope. Rotation or extension of the head may facilitate passage if the trachea seems to be kinked in any way.

Localization of the foreign body is not always as simple as it might seem. Tissue reaction, blood, secretions, and incomplete anesthesia necessitated by concomitant pulmonary disease may make identifying the foreign body a matter of repeated suction and irrigation. Overvigorous suctioning can easily impact the foreign body more distal into the bronchus, where opening the grasper jaws may not be possible. Passing a Fogarty balloon catheter beyond the foreign body and inflating the balloon may allow smooth foreign bodies to be pulled back to the point where they can be grasped with the jaws. In the rare event that distal impaction renders the foreign body not removable endoscopically, thoracotomy and bronchotomy may be necessary. On occasion, segmental or lobar resection may be the only practical alternative to removing the impacted bronchial foreign body.

ESOPHAGEAL FOREIGN BODIES

Foreign bodies are commonly swallowed. Some lodge in the esophagus. The narrowest part of the alimentary tract is the cricopharyngeus muscle or "superior constrictor" of the esophagus. This sphincter muscle is capable of relaxing to allow passage of large objects. In our experience, the majority of swallowed foreign objects that are too large

to be passed into the stomach lodge at the level of the aortic arch (Fig. 12–3). The other relatively narrow region of the esophagus is the area of the crossing left main bronchus. Esophageal anomalies, including repaired esophageal atresia, add to the chance that objects, including food that is ingested, will become lodged just above the area of anastomosis. This is due both to varying degrees of stricture at the anastomosis and to the fact that the distal esophagus does not have normal motility. Food foreign bodies are quite common after repair of esophageal atresia. Other anomalies can cause foreign bodies to lodge, including vascular rings, ectopic salivary tissue, cartilaginous rests, esophageal webs, and duplication cysts. Achalasia and peptic stricture are sometimes the cause of food foreign bodies becoming lodged in the distal esophagus. Although the lower esophageal sphincter has received a great deal of attention in children, it is really not a circular muscle and generally is not one of the limiting areas for the passage of a foreign body.

The most common symptoms of a foreign body in the esophagus are drooling, dysphagia, and pain. A majority of esophageal foreign bodies present within

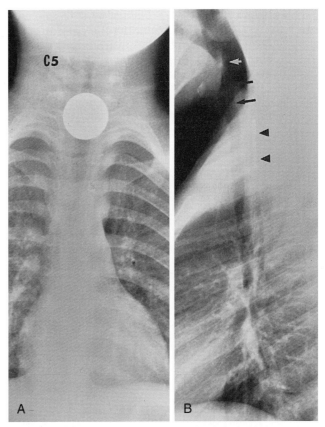

Figure 12–3. Typical for most esophageal foreign bodies, this coin lodged transversely between the aortic arch and the cricopharyngeus sphincter, not proximal to the sphincter, which has been the traditional teaching. *A*, The sphincter is at the level of C5 marked in the anteroposterior projection. *B*, In the lateral projection, the white arrow points to the epiglottis, the black arrows mark the superior and inferior limits to the sphincter, and the small triangles show the borders of the coin definitely inferior.

a few days of ingestion, although some may escape notice for weeks because the parent does not recognize the symptoms. Bleeding is a late phenomenon that may portend the ominous and possibly lethal complication of erosion or perforation into the aorta or pulmonary artery. An esophageal foreign body may erode into the lumen of the airway to produce a bronchoesophageal fistula. Chronic dysphagia or cough, low fever, or frank episodes of aspiration pneumonitis may have preceded this disastrous complication.

The radiographic demonstration of an esophageal foreign body is easy if the object is metallic or radiopaque but difficult if the object is radiolucent. The shape and the orientation help differentiate an esophageal from a tracheal foreign body, although the symptoms and the onset of the episode usually provide the best information. The long axis of a tracheal foreign body is vertically oriented, whereas the axis of an esophageal foreign body is usually transverse (Fig. 12–4). Radiolucent objects are made visible by the judicious use of contrast agents or by ultrasonography. Large swallows of barium may well obscure small esophageal foreign bodies.

The removal of a smooth esophageal foreign body that has a history of fewer than 2 days may be accomplished by using a Foley catheter passed via the nose or the mouth, distending the balloon, and then pulling the foreign body upward into the pharynx. Some pediatric surgeons prefer to perform this maneuver using fluoroscopy. We have found that fluoroscopy is not usually needed and do most of the catheter extractions in the emergency department without sedation. Once the object reaches the

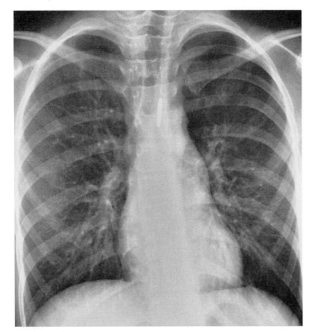

Figure 12–4. This coin on edge is in the esophagus and proves the exception to the rule in that it is lower than usual at the level of the carina and also not positioned in the transverse long axis of the esophagus. Both of these factors suggest intrinsic pathology and the need for an endoscopic examination.

pharynx, the child usually spits it out. Our experience has proved this technique to be safe and effective. We agree with others that this procedure is virtually without adverse consequences.[5]

The advent of small batteries has added the dilemma of caustic ingestion to that of the foreign body. These batteries, if electrically exhausted, may leak their caustic content and cause injury to the esophageal or intestinal wall. If there remains any "life" in the battery, the electrical current may add to the local tissue damage (see Chapter 26). Ingested batteries that are not below the stomach should be removed. Powerful, miniature magnets affixed to small catheters are available for the retrieval of some ferrous metal foreign bodies.[6] Alkaline disc batteries, although easily removed from the esophagus, are not easily found in the stomach or below. They should be followed radiographically while the patient is given cathartics or enemas to shorten the intestinal passage time.[7]

If there has been a significant delay between the decision to perform an esophagoscopy and the beginning of the operation, a repeat radiograph should be taken to determine the position of the foreign body. General endotracheal anesthesia is used so that the patient may be ventilated throughout the endoscopic removal. The same instruments may be used for esophagoscopy that were used for the bronchoscopy. The esophagus tolerates a large diameter sheath, which makes the piecemeal removal of food much easier and quicker than with the small sheath.

The esophagoscope must be inserted under direct vision through its lumen to reduce the chance of perforation. Some surgeons prefer to visualize the superior constrictor with a laryngoscope, but we feel that this is usually unnecessary. Great care is taken to protect the child's teeth from injury as the endoscope is introduced into the mouth and the posterior pharyngeal wall is visualized. The tongue is lifted with the endoscope and the cricopharyngeus is identified. Extending the neck or rotating the head usually causes the constrictor to relax and allows the endoscope to be introduced. Placing a roll under the shoulder or having an assistant place a hand under the upper back often helps to bring the lumen of the esophagus into view. The foreign body may be grasped and removed as a unit with the endoscope in the case of a coin, or a food foreign body may be removed through the endoscope, if necessary. Some objects, such as an open safety pin with the point directed cephalad, might best be grasped at the hinge, advanced into the stomach, then pulled "hinge first" into the endoscope for removal.

The integrity of the esophageal wall may be difficult to assess. A postoperative chest radiograph is advised in some cases if perforation is suspected. When a foreign body has been in the esophagus for an extended period, it may erode through the wall. It usually has also generated enough inflammatory reaction to limit the extravasation of saliva or ingested liquids. Erosion into the aorta or the trachea can create serious or fatal complications. Mediastinitis usually produces high fever, marked tachycardia, subcutaneous emphysema near the thoracic inlet, and back or neck pain.

GASTROINTESTINAL FOREIGN BODIES

Approximately 95% of foreign bodies that are ingested and reach the stomach pass the remainder of the gastrointestinal (GI) tract without incident. Exceptions include long objects such as a toothbrush, an elongated key, or a pencil. These objects are likely to become stuck within the duodenum or at the ligament of Trietz. Hat pins and nails may perforate the wall but usually dislodge and move on, with time. Shorter pins, including open safety pins, often pass without much delay and with no problem. On rare occasions, a sharp foreign body may come to rest outside the lumen of the gut with no symptoms. These may not need to be removed.

Alkaline disc batteries that have reached the stomach are able to be retrieved by endoscopy. Published guidelines exist for conservative management of these batteries already in or beyond the stomach. Radiographic proof that the battery is moving through the intestine makes observation acceptable.[7]

Bezoars are foreign bodies that may obstruct the stomach or the small intestine. They are composed of hair (trichobezoar), vegetable matter (phytobezoar), mixed matter (trichophytobezoar), and neonatal casein curd (proteinaceous) aggregations. Approximately 90% occur in girls. They are commonly seen in emotionally disturbed or retarded children. Proteinaceous bezoars usually dissolve with the oral ingestion of a pinch of papain (meat tenderizer). The dose may need to be repeated daily for a time, but too much produces gastritis. Judgment must enter into the decision as to whether or not to continue papain therapy if there is not prompt response. Bleeding, vomiting, weight loss, and pain are operative indications. Passage of the bezoar may be followed radiographically if there are minimal symptoms. Trichobezoars usually require surgical removal. Smaller, potentially obstructive tails of a gastric trichobezoar must be sought when surgical removal is undertaken.

SOFT TISSUE FOREIGN BODIES

Needles, toothpicks, splinters, and glass fragments are the most common soft tissue foreign bodies in children. They are usually found in the feet or the hands. The potential for tetanus exists with most foreign bodies, and tetanus toxoid should be administered if it has been more than 5 years since the child's previous booster. Gross contamination may occur and infection with clostridia is a possible threat to life and limb.

Most children experience pain and make the parent aware of an injury by a foreign body. There are those, however, who present with inflammation and fever or with a limp, and the presence of foreign material in a puncture wound is only a suspicion. Wooden or nonleaded glass foreign bodies in the hands and feet are radiolucent but may be demonstrated with specialized techniques such as xeroradiography, computed tomography, or magnetic resonance imaging. Ultrasonography is helpful in some cases.[8] Transillumination of tiny fingers or toes or of webspaces may help to identify a foreign body.

Splinters produce approximately one half of the foreign bodies lodged in the soft tissue of children. They are usually visible and most frequently may be removed without sedation or anesthesia. Prolonged attempts to extract a splinter from an apprehensive or terrified child is probably not the best method of treatment. Judgment is needed to decide when general anesthesia should be used. Certainly, the need for débridement or irrigation requires the patient to be anesthetized.

Multiple glass fragments may be difficult to locate and remove. The foreign material removed must be compared with the radiographically demonstrated foreign body to determine if complete removal has been accomplished. The removal of metallic foreign bodies is facilitated by the use of intraoperative C-arm fluoroscopy.

The wound produced by the entry of a foreign body or by the surgical attempt at its removal should be closed loosely, if at all. It is sometimes best to abandon the attempt to remove every tiny fragment of glass because the surgical trauma may be worse than the potential problems of leaving a fragment behind. Often, these small remnants extrude through the wound or work their way to the surface for later surgical removal. This principle is particularly applicable to glass fragments imbedded in the skin from an automobile accident.

Not all metallic or glass foreign bodies should be removed. If the patient is not symptomatic, there is little or no benefit to surgical removal.[9]

REFERENCES

1. Wood RE, Sherman JM: Pediatric flexible bronchoscopy. Ann Otol Rhinol Laryngol 89:414–416, 1980.
2. Berci G: History of endoscopy. In Berci G (ed): Endoscopy. New York, Appleton-Century-Crofts, 1976.
3. Gans SL: Pediatric Endoscopy. New York, Grune & Stratton, 1983.
4. Marzo SJ, Hotaling AJ: Airway resistance and optical resolution in pediatric rigid bronchoscopy. Ann Otol Rhinol Laryngol 104:282–287, 1995.
5. Morrow SE, Bicker SW, Kennedy AP, et al: Balloon extraction of esophageal foreign bodies in children. J Pediatr Surg 33:266–270, 1998.
6. Mayr J, Dittrich S, Triebl K: A new method for removal of metallic ferromagnetic foreign bodies. Pediatr Surg Int 12:461–462, 1997.
7. Rumack BH, Rumack CM: Disk battery ingestion. JAMA 249:2509–2511, 1983.
8. Torfing KF, Teisen HG, Skjodt T: Computed tomography, ultrasonography and plain radiography in the detection of foreign bodies. Rofo Fortschr Geb Rontgenstr Nuklearmed 149:60–62, 1988.
9. Kaiser CW, Slowick T, Spurling KP, et al: Retained foreign bodies. J Trauma 43:107–111, 1997.

13

BITES

Charles W. McGill, MD

Bite injuries occur commonly in children and adolescents. Although the incidence of various bites is probably underreported, in the United States tens of thousands of bites of various mammalian and insect species occur annually. Thousands of snake bites are reported, fewer than a third of which are poisonous.[1,2] In addition to the wounds themselves, sequelae of major importance include exposure to tetanus, rabies, and venom.

☐ Tetanus

Most bite injuries are bacteriologically contaminated, and the ubiquity of *Clostridium tetani* requires that treatment include consideration of this organism. Patients who have clean wounds with little devitalized tissue and who seek care promptly have a low risk of tetanus. Patients with dirty wounds, those with nonviable tissue, and those who delay in getting treatment for 24 hours or more have an increased risk for tetanus. Equally important to these risk factors is the immunization status of the patient before injury. Children who are current with their immunizations will have usually received three diphtheria, pertussis, and tetanus injections 2 months apart during the first year of life. Boosters are given 1 year after completion of the immunizing doses and again 4 to 5 years later when the child begins school. Boosters are required every 10 years to maintain routine tetanus prophylaxis.

The bite victim with a low-risk wound and an incomplete or uncertain immunization record should receive a dose of tetanus toxoid at the time of injury. If the patient is a child younger than 6 years, diphtheria *and* tetanus are used. The immunization course is completed with two more doses of toxoid at 2-month intervals.

The patient with a high-risk wound and an incomplete immunization history should receive 3000 to 6000 U of tetanus immune globulin in addition to the previously outlined immunization scheme. Toxoid and tetanus immune globulin should be given at separate sites so as not to neutralize each other.

Half of the tetanus immune globulin may be injected locally around the wound.

A patient who has been fully immunized and who has received a booster dose within 10 years is probably well protected. If the wound is high risk, one dose of toxoid is advisable. If the wound is more than 24 hours old, 3000 to 6000 U of tetanus immune globulin should also be given.

The antibiotic of choice to reduce the number of vegetative forms of clostridia is metronidazole or penicillin G. A 10- to 14-day course should be used if antibiotics are elected.[3]

☐ Dog and Other Mammalian Bites

Children between 5 and 14 years of age account for 40% of dog bite victims reported annually. The peak incidence is in warm weather months. Reported deaths caused by dog bite injuries have all been from hemorrhage; no deaths have resulted from rabies.

In addition to completing the tetanus management described above, one should copiously irrigate these bite wounds with saline or soap and water. The use of quaternary ammonium compounds is of no special benefit. Devitalized tissue should be débrided, and areas that are not cosmetically important should be left open. Puncture wounds anywhere are best left open. The wound should be reexamined in 24 to 48 hours.

A dog's oral flora includes streptococci, staphylococci, actinomycetes, species of *Pasteurella*, other gram-negative bacteria, and anaerobic organisms. Penicillin or cephalosporin will cover most infections, but amoxicillin plus Augmentin may be preferable because of its efficacy with *P. multocida* and *Staphylococcus aureus*.[4–6]

☐ Rabies and Postexposure Prophylaxis

A major source of concern with any mammalian bite is the risk of exposure to rabies. Because of the enforced vaccinations of domestic animals in the United States, the risk of rabies exposure from pet dogs is small. Still, decisions on whether to begin rabies treatment should be made quickly. Rabies treatment with vaccines should be considered prophylactic. Treatment must be started as soon as possible after exposure; once rabies has been contracted, the mortality in humans is exceedingly high.[4, 7]

The decision to administer postexposure prophylaxis is based on an assessment of risks, the most important of which is the likelihood the animal was rabid. Of particular importance is an understanding of which animals are most likely to carry the virus. There has been no documented transmission of rabies to humans by any rodent. Therefore, bites from rats, mice, squirrels, and chipmunks are considered low risk.[4, 7, 8] Wild animals carry the highest risk of rabies in the United States. Local knowledge of rabies carriers is important, and such information should be available from public health departments and from wildlife personnel of departments of natural resources. The risk of rabies in skunks has been estimated to be as high as 1 in 3; bats, 1 in 10; wild dogs, 1 in 100; and wild cats, 1 in 200.[7]

Abnormal behavior by the biting animal, such as unusual aggression or gait disturbances, can be a symptom of rabies and thus is indicative of a high-risk situation. Most bites by pet dogs are actually provoked, but when the animal's behavior is in question, the vaccination status becomes important. A bite from a vaccinated pet should represent a low-risk case. However, observation of the animal for 10 days is advised. There have been no reported cases of human rabies infection from animals that did not become symptomatic within this period. If the animal is to be killed to look for rabies infection, the brain must not be damaged. The presence of rabies is confirmed by studying the brain with fluorescent antibody techniques.

Wound characteristics also figure in the assessment of risk. The virus is transmitted in saliva. Therefore, scratch wounds, unless contaminated by saliva, are of low risk. Children are at greater risk of contracting rabies from an infected animal than are adults. Wounds that are in densely innervated areas and those that are close to the central nervous system are more likely to produce clinical rabies because the transmission of rabies virus to the central nervous system occurs via nerves. Wounds of the head and neck are of particular concern. The greater the amount of tissue destruction, the more likely the inoculation. Any patient having two or more of the following risk factors should be started on rabies prophylaxis[9]:

1. Age younger than 10 years
2. Bite wounds of the head and neck
3. Deep bite wounds
4. Bite by an animal whose vaccination status is in doubt

High-risk cases call for simultaneous active and passive immunization. In the United States, human diploid cell vaccine is used for active immunization. This series of intramuscular injections requires that 1 ml be given on days 0, 3, 7, 14, and 28. Deep intramuscular injection into the deltoids is preferred. Booster doses are not recommended except for repeat exposure or for those who expect to have repeated exposure to the virus.

Passive immunization is done with human rabies immune globulin. This may be omitted if the patient has previously been immunized. Human rabies immune globulin should be given simultaneously with human diploid cell vaccine if available. A dose of 20 IU human rabies immune globulin/kg body weight should be given on days 0 and 3. Half should be injected around the wound and half intramuscularly elsewhere, distant from the human diploid cell vaccine sites.[4]

☐ Snake Bites

An estimated 8000 poisonous snake bites occur annually in the United States, resulting in about 12 to 15 deaths. More than half of these are in children younger than 12 years.[1, 10]

There are four genera of venomous snakes of medical importance found wild in the United States. The five species of coral snakes (*Micrurus*) are in the family Elapidae, and the pit vipers—large rattlesnakes (*Crotalus*), pigmy rattlesnakes and ground rattlesnakes (*Sistrurus*), and cottonmouth snakes and copperheads (*Agkistrodon*)—are in the family Crotalidae.

Coral snakes differ from pit vipers. They have short fixed fangs, and they must chew the victim to envenomate.[11] They are colorful, with transversely oriented alternating bands of black, yellow or white, red, yellow, and black. The nose is black. The nonpoisonous scarlet king snake also has alternating bands. However, the king snake's bands are red, black, yellow, black, and red without adjacent red and yellow—hence the rhymes, "red on yellow kills a fellow" and "red on black won't hurt Jack."[12]

Pit vipers have two needle-like fangs through which venom is injected. Their heads are triangular, and the characteristic "pit" lies between the nostril and the eye. Venomous snakes have vertically elliptical pupils. Nonpoisonous snakes have round pupils.[13]

GENERAL CARE AND FIRST AID

General care of a suspected poisonous snake bite victim should begin with rapid transport to an adequate medical facility. The patient should be kept calm and remain as still as possible. This simple first aid is the best and safest care to provide outside the hospital. Although writings on incision and suction go back thousands of years, this practice is inefficient in removing venom and may cause more injury or risk of infection than if the wound is left alone.[14] Tourniquets do little to impede venom spread and may produce more injury from vascular compromise, if they are applied too tightly.[14] Restricting the patient's movement and muscular activity is more effective than a tourniquet in preventing the venom spread.[15] Topical cooling with ice packs is not indicated.[4, 10] Excision of the snake bite wound, if done very quickly after the bite, can remove venom but should rarely be needed.[16] Excision in the field by inexperienced hands is more likely to cause than to solve problems.

All snake bite patients should have tetanus treatment according to the guidelines given earlier. Snake bites do not require antibiotics.[17, 18] However, many physicians who care for victims of poisonous snake bite do recommend antibiotic coverage. Ampicillin or cephalothin should be adequate.[10, 13, 19]

PIT VIPER ENVENOMATION

Pit viper venom is not identical from species to species, but enough characteristics are shared that the polyvalent horse serum antivenin prepared in the United States covers all pit viper bites from snakes found in the wild. These venoms are multiple poisons—a complex of enzymes, nonenzymatic proteins, and peptides. The nonenzymatic polypeptides are the neurotoxins, cardiotoxins, and hemorrhagins. Their cumulative effect is quite toxic.

The neurotoxins are chiefly nondepolarizing agents such as curare. Cardiotoxin is a depolarizing agent with an affinity for cardiac muscle. The hemorrhagins inhibit platelet aggregation and disrupt endothelial cell junctions. Enzymes such as phospholipase A produce lysis of cells near the wound and within the bloodstream. Proteases are fibrinolytic and antithromboplastic. Amino acid esterases cause intravascular clotting by releasing procoagulant and activating factor X. Esterases do not activate or destroy factors V or VIII, so heparin is of little value in treating this form of disseminated intravascular coagulation; antivenin is required. Esterases may also release bradykinin, which is the mediator of shock seen early after envenomation.[13, 14, 19]

The effect of envenomation is directly proportional to the dose delivered. The dose is a function of the volume of venom delivered (bigger snake, more venom), the site of bite (soft tissue versus direct vascular puncture), and the size of the victim. Small victims suffer relatively greater envenomation. This explains the higher mortality in young children and the fact that small children require more antivenin than a similarly envenomated adult.

Pit vipers leave fang marks. If there is no puncture wound, there is no "bite" and therefore no chance of envenomation. Not all bites result in envenomation. If there is no swelling around the wound within 4 hours, there was likely no envenomation. Envenomation produces a local reaction that includes painful swelling at a minimum. Bleb formation, necrosis, and bleeding around the wound site are other signs of envenomation. The progression of swelling is a key observation in determining the grade of envenomation.

Systemic symptoms often begin with nausea and vomiting and progress to more life-threatening problems. Hypotension may develop from a decrease in vascular tone or from fluid shifts. Local hemorrhage in and around the wound is seen early, with intrapulmonary hemorrhage occurring as the venom spreads. Generalized hemolysis or cardiac dysrhythmias may occur.

Treatment decisions require an orderly and rapid clinical assessment followed by appropriate action. Patients with fang marks should be observed for up to 4 hours after the bite. If there has been no swelling or pain around the fang marks during this time, there was likely no envenomation. Local wound care is enough, and hospitalization may not be required.

Pain and swelling around fang marks identify a patient envenomated by a pit viper. An envenomated victim should have baseline complete blood count with platelet count, electrolytes, blood urea nitrogen, fibrinogen levels, and prothrombin time tested on admission. Blood typing and crossmatching should be done early, because systemic effects of the venom may make typing and crossmatching difficult later. A urinalysis should also be done. Laboratory tests do not determine the grade of envenomation, but they help in assessing the effects of treatment later in cases of severe envenomation.[14, 20]

Intravenous fluids should be started. Two intravenous lines should be started on the severely envenomated patient, one for antivenin and another for volume support and other drugs. The patient should not be allowed to eat or drink for the first 24 hours, because nausea and vomiting are among the earliest systemic symptoms. Input and output should be carefully monitored. An electrocardiogram is not always required for children, but most patients are admitted to an intensive care unit.

Treatment of the envenomated patient must be modified according the severity or grade of envenomation. The system of grading illustrated in Table 13–1 is probably the most commonly used.[20, 21] Local swelling may be impressive. Extremity swelling can proceed to the extent that blood flow is impeded. Aggressive antivenin use should prevent this problem. Fasciotomy may have a role in extreme cases, but for the most part more antivenin is the treatment required. Measuring compartment pressures is not helpful because the swelling is not restricted to muscle compartments. Therefore, if a fasciotomy is required, the skin and subcutaneous tissues must also be opened. Such wounds created in the face of alterations in local and systemic coagulation processes can result in significant hemorrhage.[14]

Copperhead bites result in more local than systemic symptoms because their venom is not usually as toxic as the other pit vipers. Antivenin is rarely needed for these bites.[22] Grades 2, 3, or 4 envenomation by a copperhead requires antivenin. The amount suggested in Table 13–1 is an initial esti-

TABLE 13-1. Grading Severity of Envenomation

Grade	Local Characteristics	Systemic Signs	Antivenin
0	No envenomation; fang marks but no edema	None	None
1	Fang marks with edema of 1–5 inches within 12 h	None	None
2	Fang marks with edema of 6–12 inches within 12 h	Early systemic symptoms (nausea and vomiting)	2–5 vials
3	Fang marks with edema >12 inches	Systemic symptoms and measurable defects in coagulation	5–10 vials
4	Fang marks with necrosis and bleb formation; edema to ipsilateral trunk	Hypotension; severe coagulation defects	10–20 vials

Data from McCollough NC, Gennaro JF: Treatment of venomous snake bites in the United States. Clin Toxicol 3:483–500, 1970 and Wood JJ, Hoback WW, Green TW: Treatment of snake venom poisoning with ACTH and cortisone. Virginia M Month 82:130–135, 1955.

mate. Doses may have to be repeated depending on how local or systemic symptoms respond. As with any snake bite, the small child requires more antivenin than will an adult with a similar grade envenomation. A case has been reported of a 3-year-old child who required 60 vials of antivenin during the first 11 hours of treatment.[23]

Once it is determined that a patient should receive antivenin, the required test for sensitivity to horse serum is done according to the instructions supplied with the antivenin. This is usually done as a skin test, which is a reasonable but not infallible screen for anaphylaxis; it does not address the risks of serum sickness. Anyone given more than five vials of antivenin has at least a 50% chance of developing some serum sickness symptoms in the weeks after treatment. Some physicians advocate the prophylactic use of antihistamines and steroids in postdischarge planning.[24] A patient sensitive to horse serum may still be a candidate to receive antivenin, but in such cases experts in handling anaphylaxis should be part of the treating team.

Overtreatment should obviously be avoided, but once the need for antivenin is clear, there is no benefit to proceeding slowly. The goal is to quickly neutralize the venom. After skin testing, an initial "test strength" dose of one vial in 500 ml of normal saline (a 1:50 dilution) is begun. If there are no allergic reactions after 5 minutes, the concentration should be increased by adding to the original mixture, not to exceed a 1:4 dilution. The initial dose estimate should be given within the first 2 hours if possible. All antivenin is administered intravenously; none is infiltrated around the wound. A response includes the cessation of tissue swelling, the elimination of systemic symptoms, and a return of abnormal laboratory values to normal.

CORAL SNAKE BITES

The venom of coral snake species has virtually no cytotoxins. There is minimal local tissue reaction by which to judge envenomation. Pain at the site is minimal also. A patient with sufficient local injury that suggests chewing by the snake must be assumed to have been envenomated. The clinical symptoms of envenomation may be delayed for up to 12 hours.

Coral snake venom consists mainly of neurotoxic peptides and enzymes that have a curare-like action. The baseline laboratory studies done for pit viper victims are not of value and are unnecessary. The initial symptom may be drowsiness or even euphoria. Urine and blood alcohol and toxic screens may be appropriate studies if justified by the clinical situation. As symptoms progress, there may be weakness, local fasciculations, diplopia, and slurred speech—indicative of bulbar paralysis. Once symptoms begin, progression may occur rapidly. Respiratory depression and respiratory muscle paralysis may last for days. Total recovery may take weeks.

Any patient suspected to have been envenomated must be observed for a minimum of 12 hours. Respiratory depressant drugs should be avoided. If the snake was difficult to remove from the bite site, there is a high suspicion of envenomation, and the patient should be observed for 24 hours. Some would advocate beginning antivenin in such a patient even if initial systemic symptoms are absent.[25]

Respiratory and neurologic function must be monitored closely. Peak flows and tidal volume are important parameters to watch. These patients should be intubated early if the progression of respiratory symptoms becomes worrisome. Antivenin is absolutely indicated at the first sign of symptoms. A grading scheme such as used for pit vipers does not work as well for coral snake bites. The antivenin for the coral bite is also horse serum, and similar skin testing should be done before the administration of serum. The initial dose should be five vials, even with mild signs of envenomation. This dose can be diluted in 250 ml of normal saline and delivered at 3 to 4 ml/hr as a slow drip to further test for allergic reactions. If no allergy signs appear, the infusion should be increased slowly to 120 ml/hr, which delivers two to three vials per hour. Additional dosing should be dictated by the symptom response. The response will not be as rapid or predictable as in pit viper envenomation.[11]

☐ Human Bites

The human mouth harbors a variety of pathogens, including staphylococci, streptococci, spirochetes,

Vincent's spirilla, and others. Human bite injuries are generally of three varieties: an outright bite from another person, a hand injury from striking another person's mouth, or a self-inflicted bite such as a tongue injury.

All these wounds should be carefully examined for deep tissue injury, cleansed, and débrided as necessary. Tetanus coverage should be administered, and antibiotics are required. The combination of penicillin and dicloxacillin should provide coverage for the suspected flora.[26, 27]

Exposure to viral infections by human bites is rare but possible. Hepatitis B can be transmitted by the bite of a carrier. Hepatitis B immune globulin and hepatitis B vaccine are recommended. The reverse situation of biting a carrier should not require treatment unless there is a mucosal lesion in the mouth of the biter.[28]

Although the transmission of human immunodeficiency virus by human bite is debated, there is a report of such an infection in the literature.[29, 30]

□ Spider Bites

BROWN RECLUSE

Loxosceles reclusa, the North American brown recluse spider, is a medium-sized spider of 8 to 9 mm in body length with a distinguishing dark violin-shaped spot located dorsally on the carapace. This fuses with a thin line extending forward to the abdomen. This marking accounts for the name "fiddleback" often given to this spider. The brown recluse is common in the southern and central United States. It is frequently found indoors in dry, dark areas. It may be less well known than the black widow, but it often presents a greater medical problem.[31]

The recluse venom is a composite poison containing proteases, hyaluronidase, hemolysin, and other cytotoxins that produce cell wall destruction. These effects may extend beyond local tissue to injure red blood cells and glomeruli.[32–34] *Systemic loxoscelism* is a term used to describe the distant effects of hemolysis, hemoglobinuria, renal failure, and disseminated intravascular coagulation. Systemic effects are more likely seen in small children whose relative degree of envenomation is greater.[33] Therapy for the systemic symptoms is mainly supportive. Intravenous fluids to provoke a brisk diuresis may lessen the risk of tubular injury from hemoglobinuria. Blood or frozen plasma may be needed for disseminated intravascular coagulation.[34]

The wound may go unnoticed initially, but within 3 to 4 days there is a progression from erythema to vesiculation to central necrosis. An eschar forms by 5 to 7 days. Treatment of these wounds usually involves local cleansing, antibiotics to cover staphylococci and streptococci, and pain medication. The wound is débrided only if tissue destruction is significant and only after the wound is well demar-

cated.[33] The use of dapsone and hyperbaric oxygen has been recommended, but animal model studies have shown no significant benefit.[35] The diagnosis may be in question because of the delay between injury and symptoms. A passive hemagglutination test to diagnose brown recluse bites and an older thymidine uptake lymphocyte test can be done, but neither is clinically helpful.[36, 37]

BLACK WIDOW

Black widow spiders, *Latrodectus mactans,* "the murderer," are web spinners found throughout the United States. Only the female of the five species of widow spiders is dangerous. A red hourglass-shaped spot on the abdomen identifies the spider. The venom is mainly neurotoxic, causing both local and generalized spasm. This reaction is mediated by acetylcholine depletion at motor nerve endings and catecholamine release at adrenergic nerve endings. The bite is immediately painful. The wound demarcates and forms a wheal with erythema, piloerection, and local cyanosis to produce the so-called *target lesion.*

The progression of generalized symptoms may be rapid, and the chief complaint is usually abdominal cramping rather than wound pain. Small children are more likely to have a greater systemic response than are larger children or adults. The treatment is usually symptomatic, with narcotics for pain relief and muscle relaxants such as diazepam to deal with the muscle spasm. The relief from diazepam is superior to that derived from calcium gluconate.[33] There is an antivenin (prepared from horse serum) specific for black widow envenomation. It works rapidly to relieve symptoms, and one vial is usually all that is required. It is delivered in 50 to 100 ml of 5% dextrose over 30 minutes. In a large review series of black widow bites, however, the only mortality occurred from bronchospasm in reaction to antivenin.[38]

REFERENCES

1. Litovitz TL, Felberg L, Soloway RA, et al: Annual Report of American Poison Control Centers Toxic Exposure Surveillance System. Am J Emerg Med 13:551–597, 1995.
2. Bite Wounds. In Peter G (ed): Report of the Committee on Infectious Diseases (24th ed). Elk Grove Village, IL, American Academy of Pediatrics, 1997, pp 122–126.
3. Tetanus. In Peter G (ed): Report of the Committee on Infectious Diseases (24th ed). Elk Grove Village, IL, American Academy of Pediatrics, 1997, pp 518–523.
4. Rabies. In Peter G (ed): Report of the Committee on Infectious Diseases (24th ed). Elk Grove Village, IL, American Academy of Pediatrics, 1997, pp 435–442.
5. Winkler WG: Human deaths induced by dog bites: United States 1974–75. Public Health Rep 92:425, 1977.
6. Cummings P: Antibiotics to prevent infection in patients with dog bite wounds: A meta-analysis of randomized trials. Ann Emerg Med 23:535–540, 1994.
7. Cantor SB, Clover RD, Thompson RF: A decision-analytic approach to post exposure rabies prophylaxis. Am J Public Health 84:1144–1148, 1994.
8. Rabies prevention—United States, 1991. Recommendations

of the Immunization Practices Advisory Committee (ACIP). MMWR Morb Mortal Wkly Rep 40(RR-3):1–19, 1991.

9. Robinson DA: Dog bites and rabies: An assessment of risk. Br Med J 1:1066–1067, 1976.
10. Forks TP: Evaluation and treatment of poisonous snakebites. Am Fam Physician 50:123–130, 1994.
11. Gaar GG: Assessment and management of coral and other exotic snake envenomations. J Fla Med Assoc 83:178–182, 1996.
12. Strickland NE: Snake bites: A review. J Ark Med Soc 73:69–77, 1976.
13. Van Mierop LHS: Poisonous snakebite: A review. J Fla Med Assoc 63:191–201, 1976.
14. Wingert WA: Rattlesnake bites in Southern California and rationale for recommended treatment. West J Med 148:37–44, 1988.
15. Howarth DM, Southee AE, Whyte IM: Lymphatic flow rates and first aid in simulated peripheral snake or spider envenomation. Med J Aust 16:700–701, 1994.
16. Huang TT, Lynch JB, Larson K, Lewis SR: The use of excisional therapy in the management of snakebite. Ann Surg 179:598–607, 1974.
17. Weed HG: Nonvenomous snakebite in Massachusetts: Prophylactic antibiotics are unnecessary. Ann Emerg Med 22:220–224, 1993.
18. Clark RF, Selden BS, Furbee B: The incidence of wound infection following crotalid envenomation. J Emerg Med 11:583–586, 1993.
19. Nelson BK: Snake envenomation: Incidence, clinical presentation and management. Med Toxicol Adverse Drug Exp 4:17–31, 1989.
20. Wood JT, Hoback WW, Green TW: Treatment of snake venom poisoning with ACTH and cortisone. Virginia M Month 82:130–135, 1955.
21. McCollough NC, Gennaro JF: Treatment of venomous snake bites in the United States. Clin Toxicol 3:483–500, 1970.
22. White BD, Rodgers GC, Matynumas NJ, Allen F: Copperhead snakebites reported to the Kentucky Regional Poison Control Center 1986: Epidemiology and treatment suggestions. J Ky Med Assoc 86:61–66, 1988.
23. Buntain WL: Successful venomous snakebite neutralization with massive antivenin infusion is in a child. J Trauma 23:1012–1014, 1983.
24. Jurkovich GJ, Lutherman A, McCullar K, et al: Complications of crotalid antivenin therapy. J Trauma 28:1032–1037, 1988.
25. Weisman RS, Lizarralde SS, Thompson V: Snake and spider antivenin: Risks and benefits of therapy. J Fla Med Assoc 83:192–195, 1996.
26. Ruskin JD, Laney TJ, Wendt SV, Markin RS: Treatment of mammalian bite wounds of the maxillofacial area. J Oral Maxillofac Surg 51:174–176, 1993.
27. Stewart GM, Quan L, Horton MA: Laceration management. Pediatr Emerg Care 9:247–250, 1993.
28. Report of the Committee on Infectious Diseases (24th ed). Elk Grove Village, IL, American Academy of Pediatrics, 1997, p 259.
29. Rickman KM, Rickman LS: The potential for transmission of human immunodeficiency virus through human bite. J Acquir Immune Defic Syndr 6:402–406, 1993.
30. Vidmar L, Poljak M, Tomazic J, et al: Transmission of HIV-1 by human bite [letter]. Lancet 347:1762–1763, 1996.
31. Young VL, Pin P: The brown recluse spider bite. Ann Plast Surg 20:447–452, 1988.
32. Anderson PC: What's new in loxoscelism? Mo Med 74:549–552, 1977.
33. Carbonaro PA, Janniger CK, Schwartz RA: Spider bite reactions. Cutis 56:256–259, 1995.
34. Arnold RE: Brown recluse spider bites: Five cases with a review of the literature. J Am Coll Emerg Physicians 5:262–264, 1976.
35. Hobbs GD, Anderson AR, Greene TJ, Yealy DM: Comparison of hyperbaric oxygen and dapsone therapy for loxosceles envenomation. Acad Emerg Med 3:758–761, 1996.
36. Barrett SM, Romine-Jenkins M, Blick KE: Passive hemagglutination inhibition test for diagnosis of brown recluse spider bite. Clin Chem 39:2104–2107, 1993.
37. Majeski JA, Durst GG: Necrotic arachnidism. South Med J 69:887–891, 1976.
38. Clark RF, Wethern-Kestner S, Vance MV, Gerkin R: Clinical presentation and treatment of black widow spider envenomation (163 cases). Ann Emerg Med 21:782–787, 1992.

14

BURNS

Ronald J. Sharp, MD

☐ History

The earliest writings describing treatment of burns are found in the Ebers Papyrus circa 1500 BC[1]: "A sequential treatment on the span of 5 days is vividly described; black mud on the 1st day, the dung of a calf mixed with yeast on the 2nd, dried acacia resin mixed with barley paste, cooked colocynth, and oil on the 3rd. A paste of beeswax fat, boiled papyrus with beans on the fourth day, and a mixture of colocynth, red ochre, leaves, and copper fragments on the fifth completed the varied treatment plan." The Egyptians advocated the application of plant gums and the rubbing of a frog warmed in oil on the wound to ease pain.[2, 3]

Hippocrates in 430 BC recommended melted lard mixed with resin and bitumen, spread on a piece of cloth and warmed at the fire to be used as a bandage.[3] Silver nitrate, an agent that is still in use, was first suggested in 1821.[4]

Topical treatment of burns achieved its greatest advance following the Korean War when Douglas Lindsey discovered mafenide (Sulfamylon). The discovery of silver sulfadiazine by Charles Fox in 1968 introduced a topical agent with similar efficacy but fewer side effects. These new powerful topical agents produced a significant decrease in mortality rate from burns. Use of these agents may have delayed the currently common use of early aggressive surgical coverage.[3, 5]

☐ Incidence and Epidemiology

Trauma is the leading cause of death in children. Burns are the second most common cause of accidental death in children younger than age 5 years and the most common cause of accidental death in the home.[6–10] There are 2 million burn injuries every year; 300,000 of these injuries result from the estimated 32,600,000 house fires that occur every year.[11] Children younger than age 4 years account for 50% of deaths in house fires.[12] As many as 100,000 people are hospitalized yearly for burns, and 7800 die

of their injuries. Of the 100,000 people hospitalized, 40% are younger than 15 years and 67% are male.[13] Each year, 2500 children die from burns, and 10,000 suffer severe permanent disability. Scalding is the most frequent mechanism of injury. Products associated with food preparation and consumption account for 48% of scald injuries.[14–16]

Infants are most commonly scalded during bathing. Toddlers are most frequently burned by hot liquid, food spills, or hot tap water. Hot grease spills make up a smaller percentage of toddler burns, but account for a high percentage of severe deep burns, especially to face, neck, and arms.[17] Electrical cord injuries of the mouth occur almost exclusively with this age group. Contact burns are more common in this age group and often lead to deep hand injuries.[18] The preschooler's fascination with matches and lighters results in an increased incidence of flame injury.

Adolescent and preadolescent children are more likely to experiment with the combination of fire and volatile agents. The incidence of high-voltage electrical injury increases in the teen years.[12] In England, scald injuries have shown a slight increase since the late 1980s.[19] In Denmark, by comparison, there has been a progressive decrease in the incidence of scald injuries by more than 50% since 1981 as a result of regulation and public education programs.[20, 21] Burn mortality rate has decreased significantly in most Western societies but remains high in many developing nations.[22–25]

Burn injury occurs in 10 to 20% of documented child abuse cases.[26] Abuse by burning is much more common in children younger than age 5 years, with a median age of 1.5 years. The mortality rate in abused children is significantly higher when age and burn severity are matched with accidentally burned children.[18] Tide mark burns of buttocks, perineum, and both feet are almost pathognomonic of abuse.[27] Evidence of prior abuse, bilateral symmetry, stocking-glove distribution, multiplicity of injuries, burns to the backs of the hands, and delay in seeking medical attention should alert one to the possibility that the burn was inflicted.[7, 18, 28–31] Risk factors in-

159

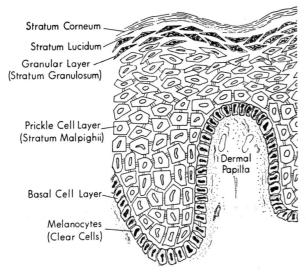

Figure 14–1. Skin, normal anatomy. (From Lewis GM, Wheeler C: Practical Dermatology [3rd ed]. Philadelphia, WB Saunders, 1967, p 3.)

the reticular dermis and the underlying fatty layer. They consist of hair follicles, eccrine sweat glands, apocrine sweat glands, and sebaceous glands. The epidermal appendages serve as a source of regenerating epidermal cells following thermal injury. They also provide a source of bacterial contamination, because the normal flora of the skin lies deep in the ducts of these structures. The skin serves as a natural barrier to invasion by bacteria. The skin desquamates continuously, carrying away organisms that may be present. The skin also has a dry outer layer that proves lethal to many viruses and gram-negative organisms. The pH of the skin normally varies between 4 and 6, retarding the growth of many bacteria. A fatty acid film exists on the skin that is fungistatic and bacteriostatic. The fact that the skin is colonized by bacteria that are not invasive serves as a means of crowding out more invasive organisms by elaborating antibiotics, competing for foodstuffs, and creating an adverse pH environment. Thermal injury destroys this vital first line of immune defense.[37–39]

clude being the youngest male child in a single parent, economically disadvantaged home. Handicaps and a history of previous burn or injury are also commonly seen.[32–35] Congenital defects can mimic abuse. They are manifest by poor weight gain, fractures, and skin lesions that often look like burns and bruises. People skilled in social evaluations must be involved with these situations.[36]

□ Anatomy

The skin is the largest organ of the body. Its presence and proper function are essential for survival.

The skin makes up approximately 15% of total body weight. The composition and thickness of skin vary tremendously from one part of the body to another, as well as by age and sex. The skin consists of five major elements: epidermis, dermal-epidermal junction, epidermal appendages, dermis, and subcutaneous tissue (Fig. 14–1). The basal layer contains the only proliferating cells within the epidermis. The basement membrane of the dermal-epidermal junction serves as a barrier to passage of macromolecules. The papillary dermis consists of fine connective tissue fibers bathed in an abundant ground substance. The papillary dermis and the deeper reticular dermis are separated by a plexus of nerves and blood vessels.

The blood supply of the skin is exceptionally rich. A 70-kg man has an average skin blood flow of 200 to 500 ml per minute. With external heating, skin blood flow may increase to as much as 7000 to 8000 ml per minute. With extreme cooling, it can decrease to as low as 20 to 50 ml per minute. This vast range of blood flow is a significant factor in moderating the severity of burn or cold injury.

The appendages of the skin are functional invaginations of the epidermis and papillary dermis into

□ Pathophysiology

Thermal injury results in a varying degree of cell death and dysfunction. The extent of injury depends on heat intensity, duration of exposure, skin thickness, and tissue conductance.[6, 40] Figure 14–2 illustrates this temperature and time relationship. A burn wound may be described as three concentric zones (Fig. 14–3). The central zone is where injury is greatest. The cells and vessels in this zone are destroyed. The zone of stasis sustains significant cellular and vessel damage. The survival of the zone of stasis depends on factors that may or may not be under the surgeon's control.[41–43] The demise of this zone may convert a partial thickness wound to a full thickness wound. The peripheral zone of hyperemia is an area of reparable damage that heals in 7 to 10 days.

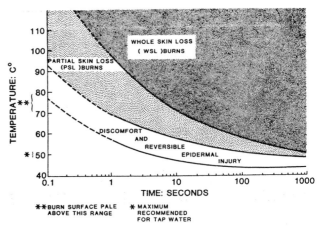

Figure 14–2. Depth of burn and function of temperature and time. (Adapted from Zawacki EB, Warden GD: In Boswich JA [ed]: The Art and Science of Burn Care. Rockville, MD, Aspen, 1987, pp 26–47.)

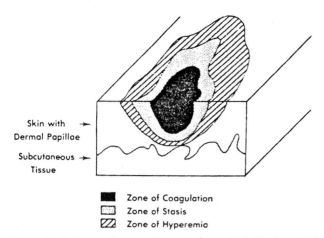

Skin with → Dermal Papillae

Subcutaneous → Tissue

■ Zone of Coagulation
▫ Zone of Stasis
▨ Zone of Hyperemia

Figure 14–3. Zones of injury. (From Achauer BM, Martinez RN: Burn wound pathophysiology and care. Crit Care Clin 1:1, 1985.)

Burns are classified as partial or full thickness.[44] Partial thickness burns are further stratified into superficial and deep. Superficial partial thickness burns extend to the basal layer of the epidermis. Blistering, erythema, and exquisite tenderness are the hallmark of this burn. A superficial partial thickness burn heals within 10 to 14 days. A deep partial thickness injury destroys the epidermis and extends for a variable depth into the dermis. The deep epidermal appendages allow some of these wounds to slowly heal over several weeks, many times with significant scarring. A full-thickness injury results in complete destruction of the epidermis, dermis, and dermal appendages. These wounds are often dry, leathery, insensate, and do not heal.[28]

The inflammatory response elicited by burn injury can be broken down into a vascular phase and a cellular phase. Initially, there is a short period of vasoconstriction followed by active vasodilatation. A marked increase in vessel permeability occurs within the burn wound. Mediators of increased permeability may include histamines, serotonins, complements, leukotrienes, prostaglandins, and oxygen radicals. Increased vascular permeability results in a rapid efflux of proteins and other serum macromolecules into the burn wound, which accounts for the edema phase of the inflammatory response. There is also an increased loss of protein into the gut lumen and wound.[45] Edema formation in nonburned tissue occurs when more than 30% body surface area is involved. The cause of this edema is disputed.[46–48] Simultaneously with the vascular response, neutrophils, monocytes, and platelets marginate and migrate into the wound. These cells release mediators that modulate vascular permeability, cellular migration, and the nonspecific and specific immune response. There is an increase in total proteolytic activity in direct proportion to the percentage of burn surface.[49] Monocytes may play a central role in modulation of the inflammatory response and may direct many phases of wound healing. Postburn hypermetabolism has been hypothesized to result from mediators released from the macrophage.[40, 50–52] A study in children who were given ibuprofen soon after burn injury demonstrated attenuation of the hypermetabolic response, possibly by decreasing basal temperature. There was no demonstrated nitrogen-sparing effect.[53] Cold stress increases the already high metabolic demands.[54]

The activated clotting and complement cascades block lymphatic drainage, stimulate cellular migration, and help modulate the vascular phase.

IMMUNE RESPONSE

When the structural integrity of the skin has been violated, the nonspecific immune system defends the breach. This second line of defense consists of cellular and serum elements. The cellular elements are neutrophils and macrophages. The serum elements consist of the coagulation-fibrinolytic system, complement, and fibronectin. Immediately following injury, the clotting cascade, the fibrinolytic system, and the complement system are activated. The C3A and C5A fragments increase vascular permeability and serve as chemoattractants to recruit circulating neutrophils and monocytes into the area. The serum factors serve as opsonins that facilitate phagocytosis of invading organisms by neutrophils and monocytes. Clotting factors seal off lymphatics and slow down efferent blood flow to localize the invading organisms and prepare them for destruction by the cellular elements.

The third line of defense is specific. It can generally be divided into thymic-derived lymphocytes and bone marrow–derived lymphocytes. The B lymphocytes are involved in the production of specific antibodies, which can attack bacteria or cells and prepare them for phagocytosis by cellular elements, or they can present them to the complement system, which can directly lyse bacteria in the absence of a phagocytic cell. The macrophage processes antigen and presents it to a T-cell lymphocyte, which is activated. This activated T cell liberates lymphokines, which stimulate the B cells to produce specific antibody. These activated T cells also have the ability to release mediators that stimulate and improve macrophage phagocytosis; accelerate the production of killer cells, which attack antibody-coated target cells; and produce cytotoxic T cells. The activity of this activated T lymphocyte is modulated by T-helper cells and T-suppressor cells. If there is an increased output of T-suppressor cells, the processing of antigen and the subsequent liberation of lymphokine is suppressed, and the immune response blunted.[55–58]

Immune suppression in burn patients is a well-documented phenomenon. Immunologic changes include decreased levels of neutrophil phagocytosis, neutrophil-killing ability, neutrophil chemotaxis, macrophage activity, lymphocyte response to mitogen stimulation, interleukin 2, fibronectin, and γ-globulin, and an increase in T-suppressor cell activity. The prospect of immune modulation and delineation of circulating immune toxins may significantly decrease deaths resulting from sepsis in burn patients.[4, 59–72]

☐ Evaluation and Classification

At the scene of injury, the burning agent must be removed as quickly as possible. In the case of chemical injury, the wound should be flushed immediately with copious amounts of water. All rings and watches should be removed from the victim's extremities to avoid a tourniquet effect. The wound should be covered and the patient kept warm during transport. In the emergency department, a burn patient should be managed as any trauma patient. Particular attention should be given to the airway if there is a history of closed-space flame injury. Upper airway obstruction, especially in smaller children, can occur rapidly. Oxygen (100%) should be administered. Intravenous (IV) access should be obtained immediately, and 20 ml of Ringer's lactate solution per kilogram body weight should be given during the first 30 minutes. Vascular access can be very difficult, especially in small children. Femoral lines are safe in children and are often easier when peripheral sites are unobtainable. Intraosseous access is ideal in the patient in shock, especially at outlying hospitals and emergency departments where expertise in venous access is limited.[73, 74] A nasogastric tube and Foley catheter should be placed in all cases of major burns. An accurate history must be taken and a detailed examination done, once the primary survey is completed and initial resuscitation started. The percentage of body surface area burned and the depth of the injury must be carefully determined. The rule of nines that is commonly used in adults is inappropriate in children. The head size of a newborn accounts for almost three times as much body surface area as it does in an adult, whereas the leg of a newborn is roughly half the percent surface area compared with an adult. Lund-Brauder charts should be used to assess the percentage of body surface involved (Fig. 14–4).[75, 76] An "accurate" dry weight must be estimated, if not measured.

Pain medication should be IV administered. Intramuscular (IM) or subcutaneous injections are ineffective and often dangerous in burn victims. Admission criteria include partial thickness burns greater than 10% or full thickness burns greater than 2%; any burns to hands, face, feet, or perineum; any inhalation injury; all electrical and chemical injuries; and all suspected cases of child abuse.[28]

Admission laboratory studies include a complete blood count (CBC), chemistry profile, urinalysis, and chest radiograph. If inhalation or electrical injury is suspected, arterial blood gas values, electrocardiography, and carboxyhemoglobin levels should be obtained.

Children with burns that do not meet hospital admission criteria can be seen as outpatients. A tetanus booster should be given to any patient who has not received one within 5 years or who cannot recall the date of last immunization. People who have not been previously immunized or who have been inadequately immunized should receive 250 units of tetanus immunoglobulin. A series of active immunizations should begin. People who do meet admission criteria should have the wounds gently washed with soap and water; all devitalized tissue and open blisters must be removed. Blisters on the palms and feet can often be left intact. Once the area has been débrided and cleaned, a generous amount of silver sulfadiazine (Silvadene) cream or other topical agent should be applied and the extremities loosely wrapped with Kerlex. Escharotomy should be considered in all circumferential burns. Escharotomies can often be carried out at the bedside, without anesthesia, using needlepoint cautery.

FLUID RESUSCITATION

Burn resuscitation formulas range from pure colloid to combinations of colloid/crystalloid to exclusively crystalloid solutions.[7, 46, 77, 78] The sodium ion is recognized as the critical element in resuscitative fluids. Volume recommendations for adult burn resuscitation cannot be transferred to children. The disparity of body surface area to weight and the higher metabolic rate in children results in significant errors when adult formulas are applied to children. A modification of the Parkland formula, giving daily maintenance fluids as Ringer's lactate Plus, 3 to 4 ml/kg/% burn, works well. Even when maintenance fluids are provided, children require substantially more fluid for the same percentage of burn compared to an adult.[79] About half of this fluid volume is calculated to be given over the first 8 hours, and the remaining half over the following 16 hours. The use of this formula makes resuscitation simple, less costly, and safer. Some centers recommend giving one half of the calculated volume over the first 4 hours, and then the other half over the remaining 20 hours. They have shown a decreased need for ventilatory support and more rapid stabilization of urine output and vital signs.[80, 81] Colloid solutions increase the cost of the resuscitation without demonstrated benefit. Hypertonic resuscitation requires less water and produces less edema, but hypernatremia, hyperosmolar coma, renal failure, and alkalosis are significant risks.[82] Central pontine myelinolysis has been described in hyperosmolar burn patients.[83] It has also been shown that the volume of fluid and sodium loss into the wound is inversely proportional to the osmolarity of the resuscitation fluid. Colloid resuscitation results in a five times greater loss of sodium in the urine and wound compared to hypertonic saline and lactated Ringer's.[84] Resuscitation formulas are guidelines. In a given situation, the child may require greater or lesser volumes depending on his or her clinical response. Deeper burns and inhalation injury may increase fluid requirements considerably.[85]

Vital signs, urine output, and mental status are

Area	Birth 1 yr.	1-4 yr.	5-9 yr.	10-14 yr.	15 yr.	Adult	2°	3°	Total	Donor Areas
Head	19	17	13	11	9	7				
Neck	2	2	2	2	2	2				
Ant. Trunk	13	13	13	13	13	13				
Post. Trunk	13	13	13	13	13	13				
R. Buttock	2½	2½	2½	2½	2½	2½				
L. Buttock	2½	2½	2½	2½	2½	2½				
Genitalia	1	1	1	1	1	1				
R. U. Arm	4	4	4	4	4	4				
L. U. Arm	4	4	4	4	4	4				
R. L. Arm	3	3	3	3	3	3				
L. L. Arm	3	3	3	3	3	3				
R. Hand	2½	2½	2½	2½	2½	2½				
L. Hand	2½	2½	2½	2½	2½	2½				
R. Thigh	5½	6½	8	8½	9	9½				
L. Thigh	5½	6½	8	8½	9	9½				
R. Leg	5	5	5½	6	6½	7				
L. Leg	5	5	5½	6	6½	7				
R. Foot	3½	3½	3½	3½	3½	3½				
L. Foot	3½	3½	3½	3½	3½	3½				
						TOTAL				

Cause of Burn _____

Date of Burn _____

Time of Burn _____

Age _____

Sex _____

Weight _____

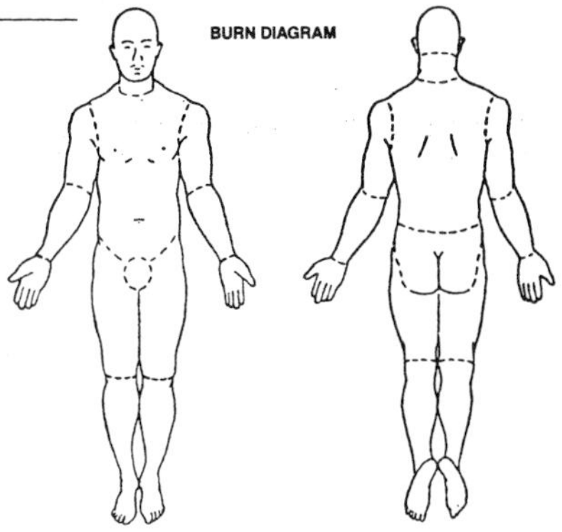

BURN DIAGRAM

Figure 14–4. Laundbrauder charts. (Adapted from Zawacki BE, Warden GD: In Boswick JA [ed]: The Art and Science of Burn Care. Rockville, MD, Aspen, 1987, pp 26–47.)

good resuscitation guidelines. Urine output should be maintained at or above 1 ml/kg/h in children weighing less than 30 kg and at least 30 to 40 ml/h in children weighing more than 30 kg. Rather than attempting to maintain central venous pressure at an arbitrary level, end organ function remains the most reliable indicator of successful resuscitation.

Capillary leak is greatest in the first 12 hours and progressively decreases over the next 12 hours. Colloid should be given during the second 24 hours, and repeated daily to keep the serum albumin at or above 2.0 g/dl. The rate of crystalloid can be reduced to maintenance levels and adjusted as indicated by urine output.[86] During the second 24 hours, 5% dextrose in one-half normal saline may be given. Tube feeding, beginning as early as 12 hours after injury, has been shown to improve gut and immune function.

☐ Nutrition

The metabolic response to a major burn can be described on a time continuum.[87] A period of relative hypometabolism lasts for the first 24 to 48 hours. This is followed by a phase of marked catabolism and massive loss of structural proteins and fat. This phase lasts as long as the wound remains open, and it is often exacerbated by episodes of infection, cold, stress, pain, anxiety, and operative procedures.[88, 89] Once the wounds are covered, metabolism enters a period of convalescence in which anabolism dominates with replenishment of body structural and visceral proteins.

The catabolic phase of burn injury is characterized by increased levels of cortisone, epinephrine, norepinephrine, glucagon, aldosterone, and antidiuretic hormone.[90] The basal metabolic rate may double. Protein-calorie malnutrition can develop rapidly in children with low body fat stores and a small muscle mass if nutritional support is not supplied.[7, 91, 92] A significant loss of protein occurs through the burn wound.

Numerous formulas have been designed to estimate caloric needs in burned children.[7, 93–96] In children, 7560 kJ/m² plus body surface burned is a commonly used formula.[86] The technology has become available to measure resting energy expenditure by indirect calorimetry.[93, 95, 97] In a study of infants and toddlers with more than 50% total body surface burns, nutritional needs could be met by supplying 120 to 200% of the measured resting metabolic rate.[96] This value is somewhat less than many of the formulas predict. This finding has been confirmed in several recent studies.[93, 98–101]

Protein should make up 20 to 25% of total calories, carbohydrates 40 to 50%, and the remaining calories should be fats.[7, 102, 103] A modular formulation has been shown to decrease postburn immune suppression, mortality, metabolic response, and hospital stay, and to enhance the gastrointestinal barrier to bacterial translocation.[104–106] This diet supplies 20% of energy needs from protein whey, 2% from arginine, 0.5% from cystine, 0.5% from histidine, and 15% from lipids. Half of the lipid calories are supplied by fish oil and the remaining 50% from safflower oil. The remaining caloric requirements are supplied by carbohydrate. A more recent study confirmed decreased immune function, more bacteremias, and worse survival rate when lower protein diets were provided.[107]

Nutrition is optimally supplied via the enteral route and requires a feeding tube in a majority of cases.[106] Gut feedings are better tolerated if the serum albumin level is maintained at or above 2.5 g/dl. This contention has recently been challenged. A recent study showed that worse outcomes and feeding intolerance did not correlate with low albumin levels.[108] If gut feedings are not tolerated, parenteral feeding is the next best option. This usually requires a central venous catheter, because adequate calories can seldom be supplied by peripheral routes.[79] Caloric intake and body weight should be monitored daily. Serum electrolytes, blood urea nitrogen (BUN), creatinine, albumin, glucose, phosphorus, calcium, hemoglobin, and hematocrit values should be monitored daily in patients on tube feedings or parenteral hyperalimentation. Urine glucose level should be monitored. Liver profile and prealbumin, transferrin, magnesium, cholesterol, and triglyceride levels should be determined weekly.

All burned children should receive at least the minimum recommended daily allowance (RDA) of vitamins, minerals, and trace elements. Vitamin C should be supplemented at 5 to 10 times the RDA, zinc at 2 times the RDA, and B vitamins at least 2 times the RDA.[102]

□ Wound Treatment

A majority (95%) of all pediatric burns are minor and can be treated in an outpatient setting. Washing and débridements of the wound are carried out twice a day. Polymyxin B sulfate (Polysporin) or Bacitracin is applied, and the wound is wrapped with gauze. These wounds heal within 10 to 14 days.[82] Superficial partial thickness minor burns can also be treated with semipermeable synthetic membranes, which simplify home care and decrease pain.[109, 110]

An obvious full thickness burn should be excised and covered with autograft as soon as the patient is hemodynamically stable. Depth of injury is often difficult to determine early, especially with scald burns, which account for a majority of pediatric burns. Early aggressive surgical closure of all burn wounds may result in loss of substantial amounts of tissue that would otherwise heal without significant scarring. Burn wounds of indeterminate depth should be treated by twice daily débridement and topical agents until the wound depth can be accurately determined, which often takes 10 to 14 days.[87] Of all the factors that lead to hypertrophic scarring, the time to wound healing or closure appears to be a major factor. Of wounds that heal between 14 and 21 days, hypertrophic scarring develops in 33%. Wounds that take longer than 21 days to heal have a 78% incidence of scarring.[111]

The ideal topical agent should be painless and nonallergenic, prevent desiccation, penetrate burn eschar, and achieve bacteriologic control; the agent should not inhibit reepithelialization or injure viable cells.[112] Silver sulfadiazine although not ideal, fills more of these requirements than almost any other agent. Its application is pain-free, has few side effects, is poorly absorbed, and has a good bacterial spectrum.[112, 113] The combination of cerium nitrate and silver sulfadiazine has been shown to be more effective in extensively burned patients. The cerium component improves gram-negative control, and the silver sulfadiazine component continues to exert good fungal and gram-positive control. Mafenide continues to be a valuable agent because it can penetrate burn eschar.[114] It has a good gram-negative and gram-positive control spectrum but no antifungal capabilities.

Several other agents are listed in Table 14–1, which indicates some of their advantages, limitations, and indications. Prostaglandin E_1 ointment has been used on superficial burns and donor sites with reported reduction of healing time and hypertrophic scarring.[115] We typically do twice daily débridement and dressing changes. A recent study showed that once-a-day débridement and dressing change cuts cost, decreases pain episodes, and results in no increased infection or morbidity. This was done in burns of 30% or less of the total body surface.[116]

Positioning is an important aspect of wound care, especially in hand injuries. Edema, inflammation, and immobility are the three great forces at work to destroy function. Exercise, elevation, proper splinting, and early closure of the wound limit disability.[1, 117] The hand should be splinted in the position of function. Elevation and active exercise of the hand should begin immediately. All joints should be exercised actively and passively several times a day.

Deep perineal burns do not require fecal or urinary diversion. A 20-year study has shown no increase in infectious complications as a result of nondiversion.[5, 118, 119]

Corneal burns should be seen by an ophthalmologist. They are treated with débridement, topical antibiotics, cycloplegia, and pressure patching.[120]

Recombinant human growth hormone at a dose of 0.2 mg/kg/day has shown accelerated wound healing, especially in donor sites. Its use was also associated with a significant decrease in hospital stay.[121]

□ Pain Management

Pain control in children is often poorly managed. The correlation between a child's perception of pain is far different than his or her nurse's perception of the pain.[122–124] Pain response varies widely among

TABLE 14-1. Topical Agents

Agent	Concentration	Application	Dressing Technique	Advantages	Limitations	Bacterial Spectrum	Indications
Silver sulfadiazine	1%	q 12 h	Open or closed	Poor absorption, rare side effects, painless, good spectrum coverage	Sensitivity in 4 to 8%, WBC count suppression, gram-negative resistance, especially *Enterobacter*, not effective in burns >60% BSA	Gram-positive cocci, gram-negative resistance including enterobacter, *Escherichia coli*, and *Candida*	First line major burns
Mafenamide	10%	q 12 h	Open or very minimally closed	Rapid eschar penetration, good bacterial spectrum	Bacterial resistance, especially *Providencia stuarti*; fungi inhibit epithelial growth, metabolic acidosis, respiratory failure, painful and rapid absorption	Broad gram-negative and gram-positive coverage, no antifungal activity, especially good against *Pseudomonas*	Invasive burn wound infections or deep burns involving small areas, such as electrical injury
Silver nitrate	1/2%	wet q 2 h	Closed	Resistance uncommon, painless	Extremely messy, hyponatremia, hypokalemia, difficult red wound, methemoglobin-emia	Gram-positive in fungi, some gram-negative	Burns < 50% BSA, for prophylaxis, sulfa-allergic individuals
Gentamycin	0.1%	q 12 h		Good gram-negative coverage, especially *Pseudomonas*	High absorption rate to toxic levels, development of resistance	Gram-negative	Small areas for short time, burn wound invasion in sulfa-allergic individuals, must monitor blood levels
Cerium nitrate-silver sulfadiazine	2.2%–1%	q 12 h	Closed	Low toxicity, poor absorption, useful in extensive burns	Same as silver sulfadiazine	Excellent gram-negative coverage, in addition to the advantages of silver sulfadiazine	Extensive burns between 60 and 80%
Povidone/iodine	1%	q 12 h	Open or closed	Good bacterial spectrum	Exudate inactivation, painful, rapid absorption with high iodine levels, metabolic acidosis	Wide	Few, may be useful in soft, difficult to excise wounds for 24 hours prior to excision
Scarlet red	5%		Closed	Painless, possible acceleration of epithelialization	Methemoglobin-emia, tanning of adjacent skin and wound, very messy	Bacteriostatic, secondary to low pH environment	Donor sites, possible use on superficial partial thickness burn in an outpatient
Nitrofurazone		q 24 h	Semiclosed	None	Inactivated by wound exudate	Limited	Small superficial burns with low infectious potential, sulfa allergies, covered meshed grafts
Neosporin/bacitracin		prn	Open or closed	Use on face, not toxic to eyes	In toxic levels on large burns		Superficial partial thickness burns in an outpatient and on facial burns treated open

BSA, body surface area; WBC, white blood cell.

patients. A recent study showed that pain severity seemed to parallel the percent of body burned.[125, 126]

Pain can be controlled by nonpharmacologic and pharmacologic means. Hypnosis, acupuncture, and transcutaneous electrical nerve stimulators (TENS) units have been found to be variably effective.[110] An adjunctive nonpharmacologic approach to pain control has been successful in children.[123] Key components of this approach include the following:

1. Before the burn dressing change, the child is told what to expect and then is kept informed as the burn dressing change progresses.
2. Emphasis is placed on the need for the child's help with the burn dressing change.
3. The choices offered to the child are appropriate and reasonable.
4. The nurse maintains control by setting reasonable time limits for the child's help with procedures.
5. The child's attention is focused on the task by being encouraged to watch, help, and look at the burned area being treated.
6. Generous praise is given for the child's help.
7. Predictability is further increased by telling the child when to expect the next burn dressing change.
8. Most importantly, no child of any age is forced to do anything that he or she clearly does not wish to do or is not ready to do.

Narcotics should be administered liberally for painful procedures and for heightened background pain. Children much prefer the oral to the IM administration. For IV use, nalbuphine (Nubain) is effective and causes little respiratory depression. If tolerance to nalbuphine occurs, morphine can be given without a withdrawal reaction. Roxanol is an effective oral form of morphine. If a longer-acting narcotic for background pain is necessary, methadone is an option. Meperidine (Demerol), even though it is a shorter-acting narcotic, can have serious toxic effects with long-term administration because of its metabolites. Fentanyl is an extremely effective narcotic analgesic that should be reserved for episodes of severe pain. The rapid development of tolerance and the high cost of fentanyl may limit its use.[127] Oral ketamine has recently been described, and has been found to be safe and effective. Children report 400% less pain and much improved sedation.[128] Nitrous oxide, patient-controlled analgesia, and epidurals are other options. New drugs for transdermal and transmucosal delivery may soon be available.[129]

☐ Surgical Management

ANESTHETIC CONSIDERATIONS

The anesthesiologist must be aware of the potential for massive and rapid blood loss. Maintenance of normal body temperature requires constant vigilance. The operating room should be heated to 85 to 90°F. Heating blankets and overhead warmers should be in place and functioning. If the child's head is not involved in the excisional procedure, it should be covered to prevent heat loss. A decrease in body temperature is almost inevitable with most major burn procedures. With careful attention to external warming and warming of all IV fluids, hypothermia can be minimized. A well-coordinated effort that shortens operating time also diminishes temperature loss. Two large-bore IV lines should be established. Depending on the clinical situation, an arterial line, a central venous line, and a urinary catheter may be indicated.

Burn patients may demonstrate altered drug sensitivity.[130] Depolarizing muscle relaxants, such as succinylcholine, may cause the rapid release of potassium. Resistance to nondepolarizing drugs, however, appears to increase with the percentage of burned surface area. Burn patients also exhibit insensitivity to thiopental, which lasts well beyond the time of complete healing of the burn wound.[96, 131–137]

Anesthesia, major débridement, grafting, and hypothermia combine to heighten metabolic stress. A marked increase occurs in catecholamine levels and a concomitant increase in urea production occurs following general anesthesia and operative procedures.[138] Limiting the operating time, the amount of blood loss, and the temperature variation helps to reduce metabolic stress.

The recovery room is an extension of the operating room. Efforts to maintain normal body temperature and ventilation are critical. Obtundation, constricting dressings, and hypothermia can combine to compromise ventilation.

OPERATIVE CONSIDERATIONS

Full thickness and deep partial thickness burns should be surgically closed. Early excision and grafting have been shown to reduce hospital stay, limit the number of painful burn débridements, and decrease overall hospital costs.[4, 139, 140] Mortality rate has been reduced from 45 to 9% in patients 17 to 30 years of age with early excision and wound closure, but there was no improvement in people older than 30 years and a seeming increase in mortality rate in children with early excision and grafting.[141]

Three techniques of excisional therapy are used.[87] The first technique is sequential excision, which involves daily débridement and once or twice weekly sessions with a guarded knife to remove more firmly adherent eschar. This maneuver results in a clean granulating bed by 2 to 3 weeks that can be skin grafted. This technique may be used in wounds of indeterminate depth.[142, 143]

The second method is primary excision to fascia. This involves excising the burn wound down to fascia, using electrocautery or heated scalpel. The blood loss is less with this type of excision, and grafting on a viable bed is assured. The judgment needed regarding the depth of the wound is not as critical. This method, therefore, can be more safely used by less experienced surgeons. This type of excision should not be used on the child's hands, face, or neck because the cosmetic deformities are significant. It is reserved for proximal limb and trunk excisions. Even in these areas, the functional and cosmetic results of primary fascial excision are often debilitating. One group who used this technique within the first 24 hours after injury in 594 children found that blood loss was halved by burn excision within this time frame. All available autograft was harvested, meshed 1 to 3 and overlaid with homograft. Areas with insufficient autograft were covered with homograft. The hospital stay and the frequency of painful dressing changes were dramatically decreased as was the incidence of infection. A significant decrease in mortality rate was not demonstrated, however.[144, 145]

The third technique is tangential excision, which involves the removal of sequential thin layers of burn eschar until a bed is reached that is clearly viable. This technique requires more surgical experience in order to judge when the depth of the excision is sufficient. The major advantage of this technique is that dermal elements can often be preserved in deep partial thickness burns, as can much of the fatty tissue in full thickness injury. If the burn depth is unknown and nonviable tissue is left, valuable autograft is lost. Tangential excision can result in massive blood loss. We routinely apply tourniquets on the extremities to limit blood loss. Subeschar clysis with epinephrine in Ringer's lactate solution limits the amount of blood loss in truncal excision. With tourniquets and epinephrine clysis, we have been able to achieve much larger excisions with an acceptable blood loss. Several studies have been done to determine the optimal time for excision in order to limit blood loss. The Shriners Burn Hospital group from Galveston has demonstrated a significant decrease in blood loss if the excision is done in the first 24 hours.[144] Other groups have shown no difference between excision done before 7 days or after.[146]

Blood loss in children can be anticipated as 3.4% of the patient's blood volume per percentage of burn excised. This can be used as a rough guide when planning blood availability for an operation.[147] A more difficult question is timing of excision in scald burns. The depth is difficult to judge in this type of injury. If excision is done before 5 days following injury, the blood loss is increased, as is the area of excision with no reduction in hospital stay. If excision is delayed until 10 to 14 days, the superficial second-degree burn is healed and one can safely excise the unhealed portions without extending the hospital stay, thereby decreasing the area of excision and decreasing the blood loss. This has been our experience, as well as that of others.[148] Facial burns that do not heal by 14 to 20 days should probably be tangentially excised and grafted. Beyond this time, the degree of hypertrophic scarring becomes excessive.[149]

Most freshly excised wounds can be immediately skin grafted. If the bleeding is severe or the surgeon is uncomfortable with the depth of the excision, the wounds can be wrapped with fine mesh gauze and bulky wet dressings and the grafting delayed for 24 hours.

Ringer's lactate solution can be injected subcutaneously into virtually any area where a graft is to be harvested, thus giving an even, firm surface from which to harvest. A roller pump can be used to inject the subcutaneous clysis, which reduces the time needed for this procedure and delivers the fluid at body temperature. Clysis of the entire back can be done in less than 10 minutes. Where smaller burns are excised, the scalp is an ideal donor site. It does not scar, is covered by hair, and avoids the often hypertrophic donor sites seen in children. The quality of graft is equal to other locations.[150] Grafts can be meshed 1:1.5 or greater, depending on the amount of autograft available, and stapled in place. Where grafts are expanded widely, such as a 1:3 or 1:4, an overlay of homograft is elected.

Meshed grafts should be covered with a fine mesh gauze and a bulky dressing. Catheters strategically placed throughout the dressings can help keep the grafts moistened with a triple antibiotic solution for the first 4 to 5 days. With this technique, graft takes are excellent. The major reasons for graft losses are inadequately excised beds, infections, or desiccations, and mechanical disruptions. Plaster casting for immobilization, especially in the smaller children, avoids many of these problems.[151]

The development of cultured epithelial cells has become commonplace. Several companies market this service. Harvest of a square centimeter of skin can be cultured and expanded to an area of more than a square meter in approximately 2 weeks. The take of these cultured cells varies widely among institutions. This technology is critical in massively burned children. Cultured cells are also being used for resurfacing scar revisions with much improved long-term results.[152, 153] Integra has recently been released. This composite membrane can be placed on a cleanly excised bed, and it effectively closes the wound. The Silastic membrane can be sequentially removed as autograft becomes available for widely meshed grafting. Very good results have been obtained with this new technology. To prevent the spread of AIDS to the patient, British surgeons have used a parent as an allograft donor to temporarily cover wounds. These allografts are safer and can be used as an overlay for widely meshed autografts or as a collagen bed for cultured cells.[154] The development of innovations such as this is critical for the survival of the massively burned child in whom donor sites are extremely limited.

RESPIRATORY INJURY

Inhalation injury is noted in 15 to 18% of burn patients admitted to hospitals but accounts for 30 to 80% of deaths from burns.[155–161] Inhalation burns result from direct heat injury or toxic chemical injury. Dry air of 500°C is cooled to almost 50°C by the time it reaches the carina. Toxic chemicals associated with inhalation injury are those that are absorbed systemically and those that cause direct injury to the tracheobronchial lining.[162] The most toxic and rapidly fatal substances are carbon monoxide and cyanide.[163] Directly toxic chemicals are numerous. Polyvinyl chloride, found in fire-retardant materials and rubber, produces aldehydes, hydrochloric acid, and chlorine. Nylon, rubber, silk, wool, and petroleum products all release ammonia. These substances, and numerous others, cause direct injury to the airway mucosa.[164, 165]

Evaluation must include a careful history. Symptoms and signs may include sore throat, hoarseness, dysphagia, cough, carbonaceous sputum production, stridor, nasal flaring, tachypnea, retractions, restlessness, confusion, or irritability. Findings may include singed nasal hairs, facial burns, and rales or wheezes on auscultation.[155, 166] A significant inhalation injury may exist in the absence of signs or symptoms and with normal laboratory data.[167] Scald injuries can result in significant airway injury in certain circumstances when the hot liquids are aspirated. A report of 13 such patients found a 25% mortality rate.[168]

Acute pulmonary insufficiency may develop in the first 24 hours. Pulmonary edema and pneumonia may follow. The most accurate means of diagnosing inhalation injury is by flexible bronchoscopy or xenon-133 scanning.[157, 165, 169]

The treatment of inhalation injury begins at the rescue scene. All patients should be given 100% oxygen, which speeds carbon monoxide elimination by a factor of 5. Humidification of inspired gas, oxygen supplementation, and good pulmonary toilet are the mainstays of treatment. Steroids have no place in the treatment of inhalation injury. Antibiotics should be given only in cases in which a documented infection is present. Indications for intubation and ventilatory support include any one of the following:

1. Increasing stridor with evidence of upper airway edema and obstruction
2. Hypoxemia
3. Inability to clear secretions
4. Inadequate ventilation unrelieved by escharotomy in a circumferential burn of the chest
5. Increased intracranial pressure from hypoxic brain injury.[167]

Inhalation injury may increase overall fluid requirements by 50%. Inadequate fluid resuscitation increases the complications of the inhalation injury, may extend the depth of the burn injury, and adds to the immunologic compromise. Inhalation injury often leads to pneumonia. Ascaris pneumonia has been described in burned children and is fatal if not diagnosed and treated. The normal life cycle of ascaris involves passage into the lung, which is usually a benign process. In the presence of an inhalation injury, it becomes a much more malignant process.[170]

Acute respiratory failure from inhalation injury and a large cutaneous burn are associated with a higher mortality rate than either condition alone. If burn wound sepsis occurs, the mortality rate doubles. Early excision and grafting has been shown to decrease mortality rate by 53% in this setting.[171] Extubation can be difficult. Heliox has been shown to facilitate extubation in this setting.[172, 173]

ELECTRICAL INJURY

Electrical burns account for less than 5% of admissions to most burn units. The energy or heat produced by electric shock is a function of voltage, amperage, and time. Tissues with high resistance, such as dry skin and bone, generate high temperatures when high voltage is applied. Muscle necrosis results from heat injury, diffuse vascular injury, and intense swelling within the fixed-muscle compartments. Vascular injury is a progressive phenomenon. Aneurysms of the aorta may develop late.

Neurologic injury may result in coma, seizures, and peripheral neuropathy. Late neurologic disability may be caused by progressive vascular occlusion and demyelinization. These abnormalities may become apparent as late as 2 years after injury. Neurologic sequelae have also been reported after low-voltage injury.[174] Bone necrosis and fractures from tetanic contraction of muscles may occur.

Low-voltage alternating current can cause ventricular fibrillation and cardiac arrest, as well as tetany of the muscles of respiration with suffocation.[175] Vigorous cardiopulmonary resuscitation should be instituted because resuscitation from electrical injury is often successful. A majority of electrical injuries in children are low voltage and usually occur in the home. There is no need to admit people with low-voltage injuries to hospitals if no abnormalities are noted on physical and laboratory examination.[176, 177] The most common injury is to the oral commissure. High temperatures from electrical arcing account for the extensive damage.[178–183]

Controversy exists regarding the best treatment for commissure injuries, that is, early versus late repair and splint versus no splint.[184–188] We have adopted a nonoperative conservative approach to these lesions with excellent long-term results. Patients with these injuries are treated as outpatients, and significant labial artery hemorrhage has never occurred. This approach is supported by other workers.[185] High-voltage electrical injury is manifested by a charred, marbleized entry point and a devastating blowout at the point of grounding (Fig. 14–5). Myoglobinuria and elevated creatine phosphokinase values indicate a deep and potentially devastating injury, often covered by viable skin.[113, 187] Ringer's lactate solution should be infused, and urine output should be established at a level of at least 1.5 to 2.0 ml/kg/h. Due to the nephrotoxic effects of myoglobin breakdown products,

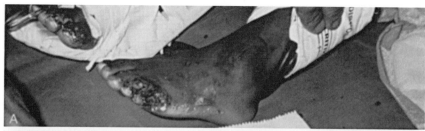

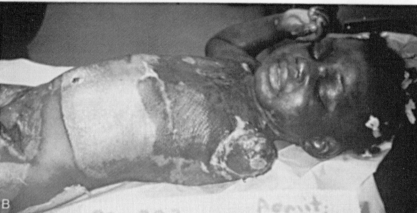

Figure 14–5. *A,* The 4-year-old victim of high-voltage electrical injury with a devastating exit site in both feet. *B,* Entry point in left upper arm resulted in its complete destruction. This child also suffered extensive flash injury from arcing, as evidenced by burns over the entire anterior thorax and groin area.

diuresis should be established with mannitol and fluid, and the urine should be alkalinized.

Muscle compartments must be carefully assessed and early fasciotomy carried out to prevent a compartment syndrome. High-voltage injury requires frequent débridement of necrotic tissue, which may be progressive. Technetium 99m stannous pyrophosphate scanning may be used to localize areas of muscle necrosis.[188] Amputations may be necessary early.[179] After these wounds have been adequately débrided and the progression of vascular thrombosis and necrosis controlled, the open wounds should be covered with split thickness skin grafts and flap rotations, and transfers deferred until everything is well healed.

BURN WOUND COVERINGS

Burn wound coverings or dressings should have at least one of the following qualifications:
1. Vapor and gas permeability
2. Adherence
3. Bacterial inhibition
4. Ability to be vascularized.

A number of burn wound coverings fill one or more of these qualifications. Coverings can be divided into synthetics and biologic dressings. The biologic dressings can be either cultured or harvested. Some workers suggest that cultured epithelial cells may be superior, in the long term, to skin grafting. Early cultured epithelial cell graft loss averages 50 to 60%. This poor percentage and the tremendous cost may limit its usefulness in less extensively burned patients. Bilayered artificial skin made of silicone bonded to a collagen base is available. The excised wound is covered with this material. As soon as

there is a good vascular take of the collagen base, which occurs at about 30 days, the silicone can be sequentially removed and a thin layer of autograft or cultured epithelial cells applied. It is possible that less contraction and scarring result from this bilayered artificial skin.

In another technique, cultured epithelial cells are placed over mechanically de-epithelialized cadaveric skin that serves as the collagen base. This technique reportedly results in less scarring and resembles normal skin. In still another technique, cultured epithelial cells are applied to a dermal membrane made from cultured human fibroblasts that are incorporated into an acellular collagen glycosaminoglycan membrane.[189]

Synthetic or biologic dressings should be carefully monitored. There are reports of toxic shock syndrome in children whose wounds are treated with synthetic wound barriers and with some xenograft material.[190] Duoderm and Biobrane are examples of synthetics that are very useful for superficial second-degree burns and donor sites. The patients are mobile, frequent painful dressings are avoided, and wound healing is prompt.[191, 192]

REHABILITATION

The two major goals of burn care are survival and limitation of physical and emotional disability. Efforts to achieve these goals are sought from the time of admission. The quality of survival depends on the ability to minimize physical and emotional disability. The entire burn team is responsible for this effort. Occupational and physical therapists are key players on the team. Several factors influence the degree of physical disability resulting from burn injury. These can be broadly classified into intrinsic and extrinsic factors. Intrinsic factors include the following:

1. Anatomic location of the burn
2. Depth of injury
3. Quality of healing
4. Genetic predisposition for scar formation
5. Physiologic contractile forces
6. Maturation
7. Age

The amount of hypertrophic scarring and the rate of healing seem to depend on depth, age, and genetics. More hypertrophic scars form in younger children than older individuals. Their scars seem to mature at a much slower rate. Extrinsic factors include the following:

1. Treatment intervention, such as early excision and grafting
2. Follow-up
3. Patient and parental compliance with the intensive therapy required to overcome physical disabilities. Positioning, active and passive range of motion exercises, and efforts to decrease edema are critical.[142, 143]

After the burn wound is completely covered, splinting, pressure garments, active and passive range of motion exercises, adaptive equipment, and adaptation to the activities of daily living must continue. Compression garments are useful in limiting hypertrophic scarring.[7] Younger children with very large burns come through burn experience remarkably well, for the most part. Their families often need as much, or more, counseling and support. Teenagers with visible scars require special attention and often have significant self-esteem problems requiring close scrutiny.[193, 194]

COMPLICATIONS

A study of 139 postburn deaths showed a 53% incidence of central nervous system complications ranging from abscesses to bleeding and infarcts.[195] A study of 224 pediatric burn admissions found a 14% infection rate. Predisposing factors included (1) a burn of more than 20% total body surface area, (2) smoke inhalation, and (3) presence of an indwelling device.[196] Fever and leukocytosis are not necessarily indicative of infection in pediatric burns. Before one resorts to use of antibiotics, other evidence of infection should be sought.[197-199]

Significant inhalation injury may not be apparent on initial evaluation. If the history is suggestive, one should be vigilant for such a condition. Hyponatremia often occurs in the first 48 hours, in part because of an increase in antidiuretic hormone output and hypotonic fluids. Evidence of a compartment syndrome should be sought, especially in circumferential injuries. Doppler pulse determination is of limited value because a significant compartment syndrome can be present long before arterial pulse is lost. Virtually all circumferential injuries require escharotomy. Fasciotomy is seldom needed except in the case of electrical injury. Circumferential thoracic burns may require escharotomy to improve ventilatory mechanics, especially in younger children. Early gut feedings may serve to maintain a normal gastric pH and prevent upper gastrointestinal bleeding.

After 7 to 10 days, burn wound sepsis becomes a major risk.[4] Severe inhalation injury and sepsis is a particularly lethal combination, resulting in multiorgan failure and death.[200] A source of sepsis that is often not considered is septic thrombophlebitis, which develops in approximately 4 to 5% of major burn patients. If this complication is untreated, the mortality rate approaches 100%. If one suspects septic thrombophlebitis, all previous IV sites should be carefully inspected. Aspiration of the site is not effective in making this diagnosis. If there is any drainage from the site, the vein should be opened directly, preferably under anesthesia. If the site is found to contain pus, the entire vein must be removed and the wound left open.

A study in 70 children reported a significant decrease in line sepsis when the practice of frequently changing lines, either by rewire or into a new site, was discontinued.[197] Another study showed that femoral lines, even through burned tissue, have no greater incidence of infection than lines in other sites.[73] Line sepsis, sinusitis, chondritis, and urosepsis from indwelling catheters must be evaluated in the septic burn patient.[4] Renal failure may result from underresuscitation, sepsis or toxic injury from myoglobin or drugs. Toxic shock syndrome can be rapidly fatal in burn cases. Early signs include sudden increase in body temperature, marked tachycardia, tachypnea, and a profound decrease in white blood cell count over a period of hours, just before the shock phase.[201] Hypertension is a postburn problem almost peculiar to children. This may begin immediately and last up to 3 months after complete closure of the wound. The cause may be excessive renin output. It can be managed with furosemide (Lasix) and hydralazine. The hypertension can be severe and, at times, can result in neurologic symptoms, if left untreated. Pulmonary embolism, a common problem in adult burn patients, is rare in children.[202] Abdominal compartment syndrome, recently reported in massively burned children, has a very poor prognosis.[203]

Once the wound is closed, itching is a significant problem in children. Children often scratch themselves so vigorously that healed donor sites and graft sites are disrupted. No effective treatment is known. Diphenhydramine and hydroxyzine (Atarax) combined with moisturizing creams and pressure garments seem to help. Children are susceptible to development of severe hypertrophic scarring.[59, 137, 204] The pressure garments and vigilant rehabilitation program help to limit this adverse event. Heterotopic calcification is also a significant problem.[205] It may be related to overzealous physical therapy with bleeding into soft tissues and subsequent calcification. Cancer in the burn scars has

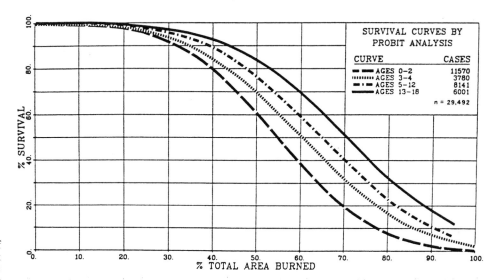

Figure 14–6. Epidemiology of burns in children. (From East MK, Jones CA, Feller I, et al: Burns in Children: Pediatric Burn Management. Chicago, Year Book, 1988, p 8.)

Epidemiology of burns in children—burned children survival by age for all heat sources, 1964–1984 (n = 29,492).

been reported. This often occurs in wounds that are chronically reopened or that heal poorly.[206]

□ Prognosis and Prevention

In 1898, it was suggested that recovery was exceptional after destruction of one third of the cutaneous surface.[3] In 1958, the LD50 remained at 30%. A study from 1978 to 1985 indicated that many factors had improved the outlook to a LD50 of 64%. Some centers, by 1991, reported that their LD50 was 90%.[4, 79] Figure 14–6 is a graphic demonstration of burn size compared with mortality rate in adults and children.[79] Although some researchers contend that burn mortality rate in children younger than 1 year of age is no different than that of the 2- to 19-year age group, this finding is not supported by data from others.[207–211] Most burn surgeons believe that the percentage of body surface burned, presence of inhalation injury, and age are the major predictors of burn survival.[212] Another recent study has shown that the percentage of fluid retention during the first 48 hours following resuscitation has a close correlation with mortality rate.[213] Another recent study of 185 burned children reported a 15% mortality rate in boys and a 3% mortality rate in girls, matched for severity. A majority of deaths in boys was found in those weighing more than the 95th percentile for their age and height.[214] Abused children have a much higher mortality rate when matched for age and severity.[215]

PREVENTION

By far, the most effective treatment of burns is prevention. In 1985, 47% of deaths from house fires were in children younger than 4 years of age. Of these deaths, three fourths could have been pre-

vented with use of residential sprinklers, operational smoke detectors, fire-safe cigarettes, and child-resistant lighters. Use of fire-safe cigarettes, which can be produced, could prevent numerous pediatric deaths. Use of smoke detectors could reduce fire deaths by almost half. Approximately 24% of scald injuries requiring admission to the hospital are a result of contact with hot tap water. These injuries could be prevented by use of antiscalding devices as well as by regulating the temperature of the water at the water heater.[12] The effectiveness of public education is well demonstrated in Denmark, where, over the past 17 years, scald injuries have been decreased by 50%.[12, 20, 21, 216] Hot grease burns make up a much smaller percentage of pediatric burns but a much larger percentage of serious burns requiring grafting.[6, 17] Hair dryers are another source of serious burns. The air at the outlet of a dryer is 110°C.[217]

Prevention programs should be targeted at high-risk areas. Census studies show a strong correlation between burn injury and poverty, frequent moves, unemployment, young children, single parents, handicapped children, older rental units, and burn injury.[32, 218] Electrical injuries in people younger than age 20 years could be largely prevented through education and proper precautions.[175]

A vital part of the burn team's responsibility is to be active in public education and legislative efforts to prevent burn injury.

REFERENCES

1. Robotti EB: The treatment of burns: An historical perspective with emphasis on the hand. Hand Clin 6:163–190, 1990.
2. Romm S: Burns in art. Clin Plast Surg 13:3–8, 1986.
3. Pinnegar MD, Pinnegar FC: History of burn care. A survey of important changes in the topical treatment of thermal injuries. Burns 12:508–517, 1986.

4. Luterman A, Dacso CC, Curreri PW: Infections in burn patients. Am J Med 81:45–52, 1986.
5. Alghanem AA, McCauley RL, Robson MC, et al: Management of pediatric perineal and genital burns: Twenty-year review. J Burn Care Rehabil 11:308–311, 1990.
6. Schubert W, Ahrenholz DH, Solem LD: Burns from hot oil and grease: A public health hazard. J Burn Care Rehabil 11:558–562, 1990.
7. Harmel RP, Vane DW, King DR: Burn care in children: Special considerations. Clin Plast Surg 13:95–105, 1986.
8. Stuart JD, Kenney JG, Morgan RF: Pediatric burns. Am Fam Physician 36:139–46, 1987.
9. Wilson DI, Bailie FB: Petrol—something nasty in the woodshed? A review of gasoline-related burns in a British burns unit. Burns 21:539–541, 1995.
10. Ryan CA, Shankowsky HA, Tredget EE: Profile of the paediatric burn patient in a Canadian burn centre. Burns 18:267–272, 1992.
11. Harvey JS, Watkins GM, Sherman RT: Emergent burn care. South Med J 77:204–214, 1984.
12. McLoughlin E, McGuire A: The causes, cost and prevention of childhood burn injuries. Am J Dis Child 144:677–683, 1990.
13. Herndon DN, Rutan RL, Rutan TC: Management of the pediatric patient with burns. J Burn Care Rehabil 14:3–8, 1993.
14. Ray JG: Burns in young children: A study of the mechanism of burns in children aged 5 years and under in the Hamilton, Ontario burn unit. Burns 21:463–466, 1995.
15. Rossignol AM, Locke JA, Burke JF: Paediatric burn injuries in New England. Burns 16:41–48, 1990.
16. Parish RA, Novack AH, Heimbach DM, et al: Pediatric patients in a regional burn center. Pediatr Emerg Care 2:165–167, 1986.
17. Murphy JT, Purdue GF, Hunt JL: Pediatric grease burn injury. Arch Surg 130:478–482, 1995.
18. Purdue GF, Hunt JL, Prescott PR: Child abuse by burning: An index of suspicion. J Trauma 28:221–224, 1988.
19. Bradshaw C, Hawkins J, Leach M, et al: A study of childhood scalds. Burns 14:21–24, 1988.
20. Elberg JJ, Schroder HA, Glent-Madsen L, et al: Burns: Epidemiology and the effect of a prevention programme. Burns 13:391–393, 1987.
21. Lyngdorf P: Epidemiology of scalds in small children. Burns 12:250–253, 1986.
22. Kalayi GD, Muhammad I: Burns in children under 3 years of age: The Zaria experience. Ann Trop Paediatr 16:243–248, 1996.
23. Kumar P, Sharma M, Chadha A: Epidemiological determinants of burns in paediatric and adolescent patients from a centre in western India. Burns 20:236–240, 1994.
24. Jie X, Ren CB: Burn injuries in the Dong Bei area of China: A study of 12,606 cases. Burns 18:288–232, 1992.
25. Mercier C, Blond MH: Epidemiological survey of childhood burn injuries in France. Burns 22:29–34, 1996.
26. Renz BM, Sherman R: Child abuse by scalding. J Med Assoc GA 81:574–578, 1992.
27. Montrey JS, Barcia PJ: Nonaccidental burns in child abuse. South Med J 78:1324–1326, 1985.
28. Coren CV: Burn injuries in children. Pediatr Ann 16:328–339, 1987.
29. Yeoh C, Nixon JW, Dickson W, et al: Patterns of scald injuries. Arch Dis Child 71:156–158, 1994.
30. Ayoub C, Pfeifer D: Burns as a manifestation of child abuse and neglect. Am J Dis Child 133:910–914, 1979.
31. Hobbs CJ: When are burns not accidental? Arch Dis Child 61:357–361, 1986.
32. Libber SM, Stayton DJ: Childhood burns reconsidered: The child, the family, and the burn injury. J Trauma 24:245–252, 1984.
33. Showers J, Garrison KM: Burn abuse: A four-year study. J Trauma 28:1581–1583, 1988.
34. Hummel RP III, Greenhalgh DG, Barthel PP, et al: Outcome and socioeconomic aspects of suspected child abuse scald burns. J Burn Care Rehabil 14:121–126, 1993.
35. Renz BM, Sherman R: Abusive scald burns in infants and children: A prospective study. Am Surg 59:329–334, 1993.
36. Wardinsky TD: Genetic and congenital defect conditions that mimic child abuse. J Fam Pract 41:377–383, 1995.
37. Holbrook KA, Byers PH, Pinnell SR: The structure and function of dermal connective tissue in normal individuals and patients with inherited connective tissue disorders. Scan Electron Microsc 4:1731–1744, 1982.
38. Lewis GM, Wheeler C: Practical Dermatology (3rd ed). Philadelphia, WB Saunders, 1967, pp 1–103.
39. Smith DJ, Robson MC, Heggers JP: Frostbite and other cold-induced injuries. In Auerbach PS, Geehr EC (eds): Management of Wilderness and Environmental Emergencies (2nd ed). St. Louis, CV Mosby, 1990, pp 101–118.
40. Cerra FB: Hypermetabolism, organ failure and metabolic support. Surgery 101:1–14, 1987.
41. Kaufman T, Newman RA, Weinberg A: Is postburn dermal ischaemia enhanced by oxygen free radicals? Burns 15:291–294, 1989.
42. Niwa Y: Lipid peroxides and superoxide dismutase (SOD) induction in skin inflammatory diseases and treatment with SOD preparations. Dermatologica 1:101–106, 1989.
43. Rockwell WB, Ehrlich HP: Fibrinolysis inhibition in human burn blister fluid. J Burn Care Rehabil 11:1–16, 1990.
44. Hendricks WM: The classification of burns [commentary]. J Am Acad Dermatol 22:838–839, 1990.
45. Matoth I, Granot E, Gorenstein A, et al: Gastrointestinal protein loss in children recovering from burns. J Pediatr Surg 26:1175–1178, 1991.
46. Rubin WD, Mani MM, Hiebert JM: Fluid resuscitation of the thermally injured patient. Current concepts with definition of clinical subsets and their specialized treatment. Clin Plast Surg 13:9–20, 1986.
47. Baxter CR: Fluid volume and electrolyte changes in the early post burn period. Clin Plast Surg 1:693–709, 1974.
48. Demling R: Fluid and electrolyte management. Critical Care Clinics 1:27–45, 1985.
49. Neely AN, Warden GD, Rieman M, et al: Components of the increased circulating proteolytic activity in pediatric burn patients. J Trauma 33:807–812, 1992.
50. Cerra F: Critical care: State of the art. Soc Crit Care Med 11:15–30, 1990.
51. Rohrich RJ: Wound healing and closure/abnormal scars/envenomation and extravasation injuries. Selected Readings in Plastic Surgery 6:1–3, 1990.
52. Moore FD, Davis CF: Monocyte activation after burns and endotoxemia. J Surg Res 46:350–354, 1989.
53. Wallace BH, Caldwell FT Jr, Cone JB: Ibuprofen lowers body temperature and metabolic rate of humans with burn injury. J Trauma 32:154–157, 1992.
54. Honeycutt D, Barrow R, Herndon D: Cold stress response in patients with severe burns after beta-blockade. J Burn Care Rehabil 13:181–186, 1992.
55. Hansbrough JF, Field TO Jr, Gadd MA, et al: Immune response modulation after burn injury: T cells and antibodies. J Burn Care Rehabil 8:509–512, 1987.
56. Deitch EA: Immunologic considerations in the burned child. In Carvajal GF, Parks DH (eds): Burns in Children: Pediatric Burn Management. Chicago, Year Book Medical Publishers, 1988, pp 195–212.
57. Moran K, Munster AM: Alterations of the host defense mechanism in burn patients. Surg Clin North Am 67:47–56, 1987.
58. Teodorczyk-Injeyan JA, Sparkes BG, Mills GB, et al: Impaired expression of interleukin-2 receptor (IL2R) in the immunosuppressed burned patient: Reversal by exogenous IL2. J Trauma 27:180–187, 1987.
59. Lazarou SA, Barbul A, Wasserkrug HL, et al: The wound is a possible source of posttraumatic immunosuppression. Arch Surg 124:1429–1431, 1989.
60. Ogle CK, Alexander JW, Nagy H, et al: The patient with burns. J Burn Care Rehabil 11:105–111, 1990.
61. Kim Y, Goldstein E, Lippert W, et al: Polymorphonuclear leukocyte motility in patients with severe burns. Burns 15:93–97, 1989.
62. Bjerknes R, Vindenes H, Laerum OD: Altered neutrophil functions in patients with large burns. J Blood Cells 16:127–141, 1990.

63. Bjerknes R, Vindenes H, Pitkanen J, et al: Altered polymorphonuclear neutrophilic granulocyte functions in patients with large burns. J Trauma 29:847–855, 1989.

64. Ferrara JJ, Dyess DL, Luterman A, et al: In vitro effects of complement inactivation upon burn-associated cell mediated immunosuppression. Am Surg 56:571–574, 1990.

65. Utoh J, Utsunomiya T, Imamura T, et al: Complement activation and neutrophil dysfunction in burned patients with sepsis—a study of two cases. Jpn J Surg 19:462–467, 1989.

66. Ferrara JJ, Peterson RD, Hester R, et al: Inhibition of lymphocyte blastogenesis caused by suppression of interleukin-2 receptor sites after thermal injury. J Burn Care Rehabil 10:119–124, 1989.

67. Klimpel GR, Herndon DH, Stein MD: Peripheral blood lymphocytes from thermal injury patients are defective in their ability to generate lymphokine-activated killer cell activity. J Clin Immunol 8:14–22, 1988.

68. Ferrara JJ, Dyess DL, Luterman A, et al: The suppressive effect of subeschar tissue fluid upon in vitro cell-mediated immunologic function. J Burn Care Rehabil 9:584–588, 1988.

69. Echinard CE: Immunity of the burned patient. Scand J Plast Reconstr Surg Hand Surg 21:317–321, 1987.

70. Ozkan AN, Hoyt DB, Ninnemann JL: Generation and activity of suppressor peptides following traumatic injury. J Burn Care Rehabil 8:527–530, 1987.

71. Asko-Seljavaara S: Granulocyte kinetics in burns. J Burn Care Rehabil 8:492–495, 1987.

72. Ninnemann JL: Trauma, sepsis and the immune response. J Burn Care Rehabil 8:462–468, 1987.

73. Goldstein AM, Weber JM, Sheridan RL: Femoral venous access is safe in burned children: An analysis of 224 catheters. J Pediatr 130:442–446, 1997.

74. Goldstein B, Doody D, Briggs S: Emergency intraosseous infusion in severely burned children. Pediatr Emerg Care 6:195–197, 1990.

75. Warden GD: Outpatient care of thermal injuries. Surg Clin North Am 67:147–157, 1987.

76. Wilson GR, Fowler CA, Housden PL: A new burn area assessment chart. Burns 13:401–405, 1987.

77. Aharoni A, Moscona R, Kremerman S, et al: Pulmonary complications in burn patients resuscitated with a low-volume colloid solution. Burns 15:281–284, 1989.

78. Graves TA, Cioffi WHG, McManus WF, et al: Fluid resuscitation of infants and children with massive thermal injury. J Trauma 28:1656–1659, 1988.

79. Merrell SW, Saffle JR, Sullivan JJ, et al: Fluid resuscitation in thermally injured children. Am J Surg 152:664–669, 1986.

80. Puffinbarger NK, Tuggle DW, Smith EI: Rapid isotonic fluid resuscitation in pediatric thermal injury. J Pediatr Surg 29:339–341, 1994.

81. Warden GD: Burn shock resuscitation. World J Surg 16:16–23, 1992.

82. Bowser-Wallace BH, Caldwell FT Jr: Fluid requirements of severely burned children up to 3 years old: Hypertonic lactated saline vs. Ringer's lactate-colloid. Burns 12:549–555, 1986.

83. McKee AC, Winkelman MD, Banker BQ: Central pontine myelinolysis in severely burned patients: Relationship to serum hyperosmolality. Neurology 38:1211–1217, 1988.

84. Bowser BH, Caldwell FT Jr: The effects of resuscitation with hypertonic vs. hypotonic vs. colloid on wound and urine fluid and electrolyte losses in severely burned children. J Trauma 23:916–923, 1983.

85. Navar PD, Saffle JR, Warden GD: Effect of inhalation injury on fluid resuscitation requirements after thermal injury. Am J Surg 150:716–720, 1985.

86. Hildreth MA, Herndon DN, Parks DH, et al: Evaluation of a caloric requirement formula in burned children treated with early excision. J Trauma 27:188–189, 1987.

87. Burke JF, Quinby WC, Bondoc CC: Primary excision and prompt grafting as routine therapy for the treatment of thermal burns in children. Hand Clin 6:305–317, 1990.

88. Bonate PL: Pathophysiology and pharmacokinetics following burn injury. Clin Pharmacokinet 18:118–130, 1990.

89. Jahoor F, Desai M, Herndon DN, et al: Dynamics of the protein metabolic response to burn injury. Metabolism 37:330–337, 1988.

90. Crum RL, Dominic W, Hansbrough JF, et al: Cardiovascular and neurohumeral responses following burn injury. Arch Surg 125:1065–1069, 1990.

91. Wolfe RR, Herndon DN, Jahoor F, et al: Effect of severe burn injury on substrate cycling by glucose and fatty acids. N Engl J Med 317:403–408, 1987.

92. Wolfe RR, Herndon DN, Peters EJ, et al: Regulation of lipolysis in severely burned children. Ann Surg 206:214–221, 1987.

93. Cunningham JJ, Lydon MK, Russell WE: Calorie and protein provision for recovery from severe burns in infants and young children. Am J Clin Nutr 51:553–557, 1990.

94. Sarubin J: Increased requirement of alcuronium in burned patients. Anaesthesist 31:392–395, 1982.

95. Matsuda T, Clark N, Hariyani GD, et al: The effect of burn wound size on resting energy expenditure. J Trauma 27:115–118, 1987.

96. Allard JP, Pichard C, Hoshino E, et al: Validation of a new formula for calculating the energy requirements of burn patients. JPEN J Parenter Enteral Nutr 14:115–118, 1990.

97. Allard JP, Jeejheebhoy KN, Whitwell J, et al: Factors influencing energy expenditure in patients with burns. J Trauma 28:199–202, 1988.

98. Gore DC, Rutan RL, Hildreth M, et al: Comparison of resting energy expenditures and caloric intake in children with severe burns. J Burn Care Rehabil 11:400–404, 1990.

99. Goran MI, Broemeling L, Herndon DN, et al: Estimating energy requirements in burned children: A new approach derived from measurements of resting energy expenditure. Am J Clin Nutr 54:35–40, 1991.

100. Trocki O, Michelini JA, Robbins ST: Evaluation of early enteral feeding in children less than 3 years old with smaller burns (8–25 percent TBSA). Burns 21:17–23, 1995.

101. Hildreth MA, Herndon DN, Desai MH, et al: Current treatment reduces calories required to maintain weight in pediatric patients with burns. J Burn Care Rehabil 11:405–409, 1990.

102. O'Neil CE, Hutsler D, Hildreth MA: Basic nutritional guidelines for pediatric burn patients. J Burn Care Rehabil 10:278–284, 1989.

103. Baxter CR: Metabolism and nutrition in burned patients. Compr Ther 13:36–42, 1987.

104. Gottschlich MM, Jenkins M, Warden GD, et al: Differential effects of three enteral regimens on selected outcome variables. Procedures Am Soc Parent Enterol Nutr 14:225–236, 1990.

105. Alexander JW, Gottschlich MM: Nutritional immunomodulation in burn patients. Crit Care Med 18:149–153, 1990.

106. Jenkins M, Gottschlich M, Alexander JW, et al: Effect of immediate enterol feeding on the hypermetabolic response following severe burn injury. 13th Clinical Congress Program Book. American Society of Parenteral Enterol Nutrition, Silver Spring, MD, 1989.

107. Alexander JW, MacMillan BG, Stinnett JD, et al: Beneficial effects of aggressive protein feeding in severely burned children. Ann Surg 192:505–517, 1980.

108. Greenhalgh DG, Housinger TA, Kagan RJ, et al: Maintenance of serum albumin levels in pediatric burn patients: a prospective, randomized trial. J Trauma 39:67–73, 1995.

109. Phillips LG, Robson MC, Smith DJ, et al: Uses and abuses of a biosynthetic dressing for partial skin thickness burns. Burns 15:254–256, 1989.

110. Patterson DR, Questad KA, Boltwood MD: Hypnotherapy as a treatment for pain in patients with burns: research and clinical considerations. J Burn Care Rehabil 8:263–268, 1987.

111. Deitch EA, Wheelahan TM, Rose MP, et al: Hypertrophic burn scars: Analysis of variables. J Trauma 23:895–898, 1983.

112. Wachtel TL: Topical antimicrobials. In Carvajal HT, Parks DH (eds). Burns in Children: Pediatric Burn Management. Chicago, Year Book Medical Publishers, 1988, pp 106–118.

113. Miller L, Hansbrough J, Slater H, et al: Sildimac: A new delivery system for silver sulfadiazine in the treatment of full-thickness burn injuries. J Burn Care Rehabil 11:35–41, 1990.

114. Monafo WW, West MA: Current treatment recommendations for topical burn therapy. Drugs 40:364–373, 1990.

115. Gunji H, Ono I, Tateshita T, et al: Clinical effectiveness of an ointment containing prostaglandin E1 for the treatment of burn wounds. Burns 22:399–405, 1996.

116. Sheridan RL, Petras L, Lydon M, Salvo PM: Once-daily wound cleansing and dressing change: Efficacy and cost. J Burn Care Rehabil 18:139–140, 1997.

117. Beasley RW: Secondary repair of burned hands. Hand Clin 6:319–341, 1990.

118. Michielsen D, Van Hee R, Neetens C, et al: Burns to the genitals and the perineum in children. Br J Urol 78:940–941, 1996.

119. Renz BM, Sherman R: Exposure of buttock burn wounds to stool in scald-abused infants and children: Stool-staining of eschar and burn wound sepsis. Am Surg 59:379–383, 1993.

120. Mannis MJ, Miller RB, Krachmer JH: Contact thermal burns of the cornea from electric curling irons. Am J Ophthalmol 98:336–339, 1984.

121. Herndon DN, Barrow RE, Kunkel KR, et al: Effects of recombinant human growth hormone on donor-site healing in severely burned children. Ann Surg 212:424–431, 1990.

122. Van der Does AJW: Patients' and nurses' ratings of pain and anxiety during burn wound care. Pain 39:95–101, 1989.

123. Osgood PF, Szyfelbein SK: Management of burn pain in children. Pediatr Clin North Am 36:1001–1013, 1989.

124. Choiniere M, Melzack R, Rondeau J, et al: The pain of burns: Characteristics and correlates. J Trauma 29:1531–1539, 1989.

125. Atchison NE, Osgood PF, Carr DB, Szyfelbein SK: Pain during burn dressing change in children: relationship to burn area, depth and analgesic regimens. Pain 47:41–45, 1991.

126. Ashburn MA: Burn pain: The management of procedure-related pain. J Burn Care Rehabil 16:365–371, 1995.

127. Lewis SM, Clelland JA, Knowles CJ, et al: Effects of auricular acupuncture-like transcutaneous electric nerve stimulation on pain levels following wound care in patients with burns: A pilot study. J Burn Care Rehabil 11:322–329, 1990.

128. Humphries Y, Melson M, Gore D: Superiority of oral ketamine as an analgesic and sedative for wound care procedures in the pediatric patient with burns. J Burn Care Rehabil 18:34–36, 1997.

129. Gaukroger PB: Paediatric analgesia. Which drug? Which dose? Drugs 41:52–59, 1991.

130. Martyn JA, Greenblatt DJ, Hagen J, et al: Alteration by burn injury of the pharmacokinetics and pharmacodynamics of cimetidine in children. Eur J Clin Pharmacol 36:361–367, 1989.

131. Mills AK, Martyn JA: Neuromuscular blockade with vecuronium in paediatric patients with burn injury. Br J Clin Pharmacol 28:155–159, 1989.

132. D'Eramo C, Stocchetti N, Vezzani A: Clinical evaluation of atracurium besylate in patients at risk: Major burns. Minerva Anestesiol 56:121–125, 1990.

133. Martyn JA, Goudsouzian NG, Matteo RS, et al: Metocurine requirements and plasma concentrations in burned paediatric patients. Br J Anaesth 55:263–268, 1983.

134. Mills AK, Martyn JA: Evaluation of atracurium neuromuscular blockade in paediatric patients with burn injury. Br J Anaesth 60:450–455, 1988.

135. Cote CJ, Petkau AJ: Thiopental requirements may be increased in children reanesthetized at least one year after recovery from extensive thermal injury. Anesth Analg 64:1156–1160, 1985.

136. Brown TC, Bell B: Electromyographic responses to small doses of suxamethonium in children after burns. Br J Anaesth 59:1017–1021, 1987.

137. McCauley RL, Beraja V, Rutan RL, et al: Longitudinal assessment of breast development in adolescent female patients with burns involving the nipple-aerolar complex. Plast Reconstr Surg 83:676–680, 1989.

138. Balogh D, Bauer M, Hortnagl H: Effect of surgery and anesthesia on the plasma catecholamine level and rate of urea production in severely burned patients. Anaesthesist 32:105–110, 1983.

139. Heimbach DM: Early burn excision and grafting. Surg Clin North Am 67:93–107, 1987.

140. Chicarilli ZN, Cuono CB, Heinrich JJ, et al: Selective aggressive burn excision for high mortality subgroups. J Trauma 26:18–25, 1986.

141. Herndon DN, Barrow RE, Rutan RL, et al: A comparison of conservative versus early excision. Therapies in severely burned patients. Ann Surg 209:547–553, 1989.

142. Clarke H, Wittpenn GP, McLeod AM, et al: Acute management of pediatric hand burns. Hand Clin 6:221–231, 1990.

143. Boswick JA: Management of the burned hands. Hand Clin 6:297–303, 1990.

144. Desai MH, Herndon DN, Broemeling L, et al: Early burn wound excision significantly reduces blood loss. Ann Surg 211:753–762, 1990.

145. Herndon DN, Parks DH: Comparison of serial debridement and autografting and early massive excision with cadaver skin overlay in the treatment of large burns in children. J Trauma 26:149–152, 1986.

146. Dye DJ: Requirements for cross-matched blood in burns surgery. Burns 19:524–528, 1993.

147. Budny PG, Regan PJ, Roberts AH: The estimation of blood loss during burns surgery. Burns 19:134–137, 1993.

148. Abston S, Bonds E, et al: The optimal time for excision of scald burns in toddlers. J Burn Care Rehabil 7:508–510, 1986.

149. Fraulin FO, Illmayer SJ, Tredget EE: Assessment of cosmetic and functional results of conservative versus surgical management of facial burns. J Burn Care Rehabil 17:19–29, 1996.

150. Martinot V, Mitchell V, Fevrier P, et al: Comparative study of split thickness skin grafts taken from the scalp. Burns 20:146–150, 1994.

151. Ricks NR, Meagher DP Jr: The benefits of plaster casting for lower-extremity burns after grafting in children. J Burn Care Rehabil 13:465–468, 1992.

152. Soeda J, Inokuchi S, Ueno S, et al: Use of cultured human epidermal allografts for the treatment of extensive partial thickness scald burn in children. Toaki J Exp Clin Med 18:65–70, 1993.

153. Gobet R, Raghunath M, Altermatt S: Efficacy of cultured epithelial autografts in pediatric burns and reconstructive surgery. Surgery 121:654–661, 1997.

154. Phipps AR, Clarke JA: The use of intermingled autograft and parental allograft skin in the treatment of major burns in children. Br J Plast Surg 44:608–611, 1991.

155. Herndon DN, Thompson PB, Hugo AL, et al: Incidence, mortality, pathogenesis and treatment of pulmonary injury. J Burn Care Rehabil 7:184–191, 1986.

156. Herndon DN, Barrow RE, Linares HA, et al: Inhalation injury in burned patients: Effects and treatment. Burns 14:349–356, 1988.

157. Waxman K: Pulmonary management. In Achauer BM (ed). Management of the Burned Patient. Norwalk, CT, Appleton & Lange, 1987, pp 149–160.

158. Deskin RWQ, McCracken MM, Hokanson JA, et al: Long-term airway sequelae in a pediatric burn population. Laryngoscope 98:721–725, 1988.

159. Shirani KZ, Pruitt BA, Mason AD: The influence of inhalation injury and pneumonia on burn mortality. Ann Surg 205:82–87, 1987.

160. Thompson PB, Herndon DN, Traber DL, et al: Effect on mortality of inhalation injury. J Trauma 26:163–165, 1986.

161. Ruddy RM: Smoke inhalation injury. Pediatr Clin North Am 41:317–336, 1994.

162. Burns TR, Greenberg SD, Cartwright J, et al: Smoke inhalation: An ultrastructural study of reaction to injury in the human alveolar wall. Environ Res 41:447–457, 1986.

163. Silverman SH, Purdue FG, Hunt JL, et al: Cyanide toxicity in burn patients. J Trauma 28:171–176, 1988.

164. Crapo RO: Causes of respiratory injury. In Haponik EF, Munster AM (eds). Respiratory Injury Smoke Inhalation and Burns. New York, McGraw-Hill, 1990, pp 47–59.

165. Parish RA: Smoke inhalation and carbon monoxide poisoning in children. Pediatr Emerg Care 2:36–39, 1986.
166. Traber DL, Herndon DN: Pathophysiology of smoke inhalation. In Haponik EF, Munster AM (eds). Respiratory Injury Smoke Inhalation and Burns. New York, McGraw-Hill, 1990, pp 61–71.
167. Blinn DL, Slater H, Goldfarb IW: Inhalation injury with burns: A lethal combination. J Emerg Med 6:471–473, 1988.
168. Hudson DA, Jones L, Rode H: Respiratory distress secondary to scalds in children. Burns 20:434–437, 1994.
169. Herndon DN, Langner F, Thompson P, et al: Pulmonary injury in burned patients. Surg Clin North Am 67:31–46, 1987.
170. Heggers JP, Muller MJ, Elwood E, et al: Ascariasis pneumonitis: A potentially fatal complication in smoke inhalation injury. Burns 21:149–151, 1995.
171. Reynolds EM, Ryan DP, Doody DP: Mortality and respiratory failure in a pediatric burn population. J Pediatr Surg 28:1326–1331, 1993.
172. Kemper KJ, Izenberg S, Marvin JA, et al: Treatment of post-extubation stridor in a pediatric patient with burns: The role of heliox. J Burn Care Rehabil 11:337–339, 1990.
173. Kemper KJ, Ritz RH, Benson MS, et al: Helium-oxygen mixture in the treatment of postextubation stridor in pediatric trauma patients. Crit Care Med 19:356–359, 1991.
174. Rosenberg DB: Neurologic sequelae of minor electric burns. Arch Phys Med Rehabil 70:914–915, 1989.
175. Gordon MWG, Reid WH, Awwaad AM: Electrical burns—incidence and prognosis in western Scotland. Burns 12:254–259, 1986.
176. Garcia CT, Smith GA, Cohen DM, et al: Electrical injuries in a pediatric emergency department. Ann Emerg Med 26:604–608, 1995.
177. Wallace BH, Cone JB, Vanderpool RD, et al: Retrospective evaluation of admission criteria for paediatric electrical injuries. Burns 21:590–593, 1995.
178. Sadove AM, Jones JE, Lynch TR, et al: Appliance therapy for perioral electrical burns: A conservative approach. J Burn Care Rehabil 9:391–395, 1988.
179. Hanumadass ML, Voora SB, Kagan RJ, et al: Acute electrical burns: A 10 year clinical experience. Burns 12:427–431, 1986.
180. Pensler JM, Rosenthal A: Reconstruction of the oral commissure after an electrical burn. J Burn Care Rehabil 11:50–53, 1990.
181. Vorhies JM: Electrical burns of the oral commissure. Angle Orthod 57:2–17, 1987.
182. Palin WE, Sadove AM, Jones JE, et al: Oral electrical burns in a pediatric population. J Oral Med 42:17–34, 1987.
183. Schneider PE: Infant commissural burn management with reverse pull headgear. Pediatr Dent 10:34–38, 1988.
184. al-Qattan MM, Gillett D, Thompson HG: Electrical burns to the oral commissure: Does splinting obviate the need for commissuroplasty? Burns 22:555–556, 1996.
185. Canady JW, Thompson SA, Bardach J: Oral commissure burns in children. Plast Reconstr Surg 97:738–755, 1996.
186. Thomas SS: Electrical burns of the mouth: Still searching for an answer. Burns 22:137–140, 1996.
187. Ahrenholz DH, Schubert W, Solem LD: Creatine kinase as a prognostic indicator in electrical injury. Surgery 104:741–747, 1988.
188. Hunt J, Lewis S, Parkey R, et al: The use of technetium-99m stannous pyrophosphate scintigraphy to identify muscle damage in acute electric burns. J Trauma 19:409–413, 1979.
189. Hergrueter CA, O'Connor NE: Skin substitutes in upper extremity burns. Hand Clin 6:239–242, 1990.
190. Egan WC, Clark WR: The toxic shock syndrome in a burn victim. Burns 14:135–138, 1988.
191. Leicht P, Siim E, Dreyer M, et al: Duoderm application on scalp donor sites in children. Burns 17:230–232, 1991.
192. Bishop JF: Pediatric considerations in the use of Biobrane in burn wound management. J Burn Care Rehabil 16:331–334, 1995.
193. Abdullah A, Blakeney P, Hunt R, et al: Visible scars and self-esteem in pediatric patients with burns. J Burn Care Rehabil 15:164–168, 1994.
194. Blakeney P, Meyer W, Moore P, et al: Psychosocial sequelae of pediatric burns involving 80% or greater total body surface area. J Burn Care Rehabil 14:684–689, 1993.
195. Winkelman MD, Galloway PG: Central nervous system complications of thermal burns. A postmortem study of 139 patients. Medicine 71:271–283, 1992.
196. Schlager T, Sadler J, Weber D, et al: Hospital-acquired infections in pediatric burn patients. South Med J 87:481–484, 1987.
197. Askew AA, Tuggle DW, Judd T, et al: Improvement in catheter sepsis rate in burned children. J Pediatr Surg 25:117–119, 1990.
198. Dacso CC, Luterman A, Curreri PW: Systemic antibiotic treatment in burned patients. Surg Clin North Am 67:57–68, 1987.
199. Parish RA, Novack AH, Heimbach DM, et al: Fever as a predictor of infection in burned children. J Trauma 27:69–71, 1987.
200. Aikawa N, Shinozawa Y, Ishibiki K, et al: Clinical analysis of multiple organ failure in burned patients. Burns 13:103–109, 1987.
201. McAllister RM, Mercer NS, Morgan BD, et al: Early diagnosis of staphylococcal toxaemia in burned children. Burns 19:22–25, 1993.
202. Purdue GF, Hunt JL: Pulmonary emboli in burned patients. J Trauma 28:218–220, 1988.
203. Greenhalgh DG, Warden GD: The importance of intra-abdominal pressure measurements in burned children. J Trauma 36:685–690, 1994.
204. Smith CJ, Smith JC, Finn MC: The possible role of mast cells (allergy) in the production of keloid and hypertrophic scarring. J Burn Care Rehabil 8:126–131, 1987.
205. Blassingame WM, Bennett GB, Helm PA, et al: Range of motion of the shoulder performed while patient is anesthetized. J Burn Care Rehabil 10:539–542, 1989.
206. Bartle EJ, Sun JH, Wang XW, et al: Cancers arising from burn scars: A literature review and report of twenty-one cases. J Burn Care Rehabil 11:46–49, 1990.
207. Tompkins RG, Remensnyder JP, Burke JF, et al: Significant reductions in mortality for children with burn injuries through the use of prompt eschar excision. Ann Surg 208:577–585, 1988.
208. Wolf SE, Rose JK, Desai MH, et al: Mortality determinants in massive pediatric burns. An analysis of 103 children with > or = 80% TBSA burns (> or = 70% full-thickness). Ann Surg 225:554–569, 1997.
209. Erickson EJ, Merrell SW, Saffle JR, et al: Differences in mortality from thermal injury between pediatric and adult patients. J Pediatr Surg 26:821–825, 1991.
210. Morrow SE, Smith DL, Cairns BA, et al: Etiology and outcome of pediatric burns. J Pediatr Surg 31:329–333, 1996.
211. Thomson PD, Bowden ML, McDonald K, et al: Survival of an infant with massive thermal injury: A case report. Burns 15:171–174, 1989.
212. Renz BM, Sherman R: The burn unit experience at Grady Memorial Hospital: 844 cases. J Burn Care Rehabil 13:426–436, 1992.
213. Carlson RG, Miller SF, Finley RK, et al: Fluid retention and burn survival. J Trauma 27:127–135, 1987.
214. Barrow RE, Herndon DN: Incidence of mortality in boys and girls after severe thermal burns. Surg Gynecol Obstet 170:295–298, 1990.
215. Durtschi MB, Kohler TR, Finley A, et al: Burn injury in infants and young children. Surg Gynecol Obstet 150:651–656, 1980.
216. Erdmann TC, Feldman KW, Rivara FP, et al: Tap water burn prevention: The effect of legislation. Pediatrics 88:572–577, 1991.
217. Prescott PR: Hair dryer burns in children. Pediatrics 86:692–697, 1990.
218. Locke JA, Rossignol AM, Boyle CM, et al: Socioeconomic factors and burn rates in persons hospitalized for burns in Massachusetts. Public Health Rep 101:389–395, 1986.

15

INITIAL HOSPITAL ASSESSMENT AND MANAGEMENT OF THE TRAUMA PATIENT

Max L. Ramenofsky, MD • Brian F. Gilchrist, MD

There is no sorrow like a parent's sorrow when his or her child has been killed or maimed by injury.[1-3] The physical and emotional pain that results from injuries to children has spurred many investigators to catalog, register, and analyze the patterns of childhood trauma.[4-8] The a priori assumption has been that understanding the dynamics of pediatric trauma will lead to the prevention of such trauma.[9, 10] Today we are cognizant of the many facets of pediatric trauma, yet trauma to children continues unabated.[11, 12] The cost to society is beyond measure, and the emotional losses are staggering.

Trauma, especially intentional trauma to the young, is a reflection of societal health. At present in the United States, there are two types of cities: the shining city atop the hill of opportunity, described by Ronald Reagan,[13] and the city of the disenfranchised and unwashed, so eloquently depicted by Mario Cuomo.[14] Trauma lurks in both these cities but in different guises. Although our nation has not been the scene of pitched battles since the War Between the States, we are now involved in what has been described as an "uncivil war."[15] This modern day war kills children with guns, knives, and drugs[16-20] in the inner city and kills with drugs, alcohol, and motor vehicles in the suburbs.[20-22] Trauma to children cannot be stopped by cerebral understanding; rather, the answer to this problem lies in the nation's ability to define its values and priorities.

☐ History

Trauma care has, in some minds, been the only benefit of warfare. Trauma care has improved most conspicuously because of lessons learned in battle. Every conflict, from Carthage to Kuwait, has re-sulted in advances in communications and transportation that have ultimately improved care to the injured, not all of whom were soldiers. The principle of total war, well articulated by General William Tecumseh Sherman, involved entire populations unrelated to combat.[23] The expanding scope of war necessitated the training of personnel who could manage complex trauma injuries in both civilians and combatants. Trauma surgeons, from Napoleon's Baron Larry to Vietnam's Norman Rich, fostered the evolution of trauma care.[24-26] Civilian trauma care now often mirrors the care of battle injuries, especially in the urban United States.

The care of injured children has quite logically followed the same evolutionary progression. Many pediatric surgeons have contributed to the development of the modern-day pediatric trauma surgeon. Although what is generally acknowledged as the first civilian trauma unit was established at Chicago's Cook County Hospital in 1968 in response to the 1966 publication of the National Academy of Science's white paper, *Accidental Death and Disability: The Neglected Disease of Modern Society*,[27] Peter Kottmeier had established the first pediatric trauma unit at King's County Hospital in Brooklyn 6 years before. The development of units that provided care for injured children lagged behind those for adults. Organized pediatric trauma care is now recognized as a significant need, because trauma is the leading cause of death and disability in the childhood age group. The American College of Surgeons (ACS) in 1990 published *Resources for Optimal Care of the Injured Patient,* which set forth the requirements for pediatric trauma centers.[28] Subsequently, two different types of pediatric trauma centers were developed: the regional resource pediatric trauma center and the adult trauma center with pediatric commitment. Most pediatric regional resource centers are located in children's hospitals,

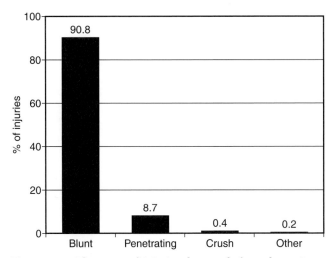

Figure 15–1. The types of injuries that result from the various injuring mechanisms (n = 77,904). (Adapted from the National Pediatric Trauma Registry Biannual Report, October 1997.)

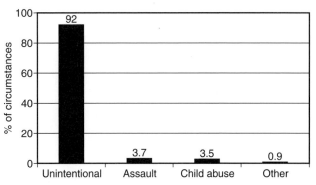

Figure 15–2. The most common form of injury in childhood is nonintentional. Assaults and child abuse are closely matched (n = 77,904). (Adapted from the National Pediatric Trauma Registry Biannual Report, October 1997.)

whereas pediatric commitment centers are part of larger adult hospital trauma centers. The ACS standards are designed to ensure that care in either type of center is equivalent.

☐ Epidemiology of Childhood Injury: The National Pediatric Trauma Registry

The epidemiology of pediatric injury has been most accurately described by the National Pediatric Trauma Registry (NPTR).[29] The NPTR first started collecting data on injured children in 1984 and has reported these data to the medical community and the public. Before the inception of the NPTR, few accurate pediatric injury data were available.

The NPTR is a database of injured children that is supported by the United States Department of Education. Currently, there are 80 medical centers

in the United States and Canada that provide data to the national center. As of October 1997, there were 77,904 patients with complete records in the registry.[30]

Reports are provided to participating centers at least twice yearly. The database is available to these institutions to use for research purposes at no cost. Examples of NPTR demographic reports are seen in Figures 15–1 to 15–8 and Table 15–1.

The mechanisms of injury identified in the NPTR reveal that the majority of injuries result from blunt mechanisms, although penetrating trauma has been increasing in large urban areas (Fig. 15–1). Nonintentional injuries are the most common form of trauma to children, followed by assaults and child abuse (Fig. 15–2). Specific mechanisms of injury are depicted in Figure 15–3. The automobile continues to represent the most lethal single element of the child's environment, accounting for 46% of all injuries in the pediatric age group.

Figure 15–4 depicts the body regions injured in children suffering trauma. Of note is the fact that nearly 50% of injured, hospitalized children have multisystem injury. The overall death rate in hospitalized children from injury is 3.2%, which is sig-

Figure 15–3. The specific mechanisms of injury. The automobile is the single greatest threat to the well-being of the child and is represented in the first four columns (n = 77,904). GSW, gunshot wound; intent., intentional; MCY, motorcycle; MVA, motor vehicle accident; SW, stab wound; unintent., unintentional. (Adapted from the National Pediatric Trauma Registry Biannual Report, October 1997.)

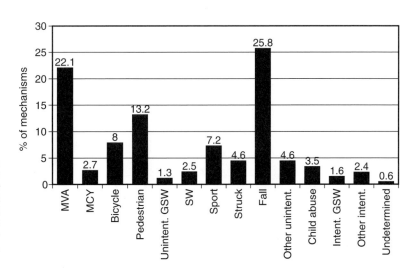

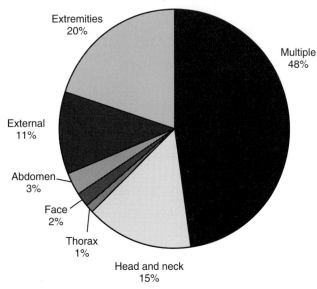

Figure 15–4. The regions of the body that have been injured. Notable is the very high frequency of multiple system injury (n = 77,904). (Adapted from the National Pediatric Trauma Registry Biannual Report, October 1997.)

TABLE 15–1. Pediatric Trauma Score

Component	Variable		
	+2	+1	−1
Size	>20 kg	10–20 kg	<10 kg
Airway status	Normal	Maintainable	Unmaintainable
CNS status	Awake	Obunded	Comatose
Systolic BP	>90 mm Hg	50–90 mm Hg	<50 mm Hg
Open wounds	None	Minor	Major or penetrating
Fractures	None	Single closed fracture	Open or multiple fractures

BP, blood pressure; CNS, central nervous system.

nificantly less than the death rate in hospitalized, injured adults. Figure 15–5 depicts the death rate in children from various, specific mechanisms.

PEDIATRIC TRAUMA SCORE. Data from the NPTR allowed the development of a pediatric trauma score (PTS). Six components were identified by multiple regression analysis as being the most predictive of death and disability:

1. Size (weight and age)
2. Respiratory status
3. Systolic blood pressure
4. Central nervous system (CNS) status
5. Open wounds
6. Presence of fractures

Each component is scored in one of three variable categories according to the severity of injury:

+2 = Minor or no injury
+1 = Major injury
−1 = Critical, potentially life-threatening injury

These points are arranged in the form of a table for ease of scoring (Table 15–1). One variable is circled for each component, and all columns are added. The PTS ranges from +12, which indicates no or minor injury, to −6, which represents a fatal injury. The lower the PTS, the more severe the injury. An inverse linear correlation exists between the PTS and mortality (Table 15–2).[31] The higher mortality rates equate with lower pediatric trauma scores.

The PTS can be used as a simple yet effective triage tool. No deaths are reported in patients with a PTS of 9 or greater. The possibility of death starts at a PTS of 8 and becomes progressively greater the lower the score (see Table 15–1). A PTS of 8 has been defined as the critical triage point.[32] The use of this scoring mechanism has resulted in 25% of patients being sent to an institution providing the highest level of care.

CAUSES OF DEATH. Head injury is known to be the major cause of death in childhood. The NPTR has also shown that although CNS injury is the one injury that most commonly results in death, it is not

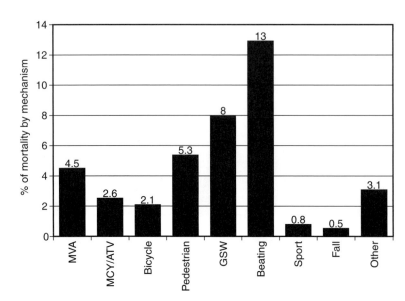

Figure 15–5. The frequency of death from the various specific injuring mechanisms. Again shown in the first four columns is the death rate from the automobile (n = 77,904). GSW, gunshot wound; MCY/ATV, motorcycle/all-terrain vehicle; MVA, motor vehicle accident. (Adapted from the National Pediatric Trauma Registry Biannual Report, October 1997.)

TABLE 15–2. Pediatric Trauma Score Cohort Distribution and Associated Mortality*

PTS Cohort	Mortality (%)	Distribution (%)
< −2	96.6	0.21
−1–0	70.9	0.78
1–2	39.3	1.49
3–4	28.1	2.54
5–6	11.7	5.45
7–8	0.9	14.63
9–10	0.1	30.56
11–12	0.0	44.3

*This table indicates the inverse linear relationship between the pediatric trauma score and mortality. Note the sharp, progressive increase in mortality at a PTS of 8. Data from 25,760 patients from the National Pediatric Trauma Registry.
PTS, pediatric trauma score.

necessarily the primary head injury that causes the death.[33, 34] Secondary CNS injury, or the injury that results when hypovolemic shock or hypoxia is not treated in a rapid and appropriate fashion, results in death as commonly as does primary CNS injury.[35]

The cerebral perfusion pressure (CPP) is defined as the difference between the mean systolic blood pressure (mSBP) and intracranial pressure (ICP). The formula $CPP = mSBP - ICP$ defines this relationship. When the CPP drops below a critical value of 70 mm Hg, either because of a decrease in the blood pressure or an increase in the intracranial pressure, perfusion of the brain decreases. Should the blood perfusing the brain have a sudden and prolonged fall in partial pressure of oxygen (PO_2), the brain, which is an obligate aerobic organ, suffers secondary injury. The optimal method of caring for the injured brain is to ensure adequate perfusion of the brain with well-oxygenated blood.

The NPTR shows that half of the deaths that have been attributed to pure CNS injury are in fact caused by a secondary CNS injury, which results from inappropriate early trauma care.

MORTALITY AND SURVIVAL. Overall mortality from injury in the pediatric age group has been well documented in the NPTR. Annually, 22,000 children die of injuries, which amounts to 1.9% of all injured children. However, 3.2% of hospitalized children die of their injuries. The difference represents those who die before entering the health care system, for example, on the scene.

Outcome assessment in pediatric trauma patients has been hampered by norms developed for adults. The science of trying to evaluate the effect of the injury itself or the effectiveness of treatment has also been limited by using mortality data. Because the mortality rate in injured children is quite low (3.2%), using mortality as a measure of outcome, which requires large numbers of children, has not provided useful information.

NPTR data, which have provided information on injury outcome defined as the number of functional limitations at the time of discharge from the hospital, have allowed much better evaluation of therapeutic intervention. Fifty-eight percent of hospitalized, injured children are discharged with no limitation of their functional activities[30] (Fig. 15–6). Thirty-four percent of children are discharged with 1 to 3 limitations and 5% with 4 to 10 limitations. Figure 15–7 provides an indication of organ-specific limitations resulting from either the injury itself or therapy of the injury. Figure 15–8 depicts the specifics of limited functions based on the number of limitations at discharge. It is evident that children who have from 4 to 10 limitations have usually had head injuries, whereas children discharged with 1 to 3 limitations usually have orthopedic injuries, which heal in time.

Finally, the 3.2% mortality among injured children compared with the 10% adult mortality rate implies that the current outcome in pediatric trauma management is satisfactory. Evaluation of outcome for the injured child is generally done by close scrutiny of the patient's chart in an attempt to identify errors in the continuum of care.

☐ Advanced Trauma Life Support Course of the American College of Surgeons

Trauma care in the United States and subsequently throughout much of the rest of the world improved dramatically in 1978. A small group of dedicated surgeons in Lincoln, Nebraska, perceived the need for a simple, reproducible, and easily taught method of trauma care by which any physician could provide lifesaving care to a critically injured patient within the first hour after an injury. The perception of this need grew out of a personal tragedy of one of the surgeons. This individual recognized that care of the injured was poorly taught in medical schools and was poorly practiced in many

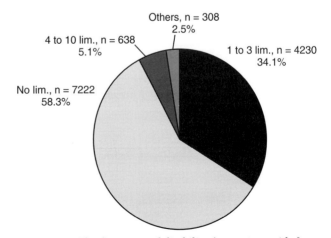

Figure 15–6. The frequency of disability (percentage with functional limitations) in a child at the time of discharge. Nearly 58% of children have no measurable disability on discharge from the hospital. The most severely disabled children are represented by 4 or more disabilities. lim., limitations. (Adapted from the National Pediatric Trauma Registry Biannual Report, October 1997.)

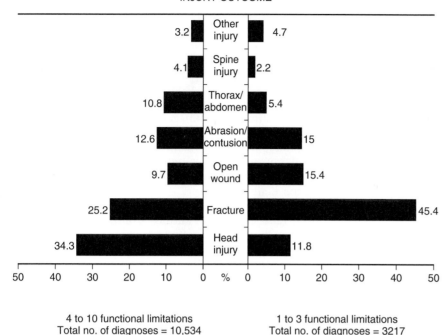

INJURY OUTCOME

4 to 10 functional limitations
Total no. of diagnoses = 10,534

1 to 3 functional limitations
Total no. of diagnoses = 3217

Figure 15–7. The specifics of the organ system disabled in the child is depicted by the number of disabilities found on discharge. (Adapted from the National Pediatric Trauma Registry Biannual Report, October 1997.)

regions of the United States. The ACS Advanced Trauma Life Support (ATLS) course for physicians was the result.[36]

The ATLS course has been taught throughout the United States and much of the developed world. More than 250,000 physicians have been trained to use the methods taught in the course. An outgrowth of ATLS is the Pre-Hospital Trauma Life Support Course of the National Association of Emergency Medical Technicians.

ATLS teaches the priorities of injury treatment based on those life-threatening injuries that kill and maim the quickest. For example, the patient does not benefit if a fractured extremity is treated in the presence of a compromised airway. The course teaches one method of stabilizing life-threatening injuries until the patient is given definitive care either in the physician's facility or elsewhere.

Priorities of treatment are temporally based on the injuries that kill the fastest. Untreated, the loss of the airway results in death in 3 to 4 minutes. If the airway is open and maintained, the inability to breathe results in death in 5 to 7 minutes. Severe, untreated, hypovolemic shock causes death in approximately 10 minutes. Thus, the simplistic use of the alphabet—ABCDE—defines the priorities of treatment:

A = Airway
B = Breathing
C = Circulation

INJURY OUTCOME

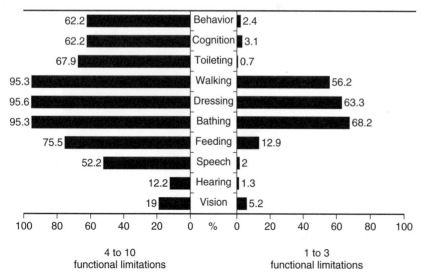

4 to 10
functional limitations

1 to 3
functional limitations

Figure 15–8. The specific disabilities noted at the time of discharge. Children with 1 to 3 disabilities have primarily orthopedic injuries that will heal in time, compared with those with 4 to 10 disabilities, which are primarily the result of head injuries. (Adapted from the National Pediatric Trauma Registry Biannual Report, October 1997.)

D = Disability (or brief neurologic status)

E = Expose (undress patient completely) and pay particular attention to the environment (avoid hypothermia from a cool room)

☐ Preplanning the Initial Assessment and Management of the Injured Child

Trauma is the quintessential surgical emergency. Traumatic incidents are unplanned and unanticipated and occur at the most inconvenient times. The trauma patient causes the orderly routine of a busy hospital to become disrupted. To minimize this disruption, a prearranged, well-conceived plan must be developed in a hospital that provides care for the injured.

An institution that elects to become an active participant in the trauma system and to treat injured children must develop a plan for providing appropriate therapy before the arrival of the first patient. The plan should include the identification, training, and provision of credentials for pediatric trauma personnel. There must also be a resuscitation area, the procurement of appropriate equipment, the installation of in-house and out-of-house communication equipment, and the participation in the local and regional emergency medical service system.[37]

There are six areas in any hospital where an injured child may be evaluated or treated:

Emergency department (resuscitation area)
Intensive care unit
Operating room
Pediatric unit
Radiology department
Rehabilitation medicine area

Within the first hour of care, the emergency department is often the most important.

Care of the trauma patient is best handled by a trauma team. A multidisciplinary trauma team is most effective in the care of an injured child. Members of the pediatric trauma team include a team leader, surgeons, emergency medicine physicians, surgical subspecialists, trauma nurses, and paramedical personnel.

The leader of the team should be a trauma surgeon, because trauma is a surgical disease and the pathophysiology of the disease is therefore most closely associated with surgical physiology. In the case of injured children, the trauma surgeon should have specific interest in pediatric trauma. The leader of the pediatric trauma team should act as the director of care. This individual is responsible for the overall evaluation of the child, ensuring that the child's evaluation and resuscitation move forward in a rapid, accurate manner. The leader is responsible for the synthesis of all incoming information and for the formulation of the short- and long-term care plans. The team leader must determine when resuscitation is adequate and when an operative procedure is needed. The team leader should coordinate the care suggested by the surgical subspecialists (e.g., orthopedics, neurosurgery), and, above all, be constantly aware of the child's overall status. The command surgeon may need to determine which operative procedure should take precedence over another, and on occasion, whether a certain procedure should be performed at all.[38]

The other members of the trauma team must be adequately trained in the care of the injured child. All specialists have generally been trained to consider the best approach to a given injury from their point of view. However, care that might be optimal for a single system injury may be disadvantageous if given in multisystem trauma. Thus, the specialist must agree to abide by the decisions of the command surgeon.

Regardless of the specialty, every member of the pediatric trauma team should have participated in the ATLS course. This type of training allows for better communication between various members of the team by ensuring that the priorities of the life-threatening injuries are well known and accepted by all. Nurses who function as members of the trauma team should have audited the ATLS course.

A designated and defined room must be available for the evaluation and resuscitation of the injured child. Generally, this room is located in the emergency department. It should be of adequate size to accommodate the trauma team and the equipment required for assessment and resuscitation.

Resuscitation rooms should have adequate lighting with operating room lights available. A method of controlling the ambient temperature for either the patient or the room is required. A large-volume, warming, rapid infusion device should be in the room at all times. Blood—specifically low-titer O, Rh-negative packed red blood cells—must be immediately available in the emergency department. Surgical supplies include sterile large-bore intravenous tubing, cutdown sets, thoracotomy sets, and thoracostomy tubes with water-seal devices.

Other equipment must include oxygen saturation and end-tidal carbon dioxide monitors in addition to multichannel physiologic monitors, an automatic blood pressure monitor, and cardiac defibrillation equipment. Equipment must be available for endotracheal intubation, cricothyroidotomy, and tracheostomy. The best available listing of required equipment is that published by the American College of Surgeons Committee on Trauma.[39]

☐ Initial Assessment of the Injured Child

THE PRIMARY SURVEY

The initial assessment of the injured child proceeds through the same ATLS steps mentioned above. However, there are a number of aspects of the ABCs that require a different approach in children. The primary survey has been designed to identify and treat life-threatening injuries.

Airway and Cervical Spine Control

When establishing an airway in a child it is imperative to assume that the cervical spine is unstable or fractured. Immobilization of the head and neck may prevent unintentional manipulation, which could result in an injury to the cervical spinal cord.

The single major life-threatening injury requiring early identification is airway obstruction. The approach to the child's airway requires knowledge of its anatomy. The supraglottic region in infancy and early childhood is quite narrow because of the presence of a large tongue and large amounts of tonsillar and adenoidal tissue. The larynx itself is small and soft and is located high and anterior in the neck. The vocal cords are oriented obliquely, with the anterior commissure being more cephalad. Occipital bossing of the head causes the supine child to lie in a slightly head-flexed position. All these factors combine to make the opening to the airway even smaller. Hyperflexion or hyperextension of the head on the neck both result in occlusion of the airway.

The first maneuver in airway management in the injured child is to clear the airway of blood, vomitus, and other material by gentle aspiration. Once the airway has been cleared, oxygen is provided regardless of the severity of injury.

The airway is opened by bringing the head slightly forward into the "sniffing" position, which draws the larynx away from its surrounding structures.

An oral airway is tolerated in the unconscious child but not in the child who is awake, because the child may vomit and aspirate. The curve of an oral airway is inserted to follow the curvature of the tongue in children. Nasopharyngeal airways are tolerable in the conscious child. Care must be taken to use the proper size tube and to ensure that the airway is passed downward to the pharynx beyond the adenoids.

If the airway can be opened and maintained by these methods, it is safe to progress to the assessment of the child's breathing. However, if the airway cannot be opened or maintained, or if there are injuries suspected by the history or physical examination that require ventilatory management, endotracheal intubation must be undertaken.

The trachea is approximately 5 cm long in a term infant. The trachea grows to 7.5 cm by 1½ years of age. The trachea and major bronchi in infancy and childhood are soft, compressible structures. The membranous trachea is thin and easily damaged. Once a child has ceased linear growth, the trachea and bronchi assume an adult structural and anatomic configuration.

Trauma centers most often use a protocol for endotracheal intubation, which is referred to as rapid sequence intubation (Fig. 15–9). This algorithm uses sedative and paralytic medications and is based on

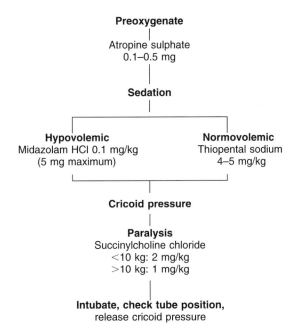

Preoxygenate
|
Atropine sulphate
0.1–0.5 mg
|
Sedation
|

Hypovolemic
Midazolam HCl 0.1 mg/kg
(5 mg maximum)

Normovolemic
Thiopental sodium
4–5 mg/kg
|
Cricoid pressure
|
Paralysis
Succinylcholine chloride
<10 kg: 2 mg/kg
>10 kg: 1 mg/kg
|
Intubate, check tube position,
release cricoid pressure

Figure 15–9. The protocol for rapid sequence intubation for the pediatric patient used in many trauma centers. (From ACS Committee on Trauma: *Advanced Trauma Life Support® Student Manual,* 1997 edition, p 294.)

the child's weight, pulse, blood pressure, and level of consciousness. Once these have been determined, the blood volume is estimated (hypovolemic vs. euvolemic), and the appropriate branch of the algorithm is selected. *Preoxygenation* is the first step, followed by administration of atropine to prevent bradycardia because the heart rate is the major determinant of the cardiac output in a child. *Sedation* is the next step. The choice of sedation medications depends on an estimate of the vascular volume. Because barbiturates such as thiopental cause hypotension in the hypovolemic patient, midazolam is the drug of choice for sedation in the hypovolemic child. The specific antidote for midazolam, flumazenil, should be immediately available. Following sedation, *cricoid pressure* must be maintained to reduce the potential complication of aspiration of gastric contents. *Paralysis* is accomplished with one of two agents. Succinylcholine is an ideal short-acting paralytic agent very suitable for intubation. If a longer period of paralysis is needed for computed tomography (CT) or other tests, vecuronium may be used. *Endotracheal intubation* is performed most often by the oral route. The tube position is verified by inspection, auscultation, and the cricoid pressure released. On occasion, if the endotracheal tube cannot be placed, bag-valve-mask ventilation may be carried out until a definitive airway can be secured. Cricoid pressure should be reinstituted at this time.

The size of the endotracheal tube is most critical when ventilation is required. *Cuffed endotracheal tubes are not used in children younger than 10 years because of the softness of the airway and the damage even a low-pressure cuff may cause.* The cricoid ring is the narrowest portion of the child's airway and serves the function of a cuff on the tube. Because of the ease with which the child's vocal cords can be damaged when an endotracheal tube is forced through the cords, a tube that easily passes the cords should be selected. The external diameter of an endotracheal tube, which is the same size as the child's small finger, is a general approximation of the appropriate tube size. There is a formula for determining tube size:

> For children older than 1 year: internal diameter of the endotracheal tube = 18 + patient's age in years ÷ 4
>
> For newborns and small infants: use a 3- to 3.5-mm tube
>
> For children in the first year of life: use a 4-mm tube

An air leak in an intubated, ventilated patient can be compensated by an increased tidal volume rather than replacement of the tube.

The endotracheal tube is easily passed too far into the trachea, resulting in mainstem bronchial intubation. Once the tube is inserted beyond the cords and secured, auscultation of the chest in both axillae is mandatory, and visual inspection of the chest helps to ensure adequate bilateral inflation of the lungs. A chest radiograph is obtained to confirm the position of the tube.

CERVICAL SPINE CONTROL. The spinal column of the child, like other portions of the bony skeleton, is softer and more pliable than that of an adult. The child's vertebrae are wedged anteriorly, the facet joints are flat, and ligamentous attachments are quite flexible. The anterior wedging gives rise to pseudosubluxation of C2 on C3 of the cervical vertebrae, which is seen only in the child (Figs. 15–10 and 15–11).

When dealing with a child's airway, a cervical spinal cord injury should be assumed. Excessive flexion or extension of the head on the neck can

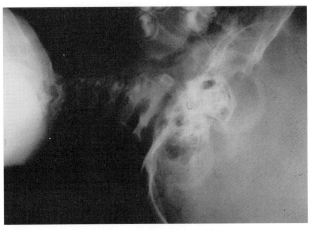

Figure 15–11. Radiograph of the same child as in Figure 15–10. The child's head has been placed in the "sniffing" position. The cervical vertebrae are now well aligned.

clearly result in damage to the spinal cord. Therefore, if it is assumed that there is a cervical spine injury, manual in-line immobilization of the head and neck should be provided when any airway is inserted. Cervical immobilization devices such as the cervical collar ("c-collar") are helpful but may not provide complete immobilization. Once a cervical collar has been applied, the entire child must be firmly attached to a long-spine board so that the head and neck do not move while the torso is immobilized.

Breathing

The chest injuries that can result in fatal cardiopulmonary compromise are:

- Tension pneumothorax
- Open pneumothorax
- Massive hemothorax
- Pericardial tamponade
- Flail chest
- Massive pulmonary contusion

Assessment of breathing in an injured child is often simple to evaluate because of the thin chest wall. Visual examination of the chest provides useful information on lung expansion. Auscultation of the lungs is best done in the child's axillae, because the chest wall is thin and these areas are the anatomic portions of the chest farthest from the major airways. Monitors are available that can accurately identify oxygen saturation and end-tidal carbon dioxide. These monitors should be used early in the primary survey.

The mediastinum of the child is mobile. Small differentials in intrapleural pressure result in the mediastinum moving to one side or the other. If sufficient displacement occurs, venous return to the heart is impeded. Thus, even a simple pneumothorax is potentially devastating to the child if not treated.

The presence of pneumothorax or hemothorax requires placement of a thoracostomy tube. A tension

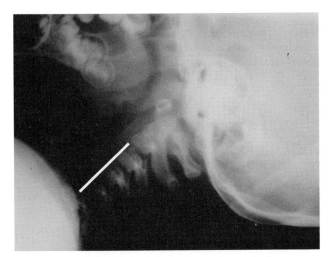

Figure 15–10. This lateral cervical spine radiograph shows pseudosubluxation of C2 on C3. Note the slight anterior displacement of C2 compared to a line drawn along the anterior borders of the seven cervical vertebral bodies *(arrow)*. Also note the slightly flexed position of the head on the neck.

pneumothorax is life threatening and requires immediate conversion of the tension to a simple pneumothorax. Pleural decompression is most efficiently achieved by the placement of an over-the-needle catheter into the second intercostal space in the midclavicular line. Relieving the tension pneumothorax in this manner allows definitive chest tube placement in a more orderly, sterile fashion. An open pneumothorax requires the placement of a chest tube and coverage of the open wound.

Treatment of flail chest in the child is aimed at treatment of the underlying pulmonary contusion. If the contusion is massive and ventilation is impaired, endotracheal intubation and mechanical ventilation are required. Inadequate ventilation because of the pain produced by a flail injury may be improved by intercostal nerve block.

Circulation

The blood volume of the child varies with age. Blood volume in the newborn is 90 ml/kg, falling to 80 ml/kg at 1 year of age, and reaching the adult value of 70 ml/kg in early adolescence.

The difference between the response of the cardiovascular system and volume loss in the very young child and the middle-aged adult is not in the mediators of the response to shock, but in the reactivity of the vessels and the heart. Aging results in atherosclerotic peripheral vascular disease and ischemic cardiac disease—both of which prevent the kind of response to hypovolemia that we see in children. Tachycardia is the simplest, clinically measurable response to the loss of 15 to 25% of the blood volume (Table 15–3). This is accompanied by a progressive decrease in cardiac output and an increase in peripheral vascular resistance. The young are able to maintain a relatively normal blood pressure in the presence of progressing hypovolemia because of the constriction of medium- to small-sized arteries. An infant or child maintains a near-normal blood pressure until the lost volume overcomes the ability of the peripheral vasculature to constrict. At this point, generally 40% blood volume loss, vascular constrictive ability is totally lost and

blood pressure rapidly falls. This is accompanied by a progressive bradycardia.

The organs of primary importance in hypovolemic shock are the heart, brain, kidneys, and skin. They can be used to monitor the volume status (see Table 15–3).

Assessment of the circulatory status of the injured patient includes an evaluation of the presence and quality of central and peripheral pulses, heart rate, capillary refill, skin color, and perfusion. Note should be made of the level of consciousness of the patient because hypovolemia results in a reduced level of consciousness (see Table 15–3). If shock is present, a urinary catheter should be inserted to monitor urine output.

Generally, direct pressure on the bleeding site is the preferred method of controlling bleeding. Blindly clamping injured tissue or using a tourniquet is not as effective. Intraabdominal bleeding from a fractured pelvis is difficult to control. Some evidence exists that the pneumatic antishock garment is of some help in controlling this type of bleeding.

Once the hemorrhage has been stopped, volume resuscitation proceeds in a much more orderly fashion. If the hemorrhage cannot be stopped, operative intervention is the most appropriate method of controlling the blood loss.

Pericardial tamponade is a condition seen primarily after penetrating thoracic injury. The signs and symptoms are typical of both hypovolemic shock and tension pneumothorax. As the pericardium fills with blood, the ability of the right side of the heart to fill is limited and, hence, cardiac output falls. At the same time, the jugular veins distend, because venous return to the right heart is impeded. Jugular venous distention is also seen in tension pneumothorax, because of the high ipsilateral intrapleural pressure. Heart tones are muffled, but Beck's triad is uncommonly seen. Treatment is by pericardiocentesis with an over-the-needle catheter, which is left in the pericardial sac for ongoing treatment on the way to the operating room.

Regardless of the estimated blood loss, large-bore intravenous lines should be inserted. Blood should

TABLE 15–3. Organ System Responses to Blood Loss in the Child

	Early (<25% Blood Volume Loss)	Prehypotensive (25% Blood Volume Loss)	Hypotensive (40% Blood Volume Loss)
Cardiac	Weak, thready pulse, increased heart rate	Increased heart rate, positive tilt test	Hypotension, tachycardia to bradycardia
CNS	Lethargic, irritable, confused, combative	Depressed level of consciousness, dulled response to pain	Comatose
Skin	Cool, clammy	Cyanotic, decreased capillary refill, cold extremities	
Kidneys	Decreased urinary output	Increased blood urea nitrogen	No urinary output
Fluid resuscitation	L/R, 20 ml/kg	L/R, 20 ml/kg (×3) PRBCs (10 ml/kg, ×1, ×2)	L/R, 20 ml/kg (×3) PRBCs (10 ml/kg) and to operating room

CNS, central nervous system; L/R, lactated Ringer's solution; PRBCs, packed red blood cells.

be drawn for typing, crossmatching, and other appropriate tests, and Ringer's lactate solution should be prepared for rapid infusion if necessary.

The sites for intravenous access in descending order of preference are as follows:

1. Percutaneous (upper extremity) peripheral
2. Interosseous
3. Venous cutdown (saphenous at the ankle)
4. Percutaneous (femoral vein)
5. Percutaneous subclavian vein
6. Percutaneous external jugular vein (cannot use with cervical collar)
7. Internal jugular vein (percutaneous or cutdown)

The initial infusion volume is based on replacing 25% of the child's blood volume. The initial bolus of 20 ml/kg of crystalloid frequently improves the child's hemodynamic status. Reassessment of the child's vital signs and peripheral perfusion will determine whether a second bolus of 20 ml/kg is needed. Continuous reassessment provides the guide to further therapy. If more volume is necessary, a third 20 ml/kg bolus is given and blood is readied for further needs.

Component therapy has replaced the use of whole blood in most hospitals today. Packed red blood cells (PRBCs) should be available in the trauma room. The initial volume of PRBCs to infuse is 10 ml/kg, which contains approximately the same oxygen-carrying capacity of 20 ml/kg whole blood. If type-specific blood is not immediately available, low-titer O-negative blood can be given. If it is necessary to use O-negative *whole blood* initially instead of O-negative PRBCs, it will be necessary to use O-negative blood or components throughout the period that the patient requires blood rather than changing to patient type-specific blood.[40] The original plasma portion of the O-negative whole blood will have provided enough antibody for massive hemolysis of transfused, type-specific blood to occur. Because the plasma is the antibody-carrying vehicle in this situation, O-negative PRBCs do not initiate this response.

The following are indications that volume resuscitation has been effective:

1. Slowing of the heart rate to less than 130 bpm with improvement in other physiologic signs
2. Increase in pulse pressure
3. Return of normal skin color
4. Increased extremity warmth
5. Clearing of the sensorium
6. Increase in systolic blood pressure (>80 mm Hg)
7. Increase in urine output to 1 to 2 ml/kg/hour (age dependent)

The child's hemodynamic response to fluid resuscitation can be categorized in one of three ways.

1. Normalization of vital signs with the use of only crystalloid fluid. This response represents the majority of children.
2. The requirement for blood in addition to crystalloid fluid to normalize the child's hemodynamic parameters.
3. A minority of children will respond only temporarily to crystalloid and blood or do not respond whatsoever. These children require operative intervention to stop the hemorrhage.

Figure 15–12 is a depiction of a resuscitation flow diagram with normal and abnormal hemodynamics. The major indication for operative intervention in the injured child is determined by the ability to rapidly and permanently correct abnormal hemodynamics.

Disability-Neurologic Assessment

The child's response to CNS injury is significantly different from that of an adult. Early responses from the injury include apnea, vomiting, and unconsciousness from even minor injury. Although these responses do occur in adults, the frequency is greater in children.

The lesions caused by the primary injury are also different qualitatively and quantitatively. Mass hemorrhagic lesions are less common in children, and simple concussions are more common. Subdural and epidural hematomas occur with a lower frequency than in adults. Children are more likely to develop subarachnoid hemorrhage manifested by headache, nuchal rigidity, and low-grade temperature elevation.

CNS injury can be mimicked by other organ system derangements. For example, the hypovolemic

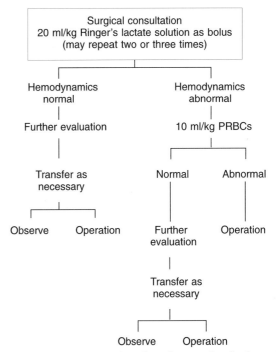

Figure 15–12. The resuscitation flow diagram for the hemodynamically normal and abnormal child. PRBCs, packed red blood cells. (From ACS Committee on Trauma: *Advanced Trauma Life Support® Student Manual,* 1997 edition, p 298.)

or hypoxic child does not manifest a normal level of consciousness. The simplest method of determining whether a child is suffering from blood volume loss or CNS injury is to normalize the ABCs.

Neurologic assessment in the primary survey is concerned with two areas: the level of consciousness and the status of the pupils. A Glasgow Coma Scale assessment is generally not done in the primary survey. The level of consciousness can be determined by evaluating the mnemonic AVPU:

A = Alert and oriented
V = Responds to verbal stimuli
P = Responds to painful stimuli
U = Unresponsive

Pupillary function is evaluated by determining their equality and responsiveness.

The treatment of primary CNS injury is initiated by assuring that the ABCs are well managed. A mild head injury can be made significantly worse by dealing directly with that injury before the ABCs of the patient have been evaluated and treated.[35]

The injured child must always be assumed to have suffered multisystem rather than single system injury. Although the CNS is the most frequently injured organ system that results in death of the child, the head injury is best treated by ensuring that the brain is well perfused with adequately oxygenated blood. Thus, the early treatment of primary head injury is actually the treatment of other organ system injuries that could result in hypoxia or hypovolemia.[33, 35]

Exposure and Environment

The injured child cannot be completely and adequately evaluated when he or she is clothed. All garments should be removed rapidly during the primary survey. The ambient temperature of the resuscitation room is important. Hypothermia in a trauma patient is often a result of ambient hypothermia and infusion of fluids that are cooler than body temperature. The sequelae of hypothermia are beyond the scope of this chapter, but adequate resuscitation is difficult if not impossible to achieve in the hypothermic patient. Thus, warmed fluids and a warm room are basic to the entire resuscitative process as well as to continuing care.

Radiographic Evaluation in the Primary Survey

Three radiographs are most appropriate to the primary survey: a lateral cervical spine study, a chest film, and an abdominal study that includes the pelvis. The lateral cervical spinal radiograph is taken with downward traction on the arms so that all seven cervical vertebrae and the top of T1 are seen (see Fig. 15–11).

Reassessment for Therapeutic Effectiveness

Throughout the entire process of trauma management the ABCs should be continually reassessed. If the basic functions addressed in the primary survey cannot be controlled, moving on to the secondary survey is ill advised. Sometimes abnormalities identified in the primary survey can only be controlled by emergent operation.

SECONDARY SURVEY

The purpose of the secondary survey is to identify coexisting injuries and other nontraumatic medical problems that may not be immediate threats to the life of the child but that, if not taken into account, could result in mortality and morbidity. As many as 10% of injuries are identified after the first 24 hours after injury. The secondary survey includes a head-to-toe physical examination, the evaluation of appropriate radiographic and other diagnostic tests, and the planning of definitive treatment.

The secondary survey examination starts at the top of the head and progresses toward the feet. In the secondary survey, there is often time to obtain a better history of the event than was obtained initially.

Head and Face

Assessment of head injuries includes the level of consciousness; the presence of lacerations, abrasions, subgaleal hematoma, and bruises near the mastoid process (Battle's sign); the presence of blood or cerebrospinal fluid draining from the ear or nose; and a detailed eye examination (to include, if possible, the cold caloric test and the doll's eyes maneuver). These assessments are accomplished by inspection, palpation, pupillary reevaluation, and cranial nerve function evaluation.

Maxillofacial trauma is not uncommon in the pediatric population. These injuries, when not associated with airway obstruction, should be treated after the patient has been completely stabilized and life-threatening injuries have been treated.

Neck

All patients with injuries above the clavicles should be assumed to have a cervical spinal injury until this diagnosis has been excluded. The neck should be protected from further injury.

Spinal cord injury without radiographic abnormality (SCIWORA) occurs in children and must be carefully evaluated both radiographically and neurologically.[41] Radiographic evidence of injury is less often found in the child, and physiologic subluxation is often misinterpreted as a cervical spinal column injury. The state of the cervical spine of the child cannot be clarified with a normal lateral cervical spine radiograph, even though seven cervical vertebrae are seen. Good presumptive evidence of a normal cervical spine includes the lack of localizing neurologic deficits, lack of tenderness or other abnormalities on neck examination, and normal findings on a lateral cervical spine radiograph. Definitive status of the cervical spine is provided by a normal physical examination of the neck, a normal neurologic examination, and a normal CT scan of the neck.

Chest

Examination of the chest should be done to reevaluate injuries identified in the primary survey and to identify other, more subtle injuries. The patient should be "log rolled" to evaluate the entire back. At this time, the back should be palpated while looking for spinal column "step-off" fractures, hematoma, or other visible injuries.

Abdomen

The abdomen can be the site of significant, occult blood loss. The child swallows large amounts of air when upset, which can cause significant gastric distention. The distension may result in a decrease in effective respiration and may mimic an intraabdominal injury.

The child's stomach is first decompressed with a nasogastric tube, unless there is an injury above the clavicles. In that case, an orogastric tube is inserted to avoid the rare possibility of inserting the tube into the cranium through a cribriform plate fracture.

Perineum and Rectum

The perineum is evaluated, and a rectal examination is performed. The inspection can reveal blood at the urethral meatus, indicating the possibility of a ruptured urethra. A rectal examination may reveal a "high-riding" prostate, indicating urethral disruption. Blood in the scrotum or labia majora may indicate a hemoperitoneum or pelvic fracture.

Extremities and Fractures

The extremities should be visually evaluated for contusions, deformities, and length discrepancies. Palpation may reveal the crepitus of a fracture. The presence and equality of pulses must be evaluated. Typical fractures in childhood include the buckle or torus and the greenstick.[42] Pelvic fractures can often be identified by exerting anterior-posterior pressure on the anterior-superior iliac spines.

Neurologic Factors

The history of the event may provide information on the level of consciousness immediately after the event, such as crying immediately or a lucid interval followed by a period of unconsciousness. Initial therapy given at the scene by the paramedics is evaluated by the trauma team.

A comprehensive neurologic examination includes a reevaluation of the patient's level of consciousness and pupillary responses as well as a motor and sensory evaluation. A Glasgow Coma Scale score is generally determined at this time. The usual

TABLE 15-4. Glasgow Coma Scale for Children

Eye Opening		Score
Spontaneous		4
Reaction to speech		3
Reaction to pain		2
No response		1
Best Verbal Response (<4 y)		
Smiles, oriented to sound, follow objects, interacts		5
Crying	Interacts	
Consolable	Inappropriate	4
Inconsistently consolable	Moaning	3
Inconsolable	Irritable, restless	2
No response	No response	1
Best Motor Response		
Spontaneous (obeys verbal command)		6
Localizes pain		5
Withdraws in response to pain		4
Abnormal flexion in response to pain (decorticate posture)		3
Abnormal extension in response to pain (decorticate posture)		2
No response		1

scale must be modified for the child younger than 4 years (Table 15–4). The scale also provides an accurate method of following the changes in the patient's level of consciousness and neurologic function.

Diagnosis and Indications for Treatment

Most diagnostic algorithms for the injured child proceed from general to specific organ system knowledge. After resuscitation and stabilization, the determination must be made of the presence of an injury followed by the specific organ injury information. For example, the first priority in the child who is suffering hypovolemic shock is to treat the shock. The second priority is to determine the exact cause of the shock. The third priority is to repair the resultant damage to permanently arrest the process.

The child with a splenic injury with intraabdominal hemorrhage and shock exemplifies these principles. The shock is treated and, when sufficiently stabilized, the child undergoes further diagnostic evaluation, most often a contrast-enhanced CT scan to identify the injured organ. The decision to operate is based on the hemodynamics and generally not on the radiographic depiction of injury to the spleen. If, however, the child cannot be stabilized, an operation should not be withheld on the chance that the spleen will cease to bleed.

In most pediatric trauma centers, the CT scan is used extensively for the evaluation of intraabdominal injury. Most CT scanners today produce such high-quality images that the degree of disruption of an injured organ, such as the spleen or liver, can be identified. Often, nonoperative management can be quite safely pursued. The surgeon should save operative intervention for those patients who do not stabilize quickly, easily, and permanently. Thus, the major indicator for operative intervention should be the inability to achieve normal hemodynamics in a reasonable length of time. As a corollary, when 40 ml/kg of blood has been given (50% blood volume loss) and the child shows any hemodynamic instability, operative intervention should be considered. Conversely, the child who becomes hemodynamically stable after volume replacement can often be managed in a nonoperative manner.[43]

On occasion, when adequate circulation cannot be maintained and the child is too unstable to go to the CT scanner, peritoneal lavage may prove useful if the site of hemorrhage has not been identified.

Risks and Benefits of Management Decisions

The risks of operative versus nonoperative management should be carefully evaluated when determining the best method of treatment in any patient. Nonoperative risks include infectious complications (non-A, non-B hepatitis, human immunodeficiency virus) from blood transfusions and the risk of failed nonoperative management.[44] Risks of operative intervention include the anesthetic risk, the infectious risk (overwhelming postsplenectomy infection) if the spleen is removed, the operative risks, and the long-term risk of bowel obstruction. The results of nonoperative treatment must be at least as safe as those of operative treatment.

Transfer Decisions

Once the primary and secondary surveys have been completed, appropriate resuscitation initiated, and presumptive and specific diagnoses determined, the decision must be made whether the child can be adequately treated in the present location or must be transferred to another facility.

☐ Injury Prevention

The term *accident* is commonly used in relation to traumatic injury. Accident denotes a random occurrence that results in injury and that is neither predictable nor preventable. Individuals and environments are sometimes known to be at high risk for injury. Injury to such individuals and in some environments are both predictable and to some extent preventable. Injury prevention has taken on new importance in today's health care market as the emphasis in health care has changed from treating illness to promoting good health.[45, 46]

Injury prevention is often described as primary, secondary, and tertiary. *Primary prevention* is aimed at eliminating a trauma incident. Examples of such efforts include stoplights at intersections, window guards to prevent falls, and fences around swimming pools to prevent drowning. *Secondary prevention* is the attempt to decrease the severity of injuries that have occurred. *Tertiary prevention* is aimed at reducing the consequences of injury after the injury has occurred. Included in this category are the development of trauma systems, such as the verification and designation of trauma centers; the development and coordination of emergency medical services, including such services for children (i.e., EMS-C grants); and rehabilitative services to decrease the degree of impairment that results from the injury.

A useful and now well-known approach to primary and secondary injury prevention has become known as the Haddon matrix.[47] According to Haddon, there are three main factors in injury occurrence:

1. The injured person or host
2. The injuring mechanism or vehicle
3. The environment in which the injury occurs

There are also three phases in which an injury and its severity can be modified:

1. The preevent phase
2. The event phase (injury)
3. The postevent phase

Table 15–5 depicts a Haddon factor-phase matrix for motor vehicle crash prevention. This matrix identifies opportunities for injury prevention as well as other causes of injury. The National Highway Traffic Safety Administration (NHTSA) has adopted this structured design, the result of which has been a sustained decrease in the number of fatalities per vehicle mile driven during the past two decades.

The effort at prevention of injury should be directed to human factors (behavioral issues), vectors of injury, or environmental factors. Implementation of prevention strategies has been done using the four Es of injury prevention: education, enforcement, engineering, and economics (incentives).

EDUCATION. The premise behind education as a method to prevent injury is based on the concept that knowledge supports a change in behavior. Thus, education is the foundation of injury prevention. Unfortunately, education by itself has not proven to be as effective as has been hoped. However, there are several exceptions to this. Mothers Against Drunk Driving (MADD) and Students Against Driving Drunk (SADD) have used education as the mainstay in their efforts to decrease the number of alcohol-related automobile crash deaths. The efforts of these two organizations have aroused the public to encourage enactment of more stringent drunk driving laws. Similarly, the public has been made aware that the use of seat belts can and will save lives in motor vehicle crashes. However, education by itself is often not enough.

ENFORCEMENT. The knowledge that a simple preventive action will decrease death and disability should an incident occur is often insufficient to convince some that they should follow this action. If a law mandating a preventive action is enacted, however, it then becomes illegal not to follow this action. For example, most states have enacted seat belt and child safety seat legislation. Where the laws are stringent enough, the public has responded by wearing seat belts and using safety seats. If, however, the

TABLE 15–5. Haddon's Factor-Phase Matrix for Motor Vehicle Crash Prevention

	Preevent	Event	Postevent
Host	Avoidance of alcohol use	Use of safety belts	Bystander delivers care
Vehicle	Antilock brakes	Air bag deploys	
Environment	Speed limits	Impact-absorbing barriers	Access to trauma system

Reproduced with the permission of the Advanced Trauma Life Support Program for Doctors (6th ed). Chicago, American College of Surgeons, 1997.

law is ineffectual or is not rigorously enforced, a portion of the public does not comply with the laws.

ENGINEERING. The implementation of engineering changes, such as the incorporation of airbags in automobiles, are often more expensive initially, but such modifications often have the greatest preventive effects. Engineering initiatives require both legislative and enforcement processes to be effective.

ECONOMIC INCENTIVES. Efforts by the federal government to link federal highway funds to the passage of motorcycle helmet laws was effective in reducing head injury fatalities: This federal mandate resulted in a 30% decrease in head injury fatalities. It is tragic that this economic incentive is no longer in effect, and it should come as no surprise that the rate of highway head injury fatalities is now comparable to the rates existing before this particular incentive.

It is clear that prevention efforts have been effective in the past and can continue to be effective with planning and implementation. The steps that should be followed are clear.[48] The problem must first be defined and the causes and risk factors identified. Interventions must then be developed and tested and the strategies for solution implemented. Finally, the results of the process must be evaluated for efficacy and altered if necessary.

☐ Trauma Centers

Organization of a trauma system allows one to place a pediatric trauma patient in an institution capable of providing the level of care appropriate to the degree of injury. It is extremely wasteful for a level I pediatric trauma center to receive large numbers of slightly injured children. Conversely, it is disastrous to have a severely injured child transported to an institution incapable of providing the indicated therapy. It is also inappropriate for a child with a life-threatening injury to be transported a long distance when a nearby institution is capable of providing lifesaving therapy. The best answer to this dilemma is the tiered level of response.

A tiered response implies adequate training of the prehospital personnel, communication links with the prehospital and in-hospital components, and rapid and safe transportation of the injured child to an appropriate treating facility. Treating facilities must have been verified as meeting certain standards of optimal care for the trauma patient by an

organization such as the ACS Verification Review Committee. Ideally, after such a verification, a local or regional designating authority should have categorized a hospital as to its treatment capabilities.

The ATLS method for physicians, when it is combined with an appropriate prehospital method such as Pre-Hospital Trauma Life Support, has the potential of providing superior care for the injured pediatric patient in a region. All personnel understand the same terminology and look for similar injuries. Patients are identified, appropriately treated in the field, and transported in optimal condition to a verified and designated trauma center.

The ideal method for decreasing mortality and morbidity from traumatic disease is to eradicate the disease. Effective, long-term prevention strategies must be developed and implemented. With time, taking into account the interests of the professionals who deal with trauma and the interests of the public on whom the ravages of injury are visited, the death and disability of traumatic disease—our most lethal and devastating childhood disease—can be brought under control.

REFERENCES

1. Wolley MM: The death of a child—the parent's perspective and advice. J Pediatr Surg 32:73–74, 1997.
2. Brown BB: Sunrise Tomorrow. Grand Rapids, MI, Fleming H. Revell, 1988, p 57.
3. Koop CE, Koop E: Sometimes Mountains Move (revised ed). Grand Rapids, MI, Zondervan Publishing House, 1995.
4. Barlow B, Niemirska M, Gandhi RP: Ten years' experience with pediatric gunshot wounds. J Pediatr Surg 17:927–931, 1982.
5. Choi E, Donoghue ER, Lifshultz BD: Deaths due to firearm injuries in children. J Forensic Sci 39:685–692, 1994.
6. Nance ML, Sing RF, Branas CC, et al: Shotgun wounds in children: Not just accidents. Arch Surg 132:58–62, 1997.
7. Bureau of Justice Statistics Crime Data Brief: Young black male victims. Publication No. NCJ-147004, December 1994.
8. Schwarz DF, Grisso JA, Miles CG, et al: A longitudinal study of injury mortality in an African-American population. JAMA 271:755–760, 1994.
9. Gallagher SS, Guyer B, Kotelchuck M, et al: A strategy for the reduction of childhood injuries in Massachusetts: SCIPP. N Engl J Med 307:1015, 1982.
10. Rouse TM, Eichelberger MR: Trends in pediatric trauma management. Surg Clin North Am 72:1347–1364, 1992.
11. Fingerhut LA, Kleinman JC, Godfrey E, et al: Firearm mortality among children, youth and young adults 1–34 years of age, trends and current status: United States, 1979–88. Monthly Vital Statistics Report 39:1–15, 1991.
12. Deaths resulting from firearm and motor vehicle injuries—United States. 1968–1991. MMWR Morb Mortal Wkly Rep 43:37–42, 1994.

13. Ronald Reagan's acceptance speech to the Republican National Convention. July 1986.
14. Mario Cuomo's endorsement speech to the Democratic National Convention. August 1986.
15. Schwab CW: Violence: America's uncivil war—presidential address, sixth scientific assembly of the Eastern Association for the Surgery of Trauma. J Trauma 35:657–665, 1993.
16. McGonigal MD, Cole J, Schwab CW, et al: Urban firearm deaths: A five-year perspective. J Trauma 35:532–536, 1993.
17. Nance ML, Stafford PW, Schwab CW: Firearm injury among urban youth during the last decade: An escalation in violence. J Pediatr Surg 32:949–952, 1997.
18. Leschoier I, DiScala C: Blunt trauma in children: Causes and outcome of head versus extracranial injury. Pediatrics 91:721–725, 1993.
19. Sells CW, Blum RW: Morbidity and mortality among US adolescents: An overview of data and trends. Am J Public Health 86:513–519, 1996.
20. Dryfoos JG: Adolescents at Risk: Prevalence and Prevention. New York, Oxford University Press, 1990.
21. Barthwell AG, Hewitt W, Jilson I: An introduction to ethnic and cultural diversity. Pediatr Clin North Am 42:431–451, 1995.
22. Johnston LD, Bachman JG, O'Malley PM: Drug Survey. Ann Arbor, University of Michigan News and Information Services, December 19, 1996, pp 11–12.
23. Perret G: Ulysses S. Grant: Soldier and President. New York, Random House, 1997, p 320.
24. Adams GW: Doctors in Blue. New York, Collier Books, 1961.
25. Blaisdell FW: Medical advances during the Civil War: Presidential address. Arch Surg 123:1045–1050, 1988.
26. Heaton LD: Army medical service activities in Vietnam. Mil Med 131:646, 1966.
27. Accidental Death and Disability: The Neglected Disease of Modern Society. Washington, DC, National Academy of Sciences/National Research Council, 1976.
28. American College of Surgeons Committee on Trauma: Resources for Optimal Care of the Injured Patient. Chicago, American College of Surgeons, 1990.
29. Tepas JJ, Ramenofsky ML, Barlow B, et al: National Pediatric Trauma Registry. J Pediatr Surg 24:156–158, 1989.
30. National Pediatric Trauma Registry Biannual Report. Boston, Tufts University School of Medicine, Research and Training Center, Rehabilitation Medicine, 1997.
31. Tepas JJ, Mollitt, DL, Talbert JL, et al: Pediatric Trauma Score as a predictor of injury severity in the injured child. J Pediatr Surg 22:14–18, 1987.
32. Ramenofsky ML, Ramenofsky MB, Jurkovich GJ, et al: The predictive validity of the Pediatric Trauma Score. J Trauma 28:1038–1042, 1988.
33. Tepas JJ, DiScala C, Ramenofsky ML, Barlow B: Mortality and head injury: The pediatric perspective. J Pediatr Surg 25:92–96, 1990.
34. Gennarelli TA, Champion HR, Sacco WJ, et al: Mortality of patients with head injury and extracranial injury treated in trauma centers. J Trauma 29:1193–1209, 1989.
35. Pugula FA, Wald SL, Shackford SR, et al: The effect of hypotension and hypoxia on children with severe head injuries. J Pediatr Surg 28:310–316, 1993.
36. Krantz BE, Bell RM, Collicott PE, et al (eds): Advanced Trauma Life Support Student Manual (6th ed). Chicago, American College of Surgeons Committee on Trauma, 1997.
37. Ramenofsky ML, Moulton SL: The pediatric trauma center. Semin Pediatr Surg 4:128–134, 1995.
38. Hoff WS, Reilly PM, Rotondo MF, et al: The importance of the command-physician in trauma resuscitation. J Trauma 43:772–777, 1997.
39. American College of Surgeons Committee on Trauma: Resources for Optimal Care of the Injured Patient. Chicago, American College of Surgeons, 1993.
40. Schwab CW, Shayne JP, Turner J: Immediate trauma resuscitation with type O uncrossmatched blood: A two-year prospective experience. J Trauma 26:897–902, 1986.
41. Pang D, Wilberger JE: Spinal cord injury without radiographic abnormality. J Neurosurg 57:114–129, 1982.
42. Rubin P: Dynamic Classification of Bone Dysplasias. Chicago, Year Book Medical, 1964.
43. Pearl RH, Wesson DE, Spence LJ, et al: Splenic injury: A 5-year update with improved results and changing criteria for conservative management. J Pediatr Surg 24:121–125, 1989.
44. Luna GK, Dellinger EP: Non-operative observation therapy for splenic injuries: A safe therapeutic option? Am J Surg 153:462–468, 1987.
45. Eastman AB, Krantz BE, Mitchell FL, et al: ACS Committee on Trauma: Injury prevention and control. In Resources for Optimal Care of the Injured Patient, American College of Surgeons, Chicago, 1997, pp 13–15.
46. Cooper A, Barlow B, Davidson L, et al: Epidemiology of pediatric trauma: Importance of population-based statistics. J Pediatr Surg 27:149–154, 1992.
47. Haddon W, Baker SP: Injury control. In Clark DW, MacMahon B (eds): Prevention and Community Medicine (2nd ed). Boston, Little, Brown & Co, 1981, pp 109–140.
48. Rivera FP: Traumatic deaths of children in the United States: Currently available prevention strategies. Pediatrics 85:456–462, 1985.

16

THORACIC TRAUMA IN CHILDREN

Gary K. Lofland, MD

In North America, trauma is the leading cause of death in patients younger than 35 years, the leading cause of death in children older than 1 year, and the third leading cause of death overall. The majority of these patients succumb before reaching a patient care facility. Thoracic injuries account for 25% of all traumatic deaths in the adult population, with aortic transection being the principal cause.[1]

☐ Epidemiologic Overview

The epidemiology of pediatric chest trauma has been extensively studied in recent decades, when the lethal nature of thoracic injuries in children became more apparent. A 1977 autopsy study represents one of the larger compilations of pediatric traumatic deaths.[2] In this study, thoracic injury was noted in 28% of children who died before receiving medical therapy. In another study, 29% of 230 children sustaining blunt trauma had thoracic injury.[3] In a study of 110 patients, 25% of the patients had major thoracic injury requiring therapy, and an additional 33% had minor to moderate chest injury not requiring therapy.[4] Thoracic injury was reported as fatal in 13 of 94 children of all ages, but the mortality was 23% in children younger than 5 years.[5] According to the same study, if two major extrathoracic systems are injured concomitantly, mortality further rises to 58%. In one study, the mortality rate of children with a thoracic injury was 26%, which may be compared to the overall mortality rate from trauma in children of 2.2%.[6] Another study of childhood trauma[6] revealed that isolated chest injury results in a mortality rate of 5.3%. If two body systems are injured, as assessed by the Abbreviated Injury Scale (AIS), the mortality rate increases to 28.6%. For injuries to three body regions, the mortality rate is 33%. Combined injuries to the head, chest, and abdomen produce a mortality rate of 38%.[6]

☐ Unique Features of Pediatric Thoracic Injuries

The pattern of injury and resultant physiologic derangement is somewhat different in a child than in an adult. Some of this difference relates to body size and proportions, and some relates to elasticity. In addition, the blood volume of the small patient is 7 to 8% of total body weight. A relatively small blood volume loss can lead to hypovolemia and shock.

The child's thorax is remarkably compliant. The bony and cartilaginous structures are pliable and will absorb kinetic energy that must be dissipated by intrathoracic structures. The child might have significant intrathoracic injury without any injury to bony structures of the chest wall. Flail chest injury is rarely seen until the child reaches adolescence.

Children sustaining trauma of any form may experience aerophagia. Gastric dilation may become massive, may compromise diaphragmatic excursion, and may compress intrathoracic structures. Nasogastric decompression of the stomach is necessary in the injured child to decrease the size of the air-filled stomach, allowing better ventilation and protection against aspiration.

It is unusual for children sustaining thoracic injury to have preexisting disease involving other organ systems. As a result, the potential for recovery is tremendous if the pathophysiology that accompanies those injuries can be reversed.

Although one usually associates injury with blunt or penetrating mechanisms, other causes of injury to intrathoracic organs exist. Injuries to the esophagus may occur as a result of foreign body ingestion or as a result of ingestion of corrosive agents. Iatrogenic injury to the esophagus may occur at the time of nasogastric intubation.

Bronchopulmonary injuries may be caused by blunt and penetrating trauma. Mechanical ventilation predisposes babies to barotrauma. This is especially true in the premature neonate.

Finally, because of the proportionally smaller size of the chest when compared with the abdomen or head in a young child, significant thoracic trauma is almost always accompanied by injury to other organ systems. These systems need to be evaluated concurrently while evaluating the potentially life-threatening intrathoracic injury.

□ Historical Aspects

The management of thoracic trauma has evolved over a period of 5000 years. The Smith Papyrus (3000 BC) contains notations about chest injuries treated by Imotep.[7] These were simple injuries treated with relatively simple techniques.

Hippocrates, writing in the 4th century BC, associated rib fractures with hemoptysis and prescribed rest and bloodletting for patients with broken ribs.[8] He also advocated stabilization of the chest wall with binding, an appropriate therapy in an age of inadequate pain control. The ancient Egyptians, Romans, and Greeks considered penetrating injuries of the chest almost uniformly fatal. In the 3rd century BC, Aristotle wrote, "The heart alone of all the viscera cannot withstand injury."[9] Galen, writing in the 2nd century AD, described packing open chest wounds suffered by gladiators in Rome.[10] Ambrose Paré in the 16th century described subcutaneous emphysema associated with chest wall injury and recommended débriding segments of broken ribs.[11] In the 17th century, Riolanus treated cardiac injuries in animals.[12] Riolanus and Scultetus described empyema as a complication of penetrating thoracic injury.[13] Scultetus also advocated drainage tubes and irrigation for established intrapleural infections, with the drainage tubes functioning largely as passive conduits. The importance of suction was recognized, however, especially in the treatment of infection. In the absence of an efficient mechanical means of aspiration, oral aspiration of wounds by professional "wound suckers" arose as a means of treating chest infections (Fig. 16–1). Anel, a military surgeon who wrote a treatise entitled *The Art of Sucking Wounds* in 1707, noted that professional wound suckers suffered (not surprisingly) from frequent oral infections.[14]

Playfair[15] developed a rudimentary water seal device to drain the pleural cavity in the 19th century. Thoracentesis, however, was associated with a high mortality rate. Dupytron of Paris, one of the leading surgeons of the day, reportedly performed thoracentesis on 50 patients with only two long-term survivors. When Dupytron subsequently developed an empyema himself, he refused thoracentesis, saying that he would "rather die by the hand of God than by that of surgeons."[16]

There was considerable debate about the treatment of injuries to the heart, with no less a figure than Theodore Billroth stating in 1885, "The surgeon who should attempt to suture a wound to the heart would lose the respect of his colleagues."[17] Despite these sentiments expressed by otherwise erudite figures, the first repairs of a penetrating cardiac wound in a human were performed in 1896 by Rehn of Frankfurt, Germany,[18] and shortly thereafter by Lucius Hill of Montgomery, Alabama.

Many of the advances in the treatment of thoracic trauma in the 20th century are the result of improvements in anesthesia, imaging, and respiratory sup-

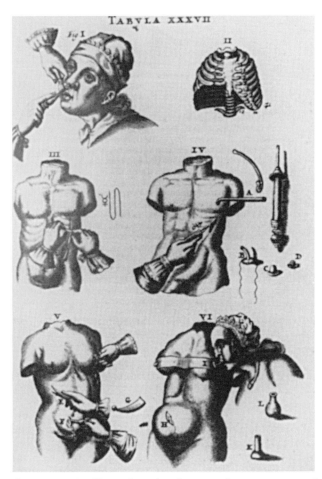

Figure 16–1. An illustration taken from a 17th century text entitled *The Surgeon's Storehouse* by Sculteteus (1674). In the lower right corner, wound sucking is demonstrated. Also illustrated are incisions for the drainage of empyema and irrigation devices.

portive care. Positive-pressure ventilation permitted more aggressive surgical management of thoracic wounds. Refinements in equipment and technique allowed for radiography of the chest, which rapidly became widely available.[19] As an outgrowth of experience with casualties during World War I, drainage of the chest for empyema became routine.[20] The development of antibiotics, which began in the 1930s, and widespread acceptance of the importance of drainage of the pleural cavity for noninfectious complications markedly improved the prognosis for both penetrating and blunt injuries. Experience with mass casualties during World War II demonstrated the efficacy of aggressive management of thoracic injuries.

Since the Korean War, the availability of cardiopulmonary bypass has allowed treatment of cardiac injuries. More recently, the development of computed tomography and magnetic resonance imaging has allowed better understanding of thoracic injuries and their management. In critical care, prolonged survival of patients with injuries that had previously been fatal has led to the formal description of the adult respiratory distress syndrome. Increasing organization of trauma care delivery, much of which was based on experience in Korea and Vietnam, and efforts at injury prevention have also reduced morbidity and mortality.[21]

Pediatric patients with thoracic injuries have benefited immensely from the military experience in the management of adults with thoracic injuries. The establishment of pediatric advanced life support and of designated pediatric trauma centers has resulted in better definition of thoracic injuries and expedited management of these injuries.

For purposes of presentation and injury classification, injuries to the chest can be divided into blunt, penetrating, and iatrogenic. Any of the chest wall structures or intrathoracic contents may be injured, and all are considered in this chapter.

☐ Initial Evaluation and Management

The initial resuscitation of patients with thoracic injuries follows the same principles as the resuscitation of any trauma patient or any patient for whom advanced cardiac life support is required. These principles are known as the "ABCs"—a popular acronym for airway, breathing, and circulation.[22, 23] Some elements of the ABCs are of particular significance for patients with thoracic injuries.

The first priority is ensuring an adequate airway.[24–26] The goal of airway management in the injured pediatric patient is optimal ventilation and oxygenation while simultaneously protecting the cervical spine. One should assume any child who sustains significant trauma has a cervical spine injury until proven otherwise. There is a 42% mortality rate associated with traumatic spinal injuries in children.[27] The cervical spine of all injured children should be managed by cervical in-line immobilization with the head in a neutral position. One should assume that cervical spine injury exists until a roentgenogram of a lateral cervical spine clearly delineates all seven cervical vertebrae to be intact. In a hemodynamically unstable child, however, when cervical radiographs cannot be obtained immediately, the neck should be immobilized both for transport and for ensurance of airway patency.

The pediatric airway is easily obstructed, especially in the child with multiple injuries and an altered level of consciousness. A loss of muscle tone in the oropharynx may cause the tongue to fall posteriorly, contributing to airway obstruction. Another cause of airway obstruction is the presence of blood, vomitus, secretions, or foreign objects in the oropharynx, larynx, or trachea. Severe injuries of the mandible or facial bones or crush injuries of the larynx or trachea also may contribute to airway obstruction. Compared with the adult, the child's tongue is proportionally larger in a smaller oral cavity, the glottic opening is more anterior and cephalad, and the trachea is shorter and narrower. These anatomic differences make the pediatric airway somewhat more difficult to manage and also more prone to iatrogenic injury by inexperienced personnel. Symptoms of upper airway obstruction are dyspnea, diminished breath sounds despite respiratory effort, retractions, dysphagia, drooling, and dysphonia.

Acute management of the obstructed airway consists first of a jaw thrust maneuver and the administration of supplemental oxygen. The jaw thrust maneuver is accomplished by placing fingers behind the angles of the mandible and lifting. The neck should remain in a neutral position; both hyperextension and flexion should be avoided. Any foreign materials in the mouth or oropharynx should be removed, either manually or by strong suction. Oral or nasopharyngeal airways are very poorly tolerated by the semi-conscious child, and they may induce gagging and vomiting. Any child who tolerates an oral or nasopharyngeal airway should be assumed to have compromised protective reflexes and therefore requires definitive airway management with an endotracheal tube. The child should be ventilated by bag valve mask with 100% oxygen until intubation is accomplished. Orotracheal intubation is the preferred approach in the injured child, as opposed to in the adult, who may tolerate nasotracheal intubation. Unlike in adults, cricothyroidotomy or tracheostomy is rarely necessary in children except when severe maxillofacial or laryngeal injury has occurred. Even in these circumstances, an oral airway can usually be established.

Tension pneumothorax may profoundly affect ventilation and perfusion. Physical signs of tension pneumothorax include acute respiratory distress or cyanosis despite adequate airway, tracheal deviation, unilateral absence of breath sounds, or diffuse breath sounds over the chest and abdomen. Both penetrating and blunt injuries may also cause hemothorax or pulmonary contusion.

Resuscitation of the child with chest trauma begins with a survey for immediate life-threatening injury using the Oslerian principles of observation, inspection, palpation and auscultation. To assess for adequate ventilation, observe symmetric chest expansion, auscultate equal breath sounds bilaterally, and evaluate the entire chest wall for signs of contusion or chest wall penetration. If ventilation or oxygenation is inadequate, reassess airway and breathing. Check for correct placement and patency of the endotracheal tube and consider the presence of pneumothorax, hemothorax, or other thoracic injury. These can be confirmed radiographically. Adequate oxygenation is present if the skin is pink centrally and oxygen saturation is 85% or greater by pulse oximetry.

When breathing remains inadequate after positive pressure ventilation, needle thoracentesis to exclude pneumothorax should be considered. One should keep in mind, however, that decompression by needle thoracentesis requires tube thoracostomy for definitive treatment. If an open pneumothorax is present, petrolatum-impregnated gauze in a sterile dressing will suffice to cover the defect, thereby reestablishing chest wall integrity. Once this is accomplished, however, a tube thoracostomy is necessary, because it is likely that the visceral pleura would have been injured, creating the potential for development of a tension pneumothorax. In the unlikely event of an unstable chest wall from flail chest, the management of any degree of respiratory compromise is endotracheal intubation and mechanical ventilation. Flail chest will usually be seen only in older children or adolescents who sustain substantial crush injuries to the chest.

Once ventilation and oxygenation are established, circulation is the next priority. Early signs of shock may be subtle in children. Normal blood volume in a child varies from 7 to 8% or 70 to 80 ml/kg body weight.[27] A volume loss that might be considered small in an adult may induce shock in a child, although hypotension may not occur until 25% of blood volume is lost. Fluid management should be aggressive and instituted early during resuscitation. An initial bolus of 20 ml/kg of lactated Ringer's solution is appropriate for any signs of shock. This volume may be repeated as necessary, even in the event of concomitant head injury. The goal of aggressive fluid resuscitation is the prevention of irreversible hypotension resistant to any resuscitative efforts, leading to multiple organ system failure and death.

If prompt improvement in the circulatory status does not occur or if signs of venous obstruction appear, the possibility of a cardiac tamponade must be entertained. Needle aspiration of the pericardial space is life saving in the presence of a pericardial tamponade. In children, cardiac tamponade may result from air trapped in the pericardial space from a bronchial injury.

The indications for proceeding with urgent thoracotomy are as follows[6]:

1. Penetrating wound to the heart or great vessels
2. Massive or continuous interpleural hemorrhage
3. Open pneumothorax with major chest wall defect
4. Aortogram confirming aortic transection
5. Massive pleural air leak suggestive of bronchial or tracheal disruption
6. Cardiac tamponade persisting after pericardiocentesis
7. Rupture of the esophagus
8. Rupture of the diaphragm
9. No palpable pulse despite cardiac massage

Whereas the need for emergency department thoracotomy is rare, the presence of a penetrating wound in the area of the mid-sternum or left sternal border and failure of the child to promptly respond to resuscitation efforts are the usual indications. Emergency department thoracotomies for blunt trauma are rarely successful and should be avoided.

□ The Management of Specific Injuries

TRAUMATIC ASPHYXIA

Traumatic asphyxia is an entity observed in children because of a flexible thorax and absence of valves in the venous system of the inferior and superior vena cava. Direct compression of the chest wall is sustained when the child is run over by a vehicle or otherwise crushed. At the time of injury, if the glottis is closed and the thoracoabdominal muscles are tensed, the increased intrathoracic pressure is transmitted through the central venous system to solid organs such as the brain, liver, spleen, and kidneys. The patient is usually disoriented, with tachypnea, hemoptysis, and respiratory insufficiency. The face and neck are cyanotic, with petechia on the head, neck, and chest. Subconjunctival and retinal hemorrhages are often present. Acute hepatomegaly secondary to transmitted caval pressure may be seen. If the patient exhibits a significant degree of pulmonary contusion, endotracheal intubation and mechanical ventilation with positive end expiratory pressure may be necessary.

SUBCUTANEOUS EMPHYSEMA

Subcutaneous emphysema occurs when the air is forced into the tissue planes of the chest. It is primarily a sign of underlying injury to ribs, pleura, intercostal muscles, bronchus, trachea, or pulmonary parenchyma. Treatment of children with subcutaneous emphysema is directed toward the primary injury, because the subcutaneous air has no physiologic effect and is spontaneously absorbed.

RIB FRACTURES

The thorax of the child is quite compliant because of the elasticity of the ribs resulting from their greater cartilage content than in adults. This compliance diffuses the force of impact, leading to fewer rib fractures than would result from a similar injury to an adult. Although splinting from the discomfort is common in children, atelectasis rarely occurs because of the propensity of children to cry.

Diagnosis of acute rib fractures is by roentgenogram or by roentgenogram plus bone scan to detect healing rib fractures in the child thought to be a victim of abuse. Multiple rib fractures should always raise the suspicion of child abuse. Rib fractures often result in intrapleural injury. Children with rib fractures are twice as likely to have a pneumothorax or hemothorax as those without. Whereas some of this may be attributable to the sharp edges of the bony fragments tearing the visceral and parietal pleura, the force required to produce a rib fracture is frequently sufficient to produce intrathoracic injury (Fig. 16–2).

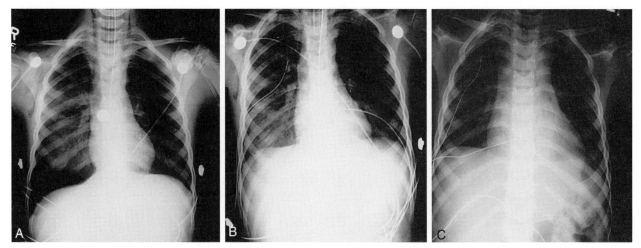

Figure 16–2. *A*, Multiple rib fractures and a pneumothorax are clearly apparent in this chest roentgenogram of a 7-year-old patient involved in a motor vehicle accident. The patient was not wearing restraints at the time of injury and had multiple other injuries. *B*, Complete reexpansion of the lung following chest tube insertion. *C*, Persistent complete expansion of the right lung and resolution of pulmonary contusion following chest tube removal.

Oral analgesics are usually sufficient to control pain, and only rarely is an intercostal nerve block necessary.

PNEUMOTHORAX

Pneumothorax may result from puncture of the lung by a rib, by a penetrating chest wall injury, by disruption of the pulmonary parenchyma, or by injury to the tracheobronchial tree.

Sucking chest wounds are relatively rare in children. When they do occur, they are most commonly associated with blast injuries, severe avulsion injuries, or close-range shotgun wounds. Sucking chest wounds can be emergently treated by covering them with an occlusive dressing, which prevents further ingress of air from the outside. Because a pneumothorax or hemopneumothorax may develop, tube thoracostomy drainage should also be done. Definitive treatment is dictated by the mechanism of injury and the response to simple therapeutic methods.

Pneumothorax is more commonly caused by air entering the pleural space via a hole in the lung. The lung is often injured on its surface by broken ribs. When the patient inspires, the hole in the lung surface opens as the lung expands, but with expiration, the hole closes. As pressure in the pleural space increases, the hole in the pulmonary surface is less and less likely to open with inspiratory effort. In most cases, the lung collapses to the point at which intrapleural air no longer accumulates with inspiration, and the pneumothorax is stable.

Sometimes, however, air continues to accumulate in the pleural space with each inspiratory effort. The fact that the hole opens with inspiration and closes with expiration produces a valve-like mechanism that causes the pneumothorax to increase in size with each respiratory cycle, producing a ten-

sion pneumothorax. Although tension pneumothorax is possible during spontaneous ventilation, it is more commonly seen when a patient is undergoing positive-pressure ventilation. Accordingly, when a patient deteriorates hemodynamically with institution of positive-pressure ventilation, the possibility of a tension pneumothorax should be considered and urgently treated.

If the pressure in the pleural space with tension pneumothorax becomes high enough, both respiration and hemodynamics are impaired. High intrapleural pressures on the side of injury minimize effective expansion of the lungs. As the pressure in the ipsilateral pleural cavity increases, the heart is pushed toward the contralateral side of the chest, venous return is compromised, and cardiac output decreases. This pathophysiology is easily and quickly reversed with decompression of the pneumothorax. Some of the physical findings associated with tension pneumothorax are identical to those seen with any pneumothorax but may be more pronounced. There are no breath sounds on the injured side, subcutaneous air may develop, and the trachea may be deviated away from the site of injury. Shock may also be present and, because there is interference with venous return to the right atrium, neck veins may be distended. Neck vein distention is not a particularly sensitive sign, however, because it may not be present in patients who are also hypovolemic.

It is almost always necessary to treat a pneumothorax resulting from blunt injury with a chest tube, particularly in patients who are also being treated with positive-pressure ventilation (Fig. 16–3). The presence of unexpanded lung and fluid in the chest can predispose the patient to the development of empyema. In addition, some element of lung function may be permanently lost if the lung is not reexpanded.

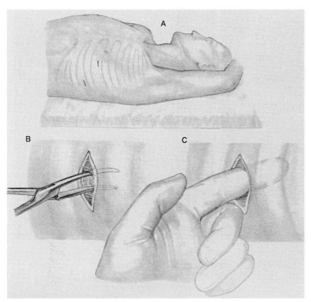

Figure 16–3. Technique for chest tube insertion. *A,* Two potential sites for chest tube insertion. The upper site is in the anterior axillary line in the fourth intercostal space. The lower site is in the fifth or sixth intercostal space in the midaxillary line. Either site allows for the chest tube to be directed either anteriorly or posteriorly. An anterior direction is preferred for pneumothorax, whereas a more posterior placement is preferred for fluid or hemothorax. *B,* After a small skin incision has been made, a Crile or Kelly clamp may be used to enlarge the incision slightly, dissect subcutaneously, and penetrate the pleural space on the anterior surface of a rib. *C,* Placement of a finger through the incision into the pleural space ensures that no pleural adhesions are present and that the pleural space has indeed been entered. Such a maneuver helps prevent placement of the tube into pulmonary parenchyma.

Tubes that are large enough to adequately drain any associated hemothorax should generally be placed in the fourth or fifth intercostal space in the midaxillary line. Small catheters, such as pigtail catheters, should be avoided. Careful insertion using an open technique should be used, especially as the hemidiaphragm is sometimes quite elevated in the chest or may even be ruptured.

HEMOTHORAX

Like pneumothorax, hemothorax is a common finding after chest trauma and frequently accompanies pneumothorax. Physical findings are not usually helpful, and the diagnosis is usually established radiographically. Hemothorax may be missed if the radiograph is taken with the patient in the supine position. A fluid level is not always appreciated, and even a large hemothorax can appear as simple elevation of the hemidiaphragm if the radiograph is taken in the upright position.

As with pneumothorax, a small traumatic hemothorax is sometimes missed on the initial chest radiograph and is seen later on the upper cuts of a computerized tomographic study or magnetic resonance study of the abdomen. One should maintain a very low threshold for tube thoracostomy. Persistent

blood in the chest increases the risk of empyema and loss of lung function and may sometimes necessitate decortication later.

Early placement of a thoracostomy tube can help greatly in the drainage of blood from the pleural cavity, but blood has a natural tendency to clot, and small amounts of residual hemothorax in a chest film taken shortly after placement of a chest tube are therefore fairly common. Usually this clot will lyse over the next several days.

When drainage from the tube is minimal and the radiographic findings demonstrate persistent hemothorax, continued attempts at drainage are rarely successful. Definitive treatment of significant hemothorax that persists beyond several days involves a limited thoracotomy, evacuation of the clot, removal of whatever organized peel has developed on the pleural surfaces, and placement of a new thoracostomy tube. This can also be accomplished thoracoscopically. It is, however, more difficult to remove peel and organized clot from the chest thoracoscopically than with a limited open technique. The role of thoracoscopy will continue to grow in the treatment of this problem.

PULMONARY CONTUSION

Some of the damage in a contused lung is the result of hemorrhage into the pulmonary parenchyma. In other areas, injury is more subtle, with damage to the pulmonary microvasculature but no extravasation of red blood cells. This range of injury is analogous to contusion in other areas of the body. Part of the fluid accumulation associated with a contusion is related to hemorrhage, but much of it is caused by extravasation of fluid from the intravascular to the extravascular space as a consequence of increased pulmonary microvascular permeability seen with a generalized inflammatory reaction. Increased permeability promotes diapedesis of inflammatory cells and diffusion of inflammatory mediators necessary to combat infection and begin repair.

In the lungs, as well as in other areas of the body, accumulation of edema fluid is a natural consequence of increased permeability. Although edema formation may help with resisting infection and initiating repair, edema certainly harms organ function. Alveoli are rendered poorly functional or nonfunctional, interfering with oxygenation and ventilation. In areas such as skeletal muscle and soft tissue, these functional side effects are of minimal importance. In the lungs, however, interstitial and alveolar edema causes arteriovenous shunting and hypoxemia.

The diagnosis of pulmonary contusion, established on the basis of radiography and blood gas analysis, can be difficult. Radiographically, pulmonary contusion appears as patchy areas of pulmonary infiltrate and is usually localized to areas of the lung that underlie obvious chest wall injury. The radiographic appearance may lag behind the loss of pulmonary function. Blood gas analyses, in the presence of an established contusion, are manifested by hypoxemia. Although other entities such as aspiration can still be confused with contusion, the distinction between the two is largely insignificant in the emergent setting because the initial treatment of each is identical.

Because pulmonary capillary membrane integrity is part of the pathogenesis of pulmonary contusion, the radiographic abnormalities may increase over the first 24 to 48 hours after injury as extravasation and edema formation occur. It may be extremely difficult to distinguish contusion from respiratory distress syndrome or from pneumonia.

Whether patients with pulmonary contusion should receive prophylactic antibiotics is controversial. The evidence that antibiotics help prevent pneumonia is not particularly convincing, and antibiotics should not be given routinely unless aspiration has occurred.

An equally contentious issue in the treatment of pulmonary contusion is fluid management. Theoretically, colloid-containing fluids should maintain intravascular osmotic pressure and discourage movement of fluid from the intravascular to the extravascular space. In actuality, the damaged pulmonary microvasculature cannot maintain a colloid osmotic gradient, and contusion is not effectively treated by this approach. Furthermore, the use of diuretics and overly stringent restriction of fluids in the acutely traumatized patient can compromise intravascular volume and perfusion, leading to dysfunction of other organ systems. Patients with pulmonary contusion should be carefully monitored, the goal being the assurance of adequate perfusion. In larger patients, pulmonary artery catheters can be placed, but this is virtually impossible in patients weighing less than 10 kg. Therefore, a balance must be struck between adequate oxygenation and tissue perfusion through careful volume administration.

INJURIES TO THE TRACHEA AND MAJOR BRONCHI

Blunt injuries of the trachea and major bronchi are rare.[28-30] The trachea can be injured anywhere along its course, but the most common locations are the neck and near the carina. Injuries to the major bronchi are usually within 2.5 cm of the carina. It is felt in adults that right-sided injuries may be more common than those on the left, but this is not proven to be true in children (Fig. 16–4).

In the neck, the pathophysiology of blunt injury to the trachea is a "clothesline" mechanism, in which sudden and violent tracheal compression occurs. Sometimes there is associated injury to the larynx or esophagus.

Several theories about the mechanism of airway injury within the chest have been proposed. One is that the chest is flattened in its anterior/posterior dimension, and the lungs, in contact with the parietal pleural of the chest wall, are stretched trans-

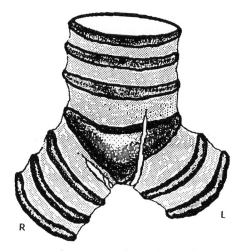

Figure 16–4. Complex injury to the trachea and main stem bronchi secondary to blunt trauma. Of note is that most such injuries are located within 2.5 cm of the carina. (From Millham FH, Rajii-Khorasani A, Birkett DF, et al: Carinal injury: Diagnosis and treatment—case report. J Trauma 31:1420, 1991.)

versely with disruption of the carina secondary to the stretching mechanism. Another theory is that chest compression against a closed glottis disrupts the airway from increased intraluminal pressure, creating a "blow-out." Because wall tension is directly proportional to the diameter of the airway, it is greatest in the larger airways, in keeping with the empiric observation that most blunt injuries to thoracic trachea or bronchi occur near the carina. A final theory about the pathogenesis of tears of the thoracic trachea and bronchi is similar to the theory for pathogenesis of tears of the thoracic aorta. According to this theory, the trachea is fixed relative to the lungs. With sudden deceleration, shear forces are generated near the carina that can disrupt the airway.

The diagnosis of blunt injury to the trachea or bronchi is sometimes missed initially because many of the associated findings are nonspecific[31] and would be identical to those findings in a patient with a pneumothorax due to pulmonary parenchymal injury. Patients who can communicate often describe dyspnea. If a laryngeal injury is present, speech may be altered or impossible. Most patients have subcutaneous emphysema, but this finding is not always present and may not become manifest until after the institution of positive-pressure ventilation.

Pneumomediastinum may be present. A large pneumothorax is another finding that can aid diagnosis. The likelihood of a major tracheobronchial injury increases if the pneumothorax is not relieved by a tube thoracostomy or if there is a massive air leak after chest tube placement. Although the previously mentioned clinical and radiographic findings suggest a major airway injury, definitive diagnosis should be made with bronchoscopy. Most patients who are stable enough to reach the hospital are stable enough to permit bronchoscopy. Both rigid and fiberoptic bronchoscopy can be used, but injuries can be missed if the bronchoscopist is not experienced.[32]

The first aim of therapy is to stabilize the airway.[33] Nonoperative management may be attempted for small injuries that are seen to encompass less than a third of the airway circumference. Short longitudinal tears of a single airway are particularly likely to be managed successfully in this way. Nonoperative management should not be attempted, even if the injury is less than a third of the circumference of the airway, if the air leak is massive and ventilation is difficult. If nonoperative treatment is attempted, ventilator management must be designed to minimize airway pressures.

Injuries to the cervical trachea should be approached via transverse neck incision. Tears to the thoracic trachea and major bronchi can be transverse or longitudinal, simple or complex. If the injury is to the distal trachea or right main stem bronchus, it should be approached via a right thoracotomy. If the injury is limited to the left main stem bronchus, a left posterior lateral thoracotomy should be used. If there is injury to only one main stem bronchus, the endotracheal tube should be positioned in the contralateral main stem bronchus to allow for ventilation of the patient while the injured side is repaired. Sometimes it is necessary to manipulate placement of the distal end of the endotracheal tube under direct vision after the chest has been opened and the airway has been visualized. Relatively simple repair techniques suffice in most patients, but some patients with complex injury involving the carina or both main stem bronchi can only be safely controlled and repaired with cardiopulmonary bypass.[33]

Major airway injuries generally should be closed with interrupted sutures, but a continuous suture can be used for longitudinal tears. Although the choice of suture is variable, there is evidence that an absorbable suture reduces the development of granulation tissue and subsequent stricture.[34, 35] After closure of the airway defect, the endotracheal tube should be positioned so that the cuff of the tube does not press against the repair. Whenever possible, a tissue flap of pleura, pericardium, or muscle should be placed over the suture line. Postoperative ventilator management should minimize airway pressures. Before extubation, the integrity of the repair can be assessed with fiberoptic bronchoscopy.

INJURIES TO GREAT VESSELS

Blunt trauma can injure the aorta or the branches of the aortic arch. Approximately 95% of patients with blunt tears of the thoracic aorta die before reaching the hospital.[36] In the small percentage who survive the initial postinjury period, bleeding is limited by the adventitia and other mediastinal tissues.[37, 38] Aortic transection in children is extraordinarily rare and does not truly begin to appear until children are of sufficient age to begin riding motorized vehicles, thereby subjecting themselves to potential deceleration injuries.

Pseudoaneurysms of the innominate, common carotid, and subclavian arteries are rare and probably related to a stretch injury. One of the more common of these injuries is disruption of a vessel at its origin from the aorta. The thoracic aorta can tear at a variety of locations, including its ascending portion and at the diaphragm. In patients who survive to reach the hospital, the most common site of disruption is just distal to the origin of the left subclavian artery at the ligamentum arteriosum. This site is the juncture of the mobile aortic arch and the immobile descending thoracic aorta tethered by the intercostal arteries. The aorta is further tethered by the ligamentum arteriosum. In sudden deceleration, the descending aorta stops with the rest of the body, while the heart and aortic arch continue moving forward. Shear force develops at the juncture of these two segments of the aorta, creating a tear.[36] Tears range from partial to complete disruption. When partial, the tear usually includes the posteriomedial aorta in the vicinity of the ligamentum arteriosum.

In most patients with tears of the thoracic aorta, there are no specific physical findings. Occasionally, blood from the aortic tear dissects distally along the course of the left subclavian artery and causes compression and spasm of that artery. The result on physical examination is diminished blood pressure in the left arm as compared with the right. Similar pathophysiology of the descending aorta can lead to differential pulses and blood pressures in the lower as compared with the upper extremities. However, these findings are uncommon and occasionally occur in the absence of a thoracic aorta tear.

Radiographic findings are often more helpful than physical examination. A widened superior mediastinal silhouette should certainly raise suspicions, but the definition of "widened" varies. Only 10 to 20% of adult patients have what is perceived to be a widened mediastinum. The low specificity can be attributed to mediastinal hematomas that occur in association with venous bleeding, a poor inspiratory effort, and supine views. Also, in a young child, a persistence of a large thymus may contribute to superior mediastinal widening. Perhaps a more sensitive radiographic indicator is deviation of the esophagus, as visualized on chest roentgenogram following passage of a nasogastric tube.

It is sometimes difficult to decide on the basis of the initial chest radiograph which patients require further study.[39] If further investigation is warranted, a decision must be made about what imaging procedure should be used. Angiography is the commonly accepted approach to the definitive diagnosis of a torn thoracic aorta. Aortography is expensive, labor intensive, and invasive, especially in younger patients. For these reasons, a less costly, less invasive, and simpler diagnostic imaging study is desirable. Computed tomography is one possibility whose advantages as an alternative to angiography are obvious.[40–42] It can be performed more quickly and is less invasive. It is also more available in more hospitals. There are also potential disadvantages. If the computed tomographic study is not definitive and the patient requires angiography anyway, more contrast agent is necessary and there is a delay in diagnosis. Also, some series have a disturbingly high percentage of false-negative results.[40, 43, 44]

Because of their propensity for rupture, traumatic pseudoaneurysms of the thoracic aorta should be treated surgically. A major complication of such repairs is the development of paraplegia as a result of spinal chord ischemia during aortic cross-clamping. Several methods have been developed to prevent this complication, and all of these methods are designed to maintain distal perfusion. None of these methods is foolproof.[45–47] A heparin-bonded Gott shunt may be used to shunt blood without an interposed pump from the proximal aorta to the distal aorta or to the femoral artery. Left heart bypass utilizes a centrifugal pump to withdraw oxygenated blood from the left atrium that is reinfused into the femoral artery or the distal thoracic aorta. Femoral-femoral cardiopulmonary bypass using an oxygenator will maintain the lower body perfusion. All of these techniques are space and time consuming and have other disadvantages. I prefer the method of femoral-femoral bypass for spinal chord protection. It is relatively easy to institute, and the cannulae do not interfere with the operative field. The bypass cannulae may be placed prior to dissection around the aorta so that if rapid aortic cross-clamping is necessary, bypass can be instituted immediately. With modern high-flow thin-wall cannulae, more than adequate bypass rates can be achieved. Body temperature can be raised or lowered, and hypertension proximal to the aortic cross-clamp can be more easily controlled.

Thoracic aortic pseudoaneurysm generally should be approached via left-sided posterolateral thoracotomy. If the pseudoaneurysm is not actively bleeding and some form of bypass is planned, the thoracotomy incision should be in place so that if aortic cross-clamping is subsequently necessary, bypass can be instituted rapidly. The aorta distal to the pseudoaneurysm should be dissected and encircled with tapes or loops. Proximal control is then obtained, first with the encirclement of the proximal left subclavian artery, and then with encirclement of the aorta between the left common carotid and left subclavian arteries. This technique of proximal control is preferred because it gives the best chance of obtaining control without entering the pseudoaneurysm and because there is often a very short cuff between the origin of the left subclavian artery and the tear. Obtaining proximal control is the most difficult part of the operation. The left recurrent laryngeal nerve loops beneath the ligamentum arteriosum or ductus arteriosus and should be protected. After proximal and distal control have been obtained, the bypass should be started, the pseudoaneurysm entered, and the free edges of the aorta

defined. Most patients require placement of a graft, but in occasional cases of partial tears, a primary repair can be done. If a graft is used, woven Dacron is the graft material of choice.

Perioperative antibiotics appropriate for skin flora are used. If there is an associated pulmonary injury with an air leak, broad-spectrum antibiotics are required. Hypertension should be rigorously controlled with cardioactive β-blocker agents rather than peripheral vasodilators.

Occasionally, patients with a remote history of trauma present with an abnormal mediastinal silhouette on a chest roentgenogram or with other symptoms such as airway compression, left recurrent laryngeal nerve compression, or compression of the left subclavian artery. Surgical repair of the chronic aortic pseudoaneurysm is indicated as outlined previously, even in asymptomatic patients. Repair of the mature aneurysm is considerably more difficult secondary to chronic scarring and the exuberant inflammatory reaction that accompanies extravasation of blood into the mediastinum.

CARDIAC INJURY

Blunt injuries of the myocardium range from mild asymptomatic contusion to cardiac rupture.[48, 49] Nonmyocardial cardiac injuries are also possible. Rupture of the pericardium can occur with or without associated cardiac injury. Laceration or thrombosis of the coronary arteries from blunt trauma is rare but possible. Diagnosis is best made by electrocardiogram and, if time permits, by coronary angiography. Treatment is selective. Repair is indicated if ischemia and myocardial dysfunction are severe and there is salvageable myocardium. Blunt rupture of the heart is not uncommon, but most patients with such a condition do not survive to reach medical attention. Occasionally, however, bleeding is controlled by tamponade, in which case the patient presents in shock from a combination of hemorrhage and cardiac tamponade.[50] However, in some patients, the admission blood pressure is normal. An admission chest radiograph reveals a wide cardiac shadow.

The mechanism of injury is probably sudden severe compression of the chest at the end of diastole. Blunt rupture occurs with equal frequency to all of the cardiac chambers, but injuries to the right atrium are associated with the most favorable prognosis because the right atrium is the low-pressure chamber and is relatively easy to access (Fig. 16–5). The prognosis of left atrial and right ventricular injuries is intermediate. Survivors of left ventricular injuries are rare.

Blunt cardiac rupture should be treated surgically (Fig. 16–6). Either sternotomy or thoracotomy can be used, with left-sided thoracotomy being the best approach for left-sided lesions, particularly of the left atrium, and sternotomy the best approach for right atrial and right ventricular lesions. Most injuries can be repaired without cardiopulmonary by-

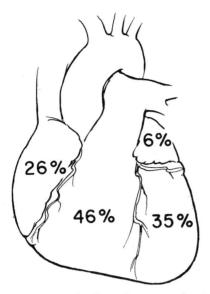

Figure 16–5. Location and relative frequency of various cardiac injuries from Baylor College of Medicine.

pass. Ruptures of the atria, particularly at the atrial appendage, can initially be controlled with a vascular clamp. Bleeding from rupture of the ventricle sometimes can be temporarily controlled by balloon tamponade using a urinary catheter placed through the defect.

Blunt trauma more frequently produces contusion of the myocardium. In experimental animals, this can lead to serious arrhythmias and cardiac pump failure. In most animals, these effects occur within seconds to minutes of the blunt injury, but the possibility of delayed manifestation of myocardial contusion is a concern.[51] There is no reliable standard for diagnosis. A number of different diagnostic tests

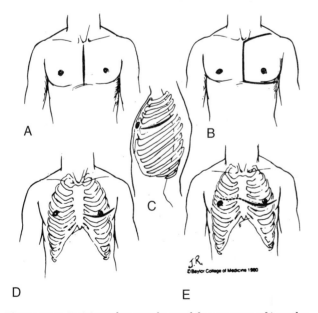

Figure 16–6. Incisions that may be used for exposure of intrathoracic injuries.

have been proposed.[52–56] For many of these tests, however, establishment of a diagnosis does not correlate with outcome in the vast majority of patients. Conversely, patients with negative results for myocardial contusion may still develop complications, possibly related to myocardial contusion. Creatinine phosphocreatine levels and echocardiography are examples of such low-sensitivity, low-specificity tests and are not helpful in diagnostic or treatment planning.

Sequelae of myocardial contusion are uncommon in patients who demonstrate hemodynamic and cardiac stability on admission.[52, 57] Obviously unstable patients declare the severity of their illness early in the emergency department course and are triaged to an intensive care setting where they receive treatment for possible myocardial contusion with monitoring, antiarrythmic drugs, and cardiac support as needed.

One of the most sensitive indicators of significance of contusion appears to be rhythm disturbances. In the presence of contusion, these will usually resolve within 48 hours. Patients without a rhythm disturbance on admission can be admitted to an unmonitored bed.[58]

Penetrating wounds of the heart are managed in a similar manner as blunt injury. If the heart is perforated by a knife, bullet, or other penetrating object, one of two pathophysiologic events may occur. Blood may leak from the heart into the adjacent pleural cavity and present as a hemothorax. This diagnosis is suspected when there is hemodynamic instability from hemorrhagic shock or persistent bleeding from a chest tube. The other possibility is that blood will accumulate in the pericardial space. For this to occur, the hole in the pericardial space must tamponade. The pericardial membrane is thick and elastic, and the hole created in it often becomes occluded, which prevents the patient from exsanguinating. Unfortunately, continued pericardial blood accumulation also leads to pericardial tamponade.

Penetrating injuries to the heart can involve any of the four chambers but are most common in the right ventricle. The right ventricle is anteriorly located and therefore more vulnerable. Because right-sided pressures are lower than left-sided pressures, the bleeding of injuries to the right side of the heart is more likely to tamponade and allow patients to survive to reach medical attention.

Many patients with penetrating injuries to the heart present with obvious hemodynamic compromise from blood loss, pericardial tamponade, or a combination of the two. When the compromise is severe enough, there are no vital signs and the patient is a candidate for emergency department thoracotomy. Regardless of whether tamponade is present, the pericardium should be opened and the heart should be visualized. This maneuver relieves tamponade, if present, and allows digital control of the cardiac wound. Attempts at suture of the heart in an emergency setting should be avoided. If sutures are not carefully placed and pledgeted, they can tear through the myocardium, enlarge the traumatic defect, and convert a salvageable wound into one that cannot be repaired.

Although many patients with penetrating cardiac injuries present in extremis, some are hemodynamically stable on presentation. In most patients, bleeding within the pericardial space produces some element of tamponade and venous return to the right heart is compromised. Administration of intravenous fluids only temporarily improves the situation.

In children, transthoracic echocardiography is extraordinarily sensitive in detecting even small amounts of pericardial fluid. Pericardiocentesis is a more invasive approach to the diagnosis of intrapericardial blood. A needle is placed in the subxyphoid position and directed toward the left shoulder at a 30- to 45-degree angle from the skin surface. While the needle is advanced, constant aspiration is maintained. If blood is aspirated, the result is positive. It is important to observe the aspirated blood for clot formation. Blood that has been aspirated from a cardiac chamber will clot, whereas, if the blood aspirated is from the pericardial sac, it is defibrinated and will not clot.

Pericardiocentesis is controversial and not without risk of injuring the heart.[59] If the result is positive, there is nothing definitive that can be done if surgical expertise is not immediately present.[60–62] Removal of only a small amount of blood from the pericardial sac may temporarily improve the hemodynamic status, but repeated aspirations may be necessary.

Creation of a subxyphoid pericardial window is another approach to treating a wound that may have injured the heart in a stable patient.[63, 64] A small subxyphoid incision is made, through which the diaphragmatic portion of the pericardial surface is grasped and incised. If a small amount of normal serous pericardial fluid is seen, the wound is closed. Hemopericardium is an indication that the patient should undergo sternotomy or thoracotomy for repair of the cardiac injury. Subxyphoid pericardial windows are both sensitive and highly specific.

One must keep in mind that many of the wounds that raise the possibility of cardiac injury also suggest underlying abdominal injury. The abdominal viscera, depending on the patient's positioning and phase of respiration at the time of injury, can rise as high as the fourth or fifth intercostal space. In many cases of penetrating precordial trauma, abdominal exploration is necessary. If a laparotomy is performed and there is concern about the possibility of a penetrating injury to the heart, it is simple to make a small hole in the diaphragmatic surface of the pericardium via laparotomy incision. Extension of the midline laparotomy into a sternotomy facilitates repair of the cardiac injury.

Either thoracotomy or sternotomy can be used to repair cardiac injuries, but sternotomy affords access to all cardiac chambers, even if some cardiac manipulation is required, whereas left thoracotomy precludes effective repair of injuries to the right side of the heart.

Repair of most cardiac injuries is straightforward. Nonabsorbable sutures should be used for repair. The type of suture is less important than the size and type of needle. An atraumatic needle should be used and should be big enough to take moderately large bites of the myocardium for approximation but not so large that there are large needle holes after the repair is done. Pledget material should be used to reinforce the repair and to prevent the sutures from pulling through the myocardium. In some wounds of the atria, a side-biting vascular clamp can be used for control during repair. Alternatively, the area of injury can be compressed with a finger while it is being sutured. Nonabsorbable sutures should be used and should be plegeted. Precise location of each initial suture is difficult in a bleeding beating heart and is not as important as getting some degree of control of the bleeding, so that refinements of the repair can be performed in a relatively bloodless field. Care always must be taken to avoid injury to coronary arteries.

DIAPHRAGM

Blunt injuries of the diaphragm are becoming more common with higher automotive speeds and increased use of seat belt restraints.[65–67] When a seat belt is in place, sudden deceleration can lead to a marked increase in intraabdominal pressure, which is transmitted to the diaphragm.

Blunt rupture of the diaphragm occurs more commonly on the left than on the right.[65] Teleologically, the liver protects the right hemidiaphragm and helps dissipate kinetic energy throughout its substance. It is also easier to make the diagnosis on the left side because radiographic findings are more obvious. Right-sided ruptures are therefore more likely to be missed because the liver prevents abdominal visceral herniation and small tears in the right side are of minimal consequence. Rarely, both hemidiaphragms are ruptured. The diaphragm can rupture in any location, but ruptures of the central tendon and the lateral attachments of the torso wall are most common. The size varies, but most of the tears that are diagnosed are at least several centimeters long. On the left side, abdominal viscera can herniate through the diaphragmatic defect, but this does not universally occur, and herniation is unlikely in patients on controlled positive-pressure ventilation.

The diagnosis of diaphragmatic rupture is usually made by either radiographic findings or incidentally discovered at the time of an operation. Herniation of hollow abdominal viscera are usually easily recognized on the radiograph, whereas solid viscera such as the liver or spleen may be interpreted as elevation of the hemidiaphragm. Bleeding from associated intraabdominal injuries is common, and when this blood leaks into the pleural cavity, it may appear as a hemothorax. Subtle blunting of the costophrenic angle and a fuzzy quality to the hemidiaphragm are common radiographic findings. Persistence of the blunting after chest tube placement and drainage of the ipsilateral pleural cavity is a clue to differentiating diaphragmatic rupture from simple hemothorax.

In some patients, bleeding from associated intraabdominal injuries is severe and manifests itself as a large hemothorax with persistent bleeding. In the absence of a definitive diagnosis of diaphragmatic rupture, the decision about whether to perform thoracotomy or laparotomy is difficult. Although thoracotomy may be appropriate on rare occasions when an intrathoracic source of hemorrhage is most likely, it is prudent to position the patient so that a laparotomy can also be done if the chest is opened and bleeding is seen to be coming through a ruptured hemidiaphragm.

It is important to inspect the diaphragm closely during exploratory laparotomy, regardless of whether the diagnosis of diaphragmatic rupture has been made preoperatively. Some of the tears are subtle and hidden by folds of the diaphragm, which can balloon and collapse with the cycle of positive pressure ventilation. When the tear is located, any herniated viscera should be returned to the abdomen and inspected for bleeding or ischemia. The rent should then be repaired. Both monofilament nonabsorbable sutures and large continuous absorbable sutures are appropriate for the repair. If not already present, a chest tube should be placed on the affected side. Drainage over the first several postoperative days is often considerable until the diaphragmatic tear has healed and become watertight.

Occasionally, the diagnosis of blunt rupture of the diaphragm is initially missed. If the hemidiaphragm is elevated in the early postinjury period and the diagnosis is suspected, computed tomography of the lower chest and upper abdomen sometimes aids diagnosis. Detection of visceral herniation can be delayed, presenting even years after the traumatic event. Herniation may be asymptomatic and only appear on a chest roentgenogram obtained incidentally, or the herniated viscera may become strangulated and cause symptoms. If the diagnosis is delayed and the patient is asymptomatic, repair can be affected by either an abdominal or a thoracic approach. If the patient is symptomatic and there is a possibility of visceral ischemia or perforation, the approach should always be through the abdomen.

REFERENCES

1. National Safety Council: Accident Facts (preliminary condensed edition). National Safety Council, March 1983.
2. Velecek FT, Weiss AD, DiMaio D, et al: Traumatic death in urban children. J Pediatr Surg 12:375–384, 1977.
3. Drew R, Perry JF, Fisher R: The expediency of peritoneal lavage for blunt trauma in children. Surg Gynecol Obstet 145:885, 1977.
4. Mayer T, Matlak M, Johnson D, et al: The modified injury severity scale in pediatric multiple trauma patients. J Pediatr Surg 15:422, 1980.
5. Smyth, BT: Chest trauma in children. J Pediatr Surg 14:41, 1979.
6. Newman KD, Eichelberger MR: The child with thoracic trauma. Current Topics in General Thoracic Surgery: An International Series. New York; Elsevier Science, 1991.
7. Breasted JH: The Edwin Smith Papyrus. Vol. 1. Chicago, University of Chicago Press, 1930.
8. Hippocrates: Works. Vol. III. Withington ET (trans). Cambridge, MA, Harvard University Press, 1959, p 307.
9. Aristotle: De Partibus Animalum. Peck A (trans). Cambridge, MA, Harvard University Press, 1937.
10. Pickard LR, Mattox KL: Thoracic Trauma: General Considerations and Indications for Thoracotomy in Trauma (2nd ed) Norwalk, CT, Appleton & Lange, 1991, p 319.
11. Paré A: Collected Works (AD 1582). Johnson I (trans). London, 1634, p 571.
12. Riolanus J: En cheiridium anatomicum et pathologicum, in quo ex naturali constituione partium, recessus, a naturale statu demonstratur; Ad usum theatri anatomici adornatum. Lugd Bat, A Wynedaerden, 1649.
13. Scultetus J: The Surgeon's Storehouse. London, Starkey, 1674, p 159.
14. Anel D: L'Art de Sucer les Plaies. Amsterdam, 1707.
15. Playfair WS: On the treatment of empyema in children. Obstet Soc London Trans 14:4, 1872.
16. Guthrie GJ: On Wounds and Injuries of the Chest. London, Rensaw and Churchill, 1848.
17. Jeger E: Die Chirurgie der Blutgefass und des Herzens. Berlin, Hirschwal, 1913, p 295.
18. Rehn L: Veber penetrierende Herzwunder und Herznaht. Arch Klin Chri 55:315, 1897.
19. Graham EA: A brief account of the development of thoracic surgery and some of its consequences. Surg Gynecol Obstet 104:241, 1957.
20. Graham EA, Bell RD: Open pneumothorax: Its reaction to the treatment of empyema. Am J Med Sci 156:839, 1918.
21. West JG, Williams MJ, Trunkey DD, Wolferth CC, Jr.: Trauma systems. Current status—future challenges. JAMA 259:3597, 1988.
22. American College of Surgeons: Advanced Trauma Life Support Course. Chicago, American College of Surgeons, 1989.
23. Wood PR, Lawler PGP: Managing the airway in cervical spine injury. A review of the Advanced Trauma Life Support protocol. Anaesthesia 47:792, 1992.
24. Barone JE, Pizzi WF, Nealon TF, Jr., Richman H: Indications for intubation in blunt chest trauma. J Trauma 26:334, 1986.
25. Grande CM, Stene JK, Bernhard WN: Airway management: Considerations in the trauma patient. Crit Care Clin 6:37, 1990.
26. Rhee KJ, Green W, Holcroft JW, Mangili JA: Oral intubation in the multiply injured patient: The risk of exacerbating spinal cord injury. Ann Emerg Med 19:511, 1990.
27. Young G, Eichelberger, MR: Initial Resuscitation of the Child with Multiple Injuries. Pediatric Emergency Medicine. Philadelphia, JB Lippincott, 1991.
28. Flynn AE, Thomas AN, Schecter WP: Acute tracheobronchial injury. J Trauma 29:1326, 1989.
29. Grover FL, Ellestad C, Arom KV, et al: Diagnosis and management of major tracheobronchial injuries. Ann Thorac Surg 28:384, 1979.
30. Symbas PN, Diorio DA, Tyras DH, et al: Penetrating cardiac wounds: Significant residual and delayed sequelae. J Thorac Cardiovasc Surg 66:526, 1973.
31. Jones WS, Mavroudis C, Richardson JD, et al: Management of tracheobronchial disruption resulting from blunt trauma. Surgery 95:319, 1984.
32. Baumgartner F, Sheppard B, de Virgilio C, et al: Tracheal and main bronchial disruptions after blunt chest trauma: Presentations and management. Ann Thorac Surg 50:569, 1990.
33. Symbas PN, Justicz AG, Ricketts RR: Rupture of the airways from blunt trauma: Treatment of complex injuries. Ann Thorac Surg 54:177, 1992.
34. Gibbons JA, Peniston RL, Diamond SS, Aaron BL: A comparison of synthetic absorbable suture with synthetic nonabsorb-

able suture for construction of tracheal anastomoses. Chest 79:340, 1981.

35. Urschel HC, Razzuk MA: Management of acute traumatic injuries of tracheobronchial tree. Surg Gynecol Obstet 136:113, 1973.

36. Feczko JD, Lynch L, Pless JE, et al: An autopsy case review of 148 nonpenetrating (blunt) injuries of the aorta. J Trauma 33:846, 1992.

37. Parmley LF, Mattingly TW, Manlow WC: Non-penetrating traumatic injury to the aorta. Circulation 17:1096, 1958.

38. Pickard LR, Mattox KL, Espada R, et al: Transection of the descending thoracic aorta secondary to blunt trauma. J Trauma 17:749, 1977.

39. Gundry SR, Burney RE, MacKenzie JR, et al: Assessment of mediastinal widening associated with traumatic rupture of the aorta. J Trauma 23:293, 1983.

40. Agee CK, Metzler MH, Churchill RJ, Mitchell FL: Computer tomographic evaluation to exclude traumatic aortic disruption. J Trauma 33:876, 1998.

41. Heiberg E, Wolverson MK, Sundaram M, Shields JB: CT in aortic trauma. AJR Am J Roentgenol 140:1119, 1983.

42. Ishikawa T, Nakajima Y, Kaji T: The role of CT in traumatic rupture of the thoracic aorta and its proximal branches. Semin Roentgenol 24:38, 1989.

43. McLean TR, Olinger GN, Thorsen MK: Computed tomography in the evaluation of the aorta in patients sustaining blunt chest trauma. J Trauma 31:254, 1991.

44. Miller FB, Richardson JD, Thomas HA: Role of CT in the diagnosis of major arterial injury after blunt thoracic trauma. Surgery 106:596, 1989a.

45. McCroskey BL, Moore EE, Moore FA, Abernathy CM: A unified approach to the torn thoracic aorta. Am J Surg 162:473, 1991.

46. Merrill WH, Lee RB, Hammon JW, Jr., et al: Surgical treatment of acute traumatic tear of the thoracic aorta. Ann Surg 207:699, 1988.

47. Van Norman GA, Pavlin EG, Eddy AC, Pavlin DJ: Hemodynamic and metabolic effects of aortic unclamping following emergency surgery for traumatic thoracic aortic tear in shunted and unshunted patients. J Trauma 31:1007, 1991.

48. Brathwaite CEM, Rodriguez A, Turney SZ, et al: Blunt traumatic cardiac rupture. Ann Surg 212:701, 1990.

49. Fulda G, Brathwaite CEM, Rodriguez A, et al: Blunt traumatic rupture of the heart and pericardium: A ten-year experience (1979–1989). J Trauma 31:167, 1991.

50. Pevec WC, Udekwu AO, Peitzman AB: Blunt rupture of the myocardium. Ann Thorac Surg 48:139, 1989.

51. Tenzer ML. The spectrum of myocardial contusion: A review. J Trauma 25:620, 1985.

52. Fabian TC, Mangiante EC, Patterson CR, et al: Myocardial contusion in blunt trauma: Clinical characteristics, means of diagnosis, and implications for patient management. J Trauma 28:50, 1988.

53. Mattox KL, Flint LM, Carrico CJ, et al: Blunt cardiac injury [editorial]. J Trauma 33:649, 1992.

54. Shapiro MJ, Yanofsky SD, Trapp J, et al: Cardiovascular evaluation in blunt thoracic trauma using transesophageal echocardiography (TEE). J Trauma 31:835, 1991.

55. Miller FB, Shumate CR, Richardson JD: Myocardial contusion. Arch Surg 124:805, 1989b.

56. Sturaitis M, McCallum D, Sutherland G, et al: Lack of significant long-term sequelae following traumatic myocardial contusion. Arch Intern Med 146:1765, 1986.

57. Wisner DH, Reed WH, Riddick RS: Suspected myocardial contusion. Triage and indications for monitoring. Ann Surg 212:82, 1990.

58. Wisner DH: A stepwise logistic regression analysis of factors affecting morbidity and mortality after thoracic trauma: Effect of epidural analgesia. J Trauma 30:799, 1990.

59. Trinkle JK, Richardson JD, Franz JL, et al: Management of flail chest without mechanical ventilation. Ann Thorac Surg 19:355, 1975.

60. Demetriades D: Cardiac penetrating injuries: Personal experience of 45 cases. Fr J Surg 71:95, 1984.

61. Ivatury RR, Rohman M, Steichen RM, et al: Penetrating cardiac injuries: Twenty-year experience. Am Surg 53:310, 1987.

62. Marshall WG, Jr., Bell JL, Kouchoukos NT: Penetrating cardiac trauma. J Trauma 24:147, 1984.

63. Jimenez E, Martin M, Krukenkamp I, Barrett J: Subxiphoid pericardiotomy versus echocardiography: A prospective evaluation of the diagnosis of occult penetrating cardiac injury. Surgery 108:676, 1990.

64. Mayor-Davies, JA, Britz RS: Subxiphoid pericardial windows—helpful in selected cases. J Trauma 30:1399, 1990.

65. Beal SL, McKennan M: Blunt diaphragm rupture. A morbid injury. Arch Surg 123:828, 1988.

66. Ilgenfritz FM, Stewart DD: Blunt trauma of the diaphragm: A 15-county, private hospital experience. Am Surg 6:334, 1992.

67. Kearney PA, Rouhana SW, Burney RE: Blunt rupture of the diaphragm: Mechanism, diagnosis and treatment. Ann Emerg Med 18:1326, 1989.

17

ABDOMINAL AND GENITOURINARY TRAUMA

Charles L. Snyder, MD

Trauma is the most common cause of death in children, and its emergent nature requires a thorough knowledge of the subject. Major trauma does not afford the luxury of long deliberation or research to determine the appropriate treatment.

Most pediatric trauma is blunt rather than penetrating. Head and extremity injuries are the most common. Organ systems that only sustain injury after significant force is applied carry the highest mortality rates. The highest mortality rates are associated with injuries to the spinal cord and the thoracic region.[1] The overall mortality rate for children admitted to the hospital with trauma is approximately 2.5%. Abdominal trauma is common in children, occurring in approximately 5% of all admissions to pediatric centers, with an attendant mortality rate of approximately 15%.[2]

Trauma is often more difficult to assess in children than adults. Afflicted patients may be nonverbal, frightened, unable to clearly communicate their symptoms, and excessively anxious. However, they are much less likely than adults to have an underlying disease process complicating their management. It is important for the examiner to proceed with assessment and treatment in an organized and orderly fashion and to be cognizant of the many pitfalls inherent in treating the traumatized child or infant. Familiarity with the pediatric advanced life support (PALS) and advanced trauma life support (ATLS) basics is essential.

Mechanisms of injury to children differ from those of adults. Understanding the mechanism of injury may help to direct the examination. Pertinent medical history should be obtained, if possible. Discrepancy between the purported mechanism of injury and the clinical findings should raise the suspicion of nonaccidental trauma.

Once the patient is stabilized, a thorough examination of the abdomen should be carried out. Passage of a nasogastric tube may facilitate the examination because significant abdominal distention from swallowed air is common in the injured child.

Inspection of the abdomen may reveal contusions and abrasions or marks from restraining devices such as lap or shoulder belts. Such findings may guide the clinician toward specific organ systems. Likewise, passage of a Foley catheter may help to decompress the bladder, improving the examination. Contraindications to catheterization include the presence of blood at the urethral meatus, a "boggy" prostate on digital rectal examination, or a pelvic fracture.

Peritoneal signs may be particularly difficult to discern in the child with lower rib fractures, contusions or abrasions of the abdominal wall, a pelvic fracture, a distended urinary bladder, or gastric dilation. The frequent presence of associated head injury and depressed sensorium may also limit the examination. Even thorough and repeated examinations at the hands of an experienced examiner, although essential, must be supplemented by additional diagnostic techniques. The evaluation of any traumatized child should include a chest radiograph and views of the abdomen and pelvis. The most useful imaging study for evaluation of the pediatric abdomen in blunt trauma is the contrast enhanced (intravenous [IV] and enteral) computed tomographic (CT) scan.

The CT scan is particularly useful in demonstrating solid organ injury and the presence of abnormal fluid collections within the peritoneal cavity. Its sensitivity in detecting hollow visceral injury is substantially lower, but such injuries occur less frequently than solid organ injuries.[3] Grading scales exist to assess the severity of solid organ injuries and are discussed later in this chapter. Contraindications to CT scan are hemodynamic instability or other major life-threatening injuries. Abdominal CT scan is a commonly obtained adjunct to the head CT in cases in which depressed sensorium limits the clinical evaluation, intraabdominal injury is suspected based on the history and physical examination, or when unexplained hypovolemia is present. Although some degree of hematuria is found in more than one half of children with abdominal trauma, isolated asymptomatic microscopic hematuria does not appear to be a significant marker for intraabdominal injury.[4, 5] The severity of the hematuria appears to correlate with the probability of an intraabdominal injury, and gross hematuria in particular may indicate an associated injury.[6] The likelihood of positive CT findings in patients with central nervous system trauma is higher for those with a Glasgow Coma scale score of 8 or less. However, the overall yield for patients with isolated head injuries in the absence of abdominal signs is low.[7]

Diagnostic peritoneal lavage (DPL), once the mainstay of the abdominal evaluation of the injured child, is infrequently necessary. However, in certain settings it may still provide useful information and may complement the CT scan. Patients with severe head injuries requiring urgent neurosurgical intervention may benefit from a rapid DPL to rule out the presence of a significant intraabdominal injury. Children with suspected hollow visceral injury, such as that seen in the lap belt complex, may also be candidates for DPL. An open technique is generally used, and the volume of lactated Ringer's solution used should be approximately 15 ml/kg body weight. Criteria for positive lavage are the presence of more than 100,000 red blood cells per high-powered field (HPF), more than 500 white blood cells per HPF, presence of bowel contents, bile, or elevated amylase.

The use of the focal abdominal sonogram for trauma (FAST) examination for adults with abdominal trauma is well documented.[8] However, the use of surgeon-directed ultrasonography (US) in the acutely injured child has not yet been clearly defined.[9]

The indications for celiotomy in children with blunt abdominal trauma include (1) shock from an intraabdominal source, (2) suspected or confirmed hollow visceral injury, (3) transfusion requirements of greater than or equal to ½ of total blood volume, (4) retroperitoneal air on CT or plain radiographs, and (5) intraperitoneal bladder rupture.

□ Penetrating Trauma

Because penetrating trauma is much less frequent than blunt trauma in children, its management may be more difficult. Concern about the high number of unnecessary laparotomies in adults with penetrating injuries has prompted a more selective approach in children.

Gunshot wounds to the abdomen, by virtue of their high associated kinetic energy, require a laparotomy. This includes gunshot wounds from below the nipples to the groin.

Stab wounds may be managed selectively in children.[10] One suggested approach uses DPL as the initial diagnostic study. If DPL is positive, laparotomy is performed. If the lavage is negative, a triple-contrast CT scan (oral, IV, and bladder contrast

agents) is done. If the CT scan is negative, the patient is observed; if the CT scan is positive, the patient undergoes celiotomy.[10] Another option for managing stab wounds includes local wound exploration before lavage. If the posterior fascia or peritoneum is intact, no further diagnostic studies other than simple observation are necessary. If peritoneal penetration is suspected, DPL is performed. Flank or back stab wounds may involve an injury to the retroperitoneum, limiting the utility of lavage. In this instance, triple-contrast CT scan may be helpful. Laparoscopy may also be a useful adjunct in such situations.

□ Abdominal Trauma

HEPATIC INJURY

The large size and strategic location of the liver account for its being, with the spleen, one of the most frequently injured solid organs in the abdomen. The right lobe, by virtue of its size and location, is injured more often than the left. The majority of pediatric liver injuries are the result of blunt trauma. In a responsive patient, diffuse abdominal pain and tenderness are usually found. Contusions, abrasions, ecchymoses, or other external signs of trauma may be visible on the abdominal wall. Signs of peritonitis are frequently present.

The standard diagnostic study is the CT scan. Hepatic injuries can be radiographically graded, but the grade does not always correlate with clinical outcome.[11] Most hepatic injuries can be managed nonoperatively.[12–14] Historically, exploratory laparotomy for liver trauma often resulted in the finding of a nonbleeding laceration. This prompted selective management of liver injuries. The primary indications for operation in a child with a liver injury are hemodynamic instability, associated injuries requiring operation, or need for transfusion of greater than or equal to ½ of the estimated blood volume. Most children at our institution with hepatic injuries are treated nonoperatively.

The nonoperative management of children with hepatic injuries usually consists of admission to the intensive care unit, strict bed rest, careful monitoring, and serial physical examinations and laboratory studies. Associated injuries are common in children with blunt hepatic trauma and may not always be recognized on initial CT scans. Complications such as hemobilia, abscess, bile peritonitis, or biliary fistula may develop either during the course of expectant management or postoperatively.

Bed rest in nonoperatively treated children at our institution is usually maintained for 7 days, but the length of time is dependent on the severity of the injury and the clinical status of the patient. Limited activities (no contact sports, no strenuous activity) are usually observed for 3 months postoperatively, again depending on the clinical circumstances. A follow-up CT scan at the conclusion of the observation period is essential in both medically and surgically managed children with liver trauma.

The primary surgical problem posed by extensive liver injuries is bleeding. Adequate exposure is essential. Vertical midline incisions are often used with thoracoabdominal or median sternotomy extension. Simple operative techniques suffice for most pediatric hepatic injuries. Bleeding often ceases before surgery. Nonexpanding hematomas can be observed. Expanding hematomas or actively bleeding lacerations require gentle exploration of the liver parenchyma and direct ligation of the bleeding site. *Resectional débridement*, consisting of removal of devitalized or injured tissue and direct suture ligation of bleeding vessels, is useful in many circumstances. Pressure is applied to the bleeding site. Gentle compression of the porta hepatis, including the portal vein and common hepatic artery, helps control bleeding.[15] Failure of this maneuver to stop the bleeding may indicate either an aberrant arterial supply or, more ominously, a retrohepatic vena caval source of bleeding (Fig. 17–1).

Although débridement of injured parenchyma or a limited segmental resection may be necessary, major anatomic liver resections should be avoided, if possible. A high mortality rate is associated with lobectomies and major anatomic resections. In the presence of significant hypothermia and coagulopathy, simply packing the abdomen is the safest alternative. The packs are usually removed in 48 to 72 hours.

Ligation of the right or left hepatic artery is rarely necessary, but it can be useful in the rare instance of bleeding from this source. Hemobilia is rare; it presents with jaundice, abdominal pain, and gastrointestinal (GI) bleeding and is due to erosion of an existing intraparenchymal hematoma into the biliary tree.[14] The treatment of hemobilia is arterial embolization; operative intervention is rarely necessary.

Hepatic vein or retrohepatic caval injuries may require either total vascular isolation of the liver or extension of the incision into a median sternotomy with placement of an atriocaval shunt.[16, 17] With the former technique, warm ischemia times of less than 1 hour are generally well tolerated. Successful use of either of these techniques requires careful preoperative planning. Large amounts of blood must be available for transfusion, a cell saver device must be ready, and an appropriately sized shunt (often simply a modified chest tube) must be available. The patient is widely prepped, and experienced surgical teams are scrubbed and ready to proceed before the abdomen is opened and any potential tamponade is released. Even with all of the aforementioned, the operative mortality of retrohepatic caval injuries remains high.[14]

SPLENIC INJURY

The spleen and liver are injured with almost equal frequency. Most splenic injuries are the result of blunt trauma. Associated injuries are frequent, occurring in up to 80% of patients.[18] Approximately one third of patients have other intraabdominal injuries, most of which do not require operative intervention. In the responsive patient, either generalized abdominal complaints or left upper quadrant pain and tenderness are usually present. Kehr's sign, diaphragmatic irritation resulting in referred pain to the left shoulder, may be present. A CT scan helps clearly delineate the extent of the splenic injury, identify the presence and amount of free intraperitoneal fluid, and detect associated injuries. However, some injuries (e.g., associated hollow visceral trauma) can be difficult or impossible to identify on the initial CT scan. A high index of suspicion is necessary.

Grading systems for CT scan analysis of splenic injury are available but are of limited clinical utility.[12, 19, 20] In children, the vast majority of splenic injuries can be managed nonoperatively.[13, 21, 22] The primary indications for operation are hemodynamic instability, suspected associated injury, or excessive transfusion requirements ($\geq$ ½ total blood volume).

The nonoperative management of splenic injury consists of a period of bed rest followed by a longer interval of limited activity. Initial admission to the ICU may be necessary for patients with severe or multiple injuries or those whose clinical status otherwise mandates such a course. Children with milder injuries may be admitted to the ward. Close observation by the nursing staff, careful monitoring, serial examinations by a single physician, and serial laboratory studies are essential. The duration of the hospitalization is somewhat controversial. We have

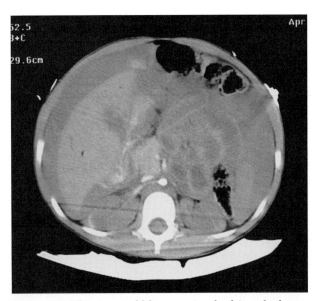

Figure 17–1. This 5-year-old boy was involved in a fatal motor vehicle accident. Computed tomography scan demonstrated massive hemoperitoneum. Extravasated intravenous contrast material is seen in the portal region. The other solid organs demonstrate minimal contrast enhancement, the aorta and cava are small, and dilated bowel loops are seen. This constellation of findings is consistent with hypoperfusion complex or shock bowel syndrome.

generally used a 7-day period of hospitalization, which varies according to the child's clinical status and the severity of the injury. Our practice has been to limit strenuous physical activity for 3 months after the injury, but the scientific basis for this is limited. Cooperative studies are currently under way to provide a more rational basis for these decisions. Given the presumed low level of compliance of the pediatric and adolescent population, the extremely low rate of recurrent bleeding or complications after standard medical management is striking.[23] Our practice is to obtain a follow-up CT scan 3 months after the injury, but the yield of such studies is low and the significance of positive findings is questionable.[24] Liver-spleen and US scans are alternative methods of follow-up.[25]

When surgery is required, bleeding may be found to have already ceased. If persistent bleeding is encountered, numerous splenorrhaphy techniques (segmental resections, mattress sutures, omental application, topical thrombin, Gelfoam and other hemostatic agents, mesh baskets) are available to control the hemorrhage without removing the spleen.[26] In the presence of multiple abdominal injuries, an unstable patient, or uncontrollable splenic bleeding, splenectomy may be necessary.[27] Such situations are uncommon in our experience.

Splenectomy is avoided primarily due to the risks of overwhelming postsplenectomy sepsis syndrome (OPSI). OPSI occurs as a result of loss of the immunologic function of the spleen. Encapsulated organisms *(Pneumococcus, Hemophilus)* are usually responsible. The precise amount of splenic tissue that must be conserved to prevent sepsis remains unknown. However, experimental studies suggest that at least one third to one half of the gland's total mass must be salvaged.[28] The risk of OPSI depends on many variables, the most important of which are the age at which the splenectomy was performed, the reason the splenectomy was performed, and the length of the interval since splenectomy. Splenectomy for trauma carries a much lower risk of OPSI than does splenectomy for hematologic disease. It is estimated that the posttraumatic splenectomy patient has nearly a 100-fold increased risk of OPSI compared with the general population. Established OPSI has a greater than 50% mortality rate.[29] Awareness of the problem, with early medical attention when symptoms develop, is essential. Prophylactic antibiotics and vaccination against encapsulated organisms are standard.

DUODENAL AND PANCREATIC INJURIES

Duodenal and pancreatic injuries occur with significantly less frequency than solid organ injuries. Injury to these areas is difficult to identify and treat.[30] The retroperitoneal location provides protection from injury but limits accessibility. The common blood supply shared by the pancreas and duodenum may pose problems for surgical management. Most injuries to these structures are the result of blunt trauma.

Crush injuries of the duodenum and pancreas, and acceleration-deceleration injuries to the duodenum, are the usual mechanisms. Associated injuries are common.

Duodenal injuries are usually identified on contrast CT examinations or via an upper GI radiograph. Perinephric air on plain radiographs and absence of the right psoas shadow are other more subtle signs. Duodenal *hematoma* may result from focal blunt trauma from bicycle handlebars or other blunt upper abdominal injury. Nonaccidental trauma should be considered in the absence of a plausible explanation for the injury. Obstructive symptoms, and consequently the diagnosis, are often delayed for several days. The classic radiologic findings consist of a "cork screw" or "coiled spring" appearance on upper GI contrast study or the identification of the hematoma on contrast CT examination.[31] In the absence of other associated injuries or another reason for laparotomy, duodenal hematomas can simply be observed. They generally resolve within 2 to 3 weeks. Failure of resolution is an indication for exploration and evacuation of the hematoma.

Most duodenal lacerations can be successfully managed by simple débridement and primary closure.[32] Serosal patch techniques can be used to buttress the repair.[33] More extensive duodenal injuries (involving >50% of the circumference of the lumen, impaired blood supply, associated bile duct-pancreatic injury) pose more of a problem. Many surgical options are available. *Pyloric exclusion* consists of closure of the injured area, tube decompression of the duodenum, dependent anterior wall gastrotomy, absorbable (polydioxanone) pursestring suture closure of the pylorus, and the creation of a gastrojejunostomy using the previously opened portion of stomach (Fig. 17–2).[34] Closed suction peritoneal drains should be placed. The pylorus reopens surprisingly rapidly, within 2 to 3 weeks. Marginal ulceration is uncommon. The *three tube technique* consists of a tube gastrostomy, a downstream jejunostomy for feeding, and another jejunostomy tube placed retrograde for drainage of the injured area, which is primarily closed.[35] *Duodenal exclusion* is simply a more radical exclusion procedure in which a truncal vagotomy, gastric antrectomy, loop gastrojejunostomy, and tube duodenostomy are combined with repair of the injured duodenum and closed suction drainage.[36] It is rarely necessary because pyloric exclusion suffices for less severe injuries and a pancreaticoduodenectomy is required for rare major combined injuries. The latter has a significant mortality rate.

Pancreatic injuries are uncommon in children, occurring in fewer than 5% of all cases of blunt pediatric trauma.[37] These injuries are difficult to detect because the early signs and symptoms are vague. In addition, initial CT findings are often minimal.[38–40] Fluid in the lesser sac may be the only abnormality identified on the scan. Associated injuries are common.

Elevation of the serum amylase level is often en-

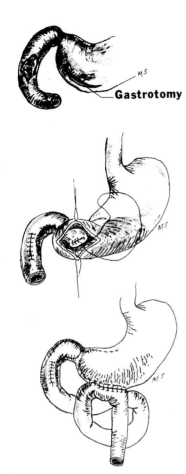

Figure 17–2. Illustration of pyloric exclusion for severe duodenal injury. The duodenal injury is repaired. A longitudinal gastrostomy is made, and the pylorus oversewn through the opening. A loop of jejunum is brought up to create a side to side anastomosis, effectively bypassing the injured segment. (From Vaughn GD III, Frazier OH, Graham DY, et al: The use of pyloric exclusion in the management of severe duodenal injuries. Am J Surg 134:785–790, 1977.)

countered in the pediatric trauma patient. This is a nonspecific finding and may not indicate pancreatic injury. Many patients proved to have significant pancreatic injury have a normal serum amylase at admission. However, persistent amylase elevations or concomitant serum lipase level elevations are much more reliable indicators of trauma to the gland.

Grading systems are available for pancreatic trauma, but their clinical utility is limited.[41] Fortunately, most (>75%) pediatric pancreatic injuries are minor, such as contusions and lacerations not involving the ductal system.[37] The majority can be managed nonoperatively.

More severe injuries require surgical repair. The general principles are conservation of as much of the pancreas as possible, identification and closure of any ductal injuries, resection of clearly devitalized tissue, and closed suction drainage. The spleen and splenic vessels should be preserved. Intraoperative pancreatography is sometimes helpful in adults, but it is of limited use in small children. If the diagnosis is delayed and ductal injury is suspected,

endoscopic retrograde cholangiopancreatography (ERCP) may be helpful in evaluating ductal continuity. Injuries to the left of the superior mesenteric vessels can be treated by resection of a portion of the tail of the gland. The duct should be identified and oversewn. Alternatively, mechanical stapling devices may be used. To conserve pancreatic tissue, a jejunal Roux-en-Y can be anastomosed to either the proximal or distal remnant of the gland. Major trauma to the head of the pancreas carries a significant morbidity rate. The principles mentioned previously for combined duodenal and pancreatic injuries apply. Major resection should rarely be necessary.

Several complications such as abscess, pancreatic ascites, pseudocyst formation, and fistula can occur after pancreatic injury. Posttraumatic pancreatitis is usually treated nonoperatively. Pancreatic fistula may occur. In contrast to the adult's, the child's pancreas is usually a healthy organ without any underlying disease. Control of the drainage, bowel rest, and IV alimentation usually result in spontaneous closure of the fistula within 1 to 2 weeks. Pancreatic abscess is treated by evacuation of any necrotic or devitalized tissue, drainage, and appropriate IV antibiotic therapy. Pancreatic pseudocyst occurs in up to one third of patients with traumatic pancreatic injury (Fig. 17–3). Asymptomatic pancreatic pseudocysts may be managed expectantly, with serial US examinations. Spontaneous resolution frequently occurs. If the patient becomes symptomatic (fever, pain, vomiting) or complications develop (enlarging mass, infection, bleeding, rupture, bowel obstruction), intervention may be necessary. In the acute phase, with a thin pseudocyst wall, external (usually percutaneous) drainage is preferred. In the chronic phase, with a thicker pseudocyst wall, standard techniques for internal drainage (Roux-en-Y or cystogastrostomy) should be used. Overall mortality rates for children with pancreatic trauma are approximately 5 to 10%, usually as a result of other injuries.[37]

HOLLOW VISCERAL INJURY

Small and large intestinal injuries are much less common than solid organ injuries in children. Hollow structures may be injured by *burst injury*, in which a rapid compressive force is applied to the distended viscus; by *shear injury*, in which a deceleration occurs near a fixed point (such as the ligament of Trietz); and by *crush injury*, in which the hollow structure is compressed against a solid surface, such as a vertebral body.

Although gastric perforation or injury is infrequent, it occurs more often in children than adults. Free air on plain films, bloody effluent from the nasogastric tube, or abnormal position of nasogastric tubes may raise the suspicion of these injuries. Installation of a small amount of air through the nasogastric tube may allow visualization of free air from a perforation. Most gastric perforations are lo-

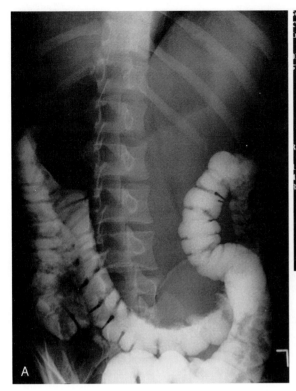

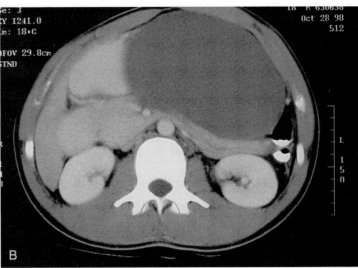

Figure 17–3. This patient was a 17-year-old boy with a vague history of blunt abdominal trauma. His initial complaints were vomiting and diarrhea, and a barium enema examination was obtained elsewhere. *A*, This study demonstrated marked extrinsic displacement of the transverse colon by a mass. *B*, A computed tomography scan was obtained, demonstrating a normal pancreas with a large thin-walled pseudocyst located anterior to the gland, displacing surrounding structures.

cated near the greater curvature of the stomach and are amenable to primary repair and closure.

Perhaps the most common setting for hollow visceral injury in children is the lap belt complex. Children present with abdominal abrasions and contusions over areas of seat or lap belt restraint devices. Peritoneal signs may be extremely difficult, if not impossible, to detect because the discomfort caused by the abdominal wall injury masks the symptoms. In addition, small tears in the bowel wall result in gradual leakage and slow progression of the symptoms and signs of peritonitis. Early findings may be normal. Only later does the patient worsen, with increasing tenderness on examination, fever, and absent intestinal function. When hollow visceral injury is suspected, initial CT scan findings may be normal, or they may demonstrate a small amount of unexplained peritoneal fluid. Serial clinical examinations, repeat CT scan in 24 to 48 hours, and diagnostic peritoneal lavage maybe useful in determining the presence of a perforated viscus in this setting. We have adopted an aggressive approach in children with lap belt injuries, feeling that the risk involved in a negative exploratory laparotomy is much less than the risk involved in a missed visceral injury.

Children with lap belt abrasions often have a triad of abdominal wall contusions or abrasions, hollow visceral injury (usually small bowel), and vertebral fracture or dislocation. The latter are usually Chance (flexion-distraction) fractures of the lumbar spine, seen in up to 50% of patients (Fig. 17–4).[42] We obtain complete spine radiographs in children with lap belt injuries. Awareness of spinal cord injury without radiographic abnormalities (SCIWORA) is also important. Nonaccidental trauma may also result in hollow visceral injuries in children. When present in such a setting, these injuries may represent a marker of increased trauma severity.[43]

The usual operative management of small intestinal injuries is either primary repair or resection with primary reanastomosis. Colonic injuries are usually treated with primary repair if the injury is limited or, alternatively, segmental resection and reanastomosis of the involved area, regardless of site. Although colostomy is rarely necessary, it may be indicated if there is excessive contamination, if there is a large amount of devitalized bowel, or if there are other major associated injuries. Exteriorization of the injured segment is another option.

Rectal injuries are uncommon in children. They may be the result of either an impalement injury, with direct penetration or perforation of the colon, or nonaccidental injury such as sexual abuse.[44, 45] Such injuries need to be carefully examined while the child is under a general anesthetic with proctoscopy or sigmoidoscopy to determine their extent. Significant penetrating injury or disruption of the rectal or anal canal requires a diverting colostomy, local débridement, and drainage of the area. With severe injury, it may be necessary to undertake definitive reconstruction at a later date. However, in most instances, primary repair is both possible and desirable.

DIAPHRAGMATIC RUPTURE, RETROPERITONEAL TRAUMA

Perhaps due to the elasticity of their tissues, traumatic diaphragmatic hernia is uncommon in chil-

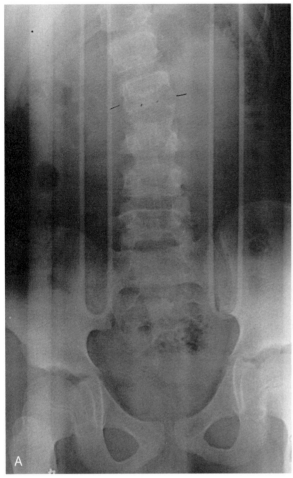

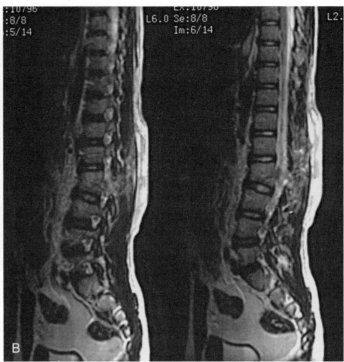

Figure 17–4. Lumbar spine Chance fracture is demonstrated in a 10-year-old boy who was a restrained front seat passenger in a motor vehicle accident. He sustained a lap belt complex injury with mesenteric avulsion and several injuries to the small and large bowel. His spinal fracture resulted in complete paraplegia. *A*, This anteroposterior spine film demonstrates the fracture. *B*, The magnetic resonance imaging scan shows a lateral view of the fracture.

dren. It usually results from blunt trauma caused by a sudden compressive force applied to the abdominal wall. The left side is far more commonly injured than the right. Associated injuries are frequent.[46] Traumatic diaphragmatic hernia is best recognized on the upright chest radiograph. A nasogastric tube may be directed into the left hemithorax. An upper GI contrast study, US, or CT scan may help confirm the diagnosis. Late presentations with bowel obstruction or perforation can occur. The treatment usually consists of simple closure of the defect through an abdominal approach. Late presentations, with extensive adhesions, may require a transthoracic approach.

The management of intraoperatively encountered retroperitoneal hematomas in children depends on the site of the hematoma and whether or not it is stable or expanding. Stable pelvic hematomas are best left undisturbed. Embolization is preferable to open procedures for expanding pelvic hematomas. Perinephric hematomas are discussed later in the chapter. Central upper retroperitoneal hematomas, particularly those involving the duodenum or pancreas, are generally explored. Proximal and distal control of vascular structures entering and exiting a hematoma is critical. Any injury to the retroperitoneal structures is identified and repaired, as discussed later in this chapter. Stable retroperitoneal

hematomas not directly overlaying vital structures may usually be left undisturbed.

□ Genitourinary Injury

RENAL TRAUMA

The kidney is the most frequently injured of the genitourinary (GU) organs in children. It is also more susceptible to injury in children than in adults; children's kidneys are larger relative to the size of their abdominal cavity; their ribs are more flexible and malleable and provide relatively less protection; and their abdominal wall musculature is generally weaker and provides less protection. Most renal injuries are the result of blunt trauma. Associated injuries are common, particularly head injuries. Most renal injuries are relatively minor: contusions, minor lacerations, hematomas; all without collecting system disruption. Grading scales are available for differentiating the severity of the injury; we have not found them useful in determining management.

The signs of renal injury are nonspecific. Contusions or abrasions of the abdominal wall, flank ecchymosis, and tenderness over the renal fossa may be present. A large hematoma or significant urinary extravasation (urinoma) may be palpable on abdominal examination. Although nonspecific, the presence of hematuria is the most common indicator of renal injury. Unfortunately, the degree of hematuria does not necessarily indicate the severity of the renal injury.[4, 6, 47] Major renal vascular injury occurs without hematuria in as many as one third of cases.[48, 49] Isolated microscopic hematuria, as an indication for radiologic investigation (CT scan), is controversial. However, microscopic hematuria associated with a significant mechanism of injury, shock, suspicious physical findings, or other major associated injuries clearly indicates a need for further studies.[4, 6]

Patients with congenital GU abnormalities, positional abnormalities, or tumors are predisposed to injury.[50, 51] The dilated system may be thin walled, enlarged, and more susceptible to trauma (Fig. 17–5). Approximately 10 to 20% of children with GU trauma have unexpected preexisting GU tract abnormalities. Unilateral renal agenesis occurs in approximately 1 in 1000 individuals.[52] Bilateral renal injury is present in nearly 1 of 10 patients with renal trauma.[53]

Most pediatric renal injuries are mild, and the management is nonoperative. As is the case with splenic and liver injuries, no clear consensus exists about the medical management of renal trauma. Generally, strict bed rest is maintained until all gross hematuria clears. Restricted activity (no contact sports, no vigorous exercise) is continued until microscopic hematuria clears.

The treatment of significant renal trauma in the stable patient is controversial. Advocates of early exploration contend that this approach reduces the

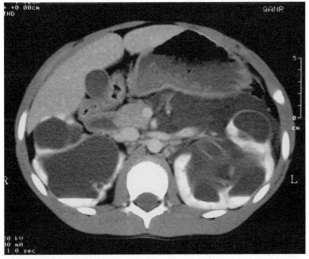

Figure 17–5. This patient is a 10-year-old boy who sustained a fall from a height of approximately 8 feet. He had no prior significant medical history. This scan demonstrates marked bilateral hydroureteronephrosis, with intravenous contrast enhancement of a rim of renal parenchyma bilaterally. In addition, just anterior to the left kidney, there is evidence of significant urinary extravasation. This patient was managed nonoperatively with serial computed tomography scans. His recovery was uneventful. Subsequent evaluation revealed massive bilateral vesicoureteral reflux.

risk of potential complications such as hematoma formation, abscess, and urinary extravasation and reduces the long-term risk of hypertension.[54–57] They also cite an earlier return of bowel function and a shorter hospitalization. Advocates of this approach report nephrectomy rates (with early surgical exploration) of less than 10%.

Conversely, those who advocate an expectant course feel that their approach markedly reduces nephrectomy rates and results in substantially fewer complications and a reduced need for laparotomy.[58–59] The injured tissue is more clearly demarcated if delayed surgery is necessary. Even significant urinary extravasation can be managed expectantly. However, if a nonoperative approach is selected, it is essential to identify and treat any associated injuries. In the absence of suspected vascular injury, we generally adopt an expectant approach.

There are few absolute indications for operation in a child with renal trauma. Patients with vital sign instability, suspected renal vascular injury, or other major associated injuries require exploration. Renal pedicle injury requires urgent operation if there is to be any chance of salvaging the kidney. The warm ischemia time in children is limited, and only a short delay from the time of injury results in irreversible damage. An aggressive approach is indicated because partial disruption of blood flow or collateral circulation may prolong parenchymal survival time. These injuries are usually the result of an acceleration or deceleration force. Associated injuries are seen in nearly half of children with renal pedicle injury.[61] Suspected renovascular injury should be evaluated with a contrast-enhanced CT scan. The kidney does not enhance, and there may be a "rim sign" resulting from peripheral collateral flow.[49] Arteriography is rarely necessary.

Most cases of main renal artery injury result in loss of the kidney.[48] Shearing or deceleration forces may result in arterial thrombosis, and salvage is not usually possible. Segmental renal artery injury can be managed expectantly or with partial nephrectomy of the involved portion of the kidney. Renal vein injuries should be repaired, if possible. Venous injuries on the left side may be treated by ligation of the renal vein near its entry into the vena cava, provided the gonadal and adrenal veins are intact to provide collateral drainage.

The operative approach to the injured kidney may be a secondary consideration if other major injuries are present. The presence of a significant perirenal hematoma is an indication for intraoperative IV pyelogram, provided the patient is stable. In a child with blunt trauma, if renal function is intact, the hematoma is stable, and there is no evidence of significant extravasation, exploration of the hematoma may not be necessary. When exploration is indicated, the first step is to control the renal artery and vein outside Gerota's fascia. This results in a lower incidence of primary nephrectomy. The injured kidney is then explored. The most immediate concern is to obtain hemostasis. Hematomas are evacuated, devitalized tissue is débrided, and collecting system injuries are primarily closed. Closed suction drains are left in place.

The long-term sequela of major pediatric renal injuries have not been precisely defined. Reports suggest that the long-term risk of hypertension or other posttraumatic complications is small.[58, 59] Minor renal injuries usually do not require long-term follow-up because late complications are rare.[62] Children with major renal injuries probably should have a follow-up study (CT or US) in the early postoperative period. Any child with a significant renal injury should also undergo at least yearly follow-up, with measurement of renal function, blood pressure, and urinalysis.[63, 64]

URETERAL INJURY

Ureteral injuries are uncommon in children. They are often difficult to identify, and a high index of suspicion is necessary. Delayed diagnosis is common and is associated with significant morbidity.[65] Hematuria is usually present but may be absent in as many as one third of children with ureteral injury.[65, 66] Occasionally, the mechanism of injury suggests the possibility of a ureteral trauma (e.g., the trajectory of gunshot wounds). Ureteral injury may be identified on contrast-enhanced CT scans.[67] However, it is usually necessary to obtain either an IV pyelogram or retrograde ureterogram (Fig. 17–6).

Ureteropelvic junction disruption, although rare, occurs more frequently in children than in adults and may be associated with preexisting renal abnormalities.[68] Deceleration injury is often the mechanism.[65, 69, 70] The right side is more commonly involved than the left.

The intraoperative identification of a ureteral injury may be difficult. Frequently, a hematoma overlies the area of injury, and palpation may provide a falsely negative impression.[65] Direct inspection of the ureter is necessary to identify injuries to this structure.

The repair of ureteral injury depends on the mechanism of injury, the site of ureteral injury, and the extent of damage. If the kidney is intact, most renal units can be preserved, even with significant ureteral injury. Proximal ureteral injuries are débrided and reconstructed, either with ureterocalicostomy or pyeloplasty. Midureteral injuries may be managed by resection, spatulation (spatulating the ureteral ends), and primary reanastomosis. If the length of the involved segment does not allow reanastomosis, then mobilization of the kidney or a psoas hitch may be necessary to allow the two ends to be approximated. Double-J stents can be placed through the site of repair. Lower ureteral injuries may be managed by a simple ureteral reimplantation. Closed suction drains are placed. Another alternative for complex injuries or those associated with other life-threatening trauma is ligation of the ureter above the level of injury, with a tube nephrostomy and delayed repair.

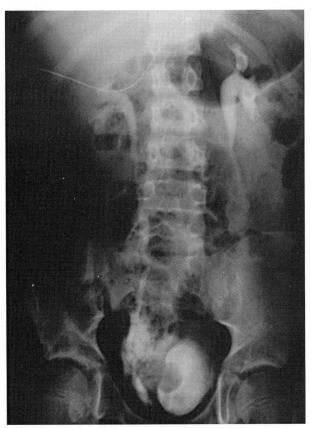

Figure 17–6. Intravenous pyelogram demonstrating extravasation of contrast material from around the distal right ureter and bladder in a 10-year-old boy who was shot in the lower abdomen and pelvis. He was found to have a penetrating injury to the distal ureter and bladder. Reimplantation of the ureter was required, and he recovered without further incident.

BLADDER INJURY

Urinary bladder injuries are uncommon in children. Bladder injuries may be classified by
- Location (intraperitoneal, extraperitoneal, or both)
- Anatomic site (trigonal or extratrigonal)
- Severity (contusion or partial thickness laceration versus rupture)
- Mechanism (blunt or penetrating)

The management of the injury depends on these variables.

Most bladder injuries in children result from blunt trauma, usually a burst injury from a sudden compressive force. The likelihood of bladder rupture increases if the bladder is full. In infants and young children, the bladder is intraabdominal, in contrast to the protected, pelvic position of the adult bladder. Associated injuries to other intraperitoneal organs are common. Pelvic fractures are found in as many as three quarters of children with bladder trauma.[71, 72]

The hallmark of bladder injury is gross hematuria. The signs and symptoms of intraperitoneal bladder rupture may be subtle and difficult to discern. Urine in the peritoneal cavity does not cause much discomfort or irritation in the first 24 to 48 hours. Intraperitoneal fluid can be difficult to detect in the acutely injured patient, and little fluid may be present soon after the injury. The presence of any degree of hematuria in association with a pelvic fracture mandates a cystogram. Although it is possible to identify bladder rupture by a triple-contrast CT scan, the best single study is a cystogram.[73] It is important to obtain oblique views with the cystogram.[74] In addition, it is essential to obtain postevacuation films because the contrast agent within the bladder may obscure the site of injury. Adequate bladder filling is important to avoid false-negative reports.[74] The degree of contrast extravasation does not accurately reflect the severity of the laceration.

Simple contusions or partial thickness lacerations usually do not require any treatment. If the patient cannot void, catheterization may be necessary. Most intraperitoneal bladder ruptures are from blunt trauma. Extraperitoneal injuries are usually secondary to pelvic fractures or penetrating injury from foreign objects. Bony spicules from the former may penetrate the bladder neck.

Extraperitoneal bladder rupture from blunt trauma can be managed with Foley catheter drainage, but intraperitoneal bladder rupture generally requires a laparotomy and layered closure of the defect.[75–77] Most authors recommend placing a suprapubic cystotomy tube in children with intraperitoneal bladder rupture. External penetrating trauma to the bladder, whether it results in intraperitoneal or extraperitoneal extravasation, should be explored because there is a significant likelihood of injury to other structures. In addition, bone fragments from a pelvic fracture lodged in the bladder wall may impede healing.

If laparotomy is necessary to treat other injuries in a child with extraperitoneal bladder rupture, the bladder can be repaired by opening the dome widely, exposing the defect, and performing a layered closure from within the bladder. This avoids dissection of a perivesical hematoma. However, this technique is rarely necessary. Combined intraperitoneal and extraperitoneal bladder injuries can occur, as well as injuries to the urethra in combination with bladder rupture.[78] Such injuries are often difficult to accurately detect, and a high degree of suspicion as well as good quality radiologic studies are necessary to identify them.

URETHRAL INJURY

Most urethral injuries result from motor vehicle accidents. Although not life-threatening, these injuries may have devastating consequences, such as impotence, stricture, and urinary incontinence. The diagnosis of urethral injury should be suspected when bloody meatal discharge is seen. Gross hematuria may be present. Inability to void is also a common symptom. Physical examination may reveal obvious contusions or abrasions. The presence of a boggy prostate or upwardly displaced prostate

gland on digital rectal examination should raise a strong suspicion of posterior urethral injury.[79]

However, rectal examination may be difficult in the anxious, injured child and radiographic studies should be obtained promptly if there is *any* suspicion of injury. It is important to avoid blindly placing urinary catheters because this may convert a partial, minor injury into a complete disruption. Instead, a retrograde urethrogram (RUG) should be obtained, injecting the contrast agent through an appropriately sized catheter, which may then be advanced into the bladder in the absence of significant injury (Fig. 17–7).

Urethral injuries may be categorized as grades 1 through 4, with grade 1 simply a mild contusion, grade 2 a stretch type of injury without disruption of the urethra, grade 3 a partial disruption, and grade 4 a complete disruption.[80] Occasionally, spasm of the sphincter musculature may limit radiographic determination of the degree of injury.

The *site* of the urethral injury is critical to management and outcome. There are two common sites of injury. One is *anterior* urethral trauma, which is usually a compression injury from the urethra being pressed against the bony pubic arch. These tend to be a result of straddle injuries or falls. They may also occur as a result of sexual manipulations or iatrogenic medical complications. Mild anterior urethral injuries may be treated without a catheter,

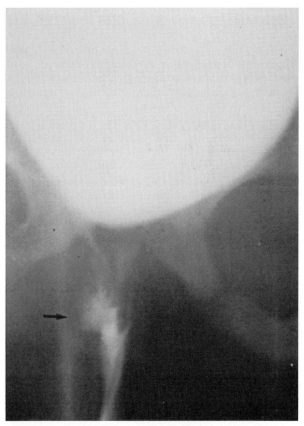

Figure 17–7. Urethral injury with extravasation *(arrow)* from disruption of the urethra associated with a pelvic fracture.

provided the patient is able to void. Moderate injuries or patients who are unable to void may require placement of a Foley catheter. More complex injuries to the anterior urethra require placement of a suprapubic catheter, with delayed repair.

The second common site of injury is the posterior urethra. *Posterior* urethral injuries are usually secondary to bony pelvis injuries or are the result of shear forces. The prostatic urethra is fixed to the pubic symphysis by the puboprostatic ligament. Shear injury may occur near this point of fixation between the prostatic and membranous urethra. As many as 1 in 20 boys with pelvic fractures suffer a posterior urethral injury. A small percentage of these children also have a bladder rupture. The most common site of urethral injuries in children is the posterior urethra.

Minor posterior urethral injuries may be managed without a urinary catheter, provided the patient can void. If the patient cannot void, it may be necessary to place a catheter. The management of more severe posterior urethral injuries in children is controversial. The rarity of the injury means that no single surgeon or institution has experience with a large series of patients. In addition, posterior urethral injuries are variable: specific anatomic locations (e.g., transprostatic) appear to carry a risk of impotence and incontinence, and even in a single anatomic site, the severity of the injury is also a significant variable.[81] Management options are diverse and include early primary realignment with or without reanastomosis, delayed primary realignment, or suprapubic tube placement followed by a definitive delayed repair 6 to 12 months later.[78, 82, 83]

Primary suture repair of the posterior urethra with realignment is an option in stable patients. In adult series, there is little evidence of benefit compared to primary realignment alone.[84] A select group of patients with injury to the bladder require immediate suturing of the injured urethra.[78]

Some authors feel that primary realignment (in stable patients) provides better long-term continence and potency.[79, 83, 85–88] It may be possible to advance a catheter at the time of the retrograde study, or it may be necessary to open the bladder for antegrade catheter passage. Another option is to place an antegrade bladder catheter while passing a catheter simultaneously through the urethral meatus. If both catheters can be identified at the site of the laceration, they can be sutured together and pulled through the injured area for primary realignment, acting as an indwelling stent. A suprapubic cystostomy tube is usually placed at the same time.

Other authors recommend initial suprapubic tube placement and primary realignment after a short delay (<2 weeks). This approach has the advantage of avoiding the acute hematoma, allowing the surgeon to operate in a stable patient, and providing a "cleaner" operative field. However, fibrosis is more common and may be significant as soon as 2 to 3 weeks after the injury.[86]

Delayed repair (usually 6 to 9 months) with initial placement of a suprapubic cystostomy tube avoids dissection in an acutely injured field. A variety of surgical approaches is available.[89, 90] Advocates of this technique feel that the risks of exacerbating the injury and potentially increasing complications is reduced. Additionally, delaying the repair allows definitive repair to be performed by a more experienced team.[91]

The incidence of incontinence and impotence appears to depend more on the nature and severity of the injury than the timing of repair.[81, 86] The overall rate of impotence in patients with major posterior urethral injury is about 1 in 3, with either primary realignment or delayed repair. The incidence of incontinence is approximately 2 in 3, again relatively similar after either early or delayed repair. However, strictures do appear to be significantly increased with the delayed repair, ranging from 89 to 96%. In contrast, the stricture rate ranges from 23 to 54% in those with early or immediate repair.[72, 81, 86] Due to this apparent benefit in reducing the stricture rate, many authors advocate primary realignment of selected posterior urethral injuries.[72]

STRADDLE INJURIES AND GENITAL TRAUMA

Perineal injuries are common in children. Most result from blunt trauma, such as a fall onto a bicycle crossbar or other hard object. In girls, straddle injuries often cause contusions or lacerations to the perineum or vagina. Small tears around the vaginal introitus or periurethral area may bleed profusely. Almost every penetrating perineal injury and all but the most minor blunt injuries should be fully evaluated under general anesthesia in the operating room. Vaginoscopy, cystourethroscope, and proctoscopy may be necessary. With either blunt or penetrating trauma, the physical perineal findings may not reflect the severity of the underlying injury.[44, 92] Traumatic rectovaginal fistula or significant rectal lacerations may require a diverting colostomy. In addition, laparotomy or laparoscopy may be necessary for penetrating vaginal trauma because injury to intraabdominal structures may occur.

In boys, straddle injuries are quite variable. Injury to the male urethra was discussed earlier. Rectal trauma may require proctoscopy or sigmoidoscopy and diverting colostomy for extensive injuries. The scrotum may expand dramatically from a hematoma. US with color-flow Doppler is useful to identify testicular fracture and verify adequate blood flow to the testicle. Because it is possible to miss epididymal injury as well as some testicular disruptions by US examination, a more aggressive approach to scrotal exploration is advocated by some.[93] Fractures of the testicle or significant hematomas should be explored under general anesthesia, the hematoma evacuated, and testicular disruption repaired.

The possibility of sexual abuse must always be kept in mind when examining children with perineal trauma. Specifically, when the details of the history do not match the physical findings, when there is a history of repeated injury, when perineal injury is associated with anal or genital condylomata, or when the affect of the child seems inappropriate, the level of suspicion should be increased. The incidence of reported sexual abuse of children is staggering and undoubtedly represents only a small portion of cases. Early involvement of an experienced sexual abuse team is critical.

REFERENCES

1. Peclet MH, Newman KD, Eichelberger MR, et al: Thoracic trauma in children: An indicator of increased mortality. J Pediatr Surg 25:961–965, 1990.
2. Eichelberger MR, Moront M: Abdominal trauma. In O'Neill JA, Rowe MI, Grosfeld JL, et al (eds): Pediatric Surgery, Vol. 1 (5th ed). St. Louis: CV Mosby, 1998, pp 261–284.
3. Sivit CJ, Eichelberger MR, Taylor GA: CT in children with rupture of the bowel caused by blunt trauma: Diagnostic efficacy and comparison with hypoperfusion complex. AJR Am J Roentgenol 163:1195–1198, 1994.
4. Taylor GA, Eichelberger MR, Potter BM: Hematuria: A marker of abdominal injury in children after blunt trauma. Ann Surg 208:688–693, 1988.
5. Taylor GA, Eichelberger MR, O'Donnell R, Bowman L: Indications for computed tomography in children with blunt abdominal trauma [published erratum appears in Ann Surg 216:99, 1992]. Ann Surg 213:212–218, 1991.
6. Knudson MM, McAninch JW, Gomez R, et al: Hematuria as a predictor of abdominal injury after blunt trauma. Am J Surg 164:482–485, 1992.
7. Taylor GA, Eich MR: Abdominal CT in children with neurologic impairment following blunt trauma: Abdominal CT in comatose children. Ann Surg 210:229–233, 1989.
8. Rozycki GS, Ochsner MG, Schmidt JA: A prospective study of surgeon-performed ultrasound as the primary adjuvant modality for injured patient assessment. J Trauma 39:492, 1995.
9. Sivit CJ, Kaufman RA: Sonography in the evaluation of children following blunt trauma: Is it to be or not to be? [commentary]. Pediatr Radiol 25:326–328, 1995.
10. Boyle EM Jr, Maier RV, Salazar JD, et al: Diagnosis of injuries after stab wounds to the back and flank. J Trauma 42:260–265, 1997.
11. Brick SH, Taylor GA, Potter BM, Eichelberger MR: Hepatic and splenic injury in children: Role of CT in the decision for laparotomy. Radiology 165:643–646, 1987.
12. Bond SJ, Eichelberger MR, Gotschall CS, et al: Nonoperative management of blunt hepatic and splenic injury in children. Ann Surg 223:286–289, 1996.
13. Coburn MC, Pfeifer J, DeLuca FG: Nonoperative management of splenic and hepatic trauma in the multiply injured pediatric and adolescent patient. Arch Surg 130:332–338, 1995.
14. Oldham KT, Guice KS, Ryckman F, et al: Blunt liver injury in childhood: Evolution of therapy and current perspective. Surgery 100:542–549, 1986.
15. Pringle JH: Notes on the arrest of hepatic hemorrhage due to trauma. Ann Surg 48:541, 1908.
16. Schrock T, Blaisdell FW, Mathewson C Jr: Management of blunt trauma to the liver and hepatic veins. Arch Surg 96:698–704, 1968.
17. Defore WW Jr, Mattox KL, Jordan GL Jr, Beall AC Jr: Management of 1,590 consecutive cases of liver trauma. Arch Surg 111:493–497, 1976.
18. Traub AC, Perry JF Jr: Injuries associated with splenic trauma. J Trauma 21:840–847, 1981.
19. Umlas SL, Cronan JJ. Splenic trauma: Can CT grading systems enable prediction of successful nonsurgical treatment? Radiology 178:481–487, 1991.
20. Ruess L, Sivit CJ, Eichelberger MR, et al: Blunt hepatic and splenic trauma in children: Correlation of a CT injury sever-

21. ity scale with clinical outcome. Pediatr Radiol 25:321–325, 1995.
21. Pearl RH, Wesson DE, Spence LJ, et al: Splenic injury: A 5-year update with improved results and changing criteria for conservative management. J Pediatr Surg 24:121–124, 1989.
22. Powell M, Courcoulas A, Gardner M, et al: Management of blunt splenic trauma: Significant differences between adults and children. Surgery 122:654–660, 1997.
23. Hunt JP, Lentz CW, Cairns BA, et al: Management and outcome of splenic injury: The results of a five-year statewide population-based study. Am Surg 62:911–917, 1996.
24. Lawson DE, Jacobson JA, Spizarny DL, Pranikoff T: Splenic trauma: Value of follow-up CT. Radiology 194:97–100, 1995.
25. Lupien C, Sauerbrei EE: Healing in the traumatized spleen: Sonographic investigation. Radiology 151:181–185, 1984.
26. Buntain WL, Gould HR: Splenic trauma in children and techniques of splenic salvage. World J Surg 9:398–409, 1985.
27. Wilson RH, Moorehead RJ: Management of splenic trauma. Injury 23:5–9, 1992.
28. Okinaga K, Giebink GS, Rich HH, et al: The effect of partial splenectomy on experimental pneumococcal bacteremia in an animal model. J Pediatr Surg 16:717–724, 1981.
29. Francke EL, Neu HC: Postsplenectomy infection. Surg Clin North Am 61:135–155, 1981.
30. Cook DE, Walsh JW, Vick CW, Brewer WH: Upper abdominal trauma: Pitfalls in CT diagnosis. Radiology 159:65–69, 1986.
31. Kleinman PK, Brill PW, Winchester P: Resolving duodenal-jejunal hematoma in abused children. Radiology 160:747–750, 1986.
32. Ivatury RR, Nallathambi M, Gaudino J, et al: Penetrating duodenal injuries: Analysis of 100 consecutive cases. Ann Surg 202:153–158, 1985.
33. Wynn M, Hill DM, Miller DR, et al: Management of pancreatic and duodenal trauma. Am J Surg 150:327–332, 1985.
34. Vaughn GD III, Frazier OH, Graham DY, et al: The use of pyloric exclusion in the management of severe duodenal injuries. Am J Surg 134:785–790, 1977.
35. Stone HH, Fabian TC: Management of duodenal wounds. J Trauma 19:334–339, 1979.
36. Berne CJ, Donovan AJ, White EJ, et al: Duodenal "diverticularization" for duodenal and pancreatic injury. Am J Surg 127:503–507, 1974.
37. Keller MS, Stafford PW, Vane DW: Conservative management of pancreatic trauma in children. J Trauma 42:1097–1100, 1997.
38. Jeffrey RB Jr, Federle MP, Crass RA: Computed tomography of pancreatic trauma. Radiology 147:491–494, 1983.
39. Sivit CJ, Eichelberger MR, Taylor GA, et al: Blunt pancreatic trauma in children: CT diagnosis. AJR Am J Roentgenol 158:1097–1100, 1992.
40. Sivit CJ, Eichelberger MR: CT diagnosis of pancreatic injury in children: Significance of fluid separating the splenic vein and the pancreas. AJR Am J Roentgenol 165:921–924, 1995.
41. Moore EE, Cogbill TH, Malangoni MA, et al: Organ injury scaling: II. Pancreas, duodenum, small bowel, colon, and rectum. J Trauma 30:1427–1429, 1990.
42. Newman KD, Bowman LM, Eichelberger MR, et al: The lap belt complex: Intestinal and lumbar spine injury in children. J Trauma 30:1133–1138, 1990.
43. Sivit CJ, Taylor GA, Eichelberger MR: Visceral injury in battered children: A changing perspective. Radiology 173:659–661, 1989.
44. Reinberg O, Yazbeck S: Major perineal trauma in children. J Pediatr Surg 24:982–984, 1989.
45. Black CT: Anorectal trauma in children. J Pediatr Surg 17:501, 1982.
46. Sukul DM, Kats E, Johannes EJ: Sixty-three cases of traumatic injury of the diaphragm. Injury 22:303–306, 1991.
47. Stein JP, Kaji DM, Eastham J, et al: Blunt renal trauma in the pediatric population: Indications for radiographic evaluation. Urology 44:406–410, 1994.
48. Carroll PR, McAninch JW, Klosterman P, Greenblatt M: Renovascular trauma: Risk assessment, surgical management, and outcome. J Trauma 30:547–552, 1990.
49. Cass AS: Renovascular injuries from external trauma: Diag-

nosis, treatment, and outcome. Urol Clin North Am 16:213–220, 1989.

50. Emanuel B, Weiss H, Gollin P: Renal trauma in children. J Trauma 17:275–278, 1977.
51. Giyanani VL, Gerlock AJ Jr, Grozinger KT, et al: Trauma of occult hydronephrotic kidney. Urology 25:8–12, 1985.
52. Ryckman FC, Noseworthy J: Developmental and positional abnormalities of the kidney. In Ashcraft KW, Holder TM (eds): Pediatric Surgery (2nd ed). Philadelphia, WB Saunders, 1993, pp 571–581.
53. McAleer IM, Kaplan GW, Scherz HC, et al: Genitourinary trauma in the pediatric patient. Urology 42:563–567, 1993.
54. Husmann DA, Gilling PJ, Perry MO, et al: Major renal lacerations with a devitalized fragment following blunt abdominal trauma: A comparison between nonoperative (expectant) versus surgical management. J Urol 150:1774–1777, 1993.
55. Cass AS: Immediate surgical management of severe renal injuries in multiply injured patients. Urology 21:140, 1983.
56. Cass AS, Luxenberg M, Gleich P: Long-term results of conservative and surgical management of blunt renal lacerations. Br J Urol 59(1): 17–20, 1987.
57. Cass AS, Cerra FB, Luxenberg M, et al: Renal failure and mortality after nephrectomy for severe trauma in multiply-injured patient: No inordinate risk. Urology 30:213–215, 1987.
58. Bass DH, Semple PL, Cywes S: Investigation and management of blunt renal injuries in children: A review of 11 years experience. J Pediatr Surg 26:196, 1991.
59. Levy JB, Baskin LS, Ewalt DH, et al: Nonoperative management of blunt pediatric major renal trauma. Urology 42:418–424, 1993.
60. Smith EM, Elder JS, Spirnak JP: Major blunt renal trauma in the pediatric population: Is a nonoperative approach indicated? J Urol 149:546–548, 1993.
61. Cass AS, Bubrick M, Luxenberg M, et al: Renal pedicle injury in patients with multiple injuries. J Trauma 25:892–896, 1985.
62. Krieger JN, Algood CB, Mason JT, et al: Urological trauma in the Pacific Northwest: Etiology, distribution, management and outcome. J Urol 132:70–73, 1984.
63. Abdalati H, Bulas DI, Sivit CJ, et al: Blunt renal trauma in children: Healing of renal injuries and recommendations for imaging follow-up. Pediatr Radiol 24:573–576, 1994.
64. Jakse G, Putz A, Gassner I, Zechmann W: Early surgery in the management of pediatric blunt renal trauma. J Urol 131:920–924, 1984.
65. Boone TB, Gilling PJ, Husmann DA: Ureteropelvic junction disruption following blunt abdominal trauma. J Urol 150:33–36, 1993.
66. Peters PC, Bright TC: Management of trauma to the urinary tract. Adv Surg 10:197–244, 1976.
67. Siegel MJ, Balfe DM: Blunt renal and ureteral trauma in childhood: CT patterns of fluid collections. AJR Am J Roentgenol 152:1043–1047, 1989.
68. Kawashima A, Sandler CM, Corriere JN Jr, et al: Ureteropelvic junction injuries secondary to blunt abdominal trauma. Radiology 205:487–492, 1997.
69. Palmer JM, Drago JR: Ureteral avulsion from non-penetrating trauma. J Urol 125:108–111, 1981.
70. Beamud-Gomez A, Martinez-Verduch M, Estornell-Moragues F, et al: Rupture of the ureteropelvic junction by nonpenetrating trauma. J Pediatr Surg 21:702–705, 1986.
71. Corriere JN Jr, Sandler CM: Mechanisms of injury, patterns of extravasation and management of extraperitoneal bladder rupture due to blunt trauma. J Urol 139:43–44, 1988.

72. Garcia VF, Sheldon CA: Genitourinary tract trauma. In O'Neill JA, Rowe MI, Grosfeld JL, et al (eds): Pediatric Surgery. Vol. 1 (5th ed). St Louis, CV Mosby, 1998, pp. 285–302.
73. Sivit CJ, Cutting JP, Eichelberger MR: CT diagnosis and localization of rupture of the bladder in children with blunt abdominal trauma: Significance of contrast material extravasation in the pelvis. AJR Am J Roentgenol 164:1243–1246, 1995.
74. Cass AS: Diagnostic studies in bladder rupture. Indications and techniques. Urol Clin North Am 16:267–273, 1989.
75. Cass AS, Luxenberg M: Features of 164 bladder ruptures. J Urol 138:743–745, 1987.
76. Cass AS, Luxenberg M: Management of extraperitoneal ruptures of bladder caused by external trauma. Urology 33:179–183, 1989.
77. Corriere JN Jr, Sandler CM: Management of extraperitoneal bladder rupture. Urol Clin North Am 16:275–277, 1989.
78. Podesta ML, Medel R, Castera R, Ruarte A: Immediate management of posterior urethral disruptions due to pelvic fracture: Therapeutic alternatives. J Urol 157:1444–1448, 1997.
79. Cass AS, Godec CJ: Urethral injury due to external trauma. Urology 11:607–611, 1978.
80. Moore EE, Cogbill TH, Jurkovich GJ, et al: Organ injury scaling, III: Chest wall, abdominal vascular, ureter, bladder, and urethra. J Trauma 33:337–339, 1992.
81. Boone TB, Wilson WT, Husmann DA: Postpubertal genitourinary function following posterior urethral disruptions in children. J Urol 148:1232–1234, 1992.
82. Boone TB, Wilson WT, Husmann DA, et al: Postpubertal genitourinary function following posterior urethral disruptions in children. J Urol 148:1232–1234, 1992.
83. Elliott DS, Barrett DM: Long-term followup and evaluation of primary realignment of posterior urethral disruptions. J Urol 157:814–816, 1997.
84. Follis HW, Koch MO, McDougal WS: Immediate management of prostatomembranous urethral disruptions. J Urol 147:1259–1262, 1992.
85. Koraitim MM: Pelvic fracture urethral injuries: Evaluation of various methods of management. J Urol 156:1288–1291, 1996.
86. Herschorn S, Thijssen A, Radomski SB: The value of immediate or early catheterization of the traumatized posterior urethra. J Urol 148:1428–1431, 1992.
87. Koch MO: Primary realignment of prostatomembranous urethral disruptions. Semin Urol 13:38–44, 1995.
88. Devine CJ Jr, Jordan GH, Devine PC: Primary realignment of the disrupted prostatomembranous urethra. Urol Clin North Am 16:291–295, 1989.
89. Senocak ME, Ciftci AO, Buyukpamukcu N, Hicsonmez A: Transpubic urethroplasty in children: Report of 10 cases with review of the literature. J Pediatr Surg 30:1319–1324, 1995.
90. Webster GD, Ramon J: Repair of pelvic fracture posterior urethral defects using an elaborated perineal approach: Experience with 74 cases. J Urol 145(4):744–748, 1991.
91. Hampel N: Posterior urethral disruption associated with pelvic fracture: The place for delayed repair. Semin Urol 13:34–37, 1995.
92. Lynch JM, Gardner MJ, Albanese CT: Blunt urogenital trauma in prepubescent female patients: More than meets the eye! Pediatr Emerg Care 11:372–375, 1995.
93. Cass AS, Luxenberg M: Testicular injuries. Urology 37:528–530, 1991.

18

HEAD INJURIES IN CHILDREN

David P. Gruber, MD •
Douglas L. Brockmeyer, MD •
Marion L. Walker, MD

The incidence of traumatic brain injury (TBI), excluding birth trauma, is approximately 200 per 100,000 children per year in the United States.[1] Head injuries can be classified with respect to their severity according to the initial Glasgow Coma Scale (GCS) score.[2] The GCS is outlined in Table 18–1. Eighty-two percent of pediatric head injuries are minor (GCS 14 to 15); 8% are moderate, and 6% are severe. Approximately 20% of survivors have significant disability.[3] Five percent of pediatric TBIs are fatal. The majority of these occur at the scene of the accident. Falls produce most of these injuries, but other important factors include motor vehicle accidents, sports, bicycle-related injuries, and assaults.[1, 4] In children younger than 1 year of age, abuse remains the most common cause of fatal traumatic cerebral injury,[2, 5] and approximately one fourth of sustained head injuries in children younger than 2 years of age are inflicted by adults.[6]

The factors contributing to cerebral trauma in children are complex and ill-defined.[7] Poverty, inner city life, and family conflict all have been associated with an increased risk of pediatric head trauma.[8] In addition, head injuries occur with greater frequency during times and seasons when children are likely to be traveling in cars or playing outdoors.[9]

□ Normal Intracranial Physiologic Relationships and Pathophysiology

The relationship between cerebral perfusion pressure (CPP), mean arterial pressure (MAP), and intracranial pressure (ICP) is described by the following equation:

$$CPP = MAP - ICP$$

Through the process of pressure autoregulation, the brain is able to maintain a constant cerebral blood flow over a wide range of MAP. This results in cerebral blood flow being independent of MAP between 50 and 150 mm Hg.

Among children with head injuries, this relationship is usually preserved, but when autoregulation is lost, cerebral blood flow will be directly reduced by fluctuations in the MAP or rising ICP. Additionally, cerebral hyperemia and vasodilation, even in the absence of macroscopic brain abnormality, can contribute to increased ICP.[10, 10a] Fifty percent of children with severe head injuries present with elevated ICP.[11]

The volume of brain, blood, and cerebrospinal fluid (CSF) is normally constant within the cranium. This relationship may be described by the Monroe-Kellie doctrine:

$$Brain\ Volume + Cerebral\ Blood\ Volume + CSF\ Volume = Constant$$

According to this equation, because the total volume of the cranial vault is constant, expansion of one compartment occurs at the expense of the others. Addition of a fourth compartment, such as an expanding mass lesion, causes compensatory changes in the other three compartments. Once these compensatory changes are exhausted, enough brain compression may occur that a cerebral herniation syndrome may manifest itself (Table 18–2). Typically, by the time a child manifests clinical signs and symptoms, all compensatory mechanisms have been exhausted and rapid neurologic deterioration may ensue.

Traumatic head injury consists of two phases. The first phase, or primary injury, represents the brain tissue damage sustained at the time of impact and is proportional to the magnitude, duration, and direction of the applied force.[12] The second phase, or secondary injury, includes intracranial or systemic events such as shock or hypoxia that occur in com-

TABLE 18-1. Glasgow Coma Scale in the Infant and Child

Glasgow Coma Scale

Sign	Score
Eye Opening	
Spontaneous	4
To verbal command	3
To pain	2
No response	1
Best Motor Response	
Obeys verbal commands	6
Localizes to pain	5
Withdraws to pain	4
Flexion response to pain	3
Extension response to pain	2
No response	1
Best Verbal Response	
Oriented	5
Confused	4
Inappropriate words	3
Nonspecific sounds	2
No response	1

Modified Glasgow Coma Scale (Infants)

Sign	Score
Eye Opening	
Spontaneous	4
To verbal command	3
To pain	2
No response	1
Best Motor Response	
Spontaneous	6
Localizes to pain	5
Withdraws to pain	4
Flexion response to pain	3
Extension response to pain	2
No response	1
Best Verbal Response	
Appropriate for age; fixes and follows; social smile	5
Cries but consolable	4
Persistently irritable	3
Restless, lethargic	2
None (no response)	1

Definitions of Pediatric Head Injuries According to Initial GCS

Head Injury	Initial GCS
Minor	13–15
Moderate	9–12
Severe	<8

bination with or in response to the primary injury.[13] Although the primary phase of injury is immediate, the secondary phase evolves over time and reaches its maximum severity hours or even days later. Nearly all strategies involved in treating children with cerebral injury aim to ameliorate the effects of secondary phase insults.[14]

PRIMARY INJURY

Primary injury includes two components. The first relates to parenchymal disruption as the brain is forced over the dural or bony protuberances of the skull base. The second component involves disruption of white matter tracts by acceleration, deceleration, and shear forces.[13] Both components occur at impact and are, therefore, not usually amenable to medical intervention. The usual mechanism in the pediatric population is the *coup injury* or the direct impact of the disrupted calvarium on the child's brain.[6]

SECONDARY INJURY

Secondary injury includes intracranial events and contributions from systemic insults that occur following the primary phase.[15] Neurons injured in the initial event may be further compromised during this period because microcirculatory disruption impairs oxygen delivery and cellular repair. Destruction of key biochemical pathways incites inflammatory processes, resulting in the formation of oxygen free radicals.[16] These free radicals are generated by arachidonic acid metabolites, mitochondria, and demarginating neutrophils.[17] Unbound iron released from extravasated red blood cells helps catalyze the formation of these compounds. The formation of oxygen free radicals leads to membrane peroxidation, which can cause large ionic shifts into and out of cells, disruption of key enzymes, and eventually neuronal death.[17]

Other important chemical mediators contributing to secondary injury include excitatory neurotransmitters such as aspartate and glutamate.[18] Uncontrolled liberation of these neurotransmitters leads to ionic shifts across neuronal membranes and ultimately to a massive influx of calcium, which causes inhibition of phosphorylation and fosters membrane hydrolysis.[19] Glutamate-induced neurotoxicity, although not completely understood, is thought to be mediated by two pathways: an early sodium-dependent process that causes neuronal swelling and a later, calcium-dependent process that promotes neuronal disintegration.

The secondary phase of injury evolves over hours to days. Although the effect of rising ICP on other cranial components is well documented, systemic insults can significantly affect patient outcome during this period in the form of hypoxia, hypercarbia, or hypotension. Hypoxia, defined as a sustained PaO$_2$ of less than 60 mm Hg, is associated with a higher mortality in children with head injuries.[15, 20] Hypotension secondary to primary cardiac injury or shock lowers CPP, promoting cerebral ischemia and thereby contributing to neuronal death.

TABLE 18-2. Cerebral Herniation Syndromes

Syndrome	Anatomic Locus
Subfalcine	From side to side underneath the falx cerebri
Transtentorial	Tentorial notch
Tonsillar	Foramen magnum

Cerebral hyperemia is also thought to be the pathologic substrate for profound neurologic deterioration that can occur following trivial head trauma. Minor head injuries can result in a transient deterioration in neurologic function consisting of headache, confusion, vomiting, cortical blindness, or seizures. This disorder is not associated with any gross structural abnormality and rapid, complete recovery usually follows. In such cases, a benign hyperemic encephalopathy mediated by hyperactivation of the trigeminovascular system is thought to be the underlying cause.[21] Treatment is conservative but in rare instances, antimigraine drugs may offer a solution to treating certain neurovascular sequelae of pediatric head injury.[22]

□ Initial Evaluation and Management

Neurologic evaluation of the head-injured child should be focused and efficient. The specific goals for evaluation are as follows:
1. Establish the level of consciousness
2. Identify any focal neurologic deficits
3. Define the anatomic substrate for these deficits
When an injured child arrives at the emergency department and multiple services are involved in his or her care, evaluation and treatment must be conducted in an organized and effective manner.

Many pediatric trauma centers have adopted protocol management strategies for the care of children with severe TBI. These protocols are multidisciplinary and strive to be evidence based. However, there is a critical lack of pediatric-specific evidence in most, if not all, avenues of clinical decision making in severe TBI. Until the data are available, unfortunately, a large portion of these protocols will remain based on data generated from adult patients. An example of one of these protocols in use at our institution is seen in Figure 18–1.

□ Neurologic Examination

For children with severe TBI, the GCS is preferably obtained prior to initiating any chemical paralysis or sedation. It is important that, following the initial neurologic evaluation, the examination be repeated when necessary to monitor trends in neurologic status. Often, a decline in neurologic status is an ominous sign and may indicate the presence of an expanding intracranial mass lesion.

The components of the neurologic examination include the initial GCS (with individual component scores), pupillary size and reactivity, respiratory rate and pattern, otologic examination for hemotympanum, brain stem reflexes (including cough and gag), and extremity response to central stimulus. Fundoscopic examination is mandatory to document the presence or absence of retinal hemorrhages in any case even remotely suspicious for nonaccidental trauma. This finding has both obvious clinical and medicolegal implications.[23]

□ Resuscitation

The fundamental goals of resuscitation in the head-injured child are the restoration of an adequate circulating blood volume, blood pressure support, adequate oxygenation, and appropriate ventilation. These goals are typically carried out within the framework of the Advanced Trauma Life Support protocol. Generally accepted normal ICP values vary according to the patient's age. In infants, normal ICP is less than 5 mm Hg. In toddlers and older children, a normal ICP is less than 10 mm Hg, and in adolescents, ICP should be less than 15 mm Hg. It is difficult to say at what point treatment for raised ICP should be initiated, but a generally accepted guideline is that sustained ICP elevations above 20 mm Hg should be managed aggressively.

Normal pressures defining adequate cerebral perfusion are also age specific. Acceptable CPPs for infants younger than 1 year of age are greater than 50 mm Hg. CPP in most children and adolescents should be at least 50 mm Hg. There is evidence in the adult neurotrauma literature that maintaining a CPP of greater than 70 mm Hg results in improved outcome. Controlling ICP and optimizing CPP are the two priorities in the neurologic resuscitation and management of a child with a TBI.[24, 25]

HYPERVENTILATION

Eucapnia, defined as a $PaCO_2$ between 35 and 40 mm Hg, is the initial therapeutic goal in the acute treatment of the head-injured child.[26] The rationale for hyperventilating patients with TBI is to avoid secondary injury related to ischemia. Recent studies of cerebral blood flow patterns shortly after brain injury demonstrate that cerebral perfusion during the 1st day following trauma is less than half that of normal individuals. These findings imply that avoiding cerebral ischemia, not managing hyperemia, is the principal goal in the first 24 hours following injury.[27–29] Aggressive hyperventilation, defined as a $PaCO_2$ less than 25 mm Hg, reduces cerebral blood flow and inconsistently reduces ICP. Prolonged hyperventilation may result in loss of autoregulation.[30] Avoiding hyperventilation in the first 24 hours following a severe head injury may improve the recovery of neurologic function.[31]

OSMOTHERAPY

Administration of intravenous mannitol has an immediate plasma-expanding effect that reduces the hematocrit and blood viscosity and increases cerebral perfusion, resulting in improved oxygen delivery.[32, 33] The beneficial effects of mannitol on elevated ICP and cerebral blood flow last between 90 minutes and 6 hours, depending on a patient's clinical condition.[34] Intermittent boluses of manni-

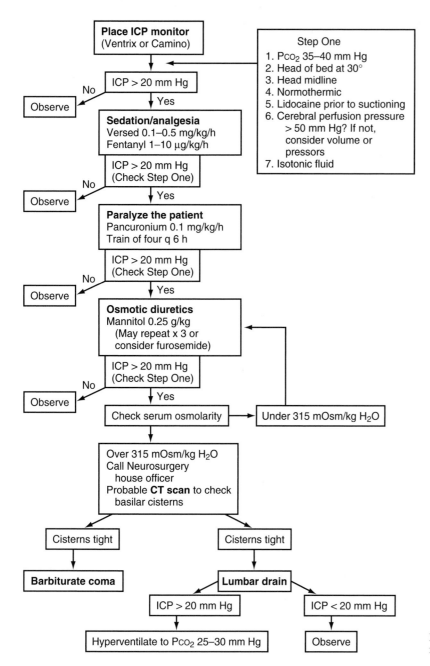

Figure 18–1. Intracranial pressure (ICP) management protocol.

tol are more efficacious than a continuous infusion.[35] The recommended dosage in the pediatric population is 0.25 g/kg given as a bolus every 4 to 6 hours. Serum osmolality is periodically measured and should be kept between 300 and 320 mOsm.

Mannitol should not be given during the initial resuscitation of an injured child with TBI unless there is a witnessed progressive neurologic decline or signs of transtentorial herniation.[26] Care must be exercised when administering mannitol because concomitant diuresis can potentiate hypotension and shock.

PRESSOR THERAPY

Head-injured patients must be adequately resuscitated to optimize their systemic perfusion pressure.[20, 36] Once an adequate circulating blood volume is achieved, pressor therapy should be considered to increase the MAP and CPP in a child with refractory ICP elevation. The drug of choice for hypertensive therapy in this setting is dopamine. Dosage begins with a bolus of a 5 to 20 µg/kg dose every 10 to 15 minutes as needed, followed by a titrated infusion of 0.1 to 0.5 µg/kg/min. Measures to ensure adequate cardiac output and euvolemia should be instituted before instituting this therapy.

☐ Neuroimaging

In the setting of TBI, the primary cerebral imaging modality is the noncontrast computed tomography (CT) scan.[37] This study adequately demonstrates most acute pathology affecting a child's skull, dura, and underlying brain. Because the secondary phase of injury may involve the development of a latent clot, contusion, or hydrocephalus, a repeat CT scan should be obtained in instances of neurologic decline, failure to improve, or unexplained rising ICP. Plain films of the skull have limited application.

Magnetic resonance imaging (MRI) enables improved evaluation of the posterior fossa and smaller paryenchymal lesions, such as shear injury, that are not well-visualized on CT scans.[37, 38] It is essential for legal documentation in cases of suspected child abuse. Because acute blood is not well-visualized on MRI, this study is best done a few days following injury. This imaging modality should be reserved for those children who are clinically stable, and it may be a better predictor of long-term functional recovery.

An adequate lateral cervical spine radiograph obtained promptly during resuscitation is mandatory. Although spinal cord injury occurs 50 to 100 times less frequently than head injury in children, an adequate cervical spine series does not rule out the possibility of significant cord compromise.[11] Twenty-five to 60% of childhood spinal cord injuries occur without radiographic abnormality.[39] We prefer to obtain full cervical spine radiographs, including flexion and extension views, before removing the cervical collar. In the unresponsive or lethargic patient, this may require obtaining the films under fluoroscopic control. MRI is the most effective screening modality for evaluating potential surgical lesions of the spinal cord; CT scanning with or without contrast agent is useful for assessing disruption of bony elements.

□ Clinical Presentation, Management, and Functional Outcome of Specific Injuries

SCALP INJURIES

Scalp injuries are frequently seen in the setting of pediatric head injury. The scalp consists of five layers. From superficial to deep, these layers include the skin, subcutaneous tissue, a musculoaponeurotic layer that contains the galea, an areolar layer rich in emissary veins, and the periosteum. The scalp also contains a dense, anastomotic blood supply. Thus, even small lacerations can bleed profusely and potentially cause shock or hypotension, especially in the infant.

After ruling out underlying cranial abnormalities, treating scalp injuries is generally uncomplicated.[40] Subgaleal hematomas and cephalhematomas rarely require operative intervention. Close inspection and probing of even small lacerations are necessary to avoid overlooking a foreign body or evidence of penetrating brain injury. Simple lacerations are reapproximated according to accepted surgical principles following irrigation and débridement. Most lac-

erations can be repaired with a single-layer closure that incorporates the galea. Infections are rare given the extensive vascular supply of the scalp, but grossly contaminated wounds may necessitate delayed closure.[13]

CONCUSSION

Concussion has been defined as an immediate and transient alteration of consciousness following head trauma.[41] The term *concussion* connotes no specific anatomic or physiologic aberrations, and the diagnosis is often made historically because most children who sustain minor head trauma are neurologically intact on presentation.

The signs and symptoms in affected children vary by age and the duration of unconsciousness. Infants are less likely to have a protracted loss of consciousness, but the incidence of posttraumatic seizures is increased within this age group. Young children are also more likely to experience delayed sequelae of somnolence, irritability, and labyrinthine disturbance.[42] Among older children, posttraumatic amnesia is common and related to the severity of the injury.[43] The constellation of these complaints, known as the *postconcussive syndrome,* is usually self-limited, but behavioral problems and difficulties with school have been described for periods of up to a year following a severe concussion.[42]

Several grading systems with attendant treatment guidelines have been promulgated for children with cerebral concussion related to sports injuries. An example of one of these grading systems along with specific management guidelines is presented in Table 18–3. Investigations remain ongoing to determine which features on a benchside examination are most important in detecting significant injuries.

For the child presenting following a concussion, the decision to obtain a head CT scan is based on the history, physical examination, and serial neurologic observations. In most cases of mild head injury, the studies are negative,[45] although one report noted a 31% incidence of abnormal CT findings in children presenting with a GCS of 12 or better.[46]

CONTUSION

Cerebral contusions are frequently seen in the pediatric trauma setting and represent areas of brain injured during the primary injury or when the cerebrum is forced over bony skull base protuberances as a result of acceleration and deceleration forces. The most common locations include the temporal, frontal, and occipital poles.[37]

Contusions present clinically during the secondary phase of injury causing neurologic decline due to mass effect, edema, or evolving hemorrhage. The characteristic radiographic findings on CT are focal, hyperdense areas surrounded by areas of hypodensity[37] (Fig. 18–2). Contusions may enlarge or coalesce over time. In these instances, surgical decompression is seldom necessary but should be

TABLE 18–3. Concussion Grading and Management of the Colorado Medical Society*

Grade	Criteria	Management Recommendations
1	No loss of consciousness Confusion without amnesia	Remove from sports contest. Examine every 5 minutes for amnesia or postconcussive symptoms at rest and with exertion. May return to contest if neither appears for at least 20 minutes.
2	No loss of consciousness Confusion with amnesia	Remove from sports contest and disallow return. Examine frequently for neurologic deficit. Reexamine the next day and permit return to practice after 1 full week without symptoms.
3	Loss of consciousness	Ambulance transport from the field to the hospital (use cervical spine precautions if indicated). Permit return to team practice only after 2 full weeks without symptoms.

*This grading scale is described in the context of an injury that occurs during a sports event such as a football game.

considered when significant mass effect or herniation threatens. Functional outcome in cerebral contusions is generally favorable but may be dictated by the location of the lesion and possibly complicated by sequelae from other injuries.[47]

INTRACEREBRAL HEMATOMA

An intracerebral hematoma is a clot of blood within the brain substance. These clots are infrequently associated with pediatric head trauma and arise during the secondary phase of injury following a cortical contusion or parenchymal laceration. Clinical presentation in afflicted children varies according to the anatomy at the affected site. Prognosis, especially for deep clots, is generally poor. Treatment in most instances is conservative, but surgical consideration is given for those children who manifest a neurologic decline or when intracranial hypertension persists despite maximum medical therapy.

EPIDURAL HEMATOMA

An epidural hematoma represents a collection of blood between the skull and the dura. Although these collections were thought to occur with low frequency in children secondary to the apposition between the dura and inner table of the calvarium,[48] one study reported a 25% incidence in a series of posttraumatic intracranial hematomas.[49]

An epidural hematoma, which can be arterial or venous, forms when disrupted vessels begin bleeding into the epidural space and dissect the dura away from the bone. Most of these collections have associated skull fractures. When the fracture extends, for example, across the middle meningeal artery, vascular disruption under arterial pressure can lead to an expanding mass and a neurosurgical emergency. As the clot grows, it usually encounters and stops at a suture line, which leads to the characteristic lentiform hyperdensity on CT scan[37] (Fig. 18–3).

In many instances, the inciting trauma might

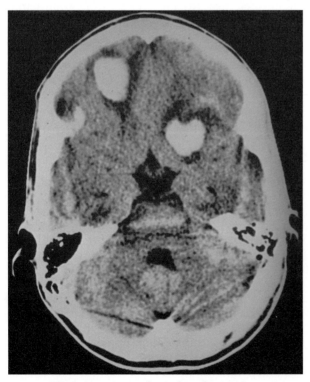

Figure 18–2. Hemorrhagic frontal contusions.

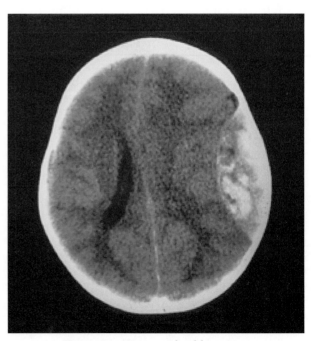

Figure 18–3. Acute epidural hematoma.

seem trivial and the child may have experienced no alteration in consciousness. Eighty-five percent of infants in a recent series had no mental status changes at the time of injury.[50] This early period is described as the "lucid interval." Although rapid clinical deterioration thereafter is common among adults, children and, in particular, infants with patent fontanels are less likely to manifest such abrupt changes unless the hematoma occurs within the posterior fossa. If the collection continues to grow, then the cerebral compensatory mechanisms are used. When these have been exhausted, herniation occurs. These intracranial changes are reflected by a deterioration in the neurologic examination. For example, the child initially may be awake and alert complaining only of a headache. As the ICP increases, the patient experiences nausea, vomiting, somnolence, and nuchal rigidity. Contralateral hemiparesis and obtundation follows, leading to posturing and ipsilateral pupillary dilation, the "blown pupil." Seizures may occur but are not commonplace in this setting.

Most symptomatic epidural hematomas are managed by emergent surgery and clot evacuation. For this reason, an early CT scan is mandatory. Burrhole drainage of these collections in the emergency department is technically difficult and not recommended except in very unusual circumstances. Indications for surgery generally incur a low threshold for intervention and include progressive clinical deterioration or radiographic evidence of an expanding clot. Nonsurgical management consists of observation and supportive care. Up to 20% of epidural hematomas may be managed without operative intervention. Outcome is integrally related to prompt institution of adequate medical therapy. In children with an isolated epidural clot and no intrinsic brain injury, two authors reported an 89% functional recovery and a 5% mortality.[51]

SUBDURAL HEMATOMA

A subdural hematoma is an extraaxial clot located between the cortical surface and the dura. Subdural hematomas are classified as acute or chronic and are frequently associated with underlying parenchymal disruption. Within the spectra of pediatric head injury, acute subdural hematomas are most common in infants, less common in toddlers and older children, but become more frequent in adolescents as injury patterns change to mirror those seen in adults.[50, 52]

Acute Subdural Hematoma

In children, most acute subdural hematomas are traumatic and result from avulsed bridging veins, from torn cortical vessels, or as a direct result of the primary injury. Subdural hematomas can occur at any site, but they are most frequently seen over the convexities. Unlike epidural hematomas, subdural

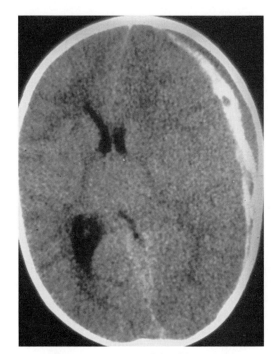

Figure 18–4. Acute subdural hematoma.

clots are not limited by sutures and can, therefore, extend over the entire hemisphere.

Clinically significant subdural hematomas are more likely to occur in a patient with a severe head injury. As these individuals usually have concomitant parenchymal pathology, the presentation is that of a child with profound neurologic injury and deterioration. Radiographic evaluation with an emergent CT scan is mandatory. Subdural clots are connoted by a hyperdense collection and may be associated with significant mass effect and edema (Fig. 18–4).

Treatment for these children begins by optimizing control of any intracranial hypertension. As an adjunct to these therapies, placement of an ICP monitor may be required. Large subdural hematomas with significant mass effect require prompt surgical extirpation, although evacuation sometimes represents only a minor component in the struggle to control intracranial hypertension. In some instances, the underlying brain may be so edematous that reapproximation of the dura and replacement of the craniotomy flap becomes impossible. The outcome in these children is less favorable than for epidural hematomas and seems to be related to the initial clinical presentation and the extent and location of parenchymal disruption.[53]

Chronic Subdural Hematoma

Chronic subdural hematomas are common problems in infancy and often present singularly as megalencephaly. As with most pediatric posttraumatic hemorrhages, males are more frequently affected. Although these collections can be seen following nonaccidental trauma or even following minor injuries, in many instances, a clear history is difficult to ascertain.[54]

The clinical presentation is often subtle. The affected child is usually younger than 2 years of age and has a history of irritability, vomiting, failure to thrive, and, possibly, seizures. The head circumference is often elevated and the anterior fontanel is open and full. Focal neurologic deficits are uncommon. In advanced cases, lethargy, dilated scalp veins, sunsetting of the eyes, papilledema, and prominent frontal bossing may be present.[55]

Most chronic subdural hematomas in children are bilateral and occur over the convexities. Although these clots are easily demonstrated on noncontrast-agent CT scans as hypodense collections, MRI imaging is used to confirm the chronicity, establish a traumatic etiology, and rule out other diagnostic possibilities[56] (Fig. 18–5).

The management of chronic subdural hematomas aims to avert progressive intracranial hypertension by removing the subdural fluid. In a majority of patients, carefully performed daily subdural taps have been shown to adequately treat this condition without operative intervention.[57] Surgical options include endoscopic irrigation of the subdural space or placement of a subdural-peritoneal shunt.[58] Craniotomy with membranectomy is not recommended. The developmental outcome in 53 children was evaluated comprehensively by two authors and found to be favorable in 72%.[59] The prognosis, however, is ultimately related to prompt resolution of intracranial hypertension and the extent of parenchymal damage incurred during the original insult.[60]

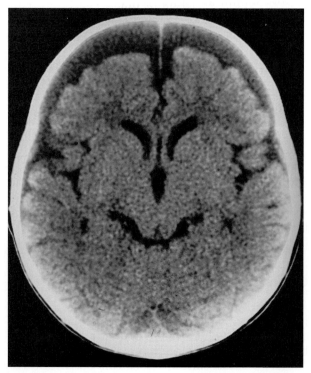

Figure 18–5. Chronic subdural hematomas following child abuse.

SUBARACHNOID HEMORRHAGE

Subarachnoid hemorrhage is the most common form of posttraumatic hemorrhage and occurs following damage to small vessels on the cortical surface, falx, or tentorium. This form of hemorrhage does not usually accompany clinically significant neurologic sequelae, although patients may develop a chemical meningitis and complain of headaches, photophobia, nuchal rigidity, and restlessness. Treatment is conservative; most individuals respond well to acetaminophen, and corticosteroids are helpful in more intransigent cases.

LINEAR, DIASTATIC, AND GROWING SKULL FRACTURES

Ninety percent of pediatric skull fractures are linear and involve the calvaria.[61] These fractures frequently occur in conjunction with concussion and contusion. Radiographic features include a dark, thin, straight course without branching on plain skull films.[37] Decisions regarding medical treatment are generally directed toward postconcussive complaints, and the expected outcome is excellent.[62]

Diastatic fractures extend into and separate a cranial suture. These are more common in children than young adults.[62] Growing skull fractures or posttraumatic leptomeningeal cysts have a distinctive appearance. This condition consists of a fracture line that widens with time, and although most are asymptomatic, the cyst may develop mass effect with associated neurologic decline. These cysts are rare, occurring in 0.6% of cases within a large series of pediatric skull fractures; they are frequently associated with a diastatic fracture and require an adjoining dural tear.[63] The mean age at injury is younger than 1 year, and 90% occur before the age of 3 years. Children present with an enlarging subgaleal mass and an antecedent history of trauma within the past 6 months. Surgical intervention is required to correct these progressive deformities.

DEPRESSED SKULL FRACTURES

Depressed skull fractures (DSFs) account for 7 to 10% of pediatric head injury hospital admissions.[64] These fractures can lead to significant problems when associated with dural tears, parenchymal disruption, or secondary formation of an intracranial hematoma. Posttraumatic epilepsy and infection are important complications. The causes of injury vary according to age and socioeconomic and cultural status.[65] Within the United States, most DSFs occur following bicycle or motor vehicle accidents; falls predominate in younger children.[64]

DSFs are characterized as either simple or compound (open), and most commonly occur over the parietal bone. Compound DSFs comprise between 42 and 90% of cases and are associated with a higher incidence of dural and cortical lacerations.[66] Given the spectrum of pathology, the clinical pre-

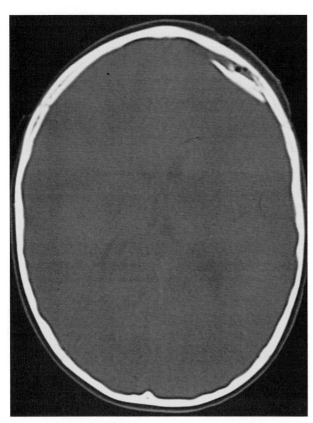

Figure 18–6. Frontal depressed skull fracture.

sentation is likewise variable and dependent on the degree of injury to the underlying brain and vascular tree. In the absence of an overt, clinically palpable depression, diagnosis can be achieved by noncontrast-agent CT evaluation with bone windows (Fig. 18–6).

Classic teaching stressed that urgent surgical elevation of the depressed bone was necessary to prevent posttraumatic epilepsy. Several studies have since shown no increase in the incidence of early posttraumatic epilepsy among patients with simple DSF.[67, 68] Late posttraumatic epilepsy, however, has been seen in 15% of patients, with a preponderance among young children.[68] This phenomenon is likely related to the degree of parenchymal disruption incurred during the primary phase of injury.

Criteria for surgical elevation of DSF include a depression that exceeds the thickness of the skull, a neurologic deficit related to compression of the underlying brain, and a spinal fluid leak secondary to a dural laceration. The presence of a compound DSF represents a relative indication for surgical intervention. Reports of compound fractures managed conservatively have been published, and no significant differences with respect to complications have been documented.[66] A contraindication to surgery exists when the fracture overlies and depresses a dural sinus. In this instance, if the patient is neurologically intact and has no evidence of a CSF leak, conservative management is recommended.

Infection rates among children with DSFs range from 2.5 to 10%.[66, 69] A missed diagnosis has been reported to play a major role in the development of posttraumatic infection. Limited prophylactic antibiotics are recommended, particularly with contaminated wounds. In a recent study of 530 cases of pediatric DSFs, an infection rate of 1.1% was reported. All of these children underwent an operation within 24 hours of presentation; bone fragments were replaced only in clean wounds. Satisfactory outcome was noted in 95% of these patients, with a mortality rate of 2.5%.[70]

BASILAR SKULL FRACTURES

Fractures of the skull base are seen in 8 to 14% of children with head trauma.[71] The diagnosis is made through a combination of distinctive clinical findings and radiographic features. Findings suggestive of a basilar skull fracture include Battle's sign (retroauricular ecchymosis without evidence of direct trauma to the mastoid) and hemotympanum. Battle's sign represents a dissection of blood through a disrupted outer table in the region of the mastoid or occipital bone. *Hemotympanum,* or blood behind the tympanic membrane, in the absence of a laceration of the external auditory canal, is caused by a fracture of the petrous bone. Periorbital ecchymosis, or "raccoon eyes," without findings suggestive of direct orbital trauma, results from the dissection of blood into the periorbita secondary to a fracture of the anterior cranial base.

Otorrhea and rhinorrhea may also occur in the presence of a basilar skull fracture. Among patients who ultimately manifest clinical evidence of a spinal fluid leak, otorrhea or rhinorrhea occurs in 60 to 70% within 48 hours of injury and is generally self-limited.[25] Meningitis occurs in 3 to 17% of children with rhinorrhea and in 4% of patients with otorrhea.[72] Prophylactic antibiotics are not recommended owing to the risk of selection of drug-resistant organisms. A spinal fluid leak in a child under age 5 is rare because the frontal sinus is not completely pneumatized until age 10 and the mastoid air cells are not developed.

When the clinical findings of a skull base fracture are suggestive but not diagnostic, radiographic studies can confirm a basilar skull fracture. Skull films are generally not helpful. A noncontrast-agent CT scan with bone windows, however, allows good visualization of the cranial base and inspection of the adjacent brain.

Treatment for the child with a basilar skull fracture is conservative, and the outcome in an isolated fracture of the skull base is excellent.[13] In the absence of infection, injury to the cranial nerves can complicate recovery. The most commonly injured cranial nerve is the olfactory tract, with 3 to 10% of children becoming permanently anosmic following a fracture of the cribriform plate.[73] Ocular paresis develops in 1 to 10% of patients following an injury to the sixth, third, or fourth cranial nerve, but 75% of affected children completely recover.[74] The facial nerve is also frequently traumatized, affecting 3 to 12% of children with a fracture of the petrous bone. Facial nerve palsies often occur in conjunction with hearing loss, dizziness, nausea, vomiting, and tinnitus following injury to the adjoining eighth nerve. Ninety percent of patients with traumatic facial nerve palsy can be expected to make a full recovery.[73]

DIFFUSE AXONAL INJURY

Diffuse axonal injury represents a significant cause of morbidity among victims of pediatric head trauma. This process occurs when rapid acceleration/deceleration and shear forces disrupt axonal pathways in the corpus callosum, deep nuclei, basal ganglia, and thalamus.[75] Shear forces preferentially affect these structures because their weight and angle of momentum vary from the rest of the cerebrum.

Affected children present with severe head injuries and usually fail to progress beyond a vegetative state. The initial CT scan often fails to demonstrate salient pathology, and interval scans may reveal evolution of petechial hemorrhages, particularly adjacent to the corpus callosum. MRI scanning represents a sensitive radiographic means of diagnosing these abnormalities[37] (Fig. 18–7). Despite aggressive rehabilitation measures, functional outcome in these children is poor.[75]

BICYCLE INJURIES

Fatal injuries following bicycle accidents involve 1000 to 1300 individuals in the United States each

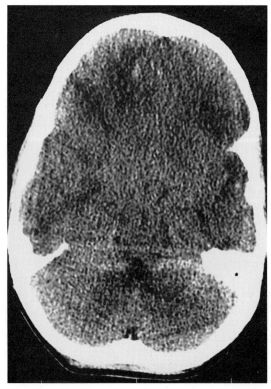

Figure 18–7. Shear injury.

year.[76] Several investigators have demonstrated that most of these bicycle-related deaths occur from head trauma, and approximately half occur in children and adolescents.[77] Most bicycle mishaps are caused by collisions with road hazards or irregularities in the road surface resulting in falls. Twenty-five percent of brain injuries in children younger than the age of 15 are the result of bicycle accidents.[3]

Numerous strategies have evolved for preventing bicycle-related head injuries, in particular, institution of community-based educational programs that encourage safe cycling practices, construction of roads that isolate bicyclists from motorists, and the use of protective helmets. According to research conducted in Seattle, Washington, children who use a helmet reduce the chance of a serious head injury by 85%.[78]

SPORTS-RELATED INJURIES

According to statistics from the National Center for Catastrophic Sports Injury Research, the four common school sports with the highest risk of head injury include football, gymnastics, ice hockey, and wrestling. Among these, based on absolute numbers, football has the highest incidence of injury, but among the very young (ages 5 to 14 years), baseball has the highest fatality rate for any youth sport with the least amount of safety equipment mandated.

As with bicycle injuries, improvement in safety equipment and school-based education programs have decreased the incidence and global severity of head injuries. Most head trauma seen by a physician historically includes a concussion or postconcussive complaints. The leading cause of death from athletic head injury remains intracranial hematoma.[79]

Second-impact syndrome consists of the rapid brain swelling and herniation that occur when an athlete sustains a head injury, such as a concussion or contusion, then has a second head injury before the symptoms associated with the first injury have resolved.[80] The second blow may be trivial; the athlete may appear stunned but usually does not lose consciousness. Within minutes of the second injury, however, the player collapses and manifests clinical evidence of cerebral herniation. The pathophysiology is thought to relate to loss of cranial autoregulation leading to vascular engorgement.[44] The mortality rate is nearly 50%, and the morbidity approaches 100%.[79] Therefore, an athlete who is symptomatic from a head injury *must not* participate in contact or collision sports until all cerebral symptoms have cleared.

CHILD ABUSE

Child abuse is the leading cause of death in children between the age of 6 and 12 months and accounts for up to 5000 deaths each year in the United States.[1, 76] The peak incidence of abuse resulting in intracranial trauma is 6 months and nearly all cases occur before the age of 2 years.[81] Infants and small children rarely sustain serious injury from accidents in the home.[23] Therefore, any brain injury with subdural or retinal hemorrhage should raise suspicions of abuse. A careful medical and social history, as well as review of all physical examination findings, is mandated.

Subdural hematomas associated with severe child abuse and head injury describe the "shaken baby syndrome."[82] Although the exact mechanism of cerebral injury in this syndrome remains controversial, one hypothesis implicates a whiplash motion of the head followed by the impact of the head on a surface.[81] The presence of a severe cranial injury in a child younger than 1 year of age who has no antecedent history of significant accidental trauma should be considered abuse until proven otherwise.

The most common CT finding in affected children is a convexity or parafalcine subdural hematoma.[37] A posterior interhemispheric collection in the absence of a history of significant accidental trauma is pathognomonic of severe child abuse.[83] MRI is the imaging modality of choice for evaluating abuse and is useful for determining the age of traumatic hematomas and examining evidence of edema or ischemia.[56]

Child abuse crosses all racial and socioeconomic lines and is diagnosed only if the physician is aware of the possibility.[81] The immediate and delayed outcome in cases of head injury from abuse is worse than with any other type of cerebral injury in childhood. The mortality rate for an abused child with an acute subdural hematoma is approximately 22% and the morbidity rate is 50% in most series.[84] Repeat abuse occurs in more than 20% of children and often leads to permanent injury or death.[81]

□ Intracranial Pressure Monitoring

The efficacy of ICP monitoring has never been subjected to the scrutiny of a clinical trial. However, a large body of evidence suggests that monitoring ICP helps in the early detection of enlarging intracranial mass lesions, limits the indiscriminate use of therapies to control ICP, and can alert the surgeon when to reduce ICP through spinal fluid drainage, thereby improving cerebral perfusion.[85, 86]

ICP monitoring devices have advanced considerably since the 1980s. Current technology allows either a parenchymal fiberoptic unit or intraventricular drain to be safely and efficiently inserted at the bedside. Subdural pressure monitors have limited application. The decision to use a specific device varies according to institution preferences. Insertion of a ventricular catheter may be complicated in a child with small ventricles, significant midline shift, or injury involving the scalp or bone. Both parenchymal monitors and ventricular drains provide consistent, reliable data, but ventricular catheters have the added advantage of being able to drain spinal fluid when other attempts at controlling intracranial hypertension fail.

The two primary indications for placement of an ICP monitor include a child with severe cerebral trauma (GCS <8) or a patient with an anticipated loss of consciousness. For example, a child presents with multiple extremity fractures coexistent with a head injury and requires urgent orthopedic operative attention. Even though the patient's cranial trauma may not immediately mandate placement of a monitor, anticipated intraoperative fluid shifts under general anesthesia and protracted loss of the neurologic examination indicate urgent placement of an ICP monitor. Insertion, however, is predicated on a normal coagulation profile.

□ Brain Death

The criteria for brain death vary among states and according to community standards. At the Primary Children's Medical Center in Salt Lake City, Utah, patients must meet the following criteria before brain death can be determined. First, the physician must determine the approximate cause of coma and ensure that no treatable conditions such as hypothermia, shock, poisoning by toxic substances, or metabolic disorders are complicating the clinical evaluation. Coma and apnea must coexist, and the patient must display a complete loss of consciousness, vocalization, and volitional activity. Absence of brain stem function must be determined according to the following criteria:

1. No pupillary light reflex
2. No corneal reflex
3. No oculocephalogyric reflex (doll's eye response)
4. No oculovestibular reflex (ice water caloric stimulation)
5. No gag or cough reflex
6. No spontaneous respirations according to standardized apnea testing protocols[87]

Two separate examinations are required to declare brain death. The interval between these evaluations is age specific, and there must be no significant change in neurologic status. Brain death may be confirmed by a lack of intracranial vascular perfusion as demonstrated by a radionuclide or cerebral angiogram. Electroencephalograms are recommended for children younger than 1 year of age when confirmation is not obtained by studies demonstrating the absence of cerebral perfusion. Appropriate communication with the parents, next of kin, or legal guardian is essential. If there are potential legal complications concerning the patient's injury, such as suspected homicide or child abuse, the removal of organ support should be delayed until consultation can be obtained with the coroner's office.

REFERENCES

1. Division of Injury Control, Center for Environmental Health and Injury Control, Centers for Disease Control: Childhood

injuries in the United States. Am J Dis Child 144:627–646, 1990.

2. Teasdale G, Jennet B: Assessment of coma and impaired consciousness. Lancet 11:81, 1974.
3. Krause JF, Fife O, Cox P, et al: Incidence, severity, and external causes of pediatric brain injury. Am J Dis Child 140:687–693, 1986.
4. Waller AE, Baker SP, Syocha A: Childhood injury deaths, national analysis and geographic variations. Am J Public Health 79:310–315, 1989.
5. Cristoffel KK: Homicide in childhood: A public health problem in need of attention. Am J Public Health 74:68–70, 1984.
6. Duhaime AC, Alario AJ, Lewander WJ, et al: Head injury in very young children: Mechanisms, injury types, and ophthalmologic findings in 100 hospitalized patients younger than 2 years of age. Pediatrics 90:179–185, 1992.
7. Jennett B: Epidemiology of head injury. J Neurol Neurosurg Psych 60:362–369, 1996.
8. Klonoff H: Head injuries in children: Predisposing factors, accident conditions, accident proneness and sequelae. Am J Public Health 61:2405–2417, 1971.
9. Krause JF, Rock A, Hemyari P: Brain injuries among infants, children, adolescents, and young adults. Am J Dis Child 144:684–691, 1990.
10. Muizelaar JP, Marmarov A, DeSalles AA, et al: Cerebral blood flow and metabolism in severely head-injured children, part 1: Relationship with GCS score, outcome, ICP, and PVI. J Neurosurg 71:63–71, 1989.
10a. Muizelaar JP, Ward JD, Marmarov A, et al: Cerebral blood flow and metabolism in severely head-injured children, part 2: Autoregulation. J Neurosurg 71:72–76, 1989.
11. Bruce DA: Head trauma. In Ashcraft KW (ed): Pediatric Surgery (2nd ed). Philadelphia, WB Saunders, 1994, pp 141–145.
12. Gennarelli TA, Thiebault LE, Adams JH, et al: Diffuse axonal injury and traumatic coma in the primate. Ann Neurol 12:564–574, 1982.
13. Allen EM, Boyer R, Cherny WB, et al: Head and spinal cord injury. In Rogers M (ed): Textbook of Pediatric Intensive Care (3rd ed). Philadelphia, Lippincott-Raven, 1996, pp 809–823.
14. Bruce DA: Head injuries in the pediatric population. Curr Probl Pediatr 20:61–107, 1990.
15. Miller JD, Becker DB: Secondary insults to the injured brain. J R Coll Surg Edinb 27:292–298, 1982.
16. Kontos HA, Povlishock JT: Oxygen radicals in brain injury. Centr Nerv Syst Trauma 3:257–263, 1986.
17. Hall E: Lipid antioxidants in acute central nervous system injury. Ann Emer Med 22:1022–1024, 1993.
18. Faden AI, Demediuk P, Panter SS, et al: The role of excitatory amino acids and NMDA receptors in traumatic brain injury. Science 244:798–800, 1989.
19. Gentile N, Mcintosh T: Antagonists of excitatory amino acids and endogenous opioid peptides in the treatment of central nervous system injury. Ann Emerg Med 22:1028–1034, 1993.
20. Chestnut RM, Marshall LF, Klanbay M, et al: The role of secondary brain injury in determining outcome from severe head injury. J Neurosurg 34:216–222, 1993.
21. Sakas DE, Whitwell HL: Neurological episodes after minor head injury and trigeminovascular activation. Med Hypotheses 48:431–435, 1997.
22. Humphrey DB, Goadsby PJ: The mode of action of sumatriptan is vascular? A debate. Cephalgia 14:401–410, 1994.
23. Wilkens B: Head injury—abuse or accident? Arch Dis Child 76:393–396, 1997.
24. McGraw CP, Howard G: The effect of mannitol on inceased intracranial pressure. Neurosurgery 13:269–271, 1983.
25. Robinson RG: Cerebrospinal fluid rhinorrhea, meningitis, and pneumocephalus due to nonmissile injuries. Aust N Z J Surg 33:312–316, 1970.
26. Brain Trauma Foundation, American Academy of Neurologic Surgeons: Guidelines for the Management of Severe Head Injury. Washington, DC, Brain Injury Association, 1995.
27. Bourma GJ, Muizelaar JP, Choi SC, et al: Cerebral circulation and metabolism after severe traumatic brain injury: The elusive roles of ischemia. J Neurosurg 75:685–693, 1991.

28. Bourma GJ, Muizelaar JP, Stringer WA, et al: Ultra early evaluation of regional cerebral blood flow in severely head-injured patients using xenon-enhanced computed tomography. J Neurosurg 77:360–368, 1992.
29. Marion DW, Darby J, Yonas H: Acute regional cerebral blood flow changes caused by severe head injuries. J Neurosurg 74:407–414, 1991.
30. Obrist WD, Langbitt TW, Jaggi JL, et al: Cerebral blood flow and metabolism in comatose patients with acute head injury: A randomized clinical trial. J Neurosurg 75:731–739, 1991.
31. Muizelaar JP, Marmarou A, Ward JP, et al: Adverse effects of prolonged hyperventilation in patients with severe head injury: A randomized clinical trial. J Neurosurg 75:731–739, 1991.
32. Israel RS, Marks JA, Moore EE, et al: Hemodynamic effect of mannitol in a canine model of concomitant increased intracranial pressure and hemorrhagic shock. Ann Emerg Med 17:560–566, 1988.
33. Kassell NF, Baumann KW, Hitchon PW, et al: The effect of high-dose mannitol on cerebral blood flow in dogs with normal intracranial pressure. Stroke 13:59–61, 1982.
34. Cruz J, Miner ME, Allen SJ, et al: Continuous monitoring of cerebral oxygenation in acute brain injury: Injection of mannitol during hyperventilation. J Neurosurg 73:725–730, 1990.
35. Cold GE: Cerebral blood flow in acute head injury: The regulation of cerebral blood flow and metabolism during the acute phase of head injury, and its significance for therapy. Acta Neurochir Suppl (Wein) 49:1–64, 1990.
36. Marmarou A, Anderson RL, Ward JD, et al: Impact of intracranial pressure instability and hypotension on outcome in patients with severe head injury. J Neurosurg 75:559–566, 1991.
37. Beckett WW, Ball WS Jr: Craniocerebral trauma. In Ball WS Jr (ed): Pediatric Neuroradiology (1st ed). Philadelphia, Lippincott-Raven, 1997, pp 443–489.
38. Orrison WW Jr, Gentry LR, Stimac LK, et al: Blinded comparison of cranial CT and MR in closed head injury evaluation. AJNR Am J Neuroradiol 15:351–356, 1994.
39. Pang D, Wilberger JE: Spinal cord injuries without radiographic abnormalities in children. J Neurosurg 57:114–129, 1982.
40. Goodrich JT: Management of scalp injuries. In Cheek WR, Marlin AE, McLone DG, et al (eds): Pediatric Neurosurgery. Surgery of the Developing Nervous System (3rd ed). Philadelphia, WB Saunders, 1994, pp 251–265.
41. Ommaya AK, Gennarelli TA: Cerebral concussion and traumatic unconsciousness: Correlations of experimental and clinical observations in blunt head injuries. Brain 97:633–654, 1974.
42. Mittenberg W, Wittner MS, Miller LJ: Postconcussion syndrome occurs in children. Neuropsychology 11:447–452, 1997.
43. Russell WR, Smith A: Post-traumatic amnesia in closed head injury. Arch Neurol 5:4, 1961.
44. Kelly JP, Nichols JS, Filley CM, et al: Concussion in sports: Guidelines for the preservation of catastrophic outcome. JAMA 266:2867–2869, 1991.
45. Carey MJ, van der Post J: Computed tomography scanning and minor head injuries. N Z Med J 107:500–501, 1994.
46. Rivara F, Tanaguchi D, Parish RA, et al: Poor prediction of positive computed tomographic scans by clinical criteria in symptomatic pediatric head trauma. Pediatrics 80:579–584, 1987.
47. Greenspan AI: Functional recovery following head injury among children. Curr Probl Pediatr 3:170–177, 1996.
48. Singounas EG, Volikas ZG: Epidural hematomas in the pediatric population. Childs Brain 11:250–254, 1984.
49. Jamieson KG, Yelland JDN: Extradural hematoma: Report of 167 cases. J Neurosurg 29:13–23, 1968.
50. Raimondi AJ, Hirschauer J: Head injury in the infant and toddler. Childs Brain 11:12, 1984.
51. Bricolo AP, Pasut LM: Extradural hematoma: Toward zero mortality. Neurosurgery 14:8–12, 1984.
52. Hahn YS, Chyung C, Barthel MJ, et al: Head injuries in

children under 36 months of age. Childs Nerv Syst 4:34, 1988.

53. Aronyk KE: Post-traumatic hematomas. In Cheek WR, Marlin AE, McLone DG, et al (eds): Pediatric Neurosurgery. Surgery of the Developing Nervous System (3rd ed). Philadelphia, WB Saunders, 1994, pp 282–284.

54. McLaurin RL: Management of chronic subdural hematomas in infancy. In O'Brian MS (ed): Pediatric Neurological Surgery. New York, Raven Press, 1978, pp 125–146.

55. Ingraham FD, Matson DD: Subdural hematoma in infancy. J Pediatr 24:1–37, 1944.

56. Ball WS Jr: Nonaccidental craniocerebral trauma (child abuse): MR imaging. Radiology 173:609, 1989.

57. McLaurin RL, Isaacs E, Lewis HP: Results of nonoperative treatment in 15 cases of infantile subdural hematoma. J Neurosurg 34:753–759, 1971.

58. Aoki N: Chronic subdural hematoma in infancy: Clinical analysis of 30 cases in the CT era. J Neurosurg 73:201–205, 1990.

59. Schulman K, Ransahoff J: Chronic subdural hematoma in infants. Am J Dis Child 39:980–1021, 1961.

60. Parent AD: Pediatric chronic subdural hematoma: A retrospective comparative analysis. Pediatr Neurosurg 18:266–271, 1992.

61. Greenberg M: Handbook of Neurosurgery (4th ed). Lakeland, FL, Greenberg Graphics, 1997, pp 721–722.

62. Mealey J: Skull fractures. In American Association of Neurological Surgeons, Section of Pediatric Neurosurgery: Pediatric Neurosurgery: Surgery of the Developing Nervous System, (1st ed). New York, Grune & Stratton, 1982, pp 289–299.

63. Ramamurthi B, Kalyanaraman S: Rationale for surgery in growing fractures of the skull. J Neurosurg 32:427–430, 1970.

64. Choux M: Incidence, diagnosis, and management of skull fractures. In Ramondi AJ, Choux M, DiRocco C (eds): Head Injuries in the Newborn and Infant. New York, Springer-Verlag, 1986, pp 163–182.

65. Steinbok P, Flodmark O, Martents D, et al: Management of simple depressed skull fractures in children. J Neurosurg 66:506–510, 1987.

66. Van Den Heever CM, Van Der Merwe DJ: Management of depressed skull fractures. J Neurosurg 71:186–190, 1989.

67. Braakman R: Depressed skull fracture: Data, treatment, and follow-up in 225 consecutive cases. J Neurol Neurosurg Psych 35:395–402, 1972.

68. Jennett B, Miller JD, Braakman R: Epilepsy after nonmissile depressed skull fracture. J Neurosurg 41:208–216, 1974.

69. Jennett B, Miller JD: Infection after depressed fractures of the skull. Implications for management of nonmissile injuries. J Neurosurg 36:333–339, 1972.

70. Ersahin Y, Matluer S, Mirzai H, et al: Pediatric depressed skull fractures: Analysis of 530 cases. Childs Nerv Syst 12:323–331, 1996.

71. Henrick EB, Harwood-Nash DC, Hudson AR: Head injuries in children. A survey of 4465 cases at the Hospital for Sick Children, Toronto, Canada. Clin Neurosurg 11:46, 1964.

72. MacGee EE, Cauthen SR, Brackett CE: Meningitis following acute traumatic cerebrospinal fistula. J Neurosurg 33:312–316, 1970.

73. Hughes BJ: The results of injury to special parts of the brain and skull. In Rowbotham GF (ed): Acute Injuries of the Head, Their Diagnosis, Treatment, Complications, and Sequelae. Baltimore, Williams & Wilkins, 1964, p 408.

74. Rucker CW: The causes of paralysis of the third, fourth, and sixth cranial nerves. Am J Ophthalmol 61:1293–1298, 1966.

75. Oppenheimer DR: Microscopic lesions of the brain following head injury. J Neurol Neurosurg Psych 61:1293–1298, 1968.

76. Division of Injury Epidemiology and Control, Center for Environmental Health, Centers for Disease Control: Bicycle-related injuries: Data from the National Electronic Injury Surveillance System. JAMA 257:3334–3337, 1987.

77. Waters EA: Should pedal cyclists wear helmets? A comparison of head injuries sustained by pedal cyclist and motor cyclists in road traffic accidents. Injury 17:372–375, 1986.

78. Thompson RS, Rivara FP, Thompson DC: A case-control study of the effectiveness of bicycle safety helmets. N Engl J Med 320:1361–1367, 1989.

79. Cantor RC: Head and spine injuries in youth sports. Clin Sports Med 14:517–533, 1995.

80. Saunders RL, Harbaugh RE: The second impact syndrome in catastrophic contact sports head trauma. JAMA 266:2867–2869, 1991.

81. Duhaime AC, Gennarelli TA, Thibault LE, et al: The shaken baby syndrome: A clinical, pathological, and biomechanical study. J Neurosurg 66:409–415, 1987.

82. Caffey J: On the theory and practice of shaking infants. Am J Dis Child 124:151, 1972.

83. Zimmerman RA, Bilaniuk LT, Bruce D, et al: CT of craniocerebral injury in the abused child. Neuroradiology 130:687, 1979.

84. Alexander R, Sato Y, Smith W, et al: Incidence of impact trauma with cranial injuries ascribed to shaking. Am J Dis Child 144:724, 1990.

85. Eisenberg HM, Gary HE Jr, Aldrich EF, et al: Initial CT findings in 753 patients with severe head injury. A report from the NIH Traumatic Coma Data Bank. J Neurosurg 73:688–698, 1990.

86. Narayan RK, Kishore PR, Becker DP, et al: Intracranial pressure: To monitor or not to monitor? A review of our experience with severe head injury. J Neurosurg 56:650–659, 1982.

87. Outwater KM, Rocknoff MA: Apnea testing to confirm brain death in children. Crit Care Med 12:357–358, 1984.

19

PEDIATRIC ORTHOPEDIC TRAUMA

Nigel Price, MD, FRCSC

Methods of treating bone and joint injuries have been known for more than 2000 years, dating back to Hippocrates. Much of the treatment for pediatric orthopedic trauma was nonoperative until the mid-20th century. Operative treatment of adults and children was avoided in favor of closed treatment.[1, 2] Modern pediatric fracture care is changing as more surgeons opt for open treatment and rigid fixation, particularly in the patient with multiple injuries.[3]

Examples of injuries being treated increasingly by operative methods include femur fractures in the older child and adolescent, supracondylar fractures of the humerus and displaced growth plate (physeal) fractures. This aggressive therapeutic approach has reduced the unacceptably high number of malunions and has permitted earlier mobilization and discharge of patients.[4] It has also allowed the patient with multiple injuries to be treated without the need for casting that has caused problems with access to body cavities and extremity compartments.

☐ Incidence and Epidemiology

Many variables such as age, season, time of day, and social factors determine the incidence of orthopedic trauma. The most common presentation of orthopedic trauma is an isolated fracture. Fractures occur more commonly in summer and in late afternoon. The percentage of patients with trauma who have a fracture is approximately 18%.

Certain trends are seen in fracture patterns. Long bone fractures in nonambulatory children are largely of nonaccidental origin and should alert the trauma surgeon to the possibility of abuse. Specific fracture types such as spiral fractures of lower extremities, long bone fractures, and physeal injuries have been identified as potentially being nonaccidental. The incidence of nonaccidental fractures appears to be rising.[5, 6]

The most common isolated accidental fractures involve the distal radius and the humerus. The tibia is more commonly fractured than the femur. Physeal injuries (those involving the growth plate) account for 22% of fractures in children. The incidence of open fractures is 3%. Multiple fractures have been reported in many series to occur in 4% of pediatric patients.[7]

Of all children's fractures, 37% occur in the home, 18 to 20% are sports related, and approximately 3 to 9% occur at school. Less than 10% occur in motor vehicle accidents (MVAs).[7, 8] The highest rates occur between the ages of 1 and 2 years and between 13 and 18 years. There is a male preponderance, with a 1.9:1 ratio in teen years. The incidence of fractures peaks at ages 15 in boys and 12 in girls.[9]

The rate of orthopedic injuries in children with multiple injuries parallels the mortality rate from injuries; approximately 10% of multiple trauma patients have fractures.[7]

Motor vehicle–related accidents account for the most deaths in children older than 1 year.[10] Accidental death rates seem to be falling, in part due to public education, safer cars, and better emergency medical care. MVA injuries are much more likely to involve multiple systems and much more likely to be fatal.[11]

Other less common causes of bone injuries include gunshot wounds, penetrating weapons, and falls. A study done at the Children's National Medical Center in Washington, D.C., showed that 13% of total admissions were trauma related.[11] The Children's Mercy Hospital experiences approximately 11% trauma related admissions (N. Felich, unpublished data, 1999).

☐ Pathophysiology

Children's bones are in a state of constant change because of growth. The method of treatment used for a given fracture varies according to the patient's age.

The immature skeleton has a very different anatomy from that of the mature skeleton. This contributes to the higher rate of fractures in children as compared with adults. These anatomic differences include the developing epiphysis, the physis (or

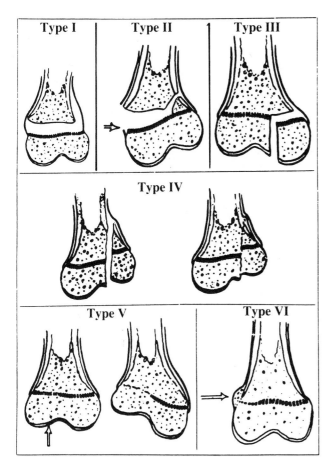

Figure 19–1. Salter classification with Rang modification. (Modified from Rang ML (ed): The Growth Plate and Its Disorders. Edinburgh, E & S Livingstone, 1969, p 139.)

growth plate), changing periosteum, and rapidly remodeling metaphyseal and diaphyseal regions. Children are more likely to suffer a fracture through the growth plate than to have a ligamentous sprain because the growth plate is the weaker structure. As the skeleton matures, a changing pattern of growth plate injuries occurs (Fig. 19–1). Salter type I injuries are more often seen in very young children, whereas types II, III, and IV injuries are seen in older children. Fifteen percent of children's fractures are physeal injuries. The metaphysis is an injury-prone area. The relatively large size of the epiphysis also has an impact on the type of joint injury.

Immature bone has a relatively thicker layer of periosteum as compared with mature bone. This layer of tissue has potent osteogenic potential. It is often partially intact after fracture and may serve as a hinge, which aids reduction and contributes to fracture stability. The periosteum also contributes to early and effective fracture healing.

Immature bone is relatively porous compared with adult bone; hence, the pattern of fracture may be different. Torus or buckle fractures are caused by compression of bone. Greenstick fractures and plastic deformation injuries are unique to children, in part because of more porous laminar bone with its thinner and softer cortex.

Children's fractures are more likely to remodel in the case of less-than-perfect anatomic alignment, especially if the injury occurs near an actively growing physis and if the fracture plane is the same as the motion of the contiguous joint; e.g., knee, wrist, ankle. Children's bones will not remodel to compensate for significant rotational malalignment or varus or valgus deformities.[12]

Fractures in children stimulate longitudinal bone growth at the epiphysis, physis, and metaphysis. In the younger age groups, some overriding of the fractured long bones is acceptable and even desirable when they are reduced.[13]

In addition to the Salter classification, there are other classifications of pediatric bone injury based on the pattern of injury and anatomic location. The site of fracture may be diaphyseal, epiphyseal, physeal, or articular. Patterns include longitudinal, transverse, oblique, spiral, impacted, bowing, greenstick, torus, pathologic, stress, and occult. A knowledge of the anatomy and fracture patterns is useful when describing injuries to other caregivers for planning treatment and in determining prognosis.

☐ Complex Extremity Injuries

Degloving injuries, open fractures, and partial amputations to upper and lower extremities are becoming increasingly common, particularly during the summer months.[14, 15] Sources of injuries include lawnmowers, recreational vehicles, trail bikes, and skateboards. Animal attacks can also create severe extremity injuries in children.[16] These injuries involve a skeletal injury associated with a variable amount of compromise to the soft tissue. The injury may range from a break in the skin to a significant muscle, periosteal, and neurovascular tissue loss.

Once the deforming force dissipates, it can be difficult to demonstrate that the fracture is truly open. It is best to assume that if a laceration or abrasion occurs near a fracture, that fracture should be treated as open.[17]

Assessment and stabilization of the patient with multiple injuries must be the first concern (see Chapter 15). The musculoskeletal injury is evaluated as part of the secondary survey. The neurovascular status of the limbs should be assessed and recorded. It is often difficult to elicit cooperation from an anxious child, but the medical records should include assessment of all motor and sensory groups and peripheral pulses. A Doppler may be used to assess the presence and quality of a pulse. Generally, it is best not to probe an open wound in the emergency department because of the risk of reactivating arterial bleeding. The size, depth, and nature of a wound and degree of contamination should be determined as much as possible without exploration. Complete assessment of the wound is

TABLE 19-1. Severity Classification
for Open Fractures

Grade	Description
I	Wound <1 cm
II	Transitional wound (1–10 cm)
III	Wound >10 cm
IIIA	Extensive soft tissue injury
IIIB	Reconstructive soft tissue
IIIC	Vascular injury

Data from Gustilo RB, Mendoza RM, Williams DN: Problems in the management of type III (severe) open fractures: A new classification of type III open fractures. J Trauma 24:747–796, 1984; Gustilo RB, Anderson JT: Prevention of infection in the treatment of 1025 open fractures of long bones. Retrospective and prospective analyses. J Bone Joint Surg Am 50:453–458, 1976.

best done in an operating room under controlled and sterile conditions.

Initial wound swabs may be taken in the emergency setting. Superficial irrigation to remove gross contamination and the initiation of broad-spectrum antibiotics should be done. The wound should be splinted above and below the fracture to immobilize contiguous joints. Radiographic assessment should include the contiguous joints and should be done in two planes. The patient's tetanus immunization status should be ascertained and augmented if necessary.

Open fractures are commonly classified according to Gustilo (Table 19–1). Operative débridement principles include the removal of obviously devitalized tissue and debris and a thorough irrigation of the wounds to minimize bacterial contamination. The amount of skin and soft tissue excised varies according to the wound. For small wounds, an ellipse of tissue including the puncture can be excised, and muscle and bone débridement can be minimal. Larger wounds need to be débrided to viable borders. Skin débridement in children can often be as little as 1 mm from the wound edge. The débridement continues layer by layer, minimizing dissection into uninvolved planes. Obviously devitalized muscles and periosteum can be sharply excised. Bone ends can be decontaminated with elevators and curettes. The amount and type of irrigation is variable, but introduction of saline by syringe or pulse lavage is appropriate. Several liters may suffice for small wounds, and up to 10 to 14 l may be used for larger wounds. Antibiotic irrigation is often used at the end of the procedure.

The goal of open fracture management is the conversion of a contaminated wound to a clean, closed wound. A small puncture wound may communicate with the periosteum or bone; therefore it is more conservative and prudent to débride and irrigate even a small puncture that communicates with bone. Orderly sequential débridement avoiding dissection in nonaffected areas is indicated. Open fractures are assumed to be contaminated, and antibiotics should be given according to the grade.

Infected wounds should be aggressively managed with serial débridement, antibiotics, drains, antibiotic-impregnated methyl methacrylate beads, and secondary wound closure.

The potential for muscle and periosteal coverage of the fracture should be assessed at the time of initial débridement. Muscle viability is best assessed by contractility and the capacity to bleed. Periosteum is a very important contributor to appositional bone growth, and it should be débrided conservatively. Extensive open fractures are increasingly being treated as aggressively as adult fractures with vascularized pedicle flaps; fewer are being treated with split thickness skin grafts.[17]

☐ Multiple Trauma

Internal or external fixation of pediatric fractures has grown in popularity to parallel improved intraoperative imaging, better hardware, and less-invasive techniques.[3] We now can manage the patient who has undergone multiple traumas much more easily with securely fixed fractures. Relative indications for internal or external fixation include displaced epiphyseal fractures, displaced intra-articular fractures, unstable fractures, fractures in a patient with multiple injuries, and open fractures with loss of muscle and soft tissue.[18]

Antibiotics are indicated for the orthopedic injury if not for the associated trauma. Cephalexin is used for grade I and II wounds, and aminoglycoside is added to grade III. Penicillin is added for soil-contaminated wounds. Antibiotics are no substitute for careful wound débridement and are used at least until the wound is stable and closed 3 to 5 days after injury.

Crushing and avulsion injuries are difficult to treat. As with other injuries, repeated irrigation and débridement and soft tissue coverage with delayed closure, split-thickness grafts, and vascularized flaps are possibilities. Degloving injuries are also treated with skin or soft tissue grafts after débridement and irrigation.

Injuries near a joint must be carefully inspected. If the joint is open, it must be thoroughly débrided and irrigated.

Traumatic amputations in childhood have a high incidence of complications (Fig. 19–2).[18] Optimal results are achieved with expectant early care of the limb. Delayed amputation is acceptable. The principles of limb salvage are

1. Preserve functional epiphyseal and physeal units.
2. Endeavor to preserve soft tissues for coverage.
3. Disarticulation is preferable to diaphyseal or metaphyseal amputation because of stump overgrowth. For very distal lower extremity injuries—often inflicted by a power mower—a delayed Syme's amputation leaves a viable heel pad over a distal stump.

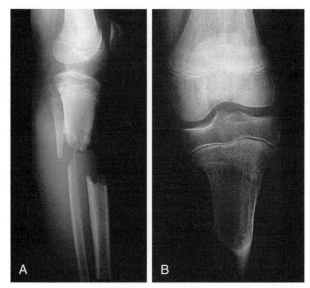

Figure 19–2. *A*, Segmental tibia and fibula fracture with subsequent below knee amputation. *B*, Stump overgrowth.

Partial amputation with bone loss necessitates thorough débridement and preservation of as much bone and periosteum as possible. Wounds are closed on a delayed basis. Chondroosseous loss from trauma is treated with the goals of preservation of limb length, maintenance of useful function of the adjacent joints and muscle groups, and fusion of the bone within 6 to 12 months.[18]

☐ Reimplantation

In cases of partial or complete traumatic amputation, the decision of whether to implant is based on the experience and expertise of the treating surgeons and the nature of the injury. Warm ischemia time greater than 10 hours or cold ischemia time greater than 20 hours is a relative contraindication to reimplantation. Clean "guillotine" amputations are easier to manage than avulsion-crush injuries. Modern techniques of nerve and vascular anastomosis ensure the best chance of healing, but the functional outcome of limb and the viability of the growth plate are often uncertain. Upper extremity reimplantation, especially thumb and distal phalanges, does well. Hand and foot reimplantations are risky, and the results less good.[19]

☐ Complications

Complications of orthopedic trauma in children can be categorized as systemic or local, early or late. Early systemic complications include hypovolemic shock and pulmonary embarrassment from fat embolism. A closed femur fracture may result in associated blood loss from the marrow or the periosteum of several hundred milliliters, which in a small child can represent up to 25% of the blood volume. The features of hemorrhagic shock are discussed

in Chapter 15; however, it should be emphasized that children generally tolerate a greater percentage of blood volume loss than adults before decompensating. Isolated orthopedic injuries in children rarely result in sufficient blood loss to produce shock unless major vessels or organs are also injured. Concurrent vascular injuries may be overlooked.[20] Most arterial injuries are evident on physical examination. A Doppler can confirm the lack of pulse. Digital subtraction angiography may be required to pinpoint the injury (Fig. 19–3). A spectrum of vascular injury is possible, even in the presence of a warm limb, if pulses are absent. Pediatric vascular injuries are usually repaired by primary anastomosis, occasionally with vein graft and rarely by prosthetic grafts. Long-term follow-up for vascular injuries is important because growth delay may not appear until years after the injury.[21]

Vasospasm in children also has been described with pediatric orthopedic trauma.[22] Careful reduction of a fracture followed by pharmacologic arterial relaxation may result in the reestablishment of good blood flow. If it does not, then radiographic investigation and surgical repair are likely necessary.

The compartment syndrome is an important sequela of limb injury and must always be considered in the trauma patient. This occurs when the intracompartmental pressure in a closed fascial space compromises the blood supply to the muscles and nerves. The initial symptoms include pain or paresthesia in the extremity, worsened with passive stretching. Important early signs include a tight compartment and a pale limb. Arterial pulse may be present despite a developing compartment syn-

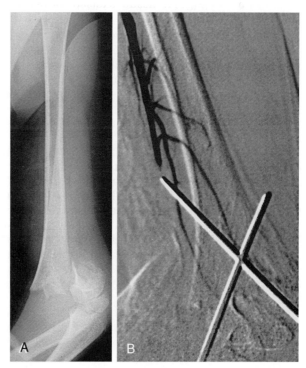

Figure 19–3. *A*, Suprachondylar humerus fracture. *B*, Pin transfixing brachial artery.

drome. All of these are crude indicators at best. Intracompartment pressures may be assessed by a variety of means.[23, 24] If the compartmental pressure is greater than 34 mm Hg, a fasciotomy should be considered in light of clinical findings. Muscle débridement may be necessary if the duration of the compromise has exceeded 8 to 10 hours. Whereas paresthesia suggests that the tissue injury is reversible, muscle injury often results in fibrotic healing, the most classic of which is called Volkmann's ischemic contracture. This is a dreaded complication of limb injury and is thought to be secondary to arterial insufficiency.

Thrombotic venous occlusion is very rare in the pediatric orthopedic injuries.[25] Peripheral nerve interruption is ideally recognized at the time of initial evaluation. Delay in nerve repair most significantly affects the return of motor function.[26] After nerve repair, sensory return may require up to 2 years.

Other less-common late complications of fractures include hypercalcemia, myositis ossificans, posttraumatic reflex dystrophy, synostosis of two contiguous bones, and pseudarthrosis.[27–29]

Specific complications related to the fracture itself include angulation, nonunion, delayed union, growth plate injury, and growth plate arrest.[27]

☐ Fracture Patterns

UPPER EXTREMITY

Most upper extremity fractures are isolated injuries and are managed by closed means. Hand fractures are usually managed by simple splinting or closed reduction and heal within 3 to 6 weeks. Less than 20% require open reduction.[30]

Injuries that require open reduction include open fractures, displaced intraarticular injuries, unstable injuries, and malaligned irreducible fractures.

Internal fixation of hand fractures usually consists of Kirschner-wires, although small screws and plates are occasionally used.

Fractures of the radius and ulna are the most common injuries in children.

The long-term prognosis is usually good with closed treatment, with 7% requiring manipulation[31] and a few having residual angulation.[32]

Open reduction and internal fixation is done when there is a failure to obtain adequate reduction by closed means. Open fracture, ipsilateral proximal fracture, comminuted interphyseal fractures, and carpal tunnel compression or compartment syndrome are other indications.[33] Complications include growth arrest and interposition of soft tissues in the fracture site.

Distal metaphyseal fractures are the most common, representing 21% of all fractures. Most are reduced closed. Immobilization in a cast for 5 to 6 weeks, with follow-up radiographs at 1 to 2 weeks, is recommended after initial reduction. Residual angulation less than 20 degrees in the plane of the fracture will remodel in children younger than 9

years, whereas only 5 degrees is acceptable in children older than 9 years.[34] Varying degrees of rotation are acceptable, as is bayonet apposition, as long as angulation is minimal and at least 2 years of growth remain.

Forearm diaphyseal fractures have less potential for remodeling and slower healing and require a more aggressive approach. Generally, closed reduction and long arm casting suffice. Internal fixation is most often done by plating or intramedullary rodding. Operative methods vary, carry low morbidity, and are especially indicated in patients older than 10 years with open fractures and irreducible injury, interposed tissue, or compartment syndrome.[35]

The Monteggia fracture dislocation of the elbow should be suspected when a proximal ulna fracture has occurred. There is an associated dislocation of the fracture of the proximal radius. The ulna fracture is reduced, followed by the radial head reduction. Close follow-up is necessary after reduction.

Radial neck and olecranon fractures are generally isolated injuries and usually respond to closed treatment. Indirect reduction of radial neck fractures and open reduction and internal fixation of olecranon fractures are required for significantly displaced irreducible injuries.

Distal humeral fractures in children are the subject of considerable discussion in the orthopedic literature. The progressive ossification pattern can make the diagnosis difficult. Contralateral elbow radiographs can clarify the normal anatomy. Displaced transphyseal injuries/condylar fractures/supracondylar fractures require closed reduction. Humeral neck and shaft fractures heal quickly and can be managed with a coadaptation splint, a thermoplastic fracture splint, or a hanging cast.

Reasons for open operative management include open fractures, irreducible closed fractures, segmental injury, vascular injury, ipsilateral multiple forearm fractures, or head injuries that require immobilization of the patient.[36] Operative methods of fixing the fracture include olecranon pin traction, plating, and external fixation. Intramedullary rodding of the humerus is seldom used.[37]

Proximal humeral fractures of metaphysis or physis have excellent healing and remodeling capacity. A sling or swath will usually suffice. Occasionally, an open reduction internal fixation is required. Most fractures of the clavicle occur within the shaft and heal and remodel uneventfully, even with significant comminution. In small children, the sling and swath will suffice, whereas highly comminuted fractures in older children do better with a figure-eight bandage. Open reduction and fixation is reserved for open fractures and neurovascular injury and occasionally for prominent bone ends. Only severe displaced fractures of the distal and the clavicle with retrosternal displacement of the proximal (medial) end need internal fixation.[38, 39]

SPINE

Significant injuries of the spine in children are uncommon compared with in adults. Spine injuries relate to the evolving anatomy of the developing spine.[40] In a traumatized spine, stability may be compromised, and care in immobilization and transportation is necessary.

Clinical evidence of the spinal injury includes pain at the fracture site, swelling, and deformity. The palpable gap in the spine is suspicious for injury. Neurologic injury may accompany the spine injury and necessitate expedient decompression of the spine. Although there is little documentation of the utility of corticosteroids in the patient younger than 13 years, many advocate the use of prophylactics (i.e., methylprednisolone) in the patient with a partial spinal cord injury.[41] A baseline clinical and neurologic evaluation is important. Loss of tendon reflexes can parallel motor loss and in the unconscious patient should raise the suspicion of spinal cord injury, especially if the loss of withdrawal is seen.[40] Spinal shock is a temporary phenomenon during which the patient has flaccid paralysis, absent deep tendon reflexes, urinary retention, and often intact sphincter tone. After hours or days, there may be a return of reflexes and a motor/sensory level. Cervical spine radiographs, including anteroposterior (AP) and odontoid views, should accompany the initial lateral views when the mechanisms of injury or findings indicate a risk of neck injury. Thoracic and lumbar spine radiographs are done when the mechanism of injury or the signs and symptoms warrant it. The trauma surgeon must be aware of the injury and need to clear the spine in conjunction with the radiologist/neurosurgeon/orthopedist familiar with pediatric spine radiographs. This should be done prior to relaxing spine precautions. A hard collar is essential until final clearance, and radiographs must be reviewed before the patient is immobilized.

The possibility of spinal cord injury without radiographic abnormality should be considered in children, especially in those younger than 8 years.[42] This is due in part to the hypermobility of the spine, relatively larger head, and weaker neck musculature in young children. Definitive care varies from Minerva casting for cervical injuries in children younger than 5 years to halo cast or brace to internal fixation and fusion.

Thoracic, lumbar, and sacral fractures are also uncommon. Spinal precautions must be adhered to and appropriate plane radiographs taken. Computed tomography scans can delineate important injuries.

Many of these injuries are caused by MVAs.[40] Thoracic fractures are often treated conservatively with rest or bracing. Thoracolumbar injuries are more likely to be unstable and may require internal fixation. Lumbar fractures become more common with advancing age. A Chance fracture is a flexion/distraction injury, most common in the upper lumbar spine suffered by an individual wearing a lap belt. There may be related visceral injuries. A ligamentous Chance fracture often requires internal fixation (Fig. 19–4).[43]

Sacral and coccygeal injuries occur through direct violence and usually require closed care. Pelvic fractures are uncommon in children but rank second to head injury in terms of complications, especially life-threatening visceral injuries. Associated injuries occur in 67% of patients with pelvic fractures, with long-term morbidity at approximately 30%.[44]

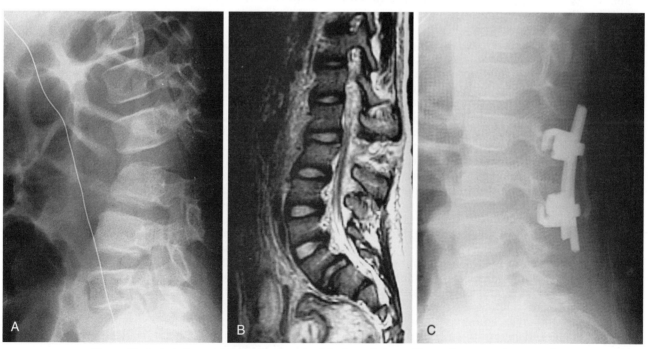

Figure 19–4. *A,* A 7-year-old girl who sustained L2-L3 soft-tissue Chance fracture with minimal neurologic deficit. *B,* Magnetic resonance image showing posterior interspinous soft-tissue disruption. *C,* Internal fixation. Child went on to full recovery.

The trauma surgeon must determine the priority of treatment and the emergency care of the child with a pelvic fracture. Patients with multiple injuries should be assumed to have a pelvic fracture until proven otherwise.

Some common signs of the pelvic fractures are Desot's sign, which is a hematoma beneath the inguinal ligament or scrotum. Roux's sign is the decreased distance from the greater trochanter to the anterior superior iliac spine on the affected side in lateral compression fractures. Earle's sign is a bony prominence or large hematoma as well as tenderness on rectal examination, indicating a significant pelvic fracture. An AP radiograph suffices as an early radiographic evaluation of the pelvis. Once other injuries have been stabilized, then a more deliberate assessment with multiple views and/or computed tomography can be done.

The mortality rate of children with pelvic fractures is between 9 and 18%.[45] Most pelvic fractures are ramis fractures and can be managed closed. Especially important are complete disruptions of the ring, which are unstable. Most of these injuries are managed by closed means; i.e., bedrest and traction. A small percent require external or internal fixation.

LOWER EXTREMITY

Hip fractures in children are rare but important injuries, usually caused by very severe trauma. The majority of these injuries require internal fixation. There is a high complication rate associated with this injury. A particularly devastating complication is avascular necrosis of the femoral neck or head.[46]

Femoral shaft fractures are common. Most of these injuries unite without complication. In the nonambulatory child, many are caused by abuse.[46] Older children generally sustain a high-energy injury, such as one that is generated in an MVA or a fall from a height. Neurovascular injury is rare with closed injuries. The incidence of neurovascular involvement rises with open or nonpenetrating injuries. Most can be treated by skin or skeletal traction followed by casting, especially in the case of an isolated injury. Internal or external fixation is being used with increasing frequency for reasons of reduced cost, psychological considerations, and avoidance of long periods of immobilization.[46]

Femur fractures in a patient 2 to 10 years old have a tendency to overgrow; therefore, these are often allowed to have overlapping segments during treatment.

Early evaluation and treatment of femur fractures includes splinting for transportation, documenting of neurovascular status, and treatment of concurrent injury. As with all fractures, children with femur fractures should have radiographic assessment of the joint above and below the fracture to rule out other injuries.

Methods of femur fracture fixation that are applicable to older children include external fixation, plating, and intermedullary rodding, using a single intermedullary nail or multiple flexible nails.

Fractures about the knee in children are more common than ligamentous injuries.[47] Younger children tend to injure the metaphysis, whereas adolescents tend to get physeal injuries. Displaced fractures around the distal femoral physis require reduction and often open or closed pinning, especially of the distal fragment if the distal fragment is anteriorly displaced and unstable. Intraarticular growth plate injuries require internal fixation if a step off of greater than 2 mm exists or if it is unstable. Growth arrest is a major long-term complication of intraarticular physeal fractures.

A variety of intraarticular fractures of the knee are possible, including tibial spine avulsions, tibial tubercle avulsions, and osteochondral injuries. Most present with an acute hemarthrosis. Temporary splinting is advisable until definitive care can be arranged. Tibial physeal injuries are rare but can be associated with a vascular injury.

Tibial shaft fractures are common in children. Most are low-impact injuries that can be treated with a long leg cast after reduction.

Indications for surgical treatment of tibial fractures include severe open injuries, failed closed treatment, and compartment syndrome. Polytrauma and ipsilateral femur fracture, which produce a floating knee, are also indications for operative management.

Ankle fractures usually involve the distal tibial and epiphyseal plates and are usually caused by an indirect injury. Intraarticular and significantly displaced open fractures need operative treatment, usually with wires or screws. Most can be managed with closed means. Often computed tomography is valuable in determining a fracture pattern if doubt exists.

Foot fractures are rare and even less commonly require surgical treatment. The most common indications for open reductions include displaced talar neck fractures and calcaneal fractures.

☐ Conclusions

Early attention by the trauma surgeon to potential skeletal injury can have important consequences on short-term outcome and avoidance of long-term disability. The trauma patient must be properly immobilized, which might include the use of a spinal board, neck immobilization, and limb splinting for obvious deformity or injury. The child's head is disproportionately large for the first 5 years of life, and this necessitates the use of a pediatric spinal board or elevation of the upper back with a blanket or cushion to maintain the correct cervical spine position. After the primary survey has been accomplished, the trauma team leader should consider obtaining AP radiographs of the pelvis and spinal column. Cervical spine films should be done with the primary survey. C-spine clearance generally requires involvement of the radiologist, orthopedist, or neurosurgeon.

It is important to assess and reassess the neurovascular status of the patient with multiple injuries to avoid the catastrophic long-term consequences of a missed vascular injury, compartment syndrome, or neurologic injury. Care of the pediatric trauma patient is evolving to resemble that of the adult polytrauma patient. Internal or external fixation techniques are being employed more frequently. Prospective outcome data are starting to emerge in the pediatric orthopedic literature. With the establishment of databases, the development of treatment algorithms, and the evaluation of treatment outcomes using validated methods, we should continue to make improvements from initial field contact to rehabilitation of the pediatric trauma patient. Prevention remains an ongoing area of concern.

REFERENCES

1. Charnley J: The Closed Treatment of Common Fractures (3rd ed). London, New York, Churchill Livingstone, 1974.
2. Blount W: Fractures in Children. Baltimore, Williams & Wilkins, 1955.
3. Green N: The evolution of pediatric trauma care [editorial]. J Pediatr Orthop 14:421–422, 1994.
4. Skaggs D: Elbow fractures in children, diagnosis and management. J Am Acad Orthop Surg 5:303–312, 1997.
5. Akbarnia B, Torg JS, Kirkpatrick J, Sussman S: Manifestations of the battered-child syndrome. J Bone Joint Surg 56A:1159, 1974.
6. Kowal-Vern A, Paxton TP, Ros SP, et al: Fracture in the under 3-year-old. Clin Pediatr 31:653, 1992.
7. Wilkins K: The Incidence of Fractures in Children. In Rockwood CA Jr, Wilkins KE, Beaty JH, et al (eds): Fractures in Children. Vol. 4. Philadelphia, Lippincott-Raven, 1996, pp 3–17.
8. Worlock P: Fracture patterns in Nottingham children. J Pediatr Orthop 6:656, 1986.
9. Landin LA: Fracture patterns in children. Acta Orthop Scand 54 (suppl 202):1, 1983.
10. Starfield B: Childhood morbidity: Comparisons, clusters and trends. Pediatrics 88:519, 1991.
11. Peclet MH, Newman KD, Lechelberger MD, et al: Preponderance of injury in children. J Pediatr Surg 25:85, 1990.
12. Ogden J: Complications of Fractures. Philadelphia, J.B. Lippincott, 1995, p 97.
13. Edvardson P, Syversen SM: Overgrowth of the femur after fracture of the shaft in childhood. J Bone Joint Surg 58B:339–346, 1976.
14. Dormans JP, Azzoni M, Davidson RS, Drummond DS: Major lower extremity lawn mower injuries in children. J Pediatr Orthop 15:78–82, 1995.
15. Hope P, Cole W: Open fractures of the tibia in children. J Bone Joint Surg 74B:546–553, 1992.
16. Kneatsey B, Condon KL: Severe dog-bite injuries introducing the concept of pack attack. A literature review and seven case reports. Injury (England), 26(1):37–41, 1995.
17. Ogden J: Open injuries and traumatic amputations. In Wickland E (ed): Skeletal Injury in the Child (2nd ed). Philadelphia, W.B. Saunders, 1990, p 199.
18. Ogden J: Open injuries and traumatic amputations. In Skeletal Injury in the Child (2nd ed). Philadelphia, W.B. Saunders, 1990, pp 220,221.
19. Sehayak R. Reimplantation in children. Orthop Trans 3:84, 1979.
20. Friedman RJ, Jupiter JB: Vascular injuries in closed extremity fractures in children. Clin Orthop 188:112, 1984.
21. Caffey J: Traumatic cupping of the metaphysis of the growing bones. Am J Res 108:451, 1978.
22. Samson R, Pasternak BM: Traumatic arterial spasm—rarity or non-entity. J Trauma 20:607, 1980.
23. Matsen FA III: Monitoring of intramuscular pressure. Surgery 79:702, 1997.
24. Mubarek SJ, Owen CA, Hargen AR, et al: Acute compartment syndromes: Diagnosis and treatment with the aid of wic catheter. J Bone Joint Surg 60A:1091, 1978.
25. Jones TRB, McIntyre MC: Venous thrombosis in infancy and childhood. Arch Dis Child 50:153, 1975.
26. Lindsay WD, Walker FG, Farmer AW: Traumatic peripheral nerve injuries in children. Plast Reconstr Surg 30:462, 1962.
27. Ogden J: Complications. In Skeletal Injury in the Child (2nd ed). Philadelphia, W.B. Saunders, 1990, pp 235–264.
28. Wilkins K: Physical and apophyseal injuries. In Rockwood CA Jr, Wilkins KE, Beaty JH, et al (eds): Fractures in Children. Philadelphia, Lippincott-Raven, 1996, pp 103–106.
29. Epps CH, Bowen JR: Physical and apophyseal injuries. In Rockwood CA Jr, Wilkins KE, Beaty JH, et al (eds): Complications in Pediatric Orthopaedic Surgery. Philadelphia, J.B. Lippincott, 1995.
30. Leonard M, Dubravcik P: Management of fractured fingers in the child. Clin Orthop 73:160–168, 1970.
31. Voto SJ, Weiner DS, Leighley B: Redisplacement after reduction of forearm fractures in children. J Pediatr Orthop 10:79–84, 1990.
32. Ghandi RK, Wilson P, Brown JM, et al: Spontaneous correction of deformity following fractures of the forearm in children. Br J Surg 50:540, 1962.
33. AAOS Monograph Series: Operative management of upper extremity fractures in children.
34. Noonan K, Price C: Forearm and distal radius fractures in children. J Am Acad Orthop Surg 6(3):146–156, 1998.
35. Noonan K, Price C: Forearm and distal radius fractures in children. J Am Acad Orthop Surg 6(3):146–156, 1998.
36. Lane RH, Foster RJ: Skeletal management of humeral shaft fractures associated with forearm fractures. Clin Orthop 195:173–177, 1985.
37. Vandergried R, Tomason J, Ward EF: Open reduction internal fixation of humeral shaft fractures. Results using AP plating techniques. J Bone Joint Surg 68A:430–433, 1986.
38. Rockwood CA, Wilkins KE, Beaty JH: Fractures in Children (4th ed). Philadelphia, Lippincott-Raven, 1996, p 952.
39. Wilkins KE: AAOS Monograph Series, Operative management of upper extremity fractures.
40. Ogden J: Spine. In Skeletal Injury in the Child (2nd ed). Philadelphia, W.B. Saunders, 1990, p 571.
41. Bracken MD, Shepard MJ, Holford TR, et al: Administration of methyprednisolone for 24 or 48 hours or uirilizad mesylate for 48 hours in the treatment of acute spinal cord injury. Results of the Third National Acute Spinal Cord Injury Randomized Control Trial. National Acute Spinal Cord Injury Study. JAMA 227:1597–1604, 1997.
42. Pollack IF, Pang D: Spinal cord injury without radiographic abnormality (SCIWORA). In Pang D (ed): Disorders of the Pediatric Spine. New York, Raven Press, 1995, pp 509–516.
43. Rumball K, Jarvis J: Seat-belt injuries of the spine in young children. J Bone Joint Surg 571–574, 1992.
44. AAOS Monograph Series. Operative treatment of lower extremity fractures, Hensinger RN, ed, 1992, p 7.
45. Rang M: Children's Fractures (2nd ed). Philadelphia, J.B. Lippincott, 1983.
46. Clinton TD, DeLee JC, Sanders R, et al: Knee ligament injuries in children. J Bone Joint Surg 61A:1195–1201, 1979.

20

CHEST WALL DEFORMITIES

Robert C. Shamberger, MD

Congenital chest wall deformities are often divided into five categories: pectus excavatum (funnel chest), pectus carinatum (pigeon breast), Poland's syndrome, sternal defects, and the miscellaneous dysplasias or the thoracic deformities in diffuse skeletal disorders. Most are not life-threatening lesions and produce limited functional abnormalities. Several of the rare lesions, such as thoracic ectopia cordis and Jeune's asphyxiating thoracic dystrophy, are almost uniformly fatal.

☐ Pectus Excavatum

Pectus excavatum is the most common chest wall deformity. The sternum is angled posteriorly toward the spine as are the lower costal cartilages (Fig. 20–1). Pectus excavatum is present in the majority (86%) of patients at birth or within the first year of life; in only a small number of patients does it appear later.[1] Pectus excavatum occurs more than three times more frequently in males than in females. The etiology of pectus excavatum is unknown, but a genetic factor exists; 37% of patients have family histories of chest wall deformities. About 15% of patients have scoliosis, and 11% have a family history of scoliosis. Pectus excavatum is seen in its most severe degree in association with Marfan's syndrome. The possibility of Marfan's syndrome must be considered in all patients with these severe deformities, especially males who also have scoliosis. Ophthalmologic evaluation should be obtained to identify subluxation of the lens, which is pathognomonic of Marfan's syndrome. An echocardiogram is also performed in patients in whom Marfan's syndrome is suspected. Dilatation of the aortic root and aortic or mitral valve regurgitation support the diagnosis of Marfan's syndrome.

Pectus excavatum is associated with congenital heart disease in 2% of patients.[1] In most, repair of the cardiac lesion is performed in infancy before it is appropriate to consider chest wall repair. In those with complex lesions requiring retrosternal conduits for repair, correction of the chest wall deformity may be required before definitive cardiac repair in order to avoid compression of the conduit by the posteriorly displaced sternum.[2]

Asthma is occasionally identified in patients with pectus excavatum and carinatum. In a review of 694 consecutive cases of chest wall deformities, a subgroup of 35 patients was identified with asthma (5.2%). This incidence of asthma was comparable to its occurrence in a general pediatric population. No evidence exists to suggest that asthma plays a causative role in chest wall deformities or that pectus deformities significantly worsen the clinical course of asthma.

The accurate assessment of the severity of a pectus excavatum deformity is important in order to identify which patients warrant surgical repair and to compare postoperative results. Several methods of grading the severity of the depression have been devised. All use ratios of the distance between the sternum and the spine and the breadth of the upper chest or the width of the chest.[3–5]

CARDIOPULMONARY EFFECTS

Some investigators have stated that pectus excavatum does not produce cardiovascular or pulmonary impairment.[6] This opinion contrasts, however, with the general clinical impression that many patients have increased stamina after surgical repair. A review has summarized the clinical studies of these patients.[7]

Many workers attribute the symptomatic impairment in pectus excavatum to a decrease in intrathoracic volume. This relationship is difficult to prove, however, with the wide range of cardiopulmonary function that exists among normal individuals. It is heavily dependent on physical training and body habitus.

One study evaluated seven patients with pectus excavatum, five of whom were symptomatic with exercise.[8] The mean total lung capacity expressed as a percentage of predicted value was 79% in the patients with pectus excavatum. The measured oxygen uptake increasingly exceeded predicted values

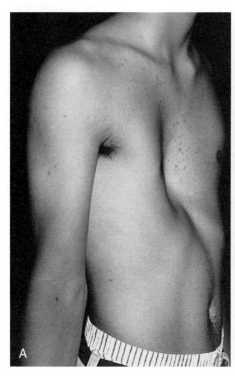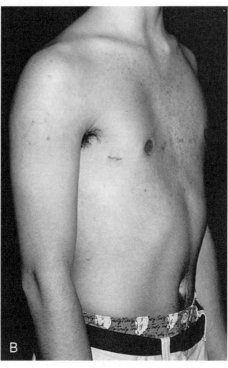

Figure 20–1. *A*, A 14.5-year-old boy with a symmetric pectus excavatum deformity before correction with a retrosternal strut. *B*, Full correction of the deformity 7 months after repair and after removal of the strut.

as the workloads approached maximum. Normal subjects and three asymptomatic patients, in contrast, had a linear response between oxygen uptake and workload. The mean oxygen uptake at maximal effort exceeded the predicted values by 25.4% in the symptomatic patients with pectus excavatum. This increased oxygen uptake suggests increased work of breathing, although the vital capacity was only mildly reduced or normal. Pulmonary function and exercise tolerance were evaluated in 14 patients with pectus excavatum before and after repair.[9] Maximal voluntary ventilation was significantly improved by repair in all patients. Exercise tolerance was also improved, as measured by total exercise time and maximal oxygen uptake. A consistent decrease occurred in heart rate at a given level of work or exercise postoperatively but with no change in oxygen consumption. Xenon Xe 133 perfusion and ventilation scintigraphy were used to study 17 patients with pectus excavatum.[10] Of 12 patients with regional ventilatory deficits, primarily in the left lower lung, 7 developed normal ventilation after surgery. Of 10 patients with regional perfusion abnormalities, also primarily in the left lower lung, 6 had normal perfusion after surgery. Of 10 patients with abnormal ventilation-to-perfusion ratios, 6 were recorded with normal ratios.

In a study of 88 patients with pectus excavatum and carinatum repaired by a technique that involved a fairly extensive chest wall dissection, pulmonary function tests before and 1 to 20 years after repair (mean, 8 years) were compared.[11] Preoperative studies were within the normal range (more than 80% of predicted) except in those subjects with both scoliosis and pectus excavatum. The postoperative values for forced expiratory volume in 1 second and vital capacity were decreased in all groups when expressed as a percentage of predicted, although the absolute values at follow-up may have been greater than at the preoperative evaluation. Radiologic evaluation of these individuals confirmed improved chest wall configuration, suggesting that the relative deterioration in pulmonary function was not the result of recurrence of the pectus deformity. An inverse relationship was found between the preoperative and postoperative function. Those individuals with less than 75% of predicted function had improved function after operation, whereas results were worse after operation if the preoperative values were greater than 75% of predicted.

Almost identical results were found in a study that evaluated 152 patients before and at a mean follow-up of 8 years after operation for pectus excavatum.[12] These physiologic results were in contrast to the subjective improvement in symptoms of the subjects and their improved chest wall configuration after repair. The decline in pulmonary function in the postoperative studies was attributed to the operation because the preoperative defect appeared to be stable regardless of the age at initial repair. Both of these studies were marred by the obvious lack of an age- and severity-matched control group without surgical treatment.

Another study reported transpulmonary and transdiaphragmatic pressures at total lung capacity in 17 individuals with pectus excavatum.[13] Preoperative and long-term follow-up evaluations were performed a mean of 12 years apart. Reduced transpulmonary and transdiaphragmatic pressures suggested the increased restrictive defect was produced by extrapulmonary rather than pulmonary factors or that surgical correction produced increased rigidity of the chest wall.

An interesting study[14] assessed 12 children with pectus excavatum measured by pulmonary function and exercise tests. Eight children underwent repair and were evaluated before and after operation. Four patients had two sets of evaluation but no operation. A decline in the total lung capacity was identified in the repaired group compared with stable values in the control group. Cardiac output and stroke volume increased appropriately with exercise before and after operation in both groups, and operation was believed to have produced no physiologically significant effect on the response to exercise.

In a large study that evaluated pulmonary function in 138 individuals before and after surgery for pectus excavatum, decrease in the vital capacity occurred during the initial 2 months postoperative, with recovery to preoperative levels by 1 year postoperative.[15] At 42 months, the values were maintained at baseline despite a significant improvement in the chest wall configuration. Similar results were found in individuals who underwent the more extensive sternal turnover technique, and these patients experienced a more significant and long-term decrease in the vital capacity.[16]

Thirty-five patients with pectus excavatum who underwent repair as teenagers or young adults (age 17.9 ± 5.6 years) were studied.[17] Preoperative evaluations were performed and repeated 1 year after operation. Preoperative total lung capacity (86.0% ± 14.4% of predicted) and vital capacity (79.7% ± 16.2%) were significantly decreased from predicted values and decreased further after operation (-9.2% ± 9.2% and -6.6% ± 10.7%, respectively). The efficiency of breathing at maximal exercise, however, improved significantly after operation. Ventilatory limitation of exercise occurred in 43% of the patients before operation, and there was a tendency toward improvement after operation. However, the group with no ventilatory limitation initially demonstrated a limitation after operation with a significant increase in oxygen consumption.

Taken together, these studies of pulmonary function during the past 4 decades have failed to document consistent improvement in pulmonary function resulting from surgical repair. Recent studies, in fact, have demonstrated deterioration in pulmonary function at long-term evaluation attributable to increased chest wall rigidity after operation. Despite this finding, workload studies have shown improvement in exercise tolerance after repair.

Cardiac catheterization was performed in six patients with moderate degrees of pectus excavatum.[18] Normal pressures were obtained with the patients at rest in the supine position. The cardiac index was normal at rest in the supine position, and the response to moderate exercise was within normal range. The response to upright exercise was below the predicted normal in two patients and at the lower limit of normal in three.

Postoperative studies were performed in three of these patients. Two achieved a higher level of exercise tolerance after surgery. The cardiac index was increased by 38%. The heart rates were unchanged, and the increase resulted from an enhanced stroke volume after surgery. First-pass radionuclide angiocardiography was used to noninvasively evaluate 13 patients with pectus excavatum, in an upright position, both at rest and during bicycle exercise.[19] Although no changes were noted in the left ventricular ejection fraction or cardiac output, either at rest or during exercise, substantial increases were observed postoperatively in both the right and left ventricular volumes, suggesting relief of cardiac compression. Workload studies were also performed on these patients. Ten of 13 were able to reach the target heart rate before surgical repair, 4 without symptoms. After operation, all but 1 patient reached the target heart rate during the exercise protocol; 9 of 13 patients reached the target heart rate without becoming symptomatic.

Results in this area of investigation at times have been in conflict. What is required is a reproducible and simply measured parameter to evaluate patients with pectus excavatum in order to assess the level of cardiopulmonary impact of the deformity.

HISTORY OF SURGICAL REPAIR

Surgical repair of pectus excavatum was first performed by Meyer and Sauerbruch in 1911 and 1913, and the methods of repair have evolved since that time.[20, 21] Ravitch in 1949 reported a technique that involved (1) excision of all deformed costal cartilages with the perichondrium, (2) division of the xiphoid from the sternum, (3) division of the intercostal bundles from the sternum, and (4) transverse sternal osteotomy. This technique allowed displacement of the sternum anteriorly with Kirschner wires.[22]

In 1957 and 1958, respectively, Baronofsky and Welch reported a technique for correction of pectus excavatum, stressing total preservation of the perichondrial sheaths of the costal cartilages and preservation of the upper intercostal bundles, a sternal osteotomy, and an anterior fixation of the sternum with silk sutures.[23, 24] Excellent results have been obtained by this method.[1] Others have used strut fixation of the sternum to guarantee early stability of the sternum in an anterior position.[25, 26] No randomized study between these two techniques has been performed to compare the long-term results of each. Two large series reported equal results from both methods: one reported 92% satisfactory results using struts in a series of 1112 patients, and the other reported 91% satisfactory results using a procedure without struts in 392 patients.[5, 27]

A method of tripod fixation is described that involves posterior sternal osteotomy, subperichondrial resection of the lower deformed costal cartilages, and oblique division of the normal second or third costal cartilages.[6] These obliquely divided cartilages are placed, overriding themselves, and are secured to support the sternum in an anterior position. In one group of 45 patients, 100% satisfactory results were reported.

A sternal turnover technique has also been described.[28, 29] It has been used primarily in Japan. In a large series, the sternum was used as a free graft that was rotated 180 degrees and secured to the costal cartilages, from which it was divided.[30] This radical approach for children with pectus excavatum has had limited general acceptance, given the alternatives and the risk of major complications, if infection occurs.

A method of elevation of the sternum with a retrosternal bar without resection or division of the costal cartilages has been reported, but confirmation of the safety and efficacy of this method awaits its replication by other centers.[31]

A variety of techniques remain in use for the surgical repair of pectus excavatum. No method is universally accepted as the optimal procedure. All have some risk for late recurrence, which plagues the management of this problem. My method of repair is shown in Figure 20–2. I currently use a retrosternal strut to achieve solid anterior fixation of the sternum, particularly in the older child or adolescent. Use of the strut also avoids the need to divide the lower perichondrial sheaths from the sternum to achieve adequate mobility. Strut fixation should be used in all children with Marfan's syndrome because of the particularly high rate of recurrence.

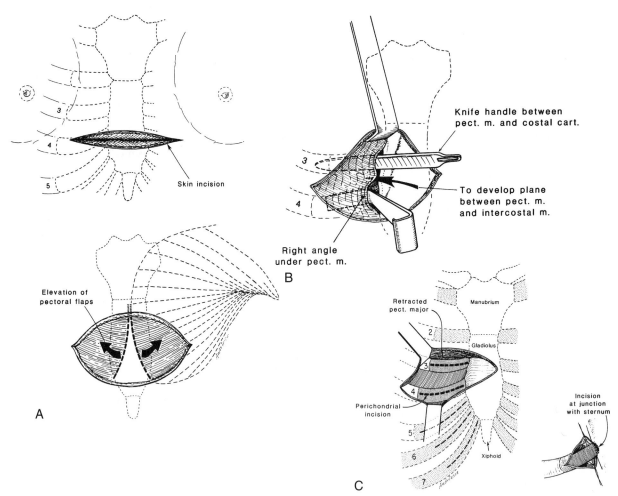

Figure 20–2. *A,* A transverse incision is placed below and well within the nipple lines at the site of the future inframammary crease. The pectoralis major muscle is elevated from the sternum along with portions of the pectoralis minor and serratus anterior muscles. *B,* The correct plane of dissection of the pectoral muscle (pect. m.) flap is defined by passing an empty knife handle directly anterior to a costal cartilage (costal cart.) after the medial aspect of the muscle is elevated with electrocautery. The knife handle is replaced with a right angle retractor, which is pulled anteriorly. The process is repeated anterior to an adjoining costal cartilage. Anterior distraction of the muscles during the dissection facilitates identification of the avascular areolar plane and avoids entry into the intercostal muscle (intercostal m.) bundles. *C,* Subperichondrial resection of the costal cartilages is achieved by incising the perichondrium anteriorly. The perichondrium is then dissected away from the costal cartilages in the bloodless plane between perichondrium and costal cartilage. Cutting back the perichondrium 90 degrees in each direction at its junction with the sternum (*inset*) facilitates visualization of the back wall of the costal cartilage.

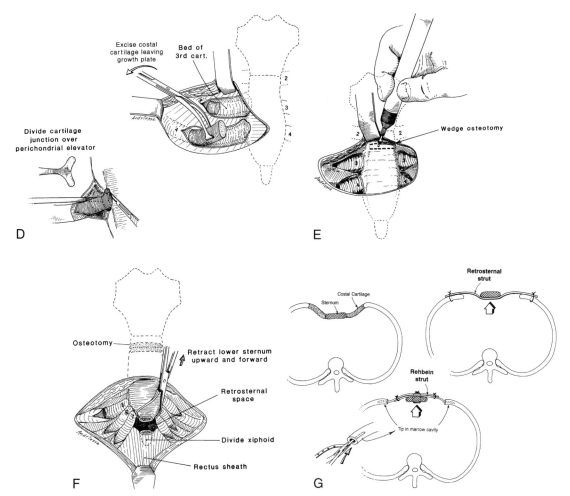

Figure 20–2 *Continued. D,* The cartilages are divided at the junction of the sternum using a knife with the Welch perichondrial elevator held posteriorly to elevate the cartilage and to protect the mediastinum (*inset*). The divided cartilage can then be held with an Allis clamp and elevated and divided laterally leaving a segment of cartilage at the costochondral junction to preserve the endochondral growth center. *E,* The sternal osteotomy is created above the level of the last deformed cartilage and the posterior angulation of the sternum, generally the third cartilage but occasionally the second. Two transverse sternal osteotomies are created through the anterior cortex with a Hall air drill, 2 to 4 mm apart. *F,* The base of the sternum and the rectus muscle flap are elevated with two towel clips and the posterior wall of the sternum is fractured. The xiphoid can be divided from the sternum with electrocautery. This maneuver allows entry into the retrosternal space, which may be required to pass the strut behind the sternum. Preservation of the attachment of the perichondrial sheaths is important to avoid an unsightly depression at the base of the sternum. *G,* A demonstration of the use of both the retrosternal struts and the Rehbein struts. The Rehbein struts are inserted into the marrow cavity (*inset*) of the third or fourth ribs and are then joined to each other medially to create a metal arch anterior to the sternum. The sternum is sewn to the arch to secure it in a forward position. The retrosternal strut is placed behind the sternum and is secured to the rib ends laterally to prevent migration.

Illustration continued on following page

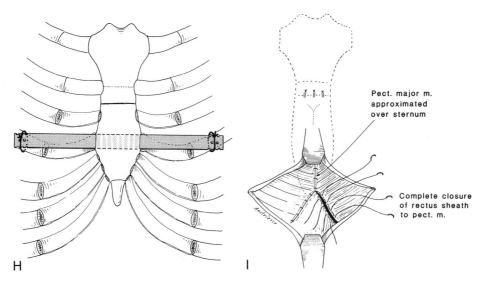

H   I

Figure 20–2 *Continued. H,* Anterior depiction of the retrosternal strut. The perichondrial sheath to either the third or fourth rib is divided at its junction with the sternum, and the retrosternal space is bluntly dissected to allow passage of the strut behind the sternum. An adequate space must be created to avoid injury to the pericardium. The strut is secured with two pericostal sutures laterally to prevent migration. *I,* The pectoral muscle flaps are secured to the midline of the sternum, advancing the flaps to obtain coverage of the entire sternum. The rectus muscle flap is then joined to the pectoral muscle flaps. (*A* to *F* and *I* from Shamberger RC, Welch KJ: Surgical repair of pectus excavatum. J Pediatr Surg 23:615–622, 1988 [*D* and *F* adapted]. *G* and *H* from Shamberger RC: Chest wall deformities. In Shields TW [ed]: General Thoracic Surgery [4th ed]. New York, Williams & Wilkins, 1994, by permission.)

Secondary repair of recurrent depressions is technically much more difficult than primary repair, because the scarred and deformed costal cartilages are often ossified. Secondary repair also is associated with greater blood loss and postoperative respiratory problems. Solid fixation of the sternum in an anterior position is crucial for acceptable results in this population. Recurrence is a frequent complication because the costal cartilages regenerate poorly after a second repair and fail to support the sternum anteriorly after removal of the struts.

RESULTS AND COMPLICATIONS

Complications after surgical repair should be limited. Pneumothorax is infrequent and requires only aspiration of the air. Pulmonary injury with continued air leak requiring a chest tube is rare. Small pneumothoraces can be safely observed. Wound infection, hematoma, or dehiscence is limited. Hemoptysis, hemopericardium, or pericardial effusion are rare. Blood transfusions are rarely required in primary repair with electrocautery but are more frequently required in secondary repair. Major recurrences are reported in large series with adequate follow-up[5, 32–34] in 5 to 10% of patients, and mild recurrences with a central hollow in the chest are reported in another 5 to 10% of patients.

Impaired chest wall growth is a recently identified complication. A deficiency in thoracic growth in children after repair of pectus excavatum was first described in 1990 and was most noticeable in children operated on during preschool years.[35] There

has been a recent additional report on three boys who presented in their teens with apparent limited growth of the ribs after resection of the costal cartilages at an early age, producing a band-like narrowing of the midchest (Fig. 20–3).[36] In some cases, the first and second ribs in which the costal cartilages have not been resected have apparent relative overgrowth, producing anterior protrusion of the upper sternum. This occurrence has been attributed to injury of the costochondral junctions, which are the longitudinal growth centers for the ribs, and to decreased growth of the sternum resulting from injury to its growth centers or vascular supply.

It has been demonstrated experimentally in 6-week-old rabbits that resection of the costal cartilages produced a marked impairment in chest growth, particularly the anterior-posterior diameter during a 5.5-month period of observation.[35] Less severe impairment occurred if only the medial three quarters of the costal cartilage was resected, leaving the growth centers at the costochondral junction. This impairment was attributed to fibrosis and scarring within the perichondrial sheaths. Perichondrial sheaths, bone, or other prosthetic tissues that cannot grow should also not be joined posterior to the sternum because they will form a band-like stricture across the chest. This complication of delayed thoracic growth was described primarily in children who underwent repair in early childhood and can be avoided by delaying surgery until the children are older. Preservation of the costochondral junction, leaving a segment of the cartilage on the osseous portion of the rib, may also minimize growth

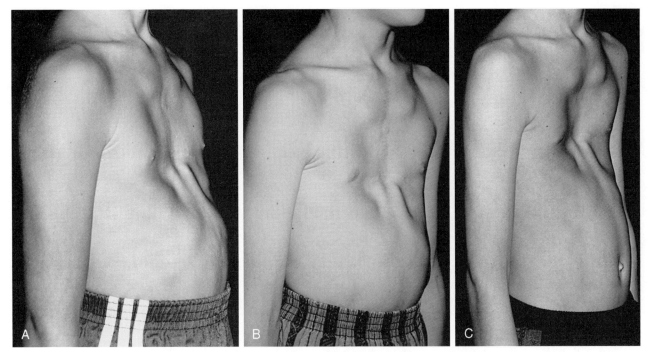

Figure 20–3. A boy who underwent repair of pectus excavatum at 4 years of age demonstrates a progressive central broad recurrence and relative overgrowth of the upper unresected costal cartilages and ribs at *(A)* 9, *(B)* 13, and *(C)* 17 years of age.

impairment. I currently delay surgery until the children have begun their pubertal growth spurt.

□ Pectus Carinatum

Pectus carinatum is a protrusion deformity of the chest that occurs less frequently than pectus excavatum and constitutes only 15% of our series of chest wall deformities. Pectus carinatum consists of a spectrum of deformities, with unilateral or bilateral involvement of the costal cartilages and with superior or inferior protrusion of the sternum. A carinate protrusion can also exist in a mixed deformity, with depression of the cartilages on one side and protrusion on the second side, with rotation of the sternum. The most common clinical presentation of this

deformity involves protrusion of the body of the sternum and symmetric protrusion of the lower costal cartilages (chondrogladiolar) (Fig. 20–4). Less frequent are the asymmetric deformities with unilateral protrusion of the costal cartilages and least frequent, the mixed deformity. The unusual superior or chondromanubrial deformity involves prominence of the manubrium and upper costal cartilages and relative depression of the gladiolus or body of the sternum (Fig. 20–5).

The etiology of pectus carinatum is unknown. Pectus carinatum occurs in excess of three times more frequently in males than females. Pectus carinatum often appears during childhood and adolescence, unlike pectus excavatum, which generally is noted at birth or within the first year of life. Pectus carinatum is noted at birth in only a third of patients

Figure 20–4. *A*, A 19-year-old man with a symmetric lower (chondrogladiolar) pectus carinatum deformity. *B*, Postoperative chest wall configuration.

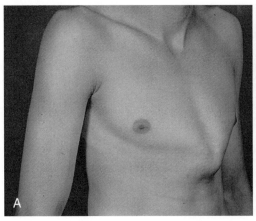
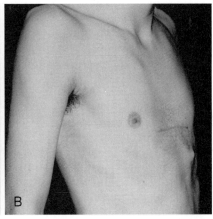

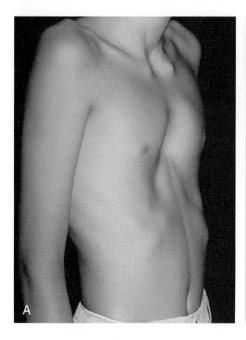
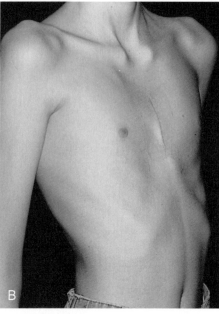

Figure 20–5. *A,* A 15-year-old boy with an upper (chondromanubrial) pectus carinatum deformity. Note the protrusion of the manubrium and the upper second and third costal cartilages and the relative posterior depression of the lower portion of the sternum. *B,* Correction of both components of the deformity seen postoperatively. (From Shamberger RC, Welch KJ: Surgical repair of pectus excavatum. J Pediatr Surg 23:615–622, 1988.)

who eventually have this deformity, and in almost half it appears after onset of the pubertal growth spurt.[37] Twenty-six percent of patients with pectus carinatum have a family history of chest wall deformities. An association with scoliosis is also noted as in pectus excavatum, with 15% of patients having scoliosis and 12% having a family history of scoliosis. Marfan's syndrome must be suspected in younger patients with pectus carinatum who have associated scoliosis or who have extremely severe degrees of the deformity.

CARDIOPULMONARY EFFECTS

Cardiopulmonary impairment by pectus carinatum has not been demonstrated. Consideration for repair of this lesion must be based solely on the severity of the deformity. Patients may complain of tenderness in the area of the protrusion resulting from frequent local trauma.

HISTORY OF SURGICAL REPAIR

The methods of repair of pectus carinatum have evolved in the four decades since correction was first performed. Ravitch reported repair of a chondromanubrial prominence in 1952, which was achieved by resecting the multiple deformed costal cartilages and by creating a double osteotomy in the sternum.[38] Later efforts included resection of the anterior portion of the sternum and even subperiosteal resection of the entire sternum.[39] These were generally sanguine and unsuccessful attempts at correction of the deformity.

Modern techniques were first employed in 1963, using subperichondrial resection of the costal cartilages and resection of the lower portion of the sternum, with advancement of the rectus muscles to the remaining sternum.[40] Subsequent methods de-

scribed in 1973 used subperichondrial resection of the prominent costal cartilages and preservation of the entire length of the sternum (Fig. 20–6). The anterior protrusion was corrected by placement of a transverse osteotomy through the anterior cortex of the sternum and fracture of the posterior cortex, allowing posterior displacement of the sternum.[41] This technique continues to be used today with excellent results (see Fig. 20–4B).[37]

RESULTS AND COMPLICATIONS

Generally, successful results are achieved with current methods of repair. Blood transfusions are rarely required. Pneumothoraces are infrequent and generally require aspiration only. Recurrence is rare and is limited to those patients who underwent surgical repair before full maturity, with unilateral resection of the involved costal cartilages. Protrusion of the contralateral cartilages may develop before full growth is achieved. Persistent deformity also occurs with inadequate initial resection of the deformity and generally involves the lower costal cartilages, which insert into the costal arch.

☐ Poland's Syndrome

Poland's syndrome is a constellation of anomalies, including absence of the pectoralis major and minor muscles, syndactyly, brachydactyly, athelia or amastia, deformed or absent ribs, absent axillary hair, and limited subcutaneous fat (Fig. 20–7). This syndrome was initially described in the French and German literature in 1826 and 1839,[42, 43] but it is named for the English medical student, Alfred Poland, who in 1841 published a partial description of the deformity as it appeared in his anatomic dissection.[44] A

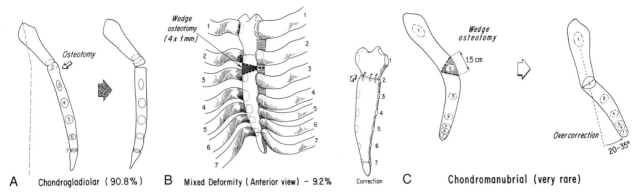

A Chondrogladiolar (90.8 %)   B Mixed Deformity (Anterior view) – 9.2%   Correction   C Chondromanubrial (very rare)

Figure 20–6. *A,* Chondrogladiolar deformity is managed with a single or double osteotomy after exposure and resection of the costal cartilages, as is performed with an excavatum deformity. This maneuver allows posterior displacement of the sternum to an orthotopic position. *B,* The mixed pectus deformity is corrected by full and symmetric resection of the third to seventh costal cartilages, followed by transverse offset (0 to 10 degrees) wedge-shaped sternal osteotomy. Closure of this defect permits both anterior displacement and rotation of the sternum. (From Shamberger RC, Welch KJ: Surgical correction of pectus carinatum. J Pediatr Surg 22:48–53, 1987.) *C,* The lateral depiction of the deformed sternum in the chondromanubrial deformity shows the future, broad, wedge-shaped sternal osteotomy placed through the anterior cortex at the obliterated sternomanubrial junction (*left*). Closure of the osteotomy after fracture of the posterior cortex achieves posterior displacement of the superior portion of the sternum, which is secured only by its attachment to the first rib. The lower portion of the sternum is overcorrected 20 to 35 degrees (*right*). (From Shamberger RC, Welch KJ: Surgical repair of pectus excavatum. J Pediatr Surg 23:615–622, 1988.)

description of the full spectrum of the deformity was summarized in 1895.[45]

Various components of the syndrome appear in each affected patient. The hand lesions are particularly variable in extent and severity of involvement. Poland's syndrome has a sporadic occurrence, estimated between 1 in 30,000 and 1 in 32,000 live births, and is rarely familial.[46, 47] The etiology of Poland's syndrome has been postulated to be abnormal migration of the embryonic tissues forming the pectoral muscles, hypoplasia of the subclavian artery, or in utero injuries. However, no cause has been established thus far.

Chest wall involvement in Poland's syndrome can vary from mild hypoplasia of the ribs and the costal cartilage on the ipsilateral side to aplasia of the anterior portion of the ribs and the entire costal cartilages (Fig. 20–8). In a series of 75 patients with Poland's syndrome, 41 had normal chest wall contours; 10 had hypoplasia of the ribs, without localized areas of depression; 16 had depression deformities of the ribs, 11 of which were major depressions; and 8 had aplasia of the ribs.[48] No correlation was found between the extent of hand deformities and chest wall deformities.

Surgical repair in Poland's syndrome is required for only a small portion of the patients—those with aplasia of the ribs or a major depression deformity (Fig. 20–9).[48] Often present in patients with major depressions are contralateral carinate protrusions of the costal cartilages (see Fig. 20–8B). These can also be corrected at the time of the repair.[49] Ravitch used

Figure 20–7. *A,* A 17-year-old boy with absence of the pectoralis major and minor muscles and mild hypoplasia of the nipple but no abnormality in the contour of the chest wall. *B,* An 8-year-old boy with aplasia of the third to fifth ribs and obliquity of the sternum. Note also the severe associated deformity of the ipsilateral hand. (From Shamberger RC, Welch KJ, Upton J III: Surgical treatment of thoracic deformity in Poland's syndrome. J Pediatr Surg 24:760–766, 1989.)

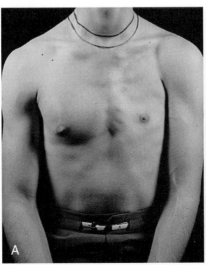

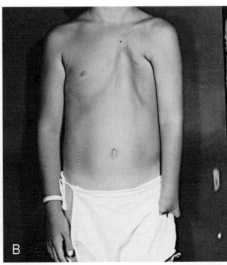

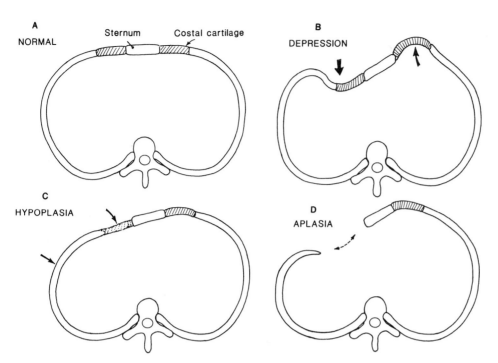

Figure 20–8. The spectrum of a rib cage abnormality in Poland's syndrome is shown. *A*, Most frequently, an entirely normal rib cage is seen with absent pectoral muscles only. *B*, Depression of the involved side of the chest wall is noted with rotation and often depression of the sternum. A carinate protrusion of the contralateral side is frequently present. *C*, Hypoplasia of the ribs on the involved side but without significant depression may be seen. It usually does not require surgical correction. *D*, Aplasia of one or more ribs is usually associated with depression of adjacent ribs on the involved side and rotation of the sternum. (From Shamberger RC, Welch KJ, Upton J III: Surgical treatment of thoracic deformity in Poland's syndrome. J Pediatr Surg 24:760–766, 1989.)

split rib grafts covered with Teflon felt for the repair.[50] Others have used latissimus dorsi muscle flaps, with placement of rib grafts.[49, 51] Chest wall reconstruction is important in females before correction of the hypoplasia or aplasia of the breast in order to provide an optimum base for augmentation (Fig. 20–10). Rotation of the latissimus dorsi muscle generally has not been used in males, but it is helpful in females for the purposes of breast reconstruction.[52]

☐ Sternal Defects

Sternal defects constitute a broad spectrum of rare deformities of the sternum, heart, and upper abdominal wall. They are best considered as four entities with limited overlap among categories, which can best be based on the tissue coverage of the heart.

THORACIC ECTOPIA CORDIS

These lesions are the classic so-called naked heart with no overlying somatic structures. The orientation of the apex of the heart is anterior and often cephalad (Fig. 20–11). Intrinsic cardiac anomalies are frequent, particularly tetralogy of Fallot, pulmonary artery stenosis, transposition of the great arteries, and ventricular septal defects.[53] An omphalocele may be present inferior to the sternal defect but does not cover the heart. Repair of these lesions has been almost universally unsuccessful, with only three reported survivors, all without intrinsic cardiac anomalies. Return of the heart to the thorax is poorly tolerated, presumably because of the torsion of the great vessels and compression of the heart. New approaches to construct the chest wall around

the anterior heart are required, if infants with thoracic ectopia cordis are to be saved.

CERVICAL ECTOPIA CORDIS

The patients with cervical ectopia cordis are distinct from the patients with thoracic ectopia cordis based only on the extent of superior displacement of the heart. Fusion between the apex of the heart and the mouth is often present. These infants have other severe congenital anomalies. None have survived.

THORACOABDOMINAL ECTOPIA CORDIS

In this group of patients, the heart is covered by an omphalocele-like membrane or thin, often pigmented, skin with an inferiorly cleft sternum (Fig. 20–12). The heart lacks the severe anterior rotation present in thoracic ectopia cordis. Intrinsic cardiac anomalies are common in these patients, most frequently tetralogy of Fallot, diverticulum of the left ventricle, and ventricular septal defects.[53] Defects in the diaphragm and pericardium along with the sternal, cardiac, and abdominal wall defects complete the anomalies associated with Cantrell's pentalogy. Repair of these lesions is much more successful than that of thoracic ectopia cordis. Initial surgical intervention must address the skin defects overlying the heart and abdominal cavity. Primary excision of the omphalocele with skin closure is preferred to avoid infection and mediastinitis, although several patients have been successfully managed by local application of topical astringents, allowing secondary epithelialization to occur. Abdominal wall coverage can be completed by mobilization of the lateral abdominal wall with

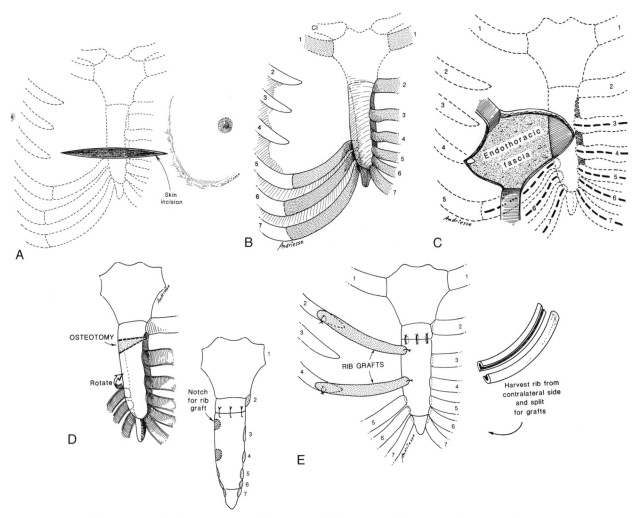

Figure 20–9. *A,* The transverse incision is placed below and within the nipples. In females, it is placed in the future inframammary crease. *B,* A schematic depiction of the deformity with rotation of the sternum, depression of the cartilages of the involved side, and carinate protrusion of the contralateral side. *C,* In cases with aplasia of the ribs, the endothoracic fascia is encountered directly below the attenuated subcutaneous tissue and pectoral fascia. The pectoral muscle flap is elevated on the contralateral side with the pectoral fascia, if present, on the involved side. Subperichondrial resection of the costal cartilages is carried out as shown by the dashed line preserving the costochondral junction. Rarely, this resection must be carried to the level of the second costal cartilage. *D,* A transverse, offset, wedge-shaped sternal osteotomy is created below the second costal cartilage. Closure of this defect with heavy silk sutures or elevation of the sternum with a strut corrects both the posterior displacement and the rotation of the sternum. *E,* In cases with rib aplasia, rib grafts are harvested from the contralateral fifth or sixth ribs, split and secured medially, with wire sutures into notches created in the sternum and with wire to the native ribs laterally. Ribs are split as shown, along their short axes to maintain maximum mechanical strength. (From Shamberger RC, Welch KJ, Upton J III: Surgical treatment of thoracic deformity in Poland's syndrome. J Pediatr Surg 24:760–766, 1989.)

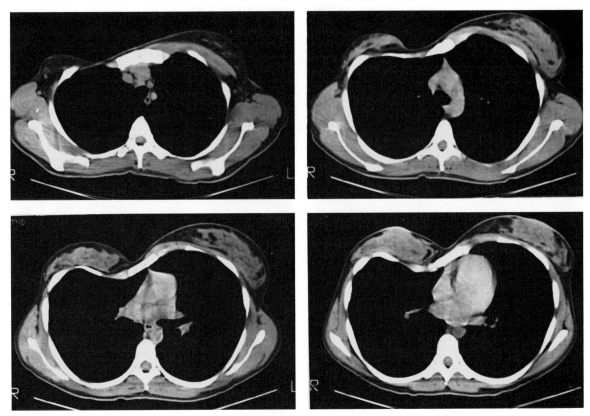

Figure 20–10. A computed tomograph of a 24-year-old woman with Poland's syndrome. Depression of the ribs on the involved side is apparent as well as a carinate protrusion of the contralateral side. Hypoplasia of the breast on the involved side is also apparent.

flaps or with prosthetic materials. Complete repair of the intracardiac defect is best performed before placement of prosthetic mesh overlying the heart.

CLEFT OR BIFID STERNUM

Cleft or bifid sternum is uniformly correctable. Patients in this group have otherwise normal hearts, partially or completely cleft sterna with normal skin coverage, and intact pericardia (Fig. 20–13). Omphalocele is not associated with cleft sternum. The defect in the sternum, if partial, involves primarily the upper sternum and manubrium. This is in contrast to thoracic ectopia cordis or thoracoabdominal ectopia cordis, in which partial defects involve primarily the lower sternum.[53] Most patients have a partially split sternum, with the xiphoid or lower

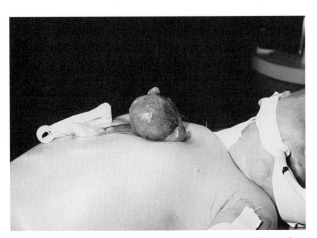

Figure 20–11. An infant with thoracic ectopia cordis with no significant abdominal wall defect present. The infant also demonstrates the characteristic high insertion of the umbilicus and anterior projection of the apex of the heart.

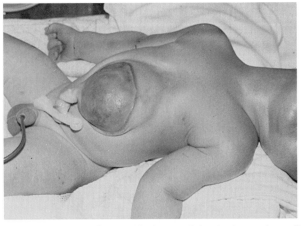

Figure 20–12. A newborn with thoracoabdominal ectopia cordis (Cantrell's pentalogy). Flaring of the lower thoracic cavity is present with a large epigastric omphalocele. The transverse septum of the diaphragm and the inferior portion of the pericardium are absent. The patient also has tetralogy of Fallot.

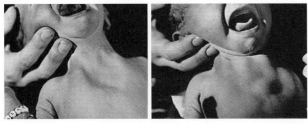

Figure 20–13. A newborn with a bifid sternum. Vigorous crying demonstrates retraction at the defect with inspiration (*left*) and protrusion with exhalation or Valsalva's maneuver (*right*).

third of the sternal body intact. Methods of repair are shown in Figure 20–14. It is important to repair these defects in infancy, when the chest wall is pliable and the sternal halves can be approximated without difficulty. When repaired in an older child, oblique chondrotomies are sometimes required to allow expansion of the chest wall to limit cardiac compression.[54]

☐ Thoracic Deformities in Diffuse Skeletal Disorders

ASPHYXIATING THORACIC DYSTROPHY (JEUNE'S SYNDROME)

Jeune, in 1954, first described a newborn with a narrow rigid chest and multiple cartilage anomalies.[55] The patient died early in the perinatal period because of respiratory insufficiency. Subsequent workers have further characterized this form of osteochondrodystrophy, which has variable skeletal involvement. Jeune's syndrome is inherited in an autosomal recessive pattern and is not associated with chromosome abnormalities.[56] Its most promi-

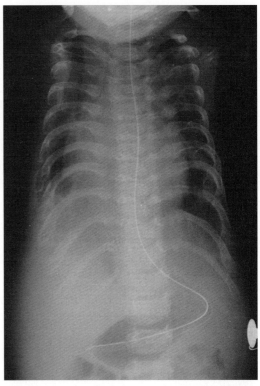

Figure 20–15. An infant with asphyxiating thoracic dystrophy (Jeune's syndrome). Radiograph shows the short horizontal ribs and the narrow thorax with limited lung volumes.

nent feature is a narrow bell-shaped thorax and a protuberant abdomen. The thorax is narrow in both the transverse and sagittal axes and has little respiratory motion because of the horizontal direction of the ribs (Fig. 20–15). The ribs are short and wide, and the splayed costochondral junctions barely reach the anterior axillary line. The costal cartilage

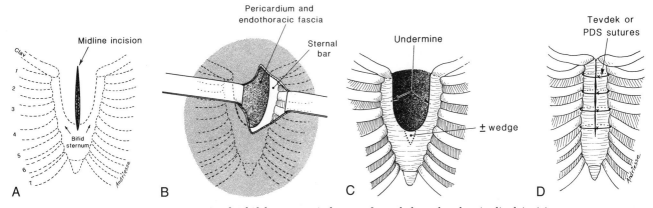

Figure 20–14. *A,* Repair of a bifid sternum is best performed through a longitudinal incision extending the length of the defect. These defects are characteristically cleft superiorly, as shown. *B,* Directly beneath the subcutaneous tissues, the sternal bars are encountered with the origin of the pectoral muscles on the lateral aspect of the bars. The endothoracic fascia and pericardium are just below these structures. *C,* The endothoracic fascia is mobilized off the sternal bars posteriorly with blunt dissection to allow safe placement of the sutures. Approximation of the sternal bars may be facilitated by excising a wedge of cartilage inferiorly. Repair is best accomplished in the neonatal period because of the flexibility of the chest wall. *D,* Closure of the defect is achieved with 2-0 Tevdek or Polydioxanone sutures. (From Shamberger RC, Welch KJ: Pediatr Surg Int 5:156–164, 1990.)

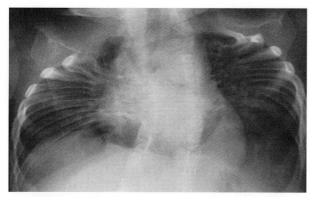

Figure 20–16. A radiograph of an infant with spondylothoracic dysplasia (Jarcho-Levin syndrome). Severe abnormality of the spine is apparent with multiple hemivertebrae and crab-like ribs, with close approximation posteriorly and splaying anteriorly.

is abundant and irregular, like a rachitic rosary. Microscopic examination of the costochondral junction reveals disorderly and poorly progressing endochondral ossification, resulting in decreased rib length.

Associated skeletal abnormalities that occur with this syndrome include short and stubby extremities, with relatively short and wide bones. The clavicles are in a fixed and elevated position, and the pelvis is small and hypoplastic with square iliac bones.

The syndrome has variable expression and degree of pulmonary impairment. The initial cases reported resulted in neonatal deaths. However, subsequent reports have documented a wide range of survival of patients with this syndrome.[57] The pathologic findings at autopsy are variable. They show a range of abnormal pulmonary development, although in most cases the bronchial development is normal and the decrease in alveolar divisions is variable.[58]

Surgical interventions for this condition have had very limited success. All have involved splitting the sternum longitudinally and widening the distance between the two sternal halves to increase the intrathoracic volume. Rib grafts, stainless steel struts, iliac bone grafts with metal plate fixation, and methyl methacrylate prostheses have all been used to maintain sternal separation. Results of these surgical attempts depend on the degree of underlying pulmonary hypoplasia.[59]

SPONDYLOTHORACIC DYSPLASIA (JARCHO-LEVIN SYNDROME)

Spondylothoracic dysplasia is an autosomal recessive deformity involving multiple vertebral and rib malformations. Death occurs in early infancy from pneumonia and respiratory failure.[60] Patients have multiple alternating hemivertebrae that affect most if not all of the thoracic and lumbar spine. The vertebral ossification centers rarely cross the midline. Multiple posterior fusions of the ribs as well as remarkable shortening of the thoracic spine result in a crab-like radiographic appearance of the

chest (Fig. 20–16). Of the patients with this syndrome, one third have associated malformations, including congenital heart disease and renal anomalies. Bone formation is normal in these patients. This syndrome has been reported primarily in Puerto Rican families (15 of 18 cases).[61]

Thoracic deformity is really secondary to the spine anomaly, which results in close posterior approximation of the origin of the ribs. Most infants with this deformity die before 15 months of age, and no surgical efforts at reconstruction have been proposed or attempted.[62]

REFERENCES

1. Shamberger RC, Welch KJ: Surgical repair of pectus excavatum. J Pediatr Surg 23:615–622, 1988.
2. Shamberger RC, Welch KJ, Castaneda AR, et al: Anterior chest wall deformities and congenital heart disease. J Thorac Cardiovasc Surg 96:427–432, 1988.
3. Haller JA Jr, Kramer SS, Lietman SA: Use of CT scans in selection of patients for pectus excavatum surgery: A preliminary report. J Pediatr Surg 22:904–906, 1987.
4. Welch KJ: Chest wall deformities. In Holder TM, Ashcraft KW (eds): Pediatric Surgery. Philadelphia, WB Saunders, 1980, pp 162–182.
5. Willital GH: Operationsindikation-Operationstechnik bei Brustkorbdeformierungen. Z Kinderchir 33:244–252, 1981.
6. Haller JA, Peters GN, Mazur D, et al: Pectus excavatum: A 20-year surgical experience. J Thorac Cardiovasc Surg 60:375–383, 1970.
7. Shamberger RC, Welch KJ: Cardiopulmonary function in pectus excavatum. Surg Gynecol Obstet 166:383–391, 1988.
8. Castile RG, Staats BA, Westbrook PR: Symptomatic pectus deformities of the chest. Am Rev Respir Dis 126:564–568, 1982.
9. Cahill JL, Lees GM, Robertson HT: A summary of preoperative and postoperative cardiorespiratory performance in patients undergoing pectus excavatum and carinatum repair. J Pediatr Surg 19:430–433, 1984.
10. Blickman JG, Rosen PR, Welch KJ, et al: Pectus excavatum in children: Pulmonary scintigraphy before and after corrective surgery. Radiology 156:781–782, 1985.
11. Derveaux L, Clarysse I, Ivanoff I, Demedts M: Preoperative and postoperative abnormalities in chest x-ray indices and in lung function in pectus deformities. Chest 95:850–856, 1989.
12. Morshuis W, Folgering H, Barentsz J, et al: Pulmonary function before surgery for pectus excavatum and at long-term follow-up. Chest 105:1646–1652, 1994.
13. Derveaux L, Ivanoff I, Rochette F, Demedts M: Mechanism of pulmonary function changes after surgical correction for funnel chest. Eur Resp J 1:823–825, 1988.
14. Wynn SR, Driscoll DJ, Ostrom NK, et al: Exercise cardiorespiratory function in adolescents with pectus excavatum. J Thorac Cardiovasc Surg 99:41–47, 1990.
15. Kaguraoka H, Ohnuki T, Itaoka T, et al: Degree of severity of pectus excavatum and pulmonary function in preoperative and postoperative periods. J Thorac Cardiovasc Surg 104:1483–1488, 1992.
16. Tanaka F, Kitano M, Shindo T, et al: Postoperative lung function in patients with funnel chest. J Jpn Assoc Thorac Surg 41:2161–2165, 1993.
17. Morshuis WJ, Folgering HT, Barentsz JO, et al: Exercise cardiorespiratory function before and one year after operation for pectus excavatum. J Thorac Cardiovasc Surg 107:1403–1409, 1994.
18. Beiser GD, Epstein SE, Stampfer M, et al: Impairment of cardiac function in patients with pectus excavatum, with improvement after operative correction. N Engl J Med 287:267–272, 1972.
19. Peterson RJ, Young WG Jr, Godwin JD, et al: Noninvasive assessment of exercise cardiac function before and after pec-

tus excavatum repair. J Thorac Cardiovasc Surg 90:251–260, 1985.

20. Meyer L: Zur chirurgischen Behandlung der angeborenen Trichterbrust. Verh Berliner Med 42:364–373, 1911.

21. Sauerbruch F: Die Chirurgie der Brustorgane. Berlin, Verlag von Julius Springer, 1920, pp 440–444.

22. Ravitch MM: The operative treatment of pectus excavatum. Ann Surg 129:429–444, 1949.

23. Baronofsky ID. Technique for the correction of pectus excavatum. Surgery 42:884–890, 1957.

24. Welch KJ: Satisfactory surgical correction of pectus excavatum deformity in childhood: A limited opportunity. J Thorac Surg 36:697–713, 1958.

25. Rehbein F, Wernicke HH: The operative treatment of the funnel chest. Arch Dis Child 32:5–8, 1957.

26. Adkins PC, Blades B: A stainless steel strut for correction of pectus excavatum. Surg Gynecol Obstet 113:111–113, 1961.

27. Hecker WCh, Procher G, Dietz HG: Results of operative correction of pigeon and funnel chest following a modified procedure of Ravitch and Haller. Z Kinderchir 34:220–227, 1981.

28. Judet J, Judet R: Thorax en entonnoir: Un procédé opératoire. Rev Orthop 40:248–257, 1954.

29. Jung A: Le traitement du thorax en entonnoir par le 'rétournement pédiculé' de la cuvette sterno-chondrale. Mem Acad Chir 82:242–249, 1956.

30. Wada J, Ikeda K, Ishida T, et al: Results of 271 funnel chest operations. Ann Thorac Surg 10:526–532, 1970.

31. Nuss D, Kelly RE Jr, Croitoru DP, Katz ME: A 10-year review of a minimally invasive technique for the correction of pectus excavatum. J Pediatr Surg 33:545–552, 1998.

32. Oelsnitz G: Fehlbildungen des Brustkorbes. Z Kinderchir 33:229–237, 1981.

33. Morshuis WJ, Mulder H, Wapperom G, et al: Pectus excavatum: A clinical study with long-term postoperative follow-up. Eur J Cardiothorac Surg 6:318–329, 1992.

34. Prévot J: Treatment of sternocostal wall malformations of the child: A series of 210 surgical corrections since 1975. Eur J Pediatr Surg 4:131–136, 1994.

35. Martinez D, Juame J, Stein T, et al. The effect of costal cartilage resection on chest wall development. Pediatr Surg Int 5:170–173, 1990.

36. Haller JA: Severe chest wall constriction from growth retardation after too extensive and too early (< 4 years) pectus excavatum repair: An alert. Ann Thorac Surg 60:1857–1864, 1995.

37. Shamberger RC, Welch KJ: Surgical correction of pectus carinatum. J Pediatr Surg 22:48–53, 1987.

38. Ravitch MM: Unusual sternal deformity with cardiac symptoms. Operative correction. J Thorac Surg 23:138–144, 1952.

39. Lester CW: Pigeon breast (pectus carinatum) and other protrusion deformities of the chest of developmental origin. Ann Surg 137:482–489, 1953.

40. Robicsek F, Sanger PW, Taylor FH, et al: The surgical treatment of chondrosternal prominence (pectus carinatum). J Thorac Cardiovasc Surg 45:691–701, 1963.

41. Welch KJ, Vos A: Surgical correction of pectus carinatum (pigeon breast). J Pediatr Surg 8:659–667, 1973.

42. Lallemand LM: Ephermérides Médicales de Montpellier. 1:144–147, 1826.

43. Froriep R: Beobachtung eines Falles Von Mangel der Brustdrauuse. Notizen aus dem Gebiete der Natur und Heilkunde 10:9–14, 1839.

44. Poland A: Deficiency of the pectoral muscles. Guys Hosp Rep 6:191–193, 1841.

45. Thomson J: On a form of congenital thoracic deformity. Teratologia 2:1–12, 1895.

46. Freire-Maia N, Chautard EA, Opitz JM, et al: The Poland syndrome—clinical and genealogical data, dermatoglyphic analysis, and incidence. Hum Hered 23:97–104, 1973.

47. McGillivray BC, Lowry RB: Poland syndrome in British Columbia: Incidence and reproductive experience of affected persons. Am J Med Genet 1:65–74, 1977.

48. Shamberger RC, Welch KJ, Upton J III: Surgical treatment of thoracic deformity in Poland's syndrome. J Pediatr Surg 24:760–766, 1989.

49. Haller JA Jr, Colombani PM, Miller D, et al: Early reconstruction of Poland's syndrome using autologous rib grafts combined with a latissimus muscle flap. J Pediatr Surg 19:423–429, 1984.

50. Ravitch MM: Atypical deformities of the chest wall—absence and deformities of the ribs and costal cartilages. Surgery 59:438–449, 1966.

51. Urschel HC Jr, Byrd HS, Sethi SM, et al: Poland's syndrome: Improved surgical management. Ann Thorac Surg 37:204–211, 1984.

52. Fodor PB, Khoury F: Latissimus dorsi muscle flap in reconstruction of congenitally absent breast and pectoralis muscle. Ann Plast Surg 4:422–425, 1980.

53. Shamberger RC, Welch KJ: Sternal defects. Pediatr Surg Int 5:156–164, 1990.

54. Sabiston DC Jr: The surgical management of congenital bifid sternum with partial ectopia cordis. J Thorac Surg 35:118–122, 1958.

55. Jeune M, Carron R, Beraud C, et al: Polychondrodystrophie avec blocage thoracique d'évolution fatale. Pediatrie 9:390–392, 1954.

56. Tahernia AC, Stamps P: "Jeune syndrome" (asphyxiating thoracic dystrophy): Report of a case, a review of the literature, and an editor's commentary. Clin Pediatr 16:903–908, 1977.

57. Kozlowski K, Masel J: Asphyxiating thoracic dystrophy without respiratory disease: Report of two cases of the latent form. Pediatr Radiol 5:30–33, 1976.

58. Williams AJ, Vawter G, Reid LM: Lung structure in asphyxiating thoracic dystrophy. Arch Pathol Lab Med 108:658–661, 1984.

59. Weber TR, Kurkchubasche AG: Operative management of asphyxiating thoracic dystrophy after pectus repair. J Pediatr Surg 33:262–265, 1998.

60. Jarcho S, Levin PM: Hereditary malformation of the vertebral bodies. Bull Johns Hopkins Hosp 62:216–226, 1938.

61. Heilbronner DM, Renshaw TS: Spondylothoracic dysplasia. J Bone Joint Surg Am 66:302–303, 1984.

62. Roberts AP, Conner AN, Tolmie JL, et al: Spondylothoracic and spondylocostal dysostosis: Hereditary forms of spinal deformity. J Bone Joint Surg Br 70:123–126, 1988.

Editorial Comment

The genesis of pectus deformities is unknown. In pectus excavatum, once the costal cartilages begin to grow inward nothing other than surgical intervention causes the chest wall to assume a normal configuration. The bent cartilages classically have been removed and the sternum brought forward so that as the cartilages regenerate, they grow from the end of the rib to the sternum, eliminating the indentation that produces the physiologic derangement in pectus excavatum. This is the standard operative procedure that Dr. Shamberger has so nicely described, a time-honored and very successful method of repair. There have been proponents of implantable bars who have argued that to support the new position of the sternum improves the ultimate structural result of the pectus excavatum repair. Most surgeons have not used such a device, believing that the risk of an infection and the need for a second procedure to remove the bar were not worth the benefit. Certainly, the results of the repair described from the Children's Hospital Medical Center speak to the efficacy of the standard procedure without implantation of any foreign materials.

The costal cartilages are, however, malleable. Based on this fact, a procedure has been reported that uses implantation of a rigid steel bar to push the sternum forward *without* removal of any cartilage.[1] After a period of 2 years, the bar is removed. The procedure is

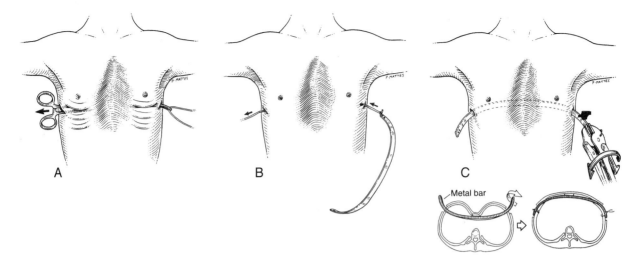

Figure 20–17. *A,* The patient is placed supine on the table with both arms extended on arm boards. The operative field is prepared from behind the midaxillary line on each side and from the clavicles to the upper abdomen. The distance from one midaxillary line to the other is measured in inches at the point of the deepest depression of the sternum. A bar is selected to correspond to this distance. The bar is bent to correspond to the desired shape of the chest, producing a bit of sternal protrusion. An incision is made on either side of the chest just anterior to the midaxillary line and deepened through the muscle layers to expose the rib. The tunnel for passage of the bar is developed using a long hemostatic forceps (provided in the instrumentation set designed for this purpose) or using a tunneling device to place implantable vascular access catheters. Care must be taken to enter the interspace and the chest at approximately the nipple line and to reduce trauma to the heart and lungs. Our preference is to use the vascular tunneling device proceeding from the patient's left side so that the sternal depression is less likely to direct the instrument into the heart. The point of the tunneling device should hug the inside of the chest wall throughout the passage. A Teflon tape is doubled and pulled through the tunnel as the instrument is withdrawn. This produces two tapes so that one may be used to pull the bar, and the other is left as a backup. We have had the bar accidentally cut the tape, and the tape has come loose as the bar is pulled through. In that instance, the remaining tape is used to once again deliver another doubled tape so that a spare always is in place. *B,* The bar is attached to the Teflon tape and brought through the substernal tunnel. It is often necessary to dilate the intercostal muscle opening and to manipulate the bar as it is being pulled, especially as it passes behind the sternum. The bar is passed with the concavity up. *C,* The bar is then grasped on each end with a Vise-Grip. The bar is turned, and the ends are slipped under the chest wall musculature. We use an absorbable suture to attach the bar to the rib at a convenient location to reduce the chance of the bar being displaced. The wounds are closed. (From Nuss D, Kelly RE Jr, Croitoru DP, Katz ME: A 10-year review of a minimally invasive technique for the correction of pectus excavatum. J Pediatr Surg 33:545–552, 1998.)

accomplished through two lateral chest wall incisions (Fig. 20–17*A–C*). The advantages of this technique compared with cartilage removal follow:

1. It does not take as long to perform
2. It does not involve a long incision on the front of the chest
3. Postoperative discomfort is considerably less and hospitalization is reduced to 2 to 3 days
4. Postoperative restriction in activity is shortened
5. Need for a clavicular splint is eliminated
6. Chest contour becomes more convex than we have seen with the best results using resection alone

The obvious disadvantage to this technique is the need for a second operation to remove the bar.

The procedure involves the "blind" passage of an instrument within the chest from one side to the other and the pulling back of the molded bar, both of which produce some anxiety on the part of the surgeon and potential risk to the thoracic contents of the patient. There has been one anecdotal report of perforation of the heart during the initial passage of the instrument to create the tunnel.

The original report of this minimally invasive technique was presented in early 1997 and included 42 patients who were all under the age of 15 years at the time of the procedure.[1] These patients were treated over a period of 10 years. Of the 30 of 42 patients who had the bar removed, excellent results were obtained in 22, good results in 4, fair results in 2, and poor results in 2. The mean follow-up was 4.2 years. These results compare favorably with our experience and that of others using the resection techniques.

Our personal experience with the bar technique consists of 62 patients who underwent surgery over a period of 22 months. None have progressed to the time for bar removal, and the ultimate result is unknown. The early results have been mixed, primarily because many of the patients were older than those reported in the original study cited. The mean age of our patients was 16 years at operation. There have been no major complications except a hemothorax in 1 patient with a previously unknown Factor VII deficiency. One patient had a pneumopericardium, and a few had minor pneumothorax, none of whom required thoracostomy. Four patients were noted to have a shift in the center of the bar cephalad 2 months postimplantation, and the bar was no longer pressing against the deepest part of the sternum. All had the bar replaced or repositioned.

The patient is often offered an epidural catheter for the postoperative pain, which seems to be very effective. All of the patients have been extubated in the operating room or the recovery room, and none have needed intensive care units. A chest radiograph is taken in the recovery room to assess the expansion of the lungs and the integrity of the pleura. Most patients are dismissed on oral pain medications on the 2nd or 3rd postoperative day.

This procedure is gaining popularity, but its long-term benefits remain to be defined.

REFERENCE

1. Nuss D, Kelly RE Jr, Croitoru DP, Katz ME: A 10-year review of a minimally invasive technique for the correction of pectus excavatum. J Pediatr Surg 33:545–552, 1998.

21

AIRWAY MALFORMATIONS AND RECONSTRUCTION

Robin T. Cotton, MD • J. Paul Willging, MD

☐ General

Feeding difficulties in a child are often a secondary sign of airway compromise. During feeding, a child's airway is challenged because of the need to coordinate the suck-swallow-breathe sequence. The effect of airway obstruction is magnified during this period of increased demand. Vocal quality can reflect possible involvement of laryngeal structures with an abnormality.

A complete head and neck examination should include an evaluation of the nasopharynx, hypopharynx, and larynx, which is easily accomplished and well tolerated, with flexible endoscopy. Any abnormality originating on or above the vocal cords can be identified. Pathology below the vocal cords requires complete endoscopic evaluation of the airway under general anesthesia.

The high-kilovolt, soft tissue radiography of the neck and chest provides the best information regarding the location and extent of an obstructing lesion.[1] Computed tomography (CT) and magnetic resonance imaging (MRI) are useful in specific circumstances following endoscopy.

For laryngeal and tracheal stenosis, the degree of maturation of the stenosis should be estimated. Active granulation tissue and acute inflammatory changes are indicative of an immature stenosis. Active lesions will change over time. Operations based on the assessment of an immature lesion may result in inadequate or excessive reconstructive procedures.

Ancillary tests are useful in the preoperative evaluation of patients with laryngotracheal pathology. Gastroesophageal reflux (GER) is a complicating factor in the postoperative healing of reconstructed airway patients.[2] Gastric emptying scans and dual pH probe studies can define the presence and extent of GER. Efficacy of medical treatments can also be assessed prior to reconstruction to ensure adequate control of the reflux. In some patients, a fundoplica-tion is required before airway reconstruction can be attempted.

Pulmonary function tests ideally provide an estimate of the pulmonary reserve of surgical candidates. Reliable data are difficult to obtain in children at the current time. However, new techniques are being developed to minimize the degree of cooperation required from a child when acquiring pulmonary function data. At present, pulmonary function testing is performed on children older than 6 years only in selective clinical situations.

Videostroboscopy allows an assessment of vocal cord function to be made. Although voice is not the major priority in airway reconstruction, maintaining maximal vocal function is important.

☐ Malformations of the Oral Cavity and Oropharynx

CONGENITAL EPULIS

The congenital epulis is a pedunculated mass, present at birth, that is usually attached to the anterior maxillary alveolar ridge of girls. Multiple lesions are not uncommon. Cellular components resemble a granular cell myoblastoma, but ultrastructural studies suggest the mass may be an ameloblastoma.[3]

A congenital epulis will be present at birth. Large lesions may be identified by prenatal ultrasonography (US). An epulis can be displaced from the mouth at birth, making it unlikely to cause airway obstruction (Fig. 21–1).

Surgical excision is required because this condition interferes with normal feeding. The pedicle is generally thin and relatively avascular. Electrocautery provides easy excision with simultaneous hemostasis. Local resection is curative.

MACROGLOSSIA

Macroglossia is a term applied to a tongue that will not fit into the oral cavity and prevents the

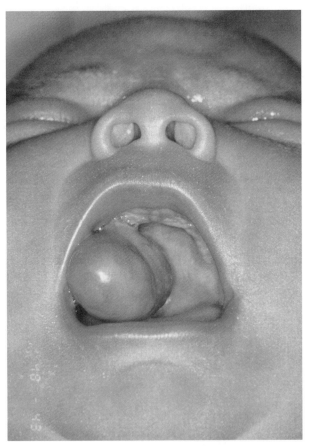

Figure 21–1. Congenital epulis arising from the upper alveolar margin.

dental arches from approximating. The primary causes of primary macroglossia are hypothyroidism, acromegaly, and Beckwith-Wiedemann syndrome. There are multiple causes of secondary macroglossia: rhabdomyosarcoma, lymphangioma, hemangioma, hereditary angioedema, angioneurotic edema, amyloidosis, neurofibromatosis, glycogen storage disease, and infection (Fig. 21–2). Management of secondary macroglossia relates to the treatment of the underlying source of the infiltration. Relative macroglossia is seen with the Pierre Robin syndrome.[4]

Macroglossia affects respiration and deglutition at an early age. Late complications relate to articulation problems and malocclusion from the altered dental arch development. There are also significant cosmetic concerns related to the chronic sialorrhea and exposed tongue. Respiratory obstruction at birth often requires a tracheotomy. Most cases of macroglossia do not present with airway obstruction.

Severe cases require tongue reduction to allow closure of the mouth. Taste and deglutition functions of the tongue must be preserved. Dental arch and malocclusion may require correction. The resection should be limited to tissue anterior to the circumvallate papilla to avoid injury to the lingual arteries and hypoglossal nerves and to preserve the sense of taste. Bleeding can be profuse. Sutures that retain their tensile strength for at least 3 weeks should be used because of the stresses generated by the tongue musculature.

Postoperative airway obstruction can be a life-threatening problem secondary to edema. An endotracheal airway should be maintained for a minimum of three days. A tracheotomy should be considered for major reduction procedures. The optimal time for surgical intervention ranges from 4 to 7 years of age.

MICROGNATHIA

Micrognathia is found in more than 60 syndromes. The ones most likely to produce airway obstruction are Treacher Collins syndrome, Hemifacial microsomia, Nager's syndrome, Pierre Robin sequence, and temporomandibular joint ankylosis.[5] Severe micrognathia may require tracheotomy for stabilization. Intubation of the airway in these cases may not be possible, necessitating that the tracheotomy be performed under mask anesthesia.

Retrognathia produces obstructive apnea, which may be managed temporarily with oral airways, Montgomery nipples, or nasopharyngeal airways. Positioning the child prone or on a side may improve air exchange in mild cases. Feeding difficulties may be the dominant symptom. The stress of feeding in the presence of a tenuous airway may

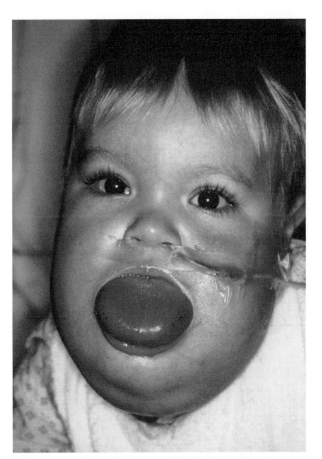

Figure 21–2. Secondary macroglossia from lymphangioma involvement of the tongue.

result in aspiration. In patients who can be managed with positioning or auxiliary airways, surgical intervention should be delayed for a week to determine if the child will be able to gain weight. Tube feedings may be required during this interval. If significant progress has not been made at the end of the first week of life, some type of surgical intervention will likely be required.

The tongue-lip adhesion is a popular surgical procedure for micrognathia but interferes with normal anterior arch formation.[6] The cosmetic appearance of the lower lip after takedown of the adhesion is often less than desirable. Hyomandibulopexy pulls the larynx superiorly, making endotracheal intubation more difficult. Both procedures require close follow-up to ensure airway patency and weight gain.

Devices that may improve the upper airway include an oral airway, a nasopharyngeal airway, and a Montgomery nipple. All require careful follow-up to ensure that the airway is being maintained. These devices may be needed for several months until adequate growth of the mandible has occurred.

The tracheotomy is the most reliable method of airway protection in micrognathia patients, but it requires the family to be trained in cardiopulmonary rescusitation and care of the cannula. The risks of tracheotomy must be balanced against the risk of airway obstruction. In our experience, tracheotomy is the preferred method of airway protection in retrognathic patients.

Gradual callus distraction is a long bone lengthening procedure that has been applied to the mandible.[7] Bidirectional double osteotomy callus distraction allows for better three-dimensional control of the lengthening procedure than the single osteotomy technique.[8] The vertical and horizontal components of the distraction can be independently manipulated. The appliance is externally pinned to the mandible, and daily distraction adjustments are made. This technique allows earlier tracheostomy decannulation and improves the overall cosmesis of the patient.[9, 10]

□ Inflammatory Lesions of the Oral Cavity and Oropharynx

Infections of the tonsils can result in airway obstruction by peritonsillar abscess formation. Older patients will tolerate needle aspiration of the abscess or incision and drainage under local anesthesia.[11] Most children are better treated with a quinsy tonsillectomy—a tonsillectomy in the presence of acute infection.[12] Removal of the tonsil serves to drain the abscess as well.

The retropharyngeal lymph nodes, which drain the nose, adenoids, nasopharynx, and paranasal sinuses, regress with age. Retropharyngeal abscesses usually occur before 5 years of age.[13] Because there is a median raphe in the retropharyngeal fascia, a peritonsillar abscess presents as a unilateral bulge on the posterior pharyngeal wall. The child will generally present with neck pain and dysphagia, fever, and torticollis with the head tilting to the uninvolved side. Lateral soft-tissue radiographs of the neck demonstrate abnormal thickening of the prevertebral soft tissues, reversal of the normal curvature of the cervical spine, and air in the retropharyngeal space if gas-producing organisms are present. CT aids in the diagnosis of retropharyngeal infection, helping in the differentiation between cellulitis and abscess.

Infections in the retropharyngeal space can be life threatening secondary to their potential to obstruct the airway. Spontaneous rupture of a retropharyngeal abscess can lead to aspiration of purulent material and the development of pneumonia and empyema.

Surgical drainage is the treatment of a retropharyngeal abscess. Cellulitis will respond to intravenous antibiotics. Endotracheal intubation from the side opposite the abscess will minimize the risk of rupturing the abscess. A direct incision over the abscess allows adequate drainage of the infection, and removal of a strip of mucosa will obviate the need for packing or drains. Young children may require overnight intubation to maintain the airway.

□ Laryngeal Malformations

LARYNGOMALACIA

Laryngomalacia has a 2-to-1 male preponderance.[14] It represents continued immaturity of the larynx, as if the fetal stage of laryngeal development has persisted. It is self-limiting but, when severe, may produce life-threatening obstructive apnea, cor pulmonale, and failure to thrive. Several anatomic features may be observed. The aryepiglottic folds are short, and often the epiglottis is excessively curled, creating an omega-shaped epiglottis. The short aryepiglottic folds result in arytenoid prolapse during inspiration. It is important to understand that there is more than one obstructing mechanism in laryngomalacia; the prolapsing cuneiform and corniculate cartilages may flop over the airway, the curled epiglottis may indraw, or there may be a combination of both. Furthermore, the supraglottic laryngeal structures may be tethered by short aryepiglottic folds, creating significant obstruction of the laryngeal inlet.

Although laryngomalacia is generally recognized as a cause of stridor and airway obstruction in infants, laryngomalacia may be manifested in older children on exercise. This exercise-induced laryngomalacia may be misdiagnosed as asthma, lack of fitness, or a functional abnormality.

Symptoms of laryngomalacia usually present within the first 2 weeks of life. A typical inspiratory fluttering noise is noted, which can be quite variable, occurring both at rest and on agitation. Expiration forces these tissues out of the airway and generally produces no noise. During quiet inspiratory effort, there may be no significant prolapse, but with increasing inspiratory effort, there is increasing obstruction, which can at times be of such a degree to allow no significant airflow (Fig. 21–3).

Stridor is frequently worse in the supine position and is lessened by neck extension. Symptoms increase over the first several months. Affected infants will maintain a normal cry without cyanosis. Whereas dyspnea is rarely experienced, feeding difficulties are quite common because of the increased respiratory demands associated with infant feeding. Gastroesophageal reflux is exacerbated by the negative intrathoracic pressure needed to inspire against a partially obstructed supraglottis. Although most patients with laryngomalacia have a benign clinical course, some infants develop severe obstruction, pectus excavatum, life-threatening cor pulmonale, obstructive apnea, and failure to thrive. Symptoms usually resolve by the age of 18 months.

Plain radiographic studies and upper airway fluoroscopy may suggest the diagnosis of laryngomalacia.[15] Contrast esophagraphy may reveal the stridor to be caused by vascular compression of the trachea and esophagus.

The mainstay of diagnosis is flexible laryngoscopy, best done in an awake child in the upright position. The scope should be passed through the nose to assess both nasal passages, the nasopharynx and supraglottic larynx. In severe cases of laryngomalacia, the vocal cords cannot be seen because of the supraglottic collapse. Airway radiographs should be obtained to look for additional abnormalities of the airway. Direct laryngoscopy in the operating room should be reserved for those cases in which a significant second lesion is suspected or when surgical intervention is being undertaken. The majority of patients with laryngomalacia require no intervention as long as growth and development are not compromised.

Obstructive apnea and failure to thrive are indications for surgical intervention. Supraglottoplasty has obviated the need for tracheotomy in many of these children and is now the preferred surgical procedure for the management of most cases of severe laryngomalacia. Direct laryngoscopy and bronchoscopy must be performed prior to the supraglottoplasty to exclude concomitant pathology contributing to airway obstruction. Tracheotomy may still be required if other obstructing mechanisms are present.

Removal of the obstructive supraglottic tissue may be achieved either with sharp dissection using laryngeal microinstruments or with the micropoint carbon dioxide (CO_2) laser.[16] It is important to be conservative in removing tissue to avoid the serious complication of supraglottic stenosis.[17, 18] Unilateral supraglottoplasty may be sufficient to relieve symptoms.[19] The patients are usually extubated the following morning. Antibiotic coverage is maintained for 5 days. Antireflux positioning and medications are recommended in the immediate postoperative period.

Aspiration and supraglottic stenosis may result from removal of too much tissue. It is essential to be conservative, even though this approach occasionally requires a second procedure to adequately correct airway compromise.

LARYNGEAL WEBS AND ATRESIA

Congenital laryngeal webs produce airway obstruction and vocal dysfunction.[20] A helpful classification of congenital laryngeal webs is presented in Table 21–1.

Vocal dysfunction may vary from aphonia to a voice that is weak, husky, or breathy. Stridor is the result of obstruction. A patient with a laryngeal web may present with croup at an early age. This diagnosis should be considered in a child with croup-like symptoms younger than 6 months.

The laryngeal web is identified by a combination of flexible laryngoscopy and direct laryngoscopy under general anesthesia. It is important to identify the thickness and the extent of the web. Careful

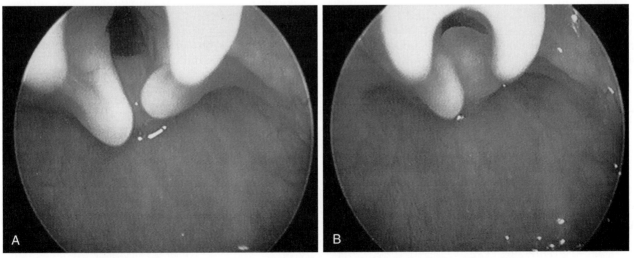

Figure 21–3. *A*, Larynx at rest. *B*, Right arytenoid prolapse into the glottis with inspiration.

TABLE 21-1. Classification of Laryngeal Webs

Type 1	Anterior web involving less than 35% of glottis Uniform thickness Negligible subglottic extension Rarely airway obstruction Slightly abnormal voice
Type 2	Anterior web involving 35–50% of glottis Moderately thick web Narrowing of the anterior subglottis Little airway obstruction Voice is husky
Type 3	Anterior web involving 50–75% of glottis Anterior web is very thick; posterior web is thin Subglottis narrowed by anterior extension of web Artificial airway frequently required Severe vocal dysfunction
Type 4	Anterior web involving 75–90% of glottis Web uniformly thick along entire extent Subglottis significantly obstructed Tracheotomy often required immediately after birth Aphonic

examination of the subglottic space is essential to determine subglottic involvement.

Treatment of congenital laryngeal webs is based on the extent of the lesion and the severity of symptoms. A type I web, which presents with no airway symptoms but only a breathy cry, is best initially managed expectantly. Definitive therapy can be delayed until the child is 3 or 4 years of age.

Type II glottic webs may be treated by incision along the margin on one vocal fold, followed by placement of a keel either endoscopically or through the thyroid lamina. A temporary tracheotomy is necessary while the keel is in position. Repeated dilation may be necessary after removal of the keel.

Type III and IV webs generally require a long-term tracheotomy and definitive therapy at 2 to 4 years of age. These webs include cricoid cartilage deformities that make the techniques of laryngotracheal reconstruction for subglottic stenosis applicable to their treatment. In severe type III and IV webs, an early, single-stage laryngotracheal reconstruction may be performed using an endotracheal tube as an airway stent, similar to the cricoid split procedure. The patient is intubated for approximately 10 days. This eliminates the need for a long-term tracheotomy, but a residual anterior web may require laryngotomy and keel placement at 3 to 4 years of age.

Complete laryngeal atresia is incompatible with life. Infants with this disorder only survive if emergency tracheotomy is carried out in the delivery room. If the child survives, then standard laryngotracheal reconstruction techniques are appropriate.

VOCAL CORD PARALYSIS

Vocal cord paralysis is the second-most common congenital laryngeal anomaly, behind laryngoma-lacia. The paralysis may be unilateral or bilateral. The cause of congenital vocal cord paralysis is neurologic. Bilateral paralysis is usually of central nervous system (CNS) etiology, whereas unilateral paralysis is caused by recurrent laryngeal nerve injury. The entire course of the recurrent laryngeal nerve must be evaluated in cases of unilateral vocal cord paralysis persisting after 2 weeks. The left recurrent laryngeal nerve is more prone to injury than the right because of the longer course the nerve takes through the neck and mediastinum. A difficult delivery with stretching of the infant's neck may produce a unilateral paralysis.

Bilateral vocal cord paralysis requires evaluation of the CNS. Head US or MRI may reveal one of a variety of problems. Deficits involving multiple cranial nerves are common in cases of bilateral vocal cord paralysis. Some cases of vocal cord paralysis have no identifiable cause. Paralysis of one or both vocal cords may occur as a complication following surgery for congenital cardiovascular or esophageal lesions. Generalized neurologic disease in infants rarely causes vocal cord paralysis.

The symptoms of unilateral vocal cord paralysis may be present at birth or may develop over the first several weeks of life. Unilateral paralysis is often well tolerated by the neonate, and delayed diagnosis is not uncommon. Airway obstruction is minimal, and stridor is apparent only with stress. A weak, hoarse, or breathy cry is commonly present. Feeding difficulties or aspiration may occur. Positioning the baby on the side of the paralyzed vocal cord during feeding may improve nutritional intake and will often improve the airway during periods of quiet respiration by allowing the affected cord to fall away from the midline.

Bilateral vocal cord paralysis presents with acute airway distress. The cry is normal, and there is a characteristic high-pitched inspiratory stridor present at rest and markedly exacerbated with agitation. Bilateral vocal cord paralysis is poorly tolerated in most neonates, and although an artificial airway is not universally necessary, emergent intubation is frequently required to stabilize the airway, followed by tracheotomy.[21]

The diagnosis of vocal cord paralysis is made by awake flexible laryngoscopy because general anesthesia affects the mobility of the cords. Direct laryngoscopy and bronchoscopy are reserved for cases of bilateral vocal cord paralysis and cases of unresolved unilateral paralysis to assess concomitant airway pathology.

The differential diagnosis of vocal cord paralysis includes cricoarytenoid joint fixation, posterior glottic web or stenosis, and infiltrative lesions of the vocal cords. For this reason, awake flexible laryngoscopy is supplemented by direct laryngoscopy under general anesthesia. After complete relaxation has been obtained, the arytenoid cartilage is carefully palpated to assess passive mobility and the true vocal cord is palpated for tone and stiffness. The posterior glottis is carefully inspected for any pathology. Complete microlaryngoscopy and bronchosopy are then performed. Laryngeal electromyography[22] and US[23] are not widely used as diagnostic adjuncts in infants.

Unilateral vocal cord paralysis from birth injury often resolves in the first few weeks of life. Bilateral vocal cord paralysis secondary to CNS pathology often improves when the neurologic problem is treated. Idiopathic vocal cord paralysis may resolve in the first few months of life. If function has not recovered by 2 years of age, it is unlikely to do so.

Surgical intervention is not often required for unilateral cord paralysis. If significant aspiration symptoms are present, vocal cord injection with Gelfoam[24] as a temporary measure or laryngeal framework surgery for a more permanent effect are possibilities.

Tracheostomy is generally, though not always, required for idiopathic bilateral vocal cord paralysis. Operative treatment of bilateral vocal cord paralysis is deferred until 2 years of age. The dilemma facing the surgeon and parents is that any procedure that involves improving the glottic airway will decrease the quality and volume of the voice. Most surgeons feel this is a worthwhile trade to eliminate the need for a lifelong tracheotomy.

SACCULAR CYSTS AND LARYNGOCELES

The ventricle is the space found between the false and true vocal cords. Congenital saccular cysts of the larynx are thought to arise in the saccule of the laryngeal ventricle. It is a mucus-filled lesion that protrudes into the supraglottic airway.[25] A laryngocele is a lesion that represents an abnormal dilation or herniation of the saccule. A laryngocele is distended by air and is palpable lateral to the larynx in the neck.[26] An anterior saccular cyst typically extends medially and posteriorly from the saccule and protrudes into the laryngeal lumen. A lateral saccular cyst typically extends posterosuperiorly into the false vocal cord and aryepiglottic fold. This is the most common presentation in infants.

Laryngoceles are rarely seen in the neonatal period. Laryngoceles can occasionally be distended with mucus or become infected (laryngopyocele). From a practical point of view a fluid-filled smooth mass distending the aryepiglottic fold may be a saccular cyst or a laryngocele. When filled with fluid, it is considered a saccular cyst; if filled with air, it is classified as a laryngocele.

Saccular cysts cause respiratory distress most often at birth and are generally diagnosed in the first few days of life. The cry may be muffled, and dysphagia may be encountered. Symptoms of laryngocele are similar, although they may present somewhat later. In addition to these symptoms, which may be worse on crying because of increased distention of air in the laryngocele, a crepitant neck mass may be felt.

Both lesions may be visible on soft-tissue radiographs or by US, CT, or MRI. The cyst content provides the most practical differentiation between saccular cyst and laryngocele. Direct laryngoscopy and bronchoscopy are performed immediately before surgical repair.

Endoscopic excision or marsupialization of the cyst is the common surgical approach to these lesions. The laser may be employed as an adjunct in marsupialization. Endoscopic dissection of the saccule to its base is followed by amputation. These methods have frequently required multiple procedures and often a concomitant tracheotomy.

Occasionally, an external laryngofissure approach has been used to remove a recurrent laryngeal cyst or a laryngocele. The current procedure of choice is a lateral cervical approach extending through the thyrohyoid membrane immediately above the alar of the thyroid cartilage. A portion of the superior alar of the thyroid cartilage may need to be removed. This allows for complete excision of the lesion and precludes the need for either a tracheotomy or multiple procedures. Short-term intubation may be required.

☐ Laryngotracheal Stenosis

Acquired subglottic stenosis (SGS) became a well-recognized entity in 1965, when long-term endotracheal intubation for ventilator support of neonates was introduced.[27] Because the cricoid cartilage is the only naturally occurring complete cartilagenous ring in the airway, an endotracheal tube that was too large or improperly secured can erode the mucosa with subsequent stenosis.

HISTORY AND PHYSICAL EXAMINATION

The history is usually "classic": Ventilator support was required for a period of days or weeks. Many times, an orotracheal tube was placed. The tube selected was as large as possible to prevent an air leak. Extubation may have been difficult, requiring several reintubations and perhaps steroids to reduce edema. After initial extubation success, the child gradually developed progressive stridor and retraction of the anterior chest wall. The child does not feed well because of respiratory distress. A tracheotomy may have been done.

Physical examination in the absence of a tracheostomy will most commonly reveal some element of malnutrition along with respiratory distress: labored breathing, retraction, and stridor. Conditions such as cleft lip and palate, choanal atresia, retrognathia, and other craniofacial anomalies must be identified. Passing a flexible suction catheter through each nare ensures nasal patency. The palate must be examined for a cleft. Auscultation over the cervical trachea may reveal restricted air movement at a particular level.

RADIOLOGIC EVALUATION

Plain radiographs of the neck may allow estimation of the length of the stenosis. The most important reason for radiographic evaluation of the airway is to rule out coexistent tracheal stenosis, long segment complete tracheal rings, and vascular compressions of the airway.

ENDOSCOPIC EVALUATION

All patients with suspected airway pathology should undergo a flexible fiberoptic nasopharyngoscopy while awake. The examination begins in the anterior nasal cavity to rule out a pyriform aperture stenosis and moves posteriorly to rule out a choanal stenosis or atresia. Hypopharyngeal visualization will assess hypopharyngeal tone. The epiglottis and arytenoid cartilages can be assessed for edema or erythema consistent with GER. Laryngomalacia may be seen. Accurate evaluation of vocal fold mobility can only be made with a flexible scope while the child is fully awake.

Rigid endoscopy remains the mainstay for the diagnosis of SGS and other tracheal pathology. Utilizing appropriate-size telescopes, bronchoscopes, and endotracheal tubes is essential and necessary.

A full-term infant with a cricoid ring less than 4 mm in diameter has SGS. A full-term infant should be able to be intubated with a 3-mm (inner diameter) endotracheal tube and still have some air leak around the tube at less than 30 cm of water pressure.

Calibration of the stenosis with an endotracheal tube is done to formulate an operative plan and to evaluate the response to treatment. The endotracheal tube that permits a leak at less than 30 cm of water pressure is considered the appropriate-size tube. The grading system for SGS[28] is shown in Figure 21–4.

Once the stenosis is identified, the length of the stenosis should be measured from its superior to inferior extent. The distance from the undersurface of the true vocal cords to the superior-most aspect of the stenosis should be measured, as should the distance from the inferior-most aspect of the stenosis to the tracheostomy tube (if present). Characteristics of the stenosis, such as an elliptical shape, prominent lateral shelves, anterior or posterior predominance, and suprastomal collapse, should be noted. Inflammatory changes or granulation tissue are indications that the scar is not mature and that operative intervention may be less successful. The trachea and bronchi must be carefully evaluated for evidence of malacia, compression, or other abnormalities that may affect the outcome of laryngotracheal reconstruction (LTR).

GASTROESOPHAGEAL REFLUX EVALUATION

At this time, the relationship between GER and SGS is not completely understood. Most surgeons feel that the evaluation of GER and appropriate management should precede LTR. If maximal medical therapy fails to control the reflux, surgical correction is necessary.[2]

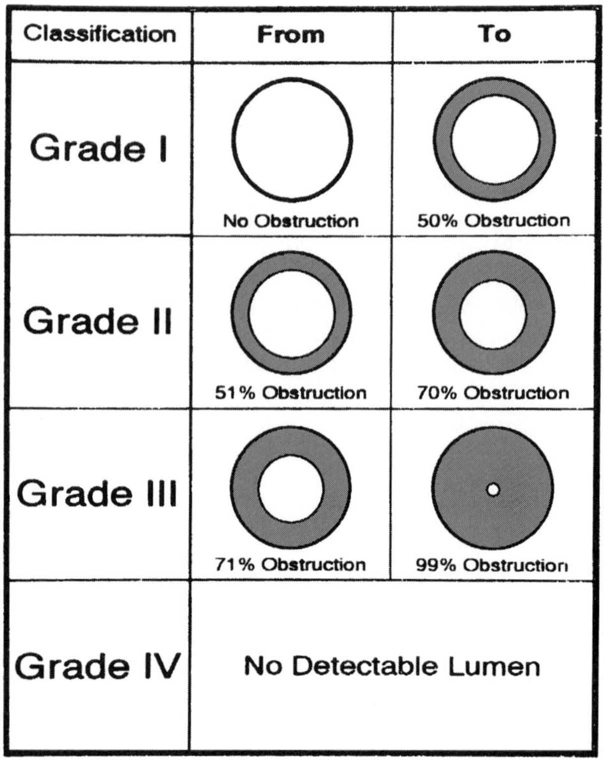

Figure 21–4. Subglottic stenosis grade classification. (From Myer CM, O'Connor DM, Cotton RT: Proposed grading system for subglottic stenosis based on endotracheal tube size. Ann Otol Rhinol Laryngol 103:319–323, 1994.)

PREOPERATIVE PLAN

The parents must be actively involved in the decision-making process and understand the long-term plan, need for long-term follow-up regardless of the surgical outcome, and potential complications with or without surgical intervention. For example, a single-stage procedure generally requires observation in intensive care for a minimum of 1 week and potentially 3 weeks. Often, children require close airway observation for an additional 1 to 2 weeks after extubation.

☐ Surgical Treatment of Laryngotracheal Stenosis

Cases of grade I or mild grade II stenosis can sometimes be observed and not require surgical intervention. If children with such conditions have only occasional and mild symptoms of stridor without retractions or feeding difficulties and have not required hospitalization for croup or airway-related illness, they may be watched closely. These are generally children who do not have tracheostomy tubes and who were intubated for only a short time earlier in life. Endoscopy and calibration must be repeated every 6 months to ensure that the airway is growing. If the airway is not growing, LTR should be considered before a tracheostomy becomes necessary.

TRACHEOTOMY

A tracheotomy may be the most appropriate initial step in safely caring for a child with SGS. It will allow the neonate time to grow and allow for bronchopulmonary dysplasia to mature. The tracheotomy will also allow for the stenosis to mature, which will improve the long-term surgical result.

Tracheostomy is not without risk. Language skills are delayed in children with a tracheotomy. For these reasons, early airway reconstruction is attractive and often the safest situation for the child.

ENDOSCOPIC APPROACHES

The use of serial dilations with or without the use of systemic steroids for the treatment of subglottic stenosis has limited application to early cases of SGS in which granulation tissue is present. Gentle dilation may minimize the formation of extensive cicatrix formation and maintain some identifiable lumen. Dilation of a firm, mature stenosis will not be of any significance in terms of enlarging the subglottic airway.

The CO_2 laser is a treatment option in highly selected cases of SGS.[29] The technique involves four quadrant incisions followed by dilation. Some cases of grade II SGS may be suitable for this modality of treatment, but great care must be undertaken not to make the original problem worse. Reconstructive surgery following laser failure becomes more difficult because of more severe scar tissue present in the subglottis. Cases of grade III and IV SGS are not amenable to laser incision and dilation.

The laser may be appropriate to treat granulation tissue that forms early as a response to intubation injury. The laser, in this situation, is used to avoid the formation of SGS.

The CO_2 laser can be helpful in some situations requiring "touch-up" procedures after LTR.

SURGICAL APPROACHES

There are many approaches to pediatric LTR, and surgeons need to be familiar with a variety of procedures to ensure the best care for their patients. Surgical reconstruction is recommended for mature SGS when conservative efforts are inappropriate or have failed. In general, grade III and IV lesions require open reconstruction. Contraindications to open reconstructive surgery include

1. An absolute contraindication to general anesthesia
2. Conditions in which even if the airway was enlarged sufficiently to allow for decannulation, the patient would still remain tracheotomy tube dependent because of aspiration or ventilation requirements
3. Conditions of severe incompetence of the esophagogastric junction that cannot be controlled medically or surgically

There are several basic approaches to alleviation of SGS, and all approaches yield comparable results when used for the correct indications.

Anterior Cricoid Split

The anterior cricoid split is indicated for neonatal acquired subglottic stenosis in the absence of other airway conditions and in the presence of adequate pulmonary reserve.[30] The concept is to avoid tracheotomy in premature children who have failed multiple extubation attempts because of subglottic pathology and in infants and children who have been extubated but continue to be symptomatic because of SGS. Interruption of the cricoid ring anteriorly allows the cartilage to spring open, thus decompressing the injured airway and allowing revascularization and reepithelization to occur. Strict criteria have been established for patient selection (Table 21–2 and Fig. 21–5).

Complications of the anterior cricoid split are unusual but can include persisting or severe SGS, wound infection, subcutaneous emphysema, pneumomediastinum, or pneumothorax.

Laryngotracheoplasty Without Cartilage Expansion

The technique of anterior cricoid split may be expanded to include a posterior cricoid split, lateral splits, or the four-quadrant split. These additional splits are not usually performed in the neonate or infant (Fig. 21–6).

Indications for a posterior split alone include SGS that is primarily posterior and has a glottic component, such as vocal fold fixation. Situations in which splits and no grafts would be considered would include in poorly controlled diabetic patients in whom the survival of cartilage graft would be questionable, or in patients who have undergone previous airway reconstructive procedures with grafts that have failed. Anterior and posterior splits are much more commonly used than lateral splits. In rare cases of severe and fibrotic stenosis, a four-quadrant split may be necessary. The lateral cuts are made at the 3 and 9 o'clock positions. The recurrent laryngeal nerves are protected by the outer peri-

TABLE 21-2. Criteria for Performing the Cricoid Split Procedure

1. At least two occasions in which extubation fails secondary to laryngeal pathology
2. Weight greater than 1500 g
3. No ventilator requirements (beyond minimal settings) for 10 days prior to proposed procedure
4. Supplemental oxygen requirements less than 35%
5. No congestive heart failure for 1 month prior to evaluation
6. No acute respiratory tract infections at the time of the evaluation
7. No antihypertensive medications for 10 days before the procedure

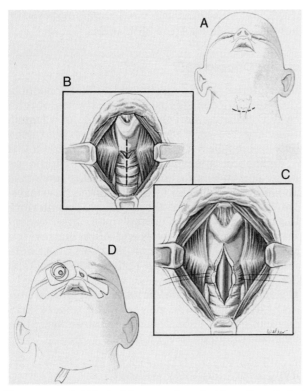

Figure 21–5. *A,* Skin incision over the cricoid cartilage. *B,* Incision through the cricoid, upper two tracheal rings, and thyroid cartilage (to the anterior commissure). *C,* Stay sutures through the cut edges of the cricoid cartilage. *D,* Wound loosely approximated with drain and nasotracheal intubation. (From Bluestone CD, Stool SE, Kenna MA: Pediatric Otolaryngology. Vol. 2 [3rd ed]. Philadelphia, WB Saunders, 1996, p 1377.)

chondrium of the cricoid cartilage.[31] Any patient undergoing posterior or lateral splits without grafting would require stenting for 6 weeks to 6 months with a Cotton-Lorenz prosthesis secured above the tracheotomy tube.

Laryngotracheoplasty with Cartilage Expansion

Augmentation of the laryngotracheal complex with a cartilage graft is required when distraction must be greater than 3 mm. The autologous cartilage is harvested at the time of LTR. Costal cartilage gives excellent rigidity and allows precise trimming and shaping specific for the individual patient's airway. It is very important to leave the perichondrium intact on the intraluminal surface to provide a surface for rapid regrowth of ciliated epithelium and to remove the perichondrium on the outer surface to allow for graft nourishment from tissue fluid.[32]

A cartilage graft placed posteriorly requires an incision sufficient to divide the fibrosis in the interarytenoid area but not high enough or deep enough to produce an iatrogenic laryngeal cleft.[33] The incision should extend inferiorly 5 to 10 mm into the membranous tracheal wall to allow for adequate distraction and comfortable placement of the graft (Fig. 21–7).

The cricoid cartilage may be augmented anteriorly, posteriorly, or both. Anterior grafts are considerably larger and thicker than grafts placed posteriorly. The anterior graft is elliptic in shape and must not extend to the level of the anterior commissure if acceptable vocal function is to be preserved. Wide flanges are preserved lateral to the inset portion of the graft to prevent prolapse of the graft into the airway. The cartilage must be treated with great care, as unnecessary suture trauma to the cartilage graft increases the likelihood of cartilage necrosis.

Posterior grafts must fit flush between the divided posterior cricoid lamina. A graft that is excessively thick will impinge on the pharynx and compromise swallowing. The elliptical graft should be carved to provide about 1 mm of distraction for each year of age, up to 1 cm. In cases of suprastomal collapse, it is sometimes necessary to place composite cartilage grafts (Fig. 21–8).

The strap muscles are closed over the anterior surface of the graft to allow for revascularization. A Penrose drain is placed underneath the strap muscles and sewn to the skin, to be removed in 48 hours assuming no air leak is present.

A postoperative chest roentgenogram is taken because of a possible pneumothorax. Antibiotics are given intravenously in the operating room and by mouth or nasogastric tube for 1 month following

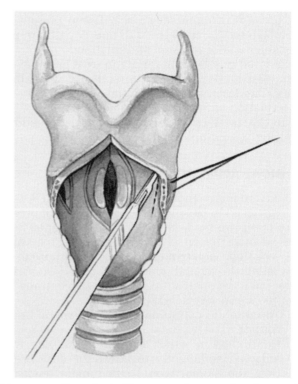

Figure 21–6. Lateral cricoid cuts may be created at the 3 and 9 o'clock positions. To protect the recurrent laryngeal nerves, the outer perichondrium must be preserved. The posterior cricoid plate may be divided to create a four quadrant split. (From Myer CM, Cotton RT, Shott SR [eds]: The Pediatric Airway: An Interdisciplinary Approach. Philadelphia, JB Lippincott, 1995, p 125.)

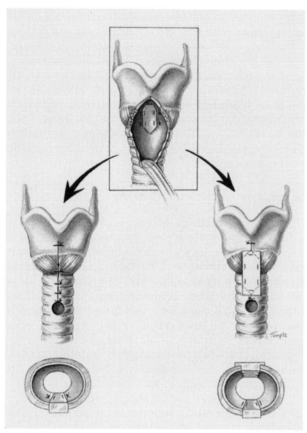

Figure 21–7. Combinations of augmentation sites are possible. The anterior and posterior grafts can be used alone or in combination. The augmentation technique is dependent on the stenosis. (From Myer CM, Cotton RT, Shott SR [eds]: The Pediatric Airway: An Interdisciplinary Approach. Philadelphia, JB Lippincott, 1995, p 127.)

surgery. If reflux is present, antireflux medication is continued for up to 1 year following surgery. Complications can include graft failure or migration, pneumonia, pneumothorax, wound infection or seroma, or subcutaneous emphysema.

Partial Cricotracheal Resection with Anastomosis

The technique of partial cricotracheal resection with primary tracheal anastomosis has been described in children.[34] The best candidates for this procedure are those with severe SGS (grade III or IV) without associated glottic pathology and a margin of a few millimeters of normal airway between the vocal folds and the stenosis. Advantages of this technique include preservation of the normal framework of the larynx, avoidance of a graft, and a nearly normal mucosal lining for the airway. Recurrent laryngeal nerve damage or anastomotic dehiscence has not been a problem in our experience.

If resection is necessary near the level of the true vocal folds, significant glottic edema should be expected, and appropriate airway management should be utilized postoperatively (tracheotomy tube or T-tube). Partial cricotracheal resection can be used for patients who have persisting stenosis following previous attempts at airway reconstruction or as the initial procedure to treat a child with a severe stenosis. If posterior glottic stenosis is also present, this technique may need to be supplemented with a posterior cricoid split and costal cartilage grafting (Fig. 21–9).

The anterior and lateral laryngotracheal anasto-

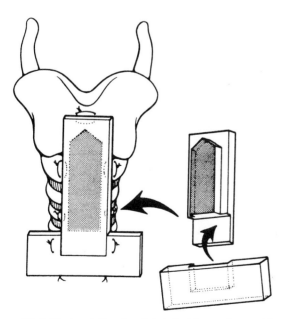

Figure 21–8. Horizontally placed interlocking graft, to add support to the suprastomal area. (From Cotton RT, Myer CM [eds]: Practical Pediatric Otolaryngology. Philadelphia, Lippincott-Raven, 1999, p 529.)

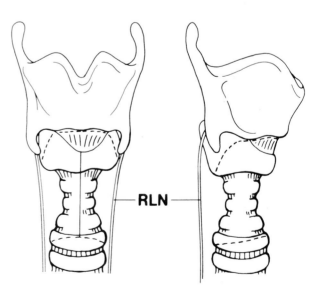

Figure 21–9. Partial cricotracheal resection. Midline vertical incision through the cricoid cartilage and upper stenotic tracheal rings. The ultimate lines of transection are indicated by the dashed lines, and determined by the stenosis. RLN, recurrent laryngeal nerve. (From Cotton RT, Myer CM [eds]: Practical Pediatric Otolaryngology. Philadelphia, Lippincott-Raven, 1999, p 531.)

mosis is created using 3-0 polypropylene (Prolene) sutures. Two or three additional tension-releasing 2-0 Prolene sutures are placed between the thyroid alae and the tracheal rings below the anastomosis. At the end of the procedure, the neck is maintained in a flexed position with three cutaneous 0 Prolene sutures placed from the chin to the chest to prohibit the child from extending the neck for 1 week postoperatively. In cases of minimal glottic involvement and in older children, a single-stage procedure with nasotracheal intubation for a period of 7 to 10 days is appropriate. In cases of moderate or severe glottic involvement and in younger children, prolonged glottic edema can be expected, so the airway is managed with a tracheotomy for a period of 4 to 6 weeks.[35]

Suprastomal Collapse

The tracheotomy cannula exerts constant forces on the anterior tracheal wall. Over time, this weakens the tracheal cartilages and promotes collapse. Granulation tissue, which universally develops on the superior aspect of the tracheotomy site, harbors bacteria that may induce a chondritis, causing a further reduction in the strength of the cartilage of the 1st and 2nd tracheal rings.[36] The granulomas should only be removed if they are significantly compromising the suprastomal airway. Repeated excision of small granuloma may lead to more aggressive recurrence. Large granulomas may be suspected if the child cannot phonate. Obstructing granulomas should be removed because of the potential for complete airway obstruction if the tube becomes blocked or displaced. Smaller granulomas should be removed just before decannulation.

Before an LTR procedure, the suprastomal area needs to be carefully assessed. It may be necessary to incorporate resection or reconstruction of the stomal area into the laryngeal repair. If an anterior graft is being performed, a second graft can be placed transversely in the trachea at the level of the suprastomal collapse. The tracheal cartilages are sewn to the undersurface of the transverse graft. The anterior laryngeal graft will then fit into a notch carved on the superior aspect of the transverse graft to prevent prolapse of the inferior aspect of the graft into the airway.

A surgical procedure may be elected to correct the suprastomal collapse as a staged procedure prior to decannulation. The softened rings may be excised in a wedge fashion with primary anastomosis, or the area can be augmented. Auricular cartilage, from the conchal bowl, has a natural curvature that conforms well to the natural contour of the trachea. Coastal cartilage can also be used for this purpose.

☐ Tracheal Stenosis

Isolated tracheal stenosis in the pediatric age group is likely to result from short-term intubation with too large an endotracheal tube or from a cuffed endotracheal tube that was overinflated. Regardless of the cause or patient age, a careful endoscopy must be performed to ascertain if the stenosis is anterior, posterior, or circumferential in nature. Calibration of the airway is imperative to allow for preoperative planning and postoperative comparison. Flexible nasopharyngoscopy should evaluate vocal fold mobility, and flexible endoscopy through the tracheotomy tube will allow assessment for possible distal tracheomalacia.

TREATMENT

Endoscopic dilation is appropriate for tracheal stenosis in the acute phase. Progressive stenosis or fixed stenosis requires more aggressive treatment. The CO_2 laser works well for short immature stenoses, those lesions that have an obvious thin lip of scar tissue, and those limited to only one quadrant of the trachea. If the lesion has failed to respond to laser therapy or involves a longer segment, open surgical intervention will be necessary.[37]

Specific cases of a predominately anterior tracheal stenosis may be best treated by a tracheoplasty with anterior cartilage expansion.

In the majority of cases, the patient can be extubated in the operating room and monitored closely in the hospital for 1 to 2 weeks. In children younger than 6 years, it is wise to wait 24 to 48 hours prior to extubation. Follow-up endoscopy is performed to assess the result.

Complications can include restenosis, anastomotic breakdown, pneumomediastinum, and wound infection.

☐ Postoperative Considerations Following Open Airway Procedures

Children who have undergone single-stage procedures must be watched especially closely for 2 weeks following extubation. Airway problems will most commonly present within this time period and may require surgical intervention. Children who have successfully undergone reconstruction and who still have a tracheotomy in place should be observed for a minimum of 48 hours plugged (trach capped) in the hospital prior to decannulation. The oxygen saturation, work of breathing, and ability to clear secretions should be monitored in these patients. These children should be observed an additional 48 hours following decannulation. All children should undergo repeat endoscopy at 4 weeks, 3 months, 6 months, 12 months, and 24 months following reconstructive surgery to identify continued growth of the airway and to identify potential problems that may be developing. Decannulation is not the only goal of reconstructive surgery. Voice quality following laryngotracheal reconstruction is an indicator of surgical success. The majority of patients who had a voice capable of communication preoperatively will have a similar or improved voice postoperatively.

□ Tracheomalacia

Chondromalacia of the trachea (tracheomalacia) represents an inability of the cartilages to keep the airway open during respiration. Primary tracheomalacia is an inherent cartilage abnormality. Secondary tracheomalacia occurs as a result of external pressure exerted on the airway from vascular abnormalities or esophageal atresia. Most cases of tracheomalacia are asymptomatic. Some children have expiratory airway noise secondary to the increased mediastinal pressures associated with exhalation. Severe cases of tracheomalacia have both inspiratory and expiratory stridor because of the complete lack of support provided to the affected tracheal segment.

Tracheomalacia is a dynamic process. Endoscopic visualization of the airway in a paralyzed, anesthetic patient will often fail to demonstrate any abnormality, whereas the same patient spontaneously ventilating will readily demonstrate the abnormality.[38] Plain radiographs may not demonstrate the lesion because of the phases of respiration. Fluoroscopy is the most reliable radiographic means of evaluating a patient for tracheomalacia.

Most children with tracheomalacia require no specific treatment, and symptoms spontaneously resolve. Tracheomalacia may be so severe that airway obstruction requires a tracheotomy. An extra-long tracheotomy cannula may be needed to provide an effective stent. Bronchomalacia, which is often associated with tracheomalacia, often improves following tracheotomy. Occasionally, bronchomalacia necessitates continuous positive airway pressure to stent the airway open during all phases of respiration.

Tracheomalacia is now being treated with expandable endoluminal stents. Exuberant granulation tissue, which may block the airway, is a known complication of stenting. The surgical removal of these stents is difficult. The long-term management of these stents as the child's airway grows is an unsettled issue. The natural history of tracheomalacia is that of spontaneous resolution. The treatment of tracheomalacia by stenting may create more tracheal problems in the future. In our opinion, the application of these devices to the pediatric airway should be discouraged.

□ Benign Laryngeal Tumors

RECURRENT RESPIRATORY PAPILLOMA

The most common benign neoplasm of the larynx is the papilloma. The adult respiratory papilloma tends to present as a solitary lesion and is responsive to treatment. In the juvenile form of the disease, multiple papillomas tend to be resistant to treatment and have the potential for life-threatening extension into the distal airway. There are no histologic differences between the juvenile and adult forms of the disease.

Juvenile papillomatosis has a predilection for the true vocal cords and the anterior commissure. Bulky lesions on the free edge of the true vocal cord or involving the anterior commissure cause hoarseness. Lesions on the superior aspect of the true vocal cords frequently obstruct the glottis. Extensive disease may present insidiously with exercise intolerance, failure to thrive, recurrent pneumonia, or sometimes acute respiratory distress (Fig. 21–10).

Juvenile papillomata occur most frequently between the ages of 2 and 5 years. The extent of disease and responsiveness to treatment cannot be correlated with age of onset. Recurrent respiratory papillomas (RRPs) are caused by the human papillomavirus (HPV). HPV-6 and HPV-11 are the most common types associated with laryngeal papilloma.[39] HPV-6$_c$ is the most common subtype and is usually associated with more extensive disease. Viral DNA has been identified in infected patients, both in areas of gross disease and in normal-appearing adjacent mucosa. A poorly understood control process is believed to be responsible for the development of distal disease as well as the eventual resolution of disease.

Much controversy centers around the association of genital papillomas and RRP. HPV-6 and HPV-11 account for 90% of genital warts. Exposure of a child to contaminated secretions in the birth canal, specifically during prolonged stage 2 labor, may infect the respiratory tract of the child.[40] Fifty percent of children with RRP have mothers with active cervical papillomas at birth. The transmission rate of the virus from an infected mother to her child is estimated to be less than 1%. Direct contact through

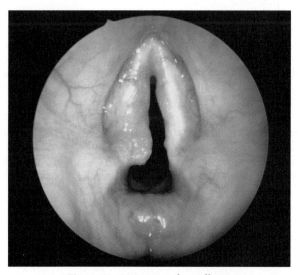

Figure 21–10. Laryngeal papilloma.

the birth canal is not the only mode of transmission, however, because HPV has been demonstrated in amniotic fluid and oral swabs taken from neonates delivered by cesarean section.

There is no universally effective treatment for RRP. Multiple combinations of medical and surgical treatment have been used, but all are ineffective in the complete eradication of disease. Antiviral agents, chemotherapeutic agents, and α-interferon have received much attention as treatments for papillomas but with variable results.

The goals of surgical management of papillomas are maintenance of the airway, preservation of vocal function, and control of papilloma growth. This disease process is not amenable to a surgical cure. The CO_2 laser has become the mainstay of treatment. The laser imparts minimal injury to normal tissue adjacent to the papilloma, but there is a 35% incidence of delayed complications consisting of webs or fixation of the false vocal cord to the true vocal cords because of overzealous laser treatment.[41]

In many cases, the natural history of papillomas is complete resolution of disease. Surgical intervention therefore must not result in long-term complications for either the voice or the airway. Complete removal of all papillomas is unrealistic and unnecessary. Maintenance of a patent airway until spontaneous regression of the lesions is the goal of surgical treatment.

Despite frequent endoscopic procedures, 21% of patients with laryngeal papilloma require tracheotomy. If a tracheotomy is required, the duration of cannulation should be less than four months if possible to minimize the risk of distal spread. Fifty percent of papilloma patients undergoing tracheotomy develop tracheal papilloma.[42]

Papilloma may extend into the tracheobronchial tree, lung parenchyma, soft tissues of the neck, and, occasionally, lymph nodes. Cytologic atypia has been described in several cases, suggesting conversion to squamous cell carcinoma.[43] Most malignancies associated with RRP occur in patients who have had previous irradiation.

Tracheal disease requires aggressive treatment. With frequent procedures, a tracheotomy may be avoided in selective cases. The CO_2 laser is ideal for these cases because the papilloma can be vaporized with minimal blood loss. Subglottiscopes can be customized to permit instrumentation to the level of the carina, obviating the need for the laser bronchoscope. In cases requiring tracheotomy, supportive care is maintained to keep the distal end of the cannula unobstructed. Vigorous chest physiotherapy and occasionally prophylactic antibiotics are required to maximize pulmonary function and minimize the incidence of pneumonia. Yearly chest radiographs should be obtained for comparison.

SUBGLOTTIC HEMANGIOMA

Subglottic hemangiomas are rarely present at birth but develop within the first 2 months of life. Fifty percent of patients with subglottic hemangioma also have cutaneous hemangioma. Eighty-five percent of subglottic hemangiomas arise in patients younger than 6 months with a 2:1 female preponderance. A rapid growth phase occurs and generally subsides by 1 year of age; a slow resolution phase occurs over a period of years. Most involuting hemangiomas show complete resolution by the time the child reaches the age of 5 years.

Agitation and excitement cause vascular engorgement, which increases the degree of airway compromise, and inspiratory stridor develops. No voice changes occur. With continued growth of the lesion, biphasic stridor develops. Acute respiratory distress is not uncommon.

Radiographic views of the neck may demonstrate an asymmetric subglottic narrowing on the anteroposterior view and a posterior subglottic mass on the lateral view. Definitive diagnosis requires microlaryngoscopy and bronchoscopy. The lesion generally is pink to blue and appears as a smooth submucosal mass with varying degrees of airway encroachment. Hemangiomas usually arise from the posterolateral aspect of the subglottis (Fig. 21–11). The lesions are generally well demarcated but in rare cases are diffuse and extend out of the larynx to involve the cervical trachea. The endoscopic appearance of the lesion generally is classic and confirms the diagnosis. The lesion is easily compressible. Biopsy is recommended only when the diagnosis is in question, such as when an atypical endoscopic appearance or aggressive behavior is present.

Subglottic hemangiomas generally require some form of surgical management. Expectant management is associated with a 50% mortality rate. The natural history of the disease is one of complete resolution with a normal functioning larynx.[44] In many instances, the best treatment modality is the placement of a tracheotomy to bypass the obstruction until the lesion spontaneously regresses. When

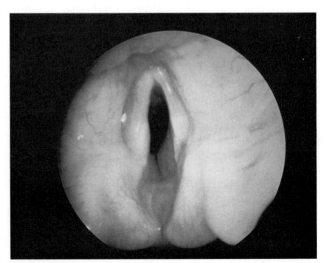

Figure 21–11. Subglottic hemangioma arising from the right posterior lateral subglottic wall.

intervention is desired, the CO_2 laser has the ability to decrease the size of the lesion, with minimal resultant edema and adjacent tissue injury. Judicious laser treatments must be performed to minimize the risk of inducing subglottic stenosis.

The CO_2 laser is most effective in the treatment of the capillary hemangioma. The cavernous hemangioma has vessels that are beyond the coagulation ability of the laser, and bleeding may become problematic.

Steroids may be useful in the treatment of subglottic hemangioma. Corticosteroids are known to occupy estradiol sites and thus inhibit any supportive function that estradiol exhibits on hemangioma growth.[45] Steroids also may sensitize the microvasculature to circulating endogenous vasoconstrictors, leading to spontaneous involution. Daily doses of dexamethasone sodium phosphate (1 mg/kg/day) for 7 days followed by a slowly tapering schedule to a minimal level administered every 72 hours may influence the proliferative phase of hemangioma development.

Steroids also may be used in conjunction with combined laser and intubation techniques when a patient is being managed without a tracheotomy. The hemangioma is treated with the CO_2 laser, and the patient is intubated postoperatively for approximately 1 week. During this period, dexamethasone sodium phosphate is administered at a dose of 1 mg/kg/day to induce involution. Repeated laser treatment is then performed as needed, and the steroids are discontinued after the first week.

LYMPHANGIOMA

Lymphangiomas are common malformations of the lymphatic system. In nearly 50% of cases, the lesion is located in the head and neck area.[46] Primary involvement of the larynx is rare; secondary involvement of the larynx by the compressive effects of the mass is more common. The lesion arises in the neonatal period in 50% of cases, 75% of cases are diagnosed within the first year of life, and 85% are identified by the age of 5 years.[47]

Lymphangiomas are divided into three morphologic groups. Lymphangioma simplex is a lesion consisting of capillary-size lymphatics. Cavernous lymphangioma are composed of dilated lymphatic spaces. Cystic hygromas contain discrete cystic spaces measuring several millimeters to many centimeters in diameter. The lesion has no malignant potential, but the invasive growth pattern decreases the potential for complete excision.

Laryngeal lymphangiomas produce airway obstruction and voice alteration. Lymphangiomas have the potential for tremendous increases in size in association with upper respiratory tract infections. Delayed recognition and treatment of lymphangiomas may lead to complications related to sudden airway compromise.

Treatment of laryngeal lymphangiomas is frustrating. The majority of patients require tracheotomy to bypass the obstruction. Complete excision of laryngeal lesions is rarely possible. Removal of the lesion should be tempered by the need to prevent long-term complications of the airway and vocal function. Various sclerosing agents have been used in an attempt to decrease the overall size and growth of lymphangioma, but the inflammatory response induced by the procedure often negates any advances achieved by the treatment. The CO_2 laser has proven the most efficacious treatment modality for laryngeal lymphangioma. The laser is used to drain the cyst, which is then vaporized, exposing the next layer of lymphangioma. Multiple procedures are most commonly required to treat laryngeal lymphangioma.

□ Inflammatory Lesions of the Larynx

Supraglottitis is an acute infectious process of the larynx. Acute airway obstruction may develop as a result of this infection and lead to a catastrophic outcome. Symptoms generally develop rapidly over 12 hours or less. The child is often between the ages of 2 and 4 years. The child complains of throat pain and odynophagia and is febrile. Symptoms progress rapidly over a few hours, with the child developing inspiratory stridor and increasing restlessness.

The physical examination demonstrates a toxic-appearing child who is generally sitting upright with the head held forward. The mouth is typically open, and the child is drooling. The child resists all attempts to lay supine. Breathing efforts are slow and deliberate. The voice is normal but may have a muffled quality. Oral inspection does not reveal any abnormality beyond the pooling of secretions. Introduction of a tongue blade may be sufficiently noxious to induce laryngospasm and should therefore be avoided.

Flexible laryngoscopy can be performed through a transnasal route if the diagnosis is in question, but care should be taken to avoid direct stimulation of the larynx.

A lateral neck roentgenogram is diagnostic for supraglottitis. A portable study taken in the emergency department is much safer than transporting the patient to the radiology suite. The "thumbprint" sign describes the marked enlargement of the epiglottis.

Once the diagnosis of supraglottitis is seriously considered, rapid intervention is required. General anesthesia induced by spontaneous ventilation allows for controlled examination and intubation. The inflammatory changes induced by supraglottitis generally do not preclude normal passage of the endotracheal tube into the trachea, but a tracheotomy tray should be immediately available should difficulties intubating the child arise. Blood and surface cultures of the epiglottis can be obtained at the time of intubation. The child should be observed and intubated in the intensive care unit until the supraglottic edema resolves, usually within 48 hours of initiating treatment. Intravenous antibiotics should be initiated after the airway is secured. Cefuroxime is generally considered the initial drug of choice for supraglottitis.[48] The most common pathogens are *Hemophilus influenzae* type B, α-hemolytic *Streptococcus*, group A β-hemolytic *Streptococcus*, *Staphylococcus aureus*, and *Streptococcus pneumoniae*. Since the introduction of the *Hemophilus* vaccine, the incidence of supraglottitis has markedly decreased. The relative incidence of bacterial agents other than *Hemophilus* has been increasing.

CROUP (VIRAL LARYNGOTRACHEOBRONCHITIS)

Croup may be distinguished clinically from epiglottitis by the slow progression of an upper respiratory infection to stridor, hoarseness, and a "barking" cough over 2 to 3 days.[49]

Radiographic studies demonstrate a normal epiglottis, with narrowing of the subglottis. The hypopharynx is frequently dilated because of the increased respiratory effort. Supportive care consisting of cool mist at home is the only care required for mild cases. In rare cases, endotracheal intubation may be required to secure the airway until the viral effects subside.

BACTERIAL TRACHEITIS (MEMBRANOUS LARYNGOTRACHEOBRONCHITIS)

Bacterial tracheitis has clinical features of both supraglottitis and croup. The disease generally follows an upper respiratory infection and is thought to be secondary to bacterial invasion of viral injured respiratory epithelium of the trachea.[50]

Patients appear toxic. There is often an antecedent history of an upper respiratory infection with a sudden deterioration over several hours. Throat pain is common, and a productive painful cough is present. Stridor, when present, is biphasic. Soft tissue radiographs of the airway demonstrate irregularities of the tracheal air column. Flexible laryngoscopy in the emergency room demonstrates a normal epiglottis, frequently edematous vocal cords, and no erythema in the subglottis. Purulent secretions can be seen in the subglottic airway, and they frequently cannot be cleared.

Bronchoscopy with débridement of the tenacious debris from the trachea and bronchi is essential and should be performed on an emergency basis. Many children require intubation postoperatively because of the degree of airway inflammation. Continued intubation allows suction access to the distal airway. The endotracheal tube should be smaller than that typically used because of the associated edema of the subglottis that typically accompanies bacterial tracheitis.

Antibiotic therapy should be initiated after the airway has been secured and cultures of the tracheal secretion obtained. *S. aureus*, *S. pneumoniae*, and *H. influenza* are the most common pathogens (Table 21–3).

☐ Pediatric Tracheotomy

Tracheotomy in children requires special attention because of the anatomic differences between the adult and pediatric larynx and trachea. The cricoid cartilage is generally the most prominent structure palpable in the anterior neck of a child. The thyroid cartilage is frequently deep to the hyoid bone, making palpation of the thyroid notch impossible. The central aspect of the anterior cricoid ring frequently overlaps the inferior edge of the thyroid cartilage in the young child, obliterating the cricothyroid membrane and making cricothyrotomy nearly impossible in children.

Tracheotomy is performed under general endotracheal anesthesia. The patient should be positioned on a shoulder roll to hyperextend the neck. The location of the cricoid should be marked. The suprasternal notch should be palpated for the presence of a high innominate artery. The midline incision can be infiltrated with xylocaine/epinephrine to diminish the anesthetic requirements of the operation.

A vertical skin incision is made midway between the cricoid cartilage and the sternal notch. Subcutaneous fat should be removed to facilitate replacement of the tracheotomy cannula in the event of accidental dislodgment prior to maturation of the stoma tract. The strap muscles are divided in the

TABLE 21-3. Comparison of Epiglottitis, Croup, and Membranous Tracheitis

Factor	Epiglottitis	Croup	Membraneous Tracheitis
Age	2–6 y	6 mo–5 y	3–7 y
Etiology	Bacterial	Viral	Bacterial
Season	Perennial	Late spring, late fall	Late spring and late fall
Recurrence	Uncommon	Common	Uncommon
Presentation	Toxic, drooling, stridor, sore throat, retractions, sitting upright	Nontoxic, not drooling, stridor, cough, retractions, supine	Toxic, cough, sore throat, hoarse voice, retractions
Onset	Rapid	Slow	Preceding viral infection
Confirmation	Endoscopic	Clinical, radiographic	Endoscopic
Therapy	Intubation, antimicrobials	Racemic epinephrine, steroids	Operative débridement, intubation, antimicrobial

midline and lateralized. The third tracheal ring will be the location of the tracheotomy incision. In the premature or young infant, the tracheal cartilages are very soft, and identification of the trachea can be difficult. The endotracheal tube or bronchoscope makes identification of the trachea easier.

Prolene traction sutures are placed in the trachea on either side of the proposed tracheal incision. These sutures are left long and labelled "left" and "right" at the completion of the procedure for easier recannulation in the early postoperative period.

With the third tracheal ring as the center of the tracheotomy incision, the airway is opened to an appropriate size to allow cannulation. A single vertical midline tracheal incision is created. Removal of tracheal cartilage is not recommended in children, as the incidence of tracheal narrowing and anterior tracheal wall collapse is higher with that technique.[51] The size of the tracheotomy tube should be judged against the tracheal lumen of the child and the specific needs of the patient. The surrounding skin edges are then sewn to the tracheotomy margins with 5-0 chromic suture. This speeds the maturation process of the stoma, further reducing the problems associated with accidental decannulation. Four sutures are used to mature the stoma.

Under direct visualization, the endotracheal tube (or bronchoscope) is retracted until the tracheotomy tube can be inserted into the airway. The tracheotomy ties are secured, with great care being taken to ensure equal tension on both sides of the neck. The traction sutures are then tied, labeled left and right, and taped to the chest in preparation for their possible use in the postoperative period.

Microlaryngoscopy and bronchoscopy are then performed to define the status of the larynx and the condition of the subglottis. The position of the tracheotomy tube can also be verified within the trachea.

The tracheotomy ties are changed on the third postoperative day to minimize manipulation of the tracheotomy tube during the most critical time of healing. The tracheotomy tube is changed on the fifth postoperative day.

A chest radiograph is always obtained immediately after tracheotomy to verify position and orientation of the tracheotomy tube within the airway and to identify complications of the procedure.

REFERENCES

1. Dunbar JS: Upper respiratory tract obstruction in infants and children. Am J Roentgen Radium Ther Nucl Med 109:227–246, 1970.
2. Walner DL, Stern Y, Gerber ME, et al: Gastroesophageal reflux in patients with subglottic stenosis. Arch Otolaryngol Head Neck Surg 124:551–555, 1998.
3. Tucker MC, Rusnock EJ, Azumi N, et al: Gingival granular cell tumors of the newborn. An ultrastructural and immunohistochemical study. Arch Pathol Lab Med 114:895–898, 1990.
4. Rizer FM, Schechter GL, Richardson MA: Macroglossia: Etiologic considerations and management techniques. Int J Pediatr Otorhinolaryngol 8:225–236, 1985.
5. Gorlin RJ, Cohen MMJ, Levin S: Orofacial clefting syndromes: General aspects. In Syndromes of the Head and Neck. Oxford, Oxford University Press, 1990, pp 700–705.
6. Hawkins DB, Simpson JV: Micrognathia and glossoptosis in the newborn. Surgical tacking of the tongue in small jaw syndromes. Clin Pediatr 13:1066–1073, 1974.
7. Ilizarov GA: The principles of the Ilizarov method. Bull Hosp Joint Dis Orthop Inst 48:1–11, 1988.
8. Klein C, Howaldt HP: Correction of mandibular hypoplasia by means of bidirectional callus distraction. J Craniofac Surg 7:258–266, 1996.
9. Losken HW, Patterson GT, Lazarou SA, Whitney T: Planning mandibular distraction: Preliminary report. Cleft Palate Craniofac J 32:71–76, 1995.
10. McCarthy JG, Schreiber J, Karp N, et al: Lengthening the human mandible by gradual distraction. Plast Reconstr Surg 89:1–8; discussion 9–10, 1992.
11. Schechter GL, Sly DE, Roper AL, Jackson RT: Changing face of treatment of peritonsillar abscess. Laryngoscope 92:657–659, 1982.
12. McCurdy JA, Jr: Peritonsillar abscess. A comparison of treatment by immediate tonsillectomy and interval tonsillectomy. Arch Otolaryngol 103:414–415, 1977.
13. Wright NL: Cervical infections. Am J Surg 113:379–386, 1967.
14. Holinger LD: Etiology of stridor in the neonate, infant and child. Ann Otol Rhinol Laryngol 89:397–400, 1980.
15. Tostevin PM, de Bruyn R, Hosni A, Evans JN: The value of radiological investigations in pre-endoscopic assessment of children with stridor. J Laryngol Otol 109:844–848, 1995.
16. Hui Y, Gaffney R, Crysdale WS: Laser aryepiglottoplasty for the treatment of neurasthenic laryngomalacia in cerebral palsy. Ann Otol Rhinol Laryngol 104:432–436, 1995.
17. Roger G, Denoyelle F, Triglia JM, Garabedian EN: Severe laryngomalacia: Surgical indications and results in 115 patients. Laryngoscope 105:1111–1117, 1995.
18. Zalzal GH, Anon JB, Cotton RT: Epiglottoplasty for the treatment of laryngomalacia. Ann Otol Rhinol Laryngol 96:72–76, 1987.
19. Kelly SM, Gray SD: Unilateral endoscopic supraglottoplasty for severe laryngomalacia. Arch Otolaryngol Head Neck Surg 121:1351–1354, 1995.
20. Cohen SR: Congenital glottic webs in children. A retrospective review of 51 patients. Ann Otol Rhinol Laryngol 121(suppl):2–16, 1985.
21. Murty GE, Shinkwin C, Gibbin KP: Bilateral vocal fold paralysis in infants: Tracheostomy or not? J Laryngol Otol 108:329–331, 1994.
22. Gartlan MG, Peterson KL, Luschei ES, et al: Bipolar hooked-wire electromyographic technique in the evaluation of pediatric vocal cord paralysis. Ann Otol Rhinol Laryngol 102:695–700, 1993.
23. Friedman EM: Role of ultrasound in the assessment of vocal cord function in infants and children. Ann Otol Rhinol Laryngol 106:199–209, 1997.
24. Levine BA, Jacobs IN, Wetmore RF, Handler SD: Vocal cord injection in children with unilateral vocal cord paralysis. Arch Otolaryngol Head Neck Surg 121:116–119, 1995.
25. Holinger LD, Barnes DR, Smid LJ, Holinger PH: Laryngocele and saccular cysts. Ann Otol Rhinol Laryngol 87:675–685, 1978.
26. Chu L, Gussack GS, Orr JB, Hood D: Neonatal laryngoceles. A cause for airway obstruction. Arch Otolaryngol Head Neck Surg 120:454–458, 1994.
27. McDonald I, Stocks J: Prolonged nasotracheal intubation. Br J Anaesth 37:161–172, 1965.
28. Myer CM III, O'Connor DM, Cotton RT: Proposed grading system for subglottic stenosis based on endotracheal tube sizes. Ann Otol Rhinol Laryngol 103:319–323, 1994.
29. Simpson GT, Healy GB, McGill T, Strong MS: Benign tumors and lesions of the larynx in children. Surgical excision by CO_2 laser. Ann Otol Rhinol Laryngol 88:479–485, 1979.
30. Cotton RT, Myer CM 3rd, Bratcher GO, Fitton CM: Anterior cricoid split, 1977–1987. Evolution of a technique. Arch Otolaryngol Head Neck Surg 114:1300–1302, 1988.

31. Drake AF, Contencin P, Narcy F, Cotton RT: Lateral cricoid cuts as an adjunctive measure to enlarge the stenotic subglottic airway: An anatomic study. lnt J Pediatr Otorhinolaryngol 18:129–137, 1989.

32. Cotton RT, Gray SD, Miller RP: Update of the Cincinnati experience in pediatric laryngotracheal reconstruction. Laryngoscope 99:1111–1116, 1989.

33. Cotton RT: The problem of pediatric laryngotracheal stenosis: A clinical and experimental study on the efficacy of autogenous cartilaginous grafts placed between the vertically divided halves of the posterior lamina of the cricoid cartilage. Laryngoscope 101:1–34,1991.

34. Monnier P, Savary M, Chapuis G: Partial cricoid resection with primary tracheal anastomosis for subglottic stenosis in infants and children. Laryngoscope 103:1273–1283, 1993.

35. Stern Y, Gerber ME, Walner DL, Cotton RT: Partial cricotracheal resection with primary anastomosis in the pediatric age group. Ann Otol Rhinol Laryngol 106:891–896, 1997.

36. Rosenfeld RM, Stool SE: Should granulomas be excised in children with long-term tracheotomy? Arch Otolaryngol Head Neck Surg 118:1323–1327, 1992.

37. Grillo HC, Dignan EF, Miura T: Experimental reconstruction of cervical trachea after circumferential resection. Surg Gynecol Obstet 122:733–738, 1966.

38. Benjamin B: Tracheomalacia in infants and children. Ann Otol Rhinol Laryngol 93:438–442, 1984.

39. Kashima HK, Kessis T, Mounts P, Shah K: Polymerase chain reaction identification of human papillomavirus DNA in CO_2 laser plume from recurrent respiratory papillomatosis. Otolaryngol Head Neck Surg 104:191–195, 1991.

40. Kashima HK, Shah F, Lyles A, et al: A comparison of risk factors in juvenile-onset and adult-onset recurrent respiratory papillomatosis. Laryngoscope 102:9–13, 1992.

41. Crockett DM, McCabe BF, Shive CJ: Complications of laser surgery for recurrent respiratory papillomatosis. Ann Otol Rhinol Laryngol 96:639–644, 1987.

42. Cole RR, Myer CM 3rd, Cotton RT: Tracheotomy in children with recurrent respiratory papillomatosis. Head Neck 11:226–230, 1989.

43. Bewtra C, Krishnan R, Lee SS: Malignant changes in nonirradiated juvenile laryngotracheal papillomatosis. Arch Otolaryngol 108:114–116, 1982.

44. Shikhani AH, Jones MM, Marsh BR, Holliday MJ: Infantile subglottic hemangiomas. An update. Ann Otol Rhinol Laryngol 95:336–347, 1986.

45. Hawkins DB, Crockett DM, Kahlstrom EJ, MacLaughlin EF: Corticosteroid management of airway hemangiomas: Long-term follow-up. Laryngoscope 94:633–637, 1984.

46. Barnhart RA, Brown AK, Jr: Cystic hygroma of the neck. Report of a case. Arch Otolaryngol 86:74–78, 1967.

47. Cohen SR, Thompson JW: Lymphangiomas of the larynx in infants and children. A surgery of pediatric lymphangioma. Ann Otol Rhinol Laryngol 127(suppl):1–20, 1986.

48. Frantz TD, Rasgon BM, Quesenberry CP, Jr: Acute epiglottitis in adults. Analysis of 129 cases. JAMA 272:1358–1360, 1994.

49. Battaglia JD. Severe croup: The child with fever and upper airway obstruction. Pediatr Rev 7:227–233, 1986.

50. Donaldson JD, Maltby CC: Bacterial tracheitis in children. J Otolaryngol 18:101–104, 1989.

51. Aberdeen E, Downes JJ: Artificial airways in children. Surg Clin North Am 54:1155–1170, 1974.

22

BRONCHOPULMONARY MALFORMATIONS

André Hebra, MD •
H. Biemann Othersen, Jr., MD •
Edward P. Tagge, MD

☐ Prenatal Ultrasound and Fetal Intervention

Since the late 1980s, dramatic improvements in prenatal ultrasonography (US) have lead to increased awareness and earlier detection of fetal pulmonary anomalies.[1] Normal fetal lung has echogenicity similar to that of the liver. As a general rule, pulmonary parenchymal lesions are diagnosed via US by the presence of abnormal echogenicity in the thorax compared with that of the normal lung or liver. Additionally, the mass effect of a lesion may produce cardiac compression or deviation.

The most common causes of an echogenic fetal chest mass include (1) congenital cystic adenomatoid malformation (CCAM); (2) pulmonary sequestration; (3) tracheal atresia; and (4) congenital diaphragmatic hernia (CDH). CCAM and CDH both produce an echogenic chest mass with cystic components. Tracheal atresia produces bilaterally enlarged and diffusely echogenic lungs in the fetus. Pulmonary sequestration, CCAM, and CDH are usually unilateral lesions. US also provides information as to the presence of other fetal abnormalities that may be important predictors of adverse outcome.

A recent review of fetal lung lesions diagnosed by prenatal US illustrated the accuracy in diagnosis when the test is performed by experienced perinatologists. Of 17 fetuses with echogenic chest masses, the prenatal diagnosis was correct in 13. The most difficult differentiation was between CCAM and CDH. Some lesions noted early in the pregnancy on US examination either disappeared[2, 3] or became significantly smaller over time.[4] A large sequestration on initial US does not necessarily predict a poor fetal or neonatal outcome.

Until recently, the option for fetuses with bronchopulmonary malformations has been expectant management with surgical resection in the neonatal or infant period or termination of pregnancy. Obviously, the former is a viable option as long as the lesions are not large enough to adversely affect fetal lung development. However, in fetuses with pulmonary malformations that will prevent development of normal lung and ultimately lead to neonatal demise, a logical approach is fetal surgery.

The role of fetal surgical therapy for CCAM, sequestration, fetal pleural effusion, and sacrococcygeal teratoma (SCT) was described in 1995.[5] Those anatomic anomalies diagnosed in utero that can be predicted to progress to nonimmune hydrops and almost certain fetal demise were the conditions considered for fetal surgical intervention. Fetal surgery was deemed justifiable if (1) the natural history of pathophysiologic features of the disease are well understood, and it is possible to predict which fetuses have a sufficiently poor prognosis to justify in utero intervention; (2) the prenatal diagnosis is accurate, and other lethal anomalies can be excluded; (3) in utero correction has been shown to be efficacious in animal models; and (4) maternal risk is proven to be acceptably low.

A poor fetal outcome, without fetal intervention, is most closely associated with hydrops, which results from vena caval obstruction or cardiac compression. The obstruction is often produced by mediastinal shift caused by a large CCAM. Pulmonary sequestration may produce fetal hydrops from either the mass effect or a tension hydrothorax resulting from serum or lymph transudation from the sequestration. Some CCAMs and sequestrations have been shown to regress spontaneously during pregnancy, suggesting that expectant management is appropriate when there is no evidence of hydrops.

Several fetal lamb models have been investigated to study the etiology of hydrops and the effects of resection on fetal outcome; not only have the results been encouraging but also these studies have led to development of the necessary surgical, anesthetic, and tocolytic techniques to allow use in humans. In order to be practical, fetal intervention must be safe for the mother and for her future reproductive potential.

The clinical experience with nine mother-fetus patients included resection of fetal CCAM (six patients) or fetal chest tube drainage (thoracoamniotic) for sequestration (three patients). All of the CCAM patients had hydrops at the time of surgery: four delivered between 26 and 34 weeks' gestation and were alive and well at 1 to 2 years; one had fetal demise 8 hours postoperatively at 21 weeks, and one died of pulmonary hypoplasia at 40 hours of age (surgery done 1 week before preterm delivery at 28 weeks). Of the patients with shunt placement, one had hydrops and was stillborn at 22 weeks' gestation, 3 days after the procedure; two had no evidence of hydrops, delivered at 23 and 38 weeks' gestation, and were alive and well at 16 months and 8 months of age, respectively. Figure 22–1 is an algorithm for the management of the fetus with a thoracic mass.

Based on this and other sporadic reports, in utero resection of these masses or pleural drainage is safe, feasible, and effective. Many challenges remain, such as (1) better maternal-fetal postoperative monitoring; (2) reliable long-term fetal intravascular access for fetal blood sampling and infusion; (3) noninvasive maternal-fetal hemodynamic assessment; (4) less-invasive methods of intervention, including fetoscopy; and (5) effective detection and treatment of preterm labor.

Definitive prenatal detection of pulmonary sequestration and CCAM and accurate delineation of these entities from CDH can be difficult at times. The majority of fetuses can be followed with serial US to monitor for worsening of fetal status as evidenced by hydrops. Unless hydrops complicates the fetal development, surgical treatment should be undertaken after birth of the fetus.

□ Bronchopulmonary Malformations

Most patients with these malformations are treated postnatally. Each condition described in this chapter is relatively rare; however, taken together, these malformations are common enough to present in most pediatric surgical practices. The developmental defects of the bronchi and lungs described here do not include those producing airway obstruction or many of the acquired lesions of the lung because both of these subjects are addressed in other chapters. The distinction between developmental malformations and acquired neonatal pulmonary lesions is often blurred. For example, cystic masses may be congenital, but when infection supervenes, the lining of the pseudostratified ciliated columnar epithelium may be destroyed, masking microscopic clues to identification. Additionally, developmental cysts may communicate with a bronchus and be misdiagnosed as a pulmonary abscess because of an air–fluid level. Because the primitive foregut is the anlage of the pulmonary system and proximal gastrointestinal (GI) tract, developmental abnormalities of the lung and GI tract are intertwined. *Congenital bronchopulmonary foregut malformations* comprise a spectrum of lesions that include anomalies such as sequestrations, foregut duplication cysts, and esophageal diverticula.[6]

CLASSIFICATION BY ORIGIN

Classification of the congenital anomalies of the tracheobronchopulmonary apparatus is extremely

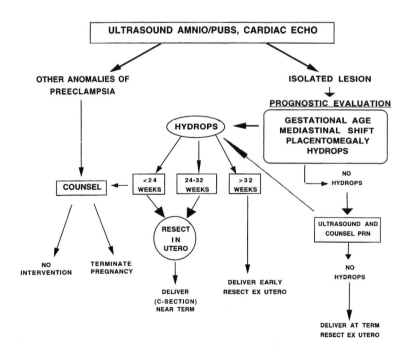

Figure 22–1. A proposed algorithm for the management of a fetus found by prenatal ultrasound to have a thoracic mass.

difficult, not only from embryologic and morphologic standpoints but also from pathologic and clinical views. Nevertheless, it is helpful to categorize the various anomalies in order to facilitate understanding of their clinical presentation and management. Table 22–1 is a list of lung anomalies according to the site of origin of the primary defect. This classification illustrates the broad spectrum of bronchopulmonary anomalies. It is important to note that complex anomalies can occur in which different developmental disorders are seen in one patient.

Pulmonary sequestration is the term applied to a pulmonary lobe or portion of a lobe that is aberrantly supplied by an anomalous artery arising from the systemic circulation and that is usually drained by anomalous veins. As an example of the anomalous nature of these lesions, they are classified under pulmonary vascular anomalies, even though

TABLE 22–1. Lung Anomalies by Site of Origin

Anomalies Derived from Developmental Disorders of the Trachea and Bronchi

Agenesis/atresia
Stenosis
Fistulas (to the esophagus or other endodermal derivatives)
Complete tracheal rings
Tracheal bronchus
Esophageal bronchus
Tracheomalacia
Bronchomalacia
Bronchial cysts
Hemangioma
Lymphangioma

Anomalies Derived from Developmental Disorders of the Pulmonary-Alveolar Parenchyma

Pulmonary agenesis (unilateral or bilateral)
Pulmonary hypoplasia (or functional immaturity at term)
Congenital pulmonary cysts
Cystic adenomatoid malformation
Congenital lobar emphysema
Pulmonary sequestration (intralobar or extralobar)
Pulmonary isomerism
Horseshoe lung

Anomalies Derived from Developmental Disorders of the Vascular Supply to the Lungs

Aberrant pulmonary arteries (e.g., vascular rings, persistent truncus arteriosus, and abnormal origin of one pulmonary artery)
Absence of one or both pulmonary arteries
Accessory arteries to the lungs (frequently associated with an accessory lobe or sequestered lung tissue)
Coarctation of the pulmonary artery
Anomalous venous drainage of the lungs
Pulmonary arteriovenous fistula
Pulmonary artery hypoplasia
Scimitar syndrome
Azygous lobe

Other Anomalies That Can Result in Pulmonary Disorders

Chest wall deformities (e.g., pectus and sternal cleft)
Phrenic nerve agenesis
Diaphragmatic hernia
Congenital chylothorax
Cardiac anomalies

they may also have a fistulous connection to the esophagus, or may contain a cystic lesion within the parenchyma. It has been proposed that sequestrations be classified into three groups: [6]
1. Without GI connection
2. With patent GI connection
3. With nonpatent GI connection

In each of the three groups, the sequestration could be intralobar or extralobar and exist with a normal diaphragm or with a diaphragmatic hernia.

We believe that such complex and cumbersome analysis is not helpful to the clinician. For that reason, this chapter provides a brief description of the embryology and a review of the most common malformations and their management with the aim of standardizing the nomenclature.

Attempts to understand these complex malformations without a clinically useful nomenclature are illustrated by this poem:

It was six men of Indostan
To learning much inclined,
Who went to see the elephant
(Though all of them were blind),
That each by observation
Might satisfy his mind.

EMBRYOLOGY

Embryologic descriptions of the lesions are addressed here only to the extent of clinical significance. Short summaries by clinicians are available,[7, 8] but a more detailed review of the significant surgical embryology of these anomalies exists.[9] Congenital lesions and other pulmonary bronchial malformations are apparently the result of abnormal development at two stages: (1) between the 3rd and 6th weeks of gestation, when the tracheal diverticulum begins as a ventral bulge from the primitive foregut at the level of the fourth somite, caudal to the pharyngeal pouches (right and left lung buds and lobar buds appear a few days later); and (2) between the 6th and 16th weeks of gestation, when rapid bronchial division beyond the subsegmental level is occurring.

CLINICAL PRESENTATION AND DIAGNOSIS

The clinical presentation of bronchopulmonary malformations is variable and dependent on several factors, such as type of malformation, size, location, communication with the airway or GI tract, and mass effect. Patients can be asymptomatic, or they may present with infection or even life-threatening respiratory failure. In many cases, unless a high index of suspicion is present, the diagnosis can be missed.

The process of diagnosis of a neonate with any degree of respiratory distress should begin with a screening chest radiograph to evaluate for the presence of an anatomic (congenital) anomaly of the lungs. Infants and children who have recurrent pulmonary infections should also be evaluated with anteroposterior and lateral chest radiographs. If an abnormality is identified, contrast esophagography, US, or computed tomography (CT) may be helpful in further defining the lesion. Occasionally, magnetic resonance imaging, angiography, or bronchoscopy may be helpful. The following is a discussion of the most common lesions.

□ Cystic Malformations

Congenital *bronchogenic cysts* can be centrally located near the pulmonary hilum or mediastinum, or they may be peripheral in location. They arise as a result of small groups of parenchymal cells that have become isolated during budding and branching to form a discrete mass of nonfunctioning pulmonary tissue. Central cysts are of early embryonic origin. They are usually solitary and asymptomatic until infection produces hemoptysis, fever, cough, or purulent secretions. These lesions are spherical and may be air filled if they communicate with the airway. If there is no communication, these cysts appear on chest radiographs as solid masses. They may be intimately related to the esophagus. Air and fluid together may be seen by air–fluid levels (Fig. 22–2A, B).

Treatment consists of simple excision. Knowledge of the natural history of these lesions justifies surgical excision even when the patient is asymptomatic. Just as thyroglossal duct cysts and preauricular cysts become infected, so may these pulmonary cysts. If bronchial communication exists, rapid enlargement of a tension cyst may produce sudden respiratory distress and may even resemble pneumothorax. Reports of malignancies arising in these congenital cysts strengthen the recommendation for their excision.[10, 11]

Peripheral *pulmonary cysts* are the result of developmental abnormalities in the 6th to 16th week of gestation and, in contrast to the central cyst, may be multiple and extensive. With multiple cysts, respiratory distress and even death may occur shortly after birth. Bronchial communication is more common with peripheral cysts. Air–fluid levels usually result from infection. The differential diagnosis includes CCAM and CDH. A chest radiograph may be the only diagnostic study necessary, especially if there is only one air–fluid level present within the mass. A congenital lung cyst, distended only with air, may be confused with congenital lobar emphysema or tension pneumothorax. Usually, delayed presentation excludes CDH from serious consideration. Compressed lung, either at the apex or base, should suggest the congenital lung cyst. In the patient with a pneumothorax, the costophrenic angle is sharp and well defined, whereas lung compressed by a cyst is seen by a meniscus in the costophrenic sulcus. Even though lobar emphysema, tension cysts, and large cystic adenomatoid malformations are sometimes clinically or radiographically indistinguishable, all require surgical correction on an urgent basis. Usually, complete removal of the abnormality can be accomplished by lobectomy.

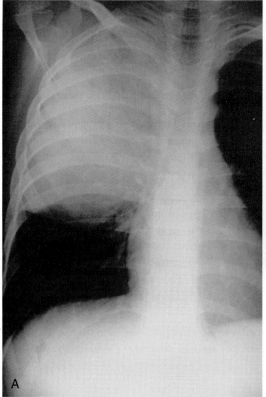

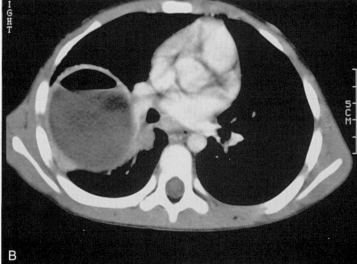

Figure 22–2. *A,* A chest radiograph of a 10-year-old child with a right upper lobe infiltrate. *B,* A chest computed tomography scan demonstrates a large bronchogenic cyst with an air–fluid level indicating bronchial communication.

The First approached the elephant,
And, happening to fall
Against his broad and sturdy side,
At once began to bawl:
"God bless me! But the elephant
Is nothing but a wall!"

CONGENITAL CYSTIC ADENOMATOID MALFORMATION

A CCAM is a multicystic mass of pulmonary tissue in which there is a proliferation of bronchial structures at the expense of alveoli. The cysts are lined by cuboidal or columnar epithelium. This disease is considered a focal pulmonary dysplasia rather than a hamartoma, although in many cases there is skeletal muscle in the cyst walls.[12] The essential feature of this disease is an overgrowth of bronchioles with almost complete suppression of alveolar development. Usually, only a single lobe is affected. The anomaly produces a multicystic rubbery malformation that becomes larger because of air and fluid trapping. The clinical picture is one of respiratory distress caused by overdistention of the involved lobe, with resulting shift of the mediastinal structures to the noninvolved side and compression of the normal lung. Anasarca, hydramnios, and even fetal death may occur.

This malformation has been subdivided into three types by its pathologic characteristics.[13] Type I includes single or multiple cysts that are more than 2 cm in diameter and that are lined by ciliated pseudostratified columnar epithelium. Structures resembling normal alveoli may lie between the cysts (Fig. 22–3A, B). Type II consists of multiple small cysts less than 1 cm in diameter that are lined by ciliated cuboidal to columnar epithelium. Respiratory bronchioles and distended alveoli may be present between these cysts, and mucous cells and cartilage are absent. This type is frequently associated with other congenital anomalies. Type III includes large and noncystic malformations that usually produce mediastinal shift. "Bronchiole-like structures are lined by ciliated cuboidal epithelium and separated by masses of alveolus-size structures lined by nonciliated cuboidal epithelium"[13] (Fig. 22–4). Few patients survive this lesion or its associated anomalies.

Types II and III may be associated with respiratory distress in the newborn period.[14] Type I, however, may appear as an asymptomatic multicystic lesion. It is important to recognize this malformation because there is a tendency for subsequent infection with life-threatening complications. CT may help differentiate these lesions.[15] In uninfected malformations, CT shows multilocular cystic masses with thin walls. Infected lesions appear complex, with a mixture of solid and cystic tissue and with variable definition of margins (Fig. 22–5A, B).

Prenatal US can distinguish individual cysts in macrocystic (type I) CCAM, whereas microcystic lesions usually have the appearance of an echogenic solid lung mass. Large cystic adenomatoid malformations frequently lead to fetal death from the development of hydrops, hypoplasia of normal lung (caused by prolonged compression in utero), and cardiac and caval compression. Thoracentesis with aspiration of the large cystic lesion in utero has been reported with very limited success. Fetal surgery with pulmonary lobectomy in utero has been successful in a few infants, allowing compensatory lung growth for the remaining lung and near-normal pulmonary function after birth.[16]

Advances in prenatal US have allowed detection of fetal pulmonary anomalies such as CCAM as early as the 12th to 14th week of intrauterine life, and careful follow-up in a few cases has demonstrated spontaneous regression. The exact mechanism by which some cystic lesions continue to grow and result in fetal death whereas others regress to complete disappearance is not known. However, it illus-

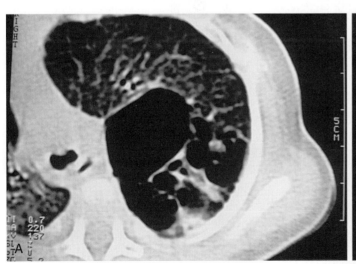 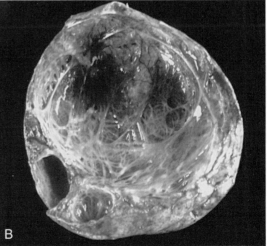

Figure 22–3. *A,* A computed tomography scan of an infant's chest demonstrating large cystic changes in the left lower lobe. *B,* A resected right lower lobe with cysts suggestive of a type I congenital cystic adenomatoid malformation.

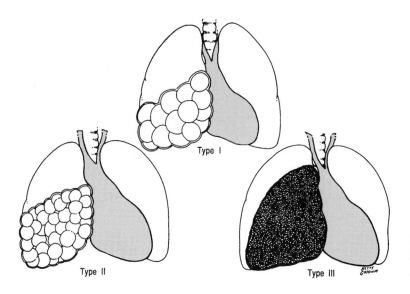

Figure 22–4. The three types of cystic adenomatoid malformation, as classically described, are showing. Detailed descriptions of the lesion are better than type classification.

trates the complex nature of these anomalies and the importance of careful monitoring when they are detected in utero.

The presence of a CCAM is an indication for surgical removal, even if the patient is asymptomatic. The treatment of choice is an anatomic lobectomy, with removal of the entire lobe containing the anomaly. However, the availability of pulmonary stapling has allowed partial lobectomy without regard to segmental planes, resulting in more conservative resection. Occasionally, an entire lung may be involved and a total pneumonectomy must be performed. The mortality in such cases is very high, and consideration may be given in selected cases to lung transplantation as a lifesaving treatment.

It is now recognized that lung hypoplasia and pulmonary hypertension can occur in neonates with large lesions. Despite successful surgical removal of the anomaly, shunting and respiratory failure may result. Such patients can be treated with extracor-

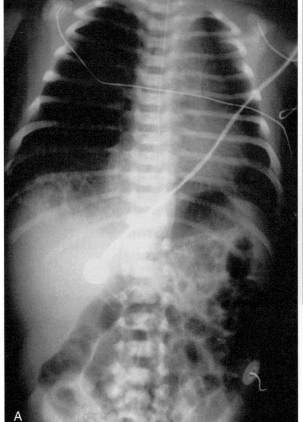

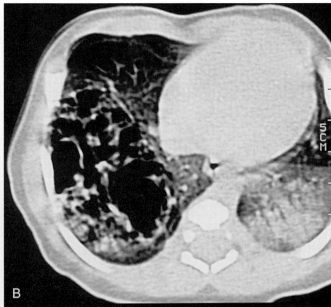

Figure 22–5. *A,* A chest radiograph of a neonate with mild respiratory distress and oxygen requirement; note the small cystic appearance of the right lower lung field overlying the diaphragm and the shifting of the mediastinum to the left. *B,* A chest computed tomography scan demonstrates multiple small and larger cysts suggestive of a type II congenital cystic adenomatoid malformation of the right lower lobe.

poreal membrane oxygenation (ECMO). A review of the Extracorporeal Life Support Organization (ELSO) Registry data from 1990 to 1997 showed that of 20 neonates with CCAM treated with ECMO, 65% required bypass after successful resection of the pulmonary lesion. There were no deaths while patients were on ECMO, but overall mortality was 25%, independent of the timing of surgical excision of the CCAM (i.e., before or after ECMO).[17]

As with any neonate with respiratory failure, the indication for ECMO in patients with CCAM should be based on the severity of the pulmonary hypertension. The mainstay of treatment remains surgical resection. However, it is important to remember that worsening of respiratory failure may follow operation for CCAM.

□ Emphysematous Lesions

CONGENITAL LOBAR EMPHYSEMA

Although described as congenital, congenital lobar emphysema (CLE) is actually postnatal overdistention of one or more lobes of a histologically normal lung, thought to result from cartilaginous deficiency in the tracheobronchial tree.[12] Other definitions include alveolar or bronchial abnormality with overdistention of one or more lobes. This condition may be caused by bronchomalacia producing check valve obstruction and air trapping within a normal-appearing lobe.[18] Pathologic studies have indicated that this condition is a symptom complex with many possible causes.[19] The obstruction causing emphysema can be the result of (1) collapse of bronchi on expiration, a form of chondromalacia that is limited to one or a few bronchi; (2) extrinsic pressure of an anomalous pulmonary artery or vein or by an abnormally large ductus arteriosus; or (3) idiopathic causes. As a rule, one third of reported cases fall into each group.[9] This lesion may also be acquired as more and more low birth weight infants undergo ventilation for long periods of time. Various forms of lobar distention may be noted with or without interstitial emphysema and bronchopulmonary dysplasia.

In CLE, the affected portion of the lung is dilated

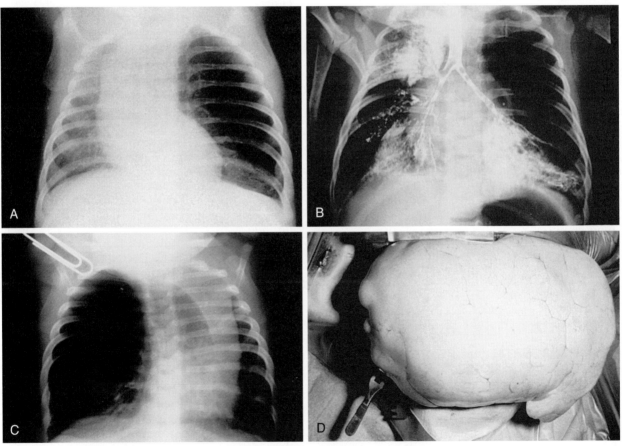

Figure 22–6. *A,* A chest radiograph of a newborn with respiratory distress. Note the overdistention (with air) of the left upper lobe with shifting of the mediastinum to the right and flattening of the left diaphragm; this must be distinguished from a tension pneumothorax. *B,* Bronchograms demonstrating the absent (or occluded) left upper lobe bronchus with compression of the left lower lobe, consistent with congenital lobar emphysema. *C,* A chest radiograph of another infant with right upper lobe emphysema. *D,* An operative view of the massively distended (emphysematous) lobe; lobectomy is difficult owing to the anatomic distortion created by the affected lobe.

to many times its actual size. The normal lobes are compressed, and the mediastinum is shifted away from the affected side (Fig. 22–6A–D). Bilateral involvement may occur but is rare. The left upper lobe is more commonly involved (47%), followed by the right middle and upper lobes (28% and 20%, respectively). Involvement of the lower lobes is unusual (less than 5%).

Diagnosis is usually not difficult by plain chest radiography, but CT and ventilation/perfusion (V/P) findings may be helpful in determining whether surgical resection would be tolerated.[20] When emphysema appears to be congenital with no evidence of other pulmonary disease, surgical lobectomy is indicated. Conservative treatment of CLE is useless and will result in progressive worsening because of compression of the normal lobes. Associated cardiac anomalies are frequent.[21] CLE may require urgent operation. In the acquired forms of lobar emphysema, nonoperative management may allow spontaneous resolution. The patient is usually in the neonatal intensive care unit and often is on a ventilator, permitting close monitoring. Selective bronchial intubation may isolate the affected lung, thereby hastening resolution.

Neonates who have CLE, usually from an idiopathic bronchial obstruction (or agenesis), can have a dramatic presentation with overdistention of the affected lobe and severe respiratory failure from lung tissue compression. The clinical and radiographic appearance mimics a tension pneumothorax. Placement of a chest tube into the emphysematous lobe can have catastrophic results. Immediate thoracotomy with lobectomy is usually lifesaving. Children may present with chronic symptoms such as dyspnea on exertion and difficulty with competitive sports. Symptoms typically worsen with rapid breathing and exertion. In cases of CLE, resection of the abnormal lobe allows normal pulmonary tissue expansion, and children show complete resolution of their symptoms.

> *The Second, feeling of the tusk,*
> *Cried: "Ho! What have we here*
> *So very round and smooth and sharp?*
> *To me 'tis mighty clear*
> *This wonder of an elephant*
> *Is very like a spear!"*

ACQUIRED NEONATAL EMPHYSEMATOUS LESIONS

Respirator therapy, particularly in premature infants, often results in interstitial emphysema, lobar emphysema, and pulmonary parenchymal cysts. These radiographic and clinical disorders may resolve spontaneously. Mediastinal shift, or compression of the surrounding normal lung, may require surgical intervention. Differentiation from congenital malformations is not difficult, because these acquired lesions occur postnatally in conjunction with ventilatory therapy (Fig. 22–7).

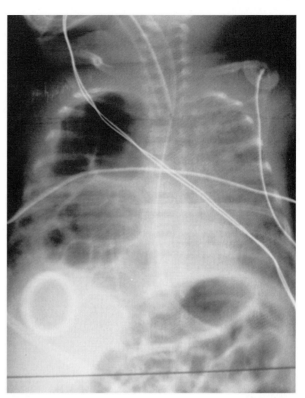

Figure 22–7. *A,* A chest radiograph of an infant with severe respiratory failure, pneumonia, and chronic changes of bronchopulmonary dysplasia. Note the cystic appearance in the right lower lung. This represents acquired pulmonary pseudocysts, and surgical excision is not indicated.

Posttraumatic pulmonary cysts may appear after pulmonary contusion or parenchymal or bronchial disruption. The lesions can be differentiated from congenital malformations because they appear after trauma in an area of pulmonary contusion. The preferred terminology for these lesions is *traumatic pulmonary pseudocysts* because the cysts do not have an epithelial lining.[22] The pathogenesis has been demonstrated experimentally to depend on airway injury, with the cystic lesions produced by the pressure of inflation and elastic recoil of the lung parenchyma.[23] If the patients with these lesions are asymptomatic and the lesions do not enlarge or produce respiratory distress, they can be observed and spontaneous resolution usually occurs. Rarely, if infection supervenes, external drainage and/or surgical excision may be required.[24]

Postinfectious pulmonary cysts (pneumatoceles) occur frequently after *Staphylococcus aureus* pneumonia. Although pneumatoceles are not the focus of this chapter, the distinction between a pneumatocele and a congenital cyst is important. With pneumatocele, there is a history of pulmonary infection with pneumonic consolidation. Subsequently, a cavitary lesion appears with a thin or nonexistent wall. Usually, the cavities contain only air (Fig. 22–8,A–D). Most regress spontaneously.

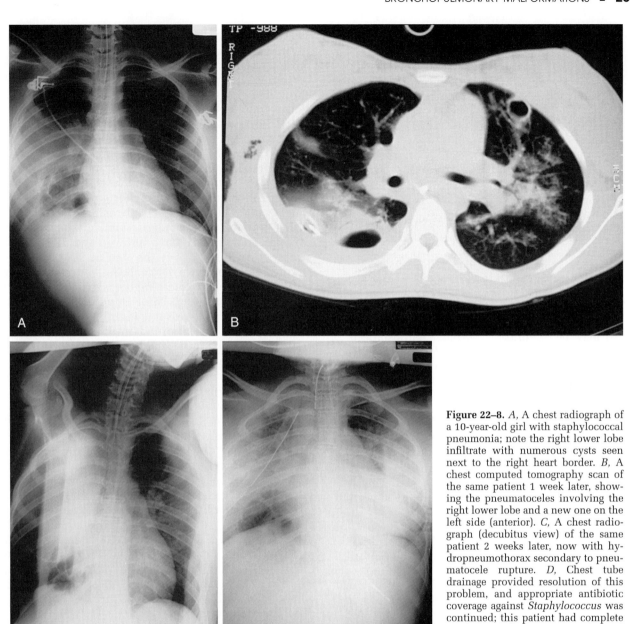

Figure 22–8. *A,* A chest radiograph of a 10-year-old girl with staphylococcal pneumonia; note the right lower lobe infiltrate with numerous cysts seen next to the right heart border. *B,* A chest computed tomography scan of the same patient 1 week later, showing the pneumatoceles involving the right lower lobe and a new one on the left side (anterior). *C,* A chest radiograph (decubitus view) of the same patient 2 weeks later, now with hydropneumothorax secondary to pneumatocele rupture. *D,* Chest tube drainage provided resolution of this problem, and appropriate antibiotic coverage against *Staphylococcus* was continued; this patient had complete resolution of the pneumonia and pneumatoceles 4 weeks after initiation of therapy.

The Third approached the animal,
And, happening to take
The squirming trunk within his hands,
Thus boldly up and spake:
"I see," quoth he, "the elephant
Is very like a snake!"

☐ Solid Bronchopulmonary Malformations

These lesions are usually irregular, not spherical, on chest radiographs. Symptoms depend on the amount of pulmonary involvement.

Pulmonary sequestration is seen as a cystic mass of nonfunctioning lung tissue that lacks an obvious communication with the tracheobronchial tree and that receives all or most of its arterial blood from the systemic circulation.[12, 25] Every conceivable combination of systemic and pulmonary arterial supply and venous drainage and of normal and abnormal pulmonary tissue has been reported in this spectrum of malformations.[26] Normal lung can be supplied by a vessel of systemic origin, and abnormal pulmonary tissue similar to that found in sequestration can exist without an anomalous blood supply.[8] Numerous case reports attest to the myriad combinations of abnormalities, including bronchogenic cysts.[27–29] As a rule, sequestrations are classified under pulmonary vascular disorders, mainly due to the observation of some form of abnormal blood supply. Although most symptoms are respiratory,

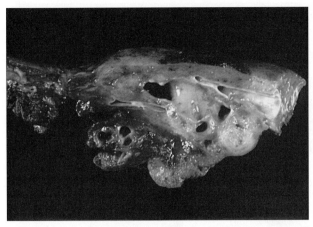

Figure 22–9. Gross appearance of a resected pulmonary lobe with sequestration of lung tissue. Note the purulent material and the chronic inflammatory changes that developed secondary to recurrent infections. Lobectomy was curative.

there may be significant cardiac manifestations of the sequestration complex, not only from the associated congenital heart defects but also from the large shunts that may develop.[30]

The communication between the sequestration and the airway is frequently absent or abnormal. Thus, infectious pulmonary symptoms are common in this nonfunctioning pulmonary tissue (Fig. 22–9). Indeed, children with unexplained recurrent pneumonias must be suspected of having sequestration, and appropriate investigation is indicated. Chest CT scan usually demonstrates the pulmonary abnormality.

Sequestrations are classified as *intralobar*, in which the abnormal tissue is contained within the normal lung, and *extralobar*, in which the sequestration is separate from the normal pulmonary lobe and outside the visceral pleura (Fig. 22–10). A malformation termed *pseudosequestration* has also been described.[31]

Intralobar sequestration is predominantly found in the lower lobes, most commonly on the left and in the posterior basilar segment. The radiographic findings range from opacification to a cystic parenchymal lesion with air fluid levels. Most often, the abnormal vascular supply is a large vessel arising from the aorta below the diaphragm. Frequently, more than one vessel supplies the sequestration, and venous drainage is via the pulmonary vein. Occasionally, the sequestration is drained to the azygos system.

A persistent mass in the lower lobe is suspicious (Fig. 22–11A–C). Angiography was considered necessary for the definitive diagnosis of pulmonary sequestration, but recent advances in US, CT with three-dimensional reconstruction, and magnetic resonance angiography have allowed the diagnosis of this condition without the use of invasive techniques. US is a noninvasive, bedside procedure, relatively inexpensive and highly sensitive and specific, particularly with color Doppler flow analysis. Once the abnormal vessel is identified, the operative resection can be planned and performed more safely. Most operative deaths have been caused by hemorrhage, when the abnormal arterial feeders were not controlled. Treatment is by lobectomy of the involved lobe, although a small percentage can be managed by segmentectomy.

Extralobar sequestration is separated from the lung by its investing pleura. It may occur in the upper thorax, the lower thorax, or the abdomen. Diagnosis is confirmed by the methods described for intralobar lesions. Usually, extralobar sequestration is asymptomatic and is discovered by accident. An asymptomatic, uninfected extralobar sequestration without cardiovascular manifestations may be simply observed. There is not usually a communication with the airway or with adjacent lung tissue. However, infection may occur by hematogenous spread of bacteria. Extralobar sequestration has been associated with other abnormalities, especially diaphragmatic hernia.[26, 28]

A condition has been described in three children in whom a diaphragmatic defect with herniation of a portion of the liver resembled the radiographic appearance of sequestration.[31] When lower lobe lesions on the right are found, radioisotope scanning of the liver or peritoneography may be helpful in delineating this abnormality, which does not require surgical repair.

Apical accessory lobe, or "tracheal lobe," is a rare form of extralobar sequestration in which the blood supply usually comes from the subclavian artery. There may be a bronchus arising directly from the trachea, hence the term *tracheal lobe.* The most common type of extralobar sequestration is the lower accessory lobe, or "Rokitansky lobe," which occurs predominantly on the left side and whose blood supply arises from the aorta. Occasionally, an abnormal bronchial communication with the esophagus, stomach, or tracheobronchial tree may be present (Fig. 22–12).

Abdominal accessory lobe indicates the presence

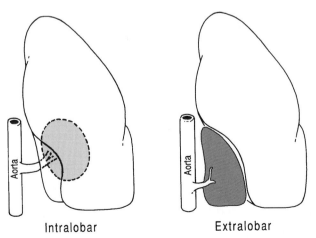

Intralobar   Extralobar

Figure 22–10. Pulmonary sequestration is illustrated. It occurs either within the lung or outside the visceral pleura.

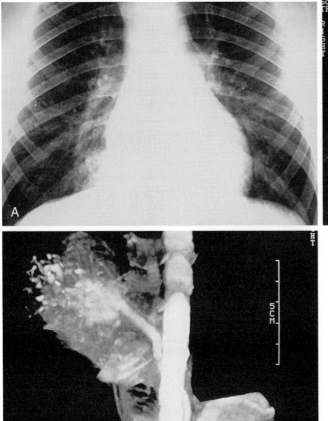

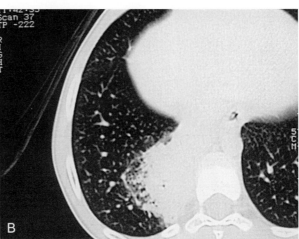

Figure 22–11. *A,* A chest radiograph of a 4-year-old child with a history of recurrent pneumonias and a right lower lobe infiltrate next to the right heart shadow. *B,* A chest computed tomography scan confirms the presence of an infiltrate in the right posterior lower lobe. *C,* Three-dimensional computed tomography scan reconstruction shows an abnormal blood vessel arising from the abdominal aorta and crossing the diaphragm to the right lower lobe.

of lung tissue below the diaphragm and is extremely rare.

> *The Fourth reached out his eager hand,*
> *And felt about the knee:*
> *"What most this wondrous beast is like*
> *Is mighty plain," quoth he;*
> *"Tis clear enough the elephant*
> *Is very like a tree."*

About half of the patients with pulmonary arteriovenous malformation (AVM) present with symptoms. The classic triad includes dyspnea on exertion, cyanosis, and clubbing of the fingers. The cyanosis occurs when at least 30% of the right ventricular output passes through the fistula without oxygenation, creating a right-to-left shunt. Clinically, a continuous murmur or bruit over the lesion may be found. Cerebrovascular symptoms may occur, and brain abscess is encountered as frequently with this condition as with congenital heart disease. The location of the malformation near the pleura can lead to hemothorax. Rupture into a bronchus produces massive hemoptysis. Radiographically, these malformations appear as round or oval, somewhat lobulated, masses of various sizes. CT of the chest demonstrates abnormal vessels, but angiography is definitive. There is a high incidence of patients with Osler-Weber-Rendu disease.[8] The malformations may also be multiple.

Treatment has been entirely by surgical resection; either lobectomy or wedge resection of the involved portion of the lung. Success in occluding the malformations using catheter embolization has been reported.[32]

Under the general category of arteriovenous malformation, a condition variously labeled *scimitar syndrome, hypogenetic lung syndrome,* and *congenital venolobar syndrome* is included. Although the term *scimitar syndrome* is short and nondescriptive, it is probably the one most commonly used. This syndrome consists of a small malformed right lung, anomalous venous return from the lung into the inferior vena cava (a left-to-right shunt), and abnormal arterial supply commonly from the systemic circulation.[8] As in many of the malformations described, a good embryologic explanation is lacking. The right lung is always malformed to some degree. The venous drainage classically appears on pulmonary radiographs as a sickle-shaped (scimitar-like) shadow in the medial aspect of the right lower lung. However, the typical appearance is seen in only one third of cases. Sometimes, the anomalous vein is small. The arterial supply to the right lung may be provided by the pulmonary or by the systemic circulation. A pulmonary artery may be absent or hypoplastic, and systemic supply may be derived from the thoracic aorta or even from below the dia-

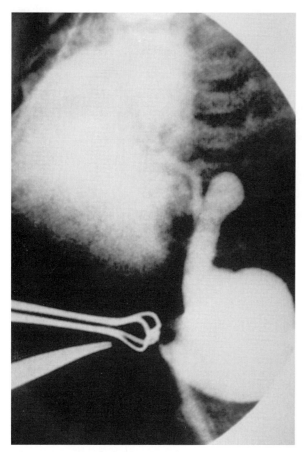

Figure 22–12. Contrast study of a neonate with esophageal atresia, pulmonary sequestration, and an abnormal communication between the distal esophagus and the sequestrated lobe.

phragm. Approximately one fourth of patients have associated cardiovascular anomalies.[8]

Radiographically, a small right hemithorax with a high right hemidiaphragm is combined with the scimitar shadow described earlier. Cardiac catheterization and angiography help to make the definitive diagnosis and to establish the abnormal arterial and venous pattern. Treatment depends on the abnormality. In the classic case, the anomalous venous drainage can be redirected to the left atrium. A pneumonectomy may be required.

The Fifth, who chanced to touch the ear,
Said: "E'en the blindest man
Can tell what this resembles most;
Deny the fact who can,
This marvel of an elephant
Is very like a fan!"

□ Miscellaneous Malformations

Unilateral agenesis of the lung is compatible with life. It may be associated with severe congenital anomalies such as those in the VATER (vertebral defects, imperforate anus, tracheoesophageal fistula, and radial and renal dysplasia) complex.[33–35] Other anomalies are common. Attempts have been made to implicate neural crest injuries in this developmental defect.[36]

Bilateral agenesis of the lungs is not compatible with life (Fig. 22–13). Agenetic lesions involve both airway and parenchymal failure of development. Aplasia is the incomplete development of the lung supplied by a rudimentary bronchus, and hypoplasia is the underdevelopment of the lung supplied by an essentially normal bronchus.[37]

It is important to note that pulmonary hypoplasia is the most common of these abnormalities. Hypoplasia may result from (1) the compression effect from an intrathoracic mass (such as CCAM, CDH, or sequestration) or an extrathoracic mass, (2) abnormal or absent fetal breathing movements (phrenic nerve abnormality), (3) decreased blood flow to the lungs, (4) primary mesodermal defect, and (5) unknown or idiopathic causes. Table 22–2 illustrates anomalies commonly associated with pulmonary hypoplasia.

The diagnosis is usually not difficult to make, but the condition may be confused with atelectasis when the opacified hemithorax is discovered late and no early chest films are available. When the right lung is absent, the heart is rotated in a clockwise direction with apparent dextrocardia. The chest on the affected side is flattened, with impaired inspiratory movement. Asymmetry of the thorax, with or without scoliosis, is a common but by no means universal finding. The correct diagnosis is

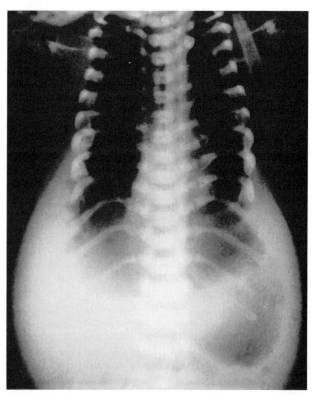

Figure 22–13. Bilateral severe pulmonary hypoplasia. Note the poorly developed chest and lung fields compared with the abdomen. This patient died shortly after birth owing to severe respiratory failure.

TABLE 22-2. Anomalies Associated
with Pulmonary Hypoplasia*

Frequent

Diaphragmatic hernia
Renal agenesis (bilateral)
Renal dysgenesis (bilateral)
Obstructive uropathy
Renal polycystic disease

Unusual

Diaphragmatic hypoplasia or eventration
Extralobar pulmonary sequestration
Hemolytic disease
Musculoskeletal abnormalities (e.g., thoracic dystrophies)
Oligohydramnios caused by prolonged amniotic fluid leakage
Chromosomal disruption, including trisomy 13, 18, and 21
Anencephaly
Scimitar syndrome

Rare

Pleural effusion
Ascites secondary to congenital infection
Thoracic neuroblastoma
Phrenic nerve agenesis
Right-sided cardiovascular malformation as with hypoplastic
  right ventricle
Gastroschisis
Upper cervical spinal cord injury
Laryngotracheoesophageal cleft

*Adapted from Stocker JT. In Dail DH, Hammar SP (eds): Pulmonary Pathology. New York, Springer-Verlag, 1988, 41–71.

rarely made on the basis of history and physical findings alone.

Treatment, of course, can be directed only toward associated anomalies, such as esophageal atresia and tracheoesophageal fistula. The prime goal in management is preservation of respiratory units. Some surgeons have advocated primary repair of the tracheoesophageal lesion,[38] whereas others would stage the repair.[39] In order to eliminate mediastinal displacement with twisting of the trachea and blood vessels, a tissue expander can be placed in the empty pleural cavity or in the extrapleural space.

□ Lobulation Anomalies

There is significant variation in the normal lung lobulation and a brief review is presented here. Three groups are used for classification purposes.

Group I—Variations of external fissures without abnormalities of bronchial branching. They are of no clinical significance. Examples include (1) cardiac lobe (separation of the left lower lobe into two), (2) dorsal lobe (superior segmentation of either the right or left lower lobes), and (3) absent fissures (the fissure between the upper and lower lobes on either side is absent in 30% of individuals, and the fissure between the upper and middle right lobes is incomplete in 56% and absent in 21%). Absence of fissures

does not indicate an alteration of the basic lobular anatomy.

Group II—Azygous lobe is not a true pulmonary lobe but a malformation of the upper lobe that occurs as a result of the aberrant azygous vein being suspended by a mesentery of pleura. It typically occurs in the apical portion of the right upper lobe. It is estimated to occur in 0.5% of the normal population.

Group III—Variations of the bronchial pattern with or without external evidence of an abnormal fissure. Rare examples include tracheal lobe, in which a segment of pulmonary tissue connects directly to the trachea without a separate blood supply, and lung duplication with separate pleural cavities. Occasionally, these patients have symptoms related to chronic infection of this lung tissue.

Pulmonary isomerism is a reversal of the normal anatomic pattern in which the right lung has two lobes and the left lobe has three. It may or may not be associated with situs inversus. Occasionally, both lungs have three lobes. The importance of this finding is that it may be associated with anomalies of the spleen and anomalous pulmonary venous return. Asplenia or polysplenia may be seen with trilobed left lung.[9]

> The Sixth no sooner had begun
> About the beast to grope,
> Then, seizing on the swinging tail
> That fell within his scope,
> "I see," quoth he, "The elephant
> Is very like a rope!"

Mesenchymal cystic hamartoma was described as a new entity in 1986. It may appear as a single cyst or as multiple bilateral nodules. The distinguishing pathologic features have been described as follows.[40]

1. Nodules less than 1 cm in diameter that are composed of primitive mesenchymal cells subdivided by a plexus of abnormally branching airways.
2. Cystic nodules between 0.5 and 1 cm in diameter that have a cambium layer of primitive mesenchymal cells and a lining of normal or metaplastic respiratory epithelium.
3. Hypertrophic systemic arteries within the walls of the cysts.

The lesions are often multicentric, and the disease follows an indolent course. Nodules occur with proliferation of mesenchymal cells and gradual transformation into cysts. Pulmonary hemorrhage, pneumothorax, or malignant transformation may result.[11]

Treatment is directed toward complications; excision of nodules is performed for diagnostic reasons. "The possible benefit of resecting nodules and cysts to preclude malignant transformation must be weighed against the multicentric nature of mesenchymal cystic hamartoma of the lung and its benign course in most patients."[40]

And so these men of Indostan
Disputed loud and long,
Each in his own opinion
Exceeding stiff and strong,
Though each was partly in the right,
And all were in the wrong!
So, oft in theologic wars
The disputants, I ween,
Rail on in utter ignorance
Of what each other mean,
And prate about an elephant
Not one of them has seen!

JOHN GODFREY SAXE

REFERENCES

1. Othersen HB: Pulmonary and bronchial malformations. In Ashcraft KW, Holder TM (eds): Pediatric Surgery (2nd ed). Philadelphia, WB Saunders, 1992, pp 176–187.
2. MacGillivray TE, Harrison MR, Goldstein RB, Adzick NS: Disappearing fetal lung lesions. J Pediatr Surg 28:1321–1325, 1993.
3. Budorick NE, Pretorius DM, Leopold GR, Stamm ER: Spontaneous improvement of intrathoracic masses diagnosed in utero. J Ultrasound Med 11:653–662, 1992.
4. King SJ, Pulling DW, Walkinshaw S: Fetal echogenic lung lesions: Prenatal ultrasound diagnosis and outcome. Pediatr Radiol 25:208–210, 1995.
5. Bullard KM, Harrison MR: Before the horse is out of the barn: Fetal surgery for hydrops. Semin Perinatol 19:462–473, 1995.
6. Gerle RD, Jaretzki A, Ashley CA, et al: Congenital bronchopulmonary-foregut malformation. N Engl J Med 278:1413–1419, 1968.
7. Shamji FM, Sachs HJ, Perkins DG: Cystic disease of the lungs. Surg Clin North Am 68:581–620, 1988.
8. Heitzman ER: Embryology of the lung and pulmonary abnormalities of developmental origin. In Heitzman ER (ed): The Lung: Radiologic-Pathologic Correlations (2nd ed). St. Louis, CV Mosby, 1984.
9. Skandalakis JE, Gray SW (eds): Embryology for Surgeons (2nd ed). Baltimore, Williams & Wilkins, 1994.
10. Sharif S, Thomas JA, Shetty N, et al: Primary pulmonary rhabdomyosarcoma in a child, with a review of literature. J Surg Oncol 38:261–264, 1988.
11. Hedland GL, Bisset GS, Bove KE: Malignant neoplasms arising in cystic hamartomas of the lung in childhood. Radiology 173:77–80, 1989.
12. Buntain WL, Isaacs H, Payne VC, et al: Lobar emphysema, cystic adenomatoid malformation, pulmonary sequestration, and bronchogenic cyst in infancy and childhood. J Pediatr Surg 9:85–93, 1974.
13. Stocker JT, Madewell JE, Drake RM: Congenital cystic adenomatoid malformation of the lung. Hum Pathol 8:155–171, 1977.
14. Gwinn JL, Barnes GR, Kaufman HJ: Radiological case of the month—cystic adenomatoid malformation of the upper lobe of the right lung. Am J Dis Child 112:61–62, 1966.
15. Shackelford GD, Siegel MJ: CT appearance of cystic adenomatoid malformations. J Comput Assist Tomogr 13:612–616, 1989.
16. Adzick NS, Harrison MR: The unborn surgical patient. Curr Probl Surg 31:9, 1994.
17. Hebra A, Nijimbaum C, Purhoit D, et al: The management of congenital cystic adenomatoid malformation of the lung in the ECMO era. J Pediatr Surg: in press.
18. Hendren WH, McKee D: Lobar emphysema of infancy. J Pediatr Surg 1:24–39, 1966.
19. Henderson R, Hislop A, Reid L: New pathological findings in emphysema of childhood. Thorax 26:195–205, 1971.
20. Markowitz RI, Mercurio MR, Vahjen GA, et al: Congenital lobar emphysema. Clin Pediatr 28:19–23, 1989.
21. Jones HC, Almond CH, Snyder HM, et al: Lobar emphysema and congenital heart disease in infancy. J Thorac Cardiovasc Surg 49:1, 1965.
22. Co ML, Rosner IK, Berkmen YM, et al: Radiological case of the month—traumatic pulmonary pseudocyst. Am J Dis Child 143:841–842, 1989.
23. Moolten SE: Mechanical production of cavities in isolated lungs. Arch Pathol Lab Med 19:825–832, 1935.
24. Kato R, Horinouchi H, Maenaka Y: Traumatic pulmonary pseudocyst. J Thorac Cardiovasc Surg 97:309–312, 1989.
25. Buntain WL, Woolley MM, Mahour GH, et al: Pulmonary sequestration in children: A 25-year experience. Surgery 81:413–420, 1977.
26. Sade RM, Clouse M, Ellis FH: The spectrum of pulmonary sequestration. Ann Thorac Surg 18:644–658, 1974.
27. Savic B, Birtel FJ, Tholen W: Lung sequestration: Report of seven cases and review of 540 published cases. Thorax 34:96–101, 1979.
28. Black TL, Fernandes ET, Wrenn EL, et al: Extralobar pulmonary sequestration and mediastinal bronchogenic cyst. J Pediatr Surg 23:999–1001, 1988.
29. Gupta SK, Abraham KA, Ganesh KM: Intralobar sequestration of upper lobe of right lung—case reports. Angiology 39:1056–1060, 1988.
30. White JJ, Donahoo JS, Ostrow PT, et al: Cardiovascular and respiratory manifestations of pulmonary sequestration in childhood. Ann Thorac Surg 18:286–294, 1974.
31. Macpherson RI, Whitehead L: Pseudosequestration. J Can Assoc Radiol 28:17–25, 1977.
32. Taylor BG, Cockerill EM, Manfredi F, Klatte EC: Therapeutic embolization of the pulmonary artery in pulmonary arteriovenous fistula. Am J Med 64:360–365, 1978.
33. Knowles S, Thomas RM, Lindenbaum RH, et al: Pulmonary agenesis as part of the VACTERL sequence. Arch Dis Child 63:723–726, 1988.
34. Davies RP, Kozlowski K, Wood BP: Radiological case of the month—right upper lobe esophageal bronchus. Am J Dis Child 143:251–253, 1989.
35. Dennis WW: Correspondence. J Pediatr Surg 23:389, 1988.
36. Osborne J, Masel J, McCredie J: A spectrum of skeletal anomalies associated with pulmonary agenesis: Possible neural crest injuries. Pediatr Radiol 19:425–432, 1989.
37. Booth JB, Berry CL: Unilateral pulmonary agenesis. Arch Dis Child 42:361–374, 1967.
38. Hoffman MA, Superina R, Wesson DE: Unilateral pulmonary agenesis with esophageal atresia and distal tracheoesophageal fistula: Report of two cases. J Pediatr Surg 24:1084–1085, 1989.
39. Black PR, Welch KJ: Pulmonary agenesis (aplasia), esophageal atresia, and tracheoesophageal fistula: A different treatment strategy. J Pediatr Surg 21:936–938, 1986.
40. Mark EJ: Mesenchymal cystic hamartoma of the lung. N Engl J Med 315:1255–1259, 1986.

23

ACQUIRED PULMONARY AND PLEURAL DISORDERS

David W. Tuggle, MD

Acquired thoracic infectious diseases are less common than in previous years due to the widespread use of early and appropriate antibiotics in the outpatient setting. However, inappropriate use of antibiotics has led to an increased number of troublesome infections with resistant organisms, resulting in increased morbidity and mortality rates for diseases that were once relatively easy to treat. Increasing numbers of immunosuppressed or immunocompromised children have been accompanied by an increased incidence of diseases that formerly were only rarely seen. An increase in tuberculosis in adults has been followed by a similar increase of the disease in children exposed to these infected adults. These changes in the patterns of thoracic diseases in children necessitates that the surgeon who treats such illnesses in children be aware of the therapeutic options.

☐ Empyema

Pleural empyema (empyema thoraces) is a serious reactive infection of the pleural space and is usually a complication of inflammation or infection adjacent to or within the chest. It rarely resolves spontaneously because host defenses are limited by the anatomy and physiology of the pleural space. Empyema may follow an infection of the lung, chest wall, or upper abdomen despite early antibiotic institution. Pleural fluid collections that lead to empyema are usually caused by pneumonia, but can arise from other disease processes.

PATHOGENESIS

Pleural effusion may develop owing to increased hydrostatic pressure or decreased oncotic pressure associated with cardiac, renal, hepatic, or metabolic disease. Pleural effusion may also result from alterations in pleural permeability resulting from inflammatory diseases, infection, toxins, malignancy,

or trauma.[1] These fluid collections are a nutritionally rich culture medium in which white blood cell (WBC) defenses are at a disadvantage. WBCs, responding to the pleural infection, require a structure on which to move in order to be effective. Bacteria in the pleural fluid are at liberty to float away, avoiding phagocytosis.[2]

Empyema develops in three stages.[3] During the acute or exudative phase, the fluid is thin, has a low WBC count, a low lactate dehydrogenase level, and normal glucose and pH levels. In the transitional or fibrinopurulent phase, the fluid becomes turbid and thick with fibrin deposition, producing a "peel" with loculations of liquid within. This process limits the expansion of the lung. The WBC and lactate dehydrogenase levels increase, while the pH and glucose levels decrease. In the third phase, an organizing stage occurs with the development of a thick fibrous peel, fibroblast proliferation, and scar formation that entraps the lung.

The death of leukocytes in the pleural effusion releases a host of intracellular constituents that are bactericidal or bacteriostatic. Many bacteria undergo autolysis in this empyema fluid, which accounts for those patients whose empyema cultures are sterile.[4] Many empyema-causing bacteria have a reduced susceptibility to β-lactam antibiotics, which is one reason that prolonged antibiotic therapy is required in patients with mature empyema. Early drainage of thin empyema fluid or decortication of gelatinous empyema collections reduces the need for prolonged antibiotic administration.

DIAGNOSIS

At least 60% of empyema cases are caused by a primary bacterial process in or near the lungs, such as pneumonia.[5] Other causes include infections in the neck, chest wall, thoracic spine, or mediastinal nodes. Postoperative empyema following surgery of the esophagus, lung, or mediastinum accounts for 20% of cases. Pneumonectomy is the procedure most likely to be associated with empyema, accounting for 2 to 12% of cases.[6] Posttraumatic empyema accounts for approximately 8% of the total cases and is usually associated with penetrating trauma, hemothorax, or hemopneumothorax. Abdominal abscesses, retained airway foreign bodies, and spontaneous or iatrogenic esophageal perforation account for the remainder.

Symptoms associated with empyema often cannot be distinguished from those of the underlying disease, that is, fever, tachycardia, tachypnea, dyspnea, and a productive cough. Patients may complain of pleuritic chest pain with heaviness in the involved hemithorax and, often, they have decreased breath sounds and dullness to percussion on the involved side. Rarely, chronic empyema can erode through the chest wall and manifest as a draining sinus or abscess (empyema necessitatis), or it can erode into the airway to form a bronchopleural fistula. Other complications of empyema include anemia, osteomyelitis of the ribs or thoracic vertebrae, pericarditis, mediastinal abscesses, and disseminated infections.

Diagnosis is often made with a simple posteroanterior and lateral chest radiograph (Figs. 23–1 and 23–2). A lateral decubitus film may show fluid layering on the involved side. An empyema can often obliterate an entire hemithorax and may cause shift of the mediastinum and trachea away from the in-

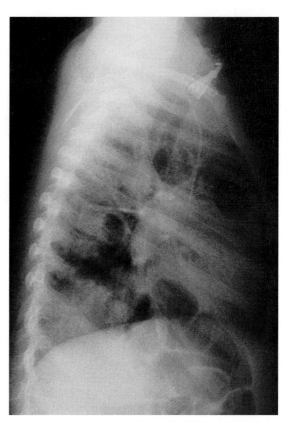

Figure 23–2. Lateral chest radiograph of the patient in Figure 23–1. There are multiple fluid collections.

volved side. The stage of empyema can be determined by using ultrasound or computed tomography (CT) scanning to identifying loculations or a thick pleural peel. CT scanning is often used to determine the difference between empyema and a lung abscess. Thoracentesis is also useful in determining the need for more definitive thoracic drainage. Empyema fluid is not commonly sterile and cultures from other sites may be needed to identify a causative organism.

THERAPY

Tube thoracostomy is effective when thin fluid collections are identified. In more advanced disease, other therapeutic options are often required. Formal thoracotomy with decortication has historically been the mainstay of treatment for late empyema, but it is often associated with significant blood loss and morbidity.[7] Earlier diagnosis and surgical intervention has led to the use of a "minithoracotomy" and, more recently, thoracoscopic decortication.[8, 9] Earlier surgery and smaller incisions have led to less patient discomfort and shorter hospital stays.

Fibrinolytic treatment of empyema was first reported in 1949 using streptokinase, but it was not often used because the quality of streptokinase formulations available was poor.[10] Enthusiasm has returned with the recent introduction of new and improved fibrinolytics. Both streptokinase and uro-

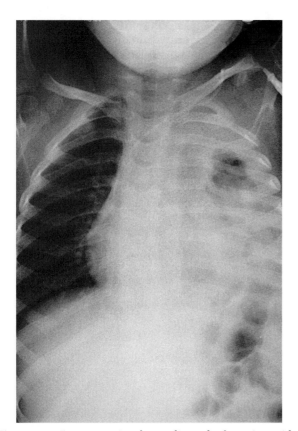

Figure 23–1. Posteroanterior chest radiograph of a patient with a multiloculated empyema of the left hemithorax. Several loculated fluid collections are noted.

kinase have been used with success in small trials and seem best suited to phase II (fibrinous) empyema cases. Streptokinase in a dose of 250,000 units in 100 ml of 0.9% saline or urokinase in a dose of 100,000 units in 100 ml of 0.9% saline may be used.[11, 12] The fluid is instilled through a chest tube and left in place with the tube clamped for 2 to 12 hours. Changing the patient's position may facilitate spread of the fibrinolytic agent. This may be repeated as often as needed, sometimes as frequently as three times per day. The typical course of treatment may last from 2 to 10 days. Little benefit from further treatment is expected when there is less than 50 ml/day chest tube drainage or when the cavity is less than 50 ml in size.

RESULTS

Lung entrapment from empyema is uncommon in the patient who receives proper and timely treatment, and pulmonary function can return to normal. The therapy should be tailored to the individual patient's needs with patient comfort and safety coming before economic considerations. Death as a result of empyema is rare. Disability from pulmonary dysfunction is an uncommon complication.

□ Pneumatocele

ETIOLOGY

A pneumatocele is a thin-walled, air-filled cyst of the lung. They are most often seen in children with *Staphylococcus aureus* pneumonia and are recognized in approximately 40% of children during the acute phase of this disease. Other pathogens that can be associated with pneumatocele formation include *Streptococcus, Haemophilus influenzae, Klebsiella, Escherichia coli,* and *Pseudomonas;* measles and tuberculosis infections are associated as well.[13]

PATHOLOGY

Pneumatoceles develop as a result of localized bronchiolar and alveolar necrosis, allowing one-way passage of air into the interstitial space and resulting in a thin-walled, air-filled intraparenchymal cyst.[14] Exotoxin released from staphylococcal organisms contributes to the extremely destructive inflammatory process. An occasional pneumatocele may compress adjacent structures, causing respiratory and cardiovascular compromise (tension pneumatocele). Pneumatocele rupture may produce a tension pneumothorax, bronchopleural fistula, or empyema.[15] A pneumatocele resulting from barotrauma can become secondarily infected. Patients being mechanically ventilated are at an increased risk of development of pneumatocele-related complications.

DIAGNOSIS

Pneumatoceles are typically diagnosed by chest radiograph. CT may provide more detail, but does not contribute to the management of an enlarging cyst. Ultrasound may also be used to evaluate a problematic or enlarging pneumatocele.[16] A pneumatocele may be confused with a pulmonary cyst. The patient's clinical course and change in the radiographic appearance over time differentiates the two conditions. Multiple pneumatoceles may be confused with a congenital diaphragmatic hernia or with congenital adenoid cystic malformation of the lung.

THERAPY

Most pneumatoceles require no treatment, although a rapidly enlarging pneumatocele may require urgent decompression to allow reexpansion of the adjacent lung.[14] When a patient has a very large cyst that is thought to be causing respiratory compromise, drainage using a chest tube or by percutaneous needle aspiration with CT or sonographic guidance is appropriate.[16] Death may result from respiratory compromise associated with multiple large pneumatoceles or ongoing fulminant pneumonia. Fatal air embolism arising from a ruptured pneumatocele has been reported.[15] Perhaps as many as 25% of pneumatoceles rupture, but most are small and do not cause a significant pneumothorax. Empyema, pneumothorax, and bronchopleural fistula, which occur secondary to cyst rupture, are uncommon and are treated by chest tube drainage and antibiotics. Thoracotomy is rarely necessary.

PROGNOSIS

The typical pneumatocele decreases in size as the pulmonary infection resolves. Approximately 45% resolve within 6 weeks and the remainder sometime within 12 months without clinical or radiographic sequelae.

□ Bronchiectasis

PATHOLOGY

Bronchiectasis is a permanent abnormal dilatation of segmental airways. Three types of bronchiectasis have been described: fusiform, cylindrical, and saccular. Of these three, only cylindrical is thought to be reversible. Bronchiectasis may be localized or diffuse. The left lower lobe tends to be most often affected, followed by the right middle lobe, then the lingula. Bronchiectasis usually involves airways of medium size.[17] The airways become obstructed by purulent exudate, the distal bronchi become inflamed, and the progress of ectatic and thick-walled airways extend to the lung periphery.[18]

ETIOLOGY

Almost all patients with bronchiectasis have an underlying chronic suppurative lung disease (acquired or congenital) that produces repeated pulmonary infection and poor clearance of bronchial secretions. This leads to destruction of the bronchial wall tissue with bronchomalacia and muscular hypertrophy.[19] With progressive disease, the lymph nodes that surround the orifice of a bronchus may become inflamed and enlarged, resulting in additional compression of the bronchus and worsening of the disease.

A number of causes can give rise to bronchiectasis (Table 23–1). Congenital bronchiectasis is rare. Undetected foreign body aspiration may be implicated in causing bronchiectasis in 3 to 16% of patients.[18] Cystic fibrosis (CF) is also a cause of bronchiectasis and is described later.[20]

DIAGNOSIS

Fever and cough are the most common symptoms in children with bronchiectasis. Even though significant amounts of purulent sputum may be produced, children often swallow it and obscure one of the more useful clinical manifestations. Physical activity or a change in position often stimulates a bout of paroxysmal coughing. Hemoptysis often occurs late in the course of the disease. Moist or musical rales may be heard in most patients. During acute exacerbations, the findings on physical examination are the same as those of pneumonia or bronchitis.[20]

A plain chest roentgenogram is the first step in the radiologic evaluation of suspected bronchiectasis.[17] Bronchography has been used to delineate the involved bronchi for consideration of a pulmonary resection. Bronchoscopy done at the time of bronchography is useful to rule out a retained foreign body. CT scan often reveals thickened and dilated airway changes of bronchiectasis and is useful for studying the pulmonary vasculature (Fig. 23–3). High-resolution CT scanning with cuts of 1.5 to 2 mm at 5- to 8-mm increments often provides the most reliable means of diagnosis and grading of disease.[21] It can also be used to monitor the patient's response to therapy. Ventilation perfusion lung scanning is sometimes helpful when attempting to

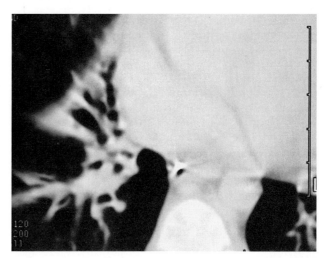

Figure 23–3. Magnified computed tomography cut of a patient with focal right middle lobe bronchiectasis. Bronchial wall thickening is present near the hilum.

define the limits of a pulmonary resection for bronchiectasis.

THERAPY

Control of the underlying cause of the bronchiectasis is the most important step in therapy. Early cases of bronchiectasis that are treated aggressively with antibiotics, good pulmonary toilet, and control of the primary disease do not require surgical intervention.[18, 20] The need for surgical intervention is often a decision best made in conjunction with pulmonologists, anesthesiologists, and surgeons. In some cases, focal bronchiectasis can best be treated with pulmonary resection. A thoracotomy in a patient with long-standing bronchiectasis reveals pleural adhesions, lobar atelectasis, and lymph node hypertrophy, all of which can make the pulmonary resection more difficult. When bronchiectasis is diffuse, resection is of little benefit and lung transplantation may be required.

PROGNOSIS

Focal bronchiectasis, when treated with a localized precise pulmonary resection, is successfully managed, as long as the underlying medical condition has been controlled.[22] Relapse may occur when some bronchiectasis remains.

☐ Lung Abscess

ETIOLOGY

A lung abscess in a child arises from a necrotizing pneumonia.[23] These infections are often a result of mixed flora with aerobic and anaerobic organisms both contributing to the inflammatory process. One or more species of anaerobic oral bacteria along with streptococci, staphylococci, or gram-negative enteric

TABLE 23–1. Causes of Bronchiectasis

Congenital	Acquired
Cystic fibrosis	Pneumonia
Congenital bronchiectasis	Foreign body
Kartagener's syndrome	Bronchitis
Pulmonary sequestration	Measles
Immune deficiencies (humoral)	Influenza
Autoimmune deficiencies	Bronchogenic tumor
Cardiovascular abnormalities	Middle lobe syndrome
Ciliary dyskinesia	Tuberculosis
	Inhalation injuries
	Cigarette smoking
	Asthma

organisms are frequently cultured from the abscess site or the airway.

CLINICAL ASPECTS

Children with severe neurologic impairment, chronic lung disease, seizure disorders, poor oral hygiene, and immune suppression are most often afflicted.[24, 25] Dependent portions of the lung are the regions most commonly affected with a lung abscess. The posterior segment of the right upper lobe and the superior segments of the right and left lower lobe are most often involved in children who are neurologically normal.

Cough, fever, tachypnea, and putrid breath are the presenting manifestations of lung abscess. A chest radiograph shows a pulmonary infiltrate around a cavity that may contain an air-fluid level (Fig. 23–4). Approximately 10% of affected children have more than one abscess.

THERAPY

Fiberoptic bronchoscopy is useful in obtaining culture material used to determine antibiotic needs. Surgical drainage is rarely necessary because most lung abscesses drain spontaneously into the bronchus and are cleared by coughing or tracheal suctioning. A 2- to 3-week course of penicillin is usu-ally effective in treating abscesses arising from oral flora. Metronidazole and clindamycin may be combined with ampicillin to provide better therapeutic effect. It may be helpful to add a β-lactamase inhibitor to cover penicillin-resistant oral bacteria, specifically anaerobes.

Percutaneous drainage of lung abscesses has been successfully used in selected cases.[14, 23, 26] Because they cough poorly, younger and more debilitated children more frequently require surgical intervention.[24, 27]

RESULTS

Successful treatment of a lung abscess usually starts with intravenous (IV) antibiotics, which are continued orally after discharge from the hospital. Gradual resolution of the abscess can be seen radiographically over several weeks. Lung abscesses occasionally recur in the site of a previous abscess if the underlying cause, such as gastroesophageal reflux in a bed-ridden patient, was not addressed. The surgical intervention necessary to prevent recurrence may not be pulmonary. Death is rare in uncomplicated cases.

☐ Chylothorax

ETIOLOGY

Traditionally, chylothorax has been divided into three broad categories. The first, congenital chylothorax, is typically found in the newborn without a history of birth trauma or other predisposing disease. It is thought to be caused by lymphatic malformations and is the most common cause of pleural effusion found in the newborn.[28] The second category, nontraumatic chylothorax, occurs in older children and includes chylothorax caused by spontaneous disorders, benign and malignant neoplasm, and various inflammatory diseases. The third category, traumatic chylothorax from surgical or nonsurgical causes, accounts for the largest number of cases and is most commonly seen in children after thoracic surgery for any reason. Child abuse has also been reported to be a cause of chylothorax.[29] A more complete classification is listed in Table 23–2.

CLINICAL ASPECTS

Nontraumatic chylothorax is of insidious onset and is associated with dyspnea and a full feeling in the chest. Traumatic or surgical chylothorax occurs more acutely and can be associated with severe respiratory embarrassment or shock. What may have been thought to be an insignificant postoperative pleural effusion may become manifest as a chylothorax when normal diet and activity are resumed. Traumatic chylothorax can occur without disruption of the main thoracic duct due to the presence of accessory lymphatic channels or malformation of

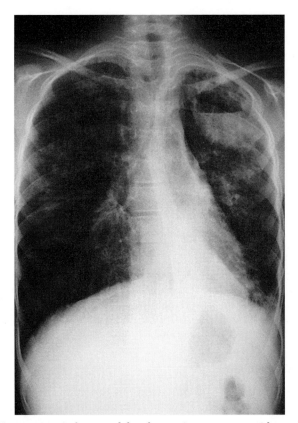

Figure 23–4. Left upper lobe abscess in a teenager with cystic fibrosis. Note the extensive pulmonary changes seen diffusely in both lungs.

TABLE 23–2. Causes of Chylothorax

Congenital	Nontraumatic
Thoracic duct hypoplasia/atresia	Spontaneous
Tracheoesophageal atresia	Forceful Valsalva (strain, cough, or vomit)
Lymphangiomatosis	
Lymphangiectasia	Subclavian/superior vena cava thrombosis
Down's syndrome	
Noonan's syndrome	Malignant neoplasm
Traumatic-Operative	Lymphoma
Cardiothoracic/esophageal procedures	Metastasis
Radical neck dissection	Miscellaneous
Transabdominal sympathectomy	Benign tumors
Diaphragmatic hernia repair	Lymphatic disorders
Subclavian or left heart catheterization	Thoracic aortic aneurysm
	Tuberculosis
Translumbar arteriography	Amyloidosis
Traumatic-Nonoperative	Sarcoidosis
Blunt trauma	Cirrhosis
Birth trauma	Pleuritis
Child abuse	Filariasis
Penetrating trauma	Lupus
	Idiopathic

Adapted from Guleserian KJ, Gilchrist BF, Luks FI, et al: Child abuse as a cause of traumatic chylothorax. J Pediatr Surg 31:1696–1697, 1996.

lymphatic pathways.[30, 31] Because chyle itself does not irritate the pleura and is bacteriostatic, its presence in the pleural space is usually painless and there is rarely fever.

DIAGNOSIS

Chylothorax can occur in either hemithorax. A chest radiograph demonstrates a pleural effusion with no distinguishing characteristics. Chyle is composed of chylomicra and lymphocytes. It is the presence of fat in the diet that leads to the chylomicra in lymph, which gives chyle its characteristic milky, turbid appearance. Thoracic duct fluid is clear in the newborn before the first feeding and in the postoperative patient until a normal diet is resumed. Clear chyle demonstrates a preponderance of lymphocytes if appropriately stained.[32]

In the older child, a chylous effusion is confirmed if the triglyceride level is more than 110 mg/dl. If the triglyceride level of pleural fluid is less than 50 mg/dl, then the fluid is likely nonchylous. A nonchylous effusion, present for more than several weeks, may appear milky and have a triglyceride level of more than 110 mg/dl. This is termed a *pseudochylothorax* and occurs in patients with none of the aforementioned risk factors. Lipoprotein electrophoresis distinguishes pseudochylothorax from a true chylothorax.

THERAPY

Treatment of chylothorax usually consists of pleural drainage on the involved side along with total enteric rest and IV alimentation. Dietary restriction of fat to only medium-chain triglycerides may reduce chyle volume and allow the leak to seal. This therapy is successful in 75 to 90% of patients. The typical duration of pleural drainage is 7 to 14 days with a mean of 12 days. Most cases with drainage persisting past 20 days are best treated by surgical ligation of the lymphatic leak.

Patients with elevated central venous pressure or superior vena cava thrombosis have a high failure rate with nonoperative therapy.[33] When surgery is required, ligation of the thoracic duct at the diaphragm may be used with or without pleurodesis. Pleurodesis alone may be ineffective with high-volume chylothorax. Thoracic duct ligation is most successful when performed on the right side. The administration of cream 1 hour before thoracotomy improves the chance that the lymphatic channel leak will be identified at thoracotomy.[33] Unilateral ligation of the lower thoracic lymphatics does not halt chyle leak in all patients because there are variations in the anatomy of the lymphatic channels. For this reason, a bilateral thoracic lymphatic ligation may occasionally be needed. Pleurodesis with fibrin glue may be an acceptable alternative to ligation in premature infants.[34]

Pleuroperitoneal shunts have been reported to have been used in the management of neonatal chylothorax with a success rate as high as 75%.[35, 36] Thoracoscopic lymphatic ligation has been reported and may be very useful in selected cases.[37] In utero drainage of chylothorax is one of the more successful fetal surgical interventions currently available.[28, 38]

RESULTS

Although there have been deaths associated with the development of chylothorax, most cases are treated successfully with pleural drainage, gut rest, and IV hyperalimentation. This treatment often results in a permanent resolution of the problem without long-term sequelae. More aggressive therapy, such as pleurodesis or thoracic duct ligation, increase morbidity but rarely cause long-term problems.

□ Cystic Fibrosis

CF is one of the most common genetic diseases affecting children. The findings of chronic obstructive pulmonary disease, pancreatic exocrine deficiency, and abnormally high sweat electrolyte concentrations are present in most patients. Transmission is autosomal recessive. Based on the incidence of diagnosis, 4% of Caucasians in the United States are estimated to be carriers of the gene.

PATHOLOGY

CF is caused by mutations in the gene for the CF transmembrane conductance regulator (CFTR).[39] All of the defined mutations in CFTR result in an abnormal transmembrane chloride channel that yields aberrant chloride secretion through defective protein production, defective protein processing, defective regulation, or defective chloride conduction. CFTR also interacts with sodium channels, resulting in increased sodium conductance. The combination of defective chloride secretion and increased sodium absorption may lead to dehydration of epithelial surface liquids and inspissated secretions—the viscid mucus seen in many CF patients.

CLINICAL ASPECTS

The pulmonary symptoms of CF may not be present at birth, and some autopsy studies suggest that the lungs are normal at birth. The first pulmonary lesion to appear is obstruction of the small airways by abnormally thick mucus secretion. Secondary to the obstruction, bronchiolitis develops. Bronchial changes precede parenchymal changes. Bronchiectasis is present in almost all patients older than 18 months of age. Very young patients can be seen with atelectasis, often involving the right upper lobe, or with severe bronchitis. The most distinctive and constant feature of pulmonary CF involvement is a chronic cough. At first, the cough may be dry, but with disease progression it becomes productive and more frequent. Sputum production is mucopurulent, wheezing is common, and allergic aspergillosis develops in some patients.

As the lung disease becomes advanced, pneumothorax and hemoptysis are frequent problems. Pneumothorax occurs secondary to rupture of apical subpleural blebs. The overall incidence is 2 to 10% and in adults may be as high as 16%. Patients have an acute onset of chest pain and shortness of breath. When a pneumothorax has occurred on one side, there is a 50% chance of pneumothorax on the contralateral side within 12 months. Blood streaking in the sputum is fairly common because there is erosion of bronchial arteries into a bronchus. Massive hemoptysis is a serious complication associated with a significant mortality rate, a high recurrence rate, and a poor prognosis. The site of bleeding may often be localized with bronchoscopy.

The overall pulmonary course of a patient with CF is characterized by chronic suppurative bronchitis with recurrent exacerbations, often following viral respiratory infections. Infection with respiratory syncytial virus may be an important cause of significant morbidity in infants less than 6 months of age. By age 10 years, 90% of patients have intermittent sputum production; by age 15 years, 90% have daily sputum production. There is progressive shortness of breath and exercise intolerance. Pulmonary involvement advances at a variable rate but eventually leads to respiratory failure, cardiac failure, or both.[40]

DIAGNOSIS

Although two thirds of cases are diagnosed by 1 year of age, 10% escape detection until adolescence or adulthood. In 85 to 90% of patients, the diagnosis is suggested owing to pulmonary symptoms, failure to thrive, a positive family history, depletion of salt, or deficiency in vitamins, protein, minerals, or calories. The diagnosis of CF should always be confirmed by documentation of an elevated sweat chloride concentration. A chloride concentration of more than 60 mEq/l is consistent with the diagnosis of CF.[41] An accurate sweat chloride test cannot be accomplished until several weeks after birth, but newborns with CF can be screened using elevated blood levels of immunoreactive trypsinogen. In utero testing of a fetus is also available.

The physical findings of CF include a barrel-shaped chest, increased use of accessory muscles of respiration, decreased growth, clubbing, pulmonary hypertrophic osteoarthropathy, and a late finding of cyanosis.[40]

Hyperinflation and bronchial wall thickening are the earliest radiographic findings in a patient with CF. Subsequently, areas of infiltrate, atelectasis, and hilar adenopathy appear. In advanced cases, segmental or lobar atelectasis, bleb formation, bronchiectasis, and pulmonary artery and right ventricular enlargement are seen.

THERAPY

The therapy for the pulmonary complications of CF is often supportive. This includes postural drainage, deep breathing, and chest percussion. Inhalational therapy is useful for treating the inspissated mucus that develops, and antibiotic therapy is used in most patients with CF of long duration. Gene therapy with delivery of wild-type CFTR through mutated viruses is currently undergoing clinical trials.[42]

Tube thoracostomy is required for pneumothorax and the resulting air leak may persist for days. Thoracoscopic stapling of blebs has been effective in stopping persistent air leak. Pulmonary resection is occasionally required for hemoptysis, localized bronchiectasis, or abscess. When pulmonary disease has reached its end stage, lung transplant has been undertaken. CF is the underlying disease in 35 to 50% of children referred for lung transplant and is the single most common indication for pediatric lung transplantation at most centers.[43]

RESULTS

The improvement in understanding infections and antibiotic therapy, pulmonary mechanics, and nutrition has dramatically lengthened the life span of children and adults with CF. There are many individuals with CF who have lived into their 40s and who lead productive lives. Their life spans have been lengthened because of the diligent care they received during childhood.

□ Pulmonary Tuberculosis

It is estimated that one third of the population of the world is infected with tuberculosis and roughly 8 to 10 million new cases occur annually.[44] An estimated 10 to 20 million persons in the United States have a tuberculosis infection. Recent surveys in large U.S. cities have detected tuberculosis infection rates from 1 to 10% in some groups of school children.[45, 46] Approximately 60% of pediatric tuberculosis cases occur in children younger than 5 years of age. Most children have acquired tuberculosis in their household settings with occasional outbreaks in schools or daycare centers.

CLINICAL ASPECTS

Up to 40% of children younger than 1 year of age with untreated tuberculosis infections will develop pulmonary disease. With increasing age, the risk of pulmonary disease decreases.[47] Primary pulmonary tuberculosis includes the lung tissue focus and the regional lymphadenopathy (Fig. 23–5). Roughly 70% of primary foci are subpleural and localized pleuritic pain is common (Fig. 23–6). Calcification of the hilar lymph nodes suggests that the infection has been present for more than 6 months. Although rare, primary tuberculosis can progress to a caseating granuloma, a complication that can result in a tension pneumatocele, bronchopleural fistula, or pyopneumothorax. Rupture into the pericardium or mediastinum has also been described. A localized pleural effusion occurs in 5 to 30% of young adults,

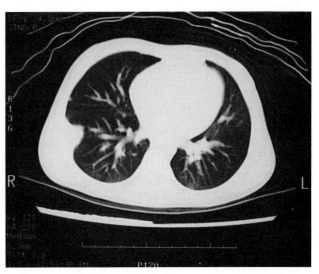

Figure 23–6. Computed tomography scan of a patient with pulmonary tuberculosis. The subpleural primary infection is noted in the periphery of the right lung field. Hilar adenopathy is present.

but effusion becomes less common with decreasing age. Chronic pulmonary tuberculosis represents endogenous reinfection from a site of previous tuberculous infection and is more likely to occur in teenagers than in younger children. The reinfection can occur in the lung, hilar nodes, or apical seedings.[48]

TREATMENT

Isoniazid has been the mainstay of medical therapy since 1952. At the usual dose of 10 mg/kg/day it has few side effects. Liver toxicity, common in adults, is infrequent in children and the peripheral neuritis seen in adults is rare in children whose pyridoxine levels remain acceptable even without supplementation.

Rifampin is a key drug in the modern management of tuberculosis. The usual dose is 10 to 15 mg/kg/day. Rifampin is metabolized in the liver and excreted by the kidneys. Rifampin, which is used almost as often as isoniazid, causes an orange-red discoloration of the urine, tears, sweat, and stool. It is available in combination with isoniazid.

Pyrazinamide was first developed in 1949 and has recently been reintroduced to treat tuberculosis. Streptomycin is used less frequently than it once was, except in cases of drug-resistant tuberculosis. Ethambutol is rarely used in children because of the possibility of optic neuritis. Para-aminosalicylic acid is used as a second-line drug. Multidrug therapy is used to prevent the emergence of resistance to isoniazid. An intensive short course of therapy has proven to be very effective in children. Isoniazid and rifampin are given for 6 months and supplemented with pyrazinamide for the first 2 months. This regimen yields cure rates approaching 100%, with relapse rates approaching 0% and a complication rate of 1%.

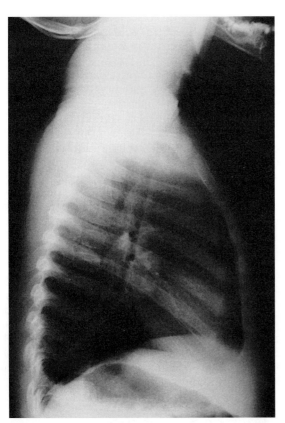

Figure 23–5. Lateral chest radiograph of a child with pulmonary tuberculosis. Note the hilar adenopathy in the center of the lung field.

RESULTS

Surgical intervention for pulmonary tuberculosis is seldom needed; however, with emerging resistant strains of pathogens, the need for surgical resection and other thoracic procedures as adjuncts to drug therapy is becoming more common.[49]

□ Atypical Mycobacterium

ETIOLOGY

There are at least 19 mycobacterium associated with human disease. These types of mycobacteria are found in ground and tap water, soil, house dust, domestic and wild animals, and birds.[44] They are not considered contagious in that person-to-person transmission is rare. The growth of these bacteria is slow, with laboratory identification taking as long as 6 to 10 weeks.

DIAGNOSIS

The most common site of clinically significant atypical mycobacterium infection occurs in the head and neck of children and is usually caused by *Mycobacterium avium-intracellulare.*[50] Excision of the lesion is curative in 95% of patients. Primary pulmonary disease resulting from atypical mycobacterium is rare, occurring most often as a complication of underlying pulmonary disease. Some children have enlarged hilar lymph nodes with endobronchial breakthrough, whereas others have more diffuse lobar disease. The onset of illness can be insidious or acute with fever, cough, or listlessness. The atypical mycobacterium can sometimes be cultured from the gastric aspirate and should be suspected in a child with the clinical picture of tuberculosis who has no known source and does not respond to antituberculosis medication.

THERAPY

Surgery generally plays an important role in the treatment of atypical mycobacterial infections. The treatment of pulmonary atypical mycobacterium infection usually requires resection of infected lung in addition to multidrug therapy for 1 to 3 years. Operative intervention is often used based on a high index of suspicion because growth of an organism in culture is often delayed or impossible.

□ Actinomycoses

Actinomycosis is a rare infection in children characterized by chronic granulomatous or suppurative inflammation and formation of external sinus tracts. This infection has a contiguous spread without regard to the usual anatomic barriers. Metastatic spread to distant sites is not uncommon. Infection occurs when these endogenous oral commensal bacteria invade tissues of the face, neck, thorax, or intestine. It is most commonly seen in individuals with chronically poor dental hygiene or diabetes.[51, 52]

ETIOLOGY

Actinomycosis may be caused by any of the bacteria in the genus *Actinomyces.* These are gram-positive, facultative or strict anaerobes. Virtually all of the organisms that cause actinomycosis have the tendency to form sulfur granules. The lesions and sulfur granules found in actinomycosis infections often reveal the presence of mixed flora, usually of oral origin. Treatment directed at the actinomycosis usually results in a cure, even if the other bacteria are resistant.

DIAGNOSIS

The three most common areas of infection involving actinomycosis are the cervicofacial, abdominal, and thoracic regions. Thoracic actinomycosis is rare in childhood. Related factors include the spread of an existing infection to the mediastinum and thorax, hematogenous seeding, inhalation of a foreign body, or inhalation or aspiration of oral bacteria. This infection can extend from the lung tissue to and through the chest wall.[53] It appears as a chronic pneumonia resistant to the usual antibiotic therapy. Lung cavitation and pleural effusion are common. Other symptoms include cough, weight loss, chest pain, and back pain. Invasion of ribs or vertebral bodies is not uncommon. Distant metastasis of infection occurs in up to 40% of patients with thoracic actinomycosis.[54]

THERAPY

The treatment of thoracic actinomycosis is with antibiotics and surgery. In mild cases, penicillin or a derivative effectively treats the symptoms with an excellent chance of cure. With more advanced disease, antibiotic therapy with drainage of abscesses, surgical resection of the involved tissue, and excision of sinus tracts is required to effect cure.[55]

□ Nocardiosis

ETIOLOGY

Nocardia is a localized or disseminated infection caused by an aerobic actinomycete. This infectious agent is found in the soil or in rotting vegetables and usually causes a pulmonary lesion that can be clinically silent or may produce chronic bronchopulmonary disease.[56] Hematogenous spread from the lungs can infect the central nervous system, bones, liver, spleen, or other soft tissues. Most reported cases of norcardiosis have occurred in immunosuppressed patients.

CLINICAL ASPECTS AND THERAPY

Nocardiosis produces suppuration with abscess formation and necrosis. Pulmonary lesions consist of multiple abscesses although a single abscess may occur. Clinical symptoms may be subtle with fever, anorexia, weight loss, cough, and dyspnea. Chest roentgenogram may show a variety of lesions, but most patients have interstitial infiltrates or bronchopneumonia. Single or combination sulfa drugs for 6 weeks are generally recommended. Metastatic abscesses during medical therapy suggest the need for surgical drainage or resection of diseased tissue.[57]

☐ Histoplasmosis

ETIOLOGY

Histoplasmosis is a common granulomatous infection caused by the fungus *Histoplasma capsulatum*. An estimated 500,000 people a year are infected with this fungus. Histoplasmosis occurs worldwide but is most common in the Ohio, Mississippi, and Missouri River valleys. Soil is contaminated by animal feces, especially those of birds and bats, which play a major role in fungal dissemination. The spores are acquired by inhalation of contaminated dust.[58]

DIAGNOSIS

Acute pulmonary histoplasmosis is occasionally seen but an asymptomatic primary infection occurs in roughly 50% of children exposed. Incubation takes 7 to 21 days and the severity of disease is related to the amount of inhaled microconidia. The presentation is similar to influenza, with headaches, fever, myalgia, malaise, and nonproductive cough. Radiography reveals patchy infiltrates and hilar adenopathy. The typical infection resolves in 3 to 10 days. For most patients, it is a self-limited disease, but occasionally disseminated histoplasmosis develop. Reinfection can occur, and calcification of these foci gives the radiologic appearance of miliary tuberculosis. Patients with immunosuppression such as AIDS infections are more susceptible to progressive or complicated *Histoplasma* pneumonia.[59]

THERAPY

Almost all cases of histoplasmosis resolve spontaneously. Treatment is indicated if the symptoms persist for more than 3 weeks or if the chest radiograph shows progression of disease. Amphotericin B is the treatment of choice for life-threatening histoplasmosis. Ketoconazole is also useful.[60] Recovery is rapid in most cases, although relapse can occur.

☐ Diffuse Pulmonary Disorders

ETIOLOGY

The lungs can be diffusely affected by a number of infectious and noninfectious conditions. Often, the cause of the diffuse pulmonary disease process is unclear and a significant effort is needed to find the cause and direct the therapy. The infectious causes of diffuse pulmonary disorders are listed in Table 23–3. An infectious agent may be difficult to isolate. When the cause is unclear, noninfectious causes should be considered (Table 23–4).

DIAGNOSIS

A culture of the upper airway often allows identification of an infectious causative agent. Special techniques may be needed to grow viral, chlamydial, fungal, and unusual bacterial organisms. Identification of an infectious agent in the upper airway of a sick patient is strong evidence that it is causing the pneumonic process. Fluorescent antibody techniques, immunoabsorbent assays, or DNA probes are used for rapid determination of the causative organism, often within hours.

Bronchoalveolar lavage, endobronchial brush biopsy, and transbronchial lung biopsy are more aggressive methods that are sometimes used to obtain specimens in more obscure cases of diffuse infectious pulmonary disorders.[61] These procedures are most useful in difficult to diagnose cases such as *Pneumocystis carinii* pneumonia. Other techniques include open lung biopsy, closed needle biopsy, and percutaneous needle aspiration. Of these, an open lung biopsy using a thoracoscopic approach is most reliable.[62] In the case of noninfectious causes of diffuse lung disease, the diagnosis can often be made based on the history. A recent exposure to noninfectious pathogens is useful. When specific testing or historical clues are insufficient, the same techniques used for infectious diseases are also useful in noninfectious cases.

TABLE 23–3. Infectious Causes of Diffuse Pulmonary Disorders

Cryptococcus infection
Aspergillosis
Streptococcus infection
Herpes simplex virus
Varicella zoster virus
Cytomegalovirus
Respiratory syncytial virus
Parainfluenza virus
Adenovirus
Mycoplasma pneumonia
Rickettsia
Chlamydia
Pneumocystis infection

TABLE 23–4. Noninfectious Causes
of Diffuse Pulmonary Disorders

Adult respiratory distress syndrome
Allergic alveolitis
Recurrent aspiration
Tracheoesophageal fistula
Pulmonary hemosiderosis
Desquamative interstitial pneumonitis
Lipoid pneumonia
Petroleum distillate ingestion
Drugs
Radiation
Graft versus host disease
Fat embolism
Systemic lupus erythematosus
Sarcoidosis
Neoplasms
Hypersensitivity pneumonitis

THERAPY

The treatment of these diffuse diseases varies with the etiology. Many of the mild cases can be managed expectantly; however, severe diffuse disease may require intensive ventilatory therapy and, in extreme cases, may even require extracorporeal life support. Antibiotics, antiviral, and antifungal agents should be used when cultures indicate a specific infectious agent. Avoiding or removing exposure in noninfectious cases may also be required. Supportive therapy should include prophylaxis in selective cases to avoid secondary bacterial infection. The long-term outcome is dependent on the causative agent involved and upon the underlying patient condition.

☐ Idiopathic Chronic Interstitial-Alveolar Pneumonitides

The term *interstitial pneumonia* describes a variety of pathologic states characterized by a diffuse inflammatory process involving the interstitium or the alveoli of the lung. Interstitial pneumonia is a nonspecific reaction to injury that can be a manifestation of infection, drugs, toxic inhalants, collagen vascular diseases, or a variety of genetic, metabolic, or inflammatory disorders. It may present as an acute or chronic pulmonary inflammatory problem. Interstitial pneumonias can be subdivided into four groups: usual interstitial pneumonia, desquamative pneumonia, lymphoid pneumonia, and giant cell pneumonia.[63]

Usual interstitial pneumonia, the most common form, presents as a patchy interstitial process and demonstrates progressive infiltration and scarring of the lung. Major signs and symptoms include tachypnea, cough, hypoxia, and failure to thrive. Respiratory failure, cardiac failure, and pneumothorax are reported complications. Associated diseases include rheumatoid arthritis, hepatitis, ulcerative colitis, thyroid disease, and systemic lupus erythematosus.

Diagnosis often requires lung biopsy. Current treatment includes high-dose corticosteroids for at least 4 to 8 weeks. Some investigators have attempted immunosuppression. Survival rates are worse when the onset is before 1 year of age, and the mortality rate for all patients, even with excellent treatment, may approach 50%.[64]

Desquamative interstitial pneumonia is less common than usual interstitial pneumonia and accounts for 10 to 25% of cases. It is characterized by hyperplasia of type 2 alveolar lining cells and the filling of distal air spaces with macrophages. There is mild alveolar thickening and sparse interstitial inflammatory infiltrate. Signs and symptoms include cough, tachypnea, dyspnea, and hypoxemia. Right ventricular hypertrophy and pulmonary hypertension are often seen. Acute lymphoblastic leukemia, glomerulonephritis with nephrotic syndrome, and trisomy 21 are often associated. There have been reported familial cases. The primary treatment is steroid therapy. The overall mortality rate in children is 35%. A rare variant of this may be chronic pneumonitis of infancy.[65]

Lymphoid interstitial pneumonia in children was rare in the past, but has become more common with the increase in AIDS cases in the pediatric population. It is a manifestation of lymphoproliferative disease involving the lung and is characterized by a prominent interstitial infiltrate of mature lymphocytes with occasional plasma cells. It can be diffuse or patchy, with presenting signs and symptoms similar to those seen in other interstitial pneumonias. Other associated diseases include those of a rheumatic or immunologic origin. Familial lymphoid pneumonia has been reported. Steroids, with or without cytologic drugs, have been used to treat this disease with generally poor results.

Giant cell interstitial pneumonia, which is rare in children, has been associated with hard-metal pneumoconiosis. It is characterized by the presence of multinucleate cells in the alveolar spaces with hyperplasia of type 2 alveolar epithelial cells and an interstitial infiltrate of lymphohistiocytic cells. The clinical presentation is similar to that of the aforementioned forms of interstitial pneumonia and its response to steroidal treatment is variable.

REFERENCES

1. Light RW: Parapneumonic effusions and empyemas. Clin Chest Med 6:55–59, 1985.
2. Wood WB Jr, Smith MR, Watson B: Studies on the mechanism of recovery in pneumococcal pneumonia IV. The mechanism of phagocytosis in the absence of antibody. J Exp Med 84:387–402, 1946.
3. Andrews NC, Parker EF, Shaw RR, et al: Management of nontuberculous empyema. Am Rev Respir Dis 85:935–936, 1962.
4. Bryant RE, Salmon C: Pleural empyema. Clin Infect Dis 22:747–764, 1996.
5. Magovern CJ, Rusch VW: Parapneumonic and post-traumatic pleural space infections. Chest Surg Clin North Am 4:561–582, 1994.
6. Light RW: Parapneumonic effusions and infections of the

pleural space. In Light RW (ed): Pleural Disease, 2nd ed. Philadelphia: Lea & Febiger, 1990, p 130.

7. Samson PC, Burford TH: Total pulmonary decortication: Its evolution and present concepts of indications and operative technique. J Thorac Surg 16:127–153, 1947.
8. Raffensberger JG, Luck SR, Shkolnik A, et al: Mini-thoracotomy and chest tube insertion for children with empyema. J Thorac Cardiovasc Surg 84:497–504, 1982.
9. Silen ML, Weber TR: Thoracoscopic debridement of loculated empyema thoracis in children. Ann Thorac Surg 59:1166–1168, 1995.
10. Tillett WS, Sherry S: The effect in patients of streptococcal fibrinolysin (streptokinase) and streptococcal desoxyribonuclease on fibrinous, purulent, and sanguinous pleural exudations. J Clin Invest 28:173–190, 1949.
11. Robinson LA, Moulton AL, Fleming WH, et al: Intrapulmonary fibrinolytic treatment of multiloculated thoracic empyemas. Ann Thorac Surg 57:803–814, 1994.
12. Moulton JS, Benkert RE, Weisiger KH, et al: Treatment of complicated pleural fluid collections with image-guided drainage and intracavitary urokinase. Chest 108:1252–1259, 1995.
13. Glustein JZ, Kaplan M: *Enterobacter cloacae* causing pneumatocele in a neonate. Acta Pediatr 83:990–991, 1994.
14. Zuhdi MK, Spear RM, Worthen HM, et al: Percutaneous catheter drainage of tension pneumatocele, secondarily infected pneumatocele, and lung abscess in children. Crit Care Med 24: 330–333, 1996.
15. Zuhdi MK, Bradley JS, Spear RM, et al: Fatal air embolism as a complication of staphylococcal pneumonia with pneumatoceles. Pediatr Infect Dis J 14:811–812, 1995.
16. Joosten KFM, Hazelzet JA, Tiddens HA, et al: Staphylococcal pneumonia in children: Will early surgical intervention lower mortality? Pediatr Pulmonol 20:83–88, 1995.
17. Barker AF, Bardanna EJ Jr: Bronchiectasis: Update of an orphan disease. Am Rev Respir Dis 137:969–978, 1988.
18. Korneich L, Horev G, Ziv N, et al: Bronchiectasis in children: Assessment by CT. Pediatr Radiol 23:120–123, 1993.
19. Reid LM: Reduction in bronchial subdivision in bronchiectasis. Thorax 5:233–247, 1950.
20. Lewiston NJ: Bronchiectasis in childhood. Pediatr Clin North Am 31:865–878, 1984.
21. Grenier P, Cordeau MP, Bergelman C: High resolution computed tomography of the airways. J Thorac Imaging 8:213–229, 1993.
22. Coleman LT, Kramer SS, Markowitz RI, et al: Bronchiectasis in children. J Thorac Imaging 10:268–279, 1995.
23. Brook I: Lung abscesses and pleural empyema in children. Adv Pediatr Infect Dis 8:159–176, 1993.
24. Bruckheimer E, Dolberg S, Shlesinger Y, et al: Primary lung abscess in infancy. Pediatr Pulmonol 19:188–191, 1995.
25. Furman AC, Jacobs J: Lung abscess in patients with AIDS. Clin Infect Dis 22:81–85, 1996.
26. van Sonnenberg E, D'Agostino HB, Casola G, et al: Lung abscess: CT-guided drainage. Radiology 178:347–351, 1991.
27. Kosloske AM, Ball WS, Butler C, Musemeche CA: Drainage of pediatric lung abscess by cough, catheter, or complete resection. J Pediatr Surg 21:596–600, 1986.
28. Watson WJ, Munson DP, Christensen MW: Bilateral fetal chylothorax: Results of unilateral in-utero therapy. Am J Perinatol 13:115–117, 1996.
29. Guleserian KJ, Gilchrist BF, Luks FI, et al: Child abuse as a cause of traumatic chylothorax. J Pediatr Surg 31:1696–1697, 1996.
30. Servelle M, Nogues C, Soulie J, et al: Spontaneous, postoperative and traumatic chylothorax. J Cardiovasc Surg (Torino) 21:475–486, 1980.
31. Skandalakis JE, Gray SW, Ricketts RR: The lymphatic system. In Skandalakis JE, Gray SW (eds): Embryology for Surgeons, 2nd ed. Baltimore: Williams & Wilkins, 1994, pp 877–897.
32. Allen EM, van Heeckeren DW, Spector ML, et al: Management of nutritional and infectious complications of postoperative chylothorax in children. J Pediatr Surg 26:1169–1174, 1991.
33. Bond SJ, Guzzetta PC, Snyder ML, et al: Management of pediatric postoperative chylothorax. Ann Thorac Surg 56:469–472, 1993.
34. Nguyen D, Tchervenkov CI: Successful management of postoperative chylothorax with fibrin glue in a premature neonate. Can J Surg 37:158–160, 1994.
35. Azizkhan RG, Canfield J, Alford BA, et al: Pleuroperitoneal shunts in the management of neonatal chylothorax. J Pediatr Surg 18:842–850, 1983.
36. Murphy MC, Newman BM, Rodgers BM: Pleuroperitoneal shunts in the management of persistent chylothorax. Ann Thorac Surg 48:195–200, 1989.
37. Graham DD, McGahren ED, Tribble CG, et al: Use of video-assisted thoracic surgery in the treatment of chylothorax. Ann Thorac Surg 57:1507–1512, 1994.
38. Petres RE, Redwine FO, Cruikshank DP: Congenital bilateral chylothorax. Antepartum diagnosis and successful intrauterine surgical management. JAMA 248:1360–1361, 1982.
39. Wagner JA, Gardner P: Toward cystic fibrosis gene therapy. Annu Rev Med 48:203–216, 1997.
40. Rosenstein BJ: Cystic fibrosis. In Oski F (ed): Principles and Practice of Pediatrics. Philadelphia: JB Lippincott, 1994, pp 1490–1500.
41. Wallis C: Diagnosing cystic fibrosis: Blood, sweat, and tears. Arch Dis Child 76:85–91, 1997.
42. Flotte TR, Carter B, Conrad CK, et al: A phase I study of adeno-associated virus-CTFR gene vector in adult CF patients with mild lung disease. Hum Gene Ther 7:1145–1159, 1996.
43. Kurland G: Pediatric lung transplantation: Indications and contraindications. Semin Thorac Cardiovasc Surg 8:277–285, 1996.
44. Preheim LC, Smith TL: Mycobacterial infections: New threats from old disease. Comp Ther 23:310–318, 1997.
45. Starke JR, Jacobs RF, Jereb J: Resurgence of tuberculosis in children. J Pediatr 120:839–855, 1992.
46. Barry MA, Shirley L, Grady MT, et al: Tuberculosis infection in urban adolescents: Results of a school-based testing program. Am J Public Health 80:439–441, 1990.
47. Starke JR. Childhood tuberculosis in the 1990s. Pediatr Ann 22:550–560, 1993.
48. Jacobs RF, Starke JR: Tuberculosis in children. Med Clin North Am 77:1335–1351, 1993.
49. Leuven MV, De Groot M, Shean KP, et al: Pulmonary resection as an adjunct in the treatment of multiple drug-resistant tuberculosis. Ann Thorac Surg 63(6):1368–1373, 1997.
50. Horsburgh CR: Advances in the prevention and treatment of *Mycobacterium avium* disease. N Engl J Med 335:428–430, 1996.
51. Brown JR: Human actinomycosis: A study of 181 subjects. Hum Pathol 4:319–330, 1973.
52. Golden N, Cohen H, Weissbrot J, et al: Thoracic actinomycosis in childhood. Clin Pediatr (Phila) 24:646–650, 1985.
53. Snape PS: Thoracic actinomycosis: An unusual childhood infection. South Med J 86:222–224, 1993.
54. Kinnear WJM, MacFarlane JT: A survey of thoracic actinomycosis. Respir Med 84:57–59, 1990.
55. Hsieh MJ, Liu HP, Chang JP, et al: Thoracic actinomycosis. Chest 104:366–370, 1993.
56. Stites DP, Glezen WP: Pulmonary nocardiosis in childhood. Am J Dis Child 114:101–105, 1967.
57. Law BJ, Marks MI: Pediatric nocardiosis. Pediatrics 70:560–565, 1982.
58. Wheat LJ: Systemic fungal infections: Diagnosis and treatment: I. Histoplasmosis. Infect Dis Clin North Am 2:841–859, 1988.
59. Byers M, Feldman S, Edwards J: Disseminated histoplasmosis as the acquired immunodeficiency syndrome-defining illness in an infant. Pediatr Infect Dis J 11:127–128, 1992.
60. Walsh TJ, Gonzalez C, Lyman CA, et al: Invasive fungal infections in children: Recent advances in diagnosis and treatment. Adv Pediatr Infect Dis 11:187–290, 1996.
61. Muntz HR, Wallace M, Lusk RP: Pediatric transbronchial lung biopsy. Ann Otol Rhinol Laryngol 101(2 pt 1):135–137, 1992.

62. Ellis ME, Spence D, Bouchama A, et al: Open lung biopsy provides a higher and more specific diagnostic yield compared to broncho-alveolar lavage in immunocompromised patients. Scand J Infect Dis 27:157–162, 1995.

63. Fan LL, Langston C: Chronic interstitial lung disease in children. State of the art review. Pediatr Pulmonol 16:184–196, 1993.

64. Fan LL, Mullen ALW, Brugman SM, et al: Clinical spectrum of chronic interstitial lung disease in children. J Pediatr 121:867–872, 1992.

65. Katzenstein ALA, Gordon LP, Oliphant M, et al: Chronic pneumonitis of infancy: A unique form of interstitial lung disease occurring in early childhood. Am J Surg Pathol 19:439–447, 1995.

24

CONGENITAL DIAPHRAGMATIC HERNIA AND EVENTRATION

Robert M. Arensman, MD •
Daniel A. Bambini, MD

Congenital diaphragmatic hernia (CDH) is one of the most challenging neonatal diagnoses faced by pediatric surgeons. Despite increased diagnostic capabilities and tremendous advances in the care and management of critically ill neonates with respiratory disease, CDH still has an overall mortality of 30 to 60% at most centers. The high mortality of CDH is directly related to the severity of lung hypoplasia induced by bowel herniation during the critical stages of fetal lung development.

Although surgery continues to play a primary role in therapy, many recent advances in the successful treatment of neonates with CDH have been nonsurgical. Early surgical intervention, once believed to be critical to survival,[1] has been largely replaced by a delayed surgical approach in which repair of the diaphragmatic defect is deferred until pulmonary hypertension and persistent fetal circulation have subsided. The improved survival of the delayed surgical approach has been modest, leading many to pursue other strategies and innovative therapies, including extracorporeal membrane oxygenation (ECMO) and fetal intervention.

Perhaps no other disease encountered by pediatric surgeons has as many therapeutic and management options as does CDH. Regardless, the optimal management strategy for neonates with congenital diaphragmatic hernia remains unknown, and the treatment of CDH continues to evolve as our understanding of the disease increases.

☐ Anatomy of the Diaphragm

The diaphragm is a dome-shaped musculotendinous structure that separates the thoracic and abdominal cavities. It is composed of fibrous and muscular parts. The fibrous central tendon is the largest single component of the diaphragm, occupies most of the anterior and central portions of the diaphragm, and accounts for approximately one third of the total diaphragmatic surface area. Crural fibers pass around the aorta and esophagus to insert at the posterior central tendon and define the apertures for the aorta and esophagus. The anatomic pattern of the crural fibers surrounding the esophageal hiatus can be highly variable.

Congenital and acquired diaphragmatic defects commonly occur at three areas of the diaphragm (Fig. 24–1). The posterolateral diaphragmatic hernia is the most common congenital diaphragmatic hernia and accounts for 85 to 90% of diaphragmatic defects presenting in the neonatal period. Bochdalek hypothesized that intrauterine rupture of the thin membrane covering the lumbocostal triangle allowed visceral herniation and was the source of the posterolateral diaphragmatic hernia. This explanation seems unlikely, and recent embryologic studies suggest that the posterolateral defect occurs as a result of failed closure of the embryonic pleuroperitoneal canal. Regardless of origin, the posterolateral diaphragmatic hernia is commonly called the Bochdalek hernia. The size of the defect can range from a small slit to the complete absence of the entire hemidiaphragm. Large defects are often circumscribed by only a thin rim of muscle tissue posteriorly. A hernia sac is present in only approximately 20% of cases. Eighty to 90% of posterolateral diaphragmatic defects occur on the left side.

A second common location of congenital diaphragmatic defects is posterior to the sternum at the anterior diaphragm. Retrosternal hernias (Morgagni's hernia) usually occur on the right side and are often identified in the midline immediately posterior to the xiphoid process. Morgagni's hernias account for only 2 to 6% of congenital diaphragmatic defects. The third common area of the diaphragm at which hernias can develop is the esophageal hiatus.

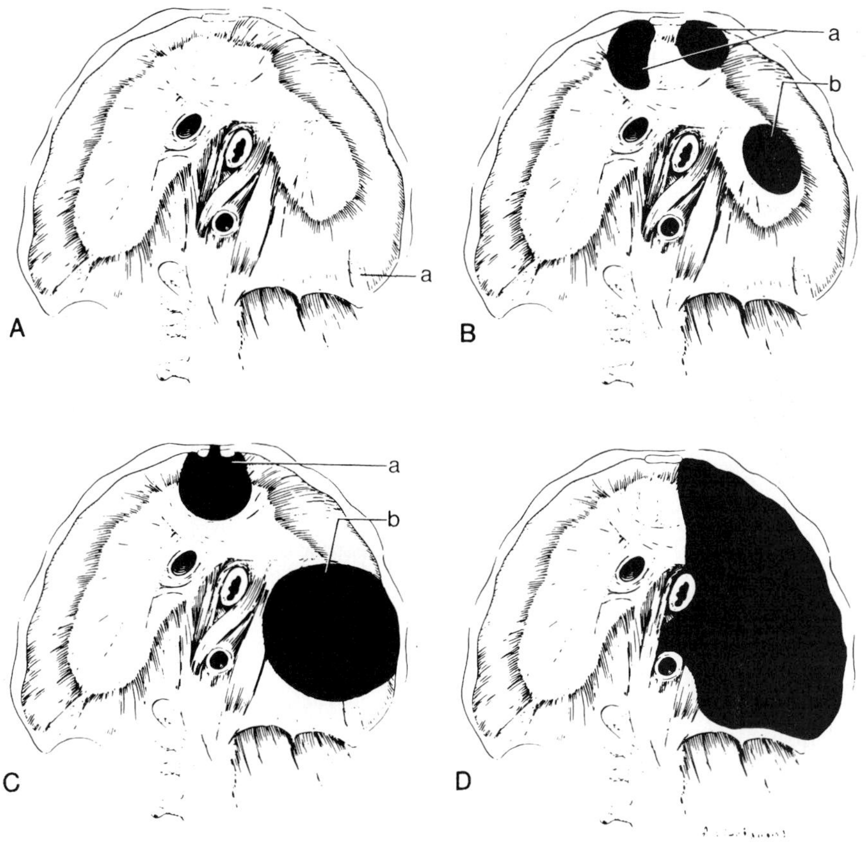

Figure 24–1. The inferior surface of the diaphragm and common locations of congenital diaphragmatic hernia. *A,* The normal diaphragm and the site (a) of the lumbosacral triangle, a potential area of weakness between diaphragmatic muscle fibers originating from the 12th rib and those originating from the lateral arcuate ligament. *B,* Retrosternal hernia (a) produced by failure of the sternal and costal contributions of the diaphragm to fuse at the site where the internal mammary artery traverses the diaphragm. Small posterolateral hernia (b) produced by failed closure of the pleuroperitoneal canal during embryologic development. *C,* Diaphragmatic defect and cleft sternum (a) associated with the pentalogy of Cantrell, which results from embryologic failure in the development of the septum transversum. Large posterolateral defect (b) with only a thin rim of posterior diaphragm. *D,* Agenesis of the left hemidiaphragm with absence of the left diaphragmatic crura.

☐ Embryology of the Diaphragm

DEVELOPMENT OF THE DIAPHRAGM AND THE DIAPHRAGMATIC HERNIA

The septum transversum fuses dorsally with the mesodermal tissue of the mediastinum surrounding the foregut; dorsolaterally, the pleuroperitoneal canals remain in continuity, connecting the pleural space and peritoneal cavity (Fig. 24–2). Closure of the pleuroperitoneal canal completes the formation of the primitive fetal diaphragm, separating the abdominal cavity from the paired pleural cavities. The mechanism by which this occurs is not completely understood.[2]

Normally, the communication through the pleuroperitoneal canals is obliterated by the 8th week of gestation. CDH has usually been attributed to a defective formation of the pleuroperitoneal membrane. Recent experimental evidence suggests that CDH results from defective development of the posthepatic mesenchymal plate, which also may play a primary role in the closure of the pleuroperitoneal canal.[3, 4] If closure of the pleuroperitoneal canal is incomplete, a posterolateral diaphragmatic defect results. Visceral herniation through the defect into the chest can occur as the intestines return to the peritoneal cavity beginning at the 10th week of gestation.

DEVELOPMENT OF THE LUNG AND PULMONARY HYPOPLASIA

Lung development is traditionally divided into four overlapping stages. The pseudoglandular stage lasts from 5 to 17 weeks and defines the period in which major bronchi and terminal bronchi are formed. The majority of respiratory bronchioles, alveolar ducts, and pulmonary vessels develop during the canalicular stage between 16 and 25 weeks. The terminal sac period begins at 24 weeks and continues until birth. Alveoli begin to develop during the alveolar stage, which begins in late fetal life and continues into childhood.

Visceral herniation during the pseudoglandular stage of development impedes and limits growth and branching of the bronchi and pulmonary vessels. Ipsilateral pulmonary hypoplasia has traditionally been attributed to the mass effect imposed by herniated viscera within the chest. The lung opposite the diaphragmatic defect is also appreciably affected if the visceral mass causes mediastinal shift and contralateral lung compression. Experimental evidence suggests that the pulmonary hypoplasia associated with CDH may not be entirely caused by the compressive effect of ectopic viscera but may be mediated by alterations in pulmonary growth factors or other mechanisms. Pulmonary hypoplasia is characterized by a decrease in pulmonary mass and weight, a reduction in bronchial divisions, and a reduction in the number of alveoli and respiratory

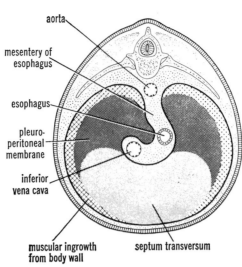

Figure 24–2. The embryologic relationship of the developing diaphragm and pleuroperitoneal canal. The septum transversum fuses posteriorly with the mediastinal mesenchyme. The pleuroperitoneal canals (white arrow) allow free communication between the pleural and peritoneal cavities. Closure of these canals is completed as the pleuroperitoneal membranes develop. The four embryologic components of the developing diaphragm are shown in cross-section. (From Skandalakis LJ, Colborn GL, Skandalakis JE: In Nyhus LM, Baker RJ, Fischer JE [eds]: Mastery of Surgery [3rd ed.] Boston, Little, Brown, 1996.)

bronchioles. In CDH, the pulmonary vascular tree is also hypoplastic, with abnormal muscularization of pulmonary arterioles. Surfactant deficiency may also be present.[5]

☐ Congenital Diaphragmatic Hernia

INCIDENCE AND EPIDEMIOLOGY

The incidence of CDH is estimated to be between 1 in 2000 and 1 in 5000 live births. Female infants are affected twice as often as males. The etiology of CDH is not known, but genetic factors may play a role because famililal cases have been reported. In familial cases, the inheritance pattern is likely multifactorial, but one epidemiologic study of 40 families with multiple siblings affected with CDH suggested an autosomal recessive pattern of inheritance. The vast majority of cases occur sporadically, and no familial link can be identified. The association of CDH with other genetic abnormalities and anomalies, including trisomies 18, 21, and 23, strongly suggests an underlying genetic etiology.

Approximately 30% of fetuses with CDH will be stillborn. Of those infants surviving to delivery, up to 30 to 50% will die before transfer to a neonatal center. Prematurity and low birth weight are associated with a significantly increased risk of perinatal mortality from CDH.[6]

PATHOPHYSIOLOGY

The pathophysiology of CDH is complex. Several interactive mechanisms are responsible for the clinical findings and pathophysiology observed in neonates with CDH (Fig. 24–3). Local and systemic factors combine to varying degrees to produce a severe, self-perpetuating cycle of hypoxia, hypercarbia, and acidosis. Therefore, therapeutic interventions should be designed to interrupt and reverse this process.

Pulmonary Hypoplasia

The lungs in newborns with CDH are hypoplastic.[7–9] The severity or degree of pulmonary hypoplasia depends on the duration and timing of visceral herniation as well as the amount of bowel within the chest.[10] Grossly, the lungs in neonates with CDH appear small. In addition, they are functionally immature and have limited capacity for gas exchange at birth.

Hypoplasia is usually more severe on the ipsilateral side, but the contralateral lung may also be

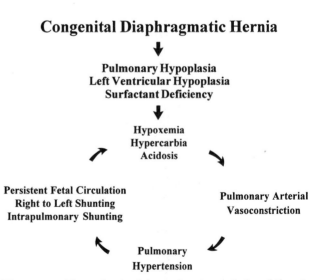

Figure 24–3. The pathophysiology of acute respiratory failure in neonates with congenital diaphragmatic hernia.

affected. Structural abnormalities of pulmonary hypoplasia may be present on the contralateral side in the absence of mediastinal shift, suggesting mechanisms other than extrinsic compression as the etiology of pulmonary hypoplasia. The number of bronchial divisions is markedly reduced in the ipsilateral and contralateral lung,[7] as are the number of mature alveoli.[11] Abnormalities of septal formation within the terminal saccules and alveolar units of the lung may also limit gas exchange at the air–capillary interface.[12] The alveoli present at birth are immature and have thickened intraalveolar septae with increased glycogen content.

Pulmonary Vascular Abnormalities

The pulmonary vasculature is abnormal in CDH with increased muscularization of pulmonary arterioles. The branching of pulmonary vessels is dramatically reduced, as is the overall cross-sectional area of the vascular bed.[9] These factors likely contribute to the increased reactivity and resistance of the pulmonary vasculature and pulmonary hypertension observed clinically in these neonates.

Persistent Pulmonary Hypertension and Persistent Fetal Circulation

Persistent pulmonary hypertension of the neonate (PPHN) and persistent fetal circulation (PFC) are common in neonates with congenital diaphragmatic hernia.[13, 14] A combination of factors, including hypoxia, acidosis, hypercarbia, and hypothermia, contribute to pulmonary hypertension, which results in a continued pattern of fetal circulation with right-to-left shunting through the ductus arteriosus and foramen ovale. Hypoxia caused by shunting further aggravates and perpetuates PPHN and PFC, which have been identified as indicators of both a poor response to treatment and overall poor prognosis.[15, 16] Vasoactive peptides, including endothelin 1, angiotensins, thromboxanes, and prostanoids, may also contribute to the pulmonary hypertension observed in neonates with CDH.[17–20]

Surfactant Deficiency

The data supporting the presence of surfactant deficiency in CDH has come largely from studies of experimental models of CDH.[5, 21] A few reports of human newborns with CDH have also suggested immaturity of the surfactant system[22, 23] and surfactant deficiency.[21, 24, 25] In contrast, a study of amniocentesis samples obtained from fetuses with prenatally diagnosed CDH failed to demonstrate a surfactant deficiency. Experimentally, exogenous surfactant administration improves pulmonary blood flow and lowers pulmonary vascular resistance. Surfactant replacement therapy has been empirically used to treat newborns with CDH, but the benefits of exogenous surfactant therapy in CDH remain unproven.[21, 26–28]

Associated Anomalies

The contribution of associated congenital anomalies in the pathophysiology and mortality of CDH must not be underestimated. Stillborn neonates with CDH have been found to have major associated anomalies in 95% of cases.[29] In a recent study, more than 60% of newborns with CDH who died during resuscitation or preoperative stabilization had associated malformations, whereas only 8% of those who survived to operation had other anomalies.[30]

Cardiac anomalies account for 63% of the anomalies identified.[31] The cardiac anomalies often exacerbate pulmonary hypertension, right-to-left shunting, and hemodynamic instability. The most common cardiac defects identified in neonates with CDH are heart hypoplasia, atrial septal defects, and ventricular septal defects. Although no single feature can be considered to be a reliable predictor of poor prognosis or nonsurvival, fetal cardiac ventricular disproportion identified before 24 weeks' gestation is associated with a 100% mortality.[32, 33] Additional anomalies with CDH include pulmonary sequestration, renal and genital anomalies, neural tube defects, and chromosomal abnormalities.[34–36]

DIAGNOSIS

The diagnosis of CDH is frequently made prenatally. At tertiary referral centers, up to 93% of neonates with CDH may be diagnosed by prenatal ultrasonography (US).[35] CDH can be identified in the human fetus as early as the 25th week of gestation.[37] Diagnosis at this early age optimizes prenatal and postnatal care of both mother and fetus and provides time for perinatal counseling, consideration of fetal surgery, or pregnancy termination.

Fetal US can accurately identify features of CDH, including bowel loops within the chest, polyhydramnios, absent or intrathoracic gastric bubble, mediastinal shift, and fetal hydrops.[38] Although suggested to be prognostic indicators of survival, none of these features can absolutely and consistently identify a fetus with a poor prognosis for survival. Prenatal diagnosis of CDH in the absence of other associated anomalies does not alter the severity of illness or survival.[39, 40]

Amniocentesis has revealed decreased lecithin-to-sphingomyelin ratios in association with CDH.[24] Chromosomal analysis of fetuses with CDH may demonstrate several chromosomal anomalies, including trisomy 18, trisomy 13, 3p microdeletion, or 12p tetrasomy.[36, 38, 40] Maternal serum alphafetoprotein (MS-AFP) levels may be reduced in CDH[41, 42] as well as with trisomy 21 and trisomy 18.[41, 42]

CLINICAL PRESENTATION

Respiratory distress, which is the common presentation of CDH, may develop immediately after birth in association with low Apgar scores or within 24 to 48 hours after an initial period of relative stability and minimal clinical signs. The initial signs include tachypnea, grunting respirations, chest retractions, pallor, cyanosis, and clinical signs of shunting and persistent fetal circulation. Physical examination reveals a scaphoid abdomen. The anterior–posterior diameter of the chest may be increased. Mediastinal shift may be detected by displacement of the point of maximal cardiac impulse away from the side of the diaphragmatic lesion. Bowel sounds may be present within the affected hemithorax. Breath sounds are decreased bilaterally from decreased tidal volume but are usually more diminished on the affected side.

The diagnosis is confirmed by chest radiography (Fig. 24–4*A, B*) performed during resuscitation. The radiographic findings of left-sided CDH include the presence of air and fluid-filled loops of bowel within the left hemithorax with mediastinal shift to the right. There will often be minimal gas within the abdomen, and the gastric bubble may be visualized within the left chest. Right-sided lesions are often harder to appreciate and appear as lobar consolidation, fluid within the chest, or diaphragmatic eventration. The findings on plain film radiography in CDH can mimic those of congenital cystic adenomatoid malformations of the lung[43] (Fig. 24–5). The differential diagnosis of CDH includes cystic adenomatoid malformation, cystic teratoma, pulmonary sequestration, bronchogenic cyst, neurogenic tumors, and primary lung sarcoma.

As many as 10% of patients with CDH will be discovered beyond the neonatal period because of acute gastrointestinal symptoms or as an incidental finding in an asymptomatic patient.[44–47] In general, late-presenting CDH has an excellent prognosis because the lung hypoplasia and pulmonary hypertension that complicate the neonate are absent. Gastric decompression proved to be lifesaving in an older child with severe respiratory and cardiopulmonary distress from massive distention of the intrathoracic stomach.[48] During fetal development, herniation of the bowel into the thorax results in both a failure of intestinal fixation and malrotation. Children with unsuspected CDH may present beyond the neonatal period with intestinal obstruction or with bowel ischemia and necrosis from volvulus.

TREATMENT

The treatment of CDH depends on the time of diagnosis, the clinical presentation, and institutional expertise. Early surgical intervention, once considered an important factor in survival, has been largely replaced by a delayed surgical approach.[49–55] Current therapeutic approaches emphasize preoperative stabilization with control of pulmonary hypertension and conventional mechanical ventilation (CMV) techniques that avoid barotrauma to an already compromised, hypoplastic pulmonary system. Therapy aimed at rescue of patients who fail CMV includes high-frequency ventilation (HFV), high-frequency oscillatory ventilation (HFOV), inhaled nitric oxide administration (NO), and ECMO.[56] Fetal diagnosis has led to fetal intervention that, although highly experimental, is available and has been performed successfully at a few centers. This approach may become more available as improvements and advances in fetal surgical techniques are made.

Although nearly 60% of fetuses diagnosed with CDH before 24 weeks' gestation will not survive,[57, 58] selection of appropriate candidates for fetal intervention has been limited by a lack of absolute indicators of poor prognosis. It is still impossible to accurately predict which fetuses will or will not

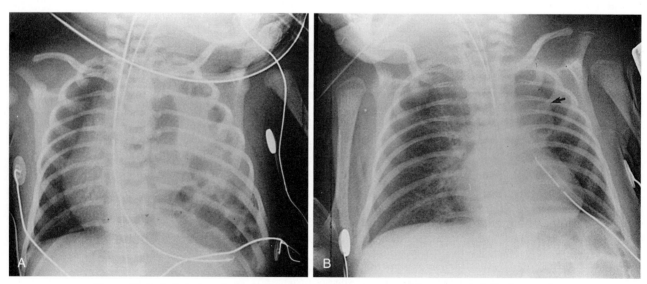

Figure 24–4. *A,* Anterioposterior chest radiography in a neonate with a congenital diaphragmatic hernia demonstrating air-filled loops of bowel within the left chest. The heart and mediastinum are shifted to the right, and the hypoplastic left lung can be seen medially. *B,* Postoperative film demonstrating hyperexpansion of the right lung with shift of the mediastinum to the left. The edge of severely hypoplastic left lung is again easily visualized *(arrow).*

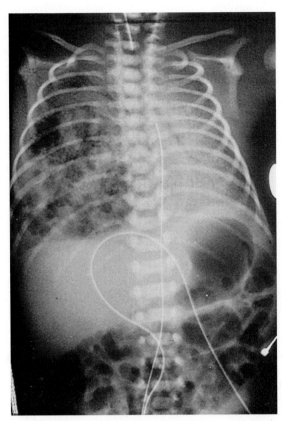

Figure 24–5. Anterioposterior chest radiograph in a neonate with a congenital cystic adenomatoid malformation (CCAM) of the right lung. The air-filled densities in the right chest closely resemble those that would result from bowel herniation into the chest. A normal bowel gas pattern within the abdomen helps to distinguish CCAM from congenital diaphragmatic hernia.

survive the gestational or neonatal period. There is no evidence that prenatal diagnosis should significantly influence decisions regarding the timing or method of delivery.

Neonates with CDH and severe respiratory distress require aggressive resuscitation. Initial interventions include endotracheal intubation, neuromuscular blockade, and positive pressure ventilation. Mask ventilation is avoided to prevent insufflation of the stomach and small bowel with air. Appropriate fluid and electrolyte management is important to ameliorate acidosis. Central venous pressure monitoring may be helpful, and a urinary catheter is generally indicated to closely monitor the adequacy of fluid resuscitation. Hypervolemia or hypovolemia should be avoided. A nasogastric tube is inserted and placed to suction to decompress the stomach and minimize bowel distension, which can compromise cardiac and pulmonary function. Echocardiography is performed early to assess associated cardiac anomalies and establish the presence and severity of pulmonary hypertension and shunting. The echocardiographic signs of pulmonary hypertension include poor contractility of the right ventricle, enlarged right heart chambers, pulmonic and tricuspid valve regurgitation, and presence of ductal shunting. Left ventricular hypoplasia

may also be identified. Pulmonary hypertension with right-to-left shunting, left ventricular dysfunction, or systemic hypotension are indications for prompt administration of inotropic agents such as dopamine (2–20 μg/kg/min), dobutamine (2–20 μg/kg/min), or epinephrine (0.1 μg/kg/min). Inotropic agents are used to augment left ventricular output and to raise systemic pressure above pulmonary pressure in order to minimize right-to-left ductal shunting. Factors that contribute to increased pulmonary vascular resistance and PPHN are avoided and quickly corrected when identified. These include hypoxia, hypercarbia, acidosis, and hypothermia. Bicarbonate is used to treat metabolic acidosis but may aggravate or increase hypercarbia.

Initial CMV using a fraction of inspired oxygen (FiO_2) of 1.0 and the lowest airway pressure possible are directed toward maintenance of preductal O_2 saturation of 90% or greater. Simultaneous preductal and postductal pulse oximetry as well as monitoring of preductal (right radial artery) and postductal (umbilical artery) blood gases aid in the assessment of ductal shunting caused by PPHN. An FiO_2 of 1.0 is commonly required to maintain adequate oxygen delivery and prevent visceral and peripheral ischemia, which cause additional acidosis and further aggravation of pulmonary hypertension. Reductions in FiO_2 should be made very gradually to prevent precipitation of PPHN.

The goals of ventilator therapy are to maintain adequate oxygenation while using techniques that minimize barotrauma to the hypoplastic and immature lungs. Barotrauma may be largely responsible for the instability of the infant and contributes to 25% of CDH deaths.[59-61] The target preductal and postductal partial pressure of oxygen (PO_2) should be at least 60 mm Hg and 40 mm Hg, respectively.

Initiation of conventional ventilator management includes pressure limited ventilation at rates of 30 to 60 breaths per minute at peak inspiratory pressures of 20 to 30 cm H_2O.[56] Positive end-expiratory pressure (PEEP) should be maintained at physiologic levels (3 to 5 cm H_2O) whenever possible, and gas flow within the ventilator circuit should be at 6 to 8 L per minute.[56] Many authors have recommended hyperventilation, hypocarbia, and alkalosis as a method to decrease ductal shunting and control PPHN in CDH.[62-64] Hyperventilation may not be necessary in the management of PPHN and may result in increased barotrauma.[65, 66] More recently, permissive hypercapnia has been suggested as a method to reduce or prevent the development of ventilator-induced lung injury.[67, 68] Permissive hypercapnia has been used in neonates with CDH and is associated with increased survival when compared with historical controls.[55, 59, 69, 70]

HFV is reserved for neonates that continue to have hypoxia and hypercarbia refractory to CMV. HFOV is more commonly used than high-frequency jet ventilation in the management of neonatal respiratory failure. HFOV can effectively reduce partial pressure of carbon dioxide (PCO_2) and induce alkalosis in neonates with CDH and may improve survival.[71, 72] However, the indications for HFOV in the management of CDH are not clearly defined. Some authors have reserved HFOV for use in those infants with hypoxia and hypercarbia ($P_{CO_2} > 60$ mm Hg) associated with high peak airway pressures (>30 cm H_2O) on CMV.[56, 73] If permissive hypercapnia replaces the long-accepted strategy of hyperventilation-induced alkalosis to manage CDH, then the benefits of HFOV become less apparent. Nevertheless, HFV permits ventilation at lower mean airway pressures[74] and may therefore reduce barotrauma.

Partial liquid ventilation has been used safely and successfully in high-risk newborns with CDH and severe respiratory distress to improve gas exchange and pulmonary compliance.[75, 76] The benefits of partial liquid ventilation with perflourocarbon in CDH are under investigation in a multicenter trial. The lungs are filled with a volume of perfluorocarbon approximately equal to functional residual capacity, and ventilation is performed at the usual CMV settings.[76] Excellent oxygenation is achieved with partial liquid ventilation at lower peak inspiratory pressures, resulting in less barotrauma.[75, 77, 79] Lung compliance is also improved by an effective reduction in alveolar surface tension.[75]

Inhaled NO, a potent and selective pulmonary vasodilator, is used for the management of severe PPHN. NO stimulates soluble guanylate cyclase within vascular endothelium to produce cyclic guanosine monophosphate, a smooth muscle relaxant. NO at doses of 6 to 80 ppm may be effective in improving postductal oxygenation, reversing ductal shunting, lowering pulmonary pressures, and improving ventilation-to-perfusion matching within the lung.[73, 80–83] Inhaled nitric oxide has been reported as being advantageous in newborn infants with CDH,[84, 85] but the clinical response to inhaled NO in other studies of neonates with CDH has been inconsistent.[80, 84–86] NO failure may be related to the severity of pulmonary hypoplasia.[73] Infants with CDH respond to lower doses of NO (<20 ppm) and may be more likely to experience rebound pulmonary hypertension if inhaled NO is weaned abruptly.[73] Dipyridamole, a phosphodiesterase inhibitor, can augment the response to inhaled NO in newborns with CDH.[87]

The pharmacologic agents tolazoline and nitroprusside have been used to induce pulmonary vasodilatation and reduce right-to-left shunting in PPHN.[62, 88] However, these agents are nonselective in their vasodilatory effects and may produce significant systemic hypotension, which may worsen shunting in these labile patients.[89, 90] For this reason, the usefulness of these agents in neonates with CDH is very limited.

Newborns with severe respiratory failure may be deficient in surfactant.[91] Replacement therapy can improve pulmonary function, reduce air leaks, and decrease the need for ECMO in neonates with PPHN associated with meconium aspiration.[92] Experimental[5, 93, 94] and clinical[21, 24, 28, 95] evidence suggests that infants with CDH are surfactant deficient and that replacement therapy might be beneficial. Some authors have questioned the presence of surfactant deficiency in human CDH.[95]

Experimentally, surfactant replacement may improve gas exchange,[94] enhance NO delivery,[93] decrease ductal shunting, and lower pulmonary vascular resistance.[26] In one randomized study, exogenous surfactant administration had no significant effect on lung compliance, duration of intubation, and oxygen requirement in neonates with CDH on extracorporeal life support.[28] Prophylactic administration of exogenous surfactant, before first breath of life in prenatally diagnosed cases, may be more effective than rescue therapy.[21, 27] The role of surfactant therapy in CDH has yet to be clearly defined.

ECMO IN CDH

ECMO is the most powerful and invasive tool for reversal of neonatal respiratory failure. ECMO is an expensive, labor-intensive technology associated with substantial morbidity and risk. ECMO has been used in the treatment and management of neonatal CDH since first reported in the late 1970s.[96] Survival in that first case series report was only 25%. Since those early years, many reports have been published suggesting that ECMO can improve survival in CDH. Overall, ECMO may have increased survival in infants with CDH by 15 to 20%. Although the results of ECMO in CDH are heavily dependent on selection criteria, survival may be as high as 69% in neonates that would otherwise have not survived without ECMO.[97] Currently, there are no absolute predictors of lethal pulmonary hypoplasia in CDH, and it is not possible to accurately predict which patients will not survive. ECMO, where available, is considered for almost all infants with CDH that cannot be managed with conventional therapy provided they have no other major lethal anomalies.

The indications for ECMO in neonates with CDH are listed in Table 24–1.[59, 70] In general, selection criteria are based on the prediction of greater than 80 to 90% mortality with maximal conventional therapy. Many predictors of survival have been proposed, including P_{CO_2}, Bohn's criteria,[98, 99] best preductal or postductal P_{O_2}, oxygenation index, and others. Although each has been applied successfully at individual institutions, none are universally applicable or accepted at other neonatal centers. Because of wide variation in management strategies and patient populations, selection criteria for ECMO should be developed in any given center based on that center's experience. The selection criteria for appropriate use of ECMO will continue to evolve as new therapies and ventilation strategies are introduced and applied.[100]

Failure of conventional therapy may be manifested by the appearance of clinical signs of barotrauma, which include interstitial or subcutaneous emphysema, pneumothorax or pneumopericardium, persistent air leaks, and high mean airway pres-

TABLE 24-1. Selection Criteria for Extracorporeal Membrane Oxygenation in Congenital Diaphragmatic Hernia

Respiratory failure refractory to maximal "conventional"
   therapy
  With oxygenation index* >40
  With acute deterioration (pH <7.15 and/or PO_2 <40 mm Hg
    for 2 h)
  Inability to hyperventilate (PCO_2 <40 mm Hg) despite
    maximal ventilation effort
  Ventilation index† >1000
  A–a O_2 gradient >600 mm Hg for >8 h (>4 h if PIP >38)
Birth weight >2000 g
Gestational age >34 weeks
Absence of intracranial hemorrhage > grade I
Absence of other congenital malformations or chromosomal
  anomalies
Preductal PO_2 <50 mm Hg for 2 h
Signs of barotrauma

*Oxygenation index = (MAP × FiO_2 × 100/postductal PO_2).
†Ventilation index = (MAP × RR).
A–a, alveolar–arterial; FiO_2, fraction of inspired oxygen; MAP, mean airway pressure; PCO_2, partial pressure of carbon dioxide; PIP, peak inspiratory pressure; PO_2, partial pressure of oxygen; RR, respiratory rate.

sures. If standard resuscitation and ventilatory techniques at an inspired oxygen concentration of 100% cannot provide preductal partial pressure of arterial oxygen (PaO_2) greater than 50 mm Hg or maintain serum pH greater than 7.15 within 1 to 2 hours, ECMO should be promptly instituted.

Arterial blood gas determinations are frequently used to determine the need for ECMO in CDH. Strict PCO_2 criteria may no longer be valid in selecting candidates for ECMO because management strategies using permissive hypercapnia may improve survival in CDH.[70] Studies correlating PCO_2 with ventilation index as a predictor of mortality were based on a strategy of hyperventilation and early surgery, both of which are losing favor.[50, 69–71] In the past, some have advocated that candidates for ECMO should have at least one preductal PO_2 of at least 80 to 100 mm Hg,[101] but many survivors have been reported who have not fulfilled this criterion.

Contraindications to ECMO include intracranial hemorrhage greater than grade I because ECMO requires systemic anticoagulation with heparin. Cranial ultrasonography is performed before initiation of ECMO and is repeated daily to assess for intracranial bleeding during the first 5 days of bypass. Neonates less than 35 weeks' gestation are at highest risk for intracranial hemorrhage. Extension of intracranial hemorrhage requires removal from ECMO.

ECMO was initially used in CDH after diaphragmatic repair.[96] More than half of newborns with CDH treated with CMV and immediate surgical repair will require postoperative ECMO.[63] Delaying the repair of CDH in newborns improves survival[102] and decreases the use of extracorporeal support.[102]

As delayed repair became more popular, preoperative stabilization with ECMO has also become more common. Consequently, preoperative stabilization using all available modalities to reverse PPHN be-

fore operative repair leads to the major problem of timing the operative repair.

The optimal time for surgical repair of the diaphragm after initiation of ECMO is controversial. Repair while on ECMO is reported to have a high rate of hemorrhagic complications,[103, 104] but refinements in surgical technique[105] and the use of antifibrinolytic agents[105, 106] have decreased these bleeding complications. Bleeding complications may also be reduced with early repair on ECMO if performed before the development of significant edema or coagulopathy.[107] Some surgeons recommend repair after resolution of pulmonary hypertension and at the point when ECMO is ready to be discontinued.[108, 109] The advantage of this approach is that ECMO can easily be reinstituted if recurrent pulmonary hypertension and respiratory failure develop postoperatively. Postoperative recurrence of respiratory failure and pulmonary hypertension may require a second course of ECMO. Survival in this group was reported at 47% in one study.[110]

A large number of pediatric surgeons prefer that the patient be weaned back to conventional ventilation and decannulated before repair of CDH. The average duration of an ECMO course in CDH is 7.9 days, and a course extending beyond 2 weeks is unusual.[107] Failure to wean from ECMO is believed to indicate lethal pulmonary hypoplasia; support may be withdrawn and operative repair of the diaphragm is not performed.[111] Overall survival in newborns with CDH managed with a delayed surgical approach and selective preoperative stabilization with ECMO can be as high as 79 to 92%.[70, 102]

SURGICAL CONSIDERATIONS AND POSTOPERATIVE MANAGEMENT

Surgical repair of a CDH should be performed efficiently and expeditiously to minimize operative stress. A transabdominal approach is preferred for most diaphragmatic defects. The abdomen is entered through an incision placed below the costal margin. This approach allows easy reduction of the viscera and excellent visualization of the diaphragmatic defect (Fig. 24–6).

Bowel, liver, and spleen are carefully reduced from the thoracic cavity. A true hernia sac may be present in up to 20% of cases and should be excised. Once the limits and extent of the diaphragmatic defect are precisely defined, the diaphragm is repaired.

Small defects are closed primarily with 2-0 or 3-0 permanent sutures with or without pledgets. Larger defects can be closed primarily but may produce a flattened diaphragm with poor respiratory excursion. In this situation, the large defect should be closed with a prosthetic patch. Polytetrafluoroethylene (1-mm thick) is a suitable material for patch closure. The patch is tailored slightly larger than the diaphragmatic defect to restore a concave shape to the reconstructed diaphragm.[112] Restoring the "dome" shape of the diaphragm helps to expand the

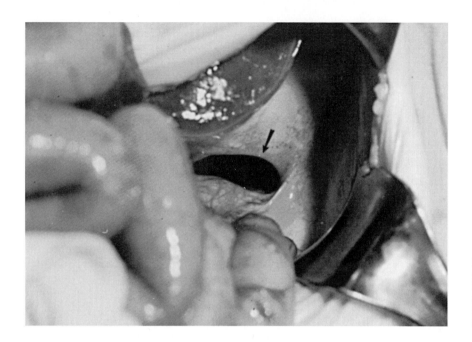

Figure 24–6. A small posterolateral diaphragmatic hernia *(arrow)* approached through a subcostal incision. The transabdominal approach allows easy reduction of the viscera and excellent visualization of the defect.

abdominal capacity and limits the overexpansion of the ipsilateral lung. Tension-free closure of the defect in this manner also prevents constriction of the thoracic cage and limits the adverse effects of closure on chest wall compliance. With very large defects there may be no apparent or easily recognizable posterior rim of diaphragm. Sutures into the abdominal wall, into the ribs, or encircling the ribs are needed to secure the prosthesis in these cases.

Before closure of the diaphragm, a chest tube is positioned and brought out through a low intercostal space. This tube can be used to adjust intrathoracic pressures to shift the mediastinum as necessary. Often it is for drainage only. Tube thoracostomy is not mandatory, and some do not use it routinely.[55] The diaphragmatic repair is inspected for hemostasis, and fibrin glue is often applied to the suture line in anticoagulated infants repaired while on ECMO.[113]

After completion of the diaphragmatic repair, the abdominal wall is stretched to increase the capacity of the abdominal cavity. The abdominal wall fascia is closed unless closure restricts ventilation, in which case only skin closure is performed. The resulting abdominal wall hernia can be repaired at a later date. An alternative is to repair the fascial defect with a prosthetic patch.[113] The skin can be mobilized and closed over the patch, avoiding a secondary ventral hernia repair.

Postoperative Care

Postoperative ventilator management continues as before diaphragmatic repair. Surgical repair of the diaphragm decreases chest compliance initially and may adversely affect peak and mean inspiratory pressures. Surgical stress can precipitate intense pulmonary vasoconstriction and recurrence of pulmonary hypertension and persistent fetal circula-

tion. If respiratory failure ensues and cannot be controlled with any of the previously discussed ventilation techniques, ECMO should be instituted.

The therapeutic goal of postoperative ventilation is to minimize barotrauma while maintaining normal pH and PCO_2. Hyperventilation has been recommended,[63] but permissive hypercapnea is gaining wider popularity. An FiO_2 of 1.0 may be required to maintain adequate oxygenation perioperatively. Rapid decreases in FiO_2 must be avoided because reductions of only 0.1 have been seen to trigger pulmonary vasospasm and recurrent pulmonary hypertension.[114]

Generally, the chest tube is connected to water seal rather than put to vacuum in the postoperative period. The lungs will gradually enlarge, displacing fluid and air within the pleural space. If air is removed from the pleural space by suction, the mediastinum will shift, allowing overdistention of the contralateral lung. Overexpansion may be a contributing factor in postoperative contralateral pneumothorax.[114]

Several nonpulmonary complications can occur in these neonates during the postoperative period.[115] These include hemorrhage, chylothorax, and adhesive intestinal obstruction. Other long-term complications associated with CDH are gastroesophageal reflux, scoliosis, and pectus deformities. Recurrent diaphragmatic hernia occurs most frequently after prosthetic patch closure.

FETAL SURGERY FOR CDH

Fetal surgical intervention is appealing as a potential method to prevent pulmonary hypoplasia, but fetal surgery exposes both fetus and mother to significant risk.[116, 117] Consequently, only fetuses with the most severe pulmonary hypoplasia should be considered potential candidates for fetal intervention.

Several early prenatal ultrasonographic findings may suggest a poor prognosis and therefore may be useful to select appropriate candidates for fetal intervention. The best ultrasonographic predictors of high mortality include early cardiac ventricular disproportion,[36] reduced lung area to head circumference ratio,[118] and hepatic herniation into the chest.[58, 119] Other findings that may be associated with a poor prognosis in CDH include polyhydramnios,[32] diagnosis before 25 weeks' gestation,[120] left ventricular hypoplasia,[35, 121] and the presence of an intrathoracic stomach.[122] None of these prenatal findings are absolutely predictive of nonsurvival with conventional postnatal therapy.

In Utero Repair of CDH

The rationale for in utero repair of CDH was initially based on experimental demonstration that reduction of herniated viscera in the fetus prevents lung hypoplasia and restores lung growth. The first clinical experience with in utero repair of CDH was reported in 1990.[119, 123] Successful repair and outcome is possible in fetuses without hepatic herniation,[123] but these fetuses have good prognosis for survival with conventional postnatal therapy[58] and therefore are not candidates for fetal surgery. Hepatic herniation into the chest is not correctable by in utero repair because reduction of the liver causes acute obstruction of the umbilical vein and fetal death.[58, 124] Although the techniques for successful open in utero surgery have been refined, in utero repair of CDH currently does not improve survival.[58, 124]

In Utero Tracheal Occlusion

The dynamics of fetal lung fluid have a dramatic effect on lung growth and maturity. Oligohydramnios and other conditions associated with a deficiency of fetal lung fluid cause pulmonary hypoplasia. Tracheal occlusion in utero can prevent pulmonary hypoplasia and can increase lung growth in these circumstances. Fetal tracheal ligation in experimental models of CDH induces lung growth,[125] reverses pulmonary hypoplasia,[125] improves lung compliance,[126, 127] and reduces herniated viscera from the chest.[125, 127] However, tracheal ligation may adversely affect type II pneumocyte development and surfactant production.[128, 129] Fetal tracheal occlusion has been successfully performed in human fetuses with CDH via both open hysterotomy[117, 130] and endoscopic[131] techniques. Although many technical problems of fetal surgery have been solved,[58] it remains a highly experimental procedure with significant risk for complications.[117, 132] Despite reversal of pulmonary hypoplasia, survival has been limited in humans.[117, 130, 131] Further experimental and clinical investigations are required before in

utero tracheal occlusion becomes a recommended therapy for CDH.

LUNG TRANSPLANTATION IN CDH

Lobar lung transplantation has been successfully used as a rescue therapy in CDH.[133] In this case report, the neonate was initially stabilized with ECMO followed by delayed repair of the diaphragm with a prosthetic patch while on ECMO. Although the neonate was successfully decannulated from ECMO, lung transplantation became necessary as a result of progressive pulmonary failure. Despite this single report, the role of lung transplantation and ECMO as a bridge to transplantation in cases of CDH with lethal pulmonary hypoplasia is not known.

OUTCOMES IN CDH

It is difficult to quantify the results of therapy and treatment of CDH owing to the tremendous variation in the strategies and techniques used to support these critically ill patients. A few points of variation between and often within institutions include differences in severity of illness, ventilation strategies (hyperventilation vs. permissive hypercapnia), ventilator type (conventional versus oscillation), availability and selection criteria of ECMO, and variable use of other pharmacologic agents (i.e., NO, surfactant). As newer and more innovative approaches to managing CDH become available, comparisons will become even more difficult.

Survival statistics in CDH are very institution-dependent. In a recent review of survival data from groups reporting between 1990 and 1995 on infants with CDH, an overall survival of 60% was reported.[134] Survival varied from 25 to 83% at the 30 reporting institutions. Prenatal diagnosis of CDH is associated with an increased mortality, but in the absence of other major anomalies, survival is probably not affected.[39] If stillbirths and infants with CDH that die before transfer to referral centers are included, overall survival from CDH is still only 40 to 60%.[40, 135, 136] CDH accounts for approximately 4 to 10% of neonatal deaths that occur from congenital anomalies.[134]

Two factors that have dramatically impacted survival in CDH have been the introduction of ECMO and the adaptation of less barotraumatic methods of ventilation, including permissive hypercapnia. The use of ECMO has generally been believed to improve overall survival by 15 to 20% at institutions using this technique. Many reports demonstrate improved survival over historical controls after introduction of ECMO in the management of CDH,[137–139] whereas others have reported no survival advantage with ECMO.[140, 141] Some surgeons have reported improvement in survival during the era of ECMO but without the use of ECMO.[51, 142, 143]

Sequelae of CDH Repair

The *pulmonary function* of survivors with CDH is favorable. Most survivors are healthy and enjoy normal lives free of respiratory problems,[144] but long-term pulmonary consequences of CDH are dependent on the severity of pulmonary hypoplasia at birth and the degree of lung injury. Infants that experience uneventful preoperative and postoperative courses will generally have normal lung function.[63] For those children who require substantial support and intervention, ventilatory impairment and thoracic deformities are demonstrated in approximately 50%, despite minimal or no pulmonary symptoms. Spirometry and diffusion studies are normal in one half of survivors, and the remainder have findings suggesting some degree of restrictive,[145, 146] obstructive,[146, 147] or combined respiratory impairment.[146]

Functional residual capacity is reduced in the newborn after repair of CDH, but investigators have reported normal lung volumes over the long term.[148, 149] Increased bronchial reactivity seen in approximately one third of survivors is more common in those patients presenting within 6 hours of birth with severe pulmonary hypoplasia and large diaphragmatic defects.[146] Pulmonary ventilation and perfusion deficiencies are more common on the side of the diaphragmatic defect,[146, 147] but diffusing capacity is typically normal. The volume of the ipsilateral lung increases with time, but this increase may be secondary to emphysematous changes.[150] Air trapping within the hypoplastic lung may appear as hyperlucent areas on chest radiography.

One third of CDH patients may have clinical and radiologic evidence of *bronchopulmonary dysplasia,* which is more common in those infants managed with prolonged mechanical ventilation and O_2 supplementation. Lung function in survivors of CDH improves with age,[151] and alveolar multiplication continues from birth until 7 or 8 years of age. Even though the hypoplastic lung may grow to be functionally normal, structurally it remains abnormal, and the number of bronchiolar and pulmonary arterial divisions is relatively fixed. It is important to note that all long-term pulmonary studies are based on survivors managed with conventional strategies (hyperventilation, alkalinization, etc). If mortality rates continue to improve with the addition of newer therapies (ECMO, NO, HFV, permissive hypercapnia), some survivors with more severe lung hypoplasia can be expected, and the long-term pulmonary sequelae may become more significant.

Gastroesophageal reflux is a common finding in patients with CDH. The incidence of gastroesophageal reflux after successful repair of CDH is reported to be 12 to 89%.[152, 153] ECMO-treated survivors may be at greatest risk.[151, 154] The gastroesophageal reflux observed in patients with CDH is part of a generalized foregut dysmotility[155, 156] that may also include esophageal ectasia and delayed gastric emptying. Esophageal ectasia and dysmotility may be the result of kinking or relative obstruction at the gastroesophageal junction that is caused when the stomach translocates into the chest.[157] Large diaphragmatic defects may compromise the esophageal

hiatus of the diaphragm, thereby destroying its contribution to the lower esophageal sphincter mechanism and predisposing to reflux. Management of gastroesophageal reflux and upper gastrointestinal dysmotility in patients with CDH is not different from the usual medical therapy, including prokinetic agents and H_2 antagonists. Antireflux surgery is not usually necessary,[156] but surgical treatment has been required in 10 to 15% of cases.[152, 158, 159]

Intestinal obstruction is a fairly common event after CDH repair and occurs in up to 20% of patients followed long-term.[115, 160] Small bowel obstruction may be caused by adhesions, midgut volvulus,[161] or recurrent herniation with incarceration.

Recurrent diaphragmatic hernia is more common with prosthetic patch repair; overall, it occurs in approximately 5 to 20% of patients.[154, 161] Patients requiring ECMO may be at a higher risk for recurrent herniation when a prosthetic patch is used to reconstruct the diaphragm,[162] particularly if the repair is performed while on bypass.

Growth retardation, failure to thrive, and *developmental delays* are common in survivors of CDH.[151] Poor growth may be caused by inadequate oral intake related to gastrointestinal dysmotility or gastroesophageal reflux. In addition, caloric requirements may be higher due to an increased work of breathing and tachypnea.[163] In survivors, 30 to 50% will be less than the fifth percentile for weight in the first year of life[154, 161, 163] despite adequate oral intake. Weight differences improve with time and may be normal for age by 2 years.[153, 156] CDH infants requiring ECMO are at greatest risk for failure to thrive.

Survivors of CDH are at increased risk for neurodevelopmental problems, including major motor disabilities[153] and developmental delays in both motor and verbal skills.[161] Neurocognitive defects are common in survivors of CDH.[164] It is difficult to separate the developmental delays that are caused by the disease process itself from those that may be caused by specific therapeutic interventions. Hyperventilation[165, 166] and ECMO are both associated with potential adverse neurologic sequelae. Hyperventilation and alkalinization therapy are often instituted to treat pulmonary hypertension but can dramatically reduce cerebral blood flow, which is sensitive to acute changes of arterial P_{CO_2} and pH.[167] Acute hyperventilation to reduce P_{CO_2} from 40 mm Hg down to 20 mm Hg can reduce cerebral perfusion by up to 50%.[167] Alkalosis reduces oxygen delivery to all body tissues by increasing hemoglobin–oxygen affinity. Consequently, hyperventilation further reduces cerebral oxygen delivery in neonates already compromised by perinatal asphyxia, hypoxemia, and cardiovascular instability. ECMO increases the risks for cerebral palsy, sensorineural hearing loss, speech and verbal skill developmental delay, vision loss, and seizure disorder.[168] The overall incidence of neurologic abnormalities in survivors of ECMO therapy is 10 to 45%.[151, 154, 161, 164, 169, 170] The hearing loss after ECMO therapy is often delayed in onset and is progressive. Significant hearing loss is detected in 4 to 28% of ECMO survivors[161, 169]; serial follow-up hearing examinations are mandatory.

☐ Retrosternal Hernia

Retrosternal hernia occurs in two forms. The most common form is called a foramen of Morgagni hernia, or parasternal hernia, and represents only 4 to 6% of congenital diaphragmatic defects.[114, 171] This diaphragmatic defect results from failure of the sternal and crural portions of the diaphragm to fuse at the site where the superior epigastric (internal mammary) artery traverses the diaphragm. Morgagni's hernias may be unilateral or bilateral, but occur unilaterally on the right side in 90% of cases. Bilateral parasternal hernias occur in 7% of cases.[171] Retrosternal hernias will often appear as a midline defect at laparotomy (Fig. 24–7). A well-defined hernia sac is usually present. The majority of these lesions are asymptomatic and are diagnosed from chest radiographs obtained in adult patients being evaluated for unrelated pulmonary symptoms.

Morgagni's hernias can be found in association with other anomalies, including congenital heart defects and trisomy 21.[172, 173] In one series, 14% of 22 infants with Morgagni's hernias also had Down's syndrome.[172] Congenital heart disease may be present in up to 58% of infants with Morgagni's hernias,[174] and cardiac tamponade is a rare presentation of this type of hernia.[175]

Children with Morgagni's hernias are more often symptomatic than adults with this lesion, presenting with recurrent respiratory infection, coughing, vomiting, or epigastric distress.[171] Intestinal obstruction[176] and ischemic bowel with necrosis[177] are possible. These hernias often contain transverse colon, omentum, liver, small bowel, stomach, or spleen. Gastrointestinal symptoms may be intermittent. Because Morgagni's hernias are at risk for incarceration and strangulation, these lesions should be repaired soon after they are discovered.

Chest radiography in the neonate with a Morgagni hernia often demonstrates a well defined air-fluid filled structure immediately behind the sternum (Fig. 24–8A, B). A lateral chest radiograph can localize this finding to the retrosternal space. Contrast studies obtained for evaluation of gastrointestinal symptoms will demonstrate small bowel, colon, and occasionally stomach within the thoracic cavity.

The second form of retrosternal hernia occurs as a component of Cantrell's pentalogy.[178] The pentalogy of Cantrell includes a constellation of congenital defects: omphalocele; inferior sternal cleft; severe cardiac defects, including thoracoabdominal ectopia cordis; diaphragmatic hernia; and pericardial defects.[179] The large diaphragmatic defect results from embryologic failure in the development of the septum transversum. Repair of this defect requires correction of cardiac defects plus diaphragmatic and abdominal wall closure. Prosthetic material is often required to repair the diaphragm.

☐ Eventration of the Diaphragm

Eventration is an abnormal elevation of diaphragm that results in paradoxical motion of the affected hemidiaphram during inspiration and expiration.[180, 181] The congenital form is characterized by an elevation of an attenuated diaphragm and results from incomplete development of the muscular portion or central tendon of the diaphragm. In cases when the diaphragm exists as only a thin membrane, the distinction from CDH with a hernia sac is arbitrary.[63] Like CDH, congenital eventration may result in pulmonary hypoplasia, but pulmonary hypertension and persistent fetal circulation are uncommon. Eventration can occur in association with other congenital anomalies, including pulmonary sequestration, congenital heart disease, tracheomalacia, cerebral agenesis, and trisomic chromosomal abnormalities.[182, 183] Congenital eventration occurs most commonly on the left side, but bilateral diaphragmatic eventration has been reported.[184–186] Large eventrations can potentially interfere with postnatal lung development.

Eventration in the neonate may be difficult to distinguish from paralysis, which is a consequence of traction injury to the nerve roots of the phrenic nerve during traumatic delivery. Brachial plexus palsy may also be present. Paralysis of the diaphragm in older infants and children is most commonly caused by iatrogenic phrenic nerve injury complicating cardiac surgery or resection of mediastinal tumors. Diaphragmatic paralysis may result from phrenic nerve injury after surgical procedures in the neck. In addition, inflammatory or neoplastic

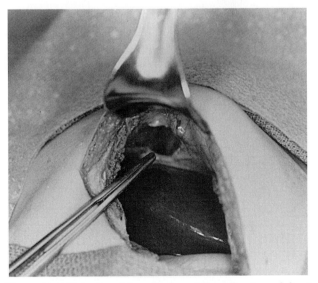

Figure 24–7. Retrosternal hernia viewed through a transabdominal incision. The bowel has been reduced, and the defect is seen immediately posterior to the xiphoid process.

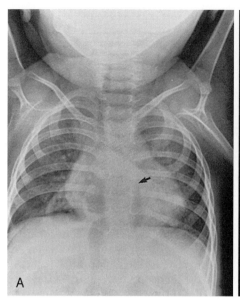
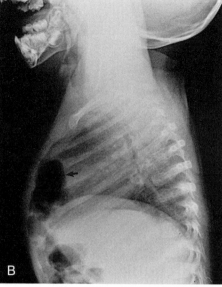

Figure 24–8. *A,* Chest radiography in a neonate with a retrosternal hernia. Anterioposterior film demonstrates air-filled loops of bowel above the diaphragm and posterior to the sternum *(arrow). B,* Lateral projection confirming the retrosternal position of the herniated viscera *(arrow).*

processes adjacent to the phrenic nerve can also cause paralysis of the diaphragm.

Although newborns with diaphragmatic eventration can be asymptomatic, most will present with respiratory distress, tachypnea, and pallor. Additional clinical signs include ipsilateral dullness to percussion and unilateral or bilateral diminished breath sounds. The maximal cardiac impulse is shifted away from the side of the lesion. Neonates with eventration often suck poorly and tire easily during feedings and subsequently fail to gain weight. Respiratory distress results from alveolar hypoventilation and paradoxical movement of the diaphragm. During inspiration, the affected hemidiaphragm rises and the mediastinum shifts toward the opposite side. Lung expansion is impaired bilaterally.

Chest radiography typically demonstrates an elevated hemidiaphragm (Fig. 24–9). If chest radiography suggests diaphragmatic eventration, the diagnosis can be confirmed by fluoroscopic or ultrasonographic demonstration of paradoxic motion of the diaphragm and mediastinal shift with inspiration and expiration. The diagnosis of eventration or paralysis may be obscured in neonates and infants who are intubated and being ventilated.[114] A dysfunctional diaphragm may be a cause for inability to wean from mechanical ventilation. Older infants and children may present with recurrent pneumonia or gastrointestinal symptoms, including intermittent vomiting, postprandial pain, dyspepsia, or gastric volvulus. Gastrointestinal complaints are more common with left-sided lesions. Computed tomography or other additional studies may be necessary to distinguish eventration from tumors, bronchogenic cysts, pulmonary sequestration or consolidation, or pleural effusions.

Initial treatment of infants with eventration includes upright positioning, supplemental oxygen, and nutritional support. Mechanical ventilation is not always necessary, but often is required to maintain adequate oxygenation and gas exchange. The indications for surgical intervention include respiratory distress requiring continued ventilatory support, recurrent pulmonary infections, and failure to thrive. Newborns with congenital eventration should undergo plication early and do not benefit from conservative management.[114, 183] Small eventrations that are clinically asymptomatic may not require surgical intervention.

The surgical treatment of a symptomatic eventration is simple plication of the diaphragm.[114, 181, 183, 187, 188] Plication improves respiratory mechanics by

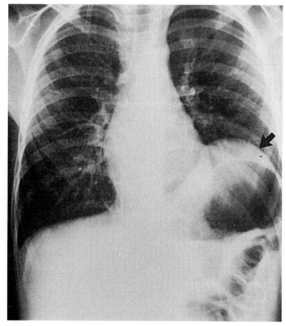

Figure 24–9. Anterioposterior chest radiograph demonstrates a large diaphragmatic eventration *(arrow).* The abdominal viscera remain beneath an intact but attenuated left hemidiaphragm.

increasing both tidal volume and maximal breathing capacity by immobilizing the plicated diaphragm to reduce its paradoxic movement and the associated contralateral shift of the mediastinum. In cases of paralysis caused by birth injury or postoperative phrenic nerve palsy, spontaneous recovery is possible; continuous positive pressure ventilation may be all that is required. Plication is indicated in patients who cannot be weaned from positive pressure ventilation after 2 to 3 weeks.[183, 187, 189, 190] Plication does not prevent return of diaphragmatic function.[187, 191] Iatrogenic phrenic nerve transection will result in permanent paralysis of the hemidiaphragm, and prophylactic plication is recommended.[114, 187, 192] Phrenic nerve repair has been successfully performed in older infants and children.[193, 194]

Plication of the diaphragm can be performed from either the transthoracic or transabdominal approach. On the right side, the operation is easiest to perform through a seventh intercostal space thoracotomy. A left-sided eventration can easily be repaired through a left subcostal incision. Bilateral eventrations are approached through a transverse upper abdominal incision. Several rows of sutures are placed to imbricate and flatten the diaphragm. Sutures are placed carefully to avoid branches of the phrenic nerve and to obtain generous bites of tissue. Resection of the diaphragm is not necessary or indicated.

The perioperative morbidity and mortality of diaphragmatic plication are low and are mostly related to complications of prolonged mechanical ventilation.[183] In infants without major anomalies or other complicating factors, early plication results in immediate improvement in pulmonary mechanics, and long-term respiratory function is excellent.[182, 187, 191]

REFERENCES

1. Gross R: Congenital hernia of the diaphragm. In Gross R (ed): The Surgery of Infancy and Childhood: Its Principles and Techniques (1st ed). Philadelphia, WB Saunders, 1953, pp 428–444.
2. Kluth D, Losty P, Schnitzer JJ, et al: Toward understanding the developmental anatomy of congenital diaphragmatic hernia. Clin Perinatol 23:655–669, 1996.
3. Iritani I: Experimental study on embryogenesis of congenital diaphragmatic hernia. Anat Embryol 169:133–139, 1984.
4. Kluth D, Keijzer R, Hertl M, et al: Embryology of congenital diaphragmatic hernia. Semin Pediatr Surg 5:224–233, 1996.
5. Glick PL, Stannard VA, Leach CL, et al: Pathophysiology of congenital diaphragmatic hernia II: The fetal lamb CDH model is surfactant deficient. J Pediatr Surg 27:382–387, 1992.
6. Puri P: Congenital diaphragmatic hernia. Curr Probl Surg 31:787–846, 1994.
7. Areechon W, Reid L: Hypoplasia of the lung with congenital diaphragmatic hernia. Br Med J 1:230–233, 1963.
8. Campanale RP, Rowland RH: Hypoplasia of the lung associated with congenital diaphragmatic hernia. Ann Surg 142:176, 1955.
9. Kitagawa M, Hislop A, Boyden EA, et al: Lung hypoplasia in congenital diaphragmatic hernia. A quantitative study of airway, artery, and alveolar development. Br J Surg 58:342–346, 1971.
10. de Lorimier A, Tierney D, Parker H: Hypoplastic lungs in
11. George DK, Cooney TP, Chiu BK, et al: Hypoplasia and immaturity of the terminal lung unit (acinus) in congenital diaphragmatic hernia. Am Rev Respir Dis 136:947–950, 1987.
12. Wilcox DT, Irish MS, Holm BA, et al: Pulmonary parenchymal abnormalities in congenital diaphragmatic hernia. Clin Perinatol 23:771–779, 1996.
13. Dibbins AW: Congenital diaphragmatic hernia: Hypoplastic lung and pulmonary vasoconstriction. Clin Perinatol 5:93–104, 1978.
14. Ein SH, Barker G, Olley P, et al: The pharmacologic treatment of newborn diaphragmatic hernia—a 2-year evaluation. J Pediatr Surg 15:384–394, 1980.
15. Vacanti J, Crone R, Murphy J, et al: The pulmonary hemodynamic response to perioperative anesthesia in the treatment of high-risk infants with congenital diaphragmatic hernia. J Pediatr Surg 19:672–679, 1984.
16. Vacanti JP, O'Rourke PP, Lillehei CW, et al: The cardiopulmonary consequences of high-risk congenital diaphragmatic hernia. Pediatr Surg Int 3:1–5, 1988.
17. Kobayashi H, Puri P: Plasma endothelin levels in congenital diaphragmatic hernia. J Pediatr Surg 29:1258–1261, 1994.
18. Bos AP, Sluiter W, Tenbrinck R, et al: Angiotensin-converting enzyme activity is increased in lungs of rats with pulmonary hypoplasia and congenital diaphragmatic hernia. Exp Lung Res 21:41–50, 1995.
19. Ford WDA, James MJ, Walsh JA: Congenital diaphragmatic hernia: Association between pulmonary vascular resistance and plasma thromboxane concentrations. Arch Dis Child 59:143–146, 1984.
20. Bos AP, Tibboel D, Hazebroek F, et al: Congenital diaphragmatic hernia: Impact of prostanoids in the perioperative period. Arch Dis Child 65:994–995, 1990.
21. Glick PL, Leach CL, Besner GE, et al: Pathophysiology of congenital diaphragmatic hernia. III: Exogenous surfactant therapy for the high-risk neonate with CDH. J Pediatr Surg 27:866–869, 1992.
22. Blackburn WR, Logsdon P, Alexander JA: Congenital diaphragmatic hernia: Studies of lung compression and structure. Am Rev Respir Dis 115:S275, 1977.
23. Wigglesworth JS, Desai R, Guerrini P: Fetal lung hypoplasia: Biochemical and structural variations and their possible significance. Arch Dis Child 56:606–615, 1981.
24. Berk C, Grundy M: 'High risk' lecithin/sphingomyelin ratios associated with neonatal diaphragmatic hernia. Case reports. Br J Obstet Gynaecol 89:250–251, 1982.
25. Hisanaga S, Shimokawa H, Kashiwabara Y, et al: Unexpectedly low lecithin/sphingomyelin ratio associated with fetal diaphragmatic hernia. Am J Obstet Gynecol 149:905–906, 1984.
26. O'Toole SJ, Karamanoukian HL, Morin FC: Surfactant decreases pulmonary vascular resistance and increases pulmonary blood flow in the fetal lamb model of congenital diaphragmatic hernia. J Pediatr Surg 31:507–511, 1996.
27. Bos AP, Tibboel D, Hazebroek FW, et al: Surfactant replacement therapy in high-risk congenital diaphragmatic hernia [letter]. Lancet 338:1279, 1991.
28. Lotze A, Knight GR, Anderson KD, et al: Surfactant (beractant) therapy for infants with congenital diaphragmatic hernia on ECMO: Evidence of persistent surfactant deficiency. J Pediatr Surg 29:407–412, 1994.
29. Butler N, Claireaux A: Congenital diaphragmatic hernia as a cause of perinatal mortality. Lancet 1:659–663, 1962.
30. Sweed Y, Puri P: The impact of associated malformations on the survival of neonates with congenital diaphragmatic hernia. Arch Dis Child 69:68–70, 1993.
31. Fauza DO, Wilson JM: Congenital diaphragmatic hernia and associated anomalies: Their incidence, identification, and impact on prognosis. J Pediatr Surg 29:1113–1117, 1994.
32. Crawford DC, Wright VM, Drake DP, et al: Fetal diaphragmatic hernia: The value of fetal echocardiography in the prediction of postnatal outcome. Br J Obstet Gynaecol 96:705–710, 1989.

fetal lambs with surgically produced congenital diaphragmatic hernia. Surgery 62:12, 1967.

33. Sharland GK, Lockhart SM, Heward AJ, et al: Prognosis in fetal diaphragmatic hernia. Am J Obstet Gynecol 166:9–13, 1991.

34. Adzick NS, Harrison MR, Glick PL, et al: Diaphragmatic hernia in the fetus: Prenatal diagnosis and outcome in 94 cases. J Pediatr Surg 20:357–361, 1985.

35. Benjamin D, Juul S, Seibert J: Congenital posterolateral diaphragmatic hernia: Associated malformations. J Pediatr Surg 23:899–903, 1988.

36. Puri P, Gorman F: Lethal non-pulmonary anomalies associated with congenital diaphragmatic hernia: Implications for early intrauterine surgery. J Pediatr Surg 19:29–32, 1984.

37. Bell M, Ternberg J: Antenatal diagnosis of congenital diaphragmatic hernia. Pediatrics 60:738–740, 1977.

38. Wilcox DT, Irish MS, Holm BA, et al: Prenatal diagnosis of congenital diaphragmatic hernia with predictors of mortality. Clin Perinatol 23:701–709, 1996.

39. Wilson JM, Fauza DO, Lund DP, et al: Antenatal diagnosis of isolated congenital diaphragmatic hernia is not an indicator of outcome. J Pediatr Surg 29:815–819, 1994.

40. Steinhorn RH, Kriesmer PJ, Green TP, et al: Congenital diaphragmatic hernia in Minnesota: Impact of antenatal diagnosis on survival. Arch Pediatr Adolesc Med 148:626–631, 1994.

41. Glick PL, Pohlson EC, Resta R, et al: Maternal serum alpha-fetoprotein is a marker for fetal anomalies in pediatric surgery. J Pediatr Surg 23:16–20, 1988.

42. Resta R, Luthy D, Kamp L, et al: Low maternal serum alpha-fetoprotein levels and congenital diaphragmatic defects. Am J Med Genet 26:991–994, 1987.

43. Campbell D, Raffensperger J: Cystic disease of the lung masquerading as diaphragmatic hernia. J Thorac Cardiovasc Surg 64:592–595, 1972.

44. Berman L, Stringer D, Ein S, et al: The late-presenting pediatric Bochdalek hernia: A 20-year review. J Pediatr Surg 23:735–739, 1988.

45. Wiseman N, MacPherson R: "Acquired" congenital diaphragmatic hernia. J Pediatr Surg 12:657–665, 1977.

46. Newman B, Afshani E, Karp M, et al: Presentation of congenital diaphragmatic hernia past the neonatal period. Arch Surg 121:813–816, 1986.

47. Weber T, Tracy T, Bailey P, et al: Congenital diaphragmatic hernia beyond infancy. Am J Surg 162:643–646, 1991.

48. Paut O, Mely L, Viard L, et al: Acute presentation of congenital diaphragmatic hernia past the neonatal period: A life threatening emergency. Can J Anaesth 43:621–625, 1996.

49. Cartlidge PH, Mann NP, Kapila L: Pre-operative stabilisation in congenital diaphragmatic hernia. Arch Dis Child 61:1226–1228, 1986.

50. Langer J, Filler R, Bohn D, et al: Timing of surgery for congenital diaphragmatic hernia: Is emergency operation necessary? J Pediatr Surg 23:731–734, 1988.

51. Charlton A, Bruce J, Davenport M: Timing of surgery in congenital diaphragmatic hernia: Low mortality after pre-operative stabilization. Anaesthesia 46:820–823, 1991.

52. Coughlin J, Drucker D, Cullen M, et al: Delayed repair of congenital diaphragmatic hernia. Am Surg 59:90–93, 1993.

53. Wilson JM, Lund DP, Lillehei CW, et al: Delayed repair and preoperative ECMO does not improve survival in high-risk congenital diaphragmatic hernia. J Pediatr Surg 27:368–372, 1992.

54. Breaux C Jr, Rouse T, Cain W, et al: Improvement in survival of patients with congenital diaphragmatic hernia utilizing a strategy of delayed repair after medical and/or extracorporeal membrane oxygenation stabilization. J Pediatr Surg 26:333–338, 1991.

55. Wung JT, Sahni R, Moffitt ST, et al: Congenital diaphragmatic hernia: Survival treated with very delayed surgery, spontaneous respiration, and no chest tubes. J Pediatr Surg 30:406–409, 1995.

56. Hirschl R: Innovative therapies in the management of newborns with congenital diaphragmatic hernia. Semin Pediatr Surg 5:256–265, 1996.

57. Harrison MR, Adzick NS, Estes JM, et al: A prospective study of the outcome for fetuses with diaphragmatic hernia. JAMA 271:382–384, 1994.

58. Mychaliska G, Bullard K, Harrison M: In utero management of congenital diaphragmatic hernia. Clin Perinatol 23:823–841, 1996.

59. Wilson J, Lund D, Lillehei C, et al: Congenital diaphragmatic hernia—a tale of two cities: The Boston experience. J Pediatr Surg 32:401–405, 1997.

60. Kolobow T, Moretti M, Fumagelli R, et al: Severe impairment in lung function induced by high peak airway pressure during mechanical ventilation. Am Rev Respir Dis 135:312–315, 1987.

61. Dreyfuss D, Sjoer P, Basset G, et al: High inflation pressure pulmonary edema: Respective effects of high airway pressure, high tidal volume, and positive end-expiratory pressure during mechanical ventilation. Am Rev Respir Dis 137:1159–1164, 1988.

62. Drummond W, Gregory G, Heymann M, et al: The independent effects of hyperventilation, tolazoline, and dopamine on infants with persistent pulmonary hypertension. J Pediatr 98:603–611, 1981.

63. de Lorimier AA: Diaphragmatic hernia. In Ashcraft KW, Holder TM (eds): Pediatric Surgery (2nd ed). Philadelphia, WB Saunders, 1993, pp 204–217.

64. Reynolds M, Luck S, Lappen R: The "critical" neonate with diaphragmatic hernia: A 21-year perspective. J Pediatr Surg 19:364–369, 1984.

65. Wung J, James L, Kilchevsky E, et al: Management of infants with severe respiratory failure and the persistence of the fetal circulation without hyperventilation. Pediatrics 76:488–494, 1985.

66. Dworetz A, Moya F, Sabo B, et al: Survival of infants with persistent pulmonary hypertension without extracorporeal membrane oxygenation. Pediatrics 84:1–6, 1989.

67. Hickling K: Low volume ventilation with permissive hypercapnia in the adult respiratory distress syndrome. Clin Intensive Care 3:67–78, 1992.

68. Hickling K, Henderson S, Jackson R: Low mortality associated with low volume pressure limited ventilation with permissive hypercapnea in severe respiratory distress syndrome. Intensive Care Med 16:372–377, 1990.

69. Wung J, Sahni R, Moffitt S, et al: Survival with congenital diaphragmatic hernia treated with delayed surgery, spontaneous respiration and no tube thoracostomy. Pediatr Res 35:261A, 1994.

70. Frenckner B, Ehren H, Granholm T, et al: Improved results in patients who have congenital diaphragmatic hernia using preoperative stabilization, extracorporeal membrane oxygenation, and delayed surgery. J Pediatr Surg 32:1185–1189, 1997.

71. Miguet D, Claris O, Lapillonne A, et al: Preoperative stabilization using high frequency oscillatory ventilation in the management of congenital diaphragmatic hernia. Crit Care Med 22:S77–S82, 1994.

72. Tamura M, Tsuchida Y, Kawano T, et al: Piston-pump-type high frequency oscillatory ventilation for neonates with congenital diaphragmatic hernia: A new protocol. J Pediatr Surg 23:478–482, 1988.

73. Bohn D, Pearl R, Irish M, et al: Postnatal management of congenital diaphragmatic hernia. Clin Perinatol 23:843–872, 1996.

74. Karl S, Ballantine T, Snider M: High-frequency ventilation at rates of 375 to 1800 cycles per minute in four neonates with congenital diaphragmatic hernia. J Pediatr Surg 18:822–828, 1983.

75. Major D, Cadenas M, Cloutier R, et al: Combined gas ventilation and perfluorochemical tracheal instillation as an alternative treatment for lethal congenital diaphragmatic hernia in lambs. J Pediatr Surg 30:1178–1182, 1995.

76. Pranikoff T, Gauger PG, Hirschl RB: Partial liquid ventilation in newborn patients with congenital diaphragmatic hernia. J Pediatr Surg 31:613–618, 1996.

77. Fuhrman BP, Paczan PR, DeFrancisis M: Perfluorocarbon-associated gas exchange. Crit Care Med 19:712–722, 1991.

78. Fuhrman BP, Hernan LJ, Holm BA, et al: Perfluorocarbon associated gas exchange (PAGE): Gas ventilation of the perfluorocarbon filled lung. Artif Cells Blood Substit Immobil Biotechnol 22:1133–1139, 1994.

79. Hirschl R, Pranikoff T, Gauger P, et al: Liquid ventilation in adults, children, and full term neonates: Preliminary report. Lancet 346:1201–1202, 1995.

80. Finer N, Etches P, Kamstra B, et al: Inhaled nitric oxide in infants referred for extracorporeal membrane oxygenation: Dose response. J Pediatr 124:302–308, 1994.

81. Kinsella JP, Abman SH: Inhalational nitric oxide therapy for persistent pulmonary hypertension of the newborn. Pediatrics 91:997–998, 1993.

82. Kinsella JP, Ivy DD, Abman SH: Inhaled nitric oxide improves gas exchange and lowers pulmonary vascular resistance in severe experimental hyaline membrane disease. Pediatr Res 36:402–408, 1994.

83. Roberts JD, Polaner DM, Lang P, et al: Inhaled nitric oxide in persistent pulmonary hypertension of the newborn. Lancet 340:818–819, 1992.

84. Dillon P, Cilley R, Hudome S, et al: Nitric oxide reversal of recurrent pulmonary hypertension and respiratory failure in an infant with CDH after successful ECMO therapy. J Pediatr Surg 30:743–744, 1995.

85. Frostell CG, Lonnqvist PA, Sonesson SE, et al: Near fatal pulmonary hypertension after surgical repair of congenital diaphragmatic hernia: Successful use of inhaled nitric oxide. Anaesthesia 48:679–683, 1993.

86. Henneberg SW, Jepsen S, Andersen PK, et al: Inhalation of nitric oxide as a treatment of pulmonary hypertension in congenital diaphragmatic hernia. J Pediatr Surg 30:853–855, 1995.

87. Kinsella J, Torielli F, Zeigler J, et al: Dipyridamole augmentation of response to nitric oxide. Lancet 346:647–648, 1995.

88. Soifer S, Clyman R, Heymann M: Effects of prostaglandin D2 on pulmonary artery pressure and oxygenation in newborn infants with persistent pulmonary hypertension. J Pediatr 112:774–777, 1988.

89. Meadow W, Bern A, Giardini G: Clinical correlates do not predict PaO_2 response after tolazoline administration in hypoxic newborns. Crit Care Med 14:548–551, 1986.

90. Ein SH, Barker G: The pharmacological treatment of newborn diaphragmatic hernia—update 1987. Pediatr Surg Int 2:341–345, 1987.

91. Lotze A, Whitsett JA, Kammerman LA, et al: Surfactant protein A concentrations in tracheal aspirate fluid from infants requiring extracorporeal membrane oxygenation. J Pediatr 116:435–440, 1990.

92. Findlay R, Taeusch H, Walther F: Surfactant replacement therapy for meconium aspiration syndrome. Pediatrics 97:48–52, 1996.

93. Karamanoukian HL, Glick PL, Wilcox DT, et al: Pathophysiology of congenital diaphragmatic hernia. VIII: Inhaled nitric oxide requires exogenous surfactant therapy in the lamb model of congenital diaphragmatic hernia. J Pediatr Surg 30:1–4, 1995.

94. Wilcox DT, Glick PL, Karamanoukian HL, et al: Pathophysiology of congenital diaphragmatic hernia. V: Effect of exogenous surfactant therapy on gas exchange and lung mechanics in the lamb congenital diaphragmatic hernia model. J Pediatr 124:289–293, 1994.

95. Sullivan KM, Hawgood S, Flake AW, et al: Amniotic fluid phospholipid analysis in the fetus with congenital diaphragmatic hernia. J Pediatr Surg 29:1020–1024, 1994.

96. German J, Gazzaniga A, Ragnar A, et al: Management of pulmonary insufficiency in diaphragmatic hernia using extracorporeal circulation with a membrane oxygenator (ECMO). J Pediatr Surg 12:905–912, 1977.

97. Heiss K, Clark R: Prediction of mortality in neonates with congenital diaphragmatic hernia treated with extracorporeal membrane oxygenation. Crit Care Med 23:1915–1919, 1995.

98. Bohn D, James I, Filler R: The relationship between $PaCO_2$ and ventilation parameters in predicting survival in congenital diaphragmatic hernia. J Pediatr Surg 19:666–671, 1984.

99. Bohn D, Tamura M, Perrin D, et al: Ventilatory predictors of pulmonary hypoplasia in congenital diaphragmatic hernia, confirmed by morphologic assessment. J Pediatr 111:423–431, 1987.

100. Wilson JM, Bower LK, Thompson JE, et al: ECMO in evolution: The impact of changing patient demographics and alternative therapies on ECMO. J Pediatr Surg 31:1116–1122, 1996.

101. van der Staak F, Thiesbrummel A, de Haan A, et al: Do we use the right entry criteria for extracorporeal membrane oxygenation in congenital diaphragmatic hernia. J Pediatr Surg 28:1003–1005, 1993.

102. Reickert C, Hirschl R, Schumacker R, et al: Effect of very delayed repair of congenital diaphragmatic hernia on survival and extracorporeal life support use. Surgery 120:766–772, 1996.

103. Lally KP, Paranka MS, Roden J, et al: Congenital diaphragmatic hernia: Stabilization and repair on ECMO. Ann Surg 216:569–573, 1992.

104. Vasquez W, Cheu H: Hemorrhagic complications and repair of congenital diaphragmatic hernias: Does timing of the repair make a difference? Data from the Extracorporeal Life Support Organization. J Pediatr Surg 29:1002–1006, 1994.

105. Wilson JM, Bower LK, Lund DP: Evolution of the technique of congenital diaphragmatic hernia repair on ECMO. J Pediatr Surg 29:1109–1112, 1994.

106. van der Staak F, de Haan A, Geven W, et al: Surgical repair of congenital diaphragmatic hernia during extracorporeal membrane oxygenation: Hemorrhagic complications and the effect of tranexamic acid. J Pediatr Surg 32:594–599, 1997.

107. Lally K: Extracorporeal membrane oxygenation in patients with congenital diaphragmatic hernia. Semin Pediatr Surg 5:249–255, 1996.

108. Sigalet DL, Tierney A, Adolph V, et al: Timing of repair of congenital diaphragmatic hernia requiring extracorporeal membrane oxygenation support. J Pediatr Surg 30:1183–1187, 1995.

109. Adolph V, Flageole H, Perreault T, et al: Repair of congenital diaphragmatic hernia after weaning from extracorporeal membrane oxygenation. J Pediatr Surg 30:349–352, 1995.

110. Lally K, Breaux C: A second course of extracorporeal membrane oxygenation in the neonate—is there a benefit? Surgery 117:175–178, 1995.

111. Atkinson J, Kitagawa H: Extracorporeal membrane oxygenation and the management of congenital diaphragmatic hernia. Pediatr Surg Int 8:200–203, 1993.

112. Bax N, Collins D: The advantages of reconstruction of the dome of the diaphragm in congenital posterolateral diaphragmatic defects. J Pediatr Surg 19:484–487, 1984.

113. Cullen M: Congenital diaphragmatic hernia: Operative considerations. Semin Pediatr Surg 5:243–248, 1996.

114. Reynolds M: Diaphragmatic anomalies. In Raffensperger JG (ed): Swenson's Pediatric Surgery. East Norwalk, CT, Appleton & Lange, 1990, pp 721–735.

115. Lund DP, Mitchell J, Kharasch V, et al: Congenital diaphragmatic hernia: The hidden morbidity. J Pediatr Surg 29:258–264, 1994.

116. Bealer J, Raisanen J, Skarsgard E, et al: The incidence and spectrum of neurological injury after open fetal surgery. J Pediatr Surg 30:1150–1154, 1995.

117. Harrison M, Adzick N, Flake A, et al: Correction of congenital diaphragmatic hernia in utero. VIII: Response of the hypoplastic lung to tracheal occlusion. J Pediatr Surg 31:1339–1348, 1996.

118. Metkus A, Filly R, Stringer M, et al: Sonographic predictors of survival in fetal diaphragmatic hernia. J Pediatr Surg 31:148–151, 1996.

119. Harrison MR, Langer JC, Adzick NS, et al: Correction of congenital diaphragmatic hernia in utero. V: Initial clinical experience. J Pediatr Surg 25:47–57, 1990.

120. Adzick NS, Vacanti JP, Lillehei CW, et al: Fetal diaphragmatic hernia: Ultrasound diagnosis and clinical outcome in 38 cases. J Pediatr Surg 24:654–657, 1989.

121. Karamanoukian HL, O'Toole SJ, Rossman JR, et al: Can cardiac weight predict lung weight in patients with congenital diaphragmatic hernia? J Pediatr Surg 31:823–825, 1996.

122. Burge DM, Atwell JD, Freeman NV: Could the stomach site help predict outcome in babies with left sided congenital diaphragmatic hernia diagnosed antenatally? J Pediatr Surg 24:567–569, 1989.

123. Harrison MR, Adzick NS, Longaker MT, et al: Successful repair in utero of a fetal diaphragmatic hernia after removal of herniated viscera from the left thorax. N Engl J Med 322:1582–1584, 1990.

124. Harrison MR, Adzick NS, Flake AW, et al: Correction of congenital diaphragmatic hernia in utero. VI: Hard-earned lessons. J Pediatr Surg 28:1411–1418, 1993.

125. DiFiore JW, Fauza DO, Slavin R, et al: Experimental fetal tracheal ligation and congenital diaphragmatic hernia: A pulmonary vascular morphometric analysis. J Pediatr Surg 30:917–924, 1995.

126. Ford W, Cool J, Parsons D, et al: Congenital diaphragmatic hernia: Lung compliance after antenatal tracheal obstruction or surgical correction of the defect. Pediatr Surg Int 11:524–529, 1996.

127. O'Toole S, Karamanoukian H, Irish M, et al: Tracheal ligation: The dark side of in utero diaphragmatic hernia treatment. J Pediatr Surg 32:407–410, 1997.

128. O'Toole S, Sharma A, Karamanoukian HL, et al: Tracheal ligation does not correct the surfactant deficiency associated with congenital diaphragmatic hernia. J Pediatr Surg 31:546–550, 1996.

129. Piedboeuf B, Laberge J, Ghitulescu G, et al: Deleterious effect of tracheal obstruction on type II pneumocytes in fetal sheep. Pediatr Res 41:473–479, 1997.

130. Flake A: Fetal surgery for congenital diaphragmatic hernia. Semin Pediatr Surg 5:266–274, 1996.

131. VanderWall K, Skarsgard E, Filly R, et al: Fetendo-clip: A fetal endoscopic tracheal clip procedure in a human fetus. J Pediatr Surg 32:970–972, 1997.

132. Graf J, Gibbs D, Adzick N, et al: Fetal hydrops after in utero tracheal occlusion. J Pediatr Surg 32:214–216, 1997.

133. Van Meurs K, Rhine W, Benitz W, et al: Lobar lung transplantation as a treatment for congenital diaphragmatic hernia. J Pediatr Surg 29:1557–1560, 1994.

134. Langham M, Kays D, Ledbetter D, et al: Congenital diaphragmatic hernia: Epidemiology and outcome. Clin Perinatol 23:671–688, 1996.

135. Torfs C, Curry C, Bateson T, et al: A population-based study of congenital diaphragmatic hernia. Teratology 46:555–565, 1992.

136. Wenstrom D, Weiner C, Hanson J: A five-year statewide experience with congenital diaphragmatic hernia. Am J Obstet Gynecol 165:838–842, 1991.

137. Heiss K, Manning P, Bartlett R, et al: Reversal of mortality for congenital diaphragmatic hernia with ECMO. Ann Surg 209:225–230, 1989.

138. Sawyer SF, Falterman KW, Goldsmith JP, et al: Improving survival in the treatment of congenital diaphragmatic hernia. Ann Thorac Surg 41:75–78, 1986.

139. Weber TR, Connors RH, Pennington DG, et al: Neonatal diaphragmatic hernia: An improving outlook with extracorporeal membrane oxygenation. Arch Surg 122:615–618, 1987.

140. Keshen T, Gursoy M, Shew S, et al: Does extracorporeal membrane oxygenation benefit neonates with congenital diaphragmatic hernia? Application of a predictive equation. J Pediatr Surg 32:818–822, 1997.

141. O'Rourke P, Lillihei C, Crone R, et al: The effect of extracorporeal membrane oxygenation (ECMO) on the survival of neonates with high risk congenital diaphragmatic hernia: 45 cases from a single institution. J Pediatr Surg 26:147–152, 1991.

142. Azarow K, Pearl R, Filler R: Congenital diaphragmatic hernia—a tale of two cities: The Toronto experience. J Pediatr Surg 32:395–400, 1997.

143. Goh D, Drake D, Brereton R, et al: Delayed surgery for congenital diaphragmatic hernia. Br J Surg 79:644–646, 1992.

144. Freyschuss U, Lannergren K, Frenkner B: Lung function after repair of congenital diaphragmatic hernia. Acta Pediatr Scand 73:589–593, 1984.

145. Reid I, Hutcherson R: Long-term follow-up of patients with congenital diaphragmatic hernia. J Pediatr Surg 11:939–942, 1976.

146. Vanamo K, Rintala R, Sovijarvi A, et al: Long-term pulmonary sequelae in survivors of congenital diaphragmatic defects. J Pediatr Surg 31:1096–1099, 1996.

147. Falconer A, Brown R, Helms P, et al: Pulmonary sequelae in survivors of congenital diaphragmatic hernia. Thorax 45:126–129, 1990.

148. Thurlbeck W, Kida K, Langston C, et al: Postnatal lung growth after repair of congenital diaphragmatic hernia. Thorax 34:338–343, 1979.

149. Wohl M, Thorne M, Strieder D, et al: The lung following repair of congenital diaphragmatic hernia. J Pediatr 90:405–414, 1977.

150. Nagaya M, Akatsuka H, Kato J, et al: Development in lung function of the affected side after repair of congenital diaphragmatic hernia. J Pediatr Surg 31:349–356, 1996.

151. D'Agostino J, Bernbaum J, Gerdes M, et al: Outcome for infants with congenital diaphragmatic hernia requiring extracorporeal membrane oxygenation: The first year. J Pediatr Surg 30:10–15, 1995.

152. Nagaya M, Akatsuka H, Kato J: Gastroesophageal reflux occurring after repair of congenital diaphragmatic hernia. J Pediatr Surg 29:1447–1451, 1994.

153. Davenport M, Rivlin E, D'Souza S, et al: Delayed surgery for congenital diaphragmatic hernia: Neurodevelopmental outcome in later childhood. Arch Dis Child 67:1353–1356, 1992.

154. van Meurs K, Robbins S, Reed V, et al: Congenital diaphragmatic hernia: Long-term outcome in neonates treated with extracorporeal membrane oxygenation. J Pediatr Surg 122:893–899, 1993.

155. Stolar C, Berdon W, Dillon P, et al: Esophageal dilitation and reflux in neonates supported with ECMO after diaphragmatic repair. AJR Am J Roentgenol 151:135–137, 1988.

156. Stolar C, Levy J, Dillon P, et al: Anatomic and functional abnormalities of the esophagus in infants surviving congenital diaphragmatic hernia. Am J Surg 159:204–207, 1990.

157. Stolar C: What do survivors of congenital diaphragmatic hernia look like when they grow up? Semin Pediatr Surg 5:275–279, 1996.

158. Kieffer J, Sapin E, Berg A, et al: Gastroesophageal reflux repair after repair of congenital diaphragmatic hernia. J Pediatr Surg 30:1330–1333, 1995.

159. Koot V, Bergmeijer J, Bos A, et al: Incidence and management of gastroesophageal reflux after repair of congenital diaphragmatic hernia. J Pediatr Surg 28:48–52, 1993.

160. Vanamo K, Rintala R, Lindahl H, et al: Long-term gastrointestinal morbidity in patients with congenital diaphragmatic defects. J Pediatr Surg 31:551–554, 1996.

161. Nobuhara K, Lund D, Mitchell J, et al: Long-term outlook for survivors of congenital diaphragmatic hernia. Clin Perinatol 23:873–887, 1996.

162. Atkinson J, Poon M: ECMO and the management of congenital diaphragmatic hernia with large diaphragmatic defects requiring a prosthetic patch. J Pediatr Surg 27:754–756, 1992.

163. Naik S, Greenough A, Zhang Y, et al: Prediction of morbidity during infancy after repair of congenital diaphragmatic hernia. J Pediatr Surg 31:1651–1654, 1996.

164. Stolar CJ, Crisafi MA, Driscoll YT: Neurocognitive outcome for neonates treated with extracorporeal membrane oxygenation: Are infants with congenital diaphragmatic hernia different? J Pediatr Surg 30:366–371, 1995.

165. Bifano E, Pfannenstiel A: Duration of hyperventilation and outcome in infants with persistent pulmonary hypertension. Pediatrics 81:657–661, 1988.

166. Marron M, Crisate M, Driscoll J, et al: Hearing and neurodevelopmental outcome in survivors of persistent pulmonary hypertension of the newborn. Pediatrics 90:392–396, 1992.

167. Brett C, Dekle M, Leonar C, et al: Developmental follow-up of hyperventilated neonates: Preliminary observations. Pediatrics 68:588–591, 1981.

168. Schumacher R, Palmer T, Roloff D, et al: Follow-up of infants treated with extracorporeal membrane oxygenation for newborn respiratory failure. Pediatrics 87:451–457, 1991.

169. Glass P, Miller M, Short B: Morbidity for survivors of extra-corporeal membrane oxygenation: Neurodevelopmental outcome at one year of age. Pediatrics 83:72–78, 1989.

170. Hofkosh D, Thompson A, Nozza R, et al: Ten years of extracorporeal membrane oxygenation: Neurodevelopmental outcome. Pediatrics 87:549–555, 1991.

171. Sarihan H, Imamoglu M, Abes M, et al: Pediatric Morgagni hernia: Report of two cases. J Cardiovasc Surg 37:195–197, 1996.

172. Pokorny W, McGill C, Halberg F: Morgagni hernia during infancy: Presentation and associated anomalies. J Pediatr Surg 19:394–397, 1984.

173. Honore L, Torfs C, Curry C: Possible association between the hernia of Morgagni and trisomy 21. Am J Med Genet 47:255–256, 1993.

174. Berman L, Stringer D, Ein S, et al: The late-presenting pediatric Morgagni hernia: A benign condition. J Pediatr Surg 24:970–972, 1989.

175. de Fonseca J, Davies M, Bolton K: Congenital hydropericardium associated with the herniation of part of the liver into the pericardial sac. J Pediatr Surg 22:851–853, 1987.

176. Kimmelstiel F, Holgerse L, Hilfer C: Retrosternal (Morgagni) hernia with small bowel obstruction secondary to a Richter's incarceration. J Pediatr Surg 22:998–1000, 1987.

177. Ozden C, Pektas O, Baskin D: Retrosternal hernia (Morgagni) with colonic perforation due to incarceration. Pediatr Surg Int 5:274–275, 1990.

178. Cantrell J, Haller J, Ravitch M: A syndrome of congenital defects involving the abdominal wall, sternum, diaphragm, pericardium and heart. Surg Gynecol Obstet 107:602–614, 1958.

179. Shamberger RC: Chest wall deformities. In Shields T, (ed): General Thoracic Surgery (4th ed). Baltimore, Williams & Wilkins, 1994, pp 529–557.

180. Symbas P, Hatcher C, Waldo W: Diaphragmatic eventration in infancy and childhood. Ann Thorac Surg 24:113–119, 1977.

181. Wayne E, Campbell J, Burrington J: Eventration of the diaphragm. J Pediatr Surg 9:643–651, 1974.

182. Sarihan H, Cay A, Akyazici R, et al: Congenital diaphragmatic eventration: Treatment and postoperative evaluation. J Cardiovasc Surg 37:173–176, 1996.

183. Smith C, Sade R, Crawford F: Diaphragmatic paralysis and eventration in infants. J Thorac Cardiovasc Surg 91:490–497, 1986.

184. Elberg J, Brok K, Pedersen S: Congenital bilateral eventration of the diaphragm in a pair of male twins. J Pediatr Surg 24:1140–1141, 1989.

185. Wayne E, Burrington J, Meyers D, et al: Bilateral eventration of the diaphragm in a neonate with congenital cytomegalic inclusion disease. J Pediatr 83:164–165, 1973.

186. Shimotake T, Jikihara R, Yanagihara J, et al: Successful management of bilateral congenital eventration of the diaphragm. Pediatr Surg Int 10:173–174, 1995.

187. Haller J, Pickard L, Tepas J: Management of diaphragmatic paralysis in infants with special emphasis on selection of patients for operative plication. J Pediatr Surg 14:779–785, 1979.

188. Kizilcan F, Tanyel F, Hicsonmez A, et al: The long-term results of diaphragmatic plication. J Pediatr Surg 28:42–44, 1993.

189. Mickell J, Oh K, Siewers R, et al: Clinical implications of postoperative unilateral phrenic nerve paralysis. J Thorac Cardiovasc Surg 76:297–304, 1978.

190. Langer J, Filler R, Coles J: Plication of the diaphragm for infants and young children with phrenic nerve palsy. J Pediatr Surg 23:749–751, 1988.

191. Stone K, Brown J, Canal D, et al: Long-term fate of the diaphragm surgically plicated during infancy and early childhood. Ann Thorac Surg 44:62–65, 1987.

192. Shoemaker R, Palmer G, Brown J: Aggressive treatment of acquired phrenic nerve paralysis in infants and small children. Ann Thorac Surg 32:250–259, 1981.

193. Brouillette R, Hahn Y, Noah Z, et al: Successful reinnervation of the diaphragm after phrenic nerve transection. J Pediatr Surg 21:63–65, 1986.

194. Merav A, Attai L, Conditt D: Successful repair of a transected phrenic nerve with restoration of diaphragmatic function. Chest 84:642–644, 1983.

25

MEDIASTINAL TUMORS

Clinton Cavett, MD

☐ Incidence and Clinical Presentation

Thoracic masses in the pediatric age group arise principally in the mediastinum, presenting a wide spectrum from congenital cysts to solid and cystic malignant tumors. Respiratory obstructive emergencies are a frequent presentation with these lesions because of their strategic location and the small caliber of the airway in children. The reported incidence of malignant mediastinal tumors in children ranges from 40% to as high as 72%.[1] The significant risk of malignancy and the high incidence of airway compromise demand urgent evaluation and diagnosis, occasionally constituting a true oncologic emergency.

Although only one third of mediastinal masses occur in children younger than 2 years of age,[2] there is an almost equal proportion of benign and malignant tumors, regardless of age. Survival rate following treatment is quite different in these groups, being reported as 88% in patients younger than 2 years of age and only 33% in patients older than 2 years of age. This difference in survival rates is principally a result of the favorable prognosis of neuroblastoma in younger children and the predominance of lymphomatous tumors in the older age group. Presentation also varies with age: younger children more typically have respiratory distress because their airways are of a smaller caliber and are more easily compressed. Nevertheless, a similar degree of respiratory distress can easily develop in older children, particularly with lymphomatous lesions, which may directly compress the distal trachea and upper bronchi.[2, 3]

☐ Classification by Region

Mediastinal masses are classically divided according to their site of origin: anterior mediastinum, middle mediastinum (visceral), and posterior or paravertebral mediastinum (Fig. 25–1). The *anterior*

mediastinum is bounded by the posterior surface of the sternum, the thoracic inlet, and the anterior surface of great vessels, heart, and pericardium. This area contains the thymus and anterior surfaces of the vascular structures, as well as a few anterior lymph nodes and the rare ectopic thyroid or parathyroid. The *middle mediastinum* contains the heart, great vessels, trachea, and bronchi and extends to the anterior border of the vertebrae, including the esophagus, the vagus and phrenic nerves, and the descending thoracic aorta. The *posterior mediastinum*, or paravertebral sulcus, is bounded

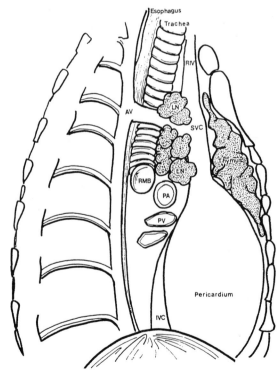

Figure 25–1. Classic anatomic divisions of the mediastinum. Note the lymphatic tissue is strategically located for varied symptoms and is most likely to cause tracheal compression when enlarged. (From Pizzo PA, Poplack DG: Principles and Practices of Pediatric Oncology [2nd ed]. Philadelphia, JB Lippincott, 1993, p. 952.)

anteriorly by the anterior surface of the vertebral bodies. Although it is not classically a part of the mediastinum, this area is included because of the predominance of neurogenic tumors in this region.[3]

A thorough knowledge of the normal structures in these three areas is requisite for the surgeon operating on these lesions. Lymph nodes, although arising principally in the middle mediastinum, can also present as pathologic lesions anteriorly and posteriorly. Cystic hygroma (lymphangioma) and other vascular masses are not confined to any specific mediastinal region.

□ Evaluation

Dyspnea, noisy breathing, or a history of dyspnea and tachypnea on exertion may indicate incipient airway compression. Weight loss, night sweats, and general malaise are also points to be evaluated in the history. Careful physical examination may detect vena cava compression with plethora of the facies, venous distention, or fullness and swelling with masses in the supraclavicular and cervical areas.

The chest radiograph, done in two views, should be the first diagnostic study done to define the nature and position of a suspected mediastinal mass. Spiral computed tomography (CT) scans with intravenous contrast are extremely helpful in providing a clear delineation of the extent and nature of a mass and its airway or vascular compromise. Magnetic resonance imaging (MRI) clearly has a place in diagnostic evaluation; however, the lengthy examination time and need for sedation in younger patients make this study unsuitable for children with significant airway compromise. However, MRI is the ideal imaging study for posterior mediastinal masses in the stable patient because any extension into the spinal

canal is clearly defined. MRI presents two limitations in evaluating the mediastinum: (1) small calcifications within a mass can be missed and (2) clusters of small lymph nodes may be misinterpreted as a single mass.[4] CT can detect small foci of calcification as in neuroblastoma and has better spatial resolution to help differentiate clustering of small nodes versus a larger mass.[5, 6] Contrast esophagogram can also reveal deviation and compression of the esophageal lumen.[7] Duplication cysts, which contain gastric mucosa, may be delineated by technetium-99m pertechnetate scintigraphy.

□ Acute Airway Obstruction During Induction of Anesthesia

Children with mediastinal masses are at risk for airway compromise, which may become life-threatening on induction of general anesthesia (Fig. 25–2).[8] In most such cases, there is an extrathoracic source from which the diagnosis can be made (e.g., cervical or supraclavicular lymph nodes) and pleural effusions from which positive cytology can be obtained. Many malignancies can be diagnosed by bone marrow aspirate. Cytology may not differentiate Hodgkin's from non-Hodgkin's lymphoma, but selective chemotherapy or radiation can begin if airway compromise precludes safe anesthesia for mediastinal biopsy. Pulmonary function studies may be useful in evaluating the degree of obstructive and restrictive deficits, and measurement of the cross-sectional area of the trachea on CT scan may be useful.[9, 10] Caution is the key, and preoperative discussions among surgeon, anesthesiologist, and oncologist are necessary to appropriately evaluate and tailor procedures to each patient. It is critical that the surgeon and anesthesiologist be aware of the potential airway obstruction that can occur in

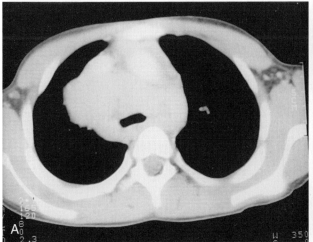 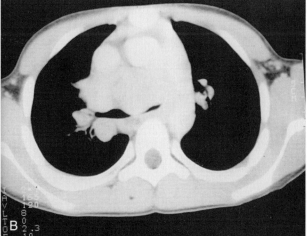

Figure 25–2. *A,* Computed tomography (CT) scan of a 12-year-old boy with dyspnea and retractions. Note the distal tracheal compression. *B,* CT scan in the same child reveals severe compression of the right mainstem bronchus and compression on the left as well. Supraclavicular node biopsy under local anesthesia provided the diagnosis of nodular sclerosing Hodgkin's disease.

patients who are even minimally symptomatic as a result of a mediastinal mass.[11] Symptomatic airway obstruction can be relieved with a short course of steroids or limited field radiation therapy, which enables thoracoscopic biopsy or uses the Chamberlain procedure to obtain nonirradiated tissue for definitive diagnosis.[12, 13] Frequently, a thorough search for extrathoracic tumor sites provides adequate data for diagnosis and direction of therapy.

☐ Tumors of the Posterior Mediastinum

Masses in the posterior mediastinum and paravertebral sulcus are most commonly *ganglioneuroma* or *neuroblastoma,* which usually arise from the sympathetic ganglia.[14] This is the principal reason for the more favorable survival rate in children younger than 2 years of age who have a mediastinal tumor. Approximately 20% of all children with ganglioneuroma and neuroblastoma have a thoracic primary tumor. See Chapter 65 for a detailed discussion of neural crest tumors.

Anterior thoracic meningocele is an extremely rare lesion. These tumors are associated with severe vertebral abnormalities. They are progressive in both size and symptoms, presenting with weakness that progresses to paraplegia. Because it is a progressive lesion, operative correction is warranted. MRI and possibly myelography are deemed the best means for evaluating these lesions.

Neurenteric cysts are very rare cystic masses found in the posterior mediastinum. They connect the central nervous system and the gastrointestinal tract, and are thought to develop very early in embryonic life as a result of failure of separation of the notochord and foregut. These lesions usually have well-differentiated muscular layers with intestinal mucosal lining, most frequently gastric. As with anterior thoracic meningocele, the diagnosis should be considered when a posterior mediastinal cystic mass is identified adjacent to spinal anomaly. Technetium-99m pertechnetate scintigraphy may confirm ectopic gastric mucosa. MRI is the diagnostic study of choice because the communication with the intraspinal mass can be seen without the need for intraspinal contrast. The gastric mucosa in these lesions produces acid that causes inflammation and bleeding. Persistent ulceration can lead to central nervous system infection and fistulization into the spinal canal, which can be devastating.[15]

☐ Tumors of the Middle Mediastinum

Middle mediastinal masses in children younger than 2 years of age are most often remnants of the embryonic foregut. Understanding their origin from a common embryonic structure helps to explain their characteristic location and composition. *Esophageal duplication cysts* are usually found arising within the esophageal wall near the carina (Fig. 25–3). As expected, there is tremendous variability in size and location in these mediastinal cystic masses. They share the muscular layer with the esophagus and often have a respiratory epithelial lining with occasional rudiments of cartilage. They may produce esophageal obstruction or erosion with bleeding.

Bronchogenic cysts are lined by respiratory epithelium and contain thick mucoid material secreted by this epithelium; many are not in close contact

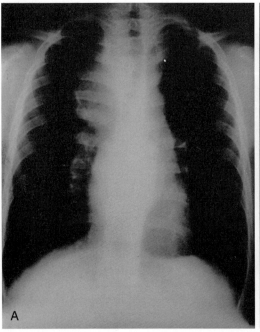

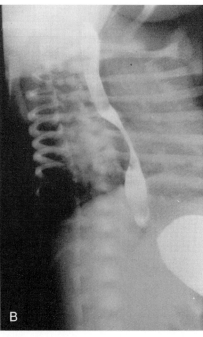

Figure 25–3. *A,* Chest radiograph in a patient with mild dyspnea revealing a right-sided mediastinal mass. *B,* Barium swallow in this patient with a mediastinal duplication cyst.

with the airway and only rarely does this anomaly communicate with the airway.

Both esophageal duplications and bronchogenic cysts are most often identified in the asymptomatic patient in whom a chest radiograph has been obtained for other reasons. Either may produce obstructive respiratory symptoms depending on the location of the cyst and its size. Infants are more likely to be seen with significant respiratory compromise for reasons already stated. Atelectasis and hyperinflation from air trapping related to compression or deviation of the affected airway can lead to an incorrect diagnosis of congenital lobar emphysema, chronic aspiration, cystic fibrosis, or congenital cystic adenomatoid malformation. Occasionally, cysts produce symptoms as a result of their strategic location, but they are too small to detect by routine chest radiograph. CT with intravenous contrast usually identifies the problem and can sometimes allow the surgeon to forego endoscopic evaluation, unless foreign body remains high in the differential diagnosis.

Treatment for either of these lesions consists of complete excision if possible. In the case of the esophageal duplication, which shares a common wall with the esophagus, the mucosal lining can be removed from the cyst to avoid major disruption of the esophageal lumen. Some esophageal lesions contain cartilage and are so obstructive that they must be excised with esophageal anastomosis (see Chapter 26).

Other enteric duplications that originate below the pylorus can present as a mass in the middle mediastinum. They may be associated with lumbar vertebral anomalies and may, therefore, be differen-

tiated from neurenteric cysts already described (Fig. 25–4). These duplications frequently contain ectopic gastric mucosa, in which case scintigraphy can be helpful in preoperative evaluation. These middle mediastinal gastrointestinal duplications, which communicate through the diaphragm or the esophageal hiatus, take their origin from the duodenum or proximal jejunum and have been labeled *thoracoabdominal duplications*.[16] The ectopic gastric mucosa may produce ulceration and perforation with empyema in the right hemithorax. These duplications are not inherently fixed to any mediastinal structures but their removal involves entry into both the chest and abdomen.

□ Tumors of the Anterior Mediastinum

The most common anterior mediastinal mass in children is *non-Hodgkin's lymphoma*, followed by *Hodgkin's disease. Germ cell neoplasms* and *mesenchymal neoplasms*, both of which are rare in children, may arise in the anterior mediastinum.[17] In a recent study of 18 patients with anterior mediastinal masses, only four were younger than 18 months of age, and the median age for the group was 7 years. Two of the four children younger than 18 months had respiratory distress, whereas none of the children in the older group had this symptom when they were first seen. Four of the 14 older children had malignant neoplasms; the remainder had benign lesions.[18]

The *normal thymus* may be mistaken for a pathologic mass on chest radiograph in the younger pa-

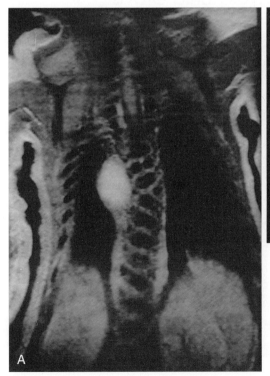

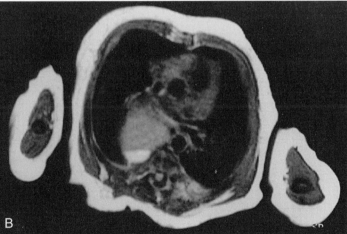

Figure 25–4. *A,* Magnetic resonance imaging (MRI) study revealing the same duplication seen in Figure 25–3. Note the associated vertebral anomalies. This T2-weighted image highlights the cystic nature of the mass (fluid filled). *B,* Transverse section on the T1-weighted MRI image shows absence of communication with the spinal canal and a fluid-fluid interface within the cyst (two fluid densities most likely representing mucus in the dependent layer). This duplication cyst was lined with gastric mucosa.

tient. The normal thymus is not a source of respiratory symptoms. It is often difficult to separate the physiologic enlargement of the infant's thymus from other anterior mediastinal masses. A 5-day course of prednisone (2 mg/kg/day) causes enough shrinkage of the normal thymus as to provide an important diagnostic tool.[18] Persistence of the mass may necessitate CT scanning in preparation for surgical biopsy. A lymphoma can diminish in size on steroid therapy as well, but lymphoma in children younger than 24 months of age is exceedingly rare.

Thymic cysts, although rare, are usually found incidentally on chest radiographs. These cysts, generally filled with cholesterol crystals and sometimes noted to have a characteristic appearance on ultrasound, can usually be resected without major difficulty.

Teratomas account for 20% of mediastinal masses in children, second only to neurogenic tumors in their frequency. The mediastinum is the second most common site for teratomas in the pediatric population. Most mediastinal teratomas originate anteriorly. Depending on their size and specific location, they may present in either hemithorax, in the middle or posterior mediastinum, in the pericardium or heart, or within lung parenchyma.

Alphafetoprotein is an effective serum tumor marker and levels are well documented for the normal newborn; carcinoembryonic antigen and human chorionic gonadotropin are markers in some tumors and should be measured preoperatively.

Mediastinal teratomas present as any other mass lesion, by incidental discovery or by symptoms of compression of contiguous structures. Respiratory symptoms are more frequent in younger patients. Calcification within the mass is highly suggestive of the diagnosis of teratoma.[19] Although it may not be seen on routine radiographs, calcification is easily recognized on CT scan or ultrasound. These two studies help to differentiate solid from cystic lesions.

Surgical removal is indicated. The approach may be through a median sternotomy or a lateral thoracotomy.[20] Most mediastinal teratomas are cystic with one germ cell layer predominating. Ectoderm is the more common cell layer seen. The blood supply is usually singular and well defined. There is no gender predominance, but the malignant lesions are almost exclusively found in male patients.

Cystic hygromas are common mediastinal abnormalities found in children. They may result from a failure of connection of lymphatic collecting channels within their drainage systems (see Chapter 74). Hygromas most commonly occur in the neck, usually in the posterior cervical triangle, and can sometimes be extremely large and invasive, creating problems because of their size and encroachment on vital structures. As many as 3% of patients with cervical cystic hygromas have extension into the superior portion of the mediastinum. Hygromas may involve all areas of the mediastinum and can extend, on rare occasions, to the diaphragm.

CT is indicated in any child whose chest radiograph suggests mediastinal extension of a cervical hygroma (Fig. 25–5). Mediastinal cystic hygroma can sometimes produce chylothorax, pericardial effusion, and chylopericardium, as well as respiratory distress from airway compression. Excision is the treatment of choice, although there may be some alternatives if that approach seems impractical (see Chapter 71). Observation has no place in the treatment of the mediastinal extension of cystic hygroma.[21]

□ Surgical Treatment of Juvenile Myasthenia Gravis

Myasthenia gravis is a disorder of the neuromuscular system presenting clinically as pathologic weakness and muscle fatigue with exercise. Only

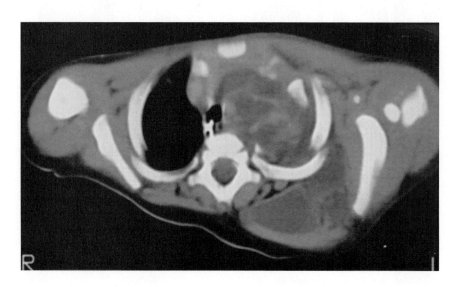

Figure 25–5. Computed tomography scan of a child with a large left, posterior cervical cystic hygroma with intrathoracic extension to the posterior mediastinum and left chest.

TABLE 25-1. Myasthenia Gravis Muscle
Strength: Osserman's Classification

I	Weakness of extraocular muscles without progression
II	Generalized weakness, bulbar and skeletal
	Mild
	Moderate
III	Acute fulminating weakness with severe bulbar manifestations
IV	Late, severe
V	Muscle atrophy

10% of patients with myasthenia gravis are children. The pathogenesis of this neuromuscular disorder is well described; the thymus produces acetylcholine receptor antibodies that block the normal binding of acetylcholine at receptor sites. These antibodies also accelerate acetylcholine degradation at the end plate. Also, thymic antigen-specific T-helper cells are believed to induce increased acetylcholine receptor antibody production by lymphocytes in the peripheral circulation.

Myasthenia gravis has been described throughout the pediatric age range, although 75% of such children are older than 10 years of age. The symptoms of myasthenia gravis can be seen in infants born to mothers with myasthenia gravis because of transplacental passage of acetylcholine receptor antibodies. These symptoms last only for a short period of time and the child fully recovers. A type of myasthenia gravis appears in infants in which the mother is not affected. These newborn patients initially have generalized weakness, but later they only show extraocular muscle symptoms of the disease, which are usually managed effectively with anticholinergic medications. Neither of these neonatal forms of myasthenia gravis benefits from thymectomy.[22]

Juvenile myasthenia gravis affects girls four times more often than boys. The symptoms are described in Table 25–1. Stage II and III patients are candidates for thymectomy. The role of median sternotomy and thymectomy is clear in juvenile cases. A better outcome is seen when thymectomy is done early in the course of the disease. Preparation for surgery includes stabilization with anticholinesterase medications and with plasmapheresis being used in refractory cases. Remission following thymectomy has been reported in 67% of pediatric patients, with improvement being reported in an additional 29%. This is in contrast to a spontaneous remission rate of 30%.[22] Early thymectomy following diagnosis is believed to allow persistent symptoms to be more easily controlled. Some patients have been reported as being able to discontinue medications as much as 7 years following thymectomy.

REFERENCES

1. Grosfeld JL, Skinner MA, Rescorla FJ, et al: Mediastinal tumors in children: Experience with 196 cases. Ann Surg Oncol 1:121–127, 1994.
2. Pokorny WJ, Sherman JO: Mediastinal masses in infants and children. J Thorac Cardiovasc Surg 68:869–875, 1974.
3. Haller JA, Mazur DO, Morgan WM: Diagnosis and management of mediastinal masses in children. J Thorac Cardiovasc Surg 58:385–393, 1969.
4. Azarow KS, Pearl RH, Surcher R, et al: Primary mediastinal masses: A comparison of adult and pediatric populations. J Thorac Cardiovasc Surg 106:67–72, 1993.
5. Siegel MJ, Nadel SN, Glazer HS, et al: Mediastinal lesions in children: Comparison of CT and MR. Radiology 160:241–244, 1986.
6. Bisset GS: Pediatric thoracic applications of magnetic resonance imaging. J Thorac Imaging 4:51–57, 1989.
7. Meza MP, Benson M, Slovis TJ: Imaging of mediastinal masses in children. Radiol Clin North Am 31:583–604, 1993.
8. Azizkhan RG, Dudgeon, DL, Buck JR, et al: Life-threatening airway obstruction as a complication to management of mediastinal masses in children. J Pediatr Surg 20:816–822, 1985.
9. King DR, Patrick LE, Ginn-Pease ME, Klopfenstein K: Pulmonary function is compromised in children with mediastinal lymphoma. J Pediatr Surg 32:292–299, 1997.
10. Shamberger RC, Holzman RS, Griscom NT, et al: CT quantitation of tracheal cross-sectional area as a guide to the surgical and anesthetic management of children with anterior mediastinal masses. J Pediatr Surg 26:138–142, 1991.
11. Robie DK, Gursoy MH, Pokorny WJ: Mediastinal tumors—airway obstruction and management. Semin Pediatr Surg 3:259–266, 1994.
12. Lange B, O'Neill JA, D'Angio G, et al: Oncologic emergencies. In Pizzo PA, Poplack DG (eds): Principles and Practice of Pediatric Oncology, 2nd ed. Philadelphia: JB Lippincott, 1993, p 953.
13. Rodgers BM: Thoracoscopic procedures in children. Semin Pediatr Surg 2:182–189, 1993.
14. Saenz NC, Schnitzer JJ, Eraklis AE, et al: Posterior mediastinal masses. J Pediatr Surg 28:172–176, 1993.
15. Alrabeeah A, Gillis DA, Giacomantonio M, et al: Neurenteric cysts—a spectrum. J Pediatr Surg 23:752–754, 1988.
16. Pokorny SJ, Goldstein IR: Enteric thoracoabdominal duplications in children. J Thorac Cardiovasc Surg 87:821–824, 1984.
17. Simpson I, Campbell PE: Mediastinal masses in childhood: A review from a paediatric pathologist's point of view. Prog Pediatr Surg 27:92–126, 1991.
18. Mullen B, Richardson JD: Primary anterior mediastinal tumors in children and adults. Ann Thorac Surg 42:338–345, 1986.
19. Carney JA, Thompson DP, Johnson CL, et al: Teratomas in children: Clinical and pathologic aspects. J Pediatr Surg 7:271–282, 1972.
20. Lakhoo K, Boyle M, Drake DP: Mediastinal teratomas: Review of 15 pediatric cases. J Pediatr Surg 28:1161–1164, 1993.
21. Curley SA, Ablin DS, Kosloske AM: Giant cystic hygroma of the posterior mediastinum. J Pediatr Surg 24:398–400, 1989.
22. Adams C, Theodorescu D, Murphy EG, et al: Thymectomy in juvenile myasthenia gravis. J Child Neurol 5:215–218, 1990.

26

THE ESOPHAGUS

Keith W. Ashcraft, MD

☐ Embryology

The embryonic foregut gives rise to the esophagus and trachea. Separation of these structures begins in the area of the carina and progresses in a cephalad direction. Because of the relatively complicated way in which the esophagus and trachea divide, lesions such as esophageal atresia (Chapter 27) and tracheal atresia (Chapter 21) may occur. Because the trachea normally contains cartilage, occasional malformations that involve the esophagus contain cartilage remnants. Cystic lesions in the wall of the esophagus may be entirely esophageal duplication cysts or bronchogenic cysts, which contain either respiratory mucosa or cartilage in their walls.

The muscular wall of the esophagus is comprised of an inner circular muscle and an outer longitudinal muscle. It has no serosal covering. The cranial one third of the esophagus is striated muscle and under voluntary control, whereas the distal two thirds of the esophagus is composed of smooth muscle and under autonomic control. The squamous mucosa of the esophagus is studded with its own intrinsic mucus glands that, in the presence of an acute obstruction, produce copious quantities of phlegm.

For purposes of surgical considerations, the esophagus can be divided into cervical, thoracic, and abdominal portions. The cervical portion is intimately attached to the larynx. The esophagus is thinnest immediately below the cricopharyngeus muscle posteriorly and is at particular risk of penetrating injury at that point. This portion of the esophagus receives its blood supply from thyrocervical vessels.

The thoracic portion of the esophagus is laterally indented by the aortic arch; it may be severely compressed by vascular ring malformations. This part of the esophagus is intimately related to the aorta and to the pericardium; therefore, these adjacent structures are subject to erosion injuries from a foreign body or to damage from caustic injury. The midportion of the esophagus has a lateral or dorsal segmental blood supply. Extensive surgical mobilization of this part of the esophagus can produce vascular insufficiency, which can adversely affect healing of an anastomosis.

The abdominal part of the esophagus is the portion that is involved with the lower esophageal sphincter (LES) mechanism (see Chapter 27). Its blood supply is received from phrenic branches and from gastric vessels and is generously supplied with blood. Lacerations of the mucosa from forceful vomiting (Boerhaave's syndrome) and the development of varicosities from portal venous obstruction are both a potential source of major blood loss. A more detailed embryologic and anatomic discussion of the esophagus is available.[1]

☐ Chemical Esophageal Injuries

The natural curiosity of children and their tendency to taste everything, coupled with the availability of certain chemicals around the house, create the setting for corrosive esophageal injury. Alkaline chemicals are much more likely to produce esophageal injury than are acid chemicals. Commercially available drain cleaners, homemade lye solutions for the same purpose, and strong dishwasher detergents are the agents that most often produce liquefaction necrosis of the esophagus.[2] Concentrated alkali solutions are slick and, when put into the mouth, slip easily into the esophagus. Liquid caustic products are contrasted in their potential for injury with dry caustic products, which tend to stick to the oral mucosa and to produce intense pain, salivation, and dilution. Often, dry caustics are spit out before they are swallowed.

In the presence of a suspected liquid caustic ingestion, esophageal damage is possible with little evidence of oral injury. Contact of the caustic agent with the esophageal mucosa produces intense spasm, which in turn exposes the entire circumference of the esophagus to the caustic agent. Liquefaction necrosis results. If the caustic dose is sufficient, the mucosa, submucosa, and muscular walls of the esophagus may be destroyed by continued liquefaction, until dilution alters the caustic agent to a near neutral pH. The marked elevation of pH at various sites around the mediastinum, as measured by a surface electrode, has been demonstrated in the cat with an intact esophagus and an opened thorax. Because of the pattern of pH changes, this is probably more of a diffusion phenomenon than a vascular dispersion. The extent of the injury both within the esophagus and into the mediastinum are probably related to the dose of hydroxyl ion.

The areas of natural closing of the esophagus are the region of the cricopharyngeus muscle, the vicinity of the aortic arch, and the LES. In these locations, a small amount of caustic may produce a circumferential burn. Often, however, the mucosal injury is extensive throughout the midportion of the esophagus as well.

Acid ingestion is much less injurious to the esophagus than alkali ingestion, unless the acid is exceedingly potent. Acid injuries more often affect the antrum of the stomach, where mucosal necrosis and mural inflammation are produced and antral stenosis results.

The sequelae of caustic ingestion in the esophagus is cicatrix in the wall of the esophagus (Fig. 26–1). The depth of the burn probably indicates the amount of scar formation that will develop and the

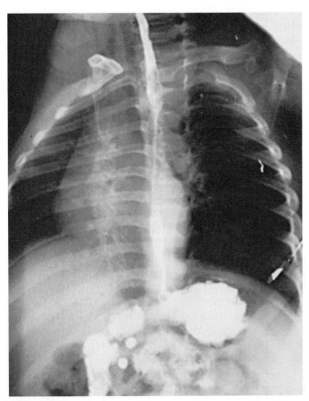

Figure 26–1. A well-established lye stricture of the esophagus is shown, with the most intense scarring from about the level of the aortic knob to the distal thoracic esophagus. The small amount of barium that passes makes it impossible to assess whether the stomach has been injured or whether the distal esophagus is also scarred from this lye injury. Both of these factors are important in the assessment and ultimate treatment of an extensive caustic stricture.

ultimate outcome of therapy. Mucosal erythema alone is usually without serious sequelae. Circumferential mucosal slough usually indicates caustic injury to the muscularis, and at best an irregular stricture will result. Similarly, full thickness injury with continuing destruction of mediastinal structures by hydroxyl ions can lead to mediastinitis and, occasionally, to perforation of the esophagus into the contiguous structures, the most disastrous result of which is the perforated aorta (Fig. 26–2).[3]

IMMEDIATE THERAPY

Unfortunately, injury to the esophagus is almost instantaneous. Unless the dose is overwhelming, what passes into the stomach is titrated with gastric acid to neutrality; thus, further injury is prevented. For many years, the first aid promulgated for toddlers who ingested lye was to induce vomiting, a process that returned the caustic to the esophageal mucosa and gave it a second chance to produce an injury. Unfortunately, any diluent or neutralizing agent must be given in such large quantities that vomiting is likely to be induced. The administration of acetic acid to neutralize the alkali is certainly emetic. Therefore, first aid is of little or no value. It may even cause further injury to the esophageal mucosa.[2]

The child is usually brought to the emergency room with a history of ingestion of "lye." Its chemical identification is of value, because certain agents that are common in the household, such as bleach, do not require endoscopy or further follow-up. Ingestion of sodium hydroxide or potassium hydroxide, either solution or powdered, or powdered detergents calls for endoscopic evaluation. The status of the oral mucosa is of little or no prognostic value in determining the presence of esophageal injury. Endoscopy, usually performed within 24 hours, reveals whether the esophagus has been injured. Linear injuries to the esophagus are of less clinical significance because, unless the burn is circumferential, the remaining unburned esophagus expands to compensate for the lateral scar. General supportive care with intravenous fluids should be given in the immediate postinjury period before determination of the extent of esophageal injury.

Rigid esophagoscopy is my choice for evaluation of the esophagus. A circumferential lesion is all that needs to be demonstrated. The length of the injury is not really important at this time.

For a long time, antibiotics were thought to prevent mediastinitis, and systemic steroids were thought to prevent the ultimate formation of esophageal stricture. It is difficult to assess the depth of injury and grade the burns as first, second, or third degree, as is done with skin burns.[4] Undoubtedly, the depth of the burn is related to the eventual scar formation, which has made the assessment of steroid therapy in the healing phase difficult. The genesis of steroid treatment stems from an experimental study of standard caustic burn injuries of the

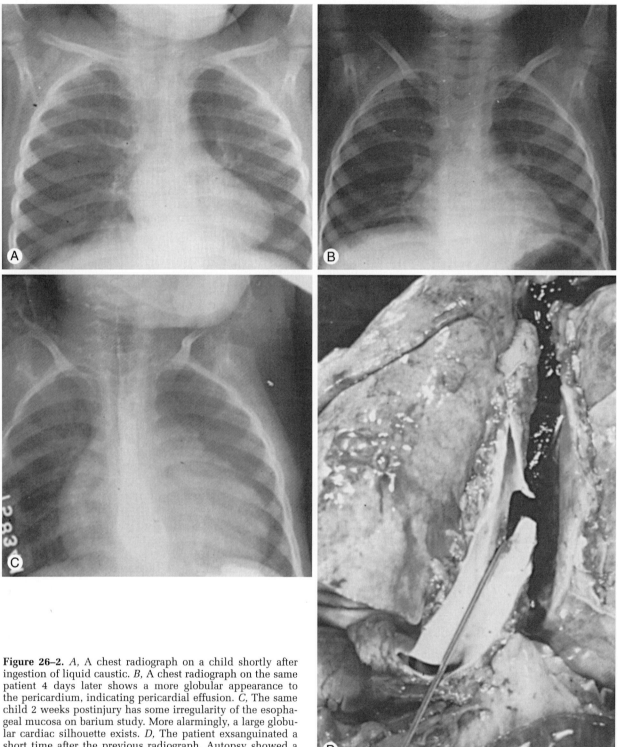

Figure 26–2. *A,* A chest radiograph on a child shortly after ingestion of liquid caustic. *B,* A chest radiograph on the same patient 4 days later shows a more globular appearance to the pericardium, indicating pericardial effusion. *C,* The same child 2 weeks postinjury has some irregularity of the esophageal mucosa on barium study. More alarmingly, a large globular cardiac silhouette exists. *D,* The patient exsanguinated a short time after the previous radiograph. Autopsy showed a massive hole eroded into the aorta.

esophagus in cats.[5] Treatment consisted of nothing, bougienage alone, steroids alone, antibiotics alone, or steroids and antibiotics. Animals treated with a combination of steroids and antibiotics lost less weight and fewer died by inanition, but the therapy did not prevent the development of strictures.

A companion clinical study included 69 patients who had endoscopically demonstrated esophageal burns and who were treated with steroids and antibiotics.[6] Eight (12%) of these patients developed strictures that responded to prolonged dilation. None required esophageal replacement. By contrast, 8 patients from other hospitals who were not treated acutely with steroids and antibiotics were referred late for esophageal replacement or prolonged dilations. The *strong impression* was that the steroid antibiotic therapy reduced the incidence of esophageal stricture but did not completely eliminate it. On the basis of these studies, steroid therapy was universally adopted, with the belief that if the steroids were not administered for a prolonged period, the treatment might be beneficial. As has been subsequently shown, there was little else to offer. Further data have suggested that, in spite of steroids and antibiotics, esophageal strictures are probably going to develop.[7] A controlled trial of steroids in children with corrosive injury of the esophagus has suggested that there is absolutely no statistically demonstrable benefit from the administration of corticosteroids in children with lye ingestion injuries.[8]

EMERGENT THERAPY FOR MASSIVE INGESTION

If the history suggests a massive ingestion of concentrated alkali[9] in a child,[10] or a suicidal ingestion of concentrated alkali in an adult or older child, immediate esophagectomy and possible gastrectomy should be considered. Whether or not this approach will prevent the aortoesophageal fistula that results from continued alkali injury to mediastinal structures is not known, but some of my own experimental data and some of the clinical data available from the treatment of adults suggest that it does.[11, 12] In accidental caustic ingestion in childhood, one of the standard approaches is to place a gastrostomy for feeding and dilation therapy. With massive caustic ingestion, the upper abdomen might be explored to assess the gastric wall, particularly its dependent portion, for evidence of caustic injury. If the caustic material ingested has been concentrated enough or voluminous enough to reach the stomach and produce a gastric wall injury, then the esophagus will be assumed to have been totally destroyed and it should be removed. If the stomach does not appear to be seriously injured, a gastrostomy alone can be established.[13]

SUBACUTE THERAPY FOR CAUSTIC INJURY

The most common approach to the subacute treatment of corrosive burns is observation to determine whether or not a stricture will develop. Most often it does.

Stenting during the healing phase has been reported to be of value both experimentally[14] and clinically, involving both children[15–18] and adults. This technique was proposed in the early 1970s but has not gained widespread acceptance. Likewise, the treatment of experimental lye burns with a β-aminopropionitrile,[19, 20] which was also postulated in the 1970s, has not gained any clinical acceptance.

ESOPHAGEAL STRICTURE THERAPY

The long-term result of most serious caustic injuries is esophageal stenosis. The treatment is discussed later.

□ Foreign Body Esophageal Injury

The most commonly ingested foreign body that can produce injury to the esophagus is the coin. Most ingested coins pass harmlessly through the gastrointestinal (GI) tract in children, many probably unbeknownst to parents. Foreign bodies and their extraction from the esophagus are discussed in Chapter 12, but the long-term sequelae of an impacted foreign body in the esophagus, producing esophageal injury, are discussed herein.

The attitude of primary care physicians and even emergency room physicians toward the ingestion of coins is varied, extending from adamant neglect[21] to immediate action of ordering plain radiographs and contrast studies.[22] Depending on the size of the child and the size of the coin, the chances of its lodging in the esophagus are variable. If the coin is sufficiently small to pass through the cricopharyngeal area, the area of the aortic knob, and the distal esophagus into the stomach, problems are unlikely at the other narrowed or angulated portions of the GI tract, namely the pylorus, the ligament of Treitz, and the ileocecal valve. Given the history of coin ingestion, a chest radiograph, including the upper abdomen, should probably be done.[23] In one study, 52 consecutive children who had swallowed coins underwent radiographic examination. Those who had symptoms underwent removal of the coins. Of 30 children who had coins in the esophagus, 9 (30%) were asymptomatic.[24] In the 3 patients whose coin had not progressed to the stomach within 24 hours, it was removed. In another almost simultaneous study in the same city, only a fraction of the patients whose parents called the emergency room to report a child's coin ingestion complied with the advice to get a radiograph; 20% of those children had coins in the esophagus. Most of the patients who had coins in the esophagus were symptomatic, with stridor or drooling.[25]

The consequences of an unrecognized esophageal foreign body, even one as smooth as a coin, can sometimes be disastrous.[26–28] Although some advise pushing the coin into the stomach,[29] most suggest using the Foley catheter to extract smooth esophageal foreign bodies.[30–32]

Esophageal injury is much more likely from sharper foreign bodies, including the detachable pop-top used on aluminum drink cans.[33, 34] Because these objects are often nearly radiolucent, diagnosis comes with the late onset of esophageal obstructive symptoms.

Tracheoesophageal fistula occasionally occurs as a result of an ingested foreign body.[35] I have had one such case. A child ingested an approximately 13-mm square plastic lattice from a badminton shuttlecock, which eroded from the esophagus into the trachea (Fig. 26–3A, B).

Of much more concern is the ingestion of the disc batteries that are used to power calculators,

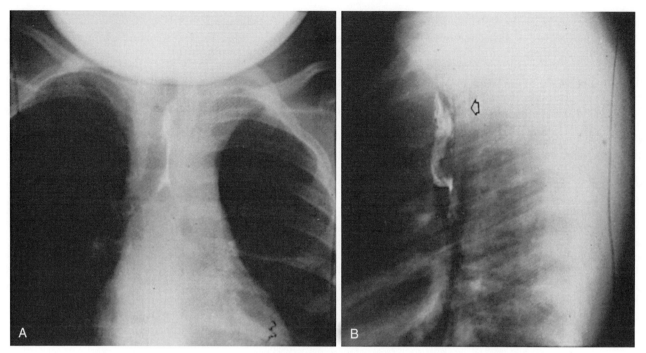

Figure 26–3. *A,* A communication between swallowed barium in the airway in a 4-year-old child with a chronic cough is demonstrated. *B,* A lateral radiograph on the same patient demonstrates a small lattice-like foreign body in the esophagus, which has eroded into the trachea. A piece of badminton shuttlecock had been ingested approximately 4 months before discovery of the acquired tracheoesophageal fistula.

watches, and other small electronic gadgets.[36, 37] These batteries may produce esophageal damage by one or all of three mechanisms: (1) pressure necrosis, (2) alkali or chemical injury from extravasation of the electrolytic agent, and (3) electrical current from a battery that is not exhausted. Some believe that dead batteries produce less injury.[38] Two instances of fatal erosion of disc batteries into the aorta have been reported.[39, 40] These two reports were among the first reports of disc battery ingestion.

Although some suggest that only batteries in the 22-mm or larger size range are dangerous, the potential for injury depends on the size of the esophagus and the ability of the battery to pass into the stomach.[36] Additionally, batteries that remain in the stomach for as little as 2 hours have produced mucosal staining and erosion. Whether this injury would have led to a gastric perforation cannot be determined. Batteries placed experimentally in normal saline quickly produce a pH of up to 12. Batteries in the esophagus for periods of days have produced extensive tracheoesophageal erosion.[37] This type of injury is reminiscent of a caustic agent, because after removal of the foreign body and presumed interruption of the pathology, progressive injury has continued in several instances.[41, 42]

Removal of the batteries from the esophagus can be accomplished by a Foley catheter[43] or by a magnetic device under radiographic control.[44] Removal from the stomach and even the upper portion of the small intestine also can be done by the magnetic device or by gastrotomy.[37]

Once the battery has passed through the pylorus, it probably will not cause further damage; however, one battery has produced a perforation in a Meckel's diverticulum on about the third day after its ingestion.[45]

Tracheoesophageal fistula or esophageal perforation resulting from foreign body injuries to the esophagus and trachea should be managed individually. The battery lesions that have produced a fistula between the trachea and the esophagus are rarely as simple to treat as they might appear to be. The extent of ultimate tissue destruction is usually more troublesome than is the erosion from simple pressure necrosis.

Iatrogenic esophageal injury may occur in the intact esophagus in the newborn[46, 47] and may be confused with unusual forms of esophageal atresia and tracheoesophageal fistula malformations. Mishaps of suctioning and intubation may also be responsible for esophageal perforation. Immediate surgical drainage can be carried out in many of these instances,[48] but the late diagnosis and exceedingly benign course in some would suggest that antibiotic coverage and nondrainage are satisfactory in selected cases.[49]

Spontaneous perforation of the esophagus has been reported in a newborn with no history of any sort of instrumentation.[50]

Other forms of iatrogenic injury include perforations of the esophagus with an instrument, such as can occur during pneumatic dilation of achalasia using a balloon dilator capable of achieving a 108F size.[51] Under the circumstance, the esophageal injury is not surprising. My esophageal perforation experience includes bougienage dilation of the esophagus in a patient undergoing treatment for a lye stricture (Fig. 26–4) and repeated balloon dilation in one patient for distal peptic stricture of the esophagus. Balloon dilation is less dangerous unless unreasonable sizes are used.[52] These extravasations drained spontaneously into the lumen of the esophagus, as evidenced by follow-up radiographs, which showed prompt clearing of extravasated contrast material. Such evidence of internal drainage, coupled with a benign clinical course, obviates the need for aggressive surgical drainage.[53]

The standard treatment, however, must remain surgical drainage for any sort of perforation of the esophagus. The signs of perforation include pain and fever. A chest radiograph rarely reveals mediastinal air early after a perforation. Up to 10% of patients may have a false-negative contrast study in the presence of perforation.[54, 55] Depending on the underlying disease process in the esophagus, primary closure may be accomplished or drainage

alone may be done.[53, 56–58] Radical resection probably should be used for the unusual situation in which the healing potential of the esophagus is questionable.[59]

Barotrauma to the esophagus usually occurs in children who bite into high-pressure devices. It can produce severe esophageal injury.[60, 61] Boerhaave's syndrome, caused by forceful vomiting, may produce an esophagopleural fistula, most commonly on the left side.[62] Primary repair and drainage should be used if the fistula is noted early.

Each esophageal perforation deserves individualized management with broad-spectrum antibiotic coverage, adequate drainage if indicated, and perhaps repair. Repair may include mobilization of surrounding tissue to support the esophageal or tracheal wall. Many patients in whom esophagus injuries occur have underlying esophageal pathology, which necessitates instrumentation. These factors complicate the treatment of esophageal perforation and, undoubtedly, play a role in the selection of therapy for the perforation.

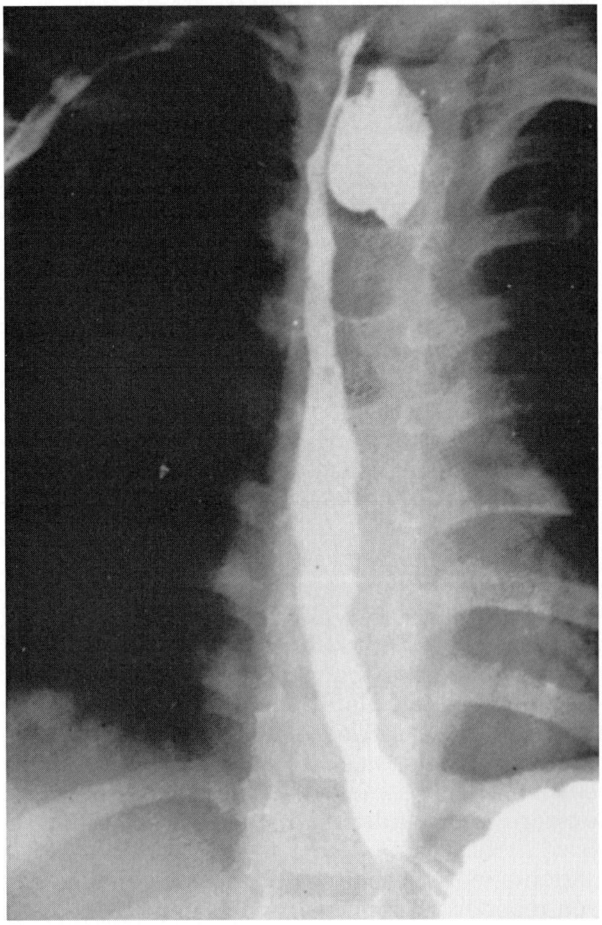

□ Congenital Esophageal Stenosis

Congenital esophageal stenosis is a lesion that is difficult to define, because early peptic strictures that have developed in children younger than 18 months have been included in this diagnosis. Those that are purely congenital stenoses, however, probably involve a remnant of respiratory cartilage in the wall.[60] Of 27 patients reviewed with congenital stenoses, most lesions were located in the distal esophagus.[63] I have seen one of these lesions and, in addition, an unusual cervical esophageal stricture that contained a large cartilaginous plaque in its posterior wall. A recent report of two cases of congenital upper esophageal stenosis did not contain cartilage: one was resected and one dilated.[64]

The diagnosis is most often made at the time of resection. These lesions are usually short but are not amenable to repeated dilations.

□ Functional Esophageal Disorders

Diffuse esophageal spasm is an uncommon condition that is also known as primary disordered motor activity.[65] The original description of this lesion is very complete.[66] A spastic pain usually occurs in the esophagus, accompanied by dysphagia. Since its early description, the pathology of diffuse esophageal spasm has been delineated as being circular muscle hypertrophy, primarily in the lower two thirds of the esophagus. The etiology is unknown.

I have had only two pediatric patients with this lesion (Fig. 26–5). One did not undergo myotomy and, when last seen, had continued intolerance of

Figure 26–4. The cervical or high thoracic perforation of the esophagus is demonstrated after dilation of caustic stricture of the esophagus. A follow-up radiograph several hours later shows complete return of the extravasated barium to the esophagus; therefore, further drainage was not undertaken. The patient eventually required esophageal replacement because of the stricture, not because of the perforation.

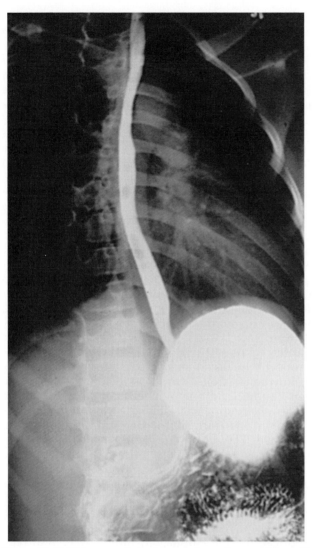

Figure 26–5. Diffuse esophageal spasm in an 8-year-old boy. He did not have gastroesophageal reflux nor did he respond well to repeated esophageal dilations. At last contact, he could take only soups and puréed foods.

foods that were not pureed. The other patient had a distal esophageal myotomy and Thal fundoplication with limited symptomatic improvement. The intrathoracic esophageal muscle would have been split during a second procedure, if necessary. Most of the reported adult patients who have undergone long myotomy have responded favorably.

SCLERODERMA

Scleroderma is an uncommon collagen disorder in children. The distal two thirds of the esophagus, which is smooth muscle, may have its normal peristalsis destroyed in the patient with scleroderma. Gastroesophageal reflux is almost universally present. Esophagitis, sometimes progressing to peptic stricture of the esophagus, occurs quite commonly in scleroderma.[67] Fundoplication has resulted in clinical improvement in many patients, despite the fact that the underlying systemic illness and the

disordered peristalsis remain unchanged. I have seen no pediatric patients with sclerodermal involvement of the esophagus. A scleroderma-like disorder of esophageal motility and lax LES pressure has recently been described in the breast-fed children of mothers who had silicone breast implants. There has been no evidence presented as to cause and effect.[68]

ESOPHAGEAL DIVERTICULUM

Diverticula of the esophagus are exceedingly rare in children. In the absence of diffuse esophageal spasm, they are rare even in adults. One child has been reported with Ehlers-Danlos syndrome, in whom diverticula in the esophagus, stomach, colon, and urinary bladder were noted.[69]

ESOPHAGEAL ACHALASIA

The etiology of achalasia is unknown. Histopathology in 24 muscle specimens from the distal esophagus revealed the complete absence of neural plexus in 2 patients and of ganglion cells in 10. However, ganglion cells were normal in 7 patients. These findings may be the result of ischemia or inflammation from esophagitis. In 5 patients, chronic inflammatory changes were present in the ganglion cells. Smooth muscle fibers appeared normal on light microscopy.[70] The patients were all children whose symptoms had their onset from age 5 days to 15 years. Achalasia, however, is primarily a disease of older people whose symptoms do not begin until adulthood. A congenital etiology is therefore unlikely. Teleologically, gastroesophageal reflux may certainly produce a spastic reaction in the lower end of the esophagus, which ultimately leads to a clinical picture resembling achalasia. Achalasia may occur in a familial pattern. In such situations, pyloric stenosis has been noted,[71] in which the initial symptoms are those of gastroesophageal reflux. A frequent cause of a delayed diagnosis of achalasia is confusion with symptoms of gastroesophageal reflux.[72]

I have one patient who presented in precisely this manner. He underwent fundoplication and was unable to swallow. Despite the fact that he had an anterior fundoplication, the wrap was taken down. Continued obstruction led to the radiographic diagnosis of achalasia. An esophagomyotomy was done with a repeat anterior fundoplication. The patient has since required pyloroplasty for what appeared, at age 5 years, to be pyloric stenosis.

By the time a patient undergoes diagnostic studies, the barium examination of the distal esophagus usually shows a large proximal esophagus with ineffectual peristalsis, a bird-beak deformity of the distal esophagus, and little contrast material passing into the stomach (Fig. 26–6). This radiographic picture is diagnostic of achalasia. In the child, manometrics are not necessary to confirm the diagnosis.

The diagnosis of achalasia may be made by bar-

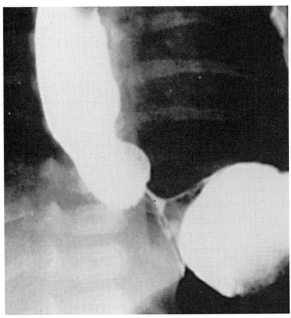

Figure 26–6. Achalasia in a 3-year-old child treated with a Heller myotomy and Thal fundoplication with an excellent result.

ium study. In adults, it is more precisely confirmed by manometric determinations. Manometry shows nonperistalsis in the body of the esophagus with little or no relaxation of the LES. [72, 73]

Monitoring of the pH in the distal esophagus may reveal the presence of gastroesophageal reflux. This study has not been done frequently in the evaluation of achalasia.

Therapy for achalasia is surgical. A calcium channel blocker (nifedipine) has been shown to reduce the LES pressure in children with demonstrated achalasia, but its effect was transient. Most likely, therefore, this treatment would not be a viable lifetime approach to the management of achalasia. [74]

Much of the literature dealing with achalasia pertains to surgery in adult patients. Comparisons of the results and the problems indicate that the management of achalasia is not much different in adults than it is in children. [75] Bougienage or balloon dilation sometimes produces good symptomatic relief, but in adults perforation rates are up to 12%. [76] Although 50% of patients were asymptomatic 4 years after dilation, 30% had symptomatic gastroesophageal reflux and 20% had dysphagia. In the discussion of this paper, it was pointed out that any operation that has a recognized 20 to 50% failure rate with a bad long-term outlook probably should not be accepted as rational therapy. [77] In a study of pneumatic dilation in both children and adults, the group least responsive to this form of therapy were the patients younger that 20 years. Successful balloon dilation resulted in symptomatic gastroesophageal reflux in a significant number of pediatric patients as well. [78]

The standard accepted surgical treatment for achalasia is the esophageal myotomy proposed by

Heller 80 years ago. Thoracic surgeons usually use a thoracic approach, and general surgeons use an abdominal approach. The basic premise is to incise both the longitudinal and circular muscle layers of the esophagus down to the submucosa, much as is done in pyloromyotomy. In young adults, the myotomy extends 5 to 10 cm above the gastroesophageal junction, a length which should be appropriately shortened in children. An international compilation of 175 pediatric patients with achalasia recently demonstrated that only 54% had surgical repair through the abdomen and that 75% of those had a concomitant fundoplication when this approach was used. Better resolution of symptoms was reported with the abdominal myotomy-fundoplication combination than with thoracic myotomy with or without fundoplication. [79]

My approach has been to perform a distal esophageal myotomy extending 2.5 to 5 cm up the esophagus and to cover the myotomy with an anterior fundoplication to prevent gastroesophageal reflux. Because myotomy alone has been complicated by symptomatic reflux, the question of the proper choice of operations for achalasia has been addressed. [80] In 19 patients who had undergone esophagomyotomy alone, esophagomyotomy plus a Nissen fundoplication, or a Nissen fundoplication alone, obstruction caused by the fundoplication was found in one third and gastroesophageal reflux in one third. The remainder had inadequate esophagomyotomies. In previously untreated patients, these investigators used a combination of esophagomyotomy and Belsey fundoplication. In those patients who were followed, 88% had a very good result documented by history, pH, and manometric studies. These investigators concluded that anterior fundoplication and esophagomyotomy were the treatments of choice for achalasia in adults. Others contend that the properly done esophagomyotomy that does not extend to the stomach is a perfectly satisfactory operation for achalasia, but that if the myotomy is extended to the stomach, a hemiwrap fundoplication is preferable to a complete wrap. [75] Many surgeons believe, as I do, that esophagomyotomy coupled with anterior fundoplication is the ideal procedure for achalasia. [70, 82–85]

In one series of 21 children, however, only 5 were reported to have had fundoplications. All of these were Nissen fundoplications with good results. [75] Another study of Nissen fundoplication in children, however, states that 50% of children who undergo esophagomyotomy for achalasia will need a fundoplication and that the Thal fundoplication is preferable. [86] In my personal experience, 26 patients have had esophagomyotomy coupled with anterior fundoplication. All had excellent long-term results.

□ Esophageal Strictures

As a practical consideration, esophageal strictures in children do not involve malignancies. The etiology of benign strictures in childhood include reflux esophagitis, corrosive ingestion, and anastomotic scarring. Anastomotic and corrosive strictures may be aggravated by the presence of gastroesophageal reflux. In many instances, therefore, the treatment program requires not only relief of the obstruction but prevention of its recurrence by correction of the gastroesophageal reflux. Anastomotic strictures are discrete and short, whereas those strictures caused by ingested corrosives are irregular and may be long. Peptic esophageal strictures are usually located in the lower one third and may be short, but nonetheless are difficult to manage.

Esophageal stenosis has been a problem for many years, and the history of its treatment by bougienage is a fascinating one.[87] Dilation to disrupt the circular scar may be more lasting when coupled with the local injection of triamcinolone to reduce the reformation of collagen linkage.[88–91]

The current techniques of dilation include the use of an indwelling string in the esophagus by which means Tucker's dilators can be passed in a retrograde manner.[92] Hurst's mercury-filled bougies, filiforms and followers, wire-guided Savary dilators, and, most recently, balloon dilation[92] can also be used. Comparisons between the tangential dilations by bougie and the radial dilations by balloon have been made. The techniques appear to be comparable, both in terms of complications and long-term outlook.[93, 94] Radial dilation with balloons is the method that I prefer.[95]

Any method of dilation carries a risk of septicemia, including the formation of brain abscess.[96] In one series, four of nine patients had *Staphylococcus aureus* in postoperative blood cultures. The investigators recommended that appropriate antibiotic coverage should be provided for patients undergoing esophageal dilation. The threat of perforation exists regardless of the method of dilation.

In addition to the anastomotic strictures that occur after the repair of esophageal atresia, strictures can occur at either end of an interposed colon. Although there are some instances in which dilation of these stenoses is effective, many times, because of acid reflux, the stricture will not be resolved by dilation alone. Dilation of a proximal esophagocolonic stricture has been reported to have resulted in the healing of a cervical fistula[97]; however, in my experience, these fistulas most often require revision or surgical resection to allow healing.

Peptic stenosis of the distal esophagus has been managed successfully by dilation and nonoperative treatment of the reflux esophagitis. Most surgeons treating this combination of lesions use dilation coupled with fundoplication to prevent further reflux.[67, 98–100] When given the choice between fundoplication and repeated dilation or a primary esophageal substitution procedure, fundoplication appears to provide better results and fewer long-term complications[101] (Fig. 26–7).

Rarely, a patient with epidermolysis presents with esophageal stricture. These patients require esopha-

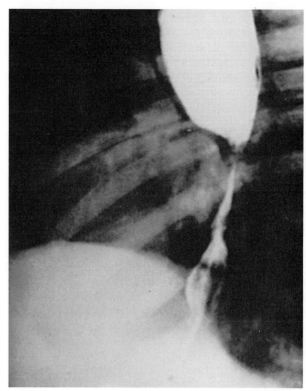

Figure 26–7. In this 8-year-old child with long-neglected reflux, a wide proximal esophagus, a tight esophageal stricture, and obvious gastric rugae about the level of the diaphragm are shown. A patient with these problems can be treated with fundoplication and dilation of the esophagus or distal esophageal replacement. The treatment depends on the ease with which dilation can be accomplished and the mobility of the esophagus. Often, the technique cannot be assessed until the time of operation. Therefore, provisions should be made for carrying out a hiatus hernia repair and fundoplication or a distal esophageal replacement by one technique or another.

geal substitution because the underlying disease process does not allow dilation of the esophagus without complete disruption of the mucosa.[102]

□ Corrosive Strictures

Corrosive strictures can be successfully dilated. One study in children has shown that adjunctive steroid injection into the scar made dilation treatment more lasting.[89] The problem with this approach to corrosive strictures is that if the esophagus continues to be used as a conduit for food, during the course of years, squamous cell carcinoma may develop at the site of injury. More than 130 patients are reported to have had squamous cell carcinoma develop at the site of corrosive injury. The usual scenario is that a child who has developed a stricture treated with bougienage for a number of years develops progressive dysphagia 20 to 40 years after the ingestion. Investigation reveals squamous cell carcinoma at the site of the major burn injury, usually at the level of the aortic arch.[103–108] In one series of 63 patients, 24 were considered surgical candidates. Only 20 underwent resection and 5 died. Of the 15 survivors, 5 were alive at 5 years. Of the radiation-treated patients, there was a 10% 5-year survival rate and a 5% 7-year survival rate. Compared with other patients who have carcinoma of the esophagus, the lesions in this group of patients are more resectable. The patients have a better prognosis, probably because dysphagia is apparent earlier because the esophagus is less distensible. The cicatrix in the esophageal wall may also prevent early local spread of the tumor.[108]

In my extensive literature search and in the experience of others,[109] not a single case of carcinoma occurred in a defunctioned esophagus after lye injury.

Given these concerns, the corrosive scarred esophagus should not be relied on as a conduit for food for the remainder of the patient's life. A substitution with its attendant difficulties is probably better than leaving the esophagus in use. Whether the defunctioned esophagus should be removed at the time of substitution remains unanswered. I have seen mucoceles develop in the residual esophagus when there was no way for the esophageal secretions to drain into the stomach, a condition that required esophagectomy.

☐ Esophageal Replacement

I have four principles of esophageal replacement:
1. The esophagus is the best conduit, provided that it functions near normally and has no malignant potential, as does a lye stricture or Barrett's esophagus.
2. A straight tract is best, avoiding as many twists and turns as possible, because esophagoscopy and dilations are frequently required. Almost all conduits function as passive tubes rather than by means of intrinsic peristaltic activity.
3. The prevention of reflux into any conduit is important; an interposition procedure that incorporates the distal normal esophagus with its gastroesophageal junction is best. This provides the opportunity for a low-resistance, anterior fundoplication.
4. Tenacity is exceedingly important. Anastomotic dilations should not be necessary except during the healing phase. Strictures should be revised surgically. Complex interpositions that do not function well can and should be rearranged to provide the straightest, lowest resistance food conduit possible.

☐ Colon Interposition

The use of the right colon as an esophageal substitute has been most popular in the United States[110] (Figs. 26–8 and 26–9). Substitution using the left colon has been more commonly done in England.[111, 112] The colon segment may be placed in an antiperistal-

tic manner[110] or in an isoperistaltic manner.[111] Some surgeons prefer intrathoracic retrohilar placement of transverse or left colon without regard to the peristaltic orientation of the colon segment.[113–117]

In a comparison study of 80 colon replacements in 79 children, 70% were placed behind the hilum in an isoperistaltic manner, and 30% were placed retrosternally. Most esophageal atresia patients with a stump of distal esophagus had that stump incorporated in the interposition. The incidence of proximal anastomotic leak was 31%, with a proximal anastomotic stricture developing in 15% of the retrohilar left colon anastomoses and in 41% of the retrosternal colon interpositions. Additionally, 60% of patients with substernal colon interposition had reflux. Only 18% of those with the retrohilar type had this problem. Five of 12 patients having substernal colon interposition required treatment of ulcers in the interposition. The investigators concluded that the retrohilar left colon interposition is preferable.[118] The function of any interposition is more satisfactory in the retrohilar position according to some because it is less tortuous.[118, 119]

In a much smaller series of 20 colon interpositions, the functional result seemed to be similar in the retrosternal compared with the intrathoracic group, but strictures requiring resection occurred only in the retrosternal interposition group.[120] More intraoperative ischemic complications of colon interposition have occurred with the right colon placed in the substernal position compared with the transverse or left colon placed behind the pulmonary hilum.[112] Perhaps this occurs because as many as 70% of patients have a right colon that lacks a marginal artery necessary to nourish the colon transplant.[121] Ischemia may result from the angulation necessary for the substernal placement.

Although one investigator reports only a 2% incidence of proximal esophageal colonic anastomotic leak,[111] most others report an incidence of this complication of approximately 30 to 33%.[119, 122, 123] Esophagocolonic leak is probably caused by technical errors or minor degrees of ischemia, but stricture formation is almost undoubtedly caused by ischemia. Repeated dilation is not often successful. Therefore, most anastomotic strictures that persist more than 6 months after the interposition procedure are ultimately going to need surgical revision. Both the management of esophageal leak and the surgical management of esophageal stricture are less difficult if the anastomosis is made in the neck. The proximal anastomosis is often at this level because of the cephalad extent of lye injury, if that is the etiology of the problem, or because of the shortened proximal pouch with isolated esophageal atresia when a cervical esophagostomy has been done.

I have had experience with one girl who had a colon interposition at age 3 years for caustic stricture. She did reasonably well in spite of repeated upper anastomotic strictures until age 18, when she developed a fistula from the conduit to the skin. The original anastomosis had been between the cervical

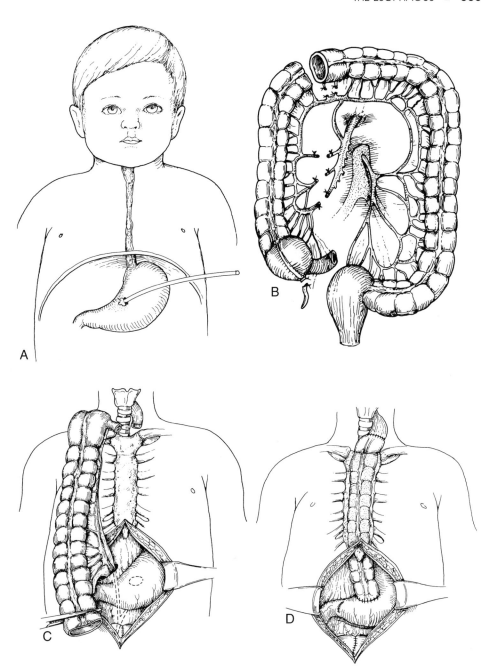

Figure 26–8. *A,* For any esophageal lesion in which a substitution procedure may be anticipated, the gastrostomy should be placed on the lesser curve at about the level of the incisura, so that a right or left colon or gastric tube interposition may be carried out without compromising the blood supply. *B,* The right colon and terminal ileum are isolated, based on blood supply from the arcades and from the middle colic artery. *C,* The colon on its pedicle is brought up through the lesser omentum and positioned substernally in an isoperistaltic fashion. *D,* Most frequently, excision of the terminal ileum and cecum is accomplished. Careful tailoring of the distal end allows a straight conduit to be anastomosed to the antrum. Pyloroplasty may or may not be added to the procedure. The incidence of significant gastrocolic reflux is reduced by a drainage procedure.

esophagus and the terminal ileum. In order to successfully treat the late esophagocutaneous fistula, the sternum was split and the tenia incised to allow lengthening of the colon segment so that the terminal ileum and cecum could be discarded. Anastomosis between the esophagus and the ascending colon was then carried out. Since that procedure, she has been without symptoms. This method of elongation of the substernal colon segment was originally described by the excision of the tenia.[124] Multiple incisions of tenia, however, are more feasible and as effective.[125]

Reflux into the colon segment occurs least when the normal distal esophagus has been used as the implantation site for the distal colonic anastomosis. Left colon placement with anastomosis of the colon

to the stomach done low on the posterior gastric wall is reputed to prevent reflux.[126] In my experience, it does not. Although it has anecdotally been reputed that an intraabdominal segment of colon of 10-cm length effectively prevents reflux, cine and manometric studies show this not to be true.[127]

The submucosal tunnel has sometimes been effective in prevention of gastrocolonic reflux,[128] as has the antireflux nipple.[129] Although the creation of a Nissen fundoplication around an anterior cologastrostomy worked well in experimental animals, it has not become a common means of preventing gastrocolonic reflux in humans. Its experimental proponent suggests that colon-to-distal-esophageal anastomosis is the best method of prevention of gastrocolonic reflux.[113, 130] Recently, experience with

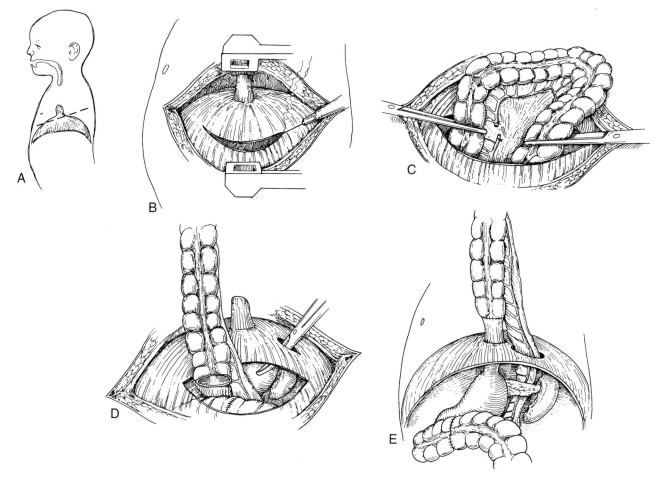

Figure 26–9. The left colon or transverse colon substitution described by Waterston is illustrated in this patient with isolated esophageal atresia. However, it works equally well for other lesions requiring esophageal replacement. *A,* A standard posterolateral left thoracotomy at about the sixth intercostal space. *B,* Incision of the diaphragm peripherally. *C,* A section of colon is isolated and its vascular pedicle is developed, usually based on the left colic artery. It may be necessary to base it on the middle colic artery, in which case this interposed colon is placed in an antiperistaltic manner. *D,* The colon and its vascular pedicle are delivered behind the spleen and pancreas and through a separate posterior opening in the diaphragm, so that the abdominal viscera do not stretch or otherwise obstruct the blood supply to this colon segment. *E,* The distal anastomosis may be made to the remnant of distal esophagus or to the posterior aspect of the stomach.

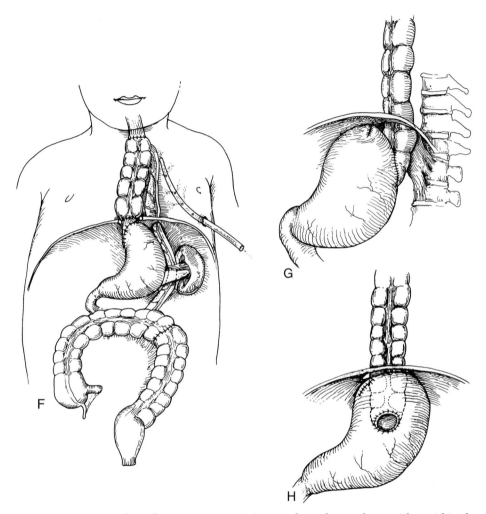

Figure 26–9 *Continued. F,* The upper anastomosis is made to the esophagus either within the mediastinum or within the neck. Adequate drainage of the pleura is necessary to prevent empyema. A fundoplication after the method of Thal may also be added to this procedure, if the distal esophagus is used. This technique reduces the amount of reflux that can interfere with the healing or that can produce ulcers in the colon. *G,* A lateral view of an alternative method of cologastrostomy with Waterston's procedure. *H,* The segment of colon is shown within the abdominal cavity, which will possibly reduce the incidence of gastrocolic reflux. In my experience, reflux is not reduced.

48 patients having a substernal, ileocolic interposition was reported, in which the ileocecal valve served as a very effective antireflux mechanism when the cecum remains within the abdomen.[131] Leaving the ileocecal valve in the upper mediastinum as an antireflux mechanism has been proposed,[132] but in my experience, this has not been effective.

The response of the distal colon-gastric anastomosis to acid has been studied, with the conclusion that the alkaline secretions of the colon tend to neutralize the acid or propel it back into the stomach before it can cause problems.[133] Clinically, such a fortuitous acid-alkali balance may occur, but it would be unreliable at best. Distal colonic ulcers have resulted from reflux of gastric acid. Most of these occurred in patients who did not undergo either pyloroplasty or pyloromyotomy to promote gastric drainage. Gastric drainage should be a part of any procedure that calls for a cologastric anastomosis.

Motor activity analysis of interposed colon (as well as other esophageal substitution conduits) has recently shown that the colon has a very satisfactory response to a bolus of food, although organized peristalsis is not seen.[134] Many older studies have demonstrated that no matter whether the colon was placed in an isoperistaltic or antiperistaltic manner, its propulsive efforts soon were lost and it came to serve mostly as a passive conduit for food.[117–119, 127] No discernible difference regarding the ability to swallow was noted in a series of 60 patients, two thirds of whom had antiperistaltic interpositions of colon. Reflux from the stomach into the distal colon segment was common in this group of patients. Complications were infrequent, possibly because of pyloroplasty.[135] Similar findings were reported in another series of 84 patients undergoing both isoperistaltic and antiperistaltic colon interpositions.[136]

A functional assessment of interposed colon with isotope-labeled milk has shown that patients who were clinically well had conduit emptying of less than 45 minutes without reflux. Those who were clinically troubled had delayed emptying of the conduit, gastrocolic reflux, or both. The function of the colon segment may be satisfactorily assessed in this way.[137]

Late complications of colon interposition include redundancy of the colon segment, which led to one instance of obstructive volvulus of the colon.[138] Ulceration of the interposed colon can penetrate into the pericardium. In my experience, a penetrating ulcer in a substernal colon interposition has produced sternal osteomyelitis, which was troublesome to treat[139] (Fig. 26–10).

Another consideration in the selection of an interposition route is the possibility of subsequent acquired heart disease, necessitating sternotomy. In those patients in whom the substernal colon interposition has been used, this approach to the heart is difficult. Similarly, the previous use of a median

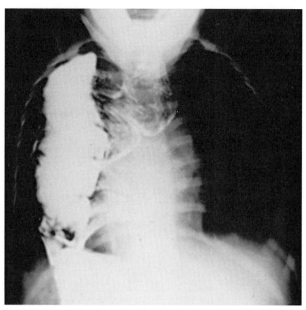

Figure 26–10. The elongation of a substernal colon is a difficult problem to manage at times, requiring careful tailoring of the distal end of the interposed colon without disrupting the blood supply to the upper portion.

sternotomy to repair the heart often necessitates an alternative route for an interposition.[140]

TIMING OF COLON INTERPOSITION

In those patients in whom esophageal atresia exists without distal tracheoesophageal fistula and in whom attempts at stretching are not considered, the colon can be interposed in the newborn period. Most pediatric surgeons, however, create a cervical esophageal fistula, place a gastrostomy, and carry out interposition sometime after the patient is 6 months of age. Some electively delay this procedure until 12 to 18 months. Both approaches have theoretic and practical advantages. Most reported experience has been with the later procedure. However, if the patient has been without oral intake for many months, once an esophageal substitution has been made he or she may not want to eat. Therefore, sham feedings by mouth should accompany gastrostomy feedings so that the patient associates a full stomach with swallowing. In patients who have experienced failed attempts at stretching, failed anastomosis of the esophagus because of long-gap esophageal atresia with fistula, or caustic injuries, the operative procedure takes place sometime after the newborn period.

Passive or active drainage must accompany any esophageal anastomosis, whether in the neck or in the chest.

My personal preference for esophageal substitution using colon is the retrohilar left or transverse colon segment placed with its vascular pedicle behind the pancreas. The distal anastomosis, whenever possible, is created using the distal stump of esophagus. In most of these patients, I also create an anterior fundoplication to enhance the LES and to prevent gastroesophageal-colonic reflux. Rather than accept a cologastric anastomosis, I prefer a gastric tube interposition placed through the esophageal hiatus with anastomosis to the upper mediastinal or cervical esophagus. In these cases, the distal esophagus stump is resected and an antireflux valve is created after the method of Toupet (see later text).

☐ Gastric Tube Esophageal Replacement

Gastric tube replacement of the esophagus became a practicality in children in the early 1970s.[142, 143] The reported experience with gastric tube esophagoplasty is much smaller than with colon interposition, perhaps because the number of patients needing esophageal substitution has diminished (Fig. 26–11). Awareness of caustic material hazards and changes in the chemical formulation of prepared drain cleaners have resulted in fewer serious ingestion injuries. Homemade lye solutions remain deadly.

Gastric tubes have become popular because they can be constructed rapidly with a stapling device. These tubes can be constructed from the antrum up or from the fundus down and can be constructed so that there is enough gastric tube to reach the neck.[143, 144] Gastric tubes can be placed substernally or behind either pulmonary hilum. In a comparison study, the functional results of gastric tubes were similar whether they were placed transthoracically or substernally; however, in my experience, the substernal placement of the gastric tube has resulted in necrosis in several patients and in an intractable stricture in one. The long-term results of gastric tube interposition are better than those of the colon interposition, and the gastric tube is simpler to construct.[143]

The gastric tube may involve peptic ulcer problems as well, both within the tube and at the junction of the gastric tube with the proximal esophagus. The ulcerations may be aggravated by stasis; therefore, some authors recommend that a pyloroplasty be done in all patients undergoing gastric tube esophageal substitutions.[143] Reflux has not been a problem if at least 6 cm of gastric tube is located within the abdomen.

My preference for a gastric tube is to place it, if at all possible, behind the hilum of the lung through the esophageal hiatus and to create a posterior (Toupet) fundoplication as illustrated in Figure 26–11. The function of such a fundoplication has been good, although in one patient it became obstructive (Fig. 26–12). I do not routinely do pyloroplasty or pyloromyotomy. I believe that the long-term course of patients having gastric tube interposition has been much more trouble-free than has the course of patients having colon interposition.

In my experience, gastric tube esophagoplasty is limited to older patients because of the percentage of stomach that must be used to create a satisfactory

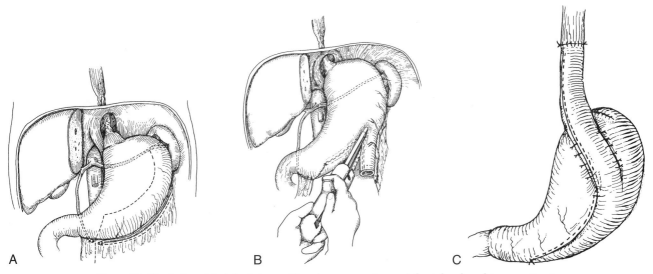

A   B   C

Figure 26–11. *A,* A gastric tube interposition, in my experience, is best developed in an antiperistaltic manner using a greater curve gastric tube. Inspection of the blood supply is important before the development of a gastric tube is begun. *B,* The tube is developed with the use of the gastrointestinal anastomosis stapling device. Iatrogenic narrowing of this tube should be avoided. A large-bore red rubber catheter can prevent this unfortunate complication. Twisting of the greater curvature, which may result in a disparity between the contributions of the posterior gastric wall and the anterior gastric wall, should also be avoided. The short gastric vessels rarely need to be divided for the creation of a satisfactory tube length. *C,* To be anastomosed to a remnant of esophagus in the mediastinum or in the neck, the gastric tube may be positioned in the anterior mediastinum substernally or through the esophageal hiatus. A posterior partial wrap, as illustrated, effectively prevents reflux of gastric content up into the gastric tube and reduces the likelihood of ulceration or anastomotic stricture.

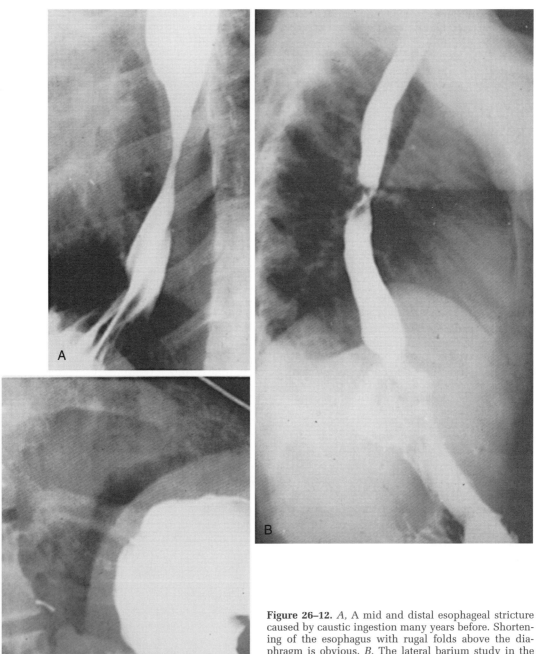

Figure 26–12. *A,* A mid and distal esophageal stricture caused by caustic ingestion many years before. Shortening of the esophagus with rugal folds above the diaphragm is obvious. *B,* The lateral barium study in the early postoperative period shows the gastric tube with some anastomotic edema in the portion of the mid-esophagus. The gastric tube has been placed through the esophageal hiatus into the posterior mediastinum. *C,* The complete absence of reflux in this interposed gastric tube can be seen with this late follow-up study. This result is probably due to the fundoplication, as illustrated in Figure 26–11*C.*

tube, which limits this technique in very small children.[145]

☐ Gastric Interposition

Mobilization of the stomach and its repositioning into the mediastinum were strictly avoided in growing children because it was believed that the patient's growth pattern would not be normal. At the Hospital for Sick Children at Great Ormond Street, London, this technique became the interposition of choice in 1981, both for infants with esophageal atresia and for older patients with caustic injury or failed repair of esophageal atresia malformations.[146] Its use in 34 patients was reported from that institution in 1987. A total of 23 patients were younger than 12 months at the time of esophagogastrostomy. Sixteen patients had the stomach moved up into the mediastinum, and 18 had the stomach placed in a transthoracic retrohilar position. A pyloromyotomy was done in 13 and a pyloroplasty in 20. Of the 31 survivors, 14 had uncomplicated recoveries and 17 had one or more postoperative complication. Many of these complications were related to the fact that the patients did not know how to feed before the interposition. One child developed a leak in the jejunostomy feeding tube and required reexploration. A jejunostomy apparently was universally used during the healing phase in these patients. Most importantly, only 6 of 23 children followed for at least a year postoperatively remained below the 30th percentile for height and weight. The others grew in a normal fashion. This experience was updated in 1995 to include a total of 83 patients. The combined mortality was 7.2%, with a 12% incidence each of an anastomotic leak and stricture. A satisfactory nutritional outcome was reported in 89%.[147]

A comparison of 112 Waterston colon interpositions done at this same institution between 1952 and 1981 revealed that the mortality was approximately the same, but the incidence of graft failure, cervical anastomotic leak, and cervical anastomotic stricture was reduced in the gastric interposition patients, and quality of life was much improved.

I have used this interposition in four patients. One had experienced a failed colon interposition and a failed gastric tube. He underwent a successful esophagogastrostomy placed through the right chest posterior to the hilum (Fig. 26–13). He has done well. Another was a 1-year-old who had his upper atretic esophagus brought out on the neck and who had no recognizable distal esophageal stump. He has been slow to eat and to maintain his nutrition. The third patient had an ulcer-destroyed substernal right colon interposition removed, which brought her stomach from the substernal position up to the cervical esophagus. After 2 years of postprandial distress and extreme inanition, the stomach was replaced in the abdomen and the left colon interposed as a retrohilar, right-sided esophageal substitute.

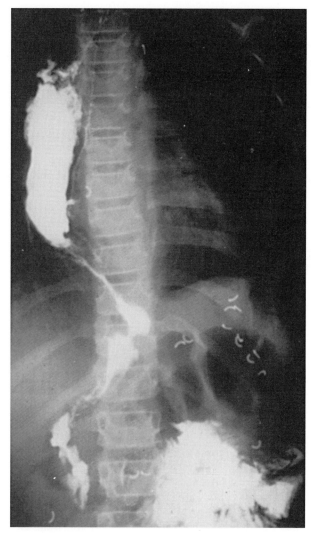

Figure 26–13. A patient who underwent an esophagogastrostomy after unsuccessful colon interposition and failed gastric tube. The patient also underwent a pyloroplasty at the time of the esophagogastrostomy.

The fourth patient had a gastric pull-up at the age of 15 years because of a very dysfunctional distal esophageal segment with Barrett's changes. He had not responded to fundoplication performed at age 4 years. There was no collateral blood supply from the left to the right gastroepiploic arteries, which precluded using a reversed gastric tube.

☐ Jejunal Substitution

The jejunum as an esophageal substitute has been much more common in adults than in children. Of 19 pediatric patients reported to have a segmental jejunal interposition placed into the midesophagus through the right chest, 12 were available for long-term follow-up: 1 developed a stricture, and 1 developed an elongation of the interposed jejunum. The surgeons preserved the distal esophagus after the method of Waterston whenever possible. The technique to harvest a 10- to 12-cm segment of jejunum required sacrifice of about 40 cm of jejunum, however. Some of the patients had nutritional problems, perhaps because of the loss of this much small intestine.[149]

The major use for jejunum has been as a free graft with microvascular anastomosis in the cervical position for adults with carcinoma. An extensive use of this procedure in 101 patients was reported with satisfactory results.[150] This procedure obviously would not be applicable to the pediatric population. I have done only one jejunal interposition between the cervical esophagus and stomach. Its early result was satisfactory. The patient was then lost to follow-up.

COMPLICATIONS OF ESOPHAGEAL SUBSTITUTION

Substitution of the esophagus carries with it a certain number of predictable complications; the most serious one is vascular insufficiency with necrosis of the interposition. This complication is most commonly seen using the colon, as mentioned earlier, and is recognized at the time of interposition as a blue, pulseless graft. Adjustment of the colon graft to relieve tension or twisting of the pedicle may be effective in improving the blood supply. Intraoperative hypotension may result in the colon graft taking on the appearance of vascular insufficiency. If the geometry of the graft and the patient's blood pressure are both satisfactory, the graft must be abandoned, because hoping that its vascularity will improve after interposition is usually in vain.

Interposition of a well-vascularized graft is sometimes followed several days later by fever, increased leukocytosis, and drainage from the proximal anastomosis. A contrast study may demonstrate that the mucosal pattern of the interposed segment is not normal. The interposition needs to be inspected and removed if necrotic. In this instance, a cervical esophagostomy should be established and a different form of substitution planned. Many investigators have reported using the left colon after failure of the right colon. I am inclined not to sacrifice that much colon and would probably resort to either gastric tube or esophagogastrostomy under the circumstances.

Proximal strictures between the esophagus and the interposition usually are the result of insufficient blood supply to the interposition. Anastomosis to a scarred esophagus also results in stricture. After a reasonable healing period, persistent strictures should be revised surgically rather than dilated repeatedly.

Ulceration in either gastric tube or interposed colon is probably the result of reflux and stasis, which may be caused by kinks or turns in the interposition or by delayed gastric emptying. The latter can be a complication of vagal injury either from the original caustic ingestion or from the surgical attempts at previous esophageal reconstruction. Whether a py-

loroplasty or a drainage procedure is necessary in all interpositions is a matter of opinion. Certainly, the elimination of sink-trap kinks in the interposition is important to prevent ulceration. Revision of the lower end of the interposed colon to eliminate redundancy must be done with great care to prevent damage to the vascular pedicle and loss of the entire graft.

One of my patients had repeated upper anastomotic strictures because of gastrocolic reflux into a substernal colon interposition placed for esophageal atresia without fistula. I detached both ends of the colon segment through a right thoracotomy and laparotomy, delivered it back into the abdominal cavity, brought it up behind the hilum of the right lung, reanastomosed it to the upper mediastinal esophagus, shortened it, anastomosed it to the distal stump of the esophagus, and performed an anterior fundoplication. An excellent outcome resulted. Such extensive revision is not often necessary but may, on occasion, turn an unsatisfactory result completely around.[151, 152]

☐ Vascular Ring

The vascular malformations that involve the aortic arch and its major branches are known as vascular rings. In this chapter, only those malformations that potentially obstruct the esophagus are discussed. The complete ring, also known as the double aortic arch, is included, as are the incomplete rings, the most common of which is the aberrant subclavian vessel crossing behind the esophagus and the transverse aortic arch that crosses behind the esophagus to descend on the side opposite the ascending aorta. The incomplete rings are often associated with a ligamentum or ductus arteriosus, which limits the space available for trachea and esophagus. The incomplete rings are an unusual cause of dysphagia but are common on barium esophagram. The other much more serious vascular ring malformation is known as the pulmonary artery sling and is often related to tracheal malformation but rarely with any esophageal symptoms.

The symptoms of vascular ring are dysphagia, for the most part. *Dysphagia lusoria* was the name attached to the symptoms attributed to the aberrant right subclavian artery, which passes behind the esophagus as it courses toward the right axilla. In fact, an aberrant right subclavian artery rarely produces dysphagia.

Because the obstruction of the esophagus is partial, the symptoms that result from vascular rings depend on how voraciously the child is eating and whether the ingested food is solid or liquid. Often, these lesions are not discovered until the child is eating table food.[153]

DIAGNOSIS

The diagnosis is established almost exclusively by barium study of the esophagus done for evalua-

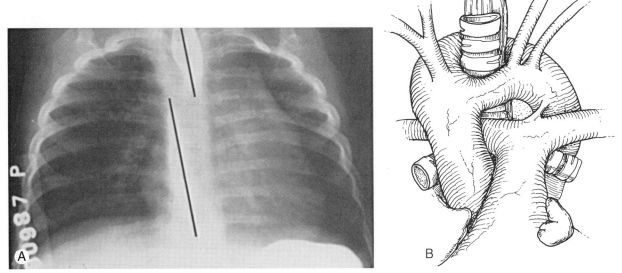

Figure 26–14. *A*, A double aortic arch demonstrated by barium esophagram. The axes of the proximal and distal portions of the esophagus are offset by the presence of a complete vascular ring. *B*, The double arch as drawn is usually narrowest on the left branch and is best approached for division through a left thoracotomy.

tion of dysphagia. The typical radiographic picture of a double aortic arch is that of an offset in the linear axis of the esophagus. It is characteristic of the double aortic arch (Fig. 26–14) and is contrasted with the indentation without offset in the axis, as in the case of aberrant right subclavian artery (Fig. 26–15). Although echocardiography,[154] digital subtraction angiography,[155] or magnetic resonance imaging[156, 157] may confirm the diagnosis, they are

rarely necessary either for diagnostic or therapeutic decisions.

SURGICAL TREATMENT

The normal formation of the aortic arch requires resorption of the dorsal fourth right arch with remolding of the right subclavian and common carotid into an innominate artery arising as the first vessel

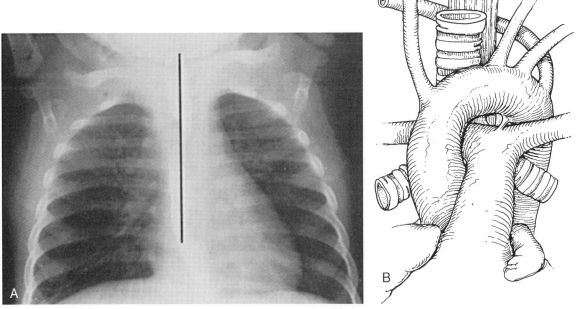

Figure 26–15. *A*, A longer postesophageal aberrant right subclavian artery is shown, which indents the esophagus but does not offset its axis. *B*, The aberrant right subclavian artery is best divided by the left thoracotomy approach.

off the arch. The double arch results when the resorptive process does not occur properly. If both arches persist, the right is almost always the larger of the two, with varying degrees of stenosis or even fibrosis of the left arch, forming the anterior portion of the ring. The right arch courses behind the esophagus. The left arch compresses the trachea and esophagus to produce the symptoms. The surgical approach to division of the vascular ring is best done through the left thorax, dividing the left arch at its narrowest point, which is either posterior to the origin of the left subclavian artery or between the ascending aorta and the origin of the left common carotid artery.[158] The ligamentum arteriosum should be divided as well to effectively relieve the esophageal obstruction. Dissection of the vessels off the trachea anteriorly and the esophagus posteriorly is usually all that is necessary to allow the trachea and the esophagus to escape the obstruction and relieve symptoms.

Although some surgeons detach the retroesophageal aberrant right subclavian artery and reimplant it on the aortic arch, most simply divide this vessel and allow the distal portion to retract across the mediastinum from behind the esophagus.[159] Thus, symptoms are relieved. Therefore, this anomaly can best be treated through a left thoracotomy as well. Other vascular or cardiac malformations are usually not associated with vascular ring. Any form of suspension of the vessels is usually not necessary after the division of the ring.

REFERENCES

1. Amoury RA: Structure and function of the esophagus in infancy and early childhood. In Ashcraft KW, Holder TM (eds): Pediatric Esophageal Surgery. Orlando, Grune & Stratton, pp 1–28, 1986.
2. Leape LL, Ashcraft KW, Scarpelli DG, et al: Hazard to health: Liquid lye. N Engl J Med 284:578–581, 1971.
3. Ashcraft KW, Padula RT: Effect of dilute corrosives on the esophagus. Pediatrics 53:226–232, 1974.
4. Webb WR, Koutras P, Ecker RR, et al: An evaluation of steroids and antibiotics in caustic burns of the esophagus. Ann Thorac Surg 9:95–102, 1970.
5. Haller JA, Bachman BA: Comparative effect of current therapy on experimental caustic burns of the esophagus. Pediatrics 34:236–245, 1964.
6. Haller JA, Andrews HG, White JJ, et al: Pathophysiology and management of acute corrosive burns of the esophagus: Results of treatment in 285 children. J Pediatr Surg 6:578–584, 1971.
7. Moazam F, Talbert JL, Miller D, et al: Caustic ingestion and its sequelae in children. South Med J 80:187–190, 1987.
8. Anderson KD, Rouse TM, Randolph JG: Controlled trial of corticosteroids in children with corrosive injury of the esophagus. N Engl J Med 323:637–640, 1990.
9. Edmonson MB: Caustic alkali ingestions by farm children. Pediatrics 79:413–416, 1987.
10. Shaw AN, Garvey J, Miller B: Lye burn requiring total gastrectomy and colon substitution for esophagus and stomach in a two-year-old boy. Surgery 65:837–844, 1969.
11. Estrera A, Taylor W, Mills LJ, et al: Corrosive burns of the esophagus and stomach: A recommendation for an aggressive surgical approach. Ann Thorac Surg 41:276–283, 1986.
12. Gago O, Ritter FN, Martel W, et al: Aggressive surgical treatment for caustic injury of the esophagus and stomach. Ann Thorac Surg 13:243–250, 1972.
13. Ashcraft KW: Correspondence. Ann Thorac Surg 14:221, 1972.
14. Reyes HM, Lin CY, Schlunk FF, et al: Experimental treatment of corrosive esophageal burns. J Pediatr Surg 9:317–327, 1974.
15. Reyes HM, Hill LJ: Modification of the experimental stent technique for esophageal burns. J Surg Res 20:65–70, 1976.
16. Hill LJ, Norberg HP, Smith MD, et al: Clinical technique and success of the esophageal stent to prevent corrosive strictures. J Pediatr Surg 11:443–450, 1976.
17. Wijburg FA, Heymans HSA, Urbanus NAM: Caustic esophageal lesions in childhood: Prevention of stricture formation. J Pediatr Surg 24:171–173, 1989.
18. Mills LJ, Estrera AS, Platt MR: Avoidance of esophageal stricture following severe caustic burns by the use of an intraluminal stent. Ann Thorac Surg 28:60–65, 1979.
19. Madden JW, Davis WM, Butler C, et al: Experimental esophageal lye burns: Correcting established strictures with beta-aminopropionitrile and bougienage. Ann Surg 178:277–284, 1973.
20. Davis WM, Madden JW, Peacock EE: A new approach to the control of esophageal stenosis. Ann Surg 176:469–476, 1972.
21. Joseph PR: The pediatric forum. Management of coin ingestion. Am J Dis Child 144:449, 1990.
22. Smith PC, Swischuk LE, Fagan CJ: An elusive and often unsuspected cause of stridor or pneumonia (the esophageal foreign body). Am J Rad Ther Nucl Med 122:80–89, 1974.
23. Foster DL: The pediatric forum. Pediatric coin ingestion. Am J Dis Child 144:450–451, 1990.
24. Schunk JE, Corneli H, Bolte R: Pediatric coin ingestions. Am J Dis Child 143:546–548, 1989.
25. Caravati EM, Bennett DL, McElwee NE: Pediatric coin ingestion: A prospective study on the utility of routine roentgenograms. Am J Dis Child 143:549–551, 1989.
26. Fernandes ET, Hollabaugh RS, Boulden T: Mediastinal mass and radiolucent esophageal foreign body. J Pediatr Surg 24:1135–1136, 1989.
27. Beal SM: Sudden infant death associated with an oesophageal problem. Med J Aust 2:91, 1979.
28. Woods I, Swan PK: Tracheal occlusion following oesophageal foreign body removal. Anaesth Intensive Care 17:356–358, 1989.
29. Bonadio WA, Jona JZ, Glicklich M, et al: Esophageal bougienage technique for coin ingestion in children. J Pediatr Surg 23:917–918, 1988.
30. Bigler FC: The use of a Foley catheter for removal of blunt foreign bodies from the esophagus. J Thorac Cardiovasc Surg 51:759–760, 1966.
31. Campbell JB, Foley CL: A safe alternative to endoscopic removal of blunt esophageal foreign bodies. Arch Otolaryngol 109:323–325, 1983.
32. Campbell JB, Condon VR: Catheter removal of blunt esophageal foreign bodies in children. Pediatr Radiol 19:361–365, 1989.
33. Burrington JD: Aluminum "pop tops": A hazard to child health. JAMA 235:2614–2617, 1976.
34. Spitz J, Hirsig J: Prolonged foreign body impaction in the oesophagus. Arch Dis Child 57:551–553, 1982.
35. Takano H, Okada A, Monden Y, et al: Unusual case of acquired benign tracheoesophageal fistula caused by an esophageal foreign body. J Thorac Cardiovasc Surg 99:755–756, 1990.
36. Litovitz TL: Button battery ingestions: A review of 56 cases. JAMA 249:2495–2500, 1983.
37. Votteler TP, Nash JC, Rutledge JC: The hazard of ingested alkaline disk batteries in children. JAMA 249:2504–2506, 1983.
38. Sigalet D, Lees G: Tracheoesophageal injury secondary to disc battery ingestion. J Pediatr Surg 23:996–998, 1988.
39. Maves MD, Carithers JS, Birck HG: Esophageal burns secondary to disc battery ingestion. Ann Otol Rhinol Laryngol 93:364–369, 1984.
40. Shabino DL, Feinberg AN: Esophageal perforation secondary to alkaline battery ingestion. J Am Coll Emerg Physicians 8:360–362, 1979.

41. Vaishnav A, Spitz L: Alkaline battery-induced tracheo-oesophageal fistula. Br J Surg 76:1045, 1989.

42. Blatnik DS, Toohill RJ, Lehman RH: Fatal complication from an alkaline battery foreign body in the esophagus. Ann Otol 86:611–615, 1977.

43. Rumack BH, Rumack CM: Disk battery ingestion. JAMA 249:2509–2511, 1983.

44. Volle E, Beyer P, Kaufmann JH: Therapeutic approach to ingested button-type batteries: Magnetic removal of ingested button-type batteries. Pediatr Radiol 19:114–118, 1989.

45. Willis GA, Ho WC: Perforation of Meckel's diverticulum by an alkaline hearing battery. Can Med Assoc J 126:497–498, 1982.

46. Wells SD, Leonidas JC, Conkle D, et al: Traumatic prevertebral pharyngoesophageal pseudodiverticulum in the newborn infant. J Pediatr Surg 9:217–222, 1974.

47. Cohen RC, Myers NA: Traumatic oesophageal pseudodiverticulum. J Pediatr Aust 23:125–127, 1987.

48. Nagaraj HS, Mullen P, Groff DB: Iatrogenic perforation of the esophagus in premature infants. Surgery 86:583–589, 1979.

49. Grosfeld JL: Discussion. In Nagaraj JS, Mullen P, Groff DB, et al: Iatrogenic perforation of the esophagus in premature infants. Surgery 86:588–599, 1979.

50. Tolstedt GE, Tudor RB: Esophagopleural fistula in a newborn infant. Arch Surg 97:780–781, 1968.

51. Adams H, Roberts GM, Smith PM: Oesophageal tears during pneumatic balloon dilatation for the treatment of achalasia. Clin Radiol 40:53–57, 1989.

52. Panieri E, Millar AJW, Rode H, et al: Iatrogenic esophageal perforation in children: Patterns of injury, presentation, management, and outcome. J Pediatr Surg 31:890–895, 1996.

53. Bolooki H: A discussion. In Attar S, Hankins JR, Suter CM, et al: Esophageal perforation: A therapeutic challenge. Ann Thorac Surg 50:50, 1990.

54. DeMeester TR: Perforation of the esophagus. Ann Thorac Surg 42:231–232, 1986.

55. Bladergroen MR, Lowe JE, Postlethwait RW: Diagnosis and recommended management of esophageal perforation and rupture. Ann Thorac Surg 42:235–239, 1986.

56. Ajalat GM, Mulder DG: Esophageal perforations. Arch Surg 119:1318–1320, 1984.

57. Cohn HE, Hubbard A, Patton G: Management of esophageal injuries. Ann Thorac Surg 48:309–314, 1989.

58. Michel L, Grillo HC, Malt RA: Esophageal perforation. Ann Thorac Surg 33:203–210, 1982.

59. Hendren WH, Henderson BM: Immediate esophagectomy for instrumental perforation of the thoracic esophagus. Ann Surg 168:997–1002, 1968.

60. Conlan AA, Wessels A, Hammond CA, et al: Pharyngo-esophageal barotrauma in children: A report of six cases. J Thorac Cardiovasc Surg 88:452–456, 1984.

61. Inculet R, Clark C, Girvan D: Boerhaave's syndrome and children: a rare and unexpected combination. J Pediatr Surg 31:1300–1301, 1996.

62. Domini R, Appignani A, Ceccarelli PL, et al: Congenital esophageal stenosis due to ectopic cartilaginous tissue: A case report. Ital J Pediatr Surg Sci 2:87–89, 1988.

63. Scherer LR, Grosfeld JL: Congenital esophageal stenosis, esophageal duplication, neurenteric cyst and esophageal diverticulum. In Ashcraft KW, Holder TM (eds): Pediatric Esophageal Surgery. Orlando, Grune & Stratton, pp 53–71, 1986.

64. Grabowski ST, Andrews DA: Upper esophageal stenosis: Two case reports. J Pediatr Surg 31:1438–1439, 1996.

65. Henderson RD, Davidson JW: Primary disordered motor activity of the esophagus (diffuse spasm). Ann Thorac Surg 18:327–336, 1974.

66. Moersch HJ, Camp JD: Diffuse spasm of the lower part of the esophagus. Ann Otorhinolaryngol 43:1165–1173, 1934.

67. Henderson RD, Henderson RF, Marryatt GV: Surgical management of 100 consecutive esophageal strictures. J Thorac Cardiovasc Surg 99:1–7, 1990.

68. Levine JJ, Ilowite NT: Sclerodermalike esophageal disease in children breast-fed by mothers with silicone breast implants. JAMA 271:213–216, 1994.

69. Toyohara T, Koneka T, Araki H, et al: Giant epiphrenic diverticulum in a boy with Ehlers-Danlos syndrome. Pediatr Radiol 19:437, 1989.

70. Nihoul-Fekete C, Bawab F, Lortat-Jacob S, et al: Achalasia of the esophagus in childhood: Surgical treatment in 35 cases with special reference to familial cases and glucocorticoid deficiency association. J Pediatr Surg 24:1060–1063, 1989.

71. Tryhus MR, Davis M, Griffith JK, et al: Familial achalasia in two siblings: Significance of possible hereditary role. J Pediatr Surg 24:292–295, 1989.

72. Rosenzweig S, Traube M: The diagnosis and misdiagnosis of achalasia. J Clin Gastroenterol 11:147–153, 1989.

73. Shoenut P, Trenholm BG, Micflikier AB, et al: Reflux patterns in patients with achalasia without operation. Ann Thorac Surg 45:303–305, 1988.

74. Smith H, Buick R, Booth I, et al: Letters to the editor. J Pediatr Gastroenterol 7:146, 1988.

75. Vane DW, Cosby K, West K, et al: Late results following esophagomyotomy in children with achalasia. J Pediatr Surg 23:515–519, 1988.

76. Sauer L, Pellegrini CA, Way LW: The treatment of achalasia. Arch Surg 124:929–932, 1989.

77. Richardson JD: Discussion. In Sauer L, Pellegrini CA, Way LW: The treatment of achalasia. Arch Surg 124:932, 1989.

78. Ponce J, Garrigues V, Pertejo V, et al: Individual prediction of response to pneumatic dilation in patients with achalasia. Dig Dis Sci 41:2135–2141, 1996.

79. Myers N, Jolley SG, Taylor R: Achalasia of the cardia in children: A worldwide survey. J Pediatr Surg 29:1375–1379, 1994

80. Little AG, Soriano A, Ferguson MK, et al: Surgical treatment of achalasia: Results with esophagomyotomy and Belsey repair. Ann Thorac Surg 45:489–494, 1988.

81. Ellis FH: Treatment of achalasia: A continuing controversy. Ann Thorac Surg 45:473, 1988.

82. Jekler J, Lhotka J: Modified Heller procedure to prevent postoperative reflux esophagitis in patients with achalasia. Am J Surg 113:251–254, 1967.

83. Skinner DB: Myotomy and achalasia. Ann Thorac Surg 37:183–184, 1984.

84. Murray GF, Battaglini JW, Keagy BA, et al: Selective application of fundoplication in achalasia. Ann Thorac Surg 37:185–188, 1984.

85. Pai GP, Ellison RG, Rubin JW, et al: Two decades of experience with modified Heller's myotomy for achalasia. Ann Thorac Surg 38:201–206, 1984.

86. Fonkalsrud E: Discussion. In Vane DW, Cosby K, West K, et al: Late results following esophagomyotomy in children with achalasia. J Pediatr Surg 23:519, 1988.

87. Bolstad DS: The management of strictures of the esophagus. Ann Otolaryngol 75:1019–1028, 1966.

88. Ashcraft KW, Holder TH: The experimental treatment of esophageal strictures by intralesional steroid injections. J Thorac Cardiovasc Surg 58:685–691, 1969.

89. Gandhi RP, Cooper A, Barlow BA: Successful management of esophageal strictures without resection or replacement. J Pediatr Surg 24:745–750, 1989.

90. Holder TH, Ashcraft KW, Leape L: The treatment of patients with esophageal strictures by local steroid injections. J Pediatr Surg 4:646–653, 1969.

91. Zein NN, Greseth JM, Perrault J: Endoscopic intralesional steroid injections in the management of refractory esophageal strictures. Gastrointest Endosc 41:596–598, 1995.

92. Fonkalsrud EW: Initial esophageal dilatation in infants with benign esophageal stricture. Surgery 59:883–885, 1966.

93. Tytgat Guido NJ: Dilation therapy of benign esophageal stenoses. World J Surg 13:142–148, 1989.

94. Shemesh E, Czerniak A: Comparison between Savary-Gilliard and balloon dilatation of benign esophageal strictures. World J Surg 14:518–522, 1990.

95. Hoffer FA, Winter HS, Fellows KE, et al: The treatment of post-operative and peptic esophageal strictures after esophageal atresia repair. Pediatr Radiol 17:454–458, 1987.

96. Golladay ES, Tepas JJ III, Pickard LR, et al: Bacteremia after

esophageal dilation: A clinical and experimental study. Ann Thorac Surg 30:19–23, 1980.

97. Musher DR, Boyd A: Esophagocolonic stricture with proximal fistulae treated by balloon dilation. Am J Gastroenterol 83:445–447, 1988.

98. Little AG, Naunheim KS, Ferguson MK, et al: Surgical management of esophageal strictures. Ann Thorac Surg 45:144–147, 1988.

99. Paulson DL: Benign stricture of the esophagus secondary to gastroesophageal reflux. Ann Surg 165:765–778, 1967.

100. Ohhama U, Tsunoda A, Nishi T, et al: Surgical treatment of reflux stricture of the esophagus. J Pediatr Surg 25:758–761, 1990.

101. Isolauri J, Nordback I, Markkula H: Surgery for reflux stricture of the oesophagus. Ann Chir Gynaecol 78:120–123, 1989.

102. Fonkalsrud EW, Ament ME: Surgical management of esophageal stricture due to recessive dystrophic epidermolysis bullosa. J Pediatr Surg 12:221–226, 1977.

103. Imre J, Kopp M: Arguments against long-term conservative treatment of oesophageal strictures due to corrosive burns. Thorax 27:594–598, 1972.

104. Kiviranta UK: Corrosion carcinoma of the esophagus: 381 cases of corrosion and nine cases of corrosion carcinoma. Acta Otolaryngol (Stockh) 42:89–95, 1952.

105. Alvarez AF, Colbert JG: Lye stricture of the esophagus complicated by carcinoma. Can J Surg 6:470–476, 1963.

106. Bigger IA, Vinson PP: Carcinoma secondary to burn of the esophagus from ingestion of lye. Surgery 28:887–889, 1950.

107. Bigelow NH: Carcinoma of the esophagus developing at the site of lye stricture. Cancer 6:1159–1164, 1953.

108. Appelqvist P, Salmo M: Lye corrosion carcinoma of the esophagus. Cancer 43:2655–2658, 1980.

109. Mansour KA, Hansen HA, Hersh T, et al: Colon interposition for advanced nonmalignant esophageal stricture: Experience with 40 patients. Ann Thorac Surg 32:584–592, 1981.

110. Gross RE, Firestone FN: Colonic reconstruction of the esophagus in infants and children. Surgery 61:955–964, 1967.

111. Belsey R, Clagett OT: Reconstruction of the esophagus with the left colon. J Thorac Cardiovasc Surg 49:33–54, 1965.

112. Kelly JP, Shackelford GD, Roper CL: Esophageal replacement with colon in children: Functional results and long-term growth. Ann Thorac Surg 36:634–644, 1983.

113. Waterston DJ: Replacement of oesophagus with colon in childhood. In Rob C, Smith R (eds): Operative Surgery. Vol. 2 (2nd ed). London, Butterworth, 1968, pp 367–374.

114. German JC, Waterston DJ: Colon interposition for the replacement of the esophagus in children. J Pediatr Surg 11:227–234, 1976.

115. Azar H, Chrispin AR, Waterston DJ: Esophageal replacement with transverse colon in infants and children. J Pediatr Surg 6:3–9, 1971.

116. Ahmad SA, Sylvester KG, Hebra A, et al: Esophageal replacement using the colon: Is it a good choice? J Pediatr Surg 31:1026–1031, 1996.

117. Choi RS, Lillehei CW, Lund DP, et al: Esophageal replacement in children who have caustic pharyngoesophageal strictures. J Pediatr Surg 32: 1083–1088, 1997.

118. Mitchell IM, Goh DW, Roberts KD, et al: Colon interposition in children. Br J Surg 76:681–686, 1989.

119. Wu M, Chiu N, Lin M, et al: Functional evaluation of esophageal substitutes. Chin Med J (Engl) 58:223–229, 1996.

120. Lindahl H, Louhimo I, Virkola K: Colon interposition or gastric tube? Follow-up study of colon-esophagus and gastric tube-esophagus patients. J Pediatr Surg 18:58–63, 1983.

121. Huang MH, Sung CY, Hsu HK, et al: Reconstruction of the esophagus with the left colon. Ann Thorac Surg 48:660–664, 1989.

122. Stone MM, Mahour GH, Weitzman JJ, et al: Esophageal replacement with colon interposition in children. Ann Surg 203:346–351, 1986.

123. West KW, Vane DW, Grosfeld JL: Esophageal replacement in children: Experience with thirty-one cases. Surgery 100:751–757, 1986.

124. Najafi H, Beattie E: Excision of teniae coli for repair of esophagocolic stricture following colon transplant: Case report. Ann Surg 162:1097–1099, 1965.

125. Lynn H: Simple method of elongating a colonic segment for esophageal replacement. J Pediatr Surg 8:391–393, 1973.

126. Belsey R: Discussion. In Kelly JP, Shackelford GD, Roper CL: Esophageal replacement with colon in children: Functional results and long-term growth. Ann Thorac Surg 36:641–642, 1983.

127. Sieber AM, Sieber WK: Colon transplants as esophageal replacement: Cineradiographic and manometric evaluation in children. Ann Surg 168:116–122, 1968.

128. Guzzetta PC, Randolph JG: Antireflux cologastric anastomosis following colonic interposition for esophageal replacement. J Pediatr Surg 21:1137–1138, 1986.

129. Larsson S, Lycke G, Radberg G: Replacement of the esophagus by a segment of colon provided with an antireflux valve. Ann Thorac Surg 48:677–682, 1989.

130. Butterfield WC, Massi J: Gastric reflux in colon interpositions: A method of treatment. J Thorac Cardiovasc Surg 64:229–234, 1972.

131. Raffensperger JG, Luck SR, Reynolds M, et al: Intestinal bypass of the esophagus. J Pediatr Surg 31:38–47, 1996.

132. Touloukian RJ, Tellides G: Retrosternal ileocolic esophageal replacement in children revisited. J Thorac Cardiovasc Surg 107:1067–1972, 1994.

133. Jones EL, Skinner DB, Demeester TR, et al: Response of the interposed human colonic segment to an acid challenge. Ann Surg 177:75–78, 1973.

134. Moreno-Osset E, Tomas-Ridocci M, Paris F, et al: Motor activity of esophageal substitute (stomach, jejunal, and colon segments). Ann Thorac Surg 41:515–519, 1986.

135. Isolauri J: Colonic interposition for benign esophageal disease. Long-term clinical and endoscopic results. Am J Surg 155:498–502, 1988.

136. Neville WE, Najem AZ: Colon replacement of the esophagus for congenital and benign disease. Ann Thorac Surg 36:626–633, 1983.

137. Sutton R, Sutton DM, Ackery DM, et al: Functional assessment of colonic interposition with Tcm-labeled milk. J Pediatr Surg 24:874–881, 1989.

138. Sterling RP, Kuykendall C, Carmichael MJ, et al: Unusual sequelae of colon interposition for esophageal reconstruction: Late obstruction requiring reoperation. Ann Thorac Surg 38:292–295, 1984.

139. Pantelides ML, Fitzgerald MD: Left ventriculo-colic fistula—a late complication of colonic interposition for the oesophagus. Postgrad Med J 64:710–712, 1988.

140. Choh JH, Balderman SC, Bingham D, et al: Parasternal intrapleural colon interposition: An alternative pathway for the colon graft. Ann Thorac Surg 31:474–477, 1981.

141. Bentley JFR: Primary colonic substitution for atresia of the esophagus. Surgery 58:731–736, 1965.

142. Anderson KD, Randolph JG: The gastric tube for esophageal replacement in children. J Thorac Cardiovasc Surg 66:333–342, 1973.

143. Cohen DH, Middleton AW, Fletcher J: Gastric tube esophagoplasty. J Pediatr Surg 9:451–460, 1974.

144. Gavrilu D: The replacement of the oesophagus by a gastric tube. In Jamieson GG (ed): Surgery of the Oesophagus. Edinburgh, Churchill Livingstone, 1988.

145. Pedersen JC, Klein RL, Andrews DA: Gastric tube as the primary procedure for pure esophageal atresia. J Pediatr Surg 31:1233–1235, 1996.

146. Spitz L, Kiely E, Sparnon T: Gastric transposition for esophageal replacement in children. Ann Surg 206:69–73, 1987.

147. Spitz L: Esophageal atresia: Past, present, and future. J Pediatr Surg 31:19–25, 1996.

148. Ravelli AM, Spitz L, Milla PJ: Gastric emptying in children with gastric transposition. J Pediatr Gastroenterol Nutr 19:403–409, 1994.

149. Saeki M, Tsuchida Y, Ogata T, et al: Long-term results of jejunal replacement of the esophagus. J Pediatr Surg 23:483–489, 1988.

150. Coleman JJ, Tan KC, Searles JM, et al: Jejunal free autograft: Analysis of complications and their resolution. Plast Reconstr Surg 84:589–595, 1989.
151. Othersen HB, Parker EF, Smith CD: The surgical management of esophageal stricture in children. Ann Surg 207:590–597, 1988.
152. Kennedy AP, Cameron BH, McGill CW: Colon patch esophagoplasty for caustic esophageal stricture. J Pediatr Surg 30:1242–1245, 1995.
153. Sigalet DL, Lagerge JM, DiLorenzo M, et al: Aortoesophageal fistula: Congenital and acquired causes. J Pediatr Surg 29:1212–1214, 1994.
154. Murdison KA, Andrews BA, Chin AJ: Ultrasonographic display of complex vascular rings. J Am Coll Cardiol 15:1645–1653, 1990.
155. Cherin MM, Pond GD, Bjelland JC, et al: Evaluation of double aortic arch and aortic coarctation by intravenous digital subtraction angiography. J Cardiovasc Surg 28:581–584, 1987.
156. Kastler B, Livolsi A, Germain P, et al: Magnetic resonance imaging in congenital heart disease of newborns: Preliminary results in 23 patients. Eur J Radiol 10:109–117, 1990.
157. van Son JAM, Julsrud PR, Hagler DJ, et al: Imaging strategies for vascular rings. Soc Thorac Surgeons 57:604–610, 1994.
158. Backer CL, Ilbawi MN, Idriss FS, et al: Vascular anomalies causing tracheoesophageal compression: Review of experience in children. J Thorac Cardiovasc Surg 97:725–731, 1989.
159. Roberts CS, Othersen HB, Sade RM, et al: Tracheoesophageal compression from aortic arch anomalies: Analysis of 30 operatively treated children. J Pediatr Surg 29:334–338, 1994.
160. Burke RP, Rosenfield HM, Wernovsky G, et al: Video-assisted thoracoscopic ring division in infants and children. J Am Coll Cardiol 25:943–947, 1995.

27

ESOPHAGEAL ATRESIA AND TRACHEOESOPHAGEAL MALFORMATIONS

Howard C. Filston, MD • Nicholas A. Shorter, MD

The surgical solution to the problem of esophageal atresia (EA) has been referred to as "the epitome of modern surgery."[1] Certainly, its evolution is an example of how incremental steps, surgical ingenuity, and sheer persistence can eventually lead to remarkable success.[2, 3] A congenital abnormality incompatible with life that was once referred to as "hopeless from the beginning" and not "of much practical importance to the surgeon" is now successfully repaired all over the world.[3] The progression from 100% mortality when it was first recognized to present overall survival rates well over 90% is a remarkable accomplishment.

☐ History

Thomas Gibson, in his 1697 book *Anatomy of Humane Bodies Epitomized*, was the first to describe the classic form of the anomaly, an infant with proximal EA and distal tracheoesophageal fistula (TEF).[2–4] No further cases were reported in the English language until the first half of the 19th century, although several were collected and reported in German.[2, 5]

The description of an infant's symptoms given in 1839 by an American physician, Thomas Hill, mirrors the earlier one by Gibson: "The infant had been noted to salivate excessively since birth, and with each feeding it would cough, become cyanotic, and regurgitate all its food."[6] Hill's report is notable also in that the infant had an imperforate anus, the first reported instance of what is now a well-known association.

Timothy Holmes, in 1869, was the first to suggest the possibility of operative treatment, but he rejected it, saying, "in any case the attempt ought not, I think, be made."[2, 3] Charles Steele, a London

surgeon, in 1888 became the first to operate on a patient with EA but without TEF.[7] Transabdominal exploration with gastrotomy was performed in the hope that only a membranous obstruction was present, which could then be perforated. This not being the case, the wounds were closed, and the child was allowed to die.

Over the next 40 years, further reports of EA, with and without fistula, continued to appear in the literature, and several infants underwent gastrostomy or jejunostomy without altering the uniformly fatal outcome. Comments by Joseph Brennemann summarize a few reported gastrostomy failures in the early part of the 20th century: "While the utter hopelessness of these cases, if untreated, justifies surgical procedures that would otherwise seem too daring; nevertheless, the physician who, after making his diagnosis of congenital atresia of the esophagus, decides to let his little patient die undisturbed, can amply justify his course."[8] On the other hand, "in these otherwise hopeless cases, however, one gives the surgeon a full range with a clear conscience."[9]

Slowly, surgeons were coming to understand the anatomy of the anomaly and were defining the necessary components of successful surgical management: control of the blind upper esophageal segment to prevent aspiration of saliva, division of the fistula to prevent regurgitation of gastric contents, provision of a route for nourishment, and potential establishment of esophageal continuity. Harry Richter was an early leading advocate of surgical intervention who unsuccessfully performed transpleural ligation of the fistula and feeding gastrostomy in two infants. In 1913 he wrote, "Direct anastomosis of the ends, with closure of the trachea, in an infant less than 1 week old is certainly a hazardous procedure. I am not certain, however, that it may not prove possible, and, if so, would be the ideal operation."[10]

The isolated "H-type" fistula was first described by Lamb in 1873[3] but was first repaired by Charles Imperatori in 1938, using a transtracheal approach.[11] The first known survivor with pure EA was born in 1935.[2, 3] A gastrostomy was performed in the newborn period by James Donovan, and esophageal continuity was eventually achieved when the patient reached age 16 by George Humphries II, using a jejunal interposition.

In 1939, both William Ladd in Boston and N. Logan Leven in St. Paul successfully managed infants with EA and a distal fistula using initial gastrostomy, followed by ligation of the fistula, cervical esophagostomy, and later esophageal substitution.[12, 13]

Thomas Lanman pioneered the use of primary anastomosis, performing the first of his five unsuccessful primary repairs in 1936. Although none of the operative patients lived from his total series of 30 treated by a variety of techniques, Lanman developed and evaluated the technique of primary anastomosis to a point where eventual success was inevitable.[14] In 1941, Cameron Haight, at the University of Michigan, achieved the first successful primary repair, using an extrapleural approach.[15] Haight had tried unsuccessfully to do the same repair in 10 children before this landmark event. An anastomotic leak occurred, but it eventually sealed. A gastrostomy was necessary. The child developed a stricture, which responded to dilation, and, after a 20-month hospitalization, eventually did well.

Haight's success was soon followed by others, both in the United States and elsewhere. Survival figures slowly improved thereafter, reaching about two of three patients in the late 1960s.[2] Today, almost 100% of infants with this once hopeless esophageal anomaly who do not have associated fatal malformations can be expected to survive and to lead nearly normal lives. It is a remarkable success story.

□ Embryology

The embryology of these anomalies is still poorly understood. It has not been possible to satisfactorily explain all the different varieties of EA/TEF malformations based on a single unifying mechanism. The uniformity of each variety, for example EA with distal TEF, suggests that the same single, definable, developmental error is responsible in each case. It is less clear whether EA and distal TEF and the other common varieties are just variations on one embryologic theme or the result of completely different ones.

The airway and the esophagus have a common progenitor. Organogenesis involves two major processes, separation and elongation, and disorders of either can potentially give rise to tracheoesophageal abnormalities.[16]

In the human embryo, at about the 19th day of gestation, the foregut exists as a tube extending from the pharynx to what will become the stomach. The ventral aspect of the foregut is destined to become the airway. Just distal to the developing pharyngeal pouches and just proximal to the developing saccular stomach a median ventral diverticulum appears at about 22 or 23 days after fertilization (3-mm embryo), eventually forming a groove in the ventral aspect of the foregut that represents the developing trachea. Elongation of the airway and esophagus occurs at the same time fusion of longitudinal ridges in the lateral walls creates a separate tubular structure of each. This process of separation begins caudally and proceeds in a cephalad direction while elongation of the trachea and esophagus occurs. Separation is complete in the normal embryo by day 36. Whatever the embryologic event that results in these abnormalities, it would be expected to occur before that time.

A number of theories have been put forth to explain the embryogenesis of EA/TEF malformations. Disturbance in the fusion process that divides the anterior trachea from the posterior esophagus has been espoused by some[17–20] and rejected by others.[21] Deficiency in cell division and mesenchymal induction has been postulated.[20, 22] There is little evidence to support or refute vascular insufficiency as a factor.[23]

Theories of external pressure by the developing heart, by aberrant vessels, or by the pneumoenteric processes were once popular but are now discounted.[20] Hyperflexion of the embryo with a resulting disturbance in foregut development has been disproved experimentally.[24]

□ Incidence and Etiology

EA occurs in between 1 in 3000 and 1 in 4500 live births.[1, 17, 25] There appears to be a slight male predominance, although this is not a universal finding and may not be true for all the varieties.[25–27]

The etiology of the disturbed embryogenesis is unknown. EA/TEF malformations have not been found to occur spontaneously in other mammals.[18] The well-known, nonrandom association with vertebral, anal, cardiac, renal, and limb abnormalities suggests a generalized disturbance in embryogenesis. It is likely that any of a number of different external insults to the fetus, if they occur during the critical period of organogenesis, can result in these abnormalities. The etiology of tracheoesophageal anomalies that occur in an otherwise normal baby may differ from that of patients in whom multiple other defects are also present.[28] Familial cases have been reported but are rare.[27]

The incidence of twinning, both monozygotic and dizygotic, appears to be higher in families with EA/TEF children than in the general population.[4, 27, 29] Monozygous twins have both been affected but, more commonly, only one has had EA/TEF, suggesting that developmental events are more important than genetic factors.

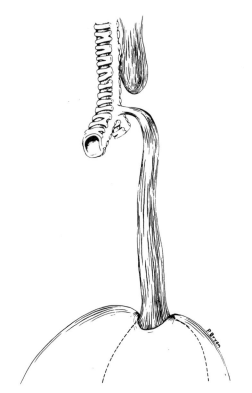

Figure 27–1. Esophageal atresia with distal tracheoesophageal fistula.

Cyclic variation of incidence, without a seasonal pattern, has been observed in one study, suggesting a possible infectious agent.[28] EA is a rare but recognized effect of thalidomide.[25] An association with the use of progesterone alone or progesterone with estrogen has been reported.[30] Esophageal defects without tracheal fistulas have been seen in the offspring of riboflavin-deficient mice,[31] and one case of TEF has been identified in the offspring of vitamin A–deficient mother rats.[32] An experimental model has recently been developed in rats using doxorubicin (Adriamycin) exposure, but the relevance of this to the etiology of such abnormalities in humans is unclear.[33] Several chromosomal deletions and duplications are associated with these anomalies, usually trisomy 18 or 21.[34]

☐ Anatomy and Classification

The first classification system for esophageal anomalies was developed by Vogt in 1929.[35] Subsequently, similar schemes were presented by Ladd,[12] Gross,[36] and others. The most detailed and exhaustive classification system is that of Kluth, which contains 10 main types of tracheoesophageal abnormalities, each with numerous subtypes, many of which are represented in the literature by only a single case.[5]

ESOPHAGEAL ATRESIA WITH DISTAL TRACHEOESOPHAGEAL FISTULA

For practical purposes, there are five major anatomic types of esophageal anomalies (a sixth, laryn-

gotracheoesophageal [LTE] cleft, is discussed later in this chapter). By far the most common form is EA with distal TEF (Fig. 27–1). This is seen in about 85% of cases.

The proximal esophagus, which is dilated and thickened, usually ends at about the level of the third thoracic vertebra. There may be a partial common wall between its anterior aspect and the posterior wall of the adjacent trachea. The blood supply to the upper pouch is excellent and comes from the thyrocervical trunk on both sides. The fistula, which is the proximal end of the much narrower distal esophageal segment, enters the membranous back wall of the lower trachea, sometimes as low as the carina. An obliterated "ligamentous remnant" of an occluded distal TEF has been recorded as a rare variant.[37] There is usually a gap between the two esophageal ends, which sometimes is wide enough to make the repair difficult. On occasion, the two ends overlap and may even have some degree of muscular continuity. The blood supply to the lower esophagus is segmental.

ISOLATED ESOPHAGEAL ATRESIA WITHOUT TRACHEOESOPHAGEAL FISTULA

Isolated EA without TEF occurs in about 3 to 5% of cases (Fig. 27–2). The position and character of the proximal esophageal pouch is similar to that in

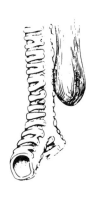

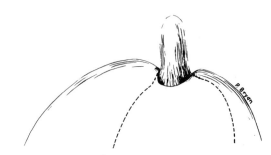

Figure 27–2. Pure esophageal atresia (without a tracheoesophageal fistula).

EA with distal TEF, but the distal pouch is usually very short. Therefore, a long gap almost always exists between the two ends, making initial primary anastomosis impossible.

ISOLATED TRACHEOESOPHAGEAL FISTULA WITHOUT ATRESIA

Three to 6% of patients have an isolated TEF without atresia (Fig. 27–3). Usually referred to as *H-type fistulas,* they are more accurately described as N-type because the tracheal end of the fistula is more cephalad than the esophageal end. These fistulas are very short and usually measure 2 to 4 mm in diameter. They are usually found at or just above the level of the thoracic inlet; therefore, most can be approached through a cervical incision. The vast majority are single, but double and triple ones have been reported.[5]

ESOPHAGEAL ATRESIA WITH PROXIMAL FISTULA

EA with proximal fistula is seen in about 2% of affected infants (Fig. 27–4). As with pure EA, the distal segment is usually short, and a long gap exists. The fistula is short and narrow, arising from the anterior wall of the upper pouch a short distance from its tip and entering directly into the trachea.

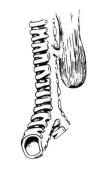

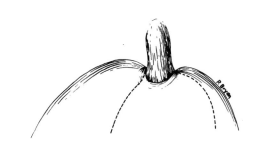

Figure 27–4. Esophageal atresia with proximal tracheoesophageal fistula.

ESOPHAGEAL ATRESIA WITH FISTULAS TO THE UPPER AND LOWER ESOPHAGEAL SEGMENTS

EA with fistulas to the upper and lower esophageal segments occurs in 3 to 5% of cases (Fig. 27–5). Increased awareness and improved diagnostic techniques have resulted in increased early recognition of proximal fistulas when they are present. The anatomy of this variant is essentially identical to that of the most common type, with the simple addition of a short, narrow fistula from the anterior aspect of the proximal pouch to the adjacent membranous trachea. A long gap is unusual.

In both types with a proximal fistula, there is usually some element of a common wall between the trachea and the esophagus in and around the site of the fistulas. These fistulas are usually identified during operative mobilization of the upper pouch or at the time of bronchoscopic evaluation prior to repair.

☐ Associated Anomalies

Associated anomalies are frequent, occurring in more than 50% of patients.[17, 25, 38–40] They are most common with pure EA and least often seen in patients with an isolated TEF.[38] Thirty to 40% of affected infants weigh less than 2500 g.[25, 41] Smaller infants have more associated anomalies than larger ones.[40] Currently, the associated anomalies usually

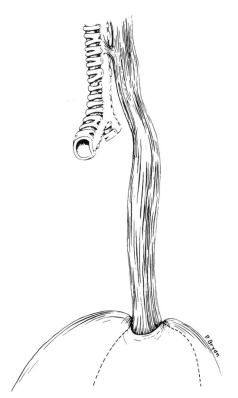

Figure 27–3. H-type tracheoesophageal fistula.

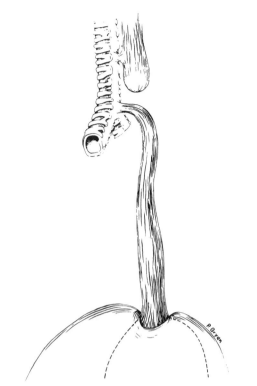

Figure 27–5. Esophageal atresia with proximal and distal tracheoesophageal fistulas.

determine survival, and their presence may alter the treatment approach.

The most frequent abnormalities are musculoskeletal, cardiovascular, gastrointestinal, and genitourinary. These can occur individually or as part of a now well-defined, nonrandom association of abnormalities known as the *VATER* (vertebral and vascular, *a*nal, *t*racheal, *e*sophageal, *r*adial, and renal) association or the *VACTERL* (vertebral, *a*nal, *c*ardiac, *t*racheal, *e*sophageal, *r*enal, and *l*imb) association.[42] Simultaneous occurrence of these other deformities is so common that all of them should be suspected in any infant with an EA/TEF abnormality.

Esophageal abnormalities can also be seen in the *CHARGE* (*c*olobomata, *h*eart disease, choanal *a*tresia, mental *r*etardation, *g*enital hypoplasia, and *e*ar anomalies with deafness) association, and have been reported in association with a number of other rare syndromes.[27] One series of 61 patients with the CHARGE association reported 10 infants with EA and TEF. All had major cardiac anomalies, mainly tetralogy of Fallot. Seven of the 10 patients had major skeletal abnormalities, most had complicated postoperative courses, and 7 of the 10 died.[43]

Rib anomalies are quite common, and they are usually associated with vertebral abnormalities. The presence of 13 pairs of ribs is a predictor of a long-gap EA.[44] Duodenal atresia, intestinal malrotation, hydrocephalus, and choanal atresia are anomalies that frequently occur with EA/TEF. There may be aortic arch and great vessel anomalies, especially with long-gap atresia.[45] There appears to be an in-

creased incidence of pyloric stenosis, which may relate to gastrostomy tube placement or may be due, in some way, to the abnormal foregut innervation that exists in these infants.[46, 47]

Tracheomalacia and disordered esophageal motility are virtually universal, although of varying clinical significance, and should not be considered as separate abnormalities.[48] Other esophageal abnormalities, such as congenital stricture due to a cartilaginous ring, have been reported.[49, 50] A recent series of 32 patients with EA reported 15 patients with anomalies of the tracheobronchial tree, including ectopic right upper lobe bronchus in 12, congenital tracheal stenosis in 4, and absent right upper lobe bronchus in 2.[51] Pulmonary agenesis or cystic adenomatoid malformation may be associated with EA/TEF.[52] The occurrence of EA and TEF with congenital diaphragmatic hernia has been reported, usually with a fatal outcome.[53]

☐ Pathophysiology

EA is incompatible with life because the infant cannot eat. If a distal TEF is present, gastric secretions gain access to the respiratory tract, leading to pneumonitis, progressive respiratory failure, and death.

The infant's respiratory status may be compromised by tracheomalacia.[54–56] In utero external pressure on the trachea from the fluid-filled, proximal esophageal pouch and decreased intraluminal pressure within the trachea due to loss of intratracheal amniotic fluid through a distal TEF have been implicated in the formation of airway malacia,[57] but it more likely represents an additional component of a generalized malformation of the trachea and esophagus.[48] There is often an absolute deficiency of tracheal cartilage and an increase in the length of the transverse muscle in the posterior tracheal wall.[58] Significant tracheomalacia has not been noted in patients with pure EA.[59]

Disordered esophageal motility is universal in patients with EA/TEF anomalies, even those with only an isolated fistula.[56, 60] Abnormal motility may partly be due to the atresia, which prevents normal propagation of esophageal muscle electrical activity, and it may, perhaps, be due to vagal nerve damage or segmental esophageal denervation during surgical mobilization.[61] However, it is mainly a consequence of abnormal development and innervation of the entire esophagus.[46, 47] Tracheal innervation abnormalities also exist in the presence of EA/TEF.[62]

☐ Symptoms and Diagnosis

The diagnosis of EA is usually not difficult. Infants with this disorder are unable to swallow their saliva and are often noted shortly after birth to have "excessive secretions," requiring suctioning. Aspiration events, either from the upper pouch or through the distal fistula may result in cough, tachypnea, and hypoxia. On occasion, this may be severe enough to require intubation and ventilation. If the infant is fed there is immediate regurgitation, usually accompanied by choking and coughing, sometimes with cyanosis.

When the suspicion of EA/TEF is raised, esophageal continuity may be demonstrated by passage of a 10 or 12 French orogastric tube. Successful passage into the stomach effectively rules out the diagnosis, although rare cases have been seen where the tube has gained access to the distal esophagus and stomach by passing by way of the trachea through the distal TEF. Radiologic confirmation of the tube's position may be desirable. If the tube does not pass beyond 9 to 13 cm from the alveolar ridge, a radiograph that includes the neck, chest, and abdomen demonstrates the atresia (Fig. 27–6). Air in the abdomen confirms the presence of a distal TEF. An abdominal "double bubble" indicates coexisting duodenal atresia. A gasless abdomen is evidence of pure atresia (Fig. 27–7), although cases are reported in which a distal TEF is present but temporarily or permanently occluded. The presence or absence of a proximal fistula is determined at the time of repair, either bronchoscopically or during mobilization of the proximal esophageal pouch.

A contrast study of the upper esophagus is rarely

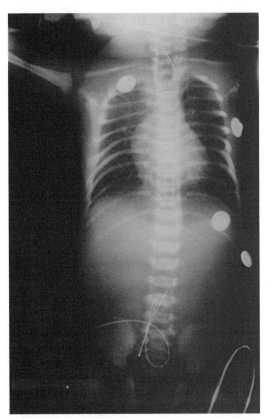

Figure 27–7. Pure esophageal atresia. There is absence of any air in the stomach or bowel. This radiographic picture is also seen in infants with esophageal atresia and a proximal tracheoesophageal fistula and in infants with a distal fistula that is plugged with mucus or is "ligamentous."

necessary. Sometimes the air-filled upper pouch is visible on plain radiographs, most easily seen on a lateral film. If a contrast study is deemed necessary, 0.5 ml of dilute barium should be instilled through the tube with the infant in an upright position. The contrast is then removed with suction. Contrast in the trachea indicates either "spill-over" aspiration or the presence of a proximal fistula or cleft.

Pharyngeal perforation by an orogastric or nasogastric tube may give the impression of esophageal obstruction.[63] A contrast study may give the impression that the esophagus is atretic, but careful examination shows that the tube does not lie in the characteristic position for EA. Usually, tube removal and antibiotics are the only therapy necessary.

Once the diagnosis of EA is confirmed, a search should be made for other components of the VACTERL association that may be present. Some are readily apparent on physical examination. Radiographs of the chest and abdomen demonstrate vertebral or rib anomalies and the contour of the heart, which may be suggestive of congenital heart disease. Additional studies should include an echocardiogram and renal ultrasonography (US). Voiding cystourethrography is usually performed at a later date.

Some cases of EA are diagnosed prenatally by US. Polyhydramnios should raise suspicion. The US finding of a small or absent stomach bubble in-

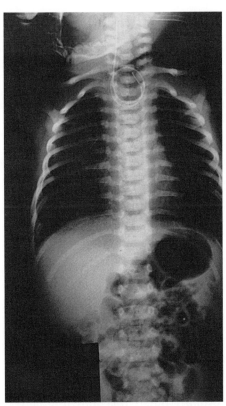

Figure 27–6. Infant with esophageal atresia and a distal tracheoesophageal fistula. The feeding tube is coiled in the upper pouch and air is present in the stomach and throughout the bowel. A fistula to the proximal esophagus might also be present, although in this case it was not.

creases the diagnostic possibility of atresia, but the positive predictive value of this combination of findings is only about 40% (56% if the stomach bubble is completely absent).[64] Amniotic fluid passes into the stomach in the presence of a distal TEF; therefore, a normal stomach bubble may be present. Even in the absence of a fistula, the stomach may be distended with gastric secretions. It is, therefore, not surprising that EA/TEF may be missed by US. Isolated EA is more likely to be detected on prenatal US. The sensitivity of the study is also about 40%.[64] Evidence indicates that those patients diagnosed prenatally have a much poorer prognosis when compared with those in whom the prenatal US is nondiagnostic.[64] Many infants diagnosed prenatally turn out to have trisomy 18.

Although recognition of an H-type fistula in infancy is now much more common than it once was, the diagnosis often is delayed. There may be choking or coughing episodes associated with feeding, but there is no impediment to the passage of a tube into the stomach. Some patients present with a history of recurrent pneumonia. Rarely, an infant on positive-pressure ventilation is noted to develop recurrent gastric overdistention as air passes by way of the fistula into the gastrointestinal tract. The diagnosis can often be made on a routine barium swallow (Fig. 27–8) or by performing a prone video esophagram with selective catheter injections along the anterior wall of the esophagus.[65]

However, a negative contrast study, or even sev-

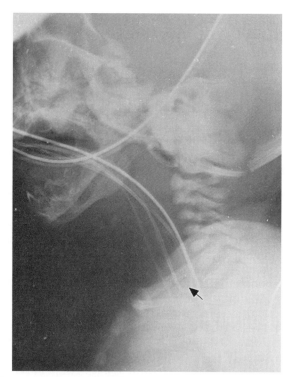

Figure 27–9. A patient with an H-type tracheoesophageal fistula. The fistula has been cannulated bronchoscopically before repair. The catheter has been retrieved esophagoscopically back out the esophagus. The *arrow* indicates the catheter in the fistula.

eral, does not exclude the presence of a fistula. If suspicion is high, rigid bronchoscopy should be performed, which has close to 100% accuracy.[66, 67] After visualization of the tracheal opening, the fistula is cannulated using a ureteral catheter, and a lateral radiograph shows the level of the fistula (Fig. 27–9). Division of the TEF should be done under the same anesthetic.

☐ Preoperative Management and Clinical Approach

ESOPHAGEAL ATRESIA WITH DISTAL TEF

Once the diagnosis has been confirmed and associated anomalies identified, a decision must be made as to whether or not the infant is a candidate for primary repair. A risk classification scheme relevant to infants with EA/TEF malformations was developed by Waterston and associates in 1962.[68] This prognostic classification took into account prematurity and other associated anomalies. It was relevant at the time it was developed, but owing to multiple factors that have changed over the ensuing decades, it has become less relevant today.

Once primary repair was shown to be possible, it soon became apparent that the presence of other abnormalities, the birth weight of the baby, and the presence of pneumonitis played significant roles in determining survival. Outcome analysis suggested

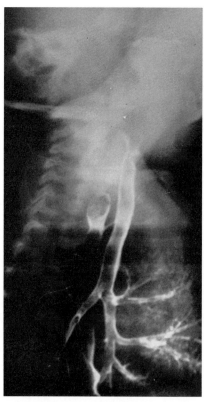

Figure 27–8. An H-type (or, more anatomically, an N-type) tracheoesophageal fistula demonstrated on barium swallow.

that immediate primary repair was not always the correct approach[68]:

Group A: Birth weight greater than 5½ lb (2500 g) and well

Group B: Birth weight 4 to 5½ lb (1800 to 2500 g) and well

Higher birth weight but moderate pneumonia or mild to moderate congenital anomaly

Group C: Birth weight less than 4 lb (1800 g)

Higher birth weight but severe pneumonia or severe congenital anomaly

Survival, in 1962, for group A patients was 95%, for group B patients was 68%, and for group C patients was 6%. For many years this system was useful in planning surgical management: group A babies usually underwent early primary repair and group B babies a delayed one, whereas group C infants were often managed with some form of staged approach. Over the years, however, refinements in surgical technique, anesthetic management, and neonatal care have improved the survival of groups B and C to the point that the current survival figures are A, 99%; B, 95%; and C, 71%.[69] Improvement in overall care has also resulted in a larger population of group C babies in more recent surgical series.[70, 71]

There is still a need, however, to identify high-risk infants based on prognostic variables and to adjust the treatment plan accordingly. Some have done this based purely on overall physiologic status.[72] When specific factors are analyzed, there is some debate about which currently have prognostic significance.

A recent study identified low birth weight (now defined as 1500 g) and the presence of major cardiac anomalies as two factors that had the greatest influence on survival. The following classification system based on these factors also results in three groups:

Group I: Birth weight greater than or equal to 1500 g *without* major cardiac disease

Group II: Birth weight less than 1500 g *or* major cardiac disease

Group III: Birth weight less than 1500 g *and* major cardiac disease[69]

Using these criteria, the survival rate for group I was 97%; for group II, 59%; and for group III, 22%. A 1997 report from Japan has confirmed the prognostic value of this system.[73] However, another study from Montreal identified only severe pulmonary dysfunction with preoperative ventilator dependence and severe associated anomalies as having prognostic value.[74] A comparison of this latter classification to that of Waterston confirmed the superior prognostic value of the Montreal classification.[75]

The physiologic state of the infant, rather than size, maturity, or the mere presence of associated anomalies, is the determining factor in treatment decisions. Infants with the more benign components of the VACTERL association tolerate primary repair. Premature infants who do not have severe respiratory distress syndrome (RDS) may undergo primary repair. On the other hand, a significant cyanotic heart anomaly with impending congestive heart failure is a major comorbid factor.

There is general agreement that a healthy near-term or full-term infant with a stable cardiovascular system and no significant pulmonary disease benefits from early division of the TEF and primary anastomosis of the esophagus. A gastrostomy is not necessary in these circumstances, but there are pediatric surgeons who favor a gastrostomy for all patients. We have found the following criteria to be useful in making the decision for primary repair:

1. Clear lungs to auscultation
2. Clear lungs by chest radiograph
3. No undefined cardiac abnormalities
4. An arterial PaO_2 of greater than 60 mm Hg in room air

Adhering to these criteria, we had no operative or early postoperative mortality and few major respiratory complications in a series of 20 patients undergoing primary repair.[76] Death occurred only in the group of patients who failed to achieve a room air PaO_2 of 60 mm Hg. Early primary repair removes the threat of aspiration pneumonia and should be the goal for each infant. As long as the TEF remains patent, the risk of reflux of gastric contents with spillage into the tracheobronchial tree is high, even when a decompression gastrostomy has been performed. In addition, secretions are difficult for the infant to clear because coughing is ineffective in the presence of a distal TEF. An unoccluded distal TEF may produce severe difficulties in ventilating the infant in the presence of reduced pulmonary compliance. Preferential passage of ventilator gases through the TEF into the stomach results in ineffectual ventilation and may lead to gastric rupture.[77]

For those infants who have cardiac disease, RDS, or severe aspiration pneumonia that would significantly increase operative risk, other approaches must be taken.[78–83] The postoperative course is much smoother and less complicated when the respiratory problems have been resolved prior to the definitive repair.

The distal TEF must be controlled to allow ventilation and to prevent further pulmonary soilage. We have advocated decompression gastrostomy under intubated general anesthesia and placement of a Fogarty balloon catheter into the fistula either translaryngeally or alongside the gastrostomy.[76, 84, 85] Fluoroscopy greatly aids transgastric placement.[77, 86] Others have proceeded with primary repair, believing that the cardiorespiratory problems can be managed postoperatively.[79, 80, 83] The staged approach of initial gastrostomy and thoracotomy with division of the fistula but delay of esophageal anastomosis has been successful for some, but it subjects the infant to two thoracotomies[80–82]; balloon occlusion has obviated the need for this, in our experience (Fig. 27–10). Placement of a gastrostomy may induce gastroesophageal reflux (GER), producing apnea, bradycardia, and aspiration pneumonia. Nevertheless, some infants, including very tiny premature infants, have

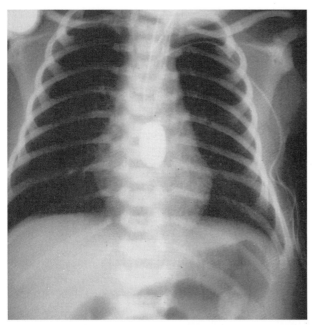

Figure 27–10. Chest radiograph showing an infant with esophageal atresia with distal tracheoesophageal fistula and a Fogarty balloon inflated in the proximal segment of the distal esophagus just beyond the tracheoesophageal fistula.

been successfully managed with initial gastrostomy, a varying period for improvement of respiratory function, and delayed primary repair.[38, 78] The definitive repair may be delayed until the infant satisfies the physiologic criteria outlined earlier, even if that involves palliative cardiac intervention.

It has been our practice to perform a bronchoscopy on all of our patients.[76] Bronchoscopy aids in defining the anatomy. Until absence of the TEF is confirmed by bronchoscopy, it should be presumed to be present. On two occasions, in our experience, when initial radiographic evaluation demonstrated a gasless abdomen suggestive of isolated EA, a mucus plug was found to be occluding the distal fistula. To have delayed repair and started gastrostomy feeding in these cases could have resulted in serious complications. Others have confirmed the observation that all distal fistulas are not readily apparent on the initial radiograph.[87, 88] In a series of 333 EA patients, 34 patients with a gasless abdomen were recorded; 25 of the 34 had EA without TEF, 4 had EA with proximal TEF, and 5 had a blocked or obliterated distal TEF.[88]

When EA with distal TEF has been confirmed, it is important to judge the gap between the proximal and the distal segments. The widest gaps are in those patients whose TEF enters the trachea at the carina. A correlation between the extent of the preoperative gap and the severity of postoperative complications has been suggested.[89] When a carinal-level TEF is confirmed at bronchoscopy, it is wise to estimate the mobility of the proximal pouch before proceeding with thoracotomy. Downward pressure of the bronchoscope in the proximal pouch using radiographic or fluoroscopic imaging facilitates the

decision as to the "bridgeability" of the gap.[90] The only gap too great to bridge, in our experience, was an infant with a carinal-level TEF, although we have had several other patients with the same anatomy who were repaired without difficulty.

If the gap seems significant, strong consideration should be given to managing these infants by delayed anastomosis, as in the patient with isolated EA. Because it usually takes at least 2 to 3 months for the proximal pouch to elongate sufficiently, initial thoracotomy with division of the TEF is probably the best approach. The proximal pouch should be left undisturbed to avoid scarring that might impede migration. We have not attempted jejunostomy feedings and transgastric balloon occlusion of the distal esophagus in such a patient, but our experience with balloon occlusion for up to 3 weeks in patients with pulmonary dysfunction suggests that it is worthy of consideration.

Occasionally, bronchoscopy reveals that the TEF enters the trachea in the region of the thoracic inlet. Repair through a cervical approach has been described for such lesions.[91, 92]

It is best to maintain spontaneous respiration until intubation is successfully completed. The surgeon may have to move quickly to bronchoscope the infant and occlude the TEF if pulmonary compliance is severely restricted.[76, 84] Rapid placement of the gastrostomy tube may avoid gastric perforation but may not resolve the problem of the inability to ventilate the infant as long as the TEF remains widely patent. Although balloon occlusion has been described both from bronchoscopic and transgastric approaches,[77, 84–86] the bronchoscopic approach provides more rapid occlusion of the TEF when compliance is severely restricted (Fig. 27–11).[84]

If balloon occlusion of the TEF is selected, it can be safely maintained for days or weeks while pulmonary deficiencies are resolved or the cardiac or neurologic anomalies are evaluated and stabilized. The nurses must be aware of the "anatomy" of the balloon catheter and its relation to the anatomy of the infant. The most significant potential complication of the balloon catheter occlusion technique is migration of the balloon catheter into the trachea with occlusion of the airway. The infant's nurses must be instructed to deflate the balloon immediately should ventilatory difficulty occur. Daily deflation of the balloon, as advocated by some, has not proved to be necessary in our patients, as long as the balloon is in the proximal segment of the distal esophagus and not directly in the fistula itself.[77, 86] No instances of injury to the esophagus by the balloon have been recognized in the 12 patients in whom we have used this technique.

Defining the anatomy of the aortic arch remains a difficult problem. The infant with a right-sided descending aorta presents the surgeon with a dilemma because the aorta will obstruct access to the esophagus from the usual right thoracotomy.[93] Plain chest radiographs and cardiac sonography have been used to define the anatomy, but neither is

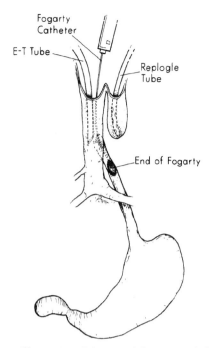

Figure 27–11. Illustration of the use of the Fogarty balloon cathe-ter to occlude the tracheoesophageal fistula. The catheter passes through the larynx alongside the endotracheal (E-T) tube, down the trachea, and through the tracheoesophageal fistula and is positioned in the proximal part of the distal esophagus. (From Filston HC, Chitwood WR Jr, Schkolne B, et al: The Fogarty balloon catheter as an aid to management of the infant with esophageal atresia and tracheoesophageal fistula complicated by severe RDS or pneumonia. J Pediatr Surg 17:149–151, 1982.)

100% dependable. If there is strong suspicion that a right arch may be present, computed tomography or magnetic resonance imaging may be necessary for accurate definition.

ISOLATED ESOPHAGEAL ATRESIA

Isolated EA is a variant that is suspected when there is a "gasless abdomen" on the plain radio-graph. However, the possibility of an occluded fis-tula should be considered. Both occlusion by mucus and complete anatomic occlusion have been de-scribed.[37, 87, 88] Bronchoscopy at the time of gastros-tomy is essential for all patients thought to have EA without distal TEF. Finding an occluded distal fis-tula usually dictates primary repair. A proximal fis-tula can also be identified by this procedure.[76, 94, 95] In a series of 170 EA/TEF patients, 13 (7.7%) had a proximal TEF, 4 of whom had only a proximal fis-tula and 9 had both proximal and distal fistulas.[94]

Management of the infant with isolated EA or with only a proximal TEF requires a quite different approach. Although at one time the wide gap was thought to require an interposition of an enteric segment, such as colon or a gastric tube, in recent years, most surgeons prefer to preserve and repair the native esophagus. Based on observations dating to the early 1960s,[87] the infant is treated with a gastrostomy through which enteral feedings may be

safely provided in the absence of a distal TEF. Be-cause amniotic fluid cannot reach the stomach through the trachea in the absence of the distal TEF, some infants with EA without distal TEF have microgastria.[96] This may make gastrostomy difficult and subsequent fundoplication impossible.

The sump tube is maintained in the proximal pouch, and with time the proximal blind-ending segment elongates into the mediastinum; 6 to 12 weeks are usually required for the migration to reach a level such that the anastomosis is possi-ble.[97–99] Some have advocated assisting the process by manual stretching of the upper pouch with bou-gies,[100–103] but this is usually unnecessary and may lead to perforation. After the gastrostomy has healed sufficiently, weekly soundings with common duct dilators, bougies, or other radiopaque devices dem-onstrate that progress is continuing and determine when repair can proceed with the expectation of successful anastomosis.[104] It is best to achieve actual overlap of the two segments at fluoroscopic evalua-tion before proceeding with repair (Fig. 27–12). Nu-merous series attest to the success of this ap-proach.[97–99, 105]

The rare fistula to the proximal pouch may tether that pouch and prevent its descent into the medias-tinum. For these infants, as well as those without a proximal fistula who fail to achieve adequate elon-gation, various maneuvers at the time of operation have been described. Circular myotomy has been the most successful maneuver; as many as three have been done in one patient.[103, 106–109] Each myot-omy adds up to a centimeter of length for the proxi-mal pouch. A significant incidence of diverticulum formation mitigates against its routine use.[110, 111] Tu-bularizing a flap of the distal aspect of the widened proximal segment may bridge an otherwise exces-

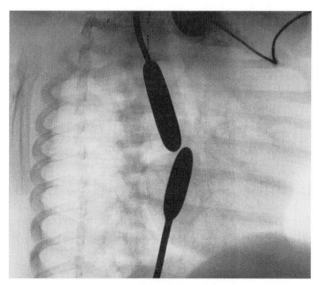

Figure 27–12. Esophageal atresia without tracheoesophageal fis-tula. Common duct dilators are used to define progressive reduc-tion in the length of the "gap." (From Filston HC, Merton DF, Kirks DR: Initial care of esophageal atresia to facilitate potential primary anastomosis. South Med J 74:1530–1533, 1981.)

sive gap.[112–114] Another maneuver involves suture approximation of the unopened ends of the proximal and distal esophageal segments with a single heavy suture that intentionally enters the lumen of each segment. The resultant esophagoesophageal fistula or stricture is dilated until a satisfactory lumen is established.[115]

If, after making every reasonable effort to achieve primary anastomosis of the native esophagus, the gap proves to be insurmountable, the distal esophagus should be closed and the proximal esophagus exteriorized in the neck as a cervical esophagostomy or "spit fistula." This is generally performed on the left side to facilitate a subsequent reconstruction with a colon segment or a gastric tube formed from the greater curvature of the stomach. Care must be taken to avoid injury to the recurrent laryngeal nerve. The details of the interposition and reconstruction procedures can be found in Chapter 26.

ISOLATED TRACHEOESOPHAGEAL FISTULA

Although increased awareness of isolated TEF has resulted in earlier diagnosis in many cases, some infants still have significant aspiration pneumonia when first diagnosed and benefit from a period of nutritional support and respiratory therapy. Placement of a gastrostomy or an orogastric tube for constant drip feedings while respiratory therapy and antibiotics are directed toward resolving the aspiration pneumonia may make the infant a better operative risk. Various endoscopic approaches have been tried to occlude the TEF including the use of Nd:YAG laser.[116] Information on these innovations is generally anecdotal, but two of three treated with the laser were reported as successful.

☐ Operative Approach

Prophylactic antibiotics are given perioperatively, and blood and fresh frozen plasma are available.

REPAIR OF ESOPHAGEAL ATRESIA WITH DISTAL TRANSESOPHAGEAL FISTULA

Once the infant meets the surgeon's criteria for safe repair, the operation should commence without undue delay to avoid aspiration and a worsening of the infant's condition. Dependable peripheral venous access is essential, but for the healthy infant, neither central venous access nor arterial access is needed. Bronchoscopy may be performed quickly in the course of anesthetizing the infant; for these cases, bronchoscopy guides the anesthesiologist in choosing the level for the endotracheal tube and directs the surgeon to the correct management of the distal esophageal segment. It is especially helpful when, as occurs not infrequently, the distal segment enters at or near the carina or high in the cervical esophagus.

Access to the mediastinum is gained through a right third or fourth interspace transpleural or extrapleural thoracotomy. The extrapleural approach adds little time to the procedure but affords the infant an added measure of protection against empyema in the event of an anastomotic leak. The pleura must be dissected well into the mediastinum; the azygos vein is an important landmark, as is the vagus nerve. The former aids identification of the mediastinum. Dividing the vein allows access to the esophagus and the trachea; the vein courses to the vena cava at the level of the distal trachea, the most frequent site for a TEF. A segment of the vein has been used to separate the TEF closure from the esophageal anastomosis to reduce recurrence of the TEF.[117] Use of this technique requires special handling of the vein at the initial dissection.

The vagus nerve enters the thorax on the lateral aspect of the esophagus and usually follows the TEF onto the distal esophagus (Fig. 27–13), facilitating identification of the distal segment. Although the proximal esophagus has an excellent intramural vascular supply and can be dissected well up into the thoracic inlet to gain extra length and mobility, the distal esophagus has a more segmental blood supply from small vessels directly off the descending aorta. Excessive mobilization of the distal segment may result in ischemia, particularly of the segment comprising the TEF. Preservation of these vessels may enable the use of the entire distal segment, preserving length and facilitating primary anastomosis.

Once the distal segment is identified, it is traced cranially until the TEF is identified. The TEF is divided close to the trachea but not so close that closure of the tracheal defect narrows the tracheal diameter (Fig. 27–14). The tracheal side of the fistula may be closed with fine silk or long-lasting absorbable interrupted or continuous sutures. Integrity of

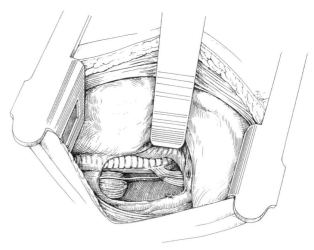

Figure 27–13. Extrapleural approach to esophageal atresia with tracheoesophageal fistula. The dissection follows the curve of the ribs to the mediastinum. The azygos vein is reflected anteriorly with the pleura after dividing the two highest intercostal veins as they enter the azygos. The vagus nerve is identified as it runs along the right side of both the proximal and distal esophageal segments. (From Holder TM, Manning PB: Esophageal atresia and tracheoesophageal fistula. Surgical Rounds 14:492–502, 1991.)

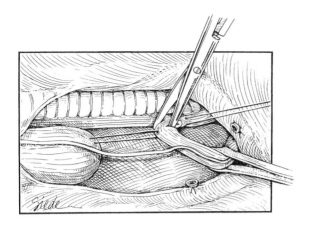

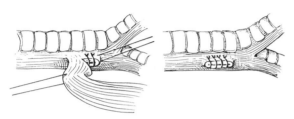

Figure 27–14. The distal esophagus is identified, looped, and carefully dissected up to its junction with the trachea, meticulously sparing the segmental vessels from the aorta. Traction sutures may be placed for gentle handling of the segments. The fistula is divided close to the trachea without narrowing its lumen. The tracheal end of the tracheoesophageal fistula is closed with continuous or interrupted sutures. Adjacent tissue, if available, is tacked over the closure. (From Holder TM, Manning PB: Esophageal and tracheoesophageal fistula. Surgical Rounds 14:492–502, 1991.)

the closure is tested by covering the suture line with warm saline solution and having the anesthesiologist inflate the airway to a sustained pressure of 40 mm Hg. Ideally, no residual pouch is left behind, but in practice, a small residual pouch frequently remains at the site of the TEF. Owing to the 8 to 10% incidence of recurrent TEF following repair, many have advocated interposing pleura or strap muscle segments between the closed TEF site and the esophageal suture line. This is not always possible, especially in smaller babies.

The proximal segment can be easily identified if the anesthesiologist pushes downward on the sump catheter in the proximal pouch. The motion of the pouch stretching into the superior mediastinum is usually obvious. Passage of a fiberoptic light has been suggested to facilitate identification but should rarely be necessary.[118] Various anastomoses have been used successfully, but a simple end-to-end approximation with fine silk sutures or long-lasting absorbable sutures works well (Fig. 27–15). Studies have shown a low incidence of stricture formation with simple interrupted anastomoses using absorbable sutures. Enthusiasm in a few centers for an end-to-side anastomosis with ligation of the TEF in continuity[119, 120] has waned with recognition of the increased incidence of recurrent TEF despite a reduced rate of stricture formation and possibly of

postoperative GER. A 1991 comparison series highlights the advantages and disadvantages of the two techniques and favors the end-to-end anastomosis.[121]

Our preference has been for the simple anastomosis with fine silk sutures (5-0 or 6-0), and our stricture rate when no leakage occurs has been negligible.[76] Careful mucosa-to-mucosa apposition is essential to avoid excessive granulation tissue formation in an area of exposed muscularis. The proximal mucosa tends to pull away from the muscularis and can be easily missed if not searched for with each suture. The distal segment may be opened in a "fish mouth" fashion to facilitate a better fit with the proximal segment if there is not sufficient length. The goal is a well-vascularized, tension-free anastomosis.

Mobilization of the proximal segment into the neck and, if necessary, one or more circular myotomies facilitates approximation.[103, 106–109] Tubularization of the proximal segment has also been described to achieve needed length.[112–114] Potential development of a diverticulum from the myotomy[110, 111] and the risk of vascular compromise in formation of the upper pouch tube flap limit their utility. If the completed anastomosis looks healthy and lies comfortably in the mediastinum without being obviously overstretched, leak and stricture formation are not likely even when the initial sutures are tied with considerable tension. We have used myotomies sparingly.

The dissection and anastomosis must be done with minimal handling of the delicate tissue of the esophagus and membranous trachea. A sizable catheter (at least an 8 or 10 French) should be passed down the distal segment to demonstrate its patency. A Silastic stent may be left in place, bridging the

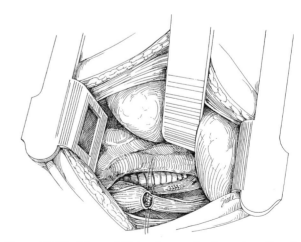

Figure 27–15. After mobilizing the proximal pouch well up into the thoracic inlet, the distal tip is incised and a meticulous mucosal-to-mucosal anastomosis accomplished with a single layer of interrupted silk or long-lasting absorbable sutures. The mucosa of the proximal segment may retract and be missed if not sought for with each suture. A Silastic stent may be left to bridge the anastomosis. A 10 French neonatal chest tube is left in the retropleural space as a drain. (From Holder TM, Manning PB: Esophageal and tracheoesophageal fistula. Surgical Rounds 14:492–502, 1991.)

anastomosis. It can be passed distally into the stomach and retrograde up the proximal segment to the oropharynx, where the anesthesiologist can secure it from the mouth until it can be brought out through the nares postoperatively.

When the procedure has been accomplished extrapleurally, a small-caliber drainage tube is attached to waterseal drainage. Should a leak occur, the drain is attached to suction, if necessary. Routine use of such a drain for a tension-free, healthy anastomosis has been questioned.[122]

If the pleural space has been entered but no injury to the visceral pleura or pulmonary parenchyma is suspected, the pleural air can be evacuated during closure of the chest. A hole in the pleura can often be closed with chromic catgut suture; if an air leak is demonstrated, an intrapleural tube should be placed and attached to low suction.

REPAIR OF ISOLATED ESOPHAGEAL ATRESIA

The operative approach to isolated EA is exactly that of repair of EA with distal TEF except that closure of the TEF is obviously not necessary. Finding the distal segment in the lower mediastinum is facilitated by passing a bougie or heavy dilator into the distal segment transgastrically. Care again must be taken to avoid devascularizing the distal segment. When overlap of the segments has been demonstrated, anastomosis is usually readily achieved (see Fig. 27–12).

If undue tension seems present, elongating procedures may be tried. We have accepted considerable tension and a high probability of leakage rather than abandon the esophagus. Leaks can usually be controlled with drainage, the defect usually heals without operative intervention, and a stricture is usually amenable to dilations. The latter are facilitated by leaving a heavy suture encased in a length of soft Silastic tubing bridging the anastomosis. The ends of the string are brought out the nose and the gastrostomy and tied in a loop to avoid dislodgment. In these cases, we do use suction on the extrapleural drain postoperatively.

REPAIR OF ISOLATED TEF

A ureteral catheter should be passed bronchoscopically through the fistula and retrieved endoscopically from the esophagus.[65] Alternatively, the catheter can be passed through the fistula into the stomach (see Fig. 27–9) with radiographic or fluoroscopic imaging to determine if the usual cervical approach is possible.

We have usually used a right-sided transverse supraclavicular incision because it avoids the thoracic duct, which is on the left side. The medial extent of the incision overlies the lateral aspect of the sternocleidomastoid muscle; it is usually unnecessary to divide the muscle. A bougie or large catheter in the esophagus aids orientation and the dissection

is carried down bluntly to the esophagus. The tracheal cartilages can be palpated. Preservation of the recurrent laryngeal nerve is essential. If the anesthesiologist tugs on the looped ureteral catheter the TEF is readily identified.

Finding the catheter in the fistula is obviously essential to ensure that the fistula has indeed been identified. It is best to cut the catheter and remove it from both structures and carefully suture closed the defects in the trachea and esophagus. Interposition of pleura, strap muscles, or sternocleidomastoid muscle lessens recurrence, but risk of recurrence is less in TEF without EA than it is with the more common variant. Layered closure without drainage is satisfactory. Early feedings are acceptable.

☐ Postoperative Care

After repair of EA with or without distal TEF, the infant may require a period of postoperative ventilator support. If there is concern that the anastomosis is under undue tension, paralysis and several days of ventilator support reduce the risk of anastomotic disruption. Secretions are a problem even in the healthiest of these infants. Ultrasonically nebulized mist that creates particle sizes of moisture that reach the distal tracheobronchial tree is essential to prevent mucus plugging and atelectasis. Before the routine use of nebulized mist, morbidity and mortality from respiratory compromise were common. Hyperextension or forceful rotation of the head can disrupt the anastomosis. Antibiotics are often continued until the anastomosis has been demonstrated to be intact and the extrapleural drain or chest tube or both have been removed. However, no data support this practice, and probably perioperative antibiotics are sufficient.

The infant is supported with intravenous fluids and peripheral parenteral nutrition until the anastomosis is proven intact and patent. We prefer to perform a contrast swallow on the 4th or 5th postoperative day, but others proceed with this as early as the 3rd day, as late as the 10th, or not at all. Oral feedings may then be initiated. If a small leak is demonstrated, the Silastic stent may serve as a means of initiating enteral feeds, but some risk of reflux and leakage of the feedings into the mediastinum exists. If a gastrostomy is present, early initiation of feedings may be possible, but reflux may aggravate a leak.

Once an intact and patent anastomosis has been demonstrated, feedings may be advanced rapidly. If other anomalies do not prolong the postoperative recovery, the infant may be discharged as soon as full feedings are tolerated and weight gain demonstrated. The infant should be seen at regular intervals to ensure continued weight gain and development and to evaluate for common complications such as GER, recurrent TEF, esophageal foreign bodies, reflex apnea, and anastomotic stenosis.

□ Complications

DYSPHAGIA

Dysfunctional peristalsis is universal in the distal esophageal segment. The esophageal "pacemaker" is in the hypopharynx and proximal esophagus, but owing to the atresia and its repair, propulsion must depend on a pacemaker in the distal segment. In most cases, the motility disturbance produces only minor clinical symptoms, even though the abnormality may be quite pronounced on a barium swallow. The child, after EA repair, experiences choking and obstructions of the esophagus by food and other foreign objects more frequently than does a normal child. Abnormal motility is most often a significant problem in patients with long-gap atresia and in those in whom oral intake must be delayed for a long period.[123]

In rare cases, the motility disturbance can result in a chronic inability to tolerate oral feedings, which can necessitate esophageal replacement. Hypogastrinemia has been noted most commonly in EA patients without a fistula and has been postulated to be a factor in the generalized intestinal dysfunction seen in these patients.[124] Some patients may manifest a state similar to familial dysautonomia with reflex apnea, bradycardia, swallowing difficulties, sweating, and episodic emesis.[125] Most preoperative studies have shown dysfunction in the distal segment, although a 1993 study suggested that the distal segment functions normally preoperatively, implicating vagus nerve injury as the source of postoperative dysfunction.[61]

Poor oral intake after EA with TEF repair may be due to associated cardiac anomalies with chronic low-grade congestive heart failure and chronic fatigue, rather than to dysfunction of the repaired esophagus. GER may also manifest itself as poor oral intake.

GASTROESOPHAGEAL REFLUX

GER is common in infants after repair of EA with or without TEF, but the perceived need for operative correction differs significantly at different centers.[73, 126, 127] When reflux occurs, acid clearance from the esophagus is delayed due to esophageal dysmotility. The role of gastrostomy in causing or aggravating GER is debated.[128] It is also unclear whether lower esophageal sphincter incompetence is part of the previously described generalized esophageal neuromotor disturbance or relates more to technical issues such as obliteration of the normal angle of His or reduction in the length of the intraabdominal esophagus by traction on the lower esophageal segment. In either event, reflux may cause significant problems and, like tracheomalacia, can be responsible for life-threatening events in the first months following repair. The increased respiratory effort due to tracheomalacia can produce increased intraabdominal pressure with resulting reflux episodes.

GER has been reported as a complication in 30 to 65% of patients.[73, 98, 126, 127, 129–132] Anastomotic tension has been implicated in its development,[133] but even when the anastomosis comes together seemingly without any tension and without any need to mobilize the distal esophageal segment, GER may occur. In some instances, GER may contribute to delayed healing of the anastomosis and to stricture formation.[134–136] Significant reflux may lead to chronic aspiration or reactive airway disease. The presenting symptoms are quite similar to those seen with recurrent TEF. The latter complication must be excluded before respiratory complications are attributed to GER.

Although some patients respond to medical management of the GER, a significantly higher percentage require operative intervention than patients with GER who did not have EA. Owing to the dysfunctional motility of the distal esophageal segment, a partial-wrap fundoplication is preferable to a complete wrap to avoid functional obstruction of the esophagus. Failure rates for the partial wrap are lower than for the complete wrap fundoplication.[137] The morbidity of complete wrap fundoplication in patients following repair of EA has been increased compared with patients in the same institution having the same fundoplication unrelated to EA.[126, 131]

ANASTOMOTIC STRICTURE

Stricture formation is common after repair of EA with or without TEF. In one series of 199 patients, 74 strictures (37%) requiring dilation were noted following repair of EA.[136] Of the 74 patients, 71 responded to dilation alone, 3 required resection or esophageal substitution, 42 had either one or two dilations, and 14 required five or more dilations. Braided silk sutures, GER, and anastomotic leak were cited as contributing to stricture formation. Anastomotic tension has been implicated in another report.[89]

With a meticulous dissection to preserve the segmental blood supply to the distal segment and careful mucosal-to-mucosal apposition of the segments, anastomotic stenosis can be avoided in most cases. We had none in 20 patients who underwent immediate or delayed primary repair of EA with distal TEF.[76]

When great tension is present or leakage occurs from the anastomosis, stenosis is likely. Stenosis is commonly present when isolated EA is repaired. Retrograde dilation guided by a transanastomotic string is the safest approach to such strictures, especially early in the course of anastomotic dilations. The Silastic tubing initially used to stent the anastomosis can be readily converted to a Silastic-covered heavy suture while performing a gastrostomy, if significant stenosis occurs. One should first ascertain that the stenosis is not just a web formed by mucosal adhesions. A web is easily ruptured with the passage of a small dilator, and the integrity of the muscular esophageal wall can be confirmed by the ease with which larger dilators can then be passed. In the 1990s, radial dilation with balloon catheters was advocated as being safer than the shearing forces applied by the passage of bougies.[138, 139] Fluoroscopic monitoring of the balloon position and the dilation enhances safety; the Silastic-covered heavy suture is still useful to guide the balloon catheter into position.

If stenosis with complete occlusion of the lumen occurs after the bridging string has been removed, double endoscopy has been advocated, passing endoscopes down from the oropharynx and up the distal esophagus from the gastrostomy. This may allow safe passage of a needle through the scar tissue with reestablishment of continuity and endoscopic enlargement by "whittling away" the scar.[115]

MAJOR ANASTOMOTIC LEAK OR DISRUPTION

Anastomotic leak has been reported in about 15% of esophageal anastomoses in large series, but only about one third of these were major leaks or anastomotic disruptions.[122, 140] Major leakage requires adequate drainage. Additional tubes or drains, including intrapleural tubes, may be needed. Major disruptions may be life-threatening events with multisystem failure related to sepsis. Fortunately, the leak is usually limited and controllable, but anastomotic stenosis should be anticipated after closure.

Complete disruptions require reanastomosis; this has been successfully accomplished acutely in the face of inflammation.[141] Partial disruptions usually produce significant stenosis as a result of healing with excessive scar tissue and late mucosal coverage. The resulting stenosis may respond to repeated dilations but may require anastomotic revision. Steroid injections sometimes soften the scar tissue and facilitate dilation to an adequate size. Complete disruption with infection may require that primary repair be abandoned; the proximal esophagus may be exteriorized as a cervical esophagostomy; the distal segment may be closed; and eventually colon, gastric tube, or jejunal interposition may be used to replace the missing esophageal segment.

RECURRENT TRACHEOESOPHAGEAL FISTULA

The published incidence of recurrent TEF is 5 to 10%.[65, 89, 120, 121, 135, 142, 143] The fistula site closure in the trachea and the esophageal anastomosis are usually in close approximation so that a small leak with resulting inflammation can rejoin the trachea and esophagus. Diagnosis of the original TEF is facilitated by telescopic bronchoscopy, which is nearly 100% accurate in the hands of experienced endoscopists. Confirmation of a recurrent TEF is more

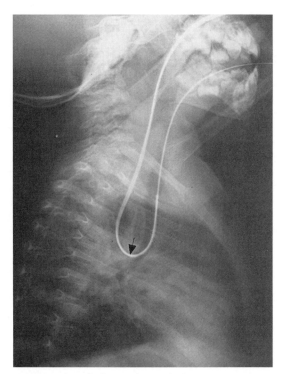

Figure 27–16. Lateral chest radiograph demonstrates a recurrent tracheoesophageal fistula that has been catheterized transesophageally with the catheter retrieved from the trachea. Tugging on the catheter during chest exploration helps to identify the recurrent fistula. (From Kirks DR, Bailey CA Jr, Currarino G: Selective catheterization of tracheoesophageal fistula. AJR Am J Roentgenol 133:763–764, 1979.)

problematic; a residual "pouch" at the site of the TEF is common.

Bronchoscopic demonstration of patency may be difficult even using small probing catheters or injections of vital dyes into the residual pouch. Careful catheter probing from the esophageal side while injecting small volumes of contrast material under fluoroscopic guidance has been most successful.[65] Passage of the catheter through the TEF from the esophagus followed by bronchoscopic retrieval greatly facilitates identification of the recurrent TEF within the scar tissue (Fig. 27–16). Pleural or pericardial flaps[144] and interposition of muscle all have been used in an attempt to prevent another recurrence. Other approaches to the recurrent TEF include endoscopic plugging with fibrin "glue."[142, 145]

TRACHEOMALACIA, AIRWAY OBSTRUCTION, VASCULAR COMPRESSION, AND REFLEX APNEA

Even after successful esophageal repair, tracheomalacia may cause frequent and prolonged respiratory infections. Due to fluttering of the tracheal wall, infants with tracheomalacia have a characteristic cry and are often described as having a "seal bark" cough. These problems usually improve with time, as the tracheal cartilage becomes stiffer and as the trachea enlarges. Tracheomalacia can produce life-threatening events or death during the first months of life.[146, 147] The combination of tracheomalacia, esophageal dysmotility, and vascular compression produces a syndrome of obstructive airway symptoms and reflex apnea. A 1990 report used cine-computed tomography to evaluate tracheomalacia after EA with TEF repair and concluded that the tracheal structure was intrinsically weakened, not just compressed, by the surrounding structures.[148]

The membranous trachea is commonly widened at the site of entry of the TEF into the trachea, and the cartilaginous "C" rings of the trachea may be flattened, decreasing the anteroposterior diameter of the trachea. Buckling of the cartilages by compression by the aorta or the innominate artery may further compromise the diameter of the airway. Innominate artery or aortic suspension may be needed (Fig. 27–17). Increased intrathoracic pressure from forced expiration or coughing may lead to complete airway occlusion. Severe degrees of these deformities may result in postoperative airway obstruction requiring continuation or reestablishment of endotracheal tube airway support.

In less severe instances, symptoms of occlusion and reflex apnea occur only with the introduction of more solid foods. Recurrent episodes require suspension of the aorta or innominate artery to the sternum to stabilize the underlying anterior tracheal wall. Use of a pericardial flap may facilitate attachment of the vessels to the sternum.[149] Reports document the success of "aortopexy" in relieving airway compression both for patients with problems after EA/TEF repair and those with vascular anomalies without EA/TEF.[149–152] Rarely, more extensive tracheal reconstruction or stenting is required.[150]

OTHER COMPLICATIONS

Even though a catheter is passed readily into the stomach at the time of initial anastomosis, distal esophageal stenosis may be present as a result of cartilaginous rings in the distal esophagus. These have been reported without association with EA,[153, 154] but the association is much more common.[49, 50, 153, 155, 156] They are thought to result from anomalous separation of the trachea and esophagus. This stenosis may be asymptomatic until solid foods are introduced, at which time the obstruction may present

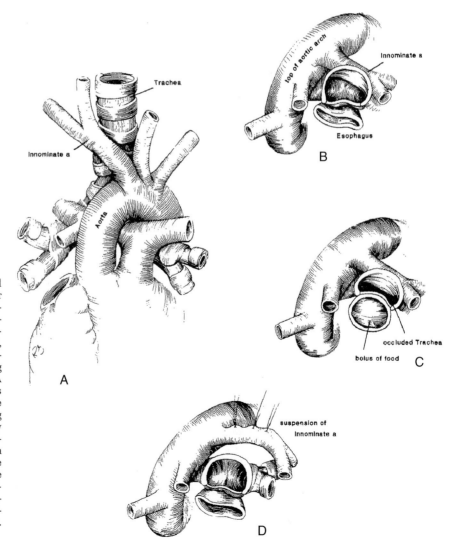

Figure 27–17. *A,* Depiction of the normal relationships of the aorta and its major branches to the trachea showing the innominate artery crossing the lower trachea producing compression of the trachea and buckling of the cartilages. *B,* "Endoscopic view" of these relationships shows the buckled arch impinging on the lumen of the distal trachea. *C,* A bolus of food in the esophagus forces the posterior membranous portion of the trachea into the tracheal lumen causing almost complete airway obliteration by the anterior compression and the posterior bulge. *D,* Suspension of the aorta and the innominate artery eliminate the anterior compression and buckling of the tracheal rings increasing the cross-sectional diameter of the trachea. (From Filston HC, Ferguson TB, Oldham HN: Airway obstruction by vascular anomalies. Ann Surg 205:541–549, 1987.)

acutely. Resection of the segment containing the ring cartilage is usually necessary because dilation is rarely successful and may result in esophageal perforation.

Chylothorax as a complication of EA repair may result from injury to the thoracic duct, which courses up the right side of the mediastinum before crossing to enter the left internal jugular vein just proximal to its entry into the subclavian vein. Chylothorax may not be appreciated immediately but may be related to scarring in the mediastinum.

Erosion of the esophagus by a chest tube has been reported in two instances, one through a myotomy site and one through the anastomosis.[157]

☐ Results

Essentially, only severe cardiac anomalies, devastating chromosomal abnormalities, and major pulmonary complications significantly affect the eventual outcome.[74] Prematurity and small size are no longer primary determinants of success or failure. Today, an infant born with EA with distal TEF who weighs more than 1500 g, is free of other life-threatening congenital anomalies, has no major chromosomal abnormalities, and has no serious preoperative pulmonary dysfunction has nearly a 100% chance of successful repair and survival.[69, 72, 74, 158, 159] Even when the physiologic derangements of prematurity complicate the picture, a combination of modern neonatal intensive care and some imaginative temporizing interventions by an experienced pediatric surgeon can sustain the infant and allow eventual successful repair.

A report of 253 patients treated between 1980 and 1987 included 8 who had no operation owing to multiple anomalies and 8 who had only gastrostomy but died of other anomalies before repair. Of the 253 patients, 38 had esophagostomy and gastrostomy for staged repair of wide gap EA, and 199 had primary repair (5 were delayed). Survival was 86% for the whole series and 89% for those treated with definitive operations.[140]

The 118 patients from Children's Mercy Hospital reported in the second edition of this text had an overall survival rate higher than 90%, confirming that complex anomalies and unmanageable pulmonary complications are the primary mortality factors.[159]

In our series of 20 patients from Duke, 18 underwent immediate and 2 delayed primary repair. There was 1 late death from complications of associated anomalies.[76] All other mortality was among the group of patients with severe chromosomal abnormalities or those whose cardiac or pulmonary disease never allowed repair. No infant died from prematurity, pneumonia, or complications of esophageal repair. Six infants who weighed less than 1500 g died: 4 had trisomy 18, and the other 2 were those with severe RDS and associated complications.

Successful primary repair of infants weighing as little as 500 g has been reported,[78, 79] and early primary repair in very premature neonates has been advocated prior to the onset of severe RDS.[80] Overall survival for the anomaly today is 70 to 85%,[76, 136, 158, 159] with survival well beyond the 90% level for those infants without preoperative physiologic derangements.

Patients with isolated EA can usually have esophagus-saving procedures by supporting them with gastrostomy feedings and proximal pouch decompression for the 6 to 12 weeks that are required for the proximal segment to elongate sufficiently to allow the segments to overlap. Two reports from one institution document a 90% survival for these children, despite the increased incidence of other anomalies associated with this variant. Waiting 3 to 4 months before attempting the anastomosis allowed primary anastomosis in 75%. One third required fundoplication for postoperative GER.[98, 99] The infant may be managed at home while awaiting lengthening of the proximal segment, obviating the cost of maintenance in the intensive care nursery. Current reports suggest that interposition operations are rarely needed today.[97–99, 105, 113, 114]

☐ Long-Term Results

As survival has become the norm, reports have begun to look at functional results in survivors.[130, 132, 135, 160, 161] In a series of 39 patients 2 to 11 years after repair of EA with TEF, 25 reported themselves to have had an excellent result, 10 were good, and 4 fair. However, esophagogastroduodenoscopy revealed 20 had esophagitis, 5 with Barrett's changes; 10 had hiatal hernias; and 3 of 9 fundoplications had failed. Only 13 esophageal biopsies were normal; 21 showed esophagitis and 3 revealed metaplasia.[130]

In another series, manometric and 24-hour pH monitoring of 22 patients who ranged in age from 12 to 22 years revealed a pattern of impaired contractility with prolonged nocturnal GER episodes with slow clearance: 72% complained of dysphagia, 59% complained of heartburn, 45% reported a foreign body requiring disimpaction, 54% had documented GER, and 31% had chronic respiratory disease.[132] Another study of physical fitness after EA/TEF repair found that exercise tolerance was reduced and time to reach maximum heart rate was shorter for patients compared with normal controls.[160] The long-term consequences of these abnormalities are not clear.

In a series of 498 patients with EA and distal TEF treated between 1948 and 1988, 50 required secondary operations.[135] Complications included 30 patients with anastomotic stricture, 15 with recurrent TEF, 4 with both, and 1 with postmyotomy diverticulum. Nine patients required esophageal replacement owing to complications and 33 had complete-wrap fundoplication.

☐ Acquired Tracheoesophageal Fistula in Infancy and Childhood

Fortunately, acquired TEF is a rare entity in childhood. A review collected only nine cases, all due to foreign body erosions, five of which resulted from the ingestion of button batteries.[162] We have seen one acquired TEF in an 8-year-old caused by a bottle rocket explosion in his mouth.

☐ Laryngotracheoesophageal Clefts

The possibility of LTE cleft as the explanation for an infant who vomited and choked with each feeding was first suggested by Richter in 1792.[163] Finlay first described a case in 1949,[164] and Pettersson performed the first successful repair of a proximal cleft and presented a classification system in 1955.[165] Since then, several hundred cases have been reported and additional classification systems have been described, none of which has been universally accepted.

ANATOMY

The LTE cleft may be limited to the supracricoid larynx (Pettersson, type I); may extend through the cricoid to the upper trachea (type II); or may involve the entire cervical trachea, sometimes extending to the carina (type III). Several cases of a more exten-

sive cleft extending into one or both bronchi have been reported (type IV)[166] (Fig. 27–18). Microgastria has been a universal association with these more extensive lesions and has complicated the repair. Up to 37% of clefts have been associated with EA and TEF.[163]

EMBRYOLOGY

The exact relationship of these entities to EA and TEF is not clear. They may be more severe forms of the disordered embryogenesis that produced EA and TEF. Failure of the septation process could explain the less extensive forms of LTE cleft but fails to explain those that involve one or both of the bronchi.[166]

DIAGNOSIS

The infant with a cleft larynx or short proximal LTE cleft may present with inspiratory stridor or with coughing or choking with feedings; the infant with an extensive cleft may quickly develop aspiration pneumonia or more severe respiratory compromise. Rigid bronchoscopy is the most accurate diagnostic test. The cleft may be missed if the integrity of the posterior wall of the larynx and trachea is not tested by pressing the bronchoscope posteriorly. A contrast esophagram cannot usually differentiate an LTE cleft from simple aspiration.

OPERATIVE APPROACH

Posterolateral and anterior transtracheal surgical approaches have been used successfully to repair

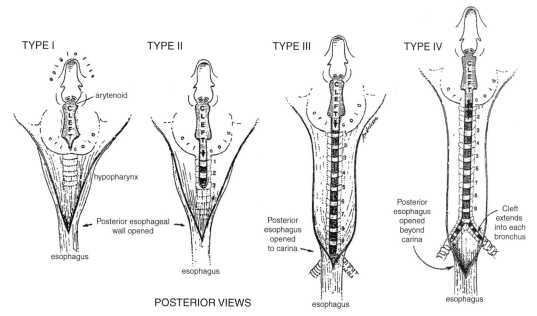

Figure 27–18. One classification of laryngeal and laryngotracheoesophageal clefts. Type I is above the cricoid, type II extends through the cricoid, type III extends well down the trachea toward the carina, and type IV extends out one or both mainstem bronchi. (From Ryan DP, Muehrcke DD, Doody DP, et al: Laryngotracheoesophageal cleft [type IV]: Management and repair of lesions beyond the carina. J Pediatr Surg 26:962–970, 1991.)

types I and II clefts. Each approach uses the adjacent esophagus to create a membranous posterior trachea and close the defect in the posterior larynx. It is essential to construct the repair in such a way as to avoid overlap of suture lines in the trachea and the remaining esophagus. An 11% recurrence rate attests to the difficulties encountered.[167]

Repair of type III clefts has been more problematic but has been achieved in a few infants.[168] For the more extensive type IV clefts, staged repair has been suggested with initial gastric division and tracheostomy with subsequent cleft repair combining thoracic and cervical approaches. Three infants reportedly survived the procedure, but two of the three eventually died.[166] The association of microgastria has complicated the management of these more extensive clefts.

RESULTS

Once a lethal lesion, laryngeal clefts are now being successfully managed with generally good outcomes.[169] Overall survival has improved from 18% before 1970 to 75% in 1990.[163] Only a few cases of success with the more extensive clefts have been reported, and the severe dysfunction of the defective tracheobronchial tree has left these children with an array of postoperative complications.[166, 168]

Acknowledgment

In the first two editions of this text, this chapter was written in part or in whole by Thomas M. Holder, MD, whose knowledge of and contributions to the topic through the years have been extensive. It has been a privilege and a challenge to produce a chapter that is worthy to follow his; except for a few additions, his work could well have continued to serve.

REFERENCES

1. Myers NA: Oesophageal atresia: The epitome of modern surgery. Ann R Coll Surg Engl 54:277–287, 1974.
2. Ashcraft KW, Holder TM: The story of esophageal atresia and tracheoesophageal fistula. Surgery 65:332–340, 1969.
3. Myers NA: The history of oesophageal atresia and tracheoesophageal fistula. Prog Ped Surg 20:106–157, 1986.
4. Haight C: Some observations on esophageal atresias and tracheo-esophageal fistulas of congenital origin. J Thorac Surg 34:141–172, 1957.
5. Kluth D: Atlas of esophageal atresia. J Pediatr Surg 11:901–919, 1976.
6. Hill TP: Congenital malformation. Boston Med Surg J 21:320–321, 1839.
7. Steele C: Case of deficient oesophagus. Lancet 2:764, 1888.
8. Brennemann J: Congenital atresia of the esophagus, with report of three cases. Am J Dis Child 5:143–150, 1913.
9. Brennemann J: Congenital atresia of the esophagus with report of four additional cases, with three necropsies. Am J Dis Child 16:143–153, 1918.
10. Richter HM: Congenital atresia of the oesophagus: An operation designed for its cure. Surg Gynecol Obstet 17:397–402, 1913.
11. Imperatori CJ: Congenital tracheoesophageal fistula without atresia of the esophagus. Arch Otolaryngol 30:352–359, 1939.
12. Ladd WE: The surgical treatment of esophageal atresia and tracheoesophageal fistulas. N Engl J Med 230:625–637, 1944.
13. Leven NL: Congenital atresia of the esophagus with tracheoesophageal fistula. J Thorac Surg 10:648–657, 1941.
14. Lanman TH: Congenital atresia of the esophagus. Arch Surg 41:1060–1083, 1940.
15. Haight C, Towsley HA: Congenital atresia of the esophagus with tracheoesophageal fistula. Surg Gynecol Obstet 76:672–688, 1943.
16. Smith EI: The early development of the trachea and esophagus in relation to atresia of the esophagus and tracheoesophageal fistula. Contrib Embryol 245:42–57, 1957.
17. de Lorimier AA, Harrison MR: Esophageal atresia: Embryogenesis and management. World J Surg 9:250–257, 1985.
18. Skandalakis JE, Gray SW, Ricketts R: The esophagus. In Skandalakis JE, Gray SW (eds): Embryology for Surgeons (2nd ed). Baltimore, Williams & Wilkins, 1994.
19. Rosenthal AH: Congenital atresia of the esophagus with tracheo-esophageal fistula. Arch Pathol 12:756–772, 1931.
20. Beasley SW: Embryology. In Beasley SW, Myers NA, Auldist AW (eds): Oesophageal Atresia. London, Chapman and Hall, 1991.
21. Kluth D, Steding G, Seidl W: The embryology of foregut malformations. J Pediatr Surg 22:389–393, 1987.
22. Gruenwald P: A case of atresia of the esophagus combined with tracheo-esophageal fistula in a 9-mm human embryo, and its embryological explanation. Anat Rec 78:293–302, 1940.
23. Kluth D, Habenicht R: The embryology of usual and unusual types of esophageal atresia. Pediatr Surg Int 2:223–227, 1987.
24. Kleckner SC, Pringle KC, Clark EB: The effect of chick embryo hyperflexion on tracheoesophageal development. J Pediatr Surg 19:340–344, 1984.
25. David TJ, O'Callaghan SE: Oesophageal atresia in the South West of England. J Med Genet 12:1–11, 1975.
26. Szendrey T, Danyi G, Czeizel A: Etiological study on isolated esophageal atresia. Hum Genet 70:51–58, 1985.
27. Bankier A, Brady J, Myers NA: Epidemiology and genetics. In Beasley SW, Myers NA, Auldist AW (eds): Oesophageal Atresia. London, Chapman and Hall, 1991.
28. Ozimek CD, Grimson RC, Aylsworth AS: An epidemiologic study of tracheoesophageal fistula and esophageal atresia in North Carolina. Teratology 25:53–59, 1982.
29. German JC, Mahour GH, Woolley MM: The twin with esophageal atresia. J Pediatr Surg 14:432–435, 1979.
30. Nora AH, Nora JJ: A syndrome of multiple congenital anomalies associated with teratogenic exposure. Arch Environ Health 30:17–21, 1975.
31. Kalter H: Congenital malformations induced by riboflavin deficiency in strains of inbred mice. Pediatrics 23:222–230, 1959.
32. Warkany J, Roth CB, Wilson JG: Multiple congenital malformations: A consideration of etiologic factors. Pediatrics 1:462–471, 1948.
33. Diez-Pardo JA, Baoquan Q, Navarro C, et al: A new rodent experimental model of esophageal atresia and tracheoesophageal fistula: Preliminary report. J Pediatr Surg 31:498–450, 1996.
34. Spitz L: Esophageal atresia: Past, present, and future. J Pediatr Surg 31:19–25, 1996.
35. Vogt EC: Congenital esophageal atresia. Am J Roentgenol 22:463–465, 1929.
36. Gross RE: The Surgery of Infancy and Childhood. Philadelphia, WB Saunders, 1953.
37. Lambrecht W, Kluth D: Esophageal atresia: A new anatomic variant with gasless abdomen. J Pediatr Surg 29:564–565, 1994.
38. Holder TM, Ashcraft KW, Sharp RJ, et al: Care of infants with esophageal atresia, tracheoesophageal fistula, and associated anomalies. J Thorac Cardiovasc Surg 94:828–835, 1987.

39. Ein SH, Shandling D, Wesson D, et al: Esophageal atresia with distal tracheoesophageal fistula: Associated anomalies and prognosis in the 1980s. J Pediatr Surg 24:1055–1059, 1989.

40. German JC, Mahour GH, Woolley MM: Esophageal atresia and associated anomalies. J Pediatr Surg 11:299–306, 1976.

41. Woolley MM: Esophageal atresia and tracheoesophageal fistula—1939 to 1979. Am J Surg 139:771–774, 1980.

42. Jones KL: Smith's Recognizable Patterns of Human Malformation (5th ed). Philadelphia, WB Saunders, 1997.

43. Kutiyanawala M, Wyse RKH, Brereton RJ, et al: Charge and esophageal atresia. J Pediatr Surg 27:558–560, 1992.

44. Kulkarni B, Rad RS, Oak S, et al: 13 pairs of ribs—a predictor of long gap atresia in tracheoesophageal fistula. J Pediatr Surg 32:1453–1454, 1997.

45. Canty TJ, Boyle EM, Linden B, et al: Aortic arch anomalies associated with long gap esophageal atresia and tracheoesophageal fistula. J Pediatr Surg 32:1587–1591, l997.

46. Nakazato Y, Landing BH, Wells TR: Abnormal Auerbach plexus in the esophagus and stomach of patients with esophageal atresia and tracheoesophageal fistula. J Pediatr Surg 21:831–837, 1986.

47. Qi BQ, Merei J, Farmer P, et al: The vagus and recurrent laryngeal nerves in the rodent experimental model of esophageal atresia. J Pediatr Surg 32:1580–1586, 1997.

48. Qi BQ, Merei J, Farmer P, et al: Tracheomalacia with esophageal atresia and tracheoesophageal fistula in fetal rats. J Pediatr Surg 32:1575–1579, 1997.

49. Neilson IR, Croitoru DP, Guttman FM, et al: Distal congenital esophageal stenosis associated with esophageal atresia. J Pediatr Surg 26:478–482, 1991.

50. Yeung CK, Spitz L, Brereton RJ, et al: Congenital esophageal stenosis due to tracheobronchial remnants: A rare but important association with esophageal atresia. J Pediatr Surg 27:852–855, 1992.

51. Usui N, Kamata S, Ishikawa S, et al: Anomalies of the tracheobronchial tree in patients with esophageal atresia. J Pediatr Surg 31:258–262, 1996.

52. Black PR, Welch KJ: Pulmonary agenesis (aplasia), esophageal atresia, and tracheoesophageal fistula: A different treatment strategy. J Pediatr Surg 21:936–938, 1986.

53. Al-Salem AH, Qaisruddin S, Qatif KKV: Concurrent left congenital diaphragmatic hernia and esophageal atresia: Case report and review of literature. J Pediatr Surg 32:772–774, 1997.

54. Spitz L, Phelan PD: Tracheomalacia. In Beasley SW, Myers NA, Auldist AW (eds): Oesophageal Atresia. London, Chapman and Hall, 1991.

55. Beasley SW: Influence of anatomy and physiology on the management of oesophageal atresia. Prog Ped Surg 27:53–61, 1991.

56. Shorr LD, Andrassy RJ: Long-term respiratory status following esophageal atresia repair. Contemp Surg 28:66–72, 1986.

57. Davies MRQ, Cywes S: The flaccid trachea and tracheoesophageal congenital anomalies. J Pediatr Surg 13:363–367, 1978.

58. Wailoo MP, Emery JL: The trachea in children with tracheo-oesophageal fistula. Histopathology 3:329–338, 1979.

59. Rideout DT, Hayashi AH, Gillis DA, et al: The absence of clinically significant tracheomalacia in patients having esophageal atresia without tracheoesophageal fistula. J Pediatr Surg 26:1303–1305, 1991.

60. Putnam TC, Lawrence RA, Wood BP, et al: Esophageal function after repair of esophageal atresia. Surg Gynecol Obstet 158:344–348, 1984.

61. Shono T, Suita S, Arima T, et al: Motility function of the esophagus before primary anastomosis in esophageal atresia. J Pediatr Surg 28:673–676, 1993.

62. Nakazato Y, Wells TR, Landing BH: Abnormal tracheal innervation in patients with esophageal atresia and tracheoesophageal fistula: Study of the intrinsic tracheal nerve plexuses by a microdissection technique. J Pediatr Surg 21:838–844, 1986.

63. Heller RM, Kirchner SG, O'Neill JA: Perforation of the pharynx in the newborn: A near look-alike for esophageal atresia. Am J Roent 129:335–337, 1977.

64. Stringer MD, McKenna KM, Goldstein RB, et al: Prenatal diagnosis of esophageal atresia. J Pediatr Surg 30:1258–1263, 1995.

65. Filston HC, Rankin JS, Kirks DR: The diagnosis of primary and recurrent tracheoesophageal fistulas: Value of selective catheterization. J Pediatr Surg 17:144–148, 1982.

66. Benjamin B, Pham T: Diagnosis of H-type tracheoesophageal fistula. J Pediatr Surg 26:667–671, 1991.

67. Gans SL, Johnson RO: Diagnosis and surgical management of "H-type" tracheoesophageal fistula in infants and children. J Pediatr Surg 12:233–236, 1977.

68. Waterston DJ, Bonham Carter RE, Aberdeen E: Oesophageal atresia: Tracheo-oesophageal fistula. Lancet 1:819–822, 1962.

69. Spitz L, Kiely EM, Morecroft JA, et al: Oesophageal atresia: At-risk groups for the 1990s. J Pediatr Surg 29:723–725, 1994.

70. Connolly B, Guiney EJ: Trends in tracheoesophageal fistula. Surg Gynecol Obstet 164:308–312, 1987.

71. Manning PB, Wesley JR, Behrendt DM, et al: Fifty years' experience with esophageal atresia and tracheoesophageal fistula. Ann Surg 204:446–451, 1986.

72. Randolph JG, Newman KD, Anderson KD: Current results in repair of esophageal atresia with tracheoesophageal fistula using physiologic status as a guide to therapy. Ann Surg 209:526–531, 1989.

73. Okada A, Usui N, Inoue M, et al: Esophageal atresia in Osaka: A review of 39 years' experience. J Pediatr Surg 32:1570–1574, 1997.

74. Poenaru D, Laberge J-M, Neilson IR, et al: A new prognostic classification for esophageal atresia. Surgery 113:426–432, 1993.

75. Teich S, Barton DP, Ginn-Pease ME, et al: Prognostic classification for esophageal atresia and tracheoesophageal fistula: Waterston versus Montreal. J Pediatr Surg 32:1075–1080, 1997.

76. Filston HC, Rankin JS, Grimm JK: Esophageal atresia. Prognostic factors and contribution of preoperative telescopic endoscopy. Ann Surg 199:532–537, 1984.

77. Richenbacher WE, Ballantine TVN: Esophageal atresia, distal tracheoesophageal fistula, and an air shunt that compromised mechanical ventilation. J Pediatr Surg 25:1216–1218, 1990.

78. Schaarschmidt K, Willital GH, Jorch G, et al: Delayed primary reconstruction of an esophageal atresia with distal esophagotracheal fistula in an infant weighing less than 500 grams. J Pediatr Surg 27:1529–1531, 1992.

79. Templeton JM, Templeton JJ, Schnaufer L, et al: Management of esophageal atresia and tracheoesophageal fistula in the neonate with severe respiratory distress syndrome. J Pediatr Surg 20:394–397, 1985.

80. Beasley SW, Myers NA, Auldist AW: Management of the premature infant with esophageal atresia and hyaline membrane disease. J Pediatr Surg 27:23–25, 1992.

81. Holcomb GW III: Survival after gastrointestinal perforation from esophageal atresia and tracheoesophageal fistula. J Pediatr Surg 28:1532–1535, 1993.

82. Alexander F, Johanningman J, Markin LW: Staged repair improves outcome of high-risk premature infants with esophageal atresia and tracheoesophageal fistula. J Pediatr Surg 28:151–154, 1993.

83. Driver CP, Bruce J: Primary reconstruction of esophageal atresia with distal tracheoesophageal fistula in a 740-gram infant. J Pediatr Surg 32:1488–1489, 1997.

84. Filston HC, Chitwood WR Jr, Schkolne B, et al: The Fogarty balloon catheter as an aid to management of the infant with esophageal atresia and tracheoesophageal fistula complicated by severe RDS or pneumonia. J Pediatr Surg 17:149–151, 1982.

85. Bloch EC, Filston HC: A thin fiberoptic bronchoscope as an aid to occlusion of the fistula in infants with tracheoesophageal fistula. Anesth Analg 67:791–793, 1988.

86. Karl HW: Control of life-threatening air leak after gastrostomy in an infant with respiratory distress syndrome and tracheoesophageal fistula. Anesthesiology 62:670–672, 1985.

87. Koop CE, Hamilton JP: Atresia of the esophagus: Increased survival with staged procedures in the poor-risk infant. Ann Surg 162:389–401, 1965.
88. Goh DW, Brereton RJ, Spitz L: Esophageal atresia with obstructed tracheoesophageal fistula and gasless abdomen. J Pediatr Surg 26:160–162, 1991.
89. McKinnon LJ, Kosloske AM: Prediction and prevention of anastomotic complications of esophageal atresia and tracheoesophageal fistula. J Pediatr Surg 25:778–781, 1990.
90. Chan KL, Saing H: Combined flexible endoscopy and fluoroscopy in the assessment of the gap between the two esophageal pouches in esophageal atresia without fistula. J Pediatr Surg 30:668–670, 1995.
91. Kemmotsu H, Joe K, Nakamura H, et al: Cervical approach for the repair of esophageal atresia. J Pediatr Surg 30:549–552, 1995.
92. Ford WDA, Freeman JK, Martin AJ: Supraclavicular approach to cervical esophageal atresia and tracheoesophageal fistula. J Pediatr Surg 20:242–243, 1985.
93. Harrison MR, Ganson BA, Mahour GH, et al: The significance of right aortic arch in repair of esophageal atresia and tracheoesophageal fistula. J Pediatr Surg 12:861–869, 1977.
94. Dudgeon DL, Morrison CW, Woolley MM: Congenital proximal tracheoesophageal fistula. J Pediatr Surg 7:614–619, 1972.
95. Yun KL, Hartman GE, Shochat SJ: Esophageal atresia with triple congenital tracheoesophageal fistulae. J Pediatr Surg 27:1527–1528, 1992.
96. Moulton SL, Bouvet M, Lynch FP: Congenital microgastria in a premature infant. J Pediatr Surg 28:1594–1595, 1992.
97. Puri P, Blake N, O'Donnell B, et al: Delayed primary anastomosis following spontaneous growth of esophageal segments in esophageal atresia. J Pediatr Surg 16:180–183, 1981.
98. Ein SH, Shandling B, Heiss K: Pure esophageal atresia: Outlook in the 1990s. J Pediatr Surg 28:1147–1150, 1993.
99. Ein SH, Shandling B: Pure esophageal atresia: A 50-year review. J Pediatr Surg 29:1208–1211, 1994.
100. Howard R, Myers NA: Esophageal atresia: A technique for elongating the upper pouch. Surgery 58:725–727, 1965.
101. Young DG: Successful primary anastomosis in oesophageal atresia after reduction of a long gap between the blind ends by bouginage of the upper pouch. Br J Surg 54:321–324, 1967.
102. Woolley MM, Leix, F, Johnston PW: Esophageal atresia types A and B: Upper pouch elongation and delayed anatomic reconstruction. J Pediatr Surg 4:148–153, 1969.
103. de Lorimier AA, Harrison MR: Long gap esophageal atresia: Primary anastomosis after esophageal elongation by bougienage and esophagomyotomy. J Thorac Cardiovasc Surg 79:138–141, 1980.
104. Filston HC, Merten DF, Kirks DR: Initial care of esophageal atresia to facilitate potential primary anastomosis. South Med J 74:1530–1533, 1981.
105. Puri P, Ninan GK, Blake NS, et al: Delayed primary anastomosis for esophageal atresia: 18 months' to 11 years' follow-up. J Pediatr Surg 27:1127–1130, 1992.
106. Livaditis A: Esophageal atresia: A method of overbridging large segmental gaps. Z Kinderchir 13:298–306, 1973.
107. Vizas D, Ein SH, Simpson JS: The value of circular myotomy for esophageal atresia. J Pediatr Surg 13:357–359, 1978.
108. Eraklis AJ, Rossello PJ, Ballantine TVN: Circular esophagomyotomy of upper pouch in primary repair of long-segment esophageal atresia. J Pediatr Surg 11:709–712, 1976.
109. Takada Y, Kent G, Filler RM: Circular myotomy and esophageal length and safe esophageal anastomosis: An experimental study. J Pediatr Surg 16:343–348, 1981.
110. Otte JB, Gianello P, Wese FX, et al: Diverticulum formation after circular myotomy for esophageal atresia. J Pediatr Surg 19:68–71, 1984.
111. Taylor RG, Myers RA: Management of a post–Livaditis-procedure oesophageal diverticulum. Pediatr Surg Int 4:238–240, 1989.
112. Gough MH: Esophageal atresia—use of an anterior flap in the difficult anastomosis. J Pediatr Surg 15:310–311, 1980.
113. Bar-Maor JA, Shoshany G, Sweed Y: Wide gap esophageal atresia: A new method to elongate the upper pouch. J Pediatr Surg 24:882–883, 1989.
114. Davenport M, Bianchi A: Early experience with oesophageal flap oesophagoplasty for repair of oesophageal atresia. Pediatr Surg Int 5:332–335, 1990.
115. Borgstein ES, Hunter DS, Youngson GG: Endoscopic restoration of esophageal continuity. J Pediatr Surg 25:1220–1223, 1990.
116. Schmittenbecher PP, Mantel K, Hofmann U, et al: Treatment of congenital TEF by endoscopic laser coagulation: Preliminary report of 3 cases. J Pediatr Surg 26–28, 1992.
117. Kosloske AM: Azygos flap technique for reinforcement of esophageal closure. J Pediatr Surg 25:793–794, 1990.
118. Hajivassiliou CA, Davis CF, Young DG: Fiberoptic localization of the upper pouch in esophageal atresia. J Pediatr Surg 32:678–679, 1997.
119. Ty R, Brunet C, Beardmore HE: A variation in the operative technique for the treatment of esophageal atresia with tracheoesophageal fistula. J Pediatr Surg 2:118–126, 1967.
120. Touloukian RJ: Reassessment of the end-to-side operation for esophageal atresia with distal tracheoesophageal fistula: 22-year experience with 68 cases. J Pediatr Surg 27:562–567, 1992.
121. Poenaru D, LaBerge J-M, Neilson IR, et al: A more than 25-year experience with end-to-end versus end-to-side repair for esophageal atresia. J Pediatr Surg 26:472–477, 1991.
122. McCallum WA, Hannon RJ, Boston VE: Prophylactic extrapleural chest drainage following repair of esophageal atresia: Is it necessary? J Pediatr Surg 27:561, 1992.
123. Hands LJ, Dudley NE: A comparison between gap-length and Waterston classification as guides to mortality and morbidity after surgery for esophageal atresia. J Pediatr Surg 21:404–406, 1986.
124. Davenport M, Merghal M, McCloy RF, et al: Hypogastrinemia and esophageal atresia. J Pediatr Surg 27:568–571, 1992.
125. Cozzi F, Myers NA, Madonna L, et al: Esophageal atresia, choanal atresia, and dysautonomia. J Pediatr Surg 26:548–552, 1991.
126. Curci MR, Dibbins AW: Problems associated with a Nissen fundoplication following tracheoesophageal fistula and esophageal atresia repair. Arch Surg 123:618–620, 1988.
127. Johnson DG, Beasley SW: Gastro-oesophageal reflux. In Beasley SW, Myers NA, Auldist AW (eds): Oesophageal Atresia. London, Chapman and Hall, 1991.
128. Black TL, Fernandez ET, Ellis DG, et al: The effect of tube gastrostomy on gastroesophageal reflux in patients with esophageal atresia. J Pediatr Surg 26:168–170, 1991.
129. Ashcraft KW, Goodwin C, Amoury RA, et al: Early recognition and aggressive treatment of gastroesophageal reflux following repair of esophageal atresia. J Pediatr Surg 12:317–321, 1977.
130. Lindahl H, Rintola R, Sariola H: Chronic esophagitis and gastric metaplasia are frequent late complications of esophageal atresia. J Pediatr Surg 28:1178–1180, 1993.
131. Wheatley MJ, Coran AG, Wesley JR: Efficacy of the Nissen fundoplication in the management of gastroesophageal reflux following esophageal atresia repair. J Pediatr Surg 28:53–55, 1993.
132. Tovar JA, Diez-Pardo JA, Murcia J, et al: Ambulatory 24-hour manometric and pH metric evidence of permanent impairment of clearance capacity in patients with esophageal atresia. J Pediatr Surg 30:1124–1231, 1995.
133. Guo W, Fonkalsrud EW, Swaniker F, et al: Relationship of esophageal anastomotic tension to the development of gastroesophageal reflux. J Pediatr Surg 32:1337–1340, 1997.
134. Peiretti R, Shandling B, Stephens CA: Resistant esophageal stenosis associated with reflux after repair of esophageal atresia. J Pediatr Surg 9:355–357, 1974.
135. Myers NA, Beasley SW, Auldist AW: Secondary esophageal surgery following repair of esophageal atresia with distal tracheoesophageal fistula. J Pediatr Surg 25:773–777, 1990.
136. Chittmittrapap S, Spitz L, Kiely EM, et al: Anastomotic stricture following repair of esophageal atresia. J Pediatr Surg 25:508–511, 1990.

137. Snyder CL, Ramachandran V, Kennedy, AP, et al: Efficacy of partial wrap fundoplication for gastroesophageal reflux after repair of esophageal atresia. J Pediatr Surg 32:1089–1092, 1997.
138. Tam PKH, Sprigg A, Cudmore RE, et al: Endoscopy-guided balloon dilatation of esophageal strictures and anastomotic strictures after esophageal replacement in children. J Pediatr Surg 26:1101–1103, 1991.
139. Allmendinger N, Hallisey MJ, Markowitz SK, et al: Balloon dilatation of esophageal strictures in children. J Pediatr Surg 31:334–336, 1996.
140. Chittmittrapap S, Spitz L, Kiely EM, et al: Anastomotic leakage following surgery for esophageal atresia. J Pediatr Surg 27:29–32, 1992.
141. Chavin K, Field G, Chandler J, et al: Save the child's esophagus: Management of major disruption after repair of esophageal atresia. J Pediatr Surg 31:48–52, 1996.
142. Wiseman NE: Endoscopic closure of recurrent tracheoesophageal fistula using Tisseel. J Pediatr Surg 30:1236–1237, 1995.
143. Ein SH, Stringer DA, Stephens CA: Recurrent tracheoesophageal fistulas: Seventeen year review. J Pediatr Surg 18:436–441, 1983.
144. Wheatley MJ, Coran AG: Pericardial flap interposition for the definitive management of recurrent tracheoesophageal fistula. J Pediatr Surg 27:1122–1126, 1992.
145. Gutierrez C, Barrios JE, Lluna J, et al: Recurrent tracheoesophageal fistula treated with fibrin glue. J Pediatr Surg 28:1567–1569, 1994.
146. Filler RM, Rossello PJ, Lebowitz RL: Life-threatening anoxic spells caused by tracheal compression after repair of esophageal atresia: Correction by surgery. J Pediatr Surg 11:739–748, 1976.
147. Schwartz MZ, Filler RM: Tracheal compression as a cause of apnea following repair of tracheoesophageal fistula: Treatment by aortopexy. J Pediatr Surg 15:842–848, 1980.
148. Kimura K, Soper RT, Kao SCS, et al: Aortosternopexy for tracheomalacia following repair of esophageal atresia: Evaluation by cine-CT and technical refinement. J Pediatr Surg 25:769–772, 1990.
149. Applebaum H, Woolley MM: Pericardial flap aortopexy for tracheomalacia. J Pediatr Surg 25:30–32, 1990.
150. Filler RM, Messineo A, Vinograd I: Severe tracheomalacia associated with esophageal atresia: Results of surgical treatment. J Pediatr Surg 27:1136–1141, 1992.
151. Roberts CS, Othersen HB Jr, Sade RM, et al: Tracheoesophageal compression from aortic arch anomalies: Analysis of 30 operatively treated children. J Pediatr Surg 29:334–338, 1994.
152. Filston HC, Ferguson TB, Oldham HN: Airway compression by vascular anomalies. Ann Surg 205:541–549, 1987.
153. Murphy SG, Yazbeck S, Russo P: Isolated congenital esophageal stenosis. J Pediatr Surg 30:1238–1241, 1995.
154. Olguner M, Ozdemir T, Akgur FM: Congenital esophageal stenosis owing to tracheobronchial remnants: A case report. J Pediatr Surg 32:1485–1487, 1997.
155. Mahour GH, Johnston PW, Gwinn JL, et al: Congenital stenosis distal to esophageal atresia. Surgery 69:936–939, 1971.
156. Spitz L: Congenital esophageal stenosis distal to associated esophageal atresia. J Pediatr Surg 8:973–974, 1973.
157. Johnson JF, Wright DR: Chest tube perforation of esophagus following repair of esophageal atresia. J Pediatr Surg 25:1227–2130, 1990.
158. Louhimo I, Lindahl H: Esophageal atresia: Primary results of 500 consecutively treated patients. J Pediatr Surg 18:217–229, 1983.
159. Holder TM: Esophageal atresia and tracheoesophageal malformations. In Ashcraft KW, Holder TM (eds): Pediatric Surgery (2nd ed). Philadelphia, WB Saunders, 1993, pp 249–269.
160. Zaccara A, Felici F, Turchetta A, et al: Physical fitness testing in children operated on for tracheoesophageal fistula. J Pediatr Surg 30:1334–1337, 1995.
161. Lindahl H, Rintala R: Long-term complications in cases of isolated esophageal atresia treated with esophageal anastomosis. J Pediatr Surg 30:1222–1223, 1995.
162. Szold A, Udassin R, Seror D, et al: Acquired tracheoesophageal fistula in infancy and childhood. J Pediatr Surg 26:672–675, 1991.
163. DuBois JJ, Pokorny WJ, Harberg FJ, et al: Current management of laryngeal and laryngotracheoesophageal clefts. J Pediatr Surg 25:855–860, 1990.
164. Finlay H: Familial congenital stridor. Arch Dis Child 24:219–223, 1949.
165. Pettersson G: Inhibited separation of larynx and upper part of trachea from oesophagus in a newborn. Acta Chir Scand 10:250–254, 1955.
166. Ryan DP, Muehrcke DD, Doody DP, et al: Laryngotracheoesophageal cleft (type IV): Management and repair of lesions beyond the carina. J Pediatr Surg 26:962–970, 1991.
167. Robie DK, Pearl RH, Gonsales C, et al: Operative strategy for recurrent laryngeal cleft: A case report and review of the literature. J Pediatr Surg 26:971–974, 1991.
168. Donahoe PK, Gee GE: Complete laryngotracheoesophageal cleft: Management and repair. J Pediatr Surg 19:143–148, 1984.
169. Cotton RT, Myer CM, Holmes DK, et al: Laryngeal and laryngotracheoesophageal clefts: Role of early surgical repair. Ann Otol Rhinol Laryngol 99:98–104, 1990.

28

GASTROESOPHAGEAL REFLUX

Jose Boix-Ochoa, MD • Claudia Marhuenda, MD

Gastroenterologists and surgeons alike continue to be vexed by a formidable array of both clinical and basic problems in the management of infants and children with gastroesophageal reflux (GER). In the 1950s, Carré made a careful and thoughtful, albeit retrospective, study of the natural history of children with GER and came to several important conclusions.[1] First, symptoms of this condition almost invariably begin within the first 6 weeks of life. Second, 60 to 65% of such infants without treatment are essentially free of symptoms and in good health by 2 years of age. The remaining have persistent and significant symptoms until at least 4 years of age, and about 4% of the total group develop esophageal strictures. Carré estimated a mortality of 5% in those without strictures, usually from inanition or infection. The patients in this study were culled largely from referrals to three small children's hospitals between 1930 and 1950, a period in which GER was little recognized in children and treated sparingly, if at all.

Since the late 1960s, GER has increasingly been recognized as a condition that affects children frequently and, at times, with serious consequences. Until the 1990s, medical treatment was relatively ineffective, and in all likelihood most of those babies and children who did become asymptomatic were taking advantage of the natural course of the disease. This left a large number who continued to have significant, at times life-threatening, complications, and surgeons eagerly rushed to fill this void. A number of effective and safe antireflux procedures were developed during these years, and by adopting one or more of these techniques, pediatric surgeons were soon performing large numbers of such operations.[2–4] Antireflux procedures now rank second or third in frequency of major operations performed by pediatric surgeons, generally to good effect. Long-term results in several large series are excellent, and complications are relatively few.[5–7] However, significant complications and failures do occur, and long-term results, although generally good, are by no means perfect.

At least two major advances in management are changing the therapeutic scenario in GER. First, of most importance, the proton pump inhibitor omeprazole has revolutionized medical treatment. This drug cures esophagitis with an effectiveness that is truly amazing in comparison with antacids, histamine-receptor antagonists, and motility-enhancing drugs. Second, antireflux operations are being performed laparoscopically in increasing numbers. Although not a fundamental change in concept, this technique shows considerable promise in terms of reducing both short-term postoperative morbidity and long-term complications such as intestinal obstruction.

In addition to these clinical advances, basic investigations have focused on mechanisms of reflux and emphasized the cause of reflux itself and the patterns and effectiveness of esophageal clearance. Much information has come from studies of lower esophageal pressure profiles in normal human beings and in patients with reflux esophagitis.[8, 9] A sophisticated manometric assembly with a sleeve sensor plus an esophageal pH electrode was used for these studies, permitting concomitant recordings of both pressure and acidity. A wide variation in the basal lower esophageal sphincter (LES) pressures was found that bore little relationship to reflux, refuting the widely held concept of a direct relationship between a low basal LES and reflux. Instead, reflux occurred most often during periods of inappropriate, complete LES relaxation. These relaxations were inappropriate in the sense that they were not secondary to esophageal peristalsis initiated by pharyngeal swallowing.

These findings have been confirmed, and the proposition that such inappropriate LES relaxations are the primary mechanism leading to reflux has been widely adopted. Additional research using similar technical approaches has expanded our knowledge of esophageal peristalsis, normal and abnormal; the role of the diaphragm in prevention of reflux; and the unsolved question of delayed gastric emptying (DGE) as important factors in this knotty puzzle. Our understanding of the multiple and complex factors controlling the esophagogastric junction has increased remarkably but remains far from complete.

☐ The Barrier

LOWER ESOPHAGEAL SPHINCTER

In 1956, as a result of the development of esophageal manometry, a high-pressure zone (HPZ) near the esophagogastric junction was described. A sphincter muscle in the lower esophagus was proposed as the mechanism for maintaining this pressure.[10] The problem with this attractive hypothesis is that there is no such anatomic structure or at least not one that can reasonably fulfill its proposed role. Meticulous dissections of the esophagus and stomach in 32 cadavers revealed an oblique gastroesophageal ring caused by a meager increase in muscle mass.[11] This ring angled upward from the lesser to the greater curvature and tapered for a few millimeters both upward toward the proximal esophagus and downward toward the stomach. This asymmetric muscle thickening is unimpressive both grossly and on microscopic examination, and it cannot reasonably account for the overall remarkable efficiency of the antireflux mechanism. Nonetheless, a well-defined HPZ does exist in the lower esophagus, referred to as the *LES*.

The propagation of esophageal peristalsis normally begins in the pharynx, progressing down the esophagus and producing, at the appropriate time, relaxation of the LES.[12] This relaxation is brief, but the mechanism results in effective and rapid passage of ingested food and saliva from the pharynx to the stomach. Presumably, afferent and efferent vagal neural pathways controlled by brain stem nuclei mediate this sequence of events.[13] The cause of the HPZ remains conjectural, but it is unlikely to be solely the result of a true muscle sphincter.[11] Patients who have had surgical removal of the distal esophagus (esophagogastrectomy) have, in manometric studies, an HPZ at the thoracoabdominal junction that relaxes on swallowing and increases with a rise in intraabdominal pressure.[14]

THE ANGLE OF HIS

The esophagus enters the stomach obliquely, forming a flap valve known as the *angle of His*. Postmortem studies demonstrated a pressure gradient across the gastroesophageal junction so that filling the stomach with water did not result in reflux into the esophagus.[15] If the angle of His was unfolded, reflux resulted. Exaggerating the angle of His increased the pressure gradient. Surgical excision of the gastric fundus in two monkeys eliminated the angle of His, but the monkeys, which did not reflux preoperatively, did not reflux after the operation, and the mean pressures in the HPZs did not

change.[16] The conclusion is that the angle of His was not an important antireflux mechanism. There remains, however, the general belief that in human beings, the angle of His plays an important role in the prevention of reflux.

LENGTH OF THE INTRAABDOMINAL ESOPHAGUS

Manometric techniques[17] were used to measure the length of the abdominal segment of the esophagus, and 24-hour pH monitoring was conducted in 266 patients with symptoms indicating possible GER. There was a direct relationship between the length of the intraabdominal esophagus and reflux. Only 38% of patients whose abdominal esophagus measured 3 cm or more refluxed, whereas 81% of those whose abdominal esophagus measured 1 cm or less refluxed. In vitro studies[18] have been conducted to determine the effect on competency of both the HPZ and the length of abdominal esophagus. An intraabdominal segment of 3 to 4.5 cm provided 100% LES competency at normal intraabdominal pressure (10 cm H_2O). Shorter lengths of intraabdominal esophagus maintained competency as intraabdominal pressure decreased. Finally, a negative intrathoracic pressure of 6 cm H_2O further improved competency at any given length of intraabdominal esophagus.

These elegant clinical and laboratory studies convincingly demonstrate the critical importance of intraabdominal esophageal length. In the one study,[18] gastroesophageal competency also improved with increases in lower esophageal pressure. For example, the 24-hour pH reflux test was abnormal in only 17.6% of those with LES pressures of 30 mm Hg or higher, but the same test was abnormal in 83.3% of those with LES pressures between 0 and 5 mg Hg. Additional studies from the same laboratory were conducted in an effort to correlate pressure in the HPZ and the length of intraabdominal esophagus.[19] A minimum pressure and a minimum length were required to prevent reflux. Reflux occurred either with a low LES pressure (0 to 5 mm Hg) or a short length of intraabdominal esophagus (<1 cm). The demonstration that low pressures may exist with an adequate length of intraabdominal esophagus discounts the direct relationship between pressure and length. This study showed that the length and pressure factors were not precisely additive, but there was an interaction effect. Surgical procedures should attempt to correct both deficiencies.

Another study of the role of the intraabdominal esophagus was novel. Esophagogastrectomies were performed in three nonrefluxing monkeys with restoration of continuity by a gastric tube.[16] Restudy with manometry after operation showed HPZs comparable with preoperative levels. In addition, relaxation of the HPZs occurred with swallowing, and reflux did not occur.

ESOPHAGEAL CLEARANCE

Although perhaps not directly involved with the antireflux barrier, prompt and efficient clearing of the esophagus by normal peristalsis is clearly necessary to avoid prolonged contact between the vulnerable esophageal mucosa and gastric contents. The sophistication and reliability of esophageal manometry have increased greatly with the modifications and the miniaturization of the manometric assemblies.[20] We now know that essentially normal esophageal peristalsis occurs in healthy preterm and term babies.[20] These patterns were found in premature newborns as young as 33 weeks' postconceptual age. Pharyngeal swallowing produced esophageal contractions 95% of the time, and of these, 70% were peristaltic and propulsive. In both infants and children, peristaltic waves ranged from 2 to 6 seconds in all age groups.[21] In newborns and infants (14 days to 11 months of age) with gentle regurgitation and with normal growth, peristaltic waves following swallowing were comparable with those of nonregurgitating infants in terms of duration, pressure, and progression.

A study of infants with significant reflux, however, shows a different picture. Thirty-four infants were evaluated for possible GER.[22] Peristalsis was normal in those with vomiting but who were otherwise healthy. In those with failure to thrive or recurrent pulmonary disease, the amplitude of the peristaltic waves was significantly reduced and the frequency of nonperistaltic contractions was significantly increased.

In another study of 60 children with documented reflux, both the frequency of propulsive peristaltic waves and their mean pressure were significantly lower than in normal controls.[23] In addition, nonpropulsive waves were more frequent. In a series of 58 adults with abnormal gastroesophageal reflux disease documented by 24-hour pH monitoring, esophageal motor function was studied by the technique of 24-hour ambulatory esophageal manometry.[24, 25] A defective LES was defined by a low basal pressure (<6 mm Hg), overall sphincter length shorter than 2 cm, or abdominal esophageal length shorter than 1 cm. Thirty-six of the 58 adults had defective LESs. Those patients with severe esophageal mucosal disease (esophagitis, stricture, Barrett's esophagus) showed impaired esophageal peristalsis that increased with the severity of the mucosal injury. Rarely was impairment of esophageal peristalsis found in the patients who had defective LESs but normal esophageal mucosa. The histology of resected esophageal specimens that were removed owing to stricture or Barrett's esophagus revealed both increased submucosal collagen and replacement of muscularis propria by collagen in comparison with specimens examined at autopsy from patients without esophageal disease. The investigators feel that the impaired peristalsis with defective clearance is caused by injury to the esophageal wall. Patients with reflux and esophagitis were compared with normal patients without reflux and to patients with reflux without mucosal inflammation.[26] The amplitude of peristaltic waves was lower in the esophagitis patients, and the degree of lowering increased with the severity of the esophagitis.

Esophageal peristalsis was studied in 27 infants with reflux, 3 to 20 months of age, by dividing the patients into those with esophagitis and those without.[27] Those with esophagitis had significantly lower amplitude of esophageal peristalsis than those with reflux alone, and nonspecific motor defects were more frequent in the first group. Most of the reflux episodes in both groups resulted from inappropriate (i.e., not associated with swallowing) relaxations of the LES, and this mechanism was more frequent in those with esophagitis.

Thus, impaired esophageal peristalsis clearly is a feature of those patients with reflux complicated by esophagitis alone or with progression to stricture or Barrett's esophagus. Whether the impairment of motor function of the esophagus is a primary element of the disease or is secondary to acid reflux is not clear, but the available evidence weighs in favor of a secondary phenomenon.

DIAPHRAGMATIC ROLE

In 1958, a comprehensive study of esophageal motility regarded the contraction of the diaphragmatic crura around the lower esophagus as an important and essential element of the antireflux barrier.[28] With the development of esophageal manometry and the demonstration of an esophageal HPZ (sphincter), this concept fell out of favor. A much more recent study reported observations of diaphragmatic activity in an elegant experimental study using cats.[29] Intrinsic pressure in the lower esophageal area corresponded to end-expiratory pressure during normal breathing (when abdominal pressure is at its lowest level). There were considerable oscillations of LES pressure that were the result of diaphragmatic activity. The frequency of these oscillations corresponded to the respiratory rate, and the highest LES pressure occurred at end inspiration, a time corresponding to peak diaphragmatic electromyographic activity. The researchers concluded that the degree of electrical activity of the diaphragm directly corresponded with the magnitude of the pressure oscillations. They theorized that because the largest gradient for reflux occurred at end inspiration and because the diaphragmatic pinch is maximal at that point, the diaphragm probably is an important factor in the antireflux barrier. They also speculated that deficiencies in this diaphragmatic activity could explain the high incidence of reflux found with chronic pulmonary diseases.

Normal human volunteers were studied using electrophysiologic techniques that focused on pressure profiles at the esophagogastric junction and the location of the LES.[30] The researchers found that the lower half of the LES is in the abdomen and that the crural diaphragm surrounds the upper half of the sphincter. The position of the crura obviously is advantageous to any antireflux actions it may have. Pressure measurements of the lower esophagus and electromyograms of the crural diaphragm were done at three periods: end expiration, 100% diaphragmatic contraction, and 50% contraction. The data from these measurements permitted conclusions that end-expiratory esophagogastric junction pressure is due to the LES, but during periods of diaphragmatic contraction, a major portion of the pressure peak results from the pinchcock crural action.

Contractions of the crural diaphragm are related to the esophagogastric pressure. These contractions correspond to respirations, and the pressure increases to a maximum during inspiration.[13] Paralysis of skeletal muscle abolishes this increase.[29] Activities that increase intraabdominal pressure result in sustained contraction of the crura and contribute to elevated pressures at the esophagogastric junction. The crura alone probably are responsible for the HPZ following esophagogastrectomies.[14]

DELAYED GASTRIC EMPTYING

A lot of attention and an equal amount of controversy since the late 1970s have centered on the role of DGE in GER. In a study of the patterns of reflux, patients who had reflux in the upright position tended to have their reflux episodes within 2 hours after a meal.[31] A radionuclide gastric emptying study in one of these patients showed significant DGE. The authors thought that pylorospasm might account for this delay, and this delay combined with active gastric contractions could raise intragastric pressure above distal esophageal pressure and result in reflux. A follow-up on this observation studied 15 patients with symptoms suggestive of GER.[32] Of the 15 patients, 12 had reflux using 24-hour pH monitoring, and 8 of the 12 had esophagitis on endoscopy. Gastric emptying was normal in those with reflux but without esophagitis and in the controls, but those with esophagitis had significant DGE. The researchers also found that reflux episodes in those with esophagitis were significantly more numerous than in those without it.

The techniques and clinical usefulness of radionuclides in the study of gastric emptying revealed that studies with radionuclide techniques showed DGE in more than 40% of patients with GER.[33] Gastric emptying in patients with reflux was studied before and after fundoplications.[34] With both liquid and solid meals, gastric emptying was significantly more rapid 6 months after fundoplication than preoperatively.

Studies have shown DGE of water in children with GER,[35] but other studies have found no significant differences in gastric emptying (using apple juice as the vehicle for the radionuclide marker) between patients with and without reflux.[36] In a separate study, the latter investigators focused on the relationship of gastric emptying to retching

symptoms occurring following antireflux surgery.[37] This proved complex. Twelve of the 66 children studied had persistent retching, and 6 of the 12 also had dumping symptoms. Those with postoperative retching and dumping had an increased effective gastric emptying; those with retching alone had decreased effective gastric emptying. Of those with decreased effective gastric emptying preoperatively, only 13% developed postoperative retching. With normal values of effective gastric emptying preoperatively, later retching is unlikely.

Experience with a large group of children treated surgically for GER has advocated pyloroplasty in conjunction with fundoplication when preoperative DGE is found.[5] In a review of 420 children treated surgically, the conclusion was that reflux and DGE were often a part of a more generalized intestinal motor disorder. Some 50% of children with symptoms of reflux also have DGE, and this percentage is much higher in those with severe mental impairment. In this report, 60 of the last 275 children who had a fundoplication also had a pyloroplasty. There were no leaks and no anastomotic obstructions in those who had pyloroplasty added and, of particular importance, no instances of persistent dumping. Again, the high risk of DGE with refluxing children who have serious mental retardation is emphasized.[38]

Evaluation of gastric emptying in 99 children with GER revealed 28 with DGE.[39] Of the 28, 21 had a gastric drainage procedure at the time of the antireflux procedure. None of these 21 had complications attributable to the drainage operation, but no mention is given of dumping symptoms. All 7 who did not have a drainage operation developed symptoms including gas bloat, gagging, and feeding difficulties. Two had a slipped or failed fundoplication and these 2, plus another 3, improved after a secondary gastric drainage procedure. Of the patients with DGE, 75% were neurologically impaired (NI).

Some reported findings in NI children with GER are totally at variance to the above.[40] Forty such patients with DGE had either fundoplication and pyloroplasty (n = 21) or fundoplication alone (n = 19). No differences between the two groups were found in incidence of recurrent symptoms, readmissions, or reoperations. Those with added pyloroplasty had significantly more postoperative complications. Another group of 58 NI children with reflux who underwent fundoplications were studied for gastric emptying preoperatively and were divided into those with DGE (n = 29) and those without DGE (n = 29). No postoperative differences in feeding tolerance, complications, or recurrent symptoms were noted; understandably, the authors of this report felt that pyloroplasty added no benefit for these children. Another retrospective study in refluxing children with neurologic disorders confirmed that pyloroplasty was of little benefit.[41]

A recently reported group of 67 children with proven GER had gastric emptying studies using radionuclide-labeled milk prior to antireflux operations.[42] In 17 with preoperative DGE, the gastric emptying became normal postoperatively, whereas 14 of the 50 with normal gastric emptying preoperatively showed DGE afterward. Because there was no way to predict which patients with normal gastric emptying preoperatively would show DGE postoperatively and because the large majority of those with DGE preoperatively demonstrate normal gastric emptying afterward, a gastric drainage operation at the time of the antireflux procedure was not felt to be warranted.

Clearly, this issue remains unsettled. Because an antireflux operation often results in more rapid gastric emptying and because many children with DGE revert to normal gastric emptying patterns following antireflux procedures, perhaps it is reasonable to delay a decision to perform a gastric drainage procedure until after the antireflux operation.

□ Breaking the Barrier

Why does GER occur? Until the 1980s, the fault was believed to be low basal pressures in the LES. On average, the basal pressure of the LES is lower in refluxing patients than in normal individuals, but there is a great deal of overlap. Surprisingly, GER is not uncommonly associated with a hypertensive LES.[43] In a study of asymptomatic people using combined continuous recordings of the esophageal pH and pressure, wide variations were found in basal lower esophageal pressures, and reflux was unrelated to the basal pressures.[8] Reflux did occur during transient drops in pressure (sphincter relaxations) not coincident with swallowing (Fig. 28–1). These inappropriate, transient LES relaxations (TLESR) occurred spontaneously or immediately following the brief period of normal relaxation stimulated by swallowing. Most of the episodes of reflux occurred within 3 hours after eating. Extending these studies to patients with symptomatic GER, more than 80%

of reflux episodes occurred during periods of TLESR.[44] Absent basal lower esophageal pressure became a significant mechanism with increasingly severe esophagitis and was associated with 23% of GER episodes in the study group with most severe esophagitis. Absence of basal lower esophageal pressure was invariably intermittent, but during periods of detectable LES pressure, episodes of reflux continued to occur due to TLESR.

These same monitoring techniques were used to study 29 children (ages 5 days to 2 years) with symptoms suggesting reflux.[45] Wide variations in lower esophageal pressures occurred over 10 to 15 minutes, ranging from 3 to 60 mm Hg, with a mean of approximately 19 mm Hg. Episodes of reflux rarely correlated with low basal LES pressures. Transient increases in intraabdominal pressure (spontaneous or induced by stress) accounted for 54% of reflux episodes, and TLESR accounted for 34%. These latter relaxations lasted 5 to 25 seconds with reflux occurring during total LES relaxation. In a later study of another group of children with reflux using esophageal pH and pressure monitoring, all patients without esophagitis and 77% of those with esophagitis had reflux episodes secondary to TLESR.[46] The remaining 23% of reflux events in those with esophagitis occurred during gradual downward drifts of LES pressure to 0. No detectable reflux occurred during the brief periods of LES relaxation related to swallowing with a normal peristaltic sequence. TLESR episodes have also been found to be the predominant mechanism of GER in 94% of premature infants.[20]

Much better data appear to be coming from the technique of continuous manometry as opposed to the pull-through method. A sleeve sensor device, which reliably measures basal sphincter pressures despite small changes in sphincter positions, is the essential feature of this method.[47] Furthermore, the assemblies can be miniaturized so that use in newborn and even premature infants is practical.

Recognition of TLESR, rather than low basal LES, as the primary mechanism of reflux clearly is a major step in our understanding of this disease. In TLESR, the drop in pressure is abrupt and profound and lasts, on average, considerably longer than the normal LES pressure drops associated with swallowing. Furthermore, and of significance, TLESR is not associated with a peristaltic wave effective in esophageal clearance; the esophageal mucosa is exposed to the noxious effects of acid gastric contents for relatively long periods. Nonetheless, the previously described parts of the antireflux barrier remain essential to the prevention of reflux, whatever the exact causative mechanism of the reflux episodes may be. Hence therapy, medical or surgical, must continue to address and correct, whenever possible, the deficiencies in the antireflux barrier mechanism.

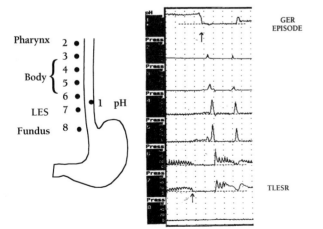

Figure 28–1. Abrupt LES relaxation not preceded by swallowing and resulting in a fall in esophageal pH in transient lower esophageal sphincter relaxation (TLESR). GER, gastroesophageal reflux; LES, lower esophageal sphincter relaxation. (Manometric trace courtesy of Prof. S. Cucchiara, University of Naples.)

□ Clinical Manifestations

Regurgitation is, by far, the most common symptom of GER in infancy. A distinctive type of regurgitation begins early in infancy, usually within the 1st week of life. The regurgitation usually is effortless and occurs with burping or when the infant is returned to his or her crib after feeding. The vomitus does not contain blood or bile. This type of vomiting, termed *chalasia*, is benign, self-limited, and rarely requires more than the simplest of treatment.[48] Occasionally, however, the regurgitation or vomiting is forceful or even projectile so that other causes, such as pyloric stenosis, must be considered. Most babies with such vomiting grow normally and do not develop other complications. Carré's study of the natural history of refluxing infants found that almost two thirds were asymptomatic by 2 years of age without treatment and that most improved before or at the time of weaning to solid foods.[1] Vomiting of this character may be considered physiologic and requires little in terms of either diagnosis or treatment.

Still, a considerable number of vomiting infants develop significant problems. Some fail to thrive and become malnourished due to the vomiting. Others refuse feedings; perhaps swallowing is painful because of esophagitis.[49] Irritability is another symptom, which, like refusal to eat, may be secondary to esophagitis and its associated discomfort. Respiratory symptoms are particularly important in babies with GER and range from coughing, wheezing, or stridor secondary to aspiration to acute life-threatening respiratory events such as apnea and near-miss sudden infant death syndrome (SIDS).[50, 51] Because many respiratory symptoms in infants obviously arise from other sources, primarily the lungs, the causal relationship between such symptoms and GER is essential to determine prior to surgical treatment.[52, 53] Gross aspiration of gastric contents obviously can produce pneumonia, but this mechanism is rare with GER. Microaspiration with acidification of the trachea is more common, leading to laryngospasm or bronchospasm. Spasm of the larynx and bronchi may also be caused by gastric acid stimulation of vagal afferents in the esophageal wall. Esophagitis probably enhances this mechanism.[50, 52]

The effects of GER on premature infants with respiratory problems have been studied.[54] Most of these infants were intubated for varying periods owing to respiratory distress syndrome or bronchopulmonary dysplasia. In the former group, GER was responsible for deteriorating pulmonary status requiring reintubation. In the latter, deterioration of pulmonary status plus failure to thrive and anorexia led to the diagnosis of GER. All improved with correction of the GER.

In children, in contrast to infants, regurgitation is less frequently seen, and the symptoms of esophagitis predominate, as with adults. Heartburn, or substernal pain, is common. The pain is increased with acid juices and relieved by antacids. There may be pain on swallowing. Some of the children also complain of dysphagia. The esophagitis may progress to stricture with severe obstructive symptoms in addition to pain. Carré's long-term study of untreated children found that about 4% developed strictures.[1] With better management, that figure is now substantially lower.

Barrett's esophagus denotes a condition of metaplasia of the squamous epithelium of the lower esophagus with replacement by columnar epithelium. Chronic injury by reflux of gastric contents onto the esophageal epithelium is thought to be responsible. Although Barrett's esophagus does not produce specific symptoms, the condition is serious owing to the potential complications of stricture, ulcer, and adenocarcinoma. More than half of the children have associated strictures.[55, 56] Neither the response to treatment nor the risk of carcinoma in these children is as yet clearly defined. These children are obviously at high risk, and vigorous treatment to control or eradicate the reflux plus long-term surveillance is imperative.

The child with Sandifer's syndrome moves his or her head, neck, and sometimes upper trunk into strange and contorted positions. Torticollis without spasm of the neck muscles is common. The neck may be extended or twisted. The movements may be more striking with eating but cease with sleep. This syndrome, although rare, is associated with GER.[57] Owing to dystonia and bizarre posturing of the head, neck, and back, some children may be misdiagnosed as having a neurologic or even a psychiatric disturbance when the problem is GER and the solution is appropriate management of the reflux.[58]

☐ Diagnosis

Diagnostic procedures other than clinical evaluation should be used when the results will strongly influence treatment or will identify complications. For the infant with frequent regurgitation but who is thriving and is otherwise well, none are needed.

RADIOLOGIC EXAMINATION

When the diagnosis of obstruction is considered or when complications of GER are present, a barium study of the esophagus, stomach, and duodenum is appropriate. In expert hands, the diagnosis of reflux itself is made with a high degree of accuracy. A skilled, experienced radiologist is essential. Associated abnormalities are relatively uncommon, but conditions such as hiatal hernia, pyloric obstruction, malrotation, or some other anatomic lesion responsible for vomiting can occasionally be clearly identified. The barium study provides important anatomic information not available by other tests. However, the study is rarely useful for quantitation of the reflux. The radiologist can also evaluate the esophagus with respect to possible structural or mucosal irregularities. Esophageal peristalsis also may be usefully evaluated together with an estimation of the efficiency of esophageal clearance. Owing to the inert nature of the barium meal, the study does not permit a critical evaluation of gastric emptying.

SCINTIGRAPHY

This technique, using a technetium isotope, would appear to have a number of advantages. Reflux is accurately demonstrated. The study can be prolonged for perhaps an hour until the isotope has left the stomach, thus permitting images to be taken while the infant is quiet and undisturbed. It can be used with meals or formulas that neutralize gastric acidity, an advantage over pH monitoring in this circumstance. Some measure of esophageal clearance is possible. Evaluation of aspiration by detection of the isotope in the lungs would be a major contribution from the technique, but, unfortunately, its sensitivity for this purpose is low.[59, 60] The technique is of use in measuring gastric emptying.

24-HOUR ESOPHAGEAL PH MONITORING

This technique was developed in the early 1970s for use in adults,[61] but it was soon adapted for children.[62, 63] A pH electrode of appropriate size is positioned transnasally at the junction of the middle and lower thirds of the esophagus (usually 2.5–3 cm above the LES). The pH is continuously measured and recorded either on a strip chart or by a computerized pH recorder. A pH of 4.0 or less denotes reflux of acid gastric contents. The frequency and duration of reflux episodes are recorded. The number of such episodes longer than 5 minutes, the longest episode, and the percentage of time with pH less than 4.0 are also determined. Finally, with the help of a parent or nurse, the relationship of reflux to a variety of activities is noted: sleeping, position, eating, and symptoms. Normal values have been determined, and a number of patterns of reflux have been demonstrated.[64–66] In the past, the study usually was performed in the hospital, but many are now being done quite satisfactorily at home. The test is the most reliable study available for finding occult episodes of reflux and for correlating reflux and symptoms.[63] The percentage of time the pH is under 4.0 (reflux index) is clinically useful as well as reliable with a sensitivity and specificity of 94% or more.[64]

The 24-hour pH monitoring study is indicated in the following several specific circumstances:

1. Infants who have respiratory symptoms (apnea, near-miss SIDS)
2. Infants who are irritable, intractably crying, and anorectic
3. Children who have reactive airway disease (asthma) or unexplained or recurrent pneumonia
4. Children who are unresponsive to medical measures and in whom the role of GER in their symptoms is uncertain

Also, the study should be done in those children who again become symptomatic after fundoplication. On the other hand, the study generally is not useful or necessary for infants with uncomplicated regurgitation, children with esophagitis already found by endoscopy and biopsy, and children with dysphagia or heartburn thought to be caused by GER. Three patterns of reflux have been described in symptomatic infants as determined by extended esophageal pH monitoring[64]: continuous, discontinuous, and mixed. Those infants with the discontinuous type rarely required a surgical antireflux operation, whereas approximately half of those with the other two types did. One should keep in mind that medical treatment at the time of this study was much less effective than in the late 1990s. Nonetheless, this study indicates that pH monitoring can be useful in sorting out infants with GER who may or may not require an antireflux procedure. Incidentally, all of the infants in this study, including normal controls, refluxed frequently in the first 2 hours following feeding (apple juice for this study).

ENDOSCOPY AND BIOPSY

Suspicion of esophagitis is the prime indication for this diagnostic technique. Irritability and anorexia in infants and heartburn or upper abdominal pain in children raise this suspicion. Dysphagia is another indication. The study is of particular value in NI children with vomiting, growth failure, and other confusing symptoms. The endoscopist may be unable to discern esophagitis on gross inspection.[67, 68] One study recorded abnormal mucosa in only 52% of children with documented reflux.[69] When the study did show inflammation, however, the finding was 100% specific, and in none of the nonrefluxing patients was mucosal inflammation found. Owing to the lack of sensitivity of esophagoscopy alone, mucosal biopsies are essential. Biopsies and microscopic diagnoses are both highly specific and sensitive (95%) in the diagnosis of esophagitis.[69, 70] The histologic criteria for esophagitis on biopsy examination are well established. Intraepithelial inflammatory cells, eosinophils particularly, plus morphometric measures of basal cell layer thickness and papillary height are highly specific for esophagitis. Clearly, the biopsy diagnosis of esophagitis is a most important finding because it demands prompt and vigorous treatment.

Esophagoscopy shows other esophageal abnormalities as well, particularly ulcer, stricture, and Barrett's esophagus. All three are severe complications of long-standing reflux and often coexist. Combining 35 patients from three separate studies on Barrett's esophagus in children, 16 strictures were identified.[71–73] The endoscopist often does not recognize the characteristic pink-red velvety appearance of Barrett's esophagus, emphasizing the importance of biopsies. The typical gross appearance of Barrett's esophagus at endoscopy occurs in only a minority of patients; the diagnosis rests on histologic biopsy examinations.[72, 73] Three types of metaplastic columnar epithelium may be identified: cardiac, fundic, and intestinal. There does appear to be some correlation between the type of columnar epithelium found and the potential for dysplasia or carcinoma.[74]

In addition to esophagitis and its complications, esophagoscopy also may show isolated patches of gastric epithelium, thought to be of congenital origin, in the proximal esophagus. Postoperative complications of repaired esophageal atresia, such as stricture or recurrent fistula, may be visualized.

MANOMETRY

Manometry is responsible for much of our knowledge concerning GER. Maturation of the LES in early infancy was first demonstrated by this technique, only to be disputed later with the advent of more sophisticated micromanometric assemblies.[4, 47] The crucial importance of TLESR to reflux changed our entire concept of the cause of GER.[8] The technique demonstrates normal and abnormal patterns of esophageal peristalsis and clearance. Pharyngeal swallowing has been shown to be the primary factor in clearing refluxed gastric fluid in the esophagus by a study using esophageal pH monitoring in conjunction with manometry.[12] Development of smaller and more sophisticated pressure transducers and recording devices has permitted 24-hour esophageal motility monitoring on an ambulatory basis. With this method, deterioration of esophageal motility has been shown to parallel increasing degrees of esophagitis secondary to reflux in adults, and its use will surely be extended to children.[75]

There is clearly a considerable potential for manometry in evaluating children with GER, but at the moment it has limited clinical roles. It cannot directly detect reflux or injury to esophageal mucosa. It does have a role in the child with a repaired esophageal atresia who develops reflux.[76] The lower esophagus in such a child characteristically has poor and disorganized peristalsis, and such an impairment is a major factor in determining treatment.

☐ Treatment

MEDICAL THERAPY

The age of the patient and the presence or absence of complications of the disease are the main determinants of treatment. Vomiting beginning in the 1st week of life characteristically is effortless, usually occurs when the infant is placed in the recumbent position after feeding, and is relieved by placing the infant in the upright position.[48] Ordinarily, there is complete and permanent relief of this reflux chalasia within a few weeks. Progressive maturation of the LES may explain the generally benign course of vomiting in these babies.[77]

Despite the effect of gravity, reflux episodes of infants in the widely used "chalasia chair" increased by four times as compared with infants lying prone.[78] Currently, the position recommended for treatment of GER is prone with the head elevated about 30 degrees.[79] Such postural therapy is not without its problems. The infant must be secured in this position so that he or she does not slide down or turn sideways. Furthermore, the prone position has been suggested as a risk factor in SIDS, although no direct causal relationship has been shown.[80] Positional therapy is effective and remains as adjunctive therapy when other measures are ineffective or the infant is beyond the age of risk for SIDS.[79]

Dietary modifications are traditional measures and often appear more helpful than they are. Frequent feedings usually are not practical for either the babies or their parents. Thickening the feedings is effective in reducing vomiting in infants.[81] Rice cereal, oatmeal, and barley can be used for this purpose. GER itself is probably not affected.

With respect to pharmacologic therapy, antacids, H2-receptor antagonists, prokinetic agents, and proton pump inhibitors are options. Antacids are effective in buffering gastric acid and may have some role in treating older children. There has been little experience with their use in infants largely owing to difficulties in the timing of administration and of side effects. H2-receptor antagonists, particularly ranitidine, are widely used and are effective in the therapy of esophagitis. These drugs increase gastric pH and reduce gastric output.[82] Ranitidine has been shown to heal esophagitis.[83]

Prokinetic agents act by increasing LES tone and improving both esophageal peristalsis and gastric emptying. Cisapride is now the drug of choice in this category because it not only is effective but also is almost completely free from serious side effects.[84] Lately, some serious side effects (cardiac arrythmia and death) have been reported in adults who were receiving cisapride. These are supposed to be produced by overdosage. The drug has been found to increase the amplitude of peristaltic contractions, increase LES pressure, and hasten gastric emptying. A significant reduction in reflux time also has been noted, and mild to moderate degrees of esophagitis are improved with its use. It also has been effective in minimizing respiratory symptoms in children with cystic fibrosis.[85, 86] Unfortunately, none of the above medications have been shown to be consistently effective in severe GER.

Omeprazole, a proton pump (or acid pump) inhibitor, is the most exciting drug to emerge for the treatment of severe GER in children. Following reports of its successful use in adults, a study was conducted in 15 children with GER complicated by esophagitis.[87] All had failed treatment with H2-receptor antagonists and prokinetic agents, and 8 were NI. Following omeprazole therapy, all showed remarkable clinical improvement. After 6 months of omeprazole therapy, the esophagitis, which had been grade 3 to 4 in most, improved to grade 0 to 1 by endoscopy and biopsy.

In another study, 22 children with GER refractory to ranitidine and cisapride were given an 8-week course of omeprazole. Improvement in symptoms occurred and endoscopy revealed healing or marked improvement in the mucosal damage.[88] However, the rate of TLESR and LES pressure drifts were not effected. Omeprazole acts by reducing gastric acidity, not by changing the mechanisms of reflux. The potency of the drug in healing esophagitis outstrips, by far, any other pharmacologic therapy introduced to date.

The dismal record of medical management of severe, complicated GER disease in children prior to omeprazole made operative therapy the only reasonable option.[89] This drug, however, has been shown to be safe and effective in the treatment of severe GER disease that has not responded to other medical therapy and that may even have failed antireflux surgery. Advocates of omeprazole therapy are critical of surgeons in terms of reporting the results of antireflux surgery and believe that patients with severe disease deserve analysis separate from those

patients with milder forms. Both fundoplication and omeprazole should be reserved for children with truly severe GER disease. Omeprazole is a reasonable choice for those who have failed antireflux surgery or who have major risk factors for surgical failure. Surgical treatment should be reserved for those who will need a lifetime of treatment and who have the greatest opportunity for surgical success.

SURGICAL THERAPY

There are several operations with proven success managing significant GER. Little difference among them is apparent in overall effectiveness. The principles of surgical procedures for GER include the following:

1. Lengthening of the intraabdominal esophagus
2. Accentuation of the angle of His
3. Increase in the pressure barrier at the esophagogastric junction
4. Approximation of the crura

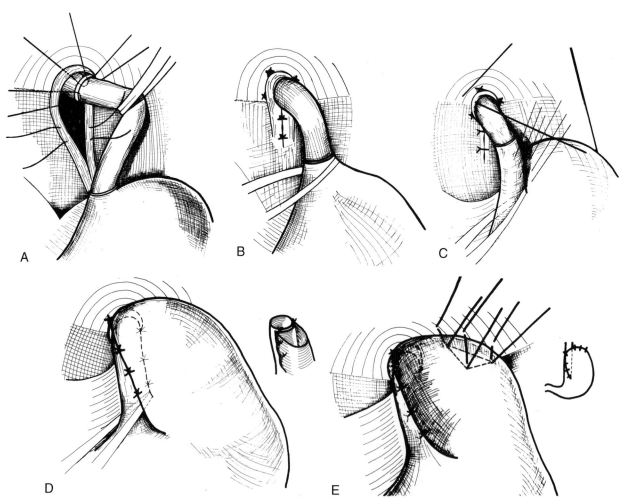

Figure 28–2. Boix-Ochoa technique. *A* and *B*, After exposure and mobilization of the distal esophagus, it is anchored to the hiatal crura to ensure as long an intraabdominal segment of esophagus as possible. The posterior pillars are closed. *C*, Restoration of the angle of His by a suture from the fundus to the right crura. *D*, The anterior plication is constructed by placing sutures between the gastric fundus and the intraabdominal esophagus. *E*, Three sutures, which suspend the fundus superiorly, are placed between the fundus and the undersurface of the left diaphragm.

The technique we prefer at the Children's Hospital in Barcelona aims to restore the normal anatomic relationships and physiologic characteristics of the lower esophageal mechanism. A length of lower esophagus is mobilized adequate for intraabdominal location, approximation of the crura posterior to the esophagus restores the size of the hiatus to normal, the esophagus is sutured to the hiatus, and a normal angle of His is created by a suture from the fundus at the level of the highest short gastric artery to the right rim of the esophageal hiatus. Sutures between the fundus and the right wall of the esophagus maintain an anterior fundoplication. Finally, the superior edge of the fundus is attached with sutures to the adjacent diaphragm to the left of the hiatus. This last step unfolds or opens up the fundus like an umbrella (Fig. 28–2A–E). By this procedure, intragastric pressure is transmitted to the intraabdominal esophagus. Additionally, unfolding the fundus buffers the effect of raised intragastric pressure (Fig. 28–3). The results of this procedure followed from 6 months to 20 years in 215 patients have been generally excellent. There are 88.4% good results. There are only 3 (1.4%) wrap failures, 10 (4.7%) who have recurrent symptoms and GER, and 12 (5.6%) who are asymptomatic but have radiologic recurrence. These results should be somewhat tempered by the fact that only 4 of the children were NI.

The Nissen fundoplication has been used much more frequently than any other operation. The lower esophagus is mobilized so that an adequate intraabdominal length is assured. By passing the fundus from left to right behind the esophagus, a 360-degree wrap is performed. This usually requires division of at least some of the short gastric vessels. The right and left margins of the wrap are sutured together anteriorly; these sutures include the anterior esophageal wall. The superior margin of the wrap is fixed to the hiatus with a few additional sutures. The wrap should be relatively short (depending on the age of the child) and constructed loosely (floppy). The wrap transmits intragastric pressure to the lower esophagus, raises the LES pressure, and acts as an effective one-way valve. A gastrostomy is often added for a vent in case the child develops gas bloat or for feedings. It is almost routinely added in NI children. Early postoperative complications are uncommon.[90, 91] Small bowel obstruction has been reported in 4 to 9% in the first 2 years after operation.[92–94] Most of these resulted from intraabdominal adhesions. A more significant problem is failure of the wrap, occurring in from 4 to 12% in the larger series.[92, 95–97] These failures usually resulted from disruption of the wrap or herniation of the wrap upward through the hiatus. Reoperation on those with a failed wrap was successful on a long-term basis in about 75 to 80%, and overall long-term good results are reported at about 90%.[90, 92]

In the Thal procedure, the lower esophagus is freed and the crura approximated posterior to the esophagus as in the previous techniques. A partial, 180-degree anterior fundal wrap is then constructed; this partial wrap attaches to the intraabdominal esophagus. Like our procedure, it is technically simpler than a Nissen procedure and has a shorter operating time. The incidence of postoperative intestinal obstruction is low (< 1%), probably due to a transverse upper abdominal incision with minimal exposure of the intestine.[6] In a series of 1150 patients, disruption of the fundoplication and recurrent GER has occurred in only 2% and with recurrent hiatal hernia in another 2%. A distinct advantage of a lesser wrap is the very low incidence of gas bloat syndrome, so that a gastrostomy is rarely done. These children are able to burp or even, when necessary, vomit. Overall good results exceed 90%.[6] In both series, the number of NI children was low, whereas in most other large series, the incidence of NI children is often 50% or higher.

Another partial wrap method is the Toupet procedure, also developed to minimize the gas bloat problem. In this operation a partial, 270-degree wrap is positioned posterior to the esophagus. The preliminary steps of the technique are identical to the previous two procedures. The Toupet procedure can be performed through an upper abdominal transverse incision, so that exposure of the intestine is largely avoided. After the crura have been approximated to restore the size of the hiatus to normal, the gastric fundus is passed posterior to the esophagus. The posterior aspect of the wrap is sutured to the right crura. The margins of the wrap on either side are then sutured to the right and left margins of the esophagus, leaving the anterior esophageal wall free. Experience with this operation in 112 patients revealed that 30% were NI.[98] The early postoperative courses were generally benign, but 2 developed intestinal obstruction. On late follow-up evaluation, the outcome was excellent in 90%. Six reoperations were necessary due to recurrent GER. Dysphagia was a temporary problem in 6 and gas bloat was not a problem.

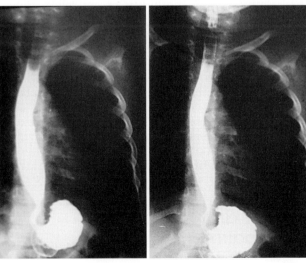

Figure 28–3. Esophagogram following the Boix-Ochoa antireflux procedure.

Laparoscopic approaches to fundoplication are being reported with increasing frequency. In 1991, the feasibility of performing Nissen fundoplication in 12 adults using a laparoscopic approach was demonstrated.[99] In rapid succession, additional reports appeared confirming the practicability and safety of this technique in adults.[100-102] To show how the pendulum has swung in some quarters vis-à-vis medical treatment, a recent report proposed laparoscopic fundoplication as a reasonable alternative to omeprazole.[103] Reports of endoscopic antireflux operations performed on children appeared soon after with documentation of both feasibility and satisfactory short-term results.[104, 105] One group's experience not only detailed the learning curve but also described a rapid drop in the percentage of cases in which conversion to an open operation was required, from 30% after the first 20 cases to a cumulative rate of 7.5% after 160 cases.[106] A similar drop in complication rate was also noted, falling from an early 12% rate to a final cumulative rate of 7.4%.

A comparison study of 212 children who had either laparoscopic or open antireflux operations over 5 years has been reported.[107] The Nissen procedure was used in almost all cases. The operative time was longer with the laparoscopic method by an average of approximately 30 minutes. Time of hospitalization averaged 3.5 days with the laparoscopic technique versus 8.1 days with the open method. There were no statistical differences in early complications between the two groups, but late complications were much more frequent in the open group (38.9% vs. 7.4%). Two thirds (143 of 212 patients) were severely NI, and the proportion of these impaired children was about the same in both groups. As has been found in most other studies of fundoplication operations, the complications occurred significantly more often in the NI than in the neurologically normal (NN). The early complications after laparoscopic Nissen were 41% in NI patients versus 17% in NN patients. The late complications occurred in 13% of NI patients and 0% of NN patients. The authors conclude that the laparoscopic technique is superior to the open method in the performance of Nissen antireflux procedures.

The results of the combined experience with antireflux operations from seven large pediatric surgical departments are encouraging.[108] A total of 7467 children were included. Significant clinical improvement was recorded in 94% of NN children and in 84.6% of the NI group. Major postoperative complications were recorded in an average of 4.2% of the NN patients and in 12.8% of the NI patients. Postoperative deaths (within 1 month of operation) were found in 0.07% of the NN patients and in 0.8% of the NI patients. Reoperation was necessary, on average, in 3.6% of the NN and 11.8% of the NI groups, respectively. These data show the significant differences between NN and NI children, but more important, they emphasize the satisfactory overall outcome in both groups. The unique problems of the NI children with GER, feeding problems, or both

are addressed in more depth in a later section on GER and neurologic impairment. In the above study, there were only minor variations in the overall results or complication and reoperation rates, irrespective of the type of antireflux procedure used.

The larger question is not which operation, but, rather, when. Until the mid-1990s, the indications for surgery were reasonably easy to define. The results of nonoperative therapy for the severe or potentially dangerous complications of reflux were generally unsatisfactory, hence failure of medical management was common in those children at the highest risk of significant morbidity or even death. As a consequence of omeprazole, the most appropriate therapy for children with severe GER is evolving, and our present concepts of the indications for surgery are changing.

Both medical and surgical treatments have advantages and drawbacks. Omeprazole does not control reflux directly; rather, omeprazole is effective by reducing gastric acidity almost to the vanishing point. This permits healing of even severe esophagitis in many children and prevents acid reflux into the esophagus, thus quite possibly preventing some of the respiratory complications. However, its effectiveness disappears when the drug is stopped; gastric acidity returns and the original problems of the disease reemerge. Hence, life-long treatment appears to be a requirement for life-long effectiveness. Fundoplication, ideally, is a one-time episode that is both effective and long lasting. Often this is true, and a number of series with long-term follow-up evaluation show highly satisfactory eventual results in more than 90% of the children.[108] These results, however, are bought at a significant price. Both short- and long-term complications as well as surgical failures do occur in significant numbers. Experience with omeprazole in children is still limited, and definitive answers to its long-term effectiveness, complications, and safety are not yet available. Critics of this large, combined study take issue with some of the data and conclusions.[109] They point to the relatively high morbidity of antireflux procedures in high-risk children such as those who are NI and those who had previous repairs of esophageal atresia. The excellent short-term results with omeprazole in these high-risk groups make the medication a viable alternative. Fundoplication is believed to be best reserved for those with proven or probable risk of aspiration from below and for the NN children whose results from surgery generally are excellent. At the least, such drug therapy may provide a considerable amount of relief and permit postponement of the decision for or against surgery for considerable time.

□ GER and Neurologic Impairment

The most difficult clinical problem in the field of GER is the overall management of the severely NI child with persistent vomiting. To begin, such vomiting is common, much more so than with normal children; 15% of institutionalized, severely retarded children had recurrent vomiting with a frequency of at least eight episodes per month.[110] Three quarters of the vomiting children were shown to have GER. Although a few prior reports had pointed out the occurrence of reflux or hiatal hernia in such children, this study strongly enforced the magnitude of the problem and paved the way for many studies and therapies designed to ameliorate it.

Earlier, such vomiting was largely felt to be psychogenic in origin or simply part of the primary neurologic disease, and little effort was made to critically investigate the cause. Perhaps for this reason, although the vomiting often began early in infancy, diagnosis was usually made relatively late. In those for whom a surgical antireflux procedure was eventually done, the average age at operation was considerably higher than for normal children. At least half of normal children have their operation in infancy, whereas retarded children's representative average and mean ages at operation were 7.5 and 5.9 years, respectively.[111, 112]

A number of manifestations or complications of the primary neurologic disease are common. This may both delay the diagnosis of and predispose the child to the development of GER. Vomiting, already mentioned, is the most common of these complications, and its misinterpretation is a major factor in delay of diagnosis. Difficulty in feeding or even refusal of feedings are frequent problems in these children, problems not uncommon with GER as well. The vast majority of the NI children are nonverbal; communication and proper identification of symptoms may be exceedingly difficult. A similar proportion also are nonambulatory; therefore, gravity as an aid to esophageal propulsion is not helpful. Increased intraabdominal pressure also probably plays a role. Scoliosis, spastic quadriplegia, and seizures all are problems in many of these children and all result in periodic elevations of intraabdominal pressure, enough to overcome the normal antireflux barrier and allow chronic reflux. Severe growth retardation is also common in these children, a complication shared with some normal children with reflux and obviously accentuated in the NI children who develop reflux.

Complications of GER itself are generally more advanced in NI children than in the normal group. Esophagitis is the most prominent of these. Esophagoscopy has been used as a major diagnostic tool in many reported studies, and esophagitis has been a common finding (66 to 100%).[113, 114] Esophageal stricture, as expected, is frequently identified.[115] Barrett's esophagus, a condition associated with both esophagitis and stricture, also has been found much more commonly in NI than in NN individuals. In one study of institutionalized adults, 26% had Barrett's esophagus changes on esophagoscopy and biopsy.[116] Another study in children and young adults found a strikingly higher incidence in the

mentally retarded group as compared with the normal group.[117] Respiratory problems, particularly repeated episodes of pneumonia, are common and almost always require hospitalization. Various investigators have documented these problems in from 35 to 85% of the patients.[110–115] One group of investigators found that 18% of the children had a history of apneic episodes prior to surgery.[118] Obviously, many of these complications, both of the disease and of GER, are interrelated, and a careful, methodical evaluation is essential when planning appropriate management. Equally obvious, most of these children have a serious and advanced degree of reflux disease.

Diagnostic studies in this group of children are basically the same as in the NN group, but a few modifications are in order. The radiologist, while performing the barium upper gastrointestinal series, must pay particular attention to the possibility of orotracheal aspiration. This is relatively common and must be appreciated prior to any surgical operation. An antireflux procedure may not be helpful if oropharyngeal aspiration is significant, and, indeed, the problem of aspiration might be worsened. Abnormal esophageal motility is relatively common, perhaps secondary to esophagitis. Hiatus hernia is more often found in NI patients than in the NN group; 51% in one study.[119] Extended esophageal pH monitoring can be accomplished as a standard method, but in some, the probe is poorly tolerated and may be pulled out at the slightest provocation. Endoscopy with biopsy is helpful as noted previously, because the incidence of esophagitis, stricture, Barrett's esophagus, and hiatus hernia is relatively high.

ENTERAL FEEDING

The provision of adequate nutrition in NI children is often the primary goal. Enteral feedings via a nasogastric tube generally were considered impractical, except as a short-term method in infants with malnutrition secondary to GER. In one study, 12 infants (11 NN) were treated with continuous infusion of formula through a small-caliber nasogastric feeding tube for 11 to 13 days. Of the 12 infants, 8 had a favorable early response with adequate weight gain and cessation of vomiting. Ten were followed 3 to 12 months, 5 of whom continued to grow normally and did not require fundoplication.[1] In this small series, the solitary NI patient did not respond.[120]

Gastrostomy is the most common long-term solution for enteral feeding. The procedure can be done by a standard Stamm gastrostomy or by the percutaneous endoscopic gastrostomy (PEG) method.[121] The Stamm gastrostomy can be done via a laparotomy or laparoscopically. PEG is a quick and simple technique and has been widely adopted, although it has some unique complications of its own.[121] A substantial number of children without prior clinical evidence of GER develop reflux after a gastrostomy, irrespective of whether the procedure is a Stamm or a PEG.[122–125] About two thirds of children who have normal studies prior to gastrostomy develop GER postoperatively, and about half eventually become symptomatic.[126] Why gastrostomy causes GER remains undetermined; widening the angle of His by pulling down the fundus during the procedure is one possible explanation. Owing to the high incidence of reflux following gastrostomy, routine antireflux operations have been recommended and practiced in a number of pediatric surgical centers. Many, however, feel that all patients referred for feeding gastrostomy should be evaluated for GER and that only those with significant clinical reflux should have a concomitant antireflux procedure. For those who develop clinical reflux postoperatively, the antireflux procedure may be done at that time.[127] Fundoplication *after* gastrostomy is a much more difficult procedure than fundoplication *with* gastrostomy.

One should realize that an antireflux operation is not necessarily mandatory in the NI child with reflux whose primary problem is nutrition. Converting bolus gastrostomy feedings to continuous feedings can dramatically resolve vomiting and result in excellent weight gain and markedly diminished pulmonary complications.[128] Another option in NI children who need a feeding gastrostomy and who have minimal to moderate reflux is to place the gastrostomy tube on the lesser curvature, thus fixing the stomach to the posterior right rectus fascia as in a Boerema anterior gastropexy. This modification was reported in nine NI children, only two of whom had moderate GER preoperatively. All did well without clinical symptoms of GER and with marked nutritional improvement. Postoperative barium studies in eight did not show reflux.[129, 130]

Still another approach in these children is to use a jejunostomy. By one technique, a percutaneous gastrostomy is established under fluoroscopic control while a small plastic tube is threaded through the gastrostomy tube and guided into the jejunum. Comparison of this technique with a Nissen fundoplication showed a strikingly lower incidence of complications in the former.[131] Obviously, this same principle could be achieved by passing the jejunal tube through a preexisting gastrostomy. One annoying problem in such methods is occasional displacement of the feeding jejunal tube upward into the stomach and the necessity for its replacement under fluoroscopic control. This technique does not directly treat the GER, and medical management must be continued. A final method along these same lines is a Roux-en-Y jejunostomy for feeding. A gastrostomy for decompression is done at the same time if one is not already in place.[132] This procedure obviously is more complex, but the results in a small series have been excellent in terms of improved nutritional status and dramatic decrease in GER symptoms.

ANTIREFLUX SURGERY

Surgical measures to correct reflux have been the standard treatment since the 1970s in both NI and NN children owing to the generally poor response to medical therapy, including upright positioning, thickening of feedings, and drugs such as H2-receptor antagonists and prokinetics. The exact percentage of NI children without demonstrable GER who receive an antireflux procedure in conjunction with a feeding gastrostomy is difficult to determine, but in one series the indication for the antireflux operation was prophylactic in 30%.[133]

All of the various antireflux surgical procedures have been used in NI children. The Nissen has been most often used, as with NN children, but the Thal operation has also been used almost exclusively in some series.[134, 135] The most vexing problem with these children is the high rate of both postoperative complications and deaths within the perioperative period as compared with NN children undergoing the same procedures. One series noted an early complication rate of 11% and a late complication rate of 26%.[136] All but one of the early complications were small bowel obstructions; more than half of the later complications were wrap herniations or wrap failure. NN children from this same institution had one third the number of early complications and less than half the rate of late complications. Reoperation for late complications was required in 19%. The Nissen fundoplication was used in about 80% of the NI children, and Thals in the remainder. Another series reported on 35 profoundly disabled children who had antireflux procedures, almost all of which were Nissens.[133] Perioperative complications, which were nonfatal, developed in 17%, and three additional complications were responsible for death. Late complications included bowel obstruction requiring laparotomy (3 patients) and recurrent GER (7 patients). A second antireflux operation was performed in 6 patients. The results of the anterior gastropexy of Boerema in 50 NI children were similar: 25 early and 9 late complications, 17 reoperations, and 2 deaths related to the operation.[137] A still larger series reported distressingly high complication rates following Nissens in 193 patients.[138] Both of the fundoplication authors questioned the advisability of continuing with operations that were designed to improve the quality of life in these children but that were plagued with numerous problems.[133, 138]

Experience using the Thal operation suggests a more optimistic picture with an 8% failure rate and an 11% complication rate.[134] The complication rate is about the same as with the NN children, but the failure rate in the NN is only 2%. In a series of Thal procedures in 141 NI children, recurrent GER or recurrent hiatal hernia required reoperation in 10%.[135] Only 6% required a later pyloroplasty due to DGE for symptoms of gagging and retching.

It is more than apparent that antireflux operations in NI children carry a considerably higher risk than in otherwise normal children. The reasons for the high incidence of wrap failure have not been clarified. Certainly, those with severe growth failure may have impaired wound healing. Chronic or periodic increased intraabdominal pressure from retching, recumbency, and seizures may be important causative factors. Because the Thal procedure permits belching and vomiting, less strain against this partial wrap may occur than against a complete wrap, hence a partial wrap may be the preferable option. These disquieting results are cause for serious consideration as to the best therapy available for these children. However, in all the series cited, most of the children were much improved, and parents and other caregivers expressed a high degree of satisfaction with the outcome. In a study that examined this important issue, feeding indices were improved and the child's comfort and quality of life were perceived to be significantly better.[139] Furthermore, the level of frustration in caring for the child was less and the quality of life for the parents as well as for the child was improved.

Reports of omeprazole therapy in NI children are not yet available. Obviously, such therapy would not reduce the necessity of some type of enteral feeding procedure, but perhaps such therapy may be able to reduce the necessity for antireflux operations.

☐ Esophageal Atresia and GER

GER following repair of esophageal atresia malformations is common. The frequency is difficult to establish precisely, but significant reflux occurs in at least 50% of these babies.[140–144] In cases of isolated esophageal atresia (no tracheoesophageal fistula [TEF]), the incidence of GER following primary repair was 100% in a series of nine infants.[145]

The cause of the GER has been assumed by many to be secondary to the repair of the esophageal atresia itself. Tension on the anastomosis with upward displacement of the lower esophageal segment may shorten the intraabdominal esophagus and widen the angle of His. Dissection of the TEF and the lower esophageal segment may damage the vagal innervation, or scarring secondary to the dissection may have the same effect. In fact, a study of 25 such children revealed that excessive tension at the anastomosis was the only factor studied that was associated with an increased incidence of GER.[143] However, most investigators in the field now believe that the cause is a primary, probably congenital, defect in the motor function of the distal esophagus.[146–149] Esophageal dysmotility, aperistalsis, nonprogressive contractions with low amplitude, and disorganized contractions all have been observed.

The long-term follow-up of 22 adolescents or young adults who had repair of esophageal atresia and distal TEF as newborns examined some of these problems.[150] The technique used was a combination of 24-hour esophageal manometry and pH monitoring on an ambulatory basis. Half had a pattern of long nocturnal episodes of reflux with very slow clearance. All had markedly diminished esophageal contractibility, disorganized propulsive activity, and

absence of acid-clearing capacity. Propulsion of ingested fluids and solids as well as clearance of refluxed fluids were accomplished largely by gravity. GER was noted in more than half of these patients, so that it is clear that the reflux noted early in life in these children persists indefinitely.

The clinical manifestations of reflux are similar in many ways to otherwise normal children with GER. Respiratory symptoms, such as recurrent pneumonia, are common, and life-threatening episodes of apnea or cyanosis may occur.[144, 151] Failure to thrive due to recurrent vomiting, dysphagia, and esophagitis is often a problem. The esophageal anastomosis may become tight, and the stricture often does not respond to dilation, presumably due to the frequent reflux of acid fluid. Esophagitis is particularly common.

Conventional medical treatment is effective in about half of the children (Fig. 28–4*A* and *B*). This includes upright positioning, thickening of the feedings, H2 blockers, and prokinetic drugs such as cisapride. Owing to dysphagia, supplemental gastrostomy feedings may be necessary. Infusion gastrostomy feedings are probably more effective than bolus because less vomiting results. Omeprazole has not been reported as treatment for these infants to date, but it surely is being tried and may be helpful because esophagitis and persistent strictures are common.

When medical measures are not effective and complications such as failure to thrive, apneic spells, recurrent pneumonia, or anastomotic strictures persist, some form of antireflux surgical procedure is necessary. Many reports document excellent results. Fifteen infants with tight anastomotic strictures failing to respond to repeated dilations were reported.[152] The cause was felt to be frequent episodes of reflux, and all were managed by an antireflux operation. The stenoses were cured in all. Another group of children was reported to have excellent but slightly less spectacular relief of stricture, vomiting, pneumonia, and dysphagia.[153] Nissen fundoplications were performed in all nine with no major complications and with relief of their reflux symptoms in all. Respiratory problems were markedly diminished and the strictures were successfully managed.

However, surgical treatment of reflux in this group of children has been, by no means, uniformly successful. The experience with fundoplications used in 14 children with GER following repair of esophageal atresia and TEF was reported to be distressing.[141] After fundoplication, half had dysphagia requiring gastrostomy supplementation, and in 5 of the 7, the dysphagia persisted beyond 1 year. All had competent fundoplications on follow-up study, but all also had absent esophageal peristalsis below the anastomosis. Another report relates similar problems using Nissen fundoplications in this scenario.[142] Only 8 of 21 of the patients had an uncomplicated postoperative course. Prolonged dysphagia occurred in 8, wrap disruption with recurrent reflux

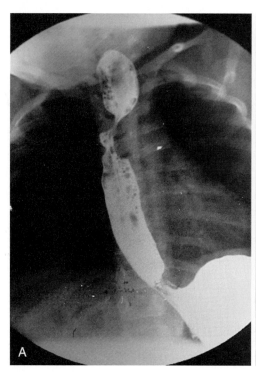
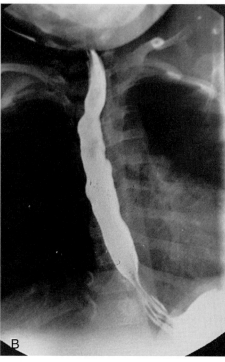

Figure 28–4. Esophagogram of a patient with esophageal atresia. *A*, Stenosis of the suture line and small hiatus hernia with reflux. *B*, Patient treated with cisapride, H2-antagonists, and bougie dilations, and, ultimately, the pH monitoring reverted to normal values. Anti-reflux surgery was not necessary.

developed in 7, and 3 died from postoperative complications. The investigators felt that the dysphagia was secondary to the inability of the defective distal esophageal motility to overcome the increased resistance of the fundoplication.

What appeared to be excellent short-term results proved to be poor long-term results with fundoplications in another report.[145] Owing to reflux, Nissen fundoplications were done in 13 children following esophageal atresia repair. All did well following the antireflux operation, and routine endoscopy 3 to 8 months later showed competent wraps in all. In 5, however, reflux later recurred and the fundal wrap was found to be disrupted. This usually occurred 1.5 to 2.5 years after the fundoplication. One child, whose wrap was intact, developed a huge dilation of the lower esophagus, presumably due to the inability of esophageal peristalsis to overcome the pressure of the wrap.

In other reports, the problems are not as severe. Reoperation was required in 18% of those children with a Nissen fundoplication and in 15% of patients who had a Thal fundoplication following esophageal atresia/TEF repair.[154, 155] Reoperation rates, of course, do indicate failure but do not necessarily reflect the total incidence of morbidity following antireflux surgery.

Obviously, the last chapter has not been written concerning the children who have successfully overcome the original problem of esophageal atresia only to develop GER. Some of the early problems of GER are life threatening or are responsible for growth failure, recurrent pneumonia, and severe esophagitis with resistant anastomotic strictures. Medical treatment alone often does not prove effec-

tive, yet antireflux surgery is beset with significant drawbacks.

☐ Esophageal Stricture and Barrett's Esophagus

Strictures of the esophagus are a severe and usually rather late complication of GER.[1] These strictures are secondary to severe esophagitis and are accompanied in some instances by Barrett's esophagus. The basic tenets of therapy are operative correction of GER so that the esophagitis may heal and dilation of the stricture.[156] The dilations may be started at diagnosis. If this can be done safely, antegrade dilations may be used. Often, however, either retrograde dilations or antegrade dilations, guided by a string, are preferred for reasons of both safety and practicability. Obviously, when the string-guided technique is used, a preliminary gastrostomy is necessary. A fine string is passed through the nose, down the esophagus, into the stomach, and out through the gastrostomy. At the times of dilation, the string is replaced with a heavier one and the upper end is drawn out through the mouth. Tucker dilators can then be passed through the stricture from above. This technique has proved to be safe and can be done without anesthesia on an outpatient basis.

Generally, dilations are ineffective until the reflux is controlled. Direct dilations of the stricture, either by finger or with Hegar dilators at laparotomy, are possible.[157] If this was not possible owing to the location or length of the stricture, Tucker dilators guided by a string (as above) were used. After the intraoperative dilation, a standard Nissen fundoplication was performed. Postoperative dilations, using the string-guided technique, were used as required.

In a series of 18 consecutive children with strictures, the results were excellent. Of the 18 children, 15 required 1 to 10 dilations over 2 to 8 months postoperatively, whereas the other 3 needed none. Dysphagia was relieved almost immediately. Mortality was nil, and there were no complications of intestinal obstruction or infection. Gas bloat did not occur. On follow-up esophagrams, complete resolution was noted in 12 and significant improvement in the remaining 6. The incidence of stricture in the GER patients was 15%, and the average age at the time of diagnosis of stricture was 5.5 years. In the overwhelming majority of reflux strictures in children, the use of antireflux operations and dilations are successful. Only in rare instances is resection required.

A large number of reports confirm the effectiveness of omeprazole in the treatment of esophagitis in children.[158–160] Perhaps the drug will eventually have a role as an adjunct in managing reflux strictures, but no reports on this use have appeared. Although its effectiveness in esophagitis is apparent, its success in truly advanced esophagitis is not as impressive; less than half of grade 4 esophagitis healed with omeprazole.[158] Recurrence seems to be inevitable when the drug is stopped.

Barrett's esophagus is a complication of esophagitis and is often accompanied by stricture. Although usually regarded as quite uncommon in childhood, the incidence has been reported at 4% and 14% of children with GER in two series.[161, 162] In another report, Barrett's esophagus was found in 25% of the children with reflux strictures.[163] In adults, progressive increase in the incidence and severity of dysplasia in the columnar epithelium has been documented on repeated endoscopic and biopsy observations over a period of years. A group of 50 adults with Barrett's esophagus were followed from 1.5 to 14 years (mean 5.2 years).[74] Low-grade dysplasia was found in only 6 at initial evaluation. At the final examination, 13 patients had dysplasia. The dysplasia was low grade in 10 and high grade in 3. Furthermore, an additional 5 patients had developed adenocarcinoma.

The progressive increase in the incidence and severity of dysplasia, together with the development of carcinoma, make Barrett's esophagus most worrisome. Two cases of carcinoma arising in Barrett's esophagus in children were reported from one institution.[161] One patient was 11 and the other 14 years of age at diagnosis of the malignancy. There is a report of an esophageal adenocarcinoma located adjacent to the esophagogastric junction in a 20-year-old woman who had repair of esophageal atresia and TEF as a newborn.[162] She was managed by an extensive resection with restoration of continuity by a colon segment interposition. The specimen did not show Barrett's epithelium, but certainly there is a reasonable possibility that Barrett's esophagus was, in fact, present at one time but was obliterated by the tumor.

How best to handle the child with reflux and Barrett's esophagus is obviously a major problem. One child, 12 years of age, was treated by antireflux operation with an excellent clinical result.[163] Two years later, on both gross endoscopic examination and histologic review, there was distinct evidence of regression with replacement of the columnar epithelium by squamous epithelium, and this regression continued over a further 3-year period. In another case, complete regression followed antireflux surgery.[164]

Generally, however, Barrett's esophagus in childhood does not regress after antireflux surgery. Five children with Barrett's esophagus who had had Nissen fundoplications were followed.[165] No evidence of regression was found on yearly follow-up endoscopic and biopsy evaluation. Another report of 11 children with Barrett's esophagus also noted lack of regression in three children following antireflux surgery.[56] Prolonged follow-up evaluation with endoscopy and biopsy are recommended if dysplastic changes are to be found and carcinoma either can be prevented or found at an early stage.[56, 72, 165] The use of endoscopic laser ablation of the epithelium has recently been reported.[166] In 17 adults with GER and Barrett's esophagus, successful antireflux operations were performed. No postoperative reflux was found by endoscopic evaluation and 24-hour pH monitoring. In 11 of these, the abnormal epithelium was then ablated using laser energy technique via an endoscope in one to eight sessions. The regenerated epithelium in the esophagus was squamous in all 11, although 2 showed intestinal metaplasia in the adjacent gastric cardia. The other 6 patients had antireflux surgery alone, and in all, the Barrett's esophagus remained unchanged.

REFERENCES

1. Carré IJ: The natural history of the partial thoracic stomach (hiatus hernia) in children. Arch Dis Child 34:344–353, 1959.
2. Nissen R: Gastropexy and fundoplication in surgical treatment of hiatal hernia. Am J Dig Dis 6:954–961, 1961.
3. Thal AP: A unified approach to surgical problems of the esophagogastric junction. Ann Surg 168:542–549, 1968.
4. Boix-Ochoa J: The physiologic approach to the management of gastric esophageal reflux. J Pediatr Surg 21:1032–1039, 1986.
5. Fonkalsrud EW, Foglia RP, Ament ME, et al: Operative treatment for the gastroesophageal syndrome in children. J Pediatr Surg 24:525–529, 1989.
6. Ashcraft KW: Gastroesophageal reflux. In Ashcraft KW, Holder TM (eds): Pediatric Surgery (2nd ed). Philadelphia, WB Saunders, 1993, pp 270–288.
7. Tunell WP, Smith EI, Carson JA: Gastroesophageal reflux in childhood: The dilemma of surgical success. Ann Surg 197:560–565, 1983.
8. Dent J, Dodds WJ, Friedman RH, et al: Mechanism of gastroesophageal reflux in recumbent asymptomatic human subjects. J Clin Invest 65:256–267, 1980.
9. Dodds WJ, Dent J, Hogan WJ, et al: Mechanisms of gastroesophageal reflux in patients with reflux esophagitis. N Engl J Med 307:1547–1552, 1982.

10. Fyke FE, Code CF, Schlegel JF: The gastroesophageal sphincter in healthy human beings. Gastroenterologia 86:135–150, 1956.

11. Liebermann-Meffert D, Allgower M, Schmid P, et al: Muscular equivalent of the lower esophageal sphincter. Gastroenterology 76:31–38, 1979.

12. Bremner RM, Hoeft SF, Costantini MD, et al: Pharyngeal swallowing. Ann Surg 218:364–370, 1993.

13. Mittal RK, Balaban DH: The esophagogastric junction. N Engl J Med 336:924–932, 1997.

14. Klein WA, Parkman HP, Dempsey DT, et al: Sphincterlike thoracoabdominal high-pressure zone after esophagogastrectomy. Gastroenterology 105:1362–1369, 1993.

15. Thor KB, Hill LD, Mercer DD, et al: Reappraisal of the flap valve mechanism in the gastroesophageal junction. Acta Chir Scand 153:25–28, 1987.

16. Moosa AR, Cooley GR, Skinner DB: Intraluminal and intraperitoneal pressures at the cardia: Effect of hormones and surgical intervention. Surg For 24:370–372, 1973.

17. Winans CS, Harris LD: Quantitation of lower esophageal sphincter competence. Gastroenterology 52:773–778, 1967.

18. DeMeester TR, Wernly JA, Bryant GH, et al: Clinical and in vitro analysis of determinants of gastroesophageal competence. Am J Surg 137:39–46, 1979.

19. O'Sullivan GC, DeMeester TR, Joelsson BE, et al: Interaction of lower esophageal sphincter pressure and length of sphincter in the abdomen as determinants of gastroesophageal competence. Am J Surg 143:40–47, 1982.

20. Omari TI, Dent J: Assessment of oesophageal motor function in children and neonates. J Japan Soc Pediatr Surg 33:25–30, 1997.

21. Gryboski JD, Thayer WR Jr, Spiro HM: Esophageal motility in infants and children. Pediatrics 31:382–395, 1983.

22. Hillemeier AC, Grill BB, McCallum R, et al: Esophageal and gastric motor abnormalities in gastroesophageal reflux during infancy. Gastroenterology 84:741–746, 1983.

23. Arana J, Tovar JA: Motor efficiency of the refluxing esophagus in basal conditions and after acid challenge. J Pediatr Surg 24:1049–1054, 1989.

24. Stein HJ, Eypasch EP, DeMeester TR, et al: Circadian esophageal motor function in patients with gastroesophageal reflux disease. Surgery 108:769–778, 1990.

25. Eypasch EP, Stein HJ, DeMeester TR, et al: A new technique to define and clarify esophageal motor disorders. Am J Surg 159:144–152, 1990.

26. Kahrilas PJ, Dodds WJ, Hogan WJ, et al: Esophageal peristaltic dysfunction in peptic esophagitis. Gastroenterology 91:897–904, 1986.

27. Cucchiara S, Staiano A, DiLorenzo G, et al: Pathophysiology of gastroesophageal reflux and distal esophageal motility in children with gastroesophageal reflux disease. J Pediatr Gastroenterol Nutr 7:830–836, 1988.

28. Ingelfinger YJ: Esophageal motility. Physiol Rev 38:533–584, 1958.

29. Boyle JT, Altschuler SM, Nixon TE, et al: Role of the diaphragm in the genesis of lower esophageal sphincter pressure in the cat. Gastroenterology 88:723–730, 1985.

30. Heine KJ, Dent J, Mittal RK: Anatomical relationship between crural diaphragm and lower esophageal sphincter: An electrophysiological study. J Gastrointest Mot 5:89–95, 1993.

31. DeMeester TR, Johnson LF, Joseph GJ, et al: Patterns of gastroesophageal reflux in health and disease. Ann Surg 184:459–470, 1976.

32. Little AG, DeMeester TR, Rezai-Zadeh K, et al: Abnormal gastric emptying in patients with gastroesophageal reflux. Surgical Forum 28:347–348, 1977.

33. Horowitz M, Cook DJ, Collins PJ, et al: The application of techniques using radionuclides to the study of gastric emptying. Surg Gynecol Obstet 155:737–744, 1982.

34. Maddern GJ, Jamieson GG: Fundoplication enhances gastric emptying. Ann Surg 201:296–299, 1985.

35. Euler AR, Byrne WJ: Gastric emptying times of water in infants and children: Comparison of those with and without gastroesophageal reflux. J Pediatr Gastroenterol Nutr 2:595–598, 1983.

36. Jolley SG, Leonard JC, Tunell WP: Gastric emptying in children with gastroesophageal reflux, I: An estimate of effective gastric emptying. J Pediatr Surg 22:923–926, 1987.

37. Jolley SG, Tunell WP, Leonard JC, et al: Gastric emptying in children with gastroesophageal reflux, II: The relationship to retching symptoms following antireflux surgery. J Pediatr Surg 22:927–930, 1987.

38. Fonkalsrud EW, Ament ME: Gastroesophageal reflux in childhood. Curr Probl Surg 33:10–70, 1996.

39. Papaila JG, Wilmot D, Grosfeld JL, et al: Increased incidence of delayed gastric emptying in children with gastroesophageal reflux. Arch Surg 124:933–936, 1989.

40. Maxson RT, Harp S, Jackson RJ, et al: Delayed gastric emptying in neurologically impaired children with gastroesophageal reflux: The role of pyloroplasty. J Pediatr Surg 29:726–729, 1994.

41. Campbell JR, Gilchrist BF, Harrison MW: Pyloroplasty in association with Nissen fundoplication in children with neurologic disorders. J Pediatr Surg 24:375–377, 1989.

42. Brown RA, Wynchank S, Rode H, et al: Is a gastric drainage procedure necessary at the time of antireflux surgery? J Pediatr Gastroenterol Nutr 25:377–380, 1997.

43. Katzka DA, Sidhu M, Castell DO: Hypertensive lower esophageal sphincter pressures and gastroesophageal reflux: An apparent paradox that is not unusual. Am J Gastroenterol 90:280–284, 1995.

44. Dent J, Holloway RH, Toouli J, et al: Mechanisms of lower esophageal incompetence in patients with symptomatic gastroesophageal reflux. Gut 29:1020–1028, 1998.

45. Werlin SL, Dodds WJ, Hogan WJ, et al: Mechanisms of gastroesophageal reflux in children. J Pediatr 97:244–249, 1980.

46. Cucchiara S, Bortolotti M, Minella R, et al: Fasting and postprandial mechanisms of gastroesophageal reflux in children with gastroesophageal reflux disease. Dig Dis Sci 38:86–92, 1993.

47. Omari T, Miki K, Fraser R, et al: Esophageal body and lower esophageal sphincter function in healthy premature infants. Gastroenterology 109:1757–1764, 1985.

48. Neuhauser EBD, Berenberg W: Cardio-esophageal relaxation as cause of vomiting in infants. Radiology 48:480–483, 1947.

49. Hyman PE. Gastroesophageal reflux: One reason why baby won't eat. J Pediatr 125(suppl):S103–s109, 1994.

50. del Rosario JF, Orenstein SR: Evaluation and management of gastroesophageal reflux and pulmonary disease. Curr Opin Pediatr 8:209–215, 1996.

51. Jolley SG, Halpern LM, Tunell WP, et al: The risk of sudden infant death from gastroesophageal reflux. J Pediatr Surg 26:691–696, 1991.

52. Jolley SG, Herbst JJ, Johnson DG, et al: Esophageal pH monitoring during sleep identifies children with respiratory symptoms from gastroesophageal reflux. Gastroenterology 80:1501–1506, 1981.

53. Andze GO, Brandt ML, St. Vil D, et al: Diagnosis and treatment of gastroesophageal reflux in 500 children with respiratory symptoms: The value of pH monitoring. J Pediatr Surg 26:295–300, 1991.

54. Hrabovsky EE, Mullett MD: Gastroesophageal reflux and the premature infant. J Pediatr Surg 21:583–587, 1986.

55. Hassall E, Weinstein WM, Ament ME: Barrett's esophagus in childhood. Gastroenterology 89:1331–1337, 1985.

56. Otherson HB Jr, Ocampo RJ, Parker EF, et al: Barrett's esophagus in children. Ann Surg 217:676–681, 1993.

57. Mandel H, Tirosh E, Berant M: Sandifer syndrome reconsidered. Acta Paediatr Scand 78:797–799, 1989.

58. Bray PF, Herbst JJ, Johnson DG, et al: Childhood gastroesophageal reflux: Neurologic and psychiatric syndromes mimicked. JAMA 237:1342–1345, 1977.

59. Fawcett HD, Hayden CK, Adams JC, et al: How useful is gastroesophageal reflux scintigraphy in suspected childhood aspiration? Pediatr Radiol 18:311–313, 1988.

60. Berdon WE, Mellins RB, Levy J: On the following paper by H.D. Fawcet, C.K. Hayden, J.C. Adams, and L.E. Swischuk: How useful is gastroesophageal reflux scintigraphy in sus-

pected childhood aspiration? Pediatr Radiol 18:309–310, 1988.

61. Johnson LF, DeMeester TR: Twenty-four hour pH monitoring of the distal esophagus: A quantitative measure of gastroesophageal reflux. Am J Gastroenterol 62:325–332, 1974.
62. Hill JL, Pelligrini CA, Burrington JD, et al: Technique and experience with 24-hour esophageal pH monitoring in children. J Pediatr Surg 12:877–887, 1977.
63. Boix-Ochoa J, Lafuente JM, Gil-Vernet JM: Twenty-four hour esophageal pH monitoring in gastroesophageal reflux. J Pediatr Surg 15:74–78, 1980.
64. Jolley SG, Herbst JJ, Johnson DG, et al: Patterns of postcibal gastroesophageal reflux in symptomatic infants. Am J Surg 138:946–950, 1979.
65. Colletti RB, Christie DL, Orenstein SR: Indications for pediatric esophageal pH monitoring. J Pediatr Gastroenterol Nutr 21:253–262, 1995.
66. Jamieson JR, Stein HJ, DeMeester TR, et al: Ambulatory 24-hour esophageal pH monitoring: Normal values, optimal thresholds, specificity, sensitivity, and reproducibility. Am J Gastroenterol 87:1102–1111, 1992.
67. Biller JA, Winter HS, Grand RJ, et al: Are endoscopic changes predictive of histologic esophagitis in children? J Pediatr 103:215–218, 1983.
68. Meyers WF, Roberts CC, Johnson DG, et al: Value of tests for evaluation of gastroesophageal reflux in children. J Pediatr Surg 20:515–520, 1985.
69. Black DD, Haggitt RC, Orenstein SR, et al: Esophagitis in infants. Gastroenterology 98:1408–1414, 1990.
70. Orenstein SR: Gastroesophageal reflux. In Wyllie R, Hyams JS (eds): Pediatric Gastrointestinal Disease. Philadelphia, WB Saunders, 1993, pp 337–369.
71. Glassman M, George D, Grill B: Gastroesophageal reflux in children. Gastroenterol Clin North Am 24:71–98, 1995.
72. Dahms BB, Rothstein FC: Barrett's esophagus in children: A consequence of chronic gastroesophageal reflux. Gastroenterology 86:318–323, 1984.
73. Cooper JE, Spitz L, Wilkins BM: Barrett's esophagus in children: A histologic and histochemical study in 11 cases. J Pediatr Surg 22:191–196, 1987.
74. Hameeteman W, Tytgat GNJ, Houthoff JH, et al: Barrett's esophagus: Development of dysplasia and adenocarcinoma. Gastroenterology 96:1249–1256, 1989.
75. Stein HJ, DeMeester TR: Indications, technique, and clinical use of ambulatory 24-hour esophageal motility monitoring in a surgical practice. Ann Surg 217:128–137, 1993.
76. Shepard R, Fenn S, Seiber WK: Evaluation of esophageal function in postoperative esophageal atresia and tracheoesophageal fistula. Surgery 59:608–617, 1966.
77. Boix-Ochoa J, Canals J: Maturation of the lower esophagus. J Pediatr Surg 11:749–756, 1976.
78. Orenstein SR, Whitington PF, Orenstein DM: The infant seat as a treatment for gastroesophageal reflux. N Engl J Med 309:760–763, 1983.
79. Vandenplas Y: A critical appraisal of current management practices for infant regurgitation. Chung Hua Cheng Hsing Shao Shang Wai Ko Tsa Chih 38:187–202, 1997.
80. Ponsonby AL, Dwyer T, Gibbons LE, et al: Factors potentiating the risk of sudden infant death syndrome associated with the prone position. N Engl J Med 329:377–382, 1993.
81. Orenstein SR, Magill HL, Brooks P: Thickening of infant feedings for therapy of gastroesophageal reflux. J Pediatr 110:181–186, 1987.
82. Kelly DA: Do H2 receptor antagonists have a therapeutic role in childhood? J Pediatr Gastroenterol Nutr 19:270–276, 1994.
83. De Angelis GL, Banchini G: Ranitidine in pediatric patients. Clin Trials J 26:370–375, 1989.
84. Vandeplas Y: Gastroesophageal reflux in children. Scand J Gastroenterol Suppl 213:31–38, 1995.
85. Cucchiara S, Staiano A, Capozzi C, et al: Cisapride for gastro-esophageal reflux and peptic esophagitis. Arch Dis Child 62:454–457, 1987.
86. Cucchiara S: Cisapride therapy for gastrointestinal disease. J Pediatr Gastroenterol Nutr 22:259–269, 1996.
87. Gunasekaran TS, Hassall EG: Efficacy and safety of omeprazole for severe gastroesophageal reflux in children. J Pediatr 123:148–154, 1993.
88. Cucchiara S, Minella R, Campanozzi A, et al: Effects of omeprazole on mechanisms of gastroesophageal reflux in childhood. Dig Dis Sci 42:293–299, 1997.
89. Hassall E: Wrap session: Is the Nissen slipping? Can medical treatment replace surgery for severe gastroesophageal disease in children? Am J Gastroenterol 90:1212–1220, 1995.
90. Leape LL, Ramenofsky ML: Surgical treatment of gastroesophageal reflux in children. Am J Dis Child 134:935–938, 1980.
91. St. Cyr JA, Ferrara TB, Thompson TR, et al: Nissen fundoplication for gastroesophageal reflux in infants. J Thorac Cardiovasc Surg 92:661–666, 1986.
92. Turnage RH, Oldham KT, Coran AG, et al: Late results of fundoplication for gastroesophageal reflux in infants and children. Surgery 105:457–464, 1989.
93. Jolley SG, Tunell WP, Hoelzer DJ, et al: Postoperative small bowel obstruction in infants and children: A problem following Nissen fundoplication. J Pediatr Surg 21:407–409, 1986.
94. Dedinsky GK, Vane DW, Black CT, et al: Complications and reoperation after Nissen fundoplication in childhood. Am J Surg 153:177–183, 1987.
95. Caniano DA, Ginn-Pease ME, King DR: The failed antireflux procedure: Analysis of risk factors and morbidity. J Pediatr Surg 25:1022–1026, 1990.
96. Price MR, Janik JS, Wayne ER, et al: Modified Nissen fundoplication for reduction of fundoplication failure. J Pediatr Surg 32:324–327, 1997.
97. Wheatley MJ, Coran AG, Wesley JR, et al: Redo fundoplication in infants and children with recurrent gastroesophageal reflux. J Pediatr Surg 26:758–761, 1991.
98. Bensoussan AL, Yazbeck S, Carceller-Blanchard A: Results and complications of Toupet partial posterior wrap: 10 years' experience. J Pediatr Surg 29:1215–1217, 1994.
99. Dallemagne B, Weerts JM, Jehaes C, et al: Laparoscopic Nissen fundoplication: Preliminary report. Surg Laparosc Endosc 1:138–142, 1991.
100. Jamieson GG, Watson DI, Britten-Jones R, et al: Laparoscopic Nissen fundoplication. Ann Surg 220:137–145, 1995.
101. Hinder RA, Filipi CJ, Wetscher A, et al: Laparoscopic Nissen fundoplication is an effective treatment for gastroesophageal reflux disease. Ann Surg 220:472–483, 1994.
102. Bittner HB, Meyers WC, Brazer SR, et al: Laparoscopic Nissen fundoplication: Operative results and short-term follow-up. Am J Surg 167:193–200, 1994.
103. Anvari M, Allen C, Borm A: Laparoscopic Nissen fundoplication is a satisfactory alternative to long-term omeprazole therapy. Br J Surg 82:938–942, 1995.
104. Lobe TE, Schropp KP, Lunsford K: Laparoscopic Nissen fundoplication in childhood. J Pediatr Surg 28:358–361, 1993.
105. Georgeson KE: Laparoscopic gastrostomy and fundoplication. Pediatr Ann 22:675–677, 1993.
106. Meehan JJ, Georgeson KE: The learning curve associated with laparoscopic antireflux surgery in infants and children. J Pediatr Surg 32:426–429, 1997.
107. Bufo AJ, Chen MK, Lobe TE, et al: Laparoscopic fundoplication in children: A superior technique. Pediatr Endosurg Innovative Techniques. 1:71–76, 1997.
108. Fonkalsrud EW, Ashcraft KW, Coran AG, et al: Surgical treatment of gastroesophageal children: A combined hospital study of 7467 patients. Pediatrics 101:419–422, 1998.
109. Hassall E: Antireflux surgery in children: Time for a harder look. Pediatrics 101:467–468, 1998.
110. Sondheimer JM, Morris BA: Gastroesophageal reflux among severely retarded children. J Pediatr 94:710–714, 1979.
111. Spitz L: Surgical treatment of gastroesophageal reflux in severely mentally retarded children. J R Soc Med 75:525–529, 1982.
112. Vane DW, Harmel RP Jr, King DR, et al: The effectiveness of Nissen fundoplication in neurologically impaired children with gastroesophageal reflux. Surgery 98:662–666, 1985.

113. Byrne WJ, Campbell M, Ashcraft E, et al: A diagnostic approach to vomiting in severely retarded patients. Am J Dis Child 137:259–262, 1983.

114. Bohmer CJM, Niezen-de Boer MC, Klinkenberg-Knol EC, et al: Gastroesophageal reflux disease in intellectually disabled individuals: Leads for diagnosis and the effect of omeprazole therapy. Am J Gastroenterol 92:1475–1479, 1997.

115. Wilkinson JD, Dudgeon DL, Sondheimer JM: A comparison of medical and surgical treatment of gastroesophageal reflux in severely retarded children. J Pediatr 99:202–205, 1981.

116. Roberts IM, Curtis RL, Madara JL: Gastroesophageal reflux and Barrett's esophagus in developmentally disabled patients. Am J Gastroenterol 81:519–523, 1986.

117. Snyder JD, Goldman H: Barrett's esophagus in children and adults: Frequent association with mental retardation. Dig Dis Sci 35:1185–1189, 1990.

118. Spitz L, Roth K, Kiely EM, et al: Operation for gastroesophageal reflux associated with severe mental retardation. Arch Dis Child 68:347–351, 1993.

119. Cameron BH, Cochran WJ, McGill CW: The uncut Collis-Nissen fundoplication: Results for 79 consecutively treated high-risk children. J Pediatr Surg 32:887–891, 1997.

120. Ferry GD, Selby M, Pietro TJ: Clinical response to short-term nasogastric feeding in infants with gastroesophageal reflux and growth failure. J Pediatr Gastroenterol Nutr 2:57–61, 1983.

121. Gauderer MWL: Percutaneous endoscopic gastrostomy: A 10 year experience with 220 children. J Pediatr Surg 26:288–294, 1991.

122. Wesley JR, Coran AG, Sarahan TM, et al: The need for evaluation of gastroesophageal reflux in brain-damaged children referred for feeding gastrostomy. J Pediatr Surg 16:866–871, 1981.

123. Mollitt DL, Golladay S, Seibert JJ: Symptomatic gastroesophageal reflux following gastrostomy in neurologically impaired patients. Pediatrics 75:1124–1126, 1985.

124. Jolley SG, Smith EI, Tunell WP: Protective antireflux operation with feeding gastrostomy. Ann Surg 201:736–740, 1985.

125. Grunow JE, Al-Hafidh A, Tunell WP: Gastroesophageal reflux following percutaneous endoscopic gastrotomy in children. J Pediatr Surg 24:42–45, 1989.

126. Langer JC, Wesson DE, Ein SH, et al: Feeding gastrostomy in neurologically impaired children: Is an antireflux procedure necessary? J Pediatr Gastroenterol Nutr 7:837–841, 1988.

127. Isch JA, Rescorla FJ, Scherer T III, et al: The development of gastroesophageal reflux after percutaneous endoscopic gastrostomy. J Pediatr Surg 32:321–323, 1997.

128. Berezin S, Schwarz SM, Halata MS, et al: Gastroesophageal reflux secondary to gastrostomy tube placement. Am J Dis Child 140:699–701, 1986.

129. Stringel G: Gastrostomy with antireflux properties. J Pediatr Surg 25:1019–1021, 1990.

130. Boerema I: Hiatus hernia: Repair by right-sided, subhepatic, anterior gastropexy. Surgery 65:884–893, 1969.

131. Albanese CT, Towbin RB, Ulman I, et al: Percutaneous gastrojejunostomy versus Nissen fundoplication for enteral feeding of the neurologically impaired child with gastroesophageal reflux. J Pediatr 123:371–375, 1993.

132. DeCou JM, Shorter NA, Karl SR: Feeding Roux-en-Y jejunostomy in the management of severely neurologically impaired children. J Pediatr Surg 28:1276–1280, 1993.

133. Smith CD, Otherson HB Jr, Gogan NJ, et al: Nissen fundoplication in children with profound neurologic disability. High risks and unmet goals. Ann Surg 215:654–659, 1992.

134. Tuggle DW, Tunell WP, Hoelzer DJ, et al: The efficacy of Thal fundoplication in the treatment of gastroesophageal reflux: The influence of central nervous system impairment. J Pediatr Surg 23:638–640, 1988.

135. Ramachandran V, Ashcraft KW, Sharp RJ, et al: Thal fundoplication in neurologically impaired children. J Pediatr Surg 31:819–822, 1996.

136. Pearl RH, Robie DK, Ein SH, et al: Complications of gastroesophageal antireflux surgery in neurologically impaired versus neurologically normal children. J Pediatr Surg 25:1169–1173, 1990.

137. Borgstein ES, Heij HA, Beugelaar JD, et al: Risks and benefits of antireflux operations in neurologically impaired children. Eur J Pediatr 153:248–251, 1994.

138. Martinez DA, Ginn-Pease ME, Caniano DA: Sequellae of antireflux surgery in profoundly disabled children. J Pediatr Surg 27:267–273, 1992.

139. O'Neill JK, O'Neill PJ, Goth-Owens T, et al: Care-giver evaluation of anti-gastroesophageal reflux procedures in neurologically impaired children: What is the real-life outcome? J Pediatr Surg 31:375–380, 1996.

140. Dalla Vecchia LK, Grosfeld JL, West KW, et al: Reoperation after Nissen fundoplication in children with gastroesophageal reflux. Experience with 130 patients. Ann Surg 226:315–323, 1997.

141. Curci MR, Dibbins AW: Problems associated with a Nissen fundoplication following tracheoesophageal fistula and esophageal atresia repair. Arch Surg 123:618–620, 1988.

142. Wheatley MJ, Coran AG, Wesley JR: Efficacy of the Nissen fundoplication in the management of gastroesophageal reflux following esophageal atresia repair. J Pediatr Surg 28:53–55, 1993.

143. Jolley SG, Johnson DG, Roberts CC, et al: Patterns of gastroesophageal reflux in children following repair of esophageal atresia and distal tracheoesophageal fistula. J Pediatr Surg 15:857–862, 1980.

144. Engum SA, Grosfeld JL, West KW, et al: Analysis of morbidity and mortality in 227 cases of esophageal atresia and/or tracheoesophageal fistula over two decades. Arch Surg 130:502–509, 1995.

145. Lindahl H, Rintala R: Long-term complications in cases of isolated esophageal atresia treated with esophageal anastomosis. J Pediatr Surg 30:1222–1223, 1995.

146. Orringer MB, Kirsh MM, Sloan H: Long-term esophageal function following repair of esophageal atresia. Ann Surg 186:436–443, 1977.

147. Duranceau A, Fisher SR, Flye MW, et al: Motor function of the esophagus after repair of esophageal atresia and tracheoesophageal fistula. Surgery 82:116–123, 1977.

148. Romeo G, Zuccarello B, Proietto F, et al: Disorders of the esophageal motor activity in atresia of the esophagus. J Pediatr Surg 22:120–124, 1987.

149. Shono T, Suita S, Arima T, et al: Motility function of the esophagus before primary anastomosis in esophageal atresia. J Pediatr Surg 28:673–676, 1993.

150. Tovar JA, Diez Pardo JA, Murcia J, et al: Ambulatory 24-hour manometric and pH metric evidence of permanent impairment of clearance capacity in patients with esophageal atresia. J Pediatr Surg 30:1224–1231, 1995.

151. Parker AF, Christie DL, Cahill JL: Incidence and significance of gastroesophageal reflux following repair of esophageal atresia and tracheoesophageal fistula and the need for antireflux procedures. J Pediatr Surg 14:5–8, 1979.

152. Pieretti R, Shandling B, Stephens CA: Resistant esophageal stenosis associated with reflux after repair of esophageal atresia: A therapeutic approach. J Pediatr Surg 9:355–357, 1974.

153. Fonkalsrud EW: Gastroesophageal fundoplication for reflux following repair of esophageal atresia: Experience with nine patients. Arch Surg 114:48–51, 1979.

154. Lindahl H, Rintala R, Louhimo I: Failure of the Nissen fundoplication to control gastroesophageal reflux in esophageal atresia patients. J Pediatr Surg 24:985–987, 1989.

155. Snyder CL, Ramachandran V, Kennedy AP, et al: Efficacy of partial wrap fundoplication for gastroesophageal reflux after repair of esophageal atresia. J Pediatr Surg 32:1089–1092, 1997.

156. Boix-Ochoa J, Rehbein F: Oesophageal stenosis due to reflux esophagitis. Arch Dis Child 40:197–199, 1965.

157. O'Neill JA Jr, Betts J, Ziegler MM, et al: Surgical management of reflux strictures of the esophagus in childhood. Ann Surg 196:453–460, 1982.

158. Hetzel DJ, Dent J, Reed WD, et al: Healing and relapse of severe peptic esophagitis after treatment with omeprazole. Gastroenterology 95:903–912, 1988.

159. Kato S, Ebina K, Fujii K, et al: Effect of omeprazole in the

treatment of refractory acid-related diseases in childhood: Endoscopic healing and 24-hour intragastric acidity. J Pediatr 128:415–421, 1996.

160. DeGiacomo C, Bawa P, Franceshi M, et al: Omeprozole for severe reflux esophagitis in children. J Pediatr Gastroenterol Nutr 24:528–532, 1997.

161. Hoeffel JC, Nihoul-Fekete C, Schmitt M: Esophageal adenocarcinoma after gastroesophageal reflux in children. J Pediatr 115:259–261, 1989.

162. Adzick NS, Fisher JH, Winter HS, et al: Esophageal adenocarcinoma 20 years after esophageal atresia repair. J Pediatr Surg 24:741–744, 1989.

163. Hassall E, Weinstein WM: Partial regression of childhood Barrett's esophagus after fundoplication. Am J Gastroenterol 87:1506–1512, 1992.

164. Nibali SC, Barresi G, Tuccari G, et al: Barrett's esophagus in an infant: A long standing history with final postsurgical regression. J Pediatr Gastroenterol Nutr 7:602–607, 1988.

165. Cheu HW, Grosfeld JL, Heifetz SA, et al: Persistence of Barrett's esophagus in children after antireflux surgery: Influence on follow-up care. J Pediatr Surg 27:260–266, 1992.

166. Salo JA, Salminen JT, Kiviluoto TA, et al: Treatment of Barrett's esophagus by endoscopic laser ablation and antireflux surgery. Ann Surg 227:40–44, 1998.

29

LESIONS OF THE STOMACH

Peter W. Dillon, MD • Robert E. Cilley, MD

☐ Hypertrophic Pyloric Stenosis

Infantile hypertrophic pyloric stenosis (PS) is the most common cause of gastric outlet obstruction in children and is one of the most frequent conditions requiring surgery in the newborn.[1]

The first report of infantile PS in 1717 included clinical as well as postmortem findings.[2] The disease was not accepted as a true entity until the description of two cases by Hirschsprung in 1888.[3] Lobker, in 1898, was the first to successfully treat a patient using a gastrojejunostomy to bypass the obstructed pylorus. Early surgical mortality rates remained high. Various extramucosal pyloroplasty techniques were reported in the early 1900s, culminating in Ramstedt's pyloromyotomy procedure in 1911, which has served as the basis for all surgical techniques since.[4]

INCIDENCE

Hypertrophic PS occurs in 1 to 3 of every 1000 live births in the United States.[5] There are reports that the incidence of PS is increasing[6] and other reports that it is declining.[7] The 4:1 male-to-female ratio remains constant. PS is more common in infants of Caucasian descent and is rare in Asian children.[8] The belief that first-born males are more frequently afflicted has been disputed.[9] A genetic contribution is supported by the fact that 19% of boys and 7% of girls whose mothers had PS as an infant also have PS. PS occurs in only 5% of boys and 2.5% of girls whose father had the disease.[10] The risk of PS is lower with older maternal age, higher maternal education, and low birth weight.[7]

As many as 7% of infants with PS have associated malformations. Three major malformations include intestinal malrotation, obstructive uropathy, and esophageal atresia. Other anomalies associated with PS include hiatal hernia and a deficiency in hepatic glucuronyl transferase activity similar to Gilbert syndrome.[11–13] The jaundice that is commonly noted with PS spontaneously resolves following surgical correction of the obstruction and reestablishment of oral feedings.

ETIOLOGY

The etiology of PS remains unknown. The lesion may be congenital or acquired. Theories explaining the etiology of PS include gastric hyperacidity leading to muscle spasm and hypertrophy,[14–16] abnormal pyloric innervation,[17–22] and abnormal motility secondary to diminished pacemaker cells.[23]

The infant with PS is usually a full-term infant who presents with the onset of nonbilious, projectile vomiting between 3 and 6 weeks of age. Premature infants comprise about 10% of the cases, whereas fewer than 4% of patients develop symptoms after 3 months of age.[1, 24] The history of vomiting varies from abrupt onset with rapid progression to gradual progression of a vomiting pattern from the first days of life. Numerous formula changes have often been made. Although rare, an infant with prolonged vomiting can present with significant weight loss and failure to thrive.

With the widespread use of newer diagnostic techniques and a greater awareness of the problem, most pediatricians and family practice physicians are able to diagnose the condition earlier in its clinical course. The classic, defining symptom of forceful or projectile vomiting can be quite impressive and difficult to ignore. The emesis usually occurs shortly after a feeding, and the infant remains constantly hungry. It is always nonbilious in nature but may be streaked with blood or appear coffee-ground in color. In one study, 66% of the patients presented with hematemesis from acid-induced esophagitis or gastritis.[25]

The diagnostic finding on physical examination is a mobile, ovoid mass, commonly referred to as an "olive," palpable in the epigastrium or right upper quadrant. In a crying, irritable infant, palpation may be difficult, and with the advent of simple and reliable diagnostic imaging modalities, there is great angst about the potential for erosion of clinical skills necessary to make the diagnosis. Patience and persistence are necessary qualities when examining an infant suspected of having PS. The chances of successfully palpating the pyloric olive are enhanced if the infant is quiet and cooperative. The examiner may see upper abdominal distention with visible gastric peristaltic waves. Gastric decompression by tube followed by a sham feeding with a pacifier dipped in formula or dextrose water may improve access to the upper abdomen.

Palpation begins in the epigastrium under the liver edge. Deep palpation just to the right of the midline reveals a firm, mobile mass approximately 2 cm in length that slides beneath the examining fingers. Given the diagnostic accuracy of ultrasonography (US), sedation for the purpose of palpation is contraindicated owing to the risk of vomiting and aspiration. Palpation of the pyloric olive obviates the need for further diagnostic evaluation.

The differential diagnosis for nonbilious emesis includes overfeeding, gastroesophageal reflux (GER), pylorospasm with delayed gastric emptying, salt-wasting adrenogenital syndrome, and elevated intracranial pressure. Anatomic abnormalities causing gastric outlet obstruction include an antral web, a pyloric or gastric duplication, a gastric neoplasm, and extrinsic gastric compression.

US or contrast upper gastrointestinal (GI) study may be done to confirm the diagnosis (Fig. 29–1). The classic radiographic contrast findings are the *string sign,* produced by contrast medium outlining the narrowed pyloric channel, and the *shoulder sign,* caused by hypertrophied muscle protruding into the gastric lumen. The pyloric channel may also appear as two parallel threads resembling rail-road tracks. The risk of aspiration of contrast medium during induction of anesthesia warrants removal of as much of the contrast agent as possible when the study is completed and aspiration of the stomach again before administration of anesthesia. Contrast studies may help identify other causes of nonbilious vomiting, such as gastric atony, delayed gastric emptying, or GER.

US is the most sensitive test to diagnose PS in the absence of a palpable olive.[26] Although it is much more operator dependent than a contrast study, it is an easier test to perform with less risk to the infant. The characteristic appearance of PS on US is on the cross-sectional axis of the pylorus with the image of a doughnut or target bull's-eye sign. Pyloric dimensions with a positive predictive value of greater than 90% are muscle thickness greater than 4 mm and pyloric channel length greater than 17 mm. Because these measurements are age dependent, 3-mm muscle thickness is diagnostic for PS in infants younger than 30 days of age.[27]

Clinical diagnosis has a sensitivity of 72%, a specificity of 97%, and a positive and negative predictive value of 98% and 61%, respectively.[28, 29] US has a sensitivity of 97%, a specificity of 100%, and a positive and negative predictive value of 100% and 98%, respectively.[30] Increased reliance on US may have a negative impact on clinical diagnostic skills. More expedient surgical treatment is possible because accurate diagnosis may be made before significant fluid and electrolyte imbalances occur.[31]

If PS is detected within 7 days of the onset of symptoms, only about 10% of patients will have severe metabolic derangements or dehydration.[31]

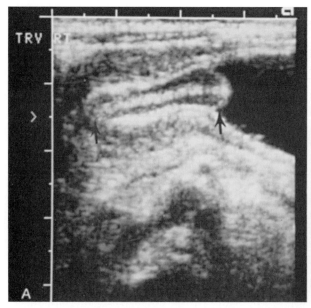 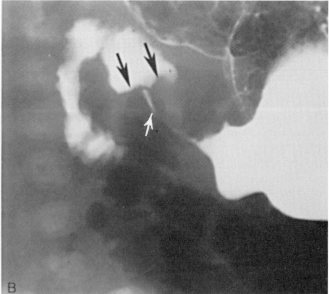

Figure 29–1. *A,* Sonogram demonstrating infant hypertrophic stenosis with an elongated pylorus (note the distance between the *arrows*) and a thickened pyloric wall with increased total diameter. *B,* Classic appearance of infant hypertrophic pyloric stenosis with a barium contrast study. Note the gastric distention, narrowed pyloric channel (*small arrow*), and fornix or "shoulder effects" of bulging hypertrophic muscle at the distal duodenal end of the pylorus (*large arrows*). (Courtesy of G.W. Taylor, MD.)

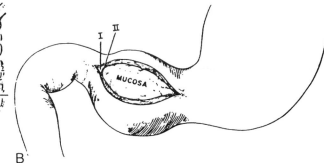

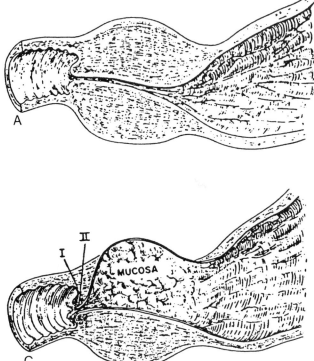

Figure 29–2. *A,* A sagittal section through hypertrophic pyloric stenosis including the distal antrum, pylorus, and proximal duodenum. Note the capping of the duodenal mucosa over the distal pylorus and the protrusion of muscle hypertrophy proximally into the distal antrum. *B,* Serosal incision and myotomy. Note extension onto the distal antrum and appearance of the duodenal mucosal "cap" (I), with the few remaining muscle fibers (II) between the pyloric mucosa and the cap. No attempt is made to divide these fibers because of the danger of duodenal mucosal perforation. *C,* Sagittal view of a complete myotomy. Note the duodenal mucosal cap (I) and the undivided distal pyloric muscle fibers (II). (From Quinby WC: Surgery 59:627, 1966.)

Prolonged vomiting produces electrolyte losses dominated by H^+ and Cl^- ions with lesser losses of Na^+ and K^+ ions. Contraction alkalosis may occur, manifested by hypochloremia and hypokalemia. As volume status is further compromised, aldosterone levels rise to increase the renal tubular absorption of Na^+ and water. As a result, potassium levels are further depleted as both K^+ and H^+ excretion in the urine are increased. Because Cl^- levels are low due to the vomiting of gastric fluid, renal tubular absorption of HCO_3^- occurs with the Na^+, thereby increasing the degree of metabolic alkalosis, in a setting of paradoxical aciduria. Alterations in magnesium and calcium levels are rarely important, but with delayed diagnosis, severe hypoglycemia and hypoalbuminemia may occur.

The infant who presents with less than 5% clinical dehydration and normal serum electrolytes can undergo surgery promptly without a substantial period of resuscitation. However, an infant with profound metabolic alkalosis and associated hypochloremia may require 48 hours or more of fluid and electrolyte replacement prior to general anesthesia. Initial fluid resuscitation should be with normal saline in boluses of 10 to 20 ml/kg. A continuous infusion of 5 or 10% dextrose in 0.45% saline should then be started at 1.5 times the calculated maintenance rate. Potassium supplementation is not added to the infusion until fluid volume is properly restored, as evidenced by adequate urine output. Potassium can then be replaced slowly with the maintenance fluids or administered in bolus form, depending on the degree of hypokalemia. Serum electrolyte levels should be rechecked every 6 to 12 hours to guide adjustments in fluid and electrolyte management. The operative treatment of PS must await correction of dehydration and restoration of near-normal serum potassium and chloride levels. Correction of the alkalosis is signaled by reduction of the serum HCO_3^- to a level below 30 mEq/dl.

Since the time of Ramstedt, the definitive treatment of PS has been the pyloromyotomy. Several incisions have been advocated, but recent studies have reported no particular advantage of one over the other.[32–36] Grossly, the hypertrophic pylorus is tan-white, has a firm consistency, and is slightly asymmetric. With palpation, the distal extent of the muscular hypertrophy can be determined, and often this junction with the normal duodenal mucosa is highlighted by a thin line visible in the seromuscular layer. Protrusion of the pyloric muscle into the duodenal bulb makes the duodenal mucosa susceptible to penetration if the incision is carried too far distally. Proximally, the boundary of the hypertrophic pylorus is not as sharply defined because the hypertrophic fibers blend with the normal muscle fibers of the anterior gastric wall (Fig. 29–2).

The initial incision of the pyloric region begins 1 to 2 mm from the pyloroduodenal junction and is carried onto the anterior gastric wall. The incision should cut little more than the serosa. The underlying firm fibers are divided using blunt dissection with a clamp, the rounded end of a scalpel handle, or a special pyloric spreader until the pyloric submucosal layer is visualized. The fibers are then mobilized for the entire length of the incision, and the wound edges are separated to allow the intact mucosa to bulge out.

The most risky point of entry into the duodenal lumen is at the pyloroduodenal boundary. All of the hypertrophied fibers at the proximal margin with the antrum should be divided, normal gastric wall thickness should be visualized, and no attempt should be made to divide the few remaining fibers at the pyloroduodenal junction. An adequate pyloromyotomy has been performed when the two halves of the hypertrophied muscle can be rocked independent of each other in opposite directions. Prior to returning the pylorus into the abdominal cavity, a check is made to ensure mucosal integrity. Leakage of air or bile signals the presence of a perforation requiring repair. No attempt should be made to arrest the venous bleeding associated with the incision because this will cease once the pylorus is returned to its anatomic position.

Laparoscopic techniques have been applied to the surgical treatment of PS.[37–41] With no significant differences reported in overall operative times, time to full feedings, and lengths of stay, the advantage of the laparoscopic approach appears to be cosmetic.[42, 43]

In most series reported by pediatric surgeons, the incidence of mucosal perforation during the course of a pyloromyotomy varies from 1 to 4%.[44, 45] This rate tends to be higher in general surgical units.[46] When a mucosal perforation is detected, there are two methods of effective repair. If the disruption is large or in the middle of the myotomy, the mucosa may be reapproximated with absorbable sutures and the muscle closed over it as a second layer. A new myotomy should then be performed a safe distance from the first site by rotating the pylorus to a suitable position. Most instances of mucosal disruption occur at the pyloroduodenal junction. Most surgeons close the mucosal defect with absorbable sutures and patch with omentum. With either technique, the outcomes have been the same.[45] Nasogastric tube decompression may be necessary for 24 to 48 hours.

Postoperative feeding regimens of infants undergoing pyloromyotomy have changed dramatically since the early 1990s because it is recognized that infants tolerate accelerated feeding schedules earlier after surgery than previously believed. Most surgeons now start graduated oral feedings 6 hours postoperatively with advancement to full feedings within 24 hours. This aggressive feeding program has resulted in significantly shorter lengths of hospitalization.[47] Measurements of gastric emptying following pyloromyotomy have shown that normal function does not return until 1 week after surgery.[48]

Postoperative complications following surgery for PS are relatively rare, although reports vary among institutions. Wound infection and dehiscence rates are approximately 1%. Persistent vomiting beyond 48 hours after surgery is a frustrating problem, with an incidence ranging from 3 to 31%.[45, 49] One must always be concerned about an incomplete myotomy, but the differential diagnosis also includes underlying GER. A younger age at diagnosis of PS is the only reported predictor of persistent postoperative vomiting.[49] In the immediate postoperative period, a contrast study to evaluate the pyloromyotomy is difficult to interpret because the radiologic appearance of the pylorus changes little from its preoperative status for some time after operation. In the absence of findings of a complete gastric outlet obstruction or a mucosal perforation, postoperative vomiting almost always subsides.

Nonoperative therapy for PS, including frequent small, liquid feedings, oral atropine,[50–53] or intravenous atropine, has been used but not widely.[54] Pyloric muscular hypertrophy was noted to resolve over 4 to 12 months. Endoscopic balloon dilation of the hypertrophied pylorus has been reported in an infant with a previously repaired giant omphalocele.[55] Although the potential risk of complete pyloric disruption exists, balloon dilation may represent a therapeutic option when direct surgical repair is not possible.

☐ Focal Foveolar Hyperplasia

Idiopathic infantile focal foveolar hyperplasia is a rare cause of gastric outlet obstruction with an unknown etiology, and it may simulate PS.[56]

Focal foveolar hyperplasia has been reported in prostaglandin E_1 therapy for infants with congenital heart disease.[57, 58] Affected infants tend to be older than would be expected with PS, with most cases reported at 2 to 3 months of age. The degree of mucosal hyperplasia that produces the pyloric channel obstruction appears to be dose related and may resolve after cessation of the drug.[58]

☐ Congenital Gastric Outlet Obstruction

Congenital gastric outlet obstructions other than PS are exceedingly rare lesions with an estimated incidence of 1 in 100,000 live births.[59] Within this group of anatomic anomalies, pyloric webs are the most common, followed by pyloric atresia, antral webs, and antral atresia.[60] The etiology of these defects is unknown. Symptoms depend on the degree of obstruction.

Antral and *pyloric webs* are circumferential membranes with a central patency composed of redundant gastric mucosa and submucosa. They cause intermittent, partial gastric obstruction. Pyloric webs appear as a windsock lesion prolapsing through the pyloric channel into the duodenum. Depending on the degree of obstruction, the diagnosis may be made at any age. Often, the symptoms are vague and nonspecific and may include epigastric pain, intermittent nonbilious vomiting, and failure to thrive.

Prolonged diagnostic delays have been reported because the symptoms are often variable and the

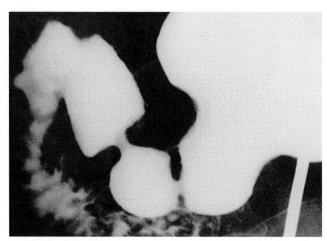

Figure 29–3. Gastric antral web in a 2-year-old child. (Courtesy of Kathleen Eggli, MD.)

obstruction is difficult to demonstrate.[61, 62] Upper GI contrast studies offer the best chance to visualize the membrane (Fig. 29–3). Often, contrast studies identify nonobstructing contraction rings in the antrum, and these structures must be differentiated from a web. The obstructing nature of the defect should then be confirmed by fiberoptic gastroscopy before embarking on surgical intervention.[63]

Surgical management of either a pyloric or antral web involves excision of a portion of the web through a transverse incision placed over the web. The exact location of the web can be determined at the time of surgery either by concomitant endoscopy or by balloon traction on the membrane following insertion of a Foley catheter through a separate gastrotomy. The incision is then closed transversely to prevent stenosis. Case reports of endoscopic balloon dilation and membrane transection have also been published, and a new technique to consider is laser ablation of the membrane.[64–67] No long-term complications of any these procedures have been reported.

Pyloric or *antral atresia* accounts for fewer than 1% of intestinal atresias. Prenatal detection is possible owing to maternal polyhydramnios, an enlarged stomach, and esophageal dilation on US.[68] Nonbilious vomiting occurs shortly after birth. Abdominal radiographs may show a dilated stomach with a gasless abdomen, and a contrast study shows complete outlet obstruction. Structurally, the atresia may be a complete membrane or a fibrotic segmental gap. Pyloric atresia is usually repaired with a gastroduodenostomy, but pyloroplasty with local excision may be effective if just a thin membrane is involved.

An unusual association of pyloric atresia has been reported with *junctional epidermolysis bullosa*,[69, 70] an autosomal recessive disease with a poor prognosis. These infants develop vesiculobullous lesions in response to minimal trauma or friction. Abnormalities in dermal basement membrane integrin expression and hemidesmosome structure have been detected. The diagnosis can be detected prenatally with fetal skin biopsies.[71–73] Almost all infants succumb to overwhelming sepsis.

□ Gastric Volvulus

Acquired or congenital abnormalities in fixation and ligamentous suspension of the stomach may predispose an infant or child to developing gastric volvulus. Two anatomic forms of gastric volvulus are possible. In children, the most common type is an organoaxial volvulus, which occurs when the line of rotation connects the gastroesophageal junction with the pylorus and allows the greater curvature of the stomach to flip up and over the lesser curve (Fig. 29–4). The less common mesentericoaxial volvulus rotates around a transverse axis line between the lesser curvature and the greater curvature of the stomach, resulting in the antrum and pyloroduodenal junction flipping up toward the gastroesophageal junction. Gastric obstruction develops in both situations. This condition has frequently been associated with diaphragmatic abnormalities such as congenital posterolateral diaphragmatic hernia, diaphragmatic eventration, esophageal hiatal hernia, and paraesophageal hernia formation.[74–77] Other associated anomalies include malrotation and asplenia syndrome (or Ivemark's syndrome).[78, 79]

Clinically, gastric volvulus is most likely to present as an acute event in infants and toddlers. Older children, particularly neurologically impaired children with a history of aerophagia, may present with chronic or recurrent episodes of volvulus. Symptoms of acute volvulus are sudden epigastric pain and persistent vomiting or retching. Abdominal or epigastric distention may be noted on physical examination, and attempted passage of a nasogastric tube may be difficult or impossible. Shock or peritonitis indicate that gastric necrosis and perforation have occurred. Chronic volvulus is much harder to diagnose because children may present with intermittent vomiting, vague epigastric abdominal pain, early satiety, and symptoms of GER.

In the acute setting, abdominal radiographs are diagnostic, demonstrating massive gastric distention, often with a solitary air-fluid level in the epigastrium or left upper quadrant. The remainder of the abdomen may be gasless. A contrast study may show a dilated esophagus with a tapered distal contour and no passage of the agent into the stomach.

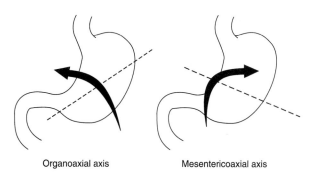

Organoaxial axis   Mesentericoaxial axis

Figure 29–4. Schematic representation of the two types of gastric volvulus with their lines of rotation.

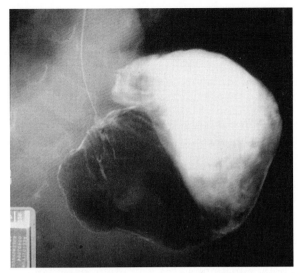

Figure 29–5. Barium contrast roentgenogram study demonstrating a mesentericoaxial gastric volvulus with the esophagogastric junction below the pylorus. (Courtesy of Kathleen Eggli, MD.)

However, the radiographic appearance of a gastric volvulus can vary depending on the degree of obstruction[80] (Fig. 29–5).

Although it is a rare problem, gastric volvulus usually presents as an acute surgical emergency requiring prompt diagnosis, resuscitation, and treatment. If is not properly recognized, the mortality is as high as 80% due to delay in recognition and treatment. The surgical mortality of 21% is due to complications of strangulation, necrosis, and perforation even if gastric volvulus is promptly treated.[74] Operative treatment involves reduction of the volvulus with repair or resection of any areas of transmural necrosis or perforation. Gastric fixation with either an anterior gastropexy or placement of a Stamm gastrostomy effectively minimizes the chance of recurrence. If the infant has concomitant GER, a fundoplication should also be constructed. A thorough inspection for associated diaphragmatic and crural abnormalities should be performed. Chronic gastric volvulus can sometimes be managed endoscopically with placement of a percutaneous gastrostomy for fixation or with laparoscopic gastropexy.[81]

☐ Congenital Microgastria

Congenital microgastria is a rare anomaly that results from an unknown impairment in foregut development. The resulting gastric structure is a hypoplastic, tubular organ with little definition or function. Reflecting an early fetal abnormality in mesodermal development, it is always associated with a variable pattern of malformations of the lung, heart, aortic arch, skeleton, and central nervous system. A number of conditions associated with microgastria have been reported including esophageal atresia, duodenal atresia, malrotation, Hirsch-

sprung's disease, imperforate anus, situs inversus viscerum, cardiac anomalies, asplenia, and skeletal anomalies.[82]

Infants with microgastria present shortly after birth with symptoms of inadequate gastric volume and intractable GER. Malnutrition, growth retardation, and failure to thrive are associated clinical problems. Due to rapid gastric emptying from the small stomach reservoir, symptoms of "dumping" with diarrhea are usually present. An upper GI contrast study shows a megaesophagus with a small stomach and profound GER.

Because symptoms of microgastria usually appear in the newborn period, initial management of this problem with continuous nasogastric or nasojejunal feedings is effective. With growth and time, graduated oral feedings can be attempted and may be tolerated. Aggressive medical therapy for GER is required. In some infants, the hypoplastic stomach may eventually enlarge enough to allow placement of a gastrostomy tube. However, if gastric feedings are not tolerated, enteral nutrition can still be supplied by means of a feeding jejunostomy.[83] Rarely is long-term parenteral nutrition required for this problem. Ultimately, if the stomach fails to grow, gastric augmentation can be considered. The best results come from the construction of a side-to-side Roux-en-Y jejunal pouch (Hunt-Lawrence pouch) to create a gastric reservoir[71–73, 84] (Fig. 29–6).

☐ Gastric Perforation

Gastric perforation is a rare abdominal catastrophe with a high mortality rate, usually occurring

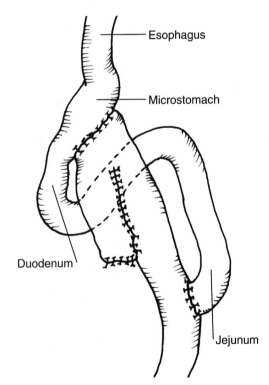

Figure 29–6. Gastric augmentation for congenital microgastria using a Roux-en-Y gastrojejunostomy with a J-pouch reservoir.

in the neonatal intensive care unit setting. Three mechanisms have been proposed: traumatic, ischemic, and spontaneous. The specific etiology of a gastric perforation may be difficult to determine because the infants are usually sick and the actual pathology yields few clues.

Most gastric perforations are due to iatrogenic trauma.[85] The most common injury is caused by vigorous nasogastric or orogastric tube placement. Perforation is usually along the greater curvature and appears as a puncture wound or a short laceration. Traumatic gastric perforation may develop as a result of severe gastric distention during the course of positive pressure ventilation during bag-mask resuscitation or mechanical ventilation for respiratory failure.[86]

The mechanism of ischemic perforation has been difficult to elucidate because these cases of perforation are associated with conditions of severe physiologic stress such as extreme prematurity, sepsis, and neonatal asphyxia. Ischemic gastric perforations have been noted in conjunction with necrotizing enterocolitis. Because gastric stress ulcers have been reported in a variety of critically ill infants, it has been proposed that these perforations result from the transmural necrosis of such ulcers.

Spontaneous gastric perforations have been reported in otherwise healthy infants, usually within the 1st week of life.[87, 88] One hypothesis is that such perforations are due to a congenital defect in the muscular wall of the stomach.[89] However, similar pathologic findings have not been noted in other reports.

Signs and symptoms of a gastric perforation are usually those of an acute abdominal catastrophe associated with sepsis and respiratory failure. The physical examination is remarkable for significant abdominal distention capable of compromising ventilatory support. An abdominal radiograph confirms the presence of massive free air within the abdomen. No other studies are necessary.

Prior to definitive surgical intervention, during the evaluation and resuscitation of the infant, needle decompression of the abdomen may be required if ventilation is compromised by the distention. Surgical repair of most perforations consists of débridement and two-layer closure of the defect. A gastrostomy may be warranted. Significant gastric resections should be avoided. Rarely, gastric perforation sites may be difficult to pinpoint. Complete visualization of the greater and lesser curvatures as well as the gastroesophageal junction and posterior wall of the stomach is then required. Instillation of air or dilute methylene blue with distention of the stomach may help locate the perforation. Due to the associated problems of sepsis and respiratory failure often found in premature infants, mortality rates for gastric perforation are high, ranging from 25 to 58%.[85, 90]

☐ Foreign Bodies

Foreign body ingestion occurs most frequently between the ages of 6 months and 3 years. Although this subject is covered in Chapter 12 there are some characteristics of gastric foreign bodies that warrant repetition. Seldom is direct surgical intervention required to treat a foreign body once it has reached the stomach.[91]

Experience has shown that certain characteristics of an object predict whether it passes out of the stomach and through the intestinal tract.[92] In general, toddlers do not pass round objects with a diameter greater than 2.5 cm or elongated objects with a width greater than 2 cm or a length greater than 5 cm. Even smaller objects, if ingested by an infant, are unlikely to move out of the stomach and should be considered for early endoscopic retrieval. Most small sharp objects, such as nails, screws, straight pins, and even safety pins pass uneventfully. Passage of any gastric foreign body can be aided by the institution of a high-fiber diet. The course of such objects should be tracked with serial radiographs every 5 to 7 days until elimination is documented. If an object remains in the stomach for 4 weeks, it should be removed endoscopically or surgically.

☐ Bezoars

Bezoars are masses of solidified organic or nonorganic material found in the stomach and small bowel. Four types of bezoars have been described based on their composition: phytobezoars, trichobezoars, lactobezoars, and miscellaneous. *Phytobezoars* are composed of plant and vegetable material such as orange pulp, celery, persimmon, pumpkin, and grass. These types of bezoars are more likely to develop in patients with poor mastication and abnormal gastric motility.[93] *Trichobezoars* consist of hair, usually the patient's own, but they can also include other nondegradable fibers including wool, nylon, and animal hair. These trichobezoars are associated with emotionally disturbed children with aberrant appetite. An unusual variant of a gastric trichobezoar has been termed the *Rapunzel syndrome* when the trichobezoar extends through the entire GI tract.[94] *Lactobezoars* form from precipitates of formula, usually in premature infants. Factors such as prematurity, high-calorie formulas containing calcium, and continuous-drip feedings are thought to contribute to their formation.[95] Several medications such as antacids and cimetidine have been found to form bezoars.[96, 97]

Bezoars are asymptomatic until they reach a critical size. Symptoms include abdominal pain, early satiety, vomiting, anorexia, and weight loss. Complete gastric obstruction and a palpable abdominal mass may be found, especially with a trichobezoar. In premature infants, a lactobezoar may present with abdominal distention, vomiting, or high gastric residuals. Abdominal radiographs and an upper GI contrast study are diagnostic, and endoscopy is then used to identify the type of bezoar (Fig. 29–7).

Therapy depends on the type and size of the bezoar. Phytobezoars can be treated with endoscopy

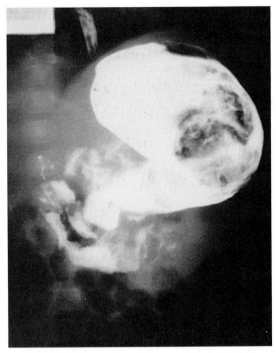

Figure 29–7. Barium contrast roentgenogram of a trichobezoar in an 8-year-old. (Courtesy of Kathleen Eggli, MD.)

and fragmentation. Techniques include physical disruption into smaller pieces followed by dissolution with saline, papain, acetylcysteine, or cellulase.[92] Lactobezoars and drug-induced bezoars seldom require endoscopic intervention and can usually be resolved with intravenous hydration and gastric decompression. Extracorporeal shock-wave lithotripsy and laser therapy have also been used. Most trichobezoars are so large that endoscopic therapy is unsuccessful and surgical extraction is required.

☐ Caustic Ingestions

Corrosive injuries causing significant damage to the stomach are unusual in children but can be seen in cases of acid or massive alkali ingestion. Most children suffering a caustic ingestion are younger than 5 years of age.[98] The most common agents ingested are commercially available liquid alkali products containing sodium hydroxide or sodium hypochlorite with a maximum concentration of 10%. Acid cleaning solutions often contain sulfuric acid, hydrochloric acid, sodium bisulfate, or hydrofluoric acid. Acids account for 15% of pediatric corrosive ingestions, producing coagulation necrosis with eschar formation, which then inhibits further acid penetration. Serious esophageal injury occurs in only 20% of acid ingestions, and the primary site of injury is the prepyloric area of the stomach.[99]

Injury assessment begins with the clinical history and an understanding of the type and the amount of substance ingested. Signs and symptoms of a caustic ingestion may include drooling, oral burns

or erythema, dysphagia, hoarseness, and substernal or epigastric abdominal pain. If oral burns are present, 30 to 50% of patients have an esophageal injury. However, the absence of an oral burn does not eliminate the possibility of an esophageal or gastric injury. Endoscopy within the first 24 hours of the ingestion is the most reliable method to evaluate the upper GI tract and to determine the degree of injury.[100]

If gastric mucosal injury is suspected following ingestion, pharmacologic blockade of intrinsic acid production should be instituted to minimize the ulcerogenic potential of the injury. Symptoms of midepigastric abdominal pain suggest a significant mucosal injury to the stomach. However, a caustic injury requiring acute surgical intervention is quite rare.[101] Development of signs and symptoms of acute peritonitis mandate urgent exploration. Because the ultimate extent of the injury may be difficult to determine in the acute setting, the initial surgical procedure should be débridement and repair of the necrotic stomach with placement of a gastrostomy tube. Ingestion of a large quantity of concentrated alkali may require a combined esophagogastrectomy with proximal diversion and a distal feeding jejunostomy. More commonly, acid gastric injuries cause prepyloric scarring that results in gastric outlet obstruction.[102] Restoration of intestinal continuity with either a gastroduodenostomy or a gastrojejunostomy following an antrectomy has been well tolerated in older children and adults.

☐ Gastric Duplications

Fewer than 4% of GI duplications are of gastric origin, and these usually occur in the antral or pyloric regions.[103, 104] Combined esophagogastric duplications are extremely rare.[105] These anomalies must be differentiated from duplications elsewhere in the GI tract that may have ectopic gastric tissue within them. Several theories have been proposed to explain the formation of these anomalies.[106–108] One third present in the newborn period, and more than half are diagnosed by 1 year of age.[109] Distal gastric duplications may simulate PS.[110] A duplication may present as a palpable mass in the midepigastrium. Rarely, cysts have been reported to cause GI bleeding and pancreatitis.[111–113]

Gastric duplications share a common outer muscular wall with the native stomach but seldom communicate with the lumen. Tubular duplications are usually found along the greater curvature in the antrum. Ectopic pancreatic tissue communicating with aberrant pancreatic ducts has been found within gastric duplications.

Plain abdominal radiographs and contrast studies are unlikely to be diagnostic. US or computed tomography may demonstrate a mass. The diagnosis can be aided by nuclear scintigraphy[114] (Figs. 29–8 and 29–9).

Surgical therapy depends on the size and the loca-

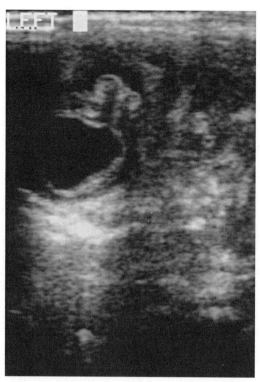

Figure 29–8. Ultrasonographic image of a tubular gastric duplication extending off of the greater curvature of the stomach. (Courtesy of Kathleen Eggli, MD.)

tion of the gastric duplication. Partial gastric resection or enucleation is the procedure of choice. For tubular lesions or those in which resection would compromise the pylorus or duodenum, stripping the mucosal lining is effective. Internal drainage procedures have been used for difficult duplications. Cyst excision may also require resection of an aberrant pancreatic lobe or drainage of a pseudocyst.

☐ Gastric Tumors

The most common gastric tumor in childhood is the teratoma, which accounts for fewer than 1% of all pediatric teratomas. Until the mid-1990s, these tumors were believed to occur exclusively in males, but there have been multiple reports of cases involving females.[115] Additionally, although originally always thought to be benign, malignant teratomas can occur as well.[116] Presenting symptoms are most often abdominal distention and a palpable mass. A gastric teratoma has produced upper GI hemorrhage as the initial symptom.[117]

Radiographic evaluation of these tumors is most effectively accomplished with either computed tomography or US. Treatment involves complete surgical resection even if a substantial gastrectomy is required owing to the potential for teratomas to recur or undergo malignant degeneration.[118]

Primary malignant tumors of the stomach are extremely rare in children and account for about 0.1% of pediatric malignancies.[119, 120] A number of reports

have described gastric lymphomas developing in children, with either Hodgkin's or non-Hodgkin's pathology.[120, 121] Presenting signs and symptoms are nonspecific and may include abdominal pain, weight loss, anorexia, a palpable abdominal mass, or gastric outlet obstruction.[122] In older patients, the incidence of gastric lymphoma is increasing, possibly as a result of chronic *Helicobacter pylori* infection.[123, 124] *H. pylori* infection induces epithelial changes of chronic gastritis that can lead to the development of low-grade mucosa-associated lymphoid tissue lymphoma, which may then evolve into high-grade lymphoma. Successful treatment of mucosa-associated lymphoid tissue lymphomas in children includes antibiotic therapy to eradicate the *H. pylori* as well as chemotherapy.[121] High-grade lymphomas are not responsive to such treatment and require surgical excision of the tumor followed by postoperative multimodal therapy.[125]

Other reported malignant tumors of the stomach include soft tissue sarcomas and ganglioneuroblastomas.[120, 126]

☐ Gastric Polyps

Gastric polyps are rare, and they seldom require surgical intervention for diagnosis or management. Solitary polyps are extremely rare, and most gastric polyps occur in association with one of the polyposis syndromes. The most common syndromes encountered are familial adenomatous polyposis, Peutz-Jeghers syndrome, and juvenile polyposis. Both juvenile polyposis and familial adenomatous polyposis have malignant potential and require lifelong repeated endoscopic surveillance of the entire GI tract.[127, 128]

Solitary gastric polyps can cause gastric outlet ob-

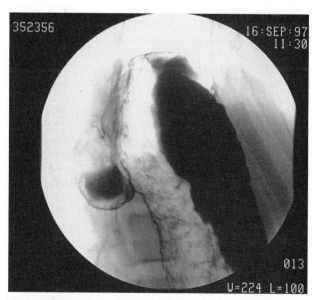

Figure 29–9. Barium contrast roentgenogram in a teenager with a symptomatic gastric diverticulum. The diverticulum originates on the posterior wall of the stomach just below the cardia.

struction and severe gastric bleeding requiring surgical intervention. Surgical procedures have included gastrotomy with simple excision of the polyp and partial gastrectomy with pyloroplasty.[129, 130]

☐ Peptic Ulcer Disease

Ulcers of the stomach and duodenum occur infrequently in children, but the incidence is clearly increasing.[131, 132] Peptic ulcer disease in children has been divided into primary or secondary categories based on the underlying pathophysiology.[133]

Primary ulcer disease occurs in children in the absence of an underlying systemic disease, acute medical illness, or extrinsic factors such as ulcerogenic medications. The ulcers are usually duodenal in location but may occur in the pyloric channel and are most often found in older children and adolescents. There is frequently a positive family history of peptic ulcer disease.[134] Primary gastric ulcers are rare.

Secondary ulcer disease develops in the setting of an underlying systemic illness or stress, or it is drug related. Head trauma, burns, sepsis, neonatal hypoxia, and certain medications (including nonsteroidal antiinflammatory medications and steroids) are recognized causes of ulcers.[135] Medical conditions reported to increase the frequency of peptic ulceration in children include systemic mastocytosis, pseudo–Zollinger-Ellison syndrome, cystic fibrosis, sickle cell disease, insulin-dependent diabetes mellitus, and gastroduodenal Crohn's disease.[136]

A significant advancement has been made in understanding the pathophysiology of primary ulcer disease in children with the identification of *H. pylori* infection as an etiologic agent.[137–139] This organism is a urease-producing, flagellated, gram-negative rod whose presence is related to chronic gastritis and duodenal ulcer disease. In *H. pylori* gastritis, the mucosa develops a chronic inflammatory infiltrate that can be severe, and antral nodularity with lymphoid hyperplasia is a characteristic finding on endoscopic biopsies. Numerous studies have confirmed the observations that *H. pylori* colonization of the gastric mucosa in this setting is associated with chronic gastritis in children.[139, 140] Additionally, there is a strong correlation between duodenal ulcer formation and *H. pylori* gastritis in the same population.[125] *H. pylori* gastritis has been reported in 90 to 100% of pediatric patients with duodenal ulcer disease.[141] If *H. pylori* was treated with antibiotic therapy and cleared from the gastric mucosa, the recurrence rate for duodenal ulcer disease was significantly reduced.[142] The most effective anti-*Helicobacter* regimen is triple therapy using a bismuth compound, tetracycline, and metronidazole for 1 to 4 weeks. Amoxicillin or ampicillin can replace tetracycline, if necessary. Only children with active gastroduodenal disease and confirmed *H. pylori* infection should be treated.

Although there is strong evidence of an association between *H. pylori* infection and antral gastritis in duodenal ulcer disease in children, there is little evidence to link such infection to gastric ulcer formation in the pediatric population.[143] Additionally, there is no evidence to implicate *H. pylori* infection in recurrent abdominal pain in children.[143, 144]

In the absence of a complication of the disease process, medical management is effective in treating gastroduodenal ulcer disease in both adults and children. Overall, approximately 80% of ulcers heal with resolution of clinical symptoms after 8 weeks of medical therapy. Pharmacologic agents effective in healing both gastric and duodenal ulcers include acid-neutralizing compounds (antacids), acid-suppressing agents (H2 blockers and proton pump blockers), and mucosal protective resins (sucralfate). Underlying conditions leading to secondary ulcer formation must also be treated. Concomitant adjuvant treatment for *H. pylori* infection is discussed earlier. Although stress ulcer prophylaxis with H2 receptor antagonists is probably effective in the pediatric population, the therapy has not been proved.[145]

Surgical intervention in children is most often indicated to manage the acute complications of peptic ulcer disease such as massive hemorrhage or perforation. Obstruction or intractability rarely develop in children. Even with significant hemorrhage the initial treatment should be medical because the majority of upper GI hemorrhage in children stops within 24 to 48 hours.[146] The indications for surgical intervention in children with persistent bleeding are ill defined and vary from a transfusion requirement of one half the calculated blood volume in 8 hours to 1 total blood volume in a 24-hour period. Most treatment strategies are derived from adult experiences.

Surgical intervention in children with peptic ulcer disease likewise is derived from adult experience. Options include truncal vagotomy and pyloroplasty, truncal vagotomy and antrectomy with either a gastroduodenostomy or gastrojejunostomy, or proximal gastric vagotomy. Little is known about the long-term implications of any of these procedures in children. For hemorrhagic ulcer disease requiring surgical intervention in infants and young children, simple oversewing of the ulcer in combination with medical therapy is indicated.[147] These ulcers are usually gastric in location and seldom require resection. In the older child, gastric ulcers are rare and usually respond to pharmacologic intervention. An ulcer with active hemorrhage in the older child is usually located in the duodenum, and surgical therapy is best accomplished with ligation of the ulcer bed and an acid-reducing surgical procedure such as a vagotomy and pyloroplasty. Consideration can be given to proximal gastric vagotomy in combination with direct surgical ligation of the ulcer. For the perforated duodenal ulcer, the technique of choice is still simple closure of the perforation with an omental patch, followed by postoperative medical therapy.

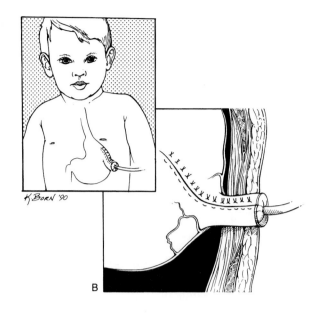

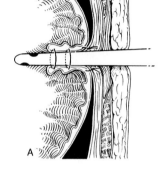

Figure 29–10. *A,* The Stamm gastrostomy with a double-pursestring inverted gastric tunnel firmly approximated to the abdominal wall tube exit site. *B,* The Janeway gastrostomy with a surgically constructed gastric pedicle tube exiting through the abdominal wall as a continent stoma.

□ Gastrostomy

A number of techniques are available for providing gastric access, and the risks and complications of each are well established (Fig. 29–10). It is now clear that the choice of a procedure should be individualized based on the health and needs of the child. There are two open surgical techniques employed in children for the placement of a gastrostomy tube. The Stamm technique is the most popular and can be done with either general or local anesthesia. The incision can either be midline or transverse. The gastrostomy tube (usually a mushroom catheter or Malecot tube) is inserted into the gastric lumen and secured with a double-pursestring suture to minimize leakage or disruption. A gastrostomy button device can also be inserted as a primary procedure. The gastrostomy site should be situated well away from the pylorus to prevent gastric outlet obstruction by the tube or the introduction of bolus feedings directly into the duodenum. The proper position of the gastrotomy on the stomach wall is debated, with its position varying anywhere from along the lesser curvature to the anterior gastric wall and the greater curvature.[148, 149]

The Janeway gastrostomy provides long-term gastric access without a continuously indwelling device such as a catheter or a button. It is established by constructing a gastric tube with a stapling device from the greater curvature or anterior gastric wall and bringing this tube through the abdominal wall as a stoma matured to the skin. Its effectiveness in children has been compromised by problems with the exposed gastric mucosa at the stoma site and the reflux of formula and gastric contents. The use of a nonrefluxing variation of this type of gastrostomy has been reported with moderate success.[150]

Percutaneous endoscopic gastrostomy (PEG) techniques are the principal invasive form of establishing enteral access in both children and adults.[151] Various modifications of this form of insertion have been proposed, including "push" and "pull" techniques.[152] Conditions considered a relative contraindication for the insertion of a PEG tube include the presence of ascites, uncorrected coagulopathy, gastric wall pathology, previous abdominal surgery, and the inability to pass an endoscope. Laparoscopic gastrostomy tube placement has been reported but is usually reserved for concomitant laparoscopic antireflux surgery.[153, 154]

Insertion of a gastrostomy tube is not a benign or risk-free procedure, and potential for complications always exists. Minor complications include skin excoriation at the gastrostomy site due to leakage of gastric contents, chronic gastrostomy site infection with yeast or bacteria, granulation tissue formation, formula leakage, gastrostomy tube dislodgment, chronic gastric erosions with bleeding, and catheter migration causing gastric outlet obstruction. Major complications include gastric, duodenal, or esophageal perforation by the catheter, gastrostomy site disruption with intraperitoneal contamination, gastric volvulus, and a persistent gastrocutaneous fistula. Depending on the type of gastrostomy, the incidence of reported complications varies between 10 and 20%.[155, 156] Almost all pediatric cancer patients who require gastrostomy tube placement can be expected to develop complications.[157]

With the development of many different types of skin-level feeding devices or buttons, patient care and comfort have been dramatically improved. Although these devices can be inserted at the time of the primary operation, their use is generally delayed until the gastrostomy site has had a chance to form and heal properly. Most surgeons arbitrarily wait 6 to 12 weeks before changing a gastrostomy tube for a button. Although rare, the major risk is disruption of the gastrostomy tract with subsequent intraperitoneal contamination that requires urgent surgical intervention. On the other hand, gastrostomy tract disruptions following button conversions of PEG tubes may occur in up to 20% of the cases. If a gastrostomy button or tube change is difficult or malposition of either type of device is suspected, a water-soluble contrast study should be obtained prior to the continued use of the device.

REFERENCES

1. Puri P, Lakshmanadass G: Hypertrophic pyloric stenosis. In Puri P (ed): Newborn Surgery. Oxford, England, Butterworth-Heinemann, 1996, pp 266–271.
2. Blair P: On the dissection of a child much emaciated. Philadelphia Transcriptions 30:631–632, 1717.
3. Hirschsprung H: Falle von angeborener Pylorus Stenose. Jb Kinderheilk 27:61, 1888.
4. Ramstedt C: Zur Operation der angeborenen Pylorus-Stenose. Med Klin 1702–1705, 1912.
5. Grant GA, McAleer JJA: Incidence of infantile hypertrophic pyloric stenosis [letter]. Lancet 1:1177, 1984.
6. Jedd MB, Melton LJ III, Griffen MR, et al: Trends in infantile hypertrophic pyloric stenosis in Olmsted County, Minnesota, 1950–1984. Paediatr Perinat Epidemiol 2:148–155, 1988.
7. Applegate MS, Druschel CM: The epidemiology of infantile hypertrophic pyloric stenosis in New York State, 1983 to 1990. Arch Pediatr Adolesc Med 149:1123–1129, 1995.
8. Klein A, Cremin BJ: Racial significance in pyloric stenosis. S Afr Med J 44:1130–1134, 1970.
9. Huguenard JR, Staples GE: Incidence of congenital hypertrophic pyloric stenosis within sibships. J Pediatr 81:45–49, 1972.
10. Carter CO, Evans KA: Inheritance of congenital hypertrophic pyloric stenosis. J Med Genet 6:233–254, 1969.
11. Pellerin D, Bertin P, Tavar JA: Gastroesophageal reflux and hypertrophic pyloric stenosis. Ann Chir Infant 15:7–14, 1974.
12. Woolley MM, Felscher BF, Asch MJ, et al: Jaundice, pyloric stenosis and hepatic glucuronyl transferase. J Pediatr Surg 9:359–363, 1974.
13. Iijima T, Okamaatsu T, Matsumura M, et al: Hypertrophic pyloric stenosis associated with hiatal hernia. J Pediatr Surg 31:277–279, 1996.
14. Miller RA: Observation on the gastric acidity during the first month of life. Arch Dis Child 16:22–27, 1941.
15. Rogers IM, Davidson DC, Lawrence J, et al: Neonatal secretion of gastrin and glucagon. Arch Dis Child 49:796–805, 1974.
16. Rogers IM: The enigma of pyloric stenosis. Some thoughts on the aetiology. Acta Paediatr 87:6–9, 1997.
17. Dieler R, Schroder JM: Myenteric plexus neuropathy in infantile hypertrophic pyloric stenosis. Acta Neuropathol (Berl) 78:649–661, 1989.
18. Okazaki T, Yamataka A, Fujiwara T, et al: Abnormal distribution of nerve terminals in infantile hypertrophic pyloric stenosis. J Pediatr Surg 29:655–658, 1994.
19. Kobayashi H, O'Brien DS, Puri P: Selective reduction in intramuscular nerve supporting cells in infantile hypertrophic pyloric stenosis. J Pediatr Surg 29:651–654, 1994.
20. Wattchow DA, Cass DT, Furness JB, et al: Abnormalities of peptide containing nerve fibers in infantile hypertrophic pyloric stenosis. Gastroenterology 92:443–448, 1987.
21. Kobayshi H, O'Briain DS, Puri P: Immunochemical characterization of neural cell adhesion molecule (NCAM), nitric oxide synthase, and neurofilament protein expression in pyloric muscle of patients with pyloric stenosis. J Pediatr Gastroenterol Nutr 20:319–325, 1995.
22. Kobayashi H, Wester T, Puri P: Age-related changes in innervation in hypertrophic pyloric stenosis. J Pediatr Surg 32:1704–1707, 1997.
23. Vanderwinden JM, Liu H, De Laet MH, et al: Study of the interstitial cells of Cajal in infantile hypertrophic pyloric stenosis. Gastroenterology 111:279–288, 1996.
24. Zhang AL, Cass DT, Dubois RS, et al: Infantile hypertrophic stenosis: A clinical review from a general hospital. J Paediatr Child Health 29:372–378, 1993.
25. Takeuchi S, Tamate S, Nakahira M, et al: Esophagitis in infants with hypertrophic pyloric stenosis: A source of hematemesis. J Pediatr Surg 28:59–62, 1993.
26. Hernanz-Schulman M, Sells LL, Ambrosino MM, et al: Hypertrophic pyloric stenosis in the infant without a palpable olive: Accuracy of sonographic diagnosis. Radiology 193:771–776, 1994.
27. Lamki N, Athey PA, Round ME, et al: Hypertrophic pyloric stenosis in the neonate—diagnostic criteria revisited. Can Assoc Radiol J 44:21–24, 1993.
28. Macdessi J, Oates RK: Clinical diagnosis of pyloric stenosis: A declining art. BMJ 306:553–555, 1993.
29. Poon TS, Zhang AL, Cartmill T, et al: Changing patterns of diagnosis and treatment of infantile hypertrophic pyloric stenosis: A clinical audit of 303 patients. J Pediatr Surg 31:1611–1615, 1996.
30. Godbole P, Sprigg A, Dickson JA, et al: Ultrasound compared with clinical examination in infantile hypertrophic pyloric stenosis. Arch Dis Child 75:335–337, 1996.
31. Chen EA, Luks FI, Gilchrist BF, et al: Pyloric stenosis in the age of ultrasonography: Fading skills, better patients? J Pediatr Surg 31:829–830, 1996.
32. Teechan EP, Garrow E: A new incision for pyloromyotomy. Int Surg 78:143–145, 1993.
33. Hingston G: Ramstedt's pyloromyotomy—what is the correct incision? N Z Med J 109:276–278, 1996.
34. Horwitz JP, Lally KP: Supraumbilical skin-fold incision for pyloromyotomy. Am J Surg 171:439–440, 1996.
35. Podevin G, Missirlu A, Branchereau S, et al: Umbilical incision for pyloromyotomy. Eur J Pediatr Surg 7:8–10, 1997.
36. Besson R, Sfeir R, Salakos C, et al: Congenital pyloric stenosis: A modified umbilical incision for pyloromyotomy. Pediatr Surg Int 12:224–225, 1997.
37. Najmaldin A, Tan HL: Early experience with laparoscopic pyloromyotomy for infantile hypertrophic pyloric stenosis. J Pediatr Surg 30:37–38, 1995.
38. Castanon J, Portilla E, Rodriquez E, et al: A new technique for laparoscopic repair of hypertrophic pyloric stenosis. J Pediatr Surg 30:1294–1296, 1995.
39. Alain JL, Grousseau D, Longis B, et al: Extramucosal pyloromyotomy by laparoscopy. Eur J Pediatr Surg 6:10–12, 1996.
40. Rothenberg SS: Laparoscopic pyloromyotomy: The slice and pull technique. Pediatr Endosurg and Innovat Tech 1:39–41, 1997.
41. Ford WD, Crameri JA, Holland AJ: The learning curve for laparoscopic pyloromyotomy. J Pediatr Surg 32:552–554, 1997.
42. Greason KL, Thompson WR, Downey EC, et al: Laparoscopic pyloromyotomy for infantile hypertrophic pyloric stenosis: Report of 11 cases. J Pediatr Surg 30:1571–1574, 1995.
43. Scorpio RJ, Tan HL, Hutson JM: Pyloromyotomy: Comparison between laparoscopic and open surgical techniques. J Laparoendosc Surg 5:81–84, 1995.
44. Royal RE, Linz DN, Gruppo DL, et al: Repair of mucosal perforation during pyloromyotomy: Surgeon's choice. J Pediatr Surg 30:1430–1432, 1995.
45. Hulka F, Harrison MW, Campbell TJ, et al: Complications of pyloromyotomy for infantile hypertrophic pyloric stenosis. Am J Surg 173:450–452, 1997.
46. Maher M, Hehir DJ, Horgan A, et al: Infantile hypertrophic pyloric stenosis: Long-term audit from a general surgical unit. Ir J Med Sci 165:115–117, 1996.
47. Georgeson KE, Corbin TJ, Griffen JW, et al: An analysis of feeding regimens after pyloromyotomy for hypertrophic pyloric stenosis. J Pediatr Surg 28:1478–1480, 1993.

48. Nour S, Mangnall Y, Dickson JA, et al: Measurement of gastric emptying in infants with pyloric stenosis using applied potential tomography. Arch Dis Child 68:484–486, 1993.

49. Luciani JL, Allai H, Polliotto S, et al: Prognostic factors of the postoperative vomiting in case of hypertrophic pyloric stenosis. Eur J Pediatr Surg 7:93–96, 1997.

50. Millin GW, Lantulli TV, Altman HS: Congenital pyloric stenosis—a controlled evaluation of medical treatment utilizing methyl-scopolamine nitrate. J Pediatr 66:649–657, 1965.

51. Day LR: Medical management of pyloric stenosis. JAMA 207:948–950, 1969.

52. Jacoby NM: Pyloric stenosis: Selective medical and surgical treatment. A survey of sixteen years' experience. Lancet 1:119–121, 1962.

53. Swift PG, Prossor JE: Modern management of pyloric stenosis—must it always be surgical? Arch Dis Child 66:667–669, 1991.

54. Nagita A, Yamaguchi J, Amemoto K, et al: Management and ultrasonographic appearance of infantile hypertrophic pyloric stenosis with intravenous atropine sulfate. J Pediatr Gastroenterol Nutr 23:172–177, 1996.

55. Ogawa Y, Higashimoto Y, Nishijima E, et al: Successful endoscopic balloon dilatation for hypertrophic pyloric stenosis. J Pediatr Surg 31:1712–1714, 1996.

56. Holland AJ, Freeman JK, Le Quesne GW, et al: Idiopathic focal foveolar hyperplasia in infants. Pediatr Surg Int 12:497–500, 1997.

57. Meercado-Deane MG, Burton EM, Brawley AV, et al: Prostaglandin-induced foveolar hyperplasia simulating pyloric stenosis in an infant with cyanotic heart disease. Pediatr Radiol 24:45–46, 1994.

58. Peled N, Dagan O, Babyn P, et al: Gastric outlet obstruction induced by prostaglandin therapy in neonates. N Engl J Med 327:505–510, 1992.

59. Cremin BJ: Neonatal pre-pyloric membrane. S Afr Med J 41:1076–1079, 1967.

60. Moore CM: Congenital gastric outlet obstruction. J Pediatr Surg 24:1241–1246, 1989.

61. Woolley MM, Gwinn JL, Mares A: Congenital partial gastric antral obstruction. Ann Surg 180:265–273, 1974.

62. Blazek F, Boeckman CR: Prepyloric antral diaphragm: Delays in treatment. J Pediatr Surg 22:948–949, 1987.

63. Schwartz SE, Rowden DR, Dudgeon DL: Antral mucosal diaphragm. Gastrointest Endoscopy 24:33–34, 1977.

64. Bjorgvinsson E, Rudzki C, Lewicki A: Antral web. Am J Gastroenterol 79:663–665, 1984.

65. Berr F, Rienmueller G, Sauerbruch T: Successful transaction of a partially obstructing antral diaphragm. Gastroenterology 89:1147–1151, 1985.

66. Kay GA, Lobe TE, Custer MD, et al: Endoscopic laser ablation of obstructing duodenal web in the newborn: A case report of limited success with criteria for patient selection. J Pediatr Surg 27:279–281, 1992.

67. Ziegler K, Schier F, Waldschmidt J: Endoscopic laser resection of a duodenal membrane. J Pediatr Surg 27:1582–1583, 1992.

68. Rizzo G, Capponi A, Arduini D, et al: Prenatal diagnosis of gastroesophageal reflux by color and pulsed Doppler ultrasonography in a case of congenital pyloric stenosis. Ultrasound Obstet Gynecol 6:290–292, 1995.

69. Valari MD, Phillips RJ, Lake BD, et al: Junctional epidermolysis bullosa and pyloric atresia: A distinct entity. Clinical and pathological studies in five patients. Br J Dermatol 133:732–736, 1995.

70. Shaw DW, Fine JD, Piacquadio DJ, et al: Gastric outlet obstruction and epidermolysis bullosa. J Am Acad Dermatol 36:304–310, 1997.

71. Neifield JP, Berman WF, Lawrence W, et al: Management of congenital microgastria with a jejunal pouch reservoir. J Pediatr Surg 15:882–885, 1980.

72. Anderson K, Guzzetta P: Treatment of congenital microgastria and dumping syndrome. J Pediatr Surg 18:747–750, 1983.

73. Velasco AF, Holcomb GW, Templeton JM Jr, et al: Management of congenital microgastria. J Pediatr Surg 25:192–197, 1990.

74. Miller DL, Pasquale MD, Seneca RP, et al: Gastric volvulus in the pediatric population. Arch Surg 126:1146–1149, 1991.

75. McIntyre RC Jr, Bensard DD, Karrer FM, et al: The pediatric diaphragm in acute gastric volvulus. J Am Coll Surg 178:234–238, 1994.

76. Leitao B, Mota CR, Enes C, et al: Acute gastric volvulus and congenital posterolateral diaphragmatic hernia. Eur J Pediatr Surg 7:106–108, 1997.

77. Yadav K, Myers NA: Paraesophageal hernia in the neonatal period—another differential diagnosis of esophageal atresia. Pediatr Surg Int 12:420–421, 1997.

78. Aoyama K, Tateishi K: Gastric volvulus in three children with asplenia syndrome. J Pediatr Surg 21:307–310, 1986.

79. Nakada K, Kawaguchi F, Wakisaka M, et al: Digestive tract disorders associated with asplenia/polysplenia syndrome. J Pediatr Surg 32:91–94, 1997.

80. Ziprowski MN, Littlewood R: Gastric volvulus in childhood. AJR Am J Roentgenol 132:921–925, 1979.

81. Cameron BH, Blair GK: Laparoscopic guided gastropexy for intermittent volvulus. J Pediatr Surg 28:1628–1629, 1993.

82. Hernaiz Driever P, Gohlich-Ratmann G, et al: Congenital microgastria, growth hormone deficiency, and diabetes insipidus. Eur J Pediatr 156:37–40, 1997.

83. Hoehner JC, Kimura K, Soper R: Congenital microgastria. J Pediatr Surg 29:1591–1593, 1994.

84. Moulton SL, Bouvet M, Lynch FP: Congenital microgastria in a premature infant. J Pediatr Surg 12:1594–1595, 1994.

85. Grosfeld JL, Molinari FM, Chaet M, et al: Gastrointestinal perforation and peritonitis in infants and children: Experience with 179 cases over ten years. Surgery 120:650–656, 1996.

86. Holcomb GW III: Survival after gastrointestinal perforation from esophageal atresia and tracheoesophageal fistula. J Pediatr Surg 28:1532–1535, 1993.

87. Roser SB, Clark CH, Elechi E: Spontaneous neonatal gastric perforation. J Pediatr Surg 17:390–394, 1982.

88. Tan CEL, Kielly EM, Agrawal M, et al: Neonatal gastrointestinal perforation. J Pediatr Surg 24:888–892, 1989.

89. Herbut PA: Congenital defect in the musculature of the stomach with rupture in a newborn. Acta Pathol 36:91, 1943.

90. Chung MT, Kuo CY, Wang JW, et al: Gastric perforation in the neonate: Clinical analysis of 12 cases. Chung Hua Min Kuo Hsiao Erh Ko I Hsueh Hui Tsa Chih 35:565–570, 1994.

91. Schwartz GF, Polsky HS: Ingested foreign bodies of the gastrointestinal tract. Am Surg 51:173–179, 1985.

92. Byrne WJ: Foreign bodies, bezoars, and caustic ingestion. Gastrointest Endosc Clin North Am 4:99–119, 1994.

93. Robles R, Parrilla P, Escamilla C, et al: Gastrointestinal bezoars. Br J Surg 81:1000–1001, 1994.

94. Seker B, Dilek ON, Karaayvaz M: Trichobezoars as a cause of gastrointestinal obstructions: The Rapunzel syndrome. Acta Gastroenterol Belg 59:166–167, 1996.

95. Kashyap S: Lactobezoar risk. Pediatrics 81:177–181, 1988.

96. Nichols T: Phytobezoar formation: A new complication of cimetidine therapy. Ann Intern Med 95:70–72, 1981.

97. Kaplan M, Ozeri Y, Agranat A, et al: Antacid bezoar in a premature infant. Am J Perinatol 12:98–99, 1995.

98. Buntain WL, Cain WC: Caustic injuries to the esophagus: A pediatric review. South Med J 74:590–598, 1981.

99. Maull KI, Scher LA, Greenfield LJ: Surgical implications of acid ingestion. Surg Gynecol Obstet 148:895–901, 1979.

100. Lowe JE, Graham DY, Bousaubin EV, et al: Corrosive injury to the stomach: The natural history and role of fiberoptic endoscope. Am J Surg 137:803–808, 1979.

101. Stiff G, Alwafi A, Rees BI, et al: Corrosive injuries of the oesophagus and stomach: Experience in management at a regional paediatric centre. Ann R Coll Surg Engl 78:119–123, 1996.

102. Hsu CP, Chen CY, Hsu NY, et al: Surgical treatment and its long-term result for caustic-induced prepyloric obstruction. Eur J Surg 163:275–279, 1997.

103. Pruksapong C, Donovan RJ, Pinit A, et al: Gastric duplication. J Pediatr Surg 14:83–85, 1979.
104. Bartels RJ: Duplication of the stomach. Case report and review of the literature. Am Surg 33:747–752, 1967.
105. Mazziotti MV, Ternberg JL: Continuous communicating esophageal and gastric duplication. J Pediatr Surg 32:775–778, 1997.
106. Lewis FT, Thyng FW: Regular occurrence of intestinal diverticula in embryos of pig, rabbit, and man. Am J Anat 7:505–519, 1908.
107. Bremer JL: Diverticula and duplications of the intestinal tract. Arch Pathol 38:132–140, 1944.
108. Bentley JF, Smith JR: Developmental posterior enteric remnants and spinal malformations. Arch Dis Child 35:76–86, 1960.
109. Wieczorek RL, Seidman I, Ransom JH, et al: Congenital duplication of the stomach: Case report and review of the English literature. Am J Gastroenterol 79:597–602, 1984.
110. Cooper S, Abrams RS, Carbaugh RA: Pyloric duplications: Review and case study. Am Surg 61:1092–1094, 1995.
111. Steyaert H, Voigt JJ, Brouet P, et al: Uncommon complication of gastric duplication in a three year old child. Eur J Pediatr Surg 7:243–244, 1997.
112. Blais C, Masse S: Preoperative ultrasound diagnosis of a gastric duplication cyst with ectopic pancreas in a child. J Pediatr Surg 30:1384–1386, 1995.
113. Moss RL, Ryan JA, Kozarek RA, et al: Pancreatitis caused by a gastric duplication communicating with an aberrant pancreatic lobe. J Pediatr Surg 31:733–736, 1996.
114. Dittrich JR, Spottswood SE, Jolles PR: Gastric duplication cyst. Scintigraphy and correlative imaging. Clin Nucl Med 22:93–96, 1997.
115. Gengler JS, Ashcraft KW, Slattery P: Gastric teratoma: The sixth reported case in a female infant. J Pediatr Surg 30:889–890, 1995.
116. Bourke CJ, Mackay AJ, Payton D: Malignant gastric teratoma: Case report. Pediatr Surg Int 12:192–193, 1997.
117. Cairo MS, Grosfeld JL, Weetman RM: Gastric teratoma: Unusual case for bleeding of the upper gastrointestinal tract in the newborn. Pediatrics 67:721–724, 1981.
118. Matsukuma S, Wada R, Daibou M, et al: Adenocarcinoma arising from gastric immature teratoma. Report of a case in an adult and a review of the literature. Cancer 75:2663–2668, 1995.
119. Mahour GH, Isaacs H Jr, Chang L: Primary malignant tumors of the stomach in children. J Pediatr Surg 15:603–608, 1980.
120. Bethel CA, Bhattacharyya N, Hutchinson C, et al: Alimentary tract malignancies in children. J Pediatr Surg 32:1004–1009, 1997.
121. Ashorn P, Lahde PL, Ruuska T, et al: Gastric lymphoma in an 11 year old boy: A case report. Med Pediatr Oncol 22:66–67, 1994.
122. Ciftci A, Tanyel FC, Kotiloglu E, et al: Gastric lymphoma causing gastric outlet obstruction. J Pediatr Surg 31:1424–1426, 1996.
123. Cogliatti SB, Schmid U, Schumacher U, et al: Primary B-cell gastric lymphoma: A clinicopathological study of 145 patients. Gastroenterology 101:1159–1170, 1991.
124. Isaacson PG: Gastric lymphoma and Helicobacter pylori. N Engl J Med 330:1310–1311, 1994.
125. Drumm B, Perez-Perez GI, Blaser MJ, et al: Intrafamilial clustering of Helicobacter pylori infection. N Engl J Med 322:359–363, 1990.
126. Sandoval C, Oiseth S, Slim M, et al: Gastric ganglioneuroblastoma: A rare finding in an infant with multifocal gangioneuroblastoma. J Pediatr Hematol Oncol 18:409–412, 1996.
127. Marcello PW, Asbun HJ, Veidenheimer MC, et al: Gastroduodenal polyps in familial adenomatous polyposis. Surg Endosc 10:418–421, 1996.
128. Desai DC, Neale KF, Talbot IC, et al: Juvenile polyposis. Br J Surg 82:14–17, 1995.
129. Kaler SG, Westman JA, Bernes SM, et al: Gastrointesinal hemorrhage associated with gastric polyps in Menkes disease. J Pediatr 122:93–95, 1993.
130. Murphy S, Shaw K, Blanchard H: Report of three gastric tumors in children. J Pediatr Surg 29:1202–1204, 1994.
131. Maki M, Ruuska T, Kuusela AL, et al: High prevalence of asymptomatic esophageal and gastric lesions in preterm infants in intensive care. Crit Care Med 21:1863–1867, 1993.
132. Mulberg AE, Linz C, Bern E, et al: Identification of nonsteroidal antiinflammatory drug-induced gastroduodenal injury in children with juvenile rheumatoid arthritis. J Pediatr 122:647–649, 1993.
133. Decklebaum RJ, Roy CC, Lusser-Lazaroff J, et al: Peptic ulcer disease: A clinical study of 73 children. CMAJ 111:225–231, 1974.
134. Kimura M, Uemara N, Sumii K, et al: Characteristics of teen-age patients with juvenile duodenal ulcer: Relation between inherited hyperpepsinogenemia I and duodenal ulcer. Scand J Gastroenterol 28:25–32, 1993.
135. Drumm B, Rhoads JM, Stringer DA, et al: Peptic ulcer disease in children: Etiology, clinical findings, and clinical course. Pediatrics 82:410–414, 1988.
136. Sherman PM: Peptic ulcer disease in children. Diagnosis, treatment and the implication of Helicobacter pylori. Gastroenterol Clin North Am 23:707–725, 1994.
137. Van Zanten SJ, Sherman P: A systemic overview of Helicobacter pylori infection as the cause of gastritis, duodenal ulcer, gastric cancer, and non-ulcer dyspepsia: Applying eight diagnostic criteria in establishing causation. CMAJ 150:177–184, 1994.
138. Van Zanten SJ, Sherman P: Helicobacter pylori: Epidemiology, diagnosis and clinical relevance. Can J Gastroenterol 7:390–395, 1993.
139. Blecker U: Helicobacter pylori–associated gastroduodenal disease in childhood. South Med J 90:570–576, 1997.
140. Cilley RE, Brighton VK: The significance of Helicobacter pylori colonization of the stomach. Semin Pediatr Surg 4:221–227, 1995.
141. Kilbridge PM, Dahms BB, Czinin SJ: Campylobacter pylori–associated gastritis and peptic ulcer disease in children. Am J Dis Child 142:1149–1152, 1988.
142. Israel DM, Hassall E: Treatment and long-term follow-up of Helicobacter pylori–associated duodenal ulcer disease in children. J Pediatr 123:53–57, 1993.
143. Macarthur C, Saunders N, Feldman W: Helicobacter pylori, gastroduodenal disease, and recurrent abdominal pain in children. JAMA 273:729–734, 1995.
144. Yoshida NR, Webber EM, Fraser RB, et al: Helicobacter pylori is not associated with nonspecific abdominal pain in children. J Pediatr Surg 31:747–749, 1996.
145. Lacroix J, Infante-Rivard C, Gauthier M, et al: Upper gastrointestinal tract bleeding acquired in a pediatric intensive care unit: Prophylaxis trial with cimetidine. J Pediatr 108:1015–1021, 1986.
146. Goyal A, Treem WR, Hyams JS: Severe upper gastrointestinal bleeding in healthy full-term neonates. Am J Gastroenterol 89:613–616, 1994.
147. Curci MR, Little K, Sieber WK, et al: Peptic ulcer disease in childhood reexamined. J Pediatr Surg 11:329–335, 1976.
148. Papaila JG, Vane DW, Colville C, et al: The effect of various types of gastrostomy on the lower esophageal sphincter. J Pediatr Surg 22:1198–1202, 1987.
149. Seekri IK, Rescorla FJ, Canal DF, et al: Lesser curvature gastrostomy reduces the incidence of postoperative gastroesophageal reflux. J Pediatr Surg 26:982–986, 1991.
150. Bianchi A, Pearse B: The non-refluxing gastrostomy: An evaluation. Pediatr Surg Int 12:494–496, 1997.
151. Marin OE, Glassman MS, Schoen BT, et al: Safety and efficacy of percutaneous endoscopic gastrostomy in children. Am J Gastroenterol 89:357–362, 1994.
152. Cromblehome TM, Jacir NN: Simplified "push" technique for percutaneous endoscopic gastrostomy in children. J Pediatr Surg 28:1393–1396, 1993.
153. Martinez-Frontanilla LA, Sartorelli KH, Haase GM, et al: Laparoscopic Thal fundoplication with gastrostomy in children. J Pediatr Surg 31:275–276, 1996.
154. Humphrey GM, Najmaldin A: Laparoscopic gastrostomy in children. Pediatr Surg Int 12:501–504, 1997.

155. Goretsky MF, Johnson N, Farrell M, et al: Alternative techniques of feeding gastrostomy in children: A critical analysis. J Am Coll Surg 182:233–240, 1996.
156. Fox VL, Abel SD, Malas S, et al: Complications following percutaneous endoscopic gastrostomy and subsequent catheter replacement in children and young adults. Gastrointest Endosc 45:64–71, 1997.
157. Mathew P, Bowman L, Williams R, et al: Complications and effectiveness of gastrostomy feedings in pediatric cancer patients. J Pediatr Hematol Oncol 18:81–85, 1996.

30

INTESTINAL ATRESIA AND STENOSIS

Alastair J. W. Millar, MBChB, FRCS, FRCS(Edin) •
Heinz Rode, MBChB, MMed(Surg), FRCS(Edin) •
Sidney Cywes, MMed(Surg), FRCS, FRCS(Edin)

Congenital defects in continuity of the intestine are morphologically divided into either stenosis or atresia and constitute one of the most common causes of neonatal intestinal obstruction.[1–5]

Pyloric atresia is rare and familial, and it has a well-documented association with epidermolysis bullosa.

Congenital duodenal atresia occurs once in approximately 2500 live births, is associated with Down's syndrome, and is more frequent in populations with a high rate of consanguinity.[6] Although first described in the 18th century, it was not until the first decade of the 20th century that the surgical treatment began with gastrojejunostomy.[7, 8] At present, duodenoduodenostomy, with or without tapering duodenoplasty, has become standard.[8–12]

Most jejunoileal atresias or stenoses result from intrauterine ischemia.[13] The incidence of jejunoileal atresia is approximately 1 in 1000 live births.[4, 14–18] The first successful surgical repair of an intestinal atresia was in 1911.[19] During 38 years (1959 to 1997), 426 babies with intestinal atresias and stenoses were treated at the Red Cross Children's Hospital in Cape Town, South Africa: 2 pyloric, 166 duodenal, 179 jejunal, 71 ileal, and 8 colonic.

Jejunoileal and colonic atresias can occur simultaneously in the same patient but rarely occur with duodenal atresia.[18, 20, 21] One of the 250 patients with small bowel atresias also had duodenal atresia, and 3 had associated colonic atresia.

☐ Pyloric Atresia

Pyloric atresia is a rare autosomal genetic defect[22, 23] in which the pyloric lumen is completely obliterated either by a diaphragm or a solid core of tissue, or there is a complete absence of the pylorus with loss of bowel continuity. Nonbilious vomiting and upper abdominal distention result. Abdominal radiograph shows a single gas bubble or air-fluid level and no distal air in the gastrointestinal (GI) tract (Fig. 30–1). Differential diagnosis includes high duodenal atresia and malrotation with volvulus of

the midgut. Gastric perforation may lead to peritonitis and toxemia.[24]

Surgical excision for membranous atresia or a side-to-side gastroduodenostomy successfully restores continuity. Gastrojejunostomy should be avoided. Long-term outcome is excellent except for those with epidermolysis bullosa.[25] We have treated two cases that were sporadic and not associated with epidermolysis. Both had a solid core of tissue and were cured by side-to-side gastroduodenostomy.

☐ Duodenal Atresia and Stenosis

ETIOLOGY

Duodenal atresia and stenosis are most commonly believed to be caused by a failure of recanalization,

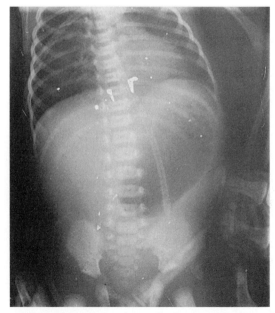

Figure 30–1. Abdominal radiograph showing a large gas-filled stomach with no distal air, typical of pyloric obstruction.

although others contest this theory.[26–29] During the 3rd week of embryonic development, the second part of the duodenum gives off biliary and pancreatic buds that lead to the formation of the hepatobiliary system and pancreas. Simultaneously, the duodenum passes through a solid phase, with its lumen being reestablished by coalescence of vacuoles between the 8th and 10th weeks. An embryologic insult during this period may lead to intrinsic webs, atresias, and stenoses.

Occasionally, the atresia is associated with pancreatic tissue that may surround the duodenum. This phenomenon is probably a failure of duodenal development rather than a true annular pancreas.[10, 30] The distal biliary tree is often abnormal and may open proximal or distal to the atresia.[31, 32] Biliary atresia, agenesis of the gallbladder, and stenosis of the common bile duct have been reported to occur in association with duodenal atresia and particularly with double atresias, a rare occurrence having a distinct familial incidence.[5, 33–36]

CLASSIFICATION

Stenosis, or incomplete obstruction, may be due to a diaphragm or web with a small opening. A thin web that has ballooned distally is referred to as a *windsock*.[37, 38] *Atresia*, or complete obstruction, may be seen with duodenal muscular continuity or with a gap that is usually filled in with pancreatic tissue (Fig. 30–2).

Prematurity, growth retardation, and coexistent malformations are common. Almost 50% of duodenal atresias are associated with some other anomaly (e.g., cardiac, genitourinary, anorectal, or, occasionally, esophageal atresia), and up to 40% have trisomy 21.[39–41]

PATHOLOGY

Although the site of obstruction is usually classified as preampullary and postampullary, the majority are periampullary. Depending on the degree of obstruction, the proximal duodenum and stomach dilate to several times their normal size. The pylorus is distended and hypertrophic. The bowel distal to the obstruction is collapsed and in cases of complete atresia, thin walled. Because the obstruction is high, it is decompressed proximally in utero, and perforation is rare.[42] Associated polyhydramnios is recorded in up to one half of cases, with premature delivery in one third.[5] Growth retardation is also common, which may imply that the fetus has been deprived of the nutritional contribution of swallowed amniotic fluid.

DIAGNOSIS

Polyhydramnios results from high intestinal obstruction because the reabsorption of amniotic fluid is disturbed. The dilated stomach and proximal duodenum may be seen on antenatal ultrasonography

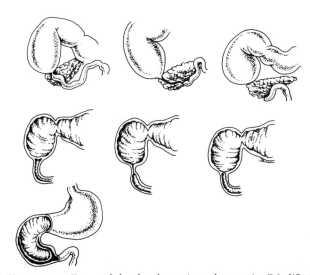

Figure 30–2. Types of duodenal atresia and stenosis. (Modified fro Irving IM, Rickham PP: Duodenal atresia and stenosis: Anular pancreas. In Rickham PP, Lister J, Irving IM [eds]: Neonatal Surgery [2nd ed]. Boston, Butterworths, 1978, p 355.)

(US), as may associated cardiac abnormalities. Most cases of duodenal atresia are detected between the 7th and 8th month of intrauterine life, but a normal US of the fetus with polyhydramnios at that time does not absolutely exclude duodenal obstruction.[43]

The vomiting of clear or bile-stained fluid usually starts within hours of birth. Distention or abnormal stooling may or may not be present. Aspiration via a nasogastric tube of more than 20 ml of gastric contents in a newborn suggests intestinal obstruction; the normal intake is less than 5 ml.[44] The diagnosis of an incomplete obstruction (stenosis or

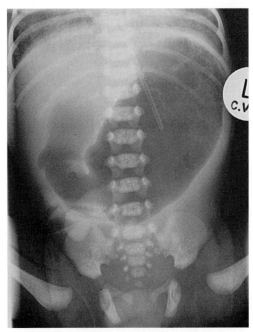

Figure 30–3. Duodenal atresia. Radiograph showing a dilated gas-filled stomach and duodenum, with a gasless distal abdomen indicating complete obstruction.

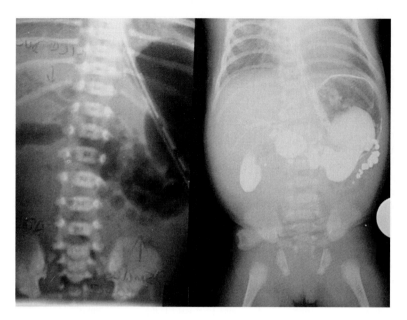

Figure 30–4. Types of biliary abnormalities in duodenal atresia.

web) may be delayed until well beyond the neonatal period.[45] Because most duodenal obstructions occur distal to the ampulla, the vomitus is bile-stained in more than two thirds. Occasionally, blood-stained vomitus results from gastritis. Abdominal distention may not be evident owing to vomiting. Delayed diagnosis may result in dehydration, hyponatremia, and hypochloremia. Jaundice, if present, is rarely obstructive and is more likely due to prematurity and dehydration.

An upright abdominal radiograph using instilled air, if necessary, as contrast, is sufficient to confirm the diagnosis (Fig. 30–3). Intestinal gas beyond the duodenum indicates incomplete obstruction. When gas is seen beyond the duodenum on the radiograph, midgut volvulus cannot be excluded and urgent exploration is mandatory. A contrast meal is required when the obstruction is incomplete to exclude malrotation and volvulus and then only if immediate operation is not possible (Fig. 30–4). Rarely, the biliary tree is air-filled, and a variety of pancreatic and biliary anomalies has been demonstrated[44] (Fig. 30–5). It has not been our practice to perform a contrast enema prior to operative treatment because

colonic atresia is rarely seen and an enema is an inexact method of determining malrotation.[46]

MANAGEMENT

Once the diagnosis has been established, gastric decompression and correction of fluid and electrolyte disturbances are begun. Other associated anomalies should be excluded. Only after the baby has been resuscitated is operative correction performed, unless malrotation and volvulus remain as possible diagnoses.

A supraumbilical transverse abdominal incision is preferred. The duodenal obstruction is exposed by mobilizing the ascending and transverse colon to the left and by identifying any associated malrotation, which occurs in approximately 30% of these patients.[5] The pancreas may appear to be annular in nature. Occasionally, an anterior portal vein may be identified. The duodenum and jejunum distal to a complete obstruction are collapsed and thin-walled compared with the hypertrophied and dilated proximal obstructed duodenum. A sufficient length of duodenum distal to the atresia is mobilized. The

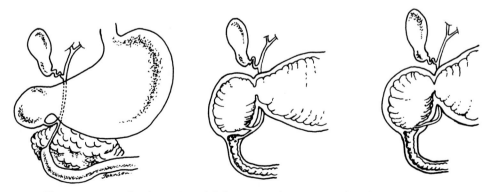

Figure 30–5. Duodenal atresia with biliary air and contrast meal outlining bile ducts.

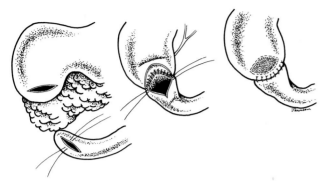

Figure 30–6. Duodenoduodenostomy.

operation preferred by most is a diamond-shaped or side-to-side duodenoduodenostomy, using a transverse incision at the inferior aspect of the proximal blind-ending bulbous part and a longitudinal incision on the distal bowel[47] (Fig. 30–6). Muscular continuity of the duodenal wall suggests a windsock deformity or diaphragm that calls for extra vigilance in the operative correction.[37, 48]

Although duodenotomy and web excision have been advocated, there is a potential for bile duct injury using this approach, which seems to have no functional advantage over duodenoduodenostomy.[32, 38, 39, 48] In some cases, a tapering duodenoplasty is performed, excising a wedge of the anterolateral aspect of the second part of the duodenum[12, 49]; this is most simply done using a GI anastomosis stapling device. One must be careful not to narrow the duodenum or injure the ampulla of Vater.[11] Ladd's procedure should be performed when needed. Postoperative nasogastric decompression instead of gastrostomy has been shown to decrease hospitalization from a mean of 20 days to 8 days.[50] Survival rates are in excess of 90%; mortality, in most cases, is due to an associated cardiac anomaly or chromosomal disorder.[39, 42]

Early postoperative complications may be associated with anastomotic leak and local sepsis. Surgical injury to the bile duct has resulted in "acquired atresia."[35] Long-term complications include alkaline reflux and peptic ulceration or duodenal stasis with blind-loop syndrome, recurrent abdominal pain, and diarrhea.[51–53] Gallstones have also been observed following duodenal atresia repair.[54] Protracted follow-up is mandatory.

PATIENT REVIEW

Over the 38-year period of 1959 to 1997, 166 infants and children with duodenal atresia or stenosis were treated at the Red Cross Children's Hospital in Cape Town. The 103 treated between 1977 and 1997 have been analyzed in detail. Of these 103 patients, maternal polyhydramnios was noted in 12.5% with stenosis and in 65% with atresia. The obstruction was due to stenosis in 21, multiple stenosis in 1, duodenal membrane in 14, single atresia in 65, and multiple atresias in 2. Thirty-six had Down's syndrome, 18 had congenital heart disease, and 8 had esophageal and anorectal anomalies (Fig. 30–7). More than 50% of those with stenosis or fenestrated membranes presented late (5 weeks to 14 years). Prematurity was much more frequent with atresia (28 [43%] of 65) as compared with incomplete obstructions (8 [23%] of 35). Only 6 patients were recorded as having a bile duct insertion proximal *and* distal to the obstruction. The 3 patients with multiple membranes were siblings and had associated immunodeficiency.[36] Neither duodenoplasty nor web excision was attempted. Gastrostomy was routinely used until 1992, when a prospective study demonstrated that time to full oral feeding was 15 days with gastrostomy patients and only 8 days in the group without gastrostomy. Ladd's procedure was performed only if the mesentery was unfixed and the residual pedicle was narrow, thus predisposing the patient to volvulus. No episodes of midgut volvulus in association with duodenal atresia have been recorded in our experience.[46] In this series, only 1 patient required reoperation, which was done at age 6 years, for chronic abdominal pain and residual megaduodenum. Tapering duodenoplasty resolved her symptoms.

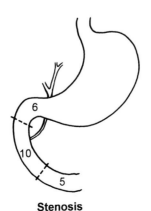

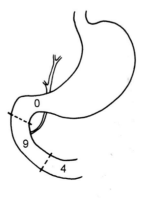

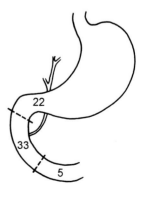

Figure 30–7. Sites of duodenal obstruction.

Stenosis
n = 21

Fenestrated membrane
n = 13

Atresia
n = 60

□ Jejunoileal Atresia and Stenosis

ETIOLOGY

Although several mechanisms have been postulated to explain the intestinal atresia malformations,[27, 28, 55, 56] the most favored theory is that of a localized intrauterine vascular accident with ischemic necrosis of the sterile bowel and subsequent resorption of the affected segment or segments[13, 40] (Fig. 30–8). This theory was based on results of an investigation of 79 children with intestinal atresia treated at The Hospital for Sick Children in London.[4]

Mesenteric vascular insults, such as ligation of a loop of intestine to simulate the effect of the volvulus, intussusception, and interference with segmental blood supply, were created in fetal dogs leading to different degrees and patterns of intraluminal obstruction, exactly reproducing the spectrum of stenosis and atresia found in people.[13, 14]

It was clearly demonstrated that devitalized segments of bowel were rapidly absorbed, the proximal and distal bowel separated from the devascularized segment and sealed to form rounded blind ends, and adhesions in the vicinity of the pathologic process disappeared unless a perforation led to meconium peritonitis. The interval between producing the ischemic insult and the birth of the experimental animals was too short to establish the histopathology of the event. Sequential histologic studies of this process in fetal rabbits showed rapid liquefaction, absorption, and resolution of necrotic tissue following vascular occlusion. Subsequently, these experimental findings were observed in several different animal models.[57–60]

These findings, together with clinical evidence of presence of bile, lanugo hair, and squamous epithelial cells from swallowed amniotic fluid distal to an atresia, support this hypothesis.[40, 59, 61, 62] In addition, evidence of intrauterine fetal intussusception, midgut volvulus, thromboembolic occlusions, transmesenteric internal hernias, and incarceration or snaring of bowel in an omphalocele or gastroschisis has been noted in people and has led to wide acceptance of this hypothesis.[1, 3, 15, 59, 62–67] In our series, the GI anomalies associated with jejunoileal atresia were mostly of such a nature as to predispose to strangulation of the fetal bowel. Anomalous fixation of the intestinal mesentery was reported in 45% of infants born with jejunoileal atresia and multiple occlusions.[4] Evidence of a "vascular accident" was present in 110 (44%) of the 250 neonates with jejunoileal atresia in our series. Malrotation or volvulus was detected in 84, exomphalos in 5, gastroschisis in 3, meconium ileus in 5, meconium peritonitis in 7, Hirschsprung's disease with proximal atresia in 5, and internal hernia in 1 neonate. Intrauterine intussusception with postnatal evidence of the intussusception and proximal atresia was seen in 2 patients and generally is responsible for 0.6 to 1.3% of atresias. The site of atresia with this etiology is usually at the ileocecal level.[68] The low prevalence of associated abnormalities is in keeping with the pattern observed in developing countries.[1]

Evidence of bowel infarction was present in 42% of 449 cases of jejunoileal atresia in a collated series.[69] The localized nature of the vascular accident occurring late in fetal life would explain the low incidence (<10%) of coexisting abnormalities of the extraabdominal organs.[14, 69] In rare instances, jejunoileal atresia has been found to be associated with esophageal, gastric, duodenal, colonic, and rectal atresias, as well as biliary atresia, meningomyelocele, and Hirschsprung's disease.[14, 15, 69–72] Methylene blue used for amniocentesis in twin pregnancies has been implicated in causing small bowel atresia.[73]

The anomaly is usually not genetically determined, although affected monozygotic twins and siblings have been described all having multiple webs.[21] There is no correlation between jejunoileal atresia and parental age or maternal disease. Although chromosomal abnormalities are relatively common in duodenal atresia, they are seen in less than 1% of more distal atresias.[2, 69]

One in three infants is significantly premature and often weighs less than is appropriate for gestational age.[69] Amniotic fluid may contribute to fetal growth, especially in the last week of gestation. Despite this,

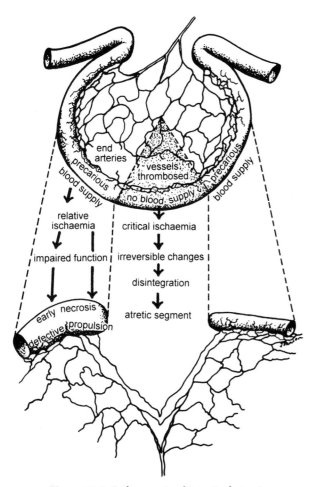

Figure 30–8. Pathogenesis of intestinal atresia.

the intrauterine growth pattern is generally not very different from other infants.

PATHOLOGY

The morphologic classification of jejunoileal atresia into three types has been of significant prognostic and therapeutic value.[40, 56, 74] Modification has retained the original classification but added a special category of type III(b) apple peel and considered multiple atresias as type IV.[17] This emphasized the importance of associated loss in intestinal length, abnormal collateral intestinal blood supply, and concomitant atresias or stenoses[75] (Fig. 30–9). The most proximal atresia determines whether it is classified as jejunal or ileal atresia. Although a single atresia is most common, multiple atretic segments may be encountered in 6 to 21% of cases.[2, 3, 69]

Stenosis

Stenosis is defined as a localized narrowing of the intestinal lumen without disruption of continuity or defect in the mesentery. At the stenotic site there is a short, narrow, somewhat rigid segment with a minute lumen where the muscularis is often irregular and the submucosa thickened. Stenosis may also take the form of a type I atresia with a fenestrated web. The small intestine is of normal length.

Atresia Type I

In *atresia type I* the obstruction is caused by a membrane or web formed by mucosa and submucosa. The proximal dilated and distal collapsed bowel are in continuity without a mesenteric defect. Increased intraluminal pressure in the proximal bowel can produce bulging of the web into the distal intestine, creating a conical transition zone, the windsock effect. The bowel length is not foreshortened.

Atresia Type II

In *atresia type II* (blind ends joined by a fibrous cord) the proximal bowel terminates in a bulbous blind end, which is connected to the collapsed distal bowel by a short fibrous cord along the edge of an intact mesentery. The proximal bowel is always dilated and hypertrophied for several centimeters and may become cyanosed as a result of ischemia

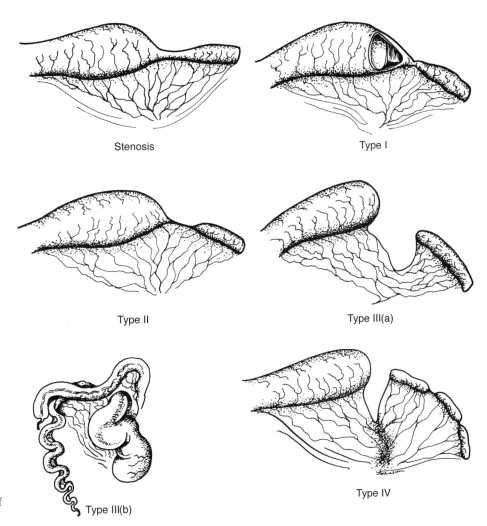

Figure 30–9. Classification of small bowel atresia.

from increased intraluminal pressure. The distal collapsed bowel commences as a blind end, which sometimes assumes a bulbous appearance owing to the remains of an intussusception. The total small bowel length is usually normal.

Atresia Type III(a)

In *atresia type III(a)* (disconnected blind ends) the atresia ends blindly both proximally and distally as in type II, but the fibrous connecting cord is absent and there is a V-shaped mesenteric defect of varying size (see Fig. 30–9). The dilated and blind-ending portion of proximal bowel is often aperistaltic and more frequently may undergo torsion or become overdistended, with necrosis and perforation as a secondary event.[4] The total length of the bowel is subnormal and variable owing to intrauterine resorption of the compromised bowel. Cystic fibrosis is commonly associated with this variety.[76]

Atresia Type III(b)

Atresia type III(b) (apple peel,[59] Christmas tree,[77] or Maypole deformity[18]) consists of a proximal jejunal atresia near the ligament of Treitz, absence of the superior mesenteric artery beyond the origin of the middle colic branch and of the dorsal mesentery, significant loss of intestinal length, and a large mesenteric defect. The distal small bowel lies free in the abdomen and assumes a helix configuration around a single perfusing vessel arising from the ileocolic or right colic arcades (Fig. 30–10). Occasionally, further type I or type II atresias are found in the bowel closest to the distal blind end. Vascularity of the distal bowel is often impaired. This type of atresia has been found in families with a pattern suggestive of an autosomal recessive mode of inheritance. It has also been encountered in siblings with identical lesions and in twins.[18, 21, 72, 78–80]

The occurrence of conventional intestinal atresia

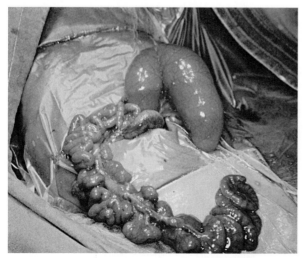
Figure 30–10. Apple-peel type III(b) atresia.

in other affected siblings, the association of multiple atresias (15%), and the discordance in a set of apparently monozygotic twins may point to more complex genetic transmission with an overall recurrence rate of 18%.[72, 81–83] Babies with this anomaly are often premature (70%), have malrotation (54%), and may develop short gut syndrome (74%) with increased morbidity (63%) and mortality (54%).[69, 72] The deformity is most likely the consequence of a proximal superior mesenteric arterial occlusion with extensive infarction of the proximal segment of the midgut on a basis of a thrombus or embolus, or of a strangulating obstruction owing to a midgut volvulus.[40, 72, 77, 84] A primary failure of development of the distal superior mesenteric artery has also been suggested as an etiologic factor, although this is unlikely because meconium is found in the bowel distal to the atresia, which indicates that the atresia was acquired after bile secretion began, which occurs around the 12th week of intrauterine life.[85]

Atresia Type IV

In *atresia type IV* there are multiple segment atresias of a combination of types I to III, often having the morphologic appearance of a string of sausages. There is a familial incidence with prematurity, a grossly shortened bowel length, and an increased mortality.[21, 78] Up to 25 separate atresias have been encountered, usually with sparing at the terminal ileum.[86] Concomitant bile duct dilation has also been described.[87] A rare autosomal recessive pattern of transmission has been documented in several neonates with multiple atresias from the stomach to the rectum. Seven babies were reported from four related French Canadian families in Quebec.[74, 88]

Multiple atresias could also be the consequence of multiple ischemia infarcts, an intrauterine inflammatory process, or a malformation of the GI tract occurring during early embryonic life.[74, 89] Pathologic findings in the familial cases would support the concept that a developmental process early in intrauterine life, and affecting the whole GI tract, may be responsible, not an ischemic or inflammatory process.[90, 91]

Based on the wide distribution of these atresias and the presence of multiple lumina, each surrounded by muscularis mucosa, the atresia may represent an example in which the solid state of epithelial proliferation took place throughout the intestine with incomplete recanalization. The recognition of familial polyatresia may be helpful in genetic counseling. Embolization of thromboplastin-rich material from a dead monozygotic fetal twin to the living one through placental vascular anastomoses could also account for single or multiple intestinal atresias.[92, 93] Multiple areas of intestinal atresias have also been seen in association with severe immunodeficiency.[36]

Among the 250 patients in our series were 29 stenoses (11.6%) and 221 atresias (88.4%). The incidence of the various types of atresias is shown in

Table 30–1. These findings are similar to surveys done in 1969 and 1971, except that there is a much higher incidence of jejunal atresias in our series.[69]

PATHOPHYSIOLOGY

The ischemic insult not only causes the morphologic abnormalities but also adversely influences the structure and subsequent function of the remaining proximal and distal bowel.[4, 13, 18, 40, 94–96] The blind-ended proximal bowel is dilated and hypertrophied with histologically normal villi, but it is without effective peristaltic activity. There is also a deficiency of mucosal enzymes and muscular adenosine triphosphatase.[18, 97] At the level of the atresia, the ganglia of the enteric nervous system are atrophic and hypocellular with minimal acetylcholinesterase activity. These changes are most likely the result of local ischemia, although obstruction per se can elicit the same but less severe morphologic and functional abnormalities.[97]

The histologic and histochemical abnormalities progressively normalize proximally, although up to 20 cm cephalad to the atretic segment, muscular hyperplasia and hypertrophy with concomitant hyperplasia of ganglia may still be observed.[94, 96, 97] The discrepancy in diameter between the lumen of the proximal and distal bowel may vary from 2 to 20 times depending on the completeness of the obstruction and its distance from the stomach.[98] These abnormalities of the proximal atretic segment may be the reason for lack of prograde movement of intraluminal contents in addition to decreased secretion and absorptive capabilities if this segment is retained when bowel continuity is restored.[40, 62, 99] The changes can be so extensive that a state of decompensation is reached, with no effective prograde movement of contents.

Canine experiments have shown that progressive obstruction of the proximal bowel results in diminished intraluminal pressure and circumferential contractions, which fail to achieve prograde movement of contents during active peristaltic activity.[95, 100] In addition, the viability of the bulbous atretic segment may be at risk, with further compromise from the excessive distention, which can lead to ischemia and perforation (9.7–20%) and allow

the transmural migration of bacteria. Histologic studies of the distal bowel have demonstrated hypertrophied, tortuous, and intertwined villi often obliterating the tiny lumen of the distal segment.[101] The apparent hypertrophy could, however, result from mucosal crowding within the unused distal lumen rather than from true villous enlargement.[102] The distal small bowel is unused and potentially normal in length and function as is the unused microcolon, although diminished contractile activity has been demonstrated.[103]

Experimental studies showing that intestinal atresia resulted from ischemic necrosis of intestine would imply precarious blood supply to the proximally dilated loop of bowel,[13, 40, 104] and postmortem injection of barium sulfate into mesenteric vessels has confirmed this suspicion.[85]

It was, however, postulated that the intestine is not ischemic at birth and becomes so only on swallowing air with subsequent distention and raised intraluminal pressure or with secondary torsion.[95] The excellent results obtained with tapering procedures without resection of the bulbous portion would support the contention that the blood and nerve supply to the bowel adjacent to the atresia is adequate.[95, 105] However, the insult may have interfered with mucosal and neural function. Defective peristalsis is commonly noticed in this area, and there is no doubt that resection of the dilated bulbous proximal end produced better results. The proximal end of the distal atretic bowel has been subjected to a similar insult and requires resection at the time of surgical correction of the atresia.[40]

Insufficient bowel length, as a result of the primary insult, excessive removal of residual bowel, or ischemic insult to the remaining bowel, as well as postoperative complications or the inappropriate use of hyperosmolar feeds or medication, can lead to a short gut syndrome with long-term sequelae for growth and development. The brown bowel syndrome has also been identified and is most likely the result of malabsorption of fat-soluble vitamins (vitamin E) resulting in lipofuscinosis of the GI tract.[106]

CLINICAL MANIFESTATIONS

Prompt recognition of intestinal atresia is essential for adequate management to be instituted.[1, 3, 4, 14, 61, 69, 70] The differentiation among atresia, intrinsic bowel obstruction, and extrinsic obstruction owing to midgut volvulus or internal hernia is the most important consideration requiring immediate diagnostic studies. In recent years, US has contributed substantially to the prenatal diagnosis of jejunoileal atresia and has improved the management of the mother and her unborn baby.[107] This is especially so in pregnancies complicated by third-trimester polyhydramnios associated with small bowel atresia, volvulus, and meconium peritonitis.[3, 69] Polyhydramnios, however, may not be present early in gestation or with distal obstruction. A family history may

TABLE 30-1. Jejunoileal Atresia and Stenosis: Red Cross Children's Hospital Experience 1959 to 1997 (n = 250)

Type	Jejunum	Ileum	Total (%)
Stenosis	17	12	29 (11.6)
Type I	43	15	58 (23.2)
Type II	15	11	26 (10.4)
Type III(a)	18	21	39 (15.6)
Type III(b)	47	—	47 (18.8)
Type IV	39	12	51 (20.4)
Total	**179**	**71**	**250**

help identify hereditary forms. A modified dominant mode of inheritance has been suggested in atresias occurring in two aunts and two nephews who were siblings.[81, 88]

Type III(b) atresia also has a familial tendency based on anomalies of intestinal rotation or fixation. A 3.4% incidence of anomalies in siblings has been reported in a large survey of children with jejunoileal atresias.[69] Familial combined duodenal and jejunoileal atresia is uncommon.[108] Bile staining and increased bile acid concentration in the amniotic fluid may indicate the presence of intestinal obstruction distal to the ampulla of Vater.[109]

Babies with atresia or stenosis usually develop bilious vomiting on the 1st day of life, but in 20% of children, it may be delayed for 2 to 3 days.[1, 2, 4, 14] The higher the obstruction, the earlier and more forceful the vomiting.[70] Dehydration, fever, unconjugated hyperbilirubinemia, and aspiration pneumonia occur with delay in diagnosis.

Abdominal distention is more pronounced with distal small bowel obstruction. Sixty to 70% of these babies fail to pass meconium on the 1st day of life.[3, 4] Although the meconium may appear normal, it is more common to find gray plugs of mucus passed via the rectum.[61] Tenderness, rigidity, edema, and erythema of the abdominal wall are signs of ischemia or peritonitis.[14] Occasionally, if ischemic distal bowel is present in type III(b) atresia, altered blood may be passed through the rectum.

Intestinal stenosis is more likely to create diagnostic difficulty. Intermittent partial obstruction or malabsorption may subside without treatment.[62, 70, 110] Investigations may initially be normal. These babies usually fail to thrive and ultimately develop complete intestinal obstruction, which requires exploration.

The diagnosis of jejunoileal atresia is by radiographic examination of the abdomen with only swallowed air as contrast.[110, 111] Swallowed air reaches the proximal bowel by 1 hour and the distal small bowel by 3 hours, where its passage is blocked.[112]

Jejunal atresia patients have a few gas-filled and fluid-filled loops of small bowel, but the remainder of the abdomen is gasless (Fig. 30–11). Air-fluid levels may be scanty or absent and may become evident only after decompression via a nasogastric tube (Fig. 30–12). Fewer air-fluid levels are evident, and there is a typical ground-glass appearance of inspissated meconium when the atresia is associated with cystic fibrosis. A limited contrast meal may be useful if intestinal stenosis is suspected.

Distal ileal atresia may be difficult to differentiate from colonic atresia because haustral markings are rarely seen in neonates. A contrast enema shows the small and large bowel distal to the obstruction; the bowel typically has an unused appearance. The rare colonic atresia that we have seen with jejunoileal atresia and malrotation of the colon may be discov-

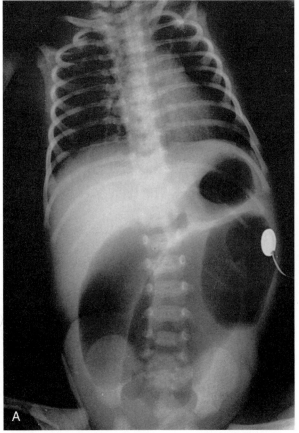

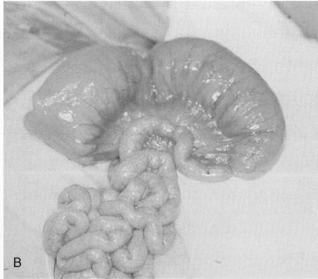

Figure 30–11. Jejunal atresia. *A,* Abdominal radiograph. *B,* Operative photograph.

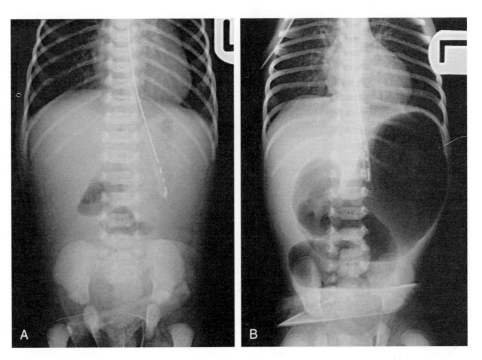

Figure 30–12. Abdominal radiograph (*A*) before and (*B*) after injection of air.

ered on this study.[14, 46, 111, 113] Omission of a diagnostic barium enema with reliance on the intraoperative injection of saline to confirm distal bowel patency may fail to identify an associated colonic or rectal atresia.[114, 115] Rotational abnormalities and volvulus were observed in 36% of our patients. If the atresia occurred late in intrauterine life, the bowel distal to the atresia may have a more normal caliber. Occasionally, air and meconium can accumulate proximal to an atresia mimicking the radiologic appearance of meconium ileus. Total colonic aganglionosis may be difficult to differentiate from atresia.[111]

Ten percent of babies with atresia have meconium peritonitis.[3, 69, 110] The perforation usually occurs proximal to the obstruction in the bulbous blind end. The radiologic appearance of a meconium pseudocyst containing a large air-fluid level is related to the late intrauterine perforation of bowel and can easily be identified on radiographs. Intraluminal calcification of meconium or intramural dystrophic calcification in the form of diffuse punctate or rounded aggregations has been reported with intestinal stenosis or atresia.[116] Meconium calcification in patients with hereditary multiple GI atresia produces a "string of pearls," which is pathognomonic of this condition.[88, 91]

The clinical and radiologic picture of jejunoileal stenosis is determined by the level and degree of stenosis, and the diagnosis may be delayed for years.[69, 70] Morphologic and functional changes in the proximal obstructed intestine vary depending on the degree of obstruction (Fig. 30–13).

DIFFERENTIAL DIAGNOSIS

Diseases that can present with symptoms and signs mimicking jejunoileal atresia include colonic atresia, midgut volvulus, meconium ileus, duplication cysts, internal hernia, ileus due to sepsis, birth trauma, maternal medications, prematurity, and hypothyroidism.[3, 14, 15, 70, 117] Special investigations, including upper GI contrast studies, contrast enema, rectal biopsy, and a delta F508 gene deletion assay or a sweat test to rule out associated cystic fibrosis, may be needed.[15, 76]

MANAGEMENT

Delay in diagnosis may lead to impairment of viability (50%), frank necrosis and perforation (10–20%) of the bulbous proximal end, fluid and electrolyte abnormalities, and increased incidence of sepsis.[4, 61, 70]

Electrolyte and volume resuscitation is started.

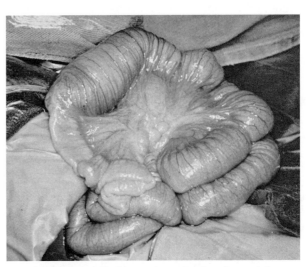

Figure 30–13. Ileal stenosis—operative photograph.

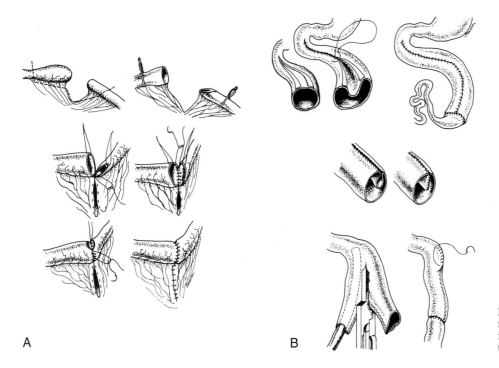

A

B

Figure 30–14. *A,* Operative technique with back resection of proximal bowel and end-to-end anastomosis. *B,* Tapering techniques.

Nasogastric or orogastric tube decompression may improve diaphragmatic excursion and prevent vomiting and aspiration.

SURGICAL CONSIDERATIONS

The operative procedure depends on the pathologic findings. Resection of the proximal dilated and hypertrophied bowel with primary end-to-end (end-to-back) anastomosis with or without tapering of the proximal bowel is most common[3, 4, 13, 14, 40, 48, 59, 61, 62, 104] (Fig. 30–14).

As recently as 1952, the surgical mortality was 80 to 90%.[14, 70] The present survival rate is approximately 90%.[4, 14, 104] Understanding that the proximal dilated and hypertrophied bowel was dysfunctional, improvement of anastomotic technique and suture material and development of total parenteral nutritional (TPN) support are the primary reasons for the greatly improved survival in the years that have followed. Appropriate management of the short bowel syndrome should lead to further improvements.

OPERATIVE CONSIDERATIONS

A transverse supraumbilical incision provides access to the abdominal contents. Intraperitoneal fluid should be sent for Gram's stain and culture. In uncomplicated cases, the bowel can easily be delivered into the wound by gentle pressure on the wound edges. Any perforation is identified and sutured before further exploration, and the abdominal cavity is irrigated with warm saline until all macroscopic debris has been removed. Division of vascularized adhesions may be required.[15] All the bowel should be exteriorized and carefully inspected to determine the site and type of obstruction and to exclude other atresias or stenoses, malrotation, or meconium ileus. Malrotation should be corrected by derotation and division of Ladd's bands.

The length of the bowel estimated to be functional should be carefully measured along the antimesenteric border because this is of prognostic significance and may determine the method of reconstruction. The patency of the bowel distal to the anastomotic site must be verified by injecting saline into the distal bowel and observing free flow into the cecum. If colonic patency has not been established preoperatively, patency of the colon must be confirmed by injection of saline either directly or via a prepositioned transrectal catheter.

If the total useable bowel length is adequate (>80 cm + ileocecal valve), the bulbous hypertrophied bowel proximal to the atresia is resected to approximately normal bowel diameter.[4, 40] In high jejunal atresia, the resection may extend into the third portion of the duodenum. The blood supply to the cut ends of the intestine must be carefully preserved.

A short segment (4 to 5 cm) of the distal atretic bowel is removed obliquely so that the mesenteric side is the longest. An incision along the antimesenteric border to create a "fish mouth" may be needed to equalize the openings for anastomosis.[18, 40, 104]

A one-layer modification of the end-to-back anastomosis using 5-0 or 6-0 monofilament absorbable sutures is preferred.[2, 4] Alternatively, an extramucosal anastomosis can be performed. Once the anastomosis has been completed, the suture line is tested for leaks and reinforcing sutures are placed as required. The mesenteric defect is repaired, taking great care not to kink the anastomosis.[18] It may be difficult at this time to close the mesenteric defect without distorting or kinking the anastomotic site.

The preserved mesentery of the resected proximal bowel can be used as a vascularized flap to close any residual defects. [118]

A similar technique is used for stenosis and intraluminal membranes. Procedures such as simple transverse enteroplasties, excision of membranes, and bypassing techniques are not recommended primarily because they fail to remove the abnormal segments of bowel, which may produce blind loop syndromes. The end-to-side ileoascending colonic anastomosis for low ileal atresia is also obsolete.[104] Neither decompression gastrostomy[119, 120] or trans-anastomotic stents are recommended.[121] Our practice is to place a nasogastric tube for decompression and to rely on short-term TPN with early introduction of graduated enteral feeding.

At completion of the operation, the bowel is carefully returned into the abdomen to avoid kinking or volvulus of the bowel.

PROGNOSTIC FACTORS

The normal small bowel length in full-term neonates is approximately 250 cm and in preterm infants is 160 to 240 cm.[104] Previous estimates that small bowel length of 100 cm or more is necessary to sustain oral intake and survival may no longer be applicable owing to the advent of TPN, special enteral diets, and pharmacologic management of short gut syndrome.[104] Nevertheless, the preservation of as much bowel length as possible at the risk of creating a poorly functioning anastomosis has little merit.[4, 69, 105, 122] In one series, an average of 15 cm (SD 13.4) of intestine proximal and 5 cm (SD 6.5) distal to the atresia was resected, with a mean of 101 cm (SD 57) of functional intestine remaining.[110]

If proximal resection is not possible, tapering or plication of the dilated bowel is indicated.[48, 100, 105, 120, 123, 124] Tapering enteroplasty as proximal as the second portion of the duodenum, if necessary, is accomplished by resecting an antimesenteric strip of the dilated proximal bowel with either suture or staple closure to ensure adequate lumen size.[124] The tapering can safely be done over a length of 35 cm.[124] The tapered bowel may be primarily anastomosed to the distal bowel or may be exteriorized as a stoma, if necessary.

Plication or infolding along the antimesenteric border is preferred by some surgeons because it conserves mucosal surface area and may facilitate the return of bowel function.[123] Plication also reduces the risk of leak from the antimesenteric suture line. More than one half of the bowel circumference may be folded into the lumen over an extended length without causing obstruction. Breakdown of the plication suture line results in a functional obstruction.[48] The plication is less likely to disrupt if a longitudinal antimesenteric seromuscular strip is resected prior to plication.[125, 126]

From 1978, when tapering was introduced into our practice, to 1997, 152 infants were treated with proximal resection and end-to-end anastomosis.

Forty (26%) had some proximal resection along with antimesenteric excision and tapering. These were predominantly done to conserve bowel length in type III(b) atresia patients or to reduce disparity in anastomotic size. Tapering was also used to correct a failed inversion plication procedure and as a secondary procedure to improve function in a persistently dilated nonfunctioning megaduodenum. Tapering was successful in all 40 children, although 1 required further proximal tapering. No anastomotic leaks were encountered. Seromuscular stripping and inversion plication were performed in 7 patients, of whom 4 required revision owing to breakdown of the plication with persistent dysfunction. Dysfunction is manifested by persistent vomiting. Contrast studies revealed a partially obstructed anastomosis with ineffective prograde movement in the dilated bowel.

Primary anastomosis may be contraindicated in cases of peritonitis, volvulus with vascular compromise, meconium ileus, and type III(b) atresia.[17, 98] Under these circumstances, exteriorization of both ends has been recommended. However, we do not favor surgical maturation of stomas because it may increase the incidence of systemic sepsis and the mortality rate.[14, 59, 61, 110, 127–130] The proximal bowel often remains dilated in spite of exteriorization, and fluid and electrolyte losses may be severe. None of the babies in our series required bowel exteriorization. Primary anastomosis has been shown to be effective with no mortality.[131]

Atresia encountered in gastroschisis may be single or multiple and may be located in either the small or large bowel.[63, 132] Rarely is the bowel suitable for primary anastomosis. Exteriorization is an option if the proximal bowel has perforated or is minimally dilated.[17, 63, 113] Identification of the atresia may be extremely difficult, and the safest course is to reduce the eviscerated bowel with the atresia left undisturbed. Primary closure of the abdominal wall or silo reduction is done. Resolution of the bowel edema then occurs, allowing safe delayed resection and anastomosis 14 to 21 days later.[63, 133]

Although isolated type I atresias are best dealt with by primary resection and end-to-end anastomosis,[69, 104] multiple diaphragms have been successfully perforated and dilated with bougies passed along the entire length of small intestine.

Reduction of the bowel with type III(b) atresia may require release of restricting bands along the free edge of the distal coiled and narrow mesentery. The potential for kinking the precarious single marginal artery and vein requires careful return of the bowel into the abdominal cavity.[77] The proximal dilated bowel should be partly resected with tapering, and limited resection of the distal bowel end may be required for questionable viability.[82, 134]

Bowel length conservation methods, such as multiple anastomoses for multiple atresias, may result in increased morbidity.[20, 61, 104] An intraluminal Silastic catheter stent can facilitate the completion of multiple primary anastomoses and serve, simultaneously, as a conduit for radiological evidence of anastomotic integrity, luminal patency, and enteral feeding.[135] Multiple atresias, which are present in as many as 18% of patients, are often localized; therefore, resection and one anastomosis is preferable.[20]

There is no place for a bowel lengthening procedure at the initial operation, but this procedure may ultimately obviate the need for prolonged TPN.[136]

POSTOPERATIVE CARE

Parenteral nutrition should begin as soon as a stable postoperative state has been reached and continued until total enteral nutrition (TEN) is established.

Paradoxically, the more proximal the atresia, the longer the period of postoperative intestinal dysfunction, necessitating nasogastric decompression. In general terms, oral intake is commenced only when the baby is alert, sucks well, has clear gastric aspirate of less than 5 ml/hour, has a soft flat abdomen, and is passing flatus or feces. Delay in function beyond 14 days may be an indication for a contrast upper GI study.[99]

Abdominal distention, vomiting, evidence of peritonitis, and a pneumoperitoneum present more than 24 hours after operation suggest an anastomotic leak, and immediate reexploration should be performed. The leaking anastomosis may be resected and reanastomosed, or it may be exteriorized.[15] It is important to reconfirm patency of the distal bowel.

A Silastic transanastomotic tube (TAT) passed via the lumen of a gastrostomy tube or transnasally allows for the early introduction of enteral feeding. TAT feeding is started 24 hours postoperatively with 1 ml iso-osmolar solution once every 4 hours and increased as tolerated. Continuous infusion of a polymeric formula should be instituted as soon as intestinal motility has returned.[62, 98, 99, 137, 138]

Improvements in quality and delivery of TPN have reduced the urgency and necessity of early TAT or oral feeding, although the judicious intraluminal deposition of expressed breast milk or iso-osmolar formula stimulates reactive hyperplasia in the residual intestinal mucosa and should enhance intestinal adaptation. Adaptation begins almost immediately after resection and continues for more than a year.[99, 139] Our experience with the gastrostomy/transanastomotic tube (GT/TAT) system revealed that TEN feedings were established at 17 days and full oral intake at an average of 25 days (14–44 days). With nasogastric decompression, with or without a transnasal TAT, full oral intake was established at an average of 20 days (16–23). Three major problems were encountered with TAT: migration into the stomach, tube blockage, and small bowel perforation. The effect of early enteral feeding on the induction of gut hormones on bowel growth, secretions, and motility; on intermediate metabolism; and, ultimately, on bowel adaptation is relatively unknown.[140–142]

Adequate oral nutrition should consist of a complete infant formula with approximately 62% carbohydrate, 18% fat, and 12% protein. Intraluminal fat is the most potent stimulus for intestinal mucosal growth, and as little as 20% of the total daily caloric requirements in the form of long-chain triglycerides is sufficient to maintain the structure and function of the small bowel.[139] The unique role of glutamine in stimulating mucosal cell growth and metabolism has not been fully determined. Caloric intake should not be less than 120 cal/kg/day. As tolerance develops, the patient's oral intake is gradually increased.

Transient GI dysfunction is frequently observed in infants with jejunal and ileal atresia and is multifactorial in etiology.[3, 4, 62, 99] Lactose intolerance, malabsorption owing to stasis with bacterial overgrowth, intestinal hurry, and diarrhea may be significant in children with short bowel syndrome following surgery for multiple atresias, surgery for the apple-peel anomaly, and loss of the ileocecal valve. These infants require a gradual transition period for the eventual goal of TEN to be reached. Regular monitoring for clinical signs and biochemical evidence of intestinal overload or intolerance is required. Disaccharide and even monosaccharide intolerance, indicative of gross intestinal brush border malfunction, should be assessed by regular biochemical evaluation of stool samples.[99] Warning signs are water-loss stools, increasing stool frequency, hematochezia, fecal-reducing substances, a falling stool pH, an increase in gastric residual volume, and rising breath hydrogen excretion levels.[99] Unintentional injury to the fragile mucosa can be caused by sugars, high-osmolality feeds, oral medications, and intestinal bacterial and viral infections. Pharmacologic control of altered GI function may hasten adaptation. Loperamide hydrochloride decreases intestinal peristaltic activity, and cholestyramine is effective in binding bile salts.[143] Cholestyramine should not be given unless water-loss stools are evident. Vitamin B_{12} and folic acid should be given regularly to the patient without a terminal ileum to prevent megaloblastic anemia.

RESULTS

Before 1952, our mortality rate for small bowel atresia was 90%, falling to 28% between 1952 and 1955.[4, 40] A change in the surgical procedure from primary anastomosis without resection to liberal resection of the blind ends and end-to-end anastomosis significantly improved the survival to 78% over the next 3 years.[40] During the 38-year period, 1959 to 1997, 250 patients with jejunoileal atresia and stenosis were admitted to our pediatric surgical service of whom 28 have died, giving an overall mortality rate of 11.2% (see Table 30–1). The highest mortality was encountered in type III(b) atresia (19.1%), accounting for 3.6% of the overall mortality (Table 30–2) Five neonates were moribund on admission with infarction of the proximal bowel owing to volvulus of the bulbous end and established peritonitis—1 type I, 1 type II, 1 type III(a), and 2 type

TABLE 30-2. Mortality Related to Type of Atresia

Type	Patients	Mortality	(%)
Stenosis	29	0	(0)
I	58	4	(6.9)
II	26	3	(11.5)
III(a)	39	7	(17.9)
III(b)	47	9	(19.1)
IV	51	5	(9.8)
Total	**250**	**28**	
Overall mortality 11.2%			

III(b)—reemphasizing the need for prompt surgical management. Six neonates died from infection related to pneumonia or peritonitis, 1 from an anastomotic leak owing to unrecognized colonic atresia. This experience and 3 deaths that have been reported due to undiagnosed colonic atresia in infants treated for jejunoileal atresia[114] have prompted us to insist on a contrast enema prior to repair of a jejunoileal atresia. Support was withdrawn from 2 patients with less than 10 cm residual small bowel. One neonate died 18 hours after birth from hemorrhagic disease. Fourteen died due to short bowel syndrome, line sepsis, and liver failure. Other researchers report that mortality is also influenced by prematurity, associated disease processes or congenital abnormalities, malrotation, postoperative volvulus and bowel infarction, and anastomotic dysfunction or leak.[14, 15, 17, 18, 69, 104, 110, 144] Owing to the small size and delicate blood supply of the distal bowel in type III(b) atresia, anastomotic leaks (15%), stricture formation (15%), and gangrene of the proximal end of the distal segment (7%) have been reported in a collected review.[72] Delay in presentation, coupled with inadequate medical facilities and nutritional support, accounted for a mortality rate of 52% in children with jejunoileal atresia.[1] A collective review of mortality from 1950 to 1997 is depicted in Table 30–3.

Short gut syndrome following surgical correction of jejunoileal atresia may be due to extensive intrauterine bowel loss, overzealous resection, operative

TABLE 30-3. Jejunoileal Atresia and Stenosis: Improvement in Survival

Authors	Years of Study	n	Survival (%)
Evans[14]	1950	1498	9.3
Gross[61]	1940–1952	71	51
Benson and colleagues[104]	1945–1959	38	55
de Lorimier[69]	1957–1966	587	65
Nixon and Tawes[18]	1956–1967	62	62
Louw[117]	1959–1967	33	94
Martin and Zerella[74]	1957–1975	59	64
Cywes and colleagues[2]	1959–1978	84	88
Danismend and colleagues[130]	1967–1981	101	77
Smith and Glasson[110]	1961–1986	84	61
Cywes and colleagues[155]	1959–1997	250	89

ischemic injury to the bowel, or postoperative complications. Short bowel syndrome is defined as residual jejunoileal length of less than 75 cm with permanent malabsorption.[145] Although many factors influence survival, long-term survival is possible in infants with an 11- to 15-cm jejunoileum and an intact ileocecal valve or with 25- to 40-cm small bowel length without an ileocecal valve.[145, 146] A survival rate of 46 to 69% can be anticipated in most infants with less than 25 cm of jejunoileum.[145–147] Careful and accurate measurement of the total residual bowel length (small bowel plus colon) is imperative to determine the infant's potential for adaptation.

The following factors must be considered in determining the final functional status of the bowel. Rapid jejunoileal growth occurs during the later stages of gestation from the mean of 115 cm at 19 to 27 gestational weeks to 248 cm at 35 to 40 weeks.[148] Postnatal growth in intestinal length can further facilitate intestinal adaptation.[147] The small intestine (digestion and assimilation areas) continues to grow and elongate most rapidly during infancy until total body length reaches about 60 cm. Thereafter, intestinal growth slows down and remains constant once 100 to 140 cm of total body length has been reached.[149] These findings emphasize the importance of maintaining overall somatic growth in these children during the period of type I intestinal adaptation until full oral intake can be achieved.[139] The dilated bowel proximal to the atresia is stretched, leading to overestimation of its functional capabilities, in contradistinction to the collapsed unused distal bowel, where the functional length is up to two times the measured length. Bowel length may also be underestimated in infants with gastroschisis.[133] Of critical importance is an intact ileocecal valve, which allows accelerated intestinal adaptation with shorter residual jejunoileal length.[138, 147] The residual bowel becomes dilated and both villus height and crypt depth increase, resulting in an increase in the absorption surface area per unit length of bowel and enhanced absorption. The adaptive response to jejunal loss is more marked than for ileal resection, and with loss of the ileocecal valve, infants are more susceptible to rapid bowel transit, malabsorption, diarrhea, and increased bacterial proliferation in the small bowel.[139] Early introduction of intraluminal feeding facilitates and hastens the period of intestinal adaptation, thereby reducing the dependency on TPN as the sole provider of adequate nutrition for growth and development.[139, 141, 146, 147]

Infants with short bowel syndrome are divided into four main functional groups: uncorrectable intestinal insufficiency, adequate bowel function for survival, adequate alimentary function for growth and development, and normal alimentary function with a degree of intestinal reserve.[2] Long-term outlook for most of these children is optimistic, although TPN-associated complications are frequent and sometimes fatal.[137, 147] Several surgical procedures have been described to improve short bowel syndrome, including interposition of colonic segments, reversal of bowel segments, and methods to increase mucosal surface area. Most are obsolete except for bowel lengthening procedures. An isoperistaltic bowel lengthening procedure has proved successful for the short-term and intermediate-term intestinal function.[136, 150–152] Intestinal transplantation is indicated when permanent dependency on TPN is expected.[153] Although intestinal transplantation in the tacrolimus immunosuppression era is feasible, morbidity and mortality remain daunting mainly due to the ongoing immunogenicity of transplanted bowel and the immunosuppression required to achieve graft acceptance. Improved survival may come with advances in immunosuppressive therapy.[154] One-year graft and patient survival in the best centers are greater than 50% both with small bowel alone and with small bowel with other visceral grafts.[153]

The 39 patients with short bowel syndrome in our series had an average small bowel length of 35 cm, 6 without an ileocecal valve. Five early deaths were due to extremely short bowel: 9 cm, 10 cm, 12 cm, 17 cm, and 22 cm. Five other early deaths were due to sepsis in patients with residual bowel, ranging from 26 cm to 50 cm. There were 4 late deaths: 2 months, 7½ months, 11 months, and 2½ years after the initial operation, all related to complications of TPN. Thus, the lack of sufficient residual bowel was responsible for 14 deaths and for considerable morbidity or a miserable quality of life in the other 25 patients. In most instances, maximal intestinal adaptation occurred within 6 to 12 months but was delayed for 18 months in 2 patients. Of the 25 survivors, 13 have developed normally, whereas 12 had delayed milestones and were below the third percentile for weight.

□ Colonic Atresia

Atresia of the colon is a rare form of intestinal atresia and comprises from 1.8% to 15% of all intestinal atresias and stenoses.[113, 114] Atresias can occur at any level, but type III lesions to the right of the splenic flexure, and type I lesions distal to the vascular watershed predominate.[113] Complicated colonic atresia with partial or complete absence of the hind gut is frequently associated with major anterior abdominal wall and genitourinary defects (i.e., vesicointestinal fissure and extrophy of the bladder) and in ischiopagus-conjoined twins.[155] Concomitant small bowel atresia, Hirschsprung's disease, and gastroschisis are not infrequently associated with colonic atresia. The atresia is most likely due to mesenteric vascular impairment or intrauterine volvulus.[13, 71, 156]

Prenatal diagnosis can be suspected on US in the presence of bowel obstruction and if the diameter of the colon is larger than expected for gestational age.[157]

These infants are usually full term and present with rapidly progressing findings of distal intestinal obstruction. Delay in diagnosis can lead to ischemia and proximal bowel perforation.

Abdominal radiographs confirm distal bowel obstruction, often with a disproportionately large loop corresponding to the ectatic and dilated proximal colonic segment.[158] This dilation can be so massive that it mimics a pneumoperitoneum (Fig. 30–15A). A contrast enema confirms colonic atresia, showing

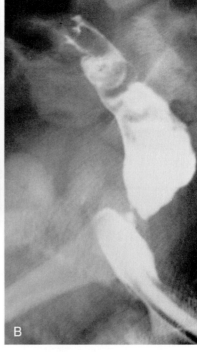

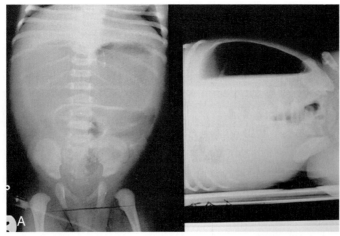

Figure 30–15. *A,* Abdominal radiograph of colonic atresia showing huge air-filled proximal colon mimicking a pneumoperitoneum. *B,* Right colonic atresia with rectal stenosis.

a small-diameter colon that terminates adjacent to the obstructed colonic segment.

The surgical approach depends on the clinical status of the patient, the level of atresia, the status of the bowel proximal to the atresia, any associated small intestinal atresia, the patency of the bowel distal to the atresia, and complications. It is important to ensure patency of the entire colon because multiple atresias and stenosis can occur and to exclude Hirschsprung's disease.[71, 159] A staged surgical approach is generally preferred, with initial resection of the dilated colon, colostomy, and distal mucous fistulas. Primary resection and anastomosis have a higher incidence of complications, usually owing to undiagnosed distal pathology.[160, 161]

Prognosis is usually excellent but depends on residual small bowel length, concomitant small bowel pathology, and associated anomalies.

PATIENT MATERIAL

We have treated eight patients with colonic atresia, excluding those with complete vesicointestinal malformations and conjoined twins. The gender incidence was equal and seven were full term. Five were type III(a), two type I, and one type II. One infant had atresia of the right colon with two further stenoses in the rectosigmoid colon (see Fig. 30–15B). Three had extensive loss of more proximal bowel owing to associated small bowel atresias, which led to short bowel syndrome in two. Four had malrotation, one had gastroschisis, and one had distal colon Hirschsprung's disease. Three had primary resection and anastomosis, all with associated small bowel atresias. In one of these patients, the colonic atresia was missed because no preoperative contrast enema had been done. Anastomotic disruption resulted in death from sepsis. Another infant with a primary anastomosis developed postoperative functional bowel obstruction, and Hirschsprung's disease of the distal colon was confirmed. Colostomy and later pull-through was required. Five had colostomy and delayed anastomosis. One of these was well for 7 months but developed protein-losing enteropathy, which was extensively investigated. Despite essentially normal contrast studies, it was only at laparotomy that a chronic 360-degree midgut volvulus was found with a completely unfixed mesentery and gross venous and lymphatic congestion. Ladd's procedure was curative.

REFERENCES

1. Adeyemi D: Neonatal intestinal obstruction in a developing tropical country: Patterns, problems, and prognosis. J Trop Pediatr 35:66, 1989.
2. Cywes S, Davies MRQ, Rode H: Congenital jejuno-ileal atresia and stenosis. S Afr Med J 57:630, 1980.
3. Grosfeld JL: Jejunoileal atresia and stenosis, section 3: The small intestine. In Ravitch MM, Welch KJ, Benson CD, et al (eds): Pediatric Surgery. Chicago, Year Book Medical, 1986, p 838.
4. Louw JH: Congenital intestinal atresia and severe stenosis in the newborn. S Afr J Science 3:109, 1952.
5. Irving IM, Rickham PP: Duodenal atresia and stenosis: Annular pancreas. In Rickham PP, Lister J, Irving IM (eds): Neonatal Surgery (2nd ed). Boston, Butterworths, 1978, p 355.
6. Al-Salem A, Khwaja S, Grant C, et al: Congenital intrinsic duodenal obstruction: Problems in the diagnosis and management. J Pediatr Surg 24:1247, 1989.
7. Calder J: Two examples of children born with preternatural conformation of the guts. Med Essay (Edinburgh) 1:203, 1733. Cited by: Kelly PM. Brit J Surg 29:245, 1941.
8. Madsen CM: Duodenal atresia—60 years of follow-up [case report]. Prog Pediatr Surg 10:61, 1977.
9. Ernst NP: A case of congenital atresia of the duodenum treated successfully by operation. BMJ 644, 1916.
10. Jackson JM: Annular pancreas and duodenal obstruction in the neonate: A review. Arch Surg 87:37, 1963.
11. Bowen J, Dickson A, Bruce J: Reconstruction for duodenal atresia: Tapered or non-tapered duodenoplasty. J Pediatr Surg 11:474, 1996.
12. Adzick NS, Harrison MR, de Lorimier AA: Tapering duodenoplasty for megaduodenum associated with duodenal atresia. J Pediatr Surg 21:311, 1986.
13. Louw JH, Barnard CN: Congenital intestinal atresia: Observations on its origin. Lancet 2:1065, 1955.
14. Evans CH: Atresias of the gastrointestinal tract. Int Abstr Surg 92:1, 1951.
15. Hays DM: Intestinal atresia and stenosis. In Ravitch M (ed): Current Problems in Surgery. Chicago, Year Book Medical, 1969, p 3.
16. World Health Organization: Congenital Malformations [bulletin]. World Health Organization, 34, 38, 1966.
17. Grosfeld JL, Ballantine TVN, Shoemaker R: Operative management of intestinal atresia and stenosis based on pathologic findings. J Pediatr Surg 14:368, 1979.
18. Nixon HH, Tawes R: Etiology and treatment of small intestinal atresia: Analysis of a series of 127 jejunoileal atresias and comparison with 62 duodenal atresias. Surgery 69:41, 1971.
19. Fockens P: Operativ geheilter Fall von kongenitaler Dünndarmatresie. Zentralbl Chir 38:532, 1911.
20. El Shafie M, Rickham PP: Multiple intestinal atresias. J Pediatr Surg 5:655, 1970.
21. Mishalany HG, Der Kaloustian VM: Familial multiple-level intestinal atresias: Report of two siblings. J Pediatr 79:124, 1971.
22. Bar-Moar JA, Nissan S, Nero P: Pyloric atresia, a hereditary congenital anomaly with autosomal recessive transmission. J Med Genet 9:70, 1972.
23. Bronsther B, Nadear MR, Abrams MW: Congenital pyloric atresia: A report of three cases and a review of the literature. Surgery 69:1, 130, 1971.
24. Burnett HA, Halpert B: Perforation of stomach of newborn infants with pyloric atresia. Arch Pathol 44:318, 1947.
25. Hayashi AH, Galliani CA, Gillis DA: Congenital pyloric atresia and junctional epidermolysis bullosa: A report of long-term survival and a review of the literature. J Pediatr Surg 11:1341, 1991.
26. Tandler J: Zur Entwicklungsgeschichte des Menschlichen Duodenums im frühen Embryonal stadiem. Gegenhaur's Morphol Jahrbuch 29:187, 190u.
27. Boyden EA, Cope JG, Bill AH: Anatomy and embryology of congenital intrinsic obstruction of the duodenum. Am J Surg 114:139, 1967.
28. Lynn HB, Espinas EE: Intestinal atresia: An attempt to relate location to embryologic processes. Arch Surg 79:357, 1959.
29. Movtosouris C: The "Solid stage" and congenital intestinal atresia. J Pediatr Surg 1:446, 1966.
30. Elliot GB, Kliman R, Elliot KA: Pancreatic annulus: A sign or a cause of duodenal obstruction? Can J Surg 11:357, 1968.
31. Gourevitch A: Duodenal atresia in the newborn. Ann R Coll Surg Engl 48:141, 1971.
32. Jona JZ: Duodenal anomalies and the ampulla of Vater. Surg Gynecol Obstet 143:565, 1976.
33. Brereton RJ, Cudmore RE, Bouton JM: Double atresia of the duodenum. Z Kinderchir 31:60, 1980.

34. Coughlin JP, Rector RE, Klein MD: Agenesis of the gallbladder in duodenal atresia: Two case reports. J Pediatr Surg 27:1304, 1992.
35. Davenport M, Saxena R, Howard E: Acquired biliary atresia. J Pediatr Surg 31:1721, 1996.
36. Moore SW, de Jongh G, Buic P, et al: Immune deficiency in familial duodenal atresia. J Pediatr Surg 31:1733, 1996.
37. Bill AH, Pope WM: Congenital duodenal diaphragm. Surgery 35:482, 1954.
38. Rowe M, Buckner D, Clatworthy HW: Wind sock web of the duodenum. Am J Surg 116:444, 1968.
39. Grosfeld JL, Rescoria FJ: Duodenal atresia and stenosis: Reassessment of treatment and outcome based on antenatal diagnosis, pathologic variance, and long-term follow-up. World J Surg 17:301, 1993.
40. Louw JH: Congenital intestinal atresia and stenosis in the newborn: Observations on its pathogenesis and treatment. Ann R Coll Surg Engl 25:209, 1959.
41. Bodian M, White LLR, Carter CO, et al: Congenital duodenal obstruction and mongolism. BMJ 1:77, 1952.
42. Fonkalsrud EW, de Lorimier AA, Hays DM: Congenital atresia and stenosis of the duodenum: A review compiled from the members of the Surgical Section of the American Academy of Pediatrics. Pediatrics 43:79, 1969.
43. Hancock BJ, Wiseman NE: Congenital duodenal obstruction: The impact of an antenatal diagnosis. J Pediatr Surg 24:1027, 1989.
44. Britton JR, Britton HL: Gastric aspirate volume at birth as an indicator of congenital intestinal obstruction. Acta Paediatr 85:945, 1995.
45. Brown RA, Millar AJW, Linegar A, et al: Fenestrated duodenal membranes: An analysis of symptoms, signs, diagnosis, and treatment. J Pediatr Surg 29:429, 1994.
46. Millar AJW, Rode H, Brown RA, et al: The deadly vomit: Malrotation and midgut volvulus: A review of 137 cases. Pediatr Surg Int 2:172, 1987.
47. Kimura L, Tsugawa C, Ogawa K, et al: Diamond-shaped anastomosis for congenital duodenal obstruction. Arch Surg 112:1262, 1977.
48. Richardson WR, Martin LW: Pitfalls in the management of the incomplete duodenal diaphragm. J Pediatr Surg 4:303, 1969.
49. de Lorimier AA, Harrison MR: Intestinal plication in the treatment of atresia. J Pediatr Surg 18:734, 1983.
50. Waever E, Nielson OH, Arnbjornsson E, et al: Operative management of duodenal atresia. Pediatr Surg Int 10:322, 1995.
51. Kokkonen ML, Kalima T, Jaaskelainen J: Duodenal atresia: Late follow-up. J Pediatr Surg 23:216, 1988.
52. Ein SH, Shandling B: The late nonfunctioning duodenal atresia repair. J Pediatr Surg 21:798, 1986.
53. Spigland N, Yazbeck S: Complications associated with surgical treatment of congenital intrinsic duodenal obstruction. J Pediatr Surg 25:1127, 1990.
54. Tchirkow G, Highman LM, Shafer AD: Cholelithiasis and cholecystitis in children after repair of congenital duodenal anomalies. Arch Surg 115:85, 1980.
55. Harris J, Kallen B, Robert E: Descriptive epidemiology of alimentary tract atresia. Teratology 52:15, 1995.
56. Bland-Sutton J: Imperforated ileum. Am J Med Sci 18:457, 1889.
57. Abrams JS: Experimental intestinal atresia. Surgery 64:185, 1968.
58. Koga Y, Hayashida Y, Ikeda K, et al: Intestinal atresia in fetal dogs produced by localized ligation of mesenteric vessels. J Pediatr Surg 10:949, 1975.
59. Santulli TV, Blanc WA: Congenital atresia of the intestine: Pathogenesis and treatment. Ann Surg 154:939, 1961.
60. Tibboel D, van der Kamp AWM, Molenaar JC: An experimental study of the effect of an intestinal perforation at various developmental stages. Z Kinderchir 37:62, 1982.
61. Gross RE: Congenital atresia of the intestine and colon. In Gross RE (ed): The Surgery of Infancy and Childhood. Philadelphia, WB Saunders, 1953, p 150.
62. Nixon HH: Intestinal obstruction in the newborn. Arch Dis Child 30:13, 1955.
63. Amoury RA, Ashcraft KW, Holder TM: Gastroschisis complicated by intestinal atresia. Surgery 82:373, 1977.
64. Grosfeld JL, Clatworthy HW Jr: The nature of ileal atresia due to intrauterine intussusception. Arch Surg 100:714, 1970.
65. Murphy DA: Internal hernias in infancy and childhood. Surgery 55:311, 1964.
66. Spriggs NI: Congenital intestinal occlusion. Guy's Hospital Report, 66:143, 1912.
67. Vassy LE, Boles ET: Iatrogenic ileal atresia secondary to clamping of an occult omphalocoele. J Pediatr Surg 10:797, 1975.
68. Todani T, Tavuchi K, Tanaka S, et al: Intestinal atresia due to intrauterine intussusception: Analysis of 24 cases in Japan. J Pediatr Surg 10:445, 1975.
69. de Lorimier AA, Fonkalsrud EW, Hays DM: Congenital atresia and stenosis of the jejunum and ileum. Surgery 65:819, 1969.
70. Lister J, Rickham PP: Intestinal atresia and stenosis, excluding the duodenum. In Rickham PP, Lister J, Irving IM (eds): Neonatal Surgery. London, Butterworths, 1978, p 381.
71. Moore SW, Rode H, Millar AJW, et al: Intestinal atresia and Hirschsprung's disease. Pediatr Surg Int 5:182, 1990.
72. Seashore JH, Collins FS, Markowitz RI, et al: Familial apple peel jejunal atresia: Surgical, genetic, and radiographic aspects. Pediatrics 80:540, 1987.
73. Nicolini U, Monni G: Intestinal obstruction in babies exposed in utero to methylene blue. Lancet 336:1258, 1990.
74. Martin LW, Zerella JT: Jejunoileal atresia: A proposed classification. J Pediatr Surg 11:399, 1976.
75. Davies MRQ, Louw JH, Cywes S, et al: The classification of congenital intestinal atresias [letter]. J Pediatr Surg 17:224, 1982.
76. Blanck C, Okmian L, Robbe H: Mucoviscidosis and intestinal atresia: A study of four cases in the same family. Acta Paediatr Scand 54:557, 1965.
77. Weitzman JJ, Vanderhoof RS: Jejunal atresia with agenesis of the dorsal mesentery with "Christmas tree" deformity of the small intestine. Am J Surg 111:443, 1966.
78. Blyth H, Dickson JAS: Apple peel syndrome: Congenital intestinal atresia. J Med Genet 6:275, 1969.
79. Mishalany HG, Najjar FB: Familial jejunal atresia: Three cases in one family. J Pediatr 73:753, 1968.
80. Olson LM, Flom LS, Kierney CMP, et al: Identical twins with malrotation and type IV jejunal atresia. J Pediatr Surg 22:1015, 1987.
81. Rickham PP, Karplus M: Familial and hereditary intestinal atresia. Helv Paediatr Acta 26:561, 1971.
82. Zerella JT, Martin LW: Jejunal atresia with absent mesentery and a helical ileum. Surgery 80:550, 1976.
83. Smith MB, Smith L, Wells JW, et al: Concurrent jejunal atresia with "apple peel" deformity in premature twins. Pediatr Surg Int 6:425, 1991.
84. Dickson JAS: Apple peel small bowel: An uncommon variant of duodenal and jejunal atresia. J Pediatr Surg 5:595, 1970.
85. Jimenez FA, Reiner L: Arteriographic findings in congenital abnormalities of the mesentery and intestine. Surg Gynecol Obstet 113:346, 1961.
86. Rittenhouse EA, Beckwith JB, Chappel JS, et al: Multiple septa of the small bowel: Description of an unusual case, with review of the literature and consideration of etiology. Surgery 71:371, 1972.
87. McHugh K, Daneman A: Multiple gastrointestinal atresias: Sonography of associated biliary abnormalities. Pediatr Radiol 21:355, 1991.
88. Guttman FM, Braun P, Garance PH, et al: Multiple atresias and a new syndrome of hereditary multiple atresias involving the gastrointestinal tract from stomach to rectum. J Pediatr Surg 8:633, 1973.
89. Tsujimoto K, Sherman FE, Ravitch MM: Experimental intestinal atresia in the rabbit fetus: Sequential pathological studies. Johns Hopkins Med J 131:287, 1972.
90. Arnal-Monreal F, Pombo F, Capdevila-Puerta A: Multiple hereditary gastrointestinal atresias: Study of a family. Acta Paediatr Scand 72:773, 1983.

91. Puri P, Guiney EJ, Carroll R: Multiple gastrointestinal atresias in three consecutive siblings: Observations on pathogenesis. J Pediatr Surg 20:22, 1985.

92. Benirschke K: Twin placenta in perinatal mortality. N Y State J Med 61:1499, 1961.

93. Braun F, Ferrier S, Berclaz J, et al: Multiple intestinal atresias and encephalomalacia in the survivor after in-utero death of a monozygous co-twin. Pediatr Surg Int 2:249, 1987.

94. Cloutier R: Intestinal smooth muscle response to chronic obstruction: Possible applications in jejunoileal atresia. J Pediatr Surg 10:3, 1975.

95. Nixon HH: An experimental study of the propulsion in isolated small intestine, and applications to surgery in the newborn. Ann R Coll Surg Engl 27:105, 1960.

96. Tepas JJ, Wyllie RG, Shermeta DW, et al: Comparison of histo-chemical studies of intestinal atresia in the human newborn and fetal lamb. J Pediatr Surg 14:376, 1979.

97. Pickard LR, Santoro S, Wyllie RG, et al: Histochemical studies of experimental fetal intestinal obstruction. J Pediatr Surg 16:256, 1981.

98. Touloukian RJ: Intestinal atresia. Clin Perinatol 5:3, 1978.

99. Haller JA, Tepas JJ, Pickard LR, et al: Intestinal atresia: Current concepts of pathogenesis, pathophysiology, and operative management. Am Surg 49:385, 1983.

100. de Lorimier AA, Norman DA, Gooding CA, et al: A model for the cinefluoroscopic and manometric study of chronic intestinal obstruction. J Pediatr Surg 8:785, 1973.

101. Touloukian RJ, Wright HK: Intrauterine villus hypertrophy with jejunoileal atresia. J Pediatr Surg 8:779, 1973.

102. Tovar JA, Sunol M, de Torre LB, et al: Mucosal morphology in experimental intestinal atresia: Studies in the chick embryo. J Pediatr Surg 26:184, 1991.

103. Doolin EJ, Ormsbee HS, Hill JL: Motility abnormalities in intestinal atresia. J Pediatr Surg 22:320, 1987.

104. Benson CD, Lloyd JR, Smith JD: Resection and primary anastomosis in the management of stenosis and atresia of the jejunum and ileum. Pediatrics 26:265, 1960.

105. Thomas CG: Jejunoplasty for the correction of jejunal atresia. Surg Gynecol Obstet 129:545, 1969.

106. Ward HC, Leake J, Millar PJ, et al: Brown bowel syndrome: A late complication of intestinal atresia. J Pediatr Surg 27:1593, 1992.

107. Lee TG, Warren BH: Antenatal ultrasonic demonstration of fetal bowel. Radiology 124:471, 1977.

108. Gross E, Aarmon Y, Abu-Dalu K, et al: Familial combined duodenal and jejunal atresia. J Pediatr Surg 31:1573, 1996.

109. Déléze G, Sidiropoulus D, Paumgartner G: Determination of bile acid concentration in human amniotic fluid for prenatal diagnosis of intestinal obstruction. Pediatrics 59:647, 1977.

110. Smith GHH, Glasson M: Intestinal atresia: Factors affecting survival. Aust N Z J Surg 59:151, 1989.

111. Cremin BJ, Cywes S, Louw JH: Small intestine. In Cremin BJ, Cywes S, Louw JH: Radiological Diagnosis of Digestive Tract Disorders in the Newborn: A Guide to Radiologists, Surgeons, and Paediatricians. London, Butterworths, 1973, pp 62–89.

112. Wasch MG, Marck A: The radiographic appearance of the gastrointestinal tract during the first day of life. J Pediatr 32:479, 1948.

113. Boles ET Jr, Vassy LE, Ralston M: Atresia of the colon. J Pediatr Surg l1:69, 1976.

114. Benson CD, Lofti MW, Brough AJ: Congenital atresia and stenosis of the colon. J Pediatr Surg 3:253, 1968.

115. Jackman S, Brereton RJ: A lesson in intestinal atresias. J Pediatr Surg 23:852, 1988.

116. Aharon M, Kleinhaus U, Lightig C: Neonatal intramural intestinal calcifications associated with bowel atresia. Am J Roentgen 130:999, 1986.

117. Louw JH: Resection and end-to-end anastomosis in the management of atresia and stenosis of the small bowel. Surgery 62:940, 1967.

118. Malcynski JT, Shorter NA, Mooney DP: The proximal mesenteric flap: A method for closing large mesenteric defects in jejunal atresia. J Pediatr Surg 29:1607, 1994.

119. Holder TM, Gross RE: Temporary gastrostomy in pediatric surgery: Experience with 187 cases. Pediatrics 26:36, 1960.

120. Howard ER, Othersen HB: Proximal jejunoplasty in the treatment of jejunoileal atresia. J Pediatr Surg 8:685, 1973.

121. Ehrenpreis TH, Sandblom PN: Duodenal atresia and stenosis. Acta Paediatr Scand 39:109, 1949.

122. Louw JH: Congenital atresia and stenosis of the small intestine: The case for resection and primary end-to-end anastomosis. S Afr J Surg 4:57, 1966.

123. Ramanujan TM: Functional capability of blind small bowel loops after intestinal remodelling techniques. Aust N Z J Surg 54:145, 1984.

124. Kimura K, Perdzynski, Soper RT: Elliptical seromuscular resection for tapering the proximal dilated bowel in duodenal or jejunal atresia. J Pediatr Surg 31:1405, 1996.

125. Weber TR, Vane DW, Grosfeld JL: Tapering enteroplasty in infants with bowel atresia and short gut. Arch Surg 117:684, 1982.

126. Kizilkan F, Tanyel FC, Hicsonmez A, et al: Modified plication technique for the treatment of intestinal atresia. Pediatr Surg Int 6:233, 1991.

127. Bishop HC, Koop CE: Management of meconium ileus, resection Roux-en-Y anastomosis, and ileostomy irrigation with pancreatic enzymes. Ann Surg 145:410, 1957.

128. Rehbein F, Halsband H: A double-tube technique for the treatment of meconium ileus and small bowel atresia. J Pediatr Surg 3:723, 1968.

129. Swenson O: End-to-end aseptic intestinal anastomosis in infants and children. Surgery 36:192, 1954.

130. Danismend EN, Frank JD, Brown ST: Morbidity and mortality in small bowel atresia: Jejuno-ileal atresia. Z Kinderchir 42:17, 1987.

131. Turncock RR, Brereton RJ, Sptiz L, et al: Primary anastomosis in apple-peel bowel syndrome. J Pediatr Surg 26:718, 1991.

132. Shah R, Woolley MM: Gastroschisis and intestinal atresia. J Pediatr Surg 26:788, 1991.

133. van Hoorn WA, Hazebroek FWJ, Molenaar JC: Gastroschisis associated with atresia—a plea for delay in resection. Z Kinderchir 40:368, 1985.

134. Waldhausen JHT, Sawin RS: Improved long-term outcome for patients with jejunoileal apple peel atresia. J Pediatr Surg 32:1307, 1997.

135. Chaet MS, Warner BW, Sheldon CA: Management of multiple jejunoileal atresias with an intraluminal Silastic stent. J Pediatr Surg 29:1604, 1982.

136. Bianchi A: Intestinal loop lengthening—a technique for increasing small intestinal length. J Pediatr Surg 15:145, 1980.

137. Thompson JS, Pinch LW, Vanderhof JA, et al: Experience with intestinal lengthening for the short bowel syndrome. J Pediatr Surg 26:721, 1991.

138. Schwartz MZ, Maeda K: Short bowel syndrome in infants and children. Pediatr Clin North Am 32:1265, 1985.

139. Dowling RH: Small bowel adaptation and its regulation. Scand J Gastroenterol, 17:53, 1982.

140. Bristol JB, Williamson RCN: Mechanisms of intestinal adaptation. Pediatr Surg Int 3(4):233, 1988.

141. Lentze MJ: Nutritional aspects of the short bowel syndrome. Pediatr Surg Int 3(5):312, 1988.

142. Gleeson MH, Bloom SR, Polak JM, et al: Endocrine tumour in kidney affecting small bowel structure, motility, and absorptive function. Gut 12:773, 1971.

143. Remmington M, Malagelada JR, Zinsmeister A, et al: Abnormalities in gastrointestinal motor activity in patients with short bowel: Effect of a synthetic opiate. Gastroenterology 85:629, 1983.

144. Louw JH, Cywes S, Davies MRQ, et al: Congenital jejuno-ileal atresia: Observations on its pathogenesis and treatment. Z Kinderchir 33:3, 1981.

145. Wilmore DW: Factors correlating with a successful outcome following extensive intestinal resection in newborn infants. J Pediatr 80:88, 1972.

146. Dorney SFA, Ament ME, Berquist WE, et al: Improved sur-

vival in very short small-bowel of infancy with use of long-term parenteral nutrition. J Pediatr 107:521, 1985.

147. Caniano DA, Starr J, Ginn-Pease ME: Extensive short-bowel syndrome in neonates: Outcome in the 1980s. Surgery 105:119, 1989.

148. Touloukian RJ, Smith GJ: Normal intestinal length in pre-term infants. J Pediatr Surg 18:720, 1983.

149. Siebert JR: Small-intestine length in infants and children. Am J Dis Child 134:593, 1980.

150. Weber TR, Powel MA: Early improvement on intestinal function after isoperistaltic bowel lengthening. J Pediatr Surg 31:61, 1996.

151. Kimura K, Soper RT: A new bowel elongating technique for the short-bowel syndrome using the isolated bowel segment Iowa models. J Pediatr Surg 28:792, 1993.

152. Chahine AA, Ricketts RR: A modification of the Bianchi intestinal lengthening procedure with a single anastomosis. J Pediatr Surg 33:1292, 1998.

153. Goulet O, Jan D, Brousse N, et al: Intestinal transplantation. J Pediatr Gastroenterol Nutr 25:1, 1997.

154. Rowe PM: Signalling an end to transplant rejection? Lancet 350:1526, 1997.

155. Cywes S, Millar AJW, Rode H, et al: Conjoined twins—the Cape Town experience. Pediatr Surg Int 12:234, 1997.

156. Erskine JM: Colonic stenosis in the newborn: The possible thromboembolic etiology of intestinal stenosis and atresia. J Pediatr Surg 5:321, 1970.

157 Anderson N, Malpas T, Robertson R: Prenatal diagnosis of colon atresia. Pediatr Radiol 23:63, 1993.

158. Winters WD, Weinberger E, Hatch EI: Atresia of the colon in neonates: Radiograph findings. AJR Am J Roentgenol 159:1273, 1992.

159. Williams MD, Burrington JD: Hirschsprung's disease complicating colon atresia. J Pediatr Surg 28:637, 1993.

160. Kim PCW, Superina RA, Ein S: Colonic atresia combined with Hirschsprung's disease: A diagnostic and therapeutic challenge. J Pediatr Surg 30:1216, 1995.

161. Pohlson EC, Hatch EI, Glick PL, et al: Individualized management of colonic atresia. Am J Surg 155:690, 1988.

31

MALROTATION

Lisa A. Clark, MD • Keith T. Oldham, MD

Normal development of the human intestine includes rotation and fixation of the embryonic midgut. These normal events were first noted by Mall[1] in 1898 and described in detail by Dott[2] in 1923. Abnormalities of rotation and fixation make up a spectrum of anatomic conditions that range in clinical importance from those in patients who are totally asymptomatic to those with catastrophic midgut volvulus and death. The clinical and anatomic features of this group of anomalies were elegantly described by William E. Ladd in his 1941 textbook entitled *Abdominal Surgery of Infancy and Childhood.*[3] Although contemporary outcomes are considerably improved, little refinement in the understanding of the basic anatomic abnormality or its technical surgical management has been possible subsequently. A thorough understanding of the embryology of the gut, particularly the midgut, is essential to comprehend the clinical presentations and operative findings associated with intestinal rotational abnormalities.[4]

☐ Embryology

The primitive gut is initially a roughly linear, tubular structure composed of endodermal tissue and centered within the embryo. The entire alimentary tract and associated digestive organs are ultimately formed from this and its derivatives. In the human, the embryonic midgut is defined as that portion of the primitive gut opening ventrally into the yolk sac. By the 5th week of gestation, the ventral opening into the yolk sac has narrowed such that it is roughly the diameter of the longitudinal gut itself, whereupon it is referred to as the omphalomesenteric duct. Disproportional growth and elongation of the midgut beginning in the 5th gestational week result in three distinct processes that relate to rotational abnormalities of the gut.

First, herniation of the primary midgut loop occurs into the base of the umbilical cord (Fig. 31–1*A* to *C*). This remains until about the 10th week of gestation. The axis of the primary midgut loop is

the superior mesenteric artery (SMA), and the omphalomesenteric duct is located at its apex. This primary loop rotates 180 degrees in a counterclockwise direction such that the proximal (prearterial) portion of the loop comes to reside posterior to the SMA. The more cranial portion of the prearterial segment and a portion of the foregut ultimately form the proximal duodenum, which is located to the right of the midline. The more distal prearterial segment passes posterior and becomes fixed to the left of the SMA. This horizontal segment forms the third and fourth portions of the duodenum and is normally attached to the posterior body wall at the ligament of Treitz to the left of the aorta. Therefore, this latter segment of the duodenum normally completes a rotational arc of 270 degrees in a counterclockwise direction from its original location.

The jejunum and proximal ileum undergo substantial elongation, forming approximately six primary intestinal loops at birth. The embryonic postarterial midgut segment gives rise to the terminal ileum, cecum, and right and proximal transverse colon. This segment also rotates 270 degrees in a counterclockwise direction, but this occurs anterior to the SMA (see Fig. 31–1*D*). Thus, the cecum is positioned initially to the left, then anterior and ultimately to the right of the SMA before becoming fixed in its final adult location in the right iliac fossa. This process is illustrated in Figure 31–1. The prearterial segment of the mature midgut extends from the duodenum to the omphalomesenteric duct remnant, and the postarterial segment is represented by the ileum and colon distal to this point, ending at the mid-transverse colon.

The second stage of midgut development is the retraction of the extracoelemic intestine. This process occurs between gestational weeks 10 and 12 as the rotation of both prearterial and postarterial segments approximates 180 degrees from the original orientation. At this point, the duodenojejunal junction has passed posterior to the SMA, most of the small bowel is to the right of the midline, and the cecum and ascending colon reside anterior to the SMA after reduction into the left abdomen.

425

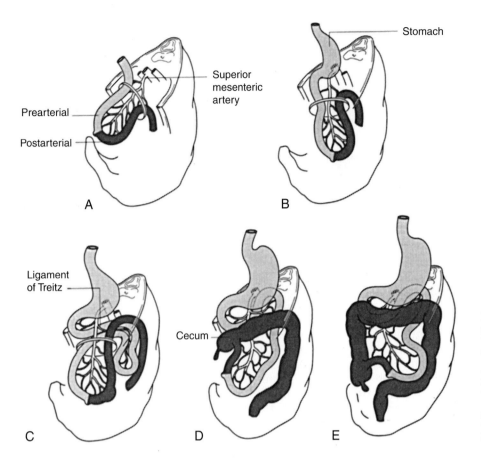

Figure 31–1. Normal midgut rotation is shown beginning in the 5th gestational week *(A)*, through completion of the process in the 12th week *(E)*. (See text.) (Adapted from Oldham KT: Pediatric abdomen. In Greenfield LJ, Mulholland M, Oldham KT, et al [eds]: Surgery: Scientific Principles and Practice. Philadelphia, Lippincott-Raven, 1997. Illustrations by Holly R. Fischer.)

Many common abnormalities of positioning occur as a result of arrested development during this 2-week period.

The final step in the normal midgut positioning process is fixation of the intestine to the posterior body wall. This occurs after the 12th week of gestation upon completion of cecal descent. Normal points of fixation include the cecum in the right iliac fossa and the duodenojejunal junction at the ligament of Treitz to the left of the aorta and anterior to the left renal vein (Fig. 31–2). The resulting oblique fixation of the intestinal mesentery is broad based and normally not at risk for volvulus. In contrast, when rotation and fixation are interrupted, the base of the mesentery is neither fixed nor broad, and the midgut may, therefore, undergo volvulus.[4] In addition to the risk of mesenteric volvulus, most individuals with rotational abnormalities have the potential for extrinsic duodenal compression and obstruction from the aberrant peritoneal bands (Ladd's bands), fixing a malpositioned cecum and colon to the posterior body wall.

The group of fixation anomalies referred to as *malrotation* results from interruption of the aforementioned embryologic events. The most common abnormalities include nonrotation, incomplete rotation, and several intermediate forms of these. More rare are mesocolic hernias and other abnormalities. Although imprecise, the term malrotation is irretrievably incorporated into the physician vocabu-

lary and is used here, as in clinical practice, to encompass the several surgically important malformations reviewed in the following paragraphs. The anatomic anomalies are quite variable and, even though a rotational abnormality may exist, by no means do all affected individuals have an anatomic configuration that will lead to symptoms or physiologic problems. Clinical symptoms discussed herein relate most importantly to either duodenal obstruction or midgut volvulus with vascular insufficiency of the bowel.

Intrinsic duodenal obstruction from a luminal web or atresia is an uncommon but well-described associated finding reported to occur in 8 to 12% of babies with rotational anomalies.[5] Therefore, eliminating this possibility is an important technical obligation either at or before the time of surgery.

NONROTATION

Nonrotation is characterized by failure of the normal counterclockwise rotation of the midgut loop around the SMA. In contrast to the normal 270-degree rotational arc, the rotation is either absent or arrested before exceeding 90 degrees (Fig. 31–3). The colon resides in the left abdomen, the cecum is at or near the midline, and the small intestine is to the right of midline. This anatomy is reported in approximately 0.2% of gastrointestinal contrast studies.[6] Midgut volvulus and extrinsic duodenal

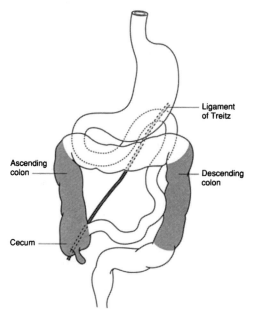

Figure 31–2. Normal oblique fixation of the midgut mesentery extends from the ligament of Treitz to the cecum in the right iliac fossa. The shaded portions of the ascending and descending colon are fixed in the retroperitoneum as well. (Adapted from Oldham KT: Pediatric abdomen. In Greenfield LJ, Mulholland M, Oldham KT, et al [eds]: Surgery: Scientific Principles and Practice. Philadelphia, Lippincott-Raven, 1997. Illustration by Holly R. Fischer.)

obstruction are significant clinical risks; the former because the SMA mesenteric vascular pedicle is narrow, and the latter because the peritoneal attachments of the abnormally positioned cecum to the posterior body wall pass anterior and lateral to the descending duodenum. The duodenojejunal juncture is more caudal and anterior than normal and it has typically failed to pass to the left of the midline. This and incomplete rotation are the most frequently encountered anomalies among patients with clinical symptoms related to malrotation. Partial duodenal obstruction from extrinsic compression by the cecal attachments to the posterior body wall is characteristic.

INCOMPLETE ROTATION

Incomplete rotation is also a relatively common positional abnormality characterized by arrest of the normal rotational process at or near 180 degrees rather than after the normal 270-degree arc (Fig. 31–4). Here the prearterial segment fails to complete the positioning posterior and to the left of the SMA. In addition, the postarterial cecum does not complete the counterclockwise rotation anterior to the SMA. The cecum typically resides in the upper abdomen, usually to the left of the SMA, and posterior body wall attachment is accomplished by peritoneal bands that potentially obstruct the duodenum as outlined earlier. A narrow SMA vascular pedicle once again provides the opportunity for midgut volvulus.

OTHER ROTATIONAL ABNORMALITIES

Mixed Rotational Abnormalities

Mixed rotational abnormalities are a more uncommon and highly variable group of anomalies in which the rotational process is arrested or disrupted with reference to either the prearterial or postarterial midgut segment. This may involve inconsequential variations such as an incompletely descended cecum, and it may involve serious anomalies at risk of mesenteric volvulus. The latter, for example, includes a phenomenon referred to as *reverse rotation*.[7] This involves some degree of midgut rotation in a clockwise direction around the SMA axis, so that the prearterial segment comes to reside anterior to the SMA rather than posterior. Therefore, the duodenum occupies an anterior position. The position of the postarterial segment is variable but can lie posterior to the SMA or within a mesocolic hernia (see later discussion). Reverse rotation with volvulus may present with obstruction of the transverse colon.

A surgeon who deals with patients who have rotational abnormalities must be familiar with the developmental basis for midgut positioning and be discerning enough to understand the variations when encountered. Although the anatomy is variable, any of these developmental abnormalities may

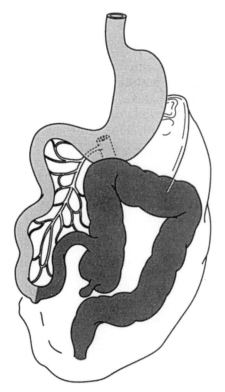

Figure 31–3. Nonrotation. The prearterial midgut *(lightly shaded)* resides on the patient's right and the postarterial segment *(darkly shaded)* is on the left. Neither segment of the midgut has undergone rotation in this illustration. (Adapted from Oldham KT: Pediatric abdomen. In Greenfield LJ, Mulholland M, Oldham KT, et al [eds]: Surgery: Scientific Principles and Practice. Philadelphia, Lippincott-Raven, 1997. Illustration by Holly R. Fischer.)

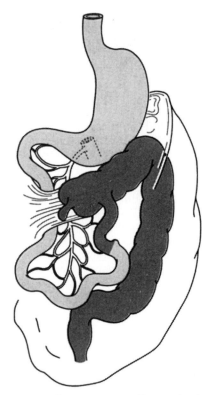

Figure 31–4. Incomplete rotation is illustrated. The prearterial midgut segment *(lightly shaded)* has failed to undergo 270-degree rotation and resides largely to the patient's right. The postarterial segment has rotated to reside anterior to the duodenum. Note that (Ladd's) bands fixing the cecum to the posterior body may compress and obstruct the duodenum.

be associated with a narrow SMA vascular pedicle as well as partial duodenal obstruction. The surgeon must correct whatever mechanical problem is encountered.

Mesocolic Paraduodenal Hernias

Mesocolic (paraduodenal) hernias are a rare but surgically important group of malformations that result from failure of fixation of either the right or left mesocolon to the posterior body wall in the normal fashion (see Fig. 31–2). These are referred to with a variety of names, including *paraduodenal hernia*. The resulting spaces offer the potential for sequestration and entrapment of the small intestine between the mesocolon and posterior body wall on either the right or left side.

A right-sided mesocolic hernia is associated with nonrotation of the prearterial midgut segment. It is characterized by small bowel entrapment posterior to the right colon and cecum. A similar phenomenon occurs on the left side; however, this is associated with normal positioning of the colon and cecum. In this latter case, entrapped small intestine is contained within a hernia sac with a neck composed of the inferior mesenteric vein and peritoneal attachments extending to the posterior body wall. As with any hernia, both right and left mesocolic hernias present potential risk for obstruction, incarceration, and strangulation of the small bowel.[8] Their surgical correction is discussed later.

ASSOCIATED ABNORMALITIES

Developmental abnormalities of midgut rotation and fixation are predictable when the intestine is malpositioned at parturition (e.g., omphalocele, gastroschisis, and congenital diaphragmatic hernia). Although the anatomy (and therefore the risk of midgut volvulus) is variable, it should be assumed that all of these patients are potentially at risk for malrotation and midgut volvulus. The duodenum and mesentery should be inspected during surgical correction of the primary lesion and a Ladd's procedure performed if the mesenteric vascular pedicle is judged narrow enough to be at risk for volvulus.

Other important associations are found in 30 to 62% of patients with malrotation.[9] Most of these relate to additional problems within the gastrointestinal tract. Up to half of patients with duodenal atresia and one third of those with jejunal atresia have associated malrotation.[10] Other anomalies are also often associated with intestinal malrotation and these are summarized in Table 31–1.[11–15] The familial occurrence of malrotation is reported, as is malrotation in both twins.[16, 17]

□ Clinical Presentation

The true incidence of rotational abnormalities of the midgut is difficult to determine. The autopsy prevalence may be as high as 0.5 to 1% of the total population, but the incidence of clinical symptoms is substantially less.[4, 18] The incidence of symptoms leading to clinical discovery is estimated at 1 in 6000 live births and the frequency among hospital admissions is about 1 in 25,000.[18, 19] Rotational abnormalities are slightly more common in boys than girls.[11, 20]

Fifty to 75% of patients with malrotation who become symptomatic do so in the first month of life, and approximately 90% of clinical symptoms occur

TABLE 31–1. Associated Anomalies

Anomaly*	%
Intestinal atresia	5–26
Imperforate anus	0–9
Cardiac anomalies	7–13
Duodenal web	1–2
Meckel's diverticulum	1–4
Hernia	0–7
Trisomy 21/mental retardation	3–10

Rare: esophageal atresia, biliary atresia, mesenteric cyst, craniosynostosis, Hirschsprung's disease, cystic duplication of stomach

*Patients with malrotation have the approximate incidence of the anomaly indicated.

in children younger than 1 year of age.[3, 11, 21] The remainder are seen later in life. Although volvulus and acute vascular insufficiency of the midgut are less common beyond the age of 1 year, these may occur at any age and this possibility remains a critical consideration as one considers the clinical approach to this problem. Among older patients, presentations also include chronic abdominal pain, weight loss or failure to thrive, chronic pancreatitis, celiac syndrome, or other relatively nonspecific gastrointestinal (GI) complaints.[11, 12] As noted, a number of patients appear asymptomatic in that the lesion is discovered incidental to other unrelated medical evaluation or at autopsy.

The symptoms with which patients with malrotation present generally result from either partial duodenal obstruction or midgut volvulus as noted earlier. The manner of presentation is age dependent (Table 31–2).[12] Duodenal obstruction is most commonly the result of extrinsic compression from Ladd's peritoneal bands as outlined. These bands are the mature derivative of the embryonic dorsal mesogastrium and serve to secure the cecum and mesocolon to the posterior body wall. Ladd's bands cross anterior and lateral to the descending duodenum, thus a postampullary site is the point of clinical obstruction and therefore bilious vomiting is characteristic. Midgut volvulus is present in approximately half of the patients who come to surgery for rotational abnormalities.[13] This often contributes additionally to duodenal obstruction at the site where the duodenal lumen is narrowed by torsion, typically in the distal duodenum. Lastly, there is a low but significant incidence of intrinsic duodenal obstruction in patients with rotational abnormalities. This may be in the form of a lumenal web, stenosis, or true atresia and is found in 8 to 12% of patients undergoing operation for malrotation.[5]

TABLE 31-2. Clinical Presentation of Patients with Malrotation Related to Age

Symptom/Sign	Age <2 mo		Age >2 mo	
	%	Duration* (d)	%	Duration* (d)
Vomiting				
Bilious	71	2	49	19
Nonbilious	25	10	49	213
Diarrhea	23	5	14	64
Abdominal pain	0	—	31	241
Constipation	6	4	23	76
Anorexia or nausea	11	14	14	35
Irritability	11	5	9	7
Apnea (intermittent)	11	2	6	75
Lethargy	9	1	9	1
Failure to thrive	6	12	23	112
Blood in stool	17	4	17	2
Fever	9	2	23	2

*Average duration of symptom.
Adapted from Powell D, Othersen HB, Smith CD: Malrotation of the intestines in children: The effect of age on presentation and therapy. J Pediatr Surg 24:777–780, 1989.

Bilious emesis is a cardinal manifestation of neonatal intestinal obstruction. This presentation demands that one consider malrotation with midgut volvulus in the differential diagnosis although it is by no means specific. Gastric and proximal duodenal distention secondary to the duodenal obstruction are important physical findings for malrotation. Early in the clinical course, relatively little air is present in the distal small bowel because of the partial duodenal obstruction. Therefore, abdominal distention is not typically present initially, although with progressive midgut ischemia and injury, ileus and small bowel distention may develop.

The most critical clinical concern with regard to malrotation and midgut volvulus is the potential for SMA pedicle torsion sufficient to develop acute vascular insufficiency to the midgut. This may be a life-threatening problem. Guaiac-positive stool or hematochezia resulting from mucosal injury is a relatively common early finding with volvulus. If transmural intestinal necrosis and frank sepsis ensue, hypotension, systemic acidosis, respiratory failure, thrombocytopenia, and other evidence of an abdominal catastrophe may be present. The outcome for midgut volvulus is time-dependent, which is the fundamental reason that signs and symptoms of neonatal intestinal obstruction must be pursued aggressively until a definitive diagnosis is obtained. Potentially, a delay of a few hours may lead to massive bowel loss. In one large series, bowel resection was required in only 15% of operative cases of malrotation.[13]

☐ Diagnosis

For neonatal intestinal obstruction or any other occasion when malrotation is included in the differential diagnosis, the imaging evaluation begins with a plain abdominal radiograph.[22] However, a patient with midgut volvulus may have a normal plain radiograph. Therefore, this is an insufficient study to rule out malrotation. Classic early plain radiographic findings of malrotation with volvulus are those of a distended stomach and proximal duodenum with a paucity of air in the distal small bowel.[23] These findings are the consequence of the partial duodenal obstruction. Although helpful, plain radiographs may not distinguish malrotation from duodenal atresia or stenosis. Therefore, if malrotation is a concern, an upper GI contrast study is necessary. Typically, malrotation with volvulus produces an incomplete obstruction of the descending or distal duodenum with the appearance of extrinsic compression and torsion, variably described as a "bird's beak," "corkscrew," or "coiled" appearance (Fig. 31–5).[23]

In contrast, duodenal atresia may occur anywhere within the duodenum but tends to be more proximal, to be completely obstructing, and to have a smoother duodenal contour, without the coiled or beak appearance; the extrinsic compression seen

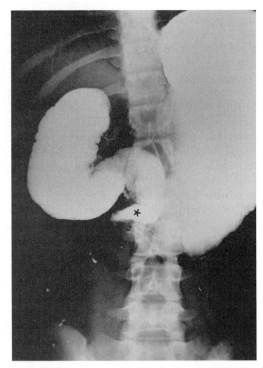

Figure 31–5. This upper gastrointestinal contrast study shows malrotation with volvulus. The "beak" is illustrated by the asterisk. Note the malposition of the distal duodenum as well. (From Oldham KT: Pediatric abdomen. In Greenfield LJ, Mulholland M, Oldham KT, et al [eds]. Surgery: Scientific Principles and Practice. Philadelphia, Lippincott-Raven, 1997.)

with malrotation is absent. Complete absence of distal air is typical of duodenal atresia, whereas diminished but discernable distal small bowel air is characteristic of malrotation. Duodenal stenosis with incomplete obstruction, particularly if located in a more distal location, may be indistinguishable from malrotation radiographically, even using intraluminal contrast. Uncertainty requires immediate operative exploration. Furthermore, radiographic differentiation of malrotation with and without midgut volvulus may be unreliable; therefore, it is potentially hazardous to defer operative exploration owing to the radiographic expectation that volvulus has not occurred.

In most circumstances, an upper GI contrast series is the definitive imaging study for rotational abnormalities (Fig. 31–6A). A well-done contrast series of the upper GI tract normally differentiates obstruction related to a rotational abnormality from intrinsic duodenal obstruction. Typically, malrotation is identified because the duodenojejunal junction is not normally located. The usual position is to the left of the midline, rising to approximately the level of the pylorus and fixed well posterior. Rather, it is anterior, low, and often midline or to the right of the midline when malrotation is compared with normal. The lateral film is very useful in assessing the anterior and posterior relationships of the duodenojejunal junction. Interpretation of an upper GI tract contrast series in this situation is somewhat subjective

and operator dependent. For maximal value, the study requires an experienced pediatric radiologist, a high-quality fluoroscopic study in the radiology suite, and direct involvement of the surgeon.

The contrast enema is helpful in evaluating children with more general concerns of neonatal intestinal obstruction, but it is less reliable with regard to malrotation because the position of the cecum and the colon are highly variable and may even appear to be normal.[24] The finding of a high right-sided or left-sided cecum is, however, abnormal and consistent with malrotation. With malrotation, the small bowel typically resides in the right abdomen and the colon and the cecum are often on the left (see Fig. 31–6B).

Other imaging studies that demonstrate axial relationships such as ultrasonography or computed tomography may periodically demonstrate evidence of malrotation.[25] The typical finding here is reversal in the relationship of the SMA to the superior mesenteric vein (SMV). Normally, the SMV is positioned to the right of the SMA. An SMA in an aberrant position, usually anterior or to the left of the SMV, suggests malrotation. If present, this finding is noteworthy but not sufficiently reliable to establish the diagnosis of malrotation with volvulus. Likewise, a normal SMA-SMV relationship does not always exclude malrotation. Even though these findings may lead to a diagnosis when found, the limitations mean that this is not generally a helpful imaging approach in the infant being evaluated acutely for neonatal intestinal obstruction.

☐ Treatment

Neonates and infants with rotational abnormalities require operative management. As previously discussed, the propensity for volvulus is greatest in newborns and infants. For the symptomatic patient, evaluation, resuscitation, and preoperative preparation should all be conducted concurrently so that a diagnosis of malrotation is followed immediately by laparotomy. The urgency is related to the fact that a delay of a few hours may determine whether ischemic midgut remains viable and, therefore, salvageable. If the midgut is not salvageable at laparotomy, survival rate is approximately 50% and has historically been achieved only with permanent or long-term parenteral hyperalimentation.[26] More recently, intestinal transplantation (with or without liver transplantation) has become an alternative, but without question, these complex approaches are to be avoided if possible.[27] There is no reason to delay surgical exploration when the clinical diagnosis is malrotation with possible midgut volvulus.

The presence of symptoms must raise the concern of volvulus; therefore, prompt exploration is warranted in all symptomatic patients. Additionally, one must always question whether a newly discovered "asymptomatic" patient is truly without complaint in that the investigations leading to this diag-

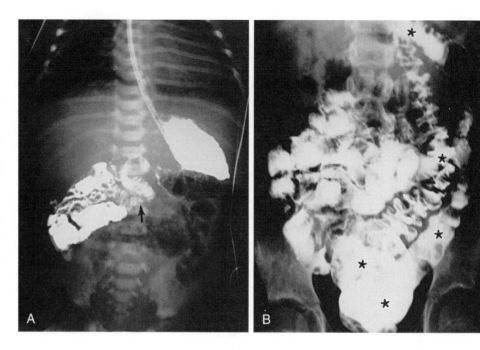

Figure 31–6. *A*, This upper gastrointestinal contrast series in a patient with malrotation without volvulus illustrates typical malposition of the duodenal-jejunal juncture *(arrow)*. This corresponds to the ligament of Treitz and is located more caudad, right, and anterior than normal. *B*, This radiograph again illustrates malrotation. The small bowel is to the right of midline, and the colon and cecum *(asterisks)* are to the left. (Adapted from Oldham KT: Pediatric abdomen. In Greenfield LJ, Mulholland M. Oldham KT, et al [eds]: Surgery: Scientific Principles and Practice. Philadelphia, Lippincott-Raven, 1997.)

nosis are not generally undertaken without some specific complaint on the part of the patient.

Preoperative preparation for symptomatic infants is not different than for any other seriously ill newborn in need of emergency laparotomy. Needs include fluid resuscitation via appropriate intravenous (IV) catheters, nasogastric decompression, possibly a urethral catheter, and aggressive medical support of critical electrolyte and respiratory needs. Broad-spectrum antibiotic coverage is appropriate as well. Most important is the necessity to proceed expeditiously to the operating room.

THE ASYMPTOMATIC PATIENT

The management of the older asymptomatic patient with malrotation is controversial.[28] Some authors believe that prompt, but nonemergent, correction should be done in the presence of known malrotation if there are not compelling medical contraindications.[10, 12, 14] The rationale includes several concerns. One is that the diagnosis of malrotation is generally not established without a GI contrast study, and, although the symptoms may be nonspecific, these patients may indeed be symptomatic without overt signs of obstruction or catastrophic vascular insufficiency. It appears as well that there is no upper limit to the age at which one is at risk for volvulus. The older child tends to be seen more often with chronic complaints and less commonly with volvulus. The risk of bowel ischemia, however, once volvulus is present, is not age dependent.[13] Careful review of the available literature, including the experience of Robert Gross, suggests that the incidence of volvulus with nonoperated malrotation is about one in three during a limited follow-up.[21]

There is no reliable imaging technique to determine whether the breadth of the SMA vascular pedicle places a particular patient at risk for volvulus. Because the potential consequences of malrotation with volvulus include death and the short bowel syndrome, and because the corrective procedure is relatively straightforward, timely repair is generally indicated. Regardless of age, incidental rotational abnormalities discovered at laparotomy should be evaluated and corrected, if necessary, when encountered, because in this circumstance, it is generally straightforward and adds no additional morbidity.

One additional dilemma is the circumstance of midgut rotational abnormalities associated with congenital heart disease in the heterotaxia syndromes.[29] In this circumstance, careful observation of the asymptomatic patient and deferral of the Ladd's procedure until the cardiac physiology is surgically stabilized appear to be appropriate.

It has been suggested that laparoscopic evaluation of the midgut mesentery and performance of a laparoscopic Ladd's procedure, if necessary, may be an alternative approach.[30, 31] Although this is described, it has not achieved widespread use and it does not offer the unrestricted visualization of the mesentery, which is so valuable.

Our general approach to an older, asymptomatic patient with malrotation is to perform a prompt, elective open abdominal exploration and Ladd's procedure when the diagnosis of malrotation is established.

□ Operative Technique

Operative repair of malrotation is achieved nearly universally using the procedure described by William E. Ladd and which bears his name.[3] Entry into the abdomen can be done via a variety of incisions, but in the infant, the authors prefer a transverse supraumbilical incision with generous exposure of the right upper quadrant. Key elements of the procedure are illustrated in Figure 31–7 and are summarized in the following paragraphs.

Following abdominal entry and rapid exploration, complete evisceration of the intestine and the mesentery is essential in order to visualize and assess the anatomic abnormality. Although it is not of physiologic importance, one often encounters some chylous ascites, apparently related to the rupture of lacteals in the twisted mesentery. This material resembles the turbid fluid encountered with intestinal infarction but it is sterile.

If present, midgut volvulus is relieved by rotating the affected small intestine opposite the direction of torsion, generally in a counterclockwise direction. The degree of torsion is variable but may involve one or more complete twists of the mesentery requiring reduction (Fig. 31–8A). Preferably, the bowel remains viable with reduction, although it is often dusky initially. A period of intraoperative warming and observation is often necessary. Assuming that the midgut is indeed viable, one proceeds as follows; if not, the infarcted intestine is resected. The principles involved in intestinal salvage include resection of the nonviable bowel, preservation of marginal tissue to preserve length, possible exteriorization, and reexploration if either the scope of the resection is excessive or the viability of the bowel cannot be adequately assessed. One of the more difficult situations is illustrated in Figure 31–

8B, in which the entire midgut is infarcted. In this situation, closure without resection and terminal care may be an appropriate approach after discussion with the family.

Having been assured of the viability of the retained bowel, recurrence of the volvulus is prevented by broadening the base of the mesenteric vascular pedicle by dividing the peritoneal bands that tether the cecum, small bowel mesentery, mesocolon, and duodenum around the base of the SMA (see Fig. 31–7C, D). Properly done, the mesenteric leaves and mesocolon open widely. With regard to the SMA pedicle, it is important to carry the dissection and division of the bands down to the SMA and SMV themselves. Much of the mesenteric broadening results in the final portion of this dissection; therefore, this should be done completely, proceeding down to the pancreas and the vessels. Clearly, injury to these structures must be meticulously avoided. Properly opened, the mesenteric pedicle is at low risk for recurrent volvulus. Postoperatively, small bowel obstruction is reported in 10% of patients or fewer, generally as a result of simple adhesion formation.[32, 33]

Concurrent with the process of broadening the SMA mesentery, Ladd's peritoneal bands must be divided to relieve any extrinsic obstruction of the duodenum. This is accomplished by meticulous and complete mobilization of the entire duodenum with division of all anterior, lateral, and posterior attachments, essentially an extensive and compulsive

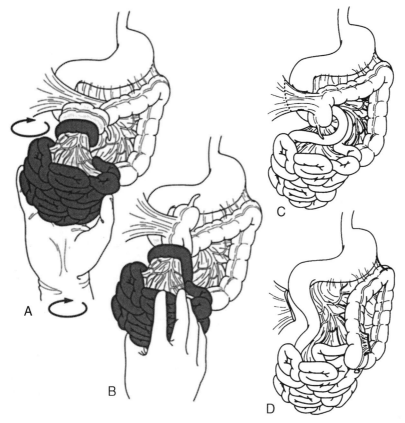

Figure 31–7. Operative correction of malrotation is illustrated. Counterclockwise detorsion is shown in *(A)* and *(B)*. The division of Ladd's cecal bands and broadening the superior mesenteric artery mesentery is shown in *(C)* and *(D)*. Note the final cecal position on the left and the incidental appendectomy. (Adapted from Oldham KT: Pediatric abdomen. In Greenfield LJ, Mulholland M, Oldham KT, et al [eds]: Surgery: Scientific Principles and Practice. Philadelphia, Lippincott-Raven, 1997. Illustrations by Holly R. Fischer.)

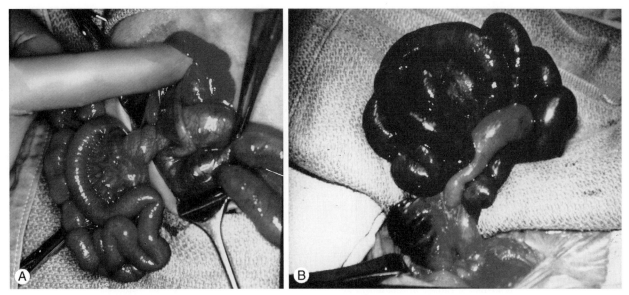

Figure 31–8. Operative photographs in two infants with malrotation and midgut volvulus. *A*, The midgut here is clearly viable although the uncorrected superior mesenteric artery vascular pedicle is less than a fingerbreadth. A Ladd's procedure as shown in Figure 31–7 is definitive therapy. *B*, The midgut here is clearly infarcted and presents a much more difficult set of decisions *(see text)*.

Kocher maneuver. Although the bands may appear relatively innocuous, compression and kinking of the neonatal duodenum may remain if they are not completely divided. The additional need to demonstrate complete duodenal lumenal patency has been discussed previously. This can be done operatively by injecting air or saline and demonstrating adequate distal progression or by passage of a catheter via a transgastric route through the entire duodenum. The latter maneuver is relatively simple owing to the mobility and position of the duodenum at this stage in the operation.

Appendectomy is considered standard because the malposition of the cecum and the attached appendix can make acute appendicitis a difficult diagnosis to make if it were to develop in the future. Because the appendix is typically normal at the time of a Ladd's procedure, the appendectomy can be done using an inversion technique to avoid entry into the GI tract.

At the conclusion of the procedure, the intestine is replaced into the abdomen without mesenteric torsion, generally, the small intestine on the right, the cecum and colon on the left. Efforts to surgically secure the mesentery by cecal or duodenal attachment to the posterior body wall have been abandoned for lack of supportive data.[32, 33]

Mesocolic hernias appear more complex, largely because they are more rare and thus unfamiliar. A right mesocolic hernia is corrected simply by dividing the lateral peritoneal attachments of the cecum and right colon to the posterior body wall, thus eliminating this potential retrocolic space. This allows the small bowel to reside in the right abdomen and the cecum and colon to occupy the left. In addition, the SMA pedicle should be broadened as much as possible using the aforementioned tech-

niques. Left mesocolic hernias are more involved technically; the elements of the procedure are to mobilize the inferior mesenteric vein, reduce the small bowel from the hernia sac, and close the neck of the mesocolic sac to eliminate the potential space. Again, the small bowel comes to reside on the right and the colon on the left when this is done. This group of anomalies is more variable and treatment must necessarily be individualized. An alternative is simply to enlarge the mesocolic space by mobilizing the left colon and opening the neck of the sac sufficiently so that no opportunity is afforded for strangulation. The final position of the intestine has no physiologic relevance; only the opportunity for entrapment, obstruction, or volvulus is important.

□ Outcomes

In Ladd's 1941 clinical summary, 8 of 35 patients with malrotation who underwent surgery died.[3] All of the surviving 27 were relieved of symptoms and there was no recurrence of the obstruction or vovulus. Contemporary results after surgical correction of malrotation are generally excellent with normal life expectancy in the absence of compromised bowel at the time of the initial procedure.[5, 13, 26] Currently, the mortality rate for the operative correction of malrotation ranges from 3 to 9% overall.[9] It is increased in patients with intestinal necrosis, prematurity, or other abnormalities.[33] Malrotation with midgut volvulus accounted for 18% of all children with shortgut syndrome in the pediatric population in one report.[34] The incidence of adhesive small bowel obstruction after surgical correction is generally between 1 and 10%.[9] Recurrent volvulus and recurrent duodenal obstruction are rare if the initial procedure is technically complete.[10]

REFERENCES

1. Mall FP: Development of the human intestine and its position in the adult. Johns Hopkins Hosp Bull 9:197–208, 1898.
2. Dott NM: Anomalies of intestinal rotation: Their embryology and surgical aspects, with report of five cases. Br J Surg 11:251, 1923.
3. Ladd WE, Gross RE: Intestinal obstruction resulting from malrotation of the intestines and colon. In Abdominal Surgery of Infancy and Childhood. Philadelphia, WB Saunders, 1941, pp 53–70.
4. Skandalakis JE, Gray SW: The small intestine. In Skandalakis JE, Gray SW (eds): Embryology for Surgeons. Philadelphia, WB Saunders, 1972, pp 129–186.
5. Firor H, Steiger E: Morbidity of rotational abnormalities of the gut beyond infancy. Cleve Clinic Q 50:303–309, 1983.
6. Kantor JL: Anomalies of the colon: Their roentgen diagnosis and clinical significance. Resume of ten years study. Radiology 23:651–662, 1934.
7. Wang C, Welch CE: Anomalies of intestinal rotation in adolescents and adults. Surgery 54:839–855, 1963.
8. Willwerth BM, Zollinger RM, Izant RJ: Congenital mesocolic (paraduodenal) hernia—embryologic basis of repair. Am J Surg 128:358–361, 1974.
9. Warner BW: Malrotation. In Oldham KT, Colombani PM, Foglia RP (eds): Surgery of Infants and Children: Scientific Principles and Practice. Philadelphia, Lippincott-Raven, 1997, pp 1229–1240.
10. Smith IE: Malrotation of the intestine. In Welch KJ, Randolph JG, Ravich MR, et al (eds): Pediatric Surgery (4th ed). Chicago, Year Book Medical, 1986, p 882.
11. Spigland N, Brandt ML, Yazbeck S: Malrotation presenting beyond the neonatal period. J Pediatr Surg 25:1139–1142, 1990.
12. Powell D, Othersen HB, Smith CD: Malrotation of the intestines in children: The effect of age on presentation and therapy. J Pediatr Surg 24:777–780, 1989.
13. Stewart DR, Colodny AL, Daggett WC: Malrotation of the bowel in infants and children: A 15 year review. Surgery 79:716–720, 1976.
14. Filston HC, Kirks DR. Malrotation—the ubiquitous anomaly. J Pediatr Surg 16:614–620, 1981.
15. Yanez R, Spitz L: Intestinal malrotation presenting outside the neonatal period. Arch Dis Child 61:682–685, 1986.
16. Burton EM, Strange ME, Pitts RM: Malrotation in twins: A rare occurrence. Pediatr Radiol 23:603–604, 1993.
17. Smith SL: Familial midgut volvulus. Surgery 72:420, 1972.
18. Estrada RL: Anomalies of Intestinal Rotation and Fixation. Springfield, IL, Charles C. Thomas, 1958.
19. Byrne WJ: Disorders of the intestines and pancreas. In Taeusch WH, Ballard RA, Avery ME (eds): Disease of the Newborn. Philadelphia, WB Saunders, 1991, p 685.
20. Schey WL, Donaldson JS, Sty JR: Malrotation of bowel: Variable patterns with different surgical considerations. J Pediatr Surg 28:96–101, 1993.
21. Gross RE: Malrotation of the intestine and colon. In The Surgery of Infancy and Childhood. Philadelphia, WB Saunders, 1953, p 192.
22. Oldham KT: Malrotation. In Greenfield LJ, Mulholland M, Oldham KT, et al (eds): Surgery: Scientific Principles and Practice, (2nd ed). Philadelphia, Lippincott-Raven, 1997, pp 2053–2057.
23. Kirks DR, Caron KH: Gastrointestinal tract. In Kirks DR (ed): Practical Pediatric Imaging (2nd ed). Philadelphia, JB Lippincott, 1991, p 710.
24. Slovis TL, Klein MD, Watts FB: Incomplete rotation of the intestine with a normal cecal position. Surgery 87:325–330, 1980.
25. Weinberger E, Winters WD, Liddell RM, et al: Sonographic diagnosis of intestinal malrotation in infants—importance of the relative positions of the superior mesenteric vein and artery. Am J Radiol 159:825–828, 1992.
26. Seashore JH, Touloukian RJ. Midgut volvulus. Arch Pediatr Adolesc Med 148:43–46, 1994.
27. Reyes J, et al: Intestinal transplantation in children [abstract]. Presented at the American Pediatric Surgical Association Annual Meeting, Naples, FL, May 1997.
28. Yanez R, Spitz L: Intestinal malrotation presenting outside the neonatal period. Arch Dis Child 61:682–685, 1986.
29. Chang J, Brueckner M, Touloukian RJ: Intestinal rotation and fixation abnormalities in heterotoxia: Early detection and management. J Pediatr Surg 28:1281–1285, 1993.
30. Gross E, Chen MK, Lobe TE: Laparoscopic evaluation and treatment of intestinal malrotation in infants. Surg Endosc 10:936–937, 1996.
31. Frantzides CT, Cziperle DJ, Spergel K, et al: Laparoscopic Ladd procedure and cecopexy in the treatment of malrotation beyond the neonatal period. Surg Laparosc Endosc 6:73–75, 1996.
32. Stauffer UG, Herman P: Comparison of late results in patients with corrected intestinal malrotation with and without fixation of the mesentery. J Pediatr Surg 15:9–12, 1980.
33. Rescorla FJ, Shedd FJ, Grosfeld JL, et al: Anomalies of intestinal rotation in childhood: Analysis of 447 cases. Surgery 108:710, 1990.
34. Warner BW, Ziegler MM: Management of the short bowel syndrome in the pediatric population. Pediatr Clin North Am 40:1335–1350, 1993.

32

MECONIUM DISEASE

Diller B. Groff, MD

The genetically determined disease cystic fibrosis (CF) is the predominant cause of meconium disease in infants.[1, 2] However, there is a spectrum of clinical conditions that share characteristics of meconium disease in CF, including meconium ileus without CF, meconium obstruction in the premature infant, and meconium plug syndrome. Hirschsprung's disease and small left colon syndrome are also associated with abnormalities of meconium.[7, 8] In newborns, meconium peritonitis is caused by the spillage of meconium into the peritoneum in the preterm or perinatal period; it may or may not be associated with CF.[9] Meconium ileus equivalent and distal intestinal obstruction syndrome are seen beyond the newborn period in patients with CF.[10] Although the meconium diseases are interrelated, they are discussed as separate entities in this chapter.

☐ Meconium Ileus History

The association between newborn bowel obstruction and pathologic changes in the pancreas was published by Landsteiner in 1905.[11] The first successful surgical treatment of meconium ileus was reported in 1948 by Hiatt and Wilson who reported survival in five of eight patients using saline irrigations of the inspissated meconium through an ileostomy.[12] In the 1950s, three successful surgical procedures were developed and reported; all of which involved resection of the dilated ileum in which the inspissated meconium was stuck. Gross used the Mikulicz (double-barrel) ileostomy with anastomosis created by a clamp crushing the common wall.[13] When the child had recovered bowel function, the stoma was closed extraperitoneally. Bishop and Koop performed an anastomosis between the proximal end of the ileum to the side of the distal ileum using the ileostomy for postoperative irrigations.[14] The stoma was closed extraperitoneally after return of bowel function allowed the child to be fed. Santulli and Blanc anastomosed the end of the distal ileum to the side of the proximal ileum so that the irrigations could be more effective proximally.[15]

Most uncomplicated meconium ileus that requires surgical intervention is currently treated without constructing an ileostomy.[16–18] Successful nonoperative treatment of uncomplicated meconium ileus using enemas with hyperosmotic contrast solutions was described by Noblett in 1969.[19] These specific treatment methods and improvements in neonatal support have increased overall 5-year survival rates from only 30% in the 1960s to near 100% in the late 1990s.[20]

☐ Incidence

Meconium ileus in the newborn is the earliest manifestation of CF and occurs in approximately 15% of CF patients. The CF gene is autosomal recessive, requiring that both parents of an affected child must be carriers. It is estimated that 3.3% of the Caucasian population in the United States are asymptomatic carriers of the CF gene.[21] There is a one in four chance that children of two carriers will have the disease. In families in which the first child with CF was born with meconium ileus, 29% of subsequent children with CF had meconium ileus. In families in which the first child with CF did not have meconium ileus, only 6% of siblings with CF would be expected to have this complication.[22]

Approximately 1200 infants with CF are born each year in the United States, an incidence of 1 in 3000 live births. Therefore, approximately 180 newborns with meconium ileus are born each year. The disease is much more rare in non-Caucasian populations: 1 in 14,000 live African American births, 1 in 25,000 live Asian births, 1 in 10,500 live Native American Aleut (Eskimo) births, and 1 in 11,500 Hispanic births.[21] However, it has been reported that meconium ileus without CF is not a rarity in Asian populations.[23]

☐ Pathogenesis

The genetic investigation of CF continues at an expanding pace since the discovery of the CF gene

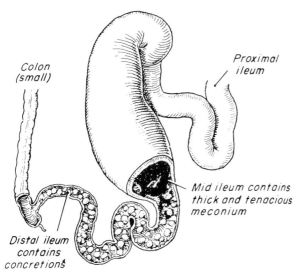

Figure 32–1. Drawing of meconium ileus. Artist depiction of obstructing pathology in meconium ileus. (From Lloyd DA: Meconium ileus. In Welch KJ, et al [eds]: Pediatric Surgery. Chicago, Mosby–Year Book, 1986, p 850.)

on chromosome 7 in 1985.[24] The most common CF marker is the mutation Δ F508, which is a deletion of phenylalanine in the DNA related to chromosome 7. The principal protein gene product in CF has been designated as the cystic fibrosis transmembrane conductance regulator (CFTCR). CFTCR is thought to be a chloride channel regulator, which is a critical component in the membrane defect in CF, but additional factors are necessary to produce meconium ileus.[25] Clinical and laboratory studies suggest that missense at codon 551 is, in combination with Δ F508, associated with a decreased incidence of meconium ileus, but clinical use of genetic information in diagnosis or screening is not currently practical.[24, 26–28]

Meconium ileus is a presentation of CF that results from abnormalities of exocrine mucous secretion, which produces thick intestinal mucus along with the viscid mucus and results in obstruction of the air passages and the pancreatic ducts. The meconium that produces obstruction in meconium ileus differs from other meconium in that it has less water content (meconium ileus, 65%; normal, 75%), lower sucrase and lactase levels, increased albumin, and decreased pancreatic enzymes.[25, 29] The thick and viscous mucous secretion is the principal contributor to the thick, sticky meconium that obstructs the intestine in meconium ileus.[26] The clinical presentation of meconium ileus results from obstruction of the distended meconium-filled small bowel, which narrows to an unused distal ileum impacted with inspissated pellets of colorless mucus (Figs. 32–1 and 32–2). The unused colon is small, containing only pellets of inspissated mucus. It is often referred to as a *microcolon*, a misnomer because it immediately distends when presented with intestinal content. Complications of prenatal perforation occur in approximately 50% of patients as a result of volvulus or distention and may result in bowel atresia, meconium peritonitis, or meconium pseudocyst (giant cystic meconium peritonitis).[1]

☐ Diagnosis

Fetal ultrasonography (US) cannot be considered to be diagnostic of meconium ileus. Echogenic bowel, often seen in the second trimester of pregnancy, does not correlate with findings in the newborn.[30]

In the newborn with uncomplicated meconium ileus, distention and bilious vomiting occur in the first 24 to 48 hours of life. There is no passage of meconium per rectum. A "doughy" mass may be seen or palpated in the abdomen (Fig. 32–3). Erythema and edema of the abdominal wall suggest the patient has complicated meconium ileus.

Roentgenographic studies are essential to estab-

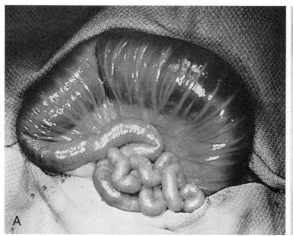
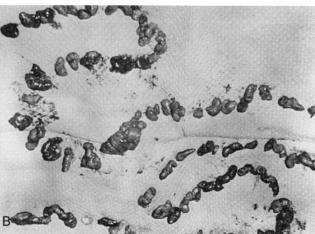

Figure 32–2. *A,* Terminal ileum with meconium ileus showing meconium-filled loop leading to inspissated pellets of meconium in terminal ileum. *B,* Pellets of inspissated meconium removed by irrigation through ileostomy at time of abdominal exploration.

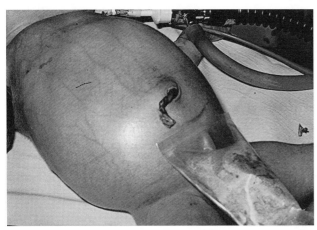

Figure 32–3. Newborn with meconium ileus not relieved by enemas. Note distention, increased vascular pattern, and suggestion of intraabdominal masses.

lish the diagnosis of meconium ileus and to differentiate it from the common conditions with similar clinical presentations: Hirschsprung's disease, small left colon syndrome, meconium plug syndrome, small bowel atresia, and functional immaturity of the intestine.[31] There is no single characteristic or set of characteristics that is radiographically pathognomonic of meconium ileus. However, meconium ileus has more variation in the bowel loop caliber, fewer air-fluid levels, more meconium mottling (ground glass appearance), and less rectal gas than neonatal Hirschsprung's or meconium plug syndrome.[32] The mixture of abnormal meconium and air bubbles is described as having a ground glass appearance, but it is not specific for meconium ileus (Fig. 32–4). Air-fluid levels typical of any intes-

tinal obstruction may be seen in meconium ileus, and perforation with meconium peritonitis or pseudocyst formation may show flecks of calcium. A significant percentage of studies in uncomplicated meconium ileus show no radiographic abnormalities.[33]

The most helpful diagnostic study is a contrast colon enema, which may also be therapeutic. A water-soluble contrast agent should be used in case the bowel is perforated in the procedure. A recent survey showed only a slightly higher therapeutic success rate using hyperosmolar solutions and wetting agents.[34] In meconium ileus, a small unused colon is seen (Fig. 32–5), whereas in neonatal Hirschsprung's disease, the colon tends to be larger in caliber and a transition zone may be present. In meconium plug syndrome, the proximal colon is usually filled with meconium, the rectum is larger, and the diagnostic enema often results in immediate passage of the meconium plug with resolution of the obstruction.

The only reliable and definitive test for CF is a pilocarpine iontophoresis sweat test.[35] Concentrations of sodium and chloride greater than 60 mEq/l are diagnostic if at least 100 mg of sweat have been collected. The newborn does not respond to pilocarpine sufficiently to produce enough sweat, so a definitive diagnosis of CF must be established later. A presumptive diagnosis of CF may be made by the parental history, clinical presentation, and roentgenographic studies. A family history of CF is present

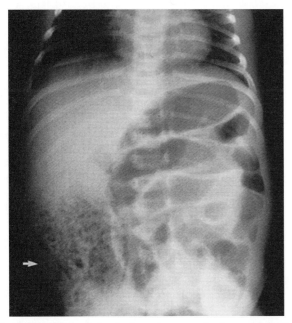

Figure 32–4. Plain abdominal roentgenograph of meconium ileus with distended loops of bowel and a mass of meconium *(arrow)* with "ground glass" appearance from mixed air and stool.

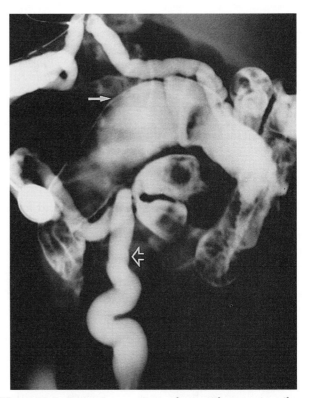

Figure 32–5. Contrast enema in newborn with meconium ileus. Note unused colon *(open arrow)* and reflux of contrast solution into dilated meconium-filled ileum *(closed arrow).*

in 10 to 30% of patients. Polyhydramnios occurs 10 to 20% of the time. The newborn is often small for gestational age, but prematurity is unusual.

□ Treatment

If meconium ileus is the diagnosis and it does not appear to be complicated by meconium peritonitis, bowel perforation, pseudocyst, or atresia, then treatment with enemas as described by Noblett to loosen the meconium is recommended.[19] Although it was thought that the use of hyperosmolar contrast solutions such as Gastrografin was necessary for success, many pediatric radiologists believe it is the hydrostatic effect that is critical in the treatment.[34] If hypertonic solutions are used, the patient must be kept well hydrated to compensate for fluid drawn into the bowel lumen. An experienced radiologist should perform this study using hand injection of the fluid with fluoroscopic control. The goal is to reflux the enema into the terminal ileum and the distal small bowel where the abnormal meconium is causing obstruction (see Fig. 32–5). If this is accomplished, the baby usually begins to pass the meconium immediately.

Performance of repeat contrast enemas or saline enemas with 1% acetylcysteine in the neonatal unit using 10- to 15-ml volumes may be necessary. Between 60 and 75% of uncomplicated meconium ileus can be relieved with this enema technique. A bowel perforation rate of 2.7% was reported in one review.[34] Because it appears that there is a higher rate of perforation when a balloon-tipped catheter is used in the rectum, only plain-tipped catheters should be inserted. If enemas are not successful, an operation is required to remove the abnormal meconium and relieve the obstruction. Simple, uncomplicated meconium ileus occurs in approximately 42% of patients with meconium ileus.[36] If only 60 to 75% are cured with enema, then operative treatment is frequently required.

□ Operative Treatment

Historically, resecting the dilated ileum and forming an ileostomy allowed recovery of neonates who otherwise would have died of the disease. With the advent of total parenteral nutrition, the addition of ventilator support, and the use of N-acetylcysteine, the performance of one or more enterotomies can enable the surgeon to relieve simple meconium ileus without the need for a stoma.[2, 16–18, 37] This is accomplished by open laparotomy, confirming the diagnosis of simple meconium ileus, then making a pursestring enterotomy in the dilated meconium-filled bowel just proximal to the inspissated meconium in the ileum (see Fig. 32–2). A 12F or 14F Foley balloon catheter or a 7F Fogerty irrigating catheter is passed into the ileum and 1 to 4% N-acetylcysteine is carefully injected proximally and distally. After a few minutes, the sticky meconium and the mucous pellets can be moved into the colon. Care is taken to avoid peritoneal contamination. Some N-acetylcysteine is left in the bowel and the enterostomy is closed. If the meconium does not yield completely to this maneuver, insertion of a T tube into the enterostomy with one arm of the tube in the proximal ileum and one in the distal ileum is a useful procedure.[18] The T tube is brought out through the abdominal wall and used to irrigate the bowel, obviating the need for an ileostomy. Total parenteral nutrition enables the child to be nourished while waiting for full recovery of bowel function.

The child should be managed as if he or she has CF, using enzymes and pulmonary toilet as directed by the physicians who will assume the child's care after recovery from operation. Clarification of the diagnosis of CF is important because simple meconium ileus can occur in otherwise normal children.[33, 38, 39] Meconium ileus has also been reported in total colon Hirschsprung's disease.[7, 39]

□ Complicated Meconium Ileus and Meconium Peritonitis

Meconium contamination of the peritoneum in utero or in the immediate perinatal period causes severe peritonitis, usually with calcification. The probable cause of meconium soilage of the peritoneum is in utero perforation of the obstructed bowel as a result of meconium ileus. However, intestinal stenosis, atresia, volvulus, internal hernia, congenital peritoneal bands, ruptured Meckel's diverticulum or appendix, and other factors may also lead to perforation and meconium peritonitis.[40] If CF is associated with the meconium peritonitis, it is termed *complicated meconium ileus.*

The presentation of meconium peritonitis in the newborn has been classified into four types[40]:
1. A *meconium pseudocyst* is formed by meconium leakage over an extended time period, resulting in a calcified pseudocapsule and calcified contents (Fig. 32–6).
2. *Adhesive meconium peritonitis* with dense fibrous adhesions of the bowel results from widespread intraperitoneal contamination; it is often associated with obstruction. Some of these newborns do not have obstruction, and evidence of meconium peritonitis may be found incidentally as intraabdominal or scrotal calcifications (Fig. 32–7).
3. *Meconium ascites* is a result of perforation near term or immediately after birth. There may be scant intraabdominal calcification.
4. *Infected meconium peritonitis* is a result of bacterial contamination of meconium after delivery.

The earliest possible diagnosis of meconium peritonitis or pseudocyst is by fetal US; however, only 22% of cases diagnosed in utero require postnatal

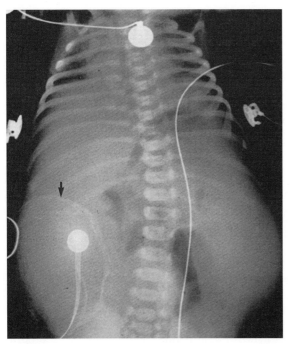

Figure 32–6. Abdominal roentgenograph in meconium peritonitis with giant pseudocyst demonstrating calcification *(arrow)* in cyst wall.

surgery.[41] The incidence of CF in prenatally diagnosed meconium peritonitis (representing complicated meconium ileus) is only about 8%.[42] Because the US diagnosis of meconium peritonitis depends on calcification, the low incidence of CF may be due to the paucity of pancreatic enzymes in the CF

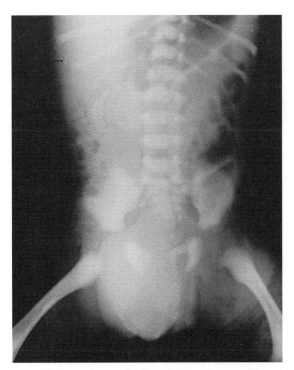

Figure 32–7. Roentgenograph of newborn with normal bowel but large scrotal calcification from meconium peritonitis.

fetus or the failure of the sticky meconium to leak out of a bowel perforation.[41, 42] When a fetus in the womb has intraabdominal calcification, the surgeon must be circumspect in predicting the need for postnatal surgery or of the possibility of CF.

The clinical presentation of the newborn with complicated meconium ileus or meconium peritonitis includes abdominal distention; a palpable mass; an erythematous, edematous abdominal wall; and occasional respiratory compromise from abdominal distention. Third space fluid losses may be severe. Surgical options include resection of the cyst and devitalized bowel with primary anastomosis or establishment of a diverting ostomy. Bowel is resected conservatively, observing the principles of bowel conservation to avoid short bowel syndrome. Simple drainage, bowel rest, total parenteral nutrition, and administration of antibiotics followed by definitive surgery in 2 to 3 weeks has been successful.[43] The outcome should be favorable in almost all infants.[44]

☐ Meconium Plug Syndrome

Meconium plug syndrome, first described in 1956,[45] is a frequent cause of neonatal intestinal obstruction. In a radiologic analysis of 133 neonates with bowel obstruction, 66% had meconium plug syndrome, 20% had meconium ileus, and 18% had Hirschsprung's disease.[33] Meconium plug syndrome is associated with maternal eclampsia, diabetes, magnesium sulfate or other tocolytic agents, prematurity, sepsis, immature neuronal function of the bowel, hypothyroidism, and other metabolic conditions, all of which produce dysmotility of the neonatal bowel.[46] Most newborns with meconium plug syndrome are ultimately found to be healthy. Approximately 14% of children with meconium plug syndrome are found to have CF, small left colon syndrome, or Hirschsprung's disease.[47–49]

The colon dysmotility allows the meconium in the left colon and rectum to become firm so that a plug is formed that cannot be passed. Characteristically, the newborn passes only some small inspissated meconium or none at all. The abdomen becomes distended. Vomiting is a late occurrence. Radiographic differentiation of meconium plug, meconium ileus, and especially Hirschsprung's disease may be difficult.

On plain abdominal roentgenogram, a patient with the meconium plug syndrome tends to have dilated bowel loops with few air-fluid levels, little bowel wall edema, and more colon and rectal gas than a patient with Hirschsprung's disease.[34] The meconium plug may be dislodged and pass after stimulation of the anus and rectum with physical examination. Passage of normal amounts of meconium often follows immediately. Despite such relief, all patients with meconium plug syndrome should have a contrast enema. Most patients with this syndrome do not pass the plug without such treatment.

The enema is performed using the same technique as in the diagnosis of meconium ileus. The enema is usually followed by passage of the plug and large amounts of meconium with relief of the obstruction (Fig. 32–8). Small saline enemas can help complete the evacuation of the meconium.

After roentgenographic diagnosis, all patients with meconium plug syndrome should have a sweat test performed at an appropriate age to rule out CF. Some surgeons recommend rectal biopsy to eliminate Hirschsprung's disease in all meconium plug newborns; others closely follow up the patient to verify that a normal stooling pattern develops and is maintained.[18, 49] Hypothyroidism should be discovered on neonatal screening. Investigation as indicated by the child's clinical course may reveal other rare associations with meconium plug syndrome.[46]

□ Meconium Ileus in Low Birth Weight Newborns

There is a meconium ileus condition reported in very low birth weight newborns (700 to 900 g) but which also occurs in babies weighing up to 1500 g.[5, 50] These premature babies have few stools in the first weeks of life or do not produce stool at all. Abdominal distention develops, leading occasionally to bowel necrosis or perforation. The risk factors include intrauterine growth retardation, maternal hypertension or eclampsia (often treated with magnesium sulfate and tocolytics), patent ductus arteriosus, hyaline membrane disease, and intraventricular hemorrhage. Immaturity of the myenteric plexus in these small newborns may also contribute to this condition.[31]

The treatment of choice in the uncomplicated patient is with fluoroscopically controlled Gastrografin enemas as in the treatment of larger infants with meconium ileus.[50] These should be performed as soon as the condition is suspected to avoid perforation and bowel necrosis. Operative manipulation to relieve these obstructions has resulted in a high rate of iatrogenic injury to the fragile bowel when trying to remove obstructing meconium.[5] This condition is self-limited and, if managed by early Gastrografin enemas, the survival rate approaches 100%.[50]

□ Meconium Ileus Equivalent

Meconium ileus equivalent, first described in 1941, is a partial or complete obstruction of the distal small bowel or colon occurring beyond the newborn period in patients with CF.[51] This condition is often referred to as *distal intestinal obstruction syndrome* and includes mild to severe colicky pain, constipation, generalized abdominal distention with pain, air-fluid levels on plain abdominal roentgenogram, and intussusception of the colon or small bowel with or without an abdominal mass.

The incidence of meconium ileus equivalent in CF is low (estimated to be 5.4 episodes per 1000 patient-years) and is almost exclusively found in older CF patients, although milder symptoms have been reported in younger children.[10, 52] The cause is probably low oral pancreatic enzyme dosage associated with a decrease in fluid intake. Strictures of the colon and small bowel requiring resection have

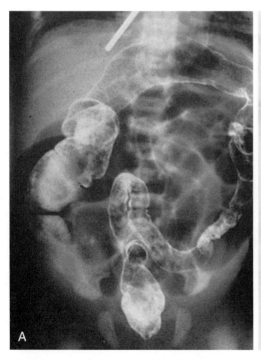
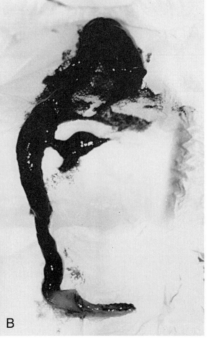

Figure 32–8. *A,* Colon study in meconium plug syndrome. Note large rectum and meconium in colon. *B,* Meconium plug passed after enema. Pale, putty-like plug was obstructing column of black normal meconium.

been associated with use of high-strength pancreatic enzyme capsules.[53] Increasing oral pancreatic enzymes or fluids is usually curative. Colonic masses of inspissated bowel contents and the associated intussusceptions can be treated with Gastrografin enemas. Operative treatment, except in cases of strictures, is rarely needed.

REFERENCES

1. Ziegler MM: Meconium ileus. Curr Probl Surg 31:731–777, 1994.
2. Docherty JG, Zaki A, Coutts JAP, et al: Meconium ileus: A review 1972–1990. Br J Surg 79:571–573, 1992.
3. Dolan TF, Touloukian RJ: Familial meconium ileus not associated with cystic fibrosis. J Pediatr Surg 9:821–824, 1974.
4. Rickham PP, Boeckman CR: Neonatal meconium obstruction in the absence of mucoviscidosis. Am J Surg 109:173–177, 1965.
5. Greenholz SK, Perez C, Wesley JR, et al: Meconium obstruction in the markedly premature infant. J Pediatr Surg 31:117–120, 1996.
6. Vinograd I, Mogle P, Pelez O, et al: Meconium disease in premature infants with very low weight. J Pediatr 103:963–966, 1983.
7. Stringer RJ, Brereton DP, Drake EM, et al: Meconium ileus due to extensive intestinal aganglionosis. J Pediatr Surg 29:501–503, 1994.
8. Stewart DR, Nixon GW, Johnson DG, et al: Neonatal small left colon syndrome. Ann Surg 186:741–745, 1977.
9. Dirkes K, Crombleholme TM, Craigo SD, et al: The natural history of meconium peritonitis diagnosed in utero. J Pediatr Surg 30:979–982, 1995.
10. Millar-Jones L, Goodchild MC: Cystic fibrosis pancreatic insufficiency and distal intestinal obstruction syndrome: A report of four cases. Acta Paediatr 84:577–578, 1995.
11. Landsteiner K: Darmverschluss durch eingeductes meconium pankreatitis. Zentralbl Allg Pathol 16:903–907, 1905.
12. Hiatt RB, Wilson PE: Celiac syndrome: Therapy of meconium ileus. Report of 8 cases with review of the literature. Surg Gynecol Obstet 87:317–327, 1948.
13. Gross RE: Intestinal obstruction in the newborn resulting from meconium ileus. In The Surgery of Infancy and Childhood: Its Principles and Techniques. Philadelphia, WB Saunders, 1953, pp 175–191.
14. Bishop HC, Koop CE: Management of meconium ileus: Resection, Roux-en-Y anastomosis and ileostomy irrigation with pancreatic enzymes. Ann Surg 145:410–414, 1957.
15. Santulli TV, Blanc WA: Congenital atresia of the intestine: Pathogenesis and treatment. Ann Surg 154:939–948, 1961.
16. Venngopal S, Shandling B: Meconium ileus: Laparotomy without resection, anastomosis or enterostomy. J Pediatr Surg 14:115–118, 1979.
17. Nguyen LT, Youssef FM, Guttman FM, et al: Meconium ileus: Is a stoma necessary? J Pediatr Surg 21:766–768, 1986.
18. Andrassy RJ, Nirgiotis JG: Meconium ileus, meconium plug syndrome, and meconium peritonitis. In Ashcraft KW, Holder TM (eds): Pediatric Surgery, 2nd ed. Philadelphia, WB Saunders, 1993, pp 331–340.
19. Noblett HR: Treatment of uncomplicated meconium ileus by Gastrografin enema: A preliminary report. J Pediatr Surg 4:190–197, 1969.
20. Del Pin CA, Czyrko C, Ziegler MM, et al: Management and survival of meconium ileus. Ann Surg 215:179–185, 1992.
21. Fitzsimmons SC: The changing epidemiology of cystic fibrosis. J Pediatr 122:1–9, 1993.
22. Allan DL, Robbie M, Phelan PD, et al: Familial occurrence of meconium ileus. Eur J Pediatr 135:291–292, 1981.
23. Ng WT, Wong MK, Kong CK, et al: Meconium ileus: A review 1972–1990 [letter]. Br J Surg 80:129, 1993.
24. Beandt AL: Genetic testing for cystic fibrosis. Pediatr Clin North Am 39:213–228, 1992.
25. Eggermont E, DeBoeck K: Small intestinal abnormalities in cystic fibrosis patients. Eur J Pediatr 150:824–828, 1991.
26. Eggermont E: Gastrointestinal manifestations in cystic fibrosis. Eur J Gastroenterol Hepatol 8:731–738. 1996.
27. Hamosh A, King T, Rosenstein BJ: Cystic fibrosis patients bearing both the common missense mutations GLY → ASP at Codon 551 and the Δ F508 mutation are clinically indistinguishable from Δ F508 homozygotes except for the decreased risk of meconium ileus. Am J Hum Genet 5l:245–250, 1992.
28. Delaney SJ, Alton EWFW, Smith SN: Cystic fibrosis mice carrying the missense mutation G551 replicates human genotype-phenotype cancellations. EMBO J 156:955–963, 1996.
29. Schwachman H, Antionowicz I: Studies on meconium. In Lebenthal E (ed): Gastroenterology and Nutrition in Infancy. New York, Raven Press, 1981, pp 83–93.
30. Sipes SL, Weiner CP, Wenstrom KD: Fetal echogenic bowel on ultrasound: Is there clinical significance? Fetal Diagn Ther 9:38–43, 1994.
31. Bisset WM: The development of motor control systems in the gastrointestinal tract of the preterm infant. In Milla PJ (ed): Disorders of Gastrointestinal Motility in Childhood. Chichester, England, John Wiley & Sons, 1988, pp 17–27.
32. Hussain SM, Meradji M, Robbin SGF, et al: Plain film diagnosis in meconium plug syndrome, meconium ileus and neonatal Hirschsprung's disease. Pediatr Radiol 21:556–559, 1991.
33. Leonidas JC, Berdon WE, Baker DH, et al: Meconium ileus and its complications: A reappraisal of plain film roentgen diagnostic criteria. Am J Roentgenol 108:598–609, 1970.
34. Kao SCS, Franken EA Jr: Nonoperative treatment of simple meconium ileus: A survey of the Society for Pediatric Radiology. Pediatr Radiol 25:97–100, 1995.
35. Gibson LE, Cooke RE: A test for concentration of electrolytes in sweat in cystic fibrosis of the pancreas utilizing pilocarpine by iontophoresis. Pediatrics 23:545–549, 1959.
36. Gross K, Desanto A, Grosfeld JL, et al: Intra-abdominal complications of cystic fibrosis. J Pediatr Surg 20:431–435, 1985.
37. Caniano DA, Beaver BL: Meconium ileus: A fifteen year experience with forty-two neonates. Surgery 102:699–702, 1987.
38. Fakhoury K, Durie PR, Levison H: Meconium ileus in the absence of cystic fibrosis. Arch Dis Child 67:1204–1206, 1992.
39. Toyosaka A, Tomimoto Y, Nose K, et al: Immaturity of the myenteric plexus is the etiology of meconium ileus without mucoviscidosis: A histopathologic study. Clin Auton Res 4:175–184, 1994.
40. Martin L. The small intestine: Meconium peritonitis. In Ravitch MM, Welch KJ, Benson DC, et al (eds): Pediatric Surgery, 3rd ed. Chicago, Year Book Medical, 1979, pp 952–955.
41. Foster MA, Nyberg DA, Mahoney BS, et al: Meconium peritonitis: Prenatal sonographic findings and their clinical significance. Radiology 165:661–665, 1987.
42. Finkel LI, Slovis TL: Meconium peritonitis, intra-peritoneal calcifications and cystic fibrosis. Pediatr Radiol 12:92–93, 1982.
43. Tanaka K, Hashizume K, Kawarasaki H: Elective surgery for cystic meconium peritonitis: Report of two cases. J Pediatr Surg 28:960–961, 1993.
44. Careskey JM, Grosfeld JL, Weber TR, el al: Giant cystic meconium peritonitis (GCMP): Improved management based on clinical and laboratory observations. J Pediatr Surg 17:482–489, 1982.
45. Clatworthy HW, Howard HW, Lloyd J: The meconium plug syndrome. Surgery 39:131–142, 1956.
46. Santulli TV: Meconium ileus. In Holder TM, Ashcraft KW (eds): Pediatric Surgery, Philadelphia, WB Saunders, 1990, pp 356–373.
47. Rosenstein BJ: Cystic fibrosis presenting with the meconium plug syndrome. Am J Dis Child 132:167–169, 1978.
48. Stewart DR, Nixon GW, Johnson DG, et al: Neonatal small left colon syndrome. Ann Surg 186:741–795, 1977.
49. Flake AW, Ryckman FC: Meconium plug syndrome. In Fanaroff AA, Martin RJ (eds): Neonatal-Perinatal Medicine, Diseases of the Fetus and Infant (5th ed). St. Louis, Mosby–Year Book, 1992, pp 1054–1055.
50. Krasna IW, Rosenfeld D, Salerno P: Is it necrotizing enteroco-

litis, meconium of prematurity, or delayed meconium plug? A dilemma in the tiny premature infant. J Pediatr Surg 31:855–858, 1996.

51. Rasor GB, Stevenson WL: Meconium ileus equivalent. Rocky Mount Med J 38:218–220, 1941.

52. Anderson HO, Hjelt K, Waever E, et al: The age related incidence of meconium ileus equivalent in a cystic fibrosis population: The impact of high energy intake. J Pediatr Gastroenterol Nutr 11:356–360, 1990.

53. Smyth RL, vanVolzen D, Smyth AR: Strictures of ascending colon in cystic fibrosis and high-strength pancreatic enzymes. Lancet 343:85–86, 1994.

33

NECROTIZING ENTEROCOLITIS

Michael G. Caty, MD •
Richard G. Azizkhan, MD

Necrotizing enterocolitis (NEC) is a disease that has appeared as a result of the successes of the modern neonatal intensive care unit (NICU). NEC was rarely described before the development of neonatal units, but it has become the most common gastrointestinal (GI) emergency in newborns.[1, 2] It is largely (>90%) a disease of premature newborns, thus its description is rarely found in the literature before 1960, when survival of small premature babies was unlikely. It is possible that some of the GI perforations reviewed by Thelander in 1939 were the result of NEC.[3] Two case reports of colon necrosis following exchange transfusion appeared in the 1950s and both of these cases had presentations similar to NEC.[4, 5] In 1959, Rossier and colleagues described 15 infants with "ulcerative-necrotic enterocolitis of the premature," giving the syndrome its descriptive name.[6] The first comprehensive description of the presentation, diagnosis, and pathology of NEC in premature infants was published in 1967.[7]

□ Incidence

NEC is the most common GI emergency in the NICU. It is characterized by a spectrum of ischemic injury to the small and large bowel, ranging from limited mucosal ischemia to total intestinal necrosis. It affects between 1 and 8% of all newborns admitted to an NICU in the United States.[8] NEC develops in 2000 to 4000 newborns annually. More than 90% of affected newborns are born prematurely. Newborns with birth weights of less than 2000 g make up 80% of NEC cases.[9] The mortality rate for NEC has been calculated to be 13 per 100,000 live births. The case fatality rate ranges from 20 to 40%.[8] NEC occurs infrequently in countries with low rates of premature birth such as Japan and Switzerland.[10]

Certain risk factors have been consistently observed in newborns with NEC: prematurity and feeding. The mean gestational age of newborns with NEC is between 30 and 32 weeks. The onset of feeding is also a consistent factor preceding NEC, although low-dose "conditioning" feedings may protect against NEC.[11] Many other "risk" factors have been identified, including asphyxia, the presence of a patent ductus arteriosus, twin gestation, exchange transfusion, umbilical artery and vein catheterization, and anemia. Despite the apparent relationships among many risk factors and NEC, most of these do not stand up to the rigor of case-control analysis.[12–14]

□ Presentation

The typical patient with NEC is a premature newborn in whom abdominal distention and bloody stools develop after enteral feedings are initiated (Fig. 33–1). The mean gestational age at onset of NEC is 31 weeks. NEC usually occurs between 3 and 12 days after birth.

An inverse relationship between gestational age

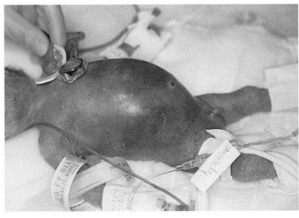

Figure 33–1. Premature newborn with necrotizing enterocolitis demonstrating distention and discoloration of the anterior abdominal wall as a result of peritonitis.

and age at onset has been demonstrated.[15] Late-onset NEC may also occur many weeks after birth. Survival rate is equivalent for both types of NEC. Although it is a rare event, a fulminant form of NEC can occur on the 1st day of life.

Although the majority of infants with NEC are premature, 7 to 13% of NEC cases develop in newborns following delivery at full term.[16] Risk factors for NEC in newborns weighing more than 2000 g include hypoglycemia, premature rupture of membranes, chorioamnionitis, exchange transfusion, and depressed Apgar scores.[17] Clinical factors that increase the suspicion for NEC in patients at all gestational ages include asphyxia, exchange transfusion, feeding intolerance, congenital heart disease, hyperviscosity, and pulmonary disease. Prenatal maternal cocaine use is considered by many to be a causative agent of NEC owing to the vasoconstrictive effect of the drug.[18, 19] In such infants, NEC presents with a particularly fulminant form, with an early onset and extensive involvement of the intestine. Other pharmacologic agents implicated in the pathogenesis of NEC have been the methylxanthines (aminophylline and theophylline), indomethacin, and vitamin E.[20–22]

Several related clinical situations warrant further discussion. These include NEC in the very low birth weight (VLBW) infant, isolated small bowel perforations, and mesenteric ischemia of the child (MIC).

The continued development of sophisticated neonatal care has resulted in increased survival for VLBW infants. VLBW infants are defined as weighing less than 1000 g and are born before or at 28 weeks' gestation. NEC presents differently in VLBW infants compared with the usual premature infant. NEC in VLBW infants presents later, has greater intestinal involvement, requires surgery more often, and has a higher mortality rate.[23, 24]

Most intestinal perforations in VLBW infants are due to NEC.[25] However, a subset of intestinal perforations in this group is due to the increasingly recognized entity of "focal GI perforation." This entity is distinguished from standard NEC. Localized intestinal perforations present with sudden abdominal distention in VLBW infants. An isolated perforation of the antimesenteric border of the ileum is the usual operative finding. Several factors distinguish VLBW infants with isolated perforations from those with NEC. VLBW infants with intestinal perforations have less hemodynamic instability, less metabolic acidosis, and improved survival rate.[26–28] The presence of umbilical artery catheters and administration of indomethacin are more common in infants with isolated perforations. Also, the pathologic finding of coagulation necrosis, which is common in NEC, is not found in resected specimens from patients with isolated perforations. Many theories exist to explain the occurrence of isolated perforations. These include embolic phenomena, inhibited local prostaglandin production, and impairment of collateral circulation to the antimesenteric surface of the bowel.

In infants with congenital heart disease, intestinal ischemia may develop and result in a clinical syndrome similar to NEC. This entity is MIC.[29] Although there are similarities between MIC and NEC, the many differences between them suggest they are distinct pathologic processes. MIC usually occurs in full-term infants with complex congenital heart disease. It may immediately follow corrective surgery or may be a consequence of low splanchnic perfusion, such as exists with the hypoplastic left heart syndrome.[29, 30] Mortality rate is high (>90%), gut involvement is usually extensive, and splanchnic ischemia is the logical proceeding pathophysiologic event.

□ Pathology

NEC results in variable degrees of ischemic necrosis of the small and large intestine of the neonate. Intestinal samples from surgical resection and autopsies show simultaneous involvement of the small intestine and colon in 44%, colon alone in 26%, and small intestine alone in 30%.[31] Whereas guaiac-positive gastric aspirates are a common clinical presentation of NEC, transmural gastric injury is rare.

The histopathologic findings of intestinal samples of patients with NEC support an ischemic basis for the disease. The most common microscopic feature is coagulation necrosis (Fig. 33–2). Other features include acute and chronic inflammation, bacterial overgrowth, and pneumatosis intestinalis. It is unusual to find thrombi in the superior mesenteric artery. Intestinal epithelial regeneration was seen in more than half of the specimens in one study.[31] This suggests that many cases of NEC are an imbalance

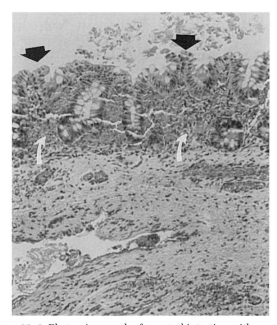

Figure 33–2. Photomicrograph of resected intestine with necrotizing enterocolitis demonstrating loss of villous tips *(black arrows)* and coagulation necrosis *(white arrows).*

between repair and injury that results in intestinal perforation and clinical deterioration.

☐ Etiology and Pathogenesis

The etiology of NEC is speculative. Epidemiologic data suggest an important role for infection, although immaturity of GI barrier function and gut motility in the premature infant may also play a role. Clinical observation and histopathologic study suggest that ischemia is the final common pathway.

Discovery of the etiology of NEC is hampered by the small number of patients affected, the variability of the clinical presentation, and the lack of representative animal models. Any theory of the origin of NEC must be reconciled with clinical and pathologic observations. The majority of neonates with NEC are premature and have been recently fed. Histology of resected specimens show coagulation necrosis. Other interesting observations are that NEC may occur in epidemics and that hygienic measures interrupt outbreaks. Circulatory disturbances, gut immunology, infection, inflammation, and feeding practices are all thought to help explain the etiology of NEC.

CIRCULATORY DISTURBANCES

Intestinal ischemia has always been thought to be an important component of NEC. Histologic evidence of intestinal necrosis provided the clinical basis for this belief. It was originally thought that perinatal asphyxia led to shunting away from the visceral circulation and subsequent ischemia.[32] This response, the Herring-Breur reflex, occurs in aquatic mammals. This theory has been discredited by the lack of evidence for asphyxia in most controlled epidemiologic studies of neonates with NEC. It is unclear whether ischemia is an initiator of NEC or is the final common pathway of a process involving infection, inflammation, and impaired mucosal immunologic defenses.

Experimental evidence concerning intrinsic control of neonatal circulation and intestinal oxygen consumption have shed light on the role of circulatory disturbances in the pathophysiology of NEC. Mesenteric vascular rings from 3-day-old swine compared to 35-day-old swine had a significant reduction in their ability to vasorelax after brief periods of ischemia.[33] The implication of this finding is that newborns may have unopposed vasoconstriction in response to minor ischemic events, leading to a cycle of worsening ischemia and tissue damage. In addition, newborn swine are more susceptible to mucosal injury following ischemia in the presence of feeding.[34] This suggests a diminished ability of newborns to increase oxygen uptake during the stress of ischemia and nutrient absorption.

INFECTION

NEC epidemics suggest an infectious agent as the etiology of the disease. Pathologic examination of resected specimens often shows bacterial overgrowth.[31] However, no predominant organism has been cultured from neonates with NEC. Blood cultures, peritoneal cultures, and intestinal cultures grow common enteric organisms such as *Klebsiella*, *Escherichia coli*, and *Clostridia* species. Case reports have documented the association of NEC with specific viruses such as rotavirus, coronavirus, and coxsackie B2. Pigbel, an illness caused by the enterotoxin of *Clostridia perfringens*, results in a clinical situation similar to NEC. The illness, which occurs in adults and children who eat tainted pork, manifests itself as abdominal distention, bloody stool, pneumatosis, and intestinal perforation.[35] Although the search for an infectious agent causing NEC is appealing, it is likely that agent-host interactions determine the occurrence of NEC in the individual patient.

GUT IMMUNOLOGY

The intestinal mucosa is a physical and immunologic barrier to intraluminal bacteria and viruses. Because NEC is largely a disease of preterm infants, the role of the immature gut must be considered. The immunologic system of the gut may be divided into specific and nonspecific components. Specific components of the immune system include B cells and T cells. Nonspecific elements include intraluminal pH, mucins, cell to cell adhesion, and gut motility. Abnormalities of both the specific and nonspecific arms of the gut immune system have been identified in the premature newborn. The immature intestine has diminished secretory immunoglobulin (IgA).[36] Clinical studies have demonstrated reduction in the incidence of NEC in at-risk neonates prophylactically given IgA.[37] Many elements of the nonspecific mucosal defenses are abnormal in the preterm infant. Gastric acid is reduced, thus raising the intraluminal pH and allowing colonization of pathogenic bacteria.[38]

In one study, acidification of formula was noted to lower the gastric pH of newborns at risk for NEC. This was associated with a lower incidence of NEC when compared to control subjects.[39] Motility is also reduced in the preterm infant. Finally, developmental differences in mucosal permeability have been demonstrated in swine fed formula instead of sow milk.[40] Breast milk has been shown to be protective against NEC in several studies. The beneficial effects of breast milk are postulated to be due to IgA, as well as other soluble factors such as lactoferrin, vitamin E, beta carotene, and platelet-activating factor (PAF) acetylhydrolase.[41, 42]

FEEDING

It is unusual for NEC to occur in the fasted neonate. Several aspects of feeding are likely to contribute to the onset of NEC. The introduction of hyperosmolar feedings provides extra sources of carbohydrate. In the presence of bacterial overgrowth, lactose is fermented to hydrogen gas, resulting in luminal distention and pneumatosis.

Both short- and long-chain fatty acids that are malabsorbed are known to increase intestinal permeability. Despite the occurrence of NEC with feeding, it is well known that the starved gut will atrophy. One solution to the problem has been the institution of hypocaloric feeding to "condition" the gut. Many studies have confirmed the efficacy of the approach in the preterm infant.[43] As discussed, expressed human milk has been shown to reduce the incidence of NEC while producing adequate weight gain.[41]

INFLAMMATION

Pathologic examination of intestinal specimens in patients with NEC reveals both acute and chronic inflammation.[31] Clinical studies have shown elevated serum tumor necrosis factor alpha (TNFα) and PAF in neonates with NEC.[44–46] PAF has been demonstrated to have a prominent role in the pathogenesis of NEC. One well-characterized model of NEC used infusions of PAF to initiate a histologically similar disease.[47] PAF acetylhydrolase, the enzyme responsible for the breakdown of PAF, is found in breast milk, suggesting another mechanism for the protective effect of breast milk. PAF is thought to exert its effects through vasoconstriction, capillary leak, increased mucosal permeability, and release of secondary mediators.[44]

SUMMARY AND SYNTHESIS

Basic science and clinical research provide many clues to the etiology of NEC. Many of these hypotheses overlap. The clinical observations of prematurity and feeding must be incorporated into any theory of the etiology of NEC. A reasonable synthesis of diverse hypotheses involves an intraluminal event provoking an extraluminal (vascular) event. It is likely that both feeding and bacterial overgrowth combine to injure an already compromised mucosal barrier. It is reasonable to suggest that this event stimulates alterations in an abnormal vascular bed that initiates ischemia. Ischemia then impairs gut motility and barrier function, and results in amplified cytokine release (Fig. 33–3).

□ Diagnosis

When considering the neonate with suspected or confirmed NEC, three diagnostic objectives must be met. First, a diagnosis should be made early in at-risk newborns. Second, neonates with NEC should have a diagnostic plan that accurately determines the need for and timing of surgical intervention. Third, newborns with NEC managed either operatively or nonoperatively should be monitored for complications of the disease.

Neonates at risk for NEC are usually premature

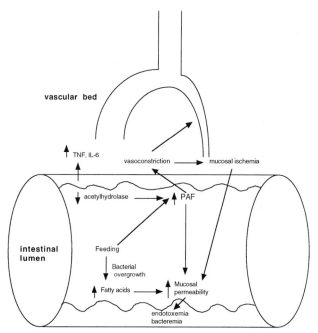

Figure 33–3. Proposed mechanism of the pathogenesis of necrotizing enterocolitis.

and have recently begun enteral feedings. Early clinical signs and symptoms are abdominal distention, heme-positive stools, high-volume gastric aspirates, and apnea. Neonates suspected of having NEC should undergo abdominal radiography with an anteroposterior and decubitus view. A left decubitus view is important to look for small amounts of free air over the liver. Suggestive radiographic findings are bowel dilation, portal venous gas, and pneumatosis intestinalis (Fig. 33–4). Pneumatosis represents intramural hydrogen gas resulting from bacterial fermentation.[48] Portal venous gas is thought to result from absorption of intramural gas into the portal circulation. Although intramural gas is thought to be pathognomonic of NEC, it is not always present, and in the appropriate clinical setting, treatment should be instituted despite its absence.

No element of laboratory data is diagnostic of NEC. Laboratory data taken in its entirety gives the clinician an impression of the severity of NEC. The white blood cell count can be elevated, normal, or low. Low values suggest sepsis, a result of complicated NEC. Thrombocytopenia and ongoing acidosis are also thought to signify complicated NEC.

Once the diagnosis of NEC is made and medical management begun, surveillance radiographs are obtained every 6 hours. Radiologic signs of bowel infarction include pneumoperitoneum, free intraperitoneal fluid, persistence of dilated loops, and diminished bowel gas with asymmetric loops.[49]

Physical findings suggestive of infarcted bowel include abdominal wall cellulitis, abdominal tenderness, and staining of the scrotum with meconium. Occasionally, a patient with NEC has no evidence of perforation yet no clinical improvement. Ultrasonography and peritoneal lavage may assist

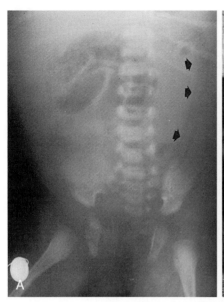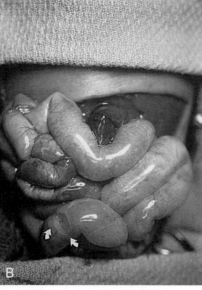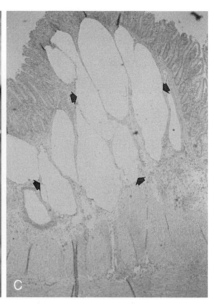

Figure 33–4. *A,* Radiographic finding of pneumatosis (*black arrows*) in newborn with proven necrotizing enterocolitis. *B,* Intraoperative photograph of pneumatosis of the small intestine identified by curved white arrows. *C,* Photomicrograph demonstrating pneumatosis in a submucosal location outlined by black arrows.

the clinician in this situation. Ultrasonography allows the detection of contained perforations and intraperitoneal fluid. Needle aspiration for peritoneal fluid is a useful diagnostic adjunct. Brown and yellow-brown fluid with organisms on Gram's stain are strongly suggestive of gangrenous bowel.[50, 51]

Following successful medical therapy or surgical intervention, the next diagnostic objective is to detect complications. The most common complication is intestinal stricture. These occur predominantly in the colon (Fig. 33–5). They present from 3 weeks to months after treatment. All neonates with NEC should undergo barium enema before stoma closure or discharge from the hospital.[52, 53] Other complications include fungal sepsis, stomal stenosis, enteric fistulae, short gut syndrome, liver abscess, wound infection, and wound dehiscence.

□ Treatment

MEDICAL TREATMENT

Treatment of established NEC begins with its recognition. Newborns with NEC without indications for surgery are managed medically. Goals of medical therapy are gut rest, reduction of enteric pathogenic bacteria, and correction of hematologic and metabolic abnormalities.

When the diagnosis of NEC is made, feedings are stopped and nasogastric suction is initiated. Limiting distention of the gut is important to prevent intestinal blood flow reductions that result from increasing intraluminal and extraluminal pressure on the gut wall. Broad-spectrum antibiotics are started to reduce pathogenic bacteria and treat any bacteremias. In most neonatal units, ampicillin, gentami-

cin, and clindamycin are administered. If resistant coagulase-negative staphylococci are important pathogens in the treating institution, then vancomycin should be substituted for ampicillin. Anaerobic coverage is important because anerobes are grown from peritoneal cultures in many newborns with perforated NEC. Thrombocytopenia and anemia are consistent components of NEC. Platelet and red blood cell transfusion are often necessary. Fluid resuscitation and bicarbonate administration are important to reverse the metabolic acidosis that often results from NEC.

Adequacy of medical treatment is judged by the clinical and radiologic response of the newborn. The newborn who continues to improve and whose radiologic abnormalities resolve is treated empirically for 7 to 10 days.

SURGICAL TREATMENT

Approximately 25 to 50% of newborns with NEC require surgical treatment. The most common indication for surgery, in our experience, is intestinal perforation as evidenced by pneumoperitoneum. Other indications include clinical deterioration, erythema of the abdominal wall, presence of portal venous gas, presence of a palpable abdominal mass, a persistent fixed loop on repeated abdominal radiographs, and a positive paracentesis. Less common indications for surgery include thrombocytopenia, a gasless abdomen with ascites, and abdominal wall tenderness. Ideally, surgery is performed when the intestine is gangrenous but not perforated.

Newborns with NEC are usually premature, often have lung disease, and may have systemic sepsis at the time of surgery. Operative therapy complements the treatment of shock, hypoxemia, and infection.

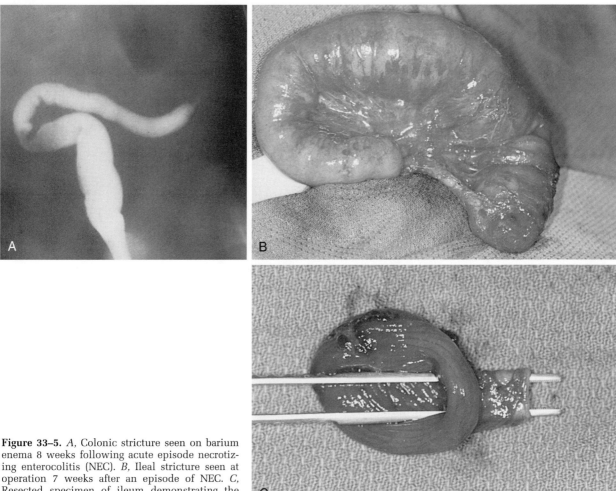

Figure 33–5. *A,* Colonic stricture seen on barium enema 8 weeks following acute episode necrotizing enterocolitis (NEC). *B,* Ileal stricture seen at operation 7 weeks after an episode of NEC. *C,* Resected specimen of ileum demonstrating the stricture.

Infants should be appropriately resuscitated to maximize their ability to withstand additional stresses associated with surgery. The need to transport the newborn, change modes of ventilation, and expose the newborn to changes in ambient temperature increases the operative risk. Cooperation among the surgical team, neonatologists, and anesthesiologists is paramount. Correction of acidosis, anemia, thrombocytopenia, and hypovolemia should precede transport to the operating room. Whereas reasonable attempts should be made to correct metabolic and hematologic abnormalities, unnecessary delays only worsen outcome. Fluid and blood resuscitation is critical, but overhydration may lead to liver disruption and death.[54]

Because the patients with NEC are typically extremely premature, measures to prevent hypothermia in the operating room must be of high priority. If possible, the operation should be performed on an open warming bed to help maintain the patient's temperature and avoid an unnecessary transfer of the patient. A rapid transition from transport monitors to the operating room monitors should be accomplished. A warming blanket should be placed underneath the infant. Wrapping of exposed extremities and the head with cellophane provides an additional insulating covering to minimize heat loss. Alternatively, the use of a wraparound air warmer is an inexpensive and effective method of keeping small infants thermoneutral during operative procedures.

The lateral aspect of the abdomen should be draped with waterproof drapes to prevent wetting of the infant during the procedure. All irrigation solutions should be kept at 38°C.

The surgeon must perform precise and expeditious surgery while minimizing the physiologic perturbations associated with the disease process and operation. Technical goals of the operation should be (1) recognition and resection of gangrenous bowel, (2) preservation of marginal and well perfused bowel, (3) establishment of diverting stomas, (4) avoidance of iatrogenic injury to the liver, and (5) minimization of physiologic perturbations in the infant.

A generous right supraumbilical transverse abdominal incision is preferred for exploration. Peritoneal fluid is sampled for Gram's stain and for aerobic and anaerobic cultures. The entire GI tract is carefully inspected for necrosis and perforations.

The operative procedure is determined by the surgical pathology and the physiology of the patient. Resectional therapy is the mainstay of the surgical treatment of NEC. Resection of only necrotic or perforated bowel is an important principle. The preservation of adequate intestinal length for growth and development is essential to avoid a lifetime of parenteral nutrition and its consequences. If possible, the ileocecal valve should be preserved. The length of viable intestine should be measured along the antimesenteric border and recorded in every case. Extensive resection of marginally viable bowel should be avoided. In infants with extensive involvement, a proximal stoma is constructed and the remaining involved bowel is left in situ.

Continued supportive treatment followed by a second look operation between 24 and 72 hours is often useful in identifying whether bowel has either progressed to frank necrosis or is viable. Improvement is often seen in dark areas that result from interstitial hemorrhage instead of gangrene. Alternative therapies include peritoneal drainage, peritoneal drainage and lavage, and the "patch, drain, and wait" method, which are described later.

FOCAL DISEASE

Resection and primary anastomosis is an option for the newborn with a single segment of involved bowel and no distal involvement (Fig. 33–6A).[55] Several authors have reported success with this technique, but complications of anastomotic leak and recurrent sepsis occur in 10%. In general, primary anastomosis without enterostomy should not be considered for those neonates with diffuse intestinal involvement, patchy areas of gangrene, or physiologic instability resulting from progressive sepsis. Multiple resections and anastomoses without diversion predispose to intestinal leaks and intraabdominal sepsis.[56, 57]

Exteriorizing the transected ends of the viable bowel is the safest method of management. A number of techniques have been successfully used, including separate or adjoining stomas. Alternatively, the distal bowel may be closed and replaced in the abdominal cavity. Surgeons who advocate a traditional approach place the proximal stoma through a separate small incision, usually in the right lower quadrant. A mucous fistula is brought out through the same incision as the proximal stoma, facilitating later stomal closure. The rationale for this technique is to minimize the risk of potential wound infections and complications.

However, in desperately ill neonates or those whose bowel is extremely short or when the mesentery is thick and nonpliable, the proximal stoma may need to be brought out through the lateral aspect of the main abdominal incision. Some authors

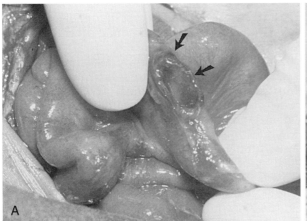
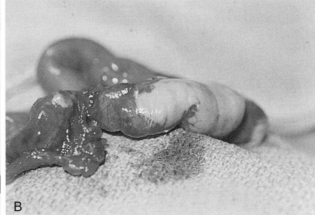
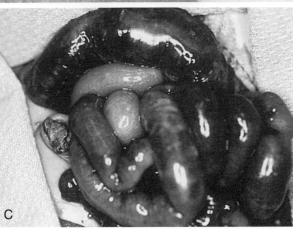

Figure 33–6. Different appearances of necrotizing enterocolitis (NEC). *A,* Isolated perforation in the distal ileum *(black arrows)* of a 26-week gestational age 650-g infant. This child had received two doses of indomethacin for a patent ductus arteriosus. *B,* Segmental necrosis of the distal ileum in a 1200-g infant with NEC. *C,* NEC totalis in a 750-g infant. More than 90% of the bowel was necrotic and the infant died.

have advocated this approach for most patients citing that there appears to be no increase in wound complications.[58] In either case, the protruding intestine is anchored to the fascia with interrupted sutures and the stoma is not matured. If viability of the stoma is in question, a small piece can be excised to observe the cut end for bleeding.

MULTISEGMENT DISEASE (>50% VIABLE BOWEL)

Multiple areas of intestinal necrosis separated by viable segments of bowel have been historically managed by resection of the individual necrotic segments and construction of multiple stomas rather than by a massive resection. Alternatively, a single stoma is placed just proximal to the highest area of necrosis and the distal segments of viable bowel are "spliced" together, thus avoiding multiple stomas. Proximal enterostomies (usually jejunum) are associated with significant fluid and electrolyte losses as well as significant peristomal skin complications.[58] Contemporary nutrition and diligent supportive care minimizes most of these problems. However, anastomotic strictures have been observed in the defunctionalized bowel. These need to be identified by preoperative GI contrast studies and repaired before enterostomy closure.

A novel technique to preserve bowel length and to avoid multiple enterostomies was recently described by Vaughan and colleagues.[60] They resected multiple areas of necrotic bowel and occluded the cut ends with surgical clips. A surgical reexploration was performed at 48 to 72 hours. Two of three infants in their series had the interrupted intestinal segments anastomosed at the second procedure. The remaining patient required resection of additional necrotic bowel and the intestinal ends were reclipped. Successful anastomosis was performed during a third operation. All three patients have done well in a 6-month to 7-year follow-up. This method of management is appealing but experience with this approach is limited.

The patient with extensive intestinal involvement and multiple perforations may benefit from the "patch, drain, and wait" method described by Moore.[61] Perforations are closed and transabdominal drains are placed. As expected, fistulae often occur, which in some patients form spontaneous stomas (Fig. 33–7). After the clinical resolution of sepsis, contrast GI radiography is essential to identify the remaining GI anatomy. These infants almost invariably require subsequent operative procedures to repair enteric fistulae and reestablish GI continuity.

NECROTIZING ENTEROCOLITIS TOTALIS (<25% VIABLE BOWEL)

NEC totalis with involvement of the entire small bowel develops in approximately 20% of patients with NEC and they have less than 25% viable bowel (see Fig. 33–6B). Treatment options include simple

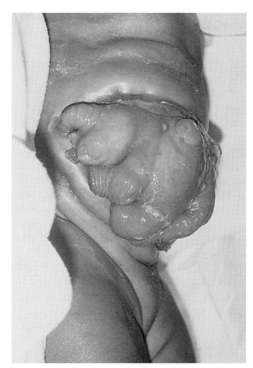

Figure 33–7. Multiple intestinal fistulae in an infant who had multiple areas of necrosis throughout the length of the intestine and initially underwent segmental resections and multiple anastomoses. These fistulae were resected and sufficient intestinal length was salvaged for the child to survive without parenteral nutrition.

closure of the abdomen, resection of all necrotic bowel with stomas, and proximal diversion without bowel resection.

Simple closure is uniformly fatal and massive resection invariably leads to short bowel syndrome. Mortality rate approaches 100% for infants weighing less than 1000 g and the few surviving larger infants have short bowel syndrome.[62] Diverting intestinal continuity by placing a high proximal enterostomy without intestinal resection may allow healing of part of the injured and ischemic bowel. This is thought to occur because the interruption of the fecal stream promotes intestinal decompression and reduces intestinal metabolic demands. Theoretically, by decreasing the bacterial load and reducing inflammatory mediators, healing of marginally viable bowel may be facilitated. Subsequent operations are usually required to resect gangrenous intestine but enough viable bowel may be salvaged to permit survival without short bowel syndrome.

PERITONEAL DRAINAGE

The technique of peritoneal drainage for NEC was first described in 1975.[63] The increasing survival of VLBW infants has prompted the introduction of this technique. Originally introduced as a temporizing procedure, several reports document its success as the sole means of operative intervention.[64]

Peritoneal drainage is ideally performed on VLBW

infants who are unstable and demonstrate either pneumoperitoneum or meconium staining of the abdominal wall.

Under local anesthesia, one or two ¼-inch Penrose drains are placed in the right and left lower quadrants. Broad-spectrum antibiotics are given and the clinical course of the newborn followed. If no improvement occurs, a laparotomy is performed. The management of the infant who stabilizes and improves on drainage alone is controversial. Some authors point to the significant number of newborns (27 to 46%) who require no other definitive treatment than drainage alone and suggest evaluation of bowel continuity with water-soluble contrast studies.[64] A more conservative approach has been to consider drain placement as the initial stabilizing procedure before laparotomy.[63]

STOMA CLOSURE

Before closure of the enterostomy, radiographic contrast studies are required to verify distal intestinal caliber and continuity. Strictures may occur up to several weeks after an NEC episode. The amount of stoma output, rate of weight gain, and length of time since operation are important factors used in determining the timing of stoma closure. Infants who are otherwise thriving and are gaining weight, with weight ranging between 2.5 and 5 kg, can have their stomas closed at 3 to 5 months of age.

However, there is no agreement on a time when enteral continuity should be operatively restored. Some patients have excessive stomal output, failure to grow, or significant stomal strictures; in these patients, early surgical closure is often warranted. When performed in less than 4 to 6 weeks, stomal closure is more technically difficult owing to residual inflammation in the bowel and peritoneal cavity. During bowel mobilization, dense vascularized adhesions obliterate the peritoneal space and increase the risk of intestinal injury. In infants with high jejunostomies and inadequate distal ileum for bile salt reabsorption, a profound secretory diarrhea may develop following restoration of enterocolonic continuity. These patients require bile salt binders such as cholestyramine to manage this complication.

☐ Outcomes

Approximately 50% of infants with NEC who receive nonoperative treatment have clinical resolution of their disease. The most common complication after medical management is intestinal stricture, usually in the colon.

Newborns with NEC who undergo operative treatment have survival rates of 44 to 87%. Complications occur in approximately half of all patients undergoing operative therapy. These include stomal stenosis, stomal retraction, intestinal strictures, enteric fistulae, short gut syndrome, intraabdominal abscess, and wound infection. Specific indications

for operation and extreme prematurity are not associated with higher complication rates. Mortality rate is higher in VLBW infants.[65]

Limited information is available to evaluate the developmental implications of NEC. Approximately 50% of the surviving infants are neurodevelopmentally normal in long-term follow-up.[66] In a small cohort of 40 NEC survivors, adverse neurodevelopmental outcomes were correlated with underlying prematurity and comorbid conditions rather than the NEC itself. At least 10% of children have GI sequelae including short bowel syndrome, fat malabsorption, or intestinal strictures.[66] As expected, the severity of any GI impairment correlates with the severity of NEC.

VLBW infants who survive NEC seem to have equivalent psychosocial development as control infants who were VLBW.[67] The severity of NEC has implications for growth and development in that surviving infants with "severe" NEC have lower adjusted body weights and head circumference.[68]

REFERENCES

1. Kosloske AM: Necrotizing enterocolitis in the neonate. Surg Gynecol Obstet 148:259–269, 1979.
2. Kliegman RM, Fanaroff AA: Necrotizing enterocotitis. N Engl J Med 310:1093–1103, 1984.
3. Thelander HE: Perforation of the gastrointestinal tract of the newborn infant. Am J Dis Child 58:371–393, 1939.
4. Corkery JJ, Dubowitz V, Lister J, et al: A colonic perforation after exchange transfusion. BMJ 4:345–349, 1968.
5. Lucey JF: Colonic perforation after exchange transfusion. N Engl J Med 280:724, 1969.
6. Rossier A, Sarrot S, Deplanque J: L'entcolite ulcero-necrotique du premature. Sem Hop Paris 35:1428–1436, 1959.
7. Touloukian RJ, Berdon WE, Amoury RA, et al: Surgical experience with necrotizing enterocolitis in the infant. J Pediatr Surg 2:389–401, 1967.
8. Kosloske AM: Epidemiology of necrotizing enterocolitis. Acta Paediatr Suppl 396:2–7, 1994.
9. Ryder RW, Shelton JD, Guinan ME: Necrotizing enterocolitis: A prospective multicenter investigation. Am J Epidemiol 112:113–123, 1980.
10. Shimura K: Necrotizing enterocolitis? A Japanese survey. NICU 3:5–7, 1990.
11. Gross SJ, Slagle TA: Feeding the low birthweight infant. Clin Perinatol 20:193–209, 1993.
12. Kanto WP, Wilson R, Breart GL, et al: Perinatal events and necrotizing enterocolitis in premature infants. Am J Dis Child 141:167–169, 1987.
13. DeCurtis M, Paone C, Vetrano G, et al: A case control study of necrotizing enterocolitis occurring over 8 years in a neonatal intensive care unit. Eur J Pediatr 146:398–400, 1987.
14. Kliegman RM, Hack M, Jones P, et al: Epidemiologic study of necrotizing enterocolitis among low birth weight infants: Absence of identifiable factors. J Pediatr 100:440–444, 1982.
15. Teasdale F, LeGuennec J-C, Bard H, et al: Neonatal necrotizing enterocolitis: The relationship of age at the time of onset and prognosis. Can Med Assoc J 123:387–390, 1980.
16. Wiswell TE, Robertson CF, Jones TA, et al: Necrotizing enterocolitis in full-term infants. A case control study. Am J Dis Child 142:532–535, 1988.
17. Martinez-Tallo E, Claure N, Bancalari E: Necrotizing enterocolitis in full-term or near-term infants: Risk factors. Biol Neonate 71:292–298, 1997.
18. Porat R, Brodsky N: Cocaine: A risk factor for necrotizing enterocolitis. J Perinatol 11:30–32, 1991.
19. Czyrko C, DelPin CA, O'Neill JA, et al: Maternal cocaine abuse and necrotizing enterocolitis: Outcome and survival. J Pediatr Surg 26:414–421, 1991.

20. Robinson MJ, Clayden GS, Smith MF: Xanthines and necrotizing enterocolitis. Arch Dis Child 55:494–495, 1980.
21. Norton ME, Merrill J, Cooper BAB, et al: Neonatal complications after administration of indomethacin for preterm labor. N Engl J Med 329:1602–1607, 1993.
22. Finer NN, Peters KL, Hayek Z, et al: Vitamin E and necrotizing enterocolitis. Pediatrics 73:387–393, 1984.
23. Rowe MI, Reblock KK, Kurkchubasche AG, et al: Necrotizing enterocolitis in the extremely low birth weight infant. J Pediatr Surg 29:987–991, 1994.
24. Snyder C, Gittes GK, Murphy JP, et al: Survival after necrotizing enterocolitis in infants weighing less than 1,000 g: 25 years' experience at a single institution. J Pediatr Surg 32:434–437, 1997.
25. Novack CM, Waffran F, Sills JH, et al: Focal intestinal perforation in the extremely low birthweight infant. J Perinatol 14:450–453, 1994.
26. Meyer CL, Payne NR, Roback SA: Spontaneous isolated intestinal perforations in neonates with birth weight < 1000 g not associated with necrotizing enterocolitis. J Pediatr Surg 26:714–717, 1991.
27. Mintz AC, Applebaum H: Focal gastrointestinal perforations not associated with necrotizing enterocolitis in very low birth weight neonates. J Pediatr Surg 28:857–860, 1993.
28. Buchheit JQ, Stewart DL: Clinical comparison of localized intestinal perforation and necrotizing enterocolitis in neonates. Pediatrics 93:32–36, 1994.
29. Hebra A, Brown MF, Hirschi RB, et al: Mesenteric ischemia in hypoplastic left heart syndrome. J Pediatr Surg 28:606–611, 1993.
30. Kleinman PK, Winchester P, Brill PW: Necrotizing enterocolitis after open heart surgery employing hypothermia and cardiopulmonary bypass. Am J Roentgenol 127:757–759, 1976.
31. Ballance WA, Dahms BB, Shenker N, et al: Pathology of neonatal necrotizing enterocolitis. J Pediatr 117(suppl):s6–s13, 1990.
32. Lloyd JR: The etiology of gastrointestinal perforation in the newborn. J Pediatr Surg 4:77–84, 1969.
33. Nowicki PT: The effects of ischemia-reperfusion on endothelial cell function in postnatal intestine. Pediatr Res 39:267–274, 1996.
34. Crissinger KD, Granger DN: Mucosal injury induced by ischemia and reperfusion in the piglet intestine: Influences of age and feeding. Gastroenterology 97:920–926, 1989.
35. Lawrence G, Walker PD: Pathogenesis of enteritis necroticans in Papua, New Guinea. Lancet 1:125–126, 1976.
36. Udall JN: Gastrointestinal host defense and necrotizing enterocolitis. J Pediatr 117(suppl):s33–s43, 1990.
37. Eibl MM, Wolf HM, Furnkranz H, et al: Prevention of necrotizing enterocolitis in low-birth-weight infants by IgA-IgG feeding. N Engl J Med 319:1–7, 1988.
38. Hyman PE, Clarke DD, Everett SL, et al: Gastric acid secretory function in preterm infants. J Pediatr 106:467–471, 1985.
39. Carrion VE, Egan E: Prevention of neonatal necrotizing enterocolitis. J Pediatr Gastroenterol Nutr 11:317–323, 1990.
40. Crissinger KD, Burney DL: Intestinal oxygenation and mucosal permeability with luminal mothers milk in developing piglets. Pediatr Res 40:269–275, 1996.
41. Lucas A, Cole TJ: Breast milk and neonatal necrotizing enterocolitis. Lancet 336:1519–1523, 1990.
42. Kliegman RM, Walker WA, Yolken RH: Necrotizing enterocolitis: Research agenda or a disease of unknown etiology and pathogenesis. Pediatr Res 34:701–708, 1993.
43. Gross SJ, Slagle TA: Feeding the low birthweight infant. Clin Perinatol 20:193–209, 1993.
44. Muguruma K, Gray PW, Tjoelker LW, et al: The central role of PAF in necrotizing enterocolitis development. Adv Expl Med Biol 407:379–382, 1997.
45. Morecraft JA, Spitz L, Hamilton PA, et al: Plasma cytokine levels in necrotizing enterocolitis. Acta Paediatr Suppl 396:18–20, 1994.
46. Amer MD, Hedlund E, Rochester J, et al: Stool PAF levels are increased following feeding and in neonatal NEC. J Pediatr (in press).
47. Hsueh W, Caplan MS, Sun X, et al: Platelet-activating factor, tumor necrosis factor, hypoxia and necrotizing enterocolitis. Acta Pediatr Suppl 396:11–17, 1994.
48. Engel RR, Virnig NL, Hunt CE: Origin of mural gas in necrotizing enterocolitis. Pediatr Res 7:292–296, 1973.
49. Fotter R, Sorantin E: Diagnostic imaging in necrotizing enterocolitis. Acta Paediatr Suppl 396:41–44, 1994.
50. Kosloske AM, Goldthorn J: Paracentesis as an aid to the diagnosis of intestinal gangrene. Arch Surg 117:571–573, 1982.
51. Kosloske AM, Lilly JR: Paracentesis and lavage for diagnosis of intestinal gangrene in neonatal necrotizing enterocolitis. J Pediatr Surg 13:315–320, 1978.
52. Janik JS, Ein SH, Mancer K: Intestinal stricture after necrotizing enterocolitis. J Pediatr Surg 16:438–443, 1981.
53. Schwartz MZ, Richardson CJ, Hayden CK, et al: Intestinal stenosis following successful medical management of necrotizing enterocolitis. J Pediatr Surg 15:890–899, 1980.
54. Vanderkolk WE, Kurz P, Daniels J, et al: Liver hemorrhage during laparotomy in patients with necrotizing enterocolitis. J Pediatr Surg 31:1063–1067, 1996.
55. Harberg FJ, Mcgill CW, Saleem MM, et al. Resection with primary anastomosis for necrotizing enterocolitis. J Pediatr Surg 18:743–746, 1983.
56. Kiesewetter WB, Taghizadeh F, Bower RJ: Necrotizing enterocolitis: Is there a place for resection and primary anastamosis? J Pediatr Surg 14:360–363, 1979.
57. Griffiths DM, Forbes DA, Pemberton PJ, et al: Primary anastomosis for necrotizing enterocolitis: A 12-year experience. J Pediatr Surg 24:515–518, 1989.
58. Albanese CT, Rowe MI: Necrotizing enterocolitis. In O'Neill JA, Rowe MI, Grosfeld JL, et al (eds): Pediatric Surgery (5th ed). St. Louis, Mosby, 1998, pp 1297–1320.
59. Musemeche CA, Kosloske AM, Ricketts RR. Enterostomy in necrotizing enterocolitis: An analysis of techniques and timing of closure. J Pediatr Surg 22:479–483, 1987.
60. Vaughan WG, Grosfeld JL, West K, et al: Avoidance of stomas and delayed anastomosis for bowel necrosis: The 'clip, and drop-back technique.' J Pediatr Surg 31:542–545, 1996.
61. Moore TC: Management of necrotizing enterocolitis by 'patch, drain, and wait.' Pediatr Surg Int 4:110–113, 1989.
62. Ricketts RR, Jerles ML: Neonatal necrotizing enterocolitis: Experience with 100 consecutive surgical patients. World J Surg 14:600–605, 1990.
63. Ein SH, Shandling B, Wesson D, et al: A 13-year experience with peritoneal drainage under local anesthesia for necrotizing enterocolitis perforation. J Pediatr Surg 25:1034–1037, 1990.
64. Morgan LJ, Shochat SJ, Hartman GE: Peritoneal drainage as primary management of perforated NEC in the very low birth weight infant. J Pediatr Surg 29:30–34, 1994.
65. Horwitz JR, Lally KP, Cheu HW, et al: Complications after surgical intervention for necrotizing enterocolitis: A multicenter review. J Pediatr Surg 30:994–999, 1995.
66. Stevenson DK, Kerner JA, Malachowski N, et al: Late morbidity among survivors of necrotizing enterocolitis. Pediatrics 66:925–927, 1980.
67. Mayr J, Fasching G, Hollwarth ME: Psychosocial and psychomotoric development of very low birthweight infants with necrotizing enterocolitis. Acta Pediatr Suppl 396:96–100, 1994.
68. Walsh MC, Kliegman RM, Hack M: Severity of necrotizing enterocolitis: Influence on outcome at 2 years of age. Pediatrics 84:804–814, 1989.

34

HIRSCHSPRUNG'S DISEASE

Alexander Holschneider, MD, PhD •
Benno M. Ure, MD, PhD

☐ Incidence

One in 5000 newborns presents with Hirschsprung's disease (HD),[1] and 70 to 80% are boys. HD is observed in all races but is less common in blacks. Siblings and offspring of familial cases have an increased risk of being afflicted. The reported incidence in these children varies from 1.5 to 17.6%[2, 3] which is 130 times higher for boys and 360 times higher for girls than in the general population.[4] HD is more likely to be transmitted by a mother with aganglionosis than by a father. As many as 12.5% of the siblings of patients with total aganglionosis of the colon (Zuelzer-Wilson syndrome) will have the same disease.[5] Associated anomalies are present in 25% of familial cases, compared with 10% in nonfamilial HD cases. One report[6] describes four families with 22 affected siblings, most of them having long segment aganglionosis. The overall incidence of neurocristopathies, including all inborn errors of the enteric nervous system (ENS) is not known. Familial cases of intestinal neuronal dysplasia (IND) are described, but the incidence of this condition or other neuronal intestinal malformations has not been reported.[7]

☐ Genetic Factors

Although Harald Hirschsprung[8] gave the first detailed description of congenital megacolon in 1888 and more than 500 papers have been published to elucidate the pathophysiology, the etiology of the disease is still not known. In recent years, attention has been focused on genetic defects.

Human beings are not the only species to suffer from aganglionosis. Aganglionosis has been observed in mice, rats, horses, cows, dogs, and cats. The rodent models pointed the way to identification of human gene defects in HD. The first description of aganglionosis in mice was published in 1957.[9] The first genetic transmission in a human being was reported in 1992.[10] A female patient with total colon aganglionosis was found to be carrying a de novo interstitial deletion of chromosome 10:46,XX,de 110q11.21-q21.2. The spotting lethal (sl) rat model has two subgroups: one with total colonic aganglionosis and a second, less numerous group in which ganglion cells extended to the proximal half of the colon.[11, 12] The lethal spotting (ls) mice have approximately 2 mm of aganglionosis,[13] whereas another strain showed a deficiency of ganglion cells over about 10 mm. Further studies in which a linkage of genes and gene "knockouts" were analyzed revealed that the *RET* knockout gene deleted on chromosome 10 was responsible for human HD.[14]

However, the high frequency of sporadic cases (80–90%), the varying expressivity in different members of an affected family, and the sex-independent differences in the extent of aganglionosis suggest that more than one gene is responsible for HD. The condition seems to have a multifactorial genesis and a complex pattern of inheritance. There might be an autosomal dominant mode of inheritance with incomplete penetrance leading to long-segment aganglionosis, and an autosomal recessive or multifactorial mode of inheritance responsible for short-segment HD.[15] In one report, the authors were able to distinguish type I (rectosigmoid HD) with multifactorial or autosomal recessive inheritance and with low penetrance from type II (aganglionosis up to the splenic flexure) autosomal dominant with incomplete penetrance.

We presently know that, three genes and three chromosome localizations are identified in the human. The *RET* gene localized to chromosome 10 (autosomal dominant), the endothelinreceptor B (*EDNRB*) gene was detected on chromosome 13 (autosomal recessive), and the endothelin 3 (*EDN 3*) gene localized to chromosome 20 (autosomal recessive). Mutations of the RET-tyrosine-kinase-receptor have been indentified in 50% of familial and 10 to 20% of sporadic cases of HD.[16] However, it has not been clarified whether the genetic defects result in neural crest cell proliferation deficiency, in migration problems of the ganglion cells, or in a peripheral microenviroment deficiency. Many questions

453

remain unanswered, and the link between genetic defects and pathophysiology has not been found.

□ Pathophysiology

The basic pathophysiology in HD is a lack of propagation of propulsive waves and an abnormal or absent relaxation of the internal anal sphincter due to aganglionosis, hypoganglionosis, or dysganglionosis of the bowel. However, innervation abnormalities in HD and allied cristopathies are not quantitative but qualitative.

PERISTALTIC REFLEX

Peristalsis consists of a reflex relaxation below and a contraction of the circular muscle layer above an intraluminal bolus (Fig. 34–1). In addition, the

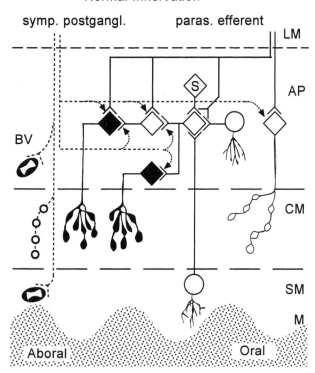

Normal Innervation

Figure 34–1. Schematic of the normal persitaltic reflex, showing the intramural plexus and the postganglionic adrenergic and preganglionic cholinergic axons entering the bowel. The sensory neurons are indicated by circles. The impulses from the mechanoreceptor cells are transmitted via interneurons *(white squares)* over cholinergic synapses to the nonadrenergic inhibitory neurons *(dark squares)*. The finely drawn neuron with white circles in its terminal axons represents a postganglionic axon. The neuron labeled S symbolizes a pacemaker neuron with spontaneous activity. Stimulation of the nonadrenergic inhibitory neurons leads to a neurogenically produced relaxation beyond the bolus. Above the bolus, a myogenically produced contraction of the circular muscle occurs (rebound excitation). The sympathetic system acts as a modulator of the acetylcholine release at the cholinergic synapses. AP, Auerbach's plexus; BV, blood vessel; CM, circular muscle; LM, longitudinal muscle; M, mucosa; S, pacemaker neuron with spontaneous activity; SM, submucosa.

longitudinal muscle layer contracts simultaneously over the bowel content, which leads to aboral propagation. The neural reflex circuit is generated by distension of the bowel and spontaneous depolarization of pacemaker cells in the smooth muscle layers. The electrical impulses are carried by cholinergic neurons to interneurons situated in the submucous and myenteric plexus. The interneurons are of nonadrenergic, noncholinergic (NANC) origin, but they depend on adenosine triphosphate, vasoactive intestinal peptide (VIP), and nitric oxide (NO) directly inhibiting the smooth muscle cells. The ganglia of the intramural plexus contain four to six ganglion cells and are modulated by cholinergic and adrenergic influences running to the ganglia and blood vessels (adrenergic fibers) via extramural neural pathways. Adrenaline modulates the acetylcholine release at cholinergic synapses. In addition to these nerve fibers and the submucous and myenteric plexus, the interstitial cells of CAJAL seem to play an important regulary role in human gut muscle function.[17]

NO has recently been recognized as a neurotransmitter that mediates relaxation of the smooth muscles of the gastrointestinal tract. It is identical to NAPDH-diaphorase, which can therefore be used as a diagnostic marker for HD. Other than NO-containing inhibitory neurons, various other peptidergic neurons storing VIP, substance P, enkephalin, neurokinin A, histidine, isoleucin, gastrin releasing peptide, and many others are involved in the peristaltic reflex. They are absent or abnormal in HD and allied disorders. Currently, the absence of NO-producing neurons is thought to be the cause of the failure of the aganglionic bowel to relax.

THE INTERNAL ANAL SPHINCTER

The internal anal sphincter is influenced by four neuronal mechanisms:
- α-Adrenergic excitatory stimuli, which travel in the hypogastric nerves and maintain the sphincter tone via alpha excitatory receptors
- β-Adrenergic inhibitory receptors relaxing the smooth muscle
- Cholinergic neurons, whose influence on the sphincter is not yet adequately known
- Nonadrenergic and noncholinergic neurons leading to internal sphincter relaxation by the mediation of NO, VIP, and other peptidergic neurons[18]

The relaxation phase of the peristaltic reflex below a fecal bolus is similar to the internal sphincter relaxation, which opens the anal channel at the beginning of defecation. Evidence of this most caudal peristaltic reflex can therefore be considered as a proof of normal neurotransmission down to the end of the gastrointestinal tract and thus exclude HD. Bowel dysfunction in HD is the result of a complex malformation of the intrinsic nerve system of the bowel, which includes the absence of cholinergic ganglia, NANC-interneurons, different peptidergic nerve fibers, and probably connective tissue structures of the bowel wall (Fig. 34–2). Cholinergic axons from the sacral parasympathetic plexus proliferate into the bowel wall and act directly with the smooth muscle cells, producing unopposed contraction. The acetylcholine released at the nerve endings is inactivated by a similar amount of acetylcholinesterase (AChE). Therefore, the staining for AChE provides a very useful diagnostic tool for HD. However, misleading results occur in 10% of cases with AChE-stained biopsies. The frequency of misleading information was highest in long-segment HD.[19] The aganglionic segment remains in permanent contraction, unable to relax due to the lack of NANC interneurons and NO, but it is elastic and able to produce some uncoordinated motility. This may allow some degree of fecal transport and could be the reason HD is sometimes diagnosed later in life. This also applies to patients with hypoganglionosis and IND who show markedly reduced neural cell adhesion molecules and NAPD-diaphorase activity.[20] Conversely, the adrenergic axons (which synapse directly on the excitatory α-receptors of the smooth muscle cells) are normal. The internal anal sphincter therefore remains permanently unable to relax.

HYPOGANGLIONOSIS

Proximal to the aganglionic segment of HD, there is generally a zone of hypoganglionosis. Hypoganglionosis can also represent an isolated disease entity. Hypoganglionosis is defined as the state in which the number of ganglion cells is reduced by a factor of 10 and the density of the nerve fibers, by a factor of 5.[21–23] AChE-positive fibers are rarely seen. The number of nerve cells in the myenteric plexus is 50% of that of normal innervated colon, and the distances between the ganglia are doubled. The mean area of the ganglia is three times smaller than in controls. However, isolated hypoganglionosis and hypoganglionosis associated with HD or IND do not differ histochemically. Hypoganglionosis sometimes involves only a short length of colon and occasionally may involve the whole bowel. As a consequence, a few ganglion cells found on microscopy of frozen section biopsies taken during an operation do not prove normal bowel innervation or guarantee normal bowel motility. In hypoganglionosis, internal sphincter relaxation is often missing or rudimentary.[24]

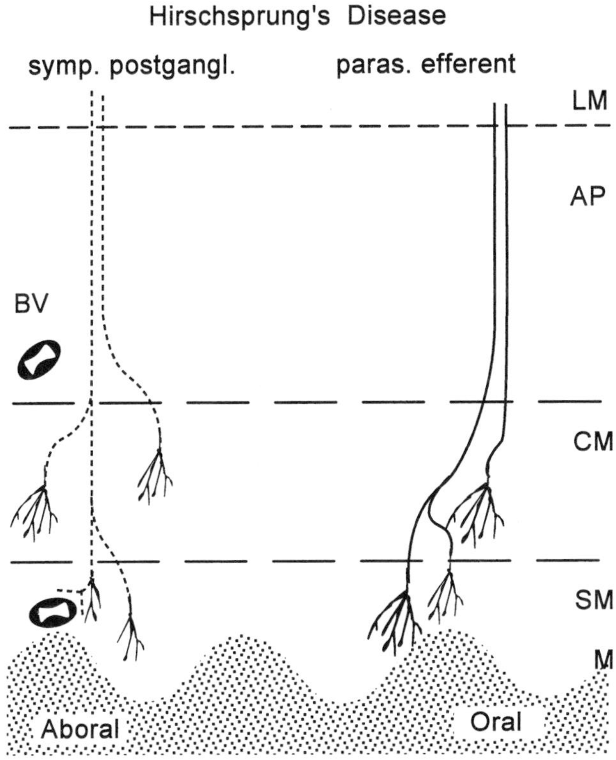

IMMATURITY OF GANGLION CELLS

Immature ganglion cells with monopolar small dentrites can be identified by lactate dehydrogenase (LDH) staining. Nerve cells in the immature ganglia have not developed a dehydrogenase-containing cytoplasm. Therefore, a differentiation between Schwann's cells and nerve cells cannot be made. The maturity of ganglion cells is most reliably determined using the succinyldehydrogenase (SDH) reaction, which tests for this specific mitochondrial enzyme. Enzyme activity is low during the first weeks of life. Maturation of ganglion cells as determined by the SDH reaction demonstrates that full maturity requires 2 to 4 years. Immaturity may be seen with IND or hypoganglionosis, and the condition may eventually cause bowel obstruction.[24] The association of hypoganglionosis and immaturity is called hypogenesis.[25, 26]

INTESTINAL NEURONAL DYSPLASIA

HD represents an abnormality of neural crest cell migration. Therefore, it is not surprising that in addition to aganglionosis and hypoganglionosis, incomplete maturation of the enteric nerve plexus or dysganglionosis can occur.[27] In 1971, IND was first described as either a separate obstructive disease or one that could coexist with classic HD.[28] IND type A (which is characterised by a malformation of the adrenergic nerve supply to the blood vessels) was distinguished from IND type B, in which the submucous plexus is involved.

The diagnosis of IND type B was based mainly on the occurrence of giant ganglia, containing on average 7 to 10, and occasionally up to 16 LDH-positive ganglion cells (Fig. 34–3). These large ganglia represent only 60% of all ganglia seen in a given case and are usually not observed in the distal rectum.[29] Moreover, the morphology of the nerve cell groups and nerve cell fibers is abnormal. They form bud-

Figure 34–2. Schematic of intramural neurons in Hirschsprung's disease. The absence of ganglion cells and interneurons and the increased adrenergic and cholinergic influence on the smooth muscle cells. AP, Auerbach's plexus; BV, blood vessel; CM, circular muscle; LM, longitudinal muscle; M, mucosa; SM, submucosa.

IND Type B

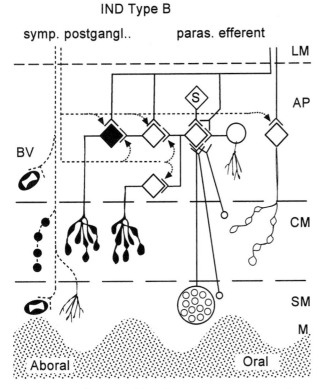

symp. postgangl.. paras. efferent

Figure 34–3. Schematic of bowel innervation in intestinal neuronal dysplasia (IND) type B. Note the increased size of ganglia, increased number of ganglion cells, increased density of ganglions, and heterotopic ganglion cells in the muscularis mucosae and lamina propria mucosae. AP, Auerbach's plexus; BV, blood vessel; CM, circular muscle; LM, longitudinal muscle; M, mucosa; S, pacemaker neuron with spontaneous activity; SM, submucosa.

like cell formations and pearlstring-like nerve fibers. Often the muscularis mucosa and sometimes the lamina propria mucosa contain heterotopic nerve cells or ganglia. The AChE activity is increased in the nerve fibers of the lamina propria but mostly normalizes at the age of 9 to 18 months. One authority believes that 40 serial sections must be investigated with LDH reaction to reliably establish the diagnosis. Thirty to 55 percent of these sections do not contain ganglia in the submucosa. Of the remainder, one in four will contain giant ganglia. At least four giant ganglia must be identified.[22] The diagnosis of IND is difficult, and these criteria generally are not accepted.[30] In children older than 4 years, IND is often associated with hypoganglionosis, hypogenesis, and heterotopia of the myenteric plexus. A recent study was performed by sending each biopsy under an anonymous code to three pediatric pathologists, who followed the criteria established by Meier-Ruge and colleagues.[31] There was an excellent consensus in the diagnosis of HD but none in the diagnosis of IND.[32, 33] It may be that this misjudgment was due to interobserver variation, differences in experience with the diagnosis, and differences in histochemical parameters for IND used. We have concluded from our studies on children

with imperforate anus that IND could also be an expression of neuromuscular hypertrophy proximal to a congenital intestinal obstruction.[34]

IND type A is characterized by a lack or immaturity of the adrenergic innervation of the myenteric plexus, arterial vessels, and mucosa (Fig. 34–4). It is very rare and observed in less than 2% of all neuronal intestinal malformations.[35, 36]

DESMOSIS OF THE COLON

Desmosis of the colon recently has been described as a cause of heterotopia of ganglion cells. The disease is characterised by a defect or a partial lack of the connective tissue net of the muscular wall of the intestine, leading to impairment of propulsive gut activity.[37]

ACQUIRED GANGLION CELL DAMAGE

Acquired aganglionosis and hypoganglionosis may be nonvascular or vascular in origin. Nonvascular causes for acquired aganglionosis include *Trypanosoma cruzi* infection (Chagas disease), vitamin B1 deficiencies, and chronic infections such as tuberculosis. Ischemic ganglion cell damage is caused by an inadequate blood supply in a pull-through segment, tension on both the arterial and venous blood supply during a pull-through procedure, or damage to

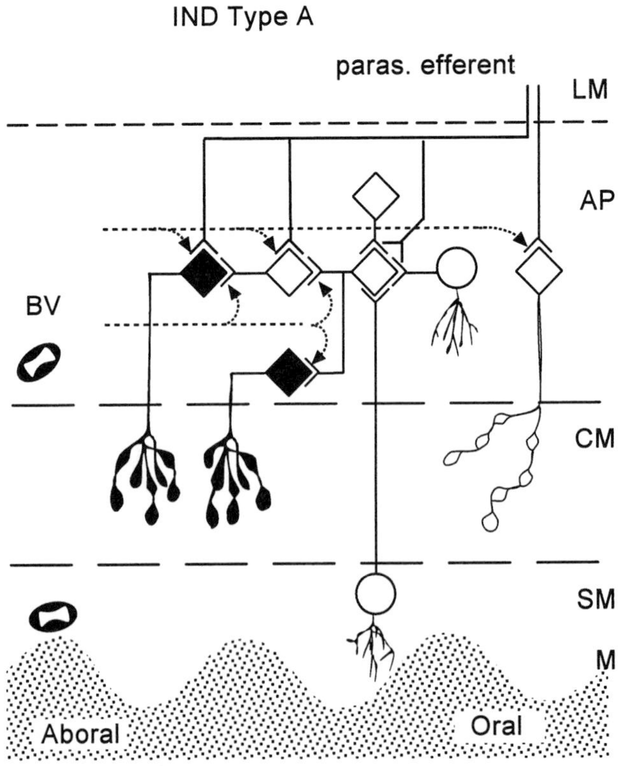

IND Type A

paras. efferent

Figure 34–4. Schematic of the bowel innervation in intestinal neuronal dysplasia (IND) type A: aplasia or hypoplasia of the sympathetic innervation of the myenteric plexus and the arterial vessels. AP, Auerbach's plexus; BV, blood vessel; CM, circular muscle; LM, longitudinal muscle; M, mucosa; SM, submucosa.

the mesenteric vessels. Five cases were analyzed, with 11 additional cases from the literature.[38] In all children, a pull-through procedure according to Swenson, Duhamel, or Soave had been performed. We know of one case of acquired hypoganglionosis.[39]

ASSOCIATED MALFORMATIONS

Associated abnormalities are present in 11 to 30% of the children with HD.[2] However, when HD patients were routinely screened by a clinical geneticist, the number with associated anomalies increased to 48%. In our recent series of 203 patients, the familial pattern was observed in 11%,[36] with 35% having associated malformations. The most common disorders were of the urogenital tract (11%), cardiovascular system (6%), and gastrointestinal system (6%), with 8% having various other malformations such as cataract, coloboma, cleft palate, and extremity or cerebral defects. Prematurity is reported in as many as 10% of the children with HD.

DOWN SYNDROME

Three percent of HD patients are reported to have Down syndrome, which is four times the incidence in the population as a whole.[40] In our series, 6% of the patients with HD had Down syndrome.[36] Constipation in Down syndrome patients also may be caused by hypothyroidism, hypotonia, or mental retardation. Therefore, difficulties in the differential diagnosis of constipation in patients with Down syndrome result in a high incidence of enterocolitis. In addition to trisomy 21, other chromosomal anomalies are associated with HD, such as deletion of chromosomes 2, 10, and 13, and partial trisomies 11 and 22.

WAARDENBURG'S AND OTHER SYNDROMES

The sympathetic ganglia of the gastrointestinal tract originate from neuroectodermal cells. These neural crest cells, especially those of the somites 4 and 5, migrate from the neural tube to the gut and contribute to the ENS. The neural crest caudal to somite 3 is primarily responsible for ENS formation in the colon. Studies indicate that ENS precursors might migrate along a ventrolateral pathway, whereas cells from the rhombencephalic neural crest down to the caudal boundary of somite 3 migrate predominantly via dorsolateral pathways to the pharngeal arches.[41] There is also some evidence of different migration pathways between the anterior and posterior vagal neural crest. While migrating to their final position in the gut, the neural crest cells receive signals from the enteric microenvironment, which indicate when and where to stop migration and to form ganglia. One of these factors might be laminin, an extracellular matrix molecule

normally present in the basal laminae of the mucosal and serosal epithelium and of the smooth muscle cells of the gut. The neural crest cells acquire a receptor for laminin while migrating to the gut. The interaction of laminin and its receptor may determine the destination of neural crest cells, but the factors that interfere with ganglion cell formation are unknown.

Waardenburg's syndrome is characterised by pigmentation anomalies caused by the fact that neural crest cells almost all form melanocytes. The syndrome is associated with inner ear deafness combined with facial abnormalities. Shah-Waardenburg's syndrome, the association of Waardenburg's syndrome with HD, is probably dependent on *SOX 10* gene mutation.[42] The mode of inheritance of Waardenburg's syndrome has been proposed as autosomal dominant.[29]

In addition to Shah-Warenburg's syndrome, several other specific pedigrees and phenotypes have been reported. HD with microcephaly, mental retardation, and facial dysmorphisms (hypertelorism, megalocornea, dense eyebrows, and anteverted ears) represents a syndrome that was eventually correlated with EDNRB *Ser 305* Asn-variant.[43] HD with congenital central hypoventilation syndrome (Haddad's syndrome)[44] is probably correlated with incomplete penetrance of *GDNF* and *RET* mutations as observed in HD and *EDN 3* gene mutation in congenital hypoventilation syndrome, "Ondine's curse." Twenty-seven percent of 161 cases with Ondine's syndrome in the literature were associated with HD.[45-47] Multiple endocrine neoplasia type II (MEN-II) is an association of medullary thyroid carcinoma, pheocromocytoma, multiple mucosal neuromas, characteristic phenotype, and, occasionally, HD. The association of pheochromocytoma, medullary thyroid carcinoma, hyperparathyroidism, and Cushing's disease is called Sipple's syndrome.[48] The association of medullary thyroid carcinoma, pheochromocytoma, and multiple ganglioneuromas is designated MEN IIA, and the combination without parathyroid disease but with severe constipation due to multiple intestinal ganglioneuromas or aganglionosis, MEN-IIB syndrome.[49] The genetic defect for these familial syndromes is not yet known.

ASSOCIATED ANOMALIES OF THE INTESTINE

Congenital atresia of the small or large intestine, meconium ileus, and imperforate anus are sometimes associated with HD, hypoganglionosis, or IND. In 1994, we reported on 19 HD patients with small bowel atresia.[34] Five also had hypoganglionosis, and 2, IND. In a recent study, just more than half of 52 patients with anorectal malformations had ENS disorders: 9 had aganglionosis in the rectal pouch specimens, 11 had hypoganglionosis, 4 had IND type B, and 3 had dysganglionosis.[50] Only in 2 patients (4%) the innervation patterns of the fistula or rectal pouch were found to be normal. Another report of 30 children with intestinal atresia who had associated HD emphasizes the association.[51]

OTHER ASSOCIATED ANOMALIES

Associated urogenital anomalies have been reported with a frequency of 23%.[1] In our series, the incidence was 11%.[36] However, it became evident that voiding problems frequently occur in patients with an enlarged rectum, which compresses the bladder neck, with subsequent bladder neck obstruction and megacystis. Bladder function in these patients may mimic that of patients with spinal lesions, and it might be difficult to wean these patients from the urinary catheter in the postoperative period.

The incidence of cardiac abnormalities in HD has been reported to range from 2 to 8%, compared with 0.5 to 1% in the normal population.[40] This pertains not only to patients with Down syndrome, who frequently have associated endocardial cushion defects. There is also a 12% incidence of associated eye abnormalities, including microphthalmia and anophthalmia.[40] We have seen a child with total intestinal HD, who also had glaucoma affecting both eyes.

☐ Clinical Presentation

Most children with HD present with intestinal obstruction or severe constipation during the neonatal period. The cardinal symptoms are failure of passage of meconium within the first 24 hours of life, abdominal distension, and vomiting. The severity of these symptoms and the degree of constipation vary considerably between patients and in individual cases. Therefore, some infants present with complete intestinal obstruction, whereas others suffer from relatively few symptoms in the first weeks or months of life. They may later present with persistent constipation, particularly in response to changes in feeding, such as weaning from the breast to cow's milk or weaning onto solids. Patients in whom HD is diagnosed later in life suffer from a long history of constipation, severe abdominal distension with a dilated drum-like belly, multiple fecal masses, and, often, enterocolitis. In some, growth impairment may occur. In these children, fecal retention and meteorism lead to secondary symptoms such as anorexia and cachexia with subsequent hypoproteinemia and anemia.

Rectal examination, a rectal tube, thermometer, or washouts may induce explosive discharge of fluid stool and gas suspicious for enterocolitis. This may lead to a remission of symptoms for a short time, then abdominal distension recurs. On rectal examination, the anal sphincter is hypertonic and the rectum is typically empty.

Diarrhea is common and was found in as many as one third of the children whose HD was diagnosed before 3 months of age.[52] It may also be considered to be a symptom of enterocolitis, which represents the most serious complication of aganglionosis. However, HD-associated enterocolitis has not been clearly defined. Whereas some authors consider diarrhea alone a mild form of enterocolitis,[53, 54] others confine enterocolitis to instances with mucosal ulceration and sepsis.[52, 55, 56]

Enterocolitis is reported to occur in 12 to 58% of patients with HD.[54, 57–60] Various hypotheses have been postulated to explain its occurrence. Fecal stasis has been suggested to result in mucosal ischemia with bacterial invasion and translocation. Furthermore, alterations in mucin components and mucosal defense mechanisms,[61–63] alterations in intestinal neuroendocrine cell populations,[64] an increased prostaglandin E1 activity,[65] and infection with *Clostridium difficile*[66] or rotavirus[67] have been suggested to cause the condition. The pathogenesis of HD-associated enterocolitis remains unclear, and patients may present with persistent symptoms even after diversion of the fecal stream by colostomy.[62, 68, 69]

Enterocolitis in its most severe form may lead to life-threatening toxic megacolon. It is characterised by fever, bile-stained vomiting, explosive diarrhea, abdominal distension, dehydration, and shock.[52, 54] Ulceration and ischemic necrosis of the mucosa above the aganglionic segment may lead to sepsis, pneumatosis, and perforation. Therefore, the possibility of underlying HD should be considered in all children with necrotizing enterocolitis. Spontaneous perforation has been reported in as many as 3% of the patients with HD.[54, 70] A strong correlation exists between the length of the aganglionic bowel and the incidence of perforation.

☐ Diagnosis

HD is suspected on the basis of history and clinical findings. The diagnosis is established by radiologic examination, anorectal manometry, and histochemical analysis of biopsy specimens.

RADIOLOGIC DIAGNOSIS

The diagnosis may be suspected when supine and erect plain abdominal radiographs show air fluid levels in the colon. In children with suspected HD, a contrast enema is routinely applied. Newborns should not have digital examination or rectal washouts prior to contrast enema, as these procedures may result in a false-negative diagnosis. In particular, in patients with suspected meconium ileus or meconium plug syndrome, a water-soluble contrast medium should always be preferred to barium to reduce the obstruction. The classic finding is that of a normal-caliber rectum or narrow distal segment, a funnel-shaped dilation at the level of the transition zone, and a marked dilation of the proximal colon. In questionable cases, retention of contrast medium in the colon for more than 24 hours may be helpful in establishing the diagnosis (Fig. 34–5).

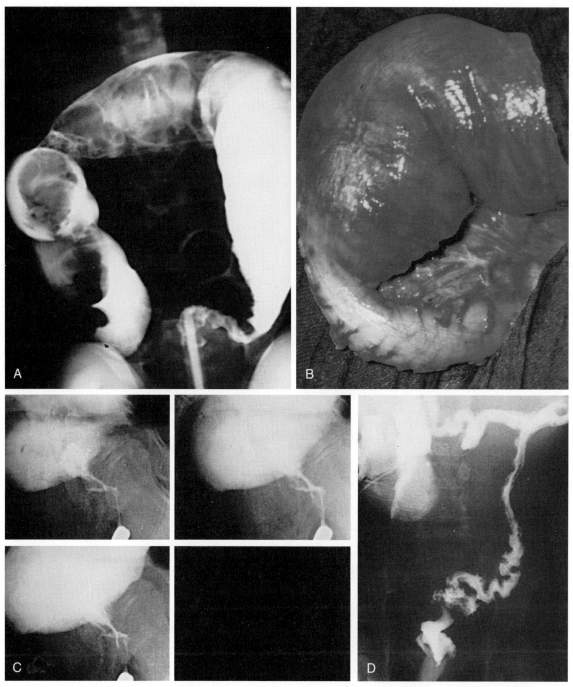

Figure 34–5. *A*, Classic radiographic finding of Hirschsprung's disease with narrow segment, short transitional zone, and proximal dilation. *B*, Intraoperative picture. *C*, Defecography showing ultrashort Hirschsprung's disease. *D*, Long-segment Hirschsprung's disease (Zuelzer-Wilson syndrome).

Contrast enema examination has been reported to be inconclusive in 10% of children with confirmed HD and in 29% of cases with HD-associated IND type B.[36] In children with total aganglionosis, the colon is not significantly narrowed and reflux into the distended ileum may be diagnostic.[71] Children with enterocolitis may show thickening of the bowel wall with mucosal irregularity and grossly distended bowel loops on plain films. In these cases, a characteristic transitional zone may not be present due to inflammatory impairment of muscular function in the normally innervated colon.

The assessment of the intestinal transit time using radiopaque markers offers an opportunity to identify the level of an eventual impairment of transport. The transit time is always prolonged in classic aganglionosis, and determining the most distal point reached by transport markers may help in identifying the level of resection. In addition, the clinical impact of associated intestinal neuronal malformations such as IND type B or hypoganglionosis can be determined.[72] No one method of evaluation of intestinal transport is generally accepted. One study used three different forms of markers given on three consecutive days with an abdominal radiograph on day 4.[73] Others rely on radiographs on days 5 or 7.[73] We give 20 markers simultaneously, repeating the abdominal radiograph every 24 hours for 3 days (Fig. 34–6). The technique can also be used in children with an enterostoma before a pull-through procedure to measure the transport from the distal stoma to the anus.

ANORECTAL ELECTROMANOMETRY

The diagnostic accuracy of anorectal manometry for HD has been reported to be as high as 85%.[36, 75–77] Normally, distension of the rectum using a balloon results in relaxation of the internal sphincter. In HD, the pressure profile of the anal canal and lower rectum in conjunction with the distending stimulus shows characteristic changes that are also occasionally found in other intestinal malformations. In children with aganglionosis, multisegmental rhythmical contractions or waves were pathognomonic (Fig. 34–7). On distension of a balloon in the rectum, no rectal or anal inhibitory response is noted. The anorectal pressure profile is sometimes elevated. Patients with hypoganglionosis or IND may also have a missing or rudimentary response.[36] However, anorectal manometry can be misleading in newborns. We believe that the normal rectosphincteric reflex is complete by the 12th day of life.[78] This reflex has not been identified in children younger than 39 weeks in gestational age or those weighing less than 2.7 kg. With these caveats, anorectal manometry

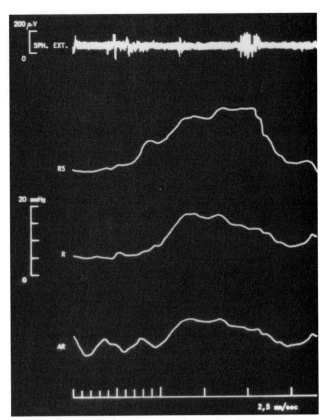

Figure 34–7. Classic electromanometric findings in a patient with Hirschsprung's disease: no internal sphincter relaxations but multisegmental mass contractions.

represents an excellent screening tool for HD and allied disorders.

RECTAL BIOPSY

HD is diagnosed by examination of rectal biopsy specimens. Since the introduction of suction biopsy techniques,[79] the procedure has become less traumatic and can be performed without anaesthesia. Suction biopsy specimens are taken at 2 cm, 3 cm, 5 cm, and, if possible, higher up above the dentate line. They may also be taken proximal and distal to a proposed stoma. However, the optimal size of a biopsy is approximately 3.5 mm in diameter to include submucosa. Perforation and bleeding due to suction biopsies have been reported in newborns. Ganglion cells in the newborn can be immature and not clearly visible without special staining techniques (LDH, SDH reaction). Small suction biopsies are not always representative for the whole involved segment. Aganglionosis may therefore be overdiagnosed at birth, leading to unnecessary resections if the definitive procedure is performed in the newborn period. Hypoganglionosis may be missed when the biopsies only contain submucous plexus. In children with suspected hypoganglionosis or heterotopia of the myenteric plexus, full-thickness biopsies are recommended (Figs. 34–8, 34–9).

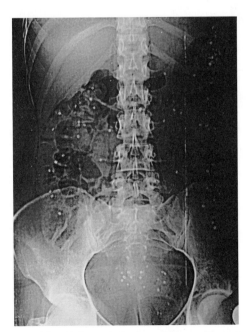

Figure 34–6. Transit-time study in a 36-year-old woman with intestinal neuronal dysplasia 11 days after ingestion of barium pellets.

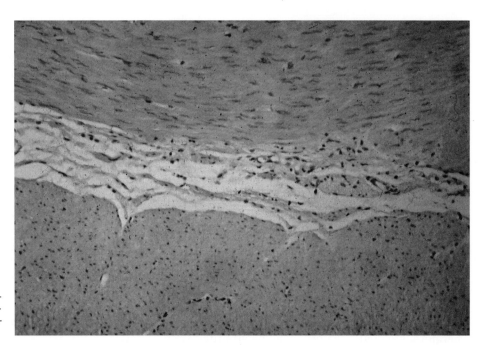

Figure 34–8. Histologic examination (hematoxylin and eosin staining): aganglionosis of the myenteric plexus.

□ Differential Diagnosis

In the newborn infant, it may be clinically difficult to differentiate between meconium plug syndrome, small left colon syndrome, HD, and allied ENS disorders. In addition, neonatal sepsis and brain injury may result in a delayed passage of meconium. However newborns and infants with symptoms of an ileus or enterocolitis should always be suspected to have HD or one of the allied disorders. In these patients, a contrast enema, histochemical examination of suction biopsies, and perhaps manometry will establish the diagnosis of aganglionosis.

Various other conditions may cause chronic constipation and intestinal obstruction in infants and children. These include inadequate dietary habits, psychological disorders, hypomotility caused by medication, and metabolic or endocrine conditions such as uremia or hypothyroidism. Other conditions that may produce constipation include disorders of the intrinsic enteric nerves (diabetes or dysautonomia), central nervous system diseases, and smooth muscle dysfunction. Intestinal smooth muscle disorders include hollow visceral myopathy syndrome and other myopathic disorders. Abnormalities of contractile proteins and connective tissue disorders such as scleroderma or dermatomyositis may also lead to persistent constipation.

Megacystis-microcolon–intestinal hypoperistalsis

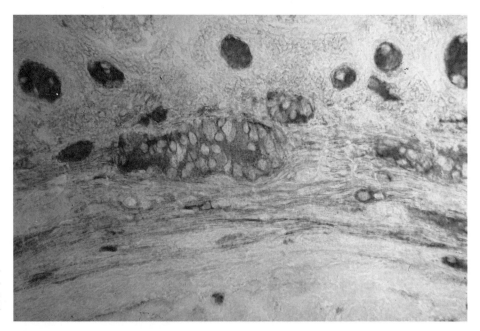

Figure 34–9. Histochemical examination: giant and heterotopic ganglion cells in the submucous plexus of a patient with intestinal neuronal dysplasia.

syndrome represents a rare cause of chronic intestinal obstruction in the newborn that is generally fatal. Degenerative changes in the smooth muscle cells with an abundant amount of connective tissue may be the cause of the disease, but the etiology remains unclear.[80] Not more than 70 cases have been described so far.[81] Abdominal distension is caused by lax abdominal musculature and a distended bladder. Characteristically incomplete intestinal rotation and microcolon with decreased peristalsis are found. Barium enema demonstration of a microcolon and ultrasonographic or intravenous urographic evidence of hydronephrosis and megacystis help to differentiate the condition from HD.

□ Management

The ENS is the brain of the intestine. Similar to the brain, it functions automatically to some degree, even when some neural mechanisms are deficient. Therefore, affected newborns may be admitted with intestinal obstruction, whereas others present later in childhood or adulthood with chronic constipation. Once symptomatic, most patients require decompression as the first step of management.

DECOMPRESSION

Decompression in the obstructed newborn is performed by introducing a nasogastric tube and by repeated emptying of the rectum using rectal tubes and irrigations. After the diagnosis is established by radiologic, electromanometric, and histochemical techniques, an appropriate stoma is established if necessary. Occasionally, patients can be managed satisfactorily over longer periods with irrigations or other conservative means to ensure daily evacuation.

COLOSTOMY

Our preference in the newborn who is obstructed by HD is to establish an enterostomy. We believe that the definitive procedures can be performed more satisfactorily outside the newborn period. In our opinion, enterostomy can only be avoided in children who are older than 3 to 5 months when the diagnosis is established.

Before performing a colostomy, a bowel washout is mandatory. Antibiotics are given intravenously 30 minutes before the operation. A urethral catheter is introduced to achieve bladder decompression during the operation and to provide postoperative drainage. We usually create a "loop" colostomy or ileostomy with a skin bridge beneath. Care should be taken not to narrow the proximal stoma, which might create a partial obstruction. Prolapse of the bowel, the second most frequent complication, can be avoided by suturing the afferent and efferent segments of the bowel loop together within the abdomen. The stoma is preferably constructed using

the right transverse colonic flexure, to be left in place during the definitive resection. It will be closed 2 weeks later. When near-total or total colectomy is necessary, the procedure is protected by an ileostomy.

A leveling end colostomy using frozen section confirmation of the level of ganglion cells is an alternative management technique. In this case, the aganglionic distal bowel is closed as a Hartmann pouch. The pull-through is not protected by a colostomy.

□ Definitive Procedures

Swenson and Bill performed the first resection of an aganglionic segment in 1948.[82] Since then, three other basic techniques have been developed (Fig. 34–10).

SWENSON'S TECHNIQUE

The patient is positioned to simultaneously provide surgical access to the abdomen and perineum. Seromuscular or full-thickness biopsies are taken to establish the proximal extent of aganglionosis by rapid staining techniques. The proximal colon and mesentery are dissected to achieve a sufficient length for reconstruction without compromising the blood supply.

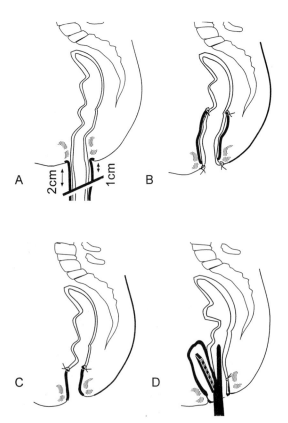

Figure 34–10. Schematic of principles of pull-through and anastomotic techniques according to Swenson (A), Soave (B), Rehbein (C), and Duhamel (D).

The peritoneal reflection at the rectosigmoid is then incised, both ureters and vas deferens are identified, and the deep pelvic dissection commenced. The dissection is performed close to the rectal wall to protect the pelvic autonomic nervous system. Division of the rectosigmoid is accomplished by a stapling device at a convenient level. A long, curved clamp is then inserted through the anus to grasp the rectosigmoid stump and invert it. The mucocutaneous line should be clearly visible. An oblique incision is made through the anterior half of the prolapsed rectum, and a clamp is inserted into the pelvis to grasp and pull through the proximal ganglionated segment through the anus. The proximal bowel wall is now divided, and an extra-anal anastomosis is performed with interrupted absorbable sutures approximating first the muscular coats and then the mucosal layers. Finally, the anastomosis is permitted to recede into the pelvis (see Fig. 34–10A).

DUHAMEL-GROB PROCEDURE

The principles of this procedure are preservation of the internal anal sphincter; opening of the retrorectal space only, followed by retrorectal pull-through of the ganglionic part of the colon; and elimination of the colorectal septum. The rectum is divided and closed just above the peritoneal reflection. Resection of the aganglionic colon is then performed. The retrorectal space is developed bluntly down to the pelvic floor. In the original Duhamel procedure,[83, 84] a long, curved forceps fitted with a small sponge is pushed into this space to evert the posterior rectal wall through the anus. The posterior half of the rectum is incised just above the dentate line. Grob[85] incised the posterior wall 1.5 to 2.5 cm above the mucocutaneous junction. The sponge can then be grasped by another curved clamp, which is pushed in a retrograde manner into the pelvis. The colon then can easily be pulled through the endoanal incision. At a level where ganglion cells have been demonstrated, the colon is transected and anastomosed to the cut edge of the rectum, creating an end-to-side colorectal anastomosis. The ultimate side-to-side anastomosis of the anterior aganglionic rectum and posterior ganglionated colon is created either by crushing the septum or by use of a long stapling device. Today, the rectocolic anastomosis is most often performed using a stapling device.[86] This technique must avoid the creation of an anterior blind rectal pouch, which will lead to retention of feces and obstruction (see Fig. 34–10D).

ANTERIOR RESECTION ACCORDING TO REHBEIN

Rehbein's technique differs from Swenson's procedure, in that the anastomosis is a low, anterior colorectal anastomosis. The pelvirectal dissection is completed, leaving the aganglionic terminal 2 to 3 cm of the rectum in infants and 4 to 5 cm in older

children. Vigorous sphincter dilation with Hegar's bougies are performed intraoperatively up to one size over the size of the stapling instrument choosen for anastomosis. We perform this bouginage under direct vision to avoid bowel rupture. Dilation of the internal anal sphincter is extremely important and must be repeated in later years because the internal anal sphincter remains aganglionic (sphincter achalasia). However, deep dissection of the upper and middle rectum decreases the resting internal anal sphincter tone.

The anastomosis may be performed using a circular end-to-end anastomosis (EEA) stapling instrument introduced through the anus[87] or by direct suture deep in the pelvis. In these cases, the anastomosis is constructed using interrupted 4-0 absorbable sutures. An extraperitoneal drain is placed, the peritoneum is closed above the anastomosis, and a transanastomotic drain is inserted through the anus. The drain can be removed after 10 to 12 days when a contrast enema shows a healed anastomosis. Gentle dilation of the anus using Hegar dilators is then commenced. The size of the dilators is gradually increased with time until the fifth finger can easily pass the anastomosis (see Fig. 34–10C).

ENDORECTAL PULL-THROUGH

The use of extramucosal dissection of the rectosigmoid was proposed[88, 89] for the treatment of high imperforate anus and was later used by Soave in HD cases to avoid primary anastomosis.[90] The first steps of the procedure are similar to the techniques described previously. After opening of the peritoneal reflection, the rectum is dissected over at least two additional centimeters extraperitoneally. Procaine hydrochloride in saline solution (0.5%) is injected between the mucosal and muscular layers of the upper rectum to facilitate the dissection. The rectal muscle is incised, and the mucosal tube is freed distally. The mucosal dissection is continued to the level of the dentate line. The progress of the dissection may be assesed by having an assistant's finger introduced into the anus. The mucosa is incised circumferentially at about 1 cm above the dentate line. Soave's procedure requires more mobilization of the colon than Rehbein's technique. The mucosal sleeve is grasped and used as a tractor to pull the colon through to the established level of ganglion cells. This pull-through may be done by attaching the mucosa to a catheter introduced transanally or by using a ring forceps. The abdominal part of the operation is completed by suturing the proximal free end of the aganglionic rectal cuff to the seromuscular layer of the pulled-through colon. The perineal stage is completed by anchoring the serosa of the colon to the everted anal canal mucosa. A Penrose drain is placed extraperitoneally between the rectal muscle sleeve and the pulled through colon.

After 10 days, when the serosa of the ganglionic colon is adherent to the rectal muscle sleeve, the protruding colon stump is amputated and a mucosa-to-mucosa anastomosis is done (see Fig. 34–10B).

Boley's procedure uses the same endorectal technique but is completed at one sitting with a primary two-layer anastomosis at the pectinate line.[91] Others have added a posterior rectal myotomy and a partial sphincterectomy to avoid anorectal dysfunction, which could result from anal sphincter achalasia.[92, 93] However, sphincteromyectomy increases the risk of fecal incontinence. Boley's procedure has become the more popular in neonates.

LAPAROSCOPIC PULL-THROUGH TECHNIQUES

Advancements in minimally invasive surgery and instrumentation have resulted in pull-through procedures being performed using laparoscopic techniques. The postulated advantages are minimal postoperative pain, more rapid return of bowel function, shorter postoperative recovery, and improved cosmetic appearance. However, the advantages of laparoscopic pull-through techniques have not yet been assessed by randomized trials comparing laparoscopy with the open technique.

Most surgeons who treat HD endoscopically have used a modified Swenson's pull-through technique,[94–96] but the Duhamel method and the Soave technique have been performed laparoscopically as well. The reported techniques were used both for primary pull-through and in patients with diverting enterostomy. Laparoscopic Swenson's pull-through is performed using three 5-mm trocars and standard laparoscopic instruments. The mesentery is mobilized laparoscopically up to the level of the inferior mesenteric artery, which may be divided in patients with a high transition zone. Dissection close to the bowel wall results in minimal bleeding. Laparoscopic pelvic dissection is extended circumferentially to the level of the prostate or cervix and the coccyx. After some transanal submucosal dissection, the smooth muscle fibers of the rectal sleeve are transsected and the colon is pulled through. The colon is transsected and sutured to the everted rectal wall.[95]

The laparoscopic Duhamel procedure is performed via four trocars.[97] After laparoscopic mobilization of the colon, the rectum is divided at the peritoneal level using a stapler. The colon is pulled through an incision made through the posterior rectal wall, and a side-to-side anastomosis is performed as usual. Two or more applications of the stapling device inserted through the anus may be necessary.

Operative times required for the laparoscopic Swenson procedure have been reported to be similar to those for the open technique.[94, 95] The duration of the Duhamel procedure was somewhat longer.[97] Most children were discharged from the hospital between postoperative days 2 and 7, which is shorter than the duration of hospital stay with using the conventional open technique. The reported rate of complications was not higher with laparoscopy.

However, the experience with the technique remains limited to special centers, and the number of patients who have undergone the procedure to date is extremely small. Laparoscopic therapy of HD represents a promising technique, particularly with refinements in instrumentation.

☐ Treatment of Total Colonic Aganglionosis

For the treatment of total colon aganglionosis, Martin[98, 99] introduced a long side-to-side anastomosis between the normal ileum and aganglionic descending colon and the rectum—essentially an extension of the Duhamel side-to-side anastomosis. Theroretically, the long aganglionic rectosigmoid segment should allow resorption of fluid and electrolytes, and recent experience has borne this out.[100] The operation should be performed at the age of 1 year, when the performing of the rectal and pelvic anastomosis is easier. A stapler is applied twice or more to create a long side-to-side anastomosis between the aganglionic rectum and the ganglionated terminal ileum.

Unfortunately, Martin's modification of Duhamel's procedure has not completely eliminated complications such as frequent and liquid stools, excoriated perineum, enterocolitis, and nighttime incontinence, which occur in as many as 60% of the patients.[101] Therefore, we prefer the Rehbein deep anterior resection in patients with total colonic aganglionosis. The persistent rectal achalasia increases transit time and the resorption capability of the ileum without increasing the frequency of enterocolitis. We use a protective ileostomy to protect the anastomosis during the healing phase. Improved bowel resorptive function has been reported by establishment of a right colon onlay patch.[102, 103]

☐ Primary Pull-Through

Primary pull-through in the newborn was introduced mostly by surgeons who prefer Boley's procedure.[104–106] They postulate that endorectal dissection is more difficult to perform in older children than in infants because of tenacious adhesions in the submucous plane caused by chronic proctitis and daily enemas. During the first 3 months of life and especially in the newborn, the rectum shows less inflammation and the dissection between the submucous layer and muscular cylinder is easy to perform. Primary endorectal pull-through usually does not require a protective colostomy, except in patients with enterocolitis. The original Soave technique is still performed at the Gaslini Institute in Genova with the second, perineal stage performed 7 to 10 days after pull-through. The dissection of the last 1 to 2 cm just above the pectineate line is difficult in the newborn, and the mucosal cylinder is very easily damaged.

A reliable histologic and histochemical diagnosis is difficult to establish in the newborn. Adaequate suction biopsies taken above the peritoneal reflection can be dangerous in newborns, and perforations have been reported in that age group. At birth, ganglion cells may be immature, and the cytoplasm may not be visualized by hematoxylin and eosin staining. Because ganglia may not mature for months or years, primary pull-through procedures may lead to excessive or inadequate resection in some newborns. The reported results of primary pull-through are not better than those of staged treatment. In a reported, series of 24 patients, 1 died, 1 developed bowel volvulus, 9 (39%) suffered from recurrent enterocolitis, and 12 (42%) were constipated.[107]

□ Postoperative Care

Some patients experience normal bowel function shortly after the operation. However, in more extented resections, frequent and liquid stools cause excoriation of the perineum. In these patients, loperamide may reduce the frequency of defecation, and kaolin-pectin suspension may help to solidify the stools. Some children develop allergic diarrhea after consuming milk products, food preservatives, nuts, strawberries, or other substances. In patients without an ileocecal valve or with a short remnant colon, cholestyramine is helpful to bind bile salts, which should be absorbed in the terminal ileum. Special diets are often necessary to improve stool consistency (i.e., bananas, carrots, blueberries) or to treat constipation (i.e., rhubarb, prune juice, bran).

□ Complications

The predominant problems after Swenson's and Duhamel's procedures are fecal incontinence and persistent constipation. The major complication following Rehbein's technique is anastomotic leakage, with subsequent stricture formation. Soave's and Boley's operations are complicated by bowel retraction, cuff abscesses, and rectal stenosis caused by the aganglionic rectal muscle cuff. However, all these methods achieve an excellent result in more than 90% of the children.[108]

EARLY COMPLICATIONS

Complications that become manifest within the first four weeks after operation are usually the result of technical errors or infection.[109] In an international study of 439 patients with HD from 16 different pediatric surgical centers, anastomotic leaks were observed in 7%, anastomotic strictures in 15%, and wound infections in 11% of the children.[108] The pulled-through colon retracted in 3% of the children who had Swenson's procedure and in 7% who

underwent Soave's technique. Rehbein's technique showed a peak in 2.8% of 176 cases.

The most frequent early complications after Swenson's and Duhamel's procedures were anastomotic leaks. A survey of the surgical section of the American Academy of Pediatrics (AAP),[110] which included more than 5000 procedures performed by 181 surgeons, revealed anastomotic leaks in 11% after Swenson's procedure and 2.4% after Duhamel's procedure. One fourth of the children with anastomotic disruption following Swenson's technique required a second pull-through, and 11% ultimately had a permanent colostomy. A collected series of 1628 procedures for HD in Japan revealed that anastomotic leaks occurred in 8% after rectosigmoidectomy (Swenson or Rehbein), 7% after Duhamel's procedure, 1% after Soave's endorectal pull-through, and 7% after a Boley procedure.[58] The data from Children's Memorial Hospital in Chicago, which include Swenson's personal experience, revealed anastomotic leaks in 5.6% of 880 patients.[70] In a smaller experience with the Duhamel procedure from another institution, only 1 of 185 patients experience a leak.[111] Fecal fistulas resulted from a leak in 6% of cases using the Swenson procedure, 3% of those utilizing a Duhamel pull-through, and 1% of those utilizing Soave's procedure.

Factors known to increase the risk of anastomotic leak are tension on the anastomosis, ischemia of the rectal cuff or distal colonic segment, incomplete anastomotic suture, and inadequate stapling. Anastomotic leaks always result in anastomotic stricture. Obstruction distal to the anastomosis increases the risk of disruption, so we advise a transanastomotic tube for the first 10 postoperative days. In case of any anastomotic leakage, an immediate enterostomy should performed. Almost all leaks heal spontaneously within 4 to 5 months.

Cuff abscess and retraction of the pull-through segment are most serious complications following Soave's and Boley's operations. Contamination of the cuff, incomplete removal of the mucosa, hemorrhage, or insufficient drainage may lead to formation of a cuff abscess or mucocoele in as many as 5% of the patients. The lower anal channel should be meticulously inspected with a speculum during the operation to prevent leaving islands of mucosa. Creating an anastomosis without any tension but with good blood supply and interrupted full-thickness sutures may help to prevent this complication.

Disturbances of micturition occur more frequently in children who undergo surgery later in life. It is sometimes difficult to wean patients from the urinary catheter placed for the short postoperative period. Dribbling, incomplete urinary control, bladder atony, and ureteric obstruction all have been reported in children after pull-through operations.[112] Voiding dysfunction occured mostly after Swenson's technique (12%) and Duhamel's technique (4%). The condition does not result from a malformation of the autonomic nerve supply to the bladder. Nerve fibers are most probably damaged during the operative procedure or by compression from the enlarged rectum before the operation.

Wound infections or intraabdominal adhesions occur at a rate comparable to those for other major abdominal operations. There is no early mortality rate for classic HD in the present day. However, for total colonic aganglionosis, the AAP Surgical Section survey conducted in the 1970s reported a mortality of 18%.[110] Current results have improved.

LATE COMPLICATIONS

Chronic constipation, enterocolitis, and encopresis represent the most relevant long-term problems. They are found more frequently during the first postoperative months and decrease within the following years. We found that 33% of the children with HD suffered from constipation shortly after the operation, but only 9% reported persistent constipation after an average of 5 years.[68] The frequency of enterocolitis and of encopresis decreased with the passage of time.

Chronic constipation mostly occurs due to anal sphincter achalasia, incomplete resection, stricture formation, and fecaloma. Persistent constipation was reported in 6% of the patients after Swenson's procedure,[113] in 10% after Duhamel's technique,[114] and in 7% after Rehbein's resection.[115]

Anal sphincter achalasia is a frequent postoperative phenomenon. In our series,[108] 32% of patients underwent repeated sphincter dilation, and 13% required sphincteromyectomy. After Rehbein's technique, sphincter dilations are part of the follow-up plan, and bouginage is performed for weeks or months until the anastomosis can no longer be detected by rectal palpation. In Swenson's technique, Duhamel's technique, and some modifications of Soave's technique, internal sphincter myectomy is part of the original procedure. We found the anorectal resting pressure profile to be increased in only 8% of the children after 5 years with no significant difference between the operative procedures used. Internal sphincter relaxations that had not been observed before treatment were present in 10% of the children at follow-up.

Incomplete resection cannot be avoided regardless of technique. Proximal to an aganglionic segment, there is always hypoganglionosis and often IND. The extent of these associated malformations varies considerably in individual patients. Short-segment aganglionosis can be associated with long-segment hypoganglionosis and vice versa. Rapid staining techniques such as hematoxylin and eosin do not allow the reliable diagnosis of either hypoganglionosis or IND.[116] One analysis of 4873 patients with HD from the literature revealed recurrent constipation in 9%.[117] In our opinion, these patients continue to suffer from constipation and/or attacks of enterocolitis due to insufficient resection of segments with hypoganglionosis or IND proximal to the aganglionosis. A second resection may be required when repeated sphincter dilations fail. We

recently reported that reoperation was necessary in 5% of 81 children.[36] Reoperation was necessary in 20 of 215 children. In another study; 9 underwent sphincteromyectomy, and 11 required a repeat pull-through.[118]

Enterocolitis was reported in the Surgical Section survey to occur in 16% of the children undergoing rectosigmoidectomy (Swenson or Rehbein), in 6% undergoing Duhamel's pull-through, in 15% undergoing the Soave technique, and in 2% undergoing the Boley procedure.[110] After Rehbein's procedure, enterocolitis was diagnosed in 10%.[36] In our international study enterocolitis was identified in 4% of the patients after rectosigmoidectomy, in 6% after anterior resection, in 13% after endorectal pull-through without anastomosis, and in 5% after retrorectal pull-through.[108] A literature review found an overall incidence of 8% in 5919 patients.[117] In 1628 Japanese patients, enterocolitis occurred in 34% after Swenson's procedure, in 14% after Duhamel's procedure, in 20% after Soave's procedure, and in 12% following Boley's operation.[58] According to published reports, the incidence of enterocolitis after repair of HD has not changed during recent years.[119]

Strictures result from anastomotic leaks, a narrow rectal muscle cuff around a pulled-through colon, or damage to the blood supply of the cuff or colon. Strictures occurred in 7% of patients having a retrorectal pull-through and 9% of patients having an endorectal pull-through.[119]

Fecal incontinence (soiling, encopresis) does not occur after Rehbein's technique[117] but occurred in 12% of the cases after Swenson's procedures, in 7% after Duhamel's technique, and in 3% following Soave's procedure. Two of 81 of our patients suffered from encopresis; both had sphincteromyectomies performed elsewhere.[36] Incontinence was noted in 9% of the children after Swenson's procedure but in only 3% after Duhamel's technique in the Japanese study.[58] Soiling was noted in 22 of 63 children after Duhamel's operation.[114] in 8% after Swenson's,[113] and in 3% after Soave's[120]; however, in this study, soiling occured in only 1% after Boley's operation. Long-segment disease is associated with a higher incidence of incontinence and soiling, which occur particularly during nighttime. Fecaloma is a complication unique to Duhamel's technique. One study reported that 17.5% of the patients developed fecal impaction and overflow incontinence.[108]

Long-term voiding dysfunction is rare and is mostly observed in older children with long-lasting chronic constipation and an enlarged rectum. These patients develop a large atonic bladder, sometimes with enlargement of the ureters and pelvis of the kidney as a result of compression of the bladder neck. The condition is mostly reversible within months after definitive repair. In a urodynamic study on 68 patients with HD, we found a spontaneous improvement of urinary incontinence from 22 to 6% within 10 years of follow-up.[121] Three children suffered from occasional enuresis, and one girl with cerebral retardation remained incontinent. Sexual dysfunction has been reported in 9% of the patients after Duhamel's procedure and in 10% after Swenson's operation.[120] The authors found dyspareunia in female patients and primary infertility, poor erections, low sperm counts, and psychosexual problems in male patients.

The late mortality compiled from published data[117] ranged from 2% after Soave's procedure to 5% after Swenson's technique and mostly involved patients with long-segment aganglionosis. Similar results were reported by the Surgical Section of the AAP,[110] with a mortality ranging from 1% for Boley's technique to 3% for Soave's two-stage procedure.

□ Ultrashort-Segment Disease

Ultrashort-segment HD is not rare. However, data on the incidence vary considerably because the term *ultrashort* is not clearly defined. One study estimated the incidence of ultrashort HD at 11 to 14% in relation to all aganglionoses.[122] Another group reported on 10 children with ultrashort segment disease out of 106 children with chronic constipation.[123] In a group of patients diagnosed with HD, short-segment disease was found in 2.6% of patients.[18] The gender ratio was estimated to be five male patients to one female one.

The postulated length of the ultrashort segment varied from 2 cm[124] to 10 cm.[125] In our opinion, the term should be restricted to the lowermost 2 to 4 cm of the anal channel above the mucocutaneous line, which means that the aganglionic segment comprises the lower half of the rectum from the dentate line upward to the third sacral vertrebra. Shorter distances restricted to the internal anal sphincter are referred to as *neurogenic anal sphincter achalasia*. Preterm newborns were found to have a 2-mm "physiologic" aganglionic zone in the myenteric plexus and an aganglionic zone of 5 mm of the submucous plexus.[126] The length of this normal zone increased with age of the baby. In contrast, another anatomic study found few ganglion cells in the internal anal sphincter, with decreasing numbers as more distal sections were studied.[127] There is not a clear definition of ultrashort segment aganglionosis or of anal sphincter achalasia, and considerable individual variation in the ganglion cell distribution in the most distal intestinal tract may exist.

The pathophysiology and symptoms of this form of the malformation are similar to classic aganglionosis. Agenesis of NO-fibers and increased AChE-activity in the lamina propria mucosae and submucous plexus (but not in the myenteric plexus) are the most important pathophysiologic parameters.[99, 128, 129] The limited extent of the disease allows for treatment with extended sphincteromyotomy. The procedures can be performed from inside the anus,[130] or from a posterior sagittal approach.[131] An ultrashort aganglionic segment can be associated with an extensive zone of hypoganglionosis leading to persistent severe chronic constipation after sphincteromyotomy.

□ Internal Anal Sphincter Achalasia

Internal anal sphincter achalasia (IASA) is defined as the inability of the internal anal sphincter to relax. IASA may represent an isolated disease of the ENS, or it may be an acquired condition of psychological (functional) origin with normal innervation patterns. However, it may also be part of HD or allied disorders (neurogenic anal sphincter achalasia).[18, 20] The inability of the sphincter to relax can be shown by electromanometry and defecography. The findings are similar to the pathognomonic signs for HD. In hypoganglionosis, IND, and ganglion cell immaturity, the relaxation reflex may be absent, rudimentary, or normal.[36]

On rectal digital examination, the sphincter is hypertonic but the rectum is impacted with stool just above the anal ring. Confirmation of the diagnosis requires biopsies taken at the mucocutaneous junction and a few centimeters above. Anal sphincter dilation under general anaesthesia may be sufficient to treat the condition. In cases with persistent constipation, sphincteromyectomy is indicated. Functional (or psychogenic or acquired) IASA is found in 95% of the cases with chronic constipation. An α receptor–blocking medication (phenoxybenzamine) in addition to psychological treatment may be helpful.[132] (See also Chapter 37.)

□ Intestinal Neuronal Dysplasia and Allied Disorders

The diagnosis of intestinal neuronal malformations has become popularized after Meier-Ruge and other investigators classified IND, hypoganglionosis, and other dysganglionoses.[28, 32, 133, 134] These malformations were found proximal to the aganglionic segment in HD,[36, 60, 135–137] and in patients with various clinical presentations such as chronic constipation,[36, 135, 138] intestinal pseudoobstruction,[139] neurofibromatosis,[140] mucoviscidosis,[36, 141] multiple endocrine neoplasia type IIb,[139] anorectal malformations,[34, 50] and small bowel atresia.[34] Numerous studies have dealt with the sequalae of these malformations, but the causal relationship between specific histologic findings and clinical symptoms remains somewhat controversial.

INTESTINAL NEURONAL DYSPLASIA TYPE A

IND type A is characterized by the paucity of sympathetic fibers and dysplasia of the submucous plexus. Clinical parasympathetic overactivity results in spasticity and ulceration of the colon.[142] The condition is extremely rare. Its dramatic clinical course is characterized by bloody stools combined with ileus.[35, 142, 143] There is unanimous agreement that children with IND type A should undergo rectosigmoidectomy or even more extended resection of the colon.[142, 143]

INTESTINAL NEURONAL DYSPLASIA TYPE B

IND type B may be associated with a great variability of symptoms. Constipation was reported in 53% of children; more significant obstruction, in 20%; colitis in 12%; and bloody stools, diarrhea, or vomiting in fewer than 10%.[144] Other associated symptoms were encopresis, enuresis, or behavioral problems.[136] It remains unclear why some children present with a dramatic clinical course such as meconium peritonitis, volvulus, or intussusception.[24, 145]

Multiple treatment plans have been suggested, including laxatives and enemas, total parenteral nutrition, sphincteromyotomy, colostomy, and partial or total resection with or without leaving IND-affected bowel in place. The results have been discordant because of the wide variations in histochemical involvement and severity of symptoms. In our experience, 25% of the patients require surgical treatment including bowel resection, temporary enterostomy, and sphincteromyotomy.[36] Another surgeon found constipation to be so severe that bowel resection was required in five of nine patients—three of whom died.[133] Posterior sphincteromyotomy was reported to be necessary in 59% of patients in one series, with a cure rate of 90% within 3 months.[143] No bowel was resected in this series. The concept of "temporary" colostomy in patients with severe symptoms is supported by a study that identified a normalization of biopsy findings after 5 years.[146] It has been postulated that patients with IND type B often spontaneously develop normal colon motility with increasing age,[35, 142, 143] but the clinical course after closure of enterostomy has only been investigated in small series.[135, 147] However, medical treatment with laxatives and enemas remains the method of first choice in children without disabling obstruction,[27, 36, 143, 146] and this may be expected to be successful in 75% of the patients.

□ Hypoganglionosis

The analysis of the intramural plexus is essential to establish the diagnosis of hypoganglionosis.[22, 23, 148] The diagnosis is often missed in patients who undergo suction biopsies. Full-thickness biopsies show a reduced number of myenteric ganglia, a low AChE activity in the lamina propria, and hypertrophy of the muscularis mucosae and circular muscle. Only small series of patients with hypoganglionosis of the myenteric plexus have been investigated so far. The symptoms were always severe, and constipation did not improve with time. Seven of nine

children in one series[24] and 11 of 12 patients in another required resection.[149]

□ Other Neuronal Intestinal Malformations

Isolated heterotopia of the myenteric plexus is extremely rare. The heterotopic neurons of the myenteric plexus in the circular and longitudinal muscles contain practically no plexus in the space between the two layers of muscle.[35] This results in severe symptoms mostly requiring bowel resection.[24, 35] The clinical significance of other intestinal malformations remains controversial. Heterotopia of the submucous plexus in the muscularis mucosa is extremely common and seems to be a normal variant.[35] It rarely requires surgical therapy in form of sphincteromyotomy. This also accounts for patients with ganglion-cell hypogenesis, immature ganglion cells, or dysganglionosis.[27, 35, 143, 150]

□ Association of Hirschsprung's Disease and Other Intestinal Neuronal Malformations

Abnormal innervation patterns may be expected in the colon proximal to an aganglionic segment in nearly all children with HD.[150] The reported incidence of associated IND type B is 20 to 75%.[36, 135–137, 143, 144, 151] Hypoganglionosis proximal to the aganglionic segment was seen in 63%, and heterotopic nerve cells of the myenteric plexus, in 20% of patients with HD.[24] It has been postulated that the acute onset of obstruction in patients with IND-associated aganglionosis indicates an additive effect of both lesions. As many as 73% of patients in whom aganglionosis was combined with IND type B presented with ileus, as compared with 32% with isolated aganglionosis.[124, 135, 136]

IND type B may be the cause of persistent constipation or obstructive symptoms after resection for HD. Nine of 16 children investigated for persistent obstructive symptoms had IND type B in one study.[112] Ten children who had enterocolitis, soiling, or constipation after resection for HD were found to have associated IND type B.[137] In another series, six of seven children underwent re-resection, because they also had IND type B.[24] As a consequence, it has been postulated that children who have HD with associated IND type B should undergo a more extended resection at the initial operation.[27] Reports of HD associated with other intestinal malformations are rare, and the clinical significance of these findings remains unclear. We reported 15 HD patients with associated heterotopia of the myenteric plexus who did not suffer significantly more frequent postoperative symptoms compared to patients with classical aganglionosis.[24]

REFERENCES

1. Ehrenpreis TH: Hirschsprung's Disease. Chicago, Year Book Medical Publishers, 1970.
2. Kaiser G, Bettex M: Clinical generalities. In Holschneider AM (ed): Hirschsprung's Disease. Stuttgart/New York, Thieme Stratton, 1982, pp 43–53.
3. Russel MB, Russel CA, Niebuhr E: Familial occurrence of Hirschsprung's disease. Clin Genetics 45:231, 1994.
4. Passarge E: Genetic heterogenicity and recurrence risk of congenital intestinal aganglionosis. Birth defects. Original article series VIII, No 2, 63. Baltimore, Williams & Wilkins, 1972.
5. Engum SA, Petrites M, Rescorla FJ, et al: Familial Hirschsprung's disease: 20 cases in 12 kindreds. J Pediatr Surg 28:1286, 1993.
6. Schiller M, Levy P, Shawa RA, et al: Familial Hirschsprung's disease. A report of 22 affected siblings in four families. J Pediatr Surg 25:322, 1990.
7. Moore SW, Kaschul ROC, Cywes S: Familial and genetic aspects of neuronal intestinal dysplasia and Hirschsprung's disease. Pediatr Surg Int 8:406, 1993.
8. Hirschsprung H: Stuhlträgheit Neugeborener infolge Dilatation und Hypertrophie des Colons. Jahresbericht Kinderheilkunde 27:1, 1888.
9. Derrick EH, St. George-Brambauer BM: Megacolon in mice. J Bact Path 73:569, 1957.
10. Martuciello G, Bjocchi M, Dodero P, et al: Total colonic aganglionosis associated with interstitial deletion of the long arm of chromosome 10. J Pediatr Surg 7:308, 1992.
11. Ikadai H, Fujita H, Agematsu Y, et al: Observation of congenital aganglionosis rat (Hirschsprung's disease rat) and its genetic analysis. Congen Anom 19:31, 1979.
12. Ikadai H, Suzufi K, Fujita H, et al: Animal models of human disease. Hirschsprung's disease. Comp Pathol Bull 13:3, 1981.
13. Lane PW, Liu HM: Association of megacolon with two recessive spotting genes in the mouse. J Hered 57:181, 1966.
14. Cass D: Animal models of aganglionosis. In Holschneider AM, Puri P (eds): Hirschsprung's Disease and Allied Disorders. London, Harwood Academic Publishers, in press.
15. Ceccherini I, Attié T, Martuciello G, et al: The molecular genetics of Hirschsprung's disease. In Holschneider AM, Puri P (eds): Hirschsprung's Disease and Allied Disorders. London, Harwood Academic Publishers, in press.
16. Pelet A, Geneste O, Edery P, et al: Various mechanisms cause RET-mediated signaling defects in Hirschsprung's disease. Presented at The Third International Meeting: Hirschsprung's Disease and Related Neurocristopathies; Evian, France, February 5–8, 1998.
17. Christensen J: Normal colonic motor function and relevant structure. In Holschneider AM, Puri P (eds): Hirschsprung's Disease and Allied Disorders. London, Harwood Academic Publishers, in press.
18. Holschneider AM: Anal sphincter achalasia and ultrashort Hirschsprung's disease. In Holschneider AM, Puri P (eds): Hirschsprung's Disease and Allied Disorders. London, Harwood Academic Publishers, in press.
19. Athow AC, Filipe MI, Drake DP: Problems and advantages of acetylcholinesterase histochemistry of rectal suction biopsies in the diagnosis of Hirschsprung's disease. J Pediatr Surg 25:520, 1990.
20. Kobayashi H, Hirakawa H, Puri P: Abnormal internal anal sphincter innervation in patients with Hirschsprung's disease and allied disorders. J Pediatr Surg 31:794, 1996.
21. Meier-Ruge W: New aspects in the pathophysiology of the hypoganglionic megacolon. Verh Dtsch Ges Pathol 53:237, 1969.
22. Meier-Ruge W: The histologic diagnosis and differential diagnosis of Hirschsprung's disease. In Holschneider AM, Puri P (eds): Hirschsprung's Disease and Allied Disorders. London, Harwood Academic Publishers, in press.
23. Meier-Ruge W, Brunner LA, Engert J, et al: A correlative morphometric and clinical investigation of hypoganglionosis of the colon. Eur J Pediatr Surg 2:67, 1999.
24. Ure BM, Holschneider AM, Schulten D, et al: Clinical impact of intestinal neuronal malformations: A prospective study in 141 patients. Pediatr Surg Int 12:377, 1997.
25. Ikeda K, Goto S, Nagasaki A, et al: Hypogenesis of intestinal ganglion cells: A rare cause of intestinal obstruction simulating aganglionosis. Z Kinderchir 43:52, 1988.
26. Munakata K, Okabe I, Morita K: Histologic studies of rectocolic aganglionosis and allied diseases. J Pediatr Surg 13:67, 1978.
27. Holschneider AM, Meier-Ruge W, Ure BM: Hirschsprung's disease and allied disorders—a review. Eur J Pediatr Surg 4:260, 1994.
28. Meier-Ruge W: Über ein Krankheitsbild mit Hirschsprung's symptomatik. Verh Dtsch Ges Pathol 55:506, 1971.
29. Badner JA, Chakravati A: Waardenburg syndrome and Hirschsprung's disease: Evidence for pleiotropic effects of a single dominant gene. Am J Med Genet 35:100, 1990.
30. Kobayashi H, Hirakawa H, Puri P: What are the diagnostic criteria for intestinal neuronal dysplasia? Pediatr Surg Int 10:459, 1995.
31. Meier-Ruge WA, Brönnimann PB, Gambazzi F, et al: Histopathological criteria for intestinal neuronal dysplasia of the submucous plexus (type B). Virchows Arch 426:549, 1995.
32. Borchard F, Meier-Ruge W, Wiebecke B, et al: Innervationsstörungen des Dickdarms—Klassifikation und Diagnostik. Pathologe 12:171, 1991.
33. Koletzko S, Jesch I, Faus-Kebetaler T, et al: Rectal biopsy for diagnosis of intestinal neuronal dysplasia in children: A prospective multicentre study on interobserver variation and clinical outcome. Gut 44:853, 1999.
34. Holschneider AM, Pfrommer W, Gerrescheim B: Results in the treatment of anorectal malformations with special regard to the histology of the rectal pouch. Eur J Pediatr Surg 4:303, 1994.
35. Meier-Ruge W: Epidemiology of congenital innervation defects of the distal colon. Virchows Archiv A Pathol Anat 420:171, 1992.
36. Ure BM, Holschneider AM, Meier-Ruge W: Neuronal intestinal malformations: A retro- and prospective study on 203 patients. Eur J Pediatr Surg 4:279, 1994.
37. Meier-Ruge W: Desmosis of the colon. A working hypothesis of primary chronic constipation. Eur J Pediatr Surg 8:299–303, 1998.
38. West KW, Grosfeld JL, Rescorla FJ, et al: Acquired aganglionosis: A rare occurrence following pull-through procedures for Hirschsprung's disease. J Pediatr Surg 25:104, 1990.
39. Dajani OM, Slim MS, Mansour A: Acquired hypoganglionosis after endorectal pullthrough procedure—a case report. Z Kinderchir 41:248, 1986.
40. Brown RA, Cywes S: Disorders and congenital malformations associated with Hirschsprung's disease. In Holschneider AM, Puri P (eds): Hirschsprung's Disease and Allied Disorders. London, Harwood Academic Publishers, in press.
41. Meyers SHC: The development of the enteric nerve system. In Holschneider AM, Puri P (eds): Hirschsprung's Disease and Allied Disorders. London, Harwood Academic Publishers, in press.
42. Pingault V, Bondurand N, Kuhlbrodt K, et al: SOX 10 mutations in patients with Waardenburg-Hirschsprung disease. Presented at The Third International Meeting: Hirschsprung's Disease and Related Neurocristopathies; Evian, France, February 5–8, 1998.
43. Brooks AS, Breubing MH, Meijers C: Spectrum of phenotypes associated with Hirschsprung's disease: An evaluation of 239 patients from a single institution. Presented at The Third International Meeting: Hirschsprung's Disease and Related Neurocristopathies; Evian, France, February 5–8, 1998.
44. Hahhad GG, Mazza NM, Defendini R, et al: Congenital failure of automatic control of ventilation, gastrointestinal motility and heart rate. Medicine (Baltimore) 57:517, 1978.
45. Elhalaby E, Coran A: Hirschsprung's disease associated with Ondine's course: Report of three cases and review of the literature. J Pediatr Surg 29:530, 1994.

46. Gaultier CI, Trang-Pham H, Dauger S, et al: Congenital central hypoventilation syndrome phenotypes. Presented at The Third International Meeting: Hirschsprung's Disease and Related Neurocristopathies; Evian, France, February 5–8, 1998.

47. Nakahara S, Yokomori K, Tamura K, et al: Hirschsprung's disease with Ondine's course: A special subgroup? J Pediatr Surg 30:1481, 1995.

48. Steiner AL, Goodman AD, Powers SR: Study of a kindred with pheochromocytoma, medullary thyroid carcinoma, hyperparathyroidism and Cushing disease: Multiple endocrine neoplasia type II. Medicine (Baltimore) 47:371, 1968.

49. Khan AH, Desjardins JG, Youssef S, et al: Gastrointestinal manifestations of Sipple syndrome in children. J Pediatr Surg 22:719, 1987.

50. Holschneider AM, Ure BM, Pfrommer W, Meier-Ruge W: Innervation patterns of the rectal pouch and fistula in anorectal malformations: A preliminary report. J Pediatr Surg 31:357, 1996.

51. Akgur FM, Tanyel FC, Buyukpamukcu N, et al: Colonic atresia and Hirschsprung's association shows further evidence for migration of enteric neurons. J Pediatr Surg 28:635, 1993.

52. Puri P, Wester T: Enterocolitis complicating Hirschsprung's disease. In Holschneier AM, Puri P (eds): Hirschsprung's Disease and Allied Disorders. London, Harwood Academic Publishers, in press.

53. Bill AH, Chapman ND: The enterocolitis of Hirschsprung's disease: Its natural history and treatment. Am J Surg 103:70–74, 1962.

54. Elhalaby EA, Coran AG, Blane CE, et al: Enterocolitis associated with Hirschsprung's disease. A clinical-radiological characterization on 168 patients. J Pediatr Surg 30:76, 1995.

55. Harrison MW, Deitz DE, Campbel JR, et al: Diagnosis and management of Hirschsprung's disease: A 25-year perspective. Am J Surg 152:49, 1986.

56. Sieber WK: Hirschsprung's disease. In Welch KJ, Randolph JG, Ravitch MM, et al (eds): Pediatric Surgery (4th ed). Chicago, Yearbook Medical Publishers, 1986, p 995.

57. Carneiro PMR, Brereton RJ, Drake DP, et al: Enterocolitis in Hirschsprung's disease. Pediatr Surg Int 7:356, 1992.

58. Ikeda K, Goto S: Diagnosis and treatment of Hirschsprung's disease in Japan: Analysis of 1628 patients. J Pediatr Surg 199:400, 1984.

59. Shanbhouge LKR, Bianchi A: Experience with primary Swenson resection and pullthrough for neonatal Hirschsprung's disease. Pediatr Surg Int 5:446, 1990.

60. Surana R, Quinn FMJ, Puri P: Evaluation of risk factors in the development of enterocolitis complicating Hirschsprung's disease. Pediatr Surg Int 9:234, 1994.

61. Akahary S, Sahwy E, Kandil W, et al: A histochemical study of the mucosubstances of the colon in cases of Hirschsprung's disease with and without enterocolitis. J Pediatr Surg 24, 1272, 1989.

62. Fujimoto T, Puri P: Persistence of enterocolitis following diversion of faecal stream in Hirschsprung's disease. A study of mucosal defense mechanisms. Pediatr Surg Int 3:141, 1988.

63. Wilson-Storey D, Scobie WG: Impaired gastrointestinal mucosal defense in Hirschsprung's disease: A clue to the pathogenesis of enterocolitis. J Pediatr Surg 24:462, 1989.

64. Soeda J, O'Brian DS, Puri P: Regional reduction in intestinal neuroendocrine cell populations in enterocolitis complicating Hirschsprung's disease. J Pediatr Surg 28:1063, 1993.

65. Lloyd-Stil JD, Demers LM: Hirschsprung's enterocolitis, prostaglandins, and response to cholestyramine. J Pediatr Surg 13:417, 1978.

66. Thomas DFM, Fernie DS, Bayston R, et al: Enterocolitis in Hirschsprung's disease: A controlled study of the etiologic role of chlostridium difficile. J Pediatr Surg 21:22, 1986.

67. Wilson-Storey D, Scobie WG, McGenity KG: Microbiological studies of the enterocolites of Hirschsprung's disease. Arch Dis Child 65:1338, 1990.

68. Lifschitz CH, Bloss R: Persistence of colitis in Hirschsprung's disease. J Pediatr Gastroenterol Nutr 4:291, 1985.

69. Teitelbaum DH, Caniano DA, Qualman SJ: The pathophysiology of Hirschsprung's associated enterocolitis: Its importance and histologic correlates. J Pediatr Surg 24:1271, 1989.

70. Sherman JO, Snyder ME, Weitzman JJ, et al: A 40-year multinational retrospective study of 880 Swenson procedures. J Pediatr Surg 24:833, 1989.

71. Blake NA: Radiological diagnosis of Hirschsprung disease and allied disorders. In Holschneider AN, Puri P (eds): Hirschsprung's Disease and Allied Disorders. London, Harwood Academic Publishers, in press.

72. Ure BM, Holschneider AM, Schulten D, et al: Intestinal transit time in children with intestinal neuronal malformations mimicking Hirschsprung's disease. Eur J Pediatr Surg 2:91, 1999.

73. Benningha MA, Büllar HA, Staalman CR, et al: Defecation disorders in children, colonic transit time versus the Barr-score. Eur J Pediatr 154:1277, 1995.

74. Papadopoulou A, Clayden GS, Booth IW: The clinical value of solid marker transit studies in childhood constipation and soiling. Eur J Pediatr 153:560, 1994.

75. Holschneider AM: Clinical and electromanometrical investigations of postoperative continence in Hirschsprung's disease. Z Kinderchir 29:39, 1980.

76. Holschneider AM: Elektromanometrie des Enddarms. Diagnostik und Therapie der Inkontinenz und der chronischen Obstipation. 2. Auflage Urban & Schwarzenberg, München Wien Baltimore, 1983.

77. Holschneider AM: Functional studies of Hirschsprung's disease and allied disorders. In Holschneider AM, Puri P (eds): Hirschsprung's Disease and Allied Disorders. London, Harwood Academic Publishers, in press.

78. Holschneider AM, Kellner E, Streibl P, et al: The development of anorectal continence and its significance in the diagnosis of Hirschsprung's disease. J Pediatr Surg 11:151, 1976.

79. Noblett HR: A rectal suction biopsy tube for use in the diagnosis of Hirschsprung's disease. J Pediatr Surg 4:406, 1969.

80. Puri P, Lake BD, Gorman F, et al: Megacystis-microcolon-intestinal hypoperistalsis syndrome: A visceral myopathy. J Pediatr Surg 18:64, 1983.

81. Puri P: Megacystis-microcolon-intestinal hypoperistalsis syndrome. In Holschneider AM, Puri P (eds): Hirschsprung's Disease and Allied Disorders. London, Harwood Academic Publishers, in press.

82. Swenson O, Bill AH: Resection of rectum and rectosigmoid with preservation of sphincter for benign spastic lesions producing megacolon. Surgery 24:212, 1948.

83. Duhamel B: Une nouvelle operation pour le megacolon congenital. L'abaissement retrorectal et transanal du colon et son application possible au traitement de quelques autres malformations. Press Med 64:2249, 1956.

84. Duhamel B: Retrorectal and transanal pullthrough procedure for the treatment of Hirschsprung's disease. Dis Colon Rectum 7:455, 1964.

85. Grob M: Intestinal obstruction in the newborn infant. Arch Dis Child 35:40, 1960.

86. Steichen FM, Spigland NA, Nunez D: The modified Duhamel operation for Hirschsprung's disease performed entirely with mechanical sutures. J Pediatr Surg 22:436, 1987.

87. Holschneider AAM, Söylet Y: Die anteriore Resektion nach Rehbein in der Behandlung des Megacolon congenitum Hirschsprung: Hand oder Stapler Anastomose. Eine vergeichende Studie. Z Kinderchir 44:216, 1989.

88. Romualdi P: Eine neue Operationstechnik für die Behandlung einiger Rectum-Missbildunger Langenbeck's Arch Dtsch Z f Chir 279:37, 1960.

89. Rehbein F: Intraabdominelle Resektion oder Rektosigmoidektomie bei der Hirschsprung'schen Krankheit. Chirurg 29:366, 1964.

90. Soave F: A new original technique for treatment of Hirschsprung's disease. Surgery 56:1007, 1964.

91. Boley SJ: New modification of the surgical treatment of Hirschsprung's disease. Surgery 56:1015, 1964.

92. Marks RM: Endorectal split sleeve pull-through procedure

for Hirschsprung's disease. Surg Gynecol Obstet 136:627, 1973.

93. Kasai M, Suzuki H, Watanabe K: Rectal myotomy with colectomy: A new radical operation for Hirschsprung's disease. J Pediatr Surg 6:36, 1971.

94. Curran TJ, Raffensperger JG: Laparoscopic Swenson's pull-through: A comparison with the open procedure. J Pediatr Surg 31:1155, 1995.

95. Georgeson KE, Fuenfer MM, Hardin WD: Primary laparoscopic pull-through for Hirschsprung's disease in infants and children. J Pediatr Surg 30:1017, 1995.

96. Hoffmann K, Schier F, Waldschmidt J: Laparoscopic Swenson's procedure in children. Eur J Pediatr Surg 6:15, 1996.

97. Bax NMA, van der Zee DC: Laparascopic removal of aganglionic bowel using the Duhamel-Martin method in five consecutive infants. Pediatr Surg Int 10:116, 1995.

98. Martin LW: Surgical management of Hirschsprung's disease involving the small intestine. Arch Surg 97:183, 1968.

99. Martin LW: Surgical management of total colonic aganglionosis. Am Surg 176:343, 1972.

100. Heath AL, Spitz L, Milla PJ: The absorptive function of colonic aganglionic intestine: Are the Duhamel and Martin procedures rational? J Pediatr Surg 20:34, 1985.

101. Ein SH, Shandling B: Long Duhamel procedure. In Holschneider AM, Puri P (eds): Hirschsprung's Disease and Allied Disorders (2nd ed). London, Harwood Academic Publishers, 1999.

102. Emslie J, Krishnamoorthy M, Allebaum H: Long-term follow up of patients treated with ileoendorectal pull-through and right colon onlay patch form total colonic aganglionosis. J Pediatr Surg 32:1542, 1997.

103. Suita S, Taguchi T, Kamimura T, et al: Total colonic aganglionosis with or without small bowel involvement: A changing profile. J Pediatr Surg 32;1537, 1997.

104. Carcassone M, Morisson-Lacombe G, LeTourneau JW: Primary corrective operation without decompression in infants less than three months of age with Hirschsprung's disease. J Pediatr Surg 17:241, 1982.

105. Cilley RE, Slatter MB, Hirschl RB, et al: Definitive treatment of Hirschsprung's disease in the newborn with a one-stage procedure. Surgery 115:551, 1994.

106. So HB, Schwartz DL, Becker JM, et al: Endorectal pull-through without preliminary colostomy in neonates with Hirschsprung's disease. J Pediatr Surg 15:470, 1980.

107. Teitelbaum DH, Drongowski RA, Chamberlain JN, et al: Long-term stooling patterns in infants undergoing primary endorectal pull-through for Hirschsprung's disease. J Pediatr Surg 32:1049, 1997.

108. Clinical and electromanometric studies of postoperative continence in Hirschsprung's disease: Relationship to the surgical procedures. In Holschneider AM (ed): Hirschsprung's Disease. Stuttgart/New York, Thieme Stratton, 1982, pp 221–241.

109. Holschneider AM: Complication after surgical treatment of Hirschsprung's disease. In Heberer G (ed): Anglo-German Coloproctology Meeting 1981. Berlin, Heidelberg, New York, Springer, 1981.

110. Kleinhaus S, Boley SJ, Sheran M, et al: Hirschsprung's disease. A survey of the members of the surgical section of the American Academy of Pediatrics. J Pediatr Surg 14:588, 1979.

111. Rescorla FJ, Morrison AM, Engles D, et al: Hirschsprung's disease—evaluation of mortality and long-term function in 260 cases. Arch Surg 127:934, 1992.

112. Moore SW, Millar AJ, Cywes S: Long-term clinical, manometric, and histological evaluation of obstructive symptoms in the postoperative Hirschsprung's patient. J Pediatr Surg 29:106, 1994.

113. Liem NT, Hau BD, Thu NX: The long-term follow up result of Swenson's operation in the treatment of Hirschsprung's disease in Vietnamese children. Eur J Pediatr Surg 14:110, 1993.

114. Heij HA, de Vries X, Bremer I, et al: Long-term anorectal function after Duhamel operation for Hirschsprung's disease. J Pediatr Surg 30:430, 1995.

115. Wester T, Hoehner J, Olsen L: Rehbein's anterior resection in Hirschsprung's disease, suing a circular stapler. Eur J Pediatr Surg 5:358, 1995.

116. Kobayashi H, Wang Y, Hirakawa H, et al: Intraoperative evaluation of extent of aganglionosis by a rapid acetylcholinesterase histochemical technique. J Pediatr Surg 30:248, 1995.

117. Joppich I: Late complications of Hirschsprung's disease. In Holschneider AM (ed): Hirschsprung's Disease. Hippokrates Stuttgart, Thieme Stratton, New York, 1982, pp 25–26.

118. Banani SA, Forootan HR, Kumar PV: Intestinal neuronal dysplasia as a cause of surgical failure in Hirschsprung's disease: A new modality for surgical management. J Pediatr Surg 31:572, 1996.

119. Snyder CL, Ashcraft KW: Late complications of Hirschsprung's disease. In Holschneider AM, Puri P (eds): Hirschsprung's Disease and Allied Disorders. London, Harwood Academic Publishers, in press.

120. Moore SW, Albertyn R, Cywes S: Clinical outcome and long-term quality of life after surgical correction of Hirschsprung's disease. J Pediatr Surg 31:1996, 1996.

121. Holschneider AM, Kraeft H, Scholtissek CH: Urodynamic Investigations of bladder disturbances in imperforate anus and Hirschsprung's disease. Z Kinderchir 35:64, 1982.

122. Meier-Ruge W, Schärli AF: The epidemiology and enzyme histotopochemical characterization of ultrashort-segment Hirschsprung's disease. Pediatr Surg Int 1:37, 1986.

123. Clayden GS, Lawson JON: Investigation and management of long-standing chronic constipation in childhood. Arch Dis Child 51:918, 1976.

124. Bettex M: Megakolon. In Zenker R, Deucher F, Schink W: Chirurgie der Gegenwart. Vol. 7. München, Berlin, Wien, Urban & Schwarzenberg, 1976.

125. Nissan S, Bar-Moar JA: Further experience in the diagnosis and surgical treatment of short-segment Hirschsprung's disease and idiopathic megacolon. J Pediatr Surg 6:738, 1971.

126. Aldrige RT, Campbell PE: Ganglion cell distribution in the normal rectum and anal canal. A basis for the diagnosis of Hirschsprung's disease by anorectal biopsy. J Pediatr Surg 3:475, 1968.

127. Müntefering H, Welskop J, Fadda B, et al: Enzymhistotopochemische Befunde bei der neurogenen Achalasie des M. Sphincter ani internus. Verh Dtsch Ges Path 70:622, 1986.

128. Meier-Ruge W: Der ultrakurze M. Hirschsprung: Ein bioptisch zuverlässig objectivierbares Krankheitsbild. Z Kinderchir 40:146–150, 1985.

129. Puri P: Hirschsprung's disease: Clinical and experimental observations. World J Surg 17:374, 1993.

130. Bentley JFR: Some new observations on megacolon in infancy and childhood with special reference to the management of megasigmoid and megarectum. Dis Colon Rectum 7:462, 1964.

131. Lynn HB: Rectal myectomy for aganglionic megacolon. Mayo Clin Proc 41:289, 1966.

132. Holschneider AM, Kraeft H: Die Wirkung von Alpha-Blockern auf den Muskulus sphincter ani internus. Z Kinderchir 30:152, 1980.

133. Munakata K, Morita K, Okabe I, et al: Clinical and histologic studies of neuronal intestinal dysplasia. J Pediatr Surg 20:231, 1985.

134. Puri P, Fujimoto T: Diagnosis of allied functional bowel disorders using monoclonal antibodies and electronmicroscopy. J Pediatr Surg 23:546, 1988.

135. Briner J, Oswald HW, Hirsig J, et al: Neuronal intestinal dysplasia—clinical and histochemical findings and its association with Hirschsprung's disease. Z Kinderchir 41:282, 1986.

136. Fadda B, Pistor G, Meier-Ruge W, et al: Symptoms, diagnosis, and therapy of neuronal intestinal dysplasia masked by Hirschsprung's disease. Pediatr Surg Int 2:76, 1987.

137. Kobayashi H, Hirakawa H, Surana R, et al: Intestinal neuronal dysplasia is a possible cause of persistent bowel symptoms after pull-through operation for Hirschsprung's disease. J Pediatr Surg 30:253, 1995.

138. Koletzko S, Ballauff A, Hadzilelimovic F, et al: Is histologi-

cal diagnosis of neuronal intestinal dysplasia related to clinical and manometric findings in constipated children? Results of a pilot study. J Pediatr Gastroenterol Nutr 17:59, 1993.

139. Navarro J, Sonsino E, Boige N, et al: Visceral neuropathies responsible for chronic intestinal pseudo-obstruction syndrome in pediatric practice: Analysis of 26 cases. J Pediatr Gastroenterol Nutr 11:179, 1990.

140. Saul RA, Sturner RA, Burger PC: Hyperplasia of the myenteric plexus: Its association with early infantile megacolon and neurofibromatosis. Am J Dis Child 136:852, 1982.

141. Wildhaber J, Seelentag WKF, Spiegel R, et al: Cystic fibrosis associated with neuronal intestinal dysplasia type B: A case report. J Pediatr Surg 31:951, 1996.

142. Fadda B, Maier WA, Meier-Ruge W, et al: Neuronal intestinal Dysplasie. Eine kritische 10-Jahres-Analyse klinischer und bioptischer Diagnostik. Z Kinderchir 38:305, 1983.

143. Schärli AF: Neuronal intestinal dysplasia. Pediatr Surg Int 7:2, 1992.

144. Csury L, Pena A: Intestinal neuronal dysplasia. Pediatr Surg Int 10:441, 1995.

145. Sacher P, Briner J, Stauffer UG: Unusual cases of neuronal intestinal dysplasia. Pediatr Surg Int 6:225, 1991.

146. Simpser E, Kahn E, Kenigsberg K, et al: Neuronal intestinal dysplasia: Quantitative diagnostic criteria and clinical management. J Pediatr Gastroenterol Nutr 12:61, 1991.

147. Rintala R, Rapola J, Louhimo I: Neuronal intestinal dysplasia. Progr Pediatr Surg 24:186, 1989.

148. Meier-Ruge W, Schärli AF, Stoss F: How to improve histopathological results in the biopsy diagnosis of gut dysganglionosis. Pediatr Surg Int 10:454, 1995.

149. Munakata K, Okabe I, Morita K: Hypoganglionosis. Pediatr Surg Int 7:8, 1992.

150. Ure BM, Holschneider AM: Treatment of intestinal neuronal malformations mimicking Hirschsprung's disease. In Holschneider AM, Puri P (eds): Hirschsprung's Disease and Allied Disorders. London, Harwood Academic Publishers, in press.

151. Hanimann B, Inderbitzin D, Briner J, et al: Clinical relevance of Hirschsprung-associated neuronal intestinal dysplasia (HANID). Eur J Pediatr Surg 2:147, 1992.

35

IMPERFORATE ANUS AND CLOACAL MALFORMATIONS

Alberto Peña, MD

□ History

Imperforate anus has been a well-known and well-recognized condition since antiquity.[1-3] For many centuries, physicians, as well as individuals who practiced medicine, created an orifice in the perineum of children with imperforate anus. Many of these children survived. Most likely, they suffered from a type of defect that would now be recognized as "low." Those with a "high" defect did not survive that kind of treatment. Amussat, in 1835, first sutured the rectal wall to the skin edges, which could be considered the first actual anoplasty.[2]

During the first 60 years of the 20th century, most surgeons performed a perineal anoplasty without a colostomy for so-called low malformations. A colostomy performed during the newborn period was followed by an abdominoperineal pull-through operation for the treatment of high malformations. The decision to create the colostomy was based mainly on the radiologic information obtained by the invertogram.[4] During the era of the abdominoperineal pull-through operation, the specific recommendation was made many times to pull the bowel as close to the sacrum as possible to avoid trauma to the genitourinary (GU) tract.

Stephens made a significant contribution to the field by performing the first objective anatomic studies of human specimens. In 1953, Stephens[5] proposed an initial sacral approach followed by an abdominoperineal operation, when necessary. The purpose of the sacral stage of the procedure was to preserve the puborectalis sling, considered a key factor in maintaining fecal continence.[5] Since then, different surgical techniques have been proposed by others.[6-9] All of the techniques had as a common denominator the protection and use of the puborectalis sling.

The posterior sagittal approach for the treatment of these defects was performed first in September 1980, and, subsequently, its description was published in 1982.[10, 11] This approach allowed direct exposure of this important anatomic area. Also, the unique opportunity arose to correlate the external appearance of the perineum with the operative findings and, subsequently, with the clinical results. Significant implications emerged in terms of terminology and classification.

□ Incidence, Types of Defects, and Terminology

Imperforate anus occurs in 1 of every 4000 to 5000 newborns.[12-14] The estimated risk for a couple having a second child with an anorectal malformation is approximately 1%.[15-17] The frequency of this defect is slightly higher in male than in female patients. The most frequent defect in male patients is imperforate anus, with a rectourethral fistula.[18] The most frequent defect in female patients is rectovestibular fistula.[18] Imperforate anus without a fistula is a rather unusual defect; it occurs in about 5% of the entire group of malformations.[18] Persistent cloaca was considered an unusual defect.[19] Instead, a high incidence of rectovaginal fistula was reported in the literature.[19] In retrospect, it seems that the presence of a cloaca is a much more common defect in female patients. Moreover, presence of a cloaca is probably the third most common defect in female patients after perineal fistulas and vestibular fistulas. In fact, rectovaginal fistula is almost a nonexistent defect, which is present in fewer than 1% of all cases.[20, 21] Probably, most patients suffering from a persistent cloaca were erroneously thought to have a rectovaginal fistula. Many of those patients underwent surgery, and the rectal component of the malformation was repaired, but the patients were left with a persistent urogenital sinus. Also, recent evidence shows that most of the rectovestibular fistulas were frequently called "rectovaginal fistula." Rectobladder-neck fistula in male patients is the only real supralevator muscle malformation and fortunately

473

TABLE 35–1. Classification of
Anorectal Malformations

Gender	Malformation	Colostomy Required
Male	Cutaneous fistula (perineal fistula)	No
	Rectourethral fistula	
	Bulbar	Yes
	Prostatic	Yes
	Rectovesical fistula	Yes
	Anorectal agenesis without fistula	Yes
	Rectal atresia	Yes
Female	Cutaneous (perineal) fistula	No
	Vestibular fistula	Yes
	Anorectal agenesis without fistula	Yes
	Rectal atresia	Yes
	Persistent cloaca	Yes

occurs in only about 10% of all male patients.[18, 20, 21] It is the only defect in male patients that requires a laparotomy in addition to the lower approach for repair.

Anorectal malformation represents a wide spectrum of defects. The terms *low*, *intermediate*, and *high* are rather arbitrary and not useful in therapeutic or prognostic terms. Within the group of anorectal malformations traditionally referred to as high, there were defects included with different therapeutic and prognostic implications. For instance, rectoprostatic fistula and rectobladder-neck fistula were both considered high, yet the first one can be repaired via posterior sagittal entry only, and the last one requires, in addition, a laparotomy. Furthermore, the prognosis for each type is completely different. Therefore, a more therapeutic-oriented classification is proposed in Table 35–1.

MALE DEFECTS

Cutaneous Fistulas

Cutaneous fistula is a low defect. The rectum is located within most of the sphincter mechanism. Only the lowest part of the rectum is anteriorly mislocated (Fig. 35–1A). Sometimes, the fistula does not open into the perineum but rather follows a subepithelial midline tract, opening somewhere

along the midline perineal raphe, scrotum, or even at the base of the penis. The diagnosis is established by perineal inspection. No further investigations are required.

Most of the time, the anal (fistula) opening is abnormally narrow (stenosis). The terms *covered anus*, *anal membrane*, and *bucket handle* malformations refer to different external manifestations of perineal fistulas.

Rectourethral Fistulas

The opening of the rectourethral fistula, the most frequent defect in the male patients,[18, 20] may be located at the lower part of the urethra (bulbar urethra; Fig. 35–1B) or at the upper urethra (prostatic urethra; Fig. 35–2A). Immediately above the fistula site, rectum and urethra share a common wall. This important anatomic fact has significant technical and surgical implications. The rectum is usually distended and surrounded laterally and posteriorly by the levator muscle. Between the rectum and the perineal skin, a portion of striated voluntary muscle called the muscle complex is present. The contraction of these muscle fibers elevates the skin of the anal dimple. At the level of the skin, a group of voluntary muscle fibers, called parasagittal fibers, are located on both sides of the midline. Lower urethral (bulbar) fistulas are usually associated with good-quality muscles, well-developed sacrum, prominent midline groove, and prominent anal dimple. Higher urethral (prostatic) fistulas are more frequently associated with poor-quality muscles, abnormally developed sacrum, and flat perineum with poor midline grooves and no visible anal dimple. However, exceptions to these rules exist. Frequently, patients pass meconium through the urethra—an unequivocal sign of rectourinary fistula.

Rectovesical Fistulas

In this defect, the rectum opens at the bladder neck (Fig. 35–2B). The patient has a poor prognosis because the levator muscle, muscle complex, and external sphincter frequently are poorly developed. The sacrum is often deformed. The entire pelvis seems to be underdeveloped (see Fig. 35–2B). The perineum is often flat, with evidence of poor muscle

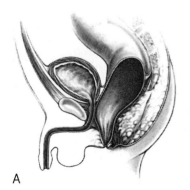
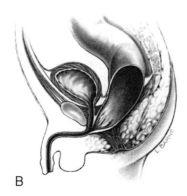

A   B

Figure 35–1. Spectrum of defects in male patients. *A*, Perineal fistula. *B*, Rectourethrobulbar fistula. (From Peña A: Atlas of Surgical Management of Anorectal Malformations. New York, Springer-Verlag, 1990, p 26. Lois Barnes, medical illustrator.)

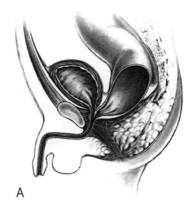
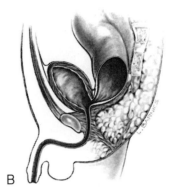

Figure 35–2. Spectrum of defects in male patients. *A*, Rectourethroprostatic fistula. *B*, Rectobladderneck fistula. (From Peña A: Atlas of Surgical Management of Anorectal Malformations. New York, Springer-Verlag, 1990, p 26. Lois Barnes, medical illustrator.)

A

B

development. About 10% of imperforate anus cases in males are in this category.[18, 20]

Anorectal Agenesis Without Fistulas

Interestingly, most patients with this unusual defect have a well-developed sacrum and good muscles. The rectum ends approximately 2 cm from the perineal skin. The patient usually has a good prognosis in terms of bowel function.[18, 20] Even when the patient does not have a communication between rectum and urethra, these two structures are separated only by a thin, common wall, which is an important anatomic detail with technical implications. About half of the patients with no fistula also suffer from Down syndrome, and more than 90% of patients with Down syndrome and imperforate anus suffer from this specific defect.[22] The fact that these patients have Down syndrome does not seem to interfere with the good prognosis in terms of bowel control for this malformation.[22]

Rectal Atresia

In this extremely unusual defect in male patients, the lumen of the rectum may be totally (atresia) or partially (stenosis) interrupted. The blind upper pouch is represented by a dilated rectum, whereas the lower portion is represented by a small anal canal, which measures approximately 1 to 2 cm deep. The structures may be separated by a thin membrane or by a dense portion of fibrous tissue.

These defects occur in approximately 1% of the entire group of malformations.[18, 20] Patients with this defect have all the necessary elements to be continent and have an excellent prognosis. Because they have a well-developed anal canal, they have normal sensation in the anorectum. Almost normal voluntary muscle structures are present.

FEMALE DEFECTS

Cutaneous (Perineal) Fistulas

From the therapeutic and prognostic points of view, this common defect is equivalent to the cutaneous fistula described in the male patients.[18, 20] The rectum is well located within the sphincter mechanism, except for its lowest portion, which is anteriorly located. Rectum and vagina are well separated (Fig. 35–3*A*).

Vestibular Fistulas

In this important defect, pediatric patients have good prognoses in terms of bowel function when properly treated. Yet in my experience, the patient is frequently referred from other institutions because of unsuccessful repairs. The bowel opens immediately behind the hymen in the vestibule of the female genitalia (Fig. 35–3*B*). Immediately above the fistula site, rectum and vagina are separated by a thin common wall. These patients usually have well-developed muscles and a normal sacrum and

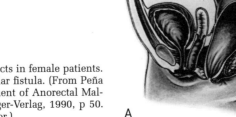
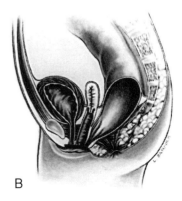

Figure 35–3. Spectrum of defects in female patients. *A*, Perineal fistula. *B*, Vestibular fistula. (From Peña A: Atlas of Surgical Management of Anorectal Malformations. New York, Springer-Verlag, 1990, p 50. Lois Barnes, medical illustrator.)

A

B

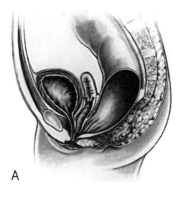

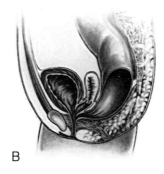

Figure 35–4. Spectrum of cloacae. *A*, Most common type of cloaca. *B*, Long common channel. (From Peña A: Atlas of Surgical Management of Anorectal Malformations. New York, Springer-Verlag, 1990, p 60. Lois Barnes, medical illustrator.)

nerves. Rarely, however, this defect is associated with a poorly developed sacrum.

Patients with vestibular fistula are frequently referred to the surgeon with an erroneous diagnosis of rectovaginal fistula. The precise diagnosis is a clinical one. A meticulous inspection of the newborn genitalia is needed for the diagnosis. A number of pediatric surgeons repair this defect without a protective colostomy. Many of these patients have a successful recovery. However, a perineal infection followed by dehiscence of the anal anastomosis and recurrence of the fistula provokes severe fibrosis that may interfere with the sphincteric mechanism. In such a case, the patient may have lost the best opportunity for an optimal functional result, because secondary operations do not render the same good prognosis as successful primary operations.[18] Thus, a protective colostomy is strongly recommended, followed by a form of limited posterior sagittal operation as a final repair.[18, 20]

The term *vaginal fistula* is frequently erroneously used in dealing with patients who actually have a vestibular fistula or a cloaca. A real vaginal fistula occurs in fewer than 1% of all cases and therefore is not considered as part of the classification proposed here.[20, 21]

Anorectal Agenesis Without Fistula

This defect in female patients carries the same therapeutic and prognostic implications as mentioned for male patients.

Persistent Cloaca

In this group of defects, the extreme in complexity of female malformations is represented. A persistent cloaca is defined as a defect in which rectum, vagina, and urinary tract meet and fuse into a single common channel (Figs. 35–4 to 35–6). The diagnosis of persistent cloaca is a clinical one. This defect should be suspected in a female infant with imperforate anus and small-looking genitalia. Careful separation of the labia discloses a single perineal orifice. The length of the common channel varies from 1 to 7 cm, which has technical and prognostic implications. Common channels longer than 3.5 cm usually represent a complex defect (see Fig. 35–4B). The mobilization of the vagina is difficult. Therefore, some form of vaginal replacement is often used during the repair. A common channel of less than 3.4 cm usually means that the defect can be repaired with a single posterior sagittal operation without opening the abdomen (see Figs. 35–4A and 35–5B). Sometimes, the rectum opens high into the dome of the vagina (see Fig. 35–5A). Therefore, a laparotomy must be part of the procedure to mobilize the bowel. Frequently, the vagina is abnormally distended and full of mucous secretions (hydrocolpos) (see Fig. 35–6A). This distended vagina compresses the trigone and therefore is frequently associated with megaureters. Such a large vagina represents a technical advantage for the repair, because more vaginal tissue facilitates its reconstruction. A frequent finding in cloacal malformations is the varying degree of vaginal and uterine septation or duplication (see Fig. 35–6B). The rectum usually opens in between the vaginas. Low cloacal malformations (see Fig. 35–5B) are usually associated with a well-developed sacrum, a normal-appearing perineum, and adequate muscles and nerves. Therefore, a good prognosis can be made.

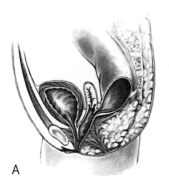

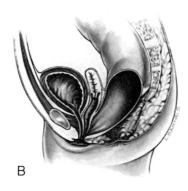

Figure 35–5. Spectrum of cloacae. *A*, High rectal implantation into the vagina. *B*, Short common channel. (From Peña A: Atlas of Surgical Management of Anorectal Malformations. New York, Springer-Verlag, 1990, p 61. Lois Barnes, medical illustrator.)

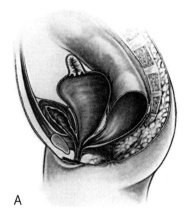
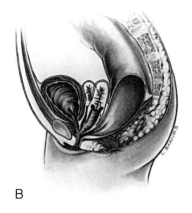

A   B

Figure 35–6. *A,* Associated hydrocolpos. *B,* Double vagina and double uterus. (From Peña A: Atlas of Surgical Management of Anorectal Malformations. New York, Springer-Verlag, 1990, p 61. Lois Barnes, medical illustrator.)

COMPLEX MALFORMATIONS

Unusual and bizarre anatomic arrangements can be seen in this group. Each case represents a different challenge to the surgeon, with different prognoses and therapeutic implications. No general guidelines can be drawn for the management of these patients. Each case must be individualized.

ASSOCIATED DEFECTS

Sacrum and Spine

Sacral deformities seem to be most frequently associated with sacrum and spine malformations. One or several sacral vertebrae may be missing. One missing vertebra does not seem to have an important prognostic implication.[18] However, more than two absent vertebrae represent a poor prognostic sign in terms of bowel continence and, sometimes, urinary control. Hemisacrum is associated with poor bowel control but is not well characterized. Other sacral abnormalities not well characterized, with implications that are not well recognized, include the presence of hemivertebrae (a higher spinal abnormality, located in the lumbar thoracic spine), asymmetric sacrum, short sacrum, and straight posteriorly protruding sacrum.

A sacral ratio has been developed to make possible a more objective evaluation of the sacrum (Fig. 35–7*A, B*). This sacral ratio in normal children is 0.77. Children with anorectal malformations suffer from different degrees of sacral hypodevelopment, and therefore, the sacral ratio varies from 0.0 to 1.0. We have never seen a patient develop good bowel control with a sacral ratio of less than 0.3.[20]

Emphasis has been placed on the diagnosis and treatment of tethered cord, which is a defect frequently associated with anorectal malformations.[23, 24] It has been assumed that the presence of tethered cord is associated with poor functional prognosis in these children. A review of our own series showed that 25% of patients with anorectal malformations suffer from tethered cord.[25] It is true that most of those children have a poor prognosis. However, the presence of tethered cord by itself coincides with the fact that those patients have very high defects, very abnormal sacrums, or spina bifida; therefore, it is very difficult to know whether the tethered cord itself produced the poor prognosis. Also, we could not find evidence that the operation to release the tethered cord changed the functional prognosis of the patient.

Genitourinary Defects

The frequency of associated GU defects varies from 20 to 54%.[26–39] The accuracy and thoroughness of the urologic evaluation may account for the reported variation. In my series, 48% of patients (55% girls and 44% boys) had associated GU anomalies.[32] These figures may not reflect the true incidence of GU defects in a broad population, because I receive referrals of children with many complex anal malformations.

The higher the malformation, the more frequent are associated urologic abnormalities. Patients with persistent cloacae or rectovesical fistulas have a 90% chance of an associated GU abnormality.[32] Conversely, children with low defects (perineal fistulas) have less than a 10% chance of an associated urologic defect. Hydronephrosis, urosepsis, and metabolic acidosis from poor renal function represent the main source of mortality and morbidity in newborns with anorectal malformations. Thus, a thorough urologic investigation is mandatory in cases of high defects. These studies may represent a higher priority than the colostomy itself. The urologic evaluation is also mandatory, although not as urgent in cases of rectovaginal and rectourethral fistulas. In cases of low defects, the urologic evaluation can be postponed and performed on an elective basis.

The urologic evaluation in every child with imperforate anus must include an ultrasonographic study of the kidneys and the entire abdomen to rule out the presence of hydronephrosis or any other obstructive process. If this study finding is abnormal, further evaluation is necessary.

☐ Initial Approach

Figure 35–8 shows a decision-making algorithm for the initial management of male patients. In more

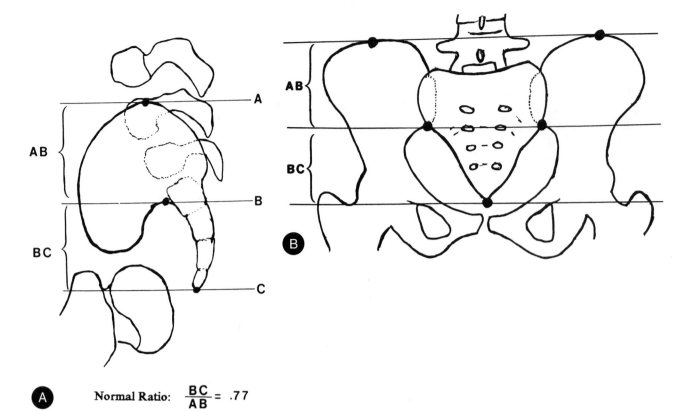

A

Normal Ratio: $\dfrac{BC}{AB} = .77$

Figure 35–7. Sacral ratios. *A*, Anterior-posterior view. *B*, Lateral view.

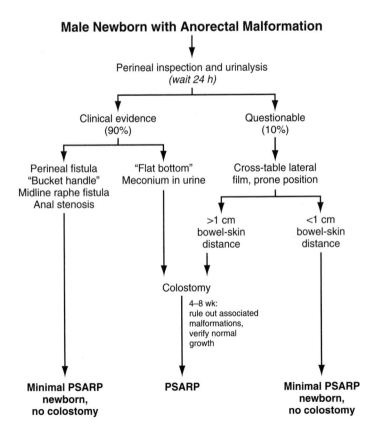

Figure 35–8. Decision-making algorithm for the management of newborn male infants with anorectal malformation. PSARP, posterior sagittal anorectoplasty.

than 80% of boys, perineal inspection allows enough clinical evidence to reach a decision about the establishment of a diverting colostomy. All those defects universally considered low are treated with a perineal anoplasty (minimal posterior sagittal anoplasty), without a protective colostomy. These defects include perineal fistula with or without a midline raphe subepithelial component, "bucket-handle" malformation below which an instrument can be passed, anal stenosis, and anal membrane.

The presence of a flat bottom or the demonstration of meconium in the urine is an indication for a diverting colostomy. Colostomy decompresses the bowel and provides protection during the healing of the subsequent total repair. After recovery from the colostomy, the patient is discharged from the hospital. If the patient is growing well and has no other associated defects (cardiac or gastrointestinal) that require treatment, the patient is readmitted at 4 to 8 weeks of age to undergo a posterior sagittal anorectoplasty. This early repair requires that the surgeon have experience in this procedure in very young infants. The operation is not as difficult in older patients. Therefore, repair of these defects is commonly done when the child is older (1 yr).

Performing the definitive repair at 1 month of age has important advantages for the patient, including less time with an abdominal stoma, less size discrepancy between proximal and distal bowel at the time of colostomy closure, simpler anal dilation, and no recognizable psychological sequelae from painful perineal maneuvers. In addition, at least theoretically, placing the rectum in the right location early in life may represent an advantage in terms of the potential for acquired local sensation.[33] All of these potential advantages of an early operation must be weighed against the possible disadvantages of an inexperienced surgeon who is not familiar with the minute anatomic structures of the pelvis of a young infant.

The urologic evaluation must be carried out before the colostomy is established in case urinary diversion is indicated. Colostomy and diversion may be done simultaneously.

Sometimes, the surgeon is unable to obtain enough clinical evidence to justify the performance of a colostomy. In this situation, which occurs in fewer than 20% of patients, an invertogram is indicated.[4] A simpler alternative is to take a cross-table, lateral roentgenogram of the infant, who is placed in a prone position with the pelvis elevated. The result of this type of radiographic study is not different from that of the traditional invertogram.[34] Either the invertogram or the cross-table radiograph must be taken after 16 to 24 hours of life. Before this, the bowel is not distended enough and the intraluminal pressure is not high enough to force air to the distal end of the gut. In addition, this waiting period may allow the passing of meconium through the urethra in cases of urethral fistula. The presence of a bowel pouch more distant than 1 cm from the anal skin represents an indication for colostomy. A rectum

located closer than 1 cm to the skin is considered a low defect. In this case, the patient most likely has a very narrow perineal fistula that has been missed by the examiners. The patient can be treated with a perineal operation without a protective colostomy.

Figure 35–9 shows a decision-making algorithm for the initial management of female patients. Perineal inspection usually provides more information in female than in male patients. The presence of a single perineal orifice means that the infant has a cloaca, and the anatomy of the urinary tract must be delineated on an emergency basis. The patient is then subjected to a colostomy and/or vaginostomy and a vesicostomy and/or any other urinary diversion, when necessary.

The final repair of this defect is called posterior sagittal anorectovaginourethroplasty, which is done usually after 3 months of age. The presence of a palpable abdominal mass in the lower abdomen in a female patient with imperforate anus is pathognomonic of hydrocolpos. The vagina must be drained through a vaginostomy tube to allow the ureters to drain well into the bladder. The presence of a vaginal or vestibular fistula that can be diagnosed by perineal inspection represents an indication for a colostomy. However, because many times those fistulas are competent and stool can pass well through them without any evidence of intestinal obstruction, the colostomy does not have to be established emergently. The patient can be discharged from the hospital. Normal growth and development can thus be verified. The colostomy is done 2 weeks prior to the repair of the vestibular fistula.

A cutaneous (perineal) fistula has the same prognostic and therapeutic implications as those discussed for male patients. A female infant with imperforate anus who fails to pass meconium through the genitalia after 24 hours of observation needs an invertogram or a cross-table lateral radiograph in the prone position. The management of these female pediatric patients must follow the same principles mentioned for male pediatric patients.

COLOSTOMY

A divided descending colostomy is ideal for the management of anorectal malformations. The completely diverting colostomy provides bowel decompression as well as protection for the final repair of the malformation. In addition, this colostomy permits the performance of a distal colostogram, which represents the most accurate diagnostic study to determine the detailed anatomy of these defects.[35] The temptation to repair these defects without a protective colostomy always exists.[36–38] Repair without a colostomy increases the risk of infection and prevents demonstration of the precise anatomy of the defect. Even though they occur infrequently, infection and dehiscence represent a serious threat to the potential continence mechanism.

A descending colostomy has definite advantages over the right or transverse colostomy.[39] A relatively

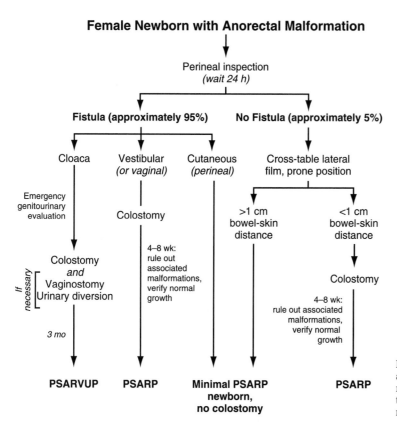

Figure 35–9. Decision-making algorithm for the management of newborn female infants with anorectal malformation; PSARP, posterior sagittal anorectoplasty; PSARVUP, posterior sagittal anorectovaginourethroplasty.

short segment of defunctionalized distal colon is left, which is important. Atrophy of the bowel distal to the colostomy may result in liquid stools for a time after colostomy closure. Mechanical cleansing of the distal colon prior to the definite repair is much less difficult when the colostomy is located in the descending portion of the colon. In the case of a large rectourethral fistula, the patient frequently passes urine into the colon. A more distal colostomy allows urine to escape through the distal stoma without significant absorption. When the patient has a proximal colostomy, the urine remains in the colon and is absorbed, increasing the incidence of metabolic acidosis. Loop colostomy permits the passage of stool from the proximal stoma into the distal bowel, which produces urinary tract infection and distal rectal pouch dilation. Prolonged distention of the rectal pouch may produce irreversible bowel wall damage, with a permanent and significant bowel hypomotility disorder, leading to severe constipation later in life. An analysis of my series demonstrated that the problem of colostomy prolapse is more frequent in loop colostomy.[39]

A colostomy created too distal in the area of the rectosigmoid interferes with the mobilization of the rectum during the pull-through.

□ Surgical Techniques for Anorectal Malformations

Many surgical techniques to repair anorectal malformations have been described. Most of these tech-

niques attempt to preserve the puborectalis sling, because it has been considered a key structure in the achievement of bowel control.[5] To avoid damage to important pelvic nerves and other pelvic structures, some workers have suggested endorectal dissection of that part of the intrapelvic intestine.[6, 8, 9] Some surgeons have advocated an anterior perineal approach to the rectourethral fistula.[40] Many different types of anoplasties to avoid the problem of rectal mucosal prolapse have been described.[41] A middle ground has been proposed between those who support a posterior sagittal approach for the management of these defects and those who oppose it.[42] The advantages of the exposure obtained by the posterior saggital approach and the recognized importance of placing the rectum accurately within the limits of the external sphincter and muscle complex are weighed against the potential damage that may result from the complete division of the muscle structures.

POSTERIOR SAGITTAL APPROACH

All anorectal malformations can be corrected by the posterior sagittal approach with or without a laparotomy. The size of the incision changes, depending on the specific defect. The patient is placed in the prone position with the pelvis elevated. The use of an electric stimulator to elicit muscle contraction during the operation is strongly recommended; these contractions serve as a guide for incising exactly in the midline, leaving an equal amount of muscle on both sides.

The incision usually starts in the middle portion of the sacrum; it is extended through the center of the external sphincter. In the case of a persistent cloaca, the incision is continued all the way to the single perineal orifice, dividing the external sphincter. Smaller incisions (limited posterior sagittal anorectoplasty) are adequate for defects such as a vestibular fistula. Low defects require a small posterior sagittal incision (minimal posterior sagittal anoplasty). The rationale of this approach is based on the fact that no important nerves or vessels cross the midline. Thus, excellent exposure is obtained without damaging important structures. In addition, a fine midline fascia plane divides the anatomy into two parts.

As part of the posterior saggital approach, the voluntary striated muscle structures are separated rather than divided. The posterior sagittal opening allows full exposure and reduces the likelihood of damage to important structures, such as the vas deferens, ectopic ureters, prostatic tissue, urethra, and seminal vesicles.

The anatomic relationship of the rectum to all of these structures is complex. The separation of the rectum from the urogenital structures represents the most delicate part of the procedure. This delicate maneuver is not simple, even under direct vision; any kind of blind maneuver exposes the patient to risk of serious injury.

About 90% of defects in boys can be repaired via the posterior sagittal approach without opening the abdomen.[18, 20] Each case has individual anatomic variants that mandate technical modifications. These changes can best be achieved with full exposure of the anatomy. An example is the size discrepancy frequently seen between an ectatic rectum and the space available for pullthrough. If the discrepancy is severe, the surgeon must tailor the rectum to fit. Forcing the rectum through a limited space risks damage to the delicate muscle complex. In addition, closure of the pelvic and perineal structures around an overly large rectum may interfere with the blood supply of the distal rectum.

A posterior sagittal approach should never be attempted without a technically adequate distal colostogram to determine the exact position of the rectum and the fistula. Attempting repair without this basic information represents a risk for potential nerve damage, damage to the seminal vesicals and prostate, ectopic ureters, and bladder dennervation.[35]

REPAIR OF SPECIFIC DEFECTS IN BOYS

Low Malformations (Cutaneous Fistula, Anal Stenosis, Anal Membrane)

Patients with low malformations have an excellent prognosis except in those cases in which the bowel was dissected unnecessarily. Simple anal dilations may be sufficient. Minimal posterior mobilization to place the fistula within the limits of the external sphincter may be necessary.

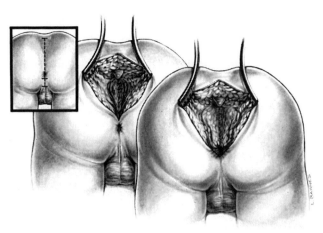

Figure 35–10. Posterior sagittal incision. Separation of parasagittal fibers and exposure of the muscle complex.

Rectourethral Fistulas

A Foley catheter is inserted through the urethra. About 25% of the time, this catheter goes into the rectum rather than into the bladder. Under these circumstances, the surgeon has two alternatives: (1) attempt the bladder catheterization again using a catheter guide or (2) relocate the catheter into the bladder under direct visualization during the operation.

The parasagittal fibers of the external sphincter as well as the muscle complex are divided exactly in the midline, using fine–needle tip cautery (Fig. 35–10). The parasagittal fibers are located on both sides of the midline just deep to the skin. They extend both posteriorly and anteriorly to the anal dimple. The muscle complex fibers represent a continuum of a voluntary muscle structure, which extends from the levator mechanism down to the skin at the anal dimple area. The muscle complex fibers run perpendicular to the parasagittal fibers. The crossing of the muscle complex fibers creates the anterior and posterior limits of the new anus (Fig. 35–11). These limits can be seen most clearly with

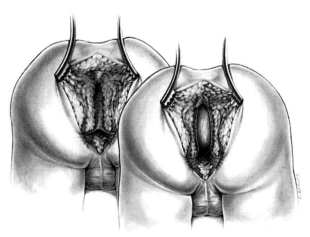

Figure 35–11. Dividing muscle complex and levator muscle. Rectum is exposed.

the use of an electric stimulator. Silk sutures temporarily mark the limits. The coccyx is split in the midline, as is the levator muscle. The levator muscle lies deep in the incision. The higher the malformation, the deeper the levator muscle is found. The levator fibers run parallel to the skin incision. The levator and muscle complex are in continuity.

We arbitrarily consider the limits between levator and muscle complex at the place where these structures create a 90-degree angle. When we finish dividing all the muscle structures, the rectum is visualized (see Fig. 35–11). In those cases of rectourethrobulbar fistulas, the bowel is prominent; it bulges through the wound. In cases of rectoprostatic fistulas, the rectum may be barely apparent. In cases of rectobladder-neck fistulas the rectum is not visible through this approach.

With rectourethral fistula, silk sutures are placed in the posterior rectal wall on both sides of the midline. The rectum is opened in the midline, and the incision is continued exactly in the midline down to the fistula site. Temporary silk sutures are placed on the edges of the opened posterior rectal wall.

The anterior rectal wall immediately above the fistula is a thin structure. No plane of separation exists between rectum and urethra in that area. Therefore, a plane of separation must be created in that common wall. For this, multiple 6-0 silk traction sutures are placed in the rectal mucosa immediately above the fistula. The rectum is then separated from the urethra, creating a submucosal plane for approximately 5 to 10 mm above the fistula site (Fig. 35–12).

The common wall between rectum and urethra is particularly thin in the midline. Laterally, both structures gradually separate. Once the rectum is fully separated, a circumferential perirectal dissection is performed to gain enough rectal length to reach the perineum. In cases of fistulas to the bulbous urethra, the dissection is rather minimal, because only a short gap exists between the rectum and the perineum. In cases of prostatic urethral fistulas the perirectal dissection is a significant one.

Frequently, the blood supply of the rectum is compromised to some degree.

The rectum has a surrounding fascia, which must be divided for mobilization. This fascia contains nerves and vessels. The implications of this denervation are unknown. One would think that this denervation might provoke some degree of pseudo-Hirschsprung's physiology. Thus, patients with higher malformations that require more dissection would be expected to suffer from more severe constipation. However, in my experience,[18, 20] patients with lower defects treated with this approach suffered more constipation than patients with higher defects.

The blood supply to the most distal part of the rectum, which is provided by intramural vessels, is usually good after the dissection has been completed. At this point, the size of the rectum can be evaluated and compared with the available space. If necessary, the rectum can be tapered, removing part of the posterior wall.

The rectal wall is reconstructed with two layers of interrupted long-lasting absorbable sutures. The anterior rectal wall is frequently damaged to some degree as a consequence of the mucosal separation between rectum and urethra. To reinforce this wall, both smooth muscle layers can be sutured together with interrupted 5-0 long-lasting absorbable sutures. The urethral fistula is sutured with the same material. Tapering of the rectum must always be done on the posterior rectal wall so that the bowel adjacent to the closed urethral fistula is normal if a recurrent rectourethral fistula is to be avoided.

The perineal body is reconstructed, bringing together the anterior limits of the external sphincter previously marked with temporary silk sutures. The rectum must be placed in front of the levator and within the limits of the muscle complex (Fig. 35–13A). Long-lasting 5-0 or 4-0 absorbable sutures are placed on the posterior edge of the levator muscle. The posterior limit of the muscle complex must also be reapproximated behind the rectum. These sutures must take part of the rectal wall to anchor it and to avoid rectal prolapse (Fig. 35–13B). The

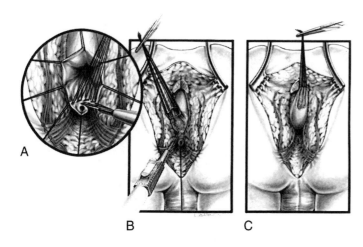

Figure 35–12. *A, B,* Separation of rectum from urethra. *C,* Rectum is completely separated.

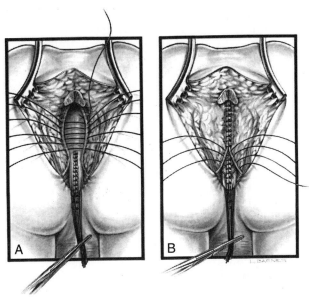

Figure 35–13. *A*, Rectum is passed in front of the levator muscle. *B*, Muscle complex sutures anchor the rectum.

posterior limit of the muscle complex is brought together behind the rectum, guided by the posterior limit of the external sphincter that was previously marked with a silk suture. We perform the anoplasty with 16 interrupted long-lasting absorbable sutures (Fig. 35–14). The wound is closed with subcuticular 5-0 absorbable monofilament. The Foley catheter is left in place for 5 days. The patient receives broad-spectrum antibiotics for 2 days.

Rectobladder-Neck Fistulas

For this repair, a total body preparation is performed. In the sterile field, the entire lower part of the patient's body is included. The initial incision is the posterior sagittal. All the muscle structures are divided in the midline. The urethra is exposed, and a rubber tube is placed through the muscle complex, where the rectum will subsequently be placed. The size of the tube should be chosen to represent the space available for the pull-through.

The wound is closed. The rubber tube is left in place to mark the path through which the rectum

will eventually be pulled. The patient is turned so that the surgeon can work simultaneously in the abdomen and in the perineum. From the abdomen, the rectosigmoid is mobilized. In this high defect, the rectobladder-neck fistula is located approximately 2 cm below the peritoneal reflection. The pelvic dissection is minimal; however, the surgeon must be careful to avoid damage to the vas deferens, which are close to the bowel in this area. The rectum is separated from the bladder neck, and the bladder end of the fistula is sutured with interrupted nonabsorbable sutures. The rubber tube is found without difficulty in the presacral space. If the rectum is much larger than the tube, the bowel must be tapered. When the bowel is mobilized enough to reach the perineum, some peripheral branches of the inferior mesenteric vessels frequently must be divided. The rectum is anchored to the rubber tube and pulled down through the pelvis (Fig. 35–15). The anoplasty is performed as previously described.

Anorectal Agenesis Without Fistulas

In these cases, the blind end of the rectum is usually located at the level of the bulbar urethra. The rectum must be carefully separated from the urethra, because both structures have a common wall even though no fistula is present. The rest of the repair must be performed as described for the rectourethral fistula type of defect.

Rectal Atresia and Stenosis

The approach to these malformations is also posterior sagittal. The upper rectal pouch is opened, as well as the little distal anal canal. An end-to-end anastomosis is performed under direct visualization, followed by a meticulous reconstruction of the muscle mechanism posterior to the rectum. The results are excellent.

REPAIR IN FEMALE PATIENTS
Perineal (Cutaneous) Fistulas

Diagnosis as well as therapeutic and prognostic implications of this defect are the same as those discussed for male defects.

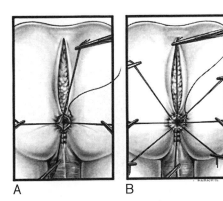
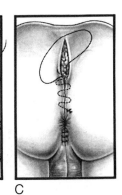

Figure 35–14. *A, B,* Anoplasty. *C,* Skin suture.

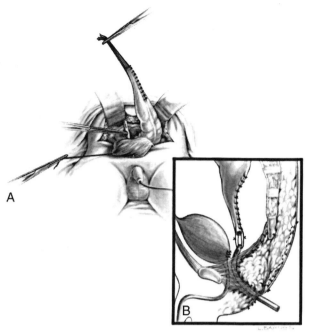

Figure 35–15. *A*, Abdominal approach for high defects (rectobladder-neck fistula). Rectum has been separated from the bladderneck. The presacral rubber tube is identified. *B*, Rectum is anchored to the rubber tube to guide the pull-through.

Vestibular Fistulas

The complexity of this defect is frequently underestimated. Multiple 5-0 silk sutures are placed at the mucocutaneous junction of the fistula. The incision used to repair this defect is shorter than the one used to repair the male rectourethral fistula. The incision continues around the fistula into the vestibule in a racket-like fashion. The rectum is dissected. The posterior part of the dissection is usually not difficult. Hemorrhoidal vessels are usually found on the lateral aspects of the rectum.

The most delicate part of this dissection is that of the anterior rectal wall (Fig. 35–16*A*). The rectum and the vagina share a common wall. The surgeon must create two walls out of one. The dissection continues cephalad until both walls (rectum and vagina) are normal. If the rectum and the vagina are not completely separated, a tense rectal anastomosis is present, which predisposes the patient to dehiscence.

Once the dissection has been completed, the perineal body is repaired (Fig. 35–16*B*). The anterior edge of the muscle complex is reapproximated, as previously described. The levator muscle is usually not exposed; therefore, it does not have to be reconstructed. The muscle complex, however, must be reconstructed posterior to the rectum. The sutures must include the posterior edge of the muscle complex and the posterior rectal wall to avoid rectal prolapse. The anoplasty is performed as previously described (Fig. 35–17).

Vaginal Fistulas

The repair of this unusual defect requires a full posterior sagittal incision. The higher the location of the fistula, the shorter the common wall is between rectum and vagina. The basic steps of the operation are the same as described for vestibular fistulas, except that the circumferential dissection of the rectum to gain length is more significant, particularly in high vaginal fistulas.

Persistent Cloacae

The repair of this group of defects is still evolving and represents the most serious technical challenge in pelvic surgery in children. The pelvis is approached through a long midsagittal incision, which extends from the middle portion of the sacrum through the external sphincter and down into the single perineal opening (Fig. 35–18). All the muscle structures are divided in the midline. In front of the levator, some visceral structure is usually found, most likely the rectum. However, because this defect is complex, the surgeon must be prepared to find bizarre anatomic arrangements of rectum and vagina.

The incision is to continue down into the single perineum orifice, which exposes the entire malformation (see Fig. 35–18). The rectum is usually the

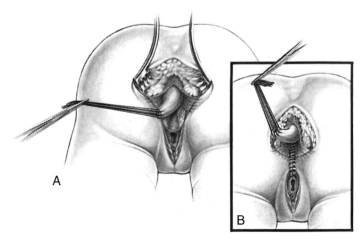

Figure 35–16. Repair of rectovestibular fistula. *A*, Rectum is completely separated from vagina. *B*, Perineal body is repaired.

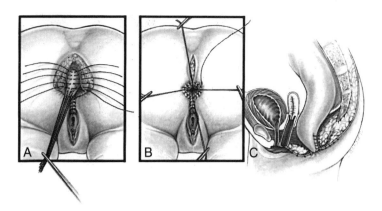

Figure 35–17. Repair of vestibular fistula. *A*, Muscle complex sutures anchor the rectum. *B*, Anoplasty. *C*, Operation is finished.

organ that lays deeper to the sphincter mechanism and should be opened. The goal of this procedure is to separate the rectum from the vagina, to pull it down and it place it within the limits of the sphincter mechanism. Until recently, the next step was to separate the vagina from the urinary tract, dissect and pull the vagina down, leave the old common channel or urogenital sinus as a neourethra and place the vagina immediately behind the neourethra. More recently, a new more valuable maneuver called "total urogenital mobilization"[43] has been incorporated as the surgical treatment of cloacae. This maneuver consists in the mobilization of both vagina and urethra together as a unit without separating them (Figs. 35–19 to 35–21). After the rectum has been separated and mobilized, multiple silk stitches are placed, taking the edge of the vagina and the common channel, to apply uniform traction on the urogenital sinus to be mobilized (see Fig. 35–20). Another series of stitches are placed across the urogenital sinus approximately 5 mm proximal to the clitoris. The urogenital sinus is totally transected between the last row of silk stitches and the clitoris. The urogenital sinus is dissected, taking advantage of the fact that there is a natural plane between it and the pubis. While applying traction

to the multiple stitches, the suspensory ligaments of the urethra and bladder neck (which are fibrous avascular bands) are divided, which immediately provides a significant mobilization of the urogenital sinus. With this relatively simple maneuver, one can gain between 2 and 3 cm of length (see Fig. 35–20 and 35–21). In probably more than 50% of all cloaca patients, this mobilization is enough to create satisfactory urethral and vaginal openings without having to separate the vagina from the urethra, the main source of urethrovaginal fistulas.[18, 20, 44] This total urogenital mobilization has the additional advantages of providing an excellent blood supply to both urethra and vagina and placing the urethral opening in a visible location to facilitate intermittent catheterization when necessary. It also provides a smooth urethra that can be catheterized easily (see Fig. 35–21). However, in a significant number of cases, this maneuver is not enough to create a good vaginal opening, and further mobilization of the vagina is necessary. For this group of patients, the traditional maneuver of separation of vagina from the urethra still has to be performed (Fig. 35–22). The advantage

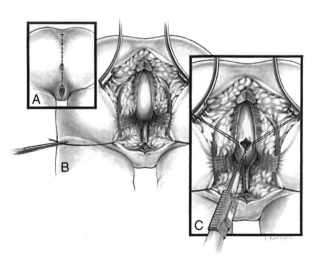

Figure 35–18. Cloaca repair. *A*, Incision. *B*, Rectum and common channel are exposed. *C*, Rectal opening.

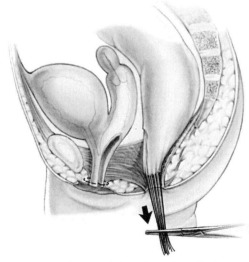

Figure 35–19. Total urogenital mobilization. Rectum separated from vagina. (From Peña A: Total urogenital mobilization—an easier way to repair cloacas. J Pediatr Surg 32:263–268, 1997. Lois Barnes, medical illustrator.)

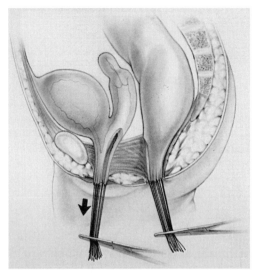

Figure 35–20. Urogenital sinus being mobilized. (From Peña A: Total urogenital mobilization—an easier way to repair cloacas. J Pediatr Surg 32:263–268, 1997. Lois Barnes, medical illustrator.)

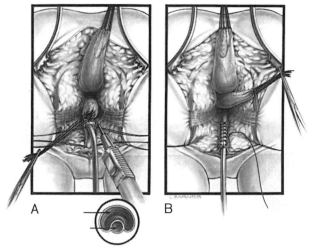

Figure 35–22. Cloaca repair. *A,* Rectum is completely separated. Vagina is being separated from the urinary tract. *B,* Rectum and vagina are separated. Reconstruction of the neourethra. (From Peña A: Atlas of Surgical Management of Anorectal Malformations. New York, Springer-Verlag, 1990, p 66. Lois Barnes, medical illustrator.)

now is that separation is done in an easier way, because the total urogenital mobilization allows that separation of vagina to be done outside the wound.

Rectum and vagina have a common wall, just as described in cases of vestibular fistula. Vagina and urinary tract also have a more extensive common wall. The vagina surrounds the urethra and the bladder neck (see Fig. 35–22). The separation of rectum and vagina is a meticulous and time-consuming maneuver, but it is simpler than separating the vagina from the urinary tract. These two structures are less elastic than the rectum, and their common wall is thin.

The separation of these structures is performed following the same principles previously described for other types of defects. Multiple 6-0 silk traction sutures are placed, taking the rectal or vaginal mucosa to facilitate this dissection. The injection of epinephrine solution also may help. The vagina is partially separated from the urinary tract. Overzealous dissection of these structures risks devascularization of the vagina or urethral injury. A 2- to 3-cm separation should be adequate. If the length of the vagina is not enough to reach the perineum, a more sophisticated vaginal reconstruction augmentation or replacement should be chosen.

The urethra is constructed utilizing the urogenital sinus. This tubularization is done over a Foley catheter, with two layers of interrupted 5-0 long-term absorbable sutures (see Fig. 35–22*B*). The electrical

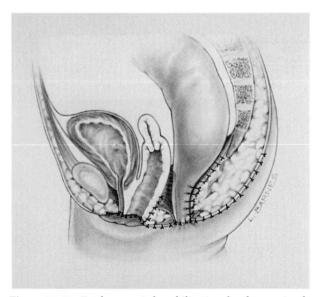

Figure 35–21. Total urogenital mobilization for the repair of a cloaca. Operation finished. (From Peña A: Total urogenital mobilization—an easier way to repair cloacas. J Pediatr Surg 32:263–268, 1997. Lois Barnes, medical illustrator.)

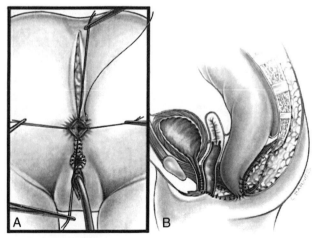

Figure 35–23. *A,* Urethra and vagina are already repaired. Anoplasty. *B,* Operation is completed. (From Peña A: Atlas of Surgical Management of Anorectal Malformations. New York, Springer-Verlag, 1990, p 69. Lois Barnes, medical illustrator.)

PERSISTENT CLOACA WITH HYDROCOLPOS, HEMIVAGINAS & HEMIUTERUS

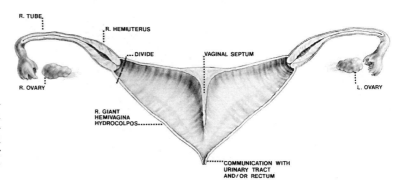

Figure 35–24. Bilateral hydrocolpos, very high vagina. Ideal anatomy to be repaired with a vaginal switch maneuver. (From Kiely EM, Peña A: Anorectal malformations. In O'Neill JA, Rowe MI, Grosfeld JL, et al. Pediatric Surgery. St. Louis, Mosby–Year Book, 1998, p 1442. Lois Barnes, medical illustrator.)

stimulator can help detect the presence of voluntary muscles located in both sides of the common channel along its entire length.

The vagina is anastomosed to the perineal skin immediately behind the urethra. In cases in which the anterior vaginal wall was damaged by the dissection, the vagina is rotated 90 degrees to leave an intact, well-vascularized, lateral vaginal wall adjacent to the urethral sutures to reduce the chance of a urethrovaginal fistula. The perineal body is then reconstructed using the previously marked limits of the external sphincter as a guideline. The rectum is reconstructed as previously described (Fig. 35–23). When the vaginal length is not adequate to reach the perineum, one of several augmentation or replacement maneuvers can be employed.

Other Alternatives for Vaginal Reconstruction

Vaginal Switch Maneuver

A significant number of cloaca patients suffer from bilateral hydrocolpos and a very long common channel (Fig. 35–24). In fact, if one measures the distance between one hemicervix and the other, it happens to be longer than the vertical length of

the vagina. To persist in trying to mobilize both hemivaginas down to the perineum requires a significant lateral dissection and therefore the sacrifice of the blood supply of both hemivaginas, which may provoke an acquired atresia due to ischemia. Under these circumstances, a vaginal switch maneuver as represented in Figure 35–25 is the best surgical alternative. One of the hemiuteri and the ipsilateral fallopian tube are resected, with particular care given to preserving the ovary. The blood supply of the hemivagina of that particular side is sacrificed. The blood supply of the contralateral hemivagina is preserved and provides good perfusion for both hemivaginas. The vaginal septum is resected, and both hemivaginas are tubularized, taking advantage of the long lateral dimension of both hemivaginas together. Then, what used to be the dome of the hemivagina where the hemiuterus was resected is turned down to the perineum. This is an excellent maneuver that can be performed only when the anatomic characteristics fulfill the requirements already mentioned.[20, 44]

Vaginal Augmentation with a Piece of Small Bowel

Vaginal augmentation with a piece of small bowel is particularly useful in cases of a long gap or a

VAGINAL RECONSTRUCTION AND SWITCH MANEUVER

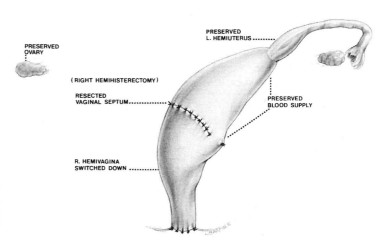

Figure 35–25. Vaginal switch maneuver. (From Kiely EM, Peña A: Anorectal malformations. In O'Neill JA, Rowe MI, Grosfeld JL, et al: Pediatric Surgery. St. Louis, Mosby–Year Book, 1998, p 1442. Lois Barnes, medical illustrator.)

total vaginal replacement.[45, 46] The abdomen must be opened, and a piece of small bowel must be selected, preserving its mesentery. The continuity of the small bowel is reestablished with an end-to-end anastomosis. Two more anastomoses are necessary: the upper one between the segment of small bowel and the upper vagina, and the lower one between the lower part of the bowel and the perineal skin.

Vaginal Dome Flap

This flap is performed in cases of a short, immobile vagina with a big dome. The large dome is used to develop a laterally based flap, which must be tubularized to reach the perineum. Sometimes this can be done through the posterior sagittal incision. With a high vagina, the abdomen must be opened to complete the separation.

POSTOPERATIVE MANAGEMENT AND COLOSTOMY CLOSURE

Postoperatively, patients generally have a smooth course. Pain is not a complaint except for those who have undergone laparotomy. In the cloaca repair, the Foley catheter remains in place for between 8 and 14 days. In patients whose newly constructed urethra is long, suprapubic drainage is established to avoid the placement of a Foley catheter. If the urethral catheter is accidentally dislodged, the patient must be observed for spontaneous complete voiding. If voiding is not possible, a percutaneous suprapubic cystostomy tube is inserted. Because reintroduction of a urethral catheter can disrupt the repair, this must be avoided.

Intravenous antibiotics are administered for 48 hours. Antibiotic ointment is locally applied for 8 to 10 days. The patient usually goes home after 3 to 4 days, except when a laparotomy is performed.

Two weeks after repair, the patient is brought to the clinic, and anal dilations are started. A dilator that fits snugly into the anus should be used. This procedure is done twice daily by the parents. Every week, the size of the dilator is increased, until the rectum reaches the desired size, which depends on the patient's age (Table 35–2). Once this desired size is reached, the colostomy may be closed. The frequency of dilations may be reduced once the parents state that the dilator goes in easily with no pain. After that, our dilation schedule is as follows:

TABLE 35–2. Size of Dilator According to Age

Age	Hegar Dilator (No.)
1–4 mo	12
4–12 mo	13
8–12 mo	14
1–3 yr	15
3–12 yr	16
>12 yr	17

At least once a day for 1 month
Every third day for 1 month
Twice a week for 1 month
Once a week for 1 month
Once a month for 3 months

Nonmanageable, severe strictures are seen in cases in which the dilation program was not done as indicated or when the blood supply of the rectum has been damaged.

After the colostomy is closed, the patient may have multiple bowel movements and may develop perineal excoriation. A "constipating diet" may be helpful in the treatment of this problem. After several weeks, the number of bowel movements decreases. By 6 months, the patient develops an individualized bowel movement pattern. A patient who has one to three bowel movements per day, remains clean in between bowel movements, and shows evidence of "feeling" or "pushing" during bowel movements usually has a good prognosis. This type of patient is trainable. A patient with multiple bowel movements or one who is passing stool constantly without showing any signs of sensation or pushing, usually has a poor functional prognosis.

FUNCTIONAL DISORDERS POSTREPAIR OF ANORECTAL MALFORMATIONS

Most patients who undergo repair of an anorectal malformation suffer from some degree of functional disorder. An abnormality in some important anatomic structures for bowel control must exist.

Fecal continence depends on three main factors:

1. *Voluntary muscle structures.* These structures are represented by the levator muscle, muscle complex, and external sphincter. Normally, they are used only for brief periods, when the rectal fecal mass reaches the anorectal area, pushed by the involuntary contraction of the rectosigmoid. This contraction occurs only in the minutes prior to defecation. These voluntary muscle structures are used only occasionally during the rest of the day and night. Patients with anorectal malformations have abnormal voluntary striated muscles with different degrees of development. However, voluntary muscles can be used only when the patient "feels" that it is necessary. For that sensation, the patient needs information that can only be derived from an intact sensory mechanism.

2. *Sensation.* Exquisite sensation in normal individuals resides in the anal canal. Except for patients with rectal atresia, most patients with these defects are born without an anal canal; therefore, this sensation does not exist or is rudimentary. Evidence exists that the distention of the rectum is felt in many of these patients, provided the rectum has been located accurately within the muscle structures. This sensation seems to be a consequence of stretching the voluntary muscle (proprioception).[47] The most important clinical implication is that

liquid stool or soft fecal material may not be felt by patients with anorectal malformations, as the rectum is not distended. Thus, to achieve some degree of sensation and bowel control, the patient must have the capacity to form solid stool.

3. *Bowel motility.* Perhaps the most important factor in fecal continence is bowel motility; however, motility has been largely underestimated. In a normal individual, the rectosigmoid remains quiet for periods (12 hours to several days), depending on specific defecation habits. During that time, sensation and voluntary muscle structures are almost not necessary because the stool remains inside the bowel if it is solid. The contraction of the rectosigmoid that occurs prior to defecation is normally felt by the patient. Voluntarily, the normal individual can relax the striated muscles, which allows the rectal content to migrate down into the highly sensitive area of the anal canal; there, accurate information is provided concerning the consistency and quality of the stool. The voluntary muscles are used to push the rectal contents back up into the rectosigmoid and to hold them if desired, until the appropriate time for evacuation.

At the time of defecation, voluntary muscle structures are relaxed. The main factor that provokes the emptying of the rectosigmoid is an involuntary massive bowel contraction, helped sometimes by Valsalva's maneuver. Most patients with anorectal malformations suffer a serious disturbance of this sophisticated bowel motility mechanism. Patients who underwent a posterior sagittal anorectoplasty or any other type of sacroperineal approach, in which the most distal part of the bowel was preserved, show evidence of an overefficient bowel reservoir (rectum). The main clinical manifestation is constipation, which seems to be more severe in patients with lower defects. Vestibular fistulas, in particular, are more prone to these problems. We suspect that an ectatic distended colon (sometimes associated with a loop colostomy that allowed fecal impaction in the blind rectal pouch) eventually leads to severe constipation. The enormously dilated rectosigmoid with normal ganglion cells behaves like a myopathic type of hypomotility disorder.

Patients with fecal incontinence who suffer from constipation are manageable with enemas. Those patients treated with techniques in which the most distal part of the bowel is resected (endorectal dissection) clinically behave as individuals without a rectal reservoir.[6, 8, 9] This is a situation equivalent to a perineal colostomy. Depending on the amount of colon resected, the patient may have loose stools, in which case medical management consists in the use of enemas plus constipating diet and medications to slow down the colon motility.

EVALUATION OF RESULTS

Each defect described here has a different prognosis. When evaluating clinical results, the error of oversimplification should be avoided. Categories such as *high*, *intermediate*, and *low*, or even *high* and *low*, do not accurately reflect the results that we have obtained, because the so-called high and intermediate defects frequently include individual malformations with differing prognoses. Patients with low defects usually have excellent results, except when technical errors have been made. Table 35–3 shows the results obtained by the author.

Patients with abnormal sacrums (more than two vertebrae missing) and flat perineum (absent muscles) suffer from fecal incontinence regardless of the type of technique used.

Because cloacae represent another spectrum of defects in themselves, they eventually will have to be subclassified on the basis of potential for continence, including quality of the sacrum, length of the common channel, and quality of the muscles. The results obtained in the surgical management of persistent cloacae are also shown in Table 35–3.

TABLE 35–3. Global Functional Results

Defect	Voluntary Bowel Movement No. of Patients	%	Soiling No. of Patients	%	Totally Continent No. of Patients	%	Constipation No. of Patients	%
Perineal fistula	15/15	100.0	0/15	0.0	15/15	100.0	4/15	26.7
Rectal atresia or stenosis	5/5	100.0	1/6	16.7	5/6	83.3	4/5	80.0
Vestibular fistula	45/48	93.8	18/47	38.3	32/45	71.1	30/47	63.8
Imperforate anus without fistula	17/20	85.0	9/22	40.9	12/17	70.6	10/21	47.6
Bulbar fistula	42/48	87.5	34/52	65.4	17/53	32.1	30/51	58.8
Prostatic fistula	39/51	76.5	46/59	77.9	11/39	28.2	30/60	50.0
Cloaca, common channel <3 cm	25/30	83.3	22/28	78.6	6/22	27.3	9/28	32.1
Cloaca, common channel >3 cm	10/17	58.8	16/18	88.9	2/9	22.2	10/19	52.7
Vaginal fistula	3/4	75.0	4/4	100.0	0/3	0.0	1/4	25.0
Bladder neck fistula	4/14	28.6	22/22	100.0	0/4	0.0	7/24	29.2

COMPLICATIONS

In my entire series of 1102 patients, 5 experienced wound infections during the immediate postoperative period. Three of these patients had a loop colostomy, which probably was not completely diverting. Fortunately, the infections affected only the skin and subcutaneous tissue. They healed secondarily, without functional sequelae. Anal strictures may be the consequence of lack of discipline in following the protocol of dilations. When trying to prevent discomfort in the patient, some surgeons dilate the anus once a week. This serious error can eventually create a severe, intractable fibrous stricture. Severe anorectal strictures occurred in 3 patients. These were correlated with devascularization of the rectum during the rectal mobilization. Dilations were more difficult than usual. One patient required a secondary operation. Tapering was not responsible for stricture in any of the patients. The patients who underwent tapering did not suffer from more constipation than those who did not.

Constipation was the most common functional disorder observed in patients who underwent posterior sagittal anorectoplasty (see Table 35–3). A possible explanation for this disorder was given earlier. Interestingly enough, the incidence of constipation almost reverses the frequency of voluntary bowel movements in our patients. This means that patients with the best prognosis (low defects) have the highest frequency of voluntary bowel movements but the worst incidence of constipation.[18, 20] Patients with very poor prognosis, such as bladder neck fistula, had a rather low incidence of constipation.[18, 20] The analysis of our series indicates that constipation seems to be directly related to the degree of rectal ectasia. Colostomies that do not allow cleansing and irrigation of the distal colon lead to megarectum. Transverse colostomies lead to dilation of the left colon and rectosigmoid. Efforts to keep the rectosigmoid as decompressed as possible from the time the colostomy is established result in better ultimate bowel function.

Urethrovaginal fistula has been the most common and feared complication in cases of persistent cloaca prior to the advent of the total urogenital mobilization maneuver.[44] The vagina can be rotated to prevent this complication. Three patients suffered from complete fibrosis (acquired atresia of the vagina), which was secondary to an excessive dissection in an attempt to mobilize a high vagina. In retrospect, one of the described vaginal replacement maneuvers should have been selected. Total urogenital mobilization has eliminated the complications of urethrovaginal fistula and vaginal ischemia.

Transient femoral nerve palsy was observed in three adolescent patients, a consequence of excessive pressure in the groin during the operation. This problem can be avoided by adequate cushioning of the patient's groin area.

During a secondary operation, one patient developed a recurrent rectourethral fistula that closed spontaneously. This particular patient had a severe pelvic inflammatory process, secondary to a foreign body left during a previous operation.

Ectopic ureteral injury and vas deferens injury occurred in two cases when a posterior sagittal dissection was used to locate a high rectum. This injury can be avoided by a distal colostogram, which should be done prior to every posterior sagittal procedure. This study allows the surgeon to know the exact location of the fistula, avoiding the risks of "exploration."

Dislodgement of the Foley catheter during the first 24 to 48 hours requires placement of a percutaneous suprapubic cystostomy if the patient is unable to void.

Postoperative bladder hypotonia occurs in patients with normal sacrums who have complex cloacae with hydrocolpos. Such patients are born with huge, hypotonic bladders. The long-term incidence of urinary incontinence in my series is shown in Table 35–4.

Neurogenic bladder has been mentioned anecdotally after a posterior sagittal operation in a patient with a normal sacrum. Surgical damage to the bladder nerves occurs if the surgeon strays from the midline plane. Also, the placement of Weitlaner's retractors deeper than necessary may compress sacral nerve branches, producing a "neurogenic" bladder.

□ Medical Management for Fecal Incontinence

For those patients who suffer from different degrees of bowel malfunction, a program of bowel management should be implemented.

With the rational administration of bowel irrigations, diets, and drugs, most patients, including those with severe fecal incontinence, are able to remain clean for 24 hours.[48] In my experience, only those patients with severe diarrhea secondary to an absent or short colon have been candidates for permanent colostomy.

TABLE 35–4. Urinary Incontinence

Type of Defect	Percentage
Rectal atresia or stenosis	0.0
Perineal fistula	0.0
Bulbar urethral fistula	0.0
Imperforate anus, no fistula	0.0
*Vestibular fistula	2.2
*Bladder neck fistula	4.3
†Cloaca, common channel <3 cm	13.8
*Prostatic fistula	18.1
†Cloaca, common channel >3 cm	66.7
Total	**9.3**

*Severe associated sacral anomaly.
†Dry with intermittent catheterization.

Patients suffering from fecal incontinence are evaluated and classified into those with constipation and those with increased bowel motility (tendency to have diarrhea). In the first group, bowel irrigations must be aggressive. A rubber tube is usually introduced high into the sigmoid to clean the bowel. This program takes advantage of the decreased bowel motility in some patients; they remain clean for the next 24 hours. No laxatives are given as part of this protocol. Those patients who suffer from increased bowel motility due to loss of the rectal reservoir or much of the colon require a constipating diet, medication to decrease the bowel motility, and a program of bowel irrigations.[48]

We adjust this treatment by trial and error over 1 week. Most patients remain clean and have an acceptable social life. Bowel management is started when the patient who is still incontinent has to go to school and all his or her classmates are already wearing regular underwear. Most patients and parents are very happy with the implementation of this program.[48] However, when the patient reaches the age of 10 to 12, he or she usually needs more independence. At that point, the creation of a continent appendicostomy (Malone procedure) is recommended.[49, 50] This operation creates a communication between the abdominal wall and the cecum through the appendix of the patient, creating a valve mechanism that allows the catheterization of the cecum but which prevents leakage of stool. This allows the patient to administer his or her own enema while sitting on the toilet. The operation consists of plicating the cecum around the native appendix of the patient and exteriorizing the appendix in the deepest portion of the umbilicus to make it inconspicuous.[50]

A significant number of patients do not have an appendix, so we then create a tubularized flap of the medial portion of the cecum and then we plicate the cecum around it. The stoma is also exteriorized through the umbilicus. Most patients who have had this operation express a great deal of satisfaction.[50]

REFERENCES

1. Aegineta P: On the imperforate anus. In Adams F (translator): The Seven Books (book 6). London, Sydenham Society, 1844, pp 405–406.
2. Amussat JZ: Gustiure d'une operation d'anus artifical pratique avec succes par un nouveau procede. Gaz Med Paris 3:735–758, 1835.
3. Roux de Brignoles JN: De l'imperforation de l'anus chez les nouveaux-nex-Rapport et discussion sur l'operation a tenter dans ces cas. Gazette Medicale de Paris 2:411–412, 1834.
4. Wangensteen OH, Rice CO: Imperforate anus: A method of determining the surgical approach. Ann Surg 92:77–81, 1930.
5. Stephens FD: Imperforate rectum: A new surgical technique. Med J Aust 1:202–206, 1953.
6. Kiesewetter WB: Imperforate anus, II: The rationale and technique of sacroabdominoperineal operation. J Pediatr Surg 2:106–117, 1967.
7. Louw JH, Cywes S, Cremin BJ: The management of anorectal agenesis. S Afr J Surg 9:21–30, 1971.
8. Rehbein F: Imperforate anus: Experiences with abdominoperineal and abdomino sacroperineal pull through procedures. J Periatr Surg 2:99–105, 1967.
9. Soave F: Surgery of rectal anomalies with preservation of the relationship between the colonic muscular sleeve and puborectal muscle. J Pediatr Surg 4:705–712, 1969.
10. deVries P, Peña A: Posterior sagittal anorectoplasty. J Pediatr Surg 17:638–643, 1982.
11. Peña A, deVries P: Posterior sagittal anorectoplasty. Important technical considerations and new applications. J Pediatr Surg 17:796–881, 1982.
12. Brenner EC: Congenital defects of the anus and rectum. Surg Gynecol Obstet 20:579–588, 1915.
13. Santulli TV: Treatment of imperforate anus and associated fistulas. Surg Gynecol Obstet 95:601–614, 1952.
14. Trusler GA, Wilkinson RH: Imperforate anus: A review of 147 cases. Can J Surg 5:169–177, 1962.
15. Anderson RC, Read SC: The likelihood of recurrence of congenital malformations. Lancet 74:175–176, 1954.
16. Cozzi F, Wilinson AW: Familial incidence of congenital malformations. Lancet 74:175–176, 1954.
17. Murken JD, Albert A: Genetic counseling in cases of anal and rectal atresia. Progr Pediatr Surg 9:115–118, 1976.
18. Peña A: Posterior sagittal anorectoplasty: Results in the management of 322 cases of anorectal malformations. Pediatr Surg Int 3:94–104, 1988.
19. Stephens FD, Smith ED: Incidence, frequency of types, etiology. In Stephens FD, Smith ED, Paul NW (eds): Anorectal Malformations in Children. Chicago, Year Book Medical, 1971, pp 160–171.
20. Peña A: Anorectal malformations. Semin Pediatr Surg 4:35–47, 1995.
21. Peña A: Advances in anorectal malformations [preface]. Semin Pediatr Surg 6:165–169, 1997.
22. Torres R, Levitt MA, Tovilla JM, et al: Anorectal malformations and Down's syndrome. J Pediatr Surg 33:194–197, 1998.
23. Warf BC, Scott RM, Barnes PD, et al: Tethered spinal cord in patients with anorectal and urogenital malformations. Pediatr Neuro Surg 19:25–30, 1993.
24. Appignani BA, Jaramillo D, Barnes PD, et al: Dysraphic myelodysplasias associated with urogenital and anorectal anomalies: Prevalence and types seen with MR imaging. AJR Am J Roentgenol, 163:1199–1203, 1994.
25. Levitt MA, Patel M, Rodriguez G, et al: The tethered spinal cord in patients with anorectal malformations. J Pediatr Surg 32:462–468, 1997.
26. Belman BA, King LR: Urinary tract abnormalities associated with imperforate anus. J Urol 108:823–824, 1972.
27. Hoekstra WJ, Scholtmeijer RJ, Molenar JC, et al: Urogenital tract abnormalities associated with congenital anorectal anomalies. J Urol 130:962–963, 1983.
28. Munn R, Schillinger JF: Urologic abnormalities found with imperforate anus. Urology 21:260–264, 1983.
29. Parrott TS: Urologic implications of anorectal malformations. Urol Clin North Am 12:13–21, 1985.
30. Wiener ES, Kiesewetter WB: Urologic abnormalities associated with imperforate anus. J Pediatr Surg 8:151–157, 1973.
31. William DI, Grant J: Urological complications of imperforate anus. Br J Urol 41:660–665, 1969.
32. Rich MA, Brock WA, Peña A: Spectrum of genitourinary malformations in patients with imperforate anus. Pediatr Surg Int 3:110–113, 1988.
33. Freeman NV, Burge DM, Soar JS, et al: Anal evoked potentials. Z Rinderchir 31:22–30, 1980.
34. Narasimharao KL, Prasad GR, Katariya K, et al: Prone crosstable lateral view: An alternative to the invertogram in imperforate anus. AJR Am J Roentgenol 140:227–229, 1983.
35. Gross GW, Wolfson PJ, Peña A: Augmented-pressure colostogram in imperforate anus with fistula. Pediatr Radiol 21:560–562, 1991.
36. Goon HK: Repair of anorectal anomalies in the neonatal period. Pediatr Surg Int 5:246–249, 1990.
37. Aluwihare APR: Primary perineal rectovaginoanoplasty for supralevator imperforateanus in female neonates. J Pediatr Surg 25:278–281, 1990.
38. Moore TC: Advantages of performing the sagittal anoplasty operation for imperforate anus at birth. J Pediatr Surg 25:276–277, 1990.
39. Wilkins S, Peña A: The role of colostomy in the management of anorectal malformations. Pediatr Surg Int 3:105–109, 1988.

40. Mollard P, Soucy P, Louis D, Meunier P: Preservation of infralevator structures in imperforate anus repair. J Pediatr Surg 24:1023–1026, 1989.

41. Nixon HH: Nixon anoplasty. In Stephens FD, Smith ED (eds): Anorectal Malformations in Children: Update 1988. Alan R. Liss, New York, 1988, pp 378–381.

42. Smith ED: Anorectal anomalies. Pediatr Surg Int 5:231–232, 1990.

43. Peña A: Total urogenital mobilization: An easier way to repair cloacas. J pediatr Surg 32:263–268, 1997.

44. Peña A: The surgical management of persistent cloaca: Results in 54 patients treated with a posterior sagittal approach. J Pediatr Surg 24:590–598, 1989.

45. Hendren WH: Repair of cloacal anomalies. Current techniques. J Pediatr Surg 21:1159–1176, 1986.

46. Hendren WH: Urogenital sinus and cloacal malformations. Semin Pediatr Surg 5:72–79, 1996.

47. Stephens FD, Smith ED: Anatomy and function of the normal rectum and anus. In Stephens FD, Smith ED, Paul NW (eds): Anorectal Malformations in Children. Chicago, Year Book Medical, 1977, pp 14–21.

48. Peña A, Guardino K, Tovilla JM, et al: Bowel management for fecal incontinence in patients with anorectal malformations. J Pediatr Surg 33:133–137, 1998.

49. Malone PS, Ransley PG, Kiely EM: Preliminary report: The antegrade continence enema. Lancet 336:1217–1218, 1990.

50. Levitt MA, Soffer SZ, Peña A: Continent appendicostomy in the bowel management of fecally incontinent children. J Pediatr Surg 32:1630–1633, 1997.

36

EXSTROPHY OF THE CLOACA

Brad W. Warner, MD • Moritz M. Ziegler, MD

Although cloacal exstrophy was first described by Littre in 1709,[1] it was not until 1960 that Rickham[2] reported the first successful reconstruction. Before this report was published, most infants with this devastating, complex malformation were allowed to die. The emotional, physical, and economic handicaps were considered too great to undertake major reconstructive efforts.

Early series of patients whose cloacal exstrophy was treated reported fairly high mortality rates. In a compiled series of patients who underwent treatment until 1970, only 6 of 19 survived.[3-7] At the Boston Children's Hospital, only 17 of 34 patients who underwent treatment from 1968 to 1976 survived the correction.[8] More encouraging reports have recently emerged, primarily owing to improved neonatal intensive care and nutritional support. In a contemporary report from the Children's Hospital of Philadelphia, 23 of 26 patients have survived long term.[9] Another report showed a survival rate of 22% between 1963 and 1978, which increased to 90% between 1979 and 1986.[10] In a 22-year experience, two workers noted an 83% survival rate among 12 infants.[11] Indeed, Rickham[2] astutely predicted that "in the next decade pediatric surgery will have to come to grips with these problems. We shall have to reexamine the contention that these children will never make useful members of society and are better left to die."

☐ Anatomy

Cloacal exstrophy, also referred to as vesicointestinal fissure, ectopic cloaca, ectopia viscerum, complicated exstrophy of the bladder, and abdominal wall fissure, is probably the most severe form of the ventral abdominal wall defects. The classic defects in cloacal exstrophy are illustrated in Figures 36–1 and 36–2. They consist of an omphalocele superiorly and exposed bowel and bladder inferiorly. The bladder is bivalved in the midline by a zone of intestinal mucosa, with each hemibladder containing a ureteral orifice. The exposed intestinal mu-cosa that sits between the hemibladders histologically represents the ileocecal area. It may contain up to four orifices.

The most superior orifice represents proximal bowel. It may be prolapsed outward, appearing as an elephant trunk-like deformity, whereas the most inferior orifice represents distal bowel. The distal bowel orifice represents the hindgut, which ends in a blind pouch and is associated with an imperforate anus. One or two appendiceal orifices are found between the proximal and distal bowel orifices.

Genital abnormalities are found in all cases. In male infants, undescended testes are present. The penis is usually bifid, with each half epispadiac and attached to widely separated pubic rami.[12] In female infants, the clitoris is divided and usually associated with a duplex vagina and bicornuate uterus.[6]

☐ Embryogenesis

An understanding of the development of cloacal exstrophy requires an appreciation of the normal

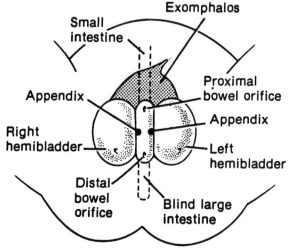

Figure 36–1. Anatomy of classic cloacal exstrophy. (From Howell C, Caldamone A, Snyder H, et al: Optimal management of cloacal exstrophy. J Pediatr Surg 18:365–369, 1983.)

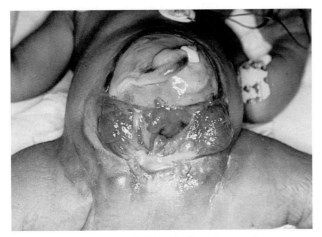

Figure 36–2. A child with cloacal exstrophy.

embryology of the cloacal region. Because the human embryo does not pass through a stage that corresponds to exstrophy, cloacal exstrophy is considered a manifestation of abnormal embryogenesis rather than an arrest in development.[13, 14]

The cloacal membrane separates the coelomic cavity from the amniotic space in early development. The membrane is first evident at the 2nd to 3rd week of gestation. At this time, the cloacal membrane is identified in the midline just caudal to the primitive streak as an area where ectoderm and endoderm are in apposition, without the ingrowth of mesoderm. By the 4th week, as the embryo and its tail elongate, the cloacal membrane forms the ventral wall of the urogenital sinus at the root of the allantois (Fig. 36–3). The unfused primordia of the genital tubercles lie cephalad and lateral to the cloacal membrane. Ultimately, these primordia enlarge and fuse in the midline superior to the cloacal membrane to form the genital tubercle.

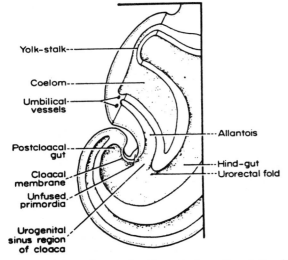

Figure 36–3. The embryo at the 4th week shows the relationship of the unfused primordia of the genital tubercle to the cloacal membrane. (From Ambrose SA, O'Brien DP III: Surgical embryology of the exstrophy-epispadias complex. Surg Clin North Am 54:1379–1390, 1974.)

Accompanying this fusion is the ingrowth of mesoderm toward the midline, thereby lengthening the area between the body stalk and cloacal membrane and allowing for the development of an intact infraumbilical body wall. At the same time, the urorectal septum develops in a medial and caudal direction, joining the primitive perineum (cloacal membrane) and dividing the cloaca into the urogenital sinus and rectum.

Two main theories explain the abnormal embryogenesis of cloacal exstrophy. The "caudal displacement" theory suggests that caudal displacement of the paired primordia of the genital tubercle, relative to the point where the urorectal fold divides the primitive cloaca into the urogenital and anal components, explains the spectrum of anomalies in the epispadias-exstrophy complex.[14] Fusion of the primordia in the midline at the point where the urorectal septum joins the cloacal membrane results in epispadias. Further caudal displacement of the primordia may result in complete bladder exstrophy. Even further caudal displacement of the primordia (caudal to the anal portion of the cloaca) results in exstrophy of both bowel and bladder-cloacal exstrophy. The spectrum of anomalies associated with varied degrees of caudal displacement of the paired primordia of the genital tubercle can be appreciated.

The other main theory proposed to explain the development of cloacal exstrophy is the "wedge effect" of an abnormally large cloacal membrane.[15] Proponents of this theory suggest that, if the genesis of abnormalities is due simply to caudal positioning of the paired primordia, lesser degrees of epispadias should be more common. However, approximately 90% of abnormalities occur at the vesical outlet. In addition, proponents suggest that, with further caudal displacement of the primordia and more severe exstrophy, the corpora should be located on the perineum or dissociated from bony attachments. However, this abnormality is rarely described.

In this theory, an abnormally large or a persisting cloacal membrane acts as a wedge to the developing structures of the abdominal wall. This explanation clarifies why the involved structures are normal but separated and why the bones are abnormal, only to the degree that might be expected from a wedge effect. With rupture of this unstable membrane by the 8th week of gestation before the descent of the urorectal septum and the fusion of the genital tubercles, a midline infraumbilical defect results, exposing bladder and bowel mucosae and producing bifid external genitalia. The timing of this theory has recently been challenged by the ultrasonographic (US) observation of an intact cloacal membrane in an 18-week gestation fetus, which then ruptured sometime before the 24th week.[16]

Evidence is provided experimentally in support of the wedge effect theory. Inert plastic grafts are placed into the area of the cloacal membranes in developing chick embryos.[17] In this study, the graft produced a wedge effect as well as a persistent cloacal membrane and resulted in varying degrees of infraumbilical defects. Many of the defects were much larger than the size of the graft. This first experimental production of exstrophy created an anomaly that normally is not seen in the chick.

Although these theories may offer explanations for the cause of the midline defects and the role of the abnormal cloacal membrane, confusion still exists regarding the cause of ileocecal prolapse and blind-ending ileocecum with associated imperforate anus.

In one theory, the hindgut, which begins at the level of Meckel's diverticulum, is greatly restricted in growth by its involvement in exstrophy.[18] The exposed bowel represents an extremely short hindgut, and the distal blind length of intestine is the persistent tailgut.

Alternatively, in another theory, a loop of midgut or hindgut prolapses between the bladder halves and becomes strangulated.[19] This theory may explain the foreshortened intestine as well as the varied intestinal plate orifices.

To explain the absence of the derivatives of the distal limb of midgut (terminal ileum, appendix, cecum, and right colon) in a patient with cloacal exstrophy, others have suggested a role for allantois-originated epithelium in the development of the distal midgut.[20] Failure of this epithelium to migrate, ascend, and align with the yolk sac or its persistence at the dome of the cloaca may play a role in the development of this type of exstrophy.

Due to the complexity associated with the development of cloacal exstrophy, not every case conforms to the classic anatomic presentation. A method of classification of the exstrophy variants has been proposed to allow for analysis of the various patterns in a more logical manner.[21]

Covered cloacal exstrophy refers to the presence of the visceral and musculoskeletal features of cloacal exstrophy but with an intact abdominal wall.[22] In our experience with two patients with covered cloacal exstrophy, in which the external appearance was of a covered bladder exstrophy, the posterior bladder was composed of ileocecal bowel on exploration. A short hindgut was present, associated with imperforate anus.

Embryologically, the lack of mesodermal migration into the infraumbilical membrane results in its disintegration, thus allowing the pelvic viscera to be open to the surface of the abdomen.[23] A covered cloacal exstrophy may result when mesoderm invades the infraumbilical membrane, preventing its breakdown, after the wedge effect of the membrane has led to separation of the pubic bones and of the lateral abdominal wall musculature. This mesodermal invasion may be incomplete or complete and may either precede or follow extroversion of the viscera. The presence of abdominal musculoskeletal defects with normal visceral development could be explained by late complete mesodermal infiltration before visceral extroversion.[24] Late and incomplete infiltration of mesoderm would account for variants,

such as the superior vesical fissure, when only the apical portion of the bladder is exstrophied or when bowel and bladder are exstrophied but confined to the subumbilical region, with normal formation of the urethra and phallus.[25]

Sequestration of segments of viscera (colon or ileum) onto the abdominal wall may occur in association with exstrophy or epispadias in both male and female patients. This sequestration might be explained by delayed mesodermal invasion with secondary (complete or incomplete) closure of the dehisced infraumbilical membrane. These segments of bowel may be useful in subsequent reconstruction of the genitourinary tract.

□ Incidence

Cloacal exstrophy represents the extreme of a spectrum of disorders ranging from epispadias to cloacal exstrophy. Epispadias, including the balanic, penile, subsymphyseal, and penopubic, accounts for 30% of the anomalies in this complex and occurs in 1 in 120,000 births.[26] Classic bladder exstrophy makes up the majority of anomalies in this group (60%) and occurs in 1 in 30,000 births. The remaining 10% of anomalies in this complex are accounted for by cloacal exstrophy and its variants, which are estimated to occur in 1 of 400,000 births. Approximately 15 new cases per year may be expected in the United States.[27] In all of these abnormalities, a male predominance exists. This predominance is more pronounced in the classic bladder exstrophy group, with a male-to-female ratio of 2.3:1, and is less prominent in the cloacal exstrophy group.[26]

□ Associated Anomalies

Aside from the usual anatomic findings in cloacal exstrophy, anomalies of other organ systems remote from the basic defect occur in up to 85% of cases (Table 36–1).[10] Abnormalities of the upper urinary tract are common. They consist of pelvic kidney, hydronephrosis, hydroureter, ureteral atresia, unilateral renal agenesis, multicystic kidney, ureteral duplication, and crossed fused ectopia. On review of several large series, such abnormalities were noted to occur in from 42 to 60% of cases.[3, 4, 10, 11, 27]

Vertebral anomalies are reported in 48 to 75% of patients.[3, 4, 10] Myelodysplasia (myelomeningocele, meningocele, lipomeningocele) is noted in 29 to 46% of patients.[10, 27] One recent report identified the presence of vertebral or spinal cord abnormalities in 16 of 17 patients who were fully evaluated.[28] The index of suspicion for this association should therefore be high. Central nervous system disorders other than myelodysplasia are relatively infrequent. Survivors have normal intelligence.[3]

Associated gastrointestinal (GI) anomalies consist of malrotation, duodenal atresia, duplication, Meck-

TABLE 36-1. Spectrum of Multiple
Anomalies of Cloacal Exstrophy

Omphalocele and abdominal wall deficiency
Split symphysis anomaly
Bladder exstrophy (open plate of mucosa)
    Two exstrophied hemibladders
    Interposed midline colonic segment
Ileocecal exstrophy
    Superior orifice prolapsed ileum
    Single or duplicate inferior-orifice, short, blind-ending
      hindgut
    Usually duplicate appendiceal stumps in intermediate
      position
Imperforate anus
Bifid external genitalia
    Diminutive penis
    Bifid clitoris and labia
    Cryptorchidism
Duplex müllerian structures
    May be exstrophied vaginas at base of bladder mucosa
    May be atretic vaginas
Myelomeningocele
Other defects
    Talipes equinovarus
    Vertebral anomalies (scoliosis)
    Renal anomalies
    Agenesis or multicystic
    Megaloureter
    Hydronephrosis
    Fusion anomalies, ectopia

From Ziegler MM, Duckett JW, Howell C: Cloacal exstrophy. In Welch KJ, Randolph JG, Ravitch MM, et al (eds): Pediatric Surgery (4th ed). Chicago, Year Book Medical, 1986, pp 764–771. By permission of Mosby, Inc.

el's diverticulum, short bowel, and absent or double appendix. In one report, such findings were present in 12 of 26 patients (46%).[10] The presence of a shortened proximal small intestine is important to recognize, because bowel preservation is one of the more important principles in the management of this condition. This problem may be more functional than real.[27] One of Rickham's original four patients died as a result of short bowel syndrome after surviving for 2 months.[2] Many other series include deaths resulting from this syndrome.

Abnormalities of the lower extremities are also noted. They consist of club feet, congenital dislocated hips, and other severe deformities. These features occur in 26 to 30% of patients.[4, 29]

The external genitalia in patients with cloacal exstrophy are invariably abnormal. In male infants, the penis and scrotum may be absent, bifid, or epispadiac. The testicles are uniformly undescended. The vas may be either absent or double. In female infants, the clitoris is bifid or absent, whereas the vagina may be absent, single, duplex, or exstrophied. Due to a failure of midline fusion of the müllerian structures in the female patient, a bifid or duplicate uterus is almost uniformly present.

□ Preoperative Evaluation

Despite multiple obvious external abnormalities, emergent surgical correction of the infant with clo-

acal exstrophy is neither wise nor indicated. The information gained by a thorough preoperative evaluation of all possible defects is extremely important toward the development of an informed and intelligent treatment plan. This information may be obtained in a relatively short period of time, such that operative intervention may take place within the first few days of life.

The major areas that require preoperative evaluation include the upper urinary tract, central nervous system, musculoskeletal deformities, and gender status. US examination of the upper urinary tracts provides important information regarding position, size, and presence or absence of kidneys. US may also detect hydronephrosis and hydroureter, which may require preoperative urinary decompression. US examination of the upper urinary tracts should be supplemented by intravenous pyelography. The last test provides useful data regarding structure and function.

The spinal cord should be evaluated by both US and plain radiographs of the lumbar and sacral spine region. The spinal US may detect the presence of myelodysplasia, tethered cord, or other abnormalities. Plain films detect missing or hemivertebrae and sacral anomalies. Additional studies such as myelography or magnetic resonance imaging may be indicated if abnormalities are suggested by the aforementioned initial studies. Cranial US should also be performed to rule out other problems, such as hydrocephalus.

Musculoskeletal defects should be carefully sought during the initial physical examination to determine whether further radiographic evaluation is needed. Every child should have a radiograph of the pelvis to detect anomalies, such as split symphysis and congenital hip dislocation.

The need for gender assignment is one of the more important and pressing issues to be dealt with during the initial evaluation. All infants should be karyotyped. The majority of male patients with cloacal exstrophy should be raised as females because the penis is usually not reconstructible for adequate sexual function. In male infants who are assigned to the female gender, orchiectomy should be performed at the time of the initial reconstruction.

In addition to the aforementioned evaluations, blood should be obtained to determine electrolyte, glucose, blood urea nitrogen, creatinine, and calcium levels; complete blood count; baseline liver function tests; and type and crossmatch. Urinalysis and chest radiographs must also be performed.

□ Treatment

Successfully managing the infant with cloacal exstrophy requires an aggressive multispecialty effort with a delegated team leader. After review of the multiple studies and determination of the anomalies to be corrected, an organized treatment plan should be designed. The plan for staged correction is formulated in concert with all consultants and includes orthopedics, neurosurgery, urology, and neonatology. The pediatric surgeon, or leader, takes the total patient into account and coordinates all consultants. The assistance of various ancillary personnel, such as enterostomal and physical therapists, social workers, family support personnel for long-term rehabilitation, and nurses, is involved. Most importantly, an overview of the entire recommended treatment plan and management options is presented to the family. Family input, support, and total agreement with the proposed plan of treatment before operative intervention cannot be overemphasized. The initial reconstruction during the neonatal period is of considerable magnitude. Ideally, it should be undertaken only at major medical centers with staff experienced in the management of patients with these anomalies. Antenatal detection of cloacal exstrophy has been reported using US.[30] This modality may facilitate the transfer of the mother to an appropriate center before delivery.

One of the important components of the initial surgical management of this condition is the determination of whether total correction will require one or more stages.[29] A one-stage reconstruction may be appropriate if the infant is in otherwise excellent condition and has favorable anatomy and minimal associated anomalies.[10] In a series of 34 patients, a one-stage reconstruction was planned in eight classic cases but performed in only four.

In general, the first operative stage (Fig. 36–4) consists of closure of the omphalocele; separation of the intestinal plate from the hemibladders with construction of a GI stoma; reapproximation of the separated bladder halves, if possible; and orchiectomy in cases of genetic males assigned to the female gender. Additional procedures may also be indicated as related to neurosurgical disorders (e.g., myelomeningocele, hydrocephalus) or orthopedic disorders (e.g., need for osteotomies, casting of lower extremities).

The second and subsequent major operative stages are usually performed when the infant has reached a weight of 20 to 25 pounds. The patient should be thriving and at reasonable operative risk. At this stage, attention is directed toward reconstruction of the bladder and/or urethra as well as the external genitalia.

CLOSURE OF THE OMPHALOCELE

Closure of the omphalocele can usually be achieved primarily, but initial placement of prosthetic material may be necessary. In one report, a temporary Silastic silo was used in closure of 2 of 15 cases.[29] From lessons learned during the correction of classic bladder exstrophy, surgical reapproximation of the pubis greatly enhances the ability to close the omphalocele.[27, 31] Therefore, the first stage of reconstruction is optimally performed within the first 48 to 72 hours of life, owing to the relative

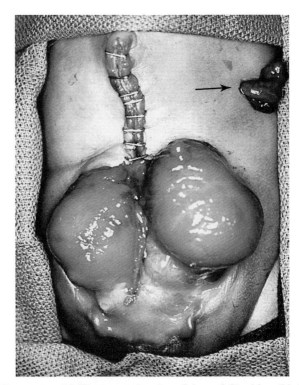

Figure 36–4. Midline approximation of the mobilized hemibladders and closure of the omphalocele. Note the terminal colostomy *(arrow)*. Closure of the bladder and bilateral iliac osteotomy will be performed at a later stage.

elasticity of the neonatal skeleton during this period.

High-tensile strength suture may be placed at each end of the pubis for reapproximation. In a patient with a huge omphalocele, the intact membrane perhaps should be left in place as a barrier for the potential staged closure. The peritoneal cavity must be entered, however, to dissect out the exstrophied bowel and bladder. This procedure usually requires a superior and an inferior extension of the incision (Fig. 36–5).

INTESTINAL TRACT

The primary goal in managing the intestinal tract in patients with cloacal exstrophy is preservation of all possible bowel, no matter how short a segment. Appendices should not be sacrificed, because appendicovesicostomy may be an option for bladder diversion during subsequent reconstructions.[32] Similarly, duplicated segments of colon may be helpful in an isoperistaltic or antiperistaltic direction to slow intestinal transit time in cases of foreshortened colon or small intestine. This extra colon may also prove useful for bladder augmentation during subsequent reconstruction.

The blind-ending colon and the exstrophied bowel plate are tubularized and approximated to the end of the ileum and brought out as an end colostomy (Fig. 36–6). Lateral placement of this

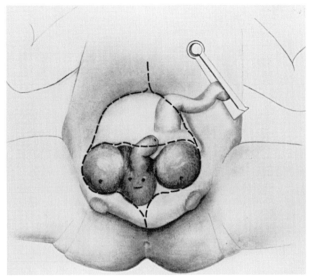

Figure 36–5. Incision for repair of cloacal exstrophy. The bladder plates will be mobilized and the abdominal cavity will be entered to repair the omphalocele. Usually, a superior and an inferior extension of the incision are required.

stoma minimizes contamination of the abdominal wall and permits the utilization of prosthetic material for closure if necessary. This small segment of bowel can enlarge considerably with time.[33]

Several series have advocated the construction of an end ileostomy for fecal diversion with preservation of the distal colon for reconstruction of the genitourinary tract.[3, 8, 34] However, the superiority of a colostomy compared with an ileostomy in the fluid, electrolyte, and nutritional management of these complex cases has become appreciated.[10, 11, 29] In a comparison of patients with cloacal exstrophy managed by terminal ileostomy or by terminal colostomy, a significantly greater number of in-hospital days were required for patients with ileostomies to treat the complications involving the GI tract. More days were also needed for parenteral nutrition in the ileostomy group.[35] In that study, no differences were noted in the total hospital days required to manage the exstrophy or the growth rates at long-term follow-up. Furthermore, the frequency of hospitalizations as a result of fluid and electrolyte disturbances in both groups was extremely rare after the age of 3 years. Thus, these children seem to ultimately adapt to terminal ileostomy at the expense of more frequent hospitalizations and prolonged intravenous nutrition during the initial management phase. Two patients were reported to require ileostomy takedown due to fluid and electrolyte problems, which were corrected following terminal colostomy.[29]

Continent reconstruction of the intestinal tract is possible but highly dependent on anatomy. In patients with simple anterior displacement of the anus, reasonable success has been achieved with perineal anoplasty.[29] Due to poor development of the perineal musculature, dismal results have been

reported in most patients following various pull-through techniques.[3, 35] Fecal continence has been reported after an anterior sagittal anoenteroplasty in a patient with a variant type of cloacal exstrophy.[36] This patient underwent reconstruction using the posterior saggital approach, which placed a tapered segment of bowel within an identifiable muscle complex.[37] Whether a significant role exists for the posterior sagittal anorectoplasty in the management of this condition remains unanswered.[29] In one large series, 6 of 20 children had rectal pull-through procedures.[38] In that report, the functional results of these procedures were not discussed. Of 26 patients reported from the Children's Hospital of Philadelphia, five patients had either posterior sagittal anorectoplasty (n = 4) or perineal anoplasty (n = 1).[9] Two of these patients are continent and one is free of soilage on a bowel management program.

URINARY TRACT

After separation of the intestinal plate from the two hemibladders, the bladder should be reapproximated posteriorly in the midline, thus converting the situation into a classic bladder exstrophy. In most cases, insufficient bladder surface is present for primary complete bladder closure. Therefore, the

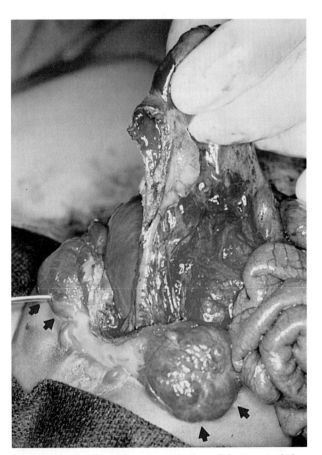

Figure 36–6. The distal bowel, consisting of the terminal ileum and the foreshortened colon, is separated from the hemibladders (arrows), tubularized, and exteriorized as a terminal colostomy.

hemibladders are approximated in the midline. Each ureteral orifice is carefully avoided. A posterior bladder wall plate is formed, which may be left exteriorized as a perineal vesicostomy, with plans for subsequent reconstruction or excision. The disadvantages of leaving the urothelium exposed include significant swelling and excoriation. These factors may contribute to urinary obstruction at the ureterovesical level as well as to difficulty during subsequent reconstruction. Primary closure of the bladder may be facilitated by using a patch of hindgut.[39] However, this technique may not be useful owing to the need to preserve all possible intestinal mucosa for the GI tract to prevent the short bowel syndrome.

Occasionally, insufficient bladder mucosa is present for bladder reconstruction by any technique. In these cases, the bladder mucosa may be excised, with preservation of the muscular layers. The remaining bladder muscularis may facilitate abdominal wall closure by allowing granulation tissue to form, with subsequent ingrowth of skin.[40] If enough bladder surface exists to construct an adequate capacity reservoir, the bladder is closed primarily by reapproximation of the anterior and posterior walls. The tubularized bladder is placed behind the approximated pubic rami, with the bladder neck draining inferiorly onto the perineum. Primary closure of the bladder has been possible in only 8 to 30% of cases in most large series.[10, 11, 29]

If primary closure can be done at the time of the initial reconstruction, simple approximation of the pubic rami may be all that is needed. When primary bladder closure is attempted beyond the first several days of life, a bilateral posterior iliac osteotomy is usually required. Recently, an anterior mid-iliac diagonal osteotomy has been proposed to provide a more functional pelvic closure.[41]

Following primary closure of the bladder, future reconstructive efforts are directed toward the establishment of continence. Many of the basic principles are used for classic bladder exstrophy. When continence is impossible, permanent urinary diversion is necessary. The variety of techniques that can achieve diversion include cutaneous ureterostomy with a cuff of bladder wall, tube vesicostomy, and construction of a conduit using either ileum or colon. Whether ileal or colon conduits should be chosen is a matter of debate. In long-term studies of ileal conduits in children with bladder exstrophy, significant delayed complications have developed over 10 to 15 years.[42, 43] Some investigators suggest that ileal conduit urinary diversion is no longer acceptable in children with a normal life expectancy.[44] Although the use of a colon conduit with nonrefluxing ureterointestinal anastomosis is attractive, a colon conduit in the patient with cloacal exstrophy whose midgut or hindgut may already be foreshortened makes this alternative less desirable.[45]

Subsequent procedures to establish urinary continence include the possible need for augmentation of the bladder, correction of the epispadias, and reconstruction of the bladder outlet. In one series, satisfactory urinary continence occurred after functional bladder closure in three of seven patients with cloacal exstrophy.[11] In another series, 17 of 20 patients are free of urinary appliances and void by intermittent catheterization.[38]

Another described technique consists of the initial construction of a colon conduit, followed by ureterovesical tubularization and anastomosis of the colon conduit to the tubularized bladder.[46] The appendix may provide continent urinary diversion with the Mitrofanoff procedure.[47] The ability to achieve urinary continence in a patient with cloacal exstrophy represents the utmost challenge to the surgeon, who must be familiar with all standard approaches and amenable to improvisation and modification. Although artificial urinary sphincters have been mentioned, no reports exist of their use in these so affected patients.

GENITALIA

Although reconstruction of the genitalia may be performed at any time, the consideration of gender assignment for male infants should be addressed immediately. Rarely, the phallus may be amenable to lengthening by partial detachment of the crura from the bony pubic rami and midline reapproximation, as described for classic bladder exstrophy.[48] Furthermore, gender assignment may not be necessary in patients in whom the surface pattern of the exstrophy consists of hemibladders that are caudal to the central bowel field. With this surface pattern, a male infant may have epispadias or a fully formed penis, which would not necessitate gender assignment.[10]

The most common situation for male infants is the presence of a phallus that is inadequate or marginally adequate for subsequent reconstruction. Such an infant should be assigned to the female gender, because the emotional consequences of an inadequate phallus may be too overwhelming. At least one patient raised as a phenotypic male may have committed suicide.[29]

The poor results with phallic reconstruction are well illustrated in a report of eight males with cloacal exstrophy who underwent such reconstruction. All patients had penile lengths that were two standard deviations below the mean. Of the four patients who have reached puberty, two have documented physiologic impotence by nocturnal penile tumescence testing. Of the other two patients capable of erection, one was unable to penetrate the vagina owing to phallic inadequacy. The other patient was married and was engaging in successful intercourse. Three patients in the series have undergone extensive psychiatric counseling owing to their feelings of sexual inadequacy.[49]

Gender-converting procedures are probably best done in the neonatal period for psychodynamic reasons. Corporal tissue should be preserved for construction of a clitoris. The hemiscrota are preserved for future labia. The abdominal testes are removed. The creation of a vagina is usually done at a later stage. Segments of small or large intestine may be utilized.

In females, the bifid clitoris and labia may be reconstructed at a later time with a fairly normal external appearance. Because the urorectal septum may prevent midline fusion of the müllerian structures, anomalies such as a septate vagina and a double uterus and tubes may be present. Vaginal exstrophy or atresia may also be present. Genital reconstruction of the female with cloacal exstrophy should be deferred to a later time to permit full evaluation of the pertinent anatomy.

MYELODYSPLASIA

About half the patients with cloacal exstrophy have a form of myelodysplasia, either as a frank myelomeningocele or lipomeningocele. Neurosurgical principles are applied as directed. They must be coordinated with the initial primary repair. Factors to consider include the need for direct repair, the timing of repair, and the need for some type of shunt. In addition, the orthopedic assessment of extremity, pelvis, and spinal deformities is important. Splinting, prosthetics, and various other orthopedic procedures are usually required as ambulation progresses.

□ Results

The management of patients with cloacal exstrophy has undergone significant change since the first successful reconstruction was reported.[2] With more series reporting excellent survival rates, the question involved in management is no longer whether the infant can survive but whether the infant will be continent of both urine and stool.[10, 11, 29] The major determinant of early mortality is the presence of associated defects (e.g., renal agenesis). Inherent in the management of these infants is the difficulty encountered with multiple operative procedures. However, the expectations for excellent outcome should remain high.

With greater experience in primary bladder closure and bladder neck reconstruction, some patients may be free of the need for urinary stomas.[38, 50] Magnetic resonance imaging and computed tomography may detect anorectal and pelvic musculature, which might facilitate pull-through procedures to eliminate the need for a GI stoma.[51] With few exceptions, male patients should undergo female gender assignment, with gonadectomy and genitoplasty early in life.

With all patients, ongoing psychologic and emotional support are required throughout reconstructive procedures, hospitalizations, and adjustments to maturation. Because the neurologic deficits, when present, are generally mild, these children have the potential for fully functional, happy, and productive lives.

REFERENCES

1. O'Neill JA: Cloacal exstrophy. In O'Neill JA, Rowe MI, Grosfeld JL, et al (eds): Pediatric Surgery (5th ed). St. Louis, Mosby–Year Book, 1998, pp 1725–1732.
2. Rickham PP: Vesico-intestinal fissure. Arch Dis Child 35:97–102, 1960.
3. Tank ES, Lindenauer SM: Principles of management of exstrophy of the cloaca. Am J Surg 119:95–98, 1970.
4. Spencer R: Exstrophia splanchnic (exstrophy of the cloaca). Surgery 57:751–766, 1965.
5. Zweiren GT, Patterson JH: Exstrophy of the cloaca: Report of a case treated surgically. Pediatrics 35:687–692, 1965.
6. Soper RT, Kilger K: Vesico-intestinal fissure. J Urol 92:490–501, 1964.
7. Graivier L: Exstrophy of the cloaca. Am Surg 34:387–390, 1968.
8. Welch KJ: Cloacal exstrophy (vesicointestinal fissure). In Ravitch MM, Welch KJ, Benson CD, et al (eds): Pediatric Surgery. Chicago, Year Book Medical, 1979, pp 802–808.
9. Davidoff AM, Hebra A, Balmer D, et al: Management of the gastrointestinal tract and nutrition in patients with cloacal exstrophy. J Pediatr Surg 31:771–773, 1996.
10. Hurwitz RS, Manzoni GAM, Ransley PG, et al: Cloacal exstrophy: A report of 34 cases. J Urol 138:1060–1064, 1987.
11. Diamond DA, Jeffs RD: Cloacal exstrophy: A 22-year experience. J Urol 133:779–782, 1985.
12. Johnston JH, Penn IA: Exstrophy of the cloaca. Br J Urol 38:302–307, 1966.
13. Pohlman AG: The development of the cloaca in human embryos. Am J Anat 12:1–26, 1911.
14. Patten BM, Barry A: The genesis of exstrophy of the bladder and epispadias. Am J Anat 90:35–53, 1952.
15. Marshall VF, Muecke EC: Variations in exstrophy of the bladder. J Urol 88:766–796, 1962.
16. Bruch SW, Adzick NS, Goldstein RB, et al: Challenging the embryogenesis of cloacal exstrophy. J Pediatr Surg 31:768–770, 1996.
17. Muecke EC: The role of the cloacal membrane in exstrophy: The first successful experimental study. J Urol 92:659–667, 1964.
18. Johnston TB: Extroversion of the bladder complicated by the presence of intestinal openings on the surface of the extroverted area. J Anat Physiol 48:89, 1913.
19. Magnus RV: Ectopia cloacae—a misnomer. J Pediatr Surg 4:511–519, 1969.
20. Zarabi CM, Rupani M: Cloacal exstrophy: A hypothesis on the allantoic origin of the distal midgut. Pediatr Pathol 4:117–124, 1985.
21. Manzoni GA, Ransley PG, Hurwitz RS: Cloacal exstrophy and cloacal exstrophy variants: A proposed system of classification. J Urol 138:1065–1068, 1987.
22. Johnston JH, Koff SA: Covered cloacal exstrophy: Another variation on the theme. J Urol 118:666–668, 1977.
23. Glenister TW: A correlation of the normal and abnormal development of the penile urethra and of the infra-umbilical abdominal wall. Br J Urol 30:117–126, 1958.
24. MacKenzie LL: Split pelvis in pregnancy. Am J Obstet Gynecol 29:255–257, 1935.
25. Koontz WW Jr, Joshi VV, Ownby R: Cloacal exstrophy with the potential for urinary control: An unusual presentation. J Urol 112:828–831, 1974.
26. Jeffs RD: Exstrophy, epispadias, and cloacal and urogenital sinus abnormalities. Pediatr Clin North Am 34:1233–1257, 1987.
27. Ziegler MM, Duckett JW, Howell C: Cloacal exstrophy. In Welch KJ, Randolph JG, Ravitch MM, et al (eds). Pediatric Surgery. Chicago, Year Book Medical, 1986, pp 764–771.
28. McLaughlin KP, Rink RC, Kalsbeck JE, et al: Cloacal exstrophy: The neurological implications. J Urol 154:782–784, 1995.

29. Howell C, Caldamone A, Snyder H, et al: Optimal management of cloacal exstrophy. J Pediatr Surg 18:365–369, 1983.

30. Meizner I, Bar-Ziv J: Prenatal ultrasonic diagnosis of cloacal exstrophy. Am J Obstet Gynecol 153:802–803, 1985.

31. Duckett JD: Newborn exstrophy closure. Presented at the American Urological Association; Kansas City, MO; May 1982.

32. Longaker MT, Harrison MR, Langer JC, et al: Appendicovesicostomy: A new technique for bladder diversion during reconstruction of cloacal exstrophy. J Pediatr Surg 24:639–641, 1989.

33. Colodny AH: Editorial comment. J Urol 133:782, 1985.

34. Sukarachana K, Sieber WK: Vesicointestinal fissure revisited. J Pediatr Surg 13:713–719, 1978.

35. Husmann DA, McLorie GA, Churchill BM, et al: Management of the hindgut in cloacal exstrophy: Terminal ileostomy versus colostomy. J Pediatr Surg 23:1107–1113, 1988.

36. Lobe TE: Fecal continence following an anterior-sagittal anoenteroplasty in a patient with cloacal exstrophy. J Pediatr Surg 19:843–845, 1984.

37. Pena A, deVries PA: Posterior sagittal anorectoplasty: Important technical considerations and new applications. J Pediatr Surg 17:796–811, 1982.

38. Lund DP, Hendren WH: Cloacal exstrophy: Experience with 20 cases. J Pediatr Surg 28:1360–1369, 1993.

39. Burbige KA, Libby C: Enterovesical cystoplasty for bladder closure in cloacal exstrophy. J Urol 137:948–950, 1987.

40. Flanigan RC, Casale AJ, McRoberts JW: Cloacal exstrophy. Urology 23:227–233, 1984.

41. McKenna PH, Khoury AE, McLorie GA, et al: Iliac osteotomy: A model to compare the options in bladder and cloacal exstrophy reconstruction. J Urol 151:182–187, 1994.

42. Jeffs RD, Schwarz GR: Ileal conduit urinary diversion in children: Computer analysis follow-up from 2 to 16 years. J Urol 114:285–288, 1975.

43. Shapiro SR, Lebowitz R, Colodny AH: Fate of 90 children with ileal conduit urinary diversion a decade later: Analysis of complications, pyelography, renal function, and bacteriology. J Urol 114:289–295, 1975.

44. MacFarlane MT, Lattimer JK, Hensle TW: Improved life expectancy for children with exstrophy of the bladder. JAMA 242:442–444, 1979.

45. Gearhart JP, Jeffs RD: Management and treatment of classic bladder exstrophy. In Ashcraft KW (ed): Pediatric Urology. Philadelphia, WB Saunders, 1990, pp 269–300.

46. Arap S, Giron AM, deGoes GM: Initial results of the complete reconstruction of bladder exstrophy. Urol Clin North Am 7:477–491, 1980.

47. Duckett JW, Snyder HM III: Continent urinary diversion: Variations on the Mitrofanoff principle. J Urol 136:58–62, 1986.

48. Johnston JH: The genital aspects of exstrophy. J Urol 113:701–705, 1975.

49. Husmann DA, McLorie GA, Churchill BM: Phallic reconstruction in cloacal exstrophy. J Urol 142:563–564, 1989.

50. Smith EA, Woodard JR, Broecker BH, et al: Current urologic management of cloacal exstrophy: Experience with 11 patients. J Pediatr Surg 32:256–262, 1997.

51. Mezzacappa PM, Price AP, Haller JO, et al: MR and CT demonstration of levator sling in congenital anorectal anomalies. J Comput Assist Tomogr 11:273–275, 1987.

37

ANORECTAL CONTINENCE AND MANAGEMENT OF CONSTIPATION

Gerard Weinberg, MD • Scott J. Boley, MD

Of the many benign disorders afflicting children, abnormal defecation often has the most disruptive effect on the family. Although enormous progress has been made in the diagnosis and management of infections and metabolic diseases, children with functional constipation remain a source of continuing frustration to themselves, their parents, and their physicians. Normal anorectal function, so frequently taken for granted, is a complex balance of three interrelated functions: (1) the transport of fecal contents from the colon into the rectum (i.e., colonic motility), (2) the intermittent, rather than continuous, evacuation of stool from the rectum (i.e., defecation), and (3) the total retention of intestinal contents between acts of defecation (i.e., continence). Social continence is not only the ability to evacuate stool intermittently but to do so only at socially appropriate times. Any alterations in the physiologic or anatomic mechanisms controlling any one of these functions can produce abnormalities that affect the others.

☐ Anatomy

Important anatomic structures involved in defecation and continence include both those with primarily a sensory role and those with primarily a motor role. The primary muscles are the internal anal sphincter (IAS), the external anal sphincter (EAS), and the puborectalis muscle; the other levator ani muscles play a less important role. The two major sites of sensation are the tension receptors in the rectal wall, especially in the adjacent puborectalis muscles, and the nerve endings in the anal mucosa, which are sensitive to pain, touch, and temperature.

The smooth muscle IAS lies one third below the dentate line and two thirds above it. The striated muscle EAS lies outside of and surrounds the IAS. The puborectalis muscle forms a sling posteriorly around the rectum. It is contiguous with the deep portion of the EAS (Fig. 37–1). These two striated

muscles are supplied by the pudendal nerve. Often acting as a unit, they are sometimes referred to as the *striated muscle complex*.[1]

INTERNAL ANAL SPHINCTER

The IAS is a smooth muscle in a tonic state of contraction. It provides at least 85% of the resting anal canal pressure.[2] The external sphincter and the puborectalis muscle provide the remainder. The tonic contraction of the IAS is primarily an intrinsic property of the smooth muscle itself, but it may be supplemented by intrinsic neural input. The IAS

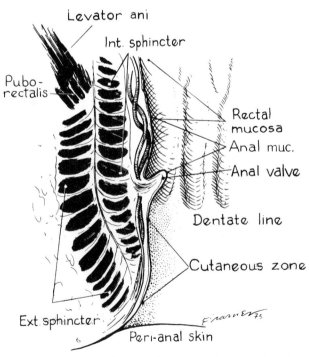

Figure 37–1. A sagittal view of the normal anorectal anatomy demonstrates the location of the internal and external anal sphincters and the puborectalis and levator ani muscles.

may be capable of slightly increased contraction, but the major change in its resting tone is relaxation in response to rectal distention. This inhibitory reflex is an intrinsic neural reflex (Fig. 37–2).[3]

The sensory receptors of the anal canal are limited to the mucosa just superior to the dentate line. In the more proximal rectum, no sensory receptors are present. Thus, the determination of whether fluid, solid stool, or gas is being passed occurs in the distal anal canal. To facilitate this discrimination, the proximal IAS relaxes, which allows the material to pass to the distal canal. The material is identified by the sensory receptors and either contained or released as appropriate.

The innervation of the smooth muscle portion of the sphincter is complex and not completely elucidated. Sympathetic innervation is supplied by both lumbar splanchnic nerves from the lumbar spinal cord and by hypogastric nerves from the inferior mesenteric ganglion. Parasympathetic innervation comes via the pelvic nerves from the sacral spinal cord.[4]

The sympathetic motor effect is primarily excitatory, but an inhibitory component may be present. α-Adrenergic stimulation is excitatory, but β-adrenergic stimulation is inhibitory. The parasympathetic nerves cause relaxation. However, cholinergic agonists actually cause excitation, whereas the cholinergic antagonist atropine produces either excitation or inhibition, depending on the experimental model.[5] Thus, excitatory innervation appears to be dual—both cholinergic and adrenergic. Both adrenergic and nonadrenergic inhibitory innervations may also be present.[6]

Intrinsic innervation of the internal sphincter also exists, which is the primary system for producing relaxation in response to rectal distention. This relaxation response occurs even in the presence of spinal anesthesia. The nerves involved lie in the intramural plexuses and the myenteric and submucosal ganglia. They are nonadrenergic and noncho-

linergic in nature.[7] Evidence suggests vasoactive intestinal polypeptide as the possible inhibitory neurotransmitter, but additional neurotransmitters may be involved.[8]

EXTERNAL ANAL SPHINCTER

The EAS muscle is a striated muscle and, hence, capable of phasic contraction. Like the IAS, the EAS may have some tonic contraction.[9] Unlike the IAS, the tonic contraction of the EAS depends exclusively on efferent nervous input. The phasic contractions are both voluntary and involuntary. The external sphincter muscle provides part of the resting tone of the sphincter complex. Depending on the situation, increased contraction of the external sphincter muscle can aid either in resisting defecation or in emptying the distal anal canal.[10]

With rectal distention, the EAS contracts reflexly—the "inflation reflex" (see Fig. 37–2), which is an extrinsic arc. The puborectalis muscle also contracts reflexly with rectal distention. The two muscles work together to enhance continence during rectal distention. After defecation, the EAS and puborectalis muscle reflexly contract, the "deflation reflex." This process empties the last part of the rectal canal.

The nervous innervation of the EAS comes exclusively from the sacral cord via the pudendal nerves. Pudendal nerve injury paralyzes the EAS.

The internal and external sphincters work together in response to rectal distention. The external sphincter contracts reflexly via extrinsic reflex pathways, whereas the internal sphincter relaxes reflexly via intrinsic reflex pathways. Spinal anesthesia blocks the external contraction but the internal sphincter relaxation is unaffected.

The reflex contraction of the external sphincter with rectal distention is one of the primary mechanisms of continence. In order to defecate, this resistance is overcome through (1) voluntarily increasing intraperitoneal and rectal pressure or (2) under normal circumstances, increasing rectal distention, which produces reflex total inhibition of the EAS and puborectalis muscles when a maximum tolerable volume is reached (Fig. 37–3).

PUBORECTALIS MUSCLE

The puborectalis muscle is the most anterior and deepest of the levator ani muscles. It forms a sling behind the rectum. The puborectalis muscle is not attached posteriorly; hence, with contraction it pulls anteriorly, forming the anorectal angle (Fig. 37–4). The other levator ani muscles are attached posteriorly; hence, they contract in a vertical plane, forming a funnel but not altering the anorectal angle. If the puborectalis muscle function is lost, incontinence almost always results regardless of the state of contraction of the internal and external anal sphincters.

The anorectal angle is normally present when any

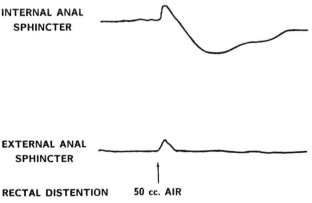

INTERNAL ANAL SPHINCTER

EXTERNAL ANAL SPHINCTER

RECTAL DISTENTION   50 cc. AIR

Figure 37–2. Anal manometric pressure tracing demonstrates normal relaxation of the internal anal sphincter in response to a 50-cc bolus of air into a balloon positioned in the rectum. The increased intraanal pressure caused by the expanding balloon is reflected in the momentary pressure elevation in the external anal sphincter pressure tracing.

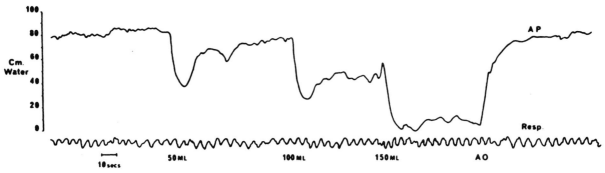

Figure 37–3. Anal manometric pressure tracing demonstrates suppression of the normal internal anal sphincter resting tone in response to increasing inflation of an intrarectal balloon. At each 50-cc increment, the anal canal pressure returns to a level below preinsufflation, until the inhibition reflex of the internal anal sphincter is totally suppressed at 150 cc. When the air in the balloon is fully withdrawn, the anal canal pressure returns to normal. (AO, air out; AP, anal pressure.) (From Lane RHS, Parks AG: Function of the anal sphincters following the colo-anal anastomosis. Br J Surg 64:599, 1977. By permission of the publisher, Butterworth-Heinemann Ltd.)

individual is erect. The puborectalis muscle is relatively relaxed during recumbency and is not needed to preserve continence. With resumption of the erect state, tonic activity of the puborectalis muscle is increased markedly, the anorectal angle is reestablished, and gross continence is maintained.

The puborectalis muscle must remain in a state of tonic contraction, a feat previously considered to be limited to smooth muscle. The puborectalis muscle is capable of both voluntary and involuntary phasic contractions that reinforce the tonic state. The muscle has two distinct types of fibers that can be differentiated biochemically, histologically, and anatomically. These fibers even develop at different stages of maturation.[11] The small "red" myocytes contain

a larger amount of myoglobin and maintain the tonic state of the sphincter, whereas the "white" cells contract the sphincter to maintain continence, even in the face of sudden increases in either intrarectal or intraabdominal pressure.

The persistent tonic state depends on a proprioceptive reflex mechanism. The sensory receptors lie within the puborectalis and levator ani muscles, with the ganglia in the lumbosacral spine. The involuntary phasic contractions are produced by a reflex arc from the puborectalis sensory receptors to the lumbosacral spinal cord and back. Transection of the cord superior to the lumbosacral region does not affect these involuntary phasic contractions. Voluntary contractions depend on cortical centers. They are abolished with cord transection.

The combination of normally functioning internal and external sphincters and the puborectalis muscle produce both gross and fine continence. Gross continence, or the ability to periodically withhold large volumes of solid or liquid feces, is a function primarily of the intact anorectal angle produced by the actions of puborectalis muscle. Fine continence, or the control of small volumes of often semisoft feces, is primarily controlled by the sphincter muscles. The critical site of fine continence is the distal 2 cm of the anal canal, that portion below the puborectalis muscle.

☐ Physiology

The nerves and muscles work to produce normal colonic motility and controlled defecation. Colonic motility produces slow transit to facilitate fluid absorption and mass movement to facilitate defecation. Three types of colonic activity exist: (1) localized segmental contractions, which slow forward movement of feces, (2) peristaltic contractions, which are primarily retrograde and slow forward movement, and (3) mass contractions, which empty long segments of the colon in a prograde fashion.

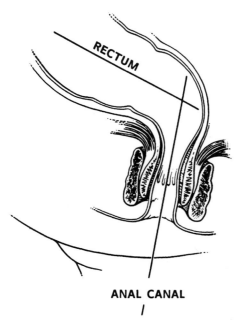

Figure 37–4. A sagittal view of the normal anal canal and rectum, which demonstrates the anorectal angle. (Modified from Pemberton JH, Kelly KA: Achieving enteric continence: Principles and applications. Mayo Clin Proc 61:586–599, 1986.)

The mass movements are not the peristaltic movements typical of the more proximal gastrointestinal tract. Rather, they are contractions of long segments of colon preceded by aboral waves of relaxation, so-called descending inhibition, which empty long segments of the colon.[12]

The process of defecation can be divided into five stages (Fig. 37–5):

1. *Stage one.* The rectal ampulla begins to fill with stool, which produces a transient reflex contraction of the external sphincter and puborectalis muscles and a relaxation of the internal sphincter. This activity can occur even before any conscious awareness of rectal distention occurs.

2. *Stage two.* The second stage occurs when the ampulla is approximately one-fourth full, which is the threshold for the awareness of stool in the rectum. At this point, a slight urge to defecate occurs, but voluntary inhibition of defecation can be prolonged. The external sphincter and puborectalis muscles are voluntarily contracted to reinforce the tonic reflex contractions. The rectum stretches, which decreases the pressure and eliminates the urge to defecate.

3. *Stage three.* The volume and the pressure in the rectum increase as more stool is pushed into it. As the urge to defecate increases in intensity, the reflex relaxation of the IAS becomes greater in degree and longer in duration. The reflex suppression of tonic contraction of the external sphincter and puborectalis muscles begins. If time and place are appropriate, the person has gone to the toilet and is ready to allow the urge to be satisfied.

4. *Stage four.* This stage involves defecation. Voluntary defecation is begun in response to the irresistible urge to defecate. Tonic activity in the internal sphincter, the external sphincter, and the puborectalis muscles is totally inhibited, and phasic activity in the striated muscle is suppressed voluntarily. The anorectal angle straightens, and the levator ani muscles fall, which leaves the rectal contents free to pass through the anal canal. Evacuation is abetted by voluntary straining and increased intraabdominal pressure.

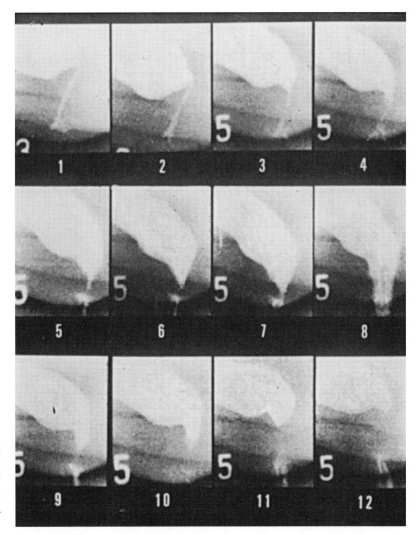

Figure 37–5. Defecogram illustrates the normal sequence of changes in the anorectum during defecation. (Modified from Kerremans R: Radio-cinematographic examination of the rectum and the anal canal in cases of rectal constipation. A radio-cinematographic and physical explanation of dyschezia. Acta Gastroenterol Belg 31:561–570, 1968.)

5. *Stage five.* The emptying of the rectal vault initiates a reflex contraction of the striated muscle—the deflation reflex. This reflex serves to empty the anal canal and initiates the return of tonic activity to the striated muscles and to the internal sphincter. The anorectal angle is reestablished, and the components of continence are again operative.

☐ Pathophysiology

Constipation can be viewed as a failure of the ability to satisfactorily undertake and complete the defecatory process. The inability may result from (1) a failure of any of the five stages of defecation, (2) a more proximal defect of colonic small intestinal or generalized motility, or (3) abnormal stool in the presence of a normal motility and defecation pattern.

Although constipation among children has been the most common disorder of anorectal function and has been recognized for thousands of years, even its definition remains a source of disagreement among physicians. Defecation patterns vary widely among normal children. A pattern that worries one child's mother may be of no concern to another. Several bowel movements a day or only one every 5 to 7 days may be normal in children older than 1 year of age. Nonetheless, constipation should be considered to be present when two or more of the following occur for an extended period of time: (1) fewer than three bowel movements per week, (2) excessive straining and pain accompanying 25% or more of bowel movements, (3) passage of hard or pellet-like stools with at least 25% of bowel movements.

During the 1st year of life, lack of a bowel movement at least every other day warrants an evaluation. In the neonatal period, any delay of passage of meconium should raise a suspicion of underlying pathologic condition and should result in vigorous investigative efforts. Although only distressed fetuses pass meconium in utero, 94 to 98% of full-term and 76% of preterm normal babies have bowel movements during the first 24 hours; 100% of full-term and 98.8% of preterm normal babies pass meconium within the first 48 hours.[13]

The problem resulting in constipation may be of major or minor importance. The causes vary in frequency by age, but in any case can be subdivided into one of five general categories: (1) changes in stool character, (2) structural problems, (3) extrinsic disorders of nerves or muscles, (4) intrinsic motility disorders, and (5) functional constipation.

ABNORMAL STOOL CHARACTER

Abnormal stool character may result from inappropriate diet. Underfeeding or insufficiency of fluid or sugar may reduce fecal bulk or produce excessively viscid or hard stools. Cystic fibrosis with its pancreatic exocrine function disturbances may cause a similar problem, as may any upper intestinal disorder that limits adequate intake, such as pyloric stenosis.

LOCAL STRUCTURAL ABNORMALITIES

Local structural abnormalities of the anorectum, including anorectal stenosis, may present actual physical barriers to normal evacuation. Even minor abnormalities, such as an anteriorly placed ectopic anus, can produce severe constipation. Those structural abnormalities may be associated with absence of the normal defecatory reflexes so that even structural corrections do not alleviate constipation.

Another commonly seen problem in infants and children that may lead to disorders of defecation are perirectal abscesses. These usually result from infection in the anal glands that enter the anus in crypts at the level of the anal valves. The pain resulting from the infection causes rectal spasm, inhibiting normal defecation. Anal fissures are painful and can cause voluntary stool withholding and result in constipation. Hard and very bulky stools may aggravate the fissure and can turn an acute problem into a chronic one. Similarly, tumors that compress or narrow the rectum interfere with normal defecation.[14]

EXTRINSIC NEUROLOGIC OR MUSCULAR ABNORMALITIES

Extrinsic neurologic or muscular abnormalities interfere with anal sensation. When the patient cannot sense a full rectum, incontinence may result from the reflex suppression of the EAS and puborectalis muscle. With the loss of the urge to defecate, constipation may lead to dilation of the rectum. Impairment of the rectal and anal reflexes, changes in sphincter tone, and neurogenic bladder often accompany neurologic defects. Constipation or incontinence may also occur. More general muscular weakness may diminish the increase in intraabdominal pressure from the diaphragm and abdominal muscles, inhibiting defecation and producing constipation. The disorders that can cause this condition include meningomyelocele, cerebral palsy, polio, or polyneuritis.

INTRINSIC MOTILITY ABNORMALITIES

Intrinsic motility abnormalities may be caused by (1) generalized causes of abnormal motility, (2) local intramural neuromuscular derangements, (3) metabolic and endocrine disturbances, including hypercalcemia, hyperkalemia, hyperparathyroidism, and abnormal thyroid function, and (4) pharmacologic agents, including phenothiazines and opiates that may slow intestinal motility at any age. This list includes drugs taken by the mother in the prenatal period. Motility abnormalities may be seen in premature infants in the absence of organic pathology, especially in those with respiratory distress, sepsis, or deranged electrolytes.

The local intramural defects run a spectrum from neurologic immaturity through classic Hirschsprung's disease to ultrashort segment aganglionosis. The most common of these causes is Hirschsprung's disease (see Chapter 34). Another entity that has been described and whose mechanism is more clearly understood is neuronal intestinal dysplasia, also known as intestinal *hyperganglionosis*. The condition is characterized by an increased number and size of ganglia in the submucosal and myenteric plexuses in conjunction with hypoplasia or aplasia of the sympathetic innervation of the myenteric plexus.[15] This disorder shares many clinical characteristics more commonly seen with Hirschsprung's disease, and, in fact, several patients have been reported as having both conditions.[16] Bowel activity is irregular and uncoordinated, resulting in ineffectual evacuation of stool. In addition, the internal sphincter is often spastic. Special nerve stains have been used to elucidate the various abnormalities that cause this condition.

Rare conditions that can affect the innervation of the anorectum include Chagas' disease and neurofibromatosis. These disorders produce constipation either by ineffective propulsive activity or by failure of the IAS to relax in response to rectal distention.

FUNCTIONAL CONSTIPATION

Functional constipation is the most common form of constipation in children. However, it almost certainly represents the combining of multiple causes under one rubric.

The classic concept of functional constipation is the conscious or subconscious suppression by the child of the urge to defecate. Eventually, the rectum dilates and remains dilated. Higher intrarectal pressures become necessary to initiate the normal defecation response. The stool volume necessary to initiate the defecation reflex is too large and often too hard to pass easily. Diminution in the sensitivity of rectal stretch receptors also occurs, which can affect the intrinsic internal sphincter relaxation response but usually does not. Rather, the conscious sensation of the urge to defecate becomes suppressed.

This discordance between the volume that produces reflex relaxation and that which causes conscious sensation has been studied. In children with a marked discrepancy between reflex relaxation and conscious sensation, encopresis often occurs. In children with a lesser discrepancy, a lower incidence of encopresis occurs. In children with no discrepancy, encopresis is rare.[17]

Loss of the urge to defecate is not the only abnormality in those with "functional constipation." Hypertonia of the puborectalis muscle has been observed, with failure to relax and straighten the anorectal angle. Not surprisingly, the child so affected also suffers from constipation. In one study of the inhibiting reflex in children considered to have functional constipation, some had failure of internal sphincter relaxation, similar to that in Hirschsprung's disease; some had relaxation of the IAS, but it was minimal; others had hypertonia of the IAS with a paradoxical hyperrelaxation when the rectum was distended.[18]

The multitude of problems that have been designated functional constipation is equaled by the number of different psychogenic problems implicated as underlying causes. Repeated use of enemas or suppositories during infancy, disturbances in parent-child relationships, early or strict toilet training, and neurodevelopmental disorders have all been cited as causes.

☐ Diagnosis

When constipation is one manifestation of a generalized disorder, its cause is usually apparent. Similarly, simple physical inspection usually enables the recognition of anorectal malformations, muscular disorders, or extrinsic neurologic defects when they are responsible for the constipation.

The major diagnostic difficulties lie in differentiating between functional constipation and intrinsic motility disorders. Features of Hirschsprung's disease that distinguish it from functional constipation include onset in infancy, absence of fecal soiling, rarity of abdominal pain, empty rectal ampulla, and, commonly, malnutrition.

The clinical presentation is not always so classic, and no one feature is pathognomonic. Especially when Hirschsprung's disease involves only a short segment, symptoms may not present until later in life. The finding of impacted stool in the rectum, and even fecal soiling in some patients, is not uncommon. In addition, some of the diseases described as intrinsic motility disorders are impossible to differentiate clinically from Hirschsprung's disease. Thus, other diagnostic modalities are necessary. The three most important of these are radiologic studies, anorectal manometry, and tissue biopsy.

In a child with Hirschsprung's disease, barium enema examination usually demonstrates a normal-sized or contracted aganglionic rectum with a transitional zone that leads to the dilated ganglionic colon. In the newborn, failure to evacuate barium within 24 hours of instillation may be the most pertinent finding. With short segment aganglionosis, the barium enema may appear similar to functional constipation, a markedly dilated rectum down to the anus.

Anorectal manometry is performed with either pressure transducers or perfused catheters. In a normal child, distention of the rectum with 10 to 30 cc of air results in reflex contraction and then relaxation of the internal sphincter, accompanied by contraction of the external sphincter. With functional constipation, there is a reduced sensation of rectal distention due to the markedly dilated rectum.

Greater volumes of air are needed to create an urge to defecate. Nevertheless, normal internal sphincter relaxation does occur with these greater volumes, and relaxation may occur even at normal volumes of air. The latter may account for the controlled passage of liquid around an impaction.

In children with Hirschsprung's disease, the internal sphincter fails to relax on rectal distention. Contraction may occur. With manometry, it is less difficult to exclude Hirschsprung's disease than to confirm its presence. Absence of internal sphincter relaxation may result from technical problems. Lack of relaxation may be found in young neonates and premature babies with normal colons, especially in those with respiratory distress syndrome, sepsis, or electrolyte disturbances (Fig. 37–6).

Anorectal manometry can be used in conjunction with electromyography in the evaluation of problems of defecation and continence from anorectal malformations and neurologic disorders. Tissue for study can be obtained by punch or suction biopsy without anesthesia or by surgical excision of a full thickness section of rectal wall with anesthesia. Specimens obtained by punch or suction techniques contain only mucosa and a portion of submucosa. About 50 to 100 sections must be examined for ganglion cells by an experienced pathologist. Full thickness sections, which are less difficult to interpret, include Auerbach's plexus.

The identification of increased acetylcholinesterase activity in superficial suction biopsies is an accurate means for diagnosing Hirschsprung's disease. This test has obviated the need for full thickness biopsies in many cases.

☐ Treatment

The treatment of most of the causes of constipation is straightforward. Metabolic and endocrine disturbances are corrected, anatomic obstructions are surgically removed, and responsible drugs are eliminated. The treatment of the two common causes of constipation, Hirschsprung's disease and functional constipation, is more complex. The management of Hirschsprung's disease is discussed in detail in Chapter 34.

Treatment of functional constipation should be approached in a systematic way. The rectum is emptied and stool reaccumulation prevented. The rectum is allowed to return to its original size. The child experiences the urge to defecate when the rectum is only mildly distended by stool entering it. The initial removal of the fecal mass can usually be aided by the administration of 5 to 10 tablespoons of mineral oil or a hypertonic phosphate enema (e.g., Fleet enema). Repeated administration may be necessary. Sufficient amounts of mineral oil should be given to cause two to four loose bowel movements each day. The dose should be titrated against the child's response—several tablespoons or more each day are commonly needed. In several instances, we have given 24 tablespoons per day of mineral oil for refractory cases. The anal discharge of oil usually indicates seepage around a still retained fecal mass, in which case the dose should be increased. To make the mineral oil more palatable and to increase compliance with the regimen, it may be refrigerated or flavored with fruit juice. The mineral oil may be taken all at once or divided into two daily portions. Administration of mineral oil may have to be continued for several months. It should be discontinued gradually. The regimen is sufficient in many cases of simple constipation.

If the child is old enough (usually older than 3 years of age), regular toilet training is started by having the patient sit on the toilet at the same time each day for 10 to 20 minutes, usually shortly after a major meal to take advantage of the gastrocolic reflex. If the child's legs do not reach the floor, a small stool should be provided so that pressure can be applied to help move the bowels.

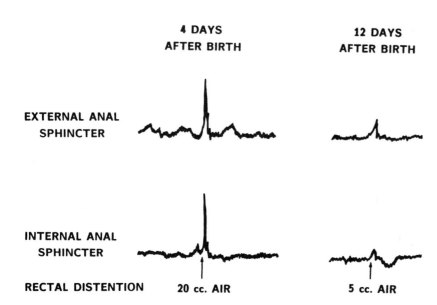

Figure 37–6. Anorectal manometric pressure tracings from a patient at 4 days of age demonstrate the absence of a normal internal sphincter relaxation in response to a transient 20-cc bolus of air into a balloon placed in the rectum. At a subsequent study done at 12 days of age, normal relaxation of the internal anal sphincter is present in response to a transient 5-cc bolus of air.

In other cases, careful exploration of family events and emotional factors that lead to the fecal retention is needed to help the family resolve parent-child conflicts and to establish sympathetic, but firm, guidelines for dealing with the patient and the patient's problems. Psychiatric referral may be helpful in some severely disturbed families. Treatment of constipation in mentally retarded children usually is unsatisfactory.

About half of all children with functional constipation contract the EAS, the puborectalis, and pelvic floor muscles during defecation attempts instead of relaxing them. Because these structures are voluntary striated muscles, they should be amenable to control and modulation by the use of biofeedback techniques.[19]

The rectum is emptied and allowed to return to a more normal size before biofeedback training is begun. A balloon, which is connected to pressure transducers, is inserted into the rectum, and the pressure tracings are displayed on a monitor. The balloon is inflated and the child is shown the pressure tracing that he or she generated in response to the rectal distention. The child is then urged to mimic defecation while the intrarectal pressures are monitored. In many of these children, the external sphincter contracts, generating a high-pressure tracing. The child is then shown a normal tracing of external sphincter relaxation during defecation. The child is then encouraged to mimic the normal tracing. Additional biofeedback reinforcement can be accomplished by adding a variety of audio and visual stimuli to the pressure apparatus. Most importantly, the child should be encouraged and rewarded when progress is made toward a normal response. This process takes time, patience, and good rapport between the child and coach. As a final step in the process, the rectal balloon is removed, and the child then practices voluntary external sphincter relaxation on command. Most children need about five sessions given at weekly intervals to achieve a satisfactory response. Biofeedback training has proven useful in children with abnormal defecation dynamics. Most of these children can learn a more normal pattern of muscle relaxation and then go on to achieve normal defecation.[20]

Anorectal myectomy or vigorous anal dilation using anesthesia has been successful in some patients who failed to respond to all of the aforementioned measures. In this procedure, a strip of rectal muscular wall, starting just below the dentate line and extending upward to the level of the puborectalis muscle, is removed. The lowest portion of the internal sphincter is not divided.[21]

☐ Anteriorly Displaced Anus

A controversial entity, which several investigators claim is a major cause of constipation, is the anteriorly displaced anus, or anterior ectopic anus. The controversy concerning this entity arises from the different definitions of the abnormality, the real relationship between the anatomic abnormality and constipation, the operation to be performed, and the incidence of the entity.[22]

In 1958, Bill and colleagues described what they considered to be a variant of the spectrum of anomalies carried under the overall term *imperforate anus*; they named this an *anteriorly placed rectal opening in the perineum,* or *ectopic anus.*[23] In 30 patients, all of the openings were in the perineum anterior to the normal anal position and the external sphincter. Some 20 years later, in two independent series, anterior anus and anterior ectopic anus were reported as a frequently unrecognized cause of constipation. One report, although not specifically stating so, appears to describe an anterior anal opening within the external sphincters.[24] The other report specifically describes an apparently normal sphincter except for its anterior ectopia.[25] In 1984, another report described a structural abnormality in seven children with anterior perineal anus, namely, the absence of a portion of the triple loop system of EASs.[26]

General agreement exists that anal openings anterior to the external sphincters, as initially described by Bill and colleagues, can produce constipation, which is relieved by operation. Most pediatric surgeons remain skeptical, however, about the importance and even the identification of anteriorly displaced anal openings within the external sphincters. One group of workers made the diagnosis of anal ectopia solely by inspection, describing an anus that is well forward of the normal location, midway between the vaginal fourchette and the tip of the coccyx. In another report, the eccentric placement of the anal opening was emphasized. Indeed, in 20% of the patients, the anus did not appear to be anteriorly displaced. An anal position index has been described based on examination of 200 newborn infants, which can be used to identify anterior displacement of the anus.[27] An abnormal index is not an indication for operation, however.

Despite specifically looking for these abnormalities in a large number of constipated children, we have not found a clearly identified anteriorly displaced anus nor an eccentrically placed anus to be common. Palpation of a posterior shelf or cul de sac behind the sphincter is the other physical finding associated with this entity. This finding is similar to the shelf that is present in the patient with the anterior ectopic anus described by Bill. In the few patients we have operated on for anterior ectopic anus, the shelf has been the most impressive finding.

A prominent posterior shelf found on barium enema has been described as indicative of this entity.[28] However, the presentations are no different from those we have seen in other children and adolescents with chronic constipation. The abnormally prominent shelf is due to a hypertrophied puborectalis muscle and is much improved within weeks of vigorous dilation of the puborectalis using anesthesia.

The operations performed for anterior ectopic anus include transplantation of the anus (a simple cut-back procedure) and posterior advancement of a mucosal flap with and without posterior sphincterotomy. We have found a simple cut-back, including the sphincter, to be effective and the simplest procedure, but care must be taken not to include the puborectalis muscle accidentally.

Anteriorly displaced anus clearly occurs, but infrequently in our experience. It is sometimes associated with chronic constipation. Some children are helped by an operation. We share the viewpoint of most pediatric surgeons, however, that this entity is an uncommon cause of chronic constipation and that children should be operated on only after a trial of medical management and careful evaluation.

REFERENCES

1. Swensen O, Bill AH: Resection of the rectum and rectosigmoid with preservation of the sphincter. Surgery 24:212–220, 1948.
2. Culver PS, Rattan S: Genesis of anal canal pressures in the opossum. Am J Physiol 251:765–771, 1986.
3. Schuster MM, Hentrix TR, Mendeloff AI: The internal and sphincter response: Manometric studies on its normal physiology, neural pathways and alteration in bowel disorders. J Clin Invest 42:196–207, 1963.
4. Aldridge RT, Campbell PE: Ganglion cell distribution in the normal rectum and anal canal. J Pediatr Surg 3:475–496, 1968.
5. Bitar Kid, Makhlow GM: Purinergic receptors on isolated smooth muscle cells. Gastroenterology 82:1018–1027, 1982.
6. Garrett JR, Howard ER, Jones W: The internal anal sphincter in the cat: A study of nervous mechanisms affecting tone and reflex activity. J Physiol 243:153–166, 1974.
7. Frenckner B, Ihre T: Influence of autonomic nerves on the internal anal sphincter in man. Gut 17:306–312, 1976.
8. Nurko S, Rattan S: Role of vasoactive intestinal polypeptide in the internal anal sphincter relaxation in the opossum. J Clin Invest 81:1146–1153 1988.
9. Christensen J: Motility of the colon. In Johnson LR (ed): Physiology of the Gastrointestinal Tract (2nd ed). New York, Raven Press, 1987.
10. Monges H, Salducci J, Nardi B, et al: Electrical activity of internal anal sphincter. In Christensen J (ed): Gastrointestinal Motility. New York, Raven Press, 1980, pp 495–502.
11. Holschneider AM: The problem of anorectal continence. Prog Pediatr Surg 9:85-97, 1976.
12. Ritchic JA: Mass peristalsis in the human colon after contact with oxyphenisatin. Gut 13:211–219, 1972.
13. Clark DA: Times of first void and first stool in 500 newborns. Pediatrics 60:457–459, 1977.
14. Loening-Baucke VA: Factors responsible for persistence of childhood constipation. J Pediatr Gastroenterol Nutr 6:915–922, 1987.
15. Munakata K, Morita K, Okabe I, et al: Clinical and histologic studies in neuronal intestinal dysplasia. J Pediatr Surg 20:231–235, 1985.
16. Fadda B, Pistor G, Meier-Ruge W, et al: Symptoms, diagnosis, and therapy of neuronal intestinal dysplasia masked by Hirschsprung's disease. Pediatr Surg Int 2:76–80, 1987.
17. Martelli H, Devroede G, Arhan P, et al: Mechanisms of idiopathic constipation: Outlet obstruction. Gastroenterology 75:623–631, 1978.
18. Meunier P, Louis D, Jaubert de Beaujeu M: Physiologic investigation of primary chronic constipation in children: Comparison with the barium enema study. Gastroenterol 87:1351–1357, 1984.
19. Loening-Baucke, VA: Modulation of abnormal defecation dynamics by biofeedback treatment in chronically constipated children with encopresis. J Pediatr 116:214–222, 1990.
20. Benninga MA, Buller HA, Taminiau JA: Biofeedback training in constipation. Arch Dis Child 68:126–129, 1993.
21. Pinho M, Yoshioka K, Keighley MRB: Long-term results of anorectal myectomy for chronic constipation. Br J Surg 76:1163–1164, 1989.
22. Ottolenghi A, Sulpasso M, Bianchi S, et al: Ectopic anus in childhood. Eur J Pediatr Surg 4:145–150, 1994.
23. Bill AH Jr, Johnson RJ, Foster RA: Anteriorly placed rectal opening in the perineum, "ectopic anus." A report of 30 cases. Ann Surg 147:173–179, 1958.
24. Hendren WH: Constipation caused by anterior location of the anus and its surgical correction. J Pediatr Surg 13:505–511, 1978.
25. Leape LL, Ramenofsky ML: Anterior ectopic anus: A common cause of constipation in children. J Pediatr Surg 13:627–630 1978.
26. Upadhyaya P: Mid-anal sphincteric malformation, cause of constipation in anterior perianal anus. J Pediatr Surg 19:183–186, 1984.
27. Bar-Maor JA, Eitan A: Determination of the normal position of the anus. J Pediatr Gastroenterol Nutr 6:559–561, 1987.
28. Reisner SH, Sivan Y, Nitzan M, et al: Determination of anterior displacement of the anus in newborn infants and children. Pediatrics 73:216-217, 1984.

38

ACQUIRED ANORECTAL DISORDERS

Keith W. Ashcraft, MD

☐ Perianal and Perirectal Abscesses

Perianal or perirectal abscesses develop primarily in infants. The abscess usually appears as a tender mass lateral to the anal opening. A history of stool abnormalities is not often noted in these children, either before development of the abscess or during its maturation. In my experience, there is approximately an equal incidence of perirectal abscess in male and female infants. Virtually all these patients are seen first when they are younger than 12 months old. However, other reports suggest that perianal abscesses are much more common in male children and are frequent in children older than age 2 years.[1]

Sitz baths (or their equivalent for the infant) are prescribed if the abscess does not appear to be fluctuant and in need of immediate drainage. Approximately one third of abscesses thus treated resolve without recurrence. Approximately two thirds require surgical drainage or drain spontaneously. Surgical drainage can be done in the infant without anesthesia or with a topical anesthetic ointment. In the child who is older than 1 year of age, the procedure usually must be done using general anesthetic, with curettage and packing of the abscess cavity. Approximately 40 to 50% of perianal abscesses progress to fistula in ano.[2]

It is unusual to find ischiorectal abscesses in children unless associated with chronic inflammatory bowel diseases.

☐ Fistula in Ano

Fistula in ano appears predominantly in male patients.[3] The child is usually seen first after two or more flare-ups of a perianal abscess that either continues to drain or to form a small pustule that ruptures only to form again.[4] The fistula is commonly located lateral to the anus rather than in the midline. Occasionally, two fistulas occur simultaneously in one child. In several patients, fistulas have occurred in a serial fashion.

An intriguing theory has been suggested that fistula in ano results from infection in abnormally deep crypts that are under the influence of androgens.[1, 3] Fistula in ano almost never follows a perianal abscess in female children.[5] The levels of circulating sex hormones have been found to be normal in adult male and female patients with idiopathic fistula in ano.[6]

The preferred surgical procedure for fistula in ano is cryptectomy or fistulectomy (rather than fistulotomy), removing the entire crypt with its granulation tissue. Hydrogen peroxide has been used as a means of identifying the associated crypt intraoperatively.[7] It has been postulated that, in addition to the fistulotomy or fistulectomy, multiple cryptotomy should be carried out to prevent serial fistulization. I have had no experience with this technique, nor have I sought to confirm the presence of abnormal crypts. The wound is left open, which provides for some distress on the part of the parents but little discomfort on the part of the child. I have not seen difficulties with healing in any of these patients, nor have I seen a recurrence of the same fistula with this approach. Suture closure has been reported to result in satisfactory healing without infection.[1]

☐ Fissure in Ano

Fissure in ano develops in toddlers whose diet changes from liquid to solid and whose stool consistency changes from soft to firm. A period of constipation often precedes a hard, bulky stool that results in a posterior midline anal tear. The discomfort associated with a fissure in ano often leads to further constipation, which, in turn, aggravates the fissure with each stool and prevents healing. Fissure in ano is usually seen in the toddler who is capable of repressing the urge to defecate due to anticipated pain. The diagnosis is made through the history of blood streaking on the stool, the child crying during bowel movements, and the recognition of a split in the skin of the anus.

Excision is rarely necessary. I prefer to manage

these patients with sitz baths and with milk of magnesia used as a stool softener. Any other form of stool softening that is effective works as well.

A fissure in ano in an older child or a teenager very often is associated with chronic inflammatory bowel disease, usually Crohn's disease (see Chapter 42).[8] The diagnosis of Crohn's disease may follow by some months the demonstration of a fissure in ano, but if the clinician is persistent, the inflammatory changes of Crohn's disease can ultimately be detected. Some of the perianal manifestations of Crohn's disease can be very destructive.[9] Treatment of Crohn's disease concomitantly with surgical treatment of the anal manifestations usually results in healing of the fissure or fistula.[10, 11] Rectourethroperineal fistula may also result from Crohn's disease and may require complex procedures for correction.[12, 13]

☐ Hemorrhoids

Hemorrhoids are uncommon in the pediatric population unless associated with portal hypertension. Formerly, extrahepatic portal vein thrombosis was the primary cause of portal hypertension, but currently the most common etiology is cystic fibrosis (CF). Rarely is it necessary to perform surgical procedures on these hemorrhoids. Symptomatic local therapy reduces the likelihood of bleeding and pruritus. Careful local hygiene is an important aspect of this treatment. Perianal skin tags can be managed with good hygiene, but if the skin tag is enlarging in a smaller child, excision is reasonable. Skin tag is rarely an indication of other disease, although it may result from a healed fissure.

Surgical treatment of hemorrhoids should be conservative. Sphincter preservation is paramount. According to Bornemeier, "The sphincter [ani] apparently can differentiate between solid, fluid, and gas. It apparently can tell when its owner has his pants on or off. No other muscle in the body is such a protector of the dignity of man, yet so ready to come to his relief. A muscle like this is worth protecting."[14]

Thrombosed hemorrhoids resulting from prolonged extrusion require incision and evacuation of clot. Little treatment exists for bleeding hemorrhoids other than to reduce portal hypertension. Cryptitis, which produces sphincter spasm and results in venous engorgement, may be successfully treated by local measures or by multiple cryptotomy.

☐ Rectal Prolapse

Rectal prolapse is relatively common in young children and usually occurs as a result of a diarrheal illness, constipation, wasting illness, or malnutrition.[15, 16] Prolapse is probably a herniation of the rectum, in most cases through a dilated levator

mechanism.[17] Straining at stool and long periods of time sitting on the toilet, due to protracted diarrhea or constipation, allows stretching of the pelvic diaphragm, the suspensory vessels, and other less well-defined suspensory structures of the rectum, resulting in prolapse.[15, 18] Sometimes, what appears to be rectal prolapse is an intussusception of the sigmoid colon.[19, 20] In these cases, an intact rectal suspension system exists, but a dilated levator mechanism produced by straining at stool, coupled with a redundant sigmoid colon, allows prolapse.[18] The pelvic diaphragm is a muscular structure. If the prolapse is prevented from recurring, the muscle fibers shorten and the situation may be self-limiting. Improvement in nutrition may also result in a spontaneous resolution of rectal prolapse.

The diagnosis is usually made by the parent who sees the rosette of rectum or sigmoid when the child complains of discomfort at the anus. Bleeding is occasionally noted as the primary symptom. The prolapse either reduces spontaneously, as the child gets off the toilet, or the parent pushes it back in. Many 3-year-old children very quickly learn to reduce their own prolapse. It generally does not recur until the next episode at stool. It is uncommon for the child to be able to produce the prolapse in the examining room. Occasionally, the prolapse can be demonstrated during a brief session on the toilet. Most often, the prolapse is not seen during examination because the patient does not relax the anus and strain sufficiently. The typical prolapse is a rosette of mucosa, sometimes slightly longer posteriorly than anteriorly (Fig. 38–1). One should be able to slip a finger alongside the prolapse and feel the

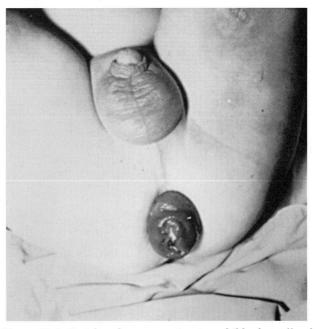

Figure 38–1. Rectal prolapse occurring in a child who suffered severe burns on his legs. Despite its being reduced repeatedly for several weeks, this prolapse continued to occur several times daily and required surgical correction.

sulcus 1 to 2 cm up inside the anus. A deeper sulcus suggests sigmoid intussusception rather than rectal prolapse. It is often difficult to clinically differentiate the two, even in the face of rectal examination at the time of prolapse or radiologic studies obtained to clarify the situation.[20]

If the child continues straining at stool once the pelvic diaphragm and rectal sphincters have been stretched, there is little chance that the prolapse will correct itself. A change in bowel habits that eliminates the persistent urge to defecate, which seems to be common in many of these children, may allow the pelvic musculature to resume its normal tone. The stretched suspensory mechanism of the rectum then has a chance to shrink, and the process may spontaneously resolve.

□ Diagnostic Studies

At least in the United States, it is probably worthwhile to investigate the patient with rectal prolapse for the possibility of CF. In personal experience with 47 patients with rectal prolapse who underwent operative treatment, only two had CF. One was a known CF patient, and the other's condition was discovered by a screening sweat test while being evaluated for rectal prolapse.

Barium enema studies are rarely of diagnostic benefit, because at the time of the barium enema the prolapse is reduced and the relationships may not appear to be abnormal at all. In several patients, my colleagues and I have demonstrated by an intraabdominal injection of water-soluble contrast material a deep sulcus of the pelvic peritoneum that extended downward, forming a "hernia sac" between the bladder and the rectum in male patients or the vagina and the rectum in female patients (Fig. 38–2). Although this herniogram may help distinguish a sigmoid intussusception from a true rectal prolapse, we have not often used it because it is an extremely uncomfortable procedure.

□ Treatment

The nonoperative treatment of rectal prolapse consists of attempts to alter the stool disorder that led to the prolapse. One of the early authorities advised against allowing the child to use the toilet or potty until the problem was resolved, suggesting that the child defecate in a squatting position on a newspaper.[15, 21] Eliminating the cause of intractable diarrhea or chronic constipation seems to be the most practical approach, but success depends on recognition of the cause. Enzymatic therapy for CF is an example of nonoperative therapy.[22]

Surgical therapy has taken a number of forms. In Europe, the Middle East, and Asia, perianal cerclage has been used frequently, because it can be done as

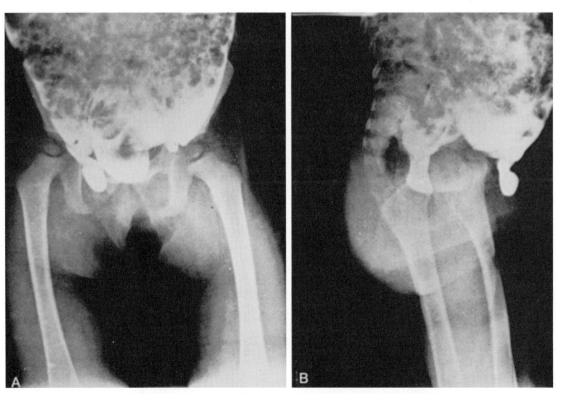

Figure 38–2. *A,* A herniogram in a child with rectal prolapse shows the overlapping sacs filled with contrast material. The right inguinal hernia sac is seen just medial to the hip joint, and the rectal prolapse extension of the peritoneum is located in the midline. *B,* A lateral view of the posterior prolapse sac and the anterior hernia sac.

an outpatient procedure. It tightens the anal outlet and prevents prolapse from recurring while the musculature of the pelvis reestablishes its more normal relationships.[23] The fact that the cerclage procedure is commonly used bespeaks its effectiveness, although erosion of the anus may occur from a wire or other suture being placed too tightly. Local infection is occasionally reported.[24]

Sclerotherapy using 30% saline, 5% phenol, or 25% glucose injected into the retrorectal space produces an inflammatory response and scar that theoretically prevents the rectum from sliding downward.[25, 26] Whatever the injection material, it sometimes must be repeated and must always be done using general anesthesia in the child owing to the associated discomfort. I do not recommend injection therapy.

Various sorts of cauterization therapy have been used for rectal prolapse, including quadrant cauterization, reduction, and taping of the buttocks.[15] Endorectal cauterization or mucosal stripping as an alternative to suspension and plication procedures may be effective by allowing restoration of the suspensory apparatus.[27, 28] There is little reason to believe rectal prolapse is due to mucosal overabundance.

An open sclerosing procedure, in which the retrorectal space is developed and packed with gauze, is done through an incision posterior to the anus but anterior to the coccyx. The gauze packing is removed gradually over a 10-day period. The packing produces enough inflammatory response that the rectum remains suspended. The major proponent of this operation has suggested that, when the sphincter mechanism is grossly stretched, a "plastic operation" may be needed to maintain the rectal suspension.[15]

Transanal suture fixation of the rectum (as described in 1909) has recently been used in a group of children with good success.[29] Its benefit probably derives from prevention of recurrent prolapse while inflammation produced by the mattress suture, which extends from the rectal lumen to the skin, produces adhesions. An extensive plication or reefing of the posterior rectal wall via coccygectomy incision has recently been reported to have good results but the potential for fistula formation from the multiple suture "bites" makes this a worrisome technique.[30]

My colleagues and I approach this lesion as if it were a true hernia. Through a natal cleft incision, we remove the coccyx, narrow the muscular hiatus, and suspend the rectum from the cut edge of the sacrum so that it cannot slide downward (Fig. 38–3).[31, 32] This maneuver immediately reestablishes the suspensory mechanism and narrows the hiatus, which are the ultimate therapeutic outcomes of all the nonoperative and operative methods of treatment. We have used this technique in 47 patients over 19 years, with 44 of them being available for follow-up from periods of 2 months to 10 years.[21] Of these patients, 34 had excellent initial results.

Three patients had mild mucosal prolapse that gradually spontaneously resolved. Four patients had recurrent "prolapse," which proved to be intussusception of the sigmoid colon. One of these required transanal resection and anastomosis.[24] One case resolved spontaneously, and two other patients underwent transabdominal sigmoid resections. In one patient, a barium study preoperatively was interpreted as normal, only later to show findings consistent with an intussusception. One case of caudal dysgenesis was a total failure.

This operation can be performed quite satisfactorily as an outpatient procedure. A modification of the posterior sagittal approach has been reported and seems to have considerable merit.[19]

☐ Rectal Trauma

Rectal trauma in pediatric patients generally occurs by one of two mechanisms. The first is an accidental impalement injury. For example, one child jumped out of a boat to put on water skis and was impaled by a hidden tree branch beneath the water. The branch entered and penetrated the anus and penetrated through the bladder into the peritoneum. Another example is that of a 12-year-old boy who was riding a bicycle that did not have a seat; he suffered a laceration of the anus from the bicycle post when he had a collision. Bicycle crossbar injuries or "monkey-bar" injuries to the perineum rarely cause anal trauma. In female patients, straddle injuries most often affect the introitus. In male patients, they affect the urethra as a crushing type of injury.

The second and most common rectal trauma is a result of sexual abuse. Digital or penile penetration of the anorectum or other instrumentation may present acutely with bleeding or bruising. The most common clinical presentation is that of a chronic stellate laceration of the anus with lymphedema (Fig. 38–4). Perianal condylomata are a common occurrence in cases of sexual abuse involving the anus.

☐ History

The patient with an accidental injury to the anus usually is seen immediately after the accident occurs. An accurate and consistent history of the mechanism of injury is needed. Evidence of sexual abuse is strengthened with a more chronic type of injury, an inconsistent history of the mechanism of injury, or no satisfactory explanation of how the condylomata came to occur. Careful questioning may reveal that a male member of the immediate family has penile condylomata. However, as many as 25% of males who carry human papillomavirus in the urethra have no external evidence of the virus.[34]

As with other forms of sexual abuse involving genital penetration in female patients or manipula-

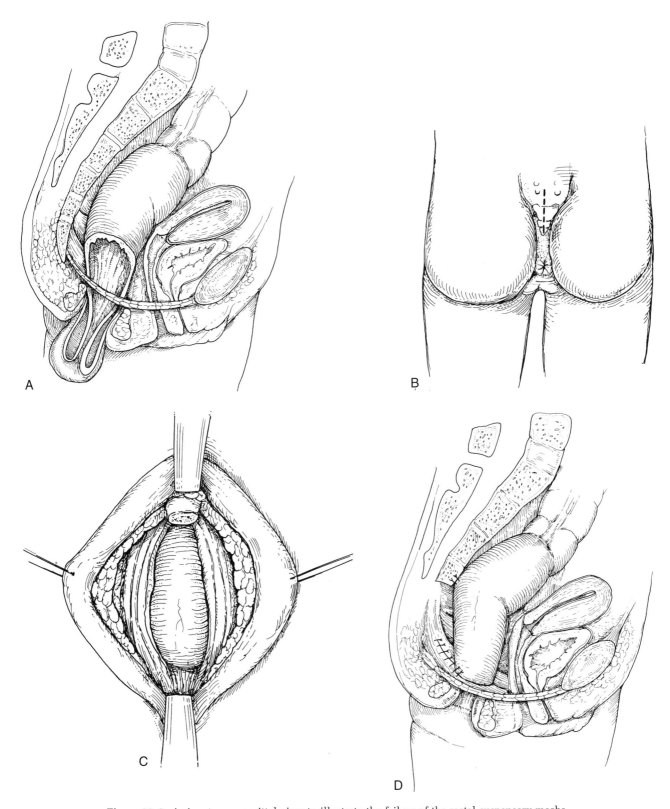

Figure 38–3. *A*, A cut-away sagittal view to illustrate the failure of the rectal suspensory mechanism to hold the rectum within the pelvis. *B*, The posterior sagittal incision for the suspension. *C*, The coccyx has been removed and the posterior rectal wall exposed. *D*, The pelvic diaphragm is closed posterior to the reduced rectum. The rectum is sutured laterally to the pelvic diaphragm. The rectum is further suspended from the cut edge of the sacrum. (*A* and *D* redrawn from Ashcraft KW, Amoury RA, Holder TM: Levator repair and posterior suspension for rectal prolapse. J Pediatr Surg 12:241–245, 1977. *B* and *C* from Ashcraft KW: Atlas of Pediatric Surgery. Philadelphia, WB Saunders, 1994, p 217.)

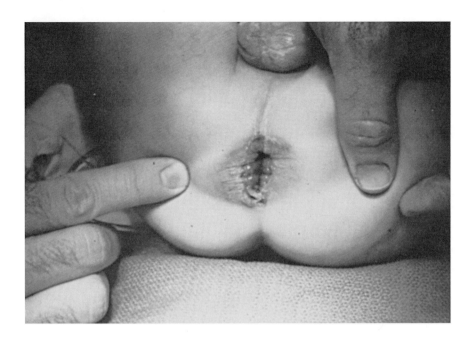

Figure 38–4. This male child was the victim of chronic sexual abuse and shows the typical stellate lacerations of the anal mucosal skin with exudate.

tion in male patients, there is often difficulty in obtaining an adequate history from the victim owing to fear, threats of retaliation, or guilt. Unexplained injuries to the rectum must be considered a manifestation of sexual abuse and must be investigated through the appropriate social service authorities.[35]

☐ Examinations

The child who has an acute traumatic rectal injury is often difficult to examine adequately owing to the associated discomfort. Penetration of a foreign object by impalement may require voiding cystourethrography followed by rectal examination and sigmoidoscopy under a general anesthetic.

The child who is sexually abused and who has either condylomata or lacerations of a more chronic nature can often be examined while awake. Making the diagnosis does not often require radiographic examination.

☐ Treatment

Treatment of penetrating rectal injuries often requires a diverting colostomy.[36] Extensive perianal lacerations are repaired at the same time to reapproximate the sphincter muscle mechanism as much as possible. Closure of the colostomy is performed once satisfactory healing is demonstrated. Some rectal injuries may be repaired primarily without fecal diversion, but the risk of a bad result producing fecal incontinence hardly seems justified.[37]

Treatment of sexual abuse lesions involves interruption of the abuse pattern, which may require removal of the child from the home environment. The anal lesions usually heal much more quickly

than the psychological trauma that has occurred with the sexual abuse. In the sexual abuse victim who may present with an acute laceration extending up the rectal wall, it is rarely necessary to do a diverting colostomy because these lacerations are not often full thickness. In two patients, however, sexual abuse resulted in laceration of the pelvic peritoneum; the resulting peritonitis caused the death of one of those patients.

REFERENCES

1. Fitzgerald RJ, Harding B, Ryan W: Fistula-in-ano in childhood: A congenital etiology. J Pediatr Surg 20:80–81, 1985.
2. Poenaru D, Yazbeck S: Anal fistula in infants: Etiology, features, management. J Pediatr Surg 28:1194–1195, 1993.
3. Shafer AD, McGlone TP, Flanagan RA: Abnormal crypts of Morgagni: The cause of perianal abscess and fistula-in-ano. J Pediatr Surg 22:203–204, 1987.
4. Ross ST: Fistula in ano. Surg Clin North Am 68:1417–1426, 1988.
5. Al-Salem AH, Laing W, Talwalker V: Fistula-in-ano in infancy and childhood. J Pediatr Surg 29:436–438, 1944.
6. Lunniss PJ, Jenkins PJ, Besser GM, et al: Gender differences in incidence of idiopathic fistula-in-ano are not explained by circulating sex hormones. Int J Colorect Dis 10:25–28, 1995.
7. Glen DL: Use of hydrogen peroxide to identify internal opening of anal fistula and perianal abscess. Aust N Z J Surg 56:433–435, 1986.
8. Sweeney L, Ritchie JK, Nichols RJ: Anal fissure in Crohn's disease. Br J Surg 75:57, 1988.
9. Markowitz J, Grancher K, Rosa J, et al: Highly destructive perianal disease in children with Crohn's disease. J Pediatr Gastroenterol Nutr 21:149–153, 1995.
10. Levien Dli, Surrell J, Mazier WP: Surgical treatment of anorectal fistula in patients with Crohn's disease. Surg Gynecol Obstet 169:133–136, 1989.
11. Bayer I, Gordon PH: Selected operative management of fistula-in-ano in Crohn's disease. Dis Colon Rectum 37:760–765, 1994.
12. Fazio VW, Jones IT, Jagelman DG, et al.: Rectourethral fistulas in Crohn's disease. Surg Gynecol Obstet 164:148–150, 1987.
13. Stamler JS, Bauer JJ, Janowitz HD: Rectourethroperineal fistula in Crohn's disease. Am J Gastroenterol 80:111–112, 1985.

14. Bornemeier WC: Sphincter protecting hemorrhoidectomy. Am J Proctol 11:48–52, 1960.
15. Lockhart-Mummery JP: Surgical procedures in general practice: Rectal prolapse. BMJ 1:345–347, 1939.
16. Severijnen R, Festen C, Van Der Staak F, et al: Rectal prolapse in children. Neth J Surg 41:149–151, 1989.
17. Moschcowitz AV: The pathogenesis, anatomy and care of prolapse of the rectum. Surg Gynecol Obstet 15:7, 1912.
18. Nigro ND: Restoration of the levator sling in the treatment of rectal procidentia. Dis Colon Rectum 1:123–127, 1958.
19. Pai GK, Pai PK: A case of congenital colonic stenosis presenting as rectal prolapse. J Pediatr Surg 25:699–700, 1990.
20. Theuerkauf FJ, Beahrs OH, Jill JR: Rectal prolapse: Causation and surgical treatment. Ann Surg 171:819–835, 1970.
21. Kopel FB: Gastrointestinal manifestations of cystic fibrosis. Gastroenterology 62:483–491, 1972.
22. Shwachman H, Redmond A, Khaw K-T: Studies in cystic fibrosis: Report of 130 patients diagnosed under 3 months of age over a 20-year period. Pediatrics 46:335–343, 1970.
23. Sempsky WT, Rosenstein BJ: The cause of rectal prolapse in children. Am J Dis Child 142:338–339, 1988.
24. Pearl RH, Ein SH, Churchill B: Posterior sagittal anorectoplasty for pediatric recurrent rectal prolapse. J Pediatr Surg 24:1100–1102, 1989.
25. Kay NRM, Zachary RB: The treatment of rectal prolapse in children with injections of 30 per cent saline solutions. J Pediatr Surg 5:334–337, 1970.
26. Wyllie GG: The injection treatment of rectal prolapse. J Pediatr Surg 14:62–64, 1979.
27. Chwals W, Brennan L, Weitzman J, et al: Transanal mucosal sleeve resection for the treatment of rectal prolapse in children. J Pediatr Surg 25:715–718, 1990.
28. Groff D, Nagaraj H: Rectal prolapse in infants and children. Am J Surg 160:531–532, 1990.
29. Schepens MA, Verhelst AA: Reappraisal of Ekehorn's rectopexy in the management of rectal prolapse in children. J Pediatr Surg 28:1494–1497, 1993.
30. Tsugawa C, Matsumoto Y, Nishijima E, et al: Posterior plication of the rectum for rectal prolapse in children. J Pediatr Surg 30:692–693, 1995.
31. Ashcraft KW, Amoury RA, Holder TM: Levator repair and posterior suspension for rectal prolapse. J Pediatr Surg 12:241–245, 1977.
32. Ashcraft KW, Garred JL, Holder TM: Rectal prolapse—17 year experience with the posterior repair and suspension. J Pediatr Surg 25:992–995, 1990.
33. Altemeier WA, Culbertson WR, Schowengerdt C, et al: Nineteen years' experience with the one-stage perineal repair of rectal prolapse. Ann Surg 173:993–1006, 1971.
34. Rosemberg SK, Husain M, Herman GE, et al: Sexually transmitted papillomaviral infection in the male: VI. Simultaneous urethral cytology-ViraPap testing of male consorts of women with genital human papillomaviral infection. Urology 36:38–41, 1990.
35. Finkel MA: Anogenital trauma in sexually abused children. Pediatrics 84:317–322, 1989.
36. Trunkey D, Hays RJ, Shired GT: Management of rectal trauma. J Trauma 13:411–415, 1973.
37. Levine JH, Longo WE, Pruitt C, et al: Management of selected rectal injuries by primary repair. Am J Surg 172:575–579, 1996.

39

INTUSSUSCEPTION

Mary E. Fallat, MD

Intussusception is a frequent cause of bowel obstruction in infants and toddlers. It was first described by Paul Barbette of Amsterdam in 1674.[1] Jonathan Hutchinson reported the first successful operation for intussusception in a 2-year-old child in 1873.[2] In 1876, Harald Hirschsprung described a systematic approach to hydrostatic reduction.[3] In the United States, Ravitch popularized the use of barium enema reduction for this problem. His 1959 monograph reviewing all aspects of intussusception remains a classic.[4]

☐ Primary Idiopathic Intussusception

PATHOGENESIS

Intussusception is the telescoping of one portion of the intestine into another. An intussusception is customarily described by the proximal portion of intestine (intussusceptum) first and the distal portion of intestine (intussuscipiens) last. More than 80% of intussusceptions are ileocolic. The ileoileal, cecocolic, colocolic, and jejunojejunal varieties occur with increasing rarity.[5] An intussusception may have an identifiable lesion that serves as a lead point, drawing the proximal bowel into the distal by peristaltic activity. In almost every patient examined at operation, marked hypertrophy of the lymphoid tissue of the ileal wall is encountered at the leading edge of the intussusceptum.[5] Intussusception occurs frequently in the wake of an upper respiratory infection or an episode of gastroenteritis, providing an etiology for hypertrophy of Peyer's patches. Adenoviruses and to a much lesser extent rotavirus have been implicated in up to 50% of cases.[5, 6] These swollen Peyer's patches protrude into the lumen of the bowel and are the likely cause of the initial invagination.

The incidence of a definite anatomic lead point ranges from 2 to 12% in reported series.[7] These include Meckel's diverticulum, the appendix, polyps, carcinoid tumors, submucosal hemorrhage resulting from Henoch-Schönlein purpura, non-Hodgkin's lymphoma, foreign bodies, ectopic pancreas or gastric mucosa, and intestinal duplication. The most common pathologic lead point is a Meckel's diverticulum. The incidence of anatomic lead points increases in proportion to age.[8]

As the mesentery of the proximal bowel is drawn into the distal bowel, it is compressed, resulting in venous obstruction, edema of the bowel wall and, if reduction does not occur, arterial insufficiency and bowel wall necrosis. Although spontaneous reduction undoubtedly occurs, the natural history of an intussusception is to progress to a fatal outcome as a result of sepsis unless the condition is recognized and appropriately treated. For many reasons, the morbidity and mortality rates have decreased dramatically at children's hospitals in North America since the mid-1940s.[7]

☐ Secondary Intussusception

Patients with cystic fibrosis are prone to intussusception, and reduction may be required on multiple occasions. It is probable that inspissated secretions and thick fecal matter in the bowel lumen act as a lead point to produce repeated intussusception in this disease. These conditions are seen in children at an average age of 9 to 12 years.[5]

☐ Incidence

Intussusception can occur at any age; however, the greatest incidence occurs in infants between 5 and 9 months of age. More than half of all cases occur within the 1st year of life, and only 10 to 25% of cases occur after the age of 2 years.[5, 9] The condition has been described in premature infants and has been postulated as the cause of small bowel atresia in some cases.[10]

Most patients are well-nourished, healthy infants. Approximately two thirds are male.[5] It seems reasonable to be more suspicious of intussusception during peaks of respiratory infection and epidemics of gastroenteritis.

☐ Clinical Presentation

Intussusception produces cramping abdominal pain, which begins acutely with signs of severe discomfort in an infant who has previously been comfortable. The child may stiffen and pull the legs up to the abdomen. Hyperextension, writhing, and breath holding may be followed by vomiting. The attack often ceases as suddenly as it started. In between attacks, the child may appear normal or fall asleep. After some time, the child may become lethargic between episodes of pain. Vomiting at some stage is almost universal, consisting of undigested food initially and later becoming bilious. Small or normal bowel movements may result initially from the straining as the colon evacuates distal to the obstruction. Later in the course, the stools may be tinged with blood. Still later in the progression of the bowel ischemia, dark red mucoid clots or "currant jelly" stools are passed.

☐ Physical Examination

The child's vital signs are usually normal early in the course of the disease. During episodes of pain, hyperperistaltic rushes may be heard.

Between episodes of cramping, the right lower quadrant may appear flat or empty. This finding is due to progression of the cecum and ileocecal portion of the intussusception into the right upper quadrant or transverse colon. During the relaxed interval between pains, a mass may be delineated almost anywhere in the abdomen. The mass is often curved because it is tethered by the blood vessels and mesentery on one side. On rectal examination, blood-stained mucus or blood may be encountered. The longer the duration of symptoms, the more likely the probability of identifying gross or occult blood. Palpation of the intussuscepted mass on bimanual examination is possible. Actual contact with the rectal examining finger is rare.

If the obstructive process has been prolonged, dehydration and bacteremia ensue, leading to tachycardia and fever. Occasionally, the child is first seen in hypovolemic or septic shock.

Prolapse of the intussusceptum through the anus is a grave sign, particularly when the intussusceptum is blue-black. Certainly rectal protrusion of an ileal lead point is an indication of extensive telescoping and severe compromise of blood supply and ischemic damage to the gut. Such a patient undoubtedly exhibits signs of systemic illness. The greatest danger in a case of prolapse of the intussusceptum is that the examiner will misdiagnose the condition and reduce what is seen to be merely a small rectal prolapse. To avoid such a tragedy, a lubricated tongue blade should be passed up along the side of the protruding mass before reduction is attempted. Prolapse of a colocolic intussusception may easily be mistaken for simple rectal prolapse. If the blade can be inserted more than a centimeter or two into the anus alongside of the mass, the diagnosis of intussusception should be made. Rectal prolapse, while producing discomfort, should not be accompanied by vomiting or signs of sepsis.

☐ Diagnostic Studies

In about half of cases, the diagnosis of intussusception can be suspected on plain abdominal radiographs (Fig. 39–1). Suggestive radiographic abnormalities on a plain film include an abdominal mass, abnormal distribution of gas and fecal contents, sparse large bowel gas, and air-fluid levels in the presence of bowel obstruction.[11] These signs are not diagnostic, however, and controversy exists over whether the limited accuracy warrants this study.[12]

☐ Ultrasonography

Ultrasonographic (US) examination of the abdomen is used in some medical centers to evaluate a

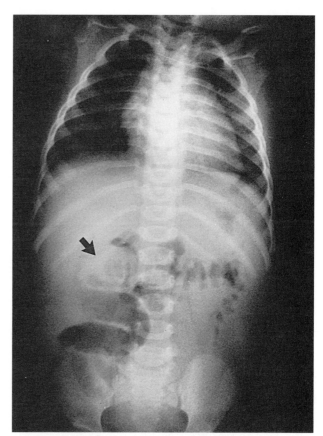

Figure 39–1. Abdominal radiograph showing dilated loops of small bowel in the right lower quadrant and a soft tissue mass density in the vicinity of the transverse colon near the hepatic flexure *(arrow).*

child with a possible intussusception. The sonographic pattern of intussusception was first reported in 1977.[13, 14] Since then, numerous studies have described the characteristic findings of a "target" lesion and a "pseudokidney" sign. The target lesion is seen on transverse section and consists of two rings of low echogenicity separated by a hyperechoic ring. The pseudokidney sign is seen on longitudinal section and appears as superimposed hypoechoic and hyperechoic layers (Fig. 39–2). This pattern represents the edematous walls of the intussusception. Successful reduction results in a smaller "donut" with an echogenic rim representing edema of the terminal ileum and ileocecal valve.

A virtue of US is that it minimizes exposure to ionizing radiation. Methods used to reduce the intussusception following diagnosis include using a sonographically guided meglumine diatrizoate enema to confirm the condition and balanced salt solution to reduce it, or using pneumatic pressure without fluoroscopic confirmation.[15, 16] US is accurate, but its use should be limited to those patients in whom there is a low index of suspicion of intussusception.[12] If a patient has the typical attacks of pain and passes currant jelly-like stools, an air or hydrostatic enema should be done.

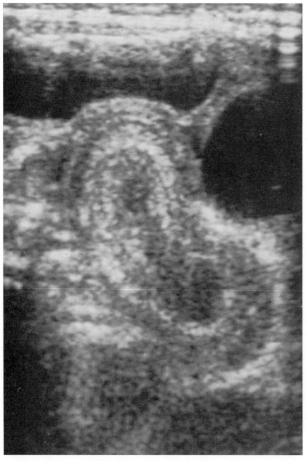

Figure 39–2. Sonogram showing the "pseudokidney" sign seen with intussusception on longitudinal section.

□ Nonoperative Management

Once the diagnosis of intussusception is considered, a nasogastric tube is inserted to decompress the stomach. Intravenous fluid resuscitation is begun. Appropriate laboratory studies are done. Contrast is the mainstay of diagnosis and the first line of reduction treatment in most centers. Few complications are reported, as long as certain guidelines are followed.

Hydrostatic or pneumatic reduction should be attempted only under controlled conditions. Evidence of peritonitis, perforation, advancing sepsis, and possible gangrenous bowel precludes enema or pneumatic reduction. This should be the surgeon's decision. The longer the history of symptoms, the greater the possibility that enema reduction will not be successful and the more dangerous it may be.

□ Hydrostatic Reduction

One of the first studies evaluating the technique of intussusception reduction using hydrostatic pressure was published in 1926.[17] These reductions were not fluoroscopically controlled using a contrast agent but were performed under anesthesia using saline solution. Fundamentals of this method of management were incorporated in the present technique of hydrostatic reduction. A lubricated straight catheter or Foley catheter is inserted into the rectum and held in place by firmly taping the buttocks together; balloon occlusion of the anus must never be used. The child is restrained. The barium is allowed to run into the rectum from a height of 3 ft above the patient. The filling of the bowel is observed fluoroscopically. Constant hydrostatic pressure is continued as long as reduction is occurring. In the absence of progress, the barium is allowed to drain. This procedure can be repeated a second or third time.

Typically, reduction of the ileum back to the area of the ileocecal valve is simple. Usually, a delay occurs at that point until a free flow of barium into the distal small bowel is seen.

The nonoperative enema technique of intussusception reduction has several obvious advantages over operative reduction, including decreased morbidity, cost, and length of hospital stay. A successful reduction is dependent on free reflux of contrast into the distal small bowel (Fig. 39–3). Hydrostatic reduction with barium under fluoroscopic guidance was the standard method until the mid-1980s.[12] Water-soluble isotonic contrast is an ideal alternative for hydrostatic reduction owing to the risk of barium extravasation with perforation.

□ Pneumatic Reduction

Adoption of the air enema or pneumatic technique has become more widespread since the late

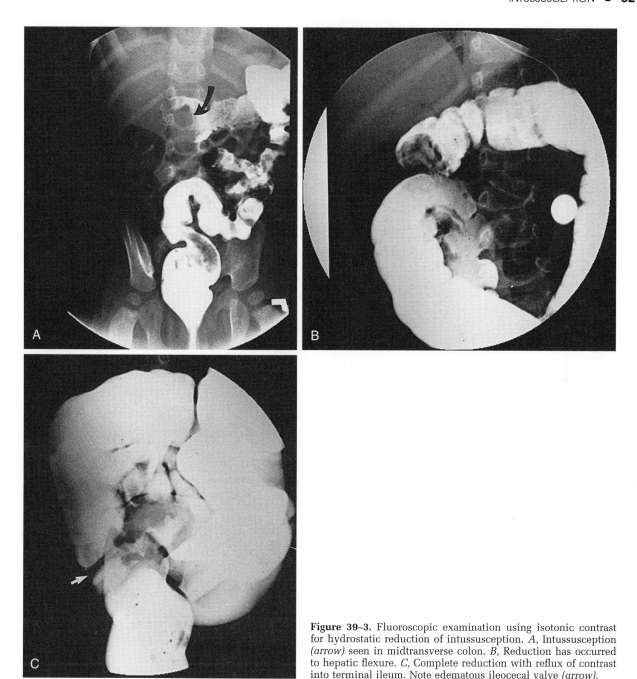

Figure 39–3. Fluoroscopic examination using isotonic contrast for hydrostatic reduction of intussusception. *A*, Intussusception *(arrow)* seen in midtransverse colon. *B*, Reduction has occurred to hepatic flexure. *C*, Complete reduction with reflux of contrast into terminal ileum. Note edematous ileocecal valve *(arrow)*.

1980s owing to the higher rates of successful reduction reported in large international series.[9] The procedure is fluoroscopically monitored as air is insufflated into the rectum. The maximum safe air pressure is 80 mm Hg for younger infants and 110 to 120 mm Hg for older infants. Advocates of the air enema believe that the method is quicker, safer, and less messy, and decreases exposure time to radiation. Accurate pressure measurements are possible and reduction rates are higher than with hydrostatic techniques (Fig. 39–4).[18] Potential drawbacks of using pneumatic reduction include the possibility of development of a tension pneumoperitoneum, poor visualization of lead points, and relatively poor visualization of the intussusception and reduction process, resulting in false-positive reductions (Fig. 39–5).[15]

Attempts at hydrostatic or pneumatic reduction are continued *as long as progress is evident.* Many knowledgeable physicians think that if the patient's general condition permits, two or three attempts at reduction should be done before abandoning the procedure.

Success rates of reduction using hydrostatic techniques between 1980 and 1991 were reported as 50 to 78% compared with 75 to 94% using pneumatic reduction between 1986 and 1991.[5] The administration of glucagon is no longer thought to be helpful as an aid in the reduction of an intussusception.[19] A second trial of hydrostatic or air reduction may

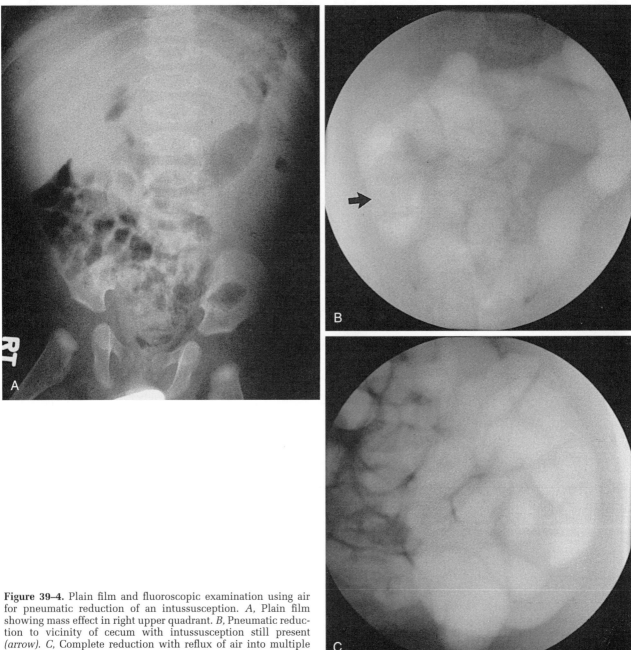

Figure 39–4. Plain film and fluoroscopic examination using air for pneumatic reduction of an intussusception. *A,* Plain film showing mass effect in right upper quadrant. *B,* Pneumatic reduction to vicinity of cecum with intussusception still present *(arrow). C,* Complete reduction with reflux of air into multiple loops of small intestine. (Courtesy of Charles Maxfield, MD.)

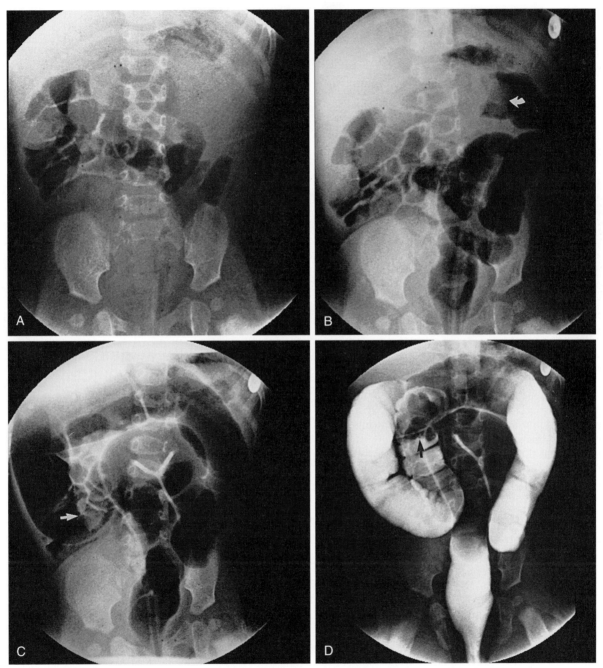

Figure 39–5. Incomplete reduction of intussusception. *A,* Scout film showing dilated loops of small intestine and little colonic gas. *B,* Pneumatic reduction to transverse colon showing intussusceptum *(arrow). C,* Further reduction with persistent filling defect *(arrow). D,* Isotonic contrast enema showing cecum in right upper quadrant and persistent intussusception *(arrow).* This child had an upper gastrointestinal series to rule out malrotation, which was normal, followed by operative reduction.

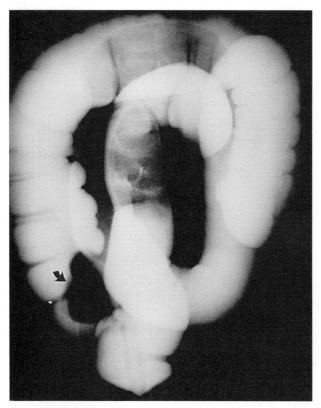

Figure 39–6. Contrast enema view following hydrostatic reduction of an intussusception to the ileocecal junction. There is a persistent filling defect *(arrow)* without free reflux into the terminal ileum.

be undertaken within a few hours if the child does not have an acute abdomen and the symptoms seem relieved but the original reduction failed to show reflux into the terminal ileum.[9] If reduction has occurred to the edematous ileocecal junction, other researchers propose only watchful waiting, with repeat study reserved for those with recurrent symptoms (Fig. 39–6).[20]

A colon perforation rate of 1 in 250 to 300 enema reductions is quoted in most large series.[18] The cause of perforation includes excessive pressure, necrotic bowel, or the revealing of an existing occult perforation.

After successful reduction under fluoroscopic monitoring, the patient should be observed for approximately 24 hours on intravenous fluids with nothing being given by mouth. The family should be advised of the possibility of recurrence, which exists regardless of whether the intussusception is reduced by enema or by operation.

□ Operative Treatment

Laparotomy is required in children with signs of shock or peritonitis and in those who have incomplete hydrostatic pressure or pneumatic reduction. Preoperative preparation includes gastric decompression, fluid resuscitation, and administration of prophylactic antibiotics.

Successful enema reduction of an intussusception does not completely exclude a lead point that might result in recurrence or that might otherwise be hazardous to the patient, and some studies suggest that the incidence of a lead point increases with age.[8] A residual intraluminal filling defect following enema reduction with terminal ileal reflux is an indication for laparotomy.[21]

A right lower quadrant muscle-splitting incision with a transverse skin incision is usually satisfactory for exposure. The involved bowel can almost always be readily reduced to this area, even when the intussusceptum has progressed to the rectosigmoid. The option of extension of the incision is available.

Gentle manipulation of the bowel is needed, pushing (rather than pulling) the lead point of the intussusceptum back toward its normal position (Fig. 39–7). When resistance to reduction reaches the point of serosal tearing, the surgeon must decide whether further attempts at reduction are likely to be fruitful or might result in intestinal rupture and contamination. As hydrostatic reduction has become more efficient, fewer patients are being operated on and the incidence of resection at operation has increased.[6]

Even when reduction is complete, the viability of the bowel may be questionable. In such cases, the application of warm saline packs may improve the circulation and relieve doubt about the necessity of resection. When serious vascular impairment has occurred, resection is usually the safest course (Fig. 39–8).

Once operative reduction has been achieved, examination for a pathologic lead point must be performed and appropriate measures must be taken.

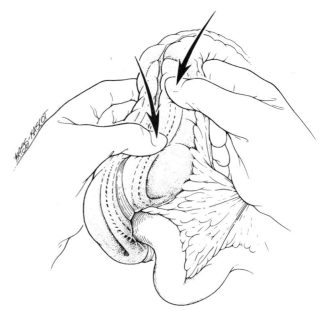

Figure 39–7. A right lower quadrant muscle-splitting incision allows for delivery of the intussusception into the wound. Gentle and continuous massage from distal to proximal usually results in reduction of the intussusception.

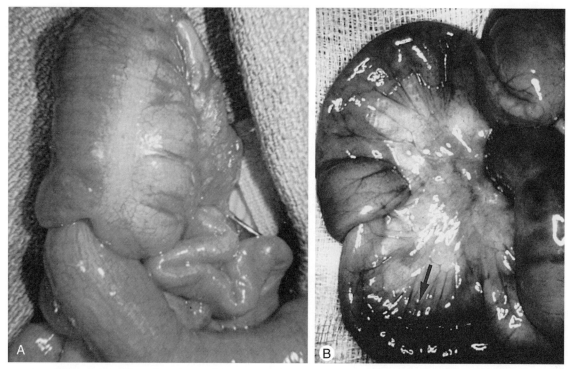

Figure 39–8. Operative views of intussusception. *A,* Exterior view of intussusception prior to reduction. *B,* Operative view of an incompletely reduced intussusception. The intestine in the lower half of the photograph has been reduced and the bowel wall is ecchymotic with at least one area of questionable viability *(arrow).*

The most concerning cases are those in which the patient is older than 2 years of age. An appendectomy is usually performed because the location of the scar suggests an appendectomy was performed.

☐ Recurrent Intussusception

Recurrent intussusception has been described in 2 to 20% of cases, with about one third occurring within 1 day and the majority within 6 months of the initial episode.[22, 23] Recurrences usually have no defined lead point, and they are less likely to occur after surgical reduction or resection. There can be multiple recurrences in the same patient. Success rates with enema reduction after one recurrence are comparable to the first episode and are better if the child did not previously require operative reduction. Patients tend to be seen earlier when suffering from recurrent intussusception, and they have fewer symptoms. Irritability and discomfort may be the only clues during the early state of a recurrence.

An overriding concern in recurrent intussusception is occult malignancy. For this reason, some investigators have recommended that recurrences be treated surgically in the following instances: (1) in a child with more than one episode of recurrence who has had no surgery to document the absence of a lead point, (2) in children older than 2 years old whose first episode was reduced by enema, and (3) in children in whom a pathologic lead point is suspected.[24] Although first recurrences are success-fully reduced by enema in most cases, the success rate diminishes with multiple recurrences and most individuals require at least a surgical reduction, if not resection.[22, 23]

☐ Postoperative Intussusception

Intussusception occurs after operations done for a variety of conditions. Thoracic as well as abdominal operations have been followed by latent intussusception. Because ileus and adhesive obstruction more frequently come to mind as a cause for intestinal obstruction, these intussusceptions are rarely diagnosed preoperatively. Most postoperative intussusceptions occur within a month of initial procedure, and an interval of about 10 days between initial operation and development of symptoms is average.[25] Contrast radiographic studies are often obtained for diagnosis and show a small bowel obstruction. Most postoperative intussusceptions are ileoileal and respond to operative reduction without resection.[25]

REFERENCES

1. Barbette P: Oeuvres Chirugiques et Anatomiques. Geneva, Francois Miege, 1674, p 522.
2. Hutchinson J: A successful case of abdominal section for intussusception. Proc R Med Chir Soc 7:195–198, 1873.
3. Hirschsprung H: Et Tilfaelde af suakut Tarminvagination. Hospitals-Tidende 3:321–327, 1876.

4. Ravitch MM: Intussusception in infants and children. Springfield, IL, Charles C. Thomas, 1959.

5. Stringer MD, Pablot SM, Brereton RJ: Paediatric intussusception. Br J Surg 79:867–876, 1992.

6. Montgomery EA, Popek EJ: Intussusception, adenovirus, and children: A brief reaffirmation. Hum Pathol 25:169–174, 1994.

7. Meier DE, Coln CE, Rescorla FJ, et al: Intussusception in children: International perspective. World J Surg 20:1035–1040, 1996.

8. Ong N, Beasley SW: The leadpoint in intussusception. J Pediatr Surg 25:640–643, 1990.

9. Guo J, Ma X, Zhou Q: Results of air pressure enema reduction of intussusception: 6,396 cases in 13 years. J Pediatr Surg 21:1201–1203, 1986.

10. Mooney DP, Steinthorsson G, Shorter NA: Perinatal intussusception in premature infants. J Pediatr Surg 31:695–697, 1996.

11. Smith DS, Bonadio WA, Losek JD, et al: The role of abdominal x-rays in the diagnosis and management of intussusception. Pediatr Emerg Care 8:325–327, 1992.

12. Daneman A, Alton DJ: Intussusception issues and controversies related to diagnosis and reduction. Radiol Clin North Am 34:743–756, 1996.

13. Burke LF, Clarke E: Ileocolic intussusception—a case report. J Clin Ultrasound 5:346–347, 1977.

14. Weissberg DL, Scheible W, Leopold GR: Ultrasonographic appearance of adult intussusception. Radiology 124:791–792, 1977.

15. Peh WCG, Khong PL, Chan KL, et al: Sonographically guided hydrostatic reduction of childhood intussusception using Hartmann's solution. AJR Am J Roentgenol 167:1237–1241, 1996.

16. Wang G, Liu XG, Zitsman JL: Nonfluoroscopic reduction of intussusception by air enema. World J Surg 19:435–438, 1995.

17. Hipsley P: Intussusception and its treatment by hydrostatic pressure: Based on an analysis of 100 consecutive cases so treated. Med J Aust 2:201–206, 1926.

18. Kirks DR: Air intussusception reduction: 'The winds of change.' Pediatr Radiol 25:89–91, 1995.

19. Franken EA, Smith WL, Chernish SNM, et al: The use of glucagon in hydrostatic reduction of intussusception: A double blind study of 30 patients. Radiology 146:687–689, 1983.

20. Ein SH, Palder SB, Alton DJ: Intussusception: Toward less surgery? J Pediatr Surg 29:433–435, 1994.

21. Ein SH, Shandling B, Reilly BJ, et al: Hydrostatic reduction of intussusceptions caused by lead points. J Pediatr Surg 21:883–886, 1986.

22. Champoux AN, Del Beccaro MA, Nazar-Stewart V: Recurrent intussusception. Arch Pediatr Adolesc Med 148:474–478, 1994.

23. Fecteau A, Flageole H, Nguyen LT, et al: Recurrent intussusception: Safe use of hydrostatic enema. J Pediatr Surg 31:859–861, 1996.

24. Beasley SW, Auldist AW, Stokes KB: Recurrent intussusception: Barium or surgery? Aust N Z J Surg 57:11–14, 1987.

25. Holcomb GW, Ross AJ, O'Neill JA: Postoperative intussusception: Increasing frequency or increasing awareness? South Med J 84:1334–1339, 1991.

40

ALIMENTARY TRACT DUPLICATIONS

Earle L. Wrenn, Jr., MD • Robert S. Hollabaugh, MD

Cystic or tubular structures lined by normal gastrointestinal mucosa and having smooth muscle walls like those of the intestine occur in proximity to all parts of the alimentary tract, from the mouth to the anus (Table 40–1).[1–8] In 1937, Ladd suggested that lesions of these types, which had previously been described under many different names, be collectively designated alimentary tract duplications.[9] Gross, in his review of a large series of duplications, further defined their clinical and pathologic features.[1]

Duplications typically lie in close proximity to the alimentary tube and frequently share a common muscular wall and a common blood supply. The usual location is dorsal to the normal intestine, that is, on the mesenteric aspect, in contrast to vitelline duct remnants, such as Meckel's diverticula, which lie on the antimesenteric aspect of the bowel. The mucosa may resemble that of the proximate alimentary viscus, but cysts lined by colonic mucosa have been found at the base of the tongue, and sinuses lined by gastric mucosa are found at the anus. Duplications are often associated with other congenital anomalies, and multiple duplications occur in the same patient. The occurrence of duplications of the alimentary tract has only rarely been reported in siblings.

Malignant tumors in duplications may develop later in life. All reported cases have been in people older than 30 years of age at diagnosis. Such tumors are rare, and although they have been reported in various gastrointestinal duplication sites, most seem to occur in colonic or presacral duplications, the majority of them being adenocarcinomas.[10]

☐ Embryology

PARTIAL TWINNING

Certain duplications appear to represent partial twinning, in particular, tubular duplications of the terminal ileum and colon.[11–16] Deformities range from complete doubling of the lower trunk and ex-

TABLE 40-1. Alimentary Tract Duplications

Reference	Number of Patients	Cervical	Mediastinal	Thoraco-abdominal	Gastric	Duodenal	Jejunal and Ileal	Colonic	Rectal
Gross[1]	68	1*	13	3	2	4	32	9	4
Sieber[2]	25†		5		4	2	16	5‡	
Houston[3]	8		1	1			6		
Basu[4]	28§		7		1	3	16	4	2
Mellish[5]	38	1	6	2	1		18	6‖	4
Grosfeld[6]	20		4	2	1		9	4	
Favara[7]	37¶	3*	4		3	4	20	4	
Wrenn	25#		3	2	1	2	12	3	4
Holcomb[8]	96**	1	20	3	8	2	47	20	
Total	**342**	**6**	**63**	**13**	**21**	**17**	**176**	**55**	**14**

*One in base of tongue.
†One patient had two duplications, one had three, one had five.
‡One patient had double appendix only—postmortem finding.
§Three patients had two duplications, one had three.
‖ One patient had double appendix only.
¶One patient had three duplications.
#Two patients each had two duplications.
**101 duplications in 96 patients.

tremities (dipygus) to mere doubling of the lower hindgut structures. Similar malformations at the opposite end range from two-headed bodies to double mouths and paired upper alimentary structures (see Chapter 76). The twinning process can result in parallel, normally functioning structures with little or no external malformations.

In most reported cases, however, associated malformations do cause symptoms. When the colon is doubled, one or both lumens often end as a fistula into the perineum or urogenital tract or as an imperforate anus. An open proximal end may allow intestinal contents to enter the obstructed segment, leading to dilation of one or both lumens. The mucosa of these duplications is normal for the particular anatomic area. The antimesenteric location of hindgut duplications is in contrast to the mesenteric location of those duplications, which may be remnants of the neurenteric canal, and suggests a different embryologic origin. Triplication of the colon has been reported and raises further uncertainty regarding the embryogenesis of these abnormalities.[17]

RESIDUA OF THE NEURENTERIC CANAL: SPLIT NOTOCORD SYNDROME

The most satisfactory of several theories of origin of other alimentary tract duplications is that which relates them to the neurenteric canal (Fig. 40–1).[18–22] Initially, the embryo has two layers: endoderm and ectoderm. Mesoderm forms between the two, but for a short while, at the primitive pit, the two layers remain in contact. A transient opening, the neurenteric canal, appears connecting the neural ectoderm with the gastrointestinal endoderm. The notocord forms in the mesoderm just caudal to the neurent-

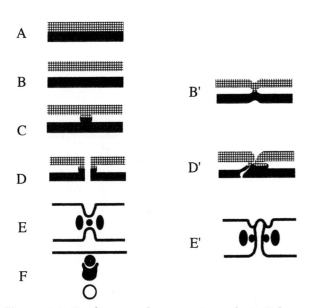

Figure 40–1. Development of neurenteric canal. *A*, Embryo—endoderm and ectoderm. *B*, Ingrowth or mesoderm. *C*, Fusion of endoderm and ectoderm. *D–D′*, Neurenteric canal and notocord. *E–E′*, Partial persistence of neurenteric canal with split notocord. *F*, Normal development.

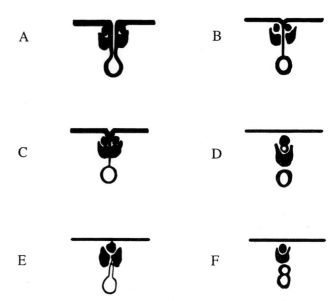

Figure 40–2. Defects resulting from persistence of portions of the neurenteric canal. *A*, Completely patent neurenteric canal forming dorsal enteric fistula. *B*, Fibrous cord with spina bifida and diastematomyelia. *C*, Dorsal midline sinus lined by gastrointestinal mucosa. *D*, Intraspinal enteric cyst. *E*, Tubular communicating duplication. *F*, Cystic duplication.

eric canal. As it migrates, the notocord is split by the persistent neurenteric canal, resulting in the development of spina bifida or other vertebral anomalies and anterior or posterior myelomeningocele. The term *split notocord syndrome* has been applied to these defects.

Possible abnormalities related to failure of regression of the neurenteric canal are complete dorsal enteric fistula, fibrous cord passing through the spinal cord as in diastematomyelia, intraspinal enteric cyst, dorsal enteric sinus, neuroenteric cyst, and enteric duplications (Fig. 40–2). The dorsal anatomic location of most duplications in relation to their normal counterparts is supportive of this theory of origin.

EMBRYONIC DIVERTICULA

Diverticula have been found in embryonic intestine that could conceivably grow into duplications; however, they were observed in numerous sites on the circumference of the bowel wall other than the mesenteric side, where duplications are found.[23] Variation of the character of the mucosal linings is not explained adequately by this theory.

DEFECTS IN RECANALIZATION

Abnormal recanalization of the intestinal lumen after the solid stage of embryologic development was believed to result in duplications.[24] Such cysts would probably not be limited to the mesenteric side of the bowel or have heterotopic mucosa. Also opposing this theory is the finding that the solid stage of development does not usually involve areas other than the duodenum in the human embryo.

☐ Diagnosis

The symptoms created by intestinal duplications depend on their type and location. A mass discovered on physical examination or radiologic examination of the chest or abdomen is a common feature. Pain is usually evidence of a complication, such as intestinal obstruction resulting from volvulus or intussusception, peptic ulceration, or perforation. Vomiting may result from these same complications or result from compression of the adjacent bowel lumen, especially in duplications of the pylorus or duodenum. Bleeding may be sudden, severe, and painless, as is seen with the more common Meckel's diverticulum. Rectal bleeding associated with severe abdominal pain is more likely to indicate intussusception or volvulus. Anemia may result from chronic blood loss into the intestine. Intrathoracic duplications can cause respiratory distress owing to compression of the tracheobronchial tree or lung, or dysphagia if the esophagus is narrowed.

Presacral enteric cysts can cause constipation or can prolapse through the anus. Persistent perineal excoriation may indicate that a gastric mucosa-lined sinus tract drains into the area. Purulent drainage from the anus or a fistula in the perineum, originating from an infected rectal duplication, may be mistaken for a perirectal abscess or fistula in ano. The diagnosis of duplication is made after multiple recurrences. No case could be found of a urinary tract fistula from a rectal duplication.[25]

Neurologic signs of spinal cord compression may result from intraspinal cysts. Myelomeningocele is present with some duplications, especially thoracic ones. Diagnostic studies, including radiography, ultrasonography, computed tomography, and nuclear magnetic resonance scans, may demonstrate a mass or displacement of normal structures. Vertebral anomalies, such as spina bifida and missing vertebrae or hemivertebrae, accompany many thoracic and abdominal duplications. A Y-shaped splitting of the lower vertebrae and sacrum is seen with many hindgut duplications, more striking when the external genitalia or other perineal structures are doubled. Such patients have septate or double urinary bladders, depending on the extent of the twinning process.

Radioisotope scans using technetium isotopes are particularly useful in the search for ectopic gastric mucosa found in tubular duplications.[26] Enteric duplications have been diagnosed on prenatal ultrasound examination.[27]

☐ Treatment

In view of the wide anatomic variations encountered with alimentary tract duplication, it is necessary to be familiar with the several surgical techniques that may be required for their management. Cystic duplications can, in most instances, be totally excised. When the cyst is in the mesentery of large or small bowel, its removal may destroy the blood supply to the adjacent bowel; therefore, the segment of normal intestine must be resected with the duplication.

Complete removal of duodenal duplications may endanger the bile ducts or pancreas. They are thus managed more safely by marsupialization of the cyst into the duodenum through an anastomosis of the common walls or by partial cystectomy and stripping of the mucosa from the residual cyst wall. The technique of mucosal stripping has been used in cystic duplications of various sites as well as in tubular duplications, as described subsequently. Tubular duplications of the hindgut may not need to be removed if they are capable of normal function.

Distal obstruction or aberrant termination of one or both lumens does require treatment. The two lumens can be joined distally to form a single channel, the distal end being left in place if it has adequate external drainage for its mucous secretions.[12] Preferably, the mucosa should be stripped from the defunctionalized segment to obliterate its lumen completely.[13, 28]

Tubular duplications of the upper gastrointestinal tract and small bowel so often contain gastric mucosa that they should be removed completely to avoid bleeding from peptic ulceration. Combined thoracoabdominal incisions may be needed for removal of intrathoracic duplications that pass through the diaphragm to communicate with the intestinal lumen. Short tubular duplications and the overlying segment of normal bowel may be managed readily by resection.

Complete resection of longer duplications lying in the mesentery would necessitate removal of too much normal bowel; thus, other techniques are required. It is possible to remove the mucosa completely by stripping it from the muscle layers of the duplication without disturbing the essential blood supply to the adjacent intestine.[29] The remaining collapsed seromuscular tube does no harm (Figs. 40–3 to 40–8). This is the treatment of choice for long tubular duplications of the bowel. Tubes of gastric mucosa longer than 70 cm in length have been removed in this fashion. One such tubular duplication was anastomosed to the stomach, where its acid secretions should have no harmful effects.[30, 31]

Rectal duplications should be excised, or the mucosa should be completely removed. Many patients have infections that initially need drainage, followed by definitive excision. Malignant tumors have been identified in later life in rectal duplications that have escaped detection in childhood. Minimal invasive procedures may be useful, especially in cystic duplications of the thorax. These can be totally excised, or the mucosal lining removed thoracoscopically, with minimal morbidity. Incomplete removal of the mucosa leads to recurrence of the lesion, however. Laparoscopic removal of localized cystic duplications in the abdomen is a reasonable approach.

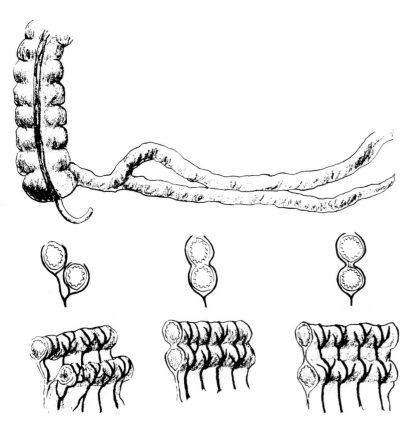

Figure 40–3. The surgical findings in a 4-month-old girl explored for melena and found to have a long tubular duplication from the ligament of Treitz to the distal ileum with an area of ulceration at the distal ileum. After resecting the area of ulceration, the duplication was anastomosed to the overlying ileum. The resected portion of the duplication was lined entirely by gastric mucosa.

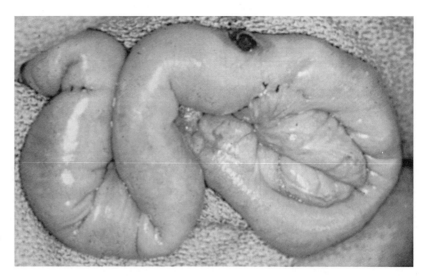

Figure 40–4. Same patient shown in Figure 40–3. She bled again 3 days later from an ulcer at the anastomosis of the duplication to the ileum.

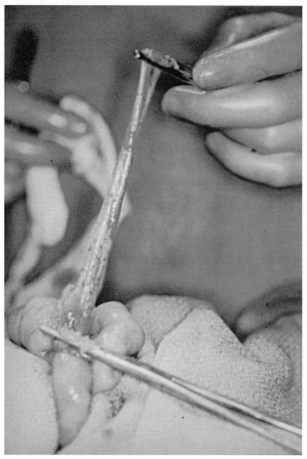

Figure 40–5. Same patient shown in Figure 40–3. At the second procedure, the mucosa was stripped from the entire length of the duplicated intestine through a series of seromuscular incisions.

□ Cervical Duplications

Only rarely are duplication cysts found in the neck.[32, 33] Intimate attachment to the esophagus may serve to differentiate them from cysts of branchial origin. A palpable mass or symptoms resulting from compression of adjacent structures should lead to the diagnosis.

□ Thoracic Duplications

Cysts, round or tube-like, occur in the posterior mediastinum, usually on the right side.[34] They may be separate from the esophagus or share a common wall with it, but they seldom communicate with its lumen. One triplication of the esophagus is reported.[35] A number of thoracic duplications communicate with the upper small intestine via an extension through the esophageal hiatus, passing behind the stomach and pancreas to join the duodenum or jejunum (Figs. 40–9 to 40–11). These duplications are commonly lined partly by gastric mucosa and lead to severe hemorrhage from peptic ulceration. Intrathoracic cysts may be large enough to produce cardiac or respiratory problems. Many thoracic duplications are associated with spinal anomalies, such as anterior or posterior spina bifida, hemivertebrae, or myelomeningocele, in which case the term *neurenteric cyst* is appropriate (Fig. 40–12).[36] Spinal anomalies occur also with gastric and small bowel duplications but less frequently.[18, 21] A severe form of this malformation is the dorsal enteric fistula, a mucosa-lined tubular structure leading from the alimentary tube to the skin of the back, passing through a bifid spinal cord and vertebral column.[37–40] Such fistulas occur more often in the thoracic area than in the lumbosacral area.

□ Duplications of the Stomach

Very large cystic duplications of the stomach may produce no symptoms except abdominal enlarge-

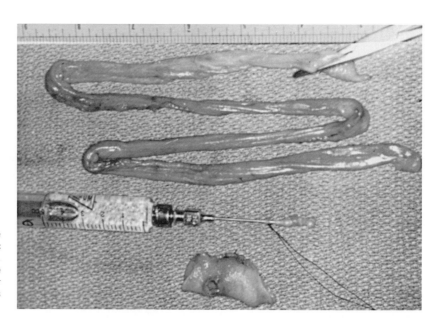

Figure 40–6. Same patient shown in Figure 40–3. Surgical specimen showing the gastric mucosal tube stripped from the duplication. The blind ending of the duplication in the vicinity of the pancreas was confirmed by inflating it with a syringe. The patient has remained well since this procedure.

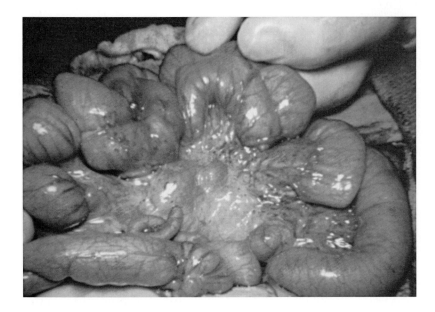

Figure 40–7. Tubular duplication of the small intestine in a 3-month-old girl with a history of blood in her stool at 6 days of age. She had occasional abdominal cramps and vomiting. She had an ulcer 10 to 12 cm proximal to the ileocecal valve.

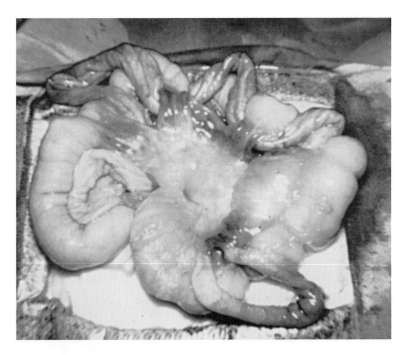

Figure 40–8. Same patient shown in Figure 40–7. Mucosal stripping of the duplication through multiple seromuscular incisions. The blood supply of the overlying normal bowel is well preserved.

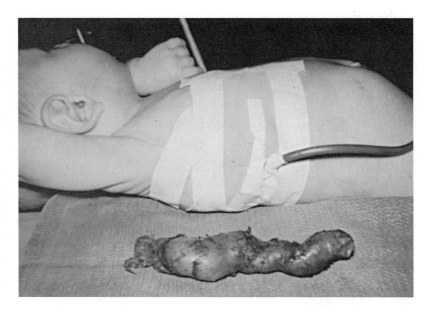

Figure 40–9. Neurenteric cyst removed from right posterior mediastinum and associated with spina bifida and anterior meningocele. This 4-month-old boy was admitted with respiratory difficulty, lethargy, and suspected leg weakness of 6 weeks' duration. Chest radiograph showed a large right posterior mediastinal mass and upper thoracic spina bifida. Myelogram showed a small anterior meningocele. At operation, a cyst was found with one locule in the midline over the area of spina bifida and in contact with the meningocele sac and a second locule forming a long, sausage-shaped cyst, extending down the right posterior mediastinum to the diaphragm. It was separate from the esophagus. The cyst was removed completely, and the narrow neck of the meningocele was ligated. No neural elements were involved. Recovery was prompt, but subsequent mental development was somewhat slowed.

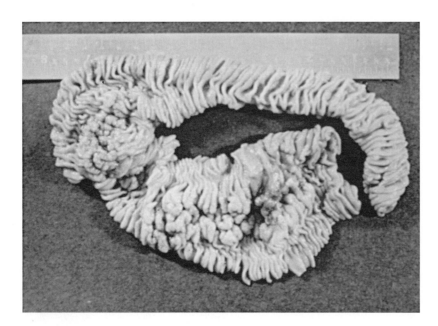

Figure 40–10. Same patient shown in Figure 40–9. Two years later, because of severe anemia and guaiac-positive stools, laparotomy was performed. An inflammatory mass in the jejunum was removed. It contained a small duplication with gastric mucosa and peptic ulceration. Anemia and guaiac-positive stools persisted. Laparotomy was repeated 2½ years later. The jejunal wall for 15 cm proximal to the previous anastomosis was slightly thicker in the mesenteric half of its circumference. That segment is pictured. The thicker area had gastric mucosa, whereas the remainder of the circumference had normal jejunal mucosa. This child has had no further gastrointestinal problems or anemia. The findings at the second laparotomy point out the need to check carefully the edges of surgical specimens containing ectopic gastric mucosa to be certain that it has all been removed. This case lends support to the neurenteric canal theory of embryogenesis of duplications and illustrates the occurrence of more than one lesion in a single patient.

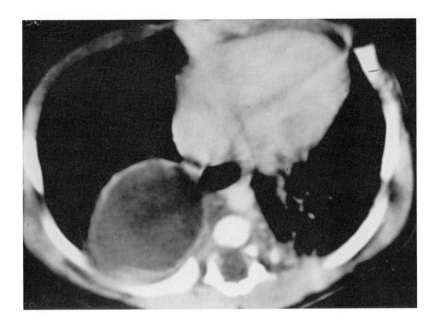

Figure 40–11. Postnatal computed topography scan showing right posterior mediastinal cyst. At 32 weeks of gestation, prenatal ultrasonography suggested right diaphragmatic hernia.

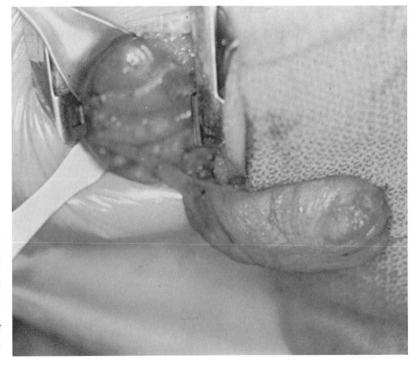

Figure 40–12. The patient in Figure 40–11 had a thoracotomy at 1 day of age to remove an enteric duplication cyst with a tubular extension passing through the diaphragm to communicate with the upper small intestine. No abdominal incision was necessary for its removal. The cyst was lined by gastric mucosa. Postoperative barium study showed no other gastrointestinal anomalies, radioisotope scan showed no residual foci of gastric mucosa, and magnetic resonance scan showed no spinal cord anomaly.

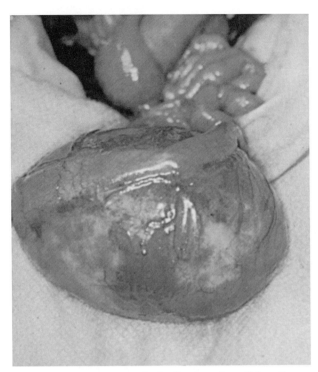

Figure 40–13. Large cystic duplication of small intestine.

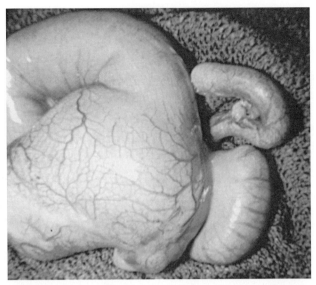

Figure 40–14. Cystic duplication of ileocecal junction. Cramping abdominal pain developed in a 3-year-old girl. Physical examination revealed a right upper quadrant abdominal mass. Barium enema showed intussusception, which was thought to be reduced, but without reflux of the contrast material into the ileum. Abdominal examination revealed the mass to be still present, and at operation, a cystic duplication of the terminal ileum near the ileocecal valve was found. This was resected and an end-to-end ileocolostomy was done.

ment, unless the gastric outlet is obstructed or rupture occurs.[41–49] Small cysts near the pylorus, in comparison, have mimicked the syndrome of hypertrophic pyloric stenosis.[43, 47] Communication with the gastric lumen has been found in one infant. In that case, the communication was thought to be secondary to perforation from peptic ulceration.

Areas of ectopic gastric mucosa are found on the tongue, in the esophagus, and in other sites outside the stomach. One series reported 16 patients in whom areas of ectopic gastric mucosa were present in the small bowel. The areas were nodular, rugose, or polypoid in appearance and 1.5 to 12 cm in length. Five areas were in the duodenum, seven in the jejunum, and four in the ileum. Although some of the patients were asymptomatic, many had complications of intestinal obstruction or hemorrhage. Heterotopic gastric mucosa in the ileum may be derived from the vitelline duct, but that origin does not seem a likely explanation for its presence elsewhere. Origin from a mechanism similar to that causing cystic and tubular duplications of the intestine appears more likely.

☐ Duplications of the Duodenum

Duplication cysts attached to the duodenal wall are less rare.[50–56] These vary greatly in size and lie, in most cases, posteromedially, fused by a common muscularis to the duodenum and partly embedded in the pancreas. No communication exists with the lumen. The mucosa often resembles that of more distal small or large intestine. Obstruction of the duodenum is the usual clinical picture. Some cysts

appear as asymptomatic masses, however. Pancreatitis has developed in patients with duodenal duplications, and perforation as a result of peptic ulceration from gastric mucosa in the duplications is a possibility.[54, 55]

☐ Enteric Duplications of the Biliary Tree

One duodenal duplication had the appearance of a double gallbladder, communicating with the lu-

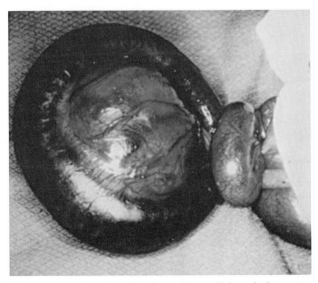

Figure 40–15. A 3-day-old infant with small bowel obstruction was found to have a perforation of the ileum resulting from volvulus of a cystic duplication.

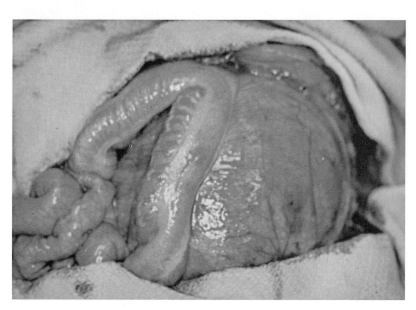

Figure 40–16. A large cystic duplication of the colon in a 2-year-old girl found at exploration for an asymptomatic midabdominal mass.

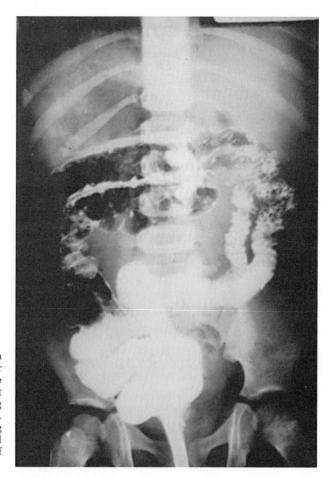

Figure 40–17. A newborn girl with imperforate anus initially had a perineal anoplasty performed. She subsequently passed part of her stools through the vagina and therefore underwent a right transverse colostomy. Four lumens in the colostomy were encountered. Contrast radiographs confirm a duplication of the colon with one lumen ending at the surgically formed anus and the other as a rectovaginal fistula. The lumen to the vagina was anastomosed to the side of that leading to the anus. The distal mucosa leading to the vagina was stripped out. The condition is consistent with the partial twinning theory of embryogenesis.

men of the bowel through the bile ducts and causing abdominal pain.[56] Boyden (personal communication, 1979) believes this case may represent a "pancreatic bladder," as has been described in cats. Another patient had a heterotopic gastric mucosal polyp in the duodenal bulb associated with congenital absence of the gallbladder and cystic duct.[57] Several other reports have been made of gastric heterotopy in the gallbladder.[58–60]

☐ Duplications of the Jejunum and Ileum

Spherical cysts in relation to the ileum form the largest group of alimentary duplications.[2, 29–31, 62] The jejunal and ileal lesions are found on the mesenteric border of the intestine, usually sharing a common muscularis. Mesenteric vessels pass over both surfaces of the duplication to supply both it and the overlying intestine (Figs. 40–13 to 40–15). Small or even very large cysts may cause no obstruction or other symptoms, unless intussusception or volvulus occurs. A freely movable mass in the abdomen may be the only abnormal finding. These lesions may be confused with mesenteric or omental cysts or cystic lymphangiomas of the mesentery, but those have endothelial rather than mucosal linings.

Tubular duplications have the same features as demonstrated in the cystic types but communicate with the lumen of the normal intestine. The length of the tubular structure varies from a few millimeters to 90 cm; at times the duplication is almost as long as the normal intestine.[29–31] The communication may be at the proximal or the distal end or at several points in between. If the only communication is at the cephalic end, the lumen may become greatly distended with intestinal content, compressing and obstructing the adjacent intestine or leading to perforation. More commonly, the communication is caudal in location, and the duplication empties readily. Gastric mucosa often lines part or all of tubular duplications; therefore, as with Meckel's diverticulum, complications due to peptic ulceration develop. Hemorrhage is most common, but perforation is also a hazard.[61, 63] Pancreatic tissue is found in the walls of some duplications.

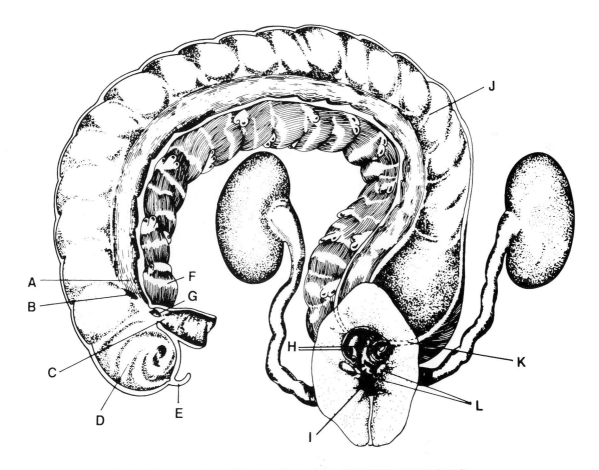

Drawing of the gross specimen of triple colon, kidneys, ureters, ectopic bladder and external genitalia:
A, first patent colon; B, aperture of first patent colon; C, ileocecal valve; D, cecum; E, appendix;
F, second patent colon; G, aperture of second patent colon; H, ureteral orifices; I, anus; J, blind colon laid open;
K, termination of blind colon; L, rudimentary labia.

Figure 40–18. Triplication of the colon with exstrophy of the bladder and genitourinary malformation. (Redrawn from Gray AW: Triplication of the large intestine. Arch Pathol 30:1215, 1940. Copyright © 1940, American Medical Association.)

□ Duplications of Colon and Rectum

Cystic duplication in the mesentery of the colon is rare (Fig. 40–16), although it is not unusual for such lesions in the small bowel mesentery to have linings of colonic mucosa.[11–16, 28, 62, 64–69] Obstruction by compression, volvulus, and intussusception are potential complications. Cystic duplications in the retrorectal and presacral space have caused partial blockage of the rectum. They must be distinguished from sacrococcygeal teratomas and anterior meningoceles. Tubular structures lying adjacent to the rectum and having a perineal opening near the anus may contain gastric mucosa that can cause perineal irritation and bleeding. A diverticulum lined by gastric mucosa entering the ventral side of the rectum has been described.[70]

A different group of defects includes tubular duplications of the hindgut. The distal ileum, cecum, appendix, and entire colon may be double and drain through a single anal orifice or through separate ones. Both lumens may be unobstructed and function normally. Not rarely, double external genitalia accompany this malformation, and the bladder may be septate or completely divided into halves. The double lumen of the colon may be seen to extend only partway from anus to cecum, with the proximal colon and ileum having developed normally. Distally, there may be imperforate anus involving one or both lumens, with the ventrally placed colon commonly ending as a rectovesical, rectourethral, or rectovaginal fistula (Fig. 40–17). When the distal opening is inadequate, that part of the colon may become massively distended or may rupture.

An association has been noted between complete duplication of the colon and extrapulmonary sequestration with esophageal communication.[69] A patient with triplication of the colon had multiple anomalies, including exstrophy of the bladder and absence of the uterus and vagina (Fig. 40–18).[17] She survived 11 months with apparently normal bowel function but died of urinary tract infection and pneumonia.

REFERENCES

1. Gross RE: The Surgery of Infancy and Childhood. Philadelphia, WB Saunders, 1953, pp 221–245.
2. Sieber WK: Alimentary tract duplication. Arch Surg 73:383–392, 1956.
3. Houston HE, Lynn HB: Duplication of the small intestine in children. Mayo Clin Proc 41:246–256, 1966.
4. Basu R, Forshall I, Rickham PP: Duplication of the alimentary tract. Br J Surg 47:477–484, 1960.
5. Mellish RWP, Koop CE: Clinical manifestations of duplication of the bowel. Pediatrics 27:397–407, 1961.
6. Grosfeld JL, O'Neill JA Jr, Clatworthy HW Jr: Enteric duplications in infancy and childhood. An 18-year review. Ann Surg 172:83–90, 1970.
7. Favara BE, Franciosi RA, Akers DR: Enteric duplications. Thirty-seven cases: A vascular theory of pathogenesis. Am J Dis Child 122:501–506, 1971.
8. Holcomb GW III, Gheissari A, O'Neill JA Jr, et al: Surgical management of alimentary tract duplications. Arch Surg 209:167–174, 1989.
9. Ladd WE: Duplications of the alimentary tract. South Med J 30:363–371, 1937.
10. Orr MM, Edwards AJ: Neoplastic change in duplication of the alimentary tract. Br J Surg 62:269–274, 1975.
11. Beach PD, Wright RH Jr, Deffer PA: Duplication of the primitive hindgut of the human being: An 8 year follow-up of a previous case report. Surgery 66:405–411, 1969.
12. Brunschwig A, Pargeon HW, Russell WA: Duplication of the entire colon and lower ileum with termination of one colon into a vaginal anus. Surgery 24:1010–1013, 1948.
13. Ravitch MM: Hindgut duplications, doubling of colon and genital urinary tracts. Ann Surg 137:588–601, 1953.
14. Rowe MI, Ravitch M, Ranninger K: Operative correction of caudal duplication (dipygus). Surgery 63:840–848, 1968.
15. Smith ED: Duplication of the anus and genitourinary tract. Surgery 66:909–921, 1969.
16. Van Zwalenburg BR: Double colon. Am J Roentgenol Radium Ther Nucl Med 68:22–27, 1952.
17. Gray AW: Triplication of the large intestine. Arch Pathol 30:1215–1222, 1940.
18. Beardmore HE, Wigglesworth FW: Vertebral anomalies and alimentary tract duplications. Pediatr Clin North Am 5:457–474, 1958.
19. Bentley JRR, Smith JR: Developmental posterior enteric remnants and spinal malformations: The split notochord syndrome. Arch Dis Child 35:76–86, 1960.
20. Burrows FGO, Sutcliff J: The split notochord syndrome. Br J Radiol 41:496–507, 1968.
21. Fallon M, Gordon ARG, Lendrum AC, et al: Mediastinal cysts of foregut origin associated with vertebral abnormalities. Br J Surg 41:520–533, 1954.
22. Faris JC, Crowe JE: The split notochord syndrome. J Pediatr Surg 10:467–472, 1975.
23. Lewis FT, Thyng FW: The regular occurrence of intestinal diverticula in embryos of the pig, rabbit, and man. Am J Anat 7:505–519, 1907.
24. Bremer JL: Diverticula and duplications of the intestinal tract. Arch Pathol 38:132–140, 1944.
25. La Quaglia MP, Feins N, Graklis A, et al: Rectal duplications. J Pediatr Surg 20:980–984, 1990.
26. Schwesinger WH, Croom RD III, Habibian MR: Diagnosis of an enteric duplication with pertechnetate 99mTc scanning. Ann Surg 181:428–430, 1975.
27. Bidewell JK, Nelson A: Prenatal ultrasonic diagnosis of congenital duplication of the stomach. J Ultrasound Med 10:589–591, 1986.
28. Cooksey G, Wagget J: Tubular duplication of the rectum treated by mucosal resection. J Pediatr Surg 19:318–319, 1984.
29. Wrenn EL Jr: Tubular duplication of the small intestine. Surgery 52:494–498, 1962.
30. Jewett TC Jr: Duplication of the entire small intestine with massive melena. Ann Surg 147:239–244, 1958.
31. Jewett TC Jr: A long term follow-up on a duplication of the entire small intestine. J Pediatr Surg 18:185–188, 1983.
32. Gans SL, Lackey DA, Zuckerbraum L: Duplications of the cervical esophagus in infants and children. Surgery 63:849–852, 1968.
33. Winslow RE, Dykstra G, Scholten DJ, et al: Duplication of the cervical esophagus. An unrecognized cause of respiratory distress in infants. Am Surg 50:506–508, 1984.
34. Gross RE, Neuhauser EBD, Longino LA, et al: Thoracic duplications which originate from the intestine. Ann Surg 131:363–375, 1950.
35. Milsom J, Unger S, Alford BA, et al: Triplication of the esophagus with gastric duplication. Surgery 98:121–125, 1985.
36. Alrabeeah A, Gillis DA, Giacomantonio M, et al: Neurenteric cysts—a spectrum. J Pediatr Surg 23:752–754, 1988.
37. Bremer JL: Dorsal intestinal fistula: Accessory neurenteric canal; diastematomyelia. Arch Pathol 54:132–138, 1952.
38. Dienes J, Honti J, Leb J: Dorsal herniation of the gut: A rare manifestation of the split notochord syndrome. J Pediatr Surg 2:359–363, 1967.

39. Kheradpir MH, Ameri MR: Dorsal herniation of the gut with posterior opening of the terminal colon: A rare manifestation of the split notocord syndrome. Z Kinderchir 38:186–187, 1983.
40. Singh A, Singh R: Split notocord syndrome with dorsal enteric fistula. J Pediatr Surg 17:412–413, 1982.
41. Abrami G, Dennison WM: Duplication of the stomach. Surgery 49:794–801, 1961.
42. Bartels RJ: Duplication of the stomach. Am Surg 33:747–752, 1967.
43. Grosfeld JL, Boles ET Jr, Reiner C: Duplication of pylorus in the newborn: A rare cause of gastric outlet obstruction. J Pediatr Surg 5:365–369, 1970.
44. Knight J, Garvin PJ, Lewis E Jr: Gastric duplication presenting as a double esophagus. J Pediatr Surg 18:300–301, 1988.
45. Kremer RM, Lepoff RB, Izant RJ Jr: Duplication of the stomach. J Pediatr Surg 5:360–364, 1970.
46. Parker BC, Guthrie J, France NE, et al: Gastric duplications in infancy. J Pediatr Surg 7:294–298, 1972.
47. Ramsay GS: Enterogenous cyst of the stomach simulating hypertrophic pyloric stenosis. Br J Surg 44:632–633, 1957.
48. Lee SM, Mosenthal WT, Weismann RE: Tumorous heterotopic gastric mucosa in small intestine. Arch Surg 10:619–622, 1970.
49. Sieunarine K, Manmohansingh E: Gastric duplication cyst presenting as an acute abdomen in a child. J Pediatr Surg 24:1152, 1989.
50. Dickinson WE, Weinberg SM, Vellios F: Perforating ulcer in a duodenal duplication. Am J Surg 122:418–420, 1971.
51. Gardner CE Jr, Hart D: Enterogenous cysts of the duodenum. JAMA 104:1809–1812, 1935.
52. Leenders EL, Osman MZ, Sukarochana K: Treatment of duodenal duplication with international review. Am Surg 36:368–371, 1970.
53. Soper RT, Selke AC: Duplication cysts of the duodenum. Surgery 68:562–566, 1970.
54. Lavine JE, Harrison M, Heyman MB: Gastrointestinal duplications causing relapsing pancreatitis in children. Gastroenterology 97:1556–1558, 1989.
55. Williams WH, Hendren WH: Intrapancreatic duplication causing pancreatitis in a child. Surgery 69:708–715, 1971.
56. Wrenn EL Jr, Favara BE: Duodenal duplication (or pancreatic bladder) presenting as double gallbladder. Surgery 69:858–862, 1971.
57. Cynn WS, Rickert RR: Heterotopic mucosal polyp in the duodenal bulb associated with congenital absence of the gallbladder. Am J Gastroenterol 60:171–177, 1973.
58. Curtis LE, Sheahan DG: Heterotopic tissues in the gallbladder. Arch Pathol 88:677–683, 1969.
59. Keramidas DC, Skondras C, Anagnostou D, et al: Gastric heterotopia in the gallbladder. J Pediatr Surg 12:759–762, 1977.
60. Martinez-Urrutia MJ, Vasques Estevez J, Larrauri J, et al: Gastric heterotopy of the biliary tract. J Pediatr Surg 25:356–357, 1990.
61. Rios-Dalenz JL, Kress JW, Montgomery LG: Duplication of small intestine with perforated peptic ulcer in ectopic gastric mucosa. Arch Surg 91:863–866, 1965.
62. Jewell CT, Miller ID, Ehrlich FE: Rectal duplication: An unusual cause for an abdominal mass. Surgery 74:783–785, 1973.
63. Duffy G, Enriquez AA, Watson WC: Duplication of the ileum with heterotopic gastric mucosa, pseudomyxoma peritonei, and nonrotation of the midgut. Gastroenterology 67:341–346, 1974.
64. MacLeod JH, Purves JKB: Duplication of the rectum. Dis Colon Rectum 13:133–137, 1970.
65. McPherson AG, Trapnell JE, Airth GR: Duplication of the colon. Br J Surg 56:138–142, 1969.
66. Reid IS: Perforation in duplication of colon. Br J Surg 56:155–156, 1969.
67. Soper RT: Tubular duplication of colon and distal ileum. Surgery 63:998–1004, 1968.
68. Waldbaum RS, Glendenning AF: Tubular duplication of rectum with a rectourethral fistula. J Urol 113:876–879, 1975.
69. Flye MW, Izant RJ: Extrapulmonary sequestration with esophageal communication and complete duplication of the colon. Surgery 71:744–752, 1972.
70. Stockman JM, Young JT, Jenkins AL, et al: Duplication of the rectum containing gastric mucosa. JAMA 173:1223–1225, 1960.

41

MECKEL'S DIVERTICULUM

Charles L. Snyder, MD

Johann Meckel described the anomaly with which he is forever eponymously associated in 1809.[1] He identified its origin from the omphalomesenteric duct and suggested it as a cause of disease. His was not the first report; Fabricus Hildanus had that distinction in 1598.[2] Heterotopic mucosa was first identified within a diverticulum in 1904.[3] Charles Mayo, in 1933, described Meckel's diverticulum as "frequently suspected, often looked for, and seldom found."[4]

□ Embryology

Although the precise cause of Meckel's diverticulum remains unknown, the embryology is well described. During the 5th to 7th week of fetal life, the vitelline (omphalomesenteric) duct regresses while the functioning placenta replaces the yolk sac as the primary source of nourishment for the developing fetus. This duct connects the yolk sac and the primitive gut. Failure of regression may result in several anomalies (Fig. 41–1), the most common being Meckel's diverticulum.

□ Demographics

Meckel's diverticulum is found in approximately 1 to 2% of the population, in pooled series of tens of thousands of patients.[5–8] There is little gender predominance in incidentally discovered diverticula, but males outnumber females 3 to 4:1 in symptomatic diverticula.[9]

Meckel's diverticulum is found with increased frequency in several conditions. In one review of almost 6000 autopsies, 12% of children with esophageal atresia and 11% of children with imperforate anus had a Meckel's diverticulum.[10] In one review of children with minor omphalocele, approximately 25% were found to have Meckel's diverticula.[11]

□ Pathology

Anatomically, Meckel's diverticula are outpouchings on the antimesenteric border of the small bowel. The location is variable, and although most are within 90 cm (about 3 feet) of the ileocecal valve, as many as one third are proximal. It is recommended that at least 5 feet of small bowel be examined in older children to ensure that there is no Meckel's diverticulum.[12, 13]

These are true diverticula, composed of normal intestinal wall. Embryologically, the right and left vitelline arteries originate from the aorta: the left involutes, and the right persists as the superior mesenteric artery and supplies the diverticulum. Distal vitelline artery remnants may persist as mesodiverticular bands, extending out to the tip of the diverticulum.

Heterotopic mucosa (normal tissue in an abnormal location) is often found in Meckel's diverticula and may lead to complications. The most common types of heterotopic mucosa are gastric and pancreatic. The incidence of heterotopic mucosa depends on the reason for diverticulectomy; if incidental diverticulectomy is performed, heterotopic mucosa is identified in fewer than one fifth of specimens. However, heterotopic mucosa (commonly gastric) is usually identified in symptomatic diverticula.[14, 15]

□ Clinical Manifestations

The clinical presentation is diverse and age dependent. The "Rule of 2" is often cited: 2% of the population, fewer than 2 feet from the ileocecal valve, 2 types of heterotopic mucosa (gastric and pancreatic), younger than 2 years of age, and 2 inches long.

The primary clinical presentations are obstruction, bleeding, and inflammation. Bleeding and obstruction are the problems most frequently encountered and usually present at a slightly younger age than do the inflammatory complications. More than

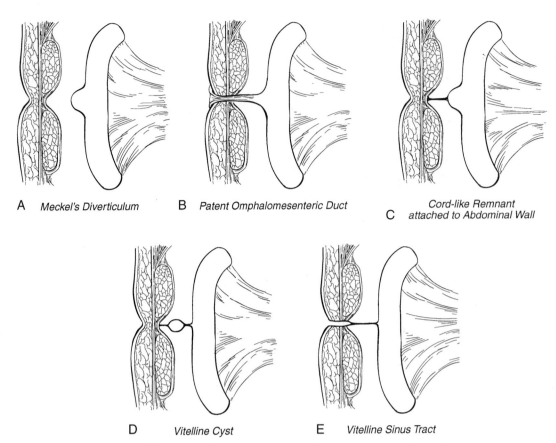

A *Meckel's Diverticulum*

B *Patent Omphalomesenteric Duct*

C *Cord-like Remnant attached to Abdominal Wall*

D *Vitelline Cyst*

E *Vitelline Sinus Tract*

Figure 41–1. *A*, Meckel's diverticulum. *B*, Patent omphalomesenteric duct. *C*, Cordlike, nonpatent fibrous tract; this may become a point of fixation for volvulus or impinge on other loops of bowel to cause an obstruction. *D*, Vitelline cyst. *E*, Blind-ending sinus tract without communication to the bowel.

three fourths of symptomatic Meckel's diverticula occur in children younger than 10 years of age. Less commonly, Meckel's diverticula can be the site of foreign body impaction, the origin of neoplasia, or even the site of parasitic infection.

OBSTRUCTION

Obstruction from Meckel's diverticulum usually is due to intussusception or volvulus. The former is more common. Intussusception in older children is more likely to be associated with a lead point such as a Meckel's diverticulum. Symptoms of obstruction—vomiting, abdominal distention, crampy pain—are usually present. The Meckel's diverticulum may be recognized on preoperative studies or at operation, or it may be found unexpectedly in the resected specimen. The diagnosis of Meckel's diverticulum should be considered in any previously healthy child without a history of prior operation who develops a bowel obstruction.

Volvulus may be due to vitelline remnants attaching to the abdominal wall and forming a focus around which the bowel twists. Alternatively, intestine may herniate under mesodiverticular bands, kinking or obstructing the bowel (Fig. 41–2).

Bowel obstruction requires rehydration, broad-spectrum antibiotics, intestinal decompression, and laparotomy. Segmental resection and reanastomosis are usually possible.

BLEEDING

Bleeding from a Meckel's diverticulum is most common in children younger than 5 years of age. Painless melena is the usual manifestation, but bleeding occasionally may be massive. Episodic bleeding is common. Meckel's diverticula can also present as an occult cause of anemia. The differential diagnosis of lower gastrointestinal bleeding in a child includes inflammatory bowel disease, intestinal polyps, duplications, and arteriovenous malformations. Peptic ulcer disease and variceal bleeding may also present in a similar fashion, but they can be distinguished via bloody nasogastric aspirates or with upper endoscopy.

The prominent role of *Helicobacter pylori* in peptic ulcer disease led to a search for this gram-negative bacterium in the heterotopic gastric mucosa of Meckel's diverticula. Several studies have failed to identify significant numbers of the organism in resected specimens.[16–18]

Suspected diverticular bleeding is an indication for radionuclide scanning. The "Meckel's scan" was

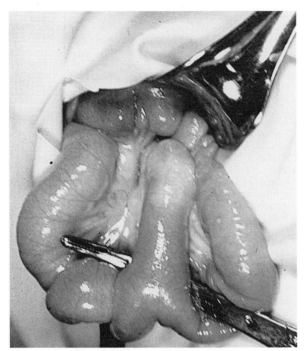

Figure 41–2. Meckel's diverticulum adherent to the small bowel mesentery at its tip, allowing adjacent loops of small bowel to herniate under the diverticulum and become obstructed.

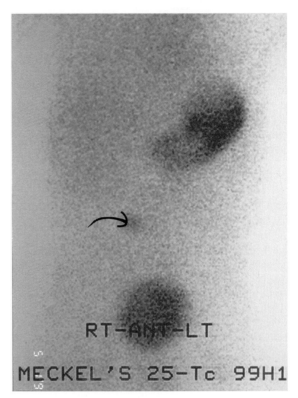

Figure 41–3. Meckel's scan of a 3-year-old boy with painless melanotic stools. The *arrow* indicates the uptake by the heterotopic mucosa in the diverticulum.

first described in 1970 by Jewett and colleagues.[19] Pertechnetate ions carrying technetium 99m are secreted into the lumen by gastric mucosal cells. The scan, therefore, requires the presence of heterotopic gastric mucosa to be positive, a condition that is usually satisfied by bleeding diverticula (Fig. 41–3). Many methods have been suggested to improve the accuracy of the scans: histamine blockers to inhibit secretion of pertechnetate, pentagastrin to stimulate uptake, glucagon to help restrict activity to the stomach, and other mechanical aids. Overall, the Meckel's scan has an accuracy of approximately 90%, a sensitivity of 85%, and a specificity of 95%.[20, 21]

The mechanism of bleeding is usually peptic ulceration due to acid production by the heterotopic gastric mucosa. The ulceration is often at the junction of the ileal and gastric mucosa, but it may be located in the normal mesenteric ileal wall opposite the diverticulum. It is important to examine this site for bleeding during diverticulectomy because merely resecting the diverticulum and leaving the ulceration may result in persistence of the bleeding (Fig. 41–4). Segmental resection is preferred in this situation. Laparoscopy has been used for both diagnosis and treatment of Meckel's diverticulum.[22]

INFLAMMATION

Meckel's diverticulitis is rarely diagnosed preoperatively. This condition is clinically similar to appendicitis. When appendicitis is suspected but not found, it is important to carefully examine the small bowel for the presence of a Meckel's diverticulum. Perforation of the diverticulum is usually the result

of peptic ulceration from heterotopic gastric mucosa. Resection of the diverticulum with or without a segment of involved intestine is usually curative.

OTHER

Carcinoid tumors have been reported in Meckel's diverticula.[23] These are generally noted in adults

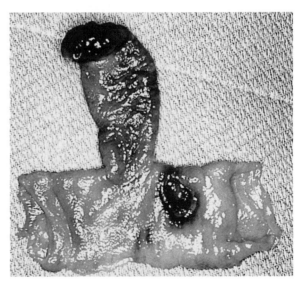

Figure 41–4. Opened segment of bowel containing a Meckel's diverticulum. Note the heterotopic mucosa at the tip as well as the ulcerated bleeding site at the base of the diverticulum.

(the mean age in 104 cases was 57 years), are relatively aggressive tumors, and biologically resemble ileal carcinoids. Leiomyomas and leiomyosarcomas have been found in Meckel's diverticula, but less commonly than carcinoids.[24]

Impacted foreign bodies are occasionally responsible for inflammation and perforation in Meckel's diverticula. The diverticulum may also be the site of parasitic infection.

□ Incidental Diverticulectomy

Incidental Meckel's diverticulectomy is controversial. Morbidity and mortality from the procedure must be weighed against the chance of a Meckel's diverticula becoming symptomatic, multiplied by the morbidity and mortality risk of acute diverticulectomy. These risks are all dependent on several variables, including age and gender of the patient and physical characteristics of the diverticulum. It is estimated that the lifetime risk of a Meckel's diverticulum becoming symptomatic is about 4 to 6%.[25, 26]

The question is perhaps more philosophic than scientific. The risk of complications (due to the diverticulectomy) with incidental diverticulectomy is probably less than 2 in 100, and the risk of complications after resection of a symptomatic diverticulum is nearly 1 in 10. Assuming resection of every diverticulum in the population at risk and comparing morbidity, incidental diverticulectomy carries the following risk:

2/100 (Population Incidence) × 2/100
 (Operative Complication Incidence) = 4/10,000

The morbidity risk of treating only symptomatic patients is as follows:

2/100 (Population Incidence) × 5/100
(Chance of Developing Symptoms) × 1/10 (Risk of
 Operative Complications) = 1/10,000

Because it is clear that not all asymptomatic diverticula will be removed, the morbidity risk of either approach is probably similar.

REFERENCES

1. Meckel J: Uber die Divertikel am Darmkanal. Archiv Physiol 9:421–453, 1809.
2. Lichtenstein ME: Meckel's diverticulum. Q Bull Northwest Univ Med 15:296–300, 1941.
3. Salzer H: Uber das Offerene Meckelesche Divertikel. Wein Klein Wochenschr 17:614–617, 1904.
4. Mayo CW: Meckel's diverticulum. Proc Mayo Clin 8:230, 1933.
5. Matsagas MI, Fatouros M, Koulouras B, et al: Incidence, complications, and management of Meckel's diverticulum. Arch Surg 130:143–146, 1995.
6. Harkins HN: Intussusception due to invaginated Meckel's diverticulum. Ann Surg 98:1070–1095, 1933.
7. Haber J: Meckel's diverticulum. Am J Surg 73:468–485, 1947.
8. Soderlund S: Meckel's diverticulum, a clinical and histologic study. Acta Chir Scand Suppl 248:213–233, 1959.
9. Androulakis JA, Gray SW, Lionakis B, et al: The sex ratio of Meckel's diverticulum. Am Surg 35:455–460, 1969.
10. Simms MH, Corkery JJ: Meckel's diverticulum: Its association with congenital malformation and the significance of atypical morphology. Br J Surg 67:216–219, 1980.
11. Nicol JW, MacKinlay GA: Meckel's diverticulum in exomphalos minor. J R Coll Surg Edinb 39:6–7, 1994.
12. Skandalakis JE, Gray SW, Ricketts R, et al: The small intestines. In Skandalakis JE, Gray SW (eds): Embryology for Surgeons (2nd ed). Baltimore, Williams & Wilkins, 1994, pp 184–241.
13. Jay GD III, Margulis RR, McGraw AB, et al: Meckel's diverticulum: A survey of one hundred and three cases. Arch Surg 61:158–169, 1950.
14. Amoury RA, Snyder CL: Meckel's diverticulum. In O'Neill J, Rowe M, Grosfeld J, et al (eds): Pediatric Surgery (5th ed). St Louis, CV Mosby, 1998, pp 1173–1185.
15. Vane DW, West KW, Grosfeld JL: Vitelline duct anomalies. Arch Surg 122:542–547, 1987.
16. Bemelman WA, Bosma A, Wiersma PH, et al: Role of *Helicobacter pylori* in the pathogenesis of complications of Meckel's diverticula. Eur J Surg 159:171–175, 1993.
17. Kumar S, Small P, Nawroz I, et al: *Helicobacter pylori* and Meckel's diverticulum. J R Coll Surg Edinb 36:225–226, 1991.
18. Fich A, Talley NJ, Shorter RG, et al: Does *Helicobacter pylori* colonize the gastric mucosa of Meckel's diverticulum? Mayo Clin Proc 65:187–191, 1990.
19. Jewett TC Jr, Duszynski DO, Allen JE: The visualization of Meckel's diverticulum with Tc^{99m}-pertechnetate. Surgery 68:567–570, 1970.
20. Sfakianakis GN, Conway JJ: Detection of ectopic gastric mucosa in Meckel's diverticulum and in other aberrations by scintigraphy, II: Indications and methods—a 10-year experience. J Nucl Med 22:732–738, 1981.
21. Sfakianakis GN, Conway JJ: Detection of ectopic gastric mucosa in Meckel's diverticulum and in other aberrations by scintigraphy, I: Pathophysiology and 10-year clinical experience. J Nucl Med 22:647–654, 1981.
22. Huang CS, Lin LH: Laparoscopic Meckel's diverticulectomy in infants: Report of three cases. J Pediatr Surg 28:1486–1489, 1993.
23. Nies C, Zielke A, Hasse C, et al: Carcinoid tumors of Meckel's diverticula. Dis Colon Rectum 35:589–596, 1992.
24. Skandalakis JE, Gray SW: Smooth muscle tumors of the alimentary tract. In Ariel IM (ed): Progress in Clinical Cancer. Vol. 1. New York, Grune & Stratton, 1965.
25. Soltero M, Bill AH: The natural history of Meckel's diverticulum found in King County, Washington, over a fifteen-year period. Am J Surg 132:168–173, 1976.
26. Cullen JJ, Kelly KA, Moir CR, et al: Surgical management of Meckel's diverticulum: An epidemiologic, population-based study [see comments]. Ann Surg 220:564–568, 1994.

42

INFLAMMATORY BOWEL DISEASE AND GASTROINTESTINAL NEOPLASMS

Eric W. Fonkalsrud, MD

Inflammatory bowel disease in children, as well as in adults, consists of ulcerative colitis (UC) and Crohn's disease. The etiology of both disorders is unknown. In most cases, differentiation between the two diseases can be made clinically, radiologically, and pathologically, although in approximately 15% of patients, it cannot be determined which disease is present, and the term "indeterminate colitis" has been applied.

Although UC is limited to the colon and rectum, Crohn's disease may involve the entire gastrointestinal (GI) tract. Although both conditions can be treated medically for relief of symptoms, only UC can be cured surgically by proctocolectomy. Crohn's disease cannot be cured, although, often, medical therapy or operation can relieve symptoms for long periods. Determination of the appropriate time for operation and the most suitable surgical procedure is often controversial.

☐ Ulcerative Colitis

UC is believed to have been first described more than 130 years ago.[1] Although the condition most often affects people after the second decade of life, at least 20% of all patients manifest initial symptoms before the age of 18 years. Men and women are afflicted with equal frequency, although the condition is more than four times as prevalent in Caucasians than African Americans, Hispanics, or Asians. UC is at least four times more common in Jews than in non-Jews.[2] The disease appears to be increasing in frequency both in the United States and Europe.

ETIOLOGY

The etiology of UC remains unknown, although several mechanisms have been suggested. Various investigators have incriminated transmissible bacteria or viruses; however, the results of studies implicating specific organisms have been inconsistent. Other investigators believe that bacteria or viruses are secondary invaders rather than primary agents.[3]

Approximately 15% of patients with UC have one or more members in the family constellation with inflammatory bowel disease. Furthermore, human leukocyte antigen (HLA)-W27 studies of patients with idiopathic ankylosing spondylitis, uveitis, and UC suggest a genetic predisposition; however, no definite predictable relationship has been determined. An immunologic response to an autologous, a bacterial, or a chemical antigen is the most attractive current etiologic theory, which is supported, in part, by clinical and laboratory characteristics of UC. Although some workers have suggested that psychological factors may be etiologic, it is not believed that there is "a premorbid personality." Psychological factors and stress may provoke relapses and contribute to the chronicity of the disease but do not necessarily initiate the disease.

PATHOLOGY

UC is primarily a disease of the rectal and colonic mucosa. The rectum is involved in more than 95% of cases and the inflammation extends proximally in a contiguous manner.[4] When the entire colon is involved (pancolitis), the most severe changes are present in the rectum and sigmoid. The characteristic microscopic feature consists of crypt abscesses, which lead to mucosal ulceration with undermining of the adjacent mucosa. Mucosal bridging and pseudopolyp formation often result. As the disease progresses, in the acute phase, the colon distends, peristalsis decreases, and the muscularis becomes thin and diffusely hemorrhagic, sometimes progressing to toxic megacolon. Conversely, with chronic UC, the colon becomes stiff, thickened, and foreshortened with atrophic mucosa and haustral fold loss, resulting in the "lead pipe" appearance on contrast enema. In remission, the mucosa may have a nearly normal microscopic appearance. Mucosal biopsy is helpful in confirming the diagnosis and assessing the activity of the disease.

CLINICAL COURSE

Approximately 4% of patients with UC experience the onset of symptoms before 10 years of age. In 17%, symptoms begin between 10 and 20 years of age.[4] The incidence of the disease reaches a peak in the middle of the third decade.

In most children, the symptoms begin insidiously with persistent diarrhea followed by the appearance of blood, mucus, and pus in the stools. Cramping lower abdominal pain and tenesmus are common. Anorexia, weight loss, and growth retardation resulting from chronic inflammation, poor appetite, and long-term corticosteroid use often develop when the disease becomes chronic. As a result, many children have feelings of inferiority and lack a desire to participate in social and physical activities. In most patients, remitting colitis with periodic relapses develops and is precipitated by emotional stress or intercurrent infection. After a few years, a permanent remission may develop in the occasional patient, but most experience chronic colitis with shorter and less frequent remissions. A single attack with complete remission occurs in less than 10% of children with UC.

In 15% of children with UC, the onset is acute and fulminating with profuse bloody diarrhea, severe abdominal cramps, fever, and occasionally sepsis, requiring prompt treatment. Most of these patients improve with medical therapy, although toxic megacolon requiring urgent operation does occasionally develop (5% of patients).[5] Children with severe UC are usually sicker, are more likely to have complete colonic involvement (pancolitis), and are less likely than adults to be cured without operation. In my experience, at least half of all children with UC eventually require colectomy.

Cancer of the colon has been reported in up to 3% of patients during the first 10 years of disease and in 20% of patients in each subsequent decade.[6] Cancer may develop even in patients with quiescent UC.

EXTRAINTESTINAL MANIFESTATIONS

Extracolonic manifestations of UC include growth retardation, failure of sexual maturation, arthralgias, skin lesions, liver disease, anemia, osteoporosis, nephrolithiasis, uveitis, and oral ulcerations. Growth retardation with delay in bone age frequently accompanies chronic colitis in adolescence. Delayed sexual maturation may be in part due to abnormally low urinary gonadotropin levels.[7]

Growth hormone levels are usually in the normal range for age.

Arthralgias occur in approximately 25% of patients with UC and most commonly involve the knees, ankles, and wrists. The joint symptoms occasionally precede the onset of intestinal symptoms and may be confused with those of juvenile rheumatoid arthritis.

The most common skin lesions include erythema nodosum and pyoderma gangrenosum, which are more common in adults. Results of liver function tests are abnormal in approximately 8% of children and may be caused by sclerosing cholangitis or fatty infiltration, approximately half the incidence seen in adults. Anemia is common and is usually the result of overt or occult blood loss in the stool. Osteoporosis and osteomalacia may occur owing to decreased calcium absorption associated with diminished uptake of fat-soluble vitamins and with increased urinary losses from steroid therapy. Nephrolithiasis occurs in approximately 5% of patients and may be largely due to inadequate fluid intake to compensate for the diarrheal losses. Uveitis is an inflammation of the iris found in less than 2% of patients. Aphthous stomatitis is common in patients with UC.

CLINICAL EXAMINATION

The child who has mild UC or is in a period of remission may have few, if any, positive findings on examination, although sigmoidoscopy may reveal friable and edematous mucosa with a thin purulent exudate. Children with chronic UC often show evidence of delayed growth in height, lack of sexual maturation, pallor, anemia, and cushingoid features from long-term steroid therapy. In 15% of pediatric cases of UC, the presentation is as an acute illness consisting of fever, dehydration, and sepsis. Pain from palpation over the sigmoid colon is common. External hemorrhoids are frequently present, but anal sinuses, fissures, and abscesses are rare. On endoscopy, the mucosa often is edematous and hemorrhagic with ulcers and has a thick purulent and often bloody exudate.

Anemia resulting from blood loss is present in two thirds of patients. The sedimentation rate is often elevated, and the prothrombin time is prolonged. The serum albumin level is usually low. Hyponatremia and hypokalemia may occur with protracted diarrhea. Stool culture findings are consistently negative for pathogenic bacteria and parasites.

Although barium enema has been used for many years to establish the extent and severity of UC, more meaningful information may be obtained from colonoscopy and flexible sigmoidoscopy. A radiographic contrast enema may show a shortened, narrow, rigid colon with loss of haustrations and pseudopolyp formation; however, the study may stimulate the acute manifestations of colitis. In acute colitis, the bowel contour may demonstrate an irregular serrated border from mucosal ulcerations. The edematous mucosae between areas of ulcerations appear as pseudopolyps. Swollen and inflamed mucosa can form symmetric defects along the borders, known as "thumbprinting."

NONOPERATIVE TREATMENT

Medical therapy for UC is nonspecific and is based on measures to provide symptomatic relief, which may be achieved in more than 90% of patients. It is doubtful, however, that the ultimate course of the disease can be altered or a cure achieved by nonoperative treatment in most patients.

Many children with mild UC localized to the rectum and sigmoid may improve for long periods with sulfasalazine (Azulfidine) therapy alone. For patients with chronic colitis in whom acute flare-ups develop, a short course of corticosteroids (prednisone) for 2 to 3 months may induce prompt disappearance of symptoms. Steroid doses are rapidly tapered, and as soon as possible alternate-day therapy is initiated. Prolonged use of prednisone is frequently associated with untoward side effects, including growth failure, osteoporosis, and cushingoid features. Steroid therapy for periods as short as 6 weeks may cause extensive permanent cutaneous striae over the trunk and proximal extremities in many adolescents, particularly girls. Rectal steroids or mesalamine (Rowasa) enemas may be combined with oral steroids for greater effectiveness.

Steroid therapy should be accompanied by administration of H2-blocking drugs (e.g., cimetidine and ranitidine or omeprazole) and, occasionally, oral antacids to reduce the incidence of peptic ulcer or gastritis. Antidiarrheal medications, such as diphenoxylate hydrochloride with atropine (Lomotil) or loperamide (Imodium), may reduce the number of bowel movements and decrease rectal spasm. They should be used with care because these drugs and opiates may occasionally induce toxic megacolon.[8] Other medications that may be of some benefit include antibiotics (metronidazole) and tranquilizers. Dietary modification is encouraged to minimize intestinal stimulants such as chocolate, vinegar, spicy foods, fresh vegetables, and nuts. Anemia and hypoalbuminemia are treated with blood transfusion or albumin infusion.

Immunosuppressive therapy (azathioprine, 6-mercaptopurine, cyclosporine) has been advocated for patients with chronic UC, but its efficacy is not universally acknowledged and the side effects may be significant. Intravenous (IV) cyclosporine therapy is rapidly effective for patients with severe corticosteroid-resistant UC, although the need for colectomy in 38 to 70% of patients within 6 months after discontinuation of cyclosporine therapy suggests that the drug merely delays colectomy.[9] Psychotherapy may help the patient with chronic UC adjust to the disease, its complications, and its therapy. More important than psychotherapy is the availability of a sympathetic and interested physician on whom the patient can rely.

During acute flare-up attacks of UC, most patients require hospitalization with IV fluid administration, bowel rest, increased steroid doses, and parenteral nutrition. This therapy provides correction of the metabolic deficit but frequently does not alter the course of the colitis. The greatest value of IV nutrition is that it reduces the surgical risk by improving nitrogen balance. Progression of the disease or failure of the patient to respond to therapy is an indication for urgent operation. When the acute attack subsides, the patient begins a bland, high-calorie diet.

OPERATIVE THERAPY

UC can be cured by removing the diseased colon and rectum. When this procedure implied a permanent ileostomy, operation was often delayed until the patient was severely ill, the risk had become high, and the complication rate excessive. Since the development of the mucosal proctectomy and ileoanal pouch procedure (IAPP), with its low risk of severe complications and good long-term functional results, serious consideration should be given to operation for any patient with chronic UC before severe disability and major complications develop.

The indications for operation in children with UC can be divided into elective and emergent categories. Indications for elective colectomy for patients with chronic disease include continued symptoms despite medical therapy, growth retardation, severe limitation of activities, and unacceptable quality of life. Emergent indications (25%) include fulminant disease refractory to medical therapy, extensive rectal bleeding, and toxic megacolon. Careful patient medical support and monitoring, including steroid therapy, have resulted in fewer children requiring emergency operation. If the indication for operation is growth failure, the diseased colon should be removed while the epiphyses are still open to allow for maximal potential growth and development. Evaluation of the child's condition should be made periodically during the course of therapy by a surgeon as well as a gastroenterologist in order to consider alternatives to long-term medical therapy.

There is increasing evidence that extensive medical therapy including steroids for UC may adversely affect healing after reconstructive surgery.[10] Aggressive medical therapy for UC has been reported to increase the need for urgent staged colectomy, with a resulting increase in morbidity, hospital stay, and cost, and a less optimal functional result.[11] Medical management should be abbreviated when disease control cannot be promptly achieved.[12]

In preparation for operation, the surgical options are discussed in detail with the patient and parents. It is helpful for the patient to speak to a person of the same sex and similar age who has undergone the operation in order to help alleviate fear as well as concern about an ileostomy and to add support to the decision for surgery. Preoperative discussion with an enterostomal therapist is helpful in preparing the child and parents for the ileostomy. A short course of parenteral hyperalimentation is used if the patient is severely malnourished. Anemia, hypoalbuminemia, and electrolyte abnormalities are corrected preoperatively. Corticosteroid therapy is maintained at an effective level to avoid an acute flare-up before operation. Oral intake is restricted to clear liquids for 48 hours before surgery. Cleansing enemas are avoided because they may stimulate an acute flare-up of the colitis. Oral antibiotics (neomycin and erythromycin) are given for 12 hours before operation and IV antibiotics (gentamicin and clindamycin) are initiated immediately before operation.

Total proctocolectomy is curative for UC, is a one-stage operation, and has been used with low morbidity and mortality rates for more than 45 years (Fig. 42–1). A major concern of children with severe UC who have been recommended for colectomy is that they will be required to wear an ileostomy appliance for life. Although the care of an ileostomy is usually easily mastered by a child, the presence of the stoma appliance often serves as a source of embarrassment during physical and social activities, and considerable time commitment is necessary to care for the ileostomy properly. Approximately 30% of patients with ileostomies experience stomal or appliance-related problems. It is estimated that the cost of ileostomy maintenance is approximately $1000 per year. Although postoperative impotence and bladder dysfunction after proctocolectomy in childhood are uncommon, these major concerns have caused many children, parents, and physicians to defer the operation until the patient is severely

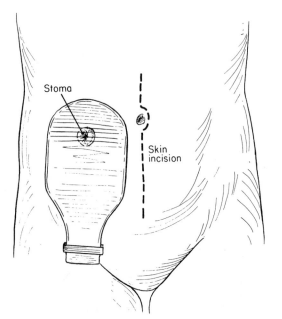

Figure 42–1. Appearance of the abdomen following one-stage proctocolectomy with permanent ileostomy.

debilitated by the colitis or steroid therapy, and this delay may manifest irreversible systemic complications.

Subtotal colectomy and preservation of the rectum with ileorectal anastomosis was performed by a few surgeons during the past, but active disease continued in the rectum in most of these patients, necessitating medical therapy and eventual surgical removal. Ileorectal anastomosis is rarely used for UC in adults or children.

Initial enthusiasm was expressed for the Kock continent ileal reservoir with nipple valve, constructed in conjunction with a flush ileostomy to obviate the need for wearing an ileostomy drainage bag.[13] Drainage is provided by inserting a siliconized catheter into the reservoir several times daily. Complications related to stasis and distention from incomplete emptying with development of chronic reservoir inflammation, as well as incompetence of the nipple valve, led to multiple reoperations and eventual removal in many patients. The procedure is currently used primarily for patients who already have a permanent ileostomy and who are severely handicapped by it.

Because UC is primarily a disease of the mucosa, a modification of the rectal mucosal stripping procedure described by Soave in 1964[14] for treatment of Hirschsprung's disease (HD) has been used with increasing frequency for the definitive treatment of UC during the past 20 years in children and adults.[15–17] Removal of the entire rectal mucosa down to the dentate line was shown not to interfere appreciably with anorectal sphincter function and the ability to discriminate between gas and liquid or solid contents. Little enthusiasm existed for clinical use of the endorectal ileal pull-through procedure until a successful outcome was reported in 15 of 17 children with a straight ileal pull-through (SP) operation in 1977.[18] Although many modifications in technique have been made during the ensuing years, the endorectal ileal pull-through has become generally accepted as the most desirable option for the surgical treatment of UC and familial polyposis. Appealing features of this operation include the absence of a permanent stoma, the lack of repeated catheterization as needed with the Kock pouch, and the development of a near-normal pattern of defecation.

Although the initial operations used a straight endorectal ileal pull-through, most patients experienced persistent stool frequency and urgency and some incontinence. The SP retains peristaltic contractions, generating spike waves down to the anal anastomosis. Most surgeons performing the pull-through procedure have, therefore, constructed an ileal reservoir above the ileoanal anastomosis to reduce peristalsis in the distal ileum and to provide an area for fecal storage. Regardless of the type of reservoir technique performed, as long as the lower 4 cm of the rectal muscle is not damaged, the anal sphincter resting pressure and the anal sphincter squeeze pressure approach normal values within 6 weeks.[19] Excessive dilation of the rectal muscle complex during mucosal proctectomy should be avoided.

Four basic pouch types have been used clinically: the S, J, lateral, and W pouches (Fig. 42–2). The S and W pouches with three or more loops must be hand sutured and require a longer operating time than the other pouches. The blood supply to the lower ileum may be partially obstructed by acute bends in the mesentery, particularly in obese patients. Pouch stasis is common in these large pouches, and an irrigating catheter is often necessary for adequate emptying. After several months, the reservoir may enlarge and the spout of the S and lateral reservoirs may elongate.

The J pouch (JP), the most common pouch currently used, is usually constructed with a stapling instrument. A major advantage is the placement of the lower end of the reservoir close to the anus without a spout. The drawback is that it is sometimes difficult to bring the side of the ileum down to the anus without tension, particularly in heavy or tall patients. Anastomosis of the side of the ileum to the anus has produced a slightly higher incidence of ileoanal strictures than an end ileal anastomosis. The double-stapled ileoanal anastomosis has been favored by several surgeons since the early 1990s owing to its technical ease and reduced rectal dissection. However, retention of the distal 2 to 3 cm of diseased rectal mucosa with persistent disease necessitates that these patients be followed up with endoscopy at least annually. Several authors have shown that the double-stapled IAPP conveys no functional advantage over the complete rectal mucosectomy and hand-sewn ileoanal anastomosis.[20] Whenever colonic carcinoma or mucosal dysplasia complicate UC, all rectal mucosa should be removed.

The early experience with pull-through operations demonstrated that a diverting ileostomy for at least 3 months minimizes the risk of pelvic infection in patients with UC. Patients who receive chronic steroids and immunosuppressive therapy are often malnourished and are at increased risk for postoperative infection, anastomotic leaks, and other complications.[10]

Since the mid-1980s, restorative proctocolectomy with IAPP has become the preferred operation for treatment of UC refractory to medical therapy. In a comprehensive review of 971 patients undergoing colectomy with IAPP, 90% rated their quality of life as excellent, with minimal deterioration over time.[21] In a review of more than 20 series of IAPP procedures with more than 3000 patients, the operative mortality rate was 0.5%.[22] Mean stool frequency was six per day; 90% of patients were continent during the day, and 60% were continent at night. Six percent required pouch removal and permanent ileostomy. Functional results in terms of stool frequency and rate of fecal continence tend to deteriorate minimally with time in patients with well-functioning pouches.[23]

CLINICAL EXPERIENCE

In 1980, we reported our clinical experience from the University of California, Los Angeles (UCLA)

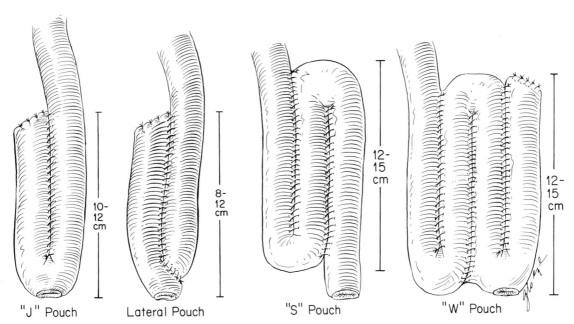

Figure 42–2. The four most frequently used pouch configurations for children undergoing restorative proctocolectomy and ileoanal pouch procedure. The J-shaped reservoir is used most frequently.

Medical Center with restorative proctocolectomy for UC and familial adenomatous polyposis (FAP) using a lateral isoperistaltic reservoir.[16] The operative technique has been modified extensively since that time.[17] The ileum is divided within 1 cm of the ileocecal valve and the mesentery is mobilized up to the origin of the superior mesenteric artery to provide suitable length for the ileum to reach the anus. Because it is rare for active UC in children to extend into the distal ileum, inflammation proximal to the ileocecal valve suggests the presence of Crohn's disease, in which case the IAPP is contraindicated. The colon, together with the omentum, is removed down to the level of the pelvic brim. The specimen is examined by the pathologist to be sure that the child does not have Crohn's disease or malignancy. The peritoneal reflection is incised circumferentially and the rectum is mobilized with electrocautery dissection downward to within 4 cm of the dentate line, at which level the full thickness of rectum is divided (Fig. 42–3A). The anus is gently dilated and a circumferential incision is made through the mucosa at the level of the dentate line. The mucosa is elevated from the underlying muscularis, with care being taken to remove all mucosa (Fig. 42–3B). Thorough hemostasis is essential.

The ileum is doubled back on itself to construct a pouch approximately 8 to 12 cm long. A small opening is made in the mesentery at the apex of the J loop. An incision is made through the antimesenteric side of the apex of the loop and the two blades of the GI anastomosis stapling instrument are inserted, one into each segment. After firing the stapling instrument, a single lumen is created between the two segments of distal ileum. A second firing of the stapling instrument is usually necessary to construct a pouch 8 to 11 cm long. The open proximal end of the J loop is then closed with a running inverting monofilament absorbable suture. The staple and suture line of the pouch is then further supported with continuous inverting seromuscular sutures of absorbable monofilament material. The ileal reservoir is then brought through the pelvis and rectal muscle canal, extending the apex of the J loop to the anus and taking care to avoid twisting the mesentery (Fig. 42–4). The full thickness of ileum is sutured to the anoderm and underlying muscularis circumferentially with interrupted absorbable stitches. The ileum is transected approximately 15 cm proximal to the upper end of the ileal pouch and the proximal end of the divided ileum is fashioned into an end ileostomy stoma. The pelvis is drained transabdominally for approximately 4 days.

IV steroids are tapered rapidly after operation, and oral prednisone can usually be discontinued within 3 weeks. Most children are discharged from the hospital by the 7th postoperative day. A Gastrografin (meglumine diatrizoate) enema radiographic study is performed within 2 months to ensure that the ileal reservoir has healed securely and there are no leaks or sinus tracts (Fig. 42–5). If a sinus tract is noted, it is marsupialized and allowed to com-

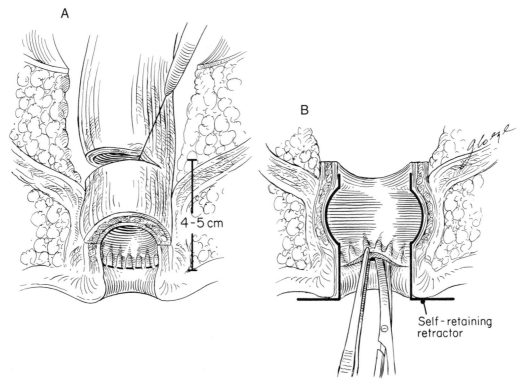

Figure 42–3. *A*, Mobilization of the rectum down to within approximately 4 cm of the dentate line at which level the rectum is completely transected with electrocautery. *B*, Transanal mobilization and resection of rectal mucosa. A circumferential incision is made through the mucosa at the level of the dentate line using needle point electrocautery. All mucosa must be removed.

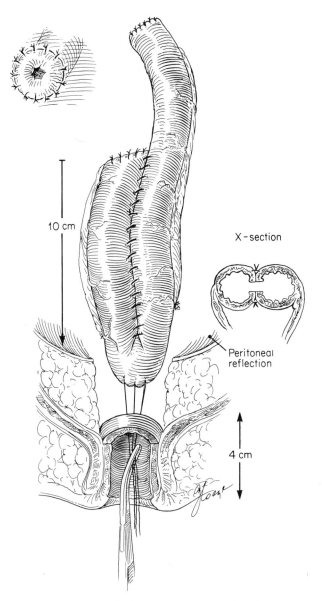

culty in establishing an optimal pattern of bowel evacuation. For any patient with a stricture of the ileoanal anastomosis, daily dilation with a No. 19 Hegar dilator is initiated by the 4th postoperative day and continued at least twice weekly during the ensuing months by the patient or parents until the stricture has resolved.

From 1980 to 1999, 132 children younger than 19 years of age—102 with UC, 20 with FAP, 9 with HD, and 1 with neuronal intestinal dysplasia—have undergone colectomy, mucosal proctectomy, and IAPP at UCLA Medical Center. During the same period, an additional 469 patients 19 years of age and older with UC or FAP underwent IAPP. Of the 132 children, 70 were girls and 62 were boys, ranging in age from 2 to 18 years (mean, 14.1 year); 13 were younger than 10 years of age.

The onset of symptoms of UC in 39 children was acute and fulminating, almost twice that in the adult patients. The duration of symptoms ranged from 3 months to 9 years (mean, 3.2 years). Thirty-seven children had missed more than 3 months of school, and 29 children had received one or more units of blood. Extracolonic manifestations of colitis were almost twice as frequent as in adults; 43 children had arthralgias.

At the time of operation, all children with UC had received prednisone and 28 had received immuno-suppressive therapy including cyclosporine, azathioprine, methotrexate, or 6-mercaptopurine. The growth of 17 children had been retarded, placing them below the 15th percentile for height. Several adolescents showed delay in bone age and sexual maturation. The diagnosis of UC was established by colonoscopy or sigmoidoscopy with mucosal biopsy in all patients. Of the 102 patients with UC, 36 had

Figure 42–4. J-shaped ileal reservoir constructed with a gastrointestinal anastomosis stapling device. Staple lines are oversewn with a second layer of continuous absorbable suture. The apex of the pouch is drawn through the rectal muscle cuff to the anus. A completely diverting end ileostomy is placed approximately 15 cm proximal to the upper end of the pouch.

pletely epithelialize before closing the ileostomy. Most children resume full physical activities within 3 weeks.

Approximately 3 months after the first operation, the child is rehospitalized for ileostomy closure and rectal dilation. When the child begins oral feedings, chocolate, vinegar salad dressings, and spicy foods are minimized in the diet to reduce diarrhea. Low-dose metronidazole (250 mg once or twice daily) is given postoperatively for approximately 6 weeks to reduce the inflammatory response in the villous folds of the ileum to fecal storage in the reservoir. Bulking agents and medications to reduce peristaltic activity are rarely necessary and may cause diffi-

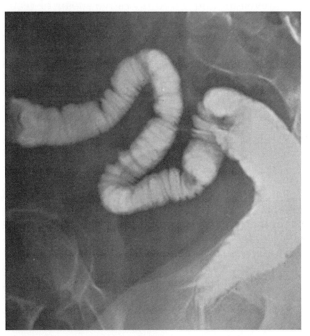

Figure 42–5. Contrast radiograph of ileal reservoir showing normal configuration 3 months after construction.

pancolitis, almost twice the frequency found in the adult patients; 7 had indeterminate colitis; 4 had dysplasia; and none had carcinoma.

A lateral ileal pouch (LP) was constructed in 62 children, 63 had a JP, and 7 had an SP. Our surgical technique has been modified extensively over the years and we have routinely used a JP from 1992 to 1999.[17]

A diverting ileostomy was used for 100 of the 102 children with UC, 9 with FAP, and 3 with HD. Eleven children with FAP, 6 with HD, 2 with UC, and 1 with neuronal intestinal dysplasia had the pull-through procedure performed in one stage. Approximately 4 months after the first operation, each patient with an ileostomy underwent closure together with rectal dilation. Low-dose metronidazole was given for approximately 6 weeks to reduce bacterial growth in the ileal pouch.

There were no perioperative deaths during the 1st year. Complications developed in 52 children (40%) following the pull-through procedure; 47 occurred in children with UC and only 5 occurred in children with FAP or HD. Pouchitis occurred in 21 children with UC, twice the rate of the adult patients. Twenty-nine of the 62 children with an LP, 8 of the 63 with a JP, and 6 of the 7 with an SP required reoperation (33% overall). Thirty-nine of the 102 UC patients had a reoperation. Thirty-four of the first 66 patients had reoperation (52%), whereas only 10 of the last 66 (15%) had reoperation. Eleven required reoperation for adhesions, internal hernia, or intussusception; 15 had abdominoperineal reconstruction with shortening of the pouch.[24] Four patients with an LP underwent transanal shortening of the spout. Six of the 7 patients with an SP underwent reconstruction to a pouch (3 to a JP) because of frequency, urgency, and soiling.[25] Two had ileostomy revision, and 2 had operative repair of rectal strictures. Ten children were given a temporary ileostomy to encourage catch-up growth due to various complications: 7 of the ileostomies have been closed. Seven children required a permanent ileostomy with pouch removal (5.3%, all with UC). Four of these patients were eventually proved to have Crohn's disease.

Fifty-seven of 65 children with an LP, 61 of the 63 with a JP, and 1 with an SP are functioning well (92%) at a mean follow-up of 7.4 years. This percentage is slightly lower than in the adult patients.

The average number of bowel movements per 24 hours at 3 months was 5.6 and at 6 months was 3.9. Fewer than 10% of children had any daytime soiling by 3 months. The rate of nocturnal soiling less than twice per week at 3 months was 18%; however, at 6 months it was only 6%. Detailed review of the last 65 patients shows that all but 3 are functioning well, indicating a decrease in the number of complications as the technique has been modified and clinical experience has increased. Although a large LP was favored in early clinical experience, it became apparent that long pouches and spouts favor stasis

with poor function. The majority of pouches in these patients have been reconstructed.

RESULTS

Pouchitis is the most common complication of pelvic pouch surgery, with complication rates of 30 to 50% being common.[26] Pouchitis is a clinical syndrome of persistent pouch inflammation associated with watery diarrhea, fever, malaise, and occasional arthralgias and other extraintestinal symptoms. Pouchitis is most common within the first 2 years after an IAPP, and episodes are more frequent and severe in children, in my experience. No pathogenic organisms are present in the stool, and the etiology remains elusive. Treatment of pouchitis begins with metronidazole and daily pouch washouts with tap water or Rowasa enemas. For persistent cases, oral mesalamine and hydrocortisone retention enemas may be added. When recalcitrant, a diverting ileostomy may become necessary. In my experience, most episodes resolve within a few weeks after therapy if there is no pouch outlet obstruction or granulomatous disease present.[27] It has become apparent that pouchitis is more common in larger reservoirs that empty only partially with each defecation. Although stenosis at the ileoanal anastomosis or lower end of the reservoir may appear to be a mild annoying problem, it can cause reservoir distention, stasis, and pouchitis if not corrected early.

Almost all complications following the IAPP are surgically correctable when recognized and treated early. Temporary ileostomy may be needed in specific patients, particularly if growth and development during adolescent years is not progressing at an optimal rate. After reservoir reconstruction has been completed and the child has resumed steady progress on the growth curve, the ileostomy may be safely closed in almost all instances. Patients with indeterminate colitis should be apprised that the risk for late pouch failure is approximately three times greater than in children with UC due to emerging Crohn's disease, as occurred in three of the patients described.

Various reservoir configurations are in clinical use with the IAPP, yielding comparable early results relating to stool frequency and continence. Fewer complications have occurred when using a short rectal muscle cuff, a short ileal reservoir, a short ileal spout (preferably no spout), and removal of all rectal mucosa down to the dentate line.[28] Long-term follow-up must be carried out to recognize some of the more insidious complications of the endorectal ileal pull-through procedure. Nonetheless, the IAPP is an excellent alternative to proctocolectomy with permanent ileostomy, ileorectal anastomosis, or the Kock pouch for the treatment of UC in childhood.

I believe that UC is a more acute and severe disease in children than in adults. Operation should be performed before the complications of the disease become severe and the medical treatment becomes complex. IAPP is the preferred operation for UC, FAP, and selected patients with HD in childhood. JP is the preferred technique owing to the simplicity of the construction and the sparsity of complications.[29] Pouch reconstruction for many types of malfunction reduces the need for pouch removal.[30]

□ Crohn's Disease

In 1932, Crohn, Ginzburg, and Oppenheimer described regional ileitis and identified it as having different characteristics from other inflammatory conditions of the small intestine.[31] Although originally believed to occur only in the ileum, it subsequently became apparent that the inflammatory process may affect any part of the alimentary tract from the mouth to the anus.[32] Lesions may be multifocal, with patches of diseased bowel separated by grossly normal segments. The colonic form of the disease was differentiated from UC by Brooke in 1959 and by Lockhart-Mummery and Morson in 1960.[32, 33] The peak onset occurs before the age of 35 years. The incidence of Crohn's disease is approximately equal in men and women, and the disease is five times more prevalent in Caucasians than in African Americans, with a marked increase in the incidence in Jews.[34] Epidemiologic studies from Norway and England indicate a gradual increase in the frequency since the 1960s.

ETIOLOGY

The etiology of Crohn's disease remains unknown, but the same causative factors suggested for UC may also be implicated.[3] Both a genetic factor and transmissible infection must be considered as likely possibilities because both are observed in patients with Crohn's disease. Because lymphangiectasia and prominent mesenteric lymphadenopathy are frequent pathologic features in Crohn's disease, obstructing lymphangitis has also been suggested as a possible etiologic factor.

PATHOLOGY

Crohn's disease is a transmural granulomatous inflammatory disorder in which the intestinal wall is thickened by submucosal edema, fibrosis, and lymphatic dilation.[4, 35] Small slit-like ulcers may appear in the mucosa, producing a cobblestone appearance. Except for the mucosa adjacent to these ulcers, the gland tubules and goblet cells are often normal. Deep fissures often occur parallel to the long axis of the intestine and are particularly notable on the mesenteric side. These ulcerations may penetrate deeply into or through the muscularis and can produce sinus tracts, fistulas, adhesions, and chronic abscesses. The characteristic epithelioid cell granulomas containing multinucleated giant cells are present in approximately 55% of cases. Granulomas are most common in the submucosa but may be found in the muscularis or in the regional lymph nodes. A few other chronic infections (e.g., tuberculosis) and fungi, *Yersinia*, and *Chlamydia* infections, among others, can also cause granulomas in the intestine. In the chronic phase, acute inflammation is replaced by fibrosis and stricture.

Often, the surgeon may estimate the extent of gross involvement of Crohn's disease at the time of operation based on the degree of intestinal thickening, the extent of fat surrounding the intestine, the increase in subserosal vascularity, or the presence of a firm stricture, although the limits of microscopic disease are usually unclear. It is not unusual to observe diseased segments of bowel interspersed between normal segments (skip areas) of involved intestine with intervening normal segments.

NATURAL HISTORY

Although Crohn's disease most often affects young adults, it is being recognized with increasing frequency in children. In a review of more than 600 cases at the Mayo Clinic, 14% of patients had symptoms before the age of 15 years.[36] In another series, 21% of 489 patients with Crohn's disease had onset before the age of 15 years.[34] The condition has been reported with increasing frequency at an earlier age and with more severe symptoms than noted previously. Medical treatment, although rarely curative, often helps to alleviate acute symptoms.[37] Presenting symptoms include weight loss (90%), abdominal pain (75%), diarrhea (67%), fever (25%), and anorexia. Extraintestinal manifestations, including arthritis, may also become apparent early in the course of the disease.

Rectal bleeding occurs less frequently with Crohn's disease than with UC, although bloody diarrhea is common with Crohn's disease of the colon. A delay in diagnosis of more than 1 year after onset of symptoms has been noted in more than two thirds of children.[38] More than one third of patients with Crohn's disease were initially believed to have non-GI disorders.

Whereas patients with UC tend to suffer from alternating remissions and relapses, children with Crohn's disease tend to have a more chronic and continuous course. Ileocolitis is the most common form of the disease requiring operation in children (55%). The colon as the only site of involvement was found in 34% of children; disease confined to the small bowel was present in 10%.[39]

EXTRAINTESTINAL MANIFESTATIONS

Most of the same extraintestinal manifestations reported with UC can occur with Crohn's disease, including growth retardation, weight loss, delayed sexual maturation, skin lesions, liver disease, uveitis, anemia, and stomatitis. Biopsy of the oral lesions may show granulomas typical of Crohn's disease. Occasionally, children with severe Crohn's disease manifest digital clubbing.

PHYSICAL EXAMINATION

Children with Crohn's disease are frequently retarded in growth and underweight for age. A tender inflammatory mass in the right lower quadrant is a common finding in patients with ileocecal disease. Perianal ulcers or sinuses are common in children with colorectal disease; indeed, perianal lesions may be the first manifestation of Crohn's disease.[40] The ulcers are often painful, may extend widely in the perineum with sinuses, and show undermining with undulant granulation tissue at the base. Occasionally, with extensive ulceration and sinuses, the perineal muscles may become damaged. Sigmoidoscopic examination is often normal in patients with small intestinal Crohn's disease, as well as in those with localized ileocolic involvement who have rectal sparing. A normal-appearing rectum with proximal colonic disease strongly suggests Crohn's disease instead of UC. In children with rectal disease, the mucosa may appear similar to that in UC, but usually it is less friable and often shows linear mucosal ulcerations.[41]

The laboratory findings in children with Crohn's disease usually indicate anemia, sedimentation rate elevation, hypoalbuminemia, IgA level increase, and prolonged prothrombin time. Vitamin B_{12} absorption may be abnormal if there is extensive distal ileal involvement. Stool cultures are consistently negative for pathogenic bacteria and parasites. The detection of antineutrophil cytoplasmic antibodies in a perinuclear fluorescence pattern in the serum of patients with inflammatory bowel disease is suggestive of UC rather than Crohn's disease, although the test is not definitive.

The radiographic appearance in Crohn's disease can show abnormalities at any site from the esophagus to the rectum, but most commonly in the distal ileum and colon. Mucosal ulcerations, intestinal fistulas, sinus tracts, or intraabdominal abscesses may be found (Fig. 42–6). Benign strictures between segments of normal-appearing intestine (skip areas) are frequently seen.

COMPLICATIONS

Internal fistulas and sinuses are characteristic of Crohn's disease and should be suspected when a flare-up of symptoms is associated with the development of persistent abdominal pain and localized abdominal tenderness and the presence of a mass. The fistula is often between the distal ileum and the right colon or sigmoid. The development of a draining sinus after an appendectomy may be an indication that the patient has Crohn's disease, although a sinogram often indicates that the internal opening is into the distal ileum and not to the base of the appendix.[42] Fistulas from the intestine to the bladder or urethra may occasionally occur. Recurrent or persistent urinary tract infections in a patient with Crohn's disease suggest obstruction of a ureter (usually the right) from an inflammatory mass or

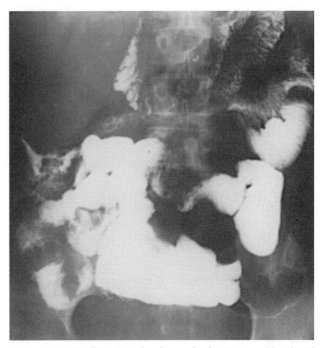

Figure 42–6. Small intestinal radiograph of a 13-year-old girl with ileocolonic Crohn's disease and enterocutaneous fistula from the terminal ileum.

enterovesical fistula; pneumaturia or fecaluria confirms the latter diagnosis.

In contrast to UC, toxic megacolon is uncommon with Crohn's disease. Free perforation into the peritoneal cavity is unusual but can occur during an acute exacerbation of chronic disease, particularly in the presence of distal obstruction. Adenocarcinoma of the small intestine in patients with Crohn's disease is slightly more common than in the general population. Most cancers occur in inflamed segments of bowel, particularly in strictures and long-standing fistulas.[43] The incidence of colorectal carcinoma is more than 20 times greater in patients with Crohn's disease than in a control population; however, it is less frequent than in patients with chronic UC.[41, 43]

NONOPERATIVE THERAPY

Most children with Crohn's disease can be managed on an ambulatory basis for long periods, with dietary modifications that include high-calorie, high-protein, low-roughage foods. Milk is eliminated for those with milk intolerance. In patients with steatorrhea, a low-fat diet with added medium-chain triglycerides is indicated. Between-meal nutritious snacks are encouraged.

Sulfasalazine is often given initially as for patients with UC, but it is often less effective. Steroids are given (1) to children in whom other medical measures have failed to achieve improvement and indications for operation are not yet present; (2) to acutely ill, toxic, hospitalized patients; (3) to patients with uncomfortable extraintestinal manifestations (e.g. arthralgias and skin lesions unresponsive to other measures); and (4) to patients with extensive enteritis considered to be inoperable.

Azathioprine (Imuran) has been used to treat chronic disease for more than three decades, even though controlled studies indicate that it is only slightly more effective than a placebo. In addition, patients receiving long-term immunosuppressive and prednisone therapy have a much higher incidence of lymphoproliferative disorders, including lymphoma, than does the general population.[44] Cyclosporine has been administered to patients unresponsive to other therapy with somewhat better results than those reported for azathioprine. Long-term therapy with these medications may produce serious side effects, such as nephrotoxicity and increased susceptibility to infections. Certain antibiotics, such as metronidazole (Flagyl), in low dosage, have been helpful in relieving symptoms in occasional patients with minimal side effects. Cholestyramine resin may be helpful in treating diarrhea after ileal resection. Addition of fish oils to the diet has been found to reduce the severity and frequency of symptoms in patients with Crohn's disease.

Hospitalization for children with Crohn's disease is advised when symptoms become severe or nutritional deficiency worsens despite therapy on an ambulatory basis. Parenteral alimentation; bowel rest; and electrolyte, vitamin, and trace element repletion may induce improvement in many patients. A sympathetic and accessible family and physician often do much to reduce the severity of the disease.

OPERATIVE THERAPY

Although the surgical treatment of Crohn's disease is rarely curative and is associated with a high frequency of recurrence, operation in selected patients may produce marked clinical improvement and make it feasible to discontinue or reduce the dosage of most medications. Operation is indicated for the complications of Crohn's disease, including intestinal obstruction; growth retardation; medical intractability; enterocutaneous, vesical, or enteric fistulas; intestinal bleeding; persistent abdominal pain; abdominal abscess; and the majority of perirectal fistulas and abscesses.[40] A judicious combination of complete bowel rest with total parenteral nutrition both before and after operation has served to reduce the complications of surgery and to restore the majority of these patients to an active life.

CLINICAL EXPERIENCE

From 1967 to 1997, 82 patients (56 boys and 26 girls) 19 years of age or younger underwent operations for Crohn's disease and its complications at the UCLA Medical Center. The median duration of symptoms before operation was 3.2 years (ranging from 3 months to 12 years). Inflammatory bowel disease was present in immediate family members (sibling, parent, uncle, or aunt) in 12 of the 82

patients (15%); 7 of these had Crohn's disease. During the same 30-year period, at least 70 children with Crohn's disease received medical therapy without operation other than for venous access.

Although Crohn's disease is generally recognized as a diffuse condition most often involving the distal small intestine and cecum, three general patterns of the condition were identified in the 82 children who underwent operation. In 45 patients, the disease was largely confined to the distal ileum and cecum or ascending colon; 29 others had primary involvement of the colon and rectum (Table 42–1). Eight children had inflammatory disease limited to a portion of the small intestine. At the time of the initial operation, the average age of those whose disease was localized to the distal ileum and cecum was 16.9 years and of those who had primary colorectal disease was 15.2 years.

Intestinal obstruction was the most frequent indication for the initial operation in children with ileocecal disease (91%), whereas only 3 of the patients with colorectal disease (10%) had intestinal obstruction. Protracted diarrhea was a prominent symptom in only 8 of the children with ileocecal disease (18%), whereas almost all of those with colorectal disease had persistent diarrhea. Rectal bleeding occurred in 11 children with colorectal disease but in only 2 with ileocecal disease. Growth retardation and delay in the development of secondary sex characteristics were present in 40% of children with ileocecal disease and in 45% of children with colorectal inflammation. Because more than half of the patients had been receiving steroid therapy longer than 2 years, it was difficult to determine whether growth retardation was due to Crohn's disease, the medical therapy, or both.

Primary or secondary enterocutaneous or enteroenteric fistulas or retroperitoneal sinuses were present in 14 of 45 patients with ileocecal disease (31%) as well as in 2 of 29 patients (7%) with colorectal inflammation. In two children, the fistulas developed within 2 years after appendectomy. Seven children with ileocecal disease had enteroenteric fistulas, including one that communicated with the bladder. Five children had enteric sinuses

TABLE 42–1. Crohn's Disease: Relation of Symptoms to Location

Symptoms	Ileocecal Disease (45 patients)		Colorectal Disease (29 patients)	
	No.	%	No.	%
Intestinal obstruction	41	91	3	10
Diarrhea	8	16	28	97
Growth failure	18	40	13	45
Enteric fistula	14	31	2	7
Anal fistula or abscess	2	4	21	71
Arthralgia	12	27	9	31

extending into the pelvis or retroperitoneal tissues. Only 1 child with colorectal disease had an internal fistula.

Anal abscesses, fistulas, or indolent fissures were often the earliest manifestation of Crohn's disease and were more than 17 times as common in children with colorectal disease as in those with ileocecal disease (Fig. 42–7). This experience is at variance with that of others who report that children with small bowel Crohn's disease had a greater frequency of perineal disease than did patients with colonic Crohn's disease.[45] Although 21 children had undergone incision and drainage of a perirectal abscess or perineal ulcer débridement, in only 3 patients was the perineal wound cured by local operative therapy. One patient underwent three perineal operations before the diagnosis of Crohn's disease was established. Most of these children with anal disease had more than one perineal drainage operation (median, 1.6) before intestinal resection was performed.

Twelve of the 45 children with ileocecal inflammation (27%) and 9 of the 29 with colorectal disease (31%) had arthralgias of the knees, hips, elbows, or shoulders at the time of operation. Nine of the 82 patients had erythema nodosum, 3 had mild uveitis, and 3 had oxalate nephrolithiasis.

Five of the 8 children with Crohn's disease confined to the small intestine underwent resection of a short segment of the ileum with reanastomosis for obstruction. None of the children had a stricturoplasty. Three other children with Crohn's disease of the ileum or cecum had the sudden onset of abdominal pain, which was diagnosed as appendicitis. Each of these patients underwent exploratory laparotomy, at which time inflammation of ileum with-

TABLE 42–2. Crohn's Disease: Major Indications for Operation (82 Children)

Indication	No. of Operations
Intestinal obstruction	45
Perianal sinus, abscess	37
Persistent diarrhea, growth failure, pain, fever	29
Recurrent small intestinal disease following previous resection	15
Enteroenteric fistula	7
Abdominal pain (undetermined cause)	7
Retroperitoneal sinus	5
Ileostomy dysfunction	4
Enterocutaneous fistula	4
TOTAL	**153**

out obstruction was found. Each had an uneventful appendectomy without bowel resection. The inflammatory disease in each patient was managed successfully by nonoperative therapy thereafter.

The primary indications for operation in the 82 children are shown in Table 42–2, although many children had more than one indication. Intestinal obstruction with resultant pain, malnutrition, and fever was the most common indication and was present before 45 of the 153 operations. Growth failure, frequently accompanied by persistent diarrhea, pain, and fever, was the indication for operation on 29 occasions. A total of 24 patients underwent 37 operations for management of perianal fistulas, sinuses, or abscesses that caused severe discomfort when accompanied by persistent rectal inflammation. Either diverting ileostomy or proctocolectomy was eventually performed on all but two of these patients. Sixteen children underwent laparotomy and intestinal resection for enteric fistulas or sinuses with or without localized abscess and obstruction. Laparotomy with resection of enteroenteric fistulas with reanastomosis was performed on 7 children. Resection of enterocutaneous fistulas was performed in 4 children, in 2 as the initial operation and in 2 after previous operations that were followed by anastomotic leaks. Five children had resection of retroperitoneal sinuses associated with ileocecal disease. Seven children with abdominal pain of undetermined etiology underwent laparotomy, 4 of whom had an appendectomy. Fifteen children required resection of recurrent small intestinal disease following previous resection.

IV hyperalimentation was used in 79 of the 82 children and was given routinely in the perioperative period to almost all of the children undergoing operation during the past 20 years. Twenty-six of the patients received parenteral nutrition for various periods on a home basis. Steroids, sulfasalazine, or both were given during the course of medical management at some time in the preoperative period in 80 of the 82 children. Most were receiving steroids at the time of operation.

A total of 153 operations were performed on the

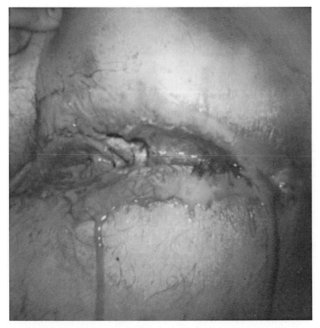

Figure 42–7. Severe multiple perirectal abscesses in a 17-year-old boy with colorectal Crohn's disease of 6 years' duration.

TABLE 42–3. Operations for Crohn's Disease (82 Children)

Type of Operation	No. of Patients
Resection of distal ileum and right colon with anastomosis	39
Drainage, débridement of perianal sinus, fistula, abscess	37
Total proctocolectomy and ileostomy	25
Small bowel resection with anastomosis or ileostomy	23
Resection of distal ileum and segment of colon with ileostomy and mucous fistula	6
Resection of distal ileum and >50% of colon with anastomosis	6
Exploratory laparotomy and appendectomy	4
Ileostomy without intestinal resection	3
Exploratory laparotomy without resection	3
Proctocolectomy with ileoanal pouch procedure	3
Colon resection with anastomosis	2
Diverting colostomy	1
Gastroenterostomy	1
TOTAL	**153**

82 children during the 30-year period of this study (Table 42–3). Drainage or débridement of perianal sinuses, fistulas, or abscesses were among the most common procedures and were performed on 37 occasions. Resection of the distal ileum and ascending colon with reanastomosis was the most common intraabdominal operation and was performed on 39 patients (Fig. 42–8). Total proctocolectomy with cutaneous ileostomy was performed on 25 patients; however, in only 14 patients was this procedure carried out as the initial operation (Fig. 42–9). The

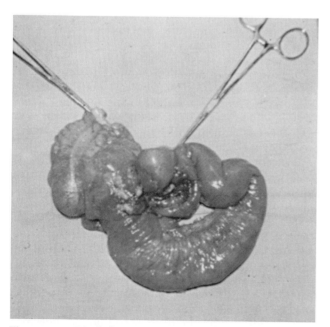

Figure 42–8. Distal ileum and ascending colon from a 16-year-old boy with localized Crohn's disease. Note the areas of obstruction and internal fistulas. An end-to-end ileocolonic anastomosis was performed.

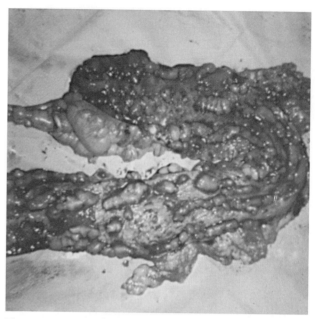

Figure 42–9. Mucosal surface of colon resected from a 13-year-old girl with severe colorectal Crohn's disease of 1.5 years' duration. Note deep ulcerations and almost complete loss of mucosa in some areas.

other 15 patients with colorectal disease previously had a diverting ileostomy or colostomy or an ileocolonic resection with or without anastomosis. Seven children with the initial diagnosis of indeterminate colitis underwent total colectomy and IAPP. In 3 of these 7 children, chronic perineal sinuses and pouchitis developed, requiring removal of the pouch and permanent ileostomy; these cases were eventually diagnosed as Crohn's disease. In our early experience, resection of the distal ileum and a segment of colon with cutaneous ileostomy and colonic mucous fistula was performed on 6 children. Resection of the distal ileum and resection of more than 50% of the colon with reanastomosis was performed in 4 patients, 2 of whom subsequently underwent total proctocolectomy.

Resection of a localized segment of ileum was performed in 16 children, in 4 as the initial operation with reanastomosis (Fig. 42–10). In 7 patients, additional distal ileum was resected within 8 years after ileostomy and proctocolectomy for localized recurrence. Ileostomy with ileal mucous fistula without intestinal resection was performed as a palliative procedure for 3 patients with colorectal disease owing to severe perianal fistulas and abscesses, pain, fever, and weight loss. Two of these patients underwent proctocolectomy within 2 years. One patient underwent colonic resection with anastomosis as a primary operation and another underwent transverse colostomy; however, recurrent disease led to subsequent proctocolectomy in both.

Eleven children with Crohn's disease who were followed up at UCLA Medical Center hospital had undergone appendectomy in other hospitals during the 6 years before resection; only 2 of these children

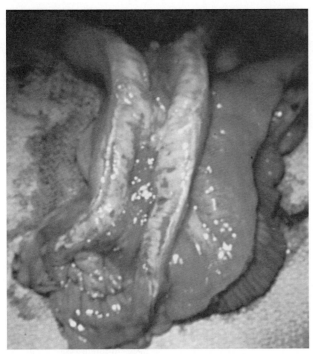

Figure 42–10. Localized stricture of the distal ileum. Note the thickened wall of the intestine and underlying mesentery.

had acute appendicitis. In 3, enteric fistulas developed later that appeared to originate in the cecum. Five patients in whom cholelithiasis and cholecystitis developed after ileal or colonic resection required cholecystectomy at a later time.

RESULTS

With follow-up ranging from 5 months to 25 years, all 82 children who underwent operation survived for more than 10 years. Recurrent inflammatory disease of the small intestine requiring reoperation occurred in 15 of the 45 children with ileocecal disease (33%). Recurrent disease occurred in each of the 15 children with colorectal disease who had a lesser operation than proctocolectomy. Nonetheless, 62% of the children had recurrence even after proctocolectomy, and 9 of these 25 patients required further operation. In 3 of the 5 patients with primary ileal disease who underwent intestinal resection, recurrent disease subsequently developed, although only 1 patient underwent reoperation.

In most cases, the recurrent disease was successfully managed with sulfasalazine, steroid therapy, bowel rest with partial or total parenteral nutrition, or metronidazole therapy for varying periods. Steroids did not appear to increase the incidence of postoperative complications. In children who had primary colorectal involvement, recurrent disease in the small intestine was occasionally severe, extending to the duodenum in one patient and associated with internal fistulas in three. In contrast, recurrent disease was more localized and milder in children with primary ileocecal involvement. Five

patients required reoperation due to persistent perineal sinus following proctocolectomy. Three patients needed reoperation because an enterocutaneous fistula developed. Seven other children required resection of a short segment of distal ileum with revision of the ileostomy stoma.

COMMENTS

Removal of the symptomatic diseased intestine with reanastomosis is the optimal operative procedure for treatment of Crohn's disease whenever feasible. Whereas previously it was common practice to resect several centimeters of normal intestine both proximal and distal to the involved intestine, many studies[46, 47] have clearly shown that reanastomosis of intestine containing mild disease rarely interferes with healing and is less likely to lead to a short intestine syndrome than if larger resections are performed. Skip areas of involved small intestine are usually not resected unless they cause obstruction or other symptoms. In my practice, we perform all anastomoses in two layers with interrupted absorbable suture. Although stricturoplasty has been reported to benefit adult patients with multiple small intestinal segments of stricture to avoid multiple resections and possible subsequent short bowel syndrome, little experience has been reported with this technique in children.[40, 48]

Colectomy with ileosigmoid anastomosis may be performed in children with mild rectal involvement who do not have perianal sinuses or fistulas. Even in this small group of patients, recurrent inflammation in the ileum requiring subsequent operation is common. IAPP and continent ileostomy (Kock pouch) are contraindicated due to the high frequency of recurrent disease in the distal ileum, although my colleagues and I continue to perform restorative proctocolectomy for patients with indeterminate colitis, regardless of age.[17, 41] Resection of an inflammatory mass involving the distal ileum and cecum may endanger the right ureter, necessitating cautious dissection. Identification of the ureter before extensive dissection into the retroperitoneal tissues is highly advisable. Enterovesical fistulas are treated by resection of the diseased intestine with closure of the bladder.

Ileostomy alone or intestinal bypass operations are followed by a higher incidence of complications and a much lower degree of clinical improvement than are resectional operations, thus they are rarely performed. Internal fistulas involving intestine near the site of resection are removed along with the specimen. Fistulas to intestine at a distance from the site of resection are divided. If the distant intestine appears healthy, simple closure of the fistula is performed; if the distant bowel segment has active disease, a second resection of this area is performed.

For children who retain diseased bowel, perianal wounds often heal poorly or not at all. Simple surgical débridement is sufficient for treatment of perianal wounds and chronic infections in many cases.[45]

Medical therapy for a few months with metronidazole, mesalamine, azathioprine, 6-mercaptopurine, or cyclosporine may produce improvement for many patients with perianal disease.[49] Satisfactory healing often follows complete extirpation of the diseased proximal bowel, if the perianal lesions are well débrided. The presence of Crohn's disease in the rectal mucosa, however, greatly increases the need for a permanent stoma in patients with severe perianal disease.[50]

Appendectomy is indicated when laparotomy is performed for abdominal pain and no active inflammatory disease is identified in the cecum or distal ileum. The incidence of subsequent fistula formation in these patients is more than sixfold higher than in patients without Crohn's disease. Appendicitis is less common in children with Crohn's disease than in the normal population.

Crohn's disease of the duodenum that causes obstruction and that is refractory to medical therapy may occasionally benefit from gastrojejunostomy and vagotomy to prevent jejunal ulceration, although symptoms are likely to recur.

A reported recurrence rate of active disease of 35% within 5 years after operation, with more than half of these patients requiring additional surgery, indicates that operation is rarely curative for Crohn's disease.[51, 52] The number of sites involved with Crohn's disease is the most important factor related to increased risk of recurrence.[35] Nonetheless, operation relieves intestinal obstruction and its accompanying pain and anorexia and allows the patient to return to a more normal existence. More than half of the patients with resection and anastomosis in whom recurrent disease develops do respond to medical therapy.[53, 54] Recurrent Crohn's disease often develops proximal to an ileostomy stoma. Children with diffuse colonic inflammation experience earlier recurrence than those with predominantly small bowel disease.[55, 56] Operation for persistently symptomatic recurrent disease is necessary in approximately 30% of patients who have had a previous primary resection.[57] The second operation is likely to achieve a good result in more than 50%.

□ Polypoid Diseases of the Gastrointestinal Tract

Polypoid disorders of the GI tract in children are relatively common and include tumor-like lesions (hamartomatous, hyperplastic, lymphoid, inflammatory polyps), epithelial tumors that are adenomatous polyps (neoplasias), and a number of miscellaneous disorders that may present as polypoid masses in the lumen of the intestine (Table 42–4).[58] Intestinal polyps are less common in children than in adults. Occasional patients with intestinal polyps have associated disorders in other areas of the body and have been classified into specific polyposis syndromes (Table 42–5). Although almost all of the GI neoplasms of adulthood may occur in

TABLE 42–4. Benign Polypoid Tumors of the Colon

Tumor-Like Lesions

Hamartoma
   Juvenile polyps
   Peutz-Jeghers polyps
   Cronkhite-Canada syndrome
   Cowden's syndrome
Hyperplastic polyps
Lymphoid polyps
Inflammatory polyps (pseudopolyps), ulcerative colitis
Heterotopic tissue (gastric, pancreatic)
Lesions secondary to mucosal prolapse, colitis cystica profunda

Epithelial Tumors

Adenoma
   Familial adenomatous polyposis
   Gardner's syndrome
   Turcot syndrome
   Tubulovillous and villous tumors
Carcinoid tumors
Endocrine tumors

Nonepithelial Tumors

Leiomyoma
Lipoma
Vascular tumors (hemangioma)
Neurogenic tumors (neurofibroma, neurilemoma, ganglioneuroma)

children, juvenile and lymphoid polyps are almost unique to the pediatric age group. Villous adenomas are rare in childhood. It is also rare for a child to have a mixture of different types of polyps.

JUVENILE POLYPS

Juvenile polyps have been recognized as a distinct pathologic entity distinguishable from adenomas and other polypoid lesions of the colon since the early 1960s. Although juvenile polyps are clearly benign lesions, the practice of equating intestinal polyps with adenoma has been so deeply ingrained that treatment of juvenile polyps has often been unclear and occasionally unnecessarily radical. Juvenile polyps, either single or multiple, are currently regarded as benign lesions usually bearing no relation to adenomatous polyps.

Pathology

Juvenile polyps, which are also regarded as mucus retention, inflammatory, or cystic polyps, are the most common type of polypoid lesion found in the GI tract in children; they account for more than 90% of colonic polyps in children younger than 10 years of age. They are generally pedunculated, but occasionally are sessile, particularly when small, and they are composed of dilated glands filled with mucus and inspissated inflammatory debris, giving them a cystic appearance (Fig. 42–11).[58] Ultrastructural and tissue culture studies support the hamartomatous nature of these lesions. The polyps are uniformly smooth, glistening, and reddish, ranging

TABLE 42–5. Gastrointestinal Polyposis Syndromes

Syndrome	Histology	Distribution	Malignant Potential	Other Manifestations	Genetic Mechanism
Familial polyposis	150–5000 adenomas	Colorectum	High	Gastric and duodenal polyps; desmoid tumors; included in many syndromes	AD
Gardner's syndrome	25–200 scattered adenomas	Colorectum, occasionally esophagus, stomach, small bowel	High	Osteomas, epidermoid cysts, fibromas, desmoid tumors, mesenteric fibromatosis, dental abnormalities	AD
Turcot syndrome	Scattered adenomas	Colorectum	High	Central nervous system tumors	AR
Familial discrete polyps	1–6 adenomas	Colorectum	High	None	AD
Peutz-Jeghers syndrome	Hamartomas	Entire GI tract, mainly stomach, small bowel, colorectum	Low or absent	Pigmentation of lips and skin	AD
Juvenile polyposis	Most hamartomas, few adenomas	Entire GI tract, most in colorectum	Low	Anemia, protein-losing enteropathy	Some familial
Cowden's syndrome	Multiple hamartomas	Entire GI tract	None in GI tract; breast and thyroid cancer	Warty papules on mucosa and skin, multiple malformations	AD
Basal cell nevus syndrome	Multiple hamartomas	Stomach	None from GI tract, skin cancer	Benign mesenteric cysts	AD
Neurofibromatosis	Submucosal neurofibromas	Entire GI tract	Occasional sarcomatous degeneration	Von Recklinghausen's disease, café-au-lait spots	AD
Cronkhite-Canada syndrome	Thickened mucosa, likened to juvenile polyps	Stomach, small bowel, colon	Low	Skin pigmentation, nail atrophy, alopecia, protein-losing enteropathy	Sporadic, probably nongenetic

AD, autosomal dominant; AR, autosomal recessive; GI, gastrointestinal.
Modified from Gardner EJ, Burt RW, Freston JW: Gastrointestinal polyposis: Syndromes and genetic mechanisms. West J Med 132:488–499, 1980.

from a few millimeters to several centimeters in diameter.[59] The average juvenile polyp is approximately 1 cm in diameter and has a thin stalk covered by normal colonic mucosa, which may be ulcerated on the surface. The eroded surface is often replaced by proliferating granulation tissue. In areas adjacent to the erosions, the regenerating epithelium occasionally may show cytologic atypism.

The etiology of juvenile polyps is unknown but has been attributed to hereditary, congenital, inflammatory, allergic, and neoplastic causes. The initial stage is ulceration and inflammation of the mucosa, which cause obstruction of one or more small colonic glands. The blocked gland then proliferates, branches, and dilates to give the appearance of a mucous cyst, thus exposing a larger surface of the mucosa, which, in turn, becomes ulcerated and inflamed. Granulation tissue develops on the ulcerated surface, and the cycle continues until the entire lesion is sufficiently large to extend into the intestinal lumen. Mucosal ulceration on the polyp may produce hemorrhage. The flow of the fecal stream usually causes the stalk to elongate and occasionally slough.

Approximately 70% of juvenile polyps occur in the rectum and 15% occur in the sigmoid colon, and the remainder are scattered throughout the more proximal colon to the cecum.[60] Three fourths of the patients have a single polyp, and one fourth have multiple or scattered polyps (usually >10 polyps).[59, 61] Juvenile polyps do not appear to occur in the small intestine.

Clinical Features

The incidence of juvenile polyps is undetermined, although reports from various workers suggest that they occur in approximately 1 in 1000 children. The polyps are slightly more common in boys than in girls. Juvenile polyps are most frequently seen in children between the ages of 2 and 8 years, with peak incidence at the age of 4 to 5 years, although occasional polyps have been identified during the 1st year of life.[60, 62] Juvenile polyps are rarely seen after early adolescence, although on rare occasions they have been reported in adults.

The most common symptom of juvenile polyps is intermittent bleeding caused by inflammation and mucosal ulceration. Blood loss is usually minimal, appearing as streaks of fresh blood on the outside of the stool. Bleeding from polyps in the proximal colon may be darker and mixed with the stool. On rare occasion, autoamputation may expose a feeding vessel at the base, which may produce brisk bleeding, sometimes requiring transfusion.

An occasional polyp located low in the rectum

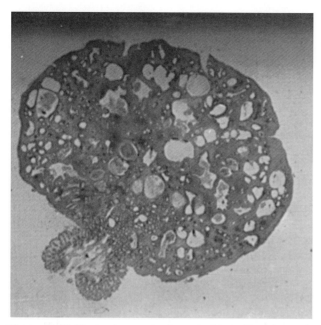

Figure 42–11. Photomicrograph of a typical juvenile polyp and a portion of the stalk. The Swiss cheese-like appearance comes from lakes of retained mucus.

may prolapse or protrude from the anus or even cause prolapse of the rectal mucosa. Children occasionally experience abdominal cramps believed to be caused by traction on the polyp during peristaltic activity; in rare instances, a polyp may initiate an intussusception. Most juvenile polyps are believed to eventually undergo autoamputation and pass into the fecal stream.[63, 64]

A low rectal polyp may occasionally be found on digital rectal examination. Fiberoptic sigmoidoscopy under heavy sedation or light general anesthesia is likely to reveal the polyps in more than 80% of children. Colonoscopy under general anesthesia provides the most thorough method of identifying juvenile polyps, although this procedure may be unnecessarily excessive for most small children. A barium enema radiographic study with air contrast is helpful for identifying pedunculated polyps of the colon in patients of all ages (Fig. 42–12). Due to the frequent difficulty of distinguishing a polyp from fecal masses in the colon lumen, the lesion should be demonstrated on two separate radiographic studies before a diagnosis of colonic polyp is made by barium enema study.

The differential diagnosis of juvenile polyps includes the common causes of rectal bleeding in young children such as anal fissures, which can be visualized; acute and chronic inflammatory bowel disease, which is usually accompanied by diarrhea; and blood dyscrasias such as Henoch-Schönlein purpura. Bleeding from Meckel's diverticulum or duplication of the intestine is usually of greater magnitude and mixed with stool. Bleeding from intussusception is usually darker and accompanied by severe cramping abdominal pain. The diagnosis of juvenile polyps is made from the history, digital rectal examination, sigmoidoscopy, and barium enema radiographs with air contrast. Laboratory studies should include a hemogram to evaluate for anemia and blood dyscrasias, as well as a stool culture and an examination for ova and parasites.

Therapy

Almost all polyps in the rectum and lower sigmoid colon can be removed through a sigmoidoscope. Many of these lesions can be drawn through the anus and removed by suture ligation of the pedicle. For higher lesions, a snare and cautery used through the sigmoidoscope can permit resection of the entire polyp.

Almost all children who have one or more polyps above the sigmoid colon have a polyp in the rectum or lower sigmoid colon that is accessible to the sigmoidoscope. In these patients, the lower polyp may be removed to verify the diagnosis of juvenile polyps. The more proximal polyps do not warrant removal unless they produce symptoms. Bleeding polyps located beyond the reach of the sigmoidoscope may require removal by colonoscopy. It is

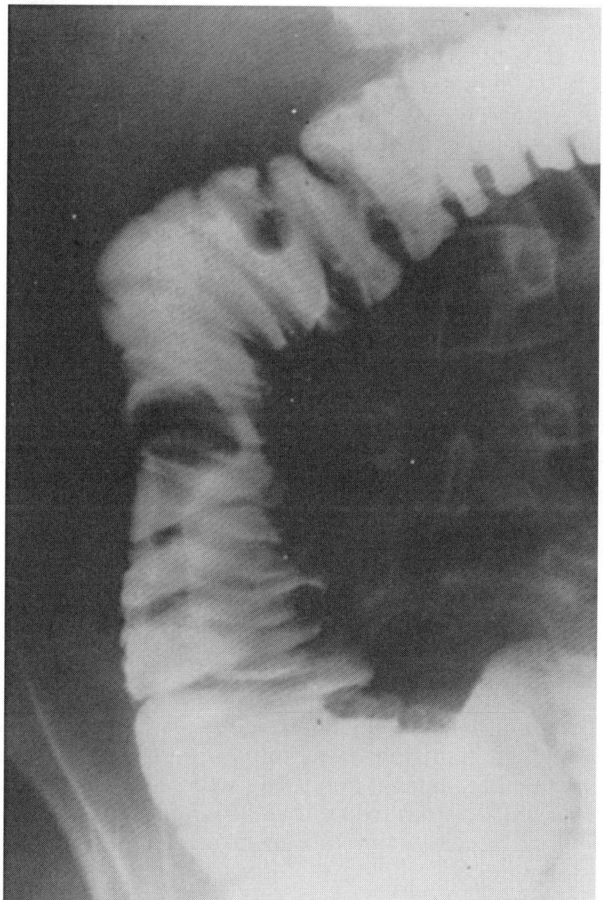

Figure 42–12. Barium enema air contrast study of the right side of the colon showing two filling defects proved at colonoscopic removal to be juvenile polyps. Note the long stalk on the larger polyp.

rarely necessary to perform a laparotomy with colotomy for removal of a juvenile polyp.[65]

Complications following endoscopic removal of juvenile polyps have been rare. Subsequent bleeding from additional or recurrent polyps occurs in approximately 5% of cases. The natural history of juvenile polyps is that they are self-limited and seem to disappear, most often during preadolescent years.

Relatives of children with juvenile polyps are at a slightly increased risk for GI cancer. Occasionally, older patients have been reported with concomitant juvenile and adenomatous polyps. Dysplasia, which may be present in individual crypts of juvenile polyps, can, on rare occasion, progress to frank cancer. Older patients with juvenile polyps containing dysplasia or adenomatous transformation should be in a clinical follow-up program to facilitate the detection of early malignancy.

FAMILIAL ADENOMATOUS POLYPOSIS COLI

FAP coli is an uncommon hereditary disorder in which innumerable premalignant adenomatous polyps of the colon develop during the early decades of life. One or more of the polyps inevitably become malignant. The incidence of its inheritance ranges from 1 in 6000 to 1 in 12,000 births.[66–68] Based on the U.S. birth rate, approximately 3000 babies are born at risk each year.[68] Varying degrees of gene penetrance seem likely, with occasional sporadic cases probably arising from spontaneous mutation. The disorder is inherited as a mendelian autosomal non–sex-linked dominant trait precisely identified on chromosome 5q21.[69, 70] Male and female patients are equally afflicted, and either sex can transmit the disease. Only those who have the disease themselves are capable of transmitting it to the next generation. In most polyposis families, one half of the children are likely to inherit the disease, the remainder being normal.

During the first decade of life, only a few afflicted patients are identified as having colonic polyps. The median age for development of these polyps is 16 years; for bowel symptoms, 29 years; and for colorectal cancer, 40 years.[71] Death resulting from malignancy occurs at a median age of 44 years.[68, 71, 72] The earliest reported appearance of polyps is at age 1 year. The youngest patient with carcinoma of the colon was diagnosed at 8 years of age.[73] It has been speculated that children in whom cancer develops at a young age may be homozygous for the polyposis gene.[66] In families in which polyposis develops early in life, cancer frequently occurs within 10 to 15 years, whereas in families in which polyposis is recognized later, the precancerous latency period is longer.

Pathology

Characteristic features of the FAP syndrome include innumerable polyps carpeting the entire colon from anus to cecum, including the appendix (Fig. 42–13). The polyps are the adult adenomatous type and may vary from 2 mm to 2 cm, but they are typically less than 1 cm in diameter. They may be sessile or pedunculated, with tubular, tubulovillous, or villous histologic features.[74]

Adenomatous polyps are benign, gland-forming neoplasms that can contain cytologically malignant cells within the basement membrane of the crypts; such areas are designated *intraepithelial carcinoma*. Extension beyond the basement membrane into the lamina propria is termed *intramucosal carcinoma*. Neither intraepithelial nor intramucosal carcinoma has a great potential for metastasis, as long as all the neoplastic tissue is removed, because there are no lymphatics in the lamina propria of the colon. When neoplastic cells are contained within the epithelial basement membrane, the term *in situ carcinoma* is used. When malignant cells extend beyond the basement membrane, the tumor is microscopically invasive. In the absence of colonic mucosal lymphatics, the risk of lymphatic invasion and nodal metastases is unlikely until the tumor invades the submucosa where lymphatics are present. Thus, carcinoma in an adenomatous polyp of the colon is

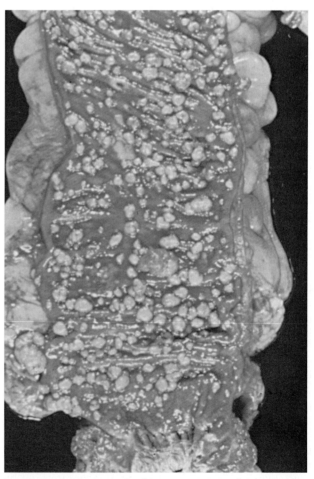

Figure 42–13. An opened colectomy specimen from a 17-year-old boy with familial adenomatous polyposis. Note the density and relative uniformity in size of the polyps.

not considered invasive until it extends through the mucosa into the submucosa. In some polyps with foci of cancer, it is difficult to determine whether malignant cells have extended into the submucosa.[75] In these instances, it is imperative to be aware of the differing histologic characteristics of normal submucosa and lamina propria.

Clinical Features

Although most patients with FAP are asymptomatic, some may experience increased stool frequency, rectal bleeding, anemia, tenesmus, and, rarely, abdominal pain. Most children are identified by surveillance studies on the basis of another member of the family having been diagnosed with FAP, often with carcinoma. The diagnosis is most frequently established by family history, sigmoidoscopic examination, and sometimes by digital rectal examination.

Colonoscopy may demonstrate a carpet of polyps covering the entire surface of the colon and rectum. Biopsy of one of the polyps establishes the diagnosis when adenomatous features are demonstrated. Although barium enema with air contrast radiographs may demonstrate many filling defects with extensive involvement of the colon, many patients with small polyps have a normal-appearing radiographic contrast enema study. When the diagnosis is established, careful investigation of all family members should be initiated. Members of the family are at high risk for developing carcinoma of the colon, because there is an inherited predisposition of the colon mucosa to undergo malignant change at an early age.

Gastric polyps are likely to develop in more than 60% of patients with FAP, although this is infrequent before the age of 18 years.[68] Most gastric polyps are hyperplastic and not precancerous, although gastric carcinoma has been reported in 2.7% of patients in a large series of FAP patients in Japan.[71, 76] Fewer than 15% of gastric polyps are adenomas. Polyps in the duodenum occur with lower frequency than those in the stomach, although they are more likely to be adenomatous and are at risk for development of carcinoma.[77, 78] Carcinoma in the duodenum and periampullary area is the most common cause of death, after colorectal cancer, in FAP patients.[79] Gastric and duodenal polyps were initially believed to occur primarily in patients with Gardner's syndrome; however, it has come to be recognized that they are a frequent occurrence in patients with FAP.

Most patients with gastric and duodenal polyps are asymptomatic, although occasional patients may experience bleeding or gastritis. Endoscopic biopsy of gastric polyps usually reveals inflammation and hyperplasia. Symptoms are often improved with antacids and H2-blocking agents; the polyps may persist for varying periods. Rarely, adenomatous polyps of the jejunum or ileum may develop in a patient with FAP.[80] Occasionally, desmoid tumors of the small intestinal mesentery or abdominal wall may occur (<8%) but less frequently than in patients with Gardner's syndrome. The relative risk of papillary carcinoma is 100 times higher in female patients with FAP compared with the general population.[81]

Therapy

Colectomy for FAP is recommended at any age if the child is symptomatic; however, operation is usually deferred until the child is between 10 and 14 years of age and is more capable of self-care following surgery. Because the major cause of death is colorectal cancer, prophylactic proctocolectomy soon after diagnosis is the recommended management. Debate has previously been concerned with whether proctocolectomy with ileostomy is more appropriate for children than colectomy with ileorectal anastomosis; however, in recent years, the IAPP has become a more favorable option. Although each of the operations has its advocates, if any rectal mucosa remains, the patient must be followed up closely with at least annual sigmoidoscopic examinations until the rectum is removed owing to the risk of carcinoma developing in the remaining rectal stump. Carcinoma develops within 10 years in 13% of patients who have the rectum preserved (ileorectal anastomosis) and within 20 years in 37%.[71, 82] Recent studies, however, indicate that administration of low-dose antiproliferative sulindac (Clinoril) is effective in reversion of adenomas in FAP patients.[83] Sulindac shows influence on tumor suppressor genes and on apoptosis markers.

Because most children with FAP, as with UC, prefer to avoid a permanent ileostomy if feasible, ileorectal anastomosis and IAPP are used most frequently. Reports of clinical experience with IAPP indicate that stool frequency, urgency, and continence are equally good, if not better, than with ileorectal anastomosis.[84, 85] Although a few surgeons recommend an SP, most surgeons use a short ileoanal pouch (JP) to reduce fecal urgency, frequency, and soiling.[17, 86, 87] Whereas most patients undergoing the IAPP for UC have fewer complications when a temporary diverting ileostomy is used, a one-stage pull-through procedure with ileal reservoir, but without ileostomy, has been performed in many children with FAP.[17] Complete rectal mucosectomy with hand-sewn ileoanal anastomosis is recommended instead of the double-stapled anastomosis because every mucosal cell carries the APC gene and is at risk for development of dysplasia or neoplasia.[85]

All 20 children with FAP who underwent colectomy and IAPP since 1980 at the UCLA Medical Center had an ileal pouch and 11 had the operation performed without a diverting ileostomy.[17] Complications in all the patients were much less frequent than in children undergoing the procedure for UC. At 1 year after surgery, the average number of bowel movements in 24 hours was 3.7. None of the children take long-term medications.

GARDNER'S SYNDROME

In 1953, Gardner and Richards described a familial form of colonic polyposis that occurred in association with osteomas of the skull and facial bones and in some instances with multiple soft tissue tumors, such as lipomas, desmoid tumors, leiomyomas, sebaceous cysts, and dental abnormalities, including multiple unerupted and supernumerary teeth and multiple dental caries.[88] Approximately 75% of involved patients have at least one extracolonic manifestation, including bone tumors (80%), inclusion cysts (35%), and desmoid tumors (18%). The longer and more scrupulously these patients are investigated, the more extracolonic manifestations are found. Some authors consider FAP and Gardner's syndrome as a continuum, with increasing extracolonic expressions of the gene inheritance developing with age.[67, 89]

As in FAP patients, gastric polyps are frequent and are usually hyperplastic or hamartomatous. Adenomatous polyps often involve the small intestine and duodenum and are premalignant. Periampullary carcinoma is the most serious and frequent extracolonic neoplasm associated with FAP and Gardner's syndrome. Pancreatic tumors develop approximately 15 years after the known onset of FAP and at an average age of 44 years. The importance of routine esophagogastroduodenoscopy in patients with FAP, and particularly in those with Gardner's syndrome, to identify duodenal neoplasms has been emphasized by many physicians.[71, 78]

Gardner's syndrome may be inherited as the expression of a single, apparently pleiotropic, dominant gene. The natural history and management of the colonic polyps in patients with this syndrome are similar to those in FAP, although there is an increased risk of carcinoma in extracolonic lesions.

Desmoid tumors of the abdominal wall or mesentery of the small intestine occur in approximately 20% of patients with Gardner's syndrome, but they also occur in patients with FAP (<9%).[90] This lesion consists of dense mature fibroblasts with scarce cell nuclei that may be localized in the skeletal muscles of the abdominal wall, or they may extend more widely when the mesentery is involved (approximately 85%).[90–92] Desmoid tumors may resemble low-grade fibrosarcomas; however, they are distinguished by a lack of mitotic activitiy.[93] Desmoid lesions are locally invasive but do not metastasize. In approximately 20% of patients, the desmoid tumor may be recognized before the diagnosis of polyposis coli is established.

Some kindred carry a high risk of development of desmoids. Desmoid tumors are recognized at a young age (mean, 30 years), but rarely in children. Women are involved approximately three times more frequently than men.[90] Most mesenteric desmoids are first recognized within 2 years after previous colectomy (>80%).[71] When present, desmoid

tumors of the mesentery may limit the surgical options, particularly IAPP, owing to fibrous contraction around the mesenteric vessels. Desmoid tumors of the small intestinal mesentery (seven) or rectus muscle (two) have subsequently developed in 9 of 71 patients in the UCLA series who underwent colectomy and IAPP for FAP.

Because desmoid tumors are not malignant, local excision without bowel resection is recommended whenever feasible; however, excision of desmoid tumors of the mesentery is rarely possible. Radiation therapy has not been effective. Clinical improvement has been observed in several patients with desmoid tumors of the mesentery following extended courses of therapy with tamoxifen and sulindac.[94] The mechanism of action of these drugs is unclear, but estrogen blockade may reduce genetic transcription in tumor growth and inhibition of prostaglandin synthesis. Other chemotherapeutic drugs have been used in patients with persistent desmoid tumors with variable success.[95] Despite many types of therapy, desmoid tumors may cause progressive contracture and eventually intestinal obstruction that may be surgically uncorrectable and lead to death in 20%.[90] Several patients, however, have lived for many years (>70%) with desmoid tumors with minimal symptoms or limitations. Surgery for FAP in a child with another family member who has a desmoid and whose average familial age of colorectal carcinoma is high and in whom the polyp density is sparse might be deferred until approximately age 20 years.[71]

ADENOMATOUS POLYPS

Adenomatous polyps are rare in children except in FAP. The adenomatous polyp, often referred to as the "adult" or "neoplastic" polyp, consists of a proliferation of glandular elements with much branching and little stroma and connective tissue. There is usually little evidence of the inflammation that is frequently seen in juvenile polyps. The epithelium is often multilayered with atypism, mitotic figures, and hyperchromatic nuclei. When a solitary adenoma is identified in a child, extensive investigation should be undertaken to clearly determine whether FAP is present. Careful follow-up of the patient as well as investigation of family members is recommended.

FAMILIAL JUVENILE ADENOMATOUS POLYPOSIS

When there are multiple colonic polyps, the patient may have *juvenile polyposis syndrome*. This rare condition consists of multiple mucosal retention polyps throughout the colon and GI tract with approximately one third of patients having family members involved (Fig. 42–14).[96] Colonic carcinoma in family members is common. These patients occasionally experience protein-losing enteropathy, severe bleeding, anemia, and intussusception, and they may require extensive resuscitation. In some

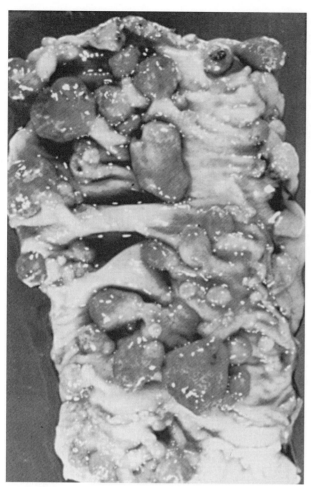

Figure 42–14. A short segment of resected sigmoid colon that contained 37 juvenile polyps. This 15-year-old girl had recurrent gross rectal bleeding cured by sleeve resection.

patients, mucosal atypia, adenomatous changes, or even carcinoma may develop, indicating that close long-term follow-up is necessary.[63, 71]

The rare association of juvenile hyperplastic and adenomatous intestinal polyps has been recognized but only in the familial juvenile polyposis syndrome. Histologic demonstration of juvenile polyps in infants with diffuse juvenile polyposis does not exclude the presence of associated adenomatous polyps. It is, therefore, recommended that multiple polyps be biopsied by endoscopy.

Because approximately half of all children with juvenile polyposis have a familial occurrence, siblings and close relatives should be evaluated. The coexistence of juvenile and adenomatous polyps has been reported only in diffuse juvenile polyposis. Although a conservative approach is used in the treatment of children with single or scattered juvenile polyps, children with diffuse juvenile polyposis should undergo early resection.

PEUTZ-JEGHERS SYNDROME

The association of intestinal polyps with abnormal mucocutaneous pigmentation was first de-

scribed by Peutz in 1921, when he called attention to the hereditary aspects of the condition.[97] In 1949, Jeghers and associates defined the syndrome and analyzed 22 cases, 10 of their own.[98] In subsequent years, additional information has accumulated regarding the increased incidence of malignancy in the GI tract and elsewhere in patients with intestinal polyposis associated with mucocutaneous pigmentation.

Pathology

Peutz-Jeghers syndrome is characterized by GI polyps and circumoral buccal or lingual pigmented lesions that also may be found on the palms and soles (Fig. 42–15). The lesions resemble freckles but do not show seasonal change and are present in areas where freckles are normally absent, such as near the mouth, the palms, and buccal mucosa.[99] The mucocutaneous lesions vary from light brown to black and may be linear, oval, or irregular. They are usually small (<5 mm), flat, without hair, and do not coalesce. Microscopically, the pigment is present in vertical bands in the basal layer of the epidermis; however, the pigmented cells are not melanoblasts. The relationship of mucocutaneous pigmentation to polyposis is unknown; the intestinal polyps are not pigmented. In occasional patients, melanin spots of the lips and skin become less prominent after puberty, whereas those of the buccal mucosa remain.

Polypoid lesions with Peutz-Jeghers syndrome occur most frequently in the small intestine (90%), but they may also occur in the nasal cavity, esophagus, stomach, colon, rectum, urinary bladder, and bronchus. The polyps are usually multiple and widely scattered. The size may vary from a few millimeters to several centimeters (Fig. 42–16). Approximately one third of patients have polyps in the rectum and colon. Only a rare Peutz-Jeghers patient with an isolated polyp has been reported.

The polyps are hamartomatous, not adenomatous, and are not regarded as precancerous. Nonetheless, carcinoma has, on rare occasion, been reported with this syndrome.[100] In approximately 5% of female patients with Peutz-Jeghers syndrome, ovarian neoplasms develop, half of which are sex cord tumors with a high percentage being hormonally active. Cutaneous fibroblasts from patients with Peutz-Jeghers syndrome are reported to be five times more susceptible to transformation with murine sarcoma virus than are those from normal individuals.

Clinical Features

Peutz-Jeghers syndrome is uncommon, the sex distribution is approximately equal, and the condition has been described in all racial groups. A family history is present in half of the patients. The syndrome is an autosomal dominant genetic abnormality. Approximately half of the descendants of patients with the syndrome are afflicted.

Although Peutz-Jeghers syndrome is often diag-

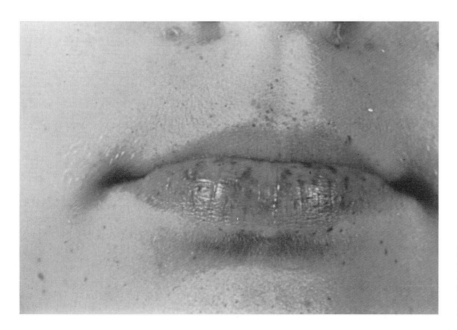

Figure 42–15. Brownish black melanin spots on the lips of an 8-year-old girl with Peutz-Jeghers syndrome. Note the ordinary freckles on the face, which are common in this syndrome but not specific for it.

nosed in childhood, the mean age at the time of diagnosis is 29 years.[99] The condition is rarely detected in infants younger than 1 year of age. The primary features of the syndrome are a frequent

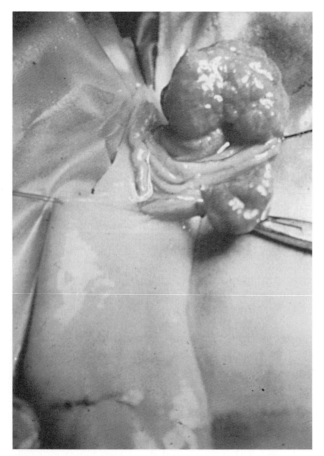

Figure 42–16. A typical Peutz-Jeghers colonic polyp. Note its lobulated surface, which is different from the juvenile polyp shown in Figure 42–11.

occurrence in family members; mucocutaneous pigmentation; GI polyposis; repeated episodes of abdominal pain caused by intussusception, melena, or occult blood loss from the intestine; and anemia. The pigmented spots are distinctive and when present should lead to investigation for intestinal polyps. Pigmentation is often the initial manifestation with abdominal symptoms rarely becoming apparent before the age of 6 to 8 years.[101]

Partial intestinal obstruction characterized by recurrent attacks of crampy abdominal discomfort caused by transient intussusception is characteristic. Plain radiographs often demonstrate dilated small bowel with air-fluid levels. Complete obstruction is uncommon, and most episodes of intussusception resolve spontaneously. The episodes of obstruction occur periodically, with intervals of quiescence lasting months to years. Occult GI bleeding with secondary anemia occurs in approximately one third of patients. Occasional patients manifest growth failure.

Barium enema radiographs with air contrast and sigmoidoscopy or colonoscopic examination identifies the 30 to 35% of patients who have rectal and colonic involvement. Gastroscopy is helpful in identifying the relatively uncommon gastric polyp. Upper GI series with small bowel follow-through sometimes allows visualization of small bowel polyps or transient ileal intussusception.

Therapy

Surgery is not often needed for the treatment of Peutz-Jeghers syndrome. The patient and family should be advised regarding the occasional necessity to operate for unreducible intussusception or for prolonged or extensive intestinal bleeding. Enterotomies to remove large bleeding polyps in either the small or large intestine are occasionally necessary, and some patients require multiple operations. Intestinal resection should be avoided if possible. The prognosis for patients with Peutz-Jeghers syndrome is good, and most patients live into advanced adult life. Although rare, death may result from the complications of intussusception, blood loss, and the necessary operations for treatment.

Peutz-Jeghers polyps are generally regarded as benign hamartomatous lesions, although coincidental adenomatous and hamartomatous polyps have occasionally been observed in the small intestine, colon, and stomach. In the long term, Peutz-Jeghers syndrome does carry a slightly increased risk of intestinal carcinoma, presumably from the associated adenomatous polyps. The small number of patients with this syndrome and the long interval between diagnosis and the appearance of cancer (approximately 25 years) have made it difficult to establish a clear relationship. Currently, it is believed that patients with Peutz-Jeghers syndrome have an increased risk for developing cancer both inside and outside the GI tract.[102, 103] The high frequency of extraintestinal cancer in patients with Peutz-Jeghers syndrome, including carcinoma of the pancreas, breast, lung, uterus, ovary, and multiple myeloma, has been emphasized. Routine breast and gynecologic examination in patients with this syndrome should be encouraged. The benefit of screening for less accessible malignant tumors such as pancreatic cancer is uncertain.

HYPERPLASTIC (METAPLASTIC) POLYPS

Unlike hamartomatous polyps, hyperplastic polyps develop from a focal abnormality in cell replication, resulting in an expansion of the proliferative zone of the glandular crypt. The cells lining individual crypts differentiate and mature as a true hyperplastic process, as distinguished from the neoplastic proliferation that occurs in adenomas. The increased cellular proliferation produces a visible polyp with microscopic intraluminal infoldings. Hyperplastic polyps are typically small (<0.5 cm) and sessile and have sharply marginated mucosal elevations composed of parallel crypts aligned perpendicular to the mucosa.

A helpful feature in diagnosing these polyps is a thickened collagen table beneath the mucosal surface epithelium near the opening of the crypt, which stains positively with P-amino salicylic acid. Although hyperplastic features may occasionally be found in adenomas larger than 2 cm, the risk for hyperplastic epithelial changes to progress to adenomas or frank cancers has not yet been established. No case of carcinoma developing in a purely hyperplastic polyp has been documented.

LYMPHOID POLYPOSIS (LYMPHOID NODULAR HYPERPLASIA)

Hyperplastic submucosal colonic lymphoid tissue may occasionally progress to pseudopolypoid lesions that may ulcerate and cause rectal bleeding. The hyperplasia is likely to be a part of a nonspecific response to infection. Submucosal lymphoid tissue is prominent in children, particularly in the distal ileum where it is termed *Peyer's patches*.[104, 105] These nonneoplastic polyps may occur in the rectum, colon, and ileum of children as well as adults.[65] The gross appearance is that of firm, round, submucosal nodules that are smooth or lobulated and occasionally ulcerated on the surfaces, but they are never pedunculated. The lesions are frequently multiple, sessile, and small as seen on sigmoidoscopic examination. The histologic appearance is that of hyperplastic lymphoid follicles with large germinal centers covered by colonic mucosa.

Lymphoid polyps are common, and they are identifiable by barium air contrast enema in almost 50% of children studied.[106] Rectal bleeding is the most frequent symptom, although abdominal pain and diarrhea may occasionally occur. The peak incidence is between the ages of 1 and 3 years. Although the diagnosis is most easily established by sigmoidoscopic examination, barium enema with air contrast roentgenograms may reveal multiple small polypoid defects, relatively uniform in size and with smooth margins.

The etiology of lymphoid polyposis is undetermined, although lymphoid hyperplasia is a normal response to various stimuli including viral or bacterial infections and allergy.[104, 105] These polyps begin to appear during the 1st year of life, peak about the 3rd or 4th year, and diminish rapidly after about the 5th year. Although most lymphoid polyps are self-limiting and regress spontaneously, occasional patients may require surgical management of a recurrent intussusception. The condition should be carefully distinguished from FAP, UC, leukemic infiltrates of the bowel, and lymphoma.

CRONKHITE-CANADA SYNDROME

The Cronkhite-Canada syndrome consists of multiple hamartomatous polyps of the stomach, small intestine, and colon that appear similar to juvenile retention polyps.[68] In the originally described cases, the mucosa of virtually the entire GI tract was replaced by inflammatory polypoid lesions. Adenomatous change has also been observed in the juvenile polyps of patients with Cronkhite-Canada syndrome, and associated colorectal carcinoma has been reported in up to 20% of patients. Associated lesions include endodermal defects such as nail atrophy, alopecia, excessive skin pigmentation, and hypoproteinemia.[68]

The syndrome is rare and usually is recognized in adults, although occasionally cases in children have been reported. This fatal disorder is manifested by watery diarrhea, abdominal discomfort, and anorexia; death results from inanition. The syndrome is distinguished from other conditions associated with polyposis owing to late onset, lack of family history, and unique ectodermal features. The treatment for Cronkhite-Canada syndrome has changed from removal of the polyp-containing organ or segment to use of hyperalimentation, corticosteroids, and antiinflammatory drugs.

TURCOT'S SYNDROME

Turcot's syndrome is characterized by adenomatous polyposis occurring in conjunction with a malignant tumor of the central nervous system, most often medulloblastoma or glioblastoma.[96, 107] Other associated lesions include ependymoma and carcinoma of the thyroid.

Unlike FAP or Gardner's syndrome, Turcot's syndrome is transmitted by an autosomal recessive gene, although some workers suggest that the syndrome may be a variant of Gardner's syndrome. There is a high risk for colon cancer, which develops at a younger age than in FAP. Colonic malignancies may arise from degeneration of the polyps, or they may arise de novo in epithelium between the polyps.[108] The colonic carcinomas in this syndrome are often multicentric. Careful follow-up of the patients and their relatives is recommended.

COWDEN'S SYNDROME

Cowden's syndrome is an uncommon autosomal dominant genodermatosis first described in 1963 and subsequently called *multiple hamartoma syndrome*.[109] The ectodermal, mesodermal, and endodermal anomalies represent a clinical picture of facial trichilemmomas, acral keratoses, and oral mucosal papillomas.[68] Associated breast and thyroid nodules and GI tract hamartomatous polyps have a propensity for malignant degeneration. Colorectal lesions may include hamartomatous colonic polyps, juvenile and lipomatous polyps, multiple small inflammatory rectal polyps, ganglioneuromatous polyps, epithelioid leiomyomas of the rectum, nodular lymphoid hyperplasia of the rectum, and adenocarcinoma of the cecum.[110]

Nonintestinal abnormalities have occasionally occurred in association with Cowden's syndrome including adenoid facies, hyperkeratotic verrucous papular lesions, keratoderma of the palms and soles, thyroglossal cysts, malignant melanoma, vitiligo, pseudoacanthosis nigricans, facial hypertrichosis, dermal fibroma, trichilemmoma, scoliosis, pectus excavatum, bone cysts, supernumerary digits, high arch palate, club foot anomalies, lipomas, hemangiomas, papules of the larynx and oral mucosa, enlarged tongue, and a variety of other lesions.[111] An extensive report on this genetic disorder and its divergent manifestations is provided by Carlson and associates.[110]

NEUROFIBROMATOSIS

Neurofibromatosis type I, or von Recklinghausen's disease, may include submucosal neurofibromas in the gastrointestinal tract that may cause symptoms of abdominal pain or bleeding. The malignant transformation of submucosal neurofibromas into neurofibrosarcomas has been reported.[112]

REFERENCES

1. Wilks S, Moxon W: Lectures on Pathologic Anatomy. London, Longmans, Green and Co, 1875.
2. Platt JW, Schlesinger BE, Benson PF: Ulcerative colitis in childhood. A study of its natural history. Q J Med 29:257–277, 1960.
3. Gitnick G: Current views of the etiology of inflammatory bowel disease. Semin Pediatr Surg 3:2–7, 1994.
4. Coulson WF: Pathologic features of inflammatory bowel disease in childhood. Semin Pediatr Surg 3:8–14, 1994.
5. Adams JT: Toxic dilatation of the colon. A surgical disease. Arch Surg 106:678–682, 1973.
6. Devroede GJ, Taylor WF, Sauer WG, et al: Cancer risk and life expectancy of children with ulcerative colitis. N Engl J Med 185:17–21, 1971.
7. McCaffery TD, Khosrow N, Lawrence AM, et al: Severe growth retardation in children with inflammatory bowel disease. Pediatrics 45:386–393, 1970.
8. Garrett JM, Sauer WG, Moertel CG: Colonic motility in ulcerative colitis after opiate administration. Gastroenterology 53:93–100, 1967.
9. Lichtiger S, Present DH, Kornbluth A, et al: Cyclosporine in severe ulcerative colitis refractory to steroid therapy. N Engl J Med 330:1841–1851, 1994.
10. Orkin BA, Telander RL, Wolff BG, et al: The surgical management of children with ulcerative colitis: The old vs the new. Dis Colon Rectum 33:947–955, 1990.
11. Ferzoco SJ, Becker JM: Does aggressive medical therapy for acute ulcerative colitis result in a higher incidence of staged colectomy? Arch Surg 129:420–424, 1994.
12. Harms BA, Myers GA, Rosenfeld DJ, et al: Management of fulminant ulcerative colitis by primary restorative proctocolectomy. Dis Colon Rectum 37:971–978, 1994.
13. Beahrs O: Use of ileal reservoir following proctocolectomy. Surg Gynecol Obstet 141:363–367, 1975.
14. Soave F: A new surgical technique for treatment of Hirschsprung's disease. Surgery 56:1007–1012, 1964.
15. Parks AG, Nicholls RJ: Proctocolectomy without ileostomy for ulcerative colitis. BMJ 2:85–88, 1978.
16. Fonkalsrud EW: Total colectomy and endorectal ileal pullthrough operation with internal ileal reservoir for ulcerative colitis. Surg Gynecol Obstet 150:1–8, 1980.
17. Fonkalsrud EW: Long-term results after colectomy and ileoanal pull-through procedure in children. Arch Surg 131:881–886, 1996.
18. Martin LW, LeCoultre C, Schubert WK: Total colectomy and mucosal proctectomy with preservation of continence in ulcerative colitis. Ann Surg 186:477–482, 1977.
19. Stelzner M, Fonkalsrud EW: Assessment of anorectal function after mucosal proctectomy and endorectal ileal pullthrough for ulcerative colitis. Surgery 107:201–208, 1990.
20. McIntyre PB, Pemberton JH, Beart RW Jr, et al: Double-stapled vs hand-sewn ileal pouch-anal anastomosis in patients with chronic ulcerative colitis. Dis Colon Rectum 37:430–433, 1994.
21. Kohler LW, Pemberton JH, Hodge DO: Long-term functional results and quality of life after ileal-pouch-anal anastomosis and cholecystectomy. World J Surg 16:1126–1132, 1995.
22. Becker JM: Surgical management of inflammatory bowel disease. Curr Opin Gastroenterol 9:600–615, 1993.
23. McIntyre PB, Pemberton JH, Wolff BG, et al: Comparing functional results one year and ten years after ileal-pouch-anal anastomosis for chronic ulcerative colitis. Dis Colon Rectum 37:303–307, 1994.
24. Fonkalsrud EW, Phillips JD: Reconstruction of malfunctioning ileoanal pouch procedures as an alternative to permanent ileostomy. Am J Surg 160:245–251, 1990.
25. Fonkalsrud EW, Stelzner M, McDonald N: Construction of

an ileal reservoir in patients with a previous straight endorectal ileal pullthrough. Ann Surg 208:50–55, 1988.
26. Fazio VW: Surgery of the colon and rectum. Am J Gastroenterology 89(suppl):106–115, 1994.
27. Fonkalsrud EW: Clinical and physiologic studies with restorative proctocolectomy. Langenbecks Arch Chir Suppl Kongressbd 1118–1122, 1994.
28. Stelzner M, Fonkalsrud EW, Lichtenstein G: Significance of reservoir length in the endorectal ileal pullthrough with ileal reservoir. Arch Surg 123:1265–1268, 1988.
29. Weaver SD, Jensen L, Rothenberger DA, et al: Long-term functional analysis of the ileoanal reservoir. Dis Colon Rectum 32:275–281, 1989.
30. Galandiuk S, Scott NA, Dozois RR, et al: Ileal pouch-anal anastomosis: Reoperation for pouch-related complications. Ann Surg 212:446–454, 1990.
31. Crohn BB, Ginzburg L, Oppenheimer GD: Regional ileitis. A pathologic and clinical entity. JAMA 99:1323–1329, 1932.
32. Brooke BN: Granulomatous disease of the intestine. Lancet 2:745–749, 1959.
33. Lockhart-Mummery HE, Morson BC: Crohn's disease of the large intestine and its distinction from ulcerative colitis. Gut 1:87–105, 1960.
34. Rogers GBH, Clark LM, Kirsner JB: The epidemiologic and demographic characteristics of inflammatory bowel disease. An analysis of a computerized file of 1,400 patients. J Chronic Dis 24:743–773, 1971.
35. Block GE, Michelassi F, Tanaka M, et al: Crohn's disease. Curr Probl Surg 3:173–272, 1993.
36. VanPatter WN, Bargan JA, Dockerty MB, et al: Regional enteritis. Gastroenterology 26:347–352, 1954.
37. Report from National Cooperative Crohn's Disease Study. Presented at the Annual Meeting of the American Gastroenterologic Association; Toronto, Canada; June 1977.
38. Gryboski JD, Spiro HM: Prognosis in children with Crohn's disease. Gastroenterology 74:807–817, 1978.
39. Fonkalsrud EW, Ament ME, Fleisher D, et al: Surgical management of Crohn's disease in children. Am J Surg 138:15–21, 1979.
40. Telander RL: Surgical management of Crohn's disease in children. Curr Opin Pediatr 7:328–334, 1995.
41. Fazio VW, Wu JS: Surgical therapy for Crohn's disease of the colon and rectum. Surg Clin North Am 77:197–210, 1997.
42. Alexander-Williams J: Surgery and the management of Crohn's disease. Clin Gastroenterol 1:469–491, 1972.
43. Richards ME, Rickert RR, Nance FC: Crohn's disease associated carcinoma. Ann Surg 209:764–773, 1989.
44. Purtilo DT, Strobach RS, Okano M, et al: Epstein-Barr virus-associated lymphoproliferative disorders. Lab Invest 67:5–23, 1992.
45. Palder SB, Shandling B, Billik R, et al: Perianal complications of pediatric Crohn's disease. J Pediatr Surg 26:513–515, 1991.
46. Hamilton SR, Reese J, Pennington L, et al: The role of resection margin frozen section in the surgical management of Crohn's disease. Surg Gynecol Obstet 160:57–62, 1985.
47. Fazio VW, Marchetti F, Church JM, et al: Effect of resection margins on the recurrence of Crohn's disease in the small bowel: A randomized control trial. Ann Surg 225:324–334, 1996.
48. Fazio VW, Galandiuk S, Jagelman DG, et al: Strictureplasty in Crohn's disease. Ann Surg 210:621–625, 1989.
49. Steinhart AH, McLeod RS: Medical and surgical management of perianal Crohn's disease. Inflamm Bowel Dis 2:200–210, 1996.
50. Hurst Rd, Molinari M, Chung TP, et al: Prospective study of the features, indications and surgical treatment in 513 consecutive patients affected by Crohn's disease. Surgery 122:661–668, 1997.
51. Greenstein AJ, Sacher DB, Pasternack BS, et al: Reoperation and recurrence in Crohn's colitis and ileocolitis. N Engl J Med 293:685–690, 1975.
52. Raab Y, Bergstrom R, Ejerblad S, et al: Factors influencing recurrence in Crohn's disease. Dis Colon Rectum 39:918–925, 1996.
53. DeDombal FT, Burton I, Goligher JC: Recurrence of Crohn's disease after primary excisional therapy. Gut 12:519–527, 1971.
54. Janowitz HD: Problems in Crohn's disease: Evaluation of the results of surgical treatments. J Chronic Dis 28:63–66, 1975.
55. Griffiths AM, Nguyen P, Smith C: Growth and clinical course of children with Crohn's disease. Gut 34:939–943, 1993.
56. Telander RL, Schmeling DJ: Current surgical management of Crohn's disease in childhood. Semin Pediatr Surg 3:19–27, 1994.
57. Colcock BP: Operative technique in surgery for Crohn's disease and its relationship to recurrence. Surg Clin North Am 53:375–380, 1973.
58. Mestre JR: The changing pattern of juvenile polyps. Am J Gastroenterol 81:312–314, 1986.
59. Mazier WP, MacKeigan JM, Billingham RP, et al: Juvenile polyps of the colon and rectum. Surg Gynecol Obstet 154:829–832, 1982.
60. Holgersen LO, Miller RE, Zintel HA: Juvenile polyps of the colon. Surgery 69:288–293, 1971.
61. Euler AR, Seibert JJ: The role of sigmoidoscopy, radiographs, and colonoscopy in the diagnostic evaluation of pediatric age patients with suspected juvenile polyps. J Pediatr Surg 16:500–502, 1981.
62. Cronstedt J, Carling L, Vestergaard P: Endoscopic polypectomy in the gastrointestinal tract. Acta Med Scand 210:187–192, 1981.
63. Lipper S, Kahn LB, Sandler RS, et al: Multiple juvenile polyposis: A study of the pathogenesis of juvenile polyps and their relationship to colonic adenomas. Hum Pathol 12:804–813, 1981.
64. Grotsky HW, Rickert RR, Smith WD, et al: Familial juvenile polyposis coli. A clinical and pathologic study of a large kindred. Gastroenterology 82:494–501, 1982.
65. Louw JH: Polypoid lesions of the large bowel in children with particular reference to benign lymphoid polyposis. J Pediatr Surg 3:195–209, 1968.
66. Reed TE, Neal JV: A genetic study of multiple polyposis of the colon. Am J Hum Genet 7:236–263, 1955.
67. Jarvinen HJ, Peltokallio P, Landtman M, et al: Gardner's stigma in patients with familial adenomatous polyposis coli. Br J Surg 69:718–721, 1982.
68. Watne AL: The syndromes of intestinal polyposis. Curr Probl Surg 24:275–340, 1987.
69. Bodmer WF, Bailey CJ, Bodmer J, et al: Localization of the gene for familial adenomatous polyposis on chromosome 5. Nature 328:614–616, 1987.
70. Kinzler KW, Nilbert MC, Su L, et al: Identification of FAP locus genes from chromosome 5q21. Science 253:661–664, 1991.
71. Iwama T, Mishima Y, Utsonomiya J: The impact of familial adenomatous polyposis on the tumorigenesis and mortality at the several organs. Ann Surg 217:101–108, 1993.
72. Bussey HJR: Familial polyposis coli: Family studies, histopathology, differential diagnosis and results of treatment. Baltimore, Johns Hopkins University Press, 1975.
73. Johnson JG, Gilbert E, Zimmermann B, et al: Gardner's syndrome, colon cancer, and sarcoma. J Surg Oncol 4:354–362, 1972.
74. Rustgi AK: Hereditary gastrointestinal polyposis and non-polyposis syndromes. N Engl J Med 331:1694–1702, 1994.
75. Maghal S, Filipe ML: Ultrastructural study of the normal mucosa-adenoma-cancer sequence in the development of familial polyposis coli. J Natl Cancer Inst 60:753–758, 1978.
76. Jarvinen H, Nyberg M, Pektokallio P: Upper gastrointestinal tract polyps in familial adenomatosis coli. Gut 24:333–339, 1983.
77. Pauli RM, Pauli ME, Hall JG: Gardner syndrome and periampullary malignancy Am J Med Genet 6:205–219, 1980.
78. Church JM, McGannon E, Hull-Boiner S, et al: Gastroduodenal polyps in patients with familial adenomatous polyposis. Dis Colon Rectum 35:1170–1173, 1992.
79. Arvanitis ML, Jagelman DG, Fazio VW, et al: Mortality in patients with familial adenomatous polyposis. Dis Colon Rectum 33:639–642, 1990.

80. Duncan BR, Dohner VA, Priest JH: The Gardner syndrome: Need for early diagnosis. J Pediatr 72:497–505, 1968.

81. Bulow S, Holm NV, Mellemgaard A: Papillary thyroid carcinoma in Danish patients with familial adenomatous polyposis. Int J Colorectal Dis 3:29–31, 1988.

82. Sarre RG, Jagelman DG, McGannon E, et al: Coloectomy with ileorectal anastomosis for familial adenomatous polyposis. The risk of rectal cancer. Surgery 101:20–26, 1987.

83. Winde G, Schmid KW, Brandt B, et al: Clinical and genomic influence of sulindac on rectal mucosa in familial adenomatous polyposis. Dis Colon Rectum 40:1156–1169, 1997.

84. Dozois RR, Kelly KA, Welling DR, et al: Ileal pouch-anal anastomosis: Comparison of results in familial adenomatous polyposis and chronic ulcerative colitis. Ann Surg 210:268–273, 1989.

85. Kartheuser AH, Parc R, Penna CP, et al: Ileal pouch-anal anastomosis as the first choice operation in patients with familial adenomatous polyposis: A ten-year experience. Surgery 119:615–623, 1996.

86. Coran AG: A personal experience with 100 consecutive total colectomies and straight ileoanal endorectal pull-throughs for benign disease of the colon and rectum in children and adults. Ann Surg 212:242–248, 1990.

87. Rintala RJ, Lindahl H: Restorative proctocolectomy for ulcerative colitis in children—is the J-pouch better than the straight pullthrough? J Pediatr Surg 31:530–533, 1996.

88. Gardner EJ, Richards RC: Multiple cutaneous and subcutaneous lesions occurring simultaneously with hereditary polyposis and osteomatosis. Am J Hum Genet 5:139–147, 1953.

89. Bulow F: Clinical features of familial polyposis coli. Results of the Danish polyposis register. Dis Colon Rectum 29:102–107, 1986.

90. Jones IT, Fazio VW, Weakley FL, et al: Desmoid tumors in familial polyposis coli. Ann Surg 204:94–97, 1986.

91. McAdam WAF, Goligher JC: The occurrence of desmoids in patients with familial polyposis coli. Br J Surg 57:618–631, 1970.

92. Häyry P, Scheinin TM: The desmoid (Reitamo) syndrome: Etiology, manifestations, pathogenesis, and treatment. Curr Probl Surg 25:227–320, 1988.

93. Anthony T, Rodriguez-Bigas MA, Weber TK, et al: Desmoid tumors. J Am Coll Surg 182:369–377, 1996.

94. Klein WA, Miller HH, Anderson M, et al: The use of indomethacin, sulindac and tamoxifen for the treatment of desmoid tumors associated with familial polyposis. Cancer 60:2863–2868, 1987.

95. Schmitzler M, Cohen Z, Blackstein M, et al: Chemotherapy for desmoid tumors in association with familial adenomatous polyposis. Dis Colon Rectum 40:798–801, 1997.

96. Erbe RW: Inherited gastrointestinal polyposis syndromes. N Engl J Med 294:1101–1104, 1976.

97. Peutz JLA: On a very remarkable case of familial polyposis of mucous membrane of intestinal tract and nasopharynx accompanied by peculiar pigmentation of skin and mucous membrane. Ned Maandschr Geneesk 10:134–146, 1921.

98. Jeghers H, McKusick VA, Katz KH: Generalized intestinal polyposis and melanin spots of the oral mucosa, lips, and digits. N Engl J Med 241:993–998, 1949.

99. Dormandy TL: Gastrointestinal polyps with mucocutaneous pigmentation (Peutz-Jeghers syndrome). N Engl J Med 236:1093–1103, 1141–1146, 1957.

100. Giardiello FM, Welsh SB, Hamilton SR, et al: Increased risk of cancer in the Peutz-Jeghers syndrome. N Engl J Med 316:1511–1516, 1987.

101. Tovar JA, Eizaguirre AA, Jiminez J: Peutz-Jeghers syndrome: Is there a predisposition to the development of intestinal malignancy? Arch Surg 98:509–517, 1969.

102. Konishi F, Wyse NE, Muto T, et al: Peutz-Jeghers polyposis associated with carcinoma of the digestive organs: Report of three cases and review of the literature. Dis Colon Rectum 30:790–799, 1987.

103. Narita T, Eto T, Ito T: Peutz-Jeghers syndrome with adenomas and adenocarcinoma in colonic polyps. Am J Surg Pathol 11:76–81, 1987.

104. Atwell JD, Burge D, Wright D: Nodular lymphoid hyperplasia of the intestinal tract in infancy and childhood. J Pediatr Surg 20:25–29, 1985.

105. Alvear DT: Localized lymphoid hyperplasia: An unusual cause of rectal bleeding. Contemp Surg 25:29–33, 1984.

106. Franken EA: Lymphoid hyperplasia of the colon. Radiology 94:323–334, 1970.

107. Tithccott GA, Filler R, Sherman PM: Turcot's syndrome: A diagnostic consideration in a child with primary adenocarcinoma of the colon. J Pediatr Surg 24:1189–1191, 1989.

108. Moertel CG, Hill JR, Adson MA: Surgical management of multiple polyposis: The problem of cancer in the retained bowel segment. Arch Surg 100:521–526, 1970.

109. Lloyd KM, Dennis M: Cowden's disease: A possible new symptom complex with multiple system involvement. Ann Intern Med 58:136–142, 1963.

110. Carlson GJ, Nivatvongs S, Snover DC: Colorectal polyps and Cowden's disease (multiple hamartomas syndrome). Am J Surg Pathol 8:763–770, 1984.

111. Nuss DD, Aeling JL, Clemons DE, et al: Multiple hamartoma syndrome (Cowden's disease). Arch Dermatol 114:743–746, 1978.

112. Rutgeerts P, Hendricks H, Geboes K, et al: Involvement of the upper digestive tract by systemic neurofibromatosis. Gastrointest Endosc 27:22–25, 1981.

43

APPENDICITIS

Sigmund H. Ein, FRCSC

☐ History

For several centuries before the 18th, there were autopsy descriptions of right iliac fossa abscesses that seemed to involve the vermiform appendix. In the 18th century, some case reports of the illness were written before the patients died. The early 19th century saw some of the giants of medicine and surgery in heated debate regarding the role of the appendix in this disease process. More case reports were published that described perforation of the appendix and that speculated on the role of foreign bodies in that process. In 1886, Harvard pathologist Reginald Fitz published a paper describing the disease, which he termed "appendicitis," emphasizing that it could be diagnosed before the onset of fatal complications.[1]

Three years later, Charles McBurney published his classic paper on appendicitis with emphasis on the etiologic role of the vermiform appendix, the variability of symptoms, the diagnostic value of tenderness at what has come to be called McBurney's point, and the value of early operation.[2] What seems so clear in modern times required more than 2 centuries to sort out. The entire spectrum of appendiceal disease was described in 1905 by Howard Kelly in his book, *The Vermiform Appendix.*[3]

The etiology of appendiceal disease is luminal obstruction and the most common cause of obstruction is a fecalith, a sometimes calcified chunk of stool shaped like an olive pit. Diet apparently plays a major role in the nature of the feces, which is important in the development of a fecalith. Appendicitis is less commonly seen in developing nations where the diet is high in fiber and the stool consistency is much softer. Colitis, diverticulitis, and colon cancer likewise are diseases seen more commonly in societies where low-fiber diets result in harder stools. Not all cases of appendicitis are associated with a fecalith, but in most, some form of obstruction occurs. Lymphoid tissue, which is found in the wall of the appendix, may become hyperplastic in response to viral infections of the gut or the respiratory tract, resulting in obstruction of the lumen of the appendix.

Appendicitis has also been caused by *Yersinia, Salmonella,* and *Shigella* and, very rarely, by a foreign body.[4] The presence of an asymptomatic fecalith is probably reason enough to suspect that at some time acute appendicitis will develop. Occasionally, a patient has recurrent right lower quadrant symptoms that spontaneously regress, which may be an example of a fecalith that passes from the appendix spontaneously. There is a familial incidence of appendicitis that is difficult to explain.

The pathology of appendiceal obstruction has been elucidated mostly in the 20th century. Obstruction of the lumen is followed by distention and vascular changes, which may ultimately lead to necrosis. The appendix is a blind-ending viscus with a small lumen that harbors the gamut of colonic flora. When the mucosal barrier is broken, bacteria invade the muscular wall. The bacteria further compromise the integrity of the appendiceal wall, leading to perforation.

The mixture of pus and stool that builds up behind the obstruction may contaminate the peritoneal cavity or produce an inflammatory mass, usually composed of omentum or small bowel, which is the means by which the body attempts to wall-off or contain the infection. The contamination may be massive and may progress to an abscess. This inflammation may occupy an area away from the right iliac fossa, depending on the location of the appendix. At least one third of appendices are retrocecal or pelvic. If the bacteria extruded from the appendix have contaminated the peritoneum before the process of containment occurred, there may be generalized peritonitis or multiple abscesses.

☐ Diagnosis

The diagnosis of appendicitis is both easy and difficult. The classic clinical history of appendicitis is well known to virtually all practitioners of medicine. The length of history of acute appendicitis seldom lasts more than 36 hours. The story usually begins with abdominal *pain*, which may have been preceded by some loss of appetite or anorexia. The pain is usually periumbilical and moves over the period of 6 to 36 hours toward the right lower quadrant of the abdomen to McBurney's point. The pain is typically steady but may be colicky or cramping. It progresses steadily until appendiceal rupture, when there is a sudden decrease in the localized pain, only to be followed by the pain of peritonitis. The peritonitis may involve just the pelvis or it may be diffuse.

Most patients have some *fever* when the appendix becomes inflamed, but there is no set way to differentiate appendicitis from the myriad of other conditions that may produce pain and fever. Most of the time, however, the patient's temperature does not elevate much above 38°C until perforation occurs. At that time, there is usually an abrupt increase to 39°C or higher.

Vomiting, if present, virtually always begins after the onset of pain in the case of appendicitis. Vomiting that begins before the onset of pain is more indicative of gastroenteritis. *Diarrhea*, on the other hand, which may be mild or severe, usually only starts after the appendix has perforated and the sigmoid colon is involved in the peritonitis. Because diarrhea is such a prominent sign of gastroenteritis, it may confuse the picture and delay the diagnosis.

The signs of acute appendicitis vary from a child who looks a bit unwell and is slightly "flushed," with localized pain in the right lower quadrant, to a prostrated, dehydrated, septic infant or child lying very still and uncomfortable with his or her legs drawn up. The patient with diffuse peritonitis often has grunting respirations, whereas the patient with pneumonia often has nasal flaring, an old-fashioned but tell-tale differential sign.

The emergency department nurse can usually identify the child with early appendicitis, because he or she walks a bit bent over. If asked, the patient will almost always complain of the trip to the emergency department because the movement of transportation aggravates the peritoneal signs.

The physical examination may reveal some degree of abdominal distention, more severe with the onset of peritonitis resulting from perforation. The presence and character of the bowel sounds are directly correlated with the degree of inflammation in the abdomen. Almost all patients have some degree of muscle guarding, localized to the area of McBurney's point in early acute appendicitis. Guarding may be minimal or absent when the inflamed appendix is retrocecal, in which case the normal overlying bowel tends to cushion the tender appendix from the examiner. Guarding may be generalized with the development of generalized peritonitis. Guarding may prevent the palpation of an inflammatory mass, which is often present in the child who lies still with the right leg and hip flexed. Other classic examining maneuvers such as eliciting the psoas sign, obturator sign, and Rovsing's sign tend to be more confirmatory than diagnostic. Getting the child to jump down from the examination table or to hop may elicit tenderness not demonstrated in any other way. Often, the child with acute appendicitis will do that once but not a second time.

Although rectal examination is rarely diagnostic of appendicitis, it is often confirmatory, especially in the patient in whom a pelvic abscess has developed with a ruptured appendix. Rarely does the examiner's finger contact the inflamed appendiceal tip. The rectal examination is best done once by an experienced examiner at the end of the physical examination because it is the most invasive and embarrassing aspect of the doctor-patient encounter up to this point.

□ Laboratory

Laboratory data should be confirmatory, rather than diagnostic, in the evaluation of appendicitis. The usual finding is an elevated white blood cell (WBC) count and increased polymorphonuclear cells and bands. The WBC count is almost always between 12,000 and 20,000/mm³ in cases of acute appendicitis and between 20,000 and 30,000/mm³ after perforation has occurred. It is not rare that appendicitis is accompanied by a normal or even subnormal WBC count. In these instances, the blood smear may reveal toxic granules, suggesting that the patient may not be able to mount an immune response to the inflammatory process. A WBC count greater than 30,000/mm³ is rare and suggests some other acute infectious process.

Dehydration and the level of sepsis determine the hemoglobin levels. The presence of WBCs in the urine should not deter the operation for appendicitis if the other physical findings support that diagnosis.

□ Diagnostic Imaging

Confirmation of the diagnosis of appendicitis is frequently sought when the diagnosis is in enough doubt that operation is not immediately undertaken. Abdominal radiographs without contrast show the gamut of conditions that may be associated with appendicitis but that offer no diagnostic help. The presence of an appendicolith (Fig. 43–1) does not absolutely confirm appendicitis as the cause of the patient's illness but, when coupled with the physical findings, certainly supports it. The presence of a localized inflammatory process in the right lower quadrant, when coupled with the findings of a perforated appendix by history and by physical examination, adds credence to the diagnosis (Fig. 43–2).

A chest radiograph should be done to determine the status of the lungs because cases of right lower lobe pneumonitis can mimic the abdominal pain of acute appendicitis. The peritoneal signs of lower quadrant inflammation would not be present, how-

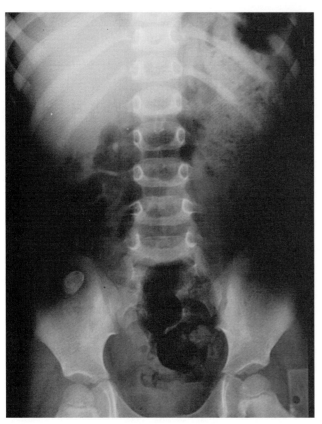

Figure 43–1. Fecalith in appendix (appendicolith) in right lower quadrant.

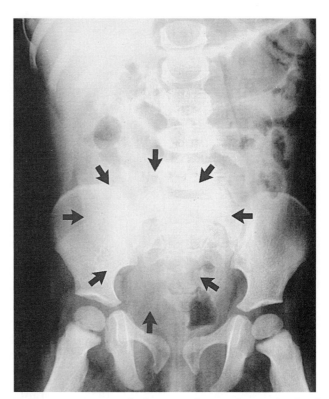

Figure 43–2. Empty right lower quadrant indicating localized inflammatory process or abscess.

ever, and a patient with radiographic pneumonitis and the physical findings of appendicitis probably has both diseases.

Contrast enema is seldom used except when the appendix cannot be "seen" by ultrasonography (US) and the diagnosis is unclear.[5] Such an inflammatory mass may resemble Crohn's disease (Fig. 43–3).[6, 7] Filling of the appendix with contrast to exclude the diagnosis of appendicitis is best done using an upper gastrointestinal series with small bowel follow-through.[8] The need for computerized tomography (CT) in the diagnosis of appendicitis is uncommon.

US has become the imaging study of choice for appendicitis. Although operator dependent, its accuracy is close to 100% for acute appendicitis. The sonographic characteristics of a 6-mm wall, a noncompressible lumen, a fecolith within the appendiceal lumen, and some surrounding peritoneal fluid are diagnostic of acute appendicitis (Fig. 43–4). Once the appendix ruptures, the aforementioned findings disappear and are replaced by peritoneal fluid and thickened bowel loops, and the diagnostic accuracy is reduced.

☐ Differential Diagnosis

Many times there is enough doubt regarding the diagnosis that the surgeon elects not to proceed with an operation. In such cases, the patient is admitted,

given intravenous fluid in lieu of oral intake, and repeatedly examined. The patient's condition invariably worsens or improves. The chances of an acute appendix rupturing under observation on a

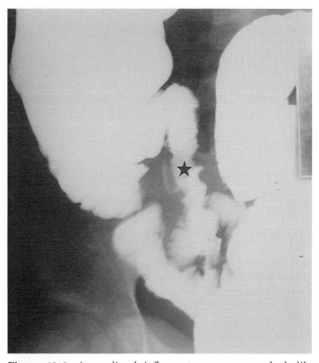

Figure 43–3. Appendiceal inflammatory mass may look like Crohn's disease of the terminal ileum *(star)* on a contrast enema.

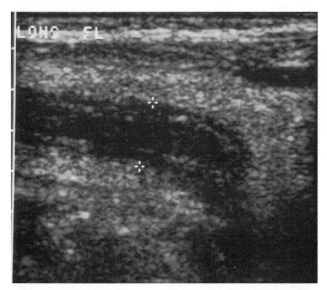

Figure 43–4. Ultrasonographic classic characteristics of acute appendicitis: 6-mm wall, dilated, noncompressible lumen, and surrounding peritoneal fluid. (Courtesy of Dr. Alan Daneman, Department of Diagnostic Imaging, The Hospital for Sick Children, Toronto, Ontario, Canada.)

pediatric surgical service is less than 1%. Table 43–1 lists entities in the differential diagnosis of acute appendicitis.[4, 6, 7, 9–16]

☐ Surgical Treatment

ACUTE APPENDICITIS

The treatment of choice for *acute* appendicitis is appendectomy.[17–20] The nonoperative treatment for acute appendicitis is discussed later.

Once the decision for operation has been made, antibiotic therapy may be started and analgesics given for the pain. It may be advisable to spend some time rehydrating the patient intravenously.

The incision of choice is either the classic McBurney or the more cosmetic transverse skin crease Rockey-Davis incision.[17] The latter incision is more easily extended if necessary.

On surgical entrance into the abdomen, the peritoneal fluid may be cultured for aerobic and anaerobic organisms. Because the antibiotic coverage is so extensive, culture and sensitivity results seldom produce a change and may not be cost effective.

The acute appendix should be handled as little as possible. The cecum can be easily found and delivered into the wound by pulling it upward toward the patient's right shoulder. Cecal attachments to the lateral abdominal wall or an incision that is too small may prevent the delivery of the cecum.

Once the cecum and terminal ileum are out of the abdominal wound, the appendix can be found where the tenia join. One third of appendices are retrocecal and are usually easily freed up by finger dissection. It is almost never necessary to remove the appendix retrograde. Omentum wrapped around

the appendix should be divided and removed along with the appendix.

The appendiceal stump may be managed in a number of ways; all techniques have their advocates. Rarely does the inflammation of an acute appendix involve the cecum to prevent a pursestring suture, if desired.

The wound is usually closed in layers. The subcutaneous tissue can be separately closed before the skin closure. Aggressive saline or antibiotic irrigation of the wound, or the dusting of cefoxitin powder has been advocated to reduce the incidence of subcutaneous wound infections (Sandler AD, Ein SH, unpublished data, 1977). A wound infection rate of 2% can be obtained with intravenous (IV) cefoxitin within 1 hour before operation coupled with the instillation of subcutaneous cefoxitin powder.

An incisional hernia with a McBurney incision is unusual, even in the presence of a wound infection.

TABLE 43-1. Differential Diagnosis for Acute Appendicitis

Abdominal migraine: History important; US; rare
Acute porphyria: History important; US; rare
Blunt abdominal trauma: Abdomen gets worse instead of better; US; rare
Cholecystitis: History and examination important; US
Constipation: History important; US; radiographs
Crohn's disease and Yersinia: Chronically ill with diarrhea[4, 6, 7]
Duodenal ulcer with perforation: History and examination; radiographs; US; rare
Familial Mediterranean fever: History important; appendectomy may help; rare
Gastroenteritis: History and examination important; US; common
Hemolytic uremic syndrome: More like ulcerative colitis; US[9]
Henoch-Schönlein purpura: History and examination; US
Intussusception: History and examination; US; more in infants; common[10, 11]
Malrotation with volvulus: History and examination; always vomit bile; radiographs
Measles: History and examination; US
Meckel's diverticulitis: "The second appendix"; a possibility
Meconium ileus equivalent: History important; cystic fibrosis; US[12]
Mesenteric adenitis: History important; US; often viral; truly rare
Mittelschmerz: History important; US; common
Omental torsion and infarction: Impossible to exclude; rare[13]
Ovarian cyst: History and examination important; US
Pancreatitis: History important; amylase; US
Pelvic inflammatory disease: Examination important; US; not rare
Pneumonia: Flaring of alae nasae; US; radiographs
Primary peritonitis: Rapid onset similar to ruptured appendix[14]
Renal colic: History and examination; US; radiographs
Sickle cell crisis: History and examination important: US; not rare
Small bowel obstruction: History and examination important; radiographs[15, 16]
Typhlitis: Immunosuppressed; appendicitis virtually impossible
Urinary tract infection: History and examination important
Viral disease (coxsackie): Headache; diarrhea; crampy; longer history

---

US, ultrasonography.

A deep wound infection may lead to incisional hernia in other instances.

PERFORATED OR RUPTURED APPENDICITIS

The incidence of perforation of the appendix is 15 to 20% in my experience. The younger the patient, the greater the chance that the appendix will be ruptured. Perforation has been reported, even in premature babies.[21] These patients are much sicker and suffer greater fluid deficits than the patient with acute appendicitis. The temperature elevation is more pronounced. After the diagnosis has been established, there should be several hours devoted to vigorous intravenous fluid resuscitation and appropriate antibiotic therapy. A nasogastric tube should be passed and the stomach decompressed both preoperatively and postoperatively. Operation is undertaken when the patient is hydrated and has begun to defervesce. The nonoperative treatment of a perforated appendix is discussed later.

The abdomen is usually entered through the same type of incision as for the acute appendectomy. On surgical entrance into the abdomen, the pus may be somewhat walled-off by the omentum or the adjacent viscera. The appendix is usually mobilized by the surgeon's finger, and it is virtually impossible to prevent pus from contaminating the wound. Once all of the pus and infected fluid have been suctioned from the area, it is not unusual to see a fecalith at the site of the perforation or lying free in the right lower quadrant. Areas of phlegmon or abscess need not be débrided, nor should any major attempt be made to remove fibrinopurulent exudate in the peritoneal cavity. In some cases, because of cecal involvement in the inflammatory process, it is unwise or impossible to do any more than ligate the base of the appendix. It is extremely unusual to not be able to find the appendix, but if this is so, it is best to place a drain and treat this inflammatory mass "nonoperatively." An abscess cavity is probably best drained with the surgeon's drainage device of choice.

There is little evidence to suggest that anything more than suctioning of pus from the four major abdominal areas is of any value in preventing postoperative infection (phlegmon or abscess). Peritoneal lavage with or without antibiotics or saline has not significantly reduced the incidence of intraabdominal sepsis.[22] In a similar fashion, attempts to "drain" the peritoneal cavity have not made any statistical difference in reducing either peritoneal or wound sepsis.[23]

The postoperative course is protracted depending on the abdominal contamination and the return of bowel function.[24] Triple antibiotic therapy should continue for a minimum of 5 days. If the patient is afebrile and passing flatus, the three antibiotics can be discontinued. Discharge on the 6th day is reasonable if the patient appears well.

The postoperative complication rate is higher in the patient with a ruptured appendix and ranges from wound infection to intraperitoneal abscess and intestinal obstruction.[23]

□ Laparoscopic Appendectomy

The value of laparoscopy in appendicitis remains debatable.[25–28] The point that seems to come out in comparative studies is that laparoscopy is at least as good as open appendectomy in general, but there does not seem to be much evidence that it is better. Nonrandomized studies might have pitfalls that alter conclusions.[26] A randomized controlled trial in 1997 showed that the laparoscopic appendectomy is at least as good as open appendectomy, with the added benefit that initial laparoscopy reduces the rate of misdiagnosis.[27] However, there are false-negative estimates made in which a "normal" appearing appendix removed at laparoscopy shows microscopic inflammation.[28] Unless an obvious cause for the patient's pain is seen laparoscopically, the appendix must be removed without regard to its appearance.

Diagnostic laparoscopy is usually performed through an umbilical trocar with one or two additional smaller trocars used if necessary.[29] For the laparoscopic appendectomy, additional trocars are placed in the right iliac fossa and suprapubically. Bipolar diathermy is used to coagulate the appendiceal mesentery. The appendix is ligated with two preknotted loops and divided with scissors. If the specimen is too large for the standard suprapubic trocar, this is replaced by a larger port or a plastic bag to prevent contact between the inflamed appendix and wound.

There have been some questions raised as to the feasibility of laparoscopy in cases of ruptured appendix, peritonitis, and abscess. One of the disadvantages of laparoscopic appendectomy is the increased operating time and the high cost. Proponents claim that this increased operating time and cost are offset by the shorter hospital stay and faster recovery. Wound infection as a complication of open appendectomy is rarely seen with the laparoscopic technique. There are no reports of postoperative adhesive bowel obstruction after laparoscopy for acute appendicitis but there is the possibility of cautery or trocar injury to the abdominal contents. Overall, laparoscopic appendectomy seems to be equal to, but not better than, open appendectomy.

□ Antibiotics and Infections

The use of antibiotics for appendicitis has changed markedly over the past 3 decades.[23, 24, 30] Before the use of antibiotics, there was a 10 to 20% wound infection and intraabdominal abscess rate in both acute and ruptured appendicitis.[23, 30] The present use of triple antibiotic therapy has reduced the overall infection rate by more than half.

The most common organisms associated with appendicitis are *Escherichia coli, Pseudomonas aeruginosa, Enterococcus, Bacteroides,* and *Streptococcus viridans,* usually occurring in mixed growth. *Bacteroides* and *Clostridium welchii* are the organisms usually cultured from the postappendectomy wound. Because all the common infecting organisms are covered with the triple antibiotic spectrum, the culture of the abdominal pus is not likely to result in many changes in management. Wound culture may reveal the rare infecting organism such as *Yersinia enterocolitica.*[4] Recommended antibiotic regimens are listed in Table 43–2.

☐ Postoperative Complications

Postoperative wound infections should be drained and not reclosed. The rare but devastating *necrotizing fasciitis* and *myositis/myonecrosis* of the anterior abdominal wall is a polymicrobial infection involving group A *Streptococcus, Staphylococcus aureus,* anaerobic organisms (e.g., *Clostridia, Bacteroides*), and *E. coli.* It may be seen once or twice in a pediatric surgeon's lifetime, but its recognition is essential because swift action is lifesaving.[31, 32] The infection occurs early in the postoperative period; fever and crepitance may not be present. Tachycardia, pallor, mottled skin, diaphoresis, and marked redness and edema of the wound point to the seriousness of the infection. The wound pain is impressive. Cutaneous gangrene is an ominous finding. A very high immature (band) leukocyte count suggests necrotizing fasciitis rather than an early wound infection. Large volumes of IV fluids are required for resuscitation to correct the oliguria. All necrotic tissue must be removed. There is a characteristic edematous plane between Scarpa's fascia and the deep muscle fascia. The extent of this plane can be determined by gentle finger dissection. The involved skin does not bleed when incised and must be débrided back to bleeding margins. The infected and necrotic subcutaneous fat has a gray, granular appearance and bleeds minimally. This process can also involve muscle and overlying soft tissues. Intraoperative Gram's stains identify the causative organism. Infectious disease and plastic surgical consultations aid in the management of antibiotic coverage and reconstruction, respectively. The abdominal wall defect resulting from débridement can be extensive and may require major reconstructive sur-

gery. If the infection originates intraabdominally from the site of the appendectomy, bowel resection and diversion are also required. This problem, although rare, leaves the patient with much morbidity and a possible risk of death.

Intraabdominal infectious problems following appendectomy are phlegmon and abscess. A *phlegmon* may be treated with the same triple antibiotic therapy that was used initially. An *abscess* must be drained by an interventional radiologist or by the surgeon through the wound or the rectum. To await spontaneous drainage is unwarranted.[33]

☐ Interval Appendectomy and Nonsurgical Treatment

Alfred Worcester wrote in 1882 concerning appendicitis: "There is only one logical treatment of the disease, namely the excision of the diseased organ as soon as the diagnosis is made."[34] Over the past 100 years, many people have taken issue with this point of view.

In the case of perforated appendicitis, it is sometimes impossible to find the appendix in the inflammatory mass that resides in the right lower abdomen. Drainage of an abscess without removal of the inflammatory phlegmon has been practiced for many years. It has also been the practice of many surgeons to go back for removal of the appendix once the phlegmon has resolved. For more than 50 years, some people have questioned the necessity of this "interval" appendectomy.[35] Many of the patients were well and had no symptoms related to the appendix. In addition, some removed appendices appeared to be normal. Some of the specimens obtained at interval appendectomy were fibrosed and others could not be found.

The rate of recurrent appendicitis in one series without interval appendectomy was 14%.[36] The recurrence is most likely to happen between 6 months and 2 years from the initial attack. The removal of an appendix involved in a second episode apparently is no more difficult than the removal of an appendix never before inflamed.

In the 1.4% of children who were seen an average of 8.7 days after onset of appendicitis symptoms and who had a localized right lower quadrant mass, symptoms were managed symptomatically, with an interval of several months before interval appendec-

TABLE 43-2. Antibiotic Coverage for Pediatric Appendicitis

Type	Drug	Preoperative	Postoperative
Suspected acute appendicitis	Cefoxitin	1 h	None if normal, or once or twice (debatable)
Ruptured appendix	Cefoxitin	With fluid resuscitation	Triples (ampicillin, metronidazole (Flagyl) or clindamycin, gentamicin) for a minimum of 5 days. If afebrile and well, discontinue; if not well, 5 more days.
Postoperative intraabdominal infection	Triple therapy	When discovered	Same as for ruptured appendix

tomy was done.[37] This approach had been used for years in adults and had been advocated for children as long as they did not have generalized peritonitis. Twenty-five percent of pediatric patients get worse while on this treatment plan, which is a definite indication for immediate appendectomy. The addition of the triple antibiotic regimen has resulted in fewer cases progressing to abscess formation. This approach becomes cost effective only if the patient has intestinal function and does not require prolonged hospitalization. Interval appendectomy requires a shorter hospitalization than does operation for perforated appendix.

A recent report of similar treatment for the ruptured appendix in the child with generalized peritonitis is encouraging.[33] Some infants and children receive their IV antibiotic therapy at home *before* "all clinical findings have returned to normal."[33] The 50% of children with a bowel obstruction will not respond to this nonoperative routine and should be operated upon. The efficacy and safety of this plan remains to be demonstrated.

Although a report in 1959 using a similar nonoperative treatment plan for acute appendicitis in children and adults has been termed "successful," there has been little or no move to adopt this approach.[36]

☐ Incidental Appendectomy

The incidental appendectomy is seldom done except in the patient having laparoscopy without other obvious causes for the right lower quadrant pain being found.

Whatever the reasons for the diminishing rate of incidental appendectomy, the reports of the appendix being used for other procedures warrants its being left in situ. The appendix may be used as a means of delivering an antegrade enema to a patient in need of prograde colonic washouts.[38] This procedure may soon be replaced by the percutaneous cecostomy, which avoids the use of the appendix.[39] Other innovative uses for the normal appendix as a conduit have been described. The appendix has been used to replace a ureter and for a ureteroplasty.[40] It has been used as a biliary conduit for cases of biliary atresia and choledochal cyst.[40] The appendix has been used as a conduit for urinary diversion in the reconstruction of cloacal exstrophy.[41] The appendix has been used as a conduit between the gallbladder and the abdominal wall in an infant with Alagille syndrome.[42] A novel use of the normal appendix in the newborn is for irrigation in a patient with meconium ileus.[43] The most common use of the normal appendix is as a conduit for continent catheterization of the bladder.[44]

☐ Special Situations

When fever develops in a child with a *ventriculoperitoneal (VP) shunt* and the child has vomiting, acute right lower quadrant pain, signs of peritonitis,

and an elevated white blood cell count, the differential diagnosis is either acute appendicitis or peritonitis resulting from an infected shunt. Our data show that acute appendicitis develops in 1 in 1100 pediatric patients with a VP shunt and 1 in 1500 children with acute appendicitis has a VP shunt, so the odds of the two existing together are rare. However, missing the correct diagnosis and treatment of appendicitis could be disastrous. US is the best diagnostic means for making this differentiation. If the US study shows that the infant or child has an inflamed appendix, the appendix is removed. If the appendix is ruptured, the lower end of the shunt must be exteriorized until all peritoneal contamination has disappeared.

Congenital malformations of the appendix are rare and range from absence to duplication to a double appendix, which is seen in gastroschisis and vesicointestinal fissure malformations.

Foreign bodies consist of bones, toothpicks, and other slender ingested objects. They may be asymptomatic or the cause of appendicitis. Appendectomy is the treatment of choice for retained appendiceal foreign bodies.

Pinworms are often described in the appendix removed from younger children. They do not cause appendicitis.

Tumors of the appendix are rare, whether benign or malignant.[19] A mucocele is probably the most common benign tumor of the appendix. It is a mucus-containing cyst that is formed distal to a lumenal obstruction. A mucocele may develop after an attack of acute appendicitis in which the appendix is not removed or after an appendectomy in which the stump is not cauterized or inverted. These mucoceles are rare but can attain a large size, and if they are uncomplicated by infection or hemorrhage, they usually remain asymptomatic. When found, they should be removed because rupture may lead to pseudomyxoma peritonei.[45]

Surgical *inversion of the appendix* into the cecum is an unusual but reported cause of an ileocolic intussusception.[11] The symptoms and signs of this presentation are typical for an intussusception by history, examination, and contrast enema.[10] A persistent cecal filling defect requires laparotomy and resection.

Carcinoid is an uncommon, potentially malignant appendiceal tumor in the pediatric population.[46] The appendiceal carcinoid is still the most common neoplasm of the gastrointestinal tract in childhood. The tumor is usually discovered incidentally by the pathologist. The appendiceal carcinoid is different from those that occur in the small bowel in that it develops from subepithelial endocrine cells and its growth is confined exclusively in the lamina propria beneath the epithelial crypt, showing no connection with the endocrine cells in the mucosal crypts of Lieberkühn (Kulchitsky's cells). Appendiceal carcinoids show strong immunoreactivity with the S-100 protein. The majority of carcinoid tumors are found in the tip of the appendix. Carcinoid syndrome (flushing or diarrhea) has not been reported in the pediatric patient with an appendiceal carcinoid. Most of the tumors are less than 1 cm in size. Whereas only one third of these carcinoid tumors are confined to the appendiceal mucosa, lymphatic invasion is common and vascular invasion rare. Residual, metastatic, or recurrent disease seldom, if ever, occurs after appendectomy in follow-up studies over many years. Based on all of these findings, a carcinoid tumor of the appendix in infants and children without metastases at the time of diagnosis appears to be a benign process, requiring only appendectomy. Right hemicolectomy should only be performed in those patients with a tumor 2 cm or greater. Those who ultimately die of their disease have metastases grossly evident at the time of diagnosis.

Adenocarcinoma of the appendix has not been reported in the pediatric patient, although earlier reports falsely classified carcinoids as grade I adenocarcinoma.[47, 48]

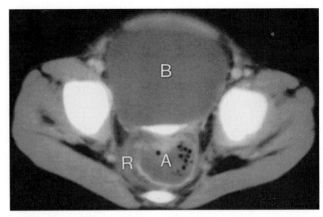

Figure 43–5. Computerized tomography cross-sectional view of the pelvis in a child with a ruptured appendix who has a pelvic abscess behind the bladder and to the left of the rectum. A, abscess; B, bladder; R, Rectum. (Courtesy of Dr. Alan Daneman, Department of Diagnostic Imaging, The Hospital for Sick Children, Toronto, Ontario, Canada.)

□ Retained Fecalith

A 1997 survey of pediatric surgeons in North America showed that the problem of the retained postappendectomy fecalith is significant, morbid, and expensive.[49] Almost 80% of pediatric patients with retained fecaliths have symptoms. Fever is present in 70% and abdominal pain in 55%. Forty-three percent are visible on radiography. An inflammatory mass or abscess is common and the treatment is surgical removal.

For the asymptomatic patient with an incidentally discovered fecalith, observation with periodic abdominal radiographs seems reasonable. If right lower quadrant pain and tenderness develops in such a child, appendectomy is certainly warranted.[50]

□ Bowel Obstruction

There are three types of bowel obstruction that are commonly associated with appendicitis:
1. Approximately 50% of neonates and infants with a ruptured appendix have a small bowel obstruction (Alloo J, Shilyansky J, Gerstle JT, et al., unpublished data, 1997). A lesser percentage of older children are seen with a similar picture. These patients cannot be treated nonoperatively and after the appropriate resuscitation they should undergo operation.
2. The most common type of bowel obstruction that occurs after appendectomy is postoperative ileus, which is often morphine-related and is usually short-lasting. Nasogastric decompression and patience are needed for bowel function to resume. The longer an obstruction carries on, the greater the chance that it is due to an intraabdominal inflammatory process. CT demonstrates the abscess, which usually must be drained (Fig. 43–5). Postoperative intussusception is rarely diagnosed before operative treatment.[51]
3. There is a 5% incidence of postoperative adhesive obstruction in children after laparotomy for any reason.[15, 16] Eighty percent of these obstructions occur within 2 years of the original operation. The later an adhesive obstruction presents, the less likely it will be relieved by decompression alone.

□ Sterility

There has been continuing concern about the possible relationship of ruptured appendicitis and infertility in female patients.[52] Tubal disease is the common cause of infertility. Most publications show that perforated appendicitis in the pediatric female has little, if any, role in subsequent infertility.[53]

□ Chronic Appendicitis (Appendiceal Fecalith Syndrome)

Chronic right lower quadrant pain in children is a problem. When associated with a fecalith, appendectomy is clearly indicated.

In the child without a visible fecalith, diagnostic laparoscopy was proposed as an alternative to laparotomy, but no abnormalities were seen at laparoscopy in more than half of the children and 40% continued to have pain.[28] Appendectomy relieves the symptoms in more than 90% of these children.

REFERENCES

1. Fitz RH: Perforating inflammation of the vermiform appendix; with special reference to its early diagnosis and treatment. Am J Med Sci 1:321–346, 1886.

2. McBurney C: Disease of the vermiform appendix. N Y Med 50:676–684, 1889.
3. Kelly HA, Hurnden E: The Vermiform Appendix. Philadelphia, WB Saunders, 1905.
4. Karmali MA, Toma S, Schiemann DA, et al: Infection caused by *Yersinia enterocolitica* serotype 0:21. J Clin Microbiol 15:596–598, 1982.
5. Hatch EI, Naffis D, Chandler NW: Pitfalls in the use of barium enema in early appendicitis in children. J Pediatr Surg 16:309–312, 1981.
6. Jacobson S: Crohn's disease of the appendix, manifested as acute appendicitis with postoperative fistula. Am J Gastroenterol 71:592–597, 1979.
7. Crohn BB, Yarnis H: Regional Ileitis (2nd ed). New York, Grune and Stratton, 1958, pp 5–22.
8. Schisgall RM: A reappraisal of the role of laparotomy for recurrent abdominal pain in children. In Brooks BJ (ed): Controversies in Pediatric Surgery. Austin, TX, University of Texas Press, 1984, pp 50–59.
9. Tapper D, Tarr P, Avner E, et al: Lessons learned in the management of hemolytic uremic syndrome in children. J Pediatr Surg 30:158–163, 1994.
10. Ein SH, Stephens CA: Intussusception: 354 cases in 10 years. J Pediatr Surg 6:16–27, 1971.
11. Krasna IH, Beardmore HE: Appendicocecal intussusception: A case report. Can J Surg 12:229–232, 1969.
12. Coughlin JP, Gauderer MWL, Stern RC, et al: The spectrum of appendiceal disease in cystic fibrosis. J Pediatr Surg 25:835–839, 1990.
13. Rich RH, Filler RM: Segmental infarction of the greater omentum: A cause of acute abdomen in childhood. Can J Surg 26:241–243, 1983.
14. Ein SH: Primary peritonitis. In Welch KJ, Randolph JG, Ravitch MM, et al (eds): Pediatric Surgery (4th ed). Chicago, Year Book Medical 1986, pp 976–978.
15. Janik JS, Ein SH, Filler RM, et al: An assessment of the surgical treatment of adhesive small bowel obstruction in infants and children. J Pediatr Surg 16:225–229, 1981.
16. Wales PM, Murphy JJ, Janzen R, et al: Adhesive small bowel obstruction in children predictions of outcome. Presented at the Meeting of the Canadian Association of Paediatric Surgeons; Banff, Alberta, Canada; October 1997.
17. Shackelford RT: Surgery of the Alimentary Tract. Philadelphia, WB Saunders, 1955, pp 2562–2567.
18. Madden JL: Atlas of Technics in Surgery. New York, Appleton & Lange, 1958, pp 310–313.
19. Shackelford RT: Surgery of the Alimentary Tract. Philadelphia, WB Saunders, 1955, pp 1352–1376.
20. Kingsley DPE: Some observations on appendectomy with particular reference to technique. Br J Surg 56:491–496, 1969.
21. Firor HV, Myers HAP: Perforating appendicitis in premature infants. Surgery 56:581–583, 1964.
22. Sherman JO, Luck SR, Borger JA: Irrigation of the peritoneal cavity for appendicitis in children: A double blind study. J Pediatr Surg 11:371–374, 1976.
23. David IB, Buck JR, Filler RM: Rational use of antibiotics for perforated appendicitis in childhood. J Pediatr Surg 17:494–500, 1982.
24. Lund DP, Murphy EA: Management of perforated appendicitis in children: A decade of aggressive treatment. J Pediatr Surg 29:1130–1134, 1994.
25. Humphrey GME, Najmaldin A: Laparoscopic appendicectomy in childhood. Pediatr Surg Int 10:86–89, 1995.
26. Karim SS, O'Regan PJ: Laparoscopic appendectomy: A review of 95 consecutive suspected cases of appendicitis. Can J Surg 38:449–453, 1995.
27. Reiertsen O, Larsen S, Trondsen E, et al: Randomized controlled trial with sequential design of laparoscopic versus conventional appendicectomy. Br J Surg 84:842–847, 1997.
28. Leape LL, Ramenofsky ML: Laparoscopy in children. Pediatrics 66:215–220, 1980.
29. Moir CR: Appendectomy: Open and laparoscopic approaches. In Spitz L, Coran AC (eds): Pediatric Surgery. London, Chapman, 1995, pp 408–410.
30. Shandling B, Ein SH, Simpson JS, et al: Perforating appendicitis and antibiotics. J Pediatr Surg 9:79–83, 1974.
31. Kosloske AM, Cushing AH, Borden TA, et al: Cellulitis and necrotizing fasciitis of the abdominal wall in pediatric patients. J Pediatr Surg 16:246–251, 1981.
32. Waldhausen JHT, Holterman MJ, Sawin RS: Surgical implications of necrotizing fasciitis in children with chicken pox. J Pediatr Surg 31:1138–1141, 1996.
33. Bufo AJ, Shah RS, Li MH, et al: Interval appendectomy for perforated appendicitis in children. Presented at the Meeting of the Surgical Section, American Academy of Pediatrics; New Orleans; November 1997.
34. McLanahan S: Further reductions in the mortality in acute appendicitis in children. Am Surg 131:853–864, 1950.
35. Ein SH, Shandling B: Is interval appendectomy necessary after rupture of an appendiceal mass? J Pediatr Surg 31:849–850, 1996.
36. Coldrey E: Five years of consecutive treatment of acute appendicitis. J Int Coll Surg 32:255–261, 1959.
37. Janik JS, Ein SH, Shandling B, et al: Nonsurgical management of appendiceal mass in late presenting children. J Pediatr Surg 15:574–576, 1980.
38. Malone PS, Ransley PG, Kiely EM: Preliminary report: The antegrade continence enema. Lancet 336:1217–1218, 1990.
39. Chait PG, Shandling B, Richards HM, et al: Fecal incontinence in children: Treatment with percutaneous cecostomy tube placement—a prospective study. Radiology 203:621–624, 1997.
40. Crombleholme TM, Harrison MR, Langer JC, et al: Biliary appendico-duodenostomy: A nonrefluxing conduit for biliary reconstruction. J Pediatr Surg 24:665–667, 1989.
41. Longaker MT, Harrison MR, Langer JC, et al: Appendicovesicostomy: A new technique for bladder diversion during reconstruction of cloacal exstrophy. J Pediatr Surg 24:639–641, 1989.
42. Gauderer MWL, Boyle JT: Cholecystoappendicostomy in a child with Alagille syndrome. J Pediatr Surg 32:166–167, 1997.
43. Fitzgerald R, Conlon K: Use of the appendix stump in the treatment of meconium ileus. J Pediatr Surg 24:899–900, 1989.
44. Mitrofanoff P: Cystostomie continente trans-appendiculare dans le traitement des vessies neurologiques. Chir Pediatr 21:297–305, 1980.
45. Byron RL Jr, Yonemoto RH, King RM, et al: The management of pseudomyxoma peritonei secondary to ruptured mucocele of the appendix. Surg Gynecol Obstet 122:1–4, 1966.
46. Moertel CL, Weiland LH, Telander RL: Carcinoid tumor of the appendix in the first two decades of life. J Pediatr Surg 25:1073–1075, 1990.
47. Otto RE, Ghislandi EV, Lorenz GA, et al: Primary appendiceal adenocarcinoma. Am J Surg 120:704–706, 1970.
48. Qureshi MA, Foley WT, Hafner CD: Adenocarcinoma of the appendix. Arch Surg 87:111–114, 1963.
49. Hunt Z, Gilchrist BF, Nguyen M, et al: Retained postappendectomy fecalith: A not uncommon occurrence. Presented at the Meeting of the American Pediatric Surgical Association; Naples, FL; May 1997.
50. Nitecki S, Karmeli R, Sarr MG: Appendiceal calculi and fecaliths as indications for appendectomy. Surg Gynecol Obstet 171:185–188, 1990.
51. Ein SH, Ferguson JM: Intussusception—the forgotten postoperative obstruction. Arch Dis Child 57:788–790, 1982.
52. Thompson WM, Lynn HB: The possible relationship of appendicitis with perforation in childhood to infertility in women. J Pediatr Surg 6:458–461, 1971.
53. Puri P, McGuiness EPJ, Guiney EJ: Fertility following perforated appendicitis in girls. J Pediatr Surg 24:547–549, 1989.

44

BILIARY TRACT DISORDERS AND PORTAL HYPERTENSION

David L. Sigalet, MD, PhD, FRCSC, MSc

Jaundice in the infant can have a wide variety of causes, many of which are relevant to pediatric surgical practice. This chapter reviews general considerations of jaundice in the infant and discusses biliary atresia, by far the most common cause of surgically correctable disease. A brief discussion of other biliary tract disorders, such as hypoplastic bile duct syndrome, inspissated bile syndrome, idiopathic perforation, and gallstones is included. The latter part of the chapter discusses portal hypertension and its treatment in children.

☐ Embryology and Development

The primordium of the liver arises from a flat plate of endodermal cells on the ventral surface of the anterior intestinal portal early during the 4th week of development.[1] The plate projects ventrally, lying close to the transverse septum just below the heart, and contains the vitelline veins, which later become the umbilical vessels. This tissue segregates from the cardiac area, and the hepatic mesoderm then stimulates developing endodermal cells to form hepatic cells. The mesodermal cells subsequently differentiate into the endothelial cells of the liver sinusoids. These veins break up into multiple plexuses, and hepatocytes proliferate around them. At 6 weeks, blood flows through the left umbilical vein and into the sinus venosus through the ductus venosus. During this time, the liver begins to bulge into the transverse septum and become a true abdominal organ. Intrahepatic ducts appear to differentiate from the hepatic cells in the region of the hilus and spread both into the liver and caudally to join the extrahepatic duct system. The duct system is complete by the 10th week. Bile canaliculi arise in situ and connect secondarily with the developing duct system. From the 6th to 10th week, the liver remodels, with the right lobe increasing in size while the left involutes. During fetal life, a significant portion of the liver is composed of hemopoietic cells, which begin to involute in the third trimester.

Areas of the hepatic duct that do not develop connections with the biliary tree may remain as hepatic cysts in later life. Lymphatic cysts can occur, especially in the falciform ligament.

The extrahepatic biliary tree develops from the hepatic diverticulum, starting at the 4th week. Demarcation of the ductal system into the gallbladder, cystic duct, hepatic duct, and pancreatic duct has occurred by the end of the 5th week. At the end of the 5th week, the ductal system has become a solid cord, which then recanalizes at the end of the 6th week, starting at the common duct and progressing into the liver. From the 5th to the 7th week, the common duct and the ventral pancreas rotate from ventral to dorsal, with fusion of the pancreatic tissue and ducts, thus establishing drainage of the body of the pancreas (dorsal pancreas) via the major duct (of Wirsung), leaving the accessory duct (of Santulli) to drain only a portion of the head of the pancreas (see Chapter 46). The common bile duct and pancreatic duct are enveloped in a common sheath of muscle fibers derived from mesenchyme of the common duct during the 11th week, which then forms the sphincter of Oddi. In roughly 75% of patients, the septum between the two ducts resorbs, creating a "common channel" where the pancreatic and common duct contents can mix; this may extend proximally outside the area of the sphincter. This may be a factor in the etiology of pancreatitis or choledochal cyst.

☐ Development of Hepatic Function

The liver begins to secrete bile in utero. Bile salts are present in the intestinal lumen after the 4th month. However, there is significant and variable immaturity in hepatic conjugation and transport of bile in the neonate.[2]

☐ Causes of Jaundice and Cholestasis in Infancy

The pediatric surgeon's involvement in the assessment and the subsequent care of the infant with jaundice varies greatly within different settings. In the community hospital, the surgeon may be called on to evaluate a wide variety of normal infants with straightforward physiologic or breast milk jaundice. Conversely, in the tertiary care setting, there may be a number of infants with total parenteral nutrition (TPN) cholestasis as well as metabolic causes that require evaluation (Table 44–1). Although surgical intervention is usually not necessary, if it is indicated, it must be done in a timely fashion. One of the most useful distinguishing features is the timing of the presentation of jaundice and whether the bilirubin is conjugated.[2]

UNCONJUGATED HYPERBILIRUBINEMIA

Unconjugated hyperbilirubinemia is a common condition in the newborn, and any process that either increases the breakdown of red cells or decreases the capacity of the liver to conjugate causes worsening of hyperbilirubinemia. An indirect bilirubin measurement greater than 1 mg/dl or a total bilirubin measurement of 3 mg/dl is abnormal.

Physiologic jaundice occurs within 2 to 4 days of delivery and disappears in 2 weeks (see Table 44–1). It is worse in stressed and premature infants. There is a significant risk of kernicterus if the indirect bilirubin exceeds 5 or total bilirubin exceeds 19 mg/dl. Prematurity lowers the threshold for treatment.[2, 3] In such cases, after blood for screening is obtained, patients are given phototherapy, which converts bilirubin IX-α into a more stable geometric isomer. Exchange transfusion is used if the bilirubin level exceeds 20 mg/dl. Such high bilirubin levels are most commonly associated with hemolytic disease in the newborn. This is much less common with the widespread use of prophylaxis for Rh-positive mothers. Typically, the baby is seen within the first few days with deep jaundice, caused by anti-Rh antibodies from the mother; these are detected with

TABLE 44-1. Causes of Jaundice and Cholestasis in Infancy

Disease	Age at Onset	Clinical Features	Diagnostic Test	Treatment
Unconjugated Hyperbilirubinemia				
Hemolytic disease	Birth–2 d	Severe jaundice, early	Positive Coombs's	Phototherapy exchange transfusion
Physiolgic jaundice	3–7 d	Increased with neonatal stress	Nonspecific	Phototherapy
Breast milk jaundice	1–8 wk	Benign	Nonspecific	D/C breast feeding ± phenobarbital
Congenital hemolytic disorders	1–8 wk	Progressive	Red cell fragility, specific tests for G6PD or pyruvate kinase levels	Variable, supportive
Metabolic	1–8 wk	Variable	Specific for disease (e.g., Crigler-Najjar, hypothyroidism)	Specific for disease
Conjugated Hyperbilirubinemia				
Inspissated bile syndrome	1st wk	Hemolytic disorders with exchange transfusion	US	Supportive, ± biliary tract irrigation
Bacterial infections	1st wk	Signs of sepsis	Blood culture + US	Supportive
Vascular cause	1st wk	Shock; congenital heart disease	US, echocardiogram	Supportive
Biliary atresia	After 1st wk	Well otherwise	US, liver biopsy, HIDA scan, open cholangiogram	Kasai portoenterostomy
Choledochal cyst	After 1st wk	May have sepsis, palpable mass	US, HIDA scan, open cholangiogram	Supportive/ reconstruction
Paucity of bile ducts	After 1st wk	Syndromatic form associated with Alagille's syndrome	US, liver biopsy, HIDA scan, open cholangiogram	Supportive/ ursodeoxycholic acid
Metabolic	After 1st wk	Varies with syndrome, galactosemia, α₁-antitrypsin deficiency, tyrosinemia, cystic fibrosis	Metabolic screening, HIDA scan, may require open cholangiogram	Specific to syndrome
Infection	After 1st wk	Generally ill	TORCH screen, HIDA scan, liver biopsy may require open cholangiogram	Specific to syndrome
Total parenteral nutrition	After 1st wk	Short gut syndrome, NEC	None specific, US, liver biopsy, HIDA	Enteral feeds
Idiopathic	After 1st wk	Systemically ill	Liver biopsy, US, HIDA scan	Supportive

D/C, discontinue; G6PD, glucose-6-phosphate dehydrogenase; HIDA, hepato-iminodiacetic acid; NEC, necrotizing enterocolitis; US, ultrasonography.

a positive Coombs test. Similar problems can result from congenital hemolytic disorders and glucose-6-phosphate dehydrogenase deficiency.

A common form of jaundice is induced by 6-α-testosterone in breast milk, which inhibits bilirubin conjugation. It typically presents on the 6th to 8th day of life and is treated by phototherapy, if indicated, as well as short-term discontinuation of breast-feeding and institution of phenobarbital treatment of the infant, until the liver matures. Other, more rare, causes include transient familial hyperbilirubinemia, metabolic diseases such as Crigler-Najjar, and global effects of systemic problems such as hypothyroidism. Most of these diseases can be ruled out by a simple history, Coombs's test, and determination of the type of hyperbilirubinemia.

CONJUGATED HYPERBILIRUBINEMIA

In general, conjugated hyperbilirubinemia is more likely to be of concern for the practicing surgeon. It can be difficult to separate the "medical" causes of jaundice from biliary atresia. The clinical presentation for the diseases listed in Table 44–1 is similar: jaundice, light-colored stools, dark urine, and hepatomegaly. Infants with this constellation of symptoms require careful evaluation; the timing of the onset of the jaundice is often useful in determining the cause (see Table 44–1). Infants with biliary atresia are often well nourished and healthy looking in contrast to most infants with "medical" causes of jaundice, in which the infants appear more sickly and have an earlier onset of symptoms.

The potential metabolic causes should prompt a careful family history. In the initial evaluation, screening tests for infectious causes (TORCH screen) and metabolic causes should be done, as should ultrasonography (US) of the biliary ductal system.[4] The US reveals mechanical problems such as a choledochal cyst, inspissated bile syndrome, and spontaneous perforation of the bile duct. If metabolic or viral causes are confirmed in the initial screening and a patent biliary system is seen on US, further investigation is not needed. In most cases, however, percutaneous liver biopsy and a hepatobiliary scan using technetium 99m iminodiacetic acid (e.g., PIPIDA) are useful. Infants should be given phenobarbital (5 mg/kg/day orally) for 5 days before the scan. If there is no excretion of the isotope by the PIPIDA scan and the biopsy shows proliferation of the bile ductules, a presumptive diagnosis of biliary atresia is made. Confirmation of the diagnosis and treatment requires an open operative cholangiogram with wedge biopsy of the liver, and a concomitant portoenterostomy. Because the outcome of the portoenterostomy is dependent on the age of the patient, with earlier operation showing improved results, often the patient is evaluated directly with intraoperative cholangiogram and biopsy, rather than waiting 5 days for the PIPIDA scan.

☐ Biliary Atresia

HISTORY

The first comprehensive review of the pathology of biliary atresia appeared in a series reported by Thomson from Edinburgh in 1891.[5] More than 20 years later, Holmes from Johns Hopkins coined the term *biliary atresia* and described the disease in more detail.[6] He introduced the term *correctable atresia* for those patients who had patent proximal ducts or bile cysts that were amenable to conventional biliary enteric anastomosis. The first successful repair with these was reported by Ladd in 1928.[7] However, few long-term successes were reported, and the majority of these children died of liver failure at age 2 or 3.

The treatment of biliary atresia was revolutionized in 1959 when Kasai and Suzuki reported their technique of hepatic portoenterostomy.[8] This report was largely ignored until the results were reported in English in 1968.[9] The addition of liver transplantation to the repertoire in recent years has allowed the salvage of those patients who are not cured by the portoenterostomy.

PATHOLOGY

The term *biliary atresia* is somewhat misleading, in that the disease is not static but rather a progressive obliteration and sclerosis of the bile ducts. The areas affected and the degree of fibrosis are variable, and presumably reflect different sites of primary involvement by the as yet unknown cause. The typical gross features fall into several patterns as shown in Figure 44–1. This disease was previously classified into "correctable" and "uncorrectable" varieties, terms that are confusing and outdated.[6] The correctable varieties refer to fibrosis in the extrahepatic duct system, with preservation of intrahepatic ducts (type C). This is very rare. It is likely that lymphatic cysts in the hepatic hilum, which are typically devoid of normal epithelial lining, were interpreted as bile ducts. Alternatively, the operative cholangiogram interpreted as showing correctable biliary atresia may have truly been either a metabolic disorder or ductal hypoplasia. The more common varieties of biliary atresia are fibrosis of the entire ductal system (type A) or fibrosis of the intrahepatic ducts with patency of the distal extrahepatic ducts (type B).

Early in the course of the disease, the liver is enlarged, firm, and green. The gallbladder may be small and filled with white mucus or it may be completely atretic.

Microscopically, the biliary tracts contain inflammatory and fibrous cells surrounding miniscule ducts that probably are remnants of the original ductal system (Fig. 44–2). The liver parenchyma is fibrotic and shows signs of cholestasis. There is proliferation of biliary neoductals. This process develops into end-stage cirrhosis if good drainage can-

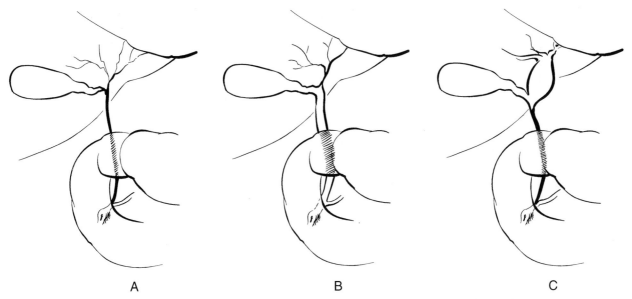

A   B   C

Figure 44–1. Common subtypes of biliary atresia. *A,* Complete obliteration of biliary ducts. *B,* Obliteration of proximal ducts with patent distal system. *C,* Patent proximal ducts with distal fibrosis (often confused with hilar cysts, which lack true epithelial lining).

not be achieved. These early changes are often non-specific and may be confused with neonatal hepatitis or metabolic diseases.

ETIOLOGY

Biliary atresia is a progressive disease. Many of these infants have definite excretion of bile at birth, which progresses to complete biliary obstruction. The incidence varies in different racial populations: the North American average is 1 in 10,000, with an apparent increase in the Native American population.[10] The etiology of biliary atresia is unclear. Various hypotheses, including viral infection and ischemic and autoimmune processes, have been proposed to explain the disease characteristics. The infantile obstructive cholangiopathy hypothesis suggests that a single process, likely viral, results in a spectrum of congenital problems, including biliary atresia, choledochal cysts, or neonatal hepatitis.[11] The suggested etiologic agent infects the liver parenchyma as well as the bile duct epithelium; the site of dominant infection determines the subsequent pathology. This is likely too general a hypothesis, because there is no apparent reason why these three diseases should have a single primary origin. More popular is the theory that a viral agent (e.g., reovirus 3) specifically infects the biliary system; this agent has been shown to cause a disease similar to biliary atresia in mice, but the results in humans have been conflicting.[12–14] Other possible causes of biliary atresia include a failure of canalization of the bile ducts, ischemia, toxic injury, or immunologic causes.[1, 15–18] Clinical observations provide clues about the etiology: the observed discordance in twins suggests an acquired defect, the rarity in stillborn and newborn infants suggests a progressive phenomenon, and the apparent clustering of cases also points to infectious etiology.[19–21] However, the insult seems to occur early in development; 15% of cases occur in association with other malformations, the most common being the polysplenia syndrome, which includes polysplenia, malrotation, preduodenal portal vein, absent vena cava, and situs inversus. This constellation of findings suggests an embryologic "event" occurs at the 6th week of gestation. The spectrum of disease as seen clinically may reflect a variety of causes, with no one cause being fundamental.

DIAGNOSIS

The initial evaluation and assessment of the patient with jaundice is discussed previously. If another diagnosis cannot be firmly established quickly, infants with cholestatic jaundice should be assessed with open biopsy and a cholangiogram. Previous fears that exploratory laparotomy would exacerbate neonatal hepatitis have not been borne out in my experience.[4]

Exploration is performed through a small laparotomy incision, planned to allow a subsequent Kasai procedure and transplantation if necessary. Coagulopathy should be corrected with vitamin K and/or fresh-frozen plasma. A nasogastric (NG) tube is placed and broad-spectrum antibiotic coverage (ampicillin/gentamicin) provided. After visualization of the liver and gallbladder, an open biopsy is done and the specimen sent for frozen section; the cholangiogram is done using a small catheter introduced into the fundus of the gallbladder and secured with a pursestring suture. In one third of cases, no gallbladder lumen can be found. Injection of 3 to 4 ml of dilute dye provides good visualization. In roughly 75% of cases of true biliary atresia,

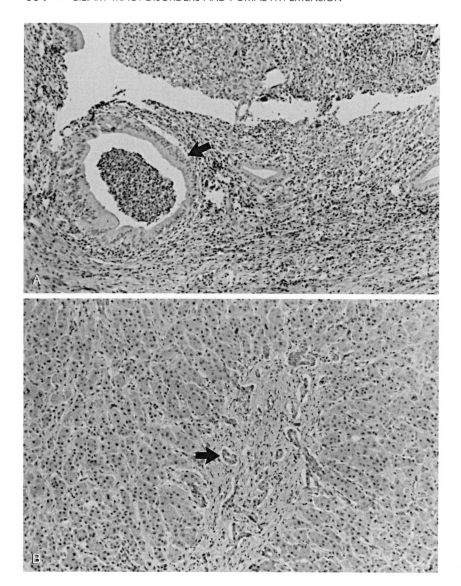

Figure 44–2. *A,* Biliary ducts in biliary atresia. Note surrounding inflammation, and inspissated material within duct lumen (*solid arrow* indicates intrahepatic duct). *B,* Liver parenchyma in biliary atresia (*solid arrow* indicates proliferating bile ductal).

the common bile duct is obliterated, so no cholangiogram is possible. The operation is directed by the gross morphology. Conversely, if the cholangiogram shows patency of the ducts from the liver to the duodenum, biliary atresia is excluded (Fig. 44–3). Syndromes such as paucity of bile duct syndrome, Alagille's syndrome, or α_1-antitrypsin deficiency are associated with small, but patent, intrahepatic ducts. Careful inspection demonstrates visualization of the intrahepatic biliary tree down to the second-generation radicals, but no further. Further operation is not necessary. Conversely, if obliterated ducts are seen or no cholangiogram is possible, a portoenterostomy is indicated.

OPERATIVE TECHNIQUE

Kasai Portoenterostomy

Once the diagnosis is confirmed, the incision is extended to a full right subcostal incision, extending to the left side. The Kasai hepatic portoenterostomy is an unusual type of anastomosis; it consists of

removal of the obliterated extrahepatic ducts, with anastomosis of the mucosa-lined intestinal conduit to the liver hilum. Success depends on bile flow from the tiny residual ducts of the fibrous remnant into the intestinal conduit.

The operation begins with mobilization of the gallbladder, following the cystic duct, to the junction with the extrahepatic duct remnants (Fig. 44–4). The common duct is divided distally and then dissected toward the hepatic hilum with traction superiorly, typically using a long silk tie around the common duct (Fig. 44–5). The cord of fibrous tissue is dissected free up to the hilum of the liver. It is important to meticulously resect the fibrous mass up to the segmental branching of the portal vein on the right and to the level of the falciform ligament on the left.[9, 22] The fibrous tissue is transected as high as possible, flush with the liver surface. There is often apparent neovascularization of the fibrous tissue, and it is important not to cauterize or ligate these vessels, because this action may damage the underlying microscopic ducts. The use of frozen

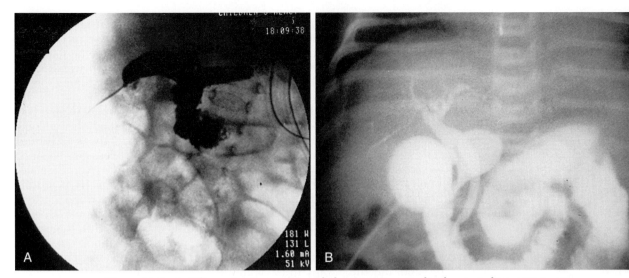

Figure 44–3. *A,* Biliary atresia, operative cholangiogram; note distal patent duct system, no intrahepatic duct seen. *B,* Hypoplastic bile duct, operative cholangiogram; note tiny intrahepatic radicals (patient had α₁-antitrypsin deficiency).

section to confirm bile ductals within the transected specimen is controversial. The demonstration of ducts with a lumen greater than 100 to 150 μm probably does indicate a greater likelihood of successful function postoperatively.[23] However, it has not been shown that aggressive dissection to achieve a larger duct size is useful, and it is likely that the severity of intrahepatic biliary disease and the associated liver damage is the most important ultimate predictor of success.[24]

The dissection and visualization of the hilum are critical. The use of a self-retaining mechanical retractor, headlight, and loupe magnification is useful. Some authorities dissect completely around the hepatic artery and portal vein branches.[22, 25] However, in my experience, this leads to a significant increase in bleeding and may ultimately be deleterious, espe-

cially if subsequent transplantation is required. Dissection of the porta to the level of the secondary branching of the portal veins does ensure that all potential bile ducts will be drained postoperatively (see Fig. 44–4).

After the transection of the fibrous mass, the operation is completed using a Roux-en-Y limb of jejunum (both limbs should be greater than 25 cm), bringing the free limb through the mesentery of the transverse colon. The anastomosis is done using an interrupted single layer of 5.0 to 6.0 monofilament polydioxanone sutures posteriorly and a running suture of the same material anteriorly. The sutures are placed in the liver parenchyma and vascular epithelium (e.g., of portal vein and hepatic artery) surrounding the fibrous cord, not in the cord itself. A Jackson-Pratt drain is placed posteriorly, and the abdominal wall is closed in layers.

Although enteric valves have been advocated to prevent bile reflux and reduce the incidence of postoperative cholangitis, I do not find these to be use-

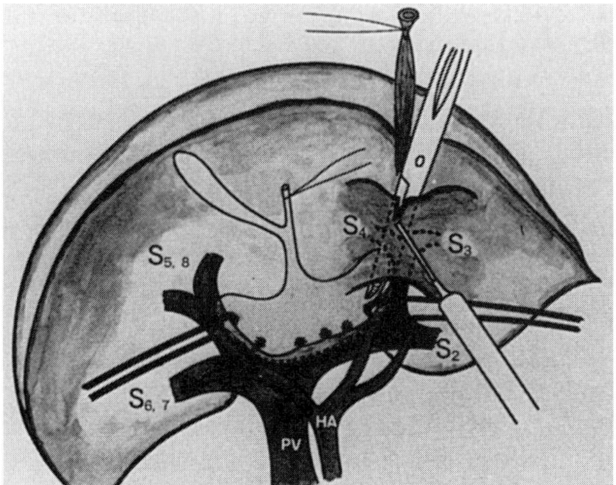

Figure 44–4. Operative landmarks during Kasai portoenterostomy showing dissection of the hilar plate to the level of the segmental branching of the portal vein on each side. HA, heptic artery; PV, portal vein; S, Couinaud segment.

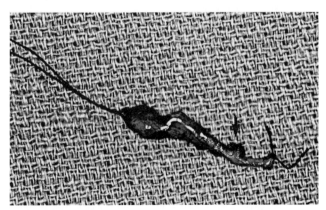

Figure 44–5. Biliary atresia, resected biliary tree. Arrow indicates ductal remnants and hepatic hilum. Silk tie is on distal common bile duct remnant.

ful, and comparative studies have shown no benefit to the procedures.[26] The use of exteriorized loops in the Roux limb have been shown to increase blood loss and morbidity if subsequent transplantation is required.

If either the proximal or distal biliary tree is patent (see Fig. 44–1, types B or C), then variations on this operation can be performed. If the gallbladder and the distal biliary system are patent, a gallbladder Kasai procedure can be performed. In this procedure, the gallbladder is dissected for anastomosis to the liver hilum. The distal common bile duct continues to function normally. Although this procedure reduces the incidence of postoperative cholangitis, the hypoplastic cystic and common duct may not accept the full volume of bile drainage initially. The gallbladder must be drained postoperatively. If the proximal bile ducts are patent but the distal common duct is obliterated, then essentially a choledochojejunostomy can be performed. This is a rare circumstance, and when encountered should theoretically have an improved outcome compared to other subtypes.

POSTOPERATIVE CARE

Postoperatively, the stomach is decompressed with an NG tube until gut function returns. Once the child resumes feeding, the Jackson-Pratt drain is also removed. Broad-spectrum antibiotics are continued for only 1 day postoperatively, but, when oral feedings begin, amoxicillin is given at a dose of 25 mg/kg/day orally. At 1 month, this regimen is switched to trimethoprim-sulfamethoxazole (Septra). Steroids are used perioperatively; glucocorticoids (Solu-Medrol) intravenously and then prednisone orally (2 mg/kg/day) are started postoperatively, continued for a month, and then slowly tapered. Both the antibiotic and steroid use are largely empiric; steroids are used both for their choleretic effect and to decrease scarring at the anastomosis.[27, 28] Phenobarbital is probably not useful. Ursodeoxycholic acid (20–40 mg/kg/day in three to four divided doses) may be useful in augmenting bile flow, but only in the presence of patent bile ducts. Bile flow results in brown or green stools soon after bowel function returns. Conversely, if stools remain acholic after the first 2 or 3 days, success is unlikely.

All children require careful postoperative followup for complications and nutrition. My colleagues and I initially use Pregestimil for all infants. If good bile excretion continues, this can be changed to a standard formula after 1 to 2 months. Both water- and fat-soluble vitamin supplements are instituted.

COMPLICATIONS

Cholangitis

Cholangitis is the most frequent complication occurring after portoenterostomy and is most common in the first 2 years. All conduits become colonized within a month of operation. Cholestasis, which occurs in all of these children because of the very small ducts, is the main risk factor for cholangitis. Typically, cholangitis does not develop in children who have no bile drainage postoperatively or in children with a gallbladder conduit.

Cholangitis presents with fever, leukocytosis, and elevations in bilirubin, signs that may also accompany any intercurrent infection in these children. Nonetheless, prompt treatment is necessary because recurring attacks cause progressive liver damage. After initial blood cultures, broad-spectrum antibiotics with good gram-negative coverage are started, and the response is usually prompt. If stools become acholic, a pulse of steroids may be useful. Recurrent attacks of cholangitis require treatment with prolonged intravenous antibiotics. However, such therapy must be monitored closely to prevent the development of continued infection with resistant organisms.

Cessation of Bile Flow

The loss of bile pigment from the stool in a patient with a well-functioning portoenterostomy is a depressing scenario in pediatric surgery. Prompt reestablishment of bile flow is imperative to avoid transplantation. The parents should be warned to report changes in stool color or signs of cholangitis. If cessation of bile flow occurs, a pulse of prednisolone is given in a dosage of 10 mg/kg twice a day.[27, 28] Steroids both augment bile flow and reduce inflammation. If bile flow is reestablished, then steroids are tapered over the next 2 weeks. If bile flow is not reestablished in 3 to 5 days, the steroids are stopped. If the child had good bile flow previously, it is reasonable to reoperate. The anterior wall of the portoenterostomy is taken down and the fibrotic portal plate is cross-hatched with a scalpel at 1-mm intervals. This theoretically reopens scarred bile ductals and allows reestablishment of bile flow.[29] However, multiple attempts at reoperation are not useful and increase the technical difficulties of subsequent transplantation.

Portal Hypertension

Portal hypertension is common following portoenterostomy, even in infants with good bile flow. On initial liver biopsy there is always some element of inflammation and scarring with fibrosis occurring in the intrahepatic parenchyma. In some children, despite good bile flow, this process continues.[30] Clinical manifestations of portal hypertension are similar to those seen in other patients, with the development of variceal bleeding, hypersplenism, and ascites. Portal hypertension and its initial treatment are discussed later. The clinical sequelae of the portal hypertension tend to subside over time, likely because of the development of spontaneous portal-systemic shunts. If portal hypertensive symptoms persist, they are due to worsening cirrhosis of the liver, and these patients require hepatic transplantation. Currently, there are few indications for shunting in patients with portal hypertension related to biliary atresia. Hypersplenism in these patients should *never* be treated by splenectomy, because subsequent transplantation will be complicated by a high sepsis rate.

NUTRITION

In patients with little or no bile drainage following portoenterostomy, attention must be paid to nutrition in general and fat absorption in particular. In these patients, vitamin supplementation and the ongoing use of a medium-chain triglyceride formula, such as Pregestimil, is necessary. As liver function worsens, growth failure intensifies, and home parenteral nutrition may be necessary while these children await transplantation.[31]

RESULTS AND PROGNOSIS

Before the introduction of the Kasai portoenterostomy, biliary atresia survival rates were less than 5% at 12 months.[32] Survival rates of greater than 50% after portoenterostomy have been reported, and, with the addition of liver transplantation, survival rates of greater than 90% should be expected.[33] Nonetheless, the disease remains a frustrating entity to treat because of the difficulty of predicting outcome and the inability to improve on the results of portoenterostomy. The major determinants of a satisfactory outcome following portoenterostomy are (1) the patient's age at operation, (2) the successful establishment of bile flow postoperatively, (3) the presence of microscopically demonstrable ductal structures in the hilum, (4) the degree of parenchymal disease at diagnosis, and (5) technical factors of the anastomosis.

The age of the infant at operation has been shown to affect outcome.[33, 34] In a series of 131 infants, the long-term survival rate was 46% in patients having portoenterostomy within the first 2½ months of life, but only 24% in patients who were operated upon at older ages. This likely reflects the ongoing cirrhosis that occurs with this disease; by 3 or 4 months of age, no ductal tissue is left and only fibrotic tissue remains. Infants who show a significant decrease in serum bilirubin and have feral signs of good bile excretion also have improved results.[10] In patients who have exteriorized shunts, the quantity of bilirubin excretion has been shown to be predictive, with daily bilirubin excretion of at least 10 mg correlating with long-term success.[35] However, in the modern era when exteriorization is not performed, this is not a useful parameter and the short-term normalization of liver function tests is the best predictor of a good result.[10]

The presence of microscopically demonstrable ducts in the hilum is somewhat controversial. Some authors have suggested that duct size is important, but not all agree.[23, 24] Probably the variation in duct size at initial operation reflects the preexisting inflammation, whereas ongoing scarring reflects inadequate drainage and ongoing inflammation.[36]

Finally, the technical aspects of the operation are important. This was demonstrated by a British survey in which patients who underwent operations at centers treating one case per year had significantly worse outcomes than those patients undergoing treatment at centers doing more than five cases per year. This likely represents factors in operative technique and experience in the postoperative management of these patients, both of which are critical to optimize outcome.[37]

LONG-TERM OUTCOME

All patients who have had portoenterostomy require careful follow-up. Patients who have poor outcomes need careful management and early referral for transplantation. Children who have had good bile flow require monitoring of nutrition and follow-up to detect signs of portal hypertension. The debate regarding the utility of the portoenterostomy procedure versus primary transplantation continues.[38, 39] In my experience, the procedures are complementary rather than competing. A significant number of patients who have had portoenterostomy will achieve long-term survival and bile drainage and thus avoid transplantation altogether. It is unclear what percentage of patients will achieve such good long-term results; in my experience, 50% of patients had an initial good response, going on to age 4 or 5 years with good bile flow. Following that, however, they have had an ongoing progression of fibrosis and portal hypertension, which have necessitated transplantation. Ultimately, less than 20% of all patients who have had a portoenterostomy survive to adulthood without a transplant. However, the technical aspects of transplantation in these patients when they are older and larger, as well as the increased availability of organs in the appropriate size range and avoidance of exposure to immunosuppressive medication during the developmental years, suggest that a primary portoenterostomy is appropriate when the patient is seen before the age of 4 months.[40] Conversely, if the child is seen after the age of 4 months with advanced cirrhosis and fibrosis, a primary transplant procedure would be appropriate.

☐ Choledochal Cyst

The initial classification of choledochal cysts was proposed by Alonso-Lej in 1959 (Fig. 44–6).[41] Cystic dilation of the common bile duct (type 1) is the most common form, whereas diverticulum of the bile duct (type 2) or choledochocele (type 3) is more rare. Subsequent classification schemes have added choledochocele with intrahepatic extension (type 4) and intrahepatic disease alone, also known as Caroli's disease.[42, 43] These lesions were once consid-

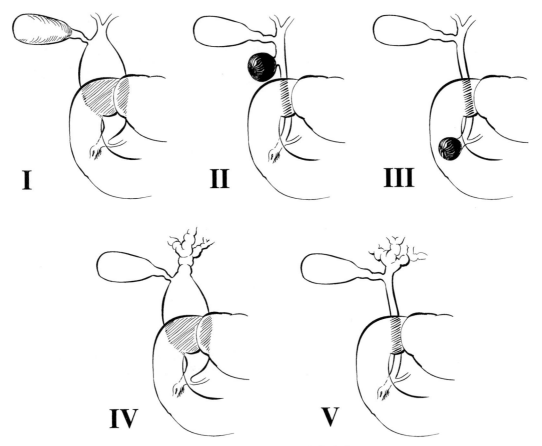

Figure 44–6. Classification of choledochal cyst.[41, 42]

PATHOGENESIS

During the development of the bile ducts, a phase of canalization occurs, which could explain the presence of subsequent ductal dilation; however, this has been difficult to substantiate. More widely accepted is the "common channel theory"; in patients with choledochal cyst, there is almost always a common channel at the junction of the distal common bile duct and pancreatic ducts. Reflux of pancreatic enzymes can occur into the common bile duct where they are activated, causing ongoing mucosal breakdown, fibrosis, and secondary cystic dilation. The widespread use of endoscopic retrograde cholangiopancreatography (ERCP) in the Japanese population has lent credence to this theory.[44, 45] In my experience, the amylase level in the fluid within the choledochal cyst is extremely elevated in all cases, and these patients often have an elevated amylase level at the time of presentation, occasionally leading to a misdiagnosis of pancreatitis. However, the common channel theory does not explain all of the clinical findings, such as the frequent segmental nature of the disease or the development of intrahepatic disease. It is possible that the classification schemes may lump together diseases that have a spectrum of embryonic and pathologic origins.

CLINICAL PRESENTATION

Choledochal cysts appear to be more common in Japan; in all races, the female-to-male ratio is roughly 4:1.[44] Patients typically are seen in the first 10 years of life, and, in my experience, Caucasian patients often have a North American Indian ancestry.

Most children have mild intermittent jaundice, often present for some time before diagnosis. The classic triad of abdominal pain, jaundice, and an abdominal mass occurs in only one third of children.[46] Pancreatitis should be actively ruled out in patients with elevated enzyme levels and pain. Patients may also have sepsis and cholangitis, or, infrequently, the cyst may rupture, causing an "acute" surgical abdomen.

Choledochal cyst presentation in infancy is often not associated with symptoms other than unremitting jaundice. In these infants, the distal obstruction can be extreme; however, the proximal ductal systems are normal or enlarged, in marked contrast to biliary atresia.

PATHOLOGY

Grossly, the typical form of type 1 choledochal cyst shows an enormously dilated common duct with a relatively thin wall; microscopically, this is entirely fibrous connective tissue, with no normal mucosa.

DIAGNOSIS

US is the best initial study for choledochal cyst. With high-resolution scanning, accurate delineation of the cyst and the intrahepatic ducts can be done. This may be the only diagnostic test that is necessary. Occasionally, the patient may require a computed tomography scan or biliary imaging with a technetium[99m] PIPIDA scan. In rare instances, percutaneous transhepatic cholangiography or ERCP may be useful. However, the ERCP may initiate pancreatitis.

TREATMENT

The treatment of choice for choledochal cyst is excision with direct anastomosis of the proximal normal bile duct to a Roux-en-Y loop of jejunum. External drainage is reserved for cases of emergent decompression in high-risk patients and should be used as a temporizing measure. Cyst enterostomy should not be done because of the high rate of stricture and the possibility of malignancy developing later.[47]

OPERATIVE TECHNIQUE

The important features of choledochal cyst resection are (1) accurate delineation of the anatomy, (2) resection of any epithelial lining in the cyst, and (3) direct anastomosis of the jejunal limb to normal, mucosa-lined biliary tree. Accordingly, I strongly recommend intraoperative cholangiography, which allows determination of the proximal extent of disease (Fig. 44–7). The body of the cyst can be resected either in total or by dissecting the inner plane of the cyst, leaving the outer fibrous shell.[46] Typically, there have been prolonged, recurrent episodes of cholangitis and the cyst wall is adherent to the adjacent portal vein; in these cases, excision of the lining mucosa is safest. Conversely, if the inflammation has not been so profound, it is better to remove the entire cyst.

It is often difficult to locate the distal common bile duct (CBD). I recommend dissection on the outside of the choledochal cyst to find the typically small distal CBD as it enters into the pancreas (see Fig. 44–8). This distal CBD is suture ligated with permanent suture. The body of the cyst is dissected proximally, resecting the gallbladder, if necessary, until the normal ductal system is encountered. If this distinction is not clear, intraoperative frozen section can be used to confirm an intact mucosal lining in the proximal duct. In the case of type 1

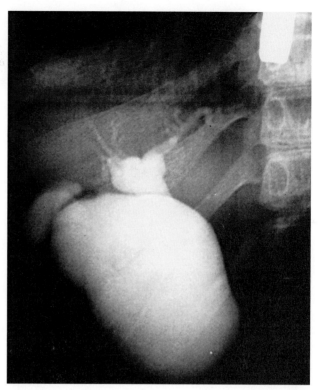

Figure 44–7. Choledochal cyst (type 1, operative cholangiogram).

cyst, the proximal ducts are then drained into a Roux-en-Y limb of jejunum. The anastomosis is done using a continuous 5-0 or 6-0 polydioxanone monofilament suture. If extensive inflammation exists, my colleagues and I have used an internal stent of a 5-French umbilical artery catheter tunneled into the jejunum limb and left across the anastomosis both to stent and decompress the hepatic ducts. This technique is also used for type 4 or type 5 cysts in which the intrahepatic ducts may be dilated. Type 5 cyst (Caroli's disease) with intrahepatic disease confined to one lobe can be resected. However, if intraparenchymal dilations exist, then recurrent stasis with stones can result. This can be a difficult situation to manage, and occasionally transhepatic stents with a U tube may be required. Type 3 choledochocele is relatively rare; the cyst is typically lined by duodenal mucosa. The choledochocele is unroofed by a transduodenal approach, and a sphincteroplasty is performed. Type 2 cyst requires resection and reanastomosis of the common duct. If the duct is very small, anastomosis over a stent may be indicated.

A Jackson-Pratt drain is used and removed once bowel function returns. Postoperatively, the patient's liver function should be followed up with serial enzyme tests. US done on an annual basis detects further bile duct changes.

RESULTS

Results are typically good, with most patients having an uncomplicated postoperative course. De-

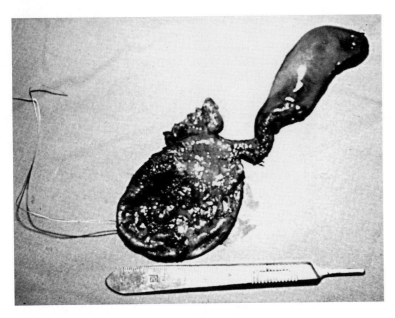

Figure 44–8. Choledochal cyst (type 1, operative specimen). Note tie on distal common duct.

layed complications include ductal stricture, cholangitis, sepsis, hepatic failure, carcinoma, and portal hypertension.[47] Patients who have had previous drainage using a bowel-to-cyst anastomosis should electively have the remaining cyst removed. The rate of malignancy is definitely lowered if cyst excision is complete.[45, 47] When incomplete excision has been performed, the incidence of cholangiocarcinoma is 2.5 to 5%, 20 times higher than that in the general population, with a survival time of less than 1 year after cancer is detected.[47]

☐ Other Biliary Tract Disorders

HYPOPLASIA OF THE BILE DUCTS

Hypoplasia of the bile ducts is impossible to distinguish from biliary atresia without an operative cholangiogram. It is not a specific diagnosis, but it is seen with a variety of hepatobiliary-biliary disorders in which diminished bile flow occurs, such as neonatal hepatitis or α_1-antitrypsin deficiency, or as a result of a true hypoplasia of the bile ducts. Such congenital paucity of the bile ducts may occur as either an isolated lesion (nonsyndromic) or as part of a more generalized problem such as Alagille's syndrome.

Typically, the biliary system can be visualized with the cholangiogram, but bile ducts after the second-generation radicals cannot be seen (see Fig. 44–3B). This may represent either atrophy caused by lack of bile flow or a true reduction in the number of bile ducts related to developmental factors. Drainage cannot be improved by surgical measures, and care must be taken during the operative exploration not to crush or damage the already small ductal structures.

Alagille's syndrome is a genetic defect that results in a typical constellation of features: peculiar facies

with a high prominent forehead and deep-set eyes, chronic cholestasis, posterior embryotoxon, butterfly-like vertebral arch defects, and heart disease—usually peripheral pulmonary stenosis. These patients often respond to supportive measures such as treatment with ursodeoxycholic acid and phenobarbital.[48] They often have hypercholesterolemia and may eventually come to liver transplantation because of ongoing hepatic scarring and the development of hepatocellular carcinoma. One feature of the disease is an intense pruritus associated with jaundice, which often makes these patients uncomfortable. Nonsymptomatic paucity of the bile ducts may be associated with liver changes similar to those in Alagille's syndrome but without the associated findings. Treatment is similar for both conditions.

INSPISSATED BILE SYNDROME

Inspissated bile syndrome occurs in infants born to mothers who have preformed antibodies directed toward the infant's red cells; typically, these are anti-Rh, but they can be due to ABO incompatibility. After the child is born, massive hemolysis occurs, resulting in jaundice and alteration in bile composition with sludge accumulating in the bile ducts. This may proceed to the point of complete obstruction or the production of calculi, which may require operative intervention. This disorder responds to simple saline irrigation, which should be done very gently via the gallbladder to minimize iatrogenic mucosal injury.[49] With modern obstetric care, this disorder is rarely seen.

IDIOPATHIC PERFORATION OF BILE DUCTS—BILE ASCITES

Bile ascites typically presents with gradually worsening abdominal distention with jaundice in the newborn infant. The disease may be associated with an episode of sepsis or ABO incompatibility; more typically, it is an isolated finding, likely related to malformation of the duct. The almost universal site of perforation is at the junction of the cystic duct with the common bile duct. US demonstration of free fluid in the abdomen suggests the diagnosis, which can be confirmed with PIPIDA scan.

At operation, sterile bile ascites and bile staining are found. An operative cholangiogram should be done, using the gallbladder. The lesion is almost always self-limiting, and the perforation seals with drainage. Aggressive operative intervention is not indicated, because the small, delicate, presumably congenitally weakened bile duct may be further damaged by attempts at anastomosis.[50]

GALLBLADDER DISEASE

Gallbladder disease in children is diagnosed with increasing frequency. This likely represents both an increased sensitivity, with the widespread use of US, and an increased incidence resulting from the modern diet of developed nations. As well, biliary disease may develop in infants supported with TPN.

HYDROPS OF THE GALLBLADDER

Acute distention of the gallbladder with edema of the gallbladder wall has been reported in association with a number of septic or shock-like states including Kawasaki disease, severe diarrhea with dehydration, hepatis, and scarlet fever.[51] The diagnosis may be suggested by a palpable gallbladder on physical examination, with only mild abnormalities identified in the liver function tests. In almost all cases, the hydrops resolves spontaneously.

ACALCULOUS CHOLECYSTITIS

Acalculous cholecystitis likely represents the progression of hydrops as described for the gallbladder and the development of secondary infection. The entity usually presents after the patient is resuscitated from a primary septic focus or shock-like disease state. Presumably, asymptomatic hydrops of the gallbladder then develops, becoming secondarily infected. Patients are often intubated in the intensive care unit setting, so early manifestations of the disease are not evident; the most common presentation is one of deterioration and signs of sepsis in a previously stable patient. If suspected, the diagnosis can be confirmed with US, which demonstrates gallbladder distention and intraluminal echogenic debris. Hepatobiliary scan shows nonfunction of the gallbladder.

Treatment in mild cases can be conservative with antibiotics. However, if the patient's condition deteriorates, then cholecystectomy is indicated. In patients who are very ill, percutaneous or open cholecystotomy may be a useful temporizing measure.

HEMOLYTIC CHOLELITHIASIS

Pigment Stones

In the past, gallstones in children occurred almost exclusively in patients with hemolytic disease such as hereditary spherocytosis, sickle cell anemia, or thalassemia. In these patients, fluctuating jaundice may occur because of the underlying hemolysis and does not necessarily mean that common duct caliculi are present. These patients are often closely followed up medically and are at known high risk of stones. If symptoms then develop, US should detect stones and cholecystectomy can be performed laparoscopically.[52, 53] An operative cholangiogram should be done. The treatment of common duct stones in these patients is controversial. Few centers possess the expertise to do laparoscopic common duct exploration by laparoscopy. In my experience, if the stones are small (<4 mm) and the common duct is not obstructed, we simply observe the patients. Other centers use ERCP preoperatively.[54] Conversely, if stones are large or a common duct obstruction is evident, we convert to an open common duct exploration.

The management of sickle cell patients has been simplified by the demonstration that a conservative transfusion regimen, which increases the preoperative hemoglobin to greater than 10 g/dl, is sufficient.[55]

In patients undergoing splenectomy for a hemolytic disorder, preoperative US to screen for gallstones should be done. If stones are present, then a combined splenectomy and cholecystectomy should be done. In patients who are undergoing a laparoscopic splenectomy, port placement is different than for the cholecystectomy, but it can be combined with the same procedure. In my practice, we have done laparoscopic cholecystectomy followed by a splenectomy done through a lateral incision with minimal dissection.

CHOLESTEROL CHOLELITHIASIS

Cholesterol gallstones appear to occur in children and adolescents because of the same pathophysiologic disturbances that cause stones in adults.[2] In most North American institutions, the incidence is increasing and has come to surpasses hemolytic disease as the leading cause of cholelithiasis in pediatric patients. The typical patient is a markedly obese young girl; the clinical symptoms are usually of vague abdominal pain, with minimal physical findings. A classic history of fatty food intolerance is often not present. The diagnosis is usually made on ultrasound, and the treatment is typically laparoscopic cholecystectomy. The technique and indications for operative cholangiogram are similar to that described for adults.[52, 53] Cholesterol stones can occur in infants on prolonged TPN or following ileal resection. Cholecystectomy is still the treatment of choice, although these patients typically have had multiple previous operations, and the laparoscopic technique may not be possible.

CONGENITAL DEFORMITIES

A variety of abnormal configuration and locations of the gallbladder have been reported; these are usually of no real clinical relevance unless they impair gallbladder emptying. In such cases, caliculi are frequent, and treatment is almost always with cholecystectomy.

☐ Portal Hypertension

Portal hypertension in children is a particularly challenging entity. There are few conditions that cause more anxiety in both parents and treating medical staff than the sight of a massive gastrointestinal bleed in a young child. The ability to diagnose and treat the conditions that cause this entity has improved greatly in recent years.

The pathophysiology of portal hypertension in children often differs distinctly from that in the adult. The dominant cause of portal hypertension in adults is cirrhosis. The fibrotic process is progressive, and liver failure often accompanies the portal hypertension. Liver transplantation is almost always required for long-term salvage. In children, portal hypertension is often due to portal vein thrombosis. Children often are seen with variceal bleeding but with satisfactory liver function. The ability of the growing child to compensate for portal vein obstruction is extraordinary, but in some instances, surgical therapy is necessary. Treatment in children with portal hypertension is not palliative, but rather it is directed to allow normal growth, development, quality of life, and longevity.

PATHOPHYSIOLOGY

Portal hypertension results from an increase in resistance to venous flow through the liver. The site of the obstruction is categorized anatomically: prehepatic, intrahepatic, or suprahepatic. The prehepatic causes of portal hypertension are relatively unique to the pediatric age group, hepatic parenchymal function is well maintained, and coagulopathy plays no role in the bleeding. Intrahepatic and suprahepatic causes typically have associated liver dysfunction, which increases the risk of bleeding resulting from coagulopathy, increases the formation of ascites, and impacts on all aspects of the child's care. The hemodynamic effects of portal venous obstruction are complex. In experimental animals, it has been shown that, in addition to portal venous obstruction, an increase in mesenteric arterial flow is required to cause an increase in portal venous pressure.[56] The interplay of these hemodynamics changes coupled with the development of collateral vessels in the growing child makes the prediction of long-term results after therapy difficult

and emphasizes the importance of long-term follow-up.[57]

SUPRAHEPATIC OBSTRUCTION

Obstruction of the hepatic vein (Budd-Chiari syndrome) is a rare cause of portal hypertension in children in North America. This syndrome may be seen in association with coagulation disorders, use of oral contraceptives, malignant disease, autoimmune disorders, and hepatic vein webs. The course is typically insidious with a long interval between the onset of hepatomegaly, abdominal pain, and ascites and the recognition of the syndrome. If symptoms develop acutely, it can be associated with severe pain, rapid liver enlargement, and liver damage with central lobular congestion and necrosis.

INTRAHEPATIC OBSTRUCTION

As in adults, portal hypertension develops in children with any form of hepatic fibrosis or cirrhosis. The number of patients seen with portal hypertension resulting from cirrhosis is increasing as survival of patients with biliary atresia improves.

Biliary atresia is the most common cause of intrahepatic obstruction leading to portal hypertension in children. Even when bile drainage has been achieved, progressive fibrosis can occur. Ongoing postsinusoidal obstruction develops as a result of parenchymal fibrosis, scarring, and formation of regenerating hepatic nodules. Typically, the degree of cirrhosis and associated liver failure parallels the degree of portal hypertension.

Congenital hepatic fibrosis characterized by hepatosplenomegaly may become apparent at age 1 to 2 years, occurring in association with a syndrome or as an isolated disease of the liver. It is most commonly associated with infantile polycystic disease. Histopathologically, the liver is infiltrated by linear fibrous bands, which produce presinusoidal obstruction. Although the liver is enlarged, hepatic function is well preserved, and portal hypertension is the most prominent symptom.[58]

A variety of other metabolic disorders can cause hepatic fibrosis and cirrhosis, including α_1-antitrypsin deficiency, cystic fibrosis, chronic active hepatitis, and side effects of chemotherapy.

PREHEPATIC OBSTRUCTION

Previously, portal vein thrombosis was the most common cause of portal hypertension noted in pediatric patients; however, the incidence appears to be decreasing.[59] Portal vein thrombosis classically develops after prolonged use of umbilical venous catheters, but in modern practice, this accounts for less than 20% of the cases of portal vein thrombosis.[60–63] Other causes include intraabdominal sepsis, severe dehydration, hypercoagulable states, and anatomic vascular abnormalities.[64–66] In general, clinical manifestations are limited to signs of portal hypertension such as variceal hemorrhage or hypersplenism but with normal liver function.

CLINICAL PRESENTATION

Variceal hemorrhage occurs most commonly from the distal esophagus. Increased portal pressure leads to dilation of the portal systemic collateral veins, the most important of which link the coronary vein to the short gastrics and the submucosal plexus of the lower esophagus. As blood flow through the system increases, esophageal varices develop, which can be frighteningly large (Fig. 44–9). The typical presentation is one of vomiting bright red blood, but melena may also occur. Retroperitoneal, periumbilical, and hemorrhoidal collaterals also develop, and although these are large, they do not tend to cause significant bleeding.[67]

After control of the acute hemorrhage, the cause of portal hypertension is sought (Fig. 44–10). In a patient without stigmata of liver disease, the diagnosis of portal vein thrombosis is by far the most likely. Physical examination typically shows an enlarged spleen and a normal-sized liver without other problems. In this situation, Doppler US is nearly 100% diagnostic. In contrast, patients with associated liver disease often are first seen with signs of liver failure. The liver is almost always firm and enlarged with signs of malnutrition, splenomegaly, ascites, and jaundice.

Occasionally, splenomegaly and hypersplenism are the first signs of portal hypertension in children. Splenic size does not correlate with the degree of venous pressure elevation but the hematologic effects of hypersplenism do correlate with the size of the spleen. All formed blood elements may be affected. Long-standing portal hypertension can cause

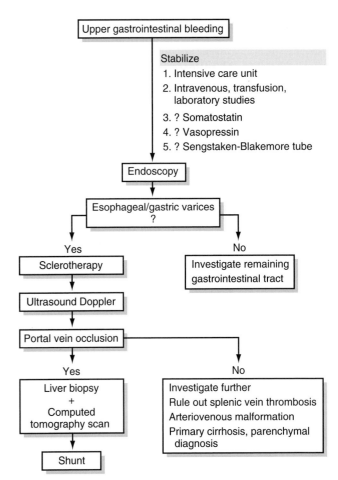

Figure 44–10. Algorithm for investigation and treatment of gastrointestinal bleeding in children.

splenic fibrosis, which then reduces the hematologic consequences. This also makes the effects of subsequent shunting less efficacious.

DIAGNOSIS AND TREATMENT

Initial management of gastrointestinal hemorrhage in children follows the same principles as in adults (see Fig. 44–10).[68, 69] Initial therapy requires volume resuscitation, an NG tube placement for diagnosis, and, if the child's condition does not stabilize, the use of octreotide therapy to reduce pressure in the portal system. Accurate monitoring of cardiovascular parameters, urine output, and frequent laboratory determination of blood counts necessitate an intensive care setting. If these conservative measures are not successful, balloon tamponade with a Sengstaken-Blakemore tube may be required. These children require tracheal intubation, sedation, and ventilation. Intragastric position of the distal balloon of the Blakemore tube is confirmed radiographically, the balloon is inflated with 20 to 30 cc of volume, and very slight tension is applied to the tube. This typically stops bleeding by tamponade of the gastric side of the varices. Once the child's condition is stabilized, endoscopic and duplex US

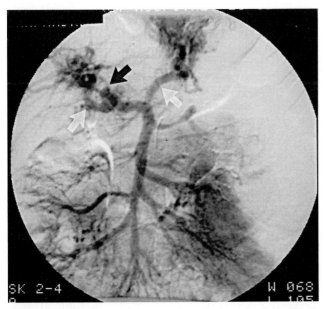

Figure 44–9. Portal vein thrombosis: mesenteric angiogram (black arrow indicates site of portal vein obstruction; white arrows indicate collaterals).

are used to delineate the status of the portal vein. US can accurately document portal venous thrombosis as well as cirrhosis with hepatofugal flow, and quantify arterial inflow. Liver function tests are done to document hepatic functional status. All patients with portal vein thrombosis should be evaluated for coagulopathy with determination of protein C, protein S, and clotting factor profile.[65]

Endoscopic varix sclerosis requires deep sedation and tracheal intubation. Short-term results are typically excellent in experienced hands.[60] Patients with acute hemorrhage are reinjected every 2 to 3 days until bleeding ceases. Patients who are not actively bleeding should have repeat endoscopy at 6-week intervals until all varices are obliterated. Nearly 100% control of bleeding can be obtained with this regimen. Minor complications include superficial esophageal ulceration, pleural effusion, and atelectasis. Very serious complications may result from varix injection. These include esophageal stricture (which can be difficult to manage), perforation, spinal cord paralysis, and systemic venous thrombosis or adult respiratory distress syndrome related to the use of excessive volumes of sclerosant.[70–72]

An alternative to sclerosants is band ligation of esophageal varices; this has fewer systemic complications, but it is equally effective in controlling bleeding.[73]

Other therapy following an acute esophageal bleed is dependent on the underlying pathophysiology. Portal hypertension resulting from intraparenchymal liver disease most likely will require liver transplantation. Once variceal bleeding occurs in these patients, the transplant evaluation is already underway. Conversely, if patients are found to have good liver function with either suprahepatic or portal venous obstruction, other surgical therapy may be appropriate. For patients who have a prehepatic cause of portal hypertension, shunt therapy should be considered after the first bleed and is indicated if repeat bleeding occurs despite sclerotherapy.[62–63] Because these patients typically have good liver function, the incidence of post-shunt encephalopathy is low.[74, 75] My choice is an H-type mesocaval shunt using autologous vein.[62, 63, 76, 77] The selective splenorenal shunt is also a satisfactory option.[78] The increased complexity of this procedure, coupled with the observations that most children at the time of shunt surgery already have hepatofugal flow in the portal vein and lose the selectivity of the distal splenorenal shunt over time, argues against its use in pediatric patients.[79]

Of special consideration are those patients who bleed from varices in the stomach, small bowel, or colon. These vessels are not amenable to sclerotherapy, and thus these patients may require earlier intervention with shunt therapy.[67]

The technical details of shunt procedures have been well described previously.[63, 77] The key feature of the H-type shunt is the use of an autologous vein graft, which provides a durable conduit, without the need for long-term anticoagulation (Fig. 44–11).

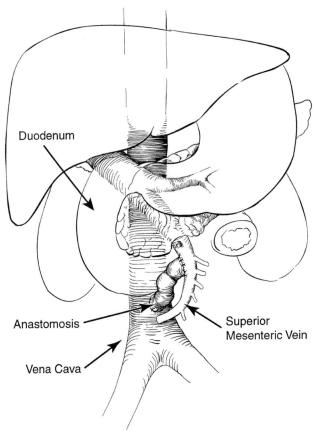

Figure 44–11. H-Type shunt procedure using autologous vein graft, operative strategy.

Most patients are out of the hospital within a week. Postoperatively, antiplatelet therapy consists of a daily pediatric aspirin tablet (80 mg), except in patients who have previously identified coagulopathy, in which case specific therapy is indicated.

The results of long-term therapy of patients with portal vein thrombosis undergoing shunt therapy has been most gratifying. Our recent experience with the H-type shunt followed up for a minimum of 2 years and an average of 6 years has shown a 100% patency rate, with no episodes of rebleeding.[62] This compares favorably with previous reports of alternative shunting procedures.[80] These children can lead a normal life with no risk of encephalopathy and with significant improvement in growth velocity.[81] In my view, shunt therapy in pediatric patients with portal vein thrombosis is underused.

Alternative Therapy

The development of transjugular intrahepatic portal systemic shunts in adult patients has led to inevitable expansion into the pediatric population.[82–84] My colleagues and I believe this option should be reserved for the short-term therapy of patients with intractable bleeding awaiting liver transplantation. In adults, the thrombosis rates are high after 6 months. This technique does not seem appropriate when long-term shunting is required.

The use of esophageal transection procedures to obliterate varices has a high rate of complications and offers no advantage over the treatment regimen previously discussed.[85, 86]

□ Ascites

Children can have severe ascites, typically associated with end-stage liver disease, and portal hypertension. The ascites may contribute to respiratory embarrassment because of elevation of the diaphragm and to malnutrition because of protein loss. Occasionally, chylous ascites may develop as a result of portal hypertension and liver disease. Long-term TPN for treatment and the use of somatostatin analogue reduce the volume of fluid produced.[87]

Initial conservative management of ascites is well described and consists of sodium and water restriction, aggressive use of loop diuretics such as furosemide, and periodic paracentesis. US guidance for paracentesis has greatly reduced the incidence of complications. Only one or two taps should be required. There are reports of the use of peritoneal-venous shunts, but this is rare in the pediatric age group. Most patients with refractory ascites require liver transplantation and therapy should be directed at preparing the patient for that procedure.

REFERENCES

1. Skandalakis JE, Gray SW: Embryology for Surgeons, 2nd ed. Baltimore, Williams & Wilkins, 1994.
2. Sherlock S: The liver in infancy and childhood. In Diseases of the Liver and Biliary System (8th ed). Oxford, Blackwell, 1989, pp 403–415.
3. Hemolytic disease of the newborn. In Nelson WE, Behrman RE, Kliegman RM (eds): Nelson's Textbook of Pediatrics (14th ed). Philadelphia, WB Saunders, 1992, pp 482–486.
4. Thaler MM, Gellis SS: Studies in neonatal hepatitis and biliary atresia, II: The effect of diagnostic laparotomy on long-term prognosis of neonatal hepatitis. Am J Dis Child 116:262–270, 1968.
5. Thomson J: On congenital obliteration of the bile ducts. Edinburgh Med J 37:523–531, 604–616, 724–735, 1891.
6. Holmes JB: Congenital obliteration of the bile ducts: Diagnosis and suggestions for treatment. Am J Dis Child 11:405–431, 1916.
7. Ladd WE: Congenital atresia and stenosis of the bile ducts. JAMA 91:1082–1085, 1928.
8. Kasai M, Suzuki S: A new operation for noncorrectable biliary atresia—hepatic portoenterostomy. Shujutsu 13:733–739, 1959.
9. Kasai M, Kimura S, Asakura Y, et al: Surgical treatment of biliary atresia. J Pediatr Surg 3:665–675, 1968.
10. Yanchar NL, Shapiro MJ, Sigalet DL: Is early response to portoenterostomy predictive of long term outcome for patients with biliary atresia? J Pediatr Surg 31:774–777, 1996.
11. Landing BH: Considerations of the pathogenesis of neonatal hepatitis, biliary atresia and choledochal cyst—the concept of infantile obstructive cholangiopathy. Prog Pediatr Surg 6:113–139, 1974.
12. Bangaru B, Morecki R, Glaser JH, et al: Comparative studies of biliary atresia in the human newborn and reovirus-induced cholangitis in weanling mice. Lab Invest 43:456, 1980.
13. Morecki R, Glaser J, Cho S, et al: Biliary atresia and reovirus type 3 infection. N Engl J Med 307:481–484, 1982.
14. Brown W, Sokol RJ, Levin M, et al: Lack of correlation between infection with reovirus 3 and extrahepatic biliary atresia or neonatal hepatitis. J Pediatr 113:670–676, 1998.
15. Pickett LK, Briggs HC: Biliary obstruction secondary to hepatic vascular ligation in fetal sheep. J Pediatr Surg 4:95–101, 1969.
16. Jenner RE, Howard ER: Unsaturated monohydroxy bile acids as a cause of idiopathic obstructive cholangiopathy. Lancet 2:1073–1074, 1975.
17. Schreiber RA, Kleinmann RE, Barksdale EM, et al: Rejection of murine congenic bile ducts: A model for immune mediated bile duct disease. Gastroenterology 102:924–930, 1992.
18. Kobayashi H, Puri P, O'Brian S, et al: Hepatic overexpression of MHC class II antigens and macrophage-associated antigens (CD68) in patients with biliary atresia of poor prognosis. J Pediatr Surg 32:590–593, 1997.
19. Strickland AD, Shannon K, Coin CD: Biliary atresia in two sets of twins. J Pediatr 107:418–420, 1985.
20. Greenholz SK, Lilly JR, Shikes RM, et al: Biliary atresia in the newborn. J Pediatr Surg 21:1147–1148, 1986.
21. Strickland AD, Shannon K: Studies in the etiology of extrahepatic biliary atresia: Time-space clustering. J Pediatr 100:749–753, 1985.
22. Toyosaka A, Okamoto E, Okasora T, et al: Extensive dissection at the porta hepatis for biliary atresia. J Pediatr Surg 29:896–899, 1994.
23. Chandra RS, Altman RP: Ductal remnants in extrahepatic biliary atresia: A histopathologic study with clinical correlation. J Pediatr 93:196–200, 1978.
24. Tan EL, Davenport M, Driver M, Howard ER: Does the morphology of the extrahepatic biliary remnants in biliary atresia influence survival? A review of 205 cases. J Pediatr Surg 29:1459–1464, 1994.
25. Ohi R, Ibrahim M: Biliary atresia. Semin Pediatr Surg 1:115–124, 1992.
26. Sartorelli KH, Holland RM, Lilly JR: The intussusception antireflux valve is ineffective in preventing cholangitis in biliary atresia. J Pediatr Surg 31:403–406, 1996.
27. Muraji T, Higashimoto Y: The improved outlook for biliary atresia with corticosteroid therapy. J Pediatr Surg 32:1103–1107, 1997.
28. Karrer FM, Lilly JR: Corticosteroid therapy in biliary atresia. J Pediatr Surg 20:693–695, 1985.
29. Freitus L, Gauthier F, Valayer J: Second operation for repair of biliary atresia. J Pediatr Surg 22:857–860, 1987.
30. Altman RP, Chandra R, Lilly JR: Ongoing cirrhosis after successful portoenterostomy with biliary atresia. J Pediatr Surg 10:685–691, 1975.
31. McDiarmid SV: Risk factors and outcomes after pediatric liver transplant. Liver Trans Surg 2(suppl 1):44–56, 1996.
32. Adelman S: Prognosis of uncorrected biliary atresia: An update. J Pediatr Surg 13:389–391, 1978.
33. Grosfeld JL, Fitzgerald JF, Predaina R, et al: The efficacy of hepatoportoenterostomy in biliary atresia. Surgery 106:692–701, 1989.
34. Lilly JR, Karrer FM, Hall RJ, et al: The surgery of biliary atresia. Ann Surg 210:289–296, 1989.
35. Ohi R, Hanamatsu M, Mochizuki I: Progress in the treatment of biliary atresia. World J Surg 9:285–293, 1985.
36. Chiba T, Kasai M, Sasano N: Histopathologic studies on intrahepatic bile ducts in the vicinity of the porta hepatis in biliary atresia. Tohoku J Exp Med 118:199–207, 1976.
37. McClement JW, Howard ER, Mowat AP: Results of surgical treatment for extrahepatic biliary atresia in the United Kingdom 1980–1982. BMJ 290:345–347, 1985.
38. Wood RP, Langnas AN, Stratta RJ, et al: Optimal therapy for patients with biliary atresia: Portoenterostomy ("Kasai" procedures) versus primary transplantation. J Pediatr Surg 25:153–160, 1990.
39. Azarow KS, Phillips JM, Sandler AD, et al: Biliary atresia: Should all patients undergo a portoenterostomy? J Pediatr Surg 32:168–174, 1997.
40. Nio M, Ohi R, Hayashi Y, et al: Current status of 21 patients who have survived more than 20 years since undergoing surgery for biliary atresia. J Pediatr Surg 31:381–384, 1996.
41. Alonso-Lej, Rever WB, Pessagno DJ: Congenital choledochal

cyst, with a report of 2, and an analysis of 94 cases. Int Abst Surg 108:1–30, 1959.

42. Flanigan DP: Biliary cyst. Ann Surg 182:635–643, 1975.

43. Caroli J: Disease of intrahepatic bile ducts. Isr J Med Sci 4:21–35, 1968.

44. Yamaguchi M: Congenital choledochal cyst. Am J Surg 140:653–657, 1980.

45. Hata Y, Sasaki F, Takahashi M, et al: Surgical treatment of congenital biliary dilatation associated with pancreaticobiliary maljunction. Surg Gynecol Obstet 178:581–587, 1993.

46. Katyal D, Lees GM: Choledochal cysts: A retrospective review of 28 patients and a review of the literature. Can J Surg 35:584–588, 1992.

47. Yamataka A, Ohshiro K, Okada Y: Complications after cyst excision with hepaticoenterostomy for choledochal cysts and their surgical management in children versus adults. J Pediatr Surg 32:1097–1102, 1997.

48. Alagille D: Alagille syndrome today. Clin Invest Med 19:325–330, 1996.

49. Cooper A, Ross AJ, O'Neill RA, et al: Resolution of intractable cholestasis associated with total parenteral nutrition following biliary irrigation. J Pediatr Surg 20:772–774, 1985.

50. Lilly JR, Weintraub WH, Altman RP: Spontaneous perforation of the extrahepatic bile ducts and bile peritonitis in infancy. Surgery 75:664–673, 1974.

51. Mercer S, Carpenter B: Surgical complications of Kawasaki disease. J Pediatr Surg 16:444–448, 1981.

52. Moir CR, Donohue JH, van Heerden JA: Laparoscopic cholecystectomy in children: Initial experience and recommendations. J Pediatr Surg 27:1066–1070, 1992.

53. Ware RE, Kinney TR, Casey JR, et al: Laparoscopic cholecystectomy in young patients with sickle hemoglobinopathies. J Pediatr 120:58–61, 1992.

54. Al-Salem AH, Nourallah H: Sequential endoscopic/laparoscopic management of cholelithiasis and choledocholithiasis in children who have sickle cell disease. J Pediatr Surg 32:1432–1435, 1997.

55. Vichinsky EP, Haberkern CM, Neumayr L, et al: A comparison of conservative and aggressive transfusion regimens in the perioperative management of sickle cell disease. N Engl J Med 333:206–213, 1995.

56. Witte CL, Tobin GR, Clark DS, et al: Relationship of splanchnic blood flow and portal venous resistance to elevated portal pressure in the dog. Gut 17:122, 1976.

57. Shaldon S, Sherlock S: Obstruction to the extrahepatic portal system in children. Lancet 1:63, 1962.

58. Alvarez F, Bernard O, Brunelle F, et al: Congenital hepatic fibrosis in children. J Pediatr 99:370–375, 1981.

59. Thompson EN, Sherlock S: The etiology of portal vein thrombosis with particular reference to the role of infection and exchange transfusion. Q J Med 33:465–480, 1964.

60. Howard E, Stringer MD, Mowat AP: Assessment of injection sclerotherapy in the management of 152 children with oesophageal varices. B J Surg 75:404–408, 1988.

61. Yadav S, Dutta KS, Sarin SK: Do umbilical vein catheterization and sepsis lead to portal vein thrombosis? A prospective, clinical, and sonographic evaluation. J Pediatr Gastroenterol Nutr 17:392–396, 1993.

62. Mayer S, Sigalet DL, Blanchard H: Portal venous decompression with H-type mesocaval shunt using autologous vein graft: A North American experience. J Pediatr Surg: in press.

63. Gauthier F, De Dreuzy O, Valayer J, et al: H-type shunt with an autologous venous graft for treatment of portal hypertension in children. J Pediatr Surg 24:1041–1043, 1989.

64. Ando H, Kaneko K, Ito F: Anatomy and etiology of extrahepatic portal vein obstruction in children leading to bleeding esophageal varices. J Am Coll Surg 183:543–547, 1996.

65. Majluf-Cruz A, Hurtado Monroy R, Sansores Garcia L, et al: The incidence of protein C deficiency in thrombosis-related portal hypertension. Am J Gastroenterol 91:976–980, 1996.

66. Pinkerton JA, Holcomb GW, Foster JH: Portal hypertension in children. Ann Surg 175:870, 1972.

67. Heaton ND, Davenport M, Howard ER: Incidence of haemorrhoids and anorectal varices in children with portal hypertension. Br J Surg 80:616–618, 1993.

68. Watanabe FD, Rosenthal P: Portal hypertension in children. Current Opinion in Pediatrics 7:533–538, 1995.

69. Rodriquez-Perez F, Groszmann RJ: Pharmacologic treatment of portal hypertension. Gastroenterol Clin North Am 21:15–40, 1992.

70. Shemesh E, Bat L: Esophageal perforation after fiberoptic endoscopic injection sclerotherapy for esophageal varices. Arch Surg 121:243–245, 1986.

71. Seidman E, Weber AM, Morin CL, et al: Spinal cord paralysis following sclerotherapy for esophageal varices. Hepatology 4:950–954, 1984.

72. Vallgren S, Sigurdsson GH, Moberger G, et al: Influence of intravenous injection of sclerosing agents on the respiratory function. Acta Chir Scand 154:271–276, 1998.

73. Hall RJ, Lilly JR, Stiegmann GV: Endoscopic esophageal varix ligation: Technique and preliminary results in children. J Pediatr Surg 23:1222–1223, 1988.

74. Alagille D, Carlier JC, Chiva M, et al: Long-term neuropsychological outcome in children undergoing portal-systemic shunts for portal vein obstruction without liver disease. J Pediatr Gastroenterol Nutr 5:861–866, 1986.

75. Alvarez F, Bernard O, Brunelle F, et al: Portal obstruction in children, I: Clinical investigation and hemorrhage risk. J Pediatr 103:696–702, 1983.

76. Bismuth H, Franco D, Alagille D: Portal diversion for portal hypertension in children. Ann Surg 192:18–24, 1980.

77. Valayer J, Hay JM, Gauthier F, et al: Shunt surgery for treatment of portal hypertension in children. World J Surg 9:258–268, 1985.

78. Evans S, Stovroff M, Heiss K, Ricketts R: Selective distal splenorenal shunts for intractable variceal bleeding in pediatric portal hypertension. J Pediatr Surg 30:1115–1118, 1995.

79. Belghiti J, Grenier P, Novel O, et al: Long-term loss of Warren's shunt selectivity: Angiographic demonstration. Arch Surg 116:1121–1124, 1981.

80. Fonkalsrud EW: Surgical management of portal hypertension in childhood. Long term results. Arch Surg 115:1042–1045, 1980.

81. Alvarez F, Bernard O, Brunelle F, et al: Portal obstruction in children, II. Results of surgical portosystemic shunts. J Pediatr 103:703–707, 1983.

82. Ring EJ, Lake JR, Roberts JP, et al: Using transjugular intrahepatic portosystemic shunts to control variceal bleeding before liver transplantation. Ann Intern Med 116:304–309, 1992.

83. Johnson SP, Leyendecker JR, Joseph FB, et al: Transjugular portosystemic shunts in pediatric patients awaiting liver transplantation. Transplantation 62:1178–1181, 1996.

84. Cao S, Monge H, Semba C, et al: Emergency transjugular intrahepatic portosystemic shunt (TIPS) in an infant: A case report. J Pediatr Surg 32:125–127, 1997.

85. Orozco H, Mercado MA, Takahashi T: Elective treatment of bleeding varices with the Sugiura operation over 10 years. Am J Surg 163:585–589, 1992.

86. Belloli G, Campobasso P: Sugiura procedure in the surgical treatment of bleeding esophageal varices in children; long-term results. J Pediatr Surg 27:1422–1426, 1992.

87. Sharpiro AM, Bain VG, Sigalet DL, et al: Rapid resolution of chylous ascites after liver transplantation using somatostatin analog and total parenteral nutrition. Transplantation 61:1410–1411, 1996.

45

SOLID ORGAN TRANSPLANTATION IN CHILDREN

Frederick C. Ryckman, MD •
Maria H. Alonso, MD

☐ Liver Transplantation

Few subspecialties have undergone the dramatic improvements in success and survival that have occurred since the 1980s in pediatric liver transplantation. In the early 1980s, survival rates of 30% limited the enthusiasm for this costly and work intense operation.

The introduction of more effective immunosuppression along with refinements in the operative and postoperative management of infants and children improved survival rates to nearly 90% in many centers specializing in pediatric transplantation. When compared to the universally fatal outcome in these patients without transplantation, it is not surprising that liver transplantation has come to be embraced as the preferred therapy for many progressive liver diseases.

With this improved survival rate has come an increasing need for transplant donor organs suitable for pediatric recipients of all ages and sizes. This wide spectrum of needs, coupled with the national shortage of transplant donor organs, has stimulated the pioneering development of surgical procedures such as reduced-size liver transplantation, "split liver" transplantation, and living donor (LD) liver transplantation. However, the excellent survival and organ availability offered by the complementary use of these transplant options cannot overshadow the need for comprehensive evaluation and selective application of liver transplantation. This chapter is an overview of the selection process, preoperative preparation, surgical options, and postoperative care in liver, renal, and pancreas transplantation.

THE SELECTION PROCESS

The primary aim of the evaluation process is to define which patients require or would benefit from orthotopic liver transplantation (OLT) and when

such therapy should be undertaken. Evaluation should be directed toward the identification of (1) progressive deterioration of hepatocellular function, (2) portal hypertension and gastrointestinal (GI) bleeding, or (3) nutritional and growth failure. Referral for transplantation should occur when progressive deterioration is noted and before the development of life-threatening complications.

INDICATIONS FOR TRANSPLANTATION

The most common clinical presentations prompting transplant evaluation in children can be classified as follows: (1) progressive primary liver disease with the expected outcome of hepatic failure, (2) stable liver disease with remarkable morbidity or known mortality, (3) hepatic-based metabolic disease, and (4) fulminant hepatic failure of known or unknown etiology. Rarely, patients with liver disease secondary to systemic illness such as cystic fibrosis or primary hepatic malignancy are seen as candidates for pediatric transplantation.

Table 45–1 reviews primary diagnoses leading to pediatric transplantation. These disease entities define the bimodal age distribution of pediatric transplant recipients. Infants and children in the first 2 years of life represent patients with biliary atresia and, occasionally, rapidly progressive hepatic failure secondary to metabolic abnormalities such as neonatal tyrosinemia and hemochromatosis. Patients with metabolic disturbances, fulminant viral hepatitis, and cirrhosis are seen for OLT as older children and adolescents.

NEONATAL CHOLESTATIC SYNDROMES
Biliary Atresia

Children with extrahepatic biliary atresia constitute at least 50% of the pediatric liver transplant population. Successful biliary drainage achieving an

TABLE 45-1. Indications for
Liver Transplantation*

Primary Diagnosis	No. of Patients	% Total
Neonatal Cholestasis	66	51
Biliary atresia	64	
Allagille's syndrome	2	
Metabolic Disease	27	21
α_1-Antitrypsin deficiency	15	
Tyrosinemia	4	
Glycogen storage disease-IV	2	
Hyperoxyluria	2	
Wilson's disease	1	
Cystic fibrosis	1	
Hemochromatosis	1	
OTC deficiency	1	
Fulminant Hepatic Failure	19	16
Non-A, non-B hepatitis	14	
Drug induced	2	
Wilson's disease	1	
X-linked LPD (Duncan's syndrome)	2	
Hepatitis	8	6
Chronic active	4	
Neonatal-cirrhosis	3	
Autoimmune	1	
Cirrhosis	7	6
Cryptogenic	5	
Short gut syndrome	2	
Tumor	1	<1
S/P hepatoblastoma	1	

*1986–1997; N = 128.

CHMC, Children's Hospital Medical Center, Cincinnati, Ohio; LPD, lymphoproliferative disease; OTC, orthotopic liver transplantation; S/P, status post.

anicteric state following the Kasai portoenterostomy is the most important factor affecting preservation of liver function and long-term survival. Primary transplantation without portoenterostomy is not recommended in patients with biliary atresia unless the initial presentation is at more than 120 days of age and the liver biopsy shows advanced cirrhosis.[1, 2] We believe that the Kasai portoenterostomy should be the primary surgical intervention for all other infants with extrahepatic biliary atresia. Patients with progressive disease following a Kasai procedure should be offered early OLT. The sequential use of these two procedures optimizes overall survival and organ use.[2, 3]

Patients with extrahepatic biliary atresia who are seen for transplantation form several cohorts. Infants with a failed Kasai have recurrent bacterial cholangitis, ascites, rapidly progressive portal hypertension, malnutrition, and progressive hepatic synthetic failure. Most require OLT within the first 2 years of life. Children with the successful establishment of biliary drainage have an improved prognosis, but this alone does not preclude the development of progressive cirrhosis with eventual portal hypertension, hypersplenism, variceal hemorrhage,

and ascites formation. These patients are seen in later childhood for OLT. Individual patients with mild hepatocellular enzyme and bilirubin elevation and mild portal hypertension can be safely observed with ongoing medical therapy. Approximately 20% of all patients do not require OLT.[4, 5]

Alagille's Syndrome

Alagille's syndrome (angiohepatic dysplasia) is an autosomal dominant genetic disorder manifest as bile duct paucity leading to progressive cholestasis and pruritus, xanthomas, malnutrition, and growth failure. Liver failure occurs late, if at all. Occasionally, severe growth retardation, hypercholesterolemia, and pruritus can compromise the patient's overall well-being to the point where transplantation is valuable.

Exact criteria for OLT are difficult to quantitate. Evaluation must include assessment for congenital cardiac disease and renal insufficiency, both of which are associated with this syndrome. Hepatocellular carcinoma has also been seen in occasional patients.[6, 7] The vast improvement in growth and nutrition and the resolution of pruritus, hypercholesterolemia, and xanthoma allow these quality of life issues to be criteria for consideration for OLT.[8–10]

Metabolic Disease

The leading indication for hepatic transplantation in older children is hepatic-based metabolic disease. In these patients, OLT is not only lifesaving but also it often accomplishes phenotypic and functional cure. A review of these diseases and their mode of presentation is given in Tables 45–2 and 45–3.

Hepatic replacement to correct the metabolic defect should be considered before other organ systems are affected and before complications develop that would preclude transplantation, such as in patients with tyrosinemia, in whom there is a high risk of hepatocellular carcinoma.[7] Although results

TABLE 45-2. Transplantation for
Metabolic Disease in Children

Wilson's disease
α_1-Antitrypsin deficiency
Crigler-Najjar syndrome (type I)
Tyrosinemia
Cystic fibrosis
Glycogen storage disease-IV
Branched chain amino acid catabolism disorders
Hemophilia A
Protoporphyria
Homozygous hypercholesterolemia
Urea cycle enzyme deficiencies
Primary hyperoxaluria
Iron storage disease

Reprinted from Balistreri WF, Ohi R, Todani T, et al: Hepatobiliary, Pancreatic and Splenic Disease in Children: Medical and Surgical Management, 1997, pp 395–399, with kind permission from Elsevier Science-NL, Sara Burgerhartstraat 25, 1055 KV Amsterdam, The Netherlands.

TABLE 45-3. Mode of Presentation*

Cirrhosis	Liver Tumor	Life-Threatening Progressive Liver Disease	Failure of Secondary Organ, Normal Liver
α₁-ATD	Tyrosinemia	Urea cycle defect	Type 1 Hyperoxalosis
Wilson's disease	GSD-1	Protein C deficiency	Hypercholesterolemia
Hemochromatosis	Galactosemia	Crigler-Najjar syndrome type 1	
Byler's disease	FHD	Niemann-Pick disease	
Cystic fibrosis	Hemochromatosis	Hemochromatosis	
Tyrosinemia	α₁-ATD	Tyrosinemia	
GSD-IV		BCAA	
FHD			
EPP			

* Classification of inherited metabolic disorders according to clinical modes of presentation.
   α₁-ATD, α₁-antitrypsin deficiency; BCAA, branched chain amino acid catabolism disorders; EPP, erythropoietic protoporphyria; FHD, fumaryl hydrolase deficiency; GSD, glycogen storage disease.
   Reprinted from Balistreri WF, Ohi R, Todani T, et al: Hepatobiliary, Pancreatic and Splenic Disease in Children: Medical and Surgical Management, 1997, pp 395–399, with kind permission from Elsevier Science-NL, Sara Burgerhartstraat 25, 1055 KV Amsterdam, The Netherlands.

of transplantation are excellent in the metabolic disease subgroup, current research efforts may show that auxiliary transplantation, orthotopic partial hepatic replacement, hepatocyte transplantation, and gene therapy may better serve this patient population in the future.[11, 12]

Fulminant Hepatic Failure

Patients with fulminant hepatic failure without recognized antecedent liver disease present diagnostic and prognostic difficulties. Rapid clinical deterioration frequently makes establishment of a primary diagnosis impossible before there is an urgent need for transplantation. Acute viral hepatitis of undefined type makes up the largest group, followed by drug toxicity and toxin exposure. Previously unrecognized metabolic disease must also be considered. The prognosis for these patients is difficult to predict, and neurologic outcome is potentially suboptimal.[13]

Use of intracranial pressure (ICP) monitoring in patients with progressive encephalopathy has allowed early recognition and directed treatment of increased intracranial pressure. Monitoring should be instituted for patients with advancing grade III encephalopathy and in all patients with grade IV encephalopathy. Intracranial monitoring is continued intraoperatively and for 24 to 48 hours after OLT because significant increases in intracranial pressure have been identified throughout the entire clinical course. Failure to maintain a cerebral perfusion pressure (mean blood pressure–ICP) of greater than 50 mm Hg and an ICP less than 20 mm Hg has been associated with very poor neurologic recovery.[14] Survival following transplantation is significantly decreased in patients who reach grade IV encephalopathy.

Efforts to identify and perform transplantation in children before this deterioration are of utmost importance. When candidates are identified before they develop irreversible neurologic abnormalities, the results of transplantation are dramatic. Hepato-cyte transplantation can provide neurologic protection during organ acquisition or while awaiting spontaneous recovery.[15]

Malignancy

Transplantation for primary hepatic malignancy is uncommon in children, thus experience is limited.[7] Transplantation for hepatoblastoma is recommended only for individuals with neoplasm confined to the liver and unresectable by conventional means after the initial administration of several chemotherapy courses. Factors associated with a favorable prognosis include (1) absence of prior surgical resection attempts, (2) unifocal rather than multifocal involvement, (3) absence of vascular invasion, and (4) fetal histology compared to anaplastic or embryonal histology. Recurrent disease accounted for 50% of postoperative mortality.[16]

Transplantation for hepatocellular carcinoma is complicated by less successful chemotherapy options and frequent extrahepatic involvement. The reported 2-year survival rates of 20 to 30% compare unfavorably to the experience with hepatoblastoma. Most deaths are due to recurrent carcinoma within the allograft or to extrahepatic tumor involvement. When primary hepatocellular carcinoma is discovered incidentally within the cirrhotic native liver at the time of hepatectomy, the overall prognosis is unaffected by the tumor.[17]

CONTRAINDICATIONS

Contraindications to transplantation include (1) serology positive for HIV, (2) primary extrahepatic unresectable malignancy, (3) malignancy metastatic to the liver, (4) progressive terminal nonhepatic disease, (5) uncontrolled systemic sepsis, and (6) irreversible neurologic injury.

Relative contraindications to transplantation that need to be individually evaluated include (1) advanced or partially treated systemic infection, (2) advanced hepatic encephalopathy (grade IV),

(3) severe psychosocial abnormalities, and (4) portal venous thrombosis extending throughout the mesenteric venous system.

PRIORITIZATION

Candidate evaluation and selection is undertaken by a multidisciplinary team who establish candidate acceptability and medical urgency and initiate preoperative intervention and education.

PREOPERATIVE PREPARATION

Efforts to correct abnormalities noted during candidate evaluation decrease both the operative risk and postoperative complications. Complications of portal hypertension and malnutrition are vigorously treated. Assessment of prior viral exposure and meticulous attention to the delivery of all normal childhood immunizations, particularly the live-virus vaccines, are imperative, if time allows, before OLT. Additionally, patients receive a one-time inoculation with pneumococcal vaccine, as well as hepatitis B vaccine. Preoperative assessment of specific cardiopulmonary reserve and hepatic vascular anatomy is also necessary.

OPERATIVE TREATMENT

Donor Options

The single factor limiting the availability of OLT is the limited supply of donor organs. The number of patients awaiting liver transplantation has increased by sevenfold since 1991. Available donor resources have not kept pace with this need. As a consequence of this donor shortage, median waiting times have increased from 39 days in 1988 to 254 days in 1995 (Fig. 45–1).

The severely limited supply of available donor organs has driven the advancement of many innovative liver transplant surgical procedures. The development of reduced-size liver transplantation allowed significant expansion of the donor pool for infants and small children. This not only improved the availability of donor organs but also allowed

access to donors with improved stability and organ function. Evolution of these operative techniques has allowed the development of both split liver transplantation and LD transplantation.

In the hands of experienced transplant teams, these procedures all have equivalent success to whole organ transplantation. Furthermore, access to these many donor options has reduced the waiting list mortality rate to less than 5%. Infants and children requiring transplantation benefit greatly by having access to all of these transplant options to minimize waiting time and optimize organ use.

Orthotopic Transplant Techniques

Donor Factors

The success of OLT has led to an increase in transplantation that has not been matched by an increase in donor volume. This increased shortage of donor organs has led to expanded efforts to use individuals of advanced age and marginal stability.

Assessment of donor organ suitability is undertaken by evaluating clinical information, static biochemical tests, and dynamic tests of hepatocellular function (Table 45–4). The clinical factors reviewed identify donors who are at the limits of age, have had prolonged intensive care hospitalization with potential sepsis, and have vasomotor instability requiring excessive vasoconstricting inotropic agents. Static biochemical tests identify preexisting functional abnormalities or organ trauma but do not serve as good benchmarks to differentiate among acceptable and poor donor allografts. Dynamic tests of hepatic function have come closer to identifying limits for organ acceptability. Indocyanine green and galactose elimination have proved to be difficult and cumbersome for rapid donor evaluation.

MEG-X (monoethylglycine-xylidide) is the primary by-product of lidocaine metabolism. Its formation is influenced by hepatic blood flow and hepatocellular function. A MEG-X measurement of less than 50 ng/ml has been correlated with increased risk of primary allograft nonfunction or allograft failure in the first 20 days following transplantation. MEG-X testing helps identify patients with good

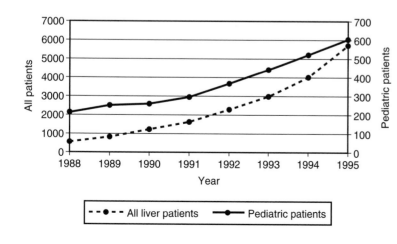

Figure 45–1. Number of patients on the United Network of Organ Sharing waiting list for liver transplantation, subdivided by all patients awaiting transplantation and pediatric patients. (Data from 1995 Annual Report, OPTN and Scientific Registry of Transplant Recipients.)

TABLE 45–4. Factors Affecting Donor Suitability

Clinical	Static Biochemical	Dynamic Functional Clearance Tests	Metabolic Tests
Donor age	Liver function tests	Indocyanine green	MEG-X
Cause of death	Prothrombin time	Galactose	
Associated injuries	Electrolytes		
Hypotension	Complete blood count		
Inotropic support	Platelet number		
Infection history	Liver biopsy		
Social history			
Donor stability			

MEG-X, monoethylglycine xylidide.
Reprinted from Balistreri WF, Ohi R, Todani T, et al: Hepatobiliary, Pancreatic and Splenic Disease in Children: Medical and Surgical Management, 1997, pp 395–399, with kind permission from Elsevier Science-NL, Sara Burgerhartstraat 25, 1055 KV Amsterdam, The Netherlands.

hepatic metabolic function who might have otherwise been excluded from donation owing to abnormal liver function tests.[18, 19] However, this test identifies donor organs whose preservation potential is limited, making them higher risk donors in situations in which prolonged ischemic preservation is anticipated. Donor liver biopsy is helpful in questionable cases to identify preexisting liver disease or donor liver steatosis.

Donor Liver Selection

Anatomic replacement of the native liver in the orthotopic position requires selection or surgical preparation of the donor liver to fill but not to exceed available space in the recipient. When using full-sized allografts, a donor weight range 15 to 20% above or below that of the recipient is usually appropriate, taking into consideration body habitus and factors that would increase recipient abdominal size such as ascites and hepatosplenomegaly.

Surgical preparation of reduced-size liver allografts is based on the anatomy of the hepatic vasculature and bile ducts.[20] Prolonged cold ischemic preservation allows the safe application of the extensive hypothermic bench surgery necessary for reduction technology. The three primary reduced-size allografts used clinically, prepared ex vivo, are the right lobe, the left lobe, and the left lateral segment.

The right lobe graft, using segments 5 to 8, can be accommodated when the weight difference is no greater than 2:1 between the donor and the recipient. The thickness of the right lobe makes this allograft of limited usefulness in small recipients. The left lobe, using segments 2 to 4, is applicable with a donor-to-recipient (D:R) disparity from 4:1 to 5:1, and a left lateral segment (segments 2 and 3) can be used with up to a 10:1 D:R weight difference. For a left or right lobe graft, the parenchymal resection follows the anatomic lobar plane through the gallbladder fossa to the vena cava.[20, 21] A crush and tie technique is preferred to achieve good closure of vascular and biliary structures. The middle hepatic vein is retained with the left lobe graft and sacrificed in the right lobe preparation. The bile duct, portal vein, and hepatic artery are divided and ligated at

the right or left confluence. The vena cava is left incorporated with the allograft in both right and left lobe preparation. Vena caval reduction by posterior caval wall resection and closure is only occasionally necessary. Resection of the inferior protruding portion of the caudate lobe is necessary during left lobe preparation to reduce the likelihood of arterial angulation, which can result in arterial thrombosis. This also facilitates shortening of the inferior vena cava to fit in a small recipient.[22]

When using left lateral segment allografts, the parenchymal dissection follows the right margin of the falciform ligament with preservation of the left hilar structures. Direct implantation of the left hepatic vein into the combined orifice of the right or middle left and middle hepatic veins in the recipient vena cava is preferred; the donor vena cava is not retained with this segmental allograft.

Biliary reconstruction in all allograft types is achieved through an end-to-side choledochojejunostomy. Primary bile duct reconstruction is not used with reduced-sized allografts owing to the risk of ischemia in the common bile duct. The bile ducts are perfused by a dense arterial plexus, which travels within the common connective tissue "vasobiliary sheath."[23] Dissection should be limited to that necessary to identify the bile duct for anastomosis.

The use of LDs has increased greatly in past years in that the safety and success of this procedure has been demonstrated. In most pediatric cases, the left lateral segment is used as the graft. In situ dissection of the left lateral segment, preserving the donor vascular integrity until the parenchymal division is completed, is undertaken as described previously. At the time of harvest, the left hepatic vein is divided from the vena cava, and the left branch of the portal vein and proper hepatic artery are removed with the allograft.[24] Vascular continuity of the portal vein branches to segment IV is maintained if possible. Recently, increased experience has been gained using the right lobe as an LD allograft for larger recipients such as adolescents and adults.[25] Cryopreservation and implantation follow standard reduced-size orthotopic liver transplant (RSOLT) techniques.

One of the critical elements of LD transplantation

is the proper selection of a donor, usually a parent or relative. This procedure is performed on the assumption that donor safety can be assured and that the donor liver status is normal. Donors should be 18 to 55 years of age, have an ABO compatible blood type, and have no acute or chronic medical condition. After a satisfactory medical and psychological examination by a physician not directly involved with the transplant program, arteriography is undertaken to assess the hepatic arterial anatomy, thereby excluding potential donors with multiple arteries to segments 2 and 3, and facilitating minimal dissection at the time of OLT.

Experience has shown that, when donors were deemed unacceptable, 90% of patients were excluded on the basis of history, examination, laboratory screening, and ABO type. Only 10% were excluded following angiography.[24, 26] Donor safety has been excellent in all LD series.[27] Efforts to extend the limits of donor acceptability have included the use of ABO incompatible LDs. Protocols to decrease preexisting isohemagglutinins by blood or plasma exchange and enhanced immunosuppression yield survival similar to ABO identical allografts.[28]

Split liver grafting involves the preparation of two allografts from a single donor. Using the aforementioned techniques, a right lobe allograft (segments 5 to 8) can be used in an adult or large child, whereas the left lateral segment allograft (segments 2 and 3) can be transplanted into a small recipient. Segment 4 is often discarded if it appears ischemic at the time of hepatic division. Vascular grafts are frequently necessary to achieve sufficient vascular length for implantation in one of the two allografts. Conventional techniques for implanting the respective allografts are then used.[29] The use of in situ division of the left lateral segment, as during LD liver procurement, has vastly improved preservation of both allografts. This technique allows the sequential harvest of the left lateral segment followed by the remaining liver with the other organs. Currently, this technique is the preferred method for split-liver donor preparation.[30, 32]

The selection of a donor segment with an appropriate parenchymal mass for adequate function is critical to success. However, the minimal mass necessary for recovery is not yet established. Any calculation must take into account loss of function following preservation damage, acute rejection, and technical problems. When the D:R weight range falls within the normal 8:1 to 10:1 ratio, risk is minimal. Estimates of donor graft to recipient body weight ratio (GRWR) may prove to be a more accurate predictor of adequate graft volume. When the GRWR is less than 0.7%, overall allograft and patient survival suffered. In extreme cases in which small-for-size grafts are used, excessive portal flow can lead to hemorrhagic necrosis of the graft. Large-for-size allografts (GRWR >5.0%) have a less deleterious effect.[29] A review of these donor anatomic options is shown in Figure 45–2.

Creative use of the techniques refined for reduced-size liver transplantation has allowed additional donor options in individual cases. Resection of the left lobe of the native liver followed by auxiliary partial orthotopic transplantation of a reduced-size left lateral segment allograft has been successfully undertaken for patients with metabolic disease (ornithine transcarbamylase deficiency, Crigler-Najjar syndrome) and fulminant hepatic failure.[33] This provides for normal hepatic synthesis and function while leaving the right lobe of the donor liver in situ. The auxiliary partial orthotopic transplantation technique has also been undertaken using an LD for similar indications.[34] Auxiliary placement of a reduced-size allograft has also been undertaken successfully for fulminant hepatic failure in patients deemed too unstable for orthotopic transplantation. In these cases, recovery of the recipient native liver function can ultimately allow discontinuation of immunosuppression and atrophy of the donor allograft if it is no longer required to supplement organ function.[35]

The Transplant Procedure

The transplant procedure is carried out through a combined upper midline-bilateral subcostal incision. Meticulous ligation of portosystemic collaterals and vascularized adhesions is necessary to avoid slow but relentless hemorrhage. Dissection of the hepatic hilum, with provision for division of the hepatic artery and portal vein above their bifurcation, allows maximal recipient vessel length to be achieved. The bile duct, when present, is divided high in the hilum to preserve the length and vasculature of the distal duct in case it is needed for later reconstruction in older recipients. Preservation of the Roux-en-Y in biliary atresia patients who have undergone Kasai portoenterostomy simplifies later biliary reconstruction. Complete mobilization of the liver, with dissection of the suprahepatic vena cava to the diaphragm and the infrahepatic vena cava to the renal veins, completes the hepatectomy.

In children with serious vascular instability who cannot tolerate caval occlusion, "piggy-back" transplantation is possible. In this procedure, the recipient vena cava is left intact and partial caval occlusion allows end-to-side implantation of a combined donor hepatic vein patch. Access to the infrarenal aorta to implant the celiac axis of the donor liver or iliac artery vascular conduits, provided by mobilizing the right colon and duodenum, is our preference for arterial reconstruction in complex allograft recipients. In recipients of a left lateral segment reduced-size allograft, the recipient vena cava is preserved and therefore not mobilized.

Control of hemorrhage is essential during the recipient hepatectomy, requiring meticulous surgical technique. Coagulation factor assays (V, VII, VIII, fibrinogen, platelets, prothrombin time, partial thromboplastin time) allow specific blood product supplementation to improve clotting function. Use of venovenous bypass is reserved for recipients who

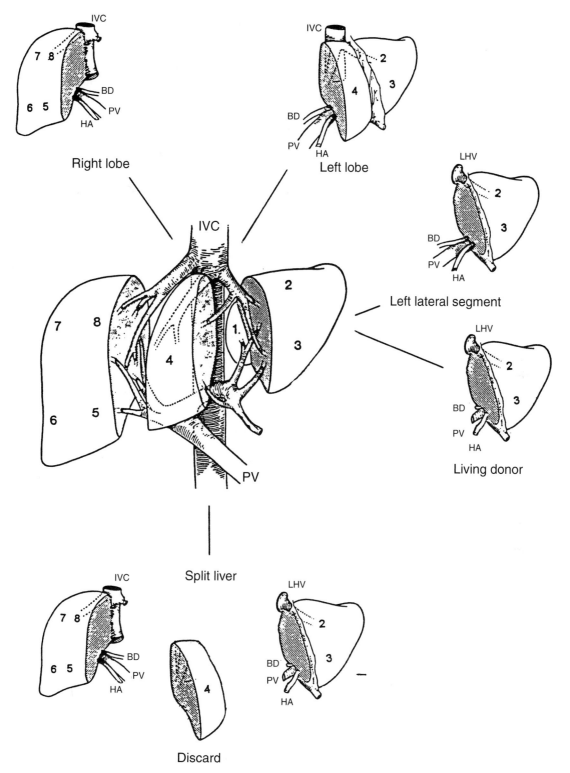

Figure 45–2. Schematic diagrams of reduced-size allografts after graft preparation. Anatomic divisions of the liver are as described by Couinaud. BD, bile duct; HA, hepatic artery; IVC, inferior vena cava; LHV, left hepatic vein; PV, pancreatic vein.

demonstrate hemodynamic instability at the time of venous interruption. Venovenous bypass is rarely necessary in patients who weigh less than 40 kg. Early institution of venovenous bypass combined with high-dose vasopressin (0.2 to 0.6 units/min) is occasionally used in patients with marked friable retroperitoneal variceal hypertension before completing hepatic mobilization.

Removal of the diseased liver is completed after vascular isolation is achieved. Retroperitoneal hemostasis is achieved before implanting the donor liver. The suprahepatic vena cava is prepared by suture ligating any large phrenic orifices and creating one caval lumen out of the hepatic vein (vena cava confluence). The donor liver is implanted using conventional vascular techniques and monofilament suture for the vascular anastomosis. In small recipients, interrupted suture techniques, monofilament dissolving suture material, and a "growth factor" knot have all been used to allow for vessel growth. When left lateral segment reduced-size grafts are used, the left hepatic vein orifice is anastomosed directly to the anterolateral surface of the infradiaphragmatic inferior vena cava (IVC) using the combined right–middle hepatic vein orifices. The left lateral segment allograft is later fixed to the undersurface of the diaphragm to prevent torsion and venous obstruction of this anastomosis. Similar fixation is not necessary with right or left lobe allograft or with whole organ transplants.

Before completing the vena caval anastomosis in all allografts, the hyperkalemic preservation solution is flushed from the graft using 500 to 800 ml of hypothermic normokalemic intravenous (IV) solutions. When using full-sized grafts, we prefer to complete all venous anastomoses before reconstructing the hepatic artery. In reduced-size allografts, the hepatic arterial anastomosis is completed before reconstructing the portal vein to improve visibility of the infrarenal aorta without placing traction on the portal vein anastomosis. We prefer to complete all anastomoses during vascular isolation before organ reperfusion, although some transplant teams reperfuse after venous reconstruction is complete.

Before reestablishing circulation to the allograft, anesthetic adjustments must be made to address the large volume of blood needed to refill the liver and the presence of hypothermic solutions released at reperfusion. Inotropic support using dopamine (5 to 10 μg/kg/min) is begun. Calcium and sodium bicarbonate are administered to combat the effects of hyperkalemia from any remaining preservation solution and systemic acidosis following aortic and vena caval occlusion. Sufficient blood volume expansion, administered as packed red blood cells to raise the central venous pressure (CVP) to 15 to 20 cm H_2O and the hematocrit to 40%, minimizes the development of hypotension on unclamping and prevents dilutional anemia. Cooperative communication between the surgical and anesthesia team facilitates a smooth sequential reestablishment of first venous and then arterial recirculation to the allograft.

Biliary reconstruction in patients with biliary atresia or in those weighing less than 25 kg is achieved through an end-to-side choledochojejunostomy using interrupted dissolving monofilament sutures. A multifenestrated Silastic internal biliary stent is placed before completing the anastomosis. In most cases, the prior Roux-en-Y can be used, with a 30 to 35 cm length being preferred. Primary bile duct reconstruction without stenting is used in older patients with whole organ allografts.

When closing the abdomen, increased intraabdominal pressure should be avoided. In many cases, avoidance of fascial closure and the use of mobilized skin flaps and running monofilament skin closure is advisable. Musculofascial abdominal closure can be completed before patient discharge.

IMMUNOSUPPRESSIVE MANAGEMENT

Most centers use an immunosuppressive protocol based on the administration of multiple complementary medications. All use corticosteroids and cyclosporine or tacrolimus. Additional antimetabolites (azathioprine, mycophenolate) are used when more antirejection treatment is needed. A sample protocol is given in Table 45–5.

TABLE 45–5. Sample Immunosuppressive Protocol

Postoperative Day	Tacrolimus: Steroid Protocol		Sequential Induction Protocol		
	Tacrolimus	Prednisolone	Prednisolone	Cyclosporine	OKT-3
0	0	15 mg/kg	3 mg/kg	0	2.5 or 5.0 mg
1	0.15 mg/kg po bid	10 mg/kg	2 mg/kg		2.5 or 5.0 mg
2	Adjust to level = 15 μg	8 mg/kg	T		2.5 or 5.0 mg
3	Adjust to level = 15 μg	6 mg/kg	A	10 mg/kg po q8–12h	2.5 or 5.0 mg
4	Adjust to level = 15 μg	4 mg/kg	P	Target level 350 ng	2.5 or 5.0 mg
5	Adjust to level = 15 μg	2 mg/kg	E	Target level 350 ng	2.5 or 5.0 mg
6	Adjust to level = 15 μg	1 mg/kg	R	Target level 350 ng	2.5 or 5.0 mg
7	Adjust to level = 15 μg	1 mg/kg	1 mg/kg/d	Target level 350 ng	2.5 or 5.0 mg
14	Adjust to level = 15 μg	1 mg/kg	0.9 mg/kg/d	Target level 350 ng	D/C if cyclosporine level adequate
28	Target level = 12 μg	0.7 mg/kg/d	0.7 mg/kg/d	Target level 350 ng	
3 mo	Target level = 10 μg	0.5 mg/kg/d	0.5 mg/kg/d	Target level 300 ng	
6 mo	Target level = 10 μg	Taper and D/C at 6–9 mo	0.3 mg/kg/d	Target level 350 ng	
12 mo	Target level = 8–10 μg	0	0.1 mg/kg/d	Target level 200–250 ng	
18 mo	Target level = 6–8 μg	0	0.1 mg/kg QOD	Target level 200–250 ng	
24 mo	Target level = 6–8 μg	0	D/C	Target level 200–250 ng	

D/C, discontinue.

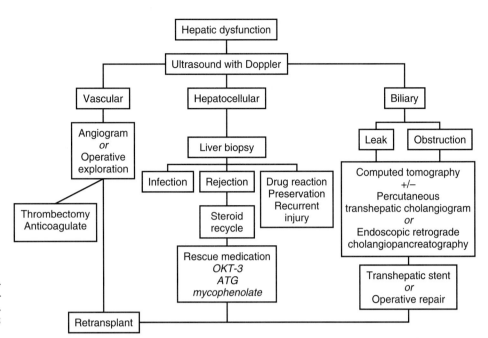

Figure 45–3. Schematic flow diagram for management of postoperative liver allograft dysfunction. ATG, antithymocyte globulin; OKT-3, monoclonal antibody.

POSTOPERATIVE COMPLICATIONS

Most postoperative complications present as cholestasis; increasing hepatocellular enzyme levels; and variable fever, lethargy, and anorexia. This nonspecific symptom complex requires specific diagnostic evaluation before instituting treatment. Therapy directed at the specific causes of allograft dysfunction is essential; empiric therapy of presumed complications is fraught with misdiagnoses, morbidity, and mortality. A flow diagram outlining this evaluation is shown in Figure 45–3.

Primary Nonfunction

Primary nonfunction (PNF) of the hepatic allograft implies the absence of metabolic and synthetic activity following transplantation. Complete nonfunction requires immediate retransplantation before irreversible coagulopathy and cerebral edema occur. Lesser degrees of allograft dysfunction occur more frequently and can be associated with several donor, recipient, and operative factors (Table 45–6).

The status of the donor liver contributes significantly to the potential for PNF. Ischemic injury secondary to anemia, hypotension, hypoxia, or direct tissue injury is often difficult to ascertain in the history of multiple trauma victims. Donor liver steatosis has also been recognized as a factor contributing to severe dysfunction or nonfunction in the donor liver. Macrovesicular steatosis on donor liver biopsy is somewhat more common in adult than pediatric donors and, when severe, is recognized grossly by the enlarged yellow, greasy consistency of the donor liver. The risk of PNF increases as the degree of fatty infiltration increases. Microscopic findings are classified as mild if less than 30% of the hepatocytes have fatty infiltration, moderate if 30 to 60% are involved, and severe if more than 60% of the hepatocytes have fatty infiltration. Livers with severe fatty infiltration should be discarded, and donors with moderate involvement are used with some concern, with the degree of steatosis and the condition of the recipient determining use of the allograft. Microvesicular steatosis is not related to PNF.

Immediate posttransplant immunologic events, such as humoral antibody-mediated hyperacute rejection, have not been unequivocally documented in liver transplantation. Initial reports suggested that a positive cytotoxic antibody crossmatch between the donor and recipient did not affect the viability or function of the allograft.[39] However, more recent experience with crossmatch positive donors has demonstrated significantly decreased allograft and patient survival.[40, 41]

The use of ABO-incompatible donors has been controversial. Allograft and patient survival rates in

TABLE 45–6. Factors Related to Primary Nonfunction

Donor Factors

Preexisting disease or injury to donor,
  anemia, hypoxia, hypotension prior to organ harvest
Donor organ steatosis (>60% macrovesicular fat)

Transplant Factors

Prolonged cold ischemic storage (>12–18 h)
Prolonged warm ischemic time at implantation
Complex vascular anastomosis requiring surgical revision
Significant size discrepancy between donor and recipient

Recipient Factors

Postreperfusion hypotension
Vascular thrombosis
Immunologic factors
ABO incompatible, positive crossmatch

---

adult recipients have not been comparable to those achieved using ABO identical or compatible donors.[42, 43] However, pediatric recipients of ABO incompatible allografts have achieved survival rates equivalent to those using ABO-compatible and ABO-identical donors, using either cadaveric donors (CDs) or LDs.[28, 44, 45]

Documentation of functional hepatic recovery is best undertaken by evaluating the ongoing hepatic output of clotting factors (V, VII) with improvement in coagulation parameters (prothrombin time, partial thromboplastin time) and the synthesis of bile. Protocol hepatic biopsies assist in the documentation of hepatic histologic and immunologic events, but they cannot accurately predict the likelihood of recovery.

Vascular Thrombosis

Hepatic artery thrombosis (HAT) occurs in children three to four times more frequently than in adult transplant series, occurring most often within the first 30 days following transplantation. Factors influencing the development of HAT are listed in Table 45–7.

HAT presents with a variable clinical picture that may include (1) fulminant allograft failure, (2) biliary disruption or obstruction, or (3) systemic sepsis. Doppler ultrasound (US) imaging has been accurate in identifying arterial thrombosis, and it is used as the primary screening modality to assess blood flow following transplantation or whenever complications arise. Acute HAT with allograft failure most often requires immediate retransplantation. Successful thrombectomy and allograft salvage is possible if reconstruction is undertaken before allograft necrosis.[46] Biliary complications are particularly common following HAT. Ischemic biliary disruption with intraparenchymal biloma formation or anastomotic disruption presents with cholestasis associated with systemic sepsis. The development of systemic septicemia or multifocal abscesses in sites of

TABLE 45–7. Factors Affecting
Vascular Thrombosis

Donor/Recipient Age/Weight

Allograft Type

Whole organ > reduced size
Living donor > reduced size

Anastomotic Anatomy

Primary hepatic artery > direct aortic

Allograft Edema—Increased Vascular Resistance

Ischemic injury secondary to prolonged
    preservation; prolonged implantation
Rejection
Fluid overload

Recipient Hypotension

Hypercoagulability

Administration of coagulation factors, fresh-frozen
    plasma
Procoagulant factor deficiencies

---

ischemic necrosis secondary to gram-negative enteric bacteria, *Enterococcus*, anaerobic bacteria, or fungi can also be seen. Antibiotic therapy directed toward these organisms, along with surgical drainage, is indicated when specific abscess sites are identified. Percutaneous drainage and biliary stenting may control bile leakage and infection until retransplantation is undertaken.

Late postoperative thrombosis can be asymptomatic or present with slowly progressive bile duct stenosis. Rarely, allograft necrosis occurs. Arterial collaterals from the Roux-en-Y limb can provide a source of revascularization of the thrombosed allograft through hilar collaterals. These collateral channels develop during the first postoperative months, making late thrombosis an often silent clinical event. Conversely, disruption of this collateral supply during operative reconstruction of the central bile ducts in patients with HAT can precipitate hepatic ischemia and parenchymal necrosis. When HAT is asymptomatic, careful follow-up alone is indicated.

Prevention of HAT requires meticulous microsurgical arterial reconstruction at the time of transplantation. Anatomic reconstruction is preferred in whole organ allografts; direct implantation of the celiac axis into the infrarenal aorta is recommended for all reduced-size liver allografts. All complex vascular reconstructions of the donor hepatic artery should be undertaken ex vivo whenever possible using microsurgical techniques before transplantation. When vascular grafts are required, they should also be directly implanted into the infrarenal aorta.[47, 48] No systemic anticoagulation was routinely used in our series, but aspirin (20 to 40 mg/day) is administered to all children for 100 days. Complex protocols administering both procoagulants and anticoagulants have also been very successful.[49]

Portal vein thrombosis is uncommon in whole organ allografts unless prior portosystemic shunting has altered the flow within the splanchnic vascular bed or unless severe portal vein stenosis in the recipient has impaired flow to the allograft. Preexisting portal vein thrombosis in the recipient can be overcome by thrombectomy, portal vein replacement, or extraanatomic venous bypass. Early thrombosis following transplantation requires immediate anastomotic revision and thrombectomy. Discrepancies in venous size imposed by reduced-size allografts can be modified to allow anastomotic construction.[48, 50] Deficiencies of anticoagulant proteins, such as protein C and S, and antithrombin III deficiency in the recipient must also be excluded as a contributing cause for vascular thrombosis.[51] Failure to recognize portal thrombosis can lead to either allograft demise or, on a more chronic basis, to significant portal hypertension with hemorrhagic sequelae or intractable ascites.

Biliary Complications

Complications related to biliary reconstruction occur in approximately 10% of pediatric liver transplant recipients. Their spectrum and treatment is determined by the status of the hepatic artery and the type of allograft used. Although whole and reduced-size allografts have an equivalent risk of biliary complications, the spectrum of complications differs.[52, 53]

Primary bile duct reconstruction is the preferred biliary reconstruction in adults, but it is less commonly used in children. It has the advantage of preserving the sphincter of Oddi, decreasing the incidence of enteric reflux and subsequent cholangitis, and not requiring an intestinal anastomosis. Early experience using primary choledochocholedochostomy without a T-tube has been favorable.[54] Late complications following any type of primary ductal reconstruction include anastomotic stricture, biliary sludge formation, and recurrent cholangitis. Endoscopic dilation and internal stenting of anastomotic strictures has been successful in early postoperative cases. Roux-en-Y choledochojejunostomy is the preferred treatment for recurrent stenosis or postoperative leak.

Roux-en-Y choledochojejunostomy is the reconstruction of choice in small children and is required in all patients with biliary atresia. Recurrent cholangitis, a theoretical risk, suggests anastomotic or intrahepatic biliary stricture formation or small bowel obstruction distal to the Roux-en-Y anastomosis. In the absence of these complications, cholangitis is uncommon.

Reconstruction of the bile ducts in patients with reduced-size allografts is more complex. Division of the bile duct in close proximity to the cut-surface margin of the allograft, with careful preservation of the biliary duct collateral circulation, decreases but does not eliminate ductal stricture formation secondary to ductal ischemia. In our early experience, in 14% of patients with left lobe reduced-size allografts, a short segmental stricture developed requiring biliary anastomotic revision (Fig. 45–4). Opera-

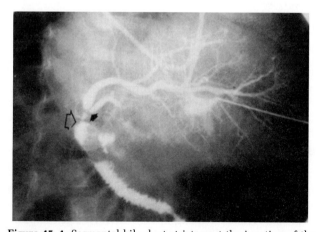

Figure 45–4. Segmental bile duct stricture at the junction of the left lateral and left medial segmental bile ducts in a left lobe reduced-size allograft. *Solid arrow,* bile duct stricture; *open arrow,* Roux-en-Y loop and bile duct anastomosis. (From Ryckman FC: Liver transplantation in children. In Suchy FJ [ed]: Liver Disease in Children. St. Louis, CV Mosby, 1994, p 941.)

tive revision of the biliary anastomosis and reimplantation of the bile ducts into the Roux-en-Y is necessary. Percutaneous transhepatic cholangiography is essential to define the intrahepatic ductal anatomy before operative revision, and temporary catheter decompression of the obstructed bile ducts allows treatment of cholangitis and elective reconstruction. Operative reconstruction is accompanied by transhepatic passage of exteriorized multifenestrated biliary ductal stents, which remain in place until reconstructive success is documented and late stenosis is unlikely. Dissection remote from the vasobiliary sheath has significantly decreased the incidence of this complication.

REJECTION

Acute Cellular Rejection

Allograft rejection is characterized by the histologic triad of endothelialitis, portal triad lymphocyte infiltration with bile duct injury, and hepatic parenchymal cell damage.[55] Allograft biopsy is essential to establish the diagnosis before treatment. The rapidity of the rejection process and its response to therapy dictates the intensity and duration of antirejection treatment.

Acute rejection occurs in approximately two thirds of patients following OLT.[56] The primary treatment of rejection is a short course of high-dose steroids. Bolus doses administered over several days with a rapid taper to baseline therapy is successful in 75 to 80% of cases.[57] When refractory or recurrent rejection occurs, antilymphocyte therapy using the monoclonal antibody OKT-3 is successful in 90% of cases.[58]

Retransplantation for refractory rejection is necessary in fulminant cases in which vascular thrombosis occurs and in cases unresponsive to treatment. In refractory cases, retransplantation should be undertaken before using multiple courses of corticosteroids or antilymphocyte agents to avoid the overwhelming risks of infection or lymphoproliferative disease. However, modern immunosuppressive treatment makes this an uncommon event.

Chronic Rejection

Uniform diagnosis and management of chronic rejection is complicated by the lack of a consistent definition or clinical course. Chronic rejection occurs in 5 to 10% of transplanted patients and occurs with equal frequency in children and adults. The primary clinical manifestation is a progressive increase in biliary ductal enzymes (alkaline phosphatase, γ-glutamyl transferase) and progressive cholestasis. This course can be initially asymptomatic or follow an unsuccessful treatment course for acute rejection. The syndrome can occur within weeks of transplantation or later in the clinical course.

Chronic rejection can follow one of two clinical forms.[59] In the first, the injury is primarily to the biliary epithelium and the clinical course is typically slowly progressive with preservation of synthetic function. Histologic evidence shows interlobular bile duct destruction in the absence of ischemic injury or the presence of hepatocellular necrosis. In full expression, this lesion is characterized as acute *vanishing bile duct syndrome* when severe ductopenia is seen in at least 20 portal tracts.[60] The eventual spontaneous resolution of nearly one half of affected patients with tacrolimus therapy has led to the development of enhanced immunosuppression protocols for this patient subgroup.[59] Retransplantation is occasionally necessary but rarely emergent.

The second subtype is characterized by the early development of progressive ischemic injury to both bile ducts and hepatocytes, leading to ductopenia and ischemic necrosis with fibrosis. The clinical picture of cholestasis is accompanied by significant synthetic dysfunction with superimposed vascular thrombosis or biliary stricture formation. The vascular endothelial injury responsible for the progressive ischemic changes is characterized by the development of subintimal foam cells or fibrointimal hypertrophy. The clinical course is relentlessly progressive and nearly always requires retransplantation. Recurrence of chronic rejection in the retransplanted allograft is common.[60]

The immunologic nature of this process is emphasized by the primary target role played by the biliary and vascular endothelium, the only tissues in the liver that express class II antigens. Other interdependent cofactors such as cytomegalovirus (CMV) infection, HLA mismatching, positive B-cell crossmatching, and differing racial demographics of the donor to recipient combination have all failed to show consistent correlation with the development of chronic rejection.[59, 60]

Infection

Infectious complications have become the most common source of morbidity and mortality following transplantation. Multiple organism infection is common as are concurrent infections by different infectious agents.

Bacterial infections occur in the immediate posttransplant period and are most often caused by gram-negative enteric organisms, *Enterococcus*, or *Staphylococcus* species. Intraabdominal abscesses or infected collections of serum along the cut surface of the reduced-size allograft are addressed with extraperitoneal or laparotomy drainage; percutaneous drainage has been unsuccessful in most cases. Intrahepatic abscesses suggest hepatic artery stenosis or thrombosis, and treatment is directed by the vascular status of the allograft and associated bile duct abnormalities. Sepsis originating at sites of invasive monitoring lines can be minimized by replacing or removing all intraoperative lines soon after transplantation. Antibacterial prophylactic antibiotics are discontinued as soon as possible to prevent the development of resistant organisms.

Fungal sepsis represents a significant potential problem in the early posttransplant period. Aggressive protocols for pretransplant prophylaxis are based on the concept that fungal infections originate from organisms colonizing the GI tract of the recipient. Selective bowel decontamination was successful in eliminating pathogenic gram-negative bacteria from the GI tract in 87% of adult patients; in all cases, *Candida* was eliminated.[61, 62] However, these protocols have not been practical in pediatric patients because there is a long waiting time for pediatric organs and the taste of the antibiotics used is poorly accepted. Fungal infection most often occurs in patients requiring multiple operative procedures and those who have had multiple antibiotic courses. Development of fungemia or urosepsis requires retinal and cardiac investigation and a search for renal fungal involvement; antifungal therapy should be undertaken. Severe fungal infection has a mortality rate greater than 80%, making early treatment essential. All patients undergoing OLT receive antifungal prophylaxis with fluconazole at our center.

The majority of early and severe viral infections are caused by viruses of the Herpesviridae family, including Epstein-Barr virus (EBV), CMV, and herpes simplex virus (HSV). The likelihood that CMV infection will develop is influenced by the preoperative CMV status of the transplant donor and recipient.[63, 64] Seronegative recipients receiving seropositive donor organs are at greatest risk, with seropositive donor to recipient combinations at the next greatest risk. Use of various immune-based prophylactic protocols including IV IgG or hyperimmune anti-CMV IgG, coupled with acyclovir or ganciclovir have all achieved success in decreasing the incidence of symptomatic CMV infection, although seroconversion in naive recipients of seropositive donor organs inevitably occurs.

The clinical diagnosis of CMV infection is suggested by the development of fever, leukopenia, maculopapular rash and hepatocellular abnormalities, respiratory insufficiency, or GI hemorrhage. Hepatic biopsy or endoscopic biopsy of colonic or gastroduodenal sites allows early diagnosis with immunohistochemical recognition. Rapid blood and urine assays for CMV can also expedite diagnosis. In suspected cases, treatment should be instituted while awaiting culture or biopsy results owing to the potential rapidity and severity of this infection in a previously naive child. The treatment of CMV has been greatly improved by the development of ganciclovir. Early treatment with IV IgG and ganciclovir is successful in most cases.

HSV syndromes, similar to those seen in nontransplant patients, require treatment with acyclovir when diagnosed.

Other viruses leading to significant posttransplant infectious complications include adenovirus hepatitis, varicella, and enterovirus-induced gastroenteritis. Recurrent viral hepatitis is an uncommon problem in pediatric transplantation, but it is commonly seen in adult patients. *Pneumocystis* infection has been nearly eliminated by the prophylactic administration of sulfamethoxazole-trimethoprim or aerosolized pentamidine.

EBV infection occurring in the perioperative period presents with a wide spectrum of disease, including a mononucleosis-like syndrome, hepatitis-simulating rejection, extranodal lymphoproliferative infiltration with bowel perforation, peritonsillar or lymph node enlargement, or encephalopathy. EBV infection can occur as a primary infection or following reactivation of a past primary infection. When serologic evidence of active infection exists, an acute reduction in immunosuppression is indicated. High-dose IV acyclovir or ganciclovir is indicated for acute clinically significant infections, and oral acyclovir should be continued until symptoms of lymphadenopathy have resolved.

Posttransplant lymphoproliferative disease (PTLD), a potentially fatal abnormal proliferation of B lymphocytes, can occur in any situation in which immunosuppression is undertaken. The importance of PTLD in pediatric liver transplantation is a result of the intensity of the immunosuppression required, its lifetime duration, and the absence of prior exposure to EBV infection in many pediatric recipients.

Multiple studies analyzing immunosuppressive therapy and the development of PTLD have shown a progressive increase in the incidence of PTLD with an increase in total immunosuppressive load.[65] No single immunosuppressive agent has been directly related to PTLD, although high-dose cyclosporine, tacrolimus, polyclonal antilymphocyte sera (MALG, ALG), and monoclonal antibodies (OKT-3) have all been implicated. Immunosuppressive strategies using these agents as sequential therapy in low doses have not produced an increase in PTLD when successful induction prevents recurrent high-dose or long duration immunotherapy for rejection. However, prolonged treatment with anti–T-cell agents and the duration, intensity, and total immunosuppressive load are the origin of the defective immunity that creates the background for neoplasia.

The second pathogenic feature influencing PTLD appears to be EBV infection. Primary or reactivation infections often precede the recognition of PTLD. Active EBV infection, whether primary or reactivation, involves the B-lymphocyte pool, causing B-cell proliferation. A simultaneous increase in cytotoxic T-cell activity is the normal primary host mechanism preventing EBV dissemination. Loss of this natural protection as a result of the administration of T-cell inhibitory immunotherapy allows polyclonal B-cell proliferation to progress. Polyclonal proliferation of B lymphocytes occurs following EBV viral replication and release. With time, transformation of a small population of cells results in a malignant monoclonal aggressive B-cell lymphoma.[66]

Most tumors seen in children are large cell lymphomas, 86% being of B-cell origin. Extranodal involvement, uncommon in primary lymphomas, is seen in 70% of PTLD cases. Extranodal sites include

central nervous system, 27%; liver, 23%; lung, 22%; kidney, 21%; intestine, 20%; and spleen, 13%. Allograft involvement is common and can mimic rejection.[66] T-cell and B-cell immunohistochemical markers of the infiltrating lymphocyte population define the B-cell infiltrate and assist in establishing an early diagnosis.

Treatment of PTLD is stratified according to the immunologic cell typing and clinical presentation.[67] Documented PTLD requires an immediate decrease in immunosuppression and institution of anti-EBV therapy. We prefer to use IV ganciclovir for initial antiviral therapy owing to the high incidence of concurrent CMV infection, but acyclovir is used for long-term treatment. Patients with polyclonal B-cell proliferation frequently show regression with this treatment. Patients with aggressive monoclonal malignancies have poor survival even with immunosuppressive reduction, acyclovir, and conventional chemotherapy or radiation therapy. These additional treatment modalities often precipitate the development of fatal systemic infection. Results with high-dose interferon alfa and IV IgG are encouraging but preliminary.[66] When treatment is successful, careful follow-up to identify recurrent disease or delayed central nervous system involvement is essential.

RETRANSPLANTATION

The vast majority of retransplantation procedures in pediatric patients are done as a result of acute allograft demise caused by HAT or PNF. Acute rejection, chronic rejection, and biliary complications are more uncommon causes. Many of these complications are associated with concurrent sepsis, which further complicates reoperation and compromises success. Survival following transplantation is directly related to prompt identification of appropriate patients and acquisition of a suitable organ. When retransplantation is promptly undertaken for acute organ failure, patient survival rate, in our experience, is 84%. However, when retransplantation is undertaken for chronic allograft failure, often complicated by multiple organ system insufficiency, the survival rate is only 50%.

Similar findings were reported by United Network of Organ Sharing (UNOS) Region I in their combined experience; patients undergoing retransplantation for acute organ failure experienced twice the overall survival rate as those undergoing retransplantation for chronic disease.[68] In addition, acute retransplantation survival was significantly influenced by the time to acquire a retransplant organ, with a greater than 3-day wait decreasing the survival rate from 52 to 20%. The overall incidence of retransplantation is 14% in our series and ranges in others' experience from 8 to 29%. This incidence is similar when primary whole organ allografts are compared to primary reduced-size allografts. Reduced-size allografts are frequently used when retransplantation is required in view of their improved availability

TABLE 45–8. Factors Affecting
Transplant Survival

Medical Status at Orthotopic Liver Transplantation
Primary Diagnosis
Age and Size
Comorbid Conditions
Encephalopathy
Infection
Multiple organ dysfunction

and their decreased incidence of allograft-threatening complications.[22, 69, 70] These findings emphasize the need for early identification of children requiring retransplantation and expeditious reoperation before the development of multisystem organ failure or sepsis.

OUTCOME FOLLOWING TRANSPLANTATION

Although the potential complications following liver transplantation are frequent and severe, the overall results are rewarding. Improvements in organ preservation, operative management, immunosuppression, and treatment of postoperative complications have all contributed to the excellent survival rate that is seen. Factors influencing the survival of children undergoing transplantation are detailed in Table 45–8. Survival rates in infants are still lower than in older children. Infants younger than 1 year of age or weighing less than 10 kg have a reported survival rate of 65 to 88% overall, an improvement over previously reported rates of 50 to 60%.[71, 72] Improved survival in these small recipients is consistent throughout all levels of medical urgency and results from a decrease in life-threatening and graft-threatening complications, such as HAT and PNF, in the reduced-size donor organ.

Patients with fulminant hepatic failure have an overall survival rate that is significantly lower than other diagnostic groups, with patients having metabolic disease having the highest survival rate. Prior surgical procedures, especially in patients who have undergone multiple reoperations, influence the incidence of complications, especially bowel perforation, but do not adversely affect overall survival. However, the most important factor determining survival is the severity of the patient's illness at the time of transplantation.[22, 73] When stratified for illness by UNOS status, emergent transplantation (UNOS Status 1) has a diminished survival rate compared to that for other patients. Present efforts to use surgically altered allografts, such as RSOLT, LD-OLT, and split liver OLT, have experienced similar survival rates as those for whole organ recipients (Fig. 45–5).[70, 74]

The increased donor availability for small recipients achieved through the use of reduced-size donor organs has also brought about a significant decrease in waiting list mortality. In our center, mortality rate for patients awaiting transplantation decreased from 29 to 2%, and similar results have been reported by other pediatric centers.[69, 70, 74] Efforts to enhance donor availability, allowing transplantation of children before they reach critical status, is essential before major improvements in postoperative survival rates can occur.

FOLLOW-UP

The overriding objective of hepatic transplantation in children is complete rehabilitation with improved quality of life. Factors contributing to the attainment of this goal include improved nutritional status with appropriate growth and development, as well as enhanced motor and cognitive skills, allowing social reintegration.

Nutrition and Growth

Optimal postoperative nutrition significantly facilitates recovery and rehabilitation. This initially

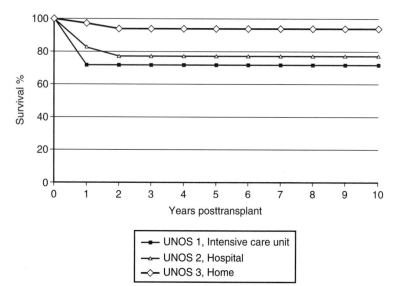

Figure 45–5. Liver transplant patient survival stratified by United Network of Organ Sharing (UNOS) status at orthotopic liver transplantation.

requires providing 100 to 130 calories/kg/day in recipients weighing less than 10 kg. Hepatic synthetic function, gut absorption, and appetite all improve following successful pediatric liver transplantation.

Despite these improvements, growth disturbances do not immediately resolve.[75, 76] In the 1st year after transplantation, very little catch-up growth occurs. During the 2nd and 3rd year after transplantation, patients usually show significant catch-up growth, with the potential for catch-up growth being directly correlated with the degree of preoperative growth retardation. Decreased corticosteroid administration improves this recovery, and the effect is further improved by the use of alternate-day steroids or complete steroid withdrawal in patients with stable allograft function 2 years following transplantation (S. H. Ryckman, Growth velocity following OLT in children, personal communication, 1996).[77] The "steroid-sparing" effects of new immunosuppressive agents, such as tacrolimus, could diminish this unwanted consequence of immune modulation.

Neuropsychological Outcome

Although most pediatric transplant recipients are returning to normal age-appropriate activities (e.g., accomplishing normal developmental milestones, re-entering school), recent studies indicate that they may be experiencing subtle functional difficulties.[78, 79] Neuropsychological function studies of children following transplantation demonstrate multiple deficits involving learning and memory, abstraction, concept formation, visual-spatial function, and motor function. The well-documented neurologic and cerebral abnormalities associated with chronic cirrhosis precede transplantation but certainly influence these results.[80, 81]

The long-term impact that transplantation has on the psychosocial and financial health of the entire family unit is also the subject of much concern. Long-term pediatric liver transplant survivors need in-depth, multicenter longitudinal studies to clarify these issues.

☐ Renal Transplantation in Infants and Children

ETIOLOGY

Acute renal failure in infants is most often the consequence of hemodynamic instability, with malperfusion or hypoxia resulting in acute tubular necrosis. Most of these patients either recover sufficient renal function for normal long-term survival or die of multisystem failure.

Chronic renal failure is uncommon in infants, with the estimate of infants with end-stage renal disease (ESRD) placed at 0.2 per million total population for infants younger than 1 year of age.[82, 83] Congenital lesions such as renal dysplasia, obstruc-

tive malformations, or complex urogenital malformation and congenital nephrosis are the most common causes of ESRD in children younger than 5 years of age, accounting for 46% of cases. Glomerulonephritis, including focal segmental glomerulosclerosis, membranoproliferative glomerulonephritis, and lupus nephritis, as well as recurrent pyelonephritis, are the leading causes of ESRD in older children (Table 45–9).[84] Hereditary causes of renal failure should be identified to plan appropriate overall treatment strategy, including evaluating other family members and providing genetic counseling when needed.

Knowledge of the etiology of the ESRD is important to allow assessment of the potential for recurrence within a transplant allograft and consideration of living related donor transplantation. Patients with a "structural/congenital" etiology without an immunologic component also enjoy better graft survival rates than those patients with "glomerulonephritis."[85]

PRETRANSPLANT MANAGEMENT

Pretransplant management is critical in infants and children with ESRD. Children with ESRD beginning in infancy or early childhood experience significant complications from growth retardation, renal osteodystrophy, and neuropsychiatric developmental delay. Recent advances in dialysis regimens, nutritional supplementation, and recombinant human erythropoietin and growth hormone have significantly improved the pretransplant management of these patients.

Dialysis

Dialysis is indicated when complications of ESRD occur despite optimal medical management, namely, hyperkalemia, volume overload, acidosis, intractable hypertension, and uremic symptoms such as vomiting. In older children, lethargy and poor school performance can signal the need for more aggressive treatment. In addition, dialysis may be necessary to facilitate the administration of adequate protein as part of an extensive nutritional resuscitation plan.

When dialysis is undertaken, the use of peritoneal dialysis is preferred for the following reasons: (1) it avoids the multiple blood transfusions associated with hemodialysis; (2) it allows a gradual correction of electrolyte abnormalities, preventing cerebral disequilibrium syndrome in small infants; and (3) it is easy to administer.

Hemodialysis can be used when there is an unsuitable peritoneal cavity secondary to prior surgery or with peritoneal infections; however, the construction and maintenance of adequate long-term vascular access sites in small infants and children is difficult. Use of centralized venous catheters rather than arteriovenous fistulas is our preferred mode for temporary hemodialysis access in children, al-

TABLE 45-9. Recipient Characteristics (North American Pediatric Renal Transplant Cooperative Study)

Diagnosis	No.	%
Obstructive uropathy	605	16.5
Aplastic/hypoplastic/dysplastic kidneys	603	16.4
Focal segmental glomerulosclerosis	426	11.6
Reflux nephropathy	209	5.7
Systemic immunologic disease	174	4.7
Chronic glomerulonephritis	160	4.4
Syndrome of agenesis of abdominal musculature	112	3.0
Congenital nephrotic syndrome	103	2.8
Hemolytic uremic syndrome	101	2.7
Polycystic kidney disease	100	2.7
Medullary cystic disease/juvenile nephronophthisis	94	2.6
Cystinosis	92	2.5
Pyelonephritis/interstitial nephritis	84	2.3
Membranoproliferative glomerulonephritis type I	84	2.3
Familial nephritis	83	2.3
Renal infarct	75	2.0
Idiopathic crescentic glomerulonephritis	65	1.8
Membranoproliferative glomerulonephritis type II	37	1.0
Oxalosis	29	0.8
Membranous nephropathy	23	0.6
Wilms' tumor	22	0.6
Drash syndrome	20	0.5
Sickle cell nephropathy	5	0.1
Diabetic nephropathy	4	0.1
Other	203	5.5
Unknown	160	4.4

though infection and vascular thrombosis complicate this therapy. Access via the internal jugular veins is preferred over subclavian routes to avoid venous occlusion from the upper extremity, which compromises later arm arteriovenous fistula sites. Although dialysis and its complications, such as infection, have a great influence on the complexity of care, they do not affect the ultimate results of renal transplantation.[86]

Nutritional Support

The need for vigorous nutritional support of the infant with uremia has been well documented by the growth retardation seen in infants and children with ESRD. The etiology of growth disturbance is multifactorial, including anorexia that leads to both protein and calorie insufficiency, renal osteodystrophy, aluminum toxicity, uremic acidosis, impaired somatomedin activity, and growth hormone and insulin resistance.[87] Because the most intense period of growth occurs during the first 2 years of life, careful nutritional support during that time is essential.

Despite extensive nutritional efforts, the mean weight at the time of transplantation for all patients was −2.2 SD below the appropriate age-adjusted and sex-adjusted mean for normal children in the recent North American Pediatric Renal Transplant Cooperative Study (NAPRTCS). Similar height deficits occurred.[86] This growth deficit was greater (−2.8 SD) in children younger than 5 years of age. Transplantation afforded a +0.8 SD increase in growth over the 1st posttransplant year; however, this accelerated growth then reaches a stable plateau. After 2 to 3 years, the mean weight values were comparable to those in normal children.[84] Children 6 years of age and older show no improvement in their height deficit 5 years after transplantation.[86] These limitations to "catch-up" growth emphasize the need for early transplantation in young ESRD patients. If epiphyseal closure has occurred (bone age >12 years), additional bone growth is often not achieved.[82, 88] Normalization of growth rarely occurs with the introduction of either hemodialysis or peritoneal dialysis.

The importance of efforts to normalize nutritional parameters is emphasized by the adverse impact of uremia on the developing nervous system in the infant. The significance of this problem was emphasized in a study in which progressive encephalopathy, developmental delay, microcephaly, hypotonia, seizures, and dyskinesia developed in 20 of 23 children with ESRD before 1 year of age.[89] All of these patients had significant growth impairment. Monitoring of the head circumference has been suggested to identify the infant at risk, with the intent to initiate dialysis, nutritional support, or transplantation if this parameter deviates from the normal curve.[82]

TRANSPLANT MANAGEMENT
Preoperative Evaluation

In preparation for transplantation, an extensive evaluation of the urinary tract and immunologic status of the patient is necessary.

The increased frequency of urinary tract abnormalities as the primary cause of ESRD in infants and children necessitates the investigation of the urinary tract for sites of obstruction, presence of ureteral reflux, and functional state and capacity of the urinary bladder.[90] This investigation is best accomplished by obtaining an IV pyelogram or US of the upper urinary tract and a voiding cystourethrogram to assess bladder and reflux parameters. Any questions related to bladder function or structure require cystometry and cystoscopy.

In patients with long-standing oliguric ESRD, the bladder capacity may appear very small. In the absence of abnormal obstructive or neuromuscular bladder pathology, adequate enlargement of the bladder in the face of normal urinary production is to be expected. Any surgical correction of urethral obstruction or augmentation of bladder size should be undertaken far in advance of undertaking transplantation. Preoperative sterilization of the urinary tract and development of unobstructed urinary outflow should be the ultimate goals of evaluation and reconstruction. Although complex anomalies of the urogenital tract often require many extensive operative procedures to augment, reconstruct, or create an acceptable lower urinary tract, virtually all such children can undergo successful reconstruction with continent urinary reservoirs without the use of intestinal conduits.[91]

Immunologic assessment includes tissue typing and panel reactive antibody analysis. Patients should be monitored periodically for the development of a positive crossmatch to their potential LD or of positive cytotoxic antibody to a panel of random donors to assess immunologic reactivity. In addition, reactivity to CMV, EBV, HSV, and hepatitis should be investigated. Childhood immunizations should be current, and immunization against hepatitis B virus instituted. Any immunizations with live virus vaccines should be given well in advance of transplantation, because their use is contraindicated in the early posttransplant period.

Selection of the appropriate donor source for transplantation is a decision for the transplant team and family to consider together. A related immediate family member LD has the advantage of a low incidence of postoperative acute tubular necrosis; improved histologic matching, leading to fewer rejection episodes and the need for less immunosuppression; and the possibility of extended organ function. In addition, any operative procedures required for recipient preparation, as well as the transplant procedure, can be scheduled around the needs of the patient, simplifying preoperative care and potentially avoiding the complications of dialysis. Parents form the majority of donors; siblings younger than 18 years of age are rarely considered unless they are identical twins. At present, 47% of children receive a related LD kidney.[86] Complete evaluation of the potential donor to exclude intrinsic renal anomalies, vascular anomalies, and systemic illness is necessary.

CD kidneys are used for 53% of renal transplants.[86] The unpredictability of donor organ availability and the need to establish a negative antibody crossmatch for CD transplantation make surgical planning impossible. The size of a potential allograft, CD or related LD, is also important. Kidneys from small adult donors can be transplanted into infants as small as 5 kg with good technical success.[92] CD organs from pediatric donors 5 years of age or older also yield an excellent survival rate. However, a progressive decrease in 1-year graft survival has been noted when kidneys from donors younger than 3 to 4 years of age have been used.[93, 94] This decrease in graft and patient survival rate is related to the donor organ source; children 2 to 5 years of age have a similar survival rate as the overall pediatric population when living related donors are used.[84, 95] Recognition of this potential risk has led to a reluctance by most centers to use donors younger than 5 years of age. An effect of donor age on graft survival has been attributed to an increased rate of both graft thrombosis and acute rejection.[84]

The decision to use a CD is often strengthened by the possibility of disease recurrence within the transplanted kidney. The incidence of disease recurrence following transplantation and the risk of graft loss are listed in Table 45–10.[96] The decision to proceed with LD transplantation in small children

TABLE 45-10. Recurrence Rates and Graft Loss from Recurrent Disease in Children

Disease	Recurrence Rate (%)	Clinical Severity	% of Those with Recurrence Whose Graft Failed
FSGS	25–30	High	40–50
MPGN type I	70	Mild	12–30
MPGN type II	100	Low	10–20
SLE	5–40	Low	5
HSP	55–85	Low–mild	5–20
HUS			
Classical	12–20	Moderate	0–10
Atypical	± 25	High	40–50

FSGS, focal segmental glomerulosclerosis; HSP, Henoch-Schönlein purpura; HUS, hemolytic uremic syndrome; MPGN, membranoproliferative glomerulonephritis; SLE, systemic lupus erythematosus.
From Fine RN, Ettenger R. In Morris PJ (ed): Kidney Transplantation: Principles and Practice (4th ed). Philadelphia, WB Saunders, 1994, p 418.

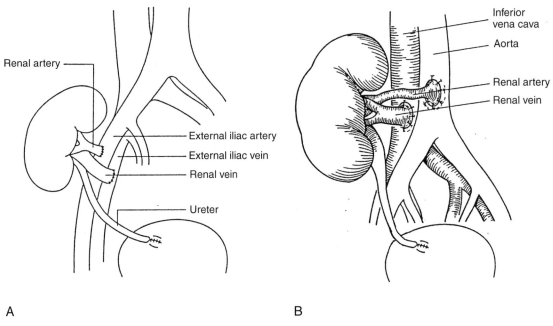

Figure 45–6. Schematic diagram of kidney transplantation. *A,* Older child and adolescent with vascular implantation into the iliac artery and vein. *B,* Transplantation in an infant with aortic and vena caval vascular anastomoses.

is also influenced by the recognized increased risk of graft failure when using related LD transplants in recipients younger than 2 years old.[86] In small infants, a CD kidney may be recommended for initial transplantation, with the use of a related LD kidney reserved for the later expected growth needs of the developing child, when the larger kidney can be more easily implanted.

Preemptive Transplantation

The desire to begin preemptive transplantation before undertaking dialysis is often fueled by the patient's or parents' desire to avoid the surgical procedures, potential infections or cardiovascular complications, and psychological impairment inherent with dialysis. A recent NAPRTCS review found 26% of primary transplantations were performed without prior dialysis.[97] Most cases used LDs rather than cadaveric sources. There was no difference in patient or graft survival in this group when compared with patients who undergo dialysis before transplantation. Preemptive transplantation is not possible when uncontrolled hypertension, massive proteinuria, or recurrent infection require prior native kidney removal or when oliguric renal failure requires immediate dialysis.[96]

Operative Procedure

Preparation for transplantation should include placing adequate large-bore IV lines and the largest Foley catheter possible. Central venous lines are used in all infants and children to ensure vascular access, hemodynamic monitoring, and a route for postoperative immunosuppressive delivery. Perioperative prophylactic antibiotics are administered. Arterial pressure monitoring lines are only necessary in small infants and patients with hemodynamic compromise, allowing preservation of future hemodialysis access sites.

Transplantation in infants and small children can be undertaken through a generous retroperitoneal approach or transabdominal placing of the allograft within the peritoneal cavity posterior to the right or left colon. An extraperitoneal approach to the retroperitoneum allows the maintenance of postoperative peritoneal dialysis and should be strongly considered when size permits. The arterial anastomosis is constructed end-to-side into the distal aorta or common iliac artery using a Carrel patch, and venous outflow of the allograft should be into the inferior vena cava or common iliac vein. Ureteral implantation using the Lich extravesical ureteroneocystostomy avoids the presence of a cystotomy and minimizes postoperative blood clots within the bladder, which may obstruct the Foley catheter. When larger donor kidneys are used in small recipients, the vessels must be shortened to avoid redundancy when the kidney is positioned in the retroperitoneum. The internal iliac artery is not used in pediatric transplants so that pelvic blood flow is preserved (Fig. 45–6). Ureteral "double-J" stents are used when small ureter size may lead to obstruction.

Anesthetic management of the infant and small child during kidney transplantation is complicated by preexisting electrolyte abnormalities and the large fluid fluxes that occur in the operating room. Intravascular blood volume must be augmented during allograft implantation to allow maintenance of normal systemic blood flow when allograft blood flow is reestablished. Perfusion of the allograft with hypothermic lactated Ringer's solution before implantation to remove any remaining hyperkalemic graft preservation solution is necessary in infants and small children to avoid massive potassium infusion with establishment of allograft perfusion. Blood volume loading to a central venous pressure of 13 to 15 cm H_2O and administration of bicarbonate, calcium, and low-dose vasopressors (dopamine 5 μg/kg/min) should be started before reperfusion of the graft.

Postoperative Management

Posttransplant management requires careful screening for technical complications, rejection, recurrence of the primary renal disease, and prevention of immunosuppression-related complications.

Frequent fluid and electrolyte monitoring is necessary immediately following transplantation because larger kidneys can excrete the equivalent of the infant's blood volume within a single hour. Careful attention to serum concentrations of calcium, phosphorus, magnesium, and electrolytes is necessary. Urine output is isovolumetrically replaced. Glucose-free urine replacement fluids minimize hyperglycemia and attendant osmotic diuresis in the recipient. Selection of appropriate electrolyte concentrations is guided by urinary electrolyte excre-tion, which is regularly monitored. Central venous filling pressures should be maintained at 7 to 10 cm H_2O to ensure adequate intravascular volume. In patients with high-output renal failure, urine losses from both the native and transplant kidneys need to be replaced to avoid hypoperfusion and thrombosis. Maintenance of catheter patency is essential, and any episode of decreased urinary output should be rapidly investigated to exclude Foley catheter occlusion and bladder distention. An algorithm for the evaluation of early postoperative oliguria is shown in Figure 45–7.

Technical Complications

Vascular thrombosis still accounts for graft loss in up to 13% of index transplants and 19% of repeat transplants in children. Graft thrombosis is significantly more frequent in children younger than 2 years of age and is directly related to the age of both the donor and the recipient. In addition, prolonged cold ischemic preservation time (>24 hours) and the related presence of acute tubular necrosis with delayed graft function also increase this risk. Prior transplantation has also been shown to be an independent risk factor. Immediate posttransplant Doppler US vascular imaging is helpful in confirming suitable allograft blood flow following abdominal closure, especially when large allografts are implanted into small recipients. Adequate hydration

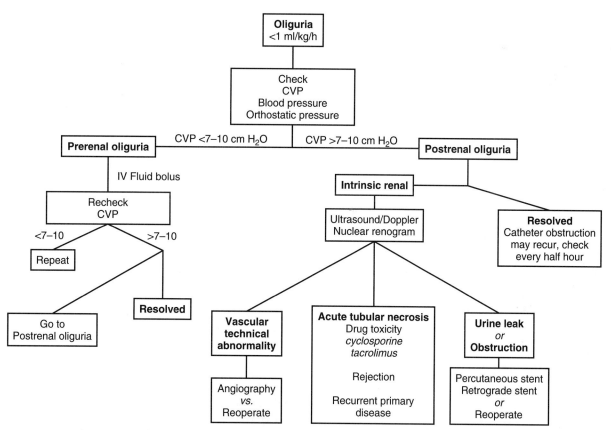

Figure 45–7. Schematic flow diagram for the management of postoperative renal allograft dysfunction and oliguria. CVP, central venous pressure; IV, intravenous.

is essential to maintain suitable perfusion; anticoagulation has not been used in most series.

Urinary leak, most often at the neocystostomy site, presents with oliguria and persisting uremia. US or nuclear imaging can be used to identify an extravesical fluid collection. Direct operative repair is necessary to prevent urinoma formation and its potential infectious complications. Urinary collections must be differentiated from lymphoceles at the transplant site. Unresolving lymphoceles are best opened into the peritoneal cavity using laparoscopic techniques.

Hypertension

Hypertension following renal transplantation is common. One month after transplantation, 72% of all patients require treatment, although this percentage decreases to 53% at 30 months. Careful attention to the pretransplant control of hypertension and dietary management improves posttransplant control. Hypertension presents a significant risk to possible renal function when using small allografts. Hypertension in the early postoperative period is most often due to fluid overload or acute rejection, but it can also originate from the native kidneys.

Preexisting hypertension is augmented by the immunosuppressive drugs cyclosporine, tacrolimus, and prednisone. The development of hypertension more than 3 months after transplantation suggests possible renal artery stenosis and warrants US Doppler flow studies for initial evaluation and arteriography in questionable cases. Transluminal angioplasty has been successful in managing the majority of these cases when recognized; surgical correction is reserved for angioplasty failures and vessels with complex arterial anastomosis.

Infection

Most long-term complications are related to infection and occur within the first 6 posttransplant months. During this time, immunosuppression is intense and susceptibility to life-threatening infection is increased. The frequent use of organs from donors who have had prior exposure to CMV and EBV in infants and children who are seronegative enhances the risk of these specific infections. Expanded use of antiviral prophylaxis using ganciclovir and acyclovir has decreased the intensity of these infections and their associated morbidity or mortality. Trimethoprim-sulfamethoxazole is used for *Pneumocystis carinii* pneumonia prophylaxis as well.

Immunosuppression

Many immunosuppressive regimens are available and all share similar strategy. Most regimens include corticosteroids, cyclosporine or tacrolimus, and azathioprine or mycophenolate. Polyclonal or monoclonal antilymphocyte antibodies are used when acute tubular necrosis (ATN) is anticipated or for retransplantation in highly presensitized patients. Significant efforts to decrease or discontinue steroids have been attempted to enhance growth and development. At 4 years after transplantation, 31% of LD and 23% of CD recipients were receiving alternate-day prednisone.[84]

Overall, half of all transplant recipients have had a bout of rejection by day 95 after transplantation.[86] The risk of rejection is similar for LD and CD recipients in the first few posttransplant weeks. The cumulative risk for a first rejection is 23%, 32%, and 38% for LD recipients versus 24%, 42%, and 51% for CD recipients at 15, 30, and 45 days, respectively.[86] Factors that increase the likelihood of rejection or long-term graft loss include receiving a graft from a CD rather than a related LD, receiving a graft from a donor younger than 5 years of age, having the graft in cold storage for more than 24 hours, being an African American recipient, and delayed graft function from acute tubular necrosis.[84] Using antirejection therapy, 52% of rejection episodes in LD recipients were reversed, 40% were partially reversed, and 4% ended in graft failure. CD recipients faired slightly poorer with 49% reversed, 45% partially reversed, and 6% failed.[86] The rate of success in treating rejection declines with each successive rejection episode.[84] Most rejection episodes can be treated with steroid administration alone (78%); monoclonal anti–T-cell agents such as orthoclone OKT-3 are needed in 32%. In patients who remain rejection free for the 1st posttransplant year, the risk of rejection in the following year is 20%.[86]

RESULTS OF RENAL TRANSPLANTATION

The overall results of renal transplantation in children are steadily improving. Overall 1-year transplant graft survival rates of 88 to 100% have been reported for LD allografts, with results for CD allografts being 50 to 72%.[82, 92, 94, 96] In the 1997 NAPRTCS report, 1-, 2-, and 5-year graft survival rates were as follows: CD, 78%, 72%, and 59%; LD, 90%, 86%, and 85%, respectively (Fig. 45–8).[86]

Chronic rejection has become the most common cause of graft failure, accounting for 27% of all graft losses.[98] With improved immunosuppressive treatments, acute rejection accounts for only 18% of failures. Recurrence of the original disease caused graft failure in 7%, and vascular thrombosis accounted for 13% of graft failures. Long-term graft survival following pediatric renal transplantation continues to deteriorate after 10 years despite low patient mortality rates. Death of the recipient with a functioning graft is an uncommon problem. When this did occur, death resulted primarily from infection (40%) or cardiovascular causes (21%). Young recipients (0 to 1 year of age) and patients with early graft failure were at the highest risk.[99] Progressive loss of renal function may be secondary to complications of hypertension, hyperfiltration, hypercholesterolemias, chronic indolent immunologic damage

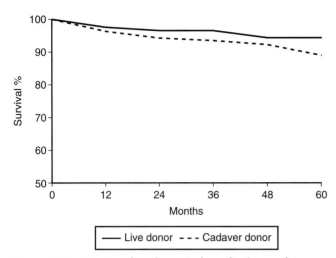

Figure 45–8. Patient and graft survival results for renal transplantation. (Data from Warady BA, Hebert D, Sullivan EK, et al: Renal transplantation, chronic dialysis, and chronic renal insufficiency in children and adolescents. Pediatr Nephrol 11:49–64, 1997.)

leading to chronic rejection, and progressive primary renal disease, which all contribute to long-term graft loss.[85, 96] Methods to circumvent this progressive graft loss will greatly improve the long-term prognosis.

The overall half-life of pediatric renal transplants is about 10 years.[100] Therefore, many recipients require second transplants in their lifetime. Overall graft survival for second transplants using LDs was equivalent to primary CD allografts.[100] The factor exerting negative influence on survival in CD grafts was donor age younger than 6 years. Improved DR matching improved graft survival. The rapidity of first allograft loss, immunologic protocol at retransplant, and race of recipient were not significant factors. Thus, use of cadaveric kidneys from young donors for these procedures is not recommended.

☐ Pancreas Transplantation in Children

Children have rarely been candidates for pancreas transplantation. In the past, the results following pancreas transplantation have not justified the risks associated with immunosuppression and operation. However, recent improvements in the operative procedure and follow-up have improved. Overall 1-year patient survival rate exceeds 90%, and graft survival with complete insulin independence exceeds 70% in patients in whom combined kidney and pancreas transplantation is undertaken. The survival rate is approximately 50% in isolated pancreas transplantation.[101, 102]

The addition of pancreas transplantation with kidney replacement for diabetic nephropathy does not subject the patient to additional immunosuppressive risks, and it is better accepted. The use of isolated pancreas transplantation is reserved for

patients who are extremely labile or experience hypoglycemic unawareness syndrome.[101] As the results of this procedure improve in the future, the role of this procedure in children will need to be reviewed.

Pancreatic islet transplantation has also become possible in children. Its role in the treatment of juvenile diabetes in childhood is still limited. This procedure has been undertaken in children following pancreatic resection when the cellular autotransplant does not require immunosuppressive treatment, with excellent results. Further expansion of this role awaits firm documentation that hypoglycemic correction retards the systemic complications of diabetes.

REFERENCES

1. Kasai M, Mochizuki I, Ohkohchi N, et al: Surgical limitation for biliary atresia: Indication for liver transplantation. J Pediatr Surg 24:851–854, 1989.
2. Ryckman F, Fisher R, Pedersen S, et al: Improved survival in biliary atresia patients in the present era of liver transplantation. J Pediatr Surg 28:382–385, 1993.
3. Otte JB, de Ville de Goyet J, Reding R, et al: Sequential treatment of biliary atresia with Kasai portoenterostomy and liver transplantation: A review [review]. Hepatology 20(1 pt 2):41S–48S, 1994.
4. Nio M, Ohi R, Hayashi Y, Endo N, et al: Current status of 21 patients who have survived more than 20 years since undergoing surgery for biliary atresia. J Pediatr Surg 31:381–384, 1996.
5. Zitelli BJ, Malatack JJ, Gartner JCJ, et al: Evaluation of the pediatric patient for liver transplantation. Pediatrics 78:559–565, 1986.
6. Riely CA: Familial intrahepatic cholestasis syndromes. In Suchy FJ (ed): Liver Disease in Children. St. Louis, CV Mosby, 1994, pp 443–459.
7. Ryckman FC, Alonso MH: Transplantation for hepatic malignancy in children. In Busuttil RW, Klintmalm GB (eds): Transplantation of the Liver. Philadelphia, WB Saunders, 1996, pp 216–226.
8. Cardona J, Houssin D, Gauthier F, et al: Liver transplantation in children with Alagille syndrome—a study of twelve cases. Transplantation 60:339–342, 1995.
9. Hoffenberg EJ, Narkewicz MR, Sondheimer JM, et al: Outcome of syndromic paucity of interlobular bile ducts (Alagille syndrome) with onset of cholestasis in infancy. J Pediatr 127:220–224, 1995.
10. Tzakis AG, Reyes J, Tepetes K, et al: Liver transplantation for Alagille's syndrome. Arch Surg 128:337–339, 1993.
11. Mito M, Kusano M, Sawa M: Hepatocyte transplantation for hepatic failure. Transplant Rev 7:35–43, 1993.
12. Jan D, Poggi F, Laurent J, et al: Liver transplantation: New indications in metabolic disorders? Transplant Proc 26:189–190, 1994.
13. Iwatsuki S, Esquivel CO, Gordon R, et al: Liver transplantation for fulminant hepatic failure. Semin Liver Dis 5:325–328, 1985.
14. Lidofsky SD, Bass NM, Prager MC, et al: Intracranial pressure monitoring and liver transplantation for fulminant hepatic failure. Hepatology 16:1–7, 1992.
15. Strom SC, Fisher RA, Thompson MT, et al: Hepatocyte transplantation as a bridge to orthotopic liver transplantation in terminal liver failure. Transplantation 63:559–569, 1997.
16. Koneru B, Flye MW, Busuttil RW, et al: Liver transplantation for hepatoblastoma. Ann Surg 213:118–121, 1991.
17. Iwatsuki S, Gordon RD, Shaw BW, et al: Role of liver transplantation in cancer therapy. Ann Surg 202:401–407, 1985.
18. Schroeder TJ, Pesce AJ, Ryckman FC, et al: Selection criteria for liver transplant donors. J Clin Lab Anal 5:275–277, 1991.

19. Karayalcin K, Mirza DR, Harrison RF, et al: The role of dynamic and morphological studies in the assessment of potential liver donors. Transplantation 57:1323–1327, 1994.

20. Broelsch CE, Emond JC, Whitington PF, et al: Application of reduced-size liver transplants as split grafts, auxiliary orthotopic grafts, and living related segmental transplants. Ann Surg 212:368–375, 1990.

21. Emond JC, Whitington PF, Thistlethwaite JR, et al: Reduced size orthotopic liver transplantation: Use in the management of children with chronic liver disease. Hepatology 10:867–872, 1989.

22. Ryckman FC, Flake AW, Fisher RA, et al: Segmental orthotopic hepatic transplantation as a means to improve patient survival and diminish waiting-list mortality. J Pediatr Surg 26:422–427, 1991.

23. de Ville de Goyet J, Otte JB: Cut-down and split liver transplantation. In Busuttil RW, Klintmalm GB (eds): Transplantation of the Liver. Philadelphia, WB Saunders, 1996, pp 481–496.

24. Broelsch CE, Whitington PF, Emond JC, et al: Liver transplantation in children from living related donors. Surgical techniques and results. Ann Surg 214:428–439, 1991.

25. Lo CM, Fan ST, Liu CL, et al: Adult-to-adult living donor liver transplantation using extended right lobe grafts. Ann Surg 226:261–270, 1997.

26. Morimoto T, Awane M, Tanaka A, et al: Analysis of functional abnormalities uncovered during preoperative evaluation of donor candidates for living-related liver transplantation. Clin Transplant 9:60–64, 1995.

27. Yamaoka Y, Morimoto T, Inamoto T, et al: Safety of the donor in living-related liver transplantation—an analysis of 100 parenteral donors. Transplantation 59:224–226, 1995.

28. Tanaka A, Tanaka K, Kitai T, et al: Living related liver transplantation across ABO blood groups. Transplantation 58:548–553, 1994.

29. Heffron TG, Emond JC: Segmental liver transplantation in children: Reduced size cadaveric, split and living related. Transplant Sci 2:28–33, 1992.

30. Rogiers X, Malago M, Gawad K, et al: In situ splitting of cadaveric livers. The ultimate expansion of a limited donor pool [review]. Ann Surg 224:331–339, 1996.

31. de Ville de Goyet J: Split liver transplantation in Europe—1988 to 1993. Transplantation 59:1371–1376, 1995.

32. Azoulay D, Astarcioglu I, Bismuth H, et al: Split-liver transplantation. The Paul Brousse Policy. Ann Surg 224:737–748, 1996.

33. Gubernatis G, Pichlmayr R, Kemnitz J, et al: Auxiliary partial orthotopic liver transplantation (APOLT) for fulminant hepatic failure: First successful case report. World J Surg 15:660–666, 1991.

34. Egawa H, Tanaka K, Inomata Y, et al: Auxiliary partial orthotopic liver transplantation from a living related donor: A report of two cases. Transplant Proc 28:1071–1072, 1996.

35. Terpstra OT, Schalm SW, Weimar W, et al: Auxiliary partial liver transplantation for end-stage chronic liver disease. N Engl J Med 319:1507–1511, 1988.

36. Todo S, Demetris AJ, Makowka L, et al: Primary non-function of hepatic allografts with pre-existing fatty infiltration. Transplantation 47:903–904, 1989.

37. D'Alessandro A, Kalayoglu M, Sollinger HW, et al: The predictive value of donor liver biopsies on the development of primary non-function after orthotopic liver transplantation. Transplantation 51:157–163, 1991.

38. Fishbein TM, Fiel MI, Emre S, et al: Use of livers with microvesicular fat safely expands the donor pool. Transplantation 64:248–251, 1997.

39. Iwatsuki S, Iwaki Y, Kano T, et al: Successful liver transplantation from crossmatch-positive donors. Transplant Proc 13:286, 1981.

40. Takaya S, Bronsther O, Iwaki Y, et al: The adverse impact on liver transplantation of using positive cytotoxic crossmatch donors. Transplantation 53:400–406, 1992.

41. Demetris AJ, Nakamura K, Yagihashi A, et al: A clinicopathological study of human liver allograft recipients harboring preformed IgG lymphocytotoxic antibodies. Hepatology 16:671–681, 1992.

42. Mor E, Skerrett D, Manzarbeitia C, et al: Successful use of an enhanced immunosuppressive protocol with plasmapheresis for ABO-incompatible mismatched grafts in liver transplant recipients. Transplantation 59:986–990, 1995.

43. Farges O, Kalil AN, Samuel D, et al: The use of ABO-incompatible grafts in liver transplantation performed in 40 patients. Transplantation 59:1124–1133, 1995.

44. Cacciarelli TV, So SK, Lim J, et al: A reassessment of ABO incompatibility in pediatric liver transplantation. Transplantation 60:757–760, 1995.

45. Yandza T, Lambert T, Alvarez F, et al: Outcome of ABO-incompatible liver transplantation in children with no specific alloantibodies at the time of transplantation. Transplantation 58:46–50, 1994.

46. Langnas AN, Marujo W, Stratta RJ, et al: Hepatic allograft rescue following arterial thrombosis. Role of urgent revascularization. Transplantation 51:86–90, 1991.

47. Stevens LH, Emond JC, Piper JB, et al: Hepatic artery thrombosis in infants. A comparison of whole livers, reduced-size grafts, and grafts from living-related donors. Transplantation 53:396–399, 1992.

48. Kirsch JP, Howard TK, Klintmalm GB, et al: Problematic vascular reconstruction in liver transplant, II: Portovenous conduits. Surgery 107:544–548, 1990.

49. Hashikura Y, Kawasaki S, Okumura N, et al: Prevention of hepatic artery thrombosis in pediatric liver transplantation. Transplantation 60:1109–1112, 1995.

50. Stieber AC, Zetti G, Todo S: The spectrum of portal vein thrombosis in liver transplantation. Ann Surg 213:199–206, 1991.

51. Harper PL, Edgar PF, Luddington RJ, et al: Protein C deficiency and portal thrombosis in liver transplantation in children. Lancet 2:924–927, 1988.

52. Heffron TG, Emond JC, Whitington PF, et al: Biliary complications in pediatric liver transplantation. A comparison of reduced-size and whole grafts. Transplantation 53:391–395, 1992.

53. Peclet MH, Ryckman FC, Pedersen SH, et al: The spectrum of bile duct complications in pediatric liver transplantation. J Pediatr Surg 29:214–219, 1994.

54. Rouch DA, Emond JC, Thistlethwaite JR, et al: Choledochocholedochostomy without a T tube or internal stent in transplantation of the liver. Surg Gynecol Obstet 170:239–244, 1990.

55. Snover DC, Sibley RK, Freese DK, et al: Orthotopic liver transplantation: A pathological study of 63 serial liver biopsies from 17 patients with special reference to the diagnostic features and natural history of rejection. Hepatology 4:1212–1222, 1984.

56. Mor E, Solomon H, Gibbs JF: Acute cellular rejection following liver transplantation: Clinical pathologic features and effect on outcome. Semin Liver Dis 12:28–40, 1992.

57. Adams DH, Neuberger JM. Treatment of acute rejection. Semin Liver Dis 12:80–88, 1992.

58. Ryckman FC, Schroeder TJ, Pedersen SH, et al: Use of monoclonal antibody immunosuppressive therapy in pediatric renal and liver transplantation. Clin Transplant 5:186–190, 1991.

59. Freese DK, Snover DC, Sharp HL, et al: Chronic rejection after liver transplantation: A study of clinical, histopathological and immunological features. Hepatology 13:882–891, 1991.

60. Ludwig J, Wiesner RH, Batts KP, et al: The acute vanishing bile duct syndrome (acute irreversible rejection) after orthotopic liver transplantation. Hepatology 7:476–483, 1987.

61. Wiesner R, Hermans PE, Rakela J, et al: Selective bowel decontamination to decrease gram negative aerobic bacterial and candida colonization and prevent infection after orthotopic liver transplantation. Transplantation 45:570, 1988.

62. Andrews W, Siegel J, Renaro T, et al: Prevention and treatment of selected fungal and viral infections in pediatric liver transplant recipients. Clin Transplant 5:204–207, 1991.

63. Patel R, Snydman DR, Rubin RH, et al: Cytomegalovirus prophylaxis in solid organ transplant recipients. Transplantation 61:1279–1289, 1996.
64. Fox AS, Tolpin MD, Baker A, et al: Seropositivity in liver transplant recipients as a predictor of cytomegalovirus disease. J Infect Dis 157:383–385, 1987.
65. Penn I: Immunosuppression: A contributing factor in lymphoma formation in immunosuppression and lymphoproliferative disorders. Roundtable report. Ortho Biotech 7–10, 1992.
66. Stephanian E, Gruber SA, Dunn DL, et al: Post-transplant lymphoproliferative disorders. Transplant Rev 5:120–129, 1991.
67. Hanto DW, Frizzera G, Gajl-Peczalska KJ, et al: Epstein-Barr virus, immunodeficiency, and B cell lymphoproliferation. Transplantation 39:461–472, 1985.
68. Washburn WK, Bradley J, Cosimi AB: A regional experience with emergency liver transplantation. Transplantation 61:235–239, 1991.
69. Esquivel CO, Nakazato P, Cox K, et al: The impact of liver reductions in pediatric liver transplantation. Arch Surg 126:1278–1285, 1991.
70. Langnas AN, Marujo WC, Inagaki M, et al: The results of reduced-size liver transplantation, including split livers, in patients with end-stage liver disease. Transplantation 53:387–391, 1992.
71. Sokal EM, Veyckemans F, de Ville de Goyet J, et al: Liver transplantation in children less than 1 year of age. J Pediatr 117:205–210, 1990.
72. Cox K, Nakazato W, Berquist W, et al: Liver transplantation in infants weighing less than 10 kilograms. Transplant Proc 23:1579–1580, 1991.
73. Bilik R, Greig P, Langer B, Superina RA: Survival after reduced-size liver transplantation is dependent on pretransplant status. J Pediatr Surg 28:1307–1311, 1993.
74. Otte JB, de Ville de Goyet, Sokal E, et al: Size reduction of the donor liver is a safe way to alleviate the shortage of size-matched organs in pediatric liver transplantation. Ann Surg 211:146–157, 1990.
75. Sarna S, Sipila I, Jalanko H, et al: Factors affecting growth after pediatric liver transplantation. Transplant Proc 26:161–164, 1994.
76. Balistreri WF, Bucuvalas JC, Ryckman FC: The effect of immunosuppression on growth and development. Liver Transplant Surg 1:64–73, 1995.
77. Chin SE, Shepherd RW, Cleghorn GJ, et al: Survival, growth, and quality of life in children after orthotopic liver transplantation: A five year experience. J Paediatr Child Health 27:380–385, 1991.
78. Zitelli BJ, Miller JW, Gartner J, et al: Changes in life-style after liver transplantation. Pediatrics 82:173–180, 1988.
79. Stewart SM, Uauy R, Waller DA, et al: Mental and motor development, social competence, and growth one year after successful pediatric liver transplantation. J Pediatr 114:574–581, 1989.
80. Stewart SM, Silver CH, Nici J, et al: Neuropsychological function in young children who have undergone liver transplantation. J Pediatr Psychol 16:569–583, 1991.
81. Tarter RE, Hays AL, Sandford SS, et al: Cerebral morphological abnormalities associated with non-alcoholic cirrhosis. Lancet 2:893–895, 1986.
82. Fine RN: Renal transplantation in children. In Morris PJ (ed): Kidney Transplantation: Principles and Practice. Orlando, Grune & Stratton, 1984, pp 509–546.
83. Potter DE, Holliday MA, Piel CF, et al: Treatment of end-stage renal disease in children: A 15 year experience. Kidney Int 18:103–109, 1980.
84. McEnery PT, Stablein DM, Arbus G, Tejani A: Renal transplantation in children: A report of the North American Pediatric Renal Transplant Cooperative Study. N Engl J Med 326:1727–1732, 1992.
85. Kashtan CE, McEnery PT, Tejani A, Stablein DM: Renal allograft survival according to primary diagnosis: A report of the North American Pediatric Renal Transplant Cooperative Study. Pediatr Nephrol 9:679–684, 1995.
86. Warady BA, Hebert D, Sullivan EK, et al: Renal transplantation, chronic dialysis, and chronic renal insufficiency in children and adolescents. The 1995 Annual Report of the North American Pediatric Renal Transplant Cooperative Study. Pediatr Nephrol 11:49–64, 1997.
87. Hanna JD, Krieg RJ, Scheinman JI, Chan JCM: Effects of uremia on growth in children. Semin Nephrol 16:230–241, 1996.
88. Grushkin CM, Fine RN: Growth in children following renal transplantation. Am J Dis Child 125:514–516, 1973.
89. Rotundo A, Nevins TE, Lipton M, et al: Progressive encephalopathy in children with chronic renal insufficiency in infancy. Kidney Int 21:486–491, 1982.
90. Najarian JS, Ascher NL, Mauer SM: Kidney transplantation. In Welch KJ, Randolph JG, Ravitch MM, et al (eds): Pediatric Surgery. Chicago, Year Book Medical, 1986, pp 360–373.
91. Sheldon CA, Gonzalez R, Burns MW, et al: Renal transplantation into the dysfunctional bladder: The role of adjunctive bladder reconstruction. J Urol 152:972–975, 1994.
92. Turcotte JG, Campbell DA, Dafoe DC, et al: Pediatric renal transplantation. In Cerilli GJ (ed): Organ Transplantation and Replacement. Philadelphia, JB Lippincott, 1988, pp 349–360.
93. Ildstad ST, Tollerud DJ, Noseworthy J, et al: The influence of donor age on graft survival in renal transplantation. J Pediatr Surg 25:134–137, 1990.
94. Ildstad ST, Tollerud DJ, Noseworthy J, et al: Renal transplantation in pediatric recipients. Transplant Proc 21:1936–1937, 1989.
95. Kim MS, Jams K, Harmon WE: Long-term patient survival in a pediatric renal transplantation program. Transplantation 51:413–417, 1991.
96. Bereket G, Fine RN: Pediatric renal transplantation. Pediatr Clin North Am 42:1603–1628, 1995.
97. Fine RN, Tejani A, Sullivan EK: Pre-emptive renal transplantation in children: Report of the North American Pediatric Renal Transplant Cooperative Study (NAPRTCS). Clin Transplant 8:474–478, 1994.
98. Tejani A, Cortes L, Stablein D: Clinical correlates of chronic rejection in pediatric renal transplantation. A report of the North American Pediatric Renal Transplant Cooperative Study. Transplantation 61:1054–1058, 1996.
99. Tejani A, Sullivan EK, Alexander S, et al: Posttransplant deaths and factors that influence the mortality rate in North American children. Transplantation 57:547–553, 1994.
100. Tejani A, Sullivan EK: Factors that impact on the outcome of second renal transplants in children. Transplantation 62:606–611, 1996.
101. Sutherland DE: The case for pancreas transplantation. Diabetes Metab 22:132–138, 1996.
102. Stratta RJ, Larsen JL, Cushing K: Pancreas transplantation for diabetes mellitus [review]. Annu Rev Med 46:281–298, 1995.

46

LESIONS OF THE PANCREAS AND SPLEEN

George K. Gittes, MD

□ Pancreas

ANATOMY AND EMBRYOLOGY

The pancreas originates in the 5th week of gestation as paired evaginations of the foregut.[1] The dorsal pancreatic bud gives rise to the body and tail of the pancreas, as well as the minor duct (Santorini) and minor papilla, and the continuation of the main duct (Wirsung) into the body and tail. The dorsal pancreas arises as a diverticulum from the dorsal aspect of the duodenal anlage. The ventral pancreatic bud arises from the biliary diverticulum and swings around the dorsal aspect of the duodenal anlage during gut rotation to give rise to the head of the pancreas, as well as the proximal portion of the main pancreatic duct (Fig. 46–1).

The two pancreatic buds fuse to form one pancreas at approximately 7 weeks' gestation, although it appears that complete fusion of the two ducts to form the main pancreatic duct is delayed until the perinatal period.[2] The endocrine component of the pancreas, the islets of Langerhans, start to differentiate before formation of the pancreatic buds in the wall of the foregut, from which the pancreas will arise.[3] The islets make up 10% of the pancreas during early embryonic and fetal life, but they decrease to less than 1% in the adult. Fetal pancreatic islets appear to play an important role in fetal homeostasis. Pancreatic acini begin to form at 12 weeks and at that time begin to accumulate organelles and zymogen granules characteristic of acinar cells. These cells do not secrete appreciable amounts of enzyme until the time of birth.[1]

The pancreas is retroperitoneal and is light pink in children. The acini can be seen with low-power loupe magnification, as can the septa dividing the lobulations. The head of the pancreas lies in the C-loop of the duodenum, and the uncinate process, emanating from the posteromedial portion of the head, projects under the superior mesenteric artery and vein. The neck of the pancreas is defined as that portion of the pancreas anterior to these vessels.[4] The body and tail, to the left of these vessels, angle sharply upward toward the hilum of the spleen. The main pancreatic duct runs along the posterior aspect of the gland and curves downward

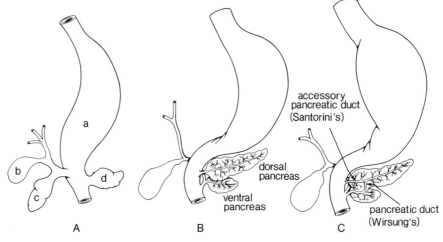

Figure 46–1. Pancreatic embryology. *A*, Stomach (a), gallbladder (b), and ventral (c) and dorsal (d) pancreatic buds develop separately at the 4th embryologic week. The pancreas develops as an evagination of the developing foregut. The dorsal bud evaginates directly off of the duodenal anlage. *B*, The ventral bud evaginates from the biliary bud and then swings around to the left with gut rotation occurring simultaneously. *C*, The main pancreatic duct of Wirsung and the minor accessory duct of Santorini are shown.

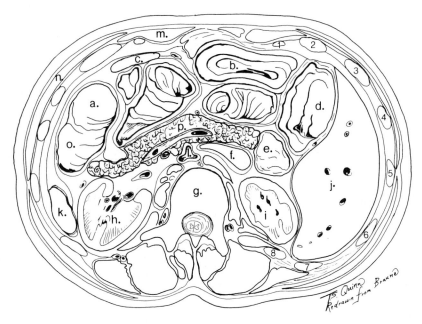

Figure 46–2. Cross-sectional anatomy of the pancreas. The pancreas lies convexly across the lumbar spine with the tail of the pancreas next to the spleen and the hilum of the left kidney. The head of the pancreas lies to the right of the spine near the hilum of the right kidney. Splenic flexure (a), transverse colon (b), stomach (c), ascending colon (d), duodenum (e), inferior vena cava (f), first lumbar vertebra (g), left kidney (h), right kidney (i), liver (j), spleen (k), aorta (l), rectus abdominis (m), external oblique (n), descending colon (o), and pancreas (p).

in the head to run alongside the common bile duct, which runs in a groove posterior to the pancreas or within the substance of the posterior gland. The main pancreatic duct and common bile duct may fuse in a "common channel" prior to entry into the duodenum.

The pancreas is quite convex, with its midportion being reflected over the anterior surface of the upper lumbar vertebrae and aorta and the lateral portions falling posteriorly toward each kidney (Fig. 46–2). The arterial supply of the pancreas is from the celiac and superior mesenteric arteries, which form the pancreaticoduodenal arcade. The pancreas also has anastomoses from the splenic artery.

CONGENITAL ANOMALIES

Ectopic pancreatic rests are frequently encountered along foregut derivatives, such as the stomach and the duodenum, as well as along the jejunum, ileum, and colon.[5] Their origin is unknown, but one possible explanation suggests an aberrant epithelial-mesenchymal interaction leading to the transdifferentiation of heterotopic embryonic epithelium into pancreatic epithelium. Ectopic rests are typically asymptomatic and are encountered incidentally at laparotomy. They can be identified as pancreatic tissue because the surface has the same granular acinar appearance. These ectopic pancreatic rests usually do not become inflamed, possibly because they contain numerous small drainage ducts rather than a large duct, which could become obstructed. Occasionally, an ectopic pancreatic rest produces obstruction or bleeding. When encountered at laparotomy, ectopic rests should probably be excised unless the excision would entail significant risk of morbidity.

Annular pancreas is thought to result from faulty rotation of the ventral pancreatic bud in its course

around the posterior aspect of the duodenal anlage. The duodenum is encircled by and obstructed with normal pancreatic tissue containing normal functioning acini, ducts, and islets of Langerhans.[6, 7] The prevailing theory of pathogenesis is that half of the ventral bud migrates anteriorly and half migrates posteriorly. The ductal drainage of this system is variable and complex. The clinical significance relates primarily to duodenal obstruction.

PANCREATITIS

Acute Pancreatitis

Acute pancreatitis is an acute inflammation of the pancreas with variable severity from mild abdominal pain, which may go undiagnosed, to fulminant necrotizing pancreatitis and death. Episodes of acute inflammation may completely resolve and then recur; in such cases, the term *acute relapsing pancreatitis* is applied to the clinical course. It is likely that there is complete interval resolution of morphology and function as opposed to the occurrence of irreversible changes in the pancreas in cases of chronic pancreatitis.

The causes of acute pancreatitis include trauma, biliary tract stone disease, choledochal cyst, ductal developmental anomalies, drugs, metabolic derangements, and infections. Most commonly, the cause is not apparent and is called "idiopathic."

Because the pancreas is fixed against the lumbar spine, trauma to the upper abdomen (classically, a bicycle handlebar) fractures the pancreas or injures the major duct at that point. Biliary stone disease, as in adults, may lead to pancreatitis from transient pancreatic duct obstruction with or without bile reflux. Choledochal cysts produce pancreatitis by pancreatic duct compression or bile reflux resulting from a long common biliary-pancreatic duct within the head of the pancreas.

Pancreas divisum is an anomaly present in 10% of the population, resulting from failure of the dorsal duct to fuse with the ventral duct. The majority of the exocrine secretions of the pancreas, including that from the entire body and tail, must drain through the small minor duct of Santorini and minor papilla into the duodenum. This relative obstruction may cause recurring episodes of pancreatitis.[8] These patients should undergo a sphincteroplasty of the minor papilla. Other rare ductal anomalies may result in obstruction and recurrent bouts of pancreatitis. Drugs that are thought to induce pancreatitis include corticosteroids and valproic acid.[9, 10] Systemic illnesses and metabolic conditions may cause pancreatitis, such as cystic fibrosis with inspissation of pancreatic secretions in the ducts, Reye's syndrome, Kawasaki's disease, hyperlipidemias, and hypercalcemia. Infections with viruses (e.g., coxsackievirus) and generalized bacterial sepsis can also cause pancreatitis.

Clearly, the pathogenesis entails the inappropriate activation of proenzymes, leading to autodigestion of the pancreas. The cellular mechanisms leading to acute pancreatitis are not known, but they are the subject of intense scientific investigation. Pancreatic enzymes can cause destruction at distant sites either by vascular dissemination or by release from the pancreas of cytokines such as tumor necrosis factor-α, free radicals such as superoxide, and vasoactive substances such as histamine and kallikrein.

The mechanism by which inappropriate activation of pancreatic enzymes occurs is not known. Possibilities include (1) reflux of duodenal enterokinase into the pancreas to activate trypsin, which then inappropriately activates other proenzymes in the pancreas; (2) ductal obstruction with extravasation of enzyme-rich ductal fluid into the parenchyma of the pancreas; or (3) fusion of lysosomes with zymogen granules inside acinar cells to allow lysosomal enzyme activation of the proenzymes. Once activated, elastase, phospholipase, and superoxide free radicals are thought to be the principal mediators of tissue damage.

Acute pancreatitis usually presents with the sudden onset of midepigastric pain associated with back pain, severe vomiting, and low-grade fever.[11, 12] The abdomen is diffusely tender with signs of peritonitis, and there is distention with a paucity of bowel sounds. In severe cases of necrotizing or hemorrhagic pancreatitis, hemorrhage may dissect from the pancreas along tissue planes, presenting as ecchymosis either in the flanks (Grey-Turner sign) or at the umbilicus (Cullen's sign) (Fig. 46–3). These ecchymoses typically take 1 to 2 days to develop.

Elevated amylase levels are helpful in the diagnosis, although normal serum amylase levels do not exclude pancreatitis from the differential diagnostic possibilities. The degree of serum amylase elevation does not correlate with severity of the disease. Amylase is excreted in urine but, as is true with glucose, tubular reabsorption results in amylase spill in the urine only after significant hyperamylasemia oc-

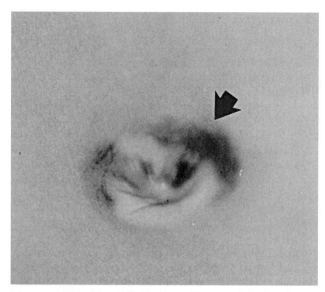

Figure 46–3. Positive Cullen's sign, with periumbilical ecchymosis *(arrow)*, in a patient with hemorrhagic pancreatitis.

curs.[13] In addition, the half-life of amylase is approximately 10 hours. Thus, moderately elevated levels of serum amylase may not be detectable in the urine.

Hyperamylasemia or hyperamylasuria may be caused by conditions other than pancreatitis, most notably salivary inflammation or trauma; intestinal disease including perforation, ischemia, necrosis, or inflammation; renal failure; and macroamylasemia. Alterations in renal excretion are compensated by measuring the ratio of clearance of amylase to creatinine. The ratio requires measurement of simultaneous spot levels of serum amylase and creatinine and urine amylase and creatinine:

$$(U_{amy}/Serum_{amy}) \times (Serum_{Cr}/Urine_{Cr})$$

Ratios over 0.03 are significant. Lipase levels have been proposed as a more specific test of pancreatic tissue damage, although intestinal perforation does cause an elevation of lipase through reabsorption via the peritoneum. Lipase is only produced in the pancreas, and its measurement is particularly helpful for distinguishing pancreatic trauma from salivary trauma.[14]

Imaging the abdomen is important as part of the evaluation of the patient with abdominal pain. In the patient with pancreatitis, plain abdominal radiographs may reveal an isolated loop of intestine in the vicinity of the inflamed pancreas, the so-called "sentinel loop." Other findings suggesting pancreatitis include local spasm of the transverse colon with proximal dilation known as the "colon cutoff" sign. Pancreatic calcifications suggest chronic pancreatitis. Plain chest roentgenograms should be performed in all patients with acute pancreatitis to look for evidence of pleural effusion and pulmonary edema.

Abdominal ultrasonography (US) may show a decrease in echogenicity of the pancreas compared with normal owing to pancreatic edema, but such a finding is not reliable in determining the diagnosis or severity.[15] The main use of US is to demonstrate gallstones as a possible cause of pancreatitis and to follow up the therapy to observe improvement in edema or peripancreatic fluid collection.

Abdominal computed tomography (CT) scan offers much better resolution than US in determining the size of the pancreas, the degree of edema, and the presence of fluid collections.[16] The size of the pancreatic duct can often be estimated much more accurately with CT than with US, and the presence of complications such as pancreatic abscess or pseudocyst may be delineated. The use of dynamic CT pancreatography has been advocated due to its ability to differentiate perfused from nonperfused (necrotic) pancreas. By using a bolus of contrast with rapid scanning in fine cuts through the pancreas, a precise assessment of the percentage of the pancreas that is either underperfused or nonperfused can be made. If necessary, CT scan can also be used for interventional procedures for diagnosis or drainage of fluid collections.

Endoscopic retrograde cholangiopancreatography (ERCP) rarely plays a role in evaluating children with acute pancreatitis. It is potentially helpful in children with severe refractory biliary pancreatitis who may have a stone impacted in the ampulla, as well as in trauma patients in whom a ductal injury is suspected or a pancreatic pseudocyst has formed.

Key features in treating patients with acute pancreatitis are aggressive fluid replacement to maintain a good urine output (2 ml/kg/h), usually measured with the aid of an indwelling urinary catheter, and, probably most importantly, a very low threshold for transferring the patient to an intensive care unit.[17, 18]

Acute pancreatitis causes diffuse tissue damage throughout the body as a result of the release of active mediators, including phospholipase A_2, elastase, histamines, kinins, kallikreins, and prostaglandins. Extracellular fluid losses can be enormous. Constant monitoring is necessary to avoid the development of severe hypovolemia. Patients with acute pancreatitis should be kept at bowel rest using nasogastric suction. Most patients receive H2 receptor antagonists to prevent exposure of the duodenal secretin-producing cells to gastric acid, which is a potent stimulator of pancreatic secretion. These antagonists may also help prevent the stress ulceration seen in patients with pancreatitis. This therapeutic regimen is logical but empiric because there have been no studies showing improvement in outcome with these interventions. Clinical trials have, however, shown improved outcome in acute pancreatitis using long-acting somatostatin analogues, and it is probably reasonable to use these analogues in moderate-to-severe cases of pancreatitis.[19]

Adequate analgesia is critical to minimize the additional stress from pain. Meperidine (Demerol) is thought to be a better analgesic in pancreatitis because morphine is well known to cause spasm of

the sphincter of Oddi, which in turn is known to increase pancreatic duct pressure and potentially worsen the pancreatitis. An important caveat is that the diagnosis of pancreatitis must be certain before giving the patient significant doses of narcotics because the ability to diagnose serious nonpancreatic problems, such as intestinal ischemia or perforated ulcer, may be lost.

As cases of severe pancreatitis progress, patients need to be followed closely for signs of the development of multiorgan system failure. Pleural effusions and pulmonary edema can progress to severe adult respiratory distress syndrome with hypoxia, requiring endotracheal intubation. The tense abdominal distention associated with pancreatitis frequently contributes to the hypoventilation. Hypocalcemia, hypomagnesemia, anemia from hemorrhage, hyperglycemia, renal failure, and late sepsis can be seen in these patients and require close monitoring. There is disagreement concerning the use of prophylactic antibiotics. In general, mild or moderate cases probably do not benefit from antibiotics. More severe cases of pancreatitis, however, may benefit because there is a high rate of sepsis, although confirmatory data in these patients are lacking.

Nutrition is critically important in the patient with pancreatitis, and an early positive nitrogen balance has been shown to improve survival rates. This need for aggressive nutrition should come in the form of early parenteral hyperalimentation. The hyperalimentation should include lipid formulations, despite the known association of hyperlipidemia and pancreatitis, although a close monitoring of the serum lipid levels should be maintained to avoid triglyceride levels over 500 mg/dl. In general, the resumption of enteral nutrition should be cautious, usually after complete resolution of abdominal pain and preferably after normalization of the serum enzyme levels.

Surgical intervention in acute pancreatitis is not often necessary. Other than for pancreatic pseudocyst or for papillotomy in the case of pancreas divisum, surgical intervention for acute pancreatitis is restricted to patients with severe necrotizing pancreatitis needing débridement or patients with pancreatic abscess.[20, 21] In some instances, pancreatitis is discovered when laparotomy is performed for a preoperative diagnosis of appendicitis (Fig. 46–4). Under this circumstance, the best course is to palpate the gallbladder for stones. If the pancreatitis is mild and gallstones are present, cholecystectomy is reasonable. If the pancreatitis is severe, the safer course is to perform a cholecystostomy, which allows later access to the biliary stones. If there are no gallstones but the patient has severe necrotizing pancreatitis, limited débridement is acceptable but simply leaving large sump drains in place is probably adequate. Early pancreatic lavage, pancreatic drainage, and pancreatic resection have not been shown to improve survival rates in cases of severe pancreatitis.

A *pancreatic abscess* may result from infection of

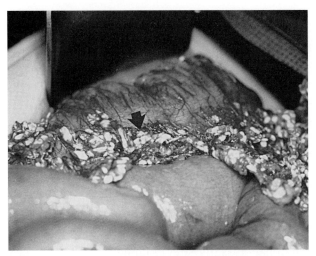

Figure 46–4. Severe peritoneal and omental fat saponification, seen as white fatty deposits *(arrow)* in a patient with acute pancreatitis. The preoperative diagnosis was acute appendicitis.

necrotic pancreatic tissue or infection of a peripancreatic fluid collection. Pancreatic abscess increases the mortality rate of pancreatitis threefold and is an absolute indication for surgical therapy.[22, 23] Differentiating a pancreatic abscess from an uninfected pancreatic fluid collection is important because pancreatitis itself can make the patient appear "septic." The diagnosis is established by Gram's stain and culture of the suspected abscess by CT-guided needle aspiration. The indication for aspiration is fever and leukocytosis persisting more than 7 to 10 days after onset of the pancreatitis. Patients shown to have pancreatic necrosis by dynamic CT pancreatography are candidates for aspiration because pancreatic necrosis usually precedes the development of a pancreatic abscess. The surgical therapy for a pancreatic abscess is débridement of clearly necrotic tissue and placement of large sump suction drains. There must be some mechanism for ongoing removal of the infected material postoperatively, either by reoperation or by the sump drains. In some cases, it is impossible to differentiate an infected pancreatic pseudocyst from an abscess. A laparotomy should be performed with sump drainage of the fluid collection.

Pancreatic pseudocyst is a complication of trauma or pancreatitis with damage to the pancreatic ductal system. The extravasated pancreatic enzymes and digested tissue are contained by the formation of a cavity composed of fibroblastic reaction and inflammation, but without epithelial lining. Pseudocysts may be acute or chronic. The acute pseudocyst has an irregular wall on CT scan, is tender, and usually shortly follows an episode of acute pancreatitis or trauma (Fig. 46–5). Chronic pseudocysts are usually spherical with a thick wall, and they are commonly seen in patients with chronic pancreatitis. The distinction between these two types of pseudocysts is important because 50% of acute pseudocysts resolve without therapy, whereas chronic

pseudocysts rarely do. An acute pseudocyst develops a thick fibrous wall in 4 to 6 weeks.

Pancreatic pseudocysts that persist require either internal drainage (preferred), excision (distal pseudocysts only), or external drainage (infected or immature cysts). A minimally invasive approach to cyst-gastrostomy was reported in which intragastric laparoscopic ports were used. Other minimally invasive strategies for pancreatic pseudocysts include transesophageal endoscopic cyst-gastrostomy and percutaneous drainage.[24] The two endoscopic procedures should be performed at institutions with significant experience with these techniques and, even then, there are serious potential risks. Percutaneous drainage is the treatment of choice for infected pseudocysts because these cysts typically have thin, weak walls not amenable to internal drainage.

The three major complications of pancreatic pseudocysts are hemorrhage, rupture, and infection. Hemorrhage, the most serious complication, usually results from pressure and erosion of the cyst into a nearby visceral vessel (e.g., splenic, gastroduodenal). These patients require emergency angiography with embolization. Rupture or infection of a pseudocyst is uncommon, and in both cases external drainage is indicated.

Pancreatic ascites in children usually follows trauma or pancreatic surgery.[25] These patients may be seen with ascites or with pancreatic pleural effusions. Free fluid results from the uncontained leakage of a major pancreatic duct. Treatment initially consists of bowel rest with hyperalimentation and use of long-acting somatostatin analogues. In many cases, ascites resolves spontaneously using this treatment. If not, ERCP should be performed to determine the site of the ductal injury. For distal duct injuries, simple distal resection is adequate, but proximal duct injury requires Roux-en-Y jejunal onlay anastomosis to preserve an adequate amount of pancreatic tissue.

Pancreatic fistula is a postoperative complication. Most low-output fistulas close spontaneously but

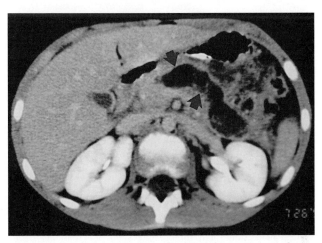

Figure 46–5. Computed tomography scan of an acute pseudocyst in a patient after a severe motor vehicle accident. The wall *(arrows)* is irregular with nonloculated fluid inside.

may drain for several months. Long-acting somato-statin analogues decrease the fistula output and accelerate the rate of closure, but they do not appear to induce closure of fistulas that would not have otherwise closed. Managing a pancreatic fistula centers around (1) maintaining adequate nutrition, with hyperalimentation if enteral feeding results in high-volume output and (2) making sure the fistula tract does not become obstructed. In fistulas that do not close, surgical intervention with a Roux-en-Y jejunostomy to the leak point is recommended.[26]

Chronic Pancreatitis

Chronic pancreatitis is distinguished from acute pancreatitis by the irreversibility of the changes associated with the inflammation.[27] Chronic pancreatitis is either *calcifying* or *obstructive*. The calcifying form, most commonly caused by hereditary pancreatitis, is more common than the obstructive form in children and is associated with intraductal pancreatic stones, pseudocysts, and a more aggressive scar formation with more significant damage (Fig. 46–6). The obstructive type of chronic pancreatitis, which is associated with anatomic obstructions (most commonly pancreas divisum), is generally less severe with less scar formation than calcifying pancreatitis. The pancreatic architecture may be partially reversible with correction of the obstruction.[28]

Chronic pancreatitis is distinctly uncommon in children, and the most common cause in North America is *hereditary* or *familial pancreatitis*.[29] The inheritance is autosomal dominant with incomplete penetrance. The clinical presentation is typically one of recurrent attacks resembling acute pancreatitis. Familial pancreatitis has no distinguishing characteristics other than pancreatic calcification and its occurrence in other family members. These patients

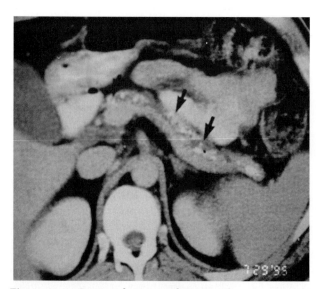

Figure 46–6. Computed tomography scan of a pancreas with chronic calcifying pancreatitis. A dilated duct can be seen within the pancreas, further supporting the diagnosis of chronic pancreatitis *(arrows)*.

typically begin to have symptoms at about 10 years of age and pancreatic insufficiency, both exocrine and endocrine, slowly develops. Such patients are at risk for developing adenocarcinoma of the pancreas.

In some patients with familial pancreatitis who have severe, intractable pain, ERCP may help locate surgically correctable lesions, such as large stones or a stricture with distal dilation of the duct. Surgical options in this form of pancreatitis include excision of localized pancreatitis, subtotal pancreatectomy, lateral pancreaticojejunostomy (modified Puestow procedure), and sphincteroplasty. Results of surgical therapy in these patients are generally disappointing.

Obstructive pancreatitis, which, in children, is due to pancreas divisum or choledochal cyst, is best treated by relieving the obstruction. The association between pancreas divisum and chronic pancreatitis remains controversial. Some patients with ductal dilation clearly improve with sphincterotomy or sphincteroplasty. Other cases may be difficult to diagnose and functional tests of duct pressure after secretin stimulation have been suggested. Surgical results in patients with functional obstruction are often not satisfying.

The diagnosis of chronic pancreatitis does not depend on amylase or lipase determination. Even though mild serum enzyme elevations are commonly seen during an exacerbation, they are not consistent and frequently are normal. The diagnosis of chronic pancreatitis relies on the characteristic pain, diminished pancreatic function, and changes in radiographic appearance. Increased stool fat, diabetes mellitus, and steatorrhea are signs of pancreatic insufficiency. Frequently on CT scan, the pancreas has microcalcifications throughout the parenchyma and calcified stones in the duct (see Fig. 46–6). Additionally, pancreatic pseudocysts or inflammation may be seen on CT scan. ERCP offers the best view of ductal anatomy and can confirm the diagnosis of pancreas divisum as a probable cause of chronic pancreatitis. Papillotomy may be done endoscopically, as well.

Therapy for chronic pancreatitis is directed toward palliation of symptoms. Initial therapy for acute exacerbation is pain control and hydration. Steatorrhea indicates the need for pancreatic enzyme replacement. In general, these patients do better with small, frequent meals. The diabetes mellitus that results from chronic pancreatitis seems to be unusually brittle with a propensity for severe hypoglycemic episodes after even low doses of insulin. This hypersensitivity to insulin may be due to loss of entire islets. Unlike autoimmune diabetes mellitus, in which there is specific destruction of the insulin-producing β-cells of the islets of Langerhans, in chronic pancreatitis, entire islets, including the glucagon-producing α-cells, are destroyed. The insulin-opposing effects of glucagon are thus lost in these patients.

Surgical or endoscopic therapy is indicated for

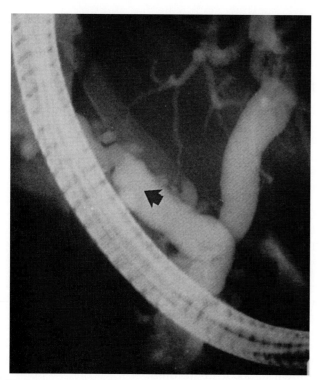

Figure 46–7. Endoscopic retrograde cholangiopancreatography in a patient with chronic pancreatitis with blockage of the biliary and pancreatic duct *(arrow)* with dilation.

bile or pancreatic duct obstruction or for pancreatic pseudocyst complications (Fig. 46–7).[30] Patients with intractable pain who do not have an identifiable anatomic problem would likely not benefit from surgical intervention. Relief of obstruction may be achieved by endoscopic sphincterotomy, ductal stenting, or open surgical drainage with Roux-en-Y lateral pancreaticojejunostomy (a modified Puestow procedure). Pancreatic resection, starting with distal resection only, but extending to subtotal or even total pancreatectomy, has been advocated for intractable pain. These patients trade sequelae of further, and perhaps complete, pancreatic insufficiency for anticipated pain relief.

FUNCTIONAL PANCREATIC DISORDERS

The causes of persistent hypoglycemia in children vary greatly with age. In newborns and infants, the major causes follow:
1. Persistent hyperinsulinemic hypoglycemia of infancy (PHHI), also called nesidioblastosis
2. Lack of substrate for gluconeogenesis (e.g., glycogen storage disease)
3. Inadequate gluconeogenic hormones (e.g., hypothyroidism or growth hormone deficiency)

In children with onset of hypoglycemia beyond 1 year of age, the causes are different, with insulinoma being the most common.

Persistent Hyperinsulinemic Hypoglycemia of Infancy

Nesidioblastosis comes from the Greek *nesidio*, meaning "island," and *blast*, meaning "new forma-

tion." Nesidioblasts are thought to be progenitor cells in the wall of pancreatic ducts, normally giving rise to islets in physiologic states requiring more islets, such as during pregnancy or after pancreatic resection. It has been postulated that these nesidioblasts overproliferate in patients with PHHI. This postulate was based on what had been thought to be atypical pathology of nesidioblastosis. However, it has been shown that the proliferation of nesidioblasts in the periductular regions of the pancreas is actually a normal variant in newborns. The defect in PHHI appears to be related to several different mutations in the β-cell in the adenosine triphosphate (ATP)-sensitive potassium channels, which normally consist of heteromultimers of the sulfonylurea receptors (SURs).[31–33] The SUR is necessary for controlling insulin release. (Oral hypoglycemic agents act by binding SUR and activating insulin release.) PHHI patients have been found to have a truncation mutation of the second nucleotide binding fold of the SUR1 of the ATP-sensitive potassium channel. Mutations in this receptor-channel prevent the normal feedback regulation of insulin production by serum glucose.

PHHI patients typically have hypoglycemia shortly after birth, although adult cases have been reported (probably not of the same origin).[34] Symptoms are those of hypoglycemia, with behavioral changes such as jitteriness and seizures. It is critical to measure serum insulin and glucose levels simultaneously because the absolute insulin level may be normal, but the ratio of insulin to blood glucose is not normal. These patients differ from insulin adenoma patients in that adenoma patients usually have high absolute insulin levels. In addition, the hyperinsulinemia of PHHI is more easily suppressed with somatostatin and somatostatin analogues.

Initial treatment of PHHI should be frequent feeding, or even a drip feeding regimen, with the addition of intravenous (IV) glucose as needed. Central venous access is advised because adequate venous access is lifesaving and high concentrations of glucose infusion may be necessary. When the glucose infusion rate necessary to prevent hypoglycemia is more than 15 mg/kg/h, PHHI is likely. When onset occurs after the newborn period, the patients may only have intermittent hypoglycemia and the diagnosis may be more difficult. Owing to the much higher incidence of insulin-producing adenoma, patients older than 1 year of age at onset of hypoglycemia should undergo evaluation, which may include exploratory laparotomy.

Initial medical treatment of PHHI should include an antisecretory drug such as diazoxide or a long-acting somatostatin analogue. Other medical therapy includes glucocorticoids to promote insulin resistance and streptozotocin (β-cell–specific toxin) to decrease the insulin-secreting population of cells. These drugs seem to be most effective treating milder cases or older children with PHHI. Medical failure to control hypoglycemia necessitates surgical resection.

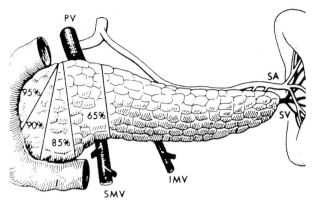

Figure 46–8. Various degrees of pancreatectomy may be indicated for persistent hyperinsulinemic hypoglycemia of infancy. Typically, a 95% pancreatectomy, as shown here, leaves behind a cuff of pancreas along the C-loop of the duodenum. IMV, inferior mesenteric vein; PV, portal vein; SA, splenic artery; SMV, superior mesenteric vein; SV, splenic vein.

Adequate surgical treatment consists of a 90 to 95% pancreatectomy, which entails leaving a residual remnant of pancreas on the common bile duct along the C-loop of the duodenum (Fig. 46–8).[35] It is important, especially in patients out of the newborn period, to closely inspect the pancreas for evidence of an insulin-producing adenoma, because finding an adenoma would allow significant preservation of pancreatic tissue and obviate potential endocrine and exocrine insufficiency. Postoperatively, these patients are often transiently hyperglycemic. All patients after resection of a large part of the pancreas are at significant risk for developing diabetes mellitus in later years. Inadequate response may necessitate further resection, prolonged adjuvant medical therapy, or special feeding regimens.

The long-term outlook for these patients depends primarily on the age of onset, which relates to severity of disease, and on expeditious diagnosis, because a late diagnosis results in a higher incidence of neurologic deficits.[36] Most patients seem to "grow out of the disease" after several years, implying diminished activity of the β-cells. This evolution may explain the development of diabetes mellitus in some of these patients during their school-age years.

Glycogen Storage Disease

Glucose-6-phosphatase deficiency (glycogen storage disease type I) classically presents as severe hypoglycemia in newborns and infants and is caused by the inability to dephosphorylate glycogen subunits into glucose.[37] The hypoglycemia becomes apparent when feedings begin to be spaced out, requiring the liver to generate glucose from glycogen stores. Diagnosed clinically by the low insulin levels and hepatomegaly, ketosis and cutaneous xanthomas develop as a result of compensatory high lipid levels, and such patients often have fasting glucose levels less than 20 mg/dl. Central venous access is needed to allow continuous infusion of highly concentrated glucose. Liver transplantation has become the treatment of choice for these patients.

Pancreatic Endocrine Tumors

The endocrine cells of the mature human pancreas are confined to the islets of Langerhans (Fig. 46–9), although pancreatic neurons are known to secrete locally active peptide hormones such as vasoactive intestinal peptide (VIP). There are four main hormones produced by islets: insulin from the centrally located β-cells, which make up more than 90% of the islet; glucagon from the peripheral mantle of α-cells; and somatostatin and pancreatic polypeptide from the δ-cells and pancreatic polypeptide (PP) cells scattered throughout. There is a small population of endocrine cells that account for production of gastrin and other peptide hormones. Currently, it is believed that pancreatic endocrine tumors arise from cells located in the islets, although there is evidence that precursor cells in the pancreatic ducts or acini may give rise to these tumors as well. Only insulinoma, gastrinoma, and VIPoma are known to occur in children.

Insulinoma is the most common pancreatic endocrine tumor in children.[38] These tumors are manifest by symptoms of hypoglycemia, including dizziness, headaches, sweating, and seizures. The classic Whipple's triad was described in patients with insulinoma and consists of the following:

1. Symptoms of hypoglycemia with fasting
2. Glucose level less than half of normal with fasting
3. Relief of symptoms with glucose administration

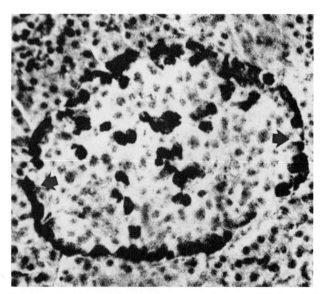

Figure 46–9. Mature islet in the pancreas. Immunohistochemical stain shows the peripheral location of the glucagon cells (α-cells, *arrows*). The insulin-producing cells (β-cells) are located in the central portion of the islet. (From Fawcett DW [ed]: Textbook of Histology. New York, Chapman & Hall, 1994, p 699.)

Patients are typically older than 4 years old, although newborns have been described with insulinoma. Ninety percent of cases are benign. Lesions are usually solitary, except in multiple endocrine neoplasia (MEN) 1 syndrome, in which there may be multiple insulinomas.

Insulinoma is diagnosed by demonstrating an insulin-to-glucose ratio of more than 1.0 (microunits of insulin per milliliter/milligrams of glucose per deciliter). Normal should be less than 0.3. Levels of insulin C-peptide should always be measured because its absence indicates exogenous administration of insulin.

Tumor localization preoperatively may be difficult.[39] Extrapancreatic insulinomas are rare, and CT scan of the pancreas with fine cuts will identify more than half of the tumors. Small hypervascular tumors may be visualized by angiographic blush, but angiography is probably not warranted with the advent of newer imaging techniques. Magnetic resonance imaging (MRI) and endoscopic US allow visualization of very small tumors. Selective portal venous sampling may help localize the tumor for blind pancreatic resections. All patients should undergo surgical resection. Tumors are pink, firm, and appear encapsulated. The tumors are usually amenable to simple enucleation. At operation, occult tumors may be localized by intraoperative US. Failure to localize the tumor by any of the aforementioned techniques is unlikely but, because insulinomas tend to be located in the tail of the pancreas, distal pancreatectomy is the best "blind" procedure. Patients with MEN 1 and multiple adenomas require a 95% pancreatectomy. Malignant insulinomas require chemotherapy, usually with the β-cell toxic drug streptozotocin.

Fetal gastrin-producing cells in the pancreas are believed to give rise to pancreatic *gastrinoma*. The pancreas is the primary source of gastrin in the fetus. After birth, the gastric antrum becomes the principal gastrin source. The Zollinger-Ellison syndrome consists of gastric hypersecretion with severe peptic ulcer disease and a gastrin-producing tumor, which classically is located in the pancreas. The pancreas is the most common site for gastrinomas, which are malignant in 65% of cases and usually produce the 17 amino acid form of gastrin. Unlike adults, children with gastrinoma have not been reported to have MEN 1.[40, 41]

The diagnosis of a gastrinoma is based on hypergastrinemia and gastric hypersecretion. Gastrin levels are usually over 500 pg/ml, but equivocal cases can be diagnosed by using 2 U/kg of IV secretin as a stimulation test. A gastrinoma responds with a 200 pg/ml or more increase in serum gastrin. Localization of gastrinomas can be difficult. These tumors may be outside the pancreas. CT scan, MRI, endoscopic US, and selective portal venous sampling have all been used to help localize tumors. Occult tumors have been shown most often to be located in the duodenum and may only be seen with duodenotomy.

The medical treatment of gastrinoma is with omeprazole, the inhibitor of acid secretion that selectively blocks the ATP-dependent hydrogen-potassium proton pump necessary for acid secretion. All patients with potentially resectable disease should undergo exploration, although most pancreatic tumors are not resectable, and only patients who undergo complete resection are cured.

NONNEOPLASTIC CYSTS

Although most cystic lesions of the pancreas are pseudocysts and acquired, *congenital cysts* may present at an early age as a symptomatic mass with compression of surrounding structures (Fig. 46–10).[42] Alternatively, these congenital cysts may be noted incidentally on physical examination or radiographic studies. Congenital cysts contain cloudy straw-colored fluid with normal pancreatic enzyme levels. The cysts are most often found in the distal pancreas and are amenable to local resection with a rim of normal pancreas. Lesions in the head of the pancreas should be internally drained with Roux-en-Y cyst-jejunostomy. Congenital duplications of the intestine may also be sequestered in the pancreas. They have a gastric mucosal lining but maintain pancreatic ductal communication. The gastric acid may cause episodes of pancreatitis. The mass is usually small and is identified only on CT scan. Surgical resection is necessary, either in the form of enucleation, distal pancreatectomy, or even pancreaticoduodenectomy.

Acquired nonneoplastic cysts of the pancreas are called *retention cysts* and seem to represent ectasia of the pancreatic ducts. The cysts contain fluid rich in pancreatic enzymes. Preoperative distinction of a

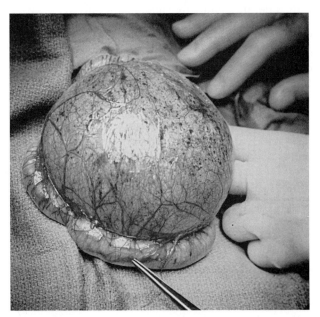

Figure 46–10. Large pancreatic cyst (retention cyst) emanating from the pancreatic parenchyma. The cyst was filled with clear fluid. (Courtesy of Howard B. Ginsburg, MD.)

retention cyst from other types of cysts or pseudocysts may be difficult. ERCP demonstrates a communication with the ductal system and may help in determining the surgical approach (resection versus Roux-en-Y cyst-jejunostomy).

PANCREATIC EXOCRINE TUMORS

The pancreatic exocrine system consists of the pancreatic ducts, centroacinar cells, and acini. Tumors arising from this system may be cystic tumors, pancreatic adenocarcinomas, or pancreatoblastomas.

Cystic Tumors

Cystic neoplasms of the pancreas are relatively rare in children.[42] There are essentially two forms:
1. Serous cystadenomas are multiloculated, microcystic tumors that are usually small and have no known malignant potential
2. Mucinous tumors (either cystadenoma or cystadenocarcinoma) consist of larger cysts filled with thick mucinous material

Mucinous cysts are typically in the tail of the pancreas and may be confused with pseudocysts. The mucinous cystadenomas have a definite malignant potential and may become quite large.

CT scan and ERCP are the best studies to delineate the location, character, and relation of the cyst to the duct. In general, all lesions should be biopsied at laparotomy. Serous tumors can be left alone if they are not causing any obstructive symptoms. Mucinous tumors must be completely excised, including the pericystic capsule, because carcinomatous recurrences of mucinous cystadenomas have been reported.

Adenocarcinoma/Pancreatoblastoma

In general, pancreatic cancers are rare in children. Ductal adenocarcinoma is the most common adult form of pancreatic cancer. Acinar cell adenocarcinoma is more often seen in children and tends to have a less aggressive behavior with a better prognosis. A variant adenocarcinoma seen in younger children and infants has been termed *pancreatoblastoma*. Pancreatoblastomas often arise in the head of the pancreas and may represent a tumor of immature duct cells. A Frantz tumor is a papillary-cystic tumor seen in girls and young women and which tends to have a benign course.[43, 44]

Therapy for all of these tumors is surgical resection. Adenocarcinomas and pancreatoblastomas often require a pancreaticoduodenectomy, but overall survival rate is much better than in adults with pancreatic cancer. Owing to this improved survival rate, aggressive resections, even with portal vein resection, seem warranted.

□ Spleen

Other than splenic trauma, surgical diseases of the spleen are mainly limited to hematologic diseases. The role of the spleen in hematologic disease is best understood with an underlying knowledge of its anatomy and function. Important new aspects of splenic surgery include splenic preservation surgery, laparoscopic approaches to the spleen, and autotransplantation.

EMBRYOLOGY, ANATOMY, AND PHYSIOLOGY

The spleen develops alongside the pancreas, from mesenchyme of the dorsal pancreatic bud and the dorsal mesogastrium, and it can be recognized in the 5th week of gestation.[45] Splenic mesenchyme gives rise to basement membrane-lined cords to form sinusoids (Fig. 46–11). The splenic filtration function is established at this time. In addition to the filtration function, the spleen also develops as a lymphoid organ with both B and T lymphocytes present by the end of the first trimester. Little is known about the factors controlling splenic development, although a patterning protein, hox11 of the homeodomain protein family, has been shown to be necessary for splenic development because hox11 knock-out mice are born without a spleen.

At birth, the formed spleen contains primarily lymphocytes with aggregations of T cells, phagocytic cells of the reticuloendothelial system, and B cells in follicles. This lymphoid aggregation (white pulp) surrounds the feeding arterioles of the spleen and is thought to function as an immune screening area to detect and process foreign antigen and antigen–antibody complexes. The red pulp, so named because there is slow flow of blood through sinusoids, which are functionally distal to the white pulp, acts as a phagocytic filtration system, digesting old or defective blood elements including spherocytes and elliptocytes, complexed foreign material and cells, and bacteria, both with and without bound specific antigens (Fig. 46–12). Of importance

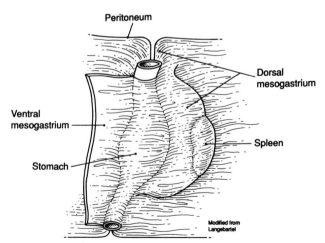

Figure 46–11. Splenic embryology. The spleen develops within the dorsal mesogastrium as it folds during gut rotation. (From Skandalakis LJ, Gray SW, Ricketts R, et al: The spleen. In Skandalakis JE, Gray SW [eds]: Embryology for Surgeons. Baltimore, Williams & Wilkins, 1994, p 336.)

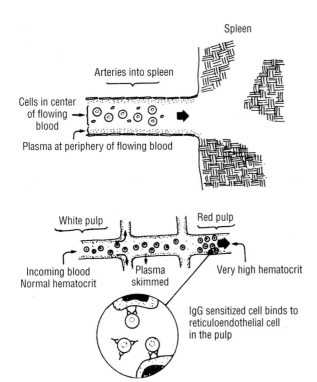

Figure 46–12. Schematic of blood flowing through the spleen. As blood flows through the arteries, acellular plasma is filtered off through the white pulp peripherally, leaving closely packed red blood cells in the red pulp where red cells can then be phagocytosed by the reticuloendothelial system if they are tagged with bound antibody. (Reprinted from Murphy WG, Kelton JG: Role of the spleen in autoimmune disorders. In Pochedly C, Sills RH, Schwartz AD [eds]: Disorders of the Spleen. New York, Dekker, 1989, p. 193, by courtesy of Marcel Dekker Inc.)

is that encapsulated bacteria in the bloodstream can only be removed by the spleen for reasons of variable antigenicity. The spleen also functions until approximately 1 to 2 months of age as a site for extramedullary hematopoiesis.[46]

Important anatomic aspects of the spleen include the ligaments, the splenic artery, and the segmental anatomy of the splenic parenchyma (Fig. 46–13). The major suspensory ligaments are the gastrosplenic and splenorenal ligaments. Laxity of these and other minor ligaments contributes to a poorly fixed, or wandering, spleen. Division of the splenorenal ligament is necessary to mobilize the spleen from the left upper quadrant. The splenic artery arises from the celiac axis and takes a tortuous and variable course to the splenic hilum. It can usually be accessed through the lesser omental sac either above or below the pancreas. Splenic collaterals allow for splenic artery ligation in the lesser sac without splenic infarct. The splenic artery divides into upper and lower pole arteries, defining surgical segments. The segmental blood supply facilitates partial splenectomy.[47]

ASPLENIA AND POLYSPLENIA

Congenital asplenia is often associated with cardiac defects, as well as other anomalies of symmetry

such as a midline liver (heterotaxy syndrome).[48, 49] The anatomy in these patients is best understood as the body having two right halves instead of a left half and a right half. These patients often have severe anomalies of cardiac looping, frequently with single ventricle anatomy. The cardiac condition is the most significant, but such an evaluation reveals evidence of asplenia such as Howell-Jolly bodies in the erythrocytes. Patients should be placed on asplenia prophylaxis (as discussed later) as soon as the diagnosis is made.

By contrast, the polysplenia syndrome may result from having two left halves of the body. The multiple spleens tend to be located along the greater curvature of the stomach. The associated cardiac anomalies are less severe than those associated with the asplenia syndrome.

ACCESSORY SPLEEN

Accessory spleens exist as small splenic nodules and are present in approximately 20% of the population. They are usually found in the splenic hilum, along the stomach, in the omentum and adjacent to the pancreas, reflecting the embryonic origin of the spleen (Fig. 46–14).[50] These nodules often resemble lymph nodes but may grow rapidly if left behind after splenectomy done for hematologic disease. This "compensatory hypertrophy" appears to be due to a factor in the blood that induces splenic growth and allows recurrence of the hematologic disorder that prompted the splenectomy.

SPLENOGONADAL FUSION

Rarely, the splenic anlage fuses with the gonadal ridge in the developing embryo.[51] As a result, ma-

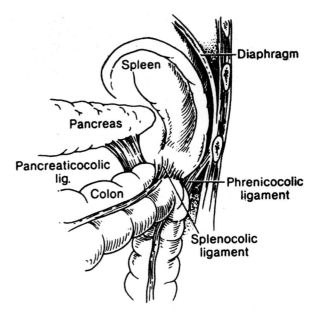

Figure 46–13. Anatomy of the spleen. Significant ligamentous attachments are to the diaphragm, left kidney, colon, and pancreas. (From Skandalakis PN, Colborn GL, Skandalakis LJ, et al: The surgical anatomy of the spleen. Surg Clin North Am 73:759, 1993.)

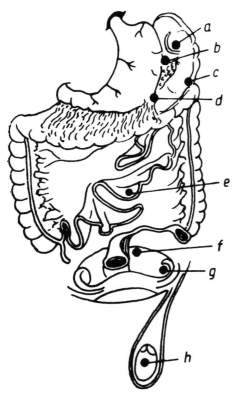

Figure 46–14. Possible locations of accessory spleens. Potential locations include *(a)* hilus of the spleen, *(b)* along the splenic vessels, *(c)* splenocolic ligament, *(d)* greater omentum, *(e)* small bowel mesentery, *(f)* pelvic wall, *(g)* adnexal region, and *(h)* left paratesticular region. (From Rudowski WJ: Accessory spleen: Clinical significance with particular reference to the recurrence of idiopathic thrombocytopenic purpura. World J Surg 9[3]:422–430, 1985.)

ture splenic tissue may be found attached to either testicle or ovary (Fig. 46–15). A fibrous cord, which may have a chain of small pieces of spleen (splenic rosary bead sign), may connect the ectopic fused spleen-gonad with the normal spleen. Splenogonadal fusion is often found associated with limb or anorectal anomalies, suggesting a global embryonic event occurring between the 5th and 8th week of embryogenesis. Boys with splenogonadal fusion typically present with an undescended testicle or a presumed hernia. In many cases, an unnecessary orchiectomy has been performed because the surgeon erroneously thought that the tissue represented a tumor. Usually, the splenic tissue can safely be dissected off the testicle or ovary.

WANDERING SPLEEN

Laxity of the splenic ligaments allows the spleen to be located anywhere in the peritoneal cavity, including the pelvis.[52, 53] The splenic pedicle may be quite long, predisposing the spleen to torsion. Full torsion may result in splenic infarction, whereas lesser degrees of twisting may produce chronic intermittent abdominal pain from ischemia. Imaging studies may suggest the absence of the spleen in the left upper quadrant and perhaps a spleen-like mass elsewhere. Splenectomy is required for a necrotic spleen and fixation for the viable spleen. Splenopexy in the left upper quadrant is possible using an absorbable mesh to avoid placing sutures through the splenic parenchyma.

CYSTIC LESIONS

Peliosis in Greek means "leaking blood" and refers to blood-filled lakes in the parenchyma of organs. These lesions occur in the spleen, usually in association with peliosis of the liver.[54] The blood-filled lakes have an endothelial lining and vary in size from 1 to 10 cm. Peliosis is of unknown origin but is often associated with steroid use or chemotherapy. The major clinical significance of peliosis is its potential to rupture either with or without trauma, which can be fatal. Treatment of incidentally discovered peliosis is uncertain.

BENIGN CYSTS

Benign cysts are rare and usually remain asymptomatic. Cysts may be unilocular or multilocular and are of variable origin. The most common forms of cyst are congenital, parasitic, or posttraumatic. The congenital cyst is usually unilocular and filled with clear fluid that may contain cholesterol crystals. The lining of these congenital cysts may be squamous (epidermoid) or endothelial. Parasitic cysts are typically ecchinococcal (hydatid) cysts. Posttraumatic cysts result from slow liquefaction of a hematoma, have a fibrous lining, and contain cloudy brown fluid. Cysts are often asymptomatic, but they may present as a mass in the left upper quadrant, sometimes with pain. Treatment is indicated for symptomatic cysts. Resection either by partial splenectomy, if feasible, or by total splenectomy is appropriate.[55] Ecchinococcal cysts should be handled carefully, similar to hepatic hydatid dis-

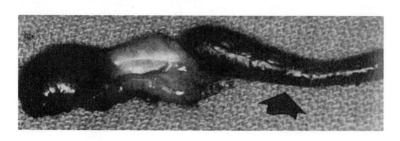

Figure 46–15. Splenogonadal fusion to the testicle. As evidenced here, orchiectomy is often mistakenly performed for suspicion of malignancy. The splenic tissue is to the right *(arrow)*. (From Balaji KC, Caldamore AA, Rabinowitz R, et al: Splenogonadal fusion. J Urol 156:854, 1996.)

ease, and if there is any question about risk of rupture, total splenectomy should be performed.

SPLENIC TUMORS

All forms of splenic tumors, other than metastases to the spleen, are rare. Hemangioma is the most common benign tumor with splenectomy frequently being necessary for large, symptomatic, or bleeding tumors.[56, 57]

SPLENIC ABSCESS

Splenic abscess is relatively rare in children. It may occur as a secondarily infected hematoma, pseudocyst, or developmental cyst. A splenic infarct resulting from a hemoglobinopathy may also become secondarily infected. Immunosuppression puts patients at risk for developing a splenic abscess from seeding during bacteremia, thus causing multiple or miliary abscesses.[58] Splenic abscess patients typically are toxic with bacteremia, fever, and left upper quadrant pleuritic pain. CT scan is usually diagnostic.

Solitary unilocular abscesses may respond well to percutaneous drainage, which also allows identification of the organism and appropriate antibiotic selection. Multiple or loculated abscesses may respond to antibiotics alone. Empiric antibiotic therapy should be started based on a presumptive diagnosis given the clinical setting. Immunosuppressed patients with multiple abscesses and negative blood cultures likely have a fungal infection. *Salmonella* species are most common in patients with hemoglobinopathy and splenic infarct. In posttraumatic infection, *Staphylococcus* and *Streptococcus* are most common. In general, failure to respond to antibiotics with or without percutaneous drainage necessitates splenectomy.

FUNCTIONAL ABNORMALITIES

Hypersplenism is defined as inappropriate sequestration of blood elements. Hypersplenism may be primary or secondary. Secondary hypersplenism is often associated with splenomegaly with simple mechanical sequestration of erythrocytes, platelets, and neutrophils. The most common cause of secondary hypersplenism in children is portal hypertension, although any cause of splenomegaly can lead to hypersplenism. Either splenic artery embolization or splenic artery ligation is adequate therapy, although splenectomy is occasionally necessary. There appear to be few sequelae from the thrombocytopenia and neutropenia that result from this form of hypersplenism. Primary hypersplenism is not a result of splenomegaly or other indirect cause. Hereditary spherocytosis (HS), hereditary elliptocytosis, and idiopathic thrombocytopenic purpura are examples of primary hypersplenism and are discussed later. Paradoxically, because the spleen can be a site of extramedullary hematopoiesis in the

disease states that produce primary hypersplenism, removal of the spleen may be detrimental.

Hyposplenism is detected by the presence of Howell-Jolly bodies in erythrocytes and increased susceptibility to infection with encapsulated organisms. Surgical splenectomy, sickle cell disease with splenic involution, or ulcerative colitis, all lead to hyposplenism. Diseases in which there is splenic parenchymal replacement, such as sarcoidosis or Gaucher's disease, may also lead to hyposplenism. The significance of hyposplenism is the risk of postsplenectomy sepsis.

HEREDITARY SPHEROCYTOSIS

Hereditary spherocytosis, or congenital hemolytic jaundice, is usually an autosomal dominant hereditary lesion, particularly common in patients of north European descent. HS is thought to be due to a deficiency of the cytoskeletal protein spectrin.[59] Spectrin deficiency allows the erythrocytes to be spheric. HS may also be sporadic or autosomal recessive. Sentinel cases in a family usually present with jaundice, anemia, and splenomegaly. Indirect hyperbilirubinemia may present in infants, whereas splenomegaly only may present very late. Without treatment in these patients, pigmented gallstones may develop, and they may suffer from acute aplastic and hemolytic crises precipitated by infections.

Owing to the abnormal shape of the erythrocytes, they are prematurely sequestered in the spleen, probably because the spheric shape prevents the normal flexibility necessary to maneuver through the cords and sinuses of the spleen.

The diagnosis of hereditary spherocytosis should be sought in patients with anemia, jaundice, or splenomegaly. The blood smear shows small spherical erythrocytes. The diagnosis is established by demonstrating increased osmotic fragility of the erythrocytes when exposed to elevated sodium concentrations. Patients suspected of having HS should also undergo Coombs's testing to rule out immune causes of hemolytic anemia.

Owing to the frequency of pigment gallstones, a routine US should be performed in all patients older than 10 years of age in whom a splenectomy is planned. For younger children, given the much lower incidence of stones, palpation of the gallbladder may be adequate. If gallstones are encountered, simultaneous cholecystectomy and splenectomy should be performed. If laparoscopic splenectomy is performed, preoperative US of the gallbladder should be performed because "palpation" for stones is unreliable. The risk of postsplenectomy sepsis is high in young children, so the current recommendation is to wait, if possible, until patients are at least 5 to 6 years old before splenectomy. Patients with severe anemia may need earlier intervention, however. There are HS patients who do not have the autosomal dominant type and who may not respond to splenectomy. These patients often have persistent episodes of anemia postoperatively. Conversely, older patients with mild anemia may not warrant splenectomy.[60]

The spleen of HS patients may be large but not technically difficult to remove, and it may be removed laparoscopically. Patients should receive pneumococcal vaccine 2 weeks preoperatively and postoperative prophylactic antibiotics. Following splenectomy, the anemia is usually cured, and these patients generally feel better and have a normal life span. Patients with autosomal recessive disease may continue to require transfusions. Pigmented gallstones may develop postoperatively, although not often enough to warrant prophylactic cholecystectomy. Anemia may also recur due to hypertrophy of residual accessory spleens; therefore, attempts to remove all accessory spleens should be made.

THE SPLEEN IN SICKLE CELL DISEASE

Patients with homozygous hemoglobin S (sickle cell disease) are prone to splenic sequestration.[61–63] As the cells pass through the spleen with its naturally hypoxic and acidotic environment, the erythrocytes sickle and are sequestered in the spleen. Often, the spleen in these patients becomes large initially, but with progressive infarction, it slowly atrophies, leading to functional autosplenectomy after approximately 10 years. In some cases, however, the spleen may persist even into adulthood.

The most common indication for splenectomy in sickle cell patients is acute splenic sequestration crisis (ASSC), in which severe anemia with splenomegaly develops with associated hypersplenism and thrombocytopenia. ASSC may be so severe that it causes circulatory collapse and death. Even though it is relatively rare, ASSC is the leading cause of death in sickle cell patients younger than 10 years old. Patients with severe attacks of ASSC should undergo splenectomy when they have recovered from the attack because there is a 40 to 50% risk of recurrence with a 20% mortality rate. Patients with less severe cases of ASSC should probably undergo splenectomy after two ASSC episodes.

Hypersplenism as a result of splenomegaly develops in many patients with sickle cell disease. Transfusion requirements dictate the need for splenectomy because these patients are at high risk for transfusion complications. Partial or subtotal splenectomy has been advocated in these patients because the risk of postsplenectomy sepsis is high in sickle cell disease. These patients should receive pneumococcal vaccine preoperatively and prophylactic antibiotics postoperatively.

IDIOPATHIC THROMBOCYTOPENIC PURPURA

As the name implies, the etiology of idiopathic thrombocytopenic purpura (ITP) is unknown. Clearly it is mediated, in the chronic form of ITP, through autoimmune binding of IgG specifically to a "platelet-associated antigen." Binding of autoanti-

body leads to reticuloendothelial platelet phagocytosis in the spleen. More than 80% of patients have *acute ITP*, a self-limited form of the disease that is treated conservatively with restricted activity, corticosteroids, and IV gammaglobulin. Medical therapy is appropriate for patients whose platelet count is less than 40,000/mm³ or in older children who are at higher risk for intracranial hemorrhage. Acute ITP occurs most frequently in children younger than 10 years old following an acute viral illness. Presenting symptoms are related to thrombocytopenia: petechiae, ecchymoses, oral or rectal bleeding, and rarely intracranial bleeding. Hepatosplenomegaly or lymphadenopathy should prompt bone marrow sampling to exclude malignancy or bone marrow dysfunction as a cause of the thrombocytopenia.

Systemic steroids quickly improve the platelet count in more than 75% of these patients, although the effects do not treat the underlying cause of the disease and do not change the ultimate course of the disease. Steroids work by inhibiting phagocytosis of the platelets and by increasing platelet production. IV gammaglobulin is thought to bind to the Fc receptor of the reticuloendothelial cells in the spleen, thereby also blocking phagocytosis. This therapy is usually given either in cases refractory to steroids or in actively bleeding patients. Although splenectomy is usually performed only in patients with chronic ITP, rare cases of acute ITP with severe bleeding complications (especially intracranial bleeding) may require emergency splenectomy.

In 10 to 20% of patients with ITP, the thrombocytopenia persists for more than 6 months. These patients are thought to have *chronic ITP*.[64] These patients require bone marrow sampling and immunologic evaluation to rule out other causes of thrombocytopenia because ITP is a diagnosis of exclusion. Like the acute form, chronic ITP is usually treated with steroids and IV gammaglobulin, but the risk and cost of these drugs used in these cases must be weighed over a long period of treatment. For this reason, other drugs and treatment modalities are under investigation, including plasmapheresis, erythrocytes with prebound IgG to attach to the Fc receptor, and cytotoxic agents.

In general, splenectomy is more commonly performed in chronic ITP than in acute ITP. Approximately 20% of chronic ITP patients require splenectomy, usually owing to medical failures. A careful intraoperative search for accessory spleens is critical to avoid long-term recurrences.[65]

THALASSEMIA

The genetic hemoglobinopathies known as *thalassemia* may be of major (homozygous), minor (heterozygous), or intermediate form. In the more severe forms, there is diffuse deposition of iron in the spleen, compounded by engorgement with destroyed red blood cells. Hypersplenism results in more erythrocyte sequestration, and transfusion requirements may escalate. These patients may benefit from splenectomy. Partial splenectomy has a particular attraction in thalassemia because postsplenectomy sepsis occurs in more than 10% of patients who have splenectomy for this disease.[66]

LEUKEMIAS AND LYMPHOMAS

The spleen is often involved with leukemic infiltrates or lymphoma.[67, 68] In non-Hodgkin's lymphoma, including small cell and large cell lymphomas, splenic involvement may lead to splenomegaly without hypersplenism. Splenectomy is not indicated in these patients. In Hodgkin's disease, the spleen may become involved with malignant cells, although rarely as a primary site. Splenomegaly may occur in Hodgkin's disease when the spleen is infiltrated with tumor, but splenectomy plays no role in the therapy of Hodgkin's disease (see Chapter 68).

Staging laparotomy for Hodgkin's disease is less frequently performed. The original rationale for staging laparotomy was to determine whether patients had disease on both sides of the diaphragm, therefore increasing the clinical stage from II to III. This upstaging from stage II to III meant that patients would then receive chemotherapy. Chemotherapy has come to be used in all stages of Hodgkin's disease to reduce the dose of radiation therapy. In addition, staging by CT scan or MRI is becoming much more precise. For these reasons, staging laparotomy/splenectomy is becoming much less frequently performed.

Chronic myelogenous leukemia is characterized by myeloid metaplasia, often leading to massive splenomegaly. In these patients, splenectomy has been performed for palliation of pain, mass-related symptoms, and secondary hypersplenism. In acute myelogenous leukemia and acute lymphoblastic leukemia, splenomegaly is less dramatic and splenectomy is rarely of benefit. Splenectomy may be detrimental in some cases because the spleen has become an important site for extramedullary hematopoiesis.

STORAGE DISEASES

Storage diseases result from the inability to properly dispose of cell breakdown products. Many of these diseases result in liver or splenic enlargement and are often incurable, with death resulting from central nervous system involvement (e.g., Niemann-Pick type 1 and mucopolysaccharidoses). Gaucher's disease is an indolent defect of the enzyme glucocerebrosidase, which results in the accumulation of glucosylceramide. Massive splenomegaly develops in these patients and may cause hypersplenism. Owing to its indolent course, splenectomy may offer considerable symptomatic relief and improvement of formed elements in the blood. Partial splenectomy may temporize symptoms but recurrence is the rule.[69, 70]

SPLENOSIS

Fragmentation of the spleen from trauma has been noted on occasion to result in *splenosis*, the growth of splenic tissue within the abdominal cavity. This observation led to the intentional implantation of small fragments of splenic tissue into the peritoneal cavity and omentum to try to avoid postsplenectomy sepsis. The function of these implants is questionable because 50% of the original splenic mass seems to be necessary for normal splenic function. These implants do not clear encapsulated bacteria as does the normal spleen, although the implants histologically appear normal. Splenosis should be treated with antibiotics in the same way asplenia is.[71, 72]

SPLENECTOMY

The operative approach to splenectomy has recently become more varied. The options, other than open, total splenectomy, include partial splenectomy, splenic embolization, splenorrhaphy, and laparoscopic splenectomy.[73–76] The traditional open splenectomy may be performed with the patient in the supine or decubitus position with transverse or left subcostal incision. For simultaneous cholecystectomy, a vertical or extended transverse incision is used. The spleen is usually first mobilized by dividing the short gastric vessels and the posterior attachments to the diaphragm. In cases of marked splenomegaly, the gastrocolic ligament can be opened laterally to allow exposure of the splenic artery along the superior aspect of the pancreas. The splenic artery can be ligated in continuity there to decrease the potential blood loss of mobilizing the large spleen.

After fully mobilizing the spleen by further detaching it from the left kidney, the spleen can then usually be brought up into the wound, allowing safe and simple division of the major hilar splenic vessels. Care must be taken to avoid damage to the tail of the pancreas, which may extend to the hilum of the spleen. Once the spleen is removed, the splenic bed should be carefully examined for persistent bleeding. Usually, a nasogastric tube is left in for gastric decompression. It has been reported that gastric distention may lead to ties slipping off the short gastric vessels after gastric distention, with subsequent exsanguinating hemorrhage. Suture ligature of the gastric end of these vessels is advised.

In patients with hemolytic anemia or ITP, and in certain cases of hypersplenism, it is critical to locate and remove any accessory spleens. Accessory spleens may often be found in the splenic hilum, lesser sac, or omentum.

Partial splenectomy and splenorrhaphy of the traumatized spleen represent surgical alternatives to total splenectomy. These procedures rely on the ability to place mattress sutures in the spleen or to place an absorbable mesh around the spleen for hemostasis. The segmental vascular anatomy of the spleen allows partial splenectomy along lines of demarcation, which follow segmental vessel ligation. These splenic salvage procedures are justified for the prevention of postsplenectomy sepsis. In trauma surgery, the advantages of splenic salvage must be weighed against the risk of bleeding and surgical delay. Splenic embolization has been used, particularly in cases of hypersplenism associated with portal hypertension in which total splenectomy is not necessary and open surgery is relatively dangerous due to enlarged portal vein collaterals. These procedures should ablate 80 to 90% of the spleen to be effective.

Laparoscopic splenectomy has become more accepted with advanced laparoscopic technical equipment, including reloadable vascular laparoscopic staples, the harmonic scalpel, and laparoscopic tissue morcellization.[77] Concomitant cholecystectomy can usually be added without difficulty. The technique uses four or five ports. The splenic hilar and short gastric vessels are stapled and the spleen is placed into a nylon bag to allow morcellization without spillage. This technique requires significantly more operative time than open splenectomy. Adequate removal of accessory spleens and removal of large spleens may limit use of this technique.

POSTSPLENECTOMY SEPSIS

The most feared complication of splenectomy is postsplenectomy sepsis (sometimes called overwhelming postsplenectomy infection).[78] Sepsis may occur within days, but usually occurs within 2 years of the splenectomy if it is going to occur at all. The risk of infection is increased in patients younger than 5 years old, with a much higher incidence in patients undergoing splenectomy for hematologic disease. Specifically, the incidence of overwhelming postsplenectomy infection after splenectomy performed for thalassemia may be more than 10%, whereas for trauma it is 1 to 2%. Considering all splenectomy patients, the incidence is 4% with a mortality rate approaching 50%.[79] The infections are typically fulminant and are most often caused by encapsulated organisms, pneumococci, *Haemophilus influenzae* B, gonococci, and *Escherichia coli*. These fulminant infections often cause meningitis and adrenal infarction with hemorrhage. The encapsulated organisms have a pathologic advantage in splenectomized patients because the circulating antibodies to these bacteria are produced in the spleen.[80]

Total splenectomy should always be avoided, if possible, but especially in patients younger than 2 years of age, owing to the markedly increased risk of postsplenectomy sepsis in this age group. If the splenectomy is elective, the polyvalent pneumococcal and *H. influenzae* B vaccines should be given preoperatively. In all patients undergoing splenectomy, even those with previous vaccinations or attempted autotransplantation, postoperative prophylactic antibiotics should be given. Penicillin is the

prophylactic most often used. The recommended length of treatment varies between 2 years and a lifetime, although the risk of postsplenectomy sepsis declines greatly 2 years after the splenectomy.[81]

REFERENCES

1. Lee PC: Functional development of the exocrine pancreas. In Lebenthal E (ed): Human Gastrointestinal Development. New York, Raven Press, 1989, p 651.
2. Dawson W, Langman J: An anatomical-radiological study on the pancreatic duct pattern in man. Anat Rec 139:59–68, 1961.
3. Gittes GK, Rutter WJ: Onset of cell-specific gene expression in the developing mouse pancreas. Proc Natl Acad Sci U S A 89:1128, 1992.
4. Bertelli E, Di Gregorio F, Bertelli L, et al: The arterial supply of the pancreas: A review. Surg Radiol Anat 17:2, 97–106, 1995.
5. Nakajima H, Kambayashi M, Okubo H, et al: Annular pancreas accompanied by an ectopic pancreas in the adult: A case report. Endoscopy 27:713, 1995.
6. Brambs HJ: Developmental anomalies and congenital diseases of the pancreas. Radiologe 36:381, 1996.
7. Skandalakis JE, Gray SW, Ricketts R, et al: The pancreas. In Skandalakis JE, Gray SW (eds): Embryology for Surgeons (2nd ed). Baltimore, Williams & Wilkins, 1994, p 381.
8. Stimee B, Korneti V, Milosavljevit T, et al: Ductal morphometry of ventral pancreas in pancreas divisum. Comparison between clinical and anatomical results. Ital J Gastroenterol 28:76–80, 1996.
9. Pescador R, Manso MA, Rebollo AJ, et al: Effect of chronic administration of hydrocortisone on the induction and evolution of acute pancreatitis induced by cerulein. Pancreas 11:165, 1995.
10. Evans RJ, Miranda RN, Jordan J, et al: Fatal acute pancreatitis caused by valproic acid. Am J Forensic Med Pathol 16:62, 1995.
11. Beger HG, Rau B, Mayer J, Pralle U: Natural course of acute pancreatitis. World J Surg 21:130, 1997.
12. Waldemar H, Buchler U, Buchler MW: Classification and severity staging of acute pancreatitis. Ann Ital Chir 66:171, 1995.
13. Levitt MD, Eckfeldt JH: Diagnosis of acute pancreatitis. In Go VLW, DiMagno EP, Gardner JD, et al (eds): The Pancreas (2nd ed). New York, Raven Press, 1993, p 613.
14. Sternby B, O'Brien JF, Zinsmeister AR, et al: What is the best biochemical test to diagnose acute pancreatitis? A prospective clinical study. Mayo Clin Proc 71:1138, 1996.
15. Panzironi G, Franceschini L, Angelini P, et al: Role of ultrasonography in the study of patients with acute pancreatitis. G Chir 18:47, 1997.
16. Fujiwara T, Takehara Y, Ichijo K, et al: Anterior extension of acute pancreatitis: CT findings. J Comput Assist Tomogr 19:963, 1995.
17. Ihse I, Andersson R, Andren-Sandberg A, et al: Conservative treatment in acute pancreatitis. Ann Ital Chir 66:181, 1995.
18. Kaufmann P, Hofmann G, Smoll KH, et al: Intensive care management of acute pancreatitis: Recognition of patients at high risk of developing severe or fatal complications. Wien Klin Wochenschr 108:9, 1996.
19. Paran H, Neufeld D, Mayo A, et al: Preliminary report of a prospective randomized study of octreotide in the treatment of severe acute pancreatitis. J Am Coll Surg 181:121, 1995.
20. Hwang TL, Chiu CT, Chen HM, et al: Surgical results for severe acute pancreatitis—comparison of the different surgical procedures. Hepatogastroenterology 42:1026, 1995.
21. Beger HG, Rau B: Necrosectomy and postoperative local lavage in necrotizing pancreatitis. Ann Ital Chir 66:209, 1995.
22. Wilson C: Management of the later complications of severe acute pancreatitis—pseudocyst, abscess and fistula. Eur J Gastroenterol Hepatol 9:117, 1997.
23. Bittner R: Clinical significance and management of pancre-

atic abscess and infected necrosis complicating acute pancreatitis. Ann Ital Chir 66:217, 1995.

24. Sharma SS: Endoscopic cystogastrostomy: Preliminary experience. Indian J Gastroenterol 14:11, 1995.

25. D'Cruz AJ, Kamath PS, Ramachandra C, et al: Pancreatic ascites in children. Acta Paediatr Jpn 37:630, 1995.

26. da Cunha JE, Machado M, Bacchella T, et al: Surgical treatment of pancreatic ascites and pancreatic pleural effusions. Hepatogastroenterology 42:748, 1995.

27. Shimizu M, Hirokawa M, Manabe T: Histological assessment of chronic pancreatitis at necropsy. J Clin Pathol 49:913, 1996.

28. Sidhu SS, Tandon RK: Chronic pancreatitis: Diagnosis and treatment. Postgrad Med J 72:327, 1996.

29. Sidhu SS, Tandon RK: The pathogenesis of chronic pancreatitis. Postgrad Med J 71:67, 1995.

30. Dite P, Zboril V, Cikankova E: Endoscopic therapy of chronic pancreatitis. Hepatogastroenterology 43:1633, 1996.

31. Kane C, Shepherd RM, Squires PE, et al: Loss of functional KATP channels in pancreatic beta-cells causes persistent hyperinsulinemic hypoglycemia of infancy. Nat Med 2:1344, 1996.

32. Thomas P, Lightner E: Mutation of the pancreatic islet inward rectifier Kir 6.2 also leads to familial persistent hyperinsulinemic hypoglycemia of infancy. Hum Mol Genet 5:1809, 1996.

33. Thomas PM, Cote GJ, Hallman DM, et al: Homozygosity mapping to chromosome 11p, of the gene for familial persistent hyperinsulinemic hypoglycemia of infancy. Am J Hum Genet 56:416, 1995.

34. al-Rabeeah A, al-Ashwal A, al-Herbish A, et al: Persistent hyperinsulinemic hypoglycemia of infancy: Experience with 28 cases. J Pediatr Surg 30:1119, 1995.

35. Soliman AT, Alsalmi I, Darwish A, et al: Growth and endocrine function after near total pancreatectomy for hyperinsulinaemic hypoglycaemia. Arch Dis Child 74:379, 1996.

36. Leibowitz G, Glaser B, Higazi AA, et al: Hyperinsulinemic hypoglycemia of infancy (nesidioblastosis) in clinical remission: High incidence of diabetes mellitus and persistent beta-cell dysfunction at long-term follow-up. J Clin Endocrinol Metab 80:386, 1995.

37. Mason JP: New insights into G6PD deficiency. Br J Haematol 94:585, 1996.

38. Grant CS: Gastrointestinal endocrine tumors. Insulinoma. Bailleres Clin Gastroenterol 10:645, 1996.

39. Angeli E, Vanzulli A, Casstrucci M, et al: Value of abdominal sonography and MR imaging at 0.5 T in preoperative detection of pancreatic insulinoma: A comparison with dynamic CT and angiography. Abdom Imaging 22:295, 1997.

40. Eire PF, Rodriguez-Pereira C, Barca-Rodriguez P, et al: Uncommon case of gastrinoma in a child. Eur J Pediatr Surg 6:173, 1996.

41. Jensen RT: Gastrointestinal endocrine tumours. Gastrinoma. Bailliers Clin Gastroenterol 10:603, 1996.

42. Brenin DR, Talamonti MS, Yang EY, et al: Cystic neoplasms of the pancreas. A clinicopathologic study, including DNA flow cytometry. Arch Surg 130:1048, 1995.

43. Murakami T, Ueki K, Kawakami H, et al: Pancreatoblastoma: Case report and review of treatment in the literature. Med Pediatr Oncol 27:193, 1996.

44. Klimstra DS, Wenig BM, Adair CF, et al: Pancreatoblastoma. A clinicopathologic study and review of the literature. Am J Surg Pathol 19:1371, 1995.

45. Skandalakis JE, Gray SW, Ricketts R: The spleen. In Skandalakis JE, Gray SW (eds): Embryology for Surgeons (2nd ed). Baltimore, Williams & Wilkins, 1994, p 381.

46. Milicevic Z, Cuschieri A, Xuereb A, et al: Stereological study of tissue compartments of the human spleen. Histol Histopathol 11:833, 1996.

47. Liu DL, Xia S, Xu W, et al: Anatomy of vasculature of 850 spleen specimens and its application in partial splenectomy. Surgery 119:27, 1996.

48. Ferlicot S, Emile JF, Le Bris JL, et al: Congenital asplenia. A childhood immune deficit often detected too late. Ann Pathol 17:44, 1997.

49. Rubino M, Van Praagh S, Kadoba K, et al: Systemic and pulmonary venous connections in visceral heterotaxy with asplenia. Diagnostic and surgical considerations based on seventy-two autopsied cases. J Thorac Cardiovasc Surg 110:641, 1995.

50. Rudowski WJ: Accessory spleen: Clinical significance with particular reference to the recurrence of idiopathic thrombocytopenic purpura. World J Surg 9:423, 1985.

51. Balaji KC, Caldarone AA, Rabinowitz R, et al: Splenogonadal fusion. J Urol 156:854, 1996.

52. Desai DC, Hebra A, Davidoff AM, et al: Wandering spleen: A challenging diagnosis. South Med J 90:439, 1997.

53. Fufiwara T, Takehara Y, Isoda H, et al: Torsion of the wandering spleen: CT and angiographic appearance. J Comput Assist Tomogr 19:84, 1995.

54. Lam KY, Chan AC, Chan TM: Peliosis of the spleen: Possible association with chronic renal failure and erythropoietin therapy. Postgrad Med J 71:493, 1995.

55. Touloukian RJ, Maharaj A, Ghoussoub R, et al: Partial decapsulation of splenic cysts: Studies on etiology and outcome. J Pediatr Surg 32:272, 1997.

56. Ramani M, Reinhold C, Semelka RC, et al: Splenic hemangiomas and hamartomas: MR imaging characteristics of 28 lesions. Radiology 202:166, 1997.

57. Velkova K, Nedeva A: Our experience in the diagnostics of liver and spleen hemangiomas. Folia Med (Plovdiv) 39:85, 1997.

58. Yelon JA, Green JD, Evans JT: Splenic abscess associated with osteomyelitis. Eur J Surg 162:913, 1996.

59. Bossi D, Russo M: Hemolytic anemias due to disorders of red cell membrane skeleton. Mol Aspects Med 17:171, 1996.

60. Tchernia G, Bader-Meunier B, Berterottiere P, et al: Effectiveness of partial splenectomy in hereditary spherocytosis. Curr Opin Hematol 4:136, 1997.

61. Lane PA: Sickle cell disease. Pediatr Clin North Am 43:639, 1996.

62. Lane PA: The spleen in children. Curr Opin Pediatr 7:36, 1995.

63. Svarch E, Vilorio P, Nordet I, et al: Partial splenectomy in children with sickle cell disease and repeated episodes of splenic sequestration. Hemoglobin 20:393, 1996.

64. Caulier MT, Darloy F, Rose C, et al: Splenic irradiation for chronic autoimmune thrombocytopenic purpura in patients with contraindications to splenectomy. Br J Haematol 91:208, 1995.

65. Najean Y, Rain JD, Billotey C: The site of destruction of autologous ^{111}In-labelled platelets and the efficiency of splenectomy in children and adults with idiopathic thrombocytopenic purpura: A study of 578 patients with 268 splenectomies. Br J Haematol 97:547, 1997.

66. Stanley P, Shen TC: Partial embolization of the spleen in patients with thalassemia. J Vasc Interv Radiol 6:137, 1995.

67. Terrosu G, Donini A, Silvestri F, et al: Laparoscopic splenectomy in the management of hematological diseases. Surgical technique and outcome of 17 patients. Surg Endosc 10:441, 1996.

68. Pui CH: Childhood leukemias—current status and future perspective. Acta Pediatr Sin 36:322, 1995.

69. Rice EO, Mifflin TE, Sakallah S, et al: Gaucher disease: Studies of phenotype, molecular diagnosis and treatment. Clin Genet 49:111, 1996.

70. Lorberboym M, Pastores GM, Kim CK, et al: Scintigraphic monitoring of reticuloendothelial system in patients with type I Gaucher disease on enzyme replacement therapy. J Nucl Med 38:890, 1997.

71. Soutter AD, Ellenbogen J, Folkman J: Splenosis is regulated by a circulating factor. J Pediatr Surg 29:1076, 1994.

72. Arzoumanian A, Rosenthal L: Splenosis. Clin Nuc Med 20:730, 1995.

73. Carroll A, Thomas P. Decision-making in surgery: Splenectomy. Br J Hosp Med 54:147, 1995.

74. Petroianu A: Subtotal splenectomy for treatment of patients with myelofibrosis and myeloid metaplasia. Int Surg 81:177, 1996.

75. Farhi DC, Ashfaq R: Splenic pathology after traumatic injury. Am J Clin Pathol 105:474, 1996.

76. Uranus S, Pfeifer J, Schauer C, et al: Laparoscopic partial splenic resection. Surg Laparosc Endosc 5:133, 1995.

77. Moores DC, McKee MA, Wang H, et al: Pediatric laparoscopic splenectomy. J Pediatr Surg 30:1201, 1995.

78. Hassan IS, Snow MH, Ong EL: Overwhelming pneumococcal sepsis in two patients splenectomized more than ten years previously. Scott Med J 41:17, 1996.

79. O'Sullivan ST, Reardon CM, O'Donnell JA, et al: "How safe is splenectomy?" Ir J Med Sci 163:374, 1994.

80. Balsalobre B, Carbonell-Tatay F: Cellular immunity in splenectomized patients. J Investig Allergol Clin Immunol 1:235, 1991.

81. Green AD, Connor MP: Prevention of post-splenectomy sepsis. Lancet 341:1034, 1993.

47

GASTROSCHISIS AND OMPHALOCELE

Barbara A. Gaines, MD • George W. Holcomb III, MD • Wallace W. Neblett III, MD

Ambroise Pare first described a newborn with an omphalocele in the 17th century. Scattered descriptions of gastroschisis and omphalocele were reported during the ensuing 200 years, but there were few survivors. In 1948, Gross described a staged repair for omphalocele, initially closing the defect with skin and later repairing the ventral hernia.[1] The next major technical advance was reported by Schuster, who described the use of a two layer temporary extraabdominal wrap of the exposed bowel.[2] Allen and Wrenn modified this technique, using a single layer of Silastic sheeting to create a bowel containing silo.[3] The bowel was gradually reduced into the abdominal cavity, and the fascial defect closed in a delayed manner.

Survival of infants with abdominal wall defects, particularly gastroschisis, would not have been possible without advances in neonatal intensive care. The introduction of total parenteral nutrition (TPN) and infant ventilators provided a means to support infants while awaiting the return of gastrointestinal (GI) function and ventilatory sufficiency. Infants born with gastroschisis or isolated omphalocele have excellent long-term survival expectations with minimal morbidity.

☐ Embryology

Gastroschisis, from the Greek word meaning "belly cleft," is a defect in the abdominal wall lateral to the intact umbilical cord. The abdominal contents herniate through this small defect (usually less than 4 cm) in utero and are free floating within the amnion. There is no peritoneal sac covering the bowel, which thereby is in direct contact with the amniotic fluid. Contact with the irritating amniotic fluid is believed to cause an intense serositis and to result in the formation of a thick peel on the serosal surface of the bowel, which may result in foreshortening (Fig. 47–1). These changes are most dramatic late in gestation.[4] Frequently, the entire small and large bowel as well as the stomach have eviscerated. The liver is rarely involved. Normal bowel rotation and fixation does not occur.

Although there is some controversy regarding the etiology of gastroschisis, it is generally thought that it is the result of a vascular accident during embryogenesis. It has been postulated that intrauterine occlusion of the right omphalomesenteric artery results in the disruption of the umbilical ring and bowel herniation.[5, 6] This hypothesis explains the right-sided predominance of the defect and its association with intestinal atresias, another defect attributable to a vascular accident in the distribution of the right omphalomesenteric artery. Other theories

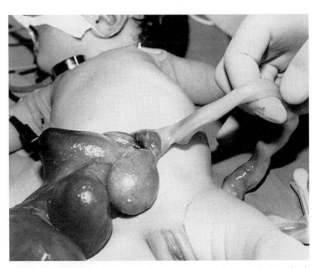

Figure 47–1. An infant with gastroschisis and matted, foreshortened intestine is depicted. Note the umbilical cord entering the abdominal wall to the left of the fascial defect.

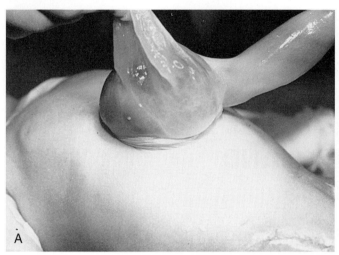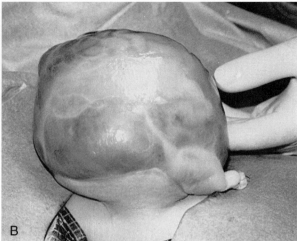

Figure 47–2. Omphaloceles vary greatly in size and complexity. *A,* Newborn with small omphalocele containing a segment of liver. Primary repair was possible. *B,* Giant omphalocele containing virtually all of the intestine and a large proportion of the liver.

postulate that the defect is the result of a ruptured hernia of the umbilical cord or of a congenital weakening of the right side of the umbilical cord.[7, 8]

An omphalocele is a central defect of the umbilical ring, through which bowel and other abdominal viscera herniate. The abdominal contents are covered with a membrane composed of an inner layer of peritoneum fused to an outer layer of amnion. Occasionally, Wharton's jelly is also found in the sac. Omphaloceles of all sizes are seen, from very small "umbilical cord hernias" to large defects that result in evisceration of the entire bowel and liver (Fig. 47–2). In cases of very large defects, the actual abdominal cavity can be small, creating difficulties when attempts are made to reduce the extracoelomic viscera. Occasionally, the omphalocele can rupture (Fig. 47–3). In this situation, the defect can be correctly identified by examination of the insertion of the umbilical cord on the remnants of the sac.

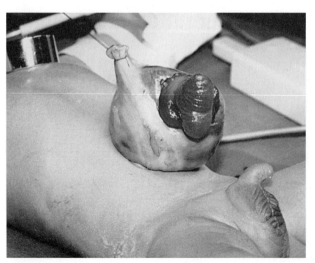

Figure 47–3. A ruptured omphalocele with a segment of intestine protruding through the torn omphalocele sac.

The primordial regions of the GI tract (foregut, midgut, and hindgut) are developmentally related to the embryologic folds of the abdominal wall. Normal development of the abdominal wall and GI tract is dependent on growth and fusion of the cephalic, caudal, and lateral folds. A failure of migration and fusion of these embryonic folds is the most widely accepted etiology of omphalocele. These events occur early in embryogenesis. Omphalocele can be associated with other midline defects, including those involving the sternum, diaphragm, and heart, as well as with bladder exstrophy and cloaca. An example is the pentalogy of Cantrell, which is associated with a failure of the cephalic embryonic fold and which results in an epigastric omphalocele, anterior diaphragmatic defect, sternal cleft, and pericardial and cardiac defects.

□ Epidemiology

Given the differences in etiology between gastroschisis and omphalocele, it is not surprising that they also differ in epidemiology. In a detailed study of gastroschisis in California, the defect was strongly associated with young maternal age, low socioeconomic status, and social instability.[9, 10] Lending support to a vascular etiology, the use of aspirin, ibuprofen, and pseudoephedrine during the first trimester was associated with an increased risk of gastroschisis.[10, 11] Alcohol, cigarette, and recreational drug use have also been shown to increase the risk of this malformation. Epidemiologic studies in Europe have confirmed the association of young maternal age with gastroschisis, with one study demonstrating an 11-fold increase in risk in mothers younger than 20 years of age.[12] Chromosomal and other anomalies are rare in patients with gastroschisis, except in cases of intestinal atresia. Babies with gastroschisis are often small for gestational age.

Environmental and social factors appear to play

less of a role in the etiology of omphalocele. Karyotype abnormalities are present in approximately 30% of affected infants, particularly trisomies 13 and 18, and less frequently trisomy 21.[13] Small defects that do not include the liver appear to have a greater incidence of chromosomal abnormalities.[14] More than half of infants with omphalocele have other major or minor malformations, with cardiac anomalies being the most common, followed by musculoskeletal, GI, and genitourinary malformations.[12, 15] There is also a close association with the Beckwith-Wiedemann syndrome (omphalocele-macroglossia-hyperinsulinism). In Great Britain, there is a strong association between omphalocele and neural tube defects, a relationship that is much rarer elsewhere.[12]

There are interesting variations in the incidence of gastroschisis and omphalocele. In the United States, Spain, and Sweden, gastroschisis has been increasing in frequency. In most of Europe, however, omphalocele is the more prevalent abdominal wall defect.[12, 16]

□ Prenatal Screening

The antenatal diagnosis of abdominal wall defects and subsequent management of the affected infant are areas of interest and controversy. Two modes of screening are routinely used: the assay of maternal serum alphafetoprotein (AFP) and fetal ultrasonography (US). AFP is measured during the second trimester of pregnancy and is useful in screening for both gastroschisis and omphalocele, although the levels in gastroschisis are statistically higher than those in omphalocele.[17] Other maternal serum markers, such as unconjugated estriol and human chorionic gonadotropin, have not proved to be clinically useful.

Fetal US performed in the second trimester of pregnancy accurately diagnoses abdominal wall defects as well as many of the associated defects. US performed during the first trimester is difficult to interpret because the midgut normally herniates into the umbilical cord during this time. The sonographic findings of gastroschisis include a small abdominal wall defect to the right of the umbilical cord with herniated bowel floating in the amniotic fluid (Fig. 47–4).[18] Omphalocele is differentiated from gastroschisis by the presence of the umbilical cord inserting into the membranous covering of the herniated bowel (Fig. 47–5). Ruptured omphaloceles can be a diagnostic dilemma, but they can generally be distinguished by the large size of the defect and liver herniation.[18] If omphalocele is suspected on prenatal US, a careful search for other anomalies is required. Amniocentesis should be performed to screen for possible chromosomal abnormalities. Parents should receive counseling from a multidisciplinary team regarding the fetus' long-term prognosis.[18] Given the low incidence of trisomies in gastroschi-

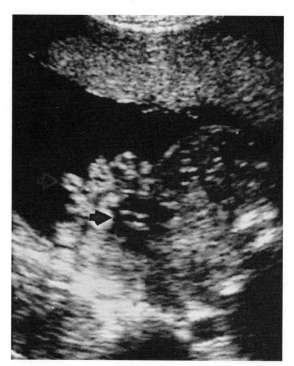

Figure 47–4. Ultrasound demonstrating a fetus with gastroschisis. Notice the loops of intestine *(open arrow)* are free floating in the amniotic cavity. Also, the umbilical cord *(solid arrow)* is seen entering the abdominal wall rather than the amniotic sac.

sis, amniocentesis is probably not justified in this population.

Antenatal discovery of a significant malformation allows for appropriate counseling of parents regarding the expected prognosis and introduces the option of elective termination of the pregnancy. Published statistics from the 21 regional registries in Europe (EUROCAT) from 1980 to 1990 indicated that 33% of fetuses diagnosed prenatally with om-

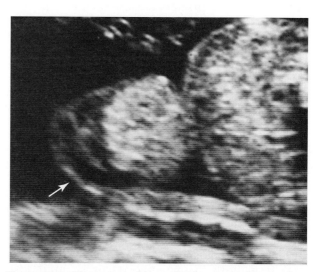

Figure 47–5. Ultrasonographic study showing a fetus with an omphalocele. The amniotic sac is seen with intestine encased within it. Also, the umbilical cord *(open arrow)* is noted to enter onto the sac rather than the abdominal wall.

phalocele and 27% of those with gastroschisis were electively aborted.[12] In a small series from North Carolina, 2 of 13 fetuses with the antenatal diagnosis of gastroschisis were electively aborted, although both these fetuses had other malformations.[19]

☐ Cesarean Section

One of the ongoing controversies regarding the perinatal care of babies with abdominal wall defects concerns the mode of delivery. Studies comparing vaginal versus cesarean delivery are subject to multiple confounding variables, including antenatal diagnosis, presence or absence of labor, regional or tertiary delivery of the infant, maternal or infant transport, and length of time to operative repair.

From a theoretical standpoint, labor could be detrimental to infants with gastroschisis for a number of reasons. First, the eviscerated bowel could be injured during the birth process, particularly in infants with an abnormal lie; second, the bowel could interfere with delivery; and third, passage of the unprotected bowel through the vagina could predispose it to infectious complications.[20] The first of these concerns appears to be well founded, and it is generally agreed that a baby with gastroschisis in the breech or transverse position should be delivered by elective section.[21] In addition, an infant with a giant omphalocele with herniation of the liver generally requires operative delivery. However, for most other infants, expert opinion is divided. One study found that babies who underwent elective cesarean delivery had less sepsis, fewer hospital days, and a shorter time to enteral feedings, whereas several other studies noted no advantage to cesarean section, and one even demonstrated a worse outcome in that group.[22–27] Many pediatric surgeons, however, believe that early planned delivery may reduce the amount of bowel "peel" and edema, which may, in turn, facilitate primary closure (Fig. 47–6).[28]

US has been used to monitor bowel wall edema and peel formation. In two separate studies, the demonstration of maximum small bowel diameter greater than 11 cm or 17 cm correlated with increased postnatal bowel complications.[29, 30] However, the determination of bowel wall thickness by US is operator dependent, and the clinical utility of this finding is still under investigation.[29]

☐ Gastroschisis

Care of the infant with gastroschisis begins at the time of birth. In many institutions, transfer of the mother to the hospital where the infant's surgery will be performed before delivery is encouraged regardless of the mode of delivery so that the elapsed time from birth to operative repair is minimized. Immediate care of the freshly delivered infant with gastroschisis centers on three areas: providing the bowel with a sterile protective covering, preventing

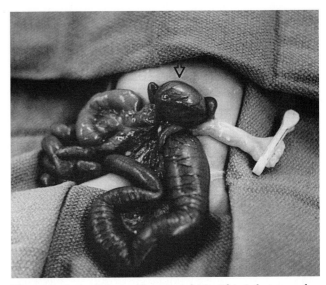

Figure 47–6. An infant with gastroschisis. This infant was electively delivered at 36 gestational weeks. Notice the distended stomach *(open arrow)*. Also, note that there is no evidence of fibrinous exudate along the intestine.

hypothermia, and ensuring adequate fluid resuscitation.

Babies with gastroschisis are often small for gestational age and are subject to large fluid and heat losses secondary to the exposed intestine. In the delivery room, the exposed viscera are protected with saline-moistened sterile wraps or a plastic "bowel bag," and the baby is placed in an infant warmer. An orogastric tube is inserted for gastric decompression and for prevention of air swallowing and aspiration.

In the neonatal intensive care unit (ICU), fluid resuscitation using isotonic fluids is initiated. These babies can require two and one half to three times the maintenance fluid volume of a normal neonate in the first 24 postnatal hours. Fluid resuscitation is continued until adequate urinary output and acid-base balance is achieved. The infant is also started on broad-spectrum antibiotic coverage.

Infants born in outlying hospitals require urgent transfer to a facility with pediatric surgical capabilities. Transport should be accomplished by a unit skilled in the care of neonatal patients with special attention paid to maintaining the infant's temperature. Full evaluation and resuscitation of the infant should occur before operative repair.

Because gastroschisis is not generally associated with major congenital defects other than intestinal atresia, infants do not require extensive evaluation before operative repair of the defect. A careful physical examination and chest radiograph should suffice.

After stabilization of the infant, operative repair is undertaken. Repair is performed in an operating suite under general anesthesia and full muscle relaxation. Recent reports suggest that regional anesthesia may be an acceptable alternative.[31, 32] Continuous epidural anesthesia has the added advantage of providing postoperative pain relief, which is especially advantageous for those infants undergoing staged repairs.[31] Many surgeons perform anal dilation and place a rectal catheter to allow irrigation and manual decompression of the colon intraoperatively. The abdomen is prepped with an iodophor-containing solution. Great care is necessary when handling the edematous intestine, and adhesions should be left intact. Although the bowel should be examined, an atresia may not be apparent. Before reduction and closure, the fascial defect can be enlarged a few centimeters. The abdominal cavity is then manually stretched and reduction of the bowel mass attempted. The umbilical artery may be used for postoperative monitoring, bringing the catheter out through a stab incision in the lower abdominal wall (Fig. 47–7).

The nature of the repair has undergone considerable evolution since the 1960s when the use of a Silastic silo was first described to provide temporary coverage of the exposed intestines.[3] Prosthetic closure is associated with an increased incidence of sepsis.[33, 34] Overly aggressive attempts at primary closure, however, can result in increased abdominal pressure, with physiologic derangements including decreased cardiac output resulting from poor venous return from caval compression, respiratory embarrassment from elevation of the diaphragms, renal failure, bowel ischemia, and decreased lower extremity perfusion. Current opinion supports a selective management, dependent on the degree of visceroabdominal disproportion and elevation of intraabdominal pressure.

How tight is too tight? This question has challenged pediatric surgeons for decades. Clinical parameters, including respiratory rate, lower extremity perfusion, and blood pressure are most frequently used, but they can be difficult to assess in an anesthetized infant. Studies in dogs have shown that elevations of intraabdominal pressure greater than 20 mm Hg markedly decrease glomerular filtration rate and renal blood flow.[35, 36] A clinical study of the hemodynamic effects of primary closure of gastroschisis and omphalocele demonstrated that significant increases in the central venous pressure and intragastric pressure (IGP) and a decrease in the cardiac output as measured using the indicator dilution technique occurred in those infants who failed primary repair.[37] They further noted that no infant with an IGP of less than 18 mm Hg or increase in central venous pressure of less than 2 mm Hg required conversion to a silo closure. Intragastric pressure less than 20 mm Hg, measured through either a fluid-filled gastrostomy or an orogastric tube, reliably predicted uncomplicated primary closure.[37–39] In addition, measurement of IGP in the ICU served as a guide to frequency of silo reduction in those infants who underwent a staged repair.

Other techniques for monitoring abdominal pressure have also been used. Using the same pressure limit of 20 mm Hg as measured through a urinary catheter led to correct treatment decisions regarding both primary and secondary closure.[40, 41] Elevation of the end tidal CO_2 greater than 50 mm Hg predicted failure of primary closure in one series.[42]

After reduction of the bowel, if primary closure is possible, the abdominal wall fascial defect may be approximated vertically or transversely in a single layer using interrupted sutures. The subcutaneous tissue and skin are closed separately. Creation of an umbilicus is possible using the technique in which the skin and subcutaneous tissue are elevated from

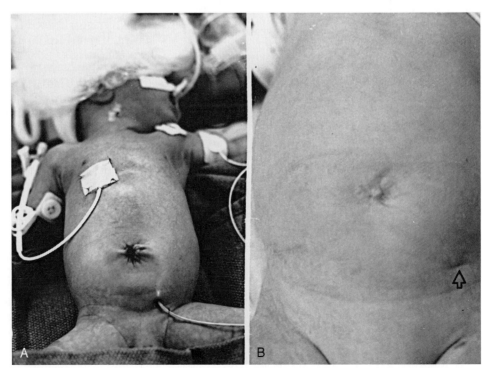

Figure 47–7. *A,* Postoperative view of an infant with gastroschisis who has undergone reduction of the intestine and primary fascial closure. It was not necessary to enlarge the fascial defect in this patient, and umbilicoplasty was easily performed. Also, note the Broviac catheter, which was placed in the right common facial vein and exteriorized on the lower chest wall. In the lower abdominal wall is an umbilical artery catheter placed through the left umbilical artery. The artery and catheter were transposed and exteriorized through a small incision in the inguinal region. *B,* the same infant at 3 months of age. Note the small incision *(open arrow)* on the lower abdominal wall where the umbilical artery catheter was exteriorized.

the fascia for approximately 1.5 cm around the defect before closure.[43] At the conclusion of the operative procedure, placement of a central venous catheter facilitates postoperative fluid administration and hyperalimentation (see Fig. 47–7).

Approximately 25% of infants are not candidates for primary closure. In this group of patients, a prosthetic, extraabdominal compartment is created for the intestines using Dacron-reinforced Silastic sheeting. The material is folded, and the double edge is sutured around the abdominal wall defect using either interrupted or continuous sutures. The walls of the silo are constructed parallel to each other, taking care to avoid creating a narrow-based cone. Long sutures are placed on the superior aspect of the silo to allow for its suspension from the infant's warmer. A sterile supportive dressing is placed around the base of the silo to prevent tilting or torsion of the enclosed viscera. Manual reduction of the silo contents is performed in the ICU at frequent intervals, with care taken to avoid excessive intraabdominal pressure (Fig. 47–8).

The silo is examined carefully during reduction procedures for signs of infection or vascular compromise of the enclosed intestine. Any suspicion of compromise necessitates removal of the prosthesis and direct inspection of the bowel. Generally, the silo can be removed and the abdominal wall closure completed within 7 to 10 days. Failure to achieve closure within 2 weeks is associated with an increased incidence of separation of the prosthesis from the abdominal wall. Antibiotics are discontinued several days after the abdominal wall is approximated.

Managing gastroschisis complicated by intestinal atresia is a difficult clinical problem and has been associated with a poor clinical outcome. Atresias can be single or multiple and involve both the small

and large intestine (Fig. 47–9). The etiology is likely vascular compromise secondary to compression at the narrow abdominal opening. If intestinal atresia is obvious, two general modes of therapy have been advocated (1) primary repair of the atresia at the time of abdominal wall closure or (2) intestinal diversion followed by delayed enteroenterostomy. Primary repair is frequently technically difficult because the bowel is thickened, edematous, and often matted. Staged repair of atresia complicating gastroschisis has been more successful. In one series, all infants survived who underwent proximal diversion either with a stoma or a long intestinal tube. Intestinal continuity was established 2 to 4 weeks later.[44] At the second procedure, the intestine appeared normal and a single layer end-to-end anastomosis could be successfully performed.

Occasionally, the intestine is so matted that atresia is not recognized or creation of a stoma is deemed impossible. In such a situation, the atretic segments can be returned to the abdomen and decompression accomplished by a long intestinal tube.[44, 45] Inadequate decompression with continued dilation of the proximal segment may lead to difficulty in performing the anastomosis later. Infants with atresias often have abnormal intestinal motility, particularly if the proximal segment is massively dilated (see Chapter 30). This may necessitate prolonged intravenous nutritional support. These babies are also at risk for short bowel syndrome resulting from loss of intestinal length in utero. Bowel lengthening techniques may improve intestinal function sufficiently to allow independence from parenteral nutrition.

Postoperative small bowel obstructions, resulting from stenotic anastomoses or adhesions, are not uncommon in these patients and may be difficult to distinguish from feeding intolerance secondary to poor intestinal motility. Small bowel enema (enteroclysis) is useful in differentiating between these two conditions.[46]

Most babies with gastroschisis can be weaned from the ventilator and extubated within 24 hours of repair. All infants have delayed intestinal function and require TPN until enteral feedings are tolerated, usually 3 to 4 weeks after abdominal closure.

Prolonged ileus is the most frequent postoperative complication in infants with gastroschisis. Sepsis, from the umbilical closure, central line, or pulmonary sources, is another frequently encountered problem. Postoperative necrotizing enterocolitis (NEC) appears to be a milder disease in the neonate with gastroschisis compared to NEC in babies with an intact abdominal wall. There does not appear to be an association between the type of closure and the development of NEC.[47] A major source of postoperative morbidity and mortality is related to TPN. Central line sepsis is not an uncommon problem. Potentially more devastating is TPN-associated cholestasis, which can lead to jaundice, cirrhosis, and, ultimately, liver failure necessitating liver transplantation.

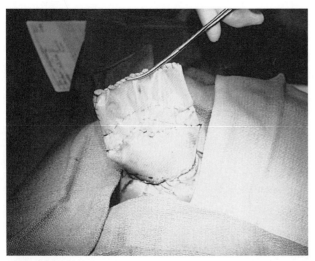

Figure 47–8. An operative view of the creation of an extraabdominal compartment (silo) for the intestines in an infant with gastroschisis. Manual reduction of the silo contents is performed in the neonatal intensive care unit once a day, which allows the abdominal cavity to slowly expand.

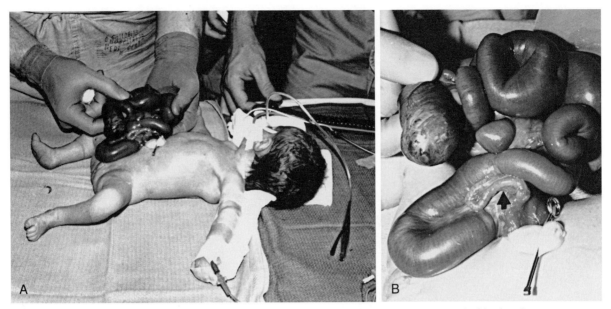

Figure 47–9. *A* and *B*, An infant with gastroschisis and colonic atresia. *B*, Note the blind ending proximal colon and the collapsed distal colon *(solid arrow).*

With modern techniques of neonatal intensive care and the variety of surgical approaches available, babies with gastroschisis have an excellent survival rate with acceptably low morbidity.

☐ Omphalocele

Managing infants with omphalocele is generally similar to managing infants with gastroschisis. The infant should be born in or rapidly transferred to a facility with neonatal intensive care and pediatric surgical capabilities. Because the herniated viscera are covered with a sac, these infants require less fluid resuscitation initially and do not lose heat as rapidly as neonates with gastroschisis.

Postoperatively, babies with surgically corrected omphalocele are not subject to the prolonged ileus seen in gastroschisis patients. If the omphalocele is ruptured, however, the baby is at risk for severe dehydration and hypothermia. Exposure to the amniotic fluid can cause a serositis and result in a prolonged postoperative ileus. As discussed previously, babies with omphalocele often have associated congenital malformations, and the initial evaluation should include a thorough physical examination, chest radiograph, and echocardiogram. An orogastric tube is placed for gastric decompression and antibiotics are administered. The omphalocele sac is wrapped in a protective dressing, with care taken to prevent mechanical trauma. Operative repair may be undertaken as soon as the infant's condition is stabilized.

Approximately 10% of patients have a giant omphalocele, in which the liver and the intestine herniate through an 8-cm to 10-cm defect. Management in these cases is difficult (Fig. 47–10). Because the anterior abdominal wall is so poorly developed, pri-

mary closure is not possible without excessive tension. A number of innovative strategies have been described to manage this complex situation. The simplest of these techniques is to promote epithelialization of the sac with secondary closure of the ensuing ventral hernia at a later date (Fig. 47–11). Various topical agents have been used, including 0.25% merbromin (Mercurochrome), silver nitrate, and silver sulfadiazine. The agent is applied to the intact sac once or twice daily and covered with an elastic dressing to apply mild compression of the sac contents. Even though this technique may require many weeks to achieve skin coverage of the defect, a recent series demonstrated that infants receiving nonoperative treatment had a shorter initial

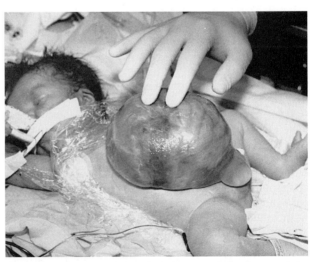

Figure 47–10. A newborn with a giant omphalocele containing liver and intestine. Primary closure is not possible in this patient, but a variety of strategies have been used to successfully manage such complex patients.

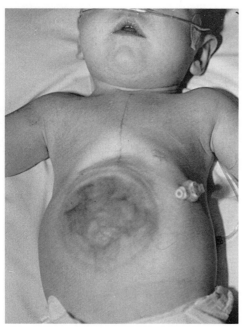

Figure 47–11. Nonoperative management of a giant epigastric omphalocele was used in this infant with pentalogy of Cantrell. Silver sulfadiazine cream was applied to the omphalocele sac during twice daily dressing changes, and gradual reduction of the viscera into the abdominal cavity was accomplished using elastic wraps to apply external pressure. The child has undergone successful repair of tetralogy of Fallot and closure of the diaphragmatic defect. Eventual repair of the ventral hernia completes the staged approach.

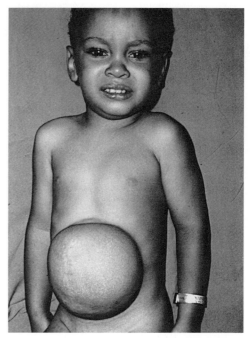

Figure 47–12. A child with a large ventral hernia following skin flap coverage of herniated liver. This technique (Gross repair) necessitates later staged hernia repair with prosthetic material but is a useful alternative in the management of giant omphaloceles.

hospitalization and time to full enteral feedings than their counterparts whose treatment was with a Silastic pouch chimney.[48]

Another nonoperative approach to the problem is to apply external pressure to the sac. Various devices including Ace wraps, Velcro binders, and a polyamide mesh glued to the skin have been described to aid in gradual reduction of the sac contents.[49, 50] Later, definitive closure of the ventral hernia is performed. Mobilization of skin flaps to cover the hernia defect, as first described by Gross,[1] has been used to provide temporary coverage of moderate to large omphaloceles. However, this technique may result in an enlarging ventral hernia because the skin sac grows and the abdominal wall musculature does not (Fig. 47–12).

With small and moderate-sized omphalocele defects, direct operative repair is undertaken. Once the patient is in the operating room, general anesthesia is induced and the abdomen and sac are washed with a povidone-iodine solution. Primary closure is attempted. In infants with small defects, direct closure of the fascia is possible (Fig. 47–13). In infants with larger defects, the sac is dissected free and the abdominal wall is manually stretched. The umbilical vessels are ligated. Abnormalities of intestinal rotation and fixation are usually present, but intestinal atresia is distinctly uncommon. Reduction of the herniated liver should be performed with care to prevent kinking of the hepatic or portal veins.

Inadvertent injury to the hepatic capsule can result in life-threatening hemorrhage. Postoperative paralysis with mechanical ventilation is usually required after abdominal closure, although significant "abdominal wall softening" generally occurs after 24 hours.[51]

The standard surgical technique for closure of an omphalocele not amenable to a primary repair is staged closure using a Silastic silo as in the patient with gastroschisis. Manual reduction of the silo contents is performed at intervals in the neonatal ICU

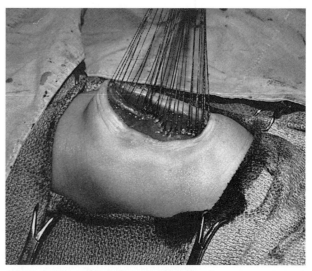

Figure 47–13. Primary fascial and skin closure is technically possible in most small and moderate-sized omphaloceles.

under sterile conditions. Failure to achieve abdominal closure within 2 weeks is associated with increased risk of infection and separation of the sac from the fascia.[33, 34, 52] Hepatic complications can also occur during reduction of large omphaloceles. A sudden increase in the level of liver enzymes may indicate acute vascular compromise of the liver. Doppler US can be used to evaluate hepatic arterial and venous flow, as well as portal flow.[53]

Once the viscera are reduced into the abdominal cavity, the infant is returned to the operating room for definitive closure. The fascia is closed with interrupted sutures, and the skin is approximated. Parenteral antibiotics are generally continued for several days after closure to prevent abdominal wall cellulitis. Prolonged ileus is not common, and enteral feeds can generally be started soon after definitive closure. Creation of an umbilicus may be desirable (see Fig. 47–7).

Infants born with a small or intermediate omphalocele have an excellent prognosis, as long as they do not have any other severe malformations. Mortality rate is considerably increased in infants with chromosomal syndromes and cardiac defects. Hospitalization averaged 51.7 days in one recent study, reflecting the importance of modern infant critical care in achieving survival in this challenging malformation.[54] The most common reason for reoperation in another series was for repair of a ventral hernia.[55] Gastroesophageal reflux is also seen with increased frequency in this patient group and may require antireflux surgery.[54]

☐ Pentalogy of Cantrell

Pentalogy of Cantrell is an unusual constellation of somatic and visceral defects of the lower thorax and upper abdomen. In this malformation, there is an upper abdominal omphalocele, a shortened or bifid lower sternum, a defect of the anterior diaphragm and parietal pericardium, and intracardiac lesions (Fig. 47–14). Lack of the anterior diaphragm results in partial herniation of the heart into the abdominal cavity. The syndrome likely occurs as the result of a failure of the lateral mesoderm to fully develop in the first weeks of embryonic development.[55] Chromosomal abnormalities, particularly trisomy 18, may also be present.[56] Survival of a child with this syndrome is uncommon owing to cardiac and respiratory compromise.

The diagnosis of pentalogy of Cantrell can be made by prenatal US. As early as the 18th week of development, the cardinal findings of ectopia cordis and omphalocele can be demonstrated.[56] In one series of fetuses in which this disorder was diagnosed prenatally, 40% were electively aborted. None of the remaining neonates survived more than 3 months postnatally.[57]

Infants who are born with this constellation of defects present a challenge to pediatric general surgeons and cardiac surgeons. The best results have

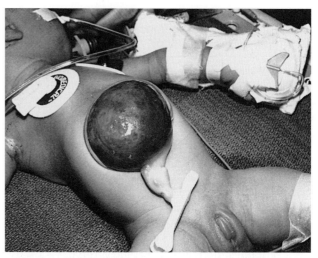

Figure 47–14. This neonate with a large epigastric omphalocele containing liver was found to have the usual additional somatic and visceral defects of pentalogy of Cantrell. Echocardiography is useful in identifying the associated cardiac anomalies.

occurred with a staged approach. Initial treatment is directed toward management of the omphalocele and possible repair of the diaphragmatic defect to separate the thoracic and abdominal cavities.[57, 58] Although primary closure of the omphalocele may be possible, often these defects are large and require either staged repair, skin flap coverage, or epithelialization of the omphalocele sac (see Fig. 47–11). Managing the intracardiac defects, which range from isolated ventricular septal defects to complex malformations including tetralogy of Fallot, is best addressed after coverage of the viscera has been achieved. The final surgical issue involves reconstruction of the chest wall to protect the heart.[58] Prosthetic materials or mobilization of native tissue can be used for this purpose.[58]

Overall, pentalogy of Cantrell is a congenital disorder associated with a high peripartum mortality rate. Those infants who do survive face multiple reconstructive procedures and prolonged hospitalization.

☐ The Vanderbilt Children's Hospital Experience

From 1988 to 1998, 101 babies with abdominal wall defects were treated at the Vanderbilt University Children's Hospital. Eighty of them had a diagnosis of gastroschisis; the remaining 21 had an omphalocele defect. There were 9 deaths in the entire group for an overall survival rate of 91%. The mortality rate in the omphalocele group was 19% (4 deaths). Two of the 4 babies who died were diagnosed with Beckwith-Wiedemann syndrome, and severe respiratory failure developed in all 4 babies. Five babies with gastroschisis died (6%). Two of them had complicated gastroschisis with either a perforation or atresia noted at the time of the origi-

TABLE 47-1. Anomalies Associated
with Omphalocele at the Vanderbilt
University Children's Hospital*

Beckwith-Wiedemann syndrome (3)	Cardiac defects:
Meckel's diverticulum (3)	Atrial septal defect
Bladder extrophy	Ventricular septal defect
Cloacal extrophy	Patent ductus
Cleft palate	Dextrocardia
	Tetralogy of Fallot
	Bicuspid aortic valve

*Associated anomalies identified in 21 patients admitted to Vanderbilt University Children's Hospital over a 10-year period.

nal repair. Seven other babies with complicated gastroschisis survived.

Most babies underwent primary repair: 73% of the gastroschisis group and 67% of those with an omphalocele. The average length of stay for those with a diagnosis of gastroschisis was 38.4 days. This was primarily the result of a prolonged ileus and dependence on parenteral nutrition. Respiratory failure was not a major problem, with babies intubated for an average of only 3.6 days. Babies with omphaloceles remained in the hospital for a longer period of time, averaging 52.6 days. The lengthy hospitalization of these babies was a result of their overall poor medical condition and respiratory failure. The average baby with an omphalocele remained on a ventilator for over 1 month.

Babies with omphaloceles also had numerous other congenital anomalies (Table 47-1). Seventy-one percent of infants with this diagnosis had at least one other defect, with a 24% incidence of cardiac anomalies. Only 9% of infants with gastroschisis had an associated defect, and no baby with gastroschisis had a major cardiac anomaly.

REFERENCES

1. Gross RE: A new method for surgical treatment of large omphaloceles. Surgery 24:277–292, 1948.
2. Schuster SR: A new method for the staged repair of large omphaloceles. Surg Gynecol Obstet 125:837–850, 1967.
3. Allen RG, Wrenn Jr EL: Silon as a sac in the treatment of omphalocele and gastroschisis. J Pediatr Surg 4:3–8, 1969.
4. Tibboel D, Vermey-Keers C, Kluck P, et al: The natural history of gastroschisis during fetal life: Development of the fibrous coating on the bowel loops. Teratology 33:267–272, 1986.
5. Hoyme HE, Higginbottom MC, Jones KL: The vascular pathogenesis of gastroschisis: Intrauterine interruption of the omphalomesenteric artery. Pediatrics 98:228–231, 1981.
6. Hoyme HE, Jones MC, Jones KL: Gastroschisis: Abdominal wall disruption secondary to early gestational interruption of the omphalomesenteric artery. Semin Perinatol 7:294–298, 1983.
7. Shaw A: The myth of gastroschisis. J Pediatr Surg 10:235–244, 1975.
8. DeVries PA: The pathogenesis of gastroschisis and omphalocele. J Pediatr Surg 15:245–251, 1980.
9. Torfs CP, Velie EM, Oechsli FW, et al: A population-based study of gastroschisis: Demographic, pregnancy, and lifestyle risk factors. Teratology 50:44–53, 1994.
10. Torfs CP, Katz EA, Bateson TF, et al: Maternal medications and environmental exposures as risk factors for gastroschisis. Teratology 54:84–92, 1996.
11. Werler MM, Michell AA, Shapiro S: First trimester maternal medication use in relation to gastroschisis. Teratology 45:361–367, 1992.
12. Calzolari E, Bianchi F, Dolk H, et al: Omphalocele and gastroschisis in Europe: A survey of 3 million births 1980–1990. Am J Med Genet 58:187–194, 1995.
13. Reddy VN, Aughton DJ, DeWitte DB, et al: Down syndrome and omphalocele: An underrecognized association. Pediatrics 93:514–515, 1994.
14. Benacerraf BR, Saltzman DH, Estroff JA, et al: Abnormal karyotype of fetuses with omphalocele: Prediction based on omphalocele contents. Obstet Gynecol 75:317–319, 1990.
15. Hughes MD, Nyberg DA, Mack LA, et al: Fetal omphalocele: Prenatal US detection of concurrent anomalies and other predictors of outcome. Radiology 173:371–376, 1989.
16. Calzolari E, Volpato S, Binachi F, et al: Omphalocele and gastroschisis: A collaborative study of five Italian congenital malformation registries. Teratology 47:47–55, 1993.
17. Saller DN, Canick JA, Palomaki GE, et al: Second-trimester maternal serum alpha-fetoprotein, unconjugated estriol, and hCG levels in pregnancies with ventral wall defects. Obstet Gynecol 84:852–855, 1994.
18. Paidas MJ, Crombleholme TM, Robertson FM: Prenatal diagnosis and management of the fetus with an abdominal wall defect. Semin Perinatol 18:196–214, 1994.
19. Chescheir NC, Azizkhan RG, Seeds JW, et al: Counseling and care for the pregnancy complicated by gastroschisis. Am J Perinat 8:323–329, 1991.
20. Meizner I: Prenatal diagnosis of anterior abdominal wall defects. Eur J Obstet Gynecol Reprod Biol 22:217–224, 1986.
21. Bagley JS, Lloyd DJ, Gray ES, et al: Small bowel injury in gastroschisis: Relation to fetal presentation. Br J Obstet Gynaecol 103:1047–1048, 1996.
22. Sakala EP, Erhard LN, White JJ: Elective cesarean section improves outcomes with gastroschisis. Am J Obstet Gynecol 169:1050–1053, 1993.
23. Bethel CAI, Seashore JH, Touloukian RJ. Cesarean section does not improve outcome in gastroschisis. J Pediatr Surg 24:1–4, 1989.
24. Lewis DF, Towers CV, Garite TJ, et al: Fetal gastroschisis and omphalocele: Is cesarean section the best mode of delivery? Am J Obstet Gynecol 163;773–775, 1990.
25. Simmons M, Georgeson KE: The effect of gestational age at birth on morbidity in patients with gastroschisis. J Pediatr Surg 31:1060–1062, 1996.
26. Sipes SL, Weiner CP, Sipes II DR, et al: Gastroschisis and omphalocele: Does either antenatal diagnosis or route of delivery make a difference in perinatal outcome? Obstet Gynecol 76:195–199, 1990.
27. Quirk Jr JG, Fortney J, Collin II HB, et al: Outcomes of newborns with gastroschisis: The effect of mode of delivery, site of delivery, and interval from birth to surgery. Am J Obstet Gynecol 174:1134–1140, 1996.
28. Lenke RR, Hatch EI Jr: Fetal gastroschisis: A preliminary report advocating the use of cesarean section. Obstet Gynecol 67:395–398, 1986.
29. Babcook CJ, Hedrick MH, Goldstein RB, et al: Gastroschisis: Can sonography of the fetal bowel accurately predict postnatal outcome? J Ultrasound Med 13:701–706, 1994.
30. Pryde PG, Bardicef M, Treadwell MC, et al: Gastroschisis: Can antenatal ultrasound predict infant outcomes? Obstet Gynecol 84:505–510, 1994.
31. Fonkalsrud EW, Smith MD, Shaw KS, et al: Selective management of gastroschisis according to the degree of visceroabdominal disproportion. Ann Surg 218:742–747, 1993.
32. Vane DW, Afajian JC, Hong AR: Spinal anesthesia for primary repair of gastroschisis: A new and safe technique for selected patients. J Pediatr Surg 29:1234–1235, 1994.
33. Ein SH, Rubin SZ: Gastroschisis: Primary closure or Silon pouch? J Pediatr Surg 15:549–552, 1980.
34. Swartz KR, Harrison MW, Campbell TJ, et al: Selective management of gastroschisis. Ann Surg 203:214–218, 1985.
35. Harmon PK, Kron IL, McLachlan HD, et al: Elevated intraabdominal pressure and renal failure. Ann Surg 196:594–597, 1982.

36. Richards WO, Scovill W, Shin B, et al: Acute renal failure associated with increased intra-abdominal pressure. Ann Surg 197:183–187, 1983.

37. Yaster M, Buck JR, Dudgeon DL, et al: Hemodynamic effects of primary closure of omphalocele/gastroschisis in human newborns. Anesthesiology 69:84–88, 1988.

38. Wesley JR, Drongowski R, Coran AG: Intragastric pressure measurement: A guide for reduction and closure of the Silastic chimney in omphalocele and gastroschisis. J Pediatr Surg 16:264–270, 1981.

39. Yaster M, Scherer TLR, Stone MM, et al: Prediction of successful primary closure of congenital abdominal wall defects using intraoperative measurements. J Pediatr Surg 24:1217–1220, 1989.

40. Lacey SR, Carris LA, Beyer III AJ, et al: Bladder pressure monitoring significantly enhances care of infants with abdominal wall defects: A prospective clinical study. J Pediatr Surg 28:1370–1375, 1993.

41. Rizzo A, Davis PC, Hamm CR, et al: Intraoperative vesical pressure measurements as a guide in the closure of abdominal wall defects. Am Surg 62:192–196, 1996.

42. Puffinbarger NK, Taylor DV, Tuggle DW, et al: End-tidal carbon dioxide for monitoring primary closure of gastroschisis. J Pediatr Surg 31:280–282, 1996.

43. Wesson DE, Baesl TJ: Repair of gastroschisis with preservation of the umbilicus. J Pediatr Surg 21:764–765, 1986.

44. Pokorny WJ, Harberg FJ, McGill CW. Gastroschisis complicated by intestinal atresia. J Pediatr Surg 16:261–263, 1981.

45. Shah R, Wooley MM: Gastroschisis and intestinal atresia. J Pediatr Surg 26:788–790, 1991.

46. Ramsden WH, Arthur RJ, Martinez D: Gastroschisis: A radiological and clinical review. Pediatr Radiol 27:166–169, 1997.

47. Oldham KT, Coran AG, Drongowski RA, et al: The development of necrotizing enterocolitis following repair of gastroschisis: A surprisingly high incidence. J Pediatr Surg 23:945–949, 1988.

48. Nuchtern JG, Baxter R, Hatch EI Jr: Nonoperative initial management versus Silon chimney for treatment of giant omphalocele. J Pediatr Surg 30:771–776, 1995.

49. DeLuca FG, Gilchrist BF, Paquette E, et al: External compression as initial management of giant omphalocele. J Pediatr Surg 31:965–967, 1996.

50. Yazbeck S: The giant omphalocele: A new approach for a rapid and complete closure. J Pediatr Surg 21:715–717, 1986.

51. Canty TG, Collins DL: Primary fascial closure in infants with gastroschisis and omphalocele: A superior approach. J Pediatr Surg 18:707–712, 1983.

52. Schwartz MZ, Tyson KR, Milliorn K, et al: Staged reduction using a Silastic sac is the treatment of choice for large congenital abdominal wall defects. J Pediatr Surg 18:713–719, 1983.

53. Skarsgard ED, Barth RA: Use of Doppler ultrasonography in the evaluation of liver blood flow during silo reduction of a giant omphalocele. J Pediatr Surg 32:733–735, 1997.

54. Dunn JCY, Fonkalsrud EW: Improved survival of infants with omphalocele. Am J Surg 173:284–287, 1997.

55. Tunnell WP, Puffinbarger NK, Tuggle DW: Abdominal wall defects in infants: Survival and implications for adult life. Ann Surg 221:525–530, 1995.

56. Cantrell JR, Haller JA, Ravitch MM: A syndrome of congenital defects involving the abdominal wall, sternum, diaphragm, pericardium, and heart. Surg Gynecol Obstet 107:602–614, 1958.

57. Ghidini A, Sirtori M, Romero R, et al: Prenatal diagnosis of pentalogy of Cantrell. J Ultrasound Med 7:567–572, 1988.

58. Abdallah HI, Marks LA, Balsara RK, et al: Staged repair of pentalogy of Cantrell with tetralogy of Fallot. Ann Thorac Surg 56:979–980, 1993.

59. Zona JZ: The surgical approach for reconstruction of the sternal and epigastric defects in children with Cantrell's deformity. J Pediatr Surg 26:702–706, 1991.

48

UMBILICAL AND OTHER ABDOMINAL WALL HERNIAS

Victor F. Garcia, MD

Abdominal wall hernias are among the most common surgical conditions found in infants and children. The clinical significance of these hernias varies from a considerable risk of strangulation to the need only to reassure a concerned parent. It is essential that the physician caring for children with abdominal wall hernias understands which of these defects need timely surgery and which simply need time. A knowledge of the natural history, anatomy, indications for operation, and timing of operative repair is essential to optimally manage abdominal wall hernias.

□ Umbilical Hernia

ETIOLOGY AND EMBRYOLOGY

The anterior wall of the embryo develops from the somatopleure of the overhanging hand and tail folds.[1] Simultaneous closure of these folds from the cranial, caudal, and lateral directions forms the umbilical ring. The ring closes by contracture after the cord is ligated and the umbilical vessels thrombose.

The development of an umbilical hernia has an embryologic as well as an anatomic basis.[2] Embryologically, failure of the recti to approximate in the midline after the return of the midgut predisposes the fetus to developing an umbilical hernia.[1] Anatomically, the umbilical ring consists of the umbilical scar, the round ligament, and the umbilical fascia. Usually, the round ligament passes over the superior margin of the umbilical ring and attaches to the inferior margin of the ring.[1] When the round ligament attaches only to the superior margin of the ring, the floor of the umbilical ring is formed only by the umbilical fascia and the peritoneum. This attenuated floor predisposes the fetus to developing an umbilical hernia.[1, 2]

INCIDENCE

Umbilical hernia is one of the most common conditions seen in infancy and childhood. The true incidence is unknown because many umbilical hernias resolve spontaneously.[3] Race and prematurity are predisposing factors. Umbilical hernias are up to 10 times more common in African Americans than in Caucasians.[4, 5] In South Africa, the racial disparity is not as marked, with umbilical hernias found in 23% of blacks compared with 19% of whites.[6] Umbilical hernias are more common in premature than full-term infants and are noted in 75 to 84% of infants weighing less than 1500 g.[4, 7, 8]

Although most umbilical hernias are isolated findings in otherwise healthy infants, a number of clinical disorders are associated with umbilical hernias, including trisomy 21, congenital hypothyroidism, mucopolysaccharidosis, and exomphalos-macroglossia-gigantism.[3]

NATURAL HISTORY

Most umbilical hernias are recognized shortly after birth. Related symptoms are rare. In some instances, the combination of a large fascial defect, redundant umbilical skin, and a straining infant results in a tense proboscis. The concerned parent should be advised that evisceration is unlikely, and continued observation is safe.

There are few definitive studies documenting the natural history of umbilical hernias.[6, 9] The general belief is that the majority regress with time. One study suggests the incidence decreases with age and complete resolution occurs by age 13.[6]

In general, the diameter and the sharpness of the fascial edge are predictors of spontaneous closure.[9, 10] Hernias with a diameter greater than 1.5 to 2.0 cm are less likely to close on their own.[3, 9] The thicker and more rounded the fascial edge, the more likely the hernia will close. Openings with a thin, sharp edge tend not to close.[2, 10]

If the hernia persists as the child approaches school age (4 to 5 years of age), it should be repaired. Earlier repair is warranted if symptoms of incarceration or recurring pain develop.[3] Repair at age 2 to 3 years is advocated if the fascial defect is greater than 2.0 cm.[11] Some consideration should be given to repairing the hernia and reducing the grotesque proboscis of skin that is seen on some young girls.

If not repaired in childhood, 10% of umbilical hernias will persist to adulthood.[12] The defect may enlarge in women during pregnancy, and there is a greater risk of incarceration in adults than in children.[3]

The risk of incarceration or strangulation of an umbilical hernia is considered rare.[6] Two studies from the 1990s, however, suggest that incarceration occurs more frequently than is generally believed.[13, 14]

OPERATIVE TECHNIQUE

Operative repair is done as an outpatient procedure under general anesthesia. The operative technique is illustrated in Figure 48–1. The redundant skin following closure of a proboscoid hernia can be managed using a pursestring stitch,[15] a V-Y plasty,[16] or an umbilicoplasty.[17]

A paraumbilical block[18] or a preincisional caudal epidural block can be used in addition to local infiltration to minimize postoperative pain.

Parents are encouraged to administer oral analgesics early in the postoperative period, before the effects of regional or local anesthesia have disappeared.

A tonsil sponge may be placed then secured with tape to compress the loose umbilical skin. There are no activity restrictions. The dressing is removed in 5 to 7 days. Complications are uncommon.

□ Epigastric Hernia

ETIOLOGY

Epigastric hernias result from defects in the interstices of the decussating fibers of the linea alba.[10] The etiology of epigastric hernias is unknown. The defects may be multiple, and they are typically elliptical with a transverse long axis. Usually, only preperitoneal fat herniates through the defect.

INCIDENCE

Epigastric hernias are seen in about 5% of children. Children present either with a visible palpable mass or with intermittent pain localized to the site of the hernia. When present, the mass is at times tender and is usually no larger than 0.5 to 1 cm. Occasionally, a defect is noted, and no mass is palpated.

The small size of the mass and the defect makes identification problematic once the child is anesthetized. Therefore, when the child is awake, the exact location of the hernia, usually in relationship to a distinct part of the umbilicus, should be noted.

Epigastric hernias do not spontaneously resolve

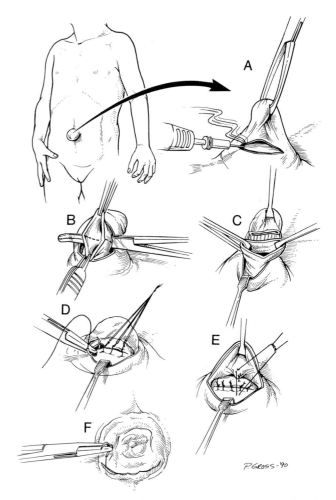

Figure 48–1. Technique of operative repair for umbilical hernia. *A,* An infraumbilical skin crease incision is made. *B,* The hernia sac is opened, leaving a portion of the sac attached to the umbilical skin for ease of subsequent umbilicoplasty. *C,* The umbilical sac has been completely divided and excised to strong fascia. *D,* The fascial defect is closed in a transverse fashion with interrupted, simple nonabsorbable sutures. *E,* The remaining umbilical sac, which is attached to the umbilical skin, is secured to the fascia with interrupted, absorbable sutures. *F,* The skin incision is closed with a subcuticular suture. Pressure dressing is placed to prevent formation of a hematoma or seroma.

and, therefore, should be repaired. A limited transverse incision is made over the defect. If herniated fat is present, it is either reduced or ligated, then excised. The defect is then closed with absorbable sutures using buried knots. The skin is closed with an absorbable subcuticular suture.

The procedure is performed on an outpatient basis. There are no postoperative limitations in activities, and complications are rare.

□ Lumbar Hernia

Lumbar hernias are rare in children. They can occur in otherwise normal babies but may be associated with lumbocostovertebral deficiency syndrome.[2] They occur through one of two areas of potential weakness: the superior or the inferior lumbar area.[19, 20]

Most congenital lumbar hernias occur in the superior lumbar triangle. This triangle is covered by the latissimus dorsi muscle and is bordered by the 12th rib, the internal oblique muscle, and the sacrospinalis muscle. Penetration of the 12th intercostal nerve and vessels in the lumbodorsal fascia in this area can cause a defect leading to the development of a hernia. The defect is usually small but eventually enlarges and may become symptomatic.

The boundaries of the inferior lumbar triangle are the latissimus dorsi posteriorly, the external oblique muscle anteriorly, and the iliac crest inferiorly.[17, 20] The defect occurs at the site of penetration of the iliohypogastric, ilioinguinal, or lumbar nerves.

A lumbar hernia presents as a bulge, usually of retroperitoneal fat. Incarceration or strangulation is rare.[2, 19, 20] Palpation may reveal a soft swelling that is easily reducible.

If the defect is not palpable, ultrasonography (US) or computed tomography (CT) may be necessary to identify the exact location of the hernia defect.

Closure of the fascial defect should be done without tension. Rarely, prosthetic material may be necessary to permit a tension-free closure of the defect.

☐ Spigelian Hernia

Spigelian hernias develop at the intersection of the linea semilunaris; the lateral border of the rectus abdominis muscle; and the linea semicircularis, the caudal termination of the posterior sheath of the rectus muscles.

The defect usually involves the transversus abdominis and internal oblique muscles but not the external oblique muscles. The spigelian hernia is, therefore, interparietal and may be difficult to diagnose.[20, 21] Spigelian hernias are more common in girls and more likely to occur on the right side than the left.[2] Examination may reveal a tender mass, usually below the umbilicus.

Although the hernia sac may be large, the defect is usually small. Pain is common, at first intermittent but often progressing to a constant, dull discomfort. Twenty percent of spigelian hernias present with strangulation.[2, 21] Diagnosis may be aided by having the cooperative child tense his or her abdominal muscles, reproducing a specific point of tenderness.

US and CT scans may identify the fascial defect within the layers of the abdominal wall. If the defect is not palpable but is noted on CT scan or US, it is advisable to mark the site of the defect using radiologic guidance.

The high risk of incarceration or strangulation makes operative repair the treatment of choice. A transverse incision is made over the mass or site of the defect as identified by US or CT scan. Once the external oblique is incised, the sac is encountered. This is dissected out and the fascial defect closed. Recurrence rate is low.

REFERENCES

1. Skandalakis JE, Gray SW, Ricketts R: The anterior abdominal wall. In Skandalakis JE, Gray SW (eds): Embryology for Surgeons (2nd ed). Baltimore, Williams & Wilkins, 1994, p 540.
2. Zinner MJ, Schwartz SI: Hernias. In Ellis H (ed): Maingot. Abdominal Operations (10th ed). Norwalk, CT, Appleton & Lange, 1997.
3. Scherer LR III, Grosfeld JL: Inguinal hernia and umbilical anomalies. Pediatr Clin North Am 40:1121, 1993.
4. Crump EP: Umbilical hernia: Occurrence of the infantile type in negro infants and children. J Pediatr 40:214, 1952.
5. Evans A: The comparative incidence of umbilical hernias in colored and white infants. J Natl Med Assoc 33:158, 1941.
6. Blumberg NA: Infantile umbilical hernia. Surg Gynecol Obstet 150:187, 1980.
7. Woods GE: Some observations on umbilical hernia in infants. Arch Dis Child 8:450, 1953.
8. Vohr BR, Rosenfield AG, Oh W: Umbilical hernia in the low-birthweight infant (less than 1500 grams). J Pediatr Surg 90:807, 1977.
9. Walker SH: The natural history of umbilical hernia. Clin Pediatr 6:29, 1967.
10. Abramson J: Epigastric, umbilical, and ventral hernia. In Cameron JL (ed): Current Surgical Therapy—3. Philadelphia, BC Decker, 1989, p 417.
11. Morgan WW, White J, Stumbough S: Prophylactic umbilical hernia repair in childhood to prevent adult incarceration. Surg Clin North Am 50:839, 1970.
12. Jackson DJ, Moglen LH: Umbilical hernia: A retrospective study. Calif Med 113:8, 1970.
13. Mawera G, Mugut GI: Umbilical hernia in Bulawayo: Some observations from a hospital-based study. Cent Afr J Med 40:319, 1994.
14. Vrsansky P, Bourdelat D: Incarcerated umbilical hernia in children. Pediatr Surg Int 12:61, 1997.
15. Cone JB, Golladay ES: Purse string closure of umbilical hernia repair. J Pediatr Surg 18:297, 1983.
16. Jamara F: Reconstruction of umbilicus by a double V-Y procedure. Plast Reconstr Surg 64:106, 1979.
17. Renya TM, Harris WH Jr, Smith SB: Surgical management of proboscoid herniae. J Pediatr Surg 22:911, 1987.
18. Courreges P, Poddevin F, Lecoutre D: Paraumbilical block: A new concept for regional anesthesia in children. Paediatr Anaesth 7:211, 1997.
19. Mehta MH, Patel RV, Mehta SG: Congenital lumbar hernia. J Pediatr Surg 27:1258, 1992.
20. Devaney K: Lumbar, obturator and spigelian hernia. In Cameron JL (ed): Current Surgical Therapy—3. Philadelphia, BC Decker, 1989, p 432.
21. Spangen L: Spigelian hernia. Surg Clin North Am 64:351, 1984.

49

GROIN HERNIAS AND HYDROCELES

Thomas R. Weber, MD • Thomas F. Tracy, Jr., MD

Hernias and hydroceles of the inguinal and scrotal regions are among the most common congenital disorders that pediatricians and pediatric surgeons manage. Affecting both male and female patients, hernias can be life-threatening or can result in the loss of a testis or an ovary or a portion of the bowel, if incarceration and strangulation occur. For these complications to be avoided, timely diagnosis and operative therapy are thus important. This chapter discusses the diagnostic methods for hernia and hydrocele detection in infants and children, the operative approaches, and the complications associated with this common pediatric surgical procedure.

☐ Embryology and Anatomy

The processus vaginalis, which gives rise to the usual pediatric indirect inguinal hernia, is present in the developing fetus at 12 weeks in utero. The processus is a peritoneal diverticulum that extends through the internal inguinal ring. As the testis descends in the 7th to 8th month of gestation, a portion of the processus attaches to the testis as it exits the abdomen and is dragged into the scrotum with the testis (Fig. 49–1).

The portion of peritoneum (processus) enveloping the testis becomes the tunica vaginalis. The remainder of the processus within the inguinal canal eventually obliterates, eliminating the communication between the scrotum and the peritoneal cavity. The exact time at which obliteration occurs is somewhat controversial. In a significant number of individuals, perhaps as many as 20%, the processus vaginalis remains asymptomatically patent throughout life.[1]

Because the testicular vessels and vas deferens are retroperitoneal structures, they exit the internal ring behind the processus; therefore, a hernia sac formed from the processus vaginalis lies anterior and slightly medial to the spermatic cord structures. The sac itself can be extremely thin or thick-walled, depending on the age of the patient, the amount of time the hernia has been symptomatic, and whether incarceration has occurred. In some cases, the hernia sac can be so thin that the testicular vessels and vas deferens appear to exit the internal ring inside the sac rather than behind it, but embryologically this is an impossibility. A diligent search always discloses a thin membrane of sac adherent anteriorly to the spermatic cord.

A patent processus is only a potential hernia and becomes an actual hernia only when bowel or other intraabdominal contents exit the peritoneal cavity into it. If only fluid leaves the peritoneal cavity, the defect is termed a *communicating hydrocele*, with a typical history of enlargement during activities that increase intraabdominal pressure (e.g., crying, straining) and shrinkage during sleep and other pe-

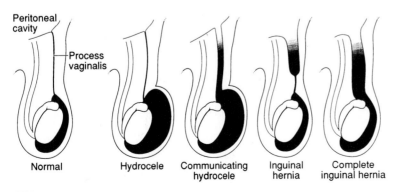

Figure 49–1. From left, configurations of hydrocele and hernia in relationship to patency of the processus vaginalis.

riods of relaxation. Because this pattern indicates a definite patent processus, most surgeons regard a communicating hydrocele as a hernia and proceed to repair.

□ Incidence

INDIRECT INGUINAL HERNIA

The incidence of *indirect inguinal hernia* in the general population of infants and children is generally unknown, because there are variations in prematurity, associated disease, and access to medical care. In carefully controlled population studies, however, the incidence approximates 1 to 5%.[2] In most series, male children with hernias outnumber female children by an 8:1 to 10:1 ratio. These figures depend on associated diseases and other factors.

Premature infants have a greatly increased risk for developing inguinal hernias. Reported incidences of 7, 17, and 30% in males and 2% in females with prematurity and low birth weight emphasize the higher risk of hernia that exists for these infants.[3–5] Associated disorders of prematurity, such as ventilator dependency, sepsis, and necrotizing enterocolitis are not associated with a greater hernia incidence.[4] This high risk of inguinal hernia, with risk of incarceration that exceeds 60% during the first 6 months of life, leads most neonatologists and pediatric surgeons to recommend repair of hernia before the infant's discharge from the hospital.[3]

ASSOCIATED DISEASES AND DISORDERS

Additional associated diseases have been found to increase both the incidence of hernia and the risk of recurrence after repair. Patients with cystic fibrosis have up to a 15% incidence of inguinal hernia. This figure is approximately eight times that of the normal population.[6] Increased intraabdominal pressure in patients with cystic fibrosis that results from chronic coughing, respiratory infection, or obstructive airway disease does not fully explain this increase, because siblings and fathers of children with cystic fibrosis are also at a greater risk for development of hernia, although to a lesser degree.[6] These greater risks are thought to be related to an altered embryogenesis of the wolffian duct structures that also leads to an absent vas deferens in male patients with cystic fibrosis.

Infants with disorders of connective tissue formation (Ehlers-Danlos syndrome) and mucopolysaccharidosis (Hunter-Hurler syndrome) are also at a higher risk for developing inguinal hernia.[7, 8] In addition, the risk of recurrence with these associated diseases exceeds 50%. A number of investigators have emphasized that recurrence of hernia in these children may be the first sign of connective tissue disease.

Children with congenital dislocation of the hip, children receiving chronic peritoneal dialysis, pre-term infants with intraventricular hemorrhage, and children with myelomeningocele who require ventriculoperitoneal shunts are also patients noted to have hernia at a frequency greater than that in the general population.[9–11]

DIRECT AND FEMORAL HERNIAS

Direct and *femoral hernias* in children are rare and constitute a small percentage of hernia defects in most series. Rarely is the diagnosis made preoperatively. In adults, direct and femoral hernias are generally believed to be acquired defects, but their origin in children remains controversial. Up to one third of children in whom direct or femoral hernias develop have had a previous indirect inguinal repair.[12] Patients with increased intraabdominal pressure and connective tissue disorders are probably at risk for these types of hernias as well.

BILATERAL HERNIA

The incidence of bilaterality of hernia in the pediatric age group has been a controversial subject for many years. This subject is important to examine for two reasons. First, a presumption exists that a negative contralateral exploration is "unnecessary surgery" and therefore should be avoided at all costs. This decision must be weighed against the risk and inconvenience of subjecting a child to a second anesthetic if contralateral hernia develops later. (An additional consideration in this regard includes the perception that the surgeon "missed" the other hernia.) Second, technical mishaps, particularly injury to the vas and vessels, can occur during contralateral exploration, just as they can occur during herniorrhaphy on the primary side. Risking such an injury for a negative exploration is questionable. However, leaving a potential hernia on the contralateral side may result in later incarceration, which carries a risk to the testis itself and strangulation and may necessitate a much larger operation that may involve bowel resection.

Numerous studies have appeared in the literature over the past 30 to 40 years regarding the incidence of bilateral hernia in children, the advisability of bilateral exploration, the incidence of later development of hernia if contralateral exploration is not performed, and the practice of most pediatric surgeons regarding these issues. Several early excellent reviews attempted to tabulate these data into workable summaries.[13–15]

The true incidence of bilateral hernia seems to depend primarily on the definition of exactly what constitutes a hernia or potential hernia. A patent processus vaginalis represents an opening from the peritoneal cavity into the inguinal canal or scrotum, but the actual potential for this structure to develop into a hernia is unknown. A contralateral patent processus vaginalis is present in 50 to 90% of cases in several operative series.[15, 16] In contrast, by using pneumoperitonography at the time of herniorrhaphy, an incidence of contralateral patency was found in 22 to 29% of cases.[17] However, additional follow-up series demonstrated only a 20% incidence of developing later hernia if the contralateral side is not explored, suggesting that clinical hernia does not subsequently develop in all patients with a patent processus.[1]

The age at presentation of the primary hernia influences the incidence of contralateral patent processus and also the incidence of subsequent contralateral hernia.[16a] The highest reported incidence of contralateral patent processus occurs in infants younger than 2 months of age (63%).[16] The incidence decreases to 41% for children aged 2 to 16 years. The high incidence of patient processus in infants corresponds to the common presentation of bilateral inguinal hernias (34%) in patients younger than 6 months old.[16a] Early data established the incidence of metachronous contralateral hernias as high as 40 to 50% for infants undergoing repair.[18, 19] More recent studies have been able to identify a much lower incidence for the development of a contralateral hernia.[16a, 19a, 19b] Overall, in one report of 548 infants and children, 8.8% developed a metachronous contralateral hernia at a median interval of 6 months (range, 4 days–7 years). The stratified incidence was found to be 12.4% in infants younger than 6 months and 10.6% in children younger than 2 years old. In other groups, analysis of the incidence of metachronous contralateral hernia was 14.8% in premature infants, 7.4% in all girls, and 27.6% in children who present with an incarcerated hernia.[16a]

Other factors that have been implicated in affecting the incidence of bilaterality of hernia in children include the gender of the patient, the side (right or left) of the primary hernia, and the presence of associated disorders or increased abdominal pressure or fluid. The incidence of bilateral hernia seems to be greater in female patients in all age groups, with reported values of 20 to 50%.[16a] This fact, combined with the observation that the injury to reproductive organs during herniorrhaphy in the female patient is probably extremely low, prompts some surgeons to advocate bilateral exploration in virtually all female patients. This practice, however, prevents a contralateral hernia in only 7% of girls.

The side of the primary hernia has been analyzed in a number of series to determine the incidence of bilateral hernia. Although a number of reports have shown a slightly higher incidence of contralateral hernia if the primary hernia is left-sided, it seems an equal number of reports have shown no significant difference in this regard. Most pediatric surgeons proceed with contralateral exploration based on other factors, such as age. Patients with associated conditions, such as ventriculoperitoneal shunts, ascites, connective tissue disorders, and cystic fibrosis, have a high enough incidence of bilaterality and the risk of subsequent anesthesia is sufficiently great to justify routine bilateral exploration.

The use of the laparoscope at the time of herniorrhaphy to assess the contralateral side is a recent innovation and has added some information regarding the incidence of bilaterality. Several series have reported that the operative approach is changed in 30 to 50% of cases (no contralateral hernia found by laparoscope) when a small scope is inserted through the hernia sac on the primary side and the contralateral internal ring is inspected.[21, 22] In addition, little difference in contralateral incidence was found with regard to patient age, gender, and associated conditions. These data are somewhat preliminary, in that the use of the laparoscope in this setting is not widespread and the reported series are small. Finally, there seems to be no reason to attempt hernia repair laparoscopically in the pediatric age group.

Based on the aforementioned data, the following recommendations regarding bilateral exploration can be made. Routine bilateral exploration is best reserved for infants and children with associated disorders, and for all patients with definite or strongly suspected bilateral clinical hernia. The risks and benefits of contralateral exploration should be proposed for higher risk groups of patients such as those with incarcerated hernias, those with a history of prematurity, or those with underlying risks of general anesthesia. Individual parents and surgeons have to balance the variation between recent data and previously reported studies to justify the need for exploration based on the potentially small difference in the overall rate of metachronous hernias. With these criteria, we believe we avoid a large number of "unnecessary" bilateral explorations and the accompanying risks of technical mishap, while ensuring that the incidence of later development of contralateral hernia is low.

HYDROCELE

Similar to hernia, the incidence of hydrocele among male infants is largely unknown. Noncommunicating hydrocele, unassociated with a patent processus vaginalis and therefore not a potential hernia, is common in male newborns and is self-limiting, usually resolving within 6 to 12 months. The persistence of hydrocele beyond 12 months of age brings on the suspicion of a communication with the abdominal cavity through a patent processus and should be regarded as a hernia. The incidence of isolated (noncommunicating) hydrocele in children older than 1 year of age is probably less than 1%.

☐ Clinical Presentation

INDIRECT INGUINAL HERNIA

The hallmark of an *indirect inguinal hernia* in a child is a groin bulge, extending toward the top of the scrotum, which is visible most frequently during periods of increased abdominal pressure (e.g., crying, laughing, straining). The hernia usually spontaneously reduces with relaxation, or it can be gently reduced manually with upward, posterior pressure directly on the mass. Caudal traction on the testicle occasionally aids in the reduction. The usual history obtained from the parents is one of recurrent groin swelling that spontaneously reduces but that is gradually enlarging or is more persistent and is becoming more difficult to reduce. Occasionally, the initial clinical presentation is one of the abrupt appearance of the hernia with incarceration. In many cases, careful questioning of the family reveals a history consistent with either a groin bulge or a communicating hydrocele.

Frequently, a patient is referred after the pediatrician or the family has seen the typical hernia bulge, but the surgeon is unable to demonstrate a definite hernia, even when such maneuvers as induced crying and laughing are used. In these cases, a reliable history, combined with palpation of a thickened cord as it crosses the pelvic tubercle or the palpable sensation of a large patent processus known as "silk glove sign," is sufficient evidence to proceed with herniorrhaphy. An alternative approach includes asking the parents to return with the child for examination when a definite bulge appears. This has been rarely successful in our experience and risks incarceration and its attendant hazards. Experienced surgeons can diagnose pediatric hernias with a high degree of accuracy by history and groin palpation. Herniograms were once proposed to aid in the diagnosis of hernia, but concerns regarding cost, complications, and gonad radiation limited enthusiasm for this technique.[23] Ultrasound of the inguinal canal and scrotum are noninvasive and often diagnostic after difficult or inconclusive examinations.

DIRECT INGUINAL HERNIA

Direct inguinal hernias in children are rare. The clinical presentation is somewhat different from that of indirect hernias. Direct hernias appear as groin masses that extend toward the femoral vessels with exertion or straining. In one third of cases, a previous indirect hernia repair on the side of the direct hernia was performed, suggesting that injury to the floor of the inguinal canal occurred during the first herniorrhaphy. Because the defect arises through the floor of the inguinal canal, medial to the epigastric vessels, the repair consists of strengthening the floor by suturing transversalis fascia or conjoined tendon to Cooper's ligament, much the same as the approach in the adult. Recurrence after such a repair in the child, in contrast to recurrence in the adult, is rare. Prosthetic material for direct hernia repair or other approaches, such as preperitoneal repair, are rarely required in the pediatric age group.

HYDROCELES

Hydroceles can be categorized into communicating and noncommunicating types. Communicating hydroceles, indicating communication with the peritoneal cavity, are hernias and should be treated as such. A typical history for this defect includes scrotal swelling that comes and goes depending on the level of activity and relaxation. Frequently, gentle pressure or squeezing reduces the hydrocele fluid from the scrotum into the peritoneal cavity, but typically the fluid abruptly reappears with increased intraabdominal pressure.

Noncommunicating hydroceles can be present at birth or can develop months or years later for no obvious reason. The usual history is one of stable size or very slow growth, without abrupt spontaneous disappearance or rapid change in size. Unless these hydroceles reach extremely large proportions, no management is indicated other than simple observation. The *abdominoscrotal hydrocele* is an unusual variant of hydrocele that requires aggressive therapy, however. A large hydrocele appears as a scrotal collection of fluid with a palpable pelvic mass on the side of the hydrocele. Frequently, pressure on the abdominal mass causes enlargement of the scrotal component.

Exactly how or why these hydroceles become so large is a matter of speculation. One explanation is that this abnormality arises as a scrotal hydrocele attached to a long processus vaginalis that is patent with the scrotum but is obliterated at the internal ring. As the processus continues to enlarge in a cephalad direction through the internal ring, a retroperitoneal component forms.[24] With continued fluid production within the hydrocele, the retroperitoneal portion enlarges proportionately greater than the scrotum, because of limited growth potential within the scrotum. Therapy of this condition consists of complete excision of all hydrocele sac components, which can usually be accomplished through a generous groin excision after evacuation of the sac. Identification of the spermatic cord in these operations can be difficult. As with all hernia procedures, the cord components must be kept in view during the dissection.

☐ Techniques of Repair

ANESTHESIA

Hernia and hydrocele operations in children usually involve outpatient (same day) surgical repair, if the child is not already hospitalized. Premature infants hospitalized at birth who are found to have hernias generally undergo repair before discharge. Nonhospitalized premature infants with hernias who are within 4 to 6 months of birth should be observed in the hospital for 24 hours after repair because of the risk of life-threatening apnea after general anesthesia (see Chapter 3). These infants, therefore, are not candidates for outpatient surgical procedures. Most term or near-term infants, however, are candidates for outpatient surgery, unless associated diseases necessitate hospitalization postoperatively.

The choice of anesthesia technique for each child should be discussed with the anesthesiologist involved, taking into account the general condition and gestational age of the infant and the experience of the staff. Most hernia repairs in children are performed using general inhalation anesthesia, which may or may not include endotracheal intubation. Local or spinal anesthesia techniques are reserved for infants with severe prematurity or associated disease that makes general anesthesia more risky. In experienced hands, spinal anesthesia can be successful in 80% of attempts in infants as small as 1500 g. In cases performed with general anesthesia, many surgeons and anesthesiologists use injections of long-acting local anesthesia within the wound edges and along the ilioinguinal nerve or in the epidural space to relieve postoperative pain.[25]

OPERATIVE TECHNIQUES

After routine sterile skin preparation and draping, a skin incision in the groin skin crease is made (Fig. 49–2). Crossing veins can be cauterized, tied, or pushed aside. Scarpa's fascia is grasped and incised with scissors, exposing the external oblique aponeurosis. Blunt dissection clears the fat from the external oblique, exposing the external inguinal ring. At this point, in both male and female patients, the hernia sac is usually seen bulging from the external ring, and the external oblique is incised. Occasionally, with extremely large or long-standing hernias, the external ring is stretched to the point where it overlaps the internal ring. Thus, opening the external oblique is unnecessary. This is especially true in female patients and premature infants. Small retractors are placed within Scarpa's fascia. The incision in the external oblique, made with either knife or scissors, can stop short of the external ring or can be made completely through the ring (Fig. 49–3). In either case, care must be taken not to injure the ilioinguinal nerve, which is usually closely adher-

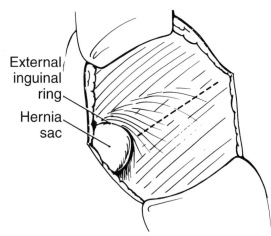

Figure 49–3. After incising and spreading Scarpa's fascia, the anterior surface of the external oblique aponeurosis is exposed. Frequently, the hernia sac can be seen bulging through the external ring. The external oblique fascia is opened in the direction of its fibers. The incision in the external oblique can be continued into the external ring or stopped before the ring fibers. Alternatively, in small infants, the external oblique can be left intact and the sac dissection can be accomplished through the external ring.

ent to the cremasteric muscle fibers, directly under the external oblique aponeurosis.

The hernia sac is found lying within the inguinal canal, anterior and slightly medial to the spermatic cord. Thus, it is usually safe to grasp the most anterior structures with a smooth forceps, delivering the sac and spermatic cord into the wound (Fig. 49–4). Careful dissection of the anterior cremasteric muscle fibers should allow the sac and attached spermatic cord to be elevated to skin level, preventing the need for dissection deep in the wound where injury to the cord structures can occur.

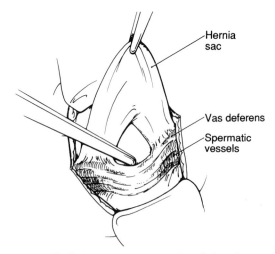

Figure 49–4. The hernia sac, anterior and medial to the spermatic cord, is grasped with a tissue forceps or hemostat and delivered into the wound. A second tissue forceps is used to dissect the cremasteric fibers away from the sac, exposing the spermatic cord. By grasping the loose tissue adjacent to the testicular artery and vein, these structures are pushed posteriorly to expose the vas deferens. The vas itself is not grasped but rather gently pushed away from the sac by a closed forceps or sponge. Care is taken to preserve the vas artery as well.

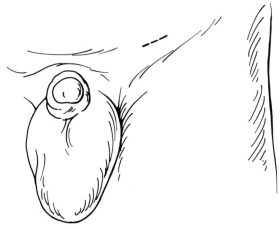

Figure 49–2. The incision *(dashed line)* for inguinal herniorrhaphy is made above the inguinal ligament in a natural skin fold.

Safe separation of the cord structures from the sac is a critical part of the herniorrhaphy. Because of the extremely small size of these structures in infants and children, many pediatric surgeons advocate intraoperative visual magnification for herniorrhaphy.

Because the spermatic vessels (artery and vein) emerge from the internal ring in the most lateral position, they are encountered first in the dissection. By carefully grasping the tissue next to the vessels, these structures are gently pushed posteriorly to free them from the sac, while the sac itself is held with another smooth forceps (see Fig. 49–4). As the vessels are dissected free, the new portions of sac that are exposed are grasped with smooth forceps, allowing the sac to rotate medially. This usually exposes the vas deferens tightly adherent to the sac. The vas itself is not grasped but rather the adjacent tissue is pushed posteriorly to free the vas from the sac. Great care and gentleness are required during the dissection to avoid injury to the vas, vas deferens artery, and spermatic vessels. In general, the testis is not delivered into the wound during this dissection, because the operative field is small and extra structures can obliterate the field and make the dissection considerably more difficult.

After the vas deferens and spermatic vessels are dissected completely away from the sac, a hemostat is passed beneath the sac and spread. The sac is doubly clamped and divided between the hemostats, only after ensuring that the vas and vessels are completely separated (Fig. 49–5). The sac is not divided if intraabdominal structures (bowel, ovary, omentum) are contained within. In these cases, the sac is opened anteriorly, with a hemostat remaining posteriorly, and the viability of the sac contents is assessed. If the sac contents are viable, reduction of these structures into the abdomen is performed with blunt forceps.

If there is incarceration with apparent nonviable

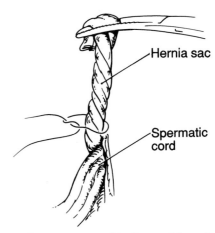

Figure 49–6. The spermatic cord is dissected from the sac to the level of the internal ring. The sac is twisted to narrow its base, as well as to reduce intraabdominal contents that may have reappeared at the inside of the internal ring. The sac is ligated with one or two transfixion sutures of nonabsorbable material.

bowel, a separate abdominal incision is usually used to aid in reduction and to fully evaluate the extent of bowel infarction. Frequently, bowel that appears nonviable in a strangulated position within a sac quickly regains evidence of viability after intraabdominal reduction. If it remains nonviable, bowel resection must be performed. Occasionally, a normal appendix is contained within a right-sided hernia sac. Although some surgeons advocate appendectomy in this setting, even a careful appendectomy increases the risk of postoperative wound infection and therefore should not be routinely performed.

After the sac is divided, the cord is completely separated proximally from the sac. The sac is twisted one to two full turns and ligated at the level of the internal ring (Fig. 49–6). The internal ring is not usually reconstructed. The distal sac can be gently dissected from the cord and removed or left in situ. If the distal sac is connected to a hydrocele, the hydrocele and testis are usually delivered into the wound and the attached cord is carefully identified. The vas deferens can take a circuitous route along the outside of the distal sac and can be injured or divided if care is not taken to identify and preserve it. It is probably better to leave a portion of the distal sac behind rather than to risk injury to the vas by overvigorous sac resection. The testis is returned to the scrotum by gentle traction on the scrotal skin to pull the gubernaculum and testis into the scrotum (Fig. 49–7). If associated undescended testis is present, concomitant orchiopexy can be performed.

The wound is closed in layers, using absorbable or nonabsorbable suture, according to the surgeon's preference. Most pediatric surgeons use subcuticular sutures for skin closure, with either flexible collodion or transparent film dressing (Op-Site, Tegaderm).

Pain relief in the postoperative period has been a

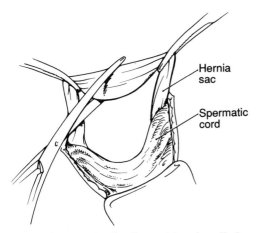

Figure 49–5. After ensuring by direct vision that all elements of the spermatic cord are completely free of the sac, the sac is palpated to assess the presence of bowel or omentum. If sac contents are present, the sac can be opened at its midpoint and the contents reduced. The sac is then clamped proximally and distally by hemostats and divided.

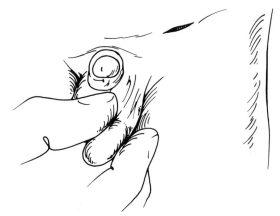

Figure 49–7. The testis is gently replaced into the scrotum, first by skin traction on the gubernaculum, then by manipulation. Pushing the testicle into the scrotum with a sharp instrument should be avoided. The external oblique, Scarpa's fascia, and skin are closed with suture of the surgeon's preference.

topic of considerable interest. Many surgeons simply provide mild oral analgesics (acetaminophen) in doses appropriate for age and weight. This method has the disadvantage of delayed onset of action. If emesis occurs, the medication may be lost in the vomitus. Acetaminophen suppositories are probably more effective for these reasons. Aspirin should be avoided owing to its anticoagulant properties.

Another method of pain relief involves injection of the skin wound edges with a long-acting local anesthetic (bupivacaine) just before suture closure. This technique is safe and probably effective, although it does not anesthetize the deeper tissue layers. To do this, an ilioinguinal nerve block should be performed before beginning the procedure or at the time of closure.

Another method of pain relief involves the caudal injection of a long-acting local agent, which presumably anesthetizes all wound layers. When performed by experienced anesthesiologists before the herniorrhaphy is begun, less anesthetic gas and medication are required during the operative procedure. The patients also awaken quicker and are ready for hospital discharge sooner. Complications can develop, however, and these must be carefully explained to the parents.[25] Informed consent is obtained before the procedure with caudal injection.

☐ Complications of Hernia and Herniorrhaphy

INCARCERATION AND STRANGULATION

An incarcerated hernia develops when the sac contents (generally, bowel in the male and ovary, fallopian tube, or bowel in the female) cannot be reduced into the peritoneal cavity nonoperatively. Incarceration occurs most frequently (70%) in infants younger than 1 year of age, with a very low incidence by 8 years of age or older. The symptoms

of incarceration include severe irritability, apparent cramping abdominal pain, and occasional vomiting, at first nonbilious but rapidly progressing to bilious or even feculent in long-standing cases, indicating strangulation. Physical findings of incarceration include a firm to fluctuant mass in the affected groin, which is usually nontender. The mass may be present only in the groin or may extend to the scrotum. Usually, there is a known hernia on the affected side. Occasionally, incarceration is the first sign or symptom of the presence of a hernia.

The pathophysiology of incarceration involves gradual swelling of the trapped organ within the closed space of the inguinal canal. This effect results in impaired venous and lymphatic drainage, thus increasing edema and pressure. Eventually, the pressure exceeds arterial perfusion pressure, and gangrene and necrosis develop. As these circulatory changes evolve, the groin mass becomes much more firm and significant tenderness develops. Skin redness and edema may appear over the mass. The infant appears much more ill. When these changes occur, the term *strangulation* is used, denoting the need for immediate operative intervention. The actual incidence of intestinal resection necessitated by incarceration in a hernia is low, ranging from 0 to 1.4%.[26]

Incarcerated hernias without evidence of strangulation can be reduced nonoperatively in 80% of cases. The advantages of such reduction include allowing time for fluid resuscitation, optimizing the preoperative status of the child, and allowing resolution of edema within the hernia sac and cord, making the subsequent herniorrhaphy technically less difficult and safer. It is highly unlikely that bowel with significant vascular compromise or necrosis can be reduced without operation.

The principles of nonoperative reduction include sedation (generally by parenterally administered medication), elevation of the lower half of the body, and application of ice to the hernia sac to attempt to reduce edema. The application of ice must be done very carefully in newborns and small premature infants to avoid hypothermia.

Intramuscular (IM) or intravenous (IV) sedation is used by most pediatric surgeons as an aid to hernia reduction. The following medications have been provided for this purpose: midazolam (Versed) 0.05 to 0.1 mg/kg IM or slowly IV; fentanyl citrate 1 to 4 μg/kg IM or slowly IV; ketamine 0.25 to 0.5 mg/kg IV or 1 to 2 mg/kg IM; and morphine sulfate 0.05 to 0.1 mg/kg IM or slowly IV.

Such potent sedatives should be given under the strict guidelines for conscious sedation and the direct supervision of a physician familiar with their possible side effects and adverse reactions. Monitoring equipment (electrocardiograph, pulse oximeter) should be used. Oxygen, suction, and resuscitation equipment must be immediately available. These medications have particular risks in the child who is premature, significantly dehydrated, or lethargic, because respiratory depression or apnea can occur.

If the hernia remains unreduced for 1 to 2 hours, including after an attempt at gentle manual reduction, urgent operative reduction and repair are necessary. Further delay would likely place the hernia sac contents, as well as the testis in the male patient, in jeopardy. The principles for repair are basically the same as those for routine herniorrhaphy, with several additions. The hernia should not be manually reduced after induction of anesthesia, so that the status of the sac contents can be assessed intraoperatively. Occasionally, the hernia reduces spontaneously before the sac is opened for inspection. Unless there is extremely bloody or foul-smelling fluid, or unless the bowel immediately inside the internal ring appears necrotic, no further intraperitoneal exploration is necessary. If the sac contents do not spontaneously reduce, the sac should be opened and the contents inspected.

If the bowel is viable, it can be reduced through the internal ring, which might require incision or dilatation with a retractor to allow reduction. Bowel with questionable viability can be wrapped in warm gauze after delivery into the wound to relieve pressure on the mesentery. If the bowel fails to recover arterial pulsations or peristalsis, if it continues to appear questionably viable, or if it appears nonviable immediately on opening the sac, bowel resection and anastomosis are required. Although some surgeons would attempt these procedures in the hernia wound, our preference is to make a separate abdominal incision, reduce the nonviable bowel into the peritoneal cavity, and perform the bowel resection and anastomosis there.

Completing the herniorrhaphy in incarcerated hernia after reduction of the sac contents can be difficult, because the edematous, friable sac tends to tear easily and because the cord structures may be obscure. Great care must be taken during the dissection to preserve the integrity of the vessels and vas deferens and to obtain a sac that will hold a transfixion suture.

The testicular blood supply is vulnerable to compression by an incarcerated or strangulated hernia, which, if prolonged, can result in testicular atrophy. The incidence of such permanent injury ranges from 2.6 to 5%.[26, 27] The incidence of finding a cyanotic testis at operation for incarcerated hernia is much greater, however (up to 29%). With relief of vascular compression by reduction and repair of the hernia, the testis generally survives. In questionable cases, the testis should not be removed but rather returned to the scrotum and herniorrhaphy completed.

RECURRENCE

Although hernia occasionally recurs, its true incidence is unclear. Recurrence rates of 0 to 1% have been reported. These series frequently fail to assess associated risk factors, however. Recurrent hernia seems to occur more in patients who are premature, have incarceration at the first operative procedure, and have associated disorders, such as inherited collagen deficiencies or peritoneal catheters for hydrocephalus or dialysis. Occasionally, recurrent hernias are of the direct type, suggesting that injury to the floor of the inguinal canal can occur at the primary herniorrhaphy.

INJURY TO SPERMATIC CORD

Injury to the spermatic vessels can take place as a result of less than ideal dissection or placement of transfixion suture. The vessels in small, premature infants are most vulnerable to injury of this type. In addition, separation of these vessels from an edematous, friable sac as a result of hernia incarceration places them at increased risk. Electrocautery should be used with extreme caution or not at all in proximity to the spermatic cord. Transmitted heat may cause thrombosis of the spermatic vessel.

The true incidence of vessel injury during herniorrhaphy, leading to testicular atrophy, is unknown. The commonly quoted figure of 1% is probably high, because the studies that gave rise to this figure did not exclude patients with incarcerated hernia, a condition in itself that can cause testicular infarction.[26] In addition, these studies were performed in an era when vigorous resection of the distal sac was practiced, putting the spermatic vessels in greater jeopardy.

Injury to the vas deferens is a definite risk during hernia repair in the male patient. A vas deferens can be injured in several ways. Experimentally, simply grasping the vas by forceps or hemostat can cause permanent occlusion.[28] Therefore, this maneuver should be carefully avoided during herniorrhaphy. Heat injury by electrocautery near the vas is also theoretically possible. The vas can be ligated during transfixion suture of the sac. Twisting the sac too tightly just before ligation can pull the vas up and into the sac, where it can be inadvertently ligated. The vas can also be divided during herniorrhaphy. This most frequently occurs during division of the sac after dissection of the vessels but can also occur during dissection or removal of the distal sac or hydrocele sac. The epididymis can also be injured, divided, or partially resected during removal of these distal sac structures.

Simple division of the vas can occur in these instances. A portion of the vas may actually be resected with the hernia sac. A resected vas should not be confused with mesonephric rests or adrenal rests, which can occasionally occur in conjunction with hernia sacs. Removal of these histologic oddities is of no consequence. Distinction of these rests from vas or epididymis is generally not problematic for an experienced pathologist.

The true incidence of vas injury is unknown. Suggestive data are found in the literature regarding (1) infertility in male patients after hernia repair and (2) the incidence of vas segments found in hernia sacs examined histologically. Several studies have examined infertility in men who have undergone previous herniorrhaphy (not necessarily in childhood, however).[29, 30] These investigators concluded that, although there is a relationship between hernia repair and infertility, only a small percentage of infertile men show such a relationship. A widely quoted series of cases of vas segments in hernia sacs demonstrated a 1.6% incidence of this histologic finding, but significant details are lacking from this experience.[14] Another unpublished series demonstrated a 1.2% incidence of vas or epididymis segments resected with hernia sacs.

The consequences of vas injury or resection are significant. Injury of vas or epididymis bilaterally almost certainly results in sterility. Even unilateral injury is unacceptable and must be avoided. The development of sperm agglutinating antibodies in postpubertal males with unilateral vas injury may also cause infertility years later.

The dilemma of how to proceed in the event of vas injury deserves some discussion. If bilateral injury occurs, the patient will be sterile unless continuity is restored in one or both sides. The optimal timing of the attempted repair is unknown, but there have been successful repairs done years after the injury.[27] The chances of reestablishing vas continuity in the infant with a tiny vas deferens are remote. Referral to a specialist with microscopic anastomotic experience seems advisable. Whether to refer a child with unilateral injury is somewhat less clear, as fertility rates may fall only 10% in prepubertal males. The later development of antisperm antibodies in adolescent boys makes referral seem appropriate. In any case, the family must be fully informed of the complication and its possible consequences, so that they may actively participate in the decision.

REFERENCES

1. Morgan EH, Anson BJ: Anatomy of region of inguinal hernia, IV: The internal surface of the parietal layers. Q Bull Northwestern Univ Med School 16:20, 1942.
2. Cox JA: Inguinal hernia of childhood. Surg Clin North Am 65:1331–1342, 1985.
3. Boocock GR, Todd PJ: Inguinal hernias are common in preterm infants. Arch Dis Child 60:669–670, 1985.
4. Powell TG, Hallows JA, Cooke RWI, et al: Why do so many small infants develop an inguinal hernia? Arch Dis Child 61:991–995, 1986.
5. Harper RG, Garcia A, Sia C: Inguinal hernia: A common problem of premature infants weighing 1000 grams or less at birth. Pediatrics 56:112–115, 1975.
6. Holsclaw DS, Shwachman H: Increased incidence of inguinal hernia, hydrocele, and undescended testicle in males with cystic fibrosis. Pediatrics 48:442–445, 1971.
7. McEntyre RL, Raffensperger JG: Surgical complications of Ehlers-Danlos syndrome in children. J Pediatr Surg 12:531–535, 1977.
8. Coran AG, Eraklis AJ: Inguinal hernia in the Hurler-Hunter syndrome. Surgery 61:302–304, 1967.
9. Uden A, Lindhagen T: Inguinal hernia in patients with congenital dislocation of the hip. Acta Orthop Scand 59:667–668, 1988.
10. Tank ES, Hatch PA: Hernias complicating chronic ambulatory peritoneal dialysis in children. J Pediatr Surg 21:41–42, 1986.
11. Moazam F, Glenn JD, Kaplan BJ, et al: Inguinal hernias after ventriculoperitoneal shunt procedures in pediatric patients. Surg Gynecol Obstet 159:570–572, 1984.
12. Fonkalsrud EW, de Lorimier AA, Clatworthy HW: Femoral and direct inguinal hernias in infants and children. JAMA 192:597, 1965.
13. Clausen EG, Jake RJ, Binkley FM: Contralateral inguinal exploration of unilateral hernia in infants and children. Surgery 44:735, 1958.
14. Sparkman RS: Bilateral exploration in inguinal hernia in juvenile patients. Surgery 51:393–406, 1962.
15. Rathauser F: Historical overview of the bilateral approach to pediatric inguinal hernias. Am J Surg 150:527–532, 1985.
16. Rowe MI, Copelson LW, Clatworthy HW: The patent processus vaginalis and the inguinal hernia. J Pediatr Surg 4:102–107, 1969.
16a. Tacket LD, Breuer CK, Luks FI, et al: Incidence of contralateral inguinal hernia: A prospective analysis. J Pediatr Surg. In press.
17. Powell RW: Intraoperative diagnostic pneumoperitoneum in pediatric patients with unilateral inguinal hernias: The Goldstein test. J Pediatr Surg 20:418–421, 1985.
18. Kieswetter WB, Parenzan L: When should hernia in the infant be treated bilaterally? JAMA 171:287, 1959.
19. Bock JE, Sobye JV: Frequency of contralateral inguinal hernia in children. Acta Chir Scand 136:707–709, 1970.
19a. Wiener ES, Touloukian RJ, Rodgers BM, et al: Hernia survey of the Section on Surgery of the American Academy of Pediatrics. J Pediatr Surg 31:1166–1169, 1996.
19b. Jona JZ: The incidence of positive contralateral inguinal exploration among preschool children—A retrospective and prospective study. J Pediatr Surg 31:656–660, 1996.
20. Holder TM, Ashcraft KW: Groin hernias and hydroceles. In Holder TM, Ashcraft KW (eds): Textbook of Pediatric Surgery. Philadelphia, WB Saunders, 1980, p 594.
21. Lobe TE, Schropp KP: Inguinal hernia in pediatrics: Initial experience with laparoscopic inguinal exploration of the asymptomatic contralateral side. J Laparoendosc Surg 2:135–140, 1992.
22. DuBois J, Jenkins JR, Egan JC: Transinguinal laparoscopic examination of the contralateral groin in pediatric herniorrhaphy. Surg Laparosc Endosc 7:384–387, 1997.
23. Jewitt TC, Kuhn JP, Allen JE: Herniography in children. J Pediatr Surg 11:451–454, 1976.
24. Khan AH, Yazbeck S: Abdominoscrotal hydrocele: A cause of abdominal mass in children: A case report and review of the literature. J Pediatr Surg 22:809–810, 1987.
25. Dalens B, Hasnaoui A: Caudal anesthesia in pediatric surgery: Success rate and adverse effects in 750 consecutive patients. Anesth Analg 58:83–89, 1989.
26. Rowe MI, Clatworthy HW: Incarcerated and strangulated hernias in children. Arch Surg 101:136–139, 1970.
27. Palmer BV: Incarcerated inguinal hernia in children. Ann R Coll Surg Eng 60:121–124, 1978.
28. Janik JS, Shandling B: The vulnerability of the vas deferens. II. The case against routine bilateral inguinal exploration. J Pediatr Surg 17:585–588, 1982.
29. Friberg J, Fritjofsson A: Inguinal herniorrhaphy and sperm-agglutinating antibodies in infertile men. Arch Androl 2:317–322, 1979.
30. Rumke P: Autospermagglutinins: A cause of infertility in men. Ann N Y Acad Sci 124:696–701, 1965.

50

UNDESCENDED TESTIS AND TESTICULAR TUMORS

Eric M. Wallen, MD • Linda M. D. Shortliffe, MD

Numerous factors interact to effect normal testicular descent (Fig. 50–1). Any abnormality in this process can result in undescended testis (UDT), also known as cryptorchidism, which carries fertility and malignancy implications. This chapter reviews the endocrine and anatomic basis of testicular descent; the diagnosis, treatment, and sequelae of UDT; and the diagnosis and management of pediatric testicular neoplasms.

☐ Embryology

Descent of the testis depends on a complex interaction of endocrine, paracrine, growth, and mechanical factors and is incompletely understood.

The gonadal tissue located on the genital ridge of the embryo is bipotential until weeks 6 and 7 of gestation, when the testis-determining SRY gene causes it to differentiate into a testis. Sertoli cells begin to produce müllerian inhibitory factor (MIF) soon thereafter, causing regression of müllerian duct structures. By the 9th week, Leydig cells produce testosterone, which stimulates development of wolffian structures including the epididymis and vas deferens. The testis passes through the inguinal canal into the scrotum during the third trimester.

Androgens, in the form of dihydrotestosterone and human chorionic gonadotropin (hCG), contribute to testicular descent. When antiandrogens are given to pregnant rats, the rate of UDT is 50%.[1–4] In humans, the frequency of UDT is increased in boys with diseases that affect androgen secretion or function.[5, 6] UDT may also be associated with blunting of the gonadotropin surge that normally occurs 60 to 90 days after birth, suggesting a primary pituitary endocrinopathy.[7] The local paracrine effects of androgens may play a more important role in the development of structures such as the epididymis than in the process of testicular descent.[8, 9]

Growth factors have recently been shown to play an important role in testicular descent.[9] Epidermal growth factor appears to act at the level of the placenta to enhance gonadotropin release, stimulating the fetal testis to secrete factors involved in descent. Descendin is an androgen-independent growth factor produced by the testis that causes gubernacular development, one of the requirements for normal descent (see Fig. 50–1).[10]

The gubernaculum testis is a mucofibrous structure with its apex at the testicle and epididymis and its base in the scrotum. It undergoes two phases, outgrowth and regression, which appear to be under separate control mechanisms.[10–13] Gubernacular outgrowth refers to a rapid swelling that occurs under the androgen-independent stimulation of descendin. Experimentally, estradiol plays an inhibitory role in outgrowth. An abnormality of either of these influences on gubernacular outgrowth could result in UDT. Gubernacular outgrowth dilates the inguinal canal, creating a pathway for testicular descent. The gubernaculum does not provide traction on the testis to cause descent; it is not anchored to the scrotum, and it does not insert onto the testis. Gubernacular regression, unlike outgrowth, requires androgen stimulation.

Mechanical and anatomic factors, including intraabdominal pressure and a patent processus vaginalis, are postulated to be requirements for normal testicular descent. According to this hypothesis, intraabdominal pressure causes protrusion of the processus vaginalis through the internal inguinal ring, transmitting abdominal pressure to the gubernaculum and initiating descent.

Factors that are probably less important in descent include MIF, estrogen, and calcitonin gene-related peptide (CGRP). The role of MIF is probably limited to removing müllerian structures, which may cause an anatomic obstruction to descent.[11, 12] High maternal levels of estradiol have been implicated in UDT; most likely this is due to a direct estrogenic effect that causes reduction of gubernacu-

663

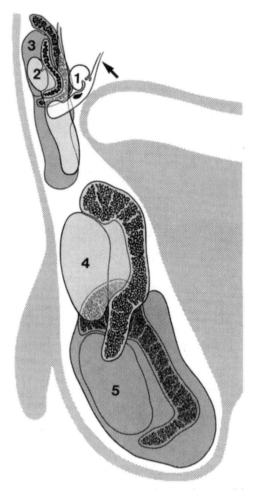

Figure 50–1. Testicular descent in human beings: (*1*) 90-mm crown-rump length (CR) (12–14 weeks of gestational age); (*2*) 125-mm CR (15–17 weeks); (*3*) 230-mm CR (24–26 weeks); (*4*) 280 mm CR (28–30 weeks); (*5*) at term. The convoluted structure is the epididymis. (Adapted from Hadziselimovic F: Embryology of testicular descent and maldescent. In Hadziselimovic F [ed]: Cryptorchidism: Management and Implications. New York, Springer-Verlag, 1983, p 23.)

lar growth.[11, 12, 14] Research done on rats has shown that CGRP is excreted by the genitofemoral nerve under androgen stimulation, causing contraction of cremasteric muscle fibers and subsequent descent of the gubernaculum, with the testis following.[15–18] The cremaster muscle is the chief component of the gubernaculum of rats, but it is entirely distinct from the gubernaculum in humans. Therefore, the role of CGRP in human testicular descent remains controversial.[9, 19, 20]

The role of the epididymis in testicular descent has also been considered. The gubernaculum inserts into the epididymis, which precedes the testis into the scrotum. Some investigators postulate that, under androgen stimulation, the gubernaculum facilitates epididymal descent, indirectly guiding the testis into the scrotum.[21] Others believe that an abnormality of the paracrine function of testosterone is responsible for epididymal anomalies and UDT but that epididymal abnormalities do not cause

UDT.[9] Epididymal anomalies are found in up to 50% of men with UDT.[22, 23]

☐ Incidence

UDT occurs in approximately 3% of boys born at term and in up to 33% of boys born prematurely. The majority of testes descend within the subsequent 12 months, resulting in an incidence of 1% undescended at 1 year.[24] The testis is unlikely to descend after this time. Series documenting the location of unilateral UDTs find at least two thirds are palpable, with most being palpable within the inguinal canal or distal to the external ring.[25] Anomalies associated with UDT include patent processus vaginalis, epididymal abnormalities, and, uncommonly, hypospadias, posterior urethral valves, and anomalies of the upper urinary tract.[26]

☐ Classification

Variability in UDT nomenclature has led to ambiguity in the literature and difficulty in comparing treatment results. The clearest classification system divides UDT into palpable and nonpalpable groups.[27] A *true undescended testis* has had its descent halted somewhere along the path of normal descent. The *ectopic undescended testis* has left the path of normal descent and can be found in the inguinal region, the perineum, the femoral canal, the penopubic area, or even the contralateral hemiscrotum. An *iatrogenic undescended testis* is a previously descended testis that has become trapped in scar tissue cephalic to the scrotum after inguinal surgery. A *retractile testis* is a normally descended testis that retracts intermittently into the inguinal canal as a result of contraction of the cremaster muscle.

Nonpalpable testes include intraabdominal testes and are further classified as *closed-ring* and *open-ring variants,* depending on the status of the internal ring. A nonpalpable testis may also be absent, or *vanishing,* secondary to intrauterine or perinatal torsion. This condition is known as *monorchia,* or *anorchia* if both testes are absent. Biopsy of the tissue at the blind-ending gonadal vessels may reveal hemosiderin and calcification.

☐ Diagnosis

A careful history and physical examination should enable distinction between a retractile testis and a low (or "gliding") UDT. Because the cremasteric reflex is weak or absent for the first 3 months of life, a diagnosis of retractile testis is suggested when a boy with documentation of normally descended testes at birth is seen later with a suspected UDT.

The diagnosis and location of UDT is determined

by a thorough, gentle physical examination performed in a warm room. The patient should be examined in both a supine and a cross-legged sitting position. The scrotum is examined for hypoplasia and for the presence of either testis. In cases of monorchia, the solitary testis may be hypertrophied. The first maneuver to locate the testis is to walk the fingers gently down the inguinal canal from the internal ring toward the scrotum. Lubricating gel may aid in reducing friction. Examining the boy who is sitting or squatting may help identify the testis. Gentle pressure on the midabdomen may help push the testis into the inguinal canal.

On physical examination, both the retractile testis and the low UDT may be manipulated into the scrotum. The retractile testis should remain in the scrotum temporarily without traction, whereas the low UDT does not remain in the scrotum. With a retractile testis, the ipsilateral hemiscrotum is fully developed, whereas in the other forms of UDT, the hemiscrotum may be underdeveloped. If there is doubt about the diagnosis of low UDT versus retractile testis, hCG injections may be helpful.[28] In response to a total of 10,000 IU of hCG administered intramuscularly over a 1- to 3-week period, a retractile testis should descend but a UDT will not.

If neither testis is palpable, anorchia must be differentiated from bilateral UDT. This can be determined by an hCG stimulation test. The baseline testosterone, follicle-stimulating hormone (FSH), and luteinizing hormone (LH) levels are measured before administration of 2000 IU of hCG daily for 3 days, with the testosterone level determined on day 6.[29] If the baseline FSH level is elevated (3 SD above the mean) in a boy younger than 9 years of age, anorchia is likely and no further evaluation is recommended. If baseline LH and FSH levels are normal and hCG stimulation results in an appropriate elevation of testosterone, testicular tissue is probably present and the patient should undergo exploration. If the testosterone level does not increase in response to hCG stimulation, however, testicular tissue may still be present, and exploration should be considered. The hCG stimulation test does not indicate whether one or both testes or functioning testicular remnants are present.[29]

Radiologic imaging is rarely helpful in locating a UDT. Multiple studies have shown that the experienced surgeon examiner has a higher sensitivity in locating a UDT than ultrasonography (US), computed tomography (CT), or magnetic resonance imaging (MRI).[30, 31] Of the options, MRI is favored.[31, 32] For the clinically impalpable testis, laparoscopy has a 95% sensitivity for locating a testis or proving it absent.[31, 33–35]

□ Fertility

A UDT and, to a lesser degree, its contralateral mate have been demonstrated to be histologically abnormal by investigators who performed bilateral testis biopsies at the time of orchiopexy.[36–38] Blunting of normal testosterone surge at 60 to 90 days may result in a lack of Leydig cell proliferation and delay in transformation of gonocytes to adult dark spermatogonia. Histopathologic changes include a decrease in the ratio of spermatogonia per tubule and Leydig cell atrophy. Clinically, patients with a history of UDT have subnormal semen analyses. Despite these abnormalities, the paternity rate of men with a history of unilateral UDT is equivalent to that of the normal population.[38–42] However, bilateral UDT results in severely impaired fertility, with paternity rates of approximately 50%, even if corrected early.[39, 42]

□ Risk of Malignancy

The risk of developing testicular cancer has been estimated to be 10 to 60 times greater for men with a history of UDT.[24] One recent large retrospective study established a 7.4-fold increased risk of malignancy over the normal population.[43] A total of 15 to 20% of the tumors arise in the normally descended contralateral testis.[44] Orchiopexy has not been shown to decrease this risk, but it does facilitate detection.[39] The incidence of carcinoma in situ (CIS) in adult men who have had an orchiopexy is 1.7%.[45] CIS is a premalignant lesion, but the natural history of CIS diagnosed in a young child at the time of orchiopexy is unknown. It has been recommended that these patients undergo repeat testis biopsy after puberty.[46]

The risk of malignancy is highest in testes originally located abdominally. Cancers arising in uncorrected abdominal testes are most frequently seminomas. Malignancies arising after successful orchiopexy, regardless of original location, are most frequently nonseminomatous germ cell tumors.[47–50]

□ Treatment: Indications and Timing

Treatment of UDT reduces the risk of torsion, facilitates examination of the testis, improves the endocrine function of the testis, and creates a normal-appearing scrotum (see Fig. 50–1). Scrotal placement of the testis may not affect the risk of malignancy or infertility.

Currently, the recommended age for a child to undergo orchiopexy is at or near 1 year of age (Fig. 50–2).[51] Repair may be undertaken earlier if a symptomatic hernia is present. The risk associated with undergoing general anesthesia after 6 months is low, and it is unlikely that a testis will descend after 1 year of age.

Authorities disagree on the management of the unilateral UDT that presents postpubertally. The endocrine function of the testis is no longer required, yet the risk of malignancy persists. The risk of death

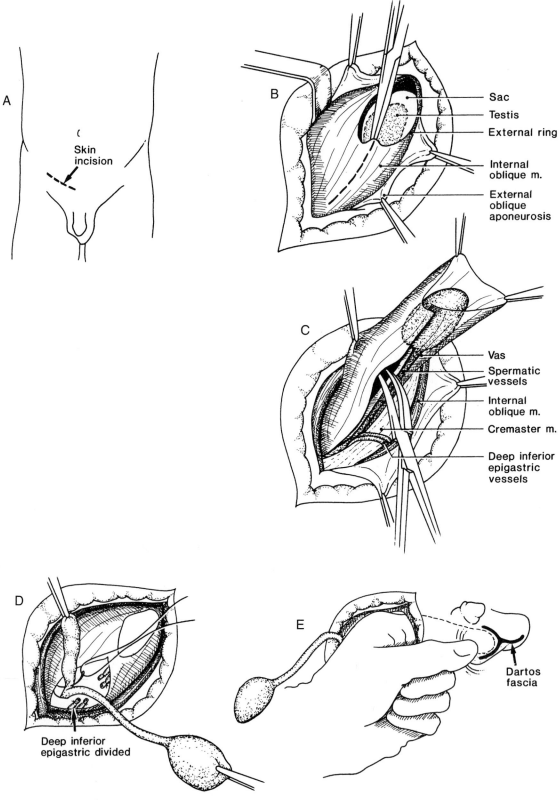

Figure 50–2. *A,* Transverse skin incision. *B,* External oblique aponeurosis is opened in the directions of its fibers with care taken to avoid the ileoinguinal nerve. *C,* The testis is delivered, and the patent processus vaginalis is opened distally near the testis. *D,* The processus vaginalis, or indirect hernia sac, is separated from the cord structures and ligated at the internal ring. Adequate cord length is usually obtained by retroperitoneal dissection of the cord contents. If additional length is required, the inferior epigastric vessels may be ligated (Prentiss maneuver), permitting medialization of the cord. *E,* A finger is passed inferiorly into the scrotum to aid in creation of a dartos pouch.

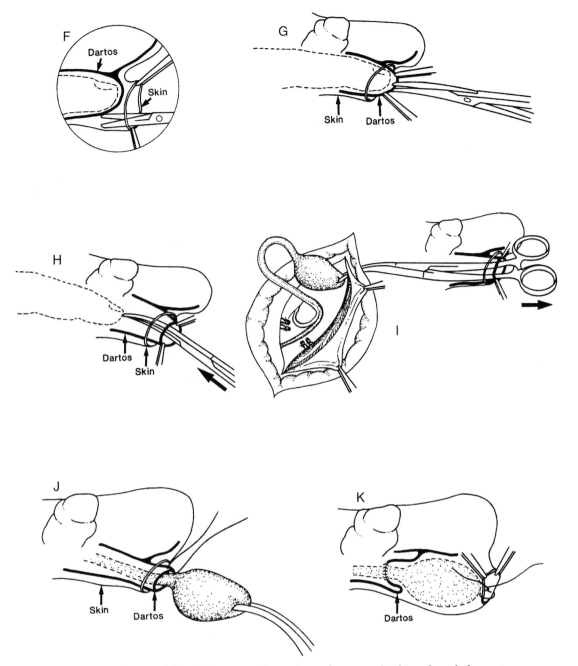

Figure 50–2 *Continued. F* to *H,* Dartos pouch creation and passage of a clamp through the scrotum into the inguinal canal. *I,* Adventitial tissue of the testis is grasped with the clamp. *J,* The testis is brought into the dartos pouch. *K,* Dartos fascia and skin are closed. (From Ellis DG: Undescended testes. In Ashcraft KW [ed]: Pediatric Urology. Philadelphia, WB Saunders, 1990, p 423.)

resulting from anesthesia and exploration was determined to be greater than the risk of death resulting from malignancy in men older than 32 years of age, but these data were compiled several decades ago before the advent of laparoscopy.[52] In light of these data, we recommend that the unilateral, palpable UDT in younger postpubertal males be brought down surgically if the testis appears normal and that it be removed if the testis is abnormally soft or small.

Management of the postpubertal unilateral intraabdominal UDT is a decision that should be made by the patient and the surgeons after consideration of the relative risks of each type of management. Given that the risk of cancer is increased and that the cord length is often short, orchiectomy is the most rational option in most cases.

☐ Treatment

The value of hormonal therapy in the treatment of UDT is controversial. Buserelin, an LH-releasing hormone agonist, is frequently used to treat UDT in

Europe. The highest success rates have been observed in cases in which the testis is at or distal to the external ring.[53–57] Trials combining buserelin and hCG have yielded higher success rates, but the testicle may not remain in the scrotum after therapy.[21, 58] Buserelin has not received Food and Drug Administration approval for the treatment of UDT in the United States.

Some authors recommend low-dose hCG therapy regardless of surgical plans to restore a normal endocrine milieu and to enhance germ cell maturation.[59] hCG may cause virilization, although lower doses do not produce this side effect.

Surgical techniques for UDT depend on whether or not the testis is palpable (Fig. 50–3). Unilateral and bilateral palpable UDT are treated the same way. For unilateral and bilateral nonpalpable UDT, definitive therapy is determined by diagnostic laparoscopy. For cases of secondary UDT, care must be taken to avoid compromise of the testicular blood supply.

PALPABLE UNDESCENDED TESTIS

The mainstay of therapy for the palpable UDT is surgical orchiopexy with creation of a subdartos pouch. The success rate, defined as a testis that remains in the scrotum and does not atrophy, is 95%.[60] Fixation is achieved by the scarring of the everted tunica vaginalis to the surrounding tissues.[61] Eversion of the tunica vaginalis eliminates the risk of torsion.[62] The placement of sutures in the tunica albuginea for scrotal fixation is generally discouraged because it causes significant testicular inflammation and may damage intratesticular vessels, especially those in the lower pole of the testis.[63–65] Biopsy of the testis at the time of surgery is controversial but may provide prognostic information regarding fertility.[38, 66]

The technique of orchiopexy with subdartos pouch is illustrated in Figure 50–2.[67–69] The operation is usually performed as an outpatient procedure using general anesthesia. The patient is supine. Intraoperative administration of an ilioinguinal nerve block with bupivacaine provides excellent postoperative analgesia. The incision should be made along one of Langer's lines, over the internal ring. The external oblique aponeurosis is incised laterally from the external ring in the direction of its fibers, avoiding injury to the ilioinguinal nerve. Once located, the testis and spermatic cord are freed. The testis and hernia sac are dissected from the canal. The tunica vaginalis is then dissected away from the vas deferens and the vessels and divided. The proximal sac is twisted, doubly suture-ligated, and amputated. Retroperitoneal dissection through the internal ring may provide additional cord length for the testis to reach the scrotum.

A tunnel is created from the inguinal canal into the scrotum using a finger or a large surgical clamp, and the scrotum is bluntly enlarged. A subdartos pouch is created by placing the finger through the tunnel and stretching the skin in a dependent portion of the scrotum. A 1-cm to 2-cm incision is made in the skin over the finger, and a hemostat is inserted just under the skin and spread both superiorly and inferiorly to create the pouch. A clamp is then placed on the surgeon's finger in this scrotal incision and its tip is guided into the inguinal canal by withdrawing the finger. The clamp is then used to grasp some adventitial tissue around the testis and guide it into the pouch. Grasping the testis or vas deferens should be avoided. Alternatively, a testicular transfixation suture may be used to deliver the testicle to the dartos pouch. Once the testis is in the dartos pouch, a suture is used to narrow the neck of the pouch to prevent testicular retraction. This suture may also be attached to the cut edge of the tunica. Testis measurements and biopsy may be performed at this time. The scrotal skin incision is closed. The external oblique aponeurosis is reapproximated with absorbable suture, and the skin and subcuticular tissue may be closed with interrupted subcuticular stitches. A collodion dressing is useful in diapered boys.

The patient is seen in the outpatient department after a few weeks for a wound check and again several months later to assess the final position and condition of the testicle. Complications of standard orchiopexy are rare but include atrophy and retraction.

UNILATERAL NONPALPABLE UNDESCENDED TESTIS

When the testis is nonpalpable, diagnostic laparoscopy through an umbilical port is useful for determining which surgical approach should be taken. If the testicular vessels are seen exiting the internal ring, an inguinal incision is used to locate the testis or testicular remnant. Orchiopexy is performed if a viable testis is found. If the vessels end blindly in the inguinal canal (vanishing testis), the tip of the vessels may be sent for pathologic examination. Remnants of testicular tissue or hemosiderin are indicative of resorption of the testis. If the vessels appear atretic or "blind-ending" as they exit the ring and laparoscopy has not been done, some clinicians have recommended no further exploration, but this is controversial.

If vessels are not seen exiting the internal ring and laparoscopy reveals an intraabdominal testis, several options are available. The Fowler-Stephens orchiopexy involves ligation of the spermatic vessels, which makes the testis dependent on the vasal and cremasteric arteries for viability.[70] For this reason, the Fowler-Stephens approach is not a good option after inguinal exploration because the blood supply to the testis may have been compromised. After ligation of the testicular vessels, which can be done laparoscopically or by laparotomy, a delay of about 6 months is recommended before orchiopexy to allow the collateral circulation to develop. The success rate of this procedure is approximately

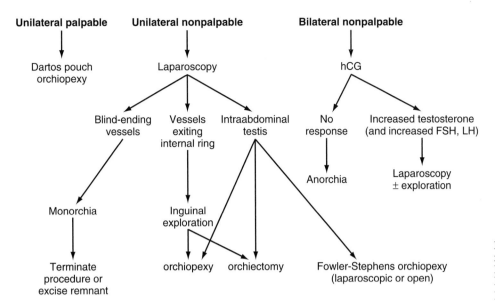

Unilateral palpable   Unilateral nonpalpable   Bilateral nonpalpable

Figure 50–3. Management algorithm for undescended testis. FSH, follicle-stimulating hormone; hCG, human chorionic gonadotropin; LH, luteinizing hormone.

80%.[71, 72] Other options for surgical management of intraabdominal testes include microvascular orchiopexy (autotransplantation) and orchiectomy.[73] More recently, successful laparoscopy-assisted orchiopexy, which involves mobilization of the testicular vessels without ligation, has been performed.[74, 75]

BILATERAL NONPALPABLE UDESCENDED TESTIS

After hCG stimulation confirms the presence of functioning testicular tissue, diagnostic laparoscopy is performed to determine surgical therapy in the same manner as for unilateral, nonpalpable UDT.

SECONDARY UNDESCENDED TESTIS

Secondary UDT is an uncommon complication of inguinal hernia repair, orchiopexy, or hydrocelectomy. Scarring from the previous procedure makes dissection difficult. The accepted surgical technique for reoperative orchiopexy minimizes the risk to the spermatic cord contents (especially the vas deferens) by mobilizing the entire cord and scar en bloc along with a strip of external oblique aponeurosis.[76] The incision is made through the previous scar, and the testis, which is usually palpable near the pubic tubercle, is exposed. A traction suture is placed through the tunica albuginea in the midtestis. Parallel incisions in the external oblique aponeurosis allow the testicle–cord–aponeurosis complex to be lifted from the canal so that a plane is developed between the spermatic cord and the inguinal floor. This dissection is carried superiorly to the internal ring, where the external oblique aponeurosis is cut to allow full mobilization of the cord and testis. Dissection continues above the scar, into the retroperitoneum, to produce sufficient length to permit placement of the testis into a dartos pouch. If more length is necessary, division of the inferior epigastric vessels allows the cord to be displaced medially.

□ Pediatric Testicular Tumors

Testicular cancer is uncommon in children, accounting for 1 to 2% of all pediatric solid tumors. Children have a much larger percentage of benign testicular lesions than adults. The peak incidence of pediatric testicular tumors occurs at 2 years of age, followed by a smaller peak during puberty.[77] Germ cell tumors comprise 65% of pediatric testicular tumors.

PRESENTATION AND DIAGNOSIS

A testis tumor typically presents as a painless scrotal mass. The differential diagnosis includes hydrocele, hernia, and tumor. A malignancy typically is nontender, does not transilluminate, and is not accompanied by an abnormal urinalysis. A hydrocele may impede an adequate testicular examination. A tumor arising in a UDT may undergo torsion and can present as acute abdominal pain. Hormonally active tumors may produce symptoms without a palpable lesion.

Testicular US should be performed if there is concern about a testicular mass. US is highly sensitive and can detect even small tumors masked by a hydrocele. Color and power Doppler US are more sensitive than gray-scale US.[78] MRI has been used to detect very small functioning Leydig cell tumors not detected by US.

Once the diagnosis of testicular cancer is made, CT has largely supplanted retroperitoneal lymph node dissection (RPLND) for the purpose of staging, but CT carries a 15 to 20% false-negative rate.[80] Either chest radiography or CT can be used to evaluate metastatic disease.

Serum tumor marker levels are valuable in both diagnosis and follow-up of testicular malignancy. Alphafetoprotein (AFP) is a glycoprotein produced by the fetal yolk sac, liver, and gastrointestinal tract, whose measurement is elevated in a variety of benign and malignant diseases including yolk sac tumors (YSTs) of the testis. The normal AFP value declines significantly in the months after birth[81]; the normal adult level of less than 10 mg/ml is not achieved until the age of 8 months.[82] The beta subunit of human chorionic gonadotropin (β-hCG) is a glycoprotein produced by embryonal carcinomas and mixed teratomas. Its half-life is 24 hours, and the normal value is less than 5 IU/l.

CARCINOMA IN SITU

CIS of the testis is a premalignant lesion. Testicular cancer is reported to develop in at least 50% of testes known to harbor CIS.[83] CIS is seen in patients with UDT and intersex disorders, conditions that are known to carry a higher risk of testicular cancer than in the general population.[84] In addition, CIS often coexists in testes that harbor a known cancer.

The natural history of CIS in prepubertal testes is unknown.[46] Testicular biopsy at the time of orchiopexy is not performed routinely; when it is done, CIS is rarely seen.[66] If biopsy of a cryptorchid testis reveals CIS, it has been recommended that the patient undergo rebiopsy postpubertally. Testicular biopsy of adults who have had a prior orchiopexy has revealed a 1.7 to 3% incidence of CIS.[45, 83] If CIS is identified, it is typically managed with annual testicular examinations and testicular US despite the reputed 50% incidence of overt carcinoma. Some European authors recommend that these patients undergo biopsy of the contralateral testis and unilateral orchiectomy; if biopsy of the remaining testis also reveals CIS, they recommend low-dose radiation treatment. The same investigators advocate routine postpubertal testis biopsy in all cases of UDT.[45, 83, 85, 86] This practice has not been routine in the United States.

GERM CELL TUMORS

The most common prepubertal testicular tumors is the YST, also known as endodermal sinus tumor, embryonal adenocarcinoma, orchidoblastoma, and Teillum's tumor.[87] Most occur within the first 2 years of life. Grossly, YSTs are firm and yellow-white. Microscopically, they are characterized by Schiller-Duval bodies and stain for AFP.[88]

Metastasis of YST to the retroperitoneum is uncommon in children (4 to 6%).[89-91] Approximately 95% of YSTs are confined to the testis. The lungs are the most common site of distant metastasis. The 5-year survival rate for YST approaches 99%.[92]

The standard diagnostic and therapeutic procedure for all testis tumors is radical inguinal orchiectomy. To minimize the risk of metastasis during manipulation, the spermatic cord is clamped or ligated immediately on entry into the inguinal canal. The role of RPLND in children with YST is controversial. Currently, most YSTs are treated with radical orchiectomy and are followed up for recurrence

by measuring AFP marker levels. If the AFP level was elevated at the time of orchiectomy and subsequently returns to normal, RPLND is not performed.

Staging of testicular tumors requires abdominopelvic CT and chest radiography, pathologic examination of the radical orchiectomy specimen, and determination of serum tumor marker levels[93] (Table 50–1). Stage I tumors are limited to the testis. They are completely resected by radical inguinal orchiectomy, after which tumor markers normalize. Patients with unknown or normal markers at diagnosis must have a negative ipsilateral RPLND for the disease to be stage I. Tumor markers, abdominal CT, and chest radiographs are done every month for a year. In the absence of recurrence, the second-year follow-up consists of serum tumor markers and chest radiograph every 2 months and a chest and abdominal CT scan every 6 months. After 2 years without recurrence, follow-up may be extended to every 6 months or yearly.[94]

Stage II disease includes those tumors with microscopic node involvement discovered by RPLND. Tumors diagnosed and treated by transscrotal orchiectomy or biopsy should also be considered stage II because resection via a transscrotal incision alters the normal lymphatic drainage of the tumor. Lymphatic drainage of the testis is to the retroperitoneal nodes, whereas the scrotum drains to the inguinal nodes. If a testicular tumor is diagnosed through a scrotal incision, ipsilateral hemiscrotectomy should be considered.[95] All patients with stage II disease

TABLE 50–1. TNM Classification of Pediatric Testis Tumors

Primary Tumor (T)

TX	Primary tumor cannot be assessed (in the absence of radical orchiectomy)
T0	Histologic scar, no evidence of primary tumor
Tis	Intratubular tumor (in situ tumor), preinvasive cancer
T1	Tumor limited to testis, including rete testis
T2	Tumor invades beyond tunica albuginea or into epididymis
T3	Tumor invades spermatic cord
T4	Tumor invades scrotum

Regional Lymph Nodes (N)

NX	Regional nodes not assessed
N0	No regional lymph node metastasis
N1	Metastasis in a single lymph node, 2 cm or less in greatest dimension
N2	Metastasis in a single lymph node, more than 2 cm but not more than 5 cm in greatest dimension, or multiple lymph nodes none more than 5 cm in greatest dimension
N3	Metastasis in a lymph node more than 5 cm in greatest dimension

Distant Metastasis (M)

MX	Presence of metastasis cannot be assessed
M0	No distant metastasis
M1	Distant metastasis

receive combination chemotherapy, although the optimal combination of agents has yet to be determined. Trials of combination chemotherapy using vincristine, dactinomycin (actinomycin D), and cyclophosphamide (VAC), with or without doxorubicin, and of bleomycin, etoposide, vinblastine, and cisplatinum in combinations have resulted in 5-year survival rates approaching 100% in patients with primary germ cell tumors of the testis.[96–98]

Stage III disease includes retroperitoneal spread seen on imaging studies and occult metastasis manifest by persistent elevation of tumor markers following orchiectomy. In children, RPLND as treatment is performed less commonly than in the past because there have been improved results with chemotherapy. Metastasis beyond the retroperitoneum or to any viscera defines stage IV disease. For both stage III and stage IV disease, chemotherapy follows the same protocols as described for stage II disease.

Teratoma is the second most common testis tumor in children.[90] Histologically, teratomas are composed of all three layers of embryonic tissue: ectoderm, endoderm, and mesoderm. Grossly, they may contain differentiated tissue such as cartilage, muscle, bone, and fat; there may also be a cystic component. In prepubertal boys, testicular teratomas follow a benign clinical course. Therefore, if US suggests teratoma in a prepubertal boy, testis-sparing enucleation can be considered.[99–101] In older boys as well as men, teratomas exhibit a propensity to metastasize and are treated with radical orchiectomy.[102]

Teratocarcinoma, or mixed germ cell tumor, accounts for 20% of pediatric germ cell tumors. Teratocarcinomas may contain any mixture of YST, embryonal carcinoma, choriocarcinoma, and seminoma.[93] Foci of choriocarcinoma confer a poorer prognosis. Eighty percent of teratocarcinomas are confined to the testis at presentation.[103] RPLND is usually performed even for stage I disease, and higher stage disease is treated by chemotherapy protocols similar to those used for adults.

Seminoma is rare in children and is treated with radical orchiectomy and retroperitoneal radiation.[104]

NON-GERM CELL TUMORS (GONADAL STROMAL TUMORS)

Leydig cell tumor is the most common non–germ cell tumor (NGCT). The peak incidence in boys occurs from 5 to 9 years of age.[105] Because these tumors produce testosterone and occasionally other androgens, patients usually have precocious puberty and a painless testicular mass. Patients may also have gynecomastia.[93] The differential diagnosis of precocious puberty also includes pituitary lesions and congenital adrenal hyperplasia. To eliminate these diagnoses, the pituitary-adrenal axis must be evaluated by assaying 17-ketosteroids and performing a dexamethasone suppression test (see Chapter 75). Reinke's crystals are the pathognomonic histologic finding in about 40% of patients with Leydig cell

tumors.[102] Currently, radical inguinal orchiectomy is the standard treatment for Leydig cell tumors, although therapy may evolve to testis-sparing enucleation because, like prepubertal teratomas, these tumors tend to follow a benign course in boys.[108]

The Sertoli cell tumor is a very rare form of NGCT and typically presents as a painless testicular mass, although a small percentage of patients may have gynecomastia. The clinical course is usually benign.

Gonadoblastoma is a form of NGCT usually seen in association with intersex disorders. The patients are typically 46XY phenotypic females with intraabdominal testes who are seen with virilization after puberty. Up to one third of patients have bilateral gonadal lesions. Whereas the clinical course is usually benign, the germ cell component of these tumors carries the risk of malignant degeneration. For this reason, early gonadectomy is recommended, especially if the patient is raised female.[109, 110]

REFERENCES

1. McMahon DR, Kramer SA, Husmann DA: Antiandrogen induced cryptorchidism in the pig is associated with failed gubernacular regression and epididymal malformations. J Urol 154(2 pt 1):553, 1995.
2. Spencer JR, Torrado T, Sanchez RS, et al: Effects of flutamide and finasteride on rat testicular descent. Endocrinology 129:741, 1991.
3. Husmann DA, McPhaul MJ: Time-specific androgen blockade with flutamide inhibits testicular descent in the rat. Endocrinology 129:1409, 1991.
4. Husmann DA, McPhaul MJ: Reversal of flutamide-induced cryptorchidism by prenatal time-specific androgens. Endocrinology 131:1711, 1992.
5. Bardin CW, Ross GT, Rifkind AB, et al: Studies of the pituitary-Leydig cell axis in young men with hypogonadotropic hypogonadism and hyposmia: Comparison with normal men, prepuberal boys, and hypopituitary patients. J Clin Invest 48:2046, 1969.
6. Santen RJ, Paulsen CA: Hypogonadotropic eunuchoidism, II: Gonadal responsiveness to exogenous gonadotropins. J Clin Endocrinol Metab 36:55, 1973.
7. Spencer JR, Vaughan ED, Imperato-McGinley J: Studies of the hormonal control of postnatal testicular descent in the rat. J Urol 149:618, 1993.
8. Jost A: Problems of fetal endocrinology: The gonadal and hypophyseal hormones. Recent Prog Horm Res 8:379, 1953.
9. Husmann DA, Levy JB: Current concepts in the pathophysiology of testicular undescent. Urology 46:267, 1995.
10. Fentener van Vlissingen JM, van Zoelen EJ, Ursem PJ, et al: In vitro model of the first phase of testicular descent: Identification of a low molecular weight factor from fetal testis involved in proliferation of gubernaculum testis cells and distinct from specified polypeptide growth factors and fetal gonadal hormones. Endocrinology 123:2868, 1988.
11. Spencer JR: The endocrinology of testicular descent. AUA Update Series XIII:94, 1994.
12. Heyns CF, Hutson JM: Historical review of theories on testicular descent (see comments). J Urol 153(3 pt 1):754, 1995.
13. Barthold JS: Cryptorchidism. In Walsh PC, Retik AB, Stamey TA, Vaughan ED Jr (eds): Campbell's Urology (6th ed). Update 11:1. Philadelphia, WB Saunders, 1994.
14. Bernstein L, Pike MC, Depue RH, et al: Maternal hormone levels in early gestation of cryptorchid males: A case-control study. Br J Cancer 58:379, 1988.
15. Yamanaka J, Metcalfe SA, Hutson JM: Demonstration of calcitonin gene-related peptide receptors in the gubernaculum by computerized densitometry. J Pediatr Surg 27:876, 1992.
16. Park WH, Hutson JM: The gubernaculum shows rhythmic

contractility and active movement during testicular descent. J Pediatr Surg 26: 615, 1991.

17. Goh DW, Middlesworth W, Farmer PJ, et al: Prenatal androgen blockade with flutamide inhibits masculinization of the genitofemoral nerve and testicular descent. J Pediatr Surg 29:836, 1994.

18. Goh DW, Momose Y, Middlesworth W, et al: The relationship among calcitonin gene-related peptide, androgens and gubernacular development in 3 animal models of cryptorchidism. J Urol 150(2 pt 2):574, 1993.

19. Heyns CF: The gubernaculum during testicular descent in the human fetus. J Anat 153:93, 1987.

20. Wensing CJ, Colenbrander B: Normal and abnormal testicular descent. Oxf Rev Reprod Biol 8:130, 1986.

21. Hadziselimovic F, Herzog B: The development and descent of the epididymis. Eur J Pediatr 152(suppl 2):S6, 1993.

22. Gill B, Kogan S, Starr S, et al: Significance of epididymal and ductal anomalies associated with testicular maldescent. J Urol 142:556, 1989.

23. Elder JS: Epididymal anomalies associated with hydrocele/hernia and cryptorchidism: Implications regarding testicular descent. J Urol 148(2 pt 2):624, 1992.

24. Pohl HG, Belman AB: The location and fate of the cryptorchid and impalpable testis. In Peppas DS, Ehrlich RM (eds): Dialogues in Pediatric Urology 20:1. Pearl River, NY, William J. Miller Associates Inc, 1997.

25. Docimo SG: The results of surgical therapy for cryptorchidism: A literature review and analysis. J Urol 154:1148, 1995.

26. Rozanski TA, Bloom DA: The undescended testis. Theory and management. Urol Clin North Am 22:107, 1995.

27. Kaplan G: Nomenclature of cryptorchidism. Eur J Pediatr 152(suppl 2):S17, 1993.

28. Rajfer J: Surgical and hormonal therapy for cryptorchidism: An overview. Horm Res 30:139, 1988.

29. Jarow JP, Berkovitz GD, Migeon CJ, et al: Elevation of serum gonadotropins establishes the diagnosis of anorchism in prepubertal boys with bilateral cryptorchidism. J Urol 136(1 pt 2):277, 1986.

30. Walker RD: Diagnosis and management of the nonpalpable undescended testicle. AUA Update Series XI(20):154, 1992.

31. Hrebinko RL, Bellinger MF: The limited role of imaging techniques in managing children with undescended testes. J Urol 150(2 pt 1):458, 1993.

32. Landa HM, Gylys-Morin V, Mattrey RF, et al: Magnetic resonance imaging of the cryptorchid testis. Eur J Pediatr 146(suppl 2):S16, 1987.

33. Bloom DA, Ayers JW, McGuire EJ: The role of laparoscopy in management of nonpalpable testes. J Urol (Paris) 94:465, 1988.

34. Froeling FM, Sorber MJ, de la Rosette JJ, et al: The nonpalpable testis and the changing role of laparoscopy. Urology 43:222, 1994.

35. Moore RG, Peters CA, Bauer SB, et al: Laparoscopic evaluation of the nonpalpable tests: A prospective assessment of accuracy. J Urol 151:728, 1994.

36. Huff DS, Hadziselimovic F, Snyder HM, et al: Histologic maldevelopment of unilaterally cryptorchid testes and their descended partners. Eur J Pediatr 152(suppl 2):S11, 1993.

37. Hadziselimovic F, Herzog B, Huff DS, et al: The morphometric histopathology of undescended testes and testes associated with incarcerated inguinal hernia: A comparative study. J Urol 146(2 pt 2):627, 1991.

38. Cendron M, Keating MA, Huff DS, et al: Cryptorchidism, orchiopexy and infertility: A critical long-term retrospective analysis. J Urol 142(2 pt 2):559, 1989.

39. Lee PA: Fertility in cryptorchidism. Does treatment make a difference? Endocrinol Metab Clin North Am 22:479, 1993.

40. Lee PA, Bellinger MF, Songer NJ, et al: An epidemiologic study of paternity after cryptorchidism: Initial results. Eur J Pediatr 152(suppl 2):S25, 1993.

41. Kogan SJ: Fertility in cryptorchidism. An overview in 1987. Eur J Pediatr 146(suppl 1):S21, 1987.

42. Chilvers C, Dudley NE, Gough MH, et al: Undescended testis: The effect of treatment on subsequent risk of subfertility and malignancy. J Pediatr Surg 21:691, 1986.

43. Pinczowski D, McLaughlin JK, Lackgren G, et al: Occurrence of testicular cancer in patients operated on for cryptorchidism and inguinal hernia. J Urol 146:1291, 1991.

44. Johnson DE, Woodhead DM, Pohl DR, et al: Cryptorchidism and testicular tumorigenesis. Surgery 63:919, 1968.

45. Skakkebaek NE, Berthelsen JG, Giwercman A, et al: Carcinoma-in-situ of the testis: Possible origin from gonocytes and precursor of all types of germ cell tumours except spermatocytoma. Int J Androl 10:19, 1987.

46. Giwercman A, Muller J, Skakkeboek NE: Cryptorchidism and testicular neoplasia. Horm Res 30:157, 1988.

47. Raja MA, Oliver RT, Badenoch D, et al: Orchidopexy and transformation of seminoma to non-seminoma [letter]. Lancet 339:930, 1992.

48. Jones BJ, Thornhill JA, O'Donnell B, et al: Influence of prior orchiopexy on stage and prognosis of testicular cancer. Eur Urol 19:201, 1991.

49. Halme A, Kellokumpu-Lehtinen P, Lehtonen T, et al: Morphology of testicular germ cell tumours in treated and untreated cryptorchidism. Br J Urol 64:78, 1989.

50. Batata MA, Whitmore WF, Chu FC, et al: Cryptorchidism and testicular cancer. J Urol 124:382, 1980.

51. American Academy of Pediatrics: Timing of elective surgery on the genitalia of male children with particular reference to the risks, benefits, and psychological effects of surgery and anesthesia. Pediatrics 97:590, 1996.

52. Farrer JH, Walker AH, Rajfer J: Management of the postpubertal cryptorchid testis: A statistical review. J Urol 134:1071, 1985.

53. Bica D, Hadziselimovic F: Buserelin treatment of cryptorchidism: A randomized, double-blind, placebo-controlled study. J Urol 148:617, 1992.

54. Bica D, Hadziselimovic F: The behavior of the epididymis, processus vaginalis and testicular descent in cryptorchid boys treated with buserelin. Eur J Pediatr 152:S38, 1993.

55. Hadziselimovic F, Buser M: Medical treatment for undescended testis [letter]. Lancet 1:1281, 1986.

56. Hadziselimovic F, Huff D, Duckett J, et al: Long-term effect of luteinizing hormone-releasing hormone analogue (buserelin) on cryptorchid testes. J Urol 138(4 pt 2):1043, 1987.

57. Hadziselimovic F, Huff D, Duckett J, et al: Treatment of cryptorchidism with low doses of buserelin over a 6-months period. Eur J Pediatr 146(suppl 2):S56, 1987.

58. Waldschmidt J, Doede T, Vygen I: The results of 9 years of experience with a combined treatment with LHRH and HCG for cryptorchidism. Eur J Pediatr 152:S34, 1993.

59. Lala R, Matarazzo P, Chiabotto P, et al: Combined therapy with LHRH and HCG in cryptorchid infants. Eur J Pediatr 152(suppl 2):S31, 1993.

60. Saw KC, Eardley I, Dennis MJ, et al: Surgical outcome of orchiopexy. I. Previously unoperated testes. Br J Urol 70:90, 1992.

61. Redman JF, Barthold JS: A technique for atraumatic scrotal pouch orchiopexy in the management of testicular torsion. J Urol 154:1511, 1995.

62. Hurren JS, Corder AP: Acute testicular torsion following orchiopexy for undescended testis (see comments). Br J Surg 79:1292, 1992.

63. Bellinger MF: Orchiopexy: An experimental study of the effect of surgical technique on testicular histology. J Urol 142:533, 1985.

64. Dixon TK, Ritchey ML, Boykin W, et al: Transparenchymal suture fixation and testicular histology in a prepubertal rat model. J Urol 148:632, 1993.

65. Jarow JP: Intratesticular arterial anatomy. J Androl 11:255, 1990.

66. Hadziselimovic F, Hecker E, Herzog B: The value of testicular biopsy in cryptorchidism. Urol Res 12:171, 1984.

67. Benson CD, Lotfi MW: The pouch technique in the surgical correction of cryptorchidism in infants and children. Surgery 62:967, 1967.

68. Koop CE: Technique of herniorrhaphy and orchiopexy. Birth Defects 13:293, 1977.

69. Rajfer J: Technique of orchiopexy. Urol Clin North Am 9:421, 1982.

70. Fowler R, Stephens FD: The role of testicular vascular anatomy in the salvage of high undescended testes. Aust N Z J Surg 29:92, 1959.

71. Kogan SJ, Houman BZ, Reda EF, et al: Orchiopexy of the high undescended testis by division of the spermatic vessels: A critical review of 38 selected transections. J Urol 141:1416, 1989.

72. Elder JS: Two-stage Fowler-Stephens orchiopexy in the management of intra-abdominal testes. J Urol 148:1239, 1992.

73. Bianchi A: Management of the impalpable testis: The role of microvascular orchidopexy. Pediatr Surg Int 5:48, 1990.

74. Bogaert GA, Kogan BA, Mevorach RA: Therapeutic laparoscopy for intra-abdominal testes. Urology 42:182, 1993.

75. Jordan GH, Winslow BH: Laparoscopic single stage and staged orchiopexy. J Urol 152:1249, 1994.

76. Cartwright PC, Velagapudi S, Snyder HM, et al: A surgical approach to reoperative orchiopexy. J Urol 149:817, 1993.

77. Li FP, Fraumeni JF: Testicular cancers in children: Epidemiologic characteristics. J Natl Cancer Inst 48:1575, 1972.

78. Luker GD, Siegel MJ: Pediatric testicular tumors: Evaluation with gray-scale and color Doppler US. Radiology 191:561, 1994.

79. Kaufman E, Akiya F, Foucar E, et al: Virilization due to Leydig cell tumor diagnosis by magnetic resonance imaging. Case management report. Clin Pediatr (Phila) 29:414, 1990.

80. Pizzocaro G, Zanoni F, Salvioni R, et al: Difficulties of a surveillance study omitting retroperitoneal lymphadenectomy in clinical stage I nonseminomatous germ cell tumors of the testis. J Urol 138:1393, 1987.

81. Brewer JA, Tank ES: Yolk sac tumors and alpha-fetoprotein in first year of life. Urology 42:79, 1993.

82. Wu JT, Book L, Sudar K: Serum alpha fetoprotein (AFP) levels in normal infants. Pediatr Res 15:50, 1981.

83. Giwercman A, Bruun E, Frimodt-Moller C, et al: Prevalence of carcinoma in situ and other histopathological abnormalities in testes of men with a history of cryptorchidism. J Urol 142: 998, 1989.

84. Wallace TM, Levin HS: Mixed gonadal dysgenesis. A review of 15 patients reporting single cases of malignant intratubular germ cell neoplasia of the testis, endometrial adenocarcinoma, and a complex vascular anomaly. Arch Pathol Lab Med 114:679, 1990.

85. Giwercman A, Grindsted J, Hansen B, et al: Testicular cancer risk in boys with maldescended testis: A cohort study. J Urol 138:1214, 1987.

86. Giwercman A, Muller J, Skakkebaek NE: Carcinoma in situ of the undescended testis. Semin Urol 6:110, 1988.

87. Kay R: Prepubertal Testicular Tumor Registry. J Urol 150(2 pt 2):671, 1993.

88. Wold LE, Kramer SA, Farrow GM: Testicular yolk sac and embryonal carcinomas in pediatric patients: Comparative immunohistochemical and clinicopathologic study. Am J Clin Pathol 81:427, 1984.

89. Bracken RB, Johnson DE, Cangir A, et al: Regional lymph nodes in infants with embryonal carcinoma of testis. Urology 11:376, 1978.

90. Brosman SA: Testicular tumors in prepubertal children. Urology 13:581, 1979.

91. Exelby PR: Testicular cancer in children. Cancer 45(suppl 7):1803, 1980.

92. Haas RJ, Schmidt P: Testicular germ-cell tumors in childhood and adolescence. World J Urol 13:203, 1995.

93. Coppes MJ, Rackley R, Kay R: Primary testicular and paratesticular tumors of childhood. Med Pediatr Oncol 22:329, 1994.

94. Connolly J, Gearhart J: Management of yolk sac tumors in children. Urol Clin North Am 20:7, 1993.

95. Giguere JK, Stablein DM, Spaulding JT, et al: The clinical significance of unconventional orchiectomy approaches in testicular cancer: A report from the Testicular Cancer Intergroup Study. J Urol 139:1225, 1988.

96. Ablin AR, Krailo MD, Ramsay NK, et al: Results of treatment of malignant germ cell tumors in 93 children: A report from the Children's Cancer Study Group. J Clin Oncol 9:1782, 1991.

97. Mann JR, Pearson D, Barrett A, et al: Results of the United Kingdom Children's Cancer Study Group's malignant germ cell tumor studies. Cancer 63:1657, 1989.

98. Haas RJ, Schmidt P, Gobel U, et al: Testicular germ cell tumors. Results of the GPO MAHO studies -82, -88, -92. Klin Padiatr 207:145, 1995.

99. Altadonna V, Snyder HM, Rosenberg HK, et al: Simple cysts of the testis in children: Preoperative diagnosis by ultrasound and excision with testicular preservation. J Urol 140:1505, 1988.

100. Ross JH, Kay R, Elder J: Testis sparing surgery for pediatric epidermoid cysts of the testis. J Urol 149:353, 1993.

101. Rushton HG, Belman AB, Sesterhenn I, et al: Testicular sparing surgery for prepubertal teratoma of the testis: A clinical and pathological study. J Urol 144:726, 1990.

102. Mostofi FK: Proceedings: Testicular tumors. Epidemiologic, etiologic, and pathologic features. Cancer 32:1186, 1973.

103. Castleberry RP, Kelly DR, Joseph DB, et al: Gonadal and extragonadal germ cell tumors. In Fernbach DJ, Vietti TJ (eds): Clinical Pediatric Oncology. St. Louis, Mosby–Year Book, 1991.

104. Perry C, Servadio C: Seminoma in childhood. J Urol 124:932, 1980.

105. Glavind K, Sondergaard G: Leydig cell tumour: Diagnosis and treatment. Case report and review. Scand J Urol Nephrol 22:343, 1988.

106. Ritchey M, Andrassy R, Kelalis P: Pediatric urologic oncology. In Gillenwater J, Grayhack J, Howards M, Ducketts J (eds): Adult and Pediatric Urology (3rd ed). St. Louis, CV Mosby, 1996.

107. Gabrilove JL, Freiberg EK, Leiter E, et al: Feminizing and non-feminizing Sertoli cell tumors. J Urol 124:757, 1980.

108. Manuel M, Katayama PK, Jones HW: The age of occurrence of gonadal tumors in intersex patients with a Y chromosome. Am J Obstet Gynecol 124:293, 1976.

109. Gourlay WA, Johnson HW, Pantzar JT, et al: Gonadal tumors in disorders of sexual differentiation. Urology 43:537, 1994.

110. Olsen MM, Caldamone AA, Jackson CL, et al: Gonadoblastoma in infancy: Indications for early gonadectomy in 46XY gonadal dysgenesis. J Pediatr Surg 23:270, 1988.

51

TESTICULAR TORSION

John Noseworthy, MD

Torsion of the testis or spermatic cord is generally considered to be the most common genitourinary tract emergency of childhood. This clinical entity is commonly referred to as "the acute scrotum,"[1–3] and it is the most serious of the conditions within the differential diagnosis of a boy with a red, swollen, and tender hemiscrotum. Mechanically produced arterial ischemia is the underlying pathophysiologic event, and prompt surgical detorsion and testicular fixation by well-established techniques are the mainstays of therapy. When diagnosis is prompt and surgery is timely, testicular salvage is the usual result. When diagnosis is delayed and treatment is expectant, the outcome is most often testicular loss. The surgical treatment is well defined; therefore, the principal challenge to the clinician is prompt and accurate diagnosis as early in the course of events as possible.

□ Differential Diagnosis

Despite increasingly sophisticated diagnostic techniques, distinguishing testicular torsion from the other causes of the acute scrotum still remains a clinical challenge.[4] The differential diagnosis of the acute scrotum is outlined in Table 51–1. The goal of this chapter is to present an approach to these patients that ensures timely surgery is not withheld due to ambiguity of diagnosis. Surgical exploration of the acutely inflamed scrotum is the accepted standard of care and should be promptly carried out if there is any doubt that testicular perfusion is compromised.[5]

□ Clinical Setting

Torsion of the testis occurs most frequently in late childhood or early adolescence, with a peak incidence at approximately 14 years of age.[6] It has been reported to occur in patients ranging from newborns to those in their seventh decade.[7] Neonatal torsion is a well-known entity, often referred to as

TABLE 51–1. Differential Diagnosis of Testicular Torsion

Major Diagnostic Categories
Torsion of the testis
Appendicular torsion
   Appendix testis
   Appendix epididymis
   Paradidymis (organ of Giraldés)
   Vas aberrans
Epididymitis/orchitis
Infections
Trauma
Minor Diagnostic Categories
Idiopathic scrotal edema
Hernia/hydrocele
Henoch/Schönlein purpura
Tumors

extravaginal torsion, and is discussed later in this chapter. Age should not be taken as a strong element in evaluating the child with the acute scrotum and should never be used to override a decision to operate when other parameters are ambiguous. Although torsion of appendicular structures seems to occur at an earlier age than does torsion of the testis, age discrepancies are not particularly strong differential elements.[8]

Testicular or scrotal pain is the primary symptom of testicular torsion, occurring in 80% or more of patients.[9] Some investigators emphasize its gradual onset.[10] Others describe the onset as abrupt.[11, 12] Our own experience favors an abrupt onset, which is a helpful distinguishing historic element favoring early surgical intervention. Abrupt, severe pain frequently leads to prompt consultation with the pediatrician or primary caregiver and early referral to the surgical specialist. Scrotal discomfort that gradually progresses to increasing pain over 12 to 24 hours is more suggestive of torsion of appendicular structures or epididymo-orchitis. Scrotal pain that radiates upward to the groin or the ipsilateral lower abdominal quadrant often accompanies testicular torsion. Severe pain of short duration, out of proportion to the inflammatory signs present on inspection, tends to occur more frequently with torsion of the testis.

Previous short-lived episodes of testicular pain accompanied by spontaneous resolution are consistent with intermittent torsion of the testicle.[13] A pattern of such episodes may constitute a strong indication for prompt surgical intervention.

Associated abdominal and gastrointestinal symptoms, such as nausea and vomiting or lower quadrant abdominal pain, as noted earlier, often accompany torsion of the testis, in contrast to the other causes of the acute scrotum. The absence of these symptoms, however, in no way excludes the diagnosis of testicular torsion because they are present in only 25% of cases.[14] Such abdominal symptoms are often confusing to the initial examiner. We have occasionally been asked to see patients with suspected appendicitis who actually have testicular torsion. The opposite situation, acute appendicitis presenting as the acute scrotum, is rare but reported.[15] We have treated one such patient presenting with severe scrotal pain who also had right lower quadrant peritoneal signs, and he was found to have acute appendicitis at laparotomy. Lower abdominal pain in the patient with an empty scrotum, with or without a mass in the groin, strongly suggests torsion of an undescended testis.

Urinary tract symptoms such as frequency, urgency, dysuria, and pyuria, and fever tend to occur more frequently in patients with epididymitis. Some patients with torsion of the testis may have mild voiding symptoms. When voiding symptoms are a significant part of the presenting complaints, a careful search for associated urinary tract infection must be made. In general, such symptoms direct the clinician away from the diagnosis of testicular torsion or appendiceal torsion and toward that of epididymitis. In a retrospective study of 238 patients with acute scrotal pain, 39% of those with epididymitis undergoing urologic evaluation were found to have structural or functional urinary tract abnormalities. Urodynamic testing of this group may help diagnose those patients with dysfunctional voiding or sphincter-detrusor dyssynergia, which results in elevated posterior urethral voiding pressures that can lead to retrograde vasal reflux and thus precipitate epididymitis.[16]

Findings on physical examination may be variable and confusing owing to limitations in the examination due to inflammatory tenderness. Scrotal erythema and scrotal wall edema may be present in all three major conditions of the acute scrotum and are not necessarily helpful in differentiating one from another. Early acute testicular torsion may not have had time to induce significant scrotal sac changes, whereas appendicular torsion of 24 to 36 hours' duration may induce obvious thickening and redness of the scrotal wall.

Localization of tenderness to particular intrascrotal structures can be helpful. Considerable patience and gentleness during examination may allow accurate distinction among localized epididymal tenderness (epididymitis), testicular tenderness (testicular torsion), and appendicular tenderness (torsion of the appendices).

Changes in intrascrotal anatomic relationships do not seem as helpful to the diagnosis as some have suggested. The findings that have been reported to increase diagnostic accuracy include the following[17]:

1. Abnormal orientation of the testis with a transverse lie in the scrotal sac
2. Anterior presentation of the epididymis
3. Elevation of the testis induced by foreshortening of the cord
4. Absence of the cremasteric reflex on the affected side

None are pathognomonic, and all have significant limitations.

When present, the "blue dot" sign of torsion of the appendix testis or appendix epididymis is clearly diagnostic.[18] On occasion, it may not be apparent owing to the accompanying edema and erythema of the scrotal wall, particularly if the process of appendicular ischemia has been present longer than 24 hours. In this circumstance, transillumination in a darkened environment can unmask the otherwise hidden necrotic appendage, creating a "black dot" floating within the glowing scrotal contents. In other circumstances, torsed appendicular structures may not be visible but may be palpable as firm, mobile, and tender nodules, even through an edema-thickened scrotal wall. Such findings are diagnostic of appendicular torsion and, if present without focal testicular tenderness, essentially preclude the need for further evaluation. One must keep in mind the variety of locations of the appendicular structures (Fig. 51–1)[19] and make a careful search of all regions of the scrotum and groin. Of particular note is the very proximal location that the paradidymal organ of Giraldés may have along the spermatic cord, in some instances arising from the cord in the distal inguinal canal, well above the testis and even above the external inguinal ring. One patient presented

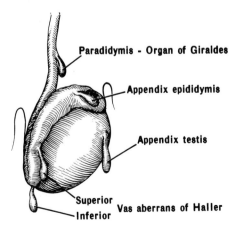

Figure 51–1. Testicular appendages. (From Rolnick D, Kawanoue S, Szanto P, et al: Anatomical incidence of testicular appendages. J Urol 100:755–756, 1968.)

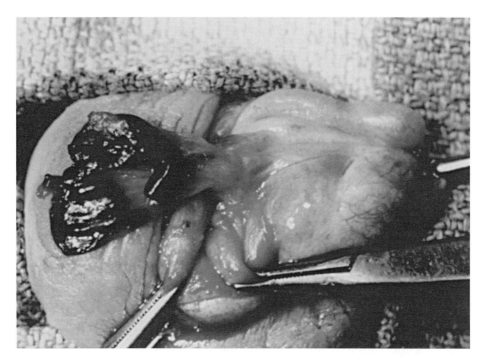

Figure 51–2. Necrotic paradidymal cyst (organ of Giraldés).

with an acute, red, and painful left groin mass suggestive of an incarcerated inguinal hernia. At exploration of the groin, an infarcted and necrotic paradidymal cyst was excised (Fig. 51–2).

In summary, the clinical presentation of the acute scrotum can be ambiguous at best, with few instances of truly pathognomonic features.[20] No constellation of findings is completely accurate. Table 51–2 includes the clinical features that typify each of the major diagnoses and that can serve as reasonable guides to their differentiation. Table 51–3 emphasizes the physical signs most consistent with the diagnosis of testicular torsion.

☐ Neonatal Torsion

Neonatal testicular torsion has a unique clinical presentation and warrants a separate discussion.

TABLE 51–2. Clinical Presentation of the Acute Scrotum

Torsion of the Testis
Acute onset
Gastrointestinal and abdominal symptoms
Focal testicular tenderness
Systemic toxicity
Previous episodes
Torsion of Appendicular Structures
Gradual onset
Absence of toxicity
"Blue dot" sign
Epididymitis
Voiding symptoms
Fever
Pyuria

True torsion of the spermatic cord from the external ring downward (extravaginal torsion) accounts for 10% or fewer of all cases of testicular infarction from torsion.[21] Although the underlying etiologic factors are not clear, it is generally believed that extravaginal torsion results either from flimsy or absent connections of the gonadal tissues to the scrotal wall, connections that occur at the time of testicular descent and shortly thereafter. These deficient or loose connections may thus permit free rotatory mobility of the testis, leading to a twisting of the gonadal vessels, with subsequent ischemic infarction. Such explanations are theoretical at best and poorly support the relatively rare occurrence of this condition. If laxity or absent tunical fixation is a principal factor leading to extravaginal torsion during or shortly after descent, one would logically expect that the incidence would be considerably higher. Thus, the underlying mechanism is not defined with any certainty. The increased incidence of testicular torsion in undescended testis, however, provides additional support for this theory because in this circumstance, the tethering attachments of the testicle are clearly abnormal and deficient.

In utero torsion is not uncommon, and a firm, apparently painless mass is often detected on initial postdelivery examination in the nursery. The scrotal skin may be discolored, ecchymotic, or edematous. In utero torsion may have occurred early enough to allow some inflammatory fixation of the infarcted gonad to the inner scrotal wall. Distinguishing neo-

TABLE 51–3. Physical Signs in Testicular Torsion

Transverse lie of testis	High-riding testis
Anterior position of epididymis	Absent cremasteric reflex

natal torsion from incarcerated hernia may necessitate urgent operation, but a salvaged testis is rarely the outcome if torsion is present. In our experience, like that of others,[22] complete infarction is generally the rule, and detorsion has not led to recovery of any such testis. The most significant indication for surgery in this setting is to provide fixation for the contralateral gonad to prevent its future loss to torsion.[23] Despite our pessimism, we do not procrastinate with management of this condition because there are reports of "testicular salvage," although long-term outcomes have not been defined.[24] We tend to agree with the viewpoint that neonatal torsion probably also accounts for the "vanishing testis" syndrome, which appears as unilateral cryptorchidism later in life.[25]

ETIOLOGIC CONSIDERATIONS

Inadequate, incomplete, or absent fixation or suspension of the testis is the underlying factor predisposing a patient to testicular torsion and infarction. Excessive freedom of movement, as provided by the flimsy or absent tunical attachments of the newborn testis; the abnormal gubernacular attachments and lack of tunical fixation in the undescended testis[26]; or the bell-clapper deformity of the intrascrotal testis of childhood[27] is considered the essential ingredient for torsion.

The term *bell-clapper deformity,* widely held as a common finding in patients with surgically proven testicular torsion, refers to the abnormally high reflection of the tunica vaginalis upward from its usual, more equatorial position about the gonad to a level of attachment to the spermatic cord itself. This arrangement of tunical attachments leaves the testicle hanging like the clapper of a bell within the tunica vaginalis, able to freely spin around the long axis of the spermatic cord. Contraction of the fibers of the cremaster muscle, initiated by events such as trauma, exercise, cold exposure, or sexual stimulation, is believed to apply a rotary force to the testis, spinning the clapper of the bell and inducing ischemia-producing cessation of gonadal arterial flow.[28]

DIAGNOSTIC TESTING

Although precise preoperative diagnosis is the goal before surgical care for the acute scrotum is begun, excessive preexploration evaluation should be avoided if delay places the testicle at any additional risk. In all instances in which the clinical presentation strongly suggests testicular torsion, surgical exploration for detorsion and fixation is mandated. Additional diagnostic tests should be set aside. However, when the clinical presentation is less clear, additional testing is often helpful.

All patients should have a complete blood count and urinalysis, including microscopic examination of the spun urinary sediment performed for baseline values. Leukocytosis may favor testicular torsion but is not specific. Pyuria suggests epididymitis and

may lead to urine culture, antibiotics, and nonoperative therapy.

Doppler Stethoscope Examination

Doppler stethoscope examinations of the scrotal blood flow have been suggested as helpful.[29] In the past, the technique had not found wide acceptance due to a high rate of false-negative findings.[30] Even with direct comparison to the asymptomatic contralateral side, scrotal wall tenderness and edema as well as local hyperemic flow tend to confuse the findings of the examination. Increasing experience with this modality and the introduction of color-coded duplex Doppler ultrasonography (US) has enhanced its role as a significant diagnostic adjunct in the acute scrotum.[31–33] Demonstration of diminished or absent arterial pulsation in the symptomatic testis, as directly compared with normal pulsatile flow in the asymptomatic testis, is strongly associated with torsion of the testicle.[34–36] We now use the data from this modality as an integral part of our preoperative evaluation of patients with the acute scrotum. Ready availability and minimal delay in obtaining the study are additional valuable aspects of its use.

Ultrasonography

US permits accurate anatomic imaging of the scrotal wall and contents in the acute scrotum, but changes in echodensity with time reduce the precision of the technique.[37] The testis may be hypoechoic with congestion and edema for the first several hours after torsion, but later it may become focally or diffusely hyperechoic, even cystic, following infarction.[38] In our experience, testicular and scrotal US is most helpful when we suspect one of the less serious causes of the acute scrotum. Traditional US images coupled with the blood flow data available from color Doppler US provide important and accurate adjunctive data for the clinician. The use of both these modalities is improving our preoperative diagnostic accuracy.[39, 40]

Scintigraphy

Nuclear testicular scintigraphy continues to be of value in the diagnosis of the acute scrotum.[41] Rapid sequential images using a technetium-99m agent with additional views employing a pinhole collimator provide the best results and the highest resolution of anatomic detail.[42]

In testicular torsion, the character of the scintigraphic image varies with the duration of ischemic insult and can be divided into three descriptive phases[43]:

Phase 1: For approximately the first 6 hours, the scintiscan blood flow to the torsed testicle does not differ markedly from the normal testis (Fig. 51–3).

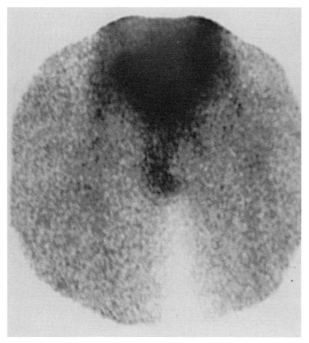

Figure 51–3. Early and midphase testicular scintigram in left testicular torsion. Note the photodeficient area in the left hemiscrotum.

Phase 2: Over the next 18 hours, the midphase scintiscan image of the involved testicle demonstrates a halo of mildly increased activity surrounding a cold center.

Phase 3: Late-phase images of an established torsion show a strongly emitting halo around a cold center.

The scintiscan image of epididymitis is manifested by markedly increased blood flow to the affected side, with no trace of a cold central area of underperfusion. A similar pattern can be seen with torsion of the appendicular structures. Such patterns of diffuse hyperperfusion strongly argue against the diagnosis of testicular torsion.

Careful application of these techniques and guidelines leads to reasonably high rates of accuracy in distinguishing testicular torsion from appendicular torsion or epididymitis. Reports of accuracy in the 90% range are not uncommon.[44] It is imperative, however, that if nuclide testicular scans are to be used in this differential diagnostic imaging, the experienced personnel and required radiopharmaceuticals must be rapidly available. It is rare to have the result of such scans available in less that 45 minutes, even under optimal conditions. The patient commonly presents to the emergency department in the evening because the red and swollen scrotum is often noted at bedtime or bath time or because the pain worsens at night. At these times, technical support is less available and 90- to 120-minute delays are not uncommon. In this circumstance, the surgeon must carefully weigh the potential risk to the testis imposed by waiting for these studies against the information to be gained. When in doubt, exploration is the safest and most appropriate action. For these reasons, we generally employ testicular imaging—specifically scintigraphy—when we suspect, on clinical grounds, that the diagnosis is epididymitis or appendicular torsion. If we are assured that scintigraphy can be completed in less than 1 hour or if the acute scrotum is of 24 hours' duration or longer, we would accept a longer delay in scintigraphy.

□ Treatment

When the diagnosis of testicular torsion is clear, manual detorsion may restore testicular blood flow. This has been done using either parenteral sedation or local anesthetic infiltration of the cord. Relief of pain seems the best endpoint, but the return of pulsatile blood flow to the testicle, as measured by Doppler stethoscope, has been used by some.[29] If manual detorsion is successful, fixation can be postponed for a short time. Prompt bilateral orchiopexy must follow, however, to protect the ipsilateral testis from early recurrence and to prophylactically secure the contralateral testis.

In most instances, acute surgical exploration for detorsion is necessary. A vertical incision in the median raphe of the scrotum allows access to both hemiscrota and is simplest to close. Paired transverse incisions oriented in the inferior scrotal rugae are acceptable as well. We prefer the raphe incision unless the torsion is called to our attention only after the infarcted testicle has undergone liquefaction or an abscess is suspected.

We treated one patient with a large scrotal abscess secondary to missed torsion when the patient presented 10 days after onset. We drained and removed the totally necrotic testis and administered broad-spectrum antibiotics. We delayed opening the contralateral hemiscrotum for testicular fixation for an additional 48 hours. This allowed the potential for infection to subside as the drainage ceased, minimizing the potential risk of infecting the contralateral scrotum.

In the usual operative scenario, detorsion of the testis cord is performed and a period of testicular observation follows. Warm, moist packs may be applied to enhance blood flow, but the ischemic insult probably induces the maximum stimulation to hyperemia. If questions about testicular viability arise, various observations have been advocated to assess potential for recovery, including active bleeding from the cut edge of the tunical albuginea, blood flow determinations by sterile Doppler probe,[29] and intravenous fluorescein staining.[45] If the testicle is viable, it must be fixed within the tunica vaginalis to prevent recurrence. Fixation of the testis requires one of two basic techniques: (1) multiple points of nonabsorbable suture anchoring the testicle within the tunica vaginalis or (2) eversion of the entire tunica vaginalis on itself to allow a large surface area for fibrous adherence of the testicle to the scrotal wall. Failing to use nonabsorbable sutures for fixation or simply reclosing the tunica vaginalis of the testis after detorsion sets the stage for potential recurrence. We prefer four-point fixation of the testis, using braided nylon sutures, and we do not close the tunica vaginalis. We do not plicate the tunical vaginalis. The same suture fixation of the contralateral testicle should be employed to prevent future torsion of the opposite testicle. The scrotal incision is closed anatomically with synthetic absorbable sutures.

An inguinal incision is used if there is any doubt about the scrotal pathology. This is particularly important when a testicular malignancy is suspected to be the cause of the scrotal swelling. The inguinal approach allows occlusion of the vascular and lymphatic components of the cord before manipulation of the testis. Failure to occlude these vessels risks venous or lymphatic spread of tumor cells. If simple torsion is found, the clamp is immediately released, detorsion performed, and fixation of the tunica albuginea is carried out through the inguinal incision. Fixation of the contralateral testicle should be done through a scrotal incision.

☐ Prognosis

If the testicle is of questionable viability, two basic concerns emerge. First, can the testicle be retained to provide an acceptable cosmetic or functional gonad? Second, will there be long-term detrimental effects from retaining the ischemically damaged testis? The duration of torsion has an effect on both the immediate salvage rates and the long-term growth of the testis.[46] Table 51–4 summarizes these data. Experimental data in dogs suggest that there is a cellular hierarchy within the testis in response to ischemia. Sertoli's cell injury was severe after as little as 4 hours of ischemia, whereas Leydig's cells were destroyed only after 10 to 12 hours of ischemia.[47] Whether these parameters apply directly to people is not known.

Several studies have demonstrated some degree of depressed spermatogenesis and infertility in men who have had sustained unilateral testicular tor-

sion,[48, 49] with the resultant degree of abnormality in semen analysis related to the duration of the ischemic injury. Whether these findings are the result of preexisting testicular abnormalities in those patients predisposed to torsion or of an autoimmune-mediated injury to the contralateral testis initiated at the time of detorsion is not yet resolved. Both human and animal study findings have been inconsistent, and results are conflicting. Thus, no clear recommendation can be made with regard to whether the testicle that has been ischemic for 12 to 24 hours should be excised or left in situ. One must be aware that the decision to leave an ischemic testis in place after an ischemic period of greater than 24 hours may not be innocuous.

In our practice we, like others,[10] tend to employ orchiectomy on an increasingly aggressive basis for torsion beyond 12 hours' duration, with the expectation that the sacrifice of one ischemic gonad is overbalanced by the long-term gains in fertility.

☐ Appendicular Torsion

When evaluation of a boy with the acute scrotum leads to the diagnosis of torsion of the appendices of the gonad, most practitioners advise expectant treatment. In most instances, bedrest, scrotal elevation or support while ambulating, and nonsteroidal antiinflammatory agents are followed by resolution of pain, tenderness, erythema, and edema.

Although some authors have admonished that appendicular torsion never requires operation, this has not been our experience. If nonoperative treatment fails to return the boy to full activity in 1 week's time, surgical excision of the necrotic appendicular structure and evacuation of the reactive hydrocele are certainly justified. In our experience, the need for operative intervention for appendicular torsion is rare, with most cases rapidly resolving over 2 to 3 days without surgery.

EPIDIDYMITIS

The antibiotic treatment of acute epididymitis is best when based on in vitro sensitivities of the causative organism. Most often, treatment is empiric because the determination of the infecting agent is difficult or impossible. In fact, urine culture findings may be negative even when a surgical diagnosis of epididymitis is made at exploration to exclude testicular torsion. It is well established that reflux of sterile urine up the vas deferens to the epididymis may induce an inflammatory response within the epididymis. Thus, the initial urinalysis and subsequent urine culture both are nondiagnostic.

The most important issue, regardless of culture-proven infection, is that the boy with acute epididymitis should have a thorough urologic evaluation to define or exclude underlying, predisposing congenital anomalies of the genitourinary tract. This evaluation should include contrast voiding cys-

TABLE 51–4. Duration of Torsion and Testicular Salvage

Duration of Torsion (h)	Testicular Salvage (%)
<6	85–97
6–12	55–85
12–24	20–80
>24	<10

Data from Smith-Harrison LI, Koontz WW Jr: Torsion of the testis: Changing concepts. In Ball TP Jr, Novicki DE, Barrett DM, et al (eds): AUA Update Series. Vol. 9 (lesson 32). Houston, American Urological Association Office of Education, 1990.

tourethrography and renal US. Ureteral ectopia, posterior urethral valves, vesicoureteral reflux, and bladder neuropathy may be related to epididymitis. Further investigation with nuclide scintigraphy, endoscopy, and other modalities such as urodynamic testing may be indicated, depending on the specific associated abnormality defined. We have treated an adolescent male who presented at age 12 years with an acute epididymitis who had a positive urine culture for *Escherichia coli.* Posterior urethral valves and reflux to the lower pole of a duplicated dysplastic left renal collecting system were found. Although such a case is not common, it illustrates the spectrum of congenital urologic diseases that may predispose boys to acute epididymitis.

REFERENCES

1. Fisher R, Walker J: The acute paediatric scrotum. Br J Hosp Med 51:290–293, 1994.
2. Kass EJ, Lundak B: The acute scrotum. Pediatr Clin North Am 44:1251–1266, 1997.
3. Noske HD, Kraus SW, Altinkilic BM, et al: Historical milestones regarding torsion of the scrotal organs. J Urol 159:13–16, 1998.
4. Rabinowitz R, Hulbert WC: Acute scrotal swelling. Urol Clin North Am 22:101–105, 1995.
5. Colodny AH: Acute urologic conditions. Pediatr Ann 23:207–210, 1994.
6. Williamson RCN: Torsion of the testis and allied conditions. Br J Surg 63:465–476, 1976.
7. Haynes BE, Bessen HA, Haynes VE: The diagnosis of testicular torsion. JAMA 249:2522–2527, 1983.
8. Jefferson RH, Perez LM, Joseph DB: Critical analysis of the clinical presentation of acute scrotum: A 9-year experience at a single institution. J Urol 158:1198–2000, 1997.
9. Leape LL: Torsion of the testis. JAMA 200:669–672, 1967.
10. Leape LL: Torsion of the testis. In Welch KJ, Randolph JG, Ravitch MM, et al (eds): Pediatric Surgery. Vol. 2 (4th ed). Chicago, Year Book Medical, 1986.
11. Klauber GT, Grannum RS: Disorders of the male external genitalia. In Kelalis PP, King LJ, Belman AB (eds): Clinical Pediatric Urology. Vol. 2 (2nd ed). Philadelphia, WB Saunders, 1985.
12. Kadish HA, Bolte RG: A retrospective review of pediatric patients with epididymitis, testicular torsion, and torsion of testicular appendages. Pediatrics 102:73–76, 1998.
13. Ransler CW, Allen TD: Torsion of the testis. Urol Clin North Am 9:245–250, 1982.
14. Workman SJ, Kogan BA: Old and new aspects of testicular torsion. Semin Urol 6:146–157, 1988.
15. Friedman SC, Sheynkin YR: Acute scrotal symptoms due to perforated appendix in children; case report and review of literature. Pediatr Emerg Care 11:181–182, 1995.
16. Lewis AG, Bukowski TP, Jarvis PD, et al: Evaluation of acute scrotum in the emergency department. J Pediatr Surg 30:277–282, 1995.
17. Ceasar RE, Kaplan GW: The incidence of the cremasteric reflex in normal boys. J Urol 15:779–780, 1994.
18. Skoglund RW, McRoberts JW, Ragde H: Torsion of the testicular appendages: Presentation of 43 new cases and a collective review. J Urol 104:604–607, 1970.
19. Rolnick D, Kawanoue S, Szanto P, et al: Anatomical incidence of testicular appendages. J Urol 100:755–756, 1968.
20. Knight PJ, Vassy LE: The diagnosis and treatment of the acute scrotum in children and adolescents. Ann Surg 200:664–673, 1984.
21. James T: Torsion of the spermatic cord in the first year of life. Br J Urol 25:56, 1953.

22. Coming DC, Hyndman CW, Deacon JSR: Intrauterine testicular torsion: Not an emergency. Urology 14:603–604, 1979.
23. Lyon RPO: Torsion of the testis in childhood: A painless emergency requiring contralateral orchiopexy. JAMA 178:702–705, 1961.
24. Jenkins GR, Noe HN, Hollabaugh RS, et al: Spermatic cord torsion in the neonate. J Urol 129:121–122, 1983.
25. Stephens FD: Embryopathology of malformations [guest editorial]. J Urol 127:13, 1982.
26. Johnston JH: The undescended testis. Arch Dis Child 40:113–122, 1965.
27. Parker RM, Robison JR: Anatomy and diagnosis of torsion of the testicle. J Urol 106:243–247, 1971.
28. Cass AS, Cass BB, Veeraraghavan K: Immediate exploration of the unilateral acute scrotum in young male subjects. J Urol 124:829–832, 1980.
29. Betts JM, Norris M, Cromie WJ, et al: Testicular detorsion using Doppler ultrasound monitoring. J Pediatr Surg 18:607–610, 1983.
30. Rodriguez DD, Rodriguez WC, Rivera JJ, et al: Doppler ultrasound versus testicular scanning in the evaluation of the acute scrotum. J Urol 135:343–346, 1981.
31. Karadeniz T, Topsakal M, Ariman A, et al: Prospective comparison of colour Doppler ultrasonography and testicular scintigraphy in acute scrotum. Int Urol Nephrol 28:543–548, 1996.
32. Schwaibold H, Fobbe F, Klau R, et al: Evaluation of acute scrotal pain by color-coded duplex sonography. Urol Int 56:96–99, 1996.
33. Suzer O, Ozcan H, Kupeli S, et al: Color Doppler imaging in the diagnosis of the acute scrotum. Eur Urol 32:457–461, 1997.
34. Luker GD, Siegel MJ: Color Doppler sonography of the scrotum in children. Am J Roentgenol 163:649–655, 1994.
35. Sanders LM, Haber S, Dembner A, et al: Significance of reversal of diastolic flow in the acute scrotum. J Ultrasound Med 13:137–139, 1994.
36. Yazbeck S, Patriquin HB: Accuracy of Doppler sonography in the evaluation of acute conditions of the scrotum in children. J Pediatr Surg 29:1270–1272, 1994.
37. Fournier GR, Laing FG, Jeffrey RB, et al: High-resolution scrotal ultrasonography: Highly sensitive but non-specific diagnostic technique. J Urol 134:490–493, 1985.
38. Hricak H, Lue T, Filly RA, et al: Experimental study of the sonographic diagnosis of testicular torsion. J Ultrasound Med 2:349–356, 1983.
39. Herbener TE: Ultrasound in the assessment of the acute scrotum. J Clin Ultrasound 24:405–421, 1996.
40. Barloon TJ, Weissman AM, Kahn D: Diagnostic imaging of patients with acute scrotal pain. Am Fam Physician 53:1734–1750, 1996.
41. Melloul M, Paz A, Lask D, et al: The value of radionuclide scrotal imaging in the diagnosis of acute testicular torsion. Br J Urol 72:628–631, 1995.
42. Fine EJ, Blaufox MD: Urologic applications of radionuclides. In Pollack HM (ed): Clinical Urography. Vol. 1. Philadelphia, WB Saunders, 1990.
43. Majd M: Nuclear medicine. In Kelalis PP, King LR, Belman AB (eds): Clinical Pediatric Urology. Vol. 1 (2nd ed). Philadelphia, WB Saunders, 1985.
44. Levu OM, Gittleman MC, Strashun AM, et al: Diagnosis of acute testicular torsion using radionuclide scanning. J Urol 129:975–977, 1983.
45. Schneider HC Jr, Kendall AR, Karafin L: Fluorescence of the testicle. Urology 5:133–136, 1975.
46. Smith-Harrison LI, Koontz WW Jr: Torsion of the testis: Changing concepts. In Ball TP Jr, Novicki DE, Barrett BM, et al (eds): AUA Update Series. Vol. 9 (lesson 32). Houston, American Urological Association Office of Education, 1990.
47. Smith GI: Cellular changes from graded testicular ischemia. J Urol 73:355–362, 1995.
48. Krarup T: The testes after torsion. Br J Urol 50:43–46, 1978.
49. Bartsch G, Frank S, Marberger H, et al: Testicular torsion: Late results with special regard to fertility and endocrine function. J Urol 124:375–378, 1980.

52

DEVELOPMENTAL AND POSITIONAL ANOMALIES OF THE KIDNEY

Douglas E. Coplen, MD

☐ Embryology

Congenital anomalies of the genitourinary (GU) tract are common and occur in 10% of the population. If other organ systems are affected, the incidence increases to 30%, and if one urinary tract anomaly is present, a second anomaly is much more likely. A complete description of the complex embryologic interactions that often result in GU anomalies is found in standard texts.[1–3] The high incidence of associated abnormalities suggests a generalized embryologic insult between the 6th and 8th week of life.

Renal development depends on the presence of the urogenital ridge that contains the nephric, gonadal, and genital duct primordia. The three distinct stages of renal development—pronephros, mesonephros, and metanephrosis—are found in the ridge. The pronephros is the mature excretory structure in primitive vertebrates. It functions only in the first 4 weeks of embryonic life in human beings.

The mesonephros functions between the 4th and 8th week. When the mesonephric tubules join the pronephric duct, the mesonephric, or wolffian duct is formed. This is the single most important structure in development of the entire urinary tract. Faulty development results in a variety of GU anomalies. The differentiation of the metanephros into the metanephric blastema is entirely dependent on normal development and cranial growth of the ureteral bud beginning in the 5th week of gestation. The bud arises from the mesonephric duct. The metanephros envelops the bud and gives rise to the renal cortex.

While the kidney differentiates between the 9th and 12th week, the metanephros ascends, rotates, and revascularizes. Ascent occurs from the 4th lumbar vertebra to the 1st lumbar or 12th thoracic vertebra as a result of both cephalad migration and caudal growth of the fetus. While the kidney ascends, the renal pelvis rotates 90 degrees from an anterior position to a medial position. The kidney is progressively supplied by arteries that are located higher on the urogenital ridge. Failure of any of these steps to occur results in anomalies of number, volume, position, and form.

☐ Abnormalities of Development

RENAL AGENESIS

The presence of a normal ureteral bud is a prerequisite to normal renal development; thus, in the vast majority of cases of renal agenesis, a ureteral bud abnormality existed during development. These include absence of the GU ridge, failure of development of the mesonephric duct, failure of ureteral bud to form off the mesonephric duct, or failure of the ureteral bud to reach the metanephros.[3] Failure of the vascular supply to invade the metanephric blastema or a primary metanephric defect also results in renal agenesis.

If there is complete failure of the GU ridge, the kidney, ureter, genital ducts, and testis are absent on the ipsilateral side. Failure of the mesonephros to form results in absence of the vas deferens and epididymis. If the ureteral bud is absent, a hemitrigone develops in the bladder; however, if there is metanephric failure, a normal trigone, vas deferens, and epididymis are present. Owing to the proximity of the müllerian and wolffian ducts, vaginal and uterine abnormalities, including complete agenesis, partial absence, and duplications, occur in conjunction with renal agenesis.[4]

Unilateral Renal Agenesis

The incidence of unilateral renal agenesis is between 1 in 500 to 1000 live births, and males predominate in a ratio of 2:1.[5] Absence is more common on the left side, and there is a familial predominance.[6] There are usually no physical signs to suggest absence of the kidney, and detection is

681

usually a result of thorough evaluation of other abnormalities detected on physical examination or in the evaluation of the newborn with multiple congenital anomalies including imperforate anus, esophageal atresia, and cardiovascular disease (e.g., VACTERL [*v*ertebral, *a*nal, *c*ardiac, *t*racheal, *e*sophageal, *r*enal, and *l*imb]).

Plain abdominal radiographs may show deviation of either the hepatic or splenic flexure that is suggestive of renal absence.[7, 8] This can be confirmed using ultrasonography (US), excretory urography, or radionuclide scans. Compensatory hypertrophy of the contralateral kidney is almost always present. Unilateral renal agenesis can also be noted on routine antenatal sonography.

Those who have a kidney removed for donor nephrectomy, as a consequence of trauma, or due to tumors, may be at higher risk for hypertension and glomerulosclerosis, but there is no evidence that patients with a congenital solitary kidney have increased susceptibility to renal disease.[9]

Bilateral Renal Agenesis

Bilateral renal agenesis occurs once in 4800 births.[10] There is a 3:1 male predominance. Nearly 40% of infants are stillborn and most do not survive more than 48 hours owing to respiratory distress secondary to pulmonary hypoplasia. Rare patients with essentially normal pulmonary function have been described.[11]

Oligohydramnios is the most common maternal or antenatal sign. Infants have a low birth weight, and respiratory distress is noted. There is a characteristic appearance to the facies consisting of a prominent skin fold beginning over the eye swinging over the medial canthus and then lateral to the cheek, a blunted nose, and low-set flattened ears.[12] The chest wall is bell shaped.

Pathologically, there is complete or partial absence of both ureters. The bladder, if present, is poorly developed because there was no urine production. The vas deferens is normal in most cases, implying that bilateral agenesis usually results from ureteral bud or metanephric abnormalities.[13] Female genitalia and duct structures are more severely affected.[14]

SUPERNUMERARY KIDNEYS

Supernumerary kidneys are extremely rare accessory organs that are distinct, encapsulated, and separated from the ipsilateral kidney.[15, 16] Attachment is, at most, by thin fibrous attachments. The kidney is reniform and usually smaller than the normal kidney. The ipsilateral kidney has the full complement of calyces and additional calyces are present in the supernumerary kidney.

This is most likely a result of induction of separate metanephric bodies, as opposed to tandem or bifid ureteral bud induction of a single metanephros.[16] An alternate explanation is fragmentation or

segmental infarction of a single metanephros. The supernumerary kidney is subserved by a branch of a bifid ureter or separate (complete duplication) ureter. It is usually located caudal to the ipsilateral kidney when there is a bifid ureter and is cranially located when there is a complete duplication. There is wide variety in ureteral anatomy, but, in most cases, the most caudal kidney has the most cranial ureteral insertion into the bladder.

Only one third of these kidneys cause a clinical problem.[16] Obstructive symptoms, calculi, infection, neoplasia, and urinary incontinence secondary to ureteral ectopia are the presenting symptoms and findings. If this is detected at the time of other imaging, elective excision of a small abnormal kidney is indicated, but if the kidney is "normal," observation with regular follow-up is advised. If the unsuspected condition is found at the time of surgery, other renal function is determined to be normal, and the kidney is small and abnormal in appearance, excision is advised.

ECTOPIA AND FUSION ANOMALIES

Multiple factors involving the ureteral buds, the metanephros, and the caudal fetal environment must interact to form ectopia and fusion anomalies (Fig. 52–1). Abnormal positioning of the kidney may be caused by arrest of development on the normal path of migration, migration beyond the normal limit, ectopia of the metanephrosis, or induction of the contralateral metanephros by a wandering ureteral bud.[17]

SIMPLE RENAL ECTOPIA

Simple renal ectopia is defined as an abnormal ipsilateral renal location and is identified by the site of termination: pelvic, lumbar, abdominal, or thoracic. It can be explained as abnormal renal ascent with normal ureteral relationships that deviate only due to incomplete rotation. The blood supply is abnormal, with multiple arteries arising from the nearest great vessel, and persistence of these abnormal vascular attachments may be the factor that prevents migration.

The simple ectopic kidney may be detected on antenatal US, but most do not cause any clinical problem and are detected incidentally. The kidney can be missed on US because the absence of a renal sinus results in absence of the typical central echo complex.[18] In a very thin patient, the kidney may be palpable as a low-lying abdominal mass. Because the kidney is often incompletely rotated, the ureteral insertion may be abnormal and predispose to hydronephrosis, infection, or calculi. Lower kidneys may be more susceptible to trauma.

Renal ectopia cranial to the normal lumbar location is rare and the kidney may be above, below, or partly through the diaphragm.[19] If the kidney is in the thorax, it is almost always on the left. The kidney is extrapleural and has no effect on pulmonary

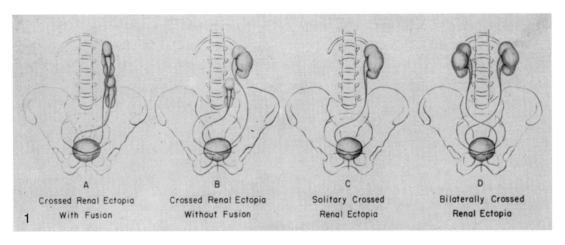

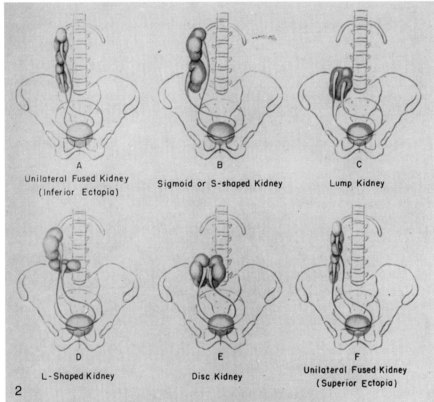

Figure 52–1. Variations of crossed renal ectopia with and without fusion. *1,* Four types of crossed ectopia without fusion. *2,* Six forms of crossed ectopia with fusion. (From Bauer SB: Anomalies of the kidney and ureteropelvic junction. In Walsh PC, Retik AB, Vaughan ED Jr, et al [eds]: Campbell's Urology [7th ed]. Philadelphia, WB Saunders, 1997, pp 1721–1722.)

function. Kidney migration is independent of and precedes development of the diaphragm and the adrenal gland, which is often caudal to the thoracic kidney. The diagnosis is usually made on the basis of an abnormal chest radiograph. There is not an association with congenital diaphragmatic hernia.

CROSSED RENAL ECTOPIA

When a kidney lies on the side opposite its ureteral insertion into the bladder, it is known as *crossed ectopia.* The spectrum of fusion anomalies is shown in Figure 52–1. Ninety percent of crossed ectopic kidneys are fused to their ipsilateral mate. Left-to-right crossover is more common, and the anomaly is more common in males. The crossed kidney is usually caudal. The kidneys usually function normally, and the ureters have normal insertion into the bladder. If an abnormality is present, it usually consists of cystic dysplasia, obstruction, or vesicoureteral reflux in the ectopic kidney.[20–22] Solitary crossed ectopia rarely occurs,[23] and these patients have a hemitrigone with an absent ureter on the side of the ectopic kidney. As with renal agenesis, the incidence of cryptorchidism and vasal, vaginal, and uterine anomalies is increased in this subset.

The embryology of crossed renal ectopia is poorly understood. Migration may occur normally but stops when the cephalad kidney reaches its normal location or when retroperitoneal structures or vessels prevent migration of the fused mass. Malalignment and abnormal rotation of the caudal end of the fetus (e.g., hemivertebra) may induce the contralateral metanephros by a ureteric bud that is abnormally directed from a medially deviated wolffian duct.[24, 25] This might explain the higher incidence of fusion anomalies in patients with cloacal exstrophy and imperforate anus.

Most of these kidneys are asymptomatic, and detection is incidental. Symptoms related to obstruction and calculi develop in the third and fourth decades.[21]

HORSESHOE KIDNEY

Horseshoe kidney is the most common of all fusion anomalies. It occurs in 1 in 400 people and is twice as common in males.[26] The abnormality is discovered clinically in all age groups, but it is more commonly identified in children owing to the high incidence of associated congenital anomalies.[27]

The abnormality occurs early in gestation, between the 4th and 6th weeks, before rotation and ascent. A change in the position of the iliac arteries might deflect the lower poles of the kidney medially, leading to contact and fusion.[28] Caudal displacement of the metanephros may cause end-on, end-to-side, or side-by-side contiguity. Midline impaction results in a symmetric horseshoe, whereas other types evolve into a wide variety of asymmetric forms.[25] Predisposing factors are agenesis of the sacral segments and high cloacal anomalies. There is an association with undescended testes, bicornuate uterus, septate vagina, and 45XO gonadal dysgenesis (Turner's syndrome).[29]

There are many variations on the basic shape of the horseshoe kidney (Fig. 52–2). The anomaly consists of two distinct renal masses that lie on either side of the midline and are attached by parenchyma or a fibrous isthmus, usually at the lower pole but occasionally at the upper pole.[30] The kidneys usually lie lower than normal kidneys, presumably because the fused isthmus' cephalad migration is stopped by the inferior mesenteric artery. Because the kidneys fail to rotate, the renal pelvis is deviated anteriorly and the axis of the pelvis is parallel to the spine or even medially deviated caudally. The lower pole calyces are closer to the midline than the upper pole calyces. Although the ureteral insertion is high and lateral owing to the incomplete rotation, insertion into the bladder is usually normal. Blood supply is anomalous, ranging from a single artery to each kidney (30%) to marked asymmetry, with vessels arising from the inferior mesenteric, iliac, and sacral vessels.

Nearly one third of all patients with a horseshoe kidney have no symptoms. The most common symptom is vague abdominal or lower back pain.

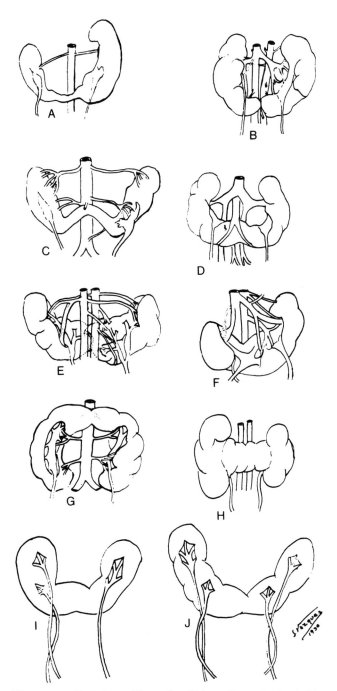

Figure 52–2. Variations of horseshoe kidney. (From Benjamin JA, Schullian DM: J Hist Med Allied Sci 5:315, 1950, after Gutierrez, 1931, by permission of Oxford University Press.)

Collecting system abnormalities are common and lead to the hydronephrosis, infection, or stone formation that is responsible for most symptoms. Ureteral duplication is present in 10%,[29] reflux is present in up to 50%,[27] and ureteropelvic junction (UPJ) obstruction causes significant hydronephrosis in up to one third of patients.[31]

Intervention is most commonly required for UPJ obstruction and its sequelae. Both intrinsic stenosis and high insertion play a role. The ureter often drapes over the parenchyma so that the standard dismembered anastomosis may not give the appropriate funneled, dependent anastomosis. A nondismembered repair may be preferred. Division of the isthmus is rarely required. The stasis in the renal pelvis predisposes the patient to renal calculi, which can be treated with extracorporeal lithotripsy, percutaneous approaches, or open surgery.

Horseshoe kidneys do appear to carry a higher risk for renal tumors.[32, 33] Most of these are renal cell carcinomas, but the incidence of Wilms' tumor is twice that expected in the general population.[34] Although the anomalous vessels can make surgical treatment of these tumors challenging, survival is related to pathology and stage.[35]

□ Cystic Abnormalities

AUTOSOMAL RECESSIVE POLYCYSTIC KIDNEY DISEASE

Autosomal recessive polycystic kidney disease (ARPKD) is usually diagnosed antenatally or in the neonate. It occurs in about 1 in 40,000 live births,[36] and the majority die in the first few days of life. It is also known as *infantile polycystic kidney disease,* but this is an inaccurate designation because the disease can present as late as 15 years of age.[37]

The disease is characterized by renal and hepatic cystic disease. The renal manifestations are variable, and ARPKD has been divided into four subtypes based on age at presentation and severity of renal disease.[38] In general, younger patients present with severe renal disease and milder liver disease, whereas those patients who present with hepatic fibrosis have milder renal disease. Despite the disease variability, a single gene locus on chromosome 6 has been identified.[39]

The clinical presentation and course are variable (Table 52–1). Neonates present with hard flank masses that do not transilluminate. Oligohydramnios is usually present, and the newborn may have respiratory distress owing to pulmonary hypoplasia. As with any newborn with an abdominal mass, the differential diagnosis includes hydronephrosis, adrenal and renal tumors, and renal vein thrombosis. The usual clinical course is death in the first 2 months of life secondary to renal or respiratory failure. If the infant survives the neonatal period, more than 90% will survive 1 year. Most have some degree of renal insufficiency, but hemodialysis may not be required until 5 years of age.[40]

Antenatal US may reveal enlarged echogenic kidneys without cysts and with diminished amniotic fluid, but even in at-risk pregnancies, the diagnosis can be missed.[36, 41] In the newborn, US reveals homogeneously hyperechogenic kidneys. The increased echogenicity arises from the tightly compacted, dilated collecting ducts. The bilaterality and homogeneity excludes most other diagnoses in the differential. If cysts are identified sonographically in the newborn, then the diagnosis of multicystic dysplastic kidney (MCDK) or autosomal dominant polycystic kidney disease (ADPKD) must be considered. Intravenous pyelography reveals radial streaking (sunburst) on delayed views.[42]

Pathologic evaluation of the kidneys reveals small subcapsular cysts that are actually fusiform dilations of the collecting tubules (Fig. 52–3). There is no clear demarcation between the cortex and the medulla. The nephron configuration is normal, suggesting that the abnormality develops after nephrogenesis.[43] In older patients the kidneys become progressively smaller as renal failure develops. All patients have hepatic disease consisting of biliary ectasia and periportal fibrosis.[44]

Treatment for ARPKD is supportive. An aggressive surgical approach that includes removal of the kidneys to treat mechanical respiratory failure has been reported.[45, 46] Patients who survive the neonatal period require treatment for systemic hypertension, renal failure, and hepatic failure. Hepatocellular dysfunction is rarely seen, but portal hypertension may require shunting. Hemodialysis and renal transplantation are eventually required in many patients.

AUTOSOMAL DOMINANT POLYCYSTIC KIDNEY DISEASE

ADPKD is the most common form of cystic disease in people and is the etiology for 10% of end-stage renal disease.[47] The incidence is approximately 1 in 500 individuals. Although most cases present in the third to fifth decade of life with flank pain, hematuria, hypertension, pyelonephritis, and progressive renal failure, the condition has been

TABLE 52-1. Blyth and Ockenden's Subdivision of Autosomal Recessive Polycystic Kidney Disease

Feature	Perinatal	Neonatal	Infantile	Juvenile
Age at presentation	At birth	<1 mo	3–6 mo	1–5 y
Presentation	Abdominal masses Normal liver	Large kidneys Large liver	Large kidneys Hepatosplenomegaly	? Renal enlargement Hepatomegaly
Course	Death by 6 wk	Death in 1st y	Some survive at least 10 y	Some survive 15 y
Renal involvement	>90%	60%	25%	<10%
Periportal fibrosis	Minimal	Mild	Moderate	Severe

Modified from Blyth H, Ockenden BG: Polycystic disease of kidneys and liver presenting in childhood. J Med Genet 8:257, 1971.

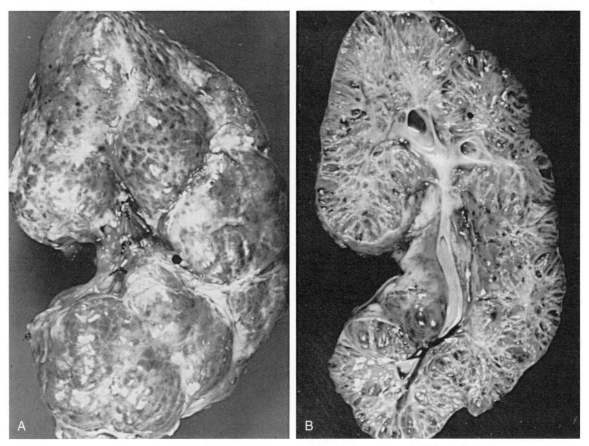

Figure 52–3. Gross appearance of autosomal recessive polycystic kidney disease.

recognized in fetuses and newborns; therefore, the historical classification as "adult" is inaccurate.[48, 49] Fewer than 10% of patients present in the first decade of life.[50]

Prenatal diagnosis is possible using both US and genetic screening.[48, 51] All USs show cystic dilations, but no data are available on the significance of prenatal US patterns and postnatal outcomes.[52] Neonates usually present due to renal enlargement. When this is the case, stillbirth or significant respiratory distress can occur. However, renal involvement is variable at birth. When families with ADPKD are screened, 80% of children diagnosed prenatally or in the 1st year of life have a normal creatinine clearance.[49] Most have hypertension, but only 20% require hemodialysis in the first 7 years of life.

In children who present after 1 year of age, early manifestations of the disease include hypertension, proteinuria, impaired renal function, and palpably enlarged kidneys. Another population is symptom-free and diagnosed sonographically as part of sibling screening. When compared with gene linkage analysis of the two ADPKD loci (chromosome 4 and 16), the overall false-negative rate for these screenings is 25%.[53]

Renal cysts are present throughout the cortex and medulla, with communications at various points along the nephron.[43] In contrast with adult kidneys,

glomeruli seem to be predominantly affected in fetal ADPKD.[48] This may explain the subset of newborns who do poorly. Hepatic disease is manifest as biliary cysts without the periportal fibrosis and portal hypertension seen in ARPKD. Associated anomalies include cysts of the liver, pancreas, spleen, and lungs as well as aneurysms of the circle of Willis (berry aneurysms) and mitral valve prolapse.

Treatment depends on renal function. Symptomatic children usually have significant renal insufficiency. Dialysis and transplantation are appropriate. Now that genetic screening is available, living related donation is appropriate.

MULTICYSTIC DYSPLASTIC KIDNEY

The pathologic finding of primitive ducts surrounded by concentric rings of connective tissue is diagnostic of renal dysplasia.[54] Primitive glomeruli and metaplastic rests of cartilage may be present but are not required for the diagnosis. Dysplasia may be total, focal, or dispersed throughout normal renal architecture. The embryogenesis may be related to defective bud formation, as is seen in some cases of severe reflux, abnormal induction of the metanephric blastema, or qualitative mesodermal abnormalities like those seen in prune-belly syndrome.[55–57] Complete urinary tract obstruction before 70 days' gestation in the fetal lamb causes dysplasia,[58, 59] but obstruction later in gestation causes only hydrone-phrosis.[60]

The MCDK represents the most extreme end of the spectrum of renal dysplasia. The kidney is composed of multiple cysts of variable sizes with little intervening stroma (Fig. 52–4). The abnormal development probably begins around the 8th week of gestation. There is no good experimental model that results in an MCDK. Complete obstruction of the ureter in conjunction with ischemia of the ureter and kidney caused by faulty vascularization during migration and differentiation of the kidney may account for the cystic dysplasia.[61] This ischemia may play a role in the involution that commonly occurs postnatally.

MCDK is the most common form of renal cystic disease in the newborn. The kidney does not have a reniform shape, and no collecting system is identifiable. The left side is most commonly involved. Prenatal US has increased the detection of MCDK. The abnormality is bilateral 20% of the time, and these newborns have the characteristic facies and pulmonary hypoplasia associated with oligohydramnios.[62] Older patients may present with an abdominal mass, abdominal pain, hematuria, or hypertension or during abdominal imaging for an unrelated condition.

It is important to distinguish between MCDK and hydronephrosis. Both may present as renal masses, and US usually differentiates the two diagnoses. The MCDK has a haphazard arrangement of separate cysts, whereas in hydronephrosis, the cysts are arranged around the periphery and communicate with each other. It is most difficult to differentiate MCDK from severe hydronephrosis. In these cases, radioisotope studies are useful because there is almost always some function in the hydronephrotic kidney, and function is rarely seen in multicystic kidneys. Multicystic dysplasia has been described in one pole of a duplex kidney and as half of a renal fusion anomaly.[63, 64]

The contralateral kidney is frequently abnormal. UPJ obstruction is found up to 12% of the time and vesicoureteral reflux is detected in up to 30% of infants.[65] Voiding cystograms should be obtained in all of these children because reflux places the only functioning kidney at risk.

If MCDK is suspected prenatally, this needs to be confirmed because congenital renal tumors have been mistakenly identified as multicystic kidneys.[66] Once the diagnosis has been made, the multicystic kidney can usually be observed unless the size of the kidney is causing symptoms or hypertension is present. The emphasis should be placed on evaluation and appropriate treatment of any abnormalities of the contralateral kidney. If there is uncertainty with respect to the diagnosis, exploration may be indicated.[67] Involution of the multicystic kidney is expected.[68, 69] The kidney may involute in the first 6 months of life, but this process may take as long as 20 years.

The major concern regarding multicystic kidneys is the potential for malignant degeneration. There is one report in the literature of malignant degeneration of a multicystic kidney.[70] Other reports describe malignancy developing in previously "unrecognized" multicystic kidneys, but most of these were probably not truly multicystic kidneys.[71] The available literature offers no proof that the incidence of tumor is higher in individuals with retained multicystic kidneys than in individuals with normal kidneys. The best approach is to follow the kidney with US. If there is increasing size at any time or no evidence of involution after 3 to 5 years, then removal may be recommended, although continued observation with US is not contraindicated.

MULTILOCULAR CYSTIC NEPHROMA

Multilocular cystic renal lesions are rare. They should not be confused with an isolated renal segment affected by multicystic kidney disease. These lesions are usually unilateral, bulky, encapsulated, and compress the surrounding normal renal parenchyma.[72, 73] The cysts do not communicate with one another or with the renal pelvis, and the septa are lined with fibrous or embryonic-type tissue. Although in children there may be a continuum from benign multilocular cyst to cystic Wilms' tumor, there is no evidence that one entity transforms into another.[74]

The majority of patients present before age 2 years or after 40 years.[73] Males predominate in the child-

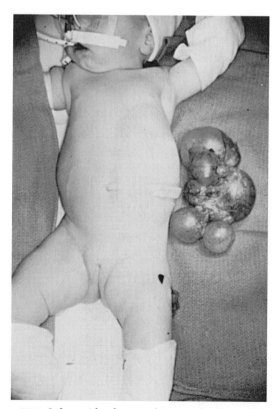

Figure 52–4. Infant with a large multicystic dysplastic kidney. A kidney was displacing the stomach and affecting nutrition.

hood group. Most present with an asymptomatic flank mass, although bleeding may occur if one of the cysts erodes into the renal pelvis.[72] US and computed tomography reveal the cystic nature of the mass and help differentiate the lesion from multicystic kidneys. The septa may enhance, but they are less dense than normal parenchyma. However, the tests cannot exclude cystic Wilms' or cystic mesoblastic nephroma.

Because malignancy cannot be excluded, the treatment for multilocular cysts is nephrectomy. Careful pathologic evaluation is required and subsequent therapy is dictated by these results. For smaller lesions, enucleation or partial nephrectomy may be performed, although there is a small risk of local recurrence.

SIMPLE CYSTS

The cause of simple cysts is unknown, but the fact that they are frequent in adults (50%) and rare in children (0.2%) suggests that they are acquired.[75] They are benign lesions located in the cortex and lined by a simple epithelium. They do not communicate with the nephron and may be single, multiple, unilateral, or bilateral. The pathogenesis is uncertain. They may be retained rudimentary glomeruli that normally undergo absorption, or they may be the result of tubular obstruction secondary to ischemia or inflammation.[76] Most do not cause any symptoms and are incidentally discovered during evaluation for other abdominal complaints.

US is the only diagnostic test required when there is an absence of internal echoes, a distinct wall with distinct margins, and good through transmission with posterior acoustic enhancement.[77] When these criteria are not met, computed tomography is the most useful adjunct. Cysts should not enhance. It is important to differentiate the simple cyst from a calyceal diverticulum and a hydrocalyx. Both of these communicate with the urinary tract and predispose to urinary tract infection and urolithiasis. Intravenous or retrograde pyelography identifies these abnormalities, if present.

Simple cysts rarely require intervention. Once malignancy has been excluded, cyst puncture or surgical unroofing is not indicated.[76] A centrally placed cyst may rarely cause hypertension or renal pelvic obstruction and require intervention.

REFERENCES

1. Moore KL: The urogenital system. In Moore KL (ed): The Developing Human: Clinically Oriented Embryology (2nd ed). Philadelphia, WB Saunders, 1977, pp 220–231.
2. Gray SW, Skandalakis JE: The kidney and ureter. In Gray SW, Skandalakis JE (eds): Embryology for Surgeons. Philadelphia, WB Saunders, 1972, pp 443–518.
3. Stephens FD: The kidney. In Stephens FD, Smith ED, Hutson JM (eds): Congenital Anomalies of the Urinary and Genital Tracts. Oxford, Isis Medical Media, 1996, pp 283–374.
4. Tarry WF, Duckett JW, Stephens FD: The Mayer-Rokitansky syndrome: Pathogenesis, classification, and management. J Urol 136:648, 1986.
5. Doroshow LW, Abeshouse BS: Congenital unilateral solitary kidney: Report of 37 cases and a review of the literature. Urol Surv 11:219, 1961.
6. Kohn G, Borns PF: The association of bilateral and unilateral renal aplasia in the same family. J Pediatr 83:95, 1973.
7. Mascatello V, Lebowitz RL: Malposition of the colon in left renal agenesis and ectopia. Radiology 120:371, 1976.
8. Curtis JA, Sadhu V, Steiner RM: Malposition of the colon in right renal agenesis, ectopia, and anterior nephrectomy. AJR Am J Roentgenol 129:845, 1977.
9. Brenner BM, Meyer TW, Hostetter TH: Dietary protein intake and the progressive nature of kidney disease: The role of hemodynamically mediated glomerular injury in the pathogenesis of progressive glomerular sclerosis in aging, renal ablation, and intrinsic renal disease. N Engl J Med 307:652, 1982.
10. Potter EL: Bilateral absence of ureters and kidneys: A report of 50 cases. Obstet Gynecol 25:3, 1965.
11. Davidson WM, Ross GIM: Bilateral absence of the kidneys and related congenital anomalies. J Pathol 68:459, 1954.
12. Potter EL: Facial characteristics in infants with bilateral renal agenesis. Am J Obstet Gynecol 51:885, 1946.
13. Ashley DJB, Mostofi FK: Renal agenesis and dysgenesis. J Urol 83:211, 1960.
14. Carpentier PJ, Potter EL: Nuclear sex and genital malformation in 48 cases of renal agenesis with special reference to nonspecific female pseudohermaphroditism. Am J Obstet Gynecol 78:235, 1959.
15. Geisinger JG: Supernumerary kidney. J Urol 38:331, 1937.
16. N'Guessan G, Stephens FD: Supernumerary kidney. J Urol 130:649, 1983.
17. Stephens FD: Renal ectopy. In Stephens FD, Smith ED, Hutson JM (eds): Congenital Anomalies of the Urinary and Genital Tracts. Oxford, Isis Medical Media, 1996, pp 322–340.
18. Barnewolt CE, Lebowitz RL: Absence of a renal sinus echo in the ectopic kidney of a child: A normal finding. Pediatr Radiol 26:318, 1996.
19. N'Guessan G, Stephens FD, Pick J: Congenital superior ectopic (thoracic) kidney. Urology 24:219, 1984.
20. Caldamone AA, Rabinowitz R: Crossed fused renal ectopia, orthotopic multicystic dysplasia, and vaginal agenesis. J Urol 126:105, 1981.
21. Gleason PE, Kelalis PP, Husmann DA, et al: Hydronephrosis in renal ectopia: Incidence, etiology, and significance. J Urol 151:1660, 1994.
22. Hertz M, Rabenstein ZJ, Shalrin N, et al: Crossed renal ectopia: Clinical and radiologic findings in 22 cases. Clin Radiol 28:339, 1977.
23. Gu LL, Alton DJ: Crossed solitary renal ectopia. Urology 38:556, 1991.
24. Maizels M, Stephens FD: Renal ectopia and congenital scoliosis. Invest Urol 17:209, 1979.
25. Cook WA, Stephens FD: Fused kidneys: Morphologic study and theory of embryogenesis. In Bergsma D, Duckett JW (eds): Urinary System Malformations in Children. New York, Alan R. Liss, 1977, p 327.
26. Campbell MF: Anomalies of the kidney. In Campbell MF, Harrison JH (eds): Urology. Philadelphia, WB Saunders, 1970, p 1447.
27. Segura JW, Kelalis PP, Burke EC: Horseshoe kidney in children. J Urol 108:333, 1972.
28. Benjamin JA, Schullian DM: Observation on fused kidneys with a horseshoe configuration: The contribution of Leonard Botallo (1564). J Hist Med 5:315, 1950.
29. Boatman DL, Kollen CP, Flocks RH: Congenital anomalies associated with horseshoe kidneys. J Urol 107:205, 1972.
30. Glenn JF: Analysis of 51 patients with horseshoe kidney. N Engl J Med 261:684, 1959.
31. Whitehouse GH: Some urographic aspects of the horseshoe kidney anomaly—a review of 59 cases. Clin Radiol 26:107, 1975.
32. Buntley D: Malignancy associated with horseshoe kidney. Urology 8:146, 1976.
33. Hohenfellner M, Schultz-Lampel D, Lampel A, et al: Tumor in the horseshoe kidney: Clinical implications and review of embryogenesis. J Urol 147:1098, 1992.

34. Mesrobian HJ, Kelalis PP, Hrabovsky E, et al: Wilms' tumor in horseshoe kidneys: A report from the national Wilms' tumor study. J Urol 133:1002, 1985.

35. Murphy DM, Zincke H: Transitional cell carcinoma in the horseshoe kidney: Report of 3 cases and review of the literature. Br J Urol 54:484, 1982.

36. Zerres K, Hansmann M, Mallman R, et al: Autosomal recessive polycystic kidney disease: Problems of prenatal diagnosis. Prenat Diagn 8:215, 1988.

37. Zerres K, Rudnik-Schoneborn S, Deget F, et al: Autosomal recessive polycystic kidney disease in 115 children: Clinical presentation, course, and influence of gender. Acta Paediatr 85:437, 1996.

38. Blyth H, Ockenden BG: Polycystic disease of kidney and liver presenting in childhood. J Med Genet 8:257, 1971.

39. Guay-Woodford LM, Mueecher G, Hopkins SD, et al: The severe perinatal form of autosomal recessive polycystic kidney disease maps to chromosome 6p21.1–p12: Implications for genetic counseling. Am J Hum Genet 56:110, 1995.

40. Cole BR, Conley SB, Stapleton FB: Polycystic kidney disease in the first year of life. J Pediatr 111:693, 1987.

41. Fong KW, Rahmani MR, Rose Th, et al: Fetal renal cystic disease: Sonographic pathologic correlation. AJR Am J Roentgenol 146:767, 1986.

42. Gagnadoux M, Habib R, Levy M, et al: Cystic renal disease in children. Adv Nephrol Necker Hosp 18:33, 1989.

43. Wilson PD, Falkenstein D: The pathology of human renal cystic disease. Curr Top Pathol 88:1, 1995.

44. Darmis F, Najum H, Mosse A, et al: Fibrose hépatique congénitale à progression clinique renal. Presse Med 78:885, 1970.

45. Bean SA, Bednarek FJ, Primack WA: Aggressive respiratory support and unilateral nephrectomy for infants with severe perinatal autosomal recessive polycystic kidney disease. J Pediatr 127:311, 1995.

46. Sumfest JM, Burns MW, Mitchell ME: Aggressive surgical and medical management of autosomal recessive polycystic kidney disease. Urology 42:309, 1993.

47. Gabow PA: Autosomal dominant polycystic kidney disease. N Engl J Med 329:332, 1993.

48. Michaud J, Russo P, Grignon A, et al: Autosomal dominant polycystic kidney disease in the fetus. Am J Med Genet 51:240, 1994.

49. Fick GM, Johnson AM, Strain JD, et al: Characteristics of very early onset autosomal dominant polycystic kidney disease. J Am Soc Nephrol 3:1863, 1993.

50. Bernstein J: Developmental abnormalities of the renal parenchyma: Renal hypoplasia and dysplasia. Pathol Annual 3:213, 1968.

51. Turco AE, Peissel B, Rossetti S, et al: Rapid DNA-based prenatal diagnosis of autosomal dominant polycystic kidney disease. Arch Pediatr Adolesc Med 148:1101, 1994.

52. Sinibaldi D, Malena S, Mingarelli R, et al: Prenatal ultrasonographic findings of dominant polycystic kidney disease and postnatal renal evolution. Am J Med Genet 65:337, 1996.

53. Gabow PA, Kimberling WJ, Strain JD, et al: Utility of ultrasonography in the diagnosis of autosomal dominant polycystic kidney disease in children. J Am Soc Nephrol 8:105, 1997.

54. Bernstein J: The morphogenesis of renal parenchymal maldevelopment (renal dysplasia). Pediatr Clin North Am 18:395, 1971.

55. Schwarz RD, Stephens FD, Cussen LJ: The pathogenesis of renal dysplasia, I: Quantification of hypoplasia and dysplasia. Invest Urol 19:94, 1981.

56. Schwarz RD, Stephens FD, Cussen LJ: The pathogenesis of renal dysplasia, II: The significance of lateral and medial ectopy of the ureteric orifice. Invest Urol 19:97, 1981.

57. Schwarz RD, Stephens FD, Cussen LJ: The pathogenesis of renal dysplasia, III: Complete and incomplete urinary obstruction. Invest Urol 19:101, 1981.

58. Beck AD: The effect of intrauterine urinary obstruction upon the development of the fetal kidney. J Urol 105:784, 1971.

59. Gonzalez R, Reinberg Y, Burke B, et al: Early bladder outlet obstruction in fetal lambs induces renal dysplasia and the prune-belly syndrome. J Pediatr Surg 25:342, 1990.

60. Harrison MR, Ross N, Noall RA, et al: Correction of congenital hydronephrosis in utero, I: The model: Fetal urethral obstruction produces hydronephrosis and pulmonary hypoplasia in fetal lambs. J Pediatr Surg 18:247, 1983.

61. Stephens FD, Cussen LJ: Renal dysgenesis: A "urologic" classification. In Stephens FD (ed): Congenital Malformations of the Urinary Tract. New York, Praeger, 1983, pp 463–475.

62. Al-Khaldi N, Watson AR, Zuccollo J, et al: Outcome of antenatally detected cystic dysplastic kidney disease. Arch Dis Child 70:520, 1994.

63. Walker RD, Fennell R, Garin E, et al: Spectrum of multicystic renal dysplasia: Diagnosis and management. Urology 11:433, 1978.

64. Corrales JG, Elder JS: Segmental multicystic kidney and ipsilateral duplication anomalies. J Urol 155:1398, 1996.

65. Flack CE, Bellinger MF: The multicystic dysplastic kidney and contralateral vesicoureteral reflux: Protection of the solitary kidney. J Urol 150:1873, 1993.

66. Oliveria-Filho AG, Carvalho MH, Sbragia-Neto L, et al: Wilms' tumor in a prenatally diagnosed multicystic kidney. J Urol 158:1926, 1997.

67. Minevich E, Wacksman J, Phipps L, et al: The importance of accurate diagnosis and early close followup in patients with suspected multicystic dysplastic kidney. J Urol 158:1301, 1997.

68. Wacksman J, Phipps L: Report of the multicystic kidney registry: Preliminary findings. J Urol 150:1870, 1993.

69. Strife JL, Souza AS, Kirks DR, et al: Multicystic dysplastic kidney in children: US follow-up. Radiology 186:785, 1993.

70. Oddone N, Marino C, Sergi C, et al: Wilms' tumor arising in a multicystic kidney. Pediatr Radiol 24:236, 1994.

71. Glassberg KI: Renal dysplasia and cystic diseases of the kidney. In Walsh PC, Vaughn ED, Wein A, et al (eds): Campbell's Urology (7th ed). Philadelphia, WB Saunders, 1997, p 1786.

72. Madewell JE, Goldman SM, Davis CJ: Multilocular cystic nephroma: A radiologic pathologic correlation of 58 patients. Radiology 146:309, 1983.

73. Castillo O, Boyle ET, Kramer SA: Multilocular cysts of the kidney: A study of 29 patients and review of the literature. Urology 37:156, 1991.

74. Joshi VV, Beckwith JB: Multilocular cyst of the kidney (cystic nephroma) and cystic partially differentiated nephroblastoma. Cancer 64:466, 1989.

75. McHugh K, Stringer DA, Hebert D, et al: Simple renal cysts in children: Diagnosis and follow-up with US. Radiology 178:383, 1991.

76. Siegel MJ, McAlister WH: Simple cysts of the kidney in children. J Urol 123:75, 1980.

77. Goldman SM, Hartman DS: The simple renal cysts. In Pollack HM (ed): Clinical Urography. Philadelphia, WB Saunders, 1990, p 1603.

53

URETERAL OBSTRUCTION AND MALFORMATIONS

Douglas E. Coplen, MD • Howard M. Snyder III, MD

Hydronephrosis and ureteral malformations are among the most common abnormalities of the urinary tract in children. Historically, these abnormalities presented with urinary tract infection, abdominal pain, or incontinence; however, with the increasing use of fetal and neonatal ultrasonography (US), they are detected before symptoms develop. Urinary tract dilation is present in 1 of 100 pregnancies, but significant uropathy is present in 1 of 500.[1] Thus, the surgeon needs to evaluate these findings critically to determine their clinical significance and whether intervention is required.

□ Ureteropelvic Junction Obstruction in Children

In ureteropelvic junction (UPJ) obstruction, there is inadequate drainage of urine from the renal pelvis into the upper ureter, resulting in hydrostatic distention of the renal pelvis and intrarenal calyces. The combination of increased intrapelvic pressure and stasis of urine in the collecting ducts results in progressive damage to the kidney.

In the past, UPJ obstruction was estimated to occur in 1 in 5000 live births, but since the advent of antenatal US, it has been recognized that the incidence is higher. UPJ obstruction is the cause of 40% of cases of neonatal hydronephrosis, placing the incidence at 1 in 1250 births.[2, 3] It is more common in males (ratio, 2:1), and two thirds of cases occur on the left side. Bilateral obstruction is present in 5 to 10% of cases; this occurs much more commonly in younger children.[4, 5]

ETIOLOGY

The narrowing at the UPJ varies from complete obstruction with associated dysplasia to a lumen indistinguishable from that of the upper ureter. Dur-

ing development of the upper ureter, the lumen of the ureteric bud solidifies with ureteral lengthening and later recanalizes.[6] Failure to recanalize adequately is thought to be the cause of most obstructions. Other causes of UPJ obstruction include ureteral valves, polyps, and leiomyomas.[7]

At surgery, the most common observation is a ureteral narrowing of variable length.[8] A high insertion of the ureter causes an angulated appearance with respect to the renal pelvis. At low volume states, peristaltic waves of urine cross the UPJ, but as the flow increases beyond a threshold, the renal pelvis dilates.[9] The dilated pelvis may kink the ureter, further increasing the pelvic pressure.[10] In 20 to 30% of patients, the ureter is draped over a lower pole vessel, although this apparent aberrancy may be secondary to incomplete renal rotation and a normal segmental vessel.[11, 12]

Histologic evaluation reveals a decrease or complete absence of smooth muscle fibers at the UPJ.[8, 13] Even when the light microscope evaluation reveals no abnormality, electron microscopy may show an increase in collagen deposition between the muscle fibers.[14] The increase in collagen is most likely the response to obstruction as opposed to its cause. Fibrosis and interruption of the smooth muscle continuity decrease myogenic conduction and transmission of the peristaltic wave.[15] Defective innervation may also play a role in the development of UPJ obstruction.[16]

UPJ obstruction can also be acquired. It has been observed at late follow-up of vesicoureteral reflux, after cutaneous ureterostomy, and after decompression of the dilated urinary tract.[17, 18] In these cases, obstruction is caused by extrinsic scarring and adhesions that cause fixed deformation and distortion of the UPJ. Vesicoureteral reflux is present in 14% of patients with UPJ obstruction,[18] and higher grades of reflux may cause obstruction (Fig. 53–1). It is important to obtain drainage films to exclude a pseudo-UPJ obstruction.

690

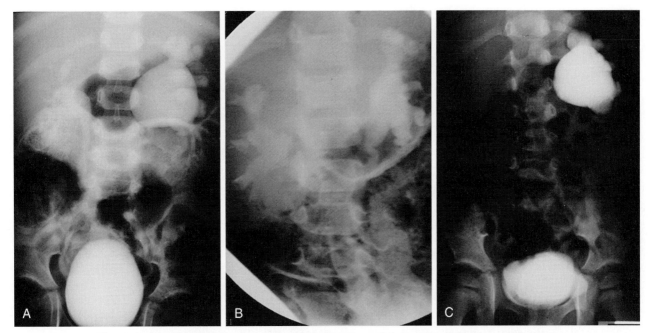

Figure 53–1. Vesicoureteral reflux and secondary ureteropelvic junction (UPJ) obstruction in a 4-year-old boy who presented with urosepsis. *A,* Excretory urogram (IVP) film with a full bladder shows typical findings of calyceal blunting and renal pelvic dilation. There is visualization of the distal ureter. *B,* Cystogram shows bilateral reflux. Note the marked discrepancy in left-sided anatomy between the IVP and cystogram and the kink just distal to the UPJ on the left side. *C,* Delayed film after cystogram shows stasis and apparent obstruction on the left side. Subsequent furosemide (Lasix) washout renal scan with a bladder catheter showed no evidence of obstruction, and the child has done well after bilateral ureteral reimplantation.

CLINICAL PRESENTATION

Most hydronephrotic kidneys are now detected prenatally. Less frequently, UPJ obstruction is detected due to an abdominal mass, urinary tract infection, association with other anomalies (i.e., VACTERL [*v*ertebral, *a*nal, *c*ardiac, *t*rachael, *e*sophageal, *r*enal, and *l*imb]), or abnormalities seen during contrast or radionuclide radiography. In older children, vague, poorly localized, cyclic or acute abdominal pain associated with nausea is common. Many of these children are initially seen by gastroenterologists. The cause of the intermittent decompensation of drainage is unclear, but renal function is almost always preserved. Hematuria after minor trauma or vigorous exercise may be a presenting feature, most likely a result of rupture of mucosal vessels in the dilated collecting system.[4] Episodic flank pain after diuresis is a common presenting feature in young adults but is uncommon in children.

DIAGNOSIS

When the diagnosis of a UPJ obstruction is suspected antenatally, the initial evaluation is performed at 10 to 14 days of life to avoid false-negative study results caused by neonatal dehydration. Bilateral UPJ obstruction is rarely associated with significant enough obstruction to cause oligohydramnios or to warrant antenatal evaluation. The newborn is placed on preventive amoxicillin (20 mg/kg once a day) pending the studies. US confirms the presence of pelvic and calyceal dilation, with variable thinning of the renal parenchyma (Fig. 53–2). The presence of corticomedullary junctions on the US is indicative of preserved function.[19, 20] The US also evaluates the contralateral kidney, bladder, and distal ureter to avoid confusion with a ureterovesical junction obstruction.

A voiding cystourethrogram is indicated in all patients who are evaluated for UPJ obstruction. Reflux increases the chance that infection will occur even in a partially obstructed system. Additionally, reflux that leads to kinking of the UPJ may be the primary disease process (see Fig. 53–1).

The excretory urogram, or intravenous pyelogram (IVP), is the traditional method used to evaluate UPJ obstruction. It reveals the anatomy but has limited use in the newborn because renal-concentrating ability does not provide adequate visualization. It is also subjective with respect to differential renal function and the degree of obstruction. The test may be indicated when more information is required regarding preoperative pelvic anatomy or to define better the level of obstruction when it is not clear from other studies.[5] In children with intermittent flank pain, IVP may be diagnostic when performed during pain.

The diuretic renogram is the most widely used and most useful technique in the evaluation of hydronephrosis, differential renal function, and drainage of kidneys.[21, 22] The study is obtained with either

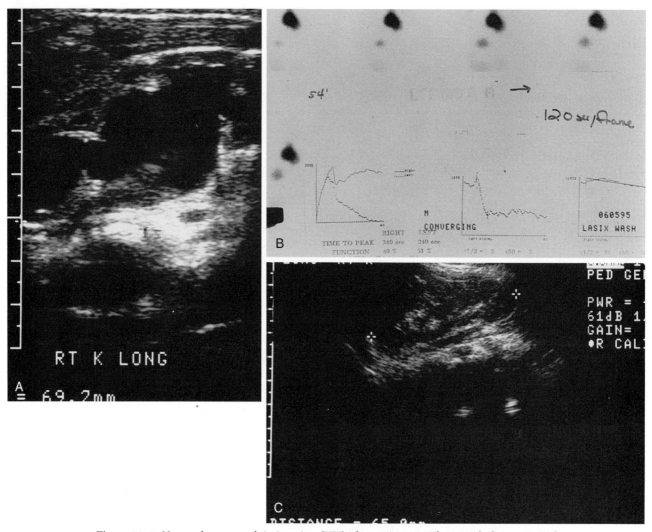

Figure 53–2. Neonatal ureteropelvic junction (UPJ) obstruction. *A,* Ultrasound shows cortical thinning, calyectasis, and renal pelvic dilation consistent with UPJ obstruction. *B,* Furosemide (Lasix) washout renal scan. Computer analysis is on the bottom. On the left side, time to peak function shows symmetric uptake in the first 2 minutes. Radionuclide drains out of the left kidney before the administration of diuretic. The half-life on the left is prolonged and was calculated to be 81 minutes. On the basis of good renal function, this was observed. *C,* Follow-up sonogram 1 year later is normal. Renal scan at this time shows symmetric function with normal washout (5 minutes).

technetium 99m-diethylenetriamine penta-acetic acid (^{99m}Tc-DTPA), whose renal clearance is by glomerular filtration, or with ^{99m}Tc-mercaptoacetyltriglycine (MAG3), whose clearance is predominately through proximal tubular secretion. MAG3 is more efficiently extracted than ^{99m}Tc-DTPA and gives better images, particularly in patients with impaired renal function.[23]

The technique for diuretic renography should be standardized.[24] Patients should be hydrated IV (15 ml/kg) 15 minutes before injection of the radionuclide. An indwelling catheter maintains an empty bladder and monitors urine output. The diuretic (1 mg/kg furosemide, not to exceed 40 mg) is not administered until the activity in the hydronephrotic kidney and renal pelvis peaks. The tracer activity is then monitored for an additional 30 minutes, and a quantitative analysis is completed.

Historically, persistence of more than 50% of the tracer in the renal pelvis 20 minutes after diuretic administration (with a half-life of more than 20 minutes) is diagnostic of obstruction. False-positive results may occur when the immature neonatal kidney fails to respond to the diuretic, when the patient is dehydrated, when the bladder is distended, or when the pelvis is significantly dilated.

Occasionally, the renal scan is equivocal, and invasive pressure flow studies may be indicated.[25] The test assumes that obstruction produces a constant restriction to outflow that necessitates elevated pressure to transport urine at high flow rates, but not all obstructions are constant. If the obstruction is intrinsic, a linear relation exists between pressure and flow. In some cases, however, the test results reflect only the response of the renal pelvis to distention and may be positive in the absence of obstruction.[10] These methods require general anesthesia in children and have limited applicability.

Retrograde urography is rarely required because a well-performed US and radionuclide study can exclude a distal obstruction.[26] Because there are risks to instrumenting the male urethra and the ureteral orifice, routine use of retrograde studies is not recommended.

MANAGEMENT

Indications for Surgery

Once a significant UPJ obstruction is defined, prompt intervention is appropriate. Ongoing ureteral obstruction is detrimental to the kidney, and in the neonatal period, early relief of obstruction maximizes functional renal development and increases the number of nephrons.[27]

The ongoing debate in the management of neonatal UPJ obstruction is the definition of significant obstruction.[28–30] A dilated renal pelvis by IVP or US may completely resolve without surgical intervention[31] (see Fig. 53–2). Such dilations can be explained by physiologic fetal polyuria and natural kinks and folds in the ureter.[32, 33]

Diuretic renography has limitations in the neonate, although using the well-tempered approach increases accuracy and applicability.[24] The standard half-life cutoff of 20 minutes for the diagnosis of significant obstruction is misleading in many cases.

Differential renal function or individual kidney uptake is the most useful information obtained during renography.[21] In the presence of an obstructive pattern on renography, many authorities believe that 35 to 40% function in the hydronephrotic kidney warrants surgical correction. However, in one series, kidneys with 25% total function improved to better than 40% of total function in all cases without surgery.[31] Even though a kidney may have greater than 40% function by renal scan, 15 to 20% eventually require surgery for diminishing function, urinary tract infection (UTI), or abdominal pain.[34, 35] Some may regain lost function.

In our opinion, a morphologic UPJ obstruction seen on US or IVP in an infant with no evidence of distal ureteral distention should be repaired if the function is below 35%. If the function is above that level, follow-up scans are obtained at 3- to 6-month intervals as clinically indicated. Deterioration in renal function then warrants surgical treatment. The ultimate concern with this approach is that delaying surgery until measurable deterioration of renal function occurs is suboptimal. In the past, urinary stasis (infection, calculi, hypertension, pain) was the indication for correction. Whether more emphasis should be placed on stasis and less on differential renal function is an unanswered question.[36] Pyeloplasty can be safely performed in the infant.[37, 38] Early intervention eliminates the indefinite period of surveillance.

When the diagnosis of significant obstruction is made in a neonate, surgery is recommended during the first 4 to 6 weeks of life. If the child presents with acute pain or infection, it is advisable to wait 1 to 2 weeks to allow for inflammation to clear. Percutaneous drainage for sepsis is rarely required preoperatively.

If the kidney functions poorly on renal scan, the best approach is renal exploration with assessment of the renal parenchyma. If the parenchyma is dysplastic, nephrectomy should be performed. Functional recovery of thinned parenchyma cannot accurately be predicted, so nephrectomy is rarely performed in infants with UPJ obstruction.

Operative Techniques

Because the flank approach is the most difficult and it is easy to commit errors of position and rotation, the anterior extraperitoneal approach or posterior lumbotomy approach is preferred. The anterior approach involves a transverse incision from the edge of the rectus to the tip of the 12th rib.[39] The retroperitoneum is entered, and the kidney may be left in situ; the UPJ is then easily exposed. In infants, this is a muscle-splitting incision with low morbidity. The posterior lumbotomy can be easily performed in infants and provides direct access to the UPJ.[40] The kidney does not require mobilization, and the ureter and renal pelvis can usually be brought up into the incision. In bilateral cases, the child does not need to be repositioned. The lumbotomy approach should not be used with a malrotated kidney or a kidney that has an intrarenal pelvis. It is more difficult in a very muscular patient. An anterior or flank approach is always preferred in reoperative cases.

The end result of any pyeloplasty is a funnel-shaped, dependent UPJ complex. Older techniques, including the Foley Y-V plasty and the Culp spiral flap, were designed to maintain the continuity of the ureter and pelvis.[41, 42] These techniques are used in unusual cases of malrotation, fusion anomalies, or long stenotic segments. The dismembered technique consistently provides the best results (Fig. 53–3).

The renal pelvis and upper ureter are mobilized, and the ureter is divided just below the obstructing segment and spatulated on its lateral border through the aperistaltic segment. If the segment is particularly long, this is identified before the renal pelvis is reduced, and a flap of renal pelvis can be created. It is usually important to resect some of the renal pelvis so that a fixed kink with obstruction does not result.

Limited handling of the pelvis and ureter is recommended.[43] Handling increases edema, and in an era when pyeloplasties are frequently performed without diversion, it is important to avoid as much trauma as is possible. Fine chromic stays allow appropriate handling of the ureter and renal pelvis. A retractor is placed only after dissection is completed so that the pyeloplasty can be more appropriately

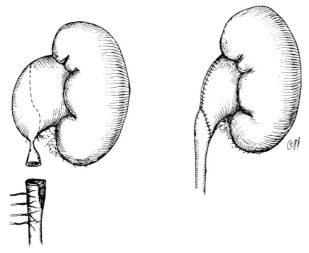

Figure 53–3. Dismembered pyeloplasty showing reduction of the renal pelvis and spatulation of the ureter, as described in the text.

designed. The anastomosis is performed with 6-0 polydioxanone or 6-0 polyglycolic acid suture. The anastomosis begins at the apex with placement of interrupted everting sutures that do not gather up ureter or pelvis and cause obstruction. After anastomosis to the dependent portion of the pelvis is completed, the remainder of the ureter and pelvis can be closed with a continuous suture, taking care to irrigate any clots from the pelvis before closure. A catheter should not be passed distally into the bladder because preoperative studies excluded a distal obstruction. Catheters only cause mucosal edema that impedes pelvic drainage or raise an obstructing mucosal flap.

Pyeloplasty can be safely performed without nephrostomy tubes or stents.[44, 45] Even if transient leakage from the anastomosis occurs, a satisfactory outcome can be expected. A Penrose drain is left near the anastomosis and can usually be removed within 48 hours of surgery, but if drainage is prolonged, the child is sent home with the drain in place.

Nephrostomy tube drainage is indicated when bilateral pyeloplasties are performed. In some small children the ureter is a thin, diaphanous structure. A nephrostomy tube is used due to the higher likelihood of postoperative obstruction. A stent is usually not required. In a poorly functioning kidney, a nephrostomy tube permits a postoperative antegrade study to demonstrate an open anastomosis. In reoperative cases, a nephrostomy is always placed because it is technically more difficult to get a watertight anastomosis.

If the UPJ obstruction is due to an aberrant lower pole vessel, the appropriate repair is to divide the ureter and perform a standard dismembered pyeloplasty. When there is an intrarenal pelvis or significant scarring in reoperative cases, a ureterocalicostomy is a useful adjunctive technique.[46] A lower pole amputation is required to prevent a postopera-

tive stricture. The ureter is spatulated and anastomosed to a lower pole calyx.

Endoscopic approaches to UPJ obstruction are now routinely used in adults.[47, 48] Their success in adults is minimally lower than in comparable open series with significantly less morbidity. The technique can be performed either percutaneously or retrograde in children using a cutting current across the aperistaltic segment.[49, 50] An indwelling ureteral stent is left for 4 to 6 weeks. The best results in children do not approach the nearly 100% success of open pyeloplasty. Because open pyeloplasty is highly successful, with minimal morbidity and a 1- to 3-day hospital stay, endopyelotomy has limited use in neonates. It does have utility in older children with good renal function and in cases in which the renal pelvis is not massively dilated. Endopyelotomy clearly has a role in secondary UPJ obstruction, in which the success approaches 100%.[49]

Uteropelvic Junction Obstruction in a Duplex Kidney

The lower pole of a duplex kidney is most commonly affected because the upper pole segment lacks a true pelvis.[51] US may not be reliable in the diagnosis because the duplex nature of the kidney may not be identified. A pyelogram or renogram shows a small nonobstructed upper segment.

The anatomy of the duplication influences the operation. If the ureter is incompletely duplicated and there is a long lower pole ureteral segment, a standard dismembered pyeloplasty can be performed. If there is a high bifurcation and a short distal segment, then the end of the renal pelvis can be anastomosed to the side of the upper pole ureter. These options can be assessed after the kidney and pelvis are exposed.

Surgical Results and Complications

The results of surgical correction have been uniformly successful when performed at pediatric surgical institutions.[26, 34, 43, 45] The rate of secondary operation is less than 1%, and the nephrectomy rate is less than 2%. The most common early complications are prolonged urinary extravasation and delayed opening of the anastomosis. When drainage continues beyond 14 days, continuity of the renal pelvis and ureter must be established with an IVP or retrograde pyelogram. If a significant leak is present, either a stent or a percutaneous nephrostomy tube should be inserted. Once diversion is instituted, the leak usually ceases within 48 hours. Late scarring at the anastomotic site is common in these situations.

Delayed opening of the anastomosis is seen most commonly with the use of a nephrostomy tube; 80% of these anastomoses open within 3 months. Secondary obstruction or failure of the primary procedure results from scarring or fibrosis, a nondependent anastomosis, ureteral angulation secondary to renal malrotation, or ureteral narrowing distal to the anastomosis. Revision can be performed through an open incision, following the same principles outlined for the initial procedure[52] or using an endoscopic approach.[49]

A postoperative functional assessment of the anastomosis should be obtained in 2 to 3 months. Further evaluation is recommended 12 to 24 months after surgery. Problems are uncommon after this time in the absence of symptoms.

□ Ureteral Abnormalities

EMBRYOLOGY

Ureteral development begins during the 4th week of gestation when the ureteral bud arises from the mesonephric duct.[53] The bud elongates, grows cephalad, and forms the ureter, renal pelvis, calyces, and collecting tubules. The distal end of the mesonephric duct from the ureteral bud to the vesicourethral tract is called the *common excretory duct* and expands in trumpet fashion into the bladder and urethra to form half of the trigone. The attachment of the ureter to the mesonephric duct switches from a posterior to an anterolateral location. With expansion and absorption of the common excretory duct into the urinary tract, the orifices of the ureteral bud and mesonephric duct become independent and move away and settle in the bladder and urethra, respectively.

Alterations in bud number, position, and time of development result in anomalies. Vesicoureteral reflux results from caudal displacement of the ureteral bud and ureteral ectopia and obstruction results from cranial displacement. Renal development and dysplasia are related to the ureteral orifice location.[54]

Ureteral Duplication

Duplication is the most common ureteral anomaly. Both sides are equally affected, and girls are affected twice as often as boys. The autopsy incidence is about 1%, but the incidence is 2 to 4% in clinical series in which pyelograms were obtained for urinary symptoms.[55, 56] Infection is the most common presentation, and many of the duplicated units show scarring or hydronephrosis on imaging studies.[57] Histologic evaluation of the kidneys shows an increased incidence of pyelonephritis and dysplasia. There is an increased incidence of infection owing to both vesicoureteral reflux and obstruction.[55]

A partial or complete duplication of the ureter occurs when a single bud branches prematurely or when two ureteral buds arise from the mesonephric duct. A bifid renal pelvis is the highest level of bifurcation and occurs in 10% of the population. Other incomplete duplications occur throughout the ureter (Fig. 53–4). When the bifurcation is near the

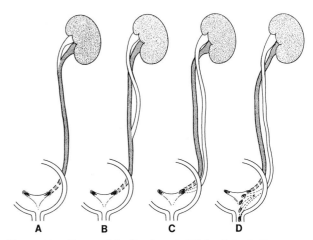

Figure 53–4. Types of duplication. *A*, Bifid pelvis. *B*, Y ureter. *C*, V ureter. *D*, Complete duplication with various ectopic orifices.

bladder, urine can pass down one limb of the duplication and then up the other side of the Y.[58] This may lead to stasis and ureteral dilation. Treatment involves either ureteral reimplantation, ureteroureterostomy, or ureteropyelostomy at the renal level.[59] An inverted Y ureter is the rarest branching anomaly[60] and presumably occurs as a result of separate ureteral buds that fuse before entering the metanephros. Treatment is directed at problems caused by the ectopic limb.

In complete duplications, reflux in the lower moiety is the most common cause of renal disease. The more caudal ureteral bud ends up laterally and cranially deviated in the bladder and has a shorter intramural tunnel. The upper pole ureter enters the bladder adjacent or distal to the lower ureter, as defined by the Weigert-Meyer law.[61] These children present with UTIs and reflux is identified in up to two thirds of children with duplicated systems who present with infection.[62] Reflux may occur into the upper pole ureter if the ureteral orifices are immediately adjacent or if the upper ureter is distally located at the level of the bladder neck without any submucosal support (Fig. 53–5).

Treatment of reflux in duplicated ureters follows the same principles as that of single-system reflux. Initial treatment includes preventive antibiotics and radiographic monitoring. Low grades of reflux are associated with the same rate of spontaneous resolution rate as single-system reflux. The distal ureters share a common blood supply, so reimplantation involves mobilization and reimplantation of the common sheath.[63] When there is associated lower pole UPJ obstruction, ipsilateral end-to-side pyeloureterostomy is an effective simultaneous management of both obstruction and reflux.[64] Even if significant scarring is present in the lower pole, reimplantation usually suffices, unless major ureteral dilation is present. In the latter case, lower pole nephroureterectomy may be indicated.

Obstructive abnormalities associated with ureteral duplication are discussed elsewhere in this chapter.

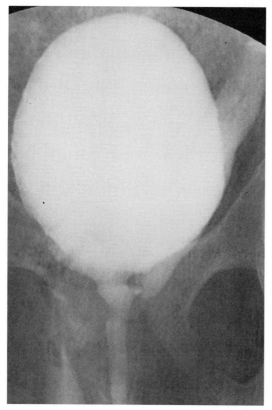

Figure 53–5. Reflux into an upper-pole ectopic ureter in the proximal urethra of a female patient who presented at 2 months with urosepsis.

Ureteral Triplication and Quadruplication

Ureteral triplication is one of the rarest anomalies of the upper urinary tract and results from either several ureteral buds or early branching. In most cases, all three ureters drain into a single orifice.[65] Triplication presents with incontinence, infection, and symptoms of obstruction and is associated with both ectopia and ureteroceles.[66, 67] Surgical treatment is individualized.

Ureteral quadruplication has been described.[68]

Retrocaval Ureter

The retrocaval or circumcaval ureter is a right ureter that passes behind the vena cava.[69] This is a result of a developmental error in the formation of the vena cava. The supracardinal vein (vena cava) lies dorsal to the developing ureter, and subcardinal veins lie ventral to the ureter. If the subcardinal vein persists as the vena cava, the ureter passes behind the vena cava and anterior to the iliac vein. If both veins persist, the ureter passes between the duplicated vena cava.[70]

Even though this is a congenital abnormality, symptoms are related to chronic ureteral obstruction and infection and rarely occur in children.[71] The radiographic appearance depends on the level of obstruction. The more common distal obstruction appears as a reversed J on IVP.[72] Less commonly, the ureter crosses at the level of the UPJ. Both of these anomalies can be confused with UPJ obstruction and should be suspected when there is pyelectasis and dilation of the upper third of the ureter.

Treatment is required only when significant obstruction or symptoms are present. Reconstruction is essentially a dismembered pyeloplasty with division of the ureter and anastomosis anterior to the vena cava, as opposed to division of the vena cava.

☐ Megaureter

Megaureter is not a diagnosis but rather a descriptive term for a dilated ureter. Normal ureteral diameter in children is rarely greater than 5 mm, and ureters larger than 7 mm can be considered megaureters.[73] The radiographic appearance of the dilated and tortuous ureter is usually striking (Fig. 53–6). Pelvicalyceal dilation and parenchymal scarring or thinning depend on the primary disease process.

Megaureters can be classified as refluxing, obstructed, and nonrefluxing nonobstructed.[74] Some ureters also have reflux and simultaneous obstruction.[75] Table 53–1 gives clinical examples of each classification. Any normal ureter dilates if the volume of urine exceeds emptying capacity,[76] and bacterial endotoxins and infection alone can cause dilation that resolves after treatment of infection.[77]

Primary obstructive megaureter is most commonly caused by a distal adynamic ureteral segment, but ureteral valves[33] and ectopic ureteral insertion also cause obstruction, as described later in this chapter. Proximal smooth muscle hypertrophy and hyperplasia are present. A normal-caliber catheter usually passes through the distal 3- to 4-cm segment, but the peristaltic wave does not propel urine across this area. The absent peristalsis is not a result of a ganglionic abnormality, as is seen in megacolon.[78] The distal ureter has a variety of histologic appearances, but the common finding is a disruption of muscular continuity that prevents muscular propulsion of urine.[14, 79–81]

As with UPJ obstruction, most megaureters are now detected antenatally, although infection is also a common presentation.[82–84] Megaureter is now the

TABLE 53–1. Classification of Megaureter, Based on the International Classification Scheme[74]

Refluxing Megaureter

Primary (congenital reflux)
Secondary (urethral valves, neurogenic bladder)

Obstructed Megaureter

Primary (adynamic segment)
Secondary (urethral obstruction, extrinsic mass, or tumor)

Nonrefluxing, Nonobstructed Megaureter

Primary (idiopathic, physiologically insignificant adynamic segment)
Secondary (polyuria, infection, postoperative residual dilation)

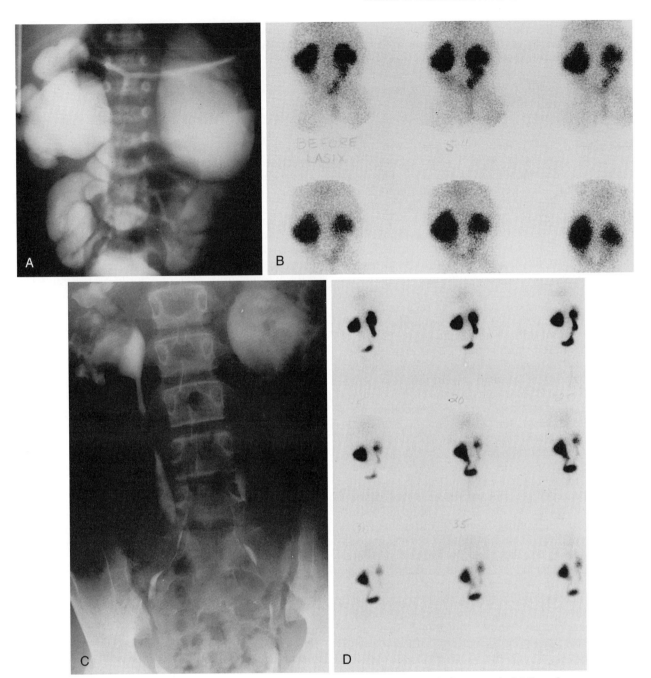

Figure 53–6. Congenital megaureter. *A*, Intravenous pyelogram (IVP) shows marked bilateral hydroureteronephrosis. *B*, Renal scan shows symmetric function and normal extraction. There is stasis bilaterally. *C*, IVP 24 months later shows marked improvement in ureteral caliber and calyceal appearance. *D*, Function is preserved on renal scan.

second most common urinary tract abnormality detected prenatally.[2] Children with this disorder typically do not have symptoms or physical or laboratory abnormalities.

Despite the variety of possibilities, standard imaging allows classification and appropriate management. The diagnosis of nonobstructed, nonrefluxing megaureter is the hardest to make and is established only when the secondary causes of megaureter have been excluded and diagnostic tests do not show obstruction. For years, it was assumed that a dilated ureter that did not reflux was obstructed,[85] but de-

velopmental ureteral dilation can be present in ureters that are not obstructed.[86]

Diagnostic imaging begins with US, which easily distinguishes megaureters from UPJ obstruction. The degree of distal ureteral dilation is often much more pronounced than the degree of renal pelvic dilation or calicectasis. A voiding cystourethrogram should be obtained in all patients. If significant reflux is present, delayed drainage films must be obtained to exclude simultaneous obstruction with a normal-caliber distal ureteral segment.

Diuretic renography or pressure–perfusion studies

are used to exclude significant obstruction. The renogram is harder to perform in patients with megaureter. Diuretic administration must be delayed because the system is so capacious and may take 60 to 90 minutes to fill. A washout time of longer than 20 minutes is indicative of obstruction.

TREATMENT

Nonoperative management is based on clearance half-time and relative renal function of the hydronephrotic and contralateral kidneys. If observation is chosen, the children are placed on preventive antibiotics and followed with serial US and renal scans. Neonatal megaureters with apparent obstruction by renography but with preserved function can be safely observed, and most become radiographically normal with time[82, 83, 87, 88] (see Fig. 53–6). Surgical correction for decreasing function or recurrent infections is indicated in only 10 to 25% of patients after up to 7 years of follow-up. Delayed evidence of obstruction after normalization of radiographs has not been seen in these children.

Initial attempts at surgical repair resulted in significant reflux and recurrent infections,[89] but when surgery is indicated, it can now be performed with high success and low morbidity. Ureteral excisional tapering with preservation of ureteral blood supply was popularized in the early 1970s.[85, 90] A longitudinal segment of ureter is excised and then closed over a 10F to 12F catheter. When the ureter is tunneled submucosally, the suture line is placed against the detrusor to decrease the chance of fistula formation. Initial repairs involved tailoring of the entire ureter, but the upper ureteral tortuosity and dilation often disappear after operation.[91] Ureteral folding techniques have been popularized because they theoretically decrease the risk of ischemic injury while achieving the decreased intraluminal diameter necessary for a successful reimplantation.[92, 93] The increased bulk is usually not a technical problem. Although dissection is usually intravesical and extravesical, solely extravesical reimplants have been described and may be associated with lower morbidity.[94] A vesicopsoas hitch is a useful adjunct that helps achieve a longer submucosal tunnel length without risking ureteral kinking.

A nonrefluxing, nonobstructed reimplantation can be achieved 85 to 95% of the time with megaureters.[84, 93] Recognized complications include persistent obstruction, reflux, and urinary extravasation. Most of these can be managed nonoperatively with drainage tubes. Lower grades of postoperative reflux often resolve.

Primary reconstruction is preferred when indicated, but temporary cutaneous diversion may be beneficial in a neonate or infant when the chance of successful reimplantation of a bulky ureter into a small bladder is reduced. Diversion may obviate the need for tailoring at the time of reimplantation. An end cutaneous ureterostomy is preferred because a high diversion may require two or more procedures for undiversion.

☐ Ectopic Ureter

An ectopic ureter is defined as one that opens at the bladder neck or more caudally rather than on the trigone. Embryologically, this results from cranial insertion of the ureteral bud on the mesonephric duct, which permits distal migration with the mesonephric duct as it is absorbed into the urogenital sinus.[55]

The incidence of ureteral ectopia is about 1 in 2000.[55] Eighty percent of ectopic ureters are reported in association with a duplicated renal system, and because clinical problems are more common in girls with ectopia, only 15% of ectopic ureters have been reported in boys.[95] Ectopia is bilateral 20% of the time.[96] Single ectopic ureters are rare but are more common in boys.[97]

ECTOPIC URETERS IN FEMALE PATIENTS

The fundamental difference between ureteral ectopia in boys and girls arises from ureteral insertion distal to the continence mechanism in girls (Fig. 53–7). About one third of ureters open at the level of the bladder neck, one third are in the vestibule around the urethral opening, and the remainder empty into the vagina, uterus, or cervix. All of these insertions are along the course of the mesonephric duct remnant (Gartner's duct).

Half of female patients present with continuous urinary incontinence despite what appears to be a normal voiding pattern.[95, 96] If the system is markedly hydronephrotic and functions poorly, leakage may occur only in the upright position and may be confused with stress incontinence. Persistent foul-smelling vaginal discharge may suggest an ectopic ureter. When the ectopic ureter is present in the urethra or the bladder neck, both obstruction and reflux are commonly present, and UTI or sepsis is the mode of presentation.

The diagnosis of ectopic ureter may be obvious or can be difficult. When there is genital ectopy, the kidney may not be visable on IVP. If there is significant hydronephrosis, the lower pole may be deviated laterally, but often there is minimal hydronephrosis, and the pyelogram may show only an absent upper pole calyx on close inspection (Fig. 53–8). US may show a dilated ectopic ureter behind the bladder. Computed tomography may be the most precise study in making this diagnosis.[98] A voiding cystourethrogram should be obtained in all patients to exclude occult reflux.[99]

The diagnosis is confirmed with physical examination, panendoscopy, and retrograde pyelography. Dyes used to stain urine may have a role. Urine in the bladder changes color, whereas poorly concentrated urine is evident as persistent clear leakage. Meticulous examination of the area around the ure-

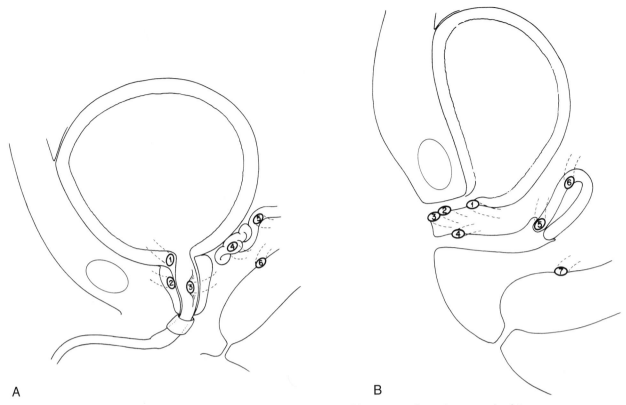

Figure 53–7. *A,* Ureteral ectopia in a male patient. Possible sites are above the external sphincter. *B,* Ureteral ectopia in a female patient, which may be located beyond the continence mechanism and produce incontinence.

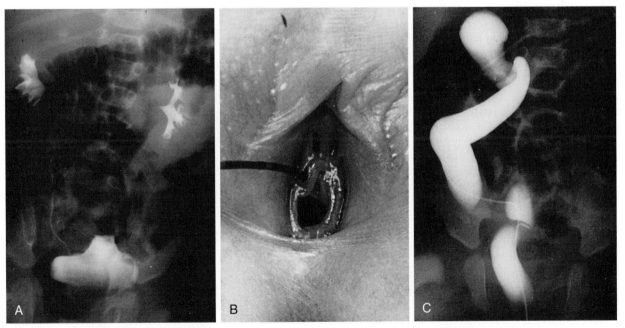

Figure 53–8. Ectopic ureter in the vaginal vestibule in a female patient. *A,* Intravenous pyelogram showing right duplication with minimal upper pole function and down and outward displacement of lower pole (drooping lily sign). *B,* Ureteral catheter in an ectopic ureter. *C,* Retrograde ureterogram.

thral meatus and vagina often reveals asymmetry or a bead of fluid coming from an opening that can be probed and injected in a retrograde fashion (see Fig. 53–8). Vaginoscopy with attention to the superior lateral aspect of the vagina may reveal a large ectopic orifice.

ECTOPIC URETER IN MALE PATIENTS

The most common sites of ectopic ureteral insertion in male patients are the posterior urethra (40 to 50%) and the seminal vesicle (20 to 60%), depending on the age at presentation.[100] Symptoms in male patients may not occur until after the onset of sexual activity and include prostatitis, seminal vesiculitis, or an infected seminal vesical cyst causing painful bowel movements. The genital insertion accounts for the common presentation with epididymitis. The male patient may present with postvoid dribbling secondary to pooling of urine in the prostatic urethra, but incontinence is never as pronounced as in the female patient.

Diagnostic testing is similar to that used in female patients. Ectopic ureters in male patients are more commonly obstructed and hydronephrotic, so US examination is often more useful. When the ectopic site of insertion is outside the urethra, it is rarely identified on endoscopic examination.

SURGICAL MANAGEMENT

Surgical treatment is dependent on the associated parenchyma.[101, 102] Single-system ectopia to the genital system usually results in poor function, and nephroureterectomy is appropriate. If the ureter is ectopic to the urethra or bladder neck, adequate function may justify ureteral reimplantation.[101] When the ectopic ureter is associated with a duplication, function of the upper pole is usually poor, and a partial nephroureterectomy is most often performed. The distal stump is left open. If function is good, a ureteropyelostomy or ureteroureterostomy can be performed to drain the ectopic system at the renal level. If this is not technically feasible, a common sheath ureteral reimplantation can be performed with tailoring of the upper pole ureter.

The distal stump rarely causes a problem in genital ectopia; however, if there is urethral or bladder neck insertion of the ectopic ureter and reflux into the ureter is identified preoperatively, excision is indicated.[102] Removal can be tedious. If the dissection plane is kept immediately adjacent to the ureter behind the bladder, the bladder neck and sphincter should not be damaged. The stump is ligated at this point. In a postpubertal female patient, this dissection can be performed transvaginally. Small stumps can be obliterated using a Bugbee electrode.

BILATERAL SINGLE ECTOPIC URETERS

Bilateral single ectopic ureter is a rare abnormality in which the altered ureteral embryologic development is associated with failure of normal bladder neck development.[103] Genital and anal anomalies are commonly present. Female patients have ureteral insertion in the distal urethra and present with infection or are noted to have continuous urinary leakage. The bladder is usually poorly developed because it has never stored urine. Male patients have somewhat larger bladders because some urine enters the bladder. However, because the bladder neck is not formed normally, they also have some degree of urinary incontinence.

The child who is incontinent with bilateral single ectopic ureter is a major reconstructive challenge and may require ureteral reimplantation, bladder neck reconstruction, and bladder augmentation if the bladder capacity is insufficient.

☐ Ureteroceles

Ureteroceles are cystic dilations of the terminal, intravesical ureter that usually have a stenotic orifice.[104–106] In children, ureteroceles are most commonly associated with the upper pole of a duplex system (80% of cases) and an ectopic orifice (60% of cases) in the urethra, whereas in adults they are usually part of a completely intravesical single system. Ureteroceles occur four to seven times more frequently in females and are more common in Caucasians. Bilateral ureteroceles are found in 10% of cases.

A single embryologic theory does not explain all ureteroceles. The most popular theory involves persistence of Chwalla's membrane at the junction of the wolffian duct and urogenital sinus.[107] Incomplete breakdown of the ureteral membrane is an obstruction that results in dilation. Abnormal development of distal ureteral musculature and delayed incorporation into the urogenital sinus have also

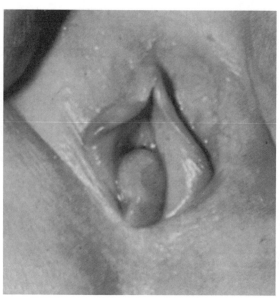

Figure 53–9. Prolapsing ectopic ureterocele.

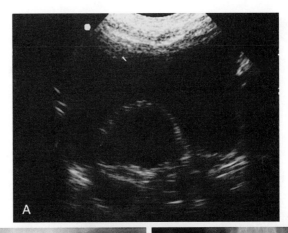

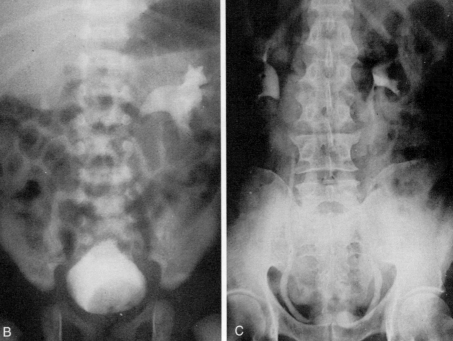

Figure 53–10. *A,* Ureterocele appearance on ultrasound. *B,* Intravenous pyelogram appearance of ureteroceles and duplication. There is downward displacement of the lower pole moiety, absent upper pole infundibulum, and lateral lower pole ureteral displacement by the dilated upperpole segment. The function of the affected unit is poor, giving a negative shadow of the nonopacified ureterocele that is present in the bladder. *C,* Single-system ureteroceles are intravesical and function well, and the ureterocele is filled with contrast, giving a cobrahead–like deformity.

been proposed as factors in ureterocele development.[108]

The classification of ureteroceles can be confusing. Pathologic description defines four types: stenotic, sphincteric, sphincterostenotic, and cecoureterocele.[108] The current recommended nomenclature classifies ureteroceles as either *intravesical* (entirely within the bladder) or *ectopic* (some portion is situated permanently at the bladder neck or in the urethra).[109]

PRESENTATION AND DIAGNOSIS

Although presentation with infection in a system with high-grade obstruction is common, antenatal detection is now achieved in up to 60% of cases.[110–112] The obstructed renal unit may be palpable in these asymptomatic infants, but most have no clinically apparent abnormality. Bladder outlet obstruction is rare because most ureteroceles decompress during micturition, but the most common cause of urethral obstruction in girls is urethral prolapse of a ureterocele (Fig. 53–9).

US reveals a well-defined cystic intravesical mass that is associated with the posterior bladder wall (Fig. 53–10). This can be followed into a dilated ureter in the bony pelvis and into upper pole hydroureteronephrosis in a duplication. The thickness and echogenicity of the renal parenchyma are often consistent with dysplasia and poor function.

IV urograms reveal typical findings (see Fig. 53–10). In adults, function is often good, and the ureterocele fills with contrast and is separated from the contrast in the bladder by a thin lucent halo. A voiding cystourethrogram is obtained in all patients. Up to 50% of the ipsilateral lower pole and 25% of the contralateral renal units have vesicoureteral reflux.[110, 113]

During cystoscopy, the bladder should be examined both when full and when completely empty because compressible ureteroceles may not be evident in a full bladder or may appear as a bladder

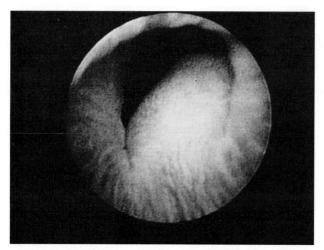

Figure 53–11. Endoscopic appearance of ureterocele.

diverticulum (Fig. 53–11). The dilated lower end of an ectopic ureter or megaureter may elevate the trigone, creating the cystoscopic, radiographic, and US appearance of a ureterocele, a so-called pseudo-ureterocele.[114]

TREATMENT OPTIONS

The goals of ureterocele treatment include control of infection, preservation of renal function, protection of normal ipsilateral and contralateral units, and maintanance of continence. The natural history of asymptomatic ureteroceles is unknown. Neonates placed on preventive antibiotics rarely develop a febrile UTI.[111, 112] Observation without prevention is rarely a good option. It should be assumed that significant urinary tract obstruction is present, and preventive antibiotics should be started.

Traditional treatment of duplex ectopic uretero-celes includes upper pole surgery through a separate flank incision, ureterocele excision, and ipsilateral lower pole ureteral reimplantation through a lower incision. The bladder-level operation may require repair of a sizable defect in the bladder base and a tapering or plication of the lower ureter. The distal extent of the ureterocele and its mucosa can often be dissected through the bladder neck. Incomplete excision may result in an obstructing urethral flap, and resection of the entire ureterocele risks damaging the bladder neck continence mechanisms. Experienced surgeons report excellent results, with low reoperation (less than 10%) and complication (less than 10%) rates.[115–117] These approaches assume that ureterocele excision is an essential component of management. However, many lower tract abnormalities detected at presentation resolve without treatment, and an absolute indication to proceed with a simultaneous bladder operation is rarely present. In older children who have absence of function on the affected side (upper and lower pole), nephroureterectomy with reconstruction of the bladder is the initial treatment of choice.

Primary upper pole partial nephroureterectomy may avoid bladder-level reconstruction and its potential risks.[110, 118, 119] Nearly all of the ureter can be removed through the flank incision, and the distal ureter is left open to facilitate decompression. The need for subsequent bladder-level surgery varies between 10% and 62%.[110, 112, 117, 119] Although up to 45% of cases of ipsilateral and contralateral reflux resolve after ureterocele decompression,[110] persistent reflux is the most common indication for a bladder-level reconstruction. Other indications for bladder-level reconstruction include ureterocele eversion acting like a diverticulum or externally compressing the bladder neck, reflux into the ureterocele, or intraluminal obstruction of the bladder neck by a cecoureterocele. The need for additional surgery is directly related to the number of renal moieties that have ureterocele or vesicoureteral reflux.[112]

Most partial nephrectomy specimens show dysplasia,[119] but some show only inflammatory and obstructive changes.[120] To preserve function, a pyeloureterostomy or ureteroureterostomy (high or low) may be performed along with distal ureterectomy and ureterocele decompression.[121] These procedures may place the lower pole system at risk in an attempt to salvage what may be a small percentage of total renal function.

Ureterocele incision is the least invasive technique of upper pole preservation. "Unroofing" of the ureterocele is advocated only as a drainage procedure for an infected system before a definitive procedure because it invariably results in reflux.[122, 123] Using a low bladder neck level ureterocele incision is the recommended technique because reflux is not inevitable (Fig. 53–12).[111, 124] A small 3F hole is made in the ureterocele just above the ureterocele base at the bladder neck. The opening is in the bladder but must also drain the ectopic urethral portion to prevent an obstructing lip at the level of the bladder neck.

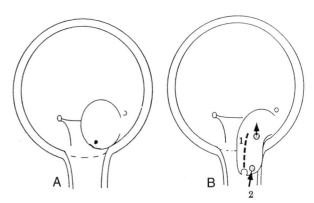

Figure 53–12. Technique for incision of ureteroceles.[111] *A*, Intravesical ureteroceles are punctured with a 3F Bugbee electrode low on the anterior wall just inside the bladder neck. *B*, Ectopic ureteroceles require drainage of the urethral segment to prevent a distal obstructing flap. This can be achieved by making a longitudinal incision across the bladder neck (1) or with two separate punctures (2).

Endoscopic incision successfully decompresses the ureterocele in 85% of cases[111, 120, 125, 126] and is the definitive procedure in more than 90% of infants with intravesical ureteroceles, whereas subsequent reconstructive surgery is required in 50 to 90% of infants with ectopic ureteroceles. Reflux into the ureterocele moiety is the most common indication for reconstruction in these infants. Decompression of the system makes this reconstruction easier.[111]

Incision should be the initial procedure in all neonates. When the ureterocele is detected before the onset of infection, appreciable function may be present after relief of obstruction.[120] Even when US shows little parenchyma, incision can be performed, and the decompressed system may require no further treatment if there is no reflux. In older children, an incision is best selected when there is associated functioning renal parenchyma, the ureterocele is intravesical, or the kidney is drained by a single system.

Single-system ureteroceles are more commonly seen in older children and adults and are associated with better function and less hydronephrosis than are found in duplex kidneys. Most often, they are incidental findings that require no treatment. Antenatally detected single-system ureteroceles may not show significant obstruction on a Lasix washout renal scan. Clinically, these behave like nonobstructed megaureters and can be followed safely with the patient on preventive antibiotics. If treatment is required, endoscopic incision is nearly always a definitive procedure.

REFERENCES

1. Thomas DFM: Fetal uropathy: Review. Br J Urol 66:225, 1990.
2. Brown T, Mandell J, Lebowitz R: Neonatal hydronephrosis in the era of sonography. Am J Radiol 148:959, 1987.
3. Mandell J, Blyth B, Peters C, et al: Structural genitourinary defects detected in utero. Radiology 178:193, 1991.
4. Williams DI, Kenawi MM: The prognosis of pelviureteric junction in childhood: A review of 190 cases. Eur Urol 2:57, 1976.
5. Snyder HM III, Lebowitz RL, Colodny AH, et al: UPJ obstruction in children. Urol Clin North Am 7:273, 1980.
6. Ruano-Gil D, Coca-Payeras A, Tejedo-Maten A: Obstruction and normal recanalization of the ureter in the human embryo: Its relation to congenital ureteric obstruction. Eur Urol 1:287, 1975.
7. Arams HJ, Buckbinder ME, Sutton AP: Benign ureteral lesions, rare causes of hydronephrosis in children. Urology 9:517–520, 1977.
8. Stephens FD: Ureterovascular hydronephrosis and the 'aberrant' renal vessels. J Urol 128:984, 1982.
9. Murnaghan GF: The dynamics of the renal pelvis and ureter with reference to congenital hydronephrosis. Br J Urol 30:321, 1958.
10. Koff SA, Hayden LJ, Cirulli C, et al: Pathophysiology of UPJ obstruction: Experimental and clinical observations. J Urol 136:336, 1986.
11. Foote JW, Blennerhassett JB, Wiglesworth FW, et al: Observations on the ureteropelvic junction. J Urol 104:252, 1970.
12. Allen TD: Congenital ureteral strictures. J Urol 104:196, 1970.
13. Starr NT, Maizels M, Chou P, et al: Microanatomy and morphometry of the hydronephrotic "obstructed" renal pelvis in asymptomatic infants. J Urol 148:519, 1992.
14. Hanna MK, Jeffs RD, Sturgess JM, et al: Ureteral structure and ultrastructure, part II: Congenital UPJ obstruction and primary obstructive megaureter. J Urol 116:725, 1976.
15. Kjurhuus JC, Nerstrom B, Gyrd-Hansen N, et al: Experimental hydronephrosis: An electrophysiologic investigation before and after release of obstruction. Acta Chir Scand Suppl 472:17, 1976.
16. Wang Y, Puri P, Hassan J, et al: Abnormal innervation and altered nerve growth factor messenger ribonucleic acid expression in ureteropelvic junction obstruction. J Urol 154:679, 1995.
17. Lebowitz RL, Blickman JG: The coexistence of UPJ obstruction and reflux. AJR Am J Roentgenol 140:231, 1983.
18. Hollowell JG, Altman HG, Snyder HM III, et al: Coexisting UPJ obstruction and vesicoureteral reflux: Diagnostic and therapeutic implications. J Urol 142:490, 1989.
19. Sanders RC, Nussbaum AR, Solez K: Renal dysplasia: Sonographic findings. Radiology 167:623, 1988.
20. Hulbert WC, Rosenberg HK, Cartwright PC, et al: The predictive value of ultrasonography in evaluation of infants with posterior urethral valves. J Urol 148:122, 1992.
21. Heyman S, Duckett JW: Extraction factor: An estimate of single kidney function in children during routine radionucleotide renography with 99m technetium diethylenetriamine pentaacetic acid. J Urol 140:780, 1988.
22. Chung S, Majd M, Rushton HG, et al: Diuretic renography in the evaluation of neonatal hydronephrosis: Is it reliable? J Urol 150:765, 1993.
23. Taylor A, Nally JV: Clinical applications of renal scintigraphy. AJR Am J Roentgenol 164:31, 1995.
24. Conway JJ: "Well-tempered" diuresis renography: Its historical development, physiological and technical pitfalls and standardized technique protocol. Semin Nucl Med 22:74, 1992.
25. Whitaker RH: The Whitaker test. Urol Clin North Am 6:529, 1979.
26. Rushton HG: Pediatric pyeloplasty: Is routine retrograde pyelography necessary? J Urol 152:604, 1994.
27. Chevalier RL, El Dahr S: The case for early relief of obstruction in young infants. In King LR (ed): Urological surgery in neonates and young infants. Philadelphia, WB Saunders, 1988, p 95.
28. Duckett JW: When to operate on neonatal hydronephrosis. Urology 42:617, 1993.
29. Woodard JR: Hydronephrosis in the neonate. Urology 42:620, 1993.
30. Blyth B, Snyder HM, Duckett JW: Antenatal diagnosis and subsequent management of hydronephrosis. J Urol 149:693, 1993.
31. Koff SA, Campbell K: Nonoperative management of unilateral neonatal hydronephrosis. 148:525, 1992.
32. Rabinowitz R, Peters MT, Byas S, et al: Measurements of fetal urine production in normal pregnancy by real-time ultrasonography. Am J Obst Gynecol 161:1264, 1989.
33. Ostling K: The genesis of hydronephrosis particularly with regard to the changes at the ureteropelvic junction. Acta Chir Scand 86:1, 1942.
34. Ransley PG, Dhillon HK, Gordon I, et al: The postnatal management of hydronephrosis diagnosed by prenatal ultrasound. J Urol 144:584, 1990.
35. Cartwright PC, Duckett JW, Keating MA, et al: Managing apparent ureteropelvic junction obstruction in the newborn. J Urol 148:1992, 1992.
36. Allen TD: The swing of the pendulum [editorial]. J Urol 148:534, 1992.
37. Wolpert JJ, Woodard JR, Parrott TS: Pyeloplasty in the young infant. J Urol 142:563, 1989.
38. Salem YH, Majd M, Rushton HG, et al: Outcome analysis of pediatric pyeloplasty as a function of patient age, presentation and differential renal function. J Urol 154:1889, 1995.
39. Duckett JW, Gibbons MD, Cromie WJ: An anterior extraperitoneal muscle-splitting approach for pediatric renal surgery. J Urol 123:79, 1980.
40. Orland SM, Snyder HM, Duckett JW: The dorsal lumbotomy incision in pediatric urological surgery. J Urol 138:963, 1987.

41. Foley FEB: A new plastic operation for stricture at the UPJ: Report of 20 cases. J Urol 38:643, 1937.

42. Culp OS, DeWeerd JH: Pelvic flap operation for certain types of ueteropelvic obstruction. Mayo Clin Proc 26:483, 1951.

43. Hendren WHH, Radhakrishnan J, Middleton AW: Pediatric pyeloplasty. J Pediatr Surg 15:133, 1980.

44. Bernstein GT, Mandell J, Lebowitz RL, et al: UPJ in the neonate. J Urol 140:1216, 1988.

45. Roth DR, Gonzales ET Jr: Management of UPJ obstruction in infants. J Urol 129:108, 1983.

46. Duckett JW, Pfister RR: Ureterocalicostomy for renal salvage. J Urol 128:98, 1982.

47. Motola JA, Badlani GH, Smith AD: Results of 212 consecutive endopyelotomies: An 8 year follow-up. J Urol 149:453, 1993.

48. Nadler RB, Rao GS, Pearle MS, et al: Acucise endopyelotomy: Assessment of long-term durability. J Urol 156:1094, 1996.

49. Figenshau RS, Clayman RV, Colberg JW, et al: Pediatric endopyelotomy: The Washington University experience. J Urol 156:2025, 1996.

50. Bogaert GA, Kogan BA, Mevorach RA, et al: Efficacy of retrograde endopyelotomy in children. J Urol 156:734, 1996.

51. Ossandon SM, Androulakakis P, Ransley PG: Surgical problems in pelviureteral junction obstruction of the lower pole moiety in incomplete duplex systems. J Urol 125:871, 1981.

52. Rohrmann D, Snyder HM, Duckett JW, et al: The operative management of recurrent ureteropelvic junction obstruction. 158:1257, 1997.

53. Brockis JG: The development of the trigone of the bladder with a report of a case of ectopic ureter. 24:192, 1952.

54. Mackie GG, Awang H, Stephens FD: The ureteric orifice: The embryologic key to radiologic status of the kidneys. J Pediatr Surg 10:473, 1975.

55. Campbell MF: Anomalies of the ureter. In Campbell MF, Harrison JH (eds): Urology (3rd ed). Philadelphia, WB Saunders, 1970, pp 1487–1670.

56. Hartman GW, Hodson CJ: The duplex kidney and related abnormalities. Clin Radiol 20:387, 1969.

57. Privett JTJ, Jeans WD, Roylance J: The incidence and importance of renal duplication. Clin Radiol 27:521, 1976.

58. Tresidder BC, Blandy JP, Murray RS: Pyelopelvic and uretero-ureteric reflux. Br J Urol 42:728, 1970.

59. Amar AD: Treatment of reflux in bifid ureters by conversion to complete duplication. J Urol 108:77, 1972.

60. Klauber GC, Reid ED: Inverted Y reduplication of the ureter. J Urol 107:362, 1972.

61. Meyer R: Normal and abnormal development of the ureter in the human embryo—a mechanisitic consideration. Anat Rec 96:355, 1946.

62. Fehrenbaker LG, Kelalis PP, Stickler GB: Vesicoureteral reflux and ureteral duplication in children. J Urol 107:862, 1972.

63. Barrett DM, Maled RS, Kelalis PP: Problems and solutions in surgical treatment of 100 consecutive ureteral duplications in children. J Urol 114:126, 1975.

64. Shelfo SW, Keller MS, Weiss RM: Ipsilateral pyeloureterostomy for managing lower pole reflux with associated ureteropelvic junction obstruction in duplex systems. J Urol 157:1420, 1997.

65. Kohri K, Nagai N, Kaneko S, et al: Bilateral trifid ureters associated with fused kidney, ureterovesical stenosis, left cryptorchidism and angioma of the bladder. J Urol 120:249, 1978.

66. Zaontz MR, Maizels M: Type I ureteral triplication: An extension of the Weiger-Meyer Law. J Urol 134:949, 1985.

67. Finkel Li, Watts FB, Cobrett DP: Ureteral triplication with a ureterocele. Pediatr Radiol 13:343, 1983.

68. Soderdahl DW, Shiraki IW, Schamber DT: Bilateral ureteral quadruplication. J Urol 116:255, 1976.

69. Considine J: Retrocaval ureter. Br J Urol 38:412, 1966.

70. Hollinshead WH: Anatomy for Surgeons (2nd ed). Vol 2. Harper & Row, 1971.

71. Resnick MI, Kursh ED: Extrinsic obstruction of the ureter. In Walsh PC, et al (eds): Campbells Urology (6th ed). Philadelphia, WB Saunders, 1992, p 540.

72. Kumar S, Bhandari M: Selection of operative procedure for circumcaval ureter (type I). Br J Urol 57:399, 1985.

73. Hellstrom M, Hjalmas K, Jacobsson B, et al: Normal ureteral diameter in infancy and childhood. Acta Radiol 26:433, 1985.

74. Stephens FD: ABC of megaureters. In Bergsma D, Duckett (eds): Birth Defects, Original Article Series. Vol 13. New York, Alan R. Liss, 1977, pp 1–8.

75. King LR: Megaloureter: Definition, diagnosis, and management. J Urol 123:222, 1980.

76. Boyd SD, Raz S, Ehrlich RM: Diabetes insipidus and nonobstructive dilation of urinary tract. Urology 16:266, 1980.

77. Kass EJ, Silver TM, Konnak JW, et al: The urographic findings in acute pyelonephritis: Non-obstructive hydronephrosis. J Urol 116:544, 1976.

78. Leibowitz S, Bodian M: A study of the vesical ganglia in children and their relationship to the megaureter megacystis syndrome and Hirschsprung's disease. J Clin Pathol 16:342, 1963.

79. Tanagho EA: Embryologic basis for lower ureteral anomalies: A hypothesis. Urology 7:451, 1976.

80. Gregoir W, Debled B: L'etiologie du reflux congenital et du mega uretere primaire. Urol Int 24:119, 1969.

81. McLaughlin AP, Pfister RC, Leadbetter WF, et al: The pathophysiology of primary megalouretere. J Urol 109:805, 1973.

82. Mollard P, Foray P, De Godoy JL, et al: Management of primary obstructive megaureter without reflux in neonates. Eur Urol 24:505, 1993.

83. Cozzi F, Madonna L, Maggi E, et al: Management of primary megaureter in infancy. J Pediatr Surg 28:1031, 1993.

84. Peters CA Mandell J, Lebowitz RL, et al: Congenital obstructed megaureters in early infancy: Diagnosis and treatment. J Urol 142:641, 1989.

85. Hendren WH: Operative repair of megaureter in children. J Urol 101:491, 1969.

86. Keating MA, Escala J, Snyder HM, et al: Changing concepts in management of primary obstructive megaureter 142:636, 1989.

87. Baskin LS, Zderic SA, Snyder HM, et al: Primary dilated megaureter: Long-term followup. J Urol 152:618, 1994.

88. Liu HY, Dhillon HK, Yeung CK, et al: Clinical outcome and management of prenatally diagnosed primary megaureters. J Urol 152:614, 1994.

89. Nesbit RM, Withycombe JF: The problem of primary megaloureter. 72:162, 1954.

90. Grégoir W: Traitement chirurgical du reflux congénital et du méga-uretère primaire. Urol Int 24:502, 1969.

91. Hendren WH: Commentary: Surgery of megaureter. In Whitehead D, Leiter E (eds): Current Operative Urology. Philadelphia, Harper & Row, 1984, pp 473–482.

92. Starr A: Ureteral plication: A new concept in uretreral tailoring for megaureter. Invest Urol 17:153, 1979.

93. Perdzynski W, Kalicinski ZH: Long-term results after megaureter folding in children. J Pediatr Surg 31:1211, 1996.

94. McLorie GA, Jayanthi VR, Kinahan TJ, et al: A modified extravesical technique for megaureter repair. Br J Urol 74:715, 1994.

95. Schulman CC: Les implantations ectopiques de l'uretère. Acta Urol Belg 40:201, 1972.

96. Malek RS, Kelalis PP, Stickler GB, et al: Observations on ureteral ectopy in children. J Urol 107:308, 1972.

97. Johnston JH, Davenport TJ: The single ectopic ureter. Br J Urol 41:428, 1969.

98. Lebowitz RL: Pediatric uroradiology. Pediatr Clin North Am 32:1353, 1985.

99. Lebowitz RL, Wyly JB: Refluxing urethral ectopic ureters: Diagnosis by the cyclic voiding cystourethrogram. AJR Am J Roentgenol 142:1263, 1984.

100. Terai A, Tsuji Y, Terachi T, et al: Ectopic ureter opening into the seminal vesicle in an infant: A case report and review of the Japanese literature. Int J Urol 2:128, 1995.

101. el Ghoneimi A, Miranda J, Truong T, et al: Ectopic ureter with complete ureteric duplication: Conservative surgical management. J Pediatr Surg 31:467, 1996.

102. Plaire JC, Pope JC, Kropp BP, et al: Management of ectopic ureters: Experience with upper tract approach. J Urol 158:1245, 1997.

103. Noseworthy J, Persky L: Spectrum of bilateral ureteral ectopia. Urology 19:489, 1982.

104. Uson AC, Lattimer JK, Melicow MM: Ureteroceles in infants and children: A report based on 44 cases. Pediatrics 27:971, 1961.

105. Mertz HO: Blind uretero-vesical protrusion. Trans Am Assoc Gen-Urin Surg. 40:180, 1948.

106. Ericson NO: Ectopic ureterocele in infants and children. Acta Chir Scand Suppl 197:8, 1954.

107. Chwalla R: The process of formation of cystic dilations of the vesical end of the ureter and of diverticula at the ureteral ostium. Urol Cutan Rev 31:499, 1927.

108. Stephens FD, Smith ED, Hutson JM: Congenital anomalies of the urinary and genital tracts. Oxford, England, Isis Medical Media, 1996, pp 243–262.

109. Glassberg KI, Braren V, Duckett JW, et al: Suggested terminology for duplex systems, ectopic ureters and ureteroceles. J Urol 132:1153–1154, 1984.

110. Caldamone AA, Snyder HM, Duckett JW: Ureteroceles in children: Follow-up of management with upper tract approach. J Urol 131:1130–1132, 1984.

111. Blyth B, Passerini-Glazel G, Camuffo C, et al: Endoscopic incision of ureteroceles: Intravesical versus ectopic. J Urol 149:556–560, 1993.

112. Husmann DA, Ewalt DH, Glenski WJ, et al: Ureterocele associated with ureteral duplication and nonfunctioning upper pole segment: Management by partial nephroureterectomy alone. J Urol 154:723–726, 1995.

113. Sen S, Beasley SW, Ahmed S, et al: Renal function and vesicoureteric reflux in children with ureteroceles. Pediatr Surg Int 7:192–194, 1992.

114. Sumfest JM, Burns MW, Mitchell ME: Pseudoureterocele: Potential for misdiagnosis of an ectopic ureter as a ureterocele. Br J Urol 75:401–405, 1995.

115. Hendren WH, Mitchell ME: Surgical correction of ureteroceles. J Urol 121:590–597, 1979.

116. Scherz HC, Kaplan GW, Packer MG, et al: Ectopic ureteroceles: Surgical management with preservation of continence—review of 60 cases. J Urol 142:538–541, 1989.

117. Mor Y, Ramon J, Raviv G, et al: A 20-year experience with treatment of ectopic ureteroceles. J Urol 147:1592–1594, 1992.

118. Cendron J, Bonhomme C: 31 Cas d'ureter abondement ectopique sons sphincterien chez l'enfant du sexe feminin. J Urol Nephrol 74:1, 1968.

119. Rickwood AMK, Reiner I, Jones M, et al: Current management of duplex-system ureteroceles: Experience with 41 patients. Br J Urol 70:196–200, 1992.

120. Monfort G, Guys JM, Coquet M, et al: Surgical management of duplex ureteroceles. J Pediatr Surg 27:634–638, 1992.

121. Huisman TK, Kaplan GW, Brock WA, et al: Ipsilateral ureteroureterostomy and pyeloureterostomy: A review of 15 years experience with 25 patients. J Urol 138:1207–1210, 1987.

122. Snyder HM, Johnston JM: Orthotopic ureteroceles in children. J Urol 119:543–546, 1978.

123. Tank ES: Experience with endoscopic incision and open unroofing of ureteroceles. J Urol 136:241–242, 1986.

124. Monfort G, Morisson-Lacombe G, Coquet M: Endoscopic treatment of ureteroceles revisited. J Urol 133:1031–1033, 1985.

125. Smith C, Gosalbez R, Parrott TS, et al: Transurethral puncture of ectopic ureteroceles in neonates and infants. J Urol 152:2110–2112, 1994.

126. Barret E, Pfister C, Dunet F, et al: [Endoscopic treatment of prenatally diagnosed ureteroceles]. Prog Urol 6:529–534, 1996.

54

URINARY TRACT INFECTION AND VESICOURETERAL REFLUX

Curtis A. Sheldon, MD • Eugene Minevich, MD • Jeffrey Wacksman, MD

□ Urinary Tract Infection

DIAGNOSIS

Although clinical signs and symptoms are important indications of childhood urinary tract infection (UTI), owing to the profound implications of UTI in children, confirmation of the diagnosis by microscopic examination and quantitative culture of a properly collected specimen is imperative. Signs and symptoms of UTI are age dependent. Neonates rarely present with findings specific to the urinary tract; lethargy, irritability, temperature instability, anorexia, emesis, or jaundice predominate. Bacteremia is common with neonatal UTI, and urine culture is an important aspect of the evaluation of neonatal sepsis.[1, 2] Older infants often present with nonspecific abdominal discomfort, emesis, diarrhea, poor weight gain, or fever. Malodorous or cloudy urine may be reported. Older children often present with dysuria. Urinary frequency, urgency, and enuresis become prevalent. Table 54–1 outlines the incidence of UTI symptoms as a function of age.[3, 4]

Analysis of a properly collected urine sample is the cornerstone of diagnosis of UTI. Errors in diagnosis occur frequently. They most commonly result from failure to confirm a clinically suspected UTI by culture or from reliance on a specimen that has been inadequately collected or mishandled. Specimens may be obtained by bag collection, clean catch, urethral catheterization, and suprapubic aspiration. Although invasive, urethral catheterization and suprapubic aspiration clearly offer the lowest risk of false-positive culture results.[5] The results of a bag specimen or clean-catch specimen are definitive only if negative. Positive findings should be confirmed using a catheter or aspiration specimen unless the clinical presentation is unequivocal. The

TABLE 54–1. Presenting Symptoms in 200 Children with Urinary Tract Infection as a Function of Age

Symptom	0-1 M	1-24 M	2-5 Y	5-12 Y
Failure to thrive, poor feeding	53%	36%	7%	0
Jaundice	44%	0	0	0
Screaming, irritability	0	13%	7%	0
Foul-smelling, cloudy urine	0	9%	13%	0
Diarrhea	18%	16%	0	0
Vomiting	24%	29%	16%	3%
Fever	11%	38%	57%	50%
Convulsions	2%	7%	9%	5%
Hematuria	0	7%	16%	6%
Frequency, dysuria	0	4%	34%	41%
Enuresis	0	0	27%	29%
Abdominal pain	0	0	23%	44%
Loin pain	12	0	0	12%
Male-to-female ratio	1:2	1:13	1:10	1:10

From Smellie JM, Hodson CJ, Edwards D, et al: Clinical and radiological features of urinary infection in childhood. Br Med J 2:1222, 1964; Bickerton MW, Duckett JW: Urinary tract infections in pediatric patients. AUA Update Service. Lesson 26. Vol 4:4, 1985.

TABLE 54-2. Criteria for Diagnosis
of Urinary Tract Infections

Method of Collection	Colony Count (Pure Culture)	Probability of Infection
Suprapubic aspiration	Gram-negative bacilli: any number	>99%
	Gram-positive cocci: >a few thousand	>99%
Catheterization	>10⁵	95%
	10⁴–10⁵	Likely
	10³–10⁴	Suspicious
	<10³	Unlikely
Clean voided (male)	>10⁵	Likely
Clean voided (female)	3 specimens >10⁵	95%
	2 specimens >10⁵	90%
	1 specimen >10⁵	80%

Modified from Hellerstein S: Recurrent urinary tract infection in children. Pediatr Infect Dis 1:275, 1982.

accuracy rate of positive findings from a bag specimen in infancy has been estimated at 7.5%,[6] whereas that of the midstream specimen varies with age: 42% in patients younger than 18 months and 71% in those 3 to 12 years of age.[7] Specimens should be either analyzed and plated immediately or placed on ice to minimize bacterial multiplication before testing.

The accepted standard for diagnosis of UTI remains the quantitative urine culture, which was based on studies of women with symptoms using early-morning voided specimens. The accepted criterion for diagnosis is a single bacterial species in greater than 10⁵ colony-forming units per milliliter.[8] The accuracy of such a positive finding on culture of a single specimen is estimated at 80%, reaching 96% when confirmed by second culture. Table 54–2 outlines the probability of infection as a function of colony count and method of collection that we use in children.[9] One must avoid applying these criteria too strictly because the colony count varies as a function of hydration and urinary frequency. One study of six untreated children with proven bacteriuria found colony counts to vary from 10³ to 10⁸ over a 24-hour period.[10]

Although clearly most accurate, urine culture results cannot provide an immediate diagnosis, and as a result, initial treatment is generally guided by urinalysis. Microscopic evaluation of a urine specimen should be done immediately on collection. This practice minimizes misleading ex vivo bacterial multiplication and deterioration of cellular elements. The identification of bacteria in an unspun urine specimen is suggestive of significant bacteriuria.[10] Pyuria (more than 10 leukocytes/mm³) is suggestive[11] but may also be seen in such instances as vaginitis, dehydration, calculi, trauma, chemical irritation, gastroenteritis, and viral immunization. Urinary Gram's stain has been found to be reliable in detecting UTI in young infants.[12]

A popular and indirect measurement of bacteriuria employs nitrite and leukocyte esterase analysis.

Nitrate, normally present in urine, is converted to nitrite in the presence of bacteria. A positive colorimetric reaction among nitrite, sulfanilic acid, and α-naphthylamine is thus indicative of bacteria, with a specificity and a positive predictive value approaching 100%.[13] The nitrate-to-nitrite reaction requires a relatively long incubation period. Thus, urinary frequency and hydration may produce a false-negative result. Inadequate dietary nitrate and infection caused by nitrite-negative organisms may also cause false-negative reactions. False-positive reactions are uncommon.[14] The combination of nitrite and leukocyte esterase is more sensitive and specific than is either by itself.[15] Overall, the combination of dipstick analysis and microscopic examination for bacteria has a sensitivity and a negative predictive value approaching 100%.[13]

CLASSIFICATION

Classification of UTIs helps to determine the need for hospital admission and parenteral antibiotic therapy as opposed to outpatient oral antibiotic therapy. An attempt is made to distinguish between upper tract (pyelonephritis) and lower tract infections. Fever, flank pain or tenderness, and leukocytosis suggest pyelonephritis and require parenteral antibiotics to minimize the risk of renal injury. Additional findings supporting parenteral antibiotic therapy include age less than 3 months, unusual pathogens, or significant urinary anomalies. After the initial stabilization, we often complete the course of parenteral antibiotics on an outpatient basis, employing home-based nursing service.

Laboratory studies designed to distinguish lower tract from upper tract UTIs include antibody-coated bacteria assay, β₂-microglobulin excretion, antibodies to Tamm-Horsfall protein, and urinary lactic dehydrogenase assay. These tests, in our opinion, are not sufficiently reliable for routine clinical use and have been previously reviewed.[16] Direct culture by ureteral catheterization or percutaneous puncture is reliable, although cumbersome, and represents excellent options in complicated clinical problems. We have found the most usable study for localizing infection to the kidney to be an isotope image during presentation of the patient with infection (Fig. 54–1).

Another important consideration regarding classification is the distinction between reinfection and relapse. Reinfection with a new organism is overwhelmingly common. Relapse with the same organism, although less common, is important because it usually implies either an ineffective therapy or a structural abnormality, such as a stone or obstruction.

EPIDEMIOLOGY

Figure 54–2 outlines the age-related and sex-related incidence of UTI. At all ages, with the exception of the neonatal period, the incidence of UTI is

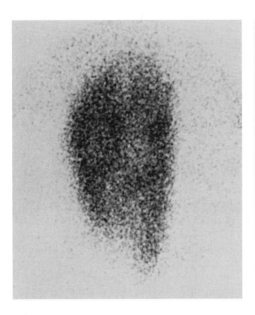
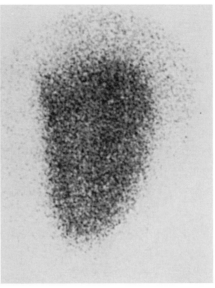

Figure 54–1. Technetium-99m DMSA scan. The magnified view of the left kidney, using a pinhole collimator, demonstrates defects in both poles that extend deep into the renal parenchyma, suggestive of acute pyelonephritis. The right kidney has an upper pole defect that may represent either acute or chronic pyelonephritis. (Courtesy of Michael J. Gelfand, MD.)

greater in females than in males. In both males and females, the incidence increases with advanced age. Although boys have one early peak in the newborn period, girls have two peaks: one is at 3 to 6 years and the other at the onset of sexual activity. The actual incidence of infection as a function of age and sex is difficult to determine from the literature. Table 54–3 summarizes available data.[9]

PATHOPHYSIOLOGY

Host Factors

The remarkable resilience of the urinary tract to bacterial infection was demonstrated in 1961.[17] Ret-

rograde inoculation of more than 10^8 bacteria in the bladder of healthy volunteers did not result in clinical infection. The establishment of clinical infection and its consequent injury to the urinary tract results from a complex interplay between host resistance and bacterial virulence. As a general rule, UTI-causing organisms originate from the feces of their host. Conceptually, four levels of defense are identifiable: periurethral, bladder, ureterovesical junction (UVJ), and renal papillae.[4] These concepts are illustrated in Figure 54–3.

Bacteria readily adhere to the vaginal mucosa to produce periurethral colonization. Replication and transurethral migration lead to infection of the bladder.[18] Healthy girls have less bacterial colonization

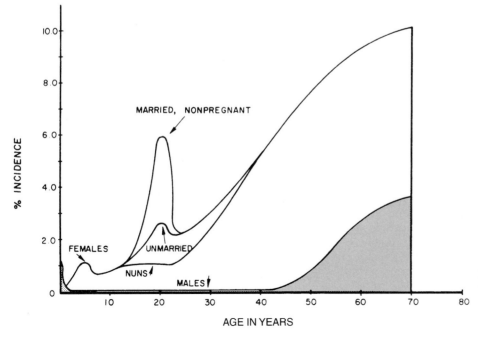

Figure 54–2. Age and sex distribution of urinary tract infection incidence. (From Devine CJ, Stecker JF: Urology in Practice. Boston, Little, Brown, 1978, p 444.)

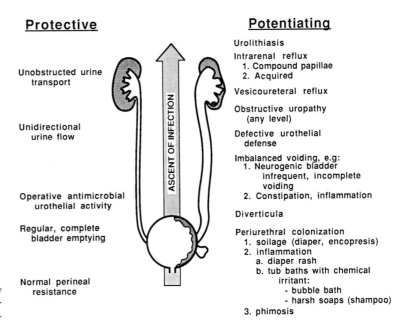

Figure 54–3. Host factors that protect the urinary tract from infection and abnormalities that potentiate the establishment of invasive bacterial infection.

of the periurethral region than do UTI-prone girls, especially before a new episode of UTI. Furthermore, the organism cultured from the introital region usually belongs to the same strain as that from the urine during the UTI that ensues. Periurethral bacterial colonization is correspondingly low in UTI patients after cessation of recurrent UTIs.[19, 20] A similar mechanism may apply to bacterial adherence in the prepuce of males.[21] This may explain why 92% of male infants younger than 6 months with UTI are uncircumcised.[22]

A number of bladder defense mechanisms help maintain a sterile urine. The most critical is the act of regular and complete voiding. The healthy bladder is capable of eliminating 99% of instilled bacteria and leaves a small residual urine that minimizes the inoculum at the onset of the following cycle.[23, 24] High intravesical pressure dynamics may also potentiate infection in children. In the absence of an elevated residual urine, uninhibited bladder contractions are associated with a high risk of recurrence of UTI, which is lessened by anticholinergic therapy.[25] Abnormal voiding habits[26] as well as constipation[26, 27] can affect the development of UTI as

well. The acid pH of urine, as well as its osmolality, further discourages bacterial growth.[28] The uroepithelial cells of healthy subjects suppress bacterial growth and are capable of killing bacteria. The uroepithelial cells secrete a mucopolysaccharide substance that, on coating the surface of the uroepithelium, provides an additional barrier to uroepithelial adherence.[24] Glycosaminoglycans are continuously shed and thus function to entrap and eliminate bacteria.

Patients with asymptomatic bacteriuria do not demonstrate all these features. Patients with recurrent UTI, after successful antireflux surgery, have defective uroepithelial defense, in contrast to those who remain sterile after reflux surgery.[29]

Abnormalities of the UVJ may allow reflux, which potentiates but is not always necessary for upper tract invasion. The anatomy of the renal papillae usually prevents intrarenal reflux (IRR) (Fig. 54–4). The papillary ducts commonly open onto the papillae with slit-like orifices that occlude with elevated intracaliceal pressure, preventing IRR. The more circular duct orifices of compound papillae fail to accomplish this goal, allowing IRR. The facts that

TABLE 54–3. Incidence of Urinary Tract Infection as a Function of Age, Sex, and Presence of Symptoms

Age	Symptomatic		Asymptomatic	
	Male	Female	Male	Female
Newborn	0.15%		1–1.4%*	
Preschool			0.2%	0.8%
	0.7%	2.8%		
School			0.03%	1–2%

*2.4 to 3.4% in premature infants.
Data compiled from multiple sources by Hellerstein S: Recurrent urinary tract infections in children. Pediatr Infect Dis 1:271, 1982.

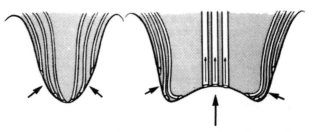

Figure 54–4. The normal oblique insertion of the collecting ducts onto the surface of simple papillae prevents intrarenal reflux *(left)*. Collecting duct insertion onto the surface of compound papillae may allow intrarenal reflux. (From Ransley PG: Intrarenal reflux: Anatomic, dynamic and radiological studies. Urol Res 5:61, 1977. Reproduced with permission of Springer-Verlag.)

compound papillae tend to occur in the upper and lower calyces and that IRR in very young children may occur at a relatively low pressure may explain the observed polar distribution of scarring and predilection to scarring noted in these children.[4] Structural abnormalities that potentiate infection include phimosis, obstructive uropathy at any level, vesicoureteral reflux (VUR), diverticula, urinary calculi or foreign bodies, and renal papillary structure.

Bacterial Factors

Several bacterial factors may potentiate UTI and are outlined in Table 54–4.[4, 29] O antigens are lipopolysaccharides that are part of the cell wall. They are thought to be responsible for many of the systemic symptoms associated with infection. Of the more than 150 strains of *Escherichia coli* identified by O antigens, 9 strains are responsible for most UTIs.

K antigens are also polysaccharides, and their presence on gram-negative bacterial capsules is considered to be an important virulence factor. They are thought to protect against phagocytosis, to inhibit the induction of a specific immune response, and to facilitate bacterial adhesion. Bacterial strains causing UTI exhibit considerably more K antigen than those isolated from the feces. Urease, a virulence factor especially prominent with *Proteus* species, permits the breakdown of urea to ammonium. This process alkalinizes the urine and facilitates stone formation. Such bacteria are generally incorporated into the stone structure, making eradication extremely difficult. Mannose-resistant pili are important adherence factors. They promote adherence to uroepithelial as well as to renal epithelial cells. This factor appears to counter the normal cleansing action of urine flow and permits tissue invasion and bacterial proliferation. That these factors truly are associated with virulence is shown in Figure 54–5.

Increasingly invasive urinary infections are asso-

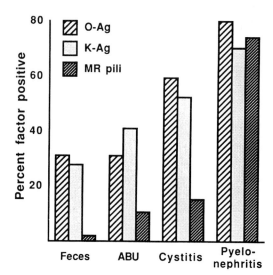

Figure 54–5. Presence of bacterial virulence factors as a function of the clinical setting. More invasive infections are associated with a high incidence of virulence factors, implicating these factors in pathogenesis. ABU, asymptomatic bacteriuria; Ag, antigen; MR, mannose resistant. (From Mannhardt W, Schofer O, Schulte-Wiserman H: Pathogenic factors in recurrent urinary tract infection and renal scar formation in children. Eur J Pediatr 145:330, 1986.)

ciated with bacteria with a high incidence of virulence factors. Figure 54–6 demonstrates the pathophysiologic changes of renal injury that may occur in the absence of significant host factors. Colonization of the feces with a virulent organism permits periurethral colonization and ultimately bladder entry. Uroepithelial adherence promotes bacterial proliferation and tissue invasion. Distortion of the UVJ and altered peristalsis allow entry into the upper tracts. Resultant distortion of the renal pyramids permits renal parenchymal invasion, which results in irreversible renal injury. This series of events is facilitated by the presence of one or more host factors (see Fig. 54–3).

INVESTIGATION

Although many patients with UTI have no serious illness, the pediatric surgeon must be cognizant of several important risks. Urinary abnormalities can be found in about half of children up to the age of 12 years who present with UTI. VUR is found in up to 35% and obstructive lesions in 8%. Nonobstructive, nonrefluxing lesions are found in 7%.[30]

Renal scars develop in about 13% of girls and 5% of boys with unspecified infection,[31] but they develop in up to 43% of kidneys involved in acute pyelonephritis.[32] Pyelonephritic scarring is responsible for 11% of cases of childhood hypertension[33] and for most cases of severe hypertension.[34] Of patients with segmental renal scars, 20% develop hypertension.[29] Although hypertension is most common with bilateral scarring, it is also seen with unilateral scarring.[35] Pyelonephritic scarring is also an important cause of end-stage renal failure in

TABLE 54–4. Bacterial Factors Potentiating Infection

O antigens (lipopolysaccharides)
   Primarily O_1, O_2, O_4, O_6, O_7, O_{11}, O_{18}, O_{35}, O_{75}
   Responsible for systemic reactions (e.g., fever, shock)
K antigens
   Primarily K_1, K_5
   Adhesive properties
   Low immunogenicity
H antigens (flagella)
   Bacterial locomotion
   Chemotaxis
Hemolysins (bacterial enzymes)
   Tissue damage
   Facilitates bacterial growth
Urease
   Alkalinizes urine
   Facilitates stone formation
P fimbriae—adherence
   Mannose sensitive (MS)
   Mannose resistant (MR)

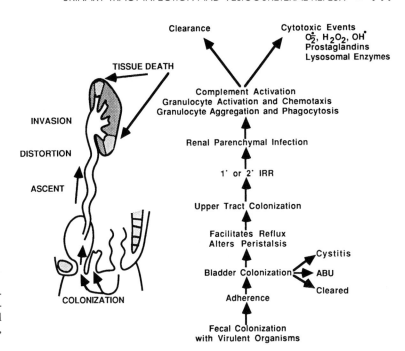

Figure 54–6. The pathogenesis of destructive infection. The process is facilitated by, but does not require, defects in the host protective factors outlined in Figure 54–3. ABU, asymptomatic bacteriuria; IRR, intrarenal reflux.

childhood and may require specific pretransplantation treatment, especially if associated with reflux.[36] Additionally, about half of patients suffer from recurrent UTI.[29]

Consequently, children of either gender should be investigated at the time of the initial infection.[4] Although controversy does persist, we investigate children with UTI with initial screening ultrasonography (US) and cyclic voiding cystography.[37] Males require contrast voiding cystourethrography (VCUG), and females are adequately evaluated by isotope VCUG, which permits a lower radiation exposure to the ovaries.[38, 39] The exception is the infant girl or the girl with suspected neurogenic bladder, ectopic ureter, or ureterocele by US. In this case, contrast VCUG is obtained.

TREATMENT

Treatment of acute UTI is dependent on clinical presentation. Patients with pyelonephritis should be treated immediately and aggressively. Prompt, effective treatment is the most important factor in preventing permanent renal injury. We prefer to initiate therapy with intravenous (IV) ampicillin and aminoglycoside after obtaining a reliable urine culture. Further therapy is dictated by culture and sensitivity findings. Patients initially may require admission to the hospital. Once afebrile, patients with otherwise uncomplicated infections with sensitive organisms may complete a 10- to 14-day course with oral antibiotics at home. Patients with resistant organisms or those with obstructions may finish the course with nursing-supervised home administration of IV antibiotics. Patients with obstruction or abscess who do not become afebrile undergo drainage percutaneously or, rarely, operatively.

Short treatment courses appear to be insufficient

for the treatment of childhood UTI[40]; therefore, we prefer a 7- to 10-day course dictated by culture and sensitivity results. Retention by the patient owing to a fear of voiding or dysuria may be managed with phenazopyridine (Pyridium) and hydration and by allowing the child to void while sitting in a tub of warm water.

Patients who have recurrent UTIs and those managed nonoperatively for VUR require long-term suppressive antibiotics. Full recovery from the urothelial injury of recurrent UTIs takes several months. As a result, irritative voiding symptoms, such as dysuria, incontinence, and frequency, may persist despite the finding of sterile urine. A propensity for recurrent UTI may also persist. Such patients generally require a minimum of 6 months of antibiotic suppression therapy to break the cycle. Table 54–5 outlines the characteristics of the three drugs we most commonly employ for suppression.

□ Vesicoureteral Reflux

VUR refers to the retrograde passage of urine from the bladder into the ureter. In 1883, reflux was first demonstrated in the experimental animal by Simblinow. In 1893, Pozzi observed reflux in people, noting retrograde urine flow from a ureteral stump at the time of nephrectomy. In 1898, Young demonstrated that VUR did not occur in normal bladders. Although VUR was first observed in the late 1800s, only since the 1950s has its clinical importance been recognized.[41] Hutch's studies, reported in 1952, demonstrated the pathophysiologic changes of VUR in the paraplegic patient. This report and the observations of Hodson in 1959, regarding the association between VUR, UTI, and pyelonephritic scarring, set the stage for the modern era of reflux management.

TABLE 54–5. Characteristics of Commonly Used Urosuppressive Antibiotics

Drug	Therapeutic Dose	Suppressive Dose	How Supplied	Comments
Nitrofurantoin	1–2 mg/kg PO qd	1 mg/kg PO qd	Suspension (5 mg/ml) Capsule (25, 50 mg)	Avoid in patients <1 mo of age Not effective if CrCl <40 ml/min Nausea common with suspension; sprinkling macrocrystals may avoid this
Trimethoprim-sulfamethoxazole	4 mg/kg trimethoprim + 20 mg/kg sulfamethoxazole PO bid	2 mg/kg trimethoprim + 10 mg/kg sulfamethoxazole PO qd	Suspension (8 mg trimethoprim + 40 mg sulfamethoxazole per ml Tablet (80 mg trimethoprim, 400 mg sulfamethoxazole)	Avoid in patients <1 mo of age Contraindicated with hyperbilirubinemia May cause blood dyscrasias and Stevens-Johnson syndrome
Amoxicillin	10 mg/kg PO tid	10 mg/kg PO qd	Suspension (25, 50 mg/ml) Drops (50 mg/ml)	Good alternative for newborns

Although most commonly diagnosed during the evaluation of the child with UTI, VUR may also be diagnosed during evaluation of the patient with hypertension, proteinuria, voiding dysfunction, or chronic renal insufficiency or during the evaluation of a sibling of a patient with VUR.

PATHOPHYSIOLOGY

Figure 54–7 depicts the various anatomic components of the competent UVJ as well as the abnormalities most often implicated in the genesis of VUR. The normal UVJ is characterized by an oblique entry of the ureter into the bladder and a length of submucosal ureter providing a high ratio of tunnel length to ureteral diameter. The anatomic configuration provides a predominantly passive valve mechanism.[42–45] As the bladder fills and the intravesical pressure rises, the resultant bladder wall tension is applied to the roof of the ureteral tunnel. The result is a compression of the ureter, which closes this structure to the retrograde passage of urine. Intermittent increases in bladder pressure, such as the act of voiding, upright posture, activity, and coughing, are met with an equal and immediate increase in resistance to retrograde urine flow. This effect is supplemented by the active effects of ureterotrigonal muscle contraction and ureteral peristalsis.[43, 46]

Marginal tunnels can be made to reflux during infection owing to UVJ distortion, loss of compliance of the valve roof, and intravesical hypertension. Excessively high intravesical pressure, as with neurovesical dysfunction (NVD) or bladder outlet obstruction (BOO), may also potentiate reflux, as may a neurogenically or structurally (e.g., diverticulum or ureterocele) weak detrusor floor. Because the submucosal ureter tends to lengthen with age, the ratio of tunnel length to ureteral diameter increases, and the propensity for reflux may disappear.[42, 43]

Of critical importance is the concept of IRR, which has been demonstrated clinically[47] and experimentally.[48] The usually oblique entry of the papillary ducts onto the surface of simple papillae inhibits IRR. In contrast, the papillary duct entrance onto compound papillae facilitates IRR (see Fig. 54–4). The critical pressure for IRR is considered to be about 35 mm Hg in compound papillae.[48, 49] Experimentally, this same pressure may cause scar formation in the absence of infection.[48, 50, 51] When oc-

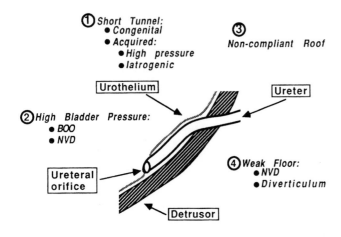

Figure 54–7. Components of the competent ureterovesical junction. The abnormalities most often implicated in the etiology of vesicoureteral reflux are outlined. BOO, bladder outlet obstruction; NVD, neurovesical dysfunction.

curring intravesically, this pressure has been associated with an increased risk of renal deterioration. Higher pressure is thought to be necessary to induce IRR in simple papillae.

The combination of infection and IRR is particularly devastating. Focal scarring appears to be explained by the different susceptibility of renal papillae to IRR. The polar distribution of compound papillae corresponds closely to the predominant occurrence of renal scarring in the upper and lower poles of the kidney.

CLASSIFICATION

A wide spectrum of VUR exists. For this reason, many attempts at classification have been advanced. Reflux has been described as low pressure, which occurs during the filling phase of the VCUG, or high pressure, which occurs only during voiding. Reflux due to a congenitally deficient UVJ is referred to as *primary reflux*, whereas reflux due to a BOO and neurogenic bladder is referred to as *secondary reflux*. Further classification includes simple reflux and complex reflux. Complex reflux includes reflux associated with megaureter, duplicated ureters, diverticulum, or ureterocele and the reflux associated with ipsilateral ureteropelvic or ureterovesical obstruction. The most clinically pertinent classification systems, however, have attempted to quantitate the degree of reflux.[52–54] At present, VUR is graded according to the international classification system diagrammed in Figure 54–8.[54] This classification system is based not only on the proximal extent of retrograde urine flow and ureteral and pelvic dilation but also on the resultant anatomy of the caliceal fornices.

Grade I VUR refers to the visualization of a nondilated ureter only, whereas grade II VUR refers to visualization of a nondilated renal pelvis and caliceal system in addition to the ureter. Grade III reflux involves mild to moderate dilation or ureteral tortuosity with mild to moderate dilation of the renal pelvis and calyces. The fornices, however, remain sharp or only minimally blunted. Once the forniceal angle is completely blunted, grade IV reflux exists. Papillary impressions in most calyces can still be

appreciated. Loss of the papillary impressions along with increased dilation and tortuosity is referred to as grade V reflux.

EPIDEMIOLOGY

The incidence of VUR in otherwise normal children has been estimated to be about 1%.[55, 56] Also apparent from these data is the fact that the incidence of VUR is also low in neonate and infant controls.

A much higher incidence of VUR, 30 to 40%, is reported in patients undergoing evaluation for UTI.[57–60] The incidence is highest in those of youngest age.[61] Thus, the infant who is most vulnerable to the combination of UTI and VUR is precisely the patient in whom this combination is most likely to occur.

Although most reflux patients are female, a few important characteristics of males with VUR require consideration. Although males account for about 14% of patients with VUR,[62] an increased incidence of VUR (30%) is found in those males presenting with UTI.[58] Despite this fact, 14% of boys with VUR have a voiding dysfunction without UTI.[62] Boys with VUR tend to present at a relatively young age (25% are younger than 3 months), and younger children tend to have the most severe degrees of reflux.[62]

The familial association of VUR was reported in 1955 in twins.[63] Since then, multiple studies have documented a significant risk of VUR in family members of patients with reflux. The reported risk of sibling reflux ranges from 27 to 34%,[64, 65] although as many as 66% of offspring of women with reflux also have VUR.[66] As a result of these studies, it has been suggested that siblings, especially those younger than 2 years, undergo screening investigation.

A particularly important subset of patients with reflux includes those who have secondary reflux. Most have NVD or BOO as the primary disease. Many patients, however, have reflux not owing to increased bladder pressure alone but rather because UVJ deficiency appears to be part of the spectrum of congenital deformity. Examples include imperforate anus,[67] ureterocele,[68] and bladder exstrophy. Al-

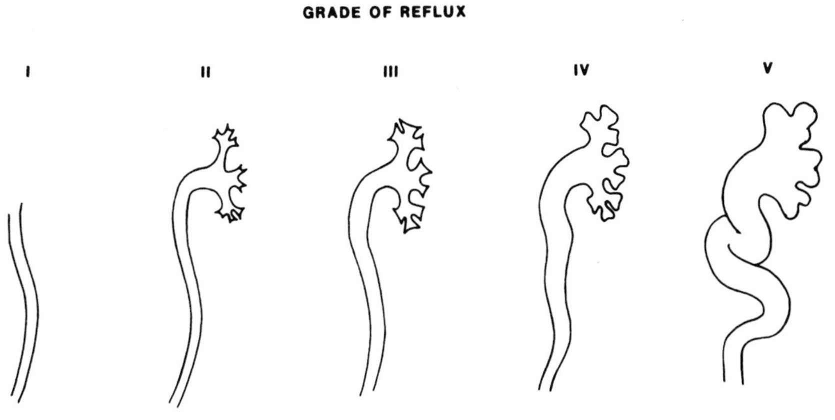

GRADE OF REFLUX

Figure 54–8. The international grading system for vesicoureteral reflux. See text for description. (From The International Reflux Committee: Medical versus surgical treatment of primary vesicoureteral reflux. Pediatrics 67:396, 1987. Reproduced by permission of *Pediatrics*.)

though a significant incidence of NVD exists in patients with imperforate anus, this is not a prerequisite to VUR.[69] The diagnosis of VUR in imperforate anus thus assumes a critical importance to the pediatric surgeon. Not only may the association of NVD potentiate increased severity of reflux and the development of infection, the presence of a rectourethral or rectovesical fistula provides the opportunity for severe urinary contamination. Consequently, we believe that patients with a rectovesical or rectourethral fistula should be managed with a completely diverting colostomy. Although many patients with posterior urethral valves (PUV) have reflux due to

or exacerbated by high intravesical pressure, as demonstrated by VUR resolution after valve ablation or vesicostomy, the incidence of VUR in PUV patients is only about 50%. Many have congenitally abnormal ureteral insertions.[70]

In addition to these structural associations, important functional associations also exist, including florid NVD, as seen in myelodysplasia,[71] and a variety of more subtle voiding disturbances.[72–74] A particularly important subset of VUR patients includes those who have uninhibited detrusor contractions (UDCs). Three important components of maturation are operative in successful toilet training. Growth

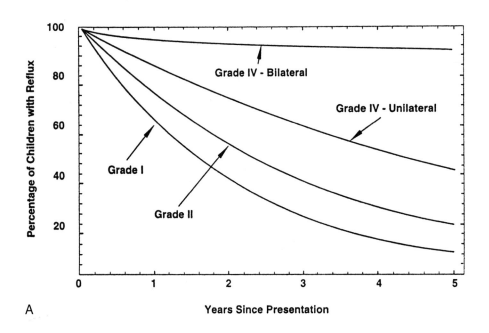

A

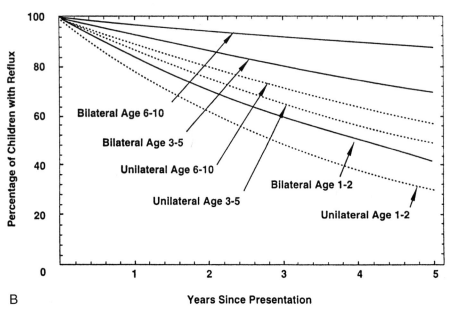

B

Figure 54–9. *A*, Percentage chance of reflux persistence, grades I, II, and IV, for 1 to 5 years after presentation *B*, Percentage chance of reflux persistence by age at presentation, grade III, for 1 to 5 years after presentation. (From American Urological Association: Report on the Management of Primary Vesicoureteral Reflux in Children. Baltimore, American Urological Association, Pediatric Vesicoureteral Reflux Clinical Guidelines Panel, 1997.)

in bladder volume and development of volitional control over the striated muscle sphincter as well as control over bladder smooth muscle are required for the infantile bladder, which empties as a simple spinal reflex, to mature. Many children with reflux and recurrent UTI have UDCs. Such involuntary or uninhibited bladder contractions are not caused by neurologic disease. Intense voluntary constriction of the striated sphincter occurs in an attempt to ensure continence and results in excessively high intravesical pressures. Pressures often exceeding 150 cm H_2O have been observed with resultant intravesical distortions, such as diverticula, saccules, trabeculations, and abnormal ureteral orifices.[75] Reflux occurred in almost half of the children studied with UDC and UTI. Abnormal ureteral orifices were seen in 30% of children without reflux.

Consequently, all patients with VUR must be screened for frequency, urgency, and incontinence, which suggest UDCs. Vincent's curtsy, a squatting maneuver spontaneously employed to prevent incontinence, is particularly suggestive.[74] That these UDCs may cause reflux is suggested by an enhanced resolution of reflux with anticholinergic drug therapy. Equally important is the potential for UDCs to cause a false-negative cystogram. During the performance of VCUG, a child is generally encouraged to void when urgency to do so occurs. In the presence of UDCs, voiding may occur prematurely, and reflux, which might otherwise occur under conditions of volitional detrusor–sphincter dyssynergia, may be masked.

DIAGNOSTIC EVALUATION

The diagnosis of VUR is accomplished by cyclic VCUG, with either contrast medium or isotope.[37, 76] Great care is taken to avoid technical factors that may themselves produce or enhance reflux. Body temperature contrast material, which is not excessively concentrated, is instilled into the bladder through a small catheter by gravity flow of modest pressure in a nonanesthetized child.

Imaging of the upper tracts (kidneys and ureters) is extremely important and may be accomplished by US, isotope renography or, rarely, IV urography (IVU). All these modalities may detect scarring, but isotope renography is particularly sensitive in our experience. US and IVU are helpful in quantitating renal growth or atrophy. Additionally, renal pelvic or ureteral folds or striations on IVU are suggestive of VUR, as is hydroureter on US, which diminishes with bladder drainage.

Cystoscopy is useful in some patients. The appearance of the ureteral orifice, tunnel length, and trabeculation or inflammation may all help determine management. Trabeculation is suggestive of NVD or BOO, which must be treated before reimplantation. Acute urothelial inflammation should be resolved before reimplantation. Patients with frequency, urgency, and incontinence and those requiring the use of Vincent's curtsy should be considered

strongly for urodynamic studies. The presence of UDCs or detrusor–sphincter dyssynergia should be resolved before consideration is given to antireflux surgery.

NATURAL HISTORY

The natural history of VUR is extremely variable, from spontaneous resolution to clinically silent scar formation to hypertension and end-stage renal failure. Numerous factors may contribute to the potential for resolution, including the patient's age, the grade of reflux, the appearance of the ureteral orifice, the length of the ureteral submucosal tunnel, and the intravesical dynamics.

The American Urological Association (AUA) Pediatric Vesicoureteral Reflux Guidelines Panel analyzed 26 reports, comprising 1987 patients with conservative follow-up, to estimate the probability of reflux resolution (Fig. 54–9).[77] In general, a lower reflux grade correlated with a better chance of spontaneous resolution. The configuration of the ureteral orifice (Fig. 54–10) may, on occasion, be helpful in predicting resolution potential.[78, 79]

Younger children are thought to have better prognoses for resolution of reflux. This occurrence may be a result of the potential for trigonal growth, but the diminishing prominence of UDCs with age is also a likely explanation.[80] Spontaneous resolution is relatively independent of grade in secondary reflux, implicating management of primary bladder

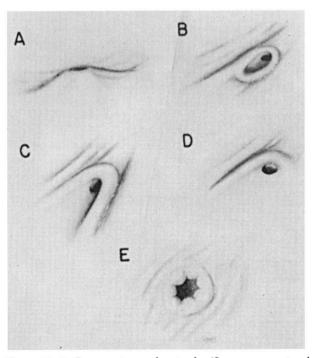

Figure 54–10. Common types of ureteral orifices as encountered endoscopically. *A,* Normal. *B,* Stadium. *C,* Horseshoe. *D,* Lateral pillar. *E,* Golf hole. (From Glassberg KI: Vesicoureteral reflux. In Goldsmith HS [ed]: Practice of Surgery. Urology. New York, Harper & Row, 1982.)

dysfunction as the primary prognostic variable[80] (Fig. 54–11).

Renal injury from VUR may take the form of focal scarring, generalized scarring with atrophy, and failure of renal growth.[81] As a result, kidneys drained by refluxing ureters should be observed not only for scarring but also for renal growth.[82] Renal growth is followed by comparisons based on standardized renal growth curves, such as that shown in Figure 54–12.

Reflux-induced renal injury is usually a result of the association of VUR with UTI.[83] In the past, it was generally considered that such injury is most likely in children younger than 2 years.[61] It is now clear, however, that the risk of renal injury from VUR extends well beyond this age.[60, 83–85] Reflux also appears to be capable of causing renal injury in the absence of UTI, owing to pressure effects from NVD and BOO. The ability of high intravesical pressure when associated with VUR to cause renal injury has been confirmed experimentally.[48, 86]

Cases in infants are encountered, however, with significant renal injury in the absence of BOO, NVD, and UTI.[87] The ureteral bud theory states that VUR associated with displacement of the ureteral orifice is associated with anomalies of renal differentiation.[88] Such ureters probably do not arise from the appropriate segment of wolffian duct and consequently make ectopic contact with the nephrogenic cord, resulting in abnormal renal development. Although such a mechanism may be present in some patients, it is now clear that congenital VUR-associated renal injury in the absence of BOO, NVD, and UTI may occur in the presence of a normally positioned ureteral orifice.[89] This finding implies that pressure effects of in utero VUR may injure the developing kidney.

In a longitudinal study of 923 children, high-pressure bladder dynamics, severity of reflux, and frequency of UTIs were the chief contributing factors in the development of new scars and the worsening of old scars.[85] Children with low-grade VUR were relatively unlikely to develop progressive renal injury, as compared with children with grade IV or V reflux (Fig. 54–13). A similar relationship is seen in children with secondary reflux (Fig. 54–14). When

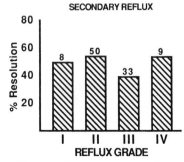

Figure 54–11. The rate of spontaneous resolution of secondary vesicoureteral reflux as a function of reflux grade. (Modified from Cohen RA, Roston MG, Belman AB, et al: Renal scarring and vesicoureteral reflux in children with myelodysplasia. Urol 144 [pt 2]:541, 1990.)

monitoring such children for progression of renal injury as an indicator of success of a therapeutic regimen, one must be cognizant of the fact that radiographic evidence of new renal injury may take 8 months to manifest.

Beyond the silent progression of renal scarring lies a spectrum of symptomatic nephropathy, most notably renal parenchymal hypertension and end-stage renal disease. The significance and predominance of reflux nephropathy as a cause of renal parenchymal hypertension has been reviewed.[90] About 30 to 65% of childhood hypertension is associated with reflux nephropathy, and it is an important cause of end-stage renal failure in children and adults.[91–93] In many affected patients, prior infection was not recognized or was first recognized at or near the time of diagnosis of end-stage renal disease.[91] Because histologic evidence of chronic pyelonephritis is found, preceding infection is likely, underscoring the silent progressive nature of renal nephropathy and the need for meticulous long-term follow-up of children with VUR. Many data exist to suggest that glomerular lesions play an important role in the progression of renal nephropathy. There is a clear association between renal nephropathy, "heavy" proteinuria, and glomerular lesions that resemble focal segmental glomerulosclerosis.[94, 95] Although the mechanisms of this disease remain uncertain, immunologic injury, macromolecular trapping with mesangial injury, vascular alterations with hypertension, and glomerular hyperfiltration have been implicated. The latter theory of glomerular hyperfiltration is presently favored.

TREATMENT

Nonoperative management of VUR is successful in most patients (Table 54–6). Such management may be considered in four stages:
1. Diagnostic evaluation
2. Avoidance of infection
3. Voiding dysfunction treatment
4. Surveillance

Diagnostic evaluation has been previously reviewed. However, it is pertinent to stress that the exclusion and treatment of voiding dysfunction and BOO is imperative. Patients with problematic UDC should undergo suppression therapy. We employ oxybutynin hydrochloride in most of these children. NVD with retentive characteristics may require intermittent catheterization. Good hydration, perineal hygiene, and bowel management are crucial and apply to all patients. With the exception of the older boy with low-grade reflux, most children require suppression antibiotics (see Table 54–5). Although generally well-tolerated, the long-term implications of chronic suppression remain incompletely investigated.

Once a nonoperative regimen is selected, the patient is committed to long-term, strict surveillance. Serial urine cultures are imperative. Renal imaging is performed every 6 to 12 months, depending on

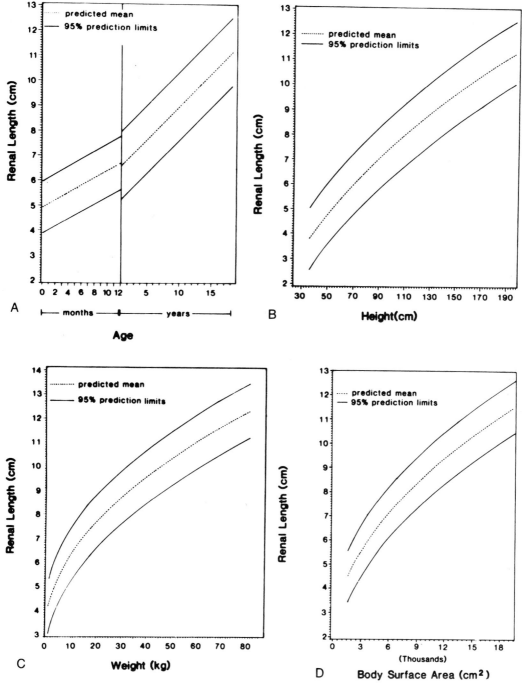

Figure 54–12. Maximal renal length as a function of *(A)* age, *(B)* height, *(C)* weight, and *(D)* body surface area. (From Han B, Babcock DS: Sonographic measurement and appearance of normal kidneys in children. AJR Am J Roentgenol 145:613, 1985.)

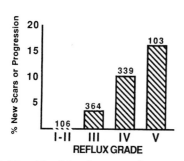

Figure 54–13. The risk of development of new scars or progression of old scars increases with increasing grades of vesicoureteral reflux. The number of ureters in each grade is indicated numerically.

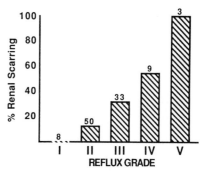

Figure 54–14. The prevalence of renal scarring as a function of reflux grade in patients with secondary reflux. Risk of renal scarring increases with increasing grades of reflux. The number of ureters in each grade is indicated numerically.

TABLE 54–6. General Guidelines for the Nonoperative Management of Vesicoureteral Reflux

Treatment

Hydration
Hygiene
　Perineal hygiene
　　Avoid harsh soaps during tub baths
　　　Bubble baths
　　　Shampoos
Bowel management
　　Avoid constipation
　　Treat encopresis
Suppressive antibiotics
Observation without antibiotics
Anticholinergics, spasmolytics

Surveillance

Urine culture
　Monthly for 3 mo after last UTI
　Thereafter, every 2 to 3 mo
Renal imaging every 6 to 12 mo
　Renal size (ultrasound, IVU)
　Focal scarring (renal scan, IVU)

Voiding cystourethrography (yearly)
　Radiographic VCUG
　　Initial (male, female suspected NVD)
　　Follow-up (NVD)
　Isotope VCUG
　　Routine surveillance
Record growth yearly (height, weight)
Blood pressure
　Routine (yearly)
　Renal scarring (quarterly)
Renal function tests
　BUN, creatinine (yearly if bilateral RN)
GFR estimated (yearly if azotemic)

$$\frac{\text{height (cm)} \times 0.55}{\text{serum creatinine}} = \text{GFR (ml/min/1.73m}^2)$$

　Maximum urine osmolality (yearly if bilateral RN)
Cystoscopy
　Done at time of antireflux surgery, otherwise rarely necessary
Urodynamic evaluation
　History of voiding dysfunction

BUN, blood urea nitrogen; GFR, glomerular filtration rate; IVU, intravenous urogram; NVD, neurovesical dysfunction; UTI, urinary tract infection; VCUG, voiding cystourethrogram.

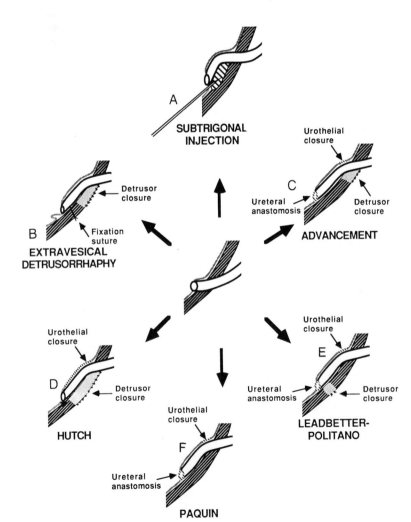

Figure 54–15. Conceptual comparison of techniques to correct reflux. A common theme is the achievement of a long length of ureter based on a strong detrusor floor and covered with compressible urothelium.

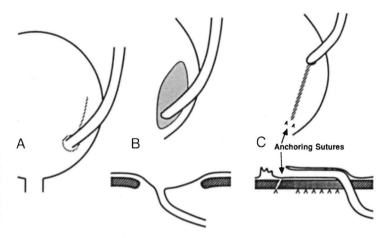

Figure 54–16. The extravesical detrusorrhaphy antireflux technique conceptually viewed from behind the bladder. *A*, The detrusor is incised. *B*, The dissection is continued until the plane between urothelium and muscle has been developed. *C*, The ureter is advanced and fixed into position with anchoring sutures. The detrusor is closed.

the age of diagnosis and the stability of the disease. Attention is directed at both renal growth and focal scarring. Voiding cystourethrography is generally performed yearly. As outlined in Table 54–7, the child's growth, renal function, and blood pressure are monitored. The role of urodynamics has been previously outlined. Cystoscopy is rarely necessary except at the time of antireflux surgery when it is done to exclude urothelial inflammation and to confirm the position and number of ureteral orifices. Otherwise, in our practice, it is generally performed to justify nonoperative therapy in marginal cases.

Patients with surgical indications, such as uncomplicated breakthrough UTIs, significant renal injury at time of initial clinical presentation, grade IV reflux, pubertal age, and failure to respond to 4 years of suppression therapy, may benefit from cystoscopy. The finding on endoscopy of a hopeless ureteral insertion favors antireflux surgery. Other indications for surgical correction of VUR, in our opinion, are progressive renal injury, documented failure of renal growth, breakthrough pyelonephritis, intolerance or noncompliance with antibiotic suppression, and informal parental request.

The AUA Pediatric Vesicoureteral Reflux Guidelines Panel published their recommendations for management of VUR in children (see Table 54–7).[77] There is still no consensus on the management of VUR in patients aged 10 years or older or on the length of time that the clinician should wait before recommending surgery. The actual decision must be carefully individualized.

The principles of antireflux reconstruction include the following:

Ureteral exposure and mobility
Meticulous preservation of blood supply
A long, capacious tunnel

In general, the ratio of tunnel length to ureteral diameter should equal or exceed 5:1. These goals can be attained by a variety of procedures, as diagrammed in Figure 54–15.

Important differences exist between these operative procedures. The following variables must be considered:

Presence or absence of ureteral anastomosis

Need for detrusor closure
Transgression of urothelium
Whether the neohiatus is fashioned by an appropriately sized detrusor incision or closure of detrusor around the ureter

Performance of a ureteral anastomosis increases the risk of postoperative obstruction, whereas the need for detrusor closure increases the risk of diverticula. Table 54–8 outlines the specific advantages and disadvantages of some representative procedures. Three of the most commonly employed procedures for primary VUR are diagrammed in Figures 54–16 through 54–18.

In general, excellent results are attainable with most open procedures. A review of 86 reports, including 6472 patients (8563 ureters), found the overall surgical success rate to be 96%.[77] Surgical success was achieved in 99% of patients with grade I disease, 99.1% with grade II, 98.3% with grade III,

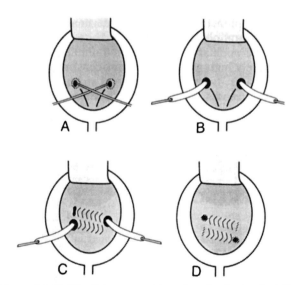

Figure 54–17. The Cohen cross-trigonal ureteral reimplantation. *A*, The ureter is intubated, and the mucosa is incised circumferentially around the ureteral orifice. *B*, The ureters are dissected from the muscular attachments and mobilized until free within the retroperitoneum. *C*, Cross-trigonal tunnels are created by scissor dissection. *D*, The ureteral anastomoses are completed.

TABLE 54–7. Recommendations for Treatment of Vesicoureteral Reflux

Recommendations were derived from a survey of preferred treatment options for 36 clinical categories of children with vesicoureteral reflux (VUR). The recommendations are classified as follows:
Guidelines = Treatments selected by 8 or 9 panel members, given the strongest recommendation language.
Preferred Options = Treatments selected by 5–7 of 9 panel members.
Reasonable Alternatives = Treatments selected by 3–4 of 9 panel members.
No Consensus = Treatments selected by no more than 2 of 9 panel members.

Treatment Recommendations for Children Without Scarring at Diagnosis

| | | Treatment | | | | | |
| | | Initial (antibiotic prophylaxis or open surgical repair) | | | Follow-Up* (continued antibiotic prophylaxis, cystography, or open surgical repair) | | |
VUR Grade Laterality	Age (y)	Guideline	Preferred Option	Reasonable Alternative	Guideline	Preferred Option	No Consensus†
I–II Unilateral or bilateral	<1	Antibiotic prophylaxis					Boys and girls
	1–5	Antibiotic prophylaxis					Boys and girls
	6–10	Antibiotic prophylaxis					Boys and girls
III–IV Unilateral or bilateral	<1	Antibiotic prophylaxis			Bilateral: Surgery if persistent	Unilateral: Surgery if persistent	
	1–5	Unilateral: Antibiotic prophylaxis	Bilateral: Antibiotic prophylaxis			Surgery if persistent	
	6–10		Unilateral: Antibiotic prophylaxis Bilateral: Surgery	Bilateral: Antibiotic prophylaxis		Surgery if persistent	
V Unilateral or bilateral	<1		Antibiotic prophylaxis		Surgery if persistent		
	1–5		Bilateral: Surgery Unilateral: Antibiotic prophylaxis	Bilateral: Antibiotic prophylaxis Unilateral: Surgery	Surgery if persistent		
	6–10	Surgery					

Table continued on opposite page

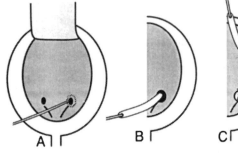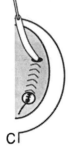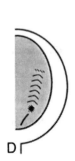

Figure 54–18. The Leadbetter-Politano ureteral reimplantation. *A*, The ureter is intubated. *B*, The ureter is mobilized. The hiatus is dilated, and the retroperitoneal ureter is mobilized. Under direct vision, the peritoneum is reflected from the outer surface of the bladder. *C*, The neohiatus is created, and the ureter is internalized into the bladder. The tunnel is created by scissor dissection, and the original hiatus is closed. *D*, The ureteral anastomosis is completed.

Treatment Recommendations for Children With Scarring at Diagnosis

Treatment

Clinical Presentation (age at presentation)		Initial (antibiotic prophylaxis or open surgical repair)			Follow-up* (continued antibiotic prophylaxis, cystography, or open surgical repair)		
VUR Grade Laterality	Age (y)	Guideline	Preferred Option	Reasonable Alternative	Guideline	Preferred Option	No Consensus†
I–II Unilateral or bilateral	<1	Antibiotic prophylaxis					Boys and girls
	1–5	Antibiotic prophylaxis					Boys and girls
	6–10	Antibiotic prophylaxis					Boys and girls
III–IV Unilateral	<1	Antibiotic prophylaxis			Girls: Surgery if persistent	Boys: Surgery if persistent	
	1–5	Antibiotic prophylaxis			Girls: Surgery if persistent	Boys: Surgery if persistent	
	6–10		Antibiotic prophylaxis		Surgery if persistent		
III–IV Bilateral	<1	Antibiotic prophylaxis			Surgery if persistent		
	1–5		Antibiotic prophylaxis	Surgery	Surgery if persistent		
	6–10	Surgery					
V Unilateral or bilateral	<1		Antibiotic prophylaxis	Surgery	Surgery if persistent		
	1–5	Bilateral: Surgery	Unilateral: Surgery			Surgery if persistent	
	6–10	Surgery					

*For patients with persistent uncomplicated reflux after extended treatment with continuous antibiotic therapy.
†No consensus was reached regarding the role of continued antibiotic prophylaxis, cystography, or surgery.
From American Urological Association: Report on the Management of Primary Vesicoureteral Reflux in Children. Baltimore, American Urological Association Pediatric Vesicoureteral Reflux Clinical Guidelines Panel, 1997.

TABLE 54-8. Specific Advantages and Disadvantages of Commonly Performed Antireflux Procedures

Procedure	Advantages	Disadvantages
Subtrigonal injection	Endoscopic procedure	Material injected: Teflon—migration, granuloma formation Collagen—uncertain durability
Extravesical detrusorrhaphy	Bladder never opened No hematuria No ureteral anastomosis Minimal bladder spasms Endoscopically accessible ureteral orifices	
Advancement: Cohen (transtrigonal) Glenn-Anderson	Avoids complications of neohiatus formation in Leadbetter-Politano reimplantation	Transtrigonal—difficult to access ureter endoscopically Glenn-Anderson—limited length of tunnel achievable
Hutch	No ureteral anastomosis Good alternative with large associated congenital diverticulum	
Leadbetter-Politano	Excellent ureteral tunnel dimensions with endoscopically accessible ureteral orifices	Risk of ureteral obstruction Risk of sigmoid colon injury with left reimplantation
Paquin	Versatility; extremely useful during complex reconstructive procedures	

98.5% with grade IV, and 80.7% with grade V. Although the morbidity rate with endoscopic correction is suggested to be less, the AUA Pediatric Vesicoureteral Reflux Guidelines Panel does not recommend this form of therapy owing to the lack of proven long-term safety and efficacy of most materials used for injection and the lack of approval of such materials by the Food and Drug Administration.[77]

We prefer the extravesical detrusorrhaphy approach.[96-98] Because the lumen of the bladder is not entered, there is no postoperative hematuria, and there are minimal bladder spasms and short hospital stay. Absence of a ureteral anastomosis decreases risk of postoperative obstruction. No ureteral stents, suprapubic tubes, or drains are employed. The Foley catheter is removed on the 1st day after unilateral surgery and on the 2nd day after a bilateral procedure. The extravesical approach for bilateral ureteral reimplantation has been questioned due to a reportedly high incidence of postoperative urinary retention.[99] In our experience with a large group of patients, we found acceptable rates of postoperative urinary retention (4%), which is transient and of minimal morbidity.[100]

Complications of ureteral reimplantation are uncommon and have been previously reviewed.[77, 101] The most common complication is de novo contralateral reflux, whereas the most common technical complications are ureteral obstruction, persistent reflux, and diverticula formation. Persistent reflux may be caused by an insufficient tunnel length–to–ureteral diameter ratio. However, the greatest risk of postoperative reflux is related to the high-pressure voiding dynamics as a result of uninhibited bladder contraction, detrusor sphincter dyssynergia, and urinary retention.

Ureteral obstruction may be due to ureteral kinking (at the neohiatus or obliterated umbilical artery), an excessively highly placed neohiatus, construction of a tight neohiatus, twisting, anastomotic stricture, devascularization, and tight tunnel. With attention directed toward the avoidance of technical complications and the selection of a procedure associated with the lowest complication rate, ureteral reimplantation remains a safe and highly successful operation.

REFERENCES

1. Hoberman A, Chao HP, Keller DM, et al: Prevalence of urinary tract infection in febrile infants. J Pediatr 123:17, 1993.
2. Visser VE, Hall RT: Urine culture in the evaluation of suspected neonatal sepsis. J Pediatr 94:635, 1979.
3. Smellie JM, Hodson CJ, Edwards D, et al: Clinical and radiological features of urinary infection in childhood. Br Med J 2:1222, 1964.
4. Bickerton MW, Duckett JW: Urinary tract infections in pediatric patients. AUA Update Series 4(26), 1985.
5. Pollack CV Jr, Pollack ES, Andrew ME: Suprapubic bladder aspiration versus urethral catheterization in ill infants: Success, efficiency and complication rates. Ann Emerg Med 23:225, 1994.
6. Edelmann CM Jr, Ogwo JE, Fine BP, et al: The prevalence of bacteriuria in full-term and premature newborn infants. J Pediatr 82:125, 1973.
7. Aronson AS, Gustafson B, Svenningsen NW: Combined suprapubic aspiration and clean voided urine examination in infants and children. Acta Paediatr Scand 62:396, 1973.
8. Iravani A: Treatment of urinary tract infections in young women. AUA Update Series 12(6), 1993.
9. Hellerstein S: Recurrent urinary tract infections in children. Pediatr Infect Dis 1:271, 1982.
10. Pryles CV, Lustik B: Laboratory diagnosis of urinary tract infection. Pediatr Clin North Am 18:233, 1971.
11. Hoberman A, Wald ER, Reynolds EA, et al: Pyuria and bacteriuria in urine specimens obtained by catheter from young children with fever. J Pediatr 124:513, 1994.
12. Lockhart GR, Lewander WJ, Cimini DM, et al: Use of urinary gram stain for detection of urinary tract infection in infants. Ann Emerg Med 25:31, 1995.
13. Lohr JA, Portilla MG, Geuder TG, et al: Making a presumptive diagnosis of urinary tract infection by using a urinalysis performed in an on-site laboratory. J Pediatr 122:22, 1993.
14. Durbin WA, Peters G: Management of urinary tract infections in infants and children. Pediatr Infect Dis 3:564, 1984.
15. Liptak GS, Campbell J, Stewart R, et al: Screening for urinary tract infection in children with neurogenic bladders. Am J Phys Med Rehabil 72:122, 1993.
16. Sheldon CA, Gonzalez R: Differentiation of upper and lower urinary tract infection: How and when? Med Clin North Am 68:321, 1984.
17. Cox CE, Hinman F: Experiments with induced bacteriuria, vesical emptying and bacterial growth in the mechanism of bladder defense to infection. J Urol 86:739, 1961.
18. Fowler J, Stamey T: Studies of introital colonization in women with recurrent urinary infections, VII: The role of bacterial adherence. J Urol 117:472, 1977.
19. Bollgren I, Winberg J: The periurethral aerobic flora in girls highly susceptible to urinary tract infections. Acta Paediatr Scand 65:81, 1976.
20. Stamey TA, Mihara G: Studies of introital colonization in women with recurrent urinary tract infection, VI: Analysis of segmented leukocytes in vaginal vestibule in relation to enterobacterial colonization. J Urol 116:72, 1976.
21. Roberts JA: Pathogenesis of nonobstructive urinary tract infections in children. J Urol 144:475, 1990.
22. Rushton HG, Majd M: Pyelonephritis in male infants: How important is the foreskin? J Urol 148:733, 1992.
23. Narden CW, Green GM, Kass EH: Antibacterial mechanisms of the urinary bladder. J Clin Invest 47:2689, 1968.
24. Parsons CL, Greenspan C, Mullholland SG: The primary antibacterial defense mechanism of the bladder. Invest Urol 13:72, 1975.
25. Koff SA, Murtagh DS: The uninhibited bladder in children: Effect of treatment on recurrence of urinary infection and on vesicoureteral reflux resolution. J Urol 130:1138, 1983.
26. Wan J, Kaplinsky R, Greenfield S: Toilet habits of children evaluated for urinary tract infection. J Urol 154:797, 1995.
27. Blethyn AJ, Jenkins HR, Roberts R, et al: Radiological evidence of constipation in urinary tract infection. Arch Dis Child 73:534, 1995.
28. Asscher AW, Sussman M, Waters WE, et al: Urine as a medium for bacterial growth. Lancet 2:1037, 1966.
29. Mannhardt W, Schofer O, Schulte-Wiserman H: Pathogenic factors in recurrent urinary tract infection and renal scar formation in children. Eur J Pediatr 145:330, 1986.
30. Smellie J, Normand I: Urinary tract infection: Clinical aspects. In Williams DI, Johnston JH (eds): Paediatric Urology. London, Butterworths, 1982, p 95.
31. Hanson L: Prognostic indicators in childhood urinary infection. Kidney Int 21:659, 1982.
32. Rushton HG, Majd M, Jantausch B, et al: Renal scarring following reflux and nonreflux pyelonephritis in children: Evaluation with 99m technetium-dimercaptosuccinic acid scintigraphy. J Urol 147:1327, 1992.
33. Wallace D, Rothwell D, Williams D: The long term follow up of surgically treated vesicoureteral reflux. Br J Urol 50:479, 1978.

34. Still J, Cottom D: Severe hypertension in childhood. Arch Dis Child 42:34, 1967.

35. Scott J: Hypertension, reflux and renal scarring. In Johnston JH (ed): Management of Vesicoureteric Reflux. Baltimore, Williams & Wilkins, 1984, p 60.

36. Sheldon CA, Geary DF, Shely EA, et al: Surgical consideration in childhood end-stage renal disease. Pediatr Clin North Am 34:1187, 1987.

37. Paltiel HJ, Rupich RC, Kiruluta HG: Enhanced detection of vesicoureteral reflux in infants and children with use of cyclic voiding cystourethrography. Radiology 184:753, 1992.

38. Conway JJ, King LR, Belman AB, et al: Detection of vesicoureteral reflux with radionuclide cystography: A comparison study with roentgenographic cystography. Am J Roentgenol Radium Ther Nucl Med 115:720, 1972.

39. Bisset GS III, Strife JL, Dunbar JS: Urography and voiding cystourethrography: Findings in girls with urinary tract infection. AJR Am J Roentgenol 148:479, 1987.

40. Johnson CE, Maslow JN, Fattlar DC, et al: The role of bacterial adhesins in the outcome of childhood urinary tract infections. Am J Dis Child 147:1090, 1993.

41. Kramer SA: Vesicoureteral reflux. In Kelalis PP, Belman AB (eds): Clinical Pediatric Urology. Philadelphia, WB Saunders, 1992, p 441.

42. King LR, Kazmi SO, Belman AB: Natural history of vesicoureteral reflux: Outcome of a trial of nonoperative therapy. Urol Clin North Am 1:441, 1974.

43. Stephens FD, Lenaghan D: Anatomical basis and dynamics of vesicoureteral reflux. J Urol 87:669, 1962.

44. Tanagho EA, Hutch JA, Meyers FH, et al: Primary vesicoureteral reflux: Experimental studies of its etiology. J Urol 93:165, 1965.

45. Young HH, Wesson MB: The anatomy and surgery of the trigone. Arch Surg 3:1, 1921.

46. Eckman H, Jacobsson B, Kock NG, et al: High diuresis, a factor in preventing vesicoureteral reflux. J Urol 95:511, 1966.

47. Rolleston GL, Maling TMJ, Hodson CJ: Intrarenal reflux and the scarred kidney. Arch Dis Child 49:531, 1974.

48. Hodson CJ, Maling TM, McManamon PJ, et al: The pathogenesis of reflux nephropathy (chronic atrophic pyelonephritis). Br J Radiol 13(suppl):1, 1975.

49. Thomsen H, Talner LB, Higgins CB: Intrarenal backflow during retrograde pyelography with graded intrapelvic pressure: A radiologic study. Invest Radiol 17:593, 1982.

50. Hodson CJ, Twohill SA: The time factor in the development of sterile reflux scarring following high pressure vesicoureteral reflux. Contr Nephrol 39:358, 1984.

51. Ransley PG, Risdon RA, Godley ML: High pressure sterile vesicoureteral reflux and renal scarring: An experimental study in the pig and minipig. Contr Nephrol 39:320, 1984.

52. Dwoskin JY, Perlmutter AD: Vesicoureteral reflux in children: A computerized review. J Urol 109:888, 1973.

53. Heikel PE, Parkkulalnen KV: Vesicoureteral reflux in children. Ann Radiol 9:1, 1966.

54. Medical versus surgical treatment of primary vesicoureteral reflux: Report of the International Reflux Study Committee. Pediatrics 67:692, 1981.

55. Ransley PG: Vesicoureteral reflux: Continuing surgical dilemma. Urology 12:246, 1978.

56. Arant BS Jr: Vesicoureteric reflux and renal injury. Am J Kidney Dis 17:491, 1991.

57. Sreenarasimhaiah V, Alon US: Uroradiologic evaluation of children with urinary tract infection: Are both ultrasonography and renal cortical scintigraphy necessary? J Pediatr 127:373, 1995.

58. Sargent MA, Stringer DA: Voiding cystourethrography in children with urinary tract infection: The frequency of vesicoureteric reflux is independent of the specialty of the physician requesting the study. AJR Am J Roentgenol 164:1237, 1995.

59. Bourchier D, Abbott GD, Maling TMJ: Radiological abnormalities in infants with urinary tract infections. Arch Dis Child 59:620, 1984.

60. Benador D, Benador N, Slosman D, et al: Are younger children at highest risk of renal sequelae after pyelonephritis? Lancet 349:17, 1997.

61. Ditchfield MR, deCampo JF, Nolan TM, et al: Risk factors in the development of early renal cortical defects in children with urinary tract infection. AJR Am J Roentgenol 162:1393, 1994.

62. Deckter RM, Roth DR, Gonzales ET: Vesicoureteral reflux in boys. J Urol 40:1089, 1988.

63. Stephens FD, Joske R, Simmons RT: Megaureter with vesico-ureteric reflux in twins. Aust N Z J Surg 24:192, 1955.

64. Noe HN: The long-term results of prospective sibling reflux screening. J Urol 148:1739, 1992.

65. Wan J, Greenfield SP, Ng M, et al: Sibling reflux: A dual center retrospective study. J Urol 156(pt 2):677, 1996.

66. Noe HN, Wyatt RJ, Peeden JN Jr, et al: The transmission of vesicoureteral reflux from parent to child. J Urol 148:1869, 1992.

67. McLorie GA, Sheldon CA, Fleisher M, et al: The genitourinary system in patients with imperforate anus. J Pediatr Surg 22:1100, 1987.

68. Churchill BM, Sheldon CA, McLorie GA: The ectopic ureterocele: A proposed practical classification based on renal unit jeopardy. J Pediatr Surg 27:497, 1992.

69. Sheldon CA, Cormier M, Crone K, et al: Occult neurovesical dysfunction in children with imperforate anus. J Pediatr Surg 26:49, 1991.

70. Henneberry MD, Stephens FD: Renal hypoplasia and dysplasia in infants with posterior urethral valves. J Urol 123:912, 1980.

71. Agarwal SK, Khoury AE, Abramson RP, et al: Outcome analysis of vesicoureteral reflux in children with myelodysplasia. J Urol 157:980, 1997.

72. Chandra M, Maddix H, McVicar M: Transient urodynamic dysfunction of infancy: Relationship to urinary tract infections and vesicoureteral reflux. J Urol 155:673, 1996.

73. Koff SA: Relationship between dysfunctional voiding and reflux. J Urol 148:1703, 1992.

74. van Gool JD, Hjalmas K, Tamminen-Mobius T, et al: Historical clues to the complex of dysfunctional voiding, urinary tract infection and vesicoureteral reflux: The International Study in Children. J Urol 148:1699, 1992.

75. Koff SA, Lapides J, Plazza DH: Association of urinary tract infections and reflux with uninhibited bladder contractions and voluntary sphincteric obstruction. J Urol 122:373, 1979.

76. Lebowitz RL: The detection and characterization of vesicoureteral reflux in child. J Urol 148:1640, 1992.

77. American Urological Association: Report on the Management of Primary Vesicoureteral Reflux in Children. Baltimore, American Urological Association, Pediatric Vesicoureteral Reflux Clinical Guidelines Panel, 1997.

78. Lyon RP, Marshall S, Tanagho EA: The ureteric orifice: Its configuration and competency. J Urol 102:504, 1969.

79. Stephens FD: Cystoscopic appearance of the ureteric orifices associated with reflux nephropathy. In Hodson J, Kincaid-Smith P (eds): Reflux Nephropathy. New York, Masson, 1979, p 121.

80. Cohen RA, Rushton HG, Belman AB, et al: Renal scarring and vesicoureteral reflux in children with myelodysplasia. J Urol 144(pt 2):541, 1990.

81. Smellie JM, Normand ICS: Reflux nephropathy in childhood. In Hodson J, Kincaid-Smith P (eds): Reflux Nephropathy. New York, Masson, 1979, p 14.

82. Claesson I, Jacobsson B, Olsson T, et al: Assessment of renal parenchymal thickness in normal children. Acta Radiol Diagn 22(3B):305, 1981.

83. Smellie JM, Ransley PG, Normand IC, et al: Development of new renal scars: A collaborative study. Br Med J 290:1957, 1985.

84. McLorie GA, McKenna PH, Jumper BM, et al: High grade vesicoureteral reflux: Analysis of observational therapy. J Urol 144(pt 2):537, 1990.

85. Shimada K, Matsui T, Ogino T, et al: Renal growth and progression of reflux nephropathy in children with vesicoureteral reflux. J Urol 140(pt 2):1097, 1988.

86. Ransley PG, Risdon RA: Reflux and renal scarring. Br J Radiol 14(suppl):1, 1978.

87. Marra G, Barbieri G, Dell'Agnola CA, et al: Congenital renal damage associated with primary vesicoureteral reflux detected prenatally in male infants. J Pediatr 124(pt 1):726, 1994.

88. Makie GG, Stephens FD: Duplex kidneys: A correlation of renal dysplasia with position of the ureteral orifice. J Urol 114:274, 1975.

89. Najmaldin A, Burge DM, Atwell JD: Reflux nephropathy secondary to intrauterine reflux. J Pediatr Surg 25:387, 1990.

90. Cortez J, Sheldon CA: Focal and diffuse renal parenchymal lesions associated with hypertension: The urologic surgeon's approach to evaluation and management. In Loggie J (ed): Pediatric and Adolescent Hypertension. Cambridge, MA, Blackwell Scientific, 1991, p 217.

91. Salvatierra O, Kountz SL, Belzer FO: Primary vesicoureteral reflux and end-stage renal disease. JAMA 226:1454, 1973.

92. McEnery PT, Alexander SR, Sullivan K, et al: Renal transplantation in children and adolescents: The 1992 annual report of the North American Pediatric Renal Transplant Cooperative Study. Pediatr Nephrol 7:711, 1993.

93. Avner ED, Chavers B, Sullivan EK, et al: Renal transplantation and chronic dialysis in children and adolescents: The 1993 annual report of the North American Pediatric Renal Transplant Cooperative Study. Pediatr Nephrol 9:61, 1995.

94. Bhathena DB, Weiss JH, Holland NH, et al: Focal and segmental glomerulosclerosis in reflux nephropathy. Am J Med 68:886, 1980.

95. Hinchliffe SA, Kreczy A, Ciftci AO, et al: Focal and segmental glomerulosclerosis in children with reflux nephropathy. Pediatr Pathol 14:327, 1994.

96. Zaontz MR, Maizels M, Sugar EC, et al: Detrusorrhaphy: Extravesical ureteral advancement to correct vesicoureteral reflux in children. J Urol 138(pt 2):947, 1987.

97. Wacksman J, Gilbert A, Sheldon CA: Results of the renewed extravesical reimplant for surgical correction of vesicoureteral reflux. J Urol 148:359, 1992.

98. Houle AM, McLorie GA, Heritz DM, et al: Extravesical nondismembered ureteroplasty with detrusorrhaphy: A renewed technique to correct vesicoureteral reflux in children. J Urol 148(pt 2):704, 1992.

99. Fung LC, McLorie GA, Jain U, et al: Voiding efficiency after ureteral reimplantation: A comparison of extravesical and intravesical techniques. J Urol 153:1972, 1995.

100. Minevich E, Aronoff D, Wacksman J, et al: Voiding dysfunction after bilateral extravesical detrusorrhaphy. J Urol 160(pt 2):1004, 1998.

101. Gibbons MD, Gonzales ET: Complications of antireflux surgery. Urol Clin North Am 10:489, 1983.

55

BLADDER AND URETHRA

Patrick C. Cartwright, MD • Brent W. Snow, MD

☐ Anatomy and Physiologic Function

The lower urinary tract consists of the bladder and urethra, which normally function as a coordinated unit to store and discharge urine from the body. Both structural and functional disorders of the bladder or urethra may be responsible for urinary incontinence, infection, discomfort or pain, and upper tract deterioration to the point of compromising renal function and threatening life. This chapter focuses on dysfunction of the bladder and urethra as a unit and on the management of such disorders.

The bladder and upper urethra are composed of bundles of smooth muscle fibers arranged in a reticular lattice, the outermost bundles being more circular and the inner bundles more longitudinal at the bladder neck.[1] The smooth muscle bundles blend into the striated muscle fibers of the external urethral sphincter, which are derived from the pelvic diaphragm. The bladder is lined by transitional epithelia, which are sensitive to irritants such as bacterial toxins and various urinary crystals. The urethra and trigone are especially sensitive, and the presence of any irritant in these areas can create significant discomfort.

Normal innervation and bladder function are intimately related: proper functioning of the lower urinary tract depends on intact autonomic and somatic nervous innervation. The detrusor muscle of the bladder proper is innervated by both sympathetic and parasympathetic fibers. Storage functions are mediated by the sympathetic component, which arises from spinal levels T10–L1 and descends through the sympathetic chain to reach the bladder. The chemical mediator of this storage process is norepinephrine, which acts on β-adrenergic receptors in the fundus of the bladder and causes muscle relaxation to aid in low-pressure storage of urine. The same sympathetic stimulus acts on predominately α-adrenergic receptors of the trigone, bladder neck, and proximal urethra to provide an increase in internal sphincter activity and further promote

continence during the storage process by maintaining outlet resistance.[2, 3]

The external urinary sphincter, innervated by the pudendal nerve, maintains a progressively increasing tone as the bladder fills. This "guarding" provides an additional continence mechanism for the storage of urine.[4] As the child develops, the external sphincter may be consciously contracted at times of urgency or stress to prevent the unwanted passage of small amounts of urine. Properly coordinated function of the external urinary sphincter relies on an intact sacral reflex arc (afferents, sacral micturition center, pudendal efferents). This should be intact and developed in normal infants but is variably functional in infants with spinal cord or pelvic lesions.

The sensation of bladder fullness initiates a response in mature human beings that causes them to seek an appropriate facility for the discharge of urine. Once that is done, the parasympathetic nervous system, with acetylcholine as the mediator, causes cholinergic fibers of the detrusor to contract and those of the proximal urethra and bladder to widen and shorten, eliminating its resistance to outflow. When coupled with relaxation of the volitional external sphincter, the bladder empties by sustained and complete contraction of the detrusor, leaving a residual urine volume in the bladder of less than 5 ml.

Spinal pathways connect the sacral micturition center with three centers in the brain stem, collectively called the *pontine micturition center*.[5] This center functions to inhibit urination and to produce external sphincter relaxation, when sustained detrusor contraction occurs. Above this level are areas of cerebral cortex, which oversee and modulate the autonomic process. It is the mature, integrated function of all these components that produces urinary continence.

Conscious control of the bladder (toilet training) is, in large part, a learned phenomenon. It requires adequate recognition by the brain that micturition would be inconvenient or socially unacceptable in a given situation. As the child grows, the bladder gains capacity, allowing for longer intervals between voiding. The approximate bladder volume in ounces may be estimated in a child as age in years plus 2. It may also be calculated by a more precise formula if needed.[6] It has been observed that the young infant voids 20 times per day, which decreases to about 10 times per day by age 3 years.[7] Along with this change, the child also learns to resist the urge to void by voluntary contraction of the external sphincter until the detrusor contraction passes and the bladder once again relaxes. Thus, toilet training depends on the development of semivoluntary detrusor sphincter dyssynergia, which at times persists as a pathologic process.[8] Finally, full bladder control relies on the child developing volitional control over the spinal micturition reflex so that he or she can initiate or inhibit detrusor contractions. Most children have attained day and night continence by 4 years of age.

The inappropriate discharge of urine (enuresis) may be in part due to immaturity of the bladder and its nervous system connections. The usual sequence of bladder development is linked to that of the bowel and is as follows:

1. Control of bowel at night
2. Control of bowel during the day
3. Control of bladder during the day
4. Control of bladder at night

Many lesions interfere with the ideal storage and emptying functions of the bladder. The application of appropriate diagnostic measures can lead to appropriate management decisions, which ultimately lead to continence and to preservation and protection of the upper urinary tract.

☐ Childhood Enuresis

Enuresis is the term used for the unintentional loss of urine beyond toilet training. The following definitions are clinically useful:

Nocturnal enuresis: nighttime (more precisely, sleep-time) incontinence
Primary nocturnal enuresis: nighttime incontinence, never been continent at night
Secondary nocturnal enuresis: nighttime incontinence following a significant dry period
Diurnal enuresis: daytime wetting after toilet training
Stress incontinence: urine leakage due to physically stressful activities such as coughing
Urge incontinence: unintentional loss of urine when bladder urgency occurs

The discussion of enuresis is divided into sections on nocturnal and diurnal enuresis, realizing that some children have both and that management strategies must therefore be melded.

NOCTURNAL ENURESIS

About 15 to 20% of children at 5 years of age continue to have bed wetting.[9] Because so many children still wet at night at this age, it is considered within the range of normal and not termed nocturnal enuresis. Night wetting, thereafter, resolves at the rate of about 15% each year, and by age 15 years, 99% of children have resolved.[10]

Etiology

Children with monosymptomatic nocturnal enuresis are, in general, physically and emotionally similar to their peers. The difference lies in their inability to awaken during sleep when their bladder is full or contracts. The etiology of this disorder is likely complex and several factors should be considered.

Genetic

Family history is often strong, with multiple members having had childhood nocturnal enuresis. If both the parents have a history of bed wetting, 77% of their offspring do. If only one parent had the problem, then 44% of the offspring exhibit the behavior. When neither parent has a history of nocturnal enuresis, then only 15% of their children have the complaint.[11]

Psychological

Psychological stress is observed to induce nocturnal enuresis in certain children. Secondary nocturnal enuresis often raises this concern. Common factors are divorce, changing of homes, birth of new sibling, trouble at school, or just starting school.

Developmental

As children grow, bladder capacity increases significantly each year at a proportion greater than urine volume produced.[12, 13] Volitional control over bladder and sphincter also may mature at variable rates and may be related to subtle delays in other areas of development (e.g., perceptual abilities, fine motor skills).[14]

Urodynamic

Studies show that enuretic episodes occur when the bladder is full, and they simulate normal awake voiding.[13] Although nocturnal enuretic patients have more nighttime unstable bladder contractions than do nonenuretic patients, the contractions are at low pressure and do not cause leakage.

When observed scientifically, night wetting appears to occur in three fashions: wetting associated with significant restlessness and visceral and somatic activity (deep respirations), wetting with a quick contraction and minimal movement, and wetting with no central nervous system response (parasomnia).

Sleep Disorders

Parents of children with nocturnal enuresis are generally convinced that these children sleep deeply and are difficult to arouse. However, controlled studies consistently find this not to be true, with enuretic patients sleeping no more deeply than age-matched controls, wetting in all stages of sleep, and showing no different awakening patterns. Wetting episodes occur randomly throughout the night.[15]

Antidiuretic Hormone

Antidiuretic hormone (ADH) is released from the pituitary in a circadian rhythm so that levels are higher at night and thus diminish urine output. Some children appear to undersecrete ADH at night; thus, by not concentrating at night, urine volume may overwhelm the bladder capacity, and bed-wetting results.[16, 17] Although some patients follow this pattern, others do not; the altered circadian patterns appear to normalize with maturation.

Evaluation

Children usually are seen by the physician when either the child becomes socially embarrassed or the parents are either "fed up" or worried that there may be other pathology. Screening evaluation should include history, physical examination, and always urinalysis. If these are normal, then no other evaluation is needed because organic disease rarely causes monosymptomatic nocturnal enuresis. Routine radiographic evaluation or cystoscopy is unwarranted. Children with an associated anomaly or problem such as urinary tract infection (UTI), evidence of sacral anomalies, or complex enuresis patterns often warrant radiographic investigation.

Treatment

The treating physician should recognize enuresis as a symptom and not a disease. Realizing that there may be more than one cause permits the physician to consider more than one treatment option. Specific treatment is generally discouraged before the age of 7 years. Certain measures are sensible in all nocturnal enuretic patients: void just before getting into bed, avoid huge fluid loads after supper, and avoid caffeine after 3:00 PM.

Enuretic Alarms

Wetting alarms are devices that fit in the underwear of the patients. When moistened, an electrical contact is made, and the alarm is sounded. This is conditioning therapy requiring a motivated patient and parents. The alarm is loud and sounds like a doorbell in the middle of the night. The parent may need to arouse the child, take him or her to the bathroom, and reset the alarm; this may occur multiple times each night.

A compilation of 16 published series showed an initial cure rate of 82%.[18] Average length of treatment to achieve dryness varied between 18 nights and 2½ months. Relapse does occur in 20 to 30% of children treated, but re-treatment can be successful.[19] In a 1995 study, 1 year after instituting nocturnal enuresis treatments, wetting alarms were shown

to give the best long-term results as compared with other treatments.[20]

Imipramine

Tricyclic antidepressants have been used for many years to treat bed wetting. The exact mechanism of action is unknown. Initial success has been reported in the 50% range. Clinical practice reveals that cessation of the treatment induces many relapses, and the longer the initial treatment the more benefit before the effect wanes. It is suggested that the medication be weaned slowly rather than stopped abruptly.

Side effects include anxiety, insomnia, dry mouth, nausea, and personality changes. An imipramine overdose can cause fatal cardiac arrhythmias and conduction blocks that are untreatable; owing to this, medication safety in the home becomes a significant issue.[21] Some suggest that imipramine may improve response rates to the enuretic alarm.

Desmopressin

Desmopressin is an analog of ADH that mimics its urine-concentrating activity without the vasopressor effect.[22] It is currently given either nasally, with a spray, or orally. The effect of desmopressin is dose dependent, usually requiring 20 to 40 µg/day for success.

Complete dryness rates vary with desmopressin and may be highest in patients with a strong bed-wetting history in the family. In three multicenter trials in the United States, response rates were reported in 24 to 35% of children who had failures associated with other forms of treatment.[23] In a study in which dose titration was watched closely, 70% dryness was reported.[24] Desmopressin may occasionally have side effects, including electrolyte changes, nasal irritation, and headaches.

Anticholinergics

Oxybutynin is the most common drug used in this category for enuresis. It is effective when day and nighttime wetting occur in the same patient but has no benefit over placebo when nighttime wetting is the only symptom.[25]

General Approach

Although many parents consider bed wetting a problem, they often do not consider it significant enough to treat, especially when medications are being considered. If therapy is desired, it is often most reasonable to begin with an enuretic alarm. This has the highest response rate, no side effects, and the lowest relapse rate. Combination therapy with imipramine may be considered when unsuccessful with the alarm. If desmopressin has proved successful in a specific patient, the patient and family may choose to keep it available and use it only on specific nights when dryness is especially desired (e.g., sleepovers, grandparents' house). Some patients do not respond to therapy, and time, reassurance, and a caring approach are all that can be offered.

DIURNAL ENURESIS

Diurnal enuresis is the undesired loss of urinary control while awake. The patient history is of paramount importance in sorting out the various categories of diurnal enuresis and is discussed later. The physical examination and evaluation should always assess for abdominal mass or tenderness, distended bladder, normal structure of genitalia, signs of spina bifida occulta, perineal sensation, sacral reflexes, gait, lower extremity reflexes, and urinalysis. Radiographic evaluation, usually voiding cystourethrogram (VCUG) and renal ultrasonography (US), are necessary in patients with UTI or complex incontinence patterns.

Unstable Bladder

Unstable bladder is by far the most common diagnosis in children with persistent daytime wetting.[26] These children have usually toilet trained but later develop increasing "accidents" associated with urgency. They describe not knowing that the bladder contraction was coming. They dash to the bathroom or try to "hold it in." Boys grab and compress the penis, and girls often cross their legs and dance around or squat with the heel compressed over the perineum (Vincent's curtsy). In our experience, children with hyperactivity disorders or a willful disposition appear prone to this dysfunctional voiding pattern.

By urodynamic studies, these children demonstrate significant unstable (unwanted) contractions during bladder filling that cause leakage before sphincter contraction (or posturing) can control it. Because these unstable contractions or spasms occur frequently during the day, there develops a retentive pattern of using the external sphincter to "hold on." When these children do get to the bathroom and try to void, the sphincter relaxes poorly or only intermittently, with resultant stop-and-go voiding, difficulty initiating, straining, and poor emptying. The elevated pressure during voiding and the poor emptying often result in secondary vesicoureteral reflux (VUR) and UTI. Finally, the overactivity of the urinary sphincter may carry over to function of the anal sphincter, and stool retention and encopresis are commonly associated findings.

Treatment

Treatment rests on managing all aspects of this condition simultaneously. Mild encopresis is treated with dietary changes or laxatives and mineral oil after initial bowel clean out. Recurring UTIs are managed with prophylactic antibiotics. Bladder instability is treated with timed voiding at frequent intervals (an alarm watch for the child is helpful) and anticholinergics such as oxybutynin, propantheline, or tolterodine.

Unfortunately, initial success is often followed by later relapse. If initial treatment is unsuccessful, it may be successful if retried later. Patients older than 8 years who fail treatment should be considered for urodynamic testing. VUR is followed in the usual manner with a high probability for resolution (80%) as bladder function improves.[27] The unstable bladder of childhood is almost always outgrown, and adults generally do not demonstrate this type of wetting problem.

Isolated Frequency Syndrome

A separate, and much less common, group of children present with fairly acute onset of urinary frequency. They appear healthy, are normal on examination, and have normal urinalysis and culture. They do not have true urgency or any wetting but feel that they must urinate frequently, sometimes every 5 to 10 minutes. They void a very small amount each time. Most sleep through the night and void a large amount on awakening. The pattern may come and go over weeks or months.

The cause is unclear but may relate to emotional stress in many cases. Careful assessment is crucial, and reassurance to parent and child is paramount. Sometimes, setting an alarm to progressively lengthen voiding intervals with a reward for success is helpful. This condition is benign and self-limited, although it may persist intermittently for months. Anticholinergics have no benefit, and further evaluation is not required.

Infrequent Voider—Lazy Bladder

On the other end of the voiding spectrum are those children who void only once or twice daily and may not go until afternoon after waking in the morning.[28] These children have developed urinary retentive behavior without any unstable bladder activity and have dilated, high-capacity, low-pressure bladders.[29] Some show an aversion to bathrooms or exhibit excessive neatness, whereas many others appear reasonably adjusted. They may be somewhat prone to UTI and stress incontinence.

Evaluation must demonstrate no neurologic cause and no structural obstruction to emptying. US can demonstrate good emptying if performed before and after voiding. A timed voiding regimen is usually required to get these children to void regularly if problems are occurring. This pattern tends to improve with maturation.

Total Incontinence and Constant Dribbling

Patients who present with total incontinence and constant dribbling of urine have a higher probability of urinary tract structural pathology and require radiographic and possibly urodynamic evaluation.

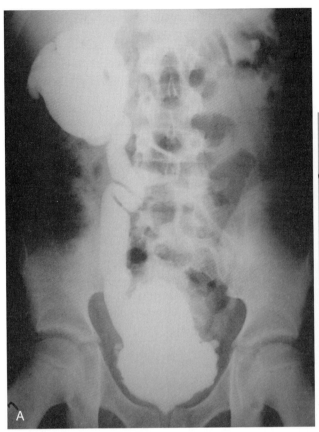

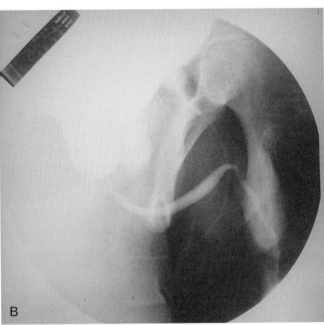

Figure 55–1. *A,* Radiograph of a typical urinary tract in a patient with Hinman's syndrome: trabeculated bladder and severe reflux. *B,* Voiding study in the same patient demonstrates dilation of the posterior urethra as a result of chronic contraction of the external sphincter during voiding.

Hinman's Syndrome

A small number of children demonstrate persistent incontinence, repeated febrile UTI, reflux, high bladder storage pressures, and very poor emptying.[30] This appears to be a deeply ingrained "learned" disorder of severe detrusor–sphincter dyssynergia. In these patients, the urinary tract has the appearance of that in a patient with neurogenic bladder. There is hydronephrosis, a trabeculated bladder, reflux, and sometimes progressive loss of renal function (Fig. 55–1).

Aggressive therapy with prophylactic antibiotics, anticholinergics, urodynamic biofeedback training, timed voiding, or intermittent catheterization may be required. Some recalcitrant cases may require bladder diversion or augmentation to avoid renal failure. As with many "functional" disorders, the severity of Hinman's syndrome tends to wane with maturation, but progressive deterioration may not permit the surgeon to wait.

☐ Neurogenic Bladder

True neurogenic dysfunction of the bladder in childhood results from acquired or congenital lesions that affect bladder innervation. Acquired lesions may occur from trauma to the brain, spinal cord, or pelvic nerves or as a result of tumor, infection, or vascular lesions affecting these same structures. Congenital lesions include spina bi-

fida and other neural tube defects (most common), degenerative neuromuscular disorders, cerebral palsy, tethered cord, sacral agenesis, imperforate anus, VACTERL (*v*ertebral, *a*nal, *c*ardiac, *t*racheal, *e*sophageal, *r*enal, and *l*imb) syndrome, and other causes.[31]

The most practical way to classify neurogenic bladder abnormalities is by a simple functional system: failure to store, failure to empty, or a combination of both.[32] Failure to store urine may be caused by the detrusor muscle itself or by the bladder outlet. Detrusor hyperactivity or poor compliance during bladder filling causes elevated bladder pressures and incontinence on this basis. Inadequate outlet resistance caused by an incompetent bladder neck or urethral sphincter mechanism can be the outlet cause of failure to store urine even if storage pressures are reasonable. Failure to empty can suggest either a bladder muscle or bladder outlet etiology as well. The hypotonic, neurogenic bladder may not generate enough pressure with detrusor contraction to empty. Alternatively, the outlet may exhibit increased resistance secondary to striated or smooth muscle sphincter dyssynergia. This classification helps to base treatment on urodynamic data.

MYELOMENINGOCELE

General

The most common cause of neurogenic bladder in childhood is the group of neural tube defects, which ranges from occult spinal dysraphism[33] to myelomeningocele.[34] Myelomeningocele is the most severe and the most common, occurring in about 1 in 1000 live births with notable geographic variations.[35, 36] The etiology is multifactorial, with a clear familial association and evidence that periconceptual folic acid supplementation (0.4 mg/day) reduces the risk by 60 to 80%.[37] Improved care of the neurosurgical aspects of this lesion since the late 1970s has increased the survival rate of children with this condition; thus, continued urologic care is of much importance. Almost all newborns with myelomeningocele have normal upper tract drainage and renal function. However, if no care is administered to the bladder, at least half of these patients show signs of upper tract deterioration or reflux within 5 years.[38] It is therefore critical that early urologic evaluation of children with myelomeningocele is undertaken.[39, 40]

Evaluation of the Newborn with Myelomeningocele

Generally, the newborn with myelomeningocele has had a thorough neurologic assessment, closure of the back defect, and possibly even ventriculoperitoneal shunting before any evaluation of the urinary tract. The level of the bony defect does not predict the functional cord level because lesions may be partial and patchy. Before discharge, renal and bladder US should be performed to evaluate parenchymal quality, the presence of hydronephrosis, and the size and emptying ability of the bladder. About 10% of patients have an abnormality on US, in which case a VCUG and an evaluation of upper tract function and drainage by renal scan should be performed. If the US is normal, other studies can probably be delayed a few months, although we prefer to proceed with VCUG before hospital discharge mainly for logistical reasons. About 10% of these patients have reflux. Children are placed on amoxicillin prophylaxis (15 mg/kg once daily), and serum creatinine is followed during the initial hospitalization period. Many children experience poor emptying for a few days or weeks after the initial back closure, and postvoid residuals should be measured before discharge from the hospital. Intermittent catheterization is begun if the residual urine is consistently greater than 15 ml. Credé's maneuver should be avoided because it is ineffective in emptying the bladder and magnifies the detrimental effects of high intravesical pressure if reflux is present.

Traditionally, urodynamic assessment of the child with myelodysplasia has been undertaken at the time of initiation of the bladder training program. Newborn urodynamic evaluation has since been shown to have prognostic value in determining which children are likely to develop upper tract dilation and VUR. Children with bladder pressures higher than 40 cm H_2O at the point of urinary leakage and those with detrusor–sphincter dyssynergia are much more likely to show upper tract deterioration or VUR.[2, 39] Other factors shown to indicate bladder "hostility" include the presence of reflux, hyperreflexic contractions, and poor detrusor compliance.[40] Therefore, early urodynamic evaluation is useful in determining the frequency of follow-up studies and the timing of initiation of bladder therapy programs.

If the radiographic evaluation is normal and no infection is present, the patient can be managed by spontaneous voiding into the diaper, especially if leak-point pressures are low. Follow-up studies are planned with urine culture and renal US at 6 months. If leak-point pressures are high or sphincter dyssynergia is present, VCUG again at 6 months is prudent. US and urine cultures should be repeated yearly if stable, with or without VCUG, depending on the relative risk of the upper tract as determined by urodynamics. If reflux or upper tract deterioration occurs at any time, intervention with clean intermittent catheterization (CIC), anticholinergic therapy, or temporary cutaneous vesicostomy may be warranted.

MANAGEMENT

Periodic reassessment of the anatomy and function of the urinary tract is key because the clinical and urodynamic picture may change with growth. Initiation of a bladder management program is generally undertaken when there is worsening reflux, upper tract dilation, or infection. If the urinary tract is stable, such management may be delayed until social continence is desired.

The cornerstone of treatment programs for neurogenic bladder in most children is CIC. Popularized in the early 1970s, CIC has revolutionized the treatment program for these children.[41] The purpose of CIC is to provide periodic low-pressure emptying of the bladder, which can prevent or improve existing deterioration of the upper tracts, including that secondary to reflux.[42, 43] In younger children, this task is performed by the caretaker. As children become older and more responsible, they themselves can assume the task. Motivation is important in adhering to a good bladder program. Therefore, it is sometimes better to wait until social pressures influence the child's desire for continence before initiating a bladder program, unless it is required for the treatment of upper tract deterioration.

CIC is associated with a high incidence of bacteriuria (when followed with serial culturing), varying greatly in different series.[44, 45] Bacteriuria is eventually found in about 60% of cases, with most patients becoming culture positive within 1 year, often with one or two symptomatic episodes per year.[46] In patients with no reflux and with normal intravesical pressure, asymptomatic bacteriuria appears to have little clinical significance. However, in patients with high pressures, reflux, or a combination of the two, the potential for upper tract deterioration increases significantly with bacteriuria.[46] Infection with urea-splitting organisms (usually *Proteus* species) is of concern owing to the potential for struvite stone formation.

Pharmacologic therapy for neurogenic bladder is usually coupled with CIC and is aimed at decreasing the pressures in the hypertonic, noncompliant bladder or increasing bladder outlet resistance to aid in gaining continence. Anticholinergic drugs, such as oxybutynin, propantheline, or tolterodine,[47] are used to lower bladder storage pressures by blocking hypertonic detrusor activity. Imipramine may also be useful alone or in combination with the anticholinergic agents because it can both relax detrusor and tighten the outlet. Inadequate vesical outlet resistance may also respond to α-adrenergic medications, such as pseudoephedrine. Often, the combination of anticholinergics, α-agonists, and CIC is required to gain adequate continence. Side effects of the anticholinergics may sometimes limit their use. Tolterodine is purported to cause fewer side effects than other anticholinergics. Instillation of oxybutynin dissolved in water directly in the bladder can lessen the side effects and still maintain a therapeutic response.[48]

Urodynamic assessment helps the clinician select medications and other modalities for neurogenic bladder and to monitor their effects.[3] This study may be elaborate in certain situations but is more often a simple measurement of the pressure–volume relationship of the bladder during filling. It is performed using a double-lumen catheter in the bladder and usually involves simultaneous assessment of external sphincter function with a perineal electrode patch. Urodynamic assessment can be performed with contrast material and monitored fluoroscopically to add information. Noting parameters such as bladder compliance, hyperreflexic contractions, leak-point pressure, stress leak-point pressure, and sphincter dyssynergia can be extremely valuable in helping to choose among treatment options. Figure 55–2 demonstrates the effect of anticholinergics in shifting the pressure–volume curve to the right and thus permitting the bladder to store more urine at any given pressure. Figure 55–3 shows

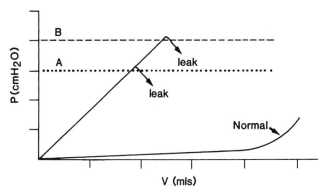

Figure 55–3. Bladder filling pressure–volume curve demonstrating the higher leak point sometimes achieved with α-adrenergic agents such as pseudoephedrine and imipramine.

the effect of α-adrenergic receptors on raising the leak-point pressure and thus permitting storage to a higher pressure.

It is crucial to understand that when bladder pressures remain greater than 35 to 40 cm H_2O, ureteral peristalsis does not effectively empty the upper tracts, and hydronephrosis and eventual renal insufficiency result. Thus, coupling cystometric data with a particular patient's estimated (or measured) hourly output permits the clinician to decide what CIC interval would keep bladder pressures in a safe range. Medications can then be sensibly adjusted to extend CIC intervals, achieve dryness, and avoid development or progression of hydronephrosis.

Transurethral electrical stimulation of the bladder has been used in several treatment centers in an effort to produce conscious urinary control in the patient with neurogenic bladder.[49] It is a time-consuming treatment program with sometimes hundreds of sessions required before a response. Although some series have shown variably encouraging results, especially concerning the improvement in bladder compliance,[49, 50] others have found the results disappointing.[51, 52] More experience is necessary, but this technique may be applicable in selected children. Selective sacral nerve root rhizotomy and electrical stimulation of the sacral nerve roots may also have some limited potential for treatment in certain children.[53–55]

In children with high bladder storage pressures and deterioration of the upper tracts who cannot be managed by CIC or pharmacologic therapy, temporary diversion with cutaneous vesicostomy may be necessary.[56, 57] Protection of the upper urinary tracts from high bladder pressures is thus accomplished until such time that other treatments can be tolerated. We reserve this treatment for infants who have serious deterioration of the upper tract and those who, for social, medical, or anatomic reasons, cannot be managed with the other aforementioned forms of medical treatment. As an alternative, some advocate urethral dilation in girls to diminish the leak-point pressure. Surprising persistence of benefit has been noted in some series.[58]

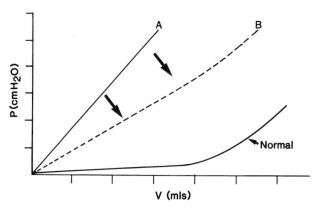

Figure 55–2. Bladder filling pressure–volume curve in a patient with a neurogenic bladder. Note the shift of the curve to the right when anticholinergics relax the detrusor, allowing for lower pressure at any given volume.

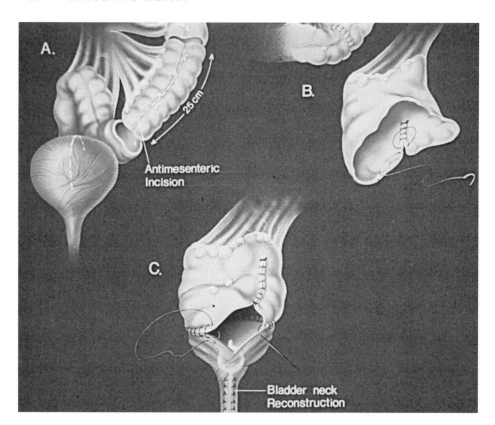

Figure 55–4. Bladder enlargement by enterocystoplasty (sigmoid) and bladder neck reconstruction. Enterocystoplasty enlarges the bladder nicely but has significant potential complications, including occasional perforation, which presents as acute abdominal pain.

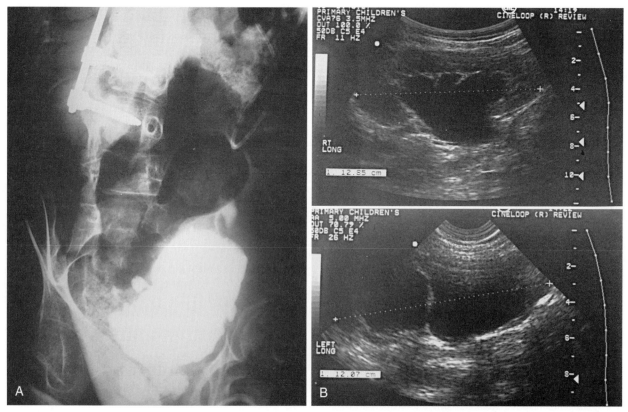

Figure 55–5. Radiograph *(A)* and ultrasound images *(B)* of a patient with spina bifida showing a small, poorly compliant bladder with worsening hydronephrosis.

SURGICAL TREATMENT

Although most patients with neurogenic bladder can be managed adequately without surgical intervention, those with reflux, poorly compliant bladder, or refractory incontinence may benefit from operative intervention.

Treatment of reflux in the neurogenic bladder is much the same as that for the normal bladder.[59] It is imperative, however, that the bladder be adequately treated for poor compliance and hyperreflexia (CIC and anticholinergics) before and after surgical intervention to diminish the high recurrence risk.[60]

In other clinical circumstances, surgical bladder augmentation or enlargement may be required. Bladder augmentation is designed to create a reservoir with good compliance and adequate capacity to store urine until it can be emptied by CIC at socially appropriate intervals. Detubularized segments of large or small bowel employed as a patch and detubularized cup on the widely opened bladder (enterocystoplasty) are the current standards for augmentation (Fig. 55–4). Other techniques for bladder augmentation include gastrocystoplasty, which has been repopularized since 1988.[61, 62] It is a technically acceptable procedure and shows advantages over enterocystoplasty with respect to a decrease in mucus formation, a possible decrease in infection rate, and maintenance of electrolyte balance in patients with renal insufficiency. Unfortunately, the hematuria-dysuria syndrome may affect up to one third of patients, which limits its applicability.[63]

Bladder autoaugmentation or detrusorectomy is an alternative augmenting technique that may prove useful in selected patients (Figs. 55–5 and 55–6).[64] The procedure involves removal of the detrusor muscle over the superior portion of the bladder, leaving the underlying bladder mucosa intact. This creates a large compliant surface, essentially a large diverticulum, which decreases bladder pressures and increases bladder capacity on filling. The advantage of this technique is that bladder epithelium is preserved and not replaced with gastrointestinal epithelium as in bowel augmentation, thus eliminating the problems associated with the secretory and absorptive functions of bowel mucosa. Long-term follow-up data on large numbers of children are lacking, but this technique appears to be a viable alternative for use in bladders with reasonable capacity and mainly poor compliance.[65] The concept has been extended to create "composite" bladders

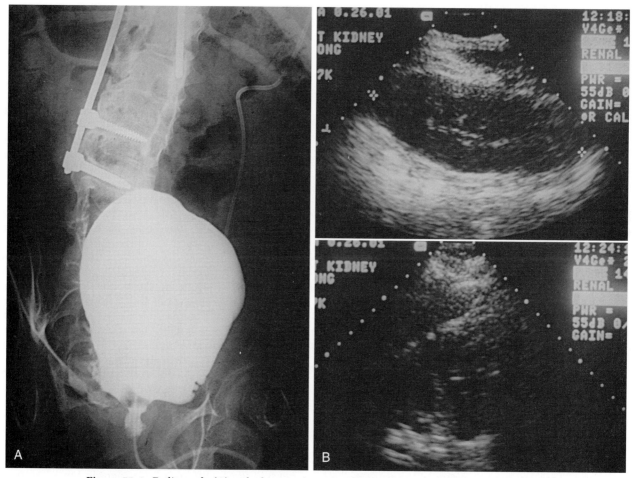

Figure 55–6. Radiograph *(A)* and ultrasound images *(B)* in the patient shown in Figure 55–5 after bladder autoaugmentation demonstrating improved bladder capacity and better compliance, which resulted in continence and diminished hydronephrosis.

by placing demucosalized bowel or stomach patches over the urothelial bulge created in autoaugmentation.[66, 67] Success rates are encouraging thus far. This concept of urothelial preservation during augmentation extends to the remarkable experimental use of cultured cells implanted onto degradable scaffolds, which can also be used to augment the bladder.[68]

Persistent incontinence, despite adequate treatment of the bladder to lower pressures and increase compliance in capacity, may require surgery on the bladder outlet to increase resistance. Bladder neck reconstructions of the Young-Dees type, which lengthen the urethra by infolding and tubularizing the trigone of the bladder, have lost some favor but still have advocates.[69] Kropp's procedure uses a tubularized anterior bladder strip reimplanted in the submucosa of the trigone to gain continence by a flap valve mechanism.[70] Continence is commonly achieved, but catheterization is sometimes difficult.[71] Sallé's procedure creates a similar (but easier to catheterize) flap valve by onlaying an anterior bladder wall flap onto a posterior incised strip up the middle of the trigone.[72] Owing to the lack of the pop-off mechanism in both these procedures, if the bladder becomes overfilled, the potential for bladder rupture of an augmented bladder or for upper tract deterioration based on high pressures is increased.

One of the more popular forms of increasing urethral resistance in the neurogenic bladder is by the pubovaginal or puboprostatic fascial sling.[73–77] This procedure has many advocates and involves securing a rectus fascial strip (or other fascial strip) around the urethra and suspending it from the anterior rectus fascia or pubis. This elevates and compresses the urethra to increase outlet resistance. Suprapubic bladder neck suspension with periurethral sutures is also advocated but has a lower success rate than the fascial sling technique, especially in the urethra that is opened widely with little resistance.

The artificial urinary sphincter works by way of a fluid-filled pressurized cuff around the urethra, which can be deflated by a pump-reservoir device that permits the urethra to open and the bladder to drain (Fig. 55–7). The artificial urinary sphincter can also be used in higher-pressure bladders in conjunction with bladder augmentation.[78] The main disadvantage is that it is a mechanical device that can erode into the urethra and malfunction over time. If the devices are left in place long enough, virtually all eventually need revision. We prefer to use autologous tissue techniques in children, when possible.

The periurethral injection of bovine collagen (Contigen) represents a simple, safe technique for enhancing urethral resistance in selected patients with myelodysplasia. It appears to be most applicable in patients requiring only a modest increase in stress leak-point pressure. Repeated treatments are usually required, but owing to the simplicity of the procedure, this may not be particularly problematic. Long-term improvement rates are only modest.[79]

In all procedures to enhance resistance at the

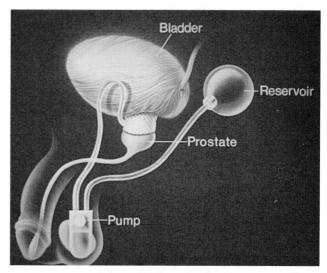

Figure 55–7. Typical artificial urinary sphincter. The scrotal pump moves fluid from the cuff to the reservoir to permit bladder emptying.

bladder outlet, it is crucial that the storage pressures of the bladder be considered simultaneously. When the bladder outlet is tightened but the bladder is unable to store increasing volumes at low pressure, hydronephrosis or reflux results. When the surgeon is considering bladder outlet surgery, it may be necessary to occlude the bladder neck with a Foley balloon during preoperative urodynamic assessment to determine how much the bladder can hold and what the storage pressures are like and thus to judge whether augmentation is needed simultaneously.

One surgical adjunct of great benefit in patients unable to self-catheterize the urethra (e.g., owing to spinal deformity, discomfort, or false passage) is the creation of a continent catheterizable stoma. This may be performed using the appendix or another small tubularized structure implanted into the bladder and anastomosed to the skin.[80] The implanted conduit can often be hidden at the base of the umbilicus (Fig. 55–8).[81] CIC may then be carried out intermittently through this segment.

Cutaneous urinary diversion by ileal or colon conduit or by cutaneous ureterostomy is considered a last resort therapy in these children. Long-term deterioration of the upper tracts is well documented in refluxing ileal conduits.[82] Some protection of the upper tracts is afforded by a nonrefluxing colon conduit, but the prognosis beyond two decades is uncertain.[83] Therefore, avoidance of diversion, if possible, is the best course in children with neurogenic bladders. All reasonable efforts should be made to maintain ureteral drainage into the bladder, if possible. Continent urinary diversion has evolved over the past several years as a popular alternative in treating incontinence. The intestinal segments for urinary reconstruction in children with neurogenic bladders generally are of neurogenic bowel as well. These children may not tolerate a loss of large segments (especially ileocecal segments) without de-

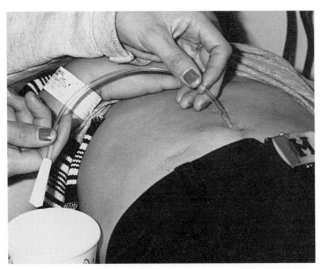

Figure 55–8. Umbilical positioning of an appendicovesicostomy permits easy access for clean intermittent catheterization; some patients can remain in their wheelchairs and drain the bladder into the toilet through a catheter extender.

veloping loose stools. In children who are dependent on constipated stools for fecal continence, loose stools may be more devastating than the original urinary incontinence; careful consideration in all such endeavors remains the key to success.

☐ Urethral Disorders

URETHRAL PROLAPSE

Urethral prolapse occurs in girls; African Americans are particularly prone to this disorder.[84] Urethral prolapse presents with dysuria and blood spotting with a bulging concentric purplish ring of prolapsed urethra seen at the urethral meatus (Fig. 55–9). Prolapse can be treated with an antiinflammatory ointment applied to the area several times a day and sitz baths. There are times when a catheter is needed temporarily. In persistent cases, excision of the prolapsing tissue with reanastomosis of the skin edges is satisfactory; a simple ligation of the prolapsing urethral epithelium over a Foley catheter, permitting necrosis, is another described option.

MEATAL STENOSIS

Meatal stenosis is the narrowing of the male urinary meatus after circumcision; it is thought to be due to exposure and irritation of the meatus in the diaper.[84, 85] For reasons that are uncertain, the stenosis is always on the ventral aspect of the meatus, causing dorsal deflection of the urinary stream that is fine and forceful. It is important for the physician to not only examine the meatus but also watch the voided urinary stream. If the stream is not narrow in caliber or is not dorsally deflected, then the meatal stenosis is not significant enough to require meatotomy. Occasionally, voiding causes the web to tear,

resulting in dysuria or a drop of blood after urination.

Meatotomy can be performed under general anesthesia but more often is performed as an office procedure. Previously, a small amount of lidocaine was injected into the ventral meatal web; some discomfort was inevitable. Since then, lidocaine (Emla) cream is applied topically and left in place for 1 hour before meatotomy. This has resulted in a painless office procedure.[85] Once anesthesia has developed, the ventral web is clamped with a hemostat; leaving this clamped for 1 minute results in adequate hemostasis. The ventral web is then snipped one half the distance to the coronal margin. Parents then spread the meatus and apply ointment daily for 4 weeks; meatal stenosis rarely recurs.

MEGALOURETHRA

Megalourethra is a rare genital anomaly causing a deformed and elongated penis occurring in two forms: fusiform and scaphoid (Fig. 55–10). These differ in embryology and appearance. Megalourethra is seen more commonly in patients with prune-belly syndrome and has been reported in association with the VATER (*v*ertebral defects, imperforate *a*nus, *tr*acheoesophageal fistula, and *r*adial and *r*enal dysplasia) syndrome.[86]

The less severe and most common form of this anomaly is the scaphoid variety, in which spongiosal tissue fails to invest the urethra.[87] The more severe fusiform variety is caused by failure of penile

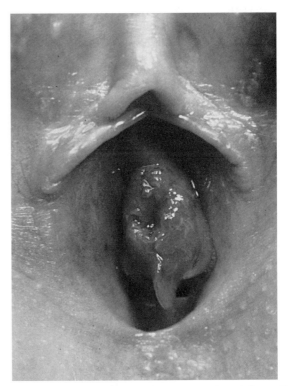

Figure 55–9. Urethral prolapse seen as a circumferential, purplish bulge at the meatus.

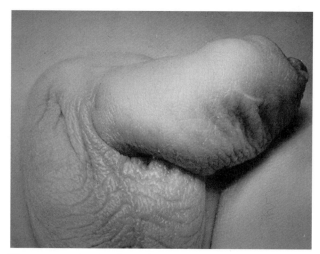

Figure 55–10. Scaphoid megalourethra in a boy with prune-belly syndrome.

mesoderm to form so that there is neither spongiosal tissue nor erectile tissue within the penis.[88] The fusiform type of megalourethra has been reported in patients with severe forms of prune-belly syndrome, stillborn fetuses, and patients with cloacal anomalies.[89, 90] Associated urologic anomalies have been reported, including megaureter, megacystis, reflux, bladder diverticula, and renal dysplasia.[90] Repair of the megalourethra relies on hypospadias techniques that tailor the urethra to a more normal size.

URETHRAL DUPLICATION

Urethral duplications occur in a wide variety of forms, with the second urethral opening located on the dorsum or ventrum of the penis or perineum.[91–93] Duplication may be complete, but incomplete forms predominate. Most commonly, the two channels form in the sagittal plane. Occasionally, side-by-side duplications occur. The urethral channel closest to the rectum is generally the more functional channel. This urethra often has more normal investing spongiosal tissue. The penile urethra is often small and poorly developed. Partial duplications that course along the penile urethra have been called *Y-type duplications*.[94] When the duplicated opening is in the perineum, it has been termed an *H-type duplication*.[95]

Treatment of urethral duplication must be individualized. When only a minor septum is present, cystoscopic division of the septum has been successful. Traditionally, with more significant duplications, efforts have been made to lengthen the posterior-most urethra to the tip of the penis (using various reconstruction techniques). Progressive dilation of the anterior urethral channel to make it functional has since been advocated.[96]

CONGENITAL URETHRAL FISTULA

A congenital urethral fistula may occur in the anterior urethra where the spongiosum has developed incompletely, permitting a small diverticulum to form that can rupture antenatally.[97] These are uncommon and difficult to repair due to the lack of spongiosal tissue surrounding the fistula.

URETHRAL STRICTURES

Most urethral strictures are acquired. Instrumentation and catheter passage by medical personnel, trauma, and inflammatory diseases are common causes. Congenital urethral strictures are rare and generally focal. Treatment can be internal urethrotomy, resection and end-to-end anastomosis, or pedicle flap urethroplasty. These strictures are usually in the bulbous urethra, with the area of embryologic joining of the bulbous urethra arising from genital folds and the posterior membranous urethra arising from the urogenital sinus. If this junction is misaligned or incompletely canalized, a discrete stricture may develop.[97]

URETHRAL ATRESIA

When urethral atresia occurs, in order to be compatible with life, a patent urachus must be present. Reconstruction can be difficult, and a Mitrofanoff catheterizable stoma may eventually be the patient's best alternative.[80]

URETHRAL DIVERTICULUM OR ANTERIOR URETHRAL VALVE

Urethral diverticula occur ventrally where the spongiosum is absent or has been thinned. The distal lip of the diverticulum functionally serves as an anterior urethral valve, blocking the urinary stream as it flows antegrade (Fig. 55–11). The diverticulum progressively fills and further compresses the urethra during urination. This valvular effect can cause marked proximal dilation.[98–100]

The diagnosis is made either by urethrogram or cystoscopy. Treatment can be accomplished by endoscopic incision of the distal lip of the diverticular neck or, if more pronounced, by open excision and closure of the urethral defect.[101] In some cases, there is a diverticulum with a narrow neck that does not function as a valve. Such a diverticulum may provide for stasis of urine and may be a site of urethral infection.

CYSTIC COWPER'S GLAND DUCTS

Cowper's glands are a pair of 5-mm glands located within the urogenital membrane. The ducts from these glands course distally and enter the ventral wall of the proximal bulbous urethra. These are the homologues of the female Bartholin's gland. Occasionally, these ducts can become occluded, producing bulbar urethral filling defects and, rarely, modest obstruction.[102] Cystoscopically, this appears to be a thin membrane over a fluid-filled cyst, sometimes called a *syringocele*.[103] Radiographically, tubular

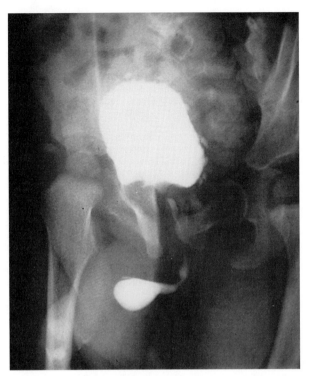

Figure 55–11. Voiding cystogram showing an anterior urethral diverticulum that functions as a valve causing outflow obstruction. Note the bladder trabeculation.

channels alongside the urethra can be seen coursing parallel to the urethra. Treatment of Cowper's duct cysts is with endoscopic unroofing and is unnecessary unless the radiographic finding is associated with clinical symptoms.

REFERENCES

1. Tanagho EA: Anatomy of the lower urinary tract. In Walsh PC, Retik AB, Stamey TA, et al (eds): Campbell's Urology. Philadelphia, WB Saunders, 1992, pp 40–51.
2. McGuire EJ, Woodside JR, Borden TA, et al: Prognostic value of urodynamic testing in myelodysplastic patients. J Urol 126:205–209, 1981.
3. Bauer SB: Urodynamics in children. In Ashcraft KW (ed): Pediatric Urology. Philadelphia, WB Saunders, 1990, pp 49–76.
4. Koff SA: Enuresis. In Walsh PC, Retik AB, Vaughan ED, et al (eds): Campbell's Urology. Philadelphia, WB Saunders, 1998, pp 2055–2068.
5. Zderic SA, Levin RM, Wein AJ: Voiding function and dysfunction. In Gillenwater JY, Grayhack JT, Howards SS, et al (eds): Adult and Pediatric Urology. St Louis, Mosby–Year Book, 1996, pp 1159–1220.
6. Kaefer M, Zurakowski D, Bauer SB, et al: Estimating normal bladder capacity in children. J Urol 158:2261–2264, 1997.
7. Goellner MH, Ziegler EE, Fomon SJ: Urination during the first three years of life. Nephron 28:174–178, 1983.
8. Allen TD, Kaplan WE, Kroovand RL: Sphincter dyssynergia. Dialog Pediatr Urol 2:1–8, 1979.
9. Miller FJW: Children who wet the bed. In Kolvin I, MacKeith RC, Meadow SR (eds): Bladder Control and Enuresis. London, W Heinemann Medical Books Ltd, 1973, pp 47–52.
10. Forsythe WI, Redmond A: Enuresis in spontaneous cure rate: Study of 1129 enuretics. Arch Dis Child 49:259–263, 1974.
11. Bakwin H: The Genetics of Enuresis. In Kolvin I, MacKeith RC, Meadow SR (eds): Bladder Control and Enuresis. London, W Heinemann Medical Books Ltd, 1973, pp 73–77.
12. Norgaard JP: Urodynamics in enuresis. I. Reservoir Function. Neurourol Urodyn 8:199–211, 1989.
13. Noorgaard JP: Pathophysiology of nocturnal enuresis. Scand J Urol Nephrol Suppl 140:1–35, 1991.
14. Jarvelin MR: Developmental history and neurological findings in enuretic children. Dev Med Child Neurol 31:728–736, 1989.
15. Norgaard JP, Hansen JH, Nielsen JB, et al: Simultaneous registration of sleep stages and bladder activity in enuresis. Urology 26:316–319, 1985.
16. Norgaard JP, Pedersen EB, Djurhuus JC: Diurnal antidiuretic hormone levels in enuretics. J Urol 134:1029–1034, 1985.
17. Puri BN: Urinary levels of antidiuretic hormone in nocturnal enuresis. Ind Pediatr 17:675–682, 1980.
18. Turner RK: Conditioning treatment of nocturnal enuresis: Present status. In Kolvin I, MacKeith RC, Meadow SR (eds): Bladder Control and Enuresis. London, W Heinemann Medical Books Ltd, 1973.
19. Morgan RTT: Relapse and therapeutic response in the conditioning treatment of enuresis: A review of recent findings on intermittent reinforcement, overlearning and stimulus intensity. Behav Res Ther 16:278–280, 1978.
20. Monda JM, Husmann DA: Primary nocturnal enuresis: A comparison among observation, imipramine, desmopressin acetate, and bed wetting alarm systems. J Urol 154:745–748, 1995.
21. Blackwell B, Currah J: Tricyclic pharmacology of nocturnal enuresis. In Kolvin I, MacKeith RC, Meadow SR (eds): Bladder Control and Enuresis. London, W Heinemann Medical Books Ltd, 1973.
22. Norgaard JP, Pedersen EB, Djurhuus JC: Diurnal antidiuretic hormone levels in enuretics. J Urol 134:1029–1033, 1985.
23. Klauber GT: Clinical efficacy and safety of desmopressin in the treatment of nocturnal enuresis. J Pediatr 114(suppl): 719–722, 1989.
24. Ritig S, Knudsen UB, Sorensen S, et al: Long term double-blind crossover study of desmopressin intranasal spray in the management of nocturnal enuresis. In Meadow SR, Canwell, Sutton, et al (eds): Desmopressin and Nocturnal Enuresis: Proceedings of an International Symposium. London, Horus Medical Publications, 1989, pp 43–54.
25. MacKeith RL, Meadow SR, Turner RK: How children become dry. In Kolvin I, MacKeith RL, Meadow SR (eds): Bladder Control in Enuresis. Philadelphia, JB Lippincott, 1973, pp 3–15.
26. Fernandes E, Vernier R, Gonzalez R: The unstable bladder in children. J Pediatr 118:831–837, 1991.
27. Koff SA, Murtagh DS: The uninhibited bladder in children: Effect of treatment on recurrence of urinary infection and vesico-ureteral reflux. J Urol 130:1158–1160, 1983.
28. DeLuca FG, Swenson O, Fisher JH, et al: The dysfunctional "lazy" bladder syndrome in children. Arch Dis Child 37:197–223, 1962.
29. Bloom DA, Seeley WW, Ritchey ML, et al: Toilet habits and continence in children: An opportunity sampling in search of normal parameters. J Urol 149:1087–1090, 1993.
30. Hinman F: Non-neurogenic neurogenic bladder (the Hinman syndrome) fifteen years later. J Urol 136:769–775, 1986.
31. Bauer SB: Neuropathology of the lower urinary tract. In Kelalis PY, King LR, Belman AB (eds): Clinical Pediatric Urology. Philadelphia, WB Saunders, 1992, pp 399–440.
32. Steers WD, Barrett DM, Wein AJ: Voiding dysfunction: Diagnosis, classification, and management. In Gillenwater JY, Grayhack JT, Howards SS, et al (eds): Adult and Pediatric Urology. St Louis, Mosby–Year Book, 1996, pp 1220–1326.
33. Mandell J, Bauer SB, Hallett M, et al: Occult spinal dysraphism: A rare but detectable cause of voiding dysfunction. Urol Clin North Am 7:349–356, 1980.
34. Kaplan WE: Management of myelomeningocele. Urol Clin North Am 12:93–101, 1985.
35. Kroovand RL: Myelomeningocele. In Walsh PC, Gittes RF, Perlmutter AD, et al (eds): Campbell's Urology. Philadelphia, WB Saunders, 1986, pp 2193–2216.

36. Bauer SB, Joseph DB: Management of the obstructed urinary tract associated with neurogenic bladder dysfunction. Urol Clin North Am 17:395–406, 1990.

37. Werler MM, Shapiro S, Mitchell AA: Periconceptual folic acid exposure and risk of occult neural tube defects. JAMA 269:1257–1263, 1993.

38. Bauer SB, Hallett M, Khoshbin S, et al: Predictive value of urodynamic evaluation in newborns with myelodysplasia. JAMA 252:650–652, 1984.

39. Wang SC, McGuire EJ, Bloom DA: A bladder pressure management system for myelodysplasia: Clinical outcome. J Urol 140:1499–1502, 1988.

40. Galloway NTM, Mekras JA, Helms M, et al: An objective score to predict upper tract deterioration in myelodysplasia. J Urol 145:535–537, 1991.

41. Lapides J, Diokno AC, Silber SJ, et al: Clean intermittent self-catheterization in the treatment of urinary tract disease. J Urol 107:458–462, 1971.

42. Klose AG, Sackett CK, Mesrobian H: Management of children with myelodysplasia: Urologic alternatives. J Urol 144:1446–1449, 1990.

43. Joseph DB, Bauer SB, Colodny AH, et al: Clean, intermittent catheterization of infants with neurogenic bladder. Pediatrics 84:78–82, 1989.

44. Cass AS: Urinary tract complications in myelomeningocele patients. J Urol 115:102–104, 1976.

45. Plunkett JM, Braren V: Clean intermittent catheterization in children. J Urol 121:469–471, 1979.

46. Klauber GT, Sant GR: Complications of intermittent catheterization. Urol Clin North Am 10:557–562, 1983.

47. Abrams P: Tolterodine, a new antimuscarinic agent: As effective but better tolerated than oxybutynin in patients with an overactive bladder. Br J Urol 81:801–810, 1998.

48. Greenfield SP, Fera M: The use of intravesical oxybutynin chloride in children with neurogenic bladder. J Urol 146:532–534, 1991.

49. Kaplan WE, Richards I: Intravesical bladder stimulation in myelodysplasia. J Urol 140:1282–1284, 1988.

50. Kaplan WE, Richards TW, Richards I: Intravesical transurethral bladder stimulation to increase bladder capacity. J Urol 142:600–602, 1989.

51. Decter RM: Transurethral electrical bladder stimulation: A follow-up report. J Urol 152:812–814, 1994.

52. Boone TB, Roehrborn CG, Hurt G: Transurethral intravesical electrotherapy for neurogenic bladder dysfunction in children: A prospective, randomized clinical trial. J Urol 148:550–553, 1992.

53. Toczek SK, McCullough DC, Garfour GW, et al: Selective sacral rootlet rhizotomy for hypertonic neurogenic bladder. J Neurosurg 42:567–574, 1975.

54. Mulcahy JJ, Young AB: Long-term follow-up of percutaneous radiofrequency sacral rhizotomy. Urology 35:76–77, 1990.

55. Tanagho EA, Schmidt RA: Electrical stimulation in the clinical management of the neurogenic bladder. J Urol 140:1331–1339, 1988.

56. Duckett JW Jr: Cutaneous vesicostomy in childhood. Urol Clin North Am 1:485–495, 1974.

57. Mandell J, Bauer SB, Colodny AH, et al: Cutaneous vesicostomy in infancy. J Urol 126:92–93, 1981.

58. Bloom DA, Knechtel JM, McGuire EJ: Urethral dilation improves bladder compliance in children with myelomeningocele and high leak point pressures. J Urol 144:430–433, 1990.

59. Jeffs RD, Jonas P, Schillinger JF: Surgical correction of vesicoureteral reflux in children with neurogenic bladder. J Urol 114:449–451, 1976.

60. Agarwal SK, McLorie GA, Grewal D, et al: Urodynamic correlates of resolution of reflux in myelomeningocele patients. J Urol 158:580–582, 1997.

61. Adams MC, Bihrle R, Rink RC: The use of stomach in urologic reconstruction. AUA Update Series. Lesson 27. 14:218–223, 1995.

62. Adams MC, Mitchell ME, Rink RC: Gastrocystoplasty: An alternative solution to the problem of urological reconstruction in the severely compromised patient. J Urol 140:1152–1156, 1988.

63. Nguyen DH, Bain MA, Salmonson KL, et al: The syndrome of dysuria and hematuria in pediatric urinary reconstruction with stomach. J Urol 150:707–709, 1993.

64. Cartwright PC, Snow BW: Bladder autoaugmentation: Early clinical experience. J Urol 142:595–598, 1989.

65. Snow BW, Cartwright PC: Bladder autoaugmentation. Urol Clin North Am 23:323–331, 1996.

66. Gonzalez R, Buson H, Reid C, et al: Seromuscular colocystoplasty lined with urothelium: Experience with 16 patients. Urology 45:124–129, 1994.

67. Dewan P, Byard R: Autoaugmentation gastrocystoplasty in a sheep model. Br J Urol 72:56–59, 1993.

68. Atala A: Tissue engineering in urologic surgery. Urol Clin North Am 25:39–50, 1998.

69. Reda EF: The use of the Young-Dees Leadbetter procedure. Dialog Pediatr Urol 14:7–8, 1991.

70. Kropp KA, Angwafo FF: Urethral lengthening and reimplantation for neurogenic incontinence in children. J Urol 135:533–536, 1986.

71. Kropp KA: Management of urethral incompetence in the patient with neurogenic bladder. Dialog Pediatr Urol 14:6–7, 1991.

72. Salle JL, McLorie GA, Bagli DJ, et al: Urethral lengthening with anterior bladder wall flap (Pippi-Salle procedure): Modifications and extended indications of the technique. J Urol 158:585–590, 1997.

73. McGuire J, Lytton B: Pubovaginal sling procedure for stress incontinence. J Urol 119:82–84, 1978.

74. Bauer SB, Peters CA, Colodny AH, et al: The use of rectus fascia to manage urinary incontinence. J Urol 142:516–519, 1989.

75. McGuire EJ, Wang C, Usitalo H, et al: Modified pubovaginal sling in girls with myelodysplasia. J Urol 135:94–96, 1986.

76. Elder JS: Periurethral and puboprostatic sling repair for incontinence in patients with myelodysplasia. J Urol 144:434–437, 1990.

77. Norbeck JC, McGuire EJ: The use of pubovaginal and puboprostatic slings. Dialog Pediatr Urol 14:3–4, 1991.

78. Gonzalez R, Nguyen DH, Koleilat N, et al: Compatibility of enterocystoplasty and the artificial urinary sphincter. J Urol 142:502–504, 1989.

79. Sundaram CP, Reinberg Y, Aliabadi HA: Failure to obtain durable results with collagen implantation in children with urinary incontinence. J Urol 157:2306–2307, 1997.

80. Mitrofanoff P: Cystostomie continente trans-appendiculaire dans le traitement des vessies neurolgiques. Chir Pediatr 21:297–301, 1980.

81. Keating MA, Rink RC, Adams MC: Appendicovesicostomy: A useful adjunct to continent reconstruction of the bladder. J Urol 149:1091–1094, 1993.

82. Cass AS, Luxenberg M, Gleich P, et al: A 22-year follow-up of ileal conduits in children with a neurogenic bladder. J Urol 132:529–531, 1984.

83. Husmann DA, McLorie GA, Churchill BM: Non refluxing colonic conduits: A long-term life-table analysis. J Urol 142:1201–1205, 1989.

84. Brown MR, Cartwright PC, Snow BW: Common office problems in pediatric urology and gynecology. Pediatr Clin North Am 44:1101–1102, 1997.

85. Cartwright PC, Snow BW, McNees DC: Office meatotomy utilizing EMLA cream as the anesthetic. J Urol 156:857–859, 1996.

86. Fernbach SK: Urethral abnormalities in male neonates with VATER association. AJR Am J Roentgenol 156:137–140, 1991.

87. Stephens FD, Smith ED, Huston JM: Congenital intrinsic lesions of the anterior urethra. In Congenital Anomalies of the Urinary and Genital Tracts. Oxford, England, Isis Medical Media, 1996, pp 119–124.

88. Dorairajan T: Defects of spongy tissue and congenital diverticula of the penile urethra. Aust N Z J Surg 32:209–214, 1963.

89. Duckett JW: The prune-belly syndrome. In Kelalis PP, King

LR, Bellman AB (eds): Clinical Pediatric Urology. Philadelphia, WB Saunders, 1976, pp 615–638.

90. Shrom SH, Cromie WJ, Duckett JW, et al: Megalourethra. Urology 17:152–156, 1981.

91. Gross RE, Moore TC: Duplication of the urethra. Arch Surg 60:749–756, 1950.

92. Das S, Brosman SA: Duplication of the male urethra. J Urol 117:452–454, 1977.

93. Woodhouse CRJ, Williams DI: Duplications of the lower urinary tract in children. Br J Urol 51:481–486, 1979.

94. Williams DE, Bloomberg S: Bifid urethra with three anal accessory tracts (Y duplication). Br J Urol 47:877–880, 1976.

95. Stephens FD, Donnellan WL: H-type urethral anal fistula. J Pediatr Surg 12:95–102, 1977.

96. Passerini-Glazal G, Araguna F, Chiozza L: P.A.D.U.A. (Posterior augmentation by dilating the urethra anterior): Procedure of treatment of severe urethral hypoplasia. J Urol 140:1247–1249, 1988.

97. Duckett JW, Snow BW: Disorders of the urethra and penis. In Walsh PC, Gittes RF, Perlmutter AD, et al (eds): Campbell's Urology (5th ed). Philadelphia, WB Saunders, 1986, pp 2000–2030.

98. Firlit CF, King LR: Anterior urethral valves in children. J Urol 108:972–975, 1972.

99. Rudhe U, Ericsson NO: Congenital urethral diverticula. Ann Radiol 13:289–295, 1970.

100. Williams DI, Retik AB: Congenital valves and diverticula of the anterior urethra. Br J Urol 41:228–233, 1969.

101. Firlit RF, Firlit CF, King LR: Obstructing anterior urethral valves in children. J Urol 119:819–821, 1978.

102. Colodny AH, Lebowitz RL: Lesions of Cowper's ducts and glands in infants and children. Urology 11:321–325, 1978.

103. Maizel M, Stephens FD, King LR, et al: Cowper's syringocele: A classification of dilatations of Cowper's gland duct based upon clinical characteristics of eight boys. J Urol 129:111–114, 1983.

56

URETHRAL VALVES

W. Hardy Hendren, MD

Ridges or small folds are found in the normal male urethra. The majority of urethral valves are probably exaggerated forms of these folds. In 1919, Dr. Hugh Young and colleagues described the basic anatomic types of urethral valves.[1] Little has been added since then, although today we can diagnose valves more easily with current radiographic techniques and can see them better with modern endoscopes.

All congenital malformations occur in a spectrum of severity. Good examples are hypospadias and cleft lip. Mild forms are usually more common than severe malformations. This occurrence is also true of urethral valves.[2] At the minimal end of the spectrum are prominent folds that do not cause obstruction. At the maximal end of the spectrum is almost complete obstruction of the urethra with massive hydronephrosis and destroyed kidneys. Severe cases are not difficult to recognize; however, mild to moderate cases of urethral valves are often not recognized and consequently remain undiagnosed.

The clinical presentation and treatment of patients with valves vary greatly, depending on the severity of urethral obstruction.

☐ Anatomy

Figure 56–1 shows the main types of urethral valves described by Young and associates in 1919.[1] Type I valves are most common. They are sail-like leaflets that arise from the crista urethralis distal to the verumontanum. The crista may be short, with the valve close to the verumontanum, or the crista may be quite long, with an elongated prostatic urethra. Valve leaflets may fill only the lower half of the endoscopic field when they are incomplete. In severe cases, however, they encircle the urethra and form a prominent diaphragm dorsally. That diaphragm can cause complete obstruction.

Type II valves are extremely rare. It is common to see folds between the upper margin of the verumon-

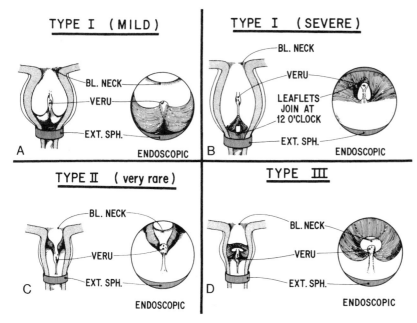

TYPE I (MILD)

BL. NECK
VERU
EXT. SPH.
A
ENDOSCOPIC

TYPE I (SEVERE)

BL. NECK
VERU
LEAFLETS JOIN AT 12 O'CLOCK
EXT. SPH.
B
ENDOSCOPIC

TYPE II (very rare)

BL. NECK
VERU
EXT. SPH.
C
ENDOSCOPIC

TYPE III

BL. NECK
VERU
EXT. SPH.
D
ENDOSCOPIC

Figure 56–1. Types of urethral valves. *A,* Mild type I valves are common in boys with voiding disturbances of urinary infections if there is vesicoureteral reflux. These valves are often overlooked radiographically and endoscopically. *B,* Severe type I valves in which the leaflets encircle the urethra and join at 12 o'clock, forming a diaphragm. This type usually is associated with the upper tract changes. *C,* Type II valves are extremely rare. They are often seen in association with severe type I valves. They seldom cause obstruction. *D,* Type III valves with diaphragm-like configuration usually occur at the level of the verumontanum (Veru), but they can be at any level of the urethra more distally. Some valves are hybrid in appearance—intermediate between type I and type II. Ext. Sph., external sphincter.

tanum and the bladder neck in normal males as well as in patients with urethral valves. I have seen only a few patients in whom type II folds appeared to cause urethral obstruction.

Type III valves are less uniform in location and appearance than are type I valves. They usually form a diaphragm-like obstruction at the level of the verumontanum. However, they can be encountered elsewhere, such as in the anterior urethra distal to the external urethral sphincter. Another obstruction that occurs in the anterior urethra is a urethral diverticulum, the distal rim of which obstructs the flow of urine.

Urethral valves occur almost exclusively in male patients. However, I have seen several cases of valves in female patients. The valves can be demonstrated by bending a malleable silver probe into a "shepherd's crook." The probe is passed into the urethra alongside the endoscope, and the surgeon pulls back on the crook to catch the valve leaflet. One of my patients had undergone previous ureteral reimplantations elsewhere twice. The operations failed because an obstructing valve distal to the bladder neck had not been appreciated. I have also observed valves in the masculinized urethra of female patients with the adrenogenital syndrome. Thus, although very rare, valves can be encountered in a female patient with outlet obstruction.

□ Symptoms

Symptoms in a male patient with urethral valves differ with the age of the patient and the severity of urethral obstruction. In pediatric patients with severe urethral valves with hydronephrosis and dilated ureters, about half present before age 1 year, usually with an abdominal mass and infection. Beyond 1 year of age, urinary tract infection is the most common presenting symptom. Curiously, a poor urinary stream is seldom noted by parents. In a review of valves of all degrees, symptoms in order of frequency included bed wetting, urinary infection, day wetting, poor stream, frequency, dribbling, hematuria, and acute urinary retention.[2]

We treated one 80-year-old man with severe type I urethral valves.[3] He did not recognize that his urinary stream was poor but did note a 20-year history of frequency and nocturia. We also treated a 20-year-old male with severe urethral valves that caused dilation of the prostatic ducts and severe bilateral hydronephrosis. The finding was discovered incidentally during investigation for hypertension. He had not noted a poor urinary stream, but he described a much more forceful stream after resection of the valves. Another adult male, who presented with failure to ejaculate during orgasm due to obstruction from valves, was treated. Unsuspected urethral valves have also been noted in adults presenting for dialysis or renal transplantation.[4]

Residual urine is not always present in male pa-

tients with valves, because the bladder, like any hollow viscus, can compensate for obstruction by muscular hypertrophy, emptying at high pressure. Great hypertrophy of the bladder can be caused by urethral valves. Even after the valves are eliminated, high intravesical pressure and noncompliance of the bladder can remain. That abnormal state can be shown by urodynamic investigation.[5, 6] Augmentation cystoplasty can be helpful for some of these "valve bladders."[7, 8]

□ Diagnosis

The first step in diagnosing urethral valves is to suspect that they may be present in a male patient of any age with a urinary infection or voiding abnormality. A widespread concept exists that valves always cause hydronephrosis. Valve cases may be missed because the clinician does not recognize that valves form a spectrum of findings. A voiding cystourethrogram is mandatory to demonstrate valves. This is done by filling the bladder through a small plastic catheter and by withdrawing the catheter when voiding begins in the patient too young to cooperate with the command to void. Radiographs from typical valve cases are shown in Figures 56–2 and 56–3. It is my experience that a pediatric radiologist who is experienced in interpreting voiding cystourethrograms will have a high degree of accuracy in diagnosing urethral valves. However, when the radiologist is less experienced, valves are often not diagnosed.

The surgeon who knows the patient, views the radiographs, and observes the endoscopic findings has a great advantage in learning to recognize urethral valve disease in all degrees of severity. Secondary radiographic findings in valve cases can include arborization of contrast medium in the prostatic ducts in some severe cases, hypertrophy of the bladder neck, trabeculation of the bladder, diverticula of the bladder, vesicoureteral reflux, and hydronephrosis. Neonatal urinary ascites occurs in some infants with valves caused by spontaneous perforation of the urinary tract.[9] Not all hydroureteronephrosis in boys with urethral valves is secondary. Some patients have concomitant disease, such as obstructive megaureter or ureteropelvic junction obstruction.

Since the advent of maternal ultrasonography, urethral valves are being diagnosed antenatally.[10–12] Antenatal diagnosis does not always benefit these infants[13, 14] and poses a risk to the mother.[15] The main value of antenatal diagnosis is that it enables early treatment after birth and before infection.

VALVE RESECTION

Destruction of the urethral valves has been facilitated by the development of modern fiberoptic miniature endoscopes. In 1919, Young and associates used a cold punch to resect valves.[1] Later, valves were resected under direct visualization by splitting

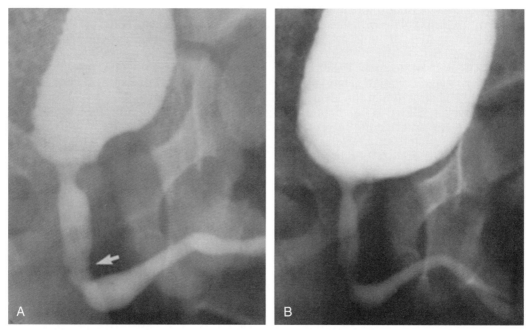

Figure 56–2. Small type I urethral valves in a 7-year-old boy with daytime and nighttime wetting. Radiograph and cystoscopy findings had previously been declared normal. *A*, Preoperative voiding cystourethrogram. A mild constriction of the prostatic urethra *(arrow)* is just proximal to the external urethral sphincter. Valve leaflets are faintly visible, arising from the verumontanum in the midprostatic urethra. Cystoscopy showed trabeculation of the bladder, prominence of the bladder neck, and small type I urethral valves arising just distal to the verumontanum and circling dorsally to form a diaphragm at 12 o'clock. This diaphragm was cut at 12 o'clock, and each leaflet was cut at 4 o'clock and 8 o'clock. The patient's symptoms of wetting stopped immediately and did not return during 12-year follow-up. *B*, Normal voiding cystourethrogram 3 months after valves were resected.

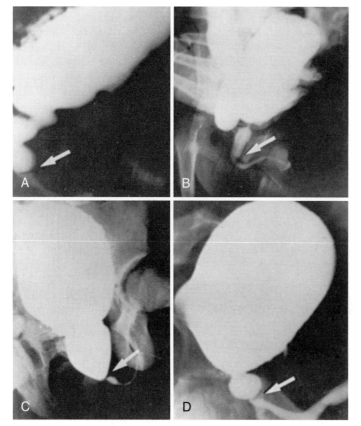

Figure 56–3. Voiding cystourethrograms of four boys with severe posterior valves. Note that although valves were present in all cases, no two radiographs are alike. *A*, A 3-month-old boy with urosepsis. *Arrow* points to level of obstruction from type I valves. The bladder neck is very prominent. Cellule formation is noted in the trigone but no reflux. *B*, A 5-year-old boy with urinary infection. *Arrow* points to obstruction between the verumontanum and the external sphincter. Elongation and widening of the prostatic urethra and marked hypertrophy of the bladder neck are observed. There is a massive vesicoureteral reflux. *C*, An 8-year-old boy with bed wetting. As in *A* and *B*, this is also a type I valve with marked obstruction just proximal to the external sphincter. Great widening of the prostatic urethra is evident but the shape is entirely different from that seen in *A* and *B*. *D*, Type III urethral valve, a diaphragm obstructing at the level of the verumontanum, in a 5-year-old boy with bed wetting, daytime wetting, and urinary frequency. The bladder does not appear trabeculated. Much better filling of the penile urethra is noted than in the other three cases.

the pubic symphysis. By today's standards, these techniques are unnecessary and are apt to lead to urinary incontinence. A pediatric resectoscope has been utilized to destroy valves, but even the smallest resectoscope is large for an infant's urethra. Therefore, its use may require perineal urethrostomy. A perineal urethrostomy is close to the external urethral sphincter. I have seen several cases in which perineal urethrostomy damaged the external urethral sphincter from stricture or from cutting the sphincter itself. Valves can be cut by passing a hooked electrode in the urethra, engaging the valve with fluoroscopic control, and cutting it with diathermy.[16, 17] However, I cannot subscribe to any blind technique when direct visualization is possible with currently available endoscopes, which are as small as 7.5 French. Destroying valves through a suprapubic cystostomy has been described,[18] but the natural curve of the male urethra makes it difficult to visualize the most important part of the valve—namely, its confluence at 12 o'clock. If the infant is very small, so that the urethra will not accept the smallest endoscope, temporary vesicostomy is reasonable, deferring valve ablation until the infant is several months of age. There is absolutely no justification for attempting endoscopic resection of valves with oversized equipment that can cause urethral stricture.[19]

Prompted by seeing many cases of urethral valves missed both radiographically and endoscopically, I made a film that depicts the spectrum of urethral valves and their treatment.[20] I use the wire stylette of a No. 3 woven ureteral catheter to which an electrode cord is attached. There must be no side holes in the catheter sheath; otherwise, the current can arc to the endoscope lens and destroy it. A larger endoscope sheath can be employed to allow better water flow in older male patients. Cutting current is applied in very short bursts. Valves are best seen with the bladder full. By manipulating the water inflow or outflow through a drainage tube attached to the endoscope, bubbles can be cleared away during valve fulguration.

Figure 56–4 shows destruction of severe urethral valves. After the anatomy is studied endoscopically, the electrode is introduced to cut the dorsal conflu-

SEVERE TYPE I VALVES

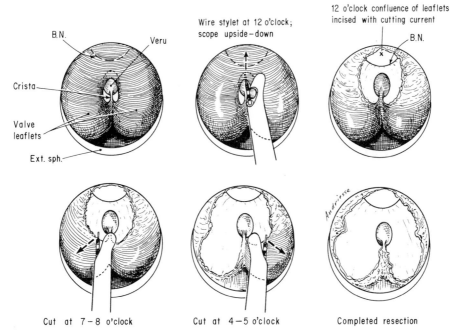

Figure 56–4. Technique for resecting severe type I urethral valves. The valves are visualized with the bladder full and the irrigating reservoir about 3 feet above the patient to distend the prostatic urethra. A 3-French urethral catheter and its wire stylette are used as a cutting electrode, with a cautery unit attached to the distal end of the wire. A length of wire a few millimeters beyond the end of the catheter acts as a cutting electrode. When the electrode is advanced into the field of vision, the endoscope should be in the bladder to avoid inadvertently puncturing the side wall of the urethra. When the electrode is in view, using the 30-degree lens, the endoscope is withdrawn until the valve is reached. The endoscope is turned 180 degrees so that the electrode can incise the 12 o'clock confluence of the leaflets. Very brief applications of cutting current are used.

The dorsal diaphragm is incised up to its point of attachment on the roof of the urethra. In some cases, only the 12 o'clock cut is necessary. If prominent leaflets remain, each can be cut—the right one at 7 to 8 o'clock and the left one at 4 to 5 o'clock. After this method of destroying valves, there is a cloverleaf-shaped defect, with an intact verumontanum (Veru), bladder neck (BN), and external sphincter (Ext. Sph.).

ence of the valve leaflets at 12 o'clock. This dorsal, diaphragm-like confluence of the valves inserts close to the external urethral sphincter. Cutting too far distally with the electrode can destroy the sphincter. The bases of the valve leaflets are then incised with the cutting electrode, the left at 4 to 5 o'clock and the right at 7 to 8 o'clock. This creates a cloverleaf defect where the valves were located. In less severe cases, cutting the leaflets at 4 to 5 o'clock and 7 to 8 o'clock will suffice. We do not use a cutting loop to destroy valves. The concept of hooking the leaflet with a cutting loop and pulling the loop toward the operator, as in transurethral resection of the prostate, is unnecessary and apt to injure the urethral sphincter. Valve resection should not touch the verumontanum, the sphincter, or the bladder neck. Formerly, we incised the bladder neck at 6 o'clock if it was extremely prominent. However, that is not done today because it can cause incontinence and retrograde ejaculation in later life.

SPECIFIC CASE STUDIES

Although the actual technique of valve destruction has just been described, this does not give an appreciation of the overall treatment needed for many of these cases. The older boy, with mild-to-moderate urethral valves discovered after investigation for urinary infection or abnormal wetting, undergoes a straightforward treatment. The valves are destroyed endoscopically as an outpatient procedure. The patient is discharged home 2 hours later without a catheter. Follow-up cystogram is obtained 3 to 4 months later to demonstrate the changed appearance of the urethra. Vesicoureteral reflux is common in these patients and will often disappear after urethral obstruction is relieved. If reflux does not disappear in time, ureteral reimplantation is performed.

Most challenging, however, is the young infant with severe hydronephrosis and uremia secondary to urethral valves. It is common for these patients to present with sepsis, dehydration, and acidosis. If the bladder and kidneys are palpable, urethral valves are most likely the cause. Twenty years ago, infants were treated with immediate open drainage by a variety of techniques, including loop cutaneous ureterostomy, ring ureterostomy, end ureterostomy, pyelostomy, and vesicostomy.[21–28] Although recently recommended,[29] in my opinion and that of others,[30, 31] this approach is seldom indicated today. A 5-French plastic infant feeding catheter is passed through the urethra into the bladder to initiate drainage. Appropriate antibiotics and intravenous therapy are administered to correct the precarious metabolic state. A nephrologist participates in this effort. When metabolic homeostatis is achieved, appropriate diagnostic studies can be performed. These studies include cystography, ultrasound examination, intravenous pyelography (IVP), and radionuclide scan for renal function. In some cases, one kidney has excellent

function and the other may have no function. Endoscopic resection is delayed until the infant has improved, so that general anesthesia does not pose a high risk. This preoperative preparation may take several days or longer.

Controversy exists among surgeons with equal experience regarding treatment of dilated ureters, with or without massive vesicoureteral reflux—whether to repair them or practice "watchful waiting."[32–36] During the 1st year of life, renal function normally increases. The normal neonate has a creatinine clearance level that is about 20% that of the adult. Renal function reaches adult values of 100 to 120 l/m^2 of body surface area (BSA) per day at about age 1 year. If there is obstructive uropathy, its repair early in the 1st year of life may yield greater function than if corrected later. Therefore, if there is massive reflux or ureteral obstruction in these infants after valve ablation, I believe further surgery should be considered. Temporary drainage has been used by many surgeons, but that introduces other technical problems to be solved in the future.[37] Therefore, I have preferred to correct reflux and obstruction.[38, 39] The problem is to decide which child can be reasonably observed and which should undergo a corrective operation. This decision can be guided by blood chemical values, presence or absence of urinary infection, improvement or lack of improvement in findings at the radiographic examination, and creatinine clearance values. A nadir serum creatinine level in the 1st year of life less than 0.8 mg/dl is predictive of continuing adequate renal function with growth.[40]

However, among my own cases of boys presenting before 1 year of age were some who ultimately developed renal failure, despite having serum creatinine levels in the "favorable" range. We found that prognosis correlates better with creatinine clearance rather than serum creatinine level. In general, clearance above 33 l/m^2 BSA/day was associated with a satisfactory long-term prognosis. Ureteral reimplantation into a small, hypertrophied bladder, especially if the ureter requires tapering, is much more difficult than ureteral reimplantation into a normal or almost normal bladder. The following cases illustrate various parts of the clinical spectrum of urethral valves. Other cases have been described previously.[2, 38, 39]

Case 1 (Fig. 56–5): Ablation of Urethral Valves with No Further Treatment

This 13-year-old boy had no history of urologic complaints but developed acute urinary retention after a blow to the lower abdomen by a basketball. After catheterization, he was referred for investigation, which showed typical urethral valves and bilateral reflux. The valves were resected endoscopically. Postoperatively, he voided with a strong urinary stream and stated that he had not been aware that it had been abnormal previously. The

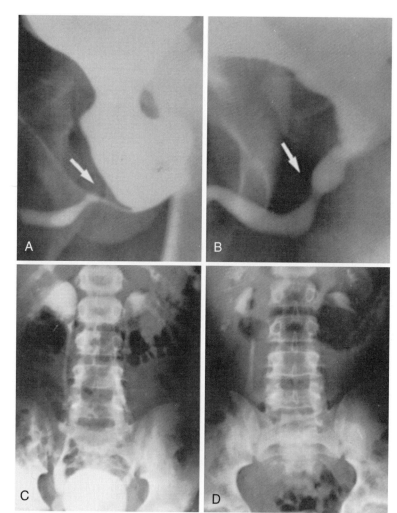

Figure 56–5. Case 1. Urethral valves in a 13-year-old boy who developed acute urinary retention after being struck in the lower abdomen by a basketball. *A,* Preoperative voiding cystourethrogram shows obvious type I valves *(arrow)* obstructing prostatic urethra. Note the very dilated prostatic urethra. *B,* Voiding study 2½ years after endoscopic resection of valves. *Arrow* indicates level at which the valve was resected. *C,* Preoperative intravenous pyelogram (IVP). Note mild dilation of both ureters. Moderate reflux was noted bilaterally, which disappeared on later study. *D,* Subsequent IVP, taken 2½ years after resection of valves, shows normal upper tracts and ureters. No reflux is seen on cystogram.

vesicoureteral reflux disappeared on follow-up study. There have been no urologic complaints during 23 years of follow-up.

COMMENT. Moderate reflux will disappear in about 50% of cases. If the ureteral orifice looks normal endoscopically, reflux is more apt to disappear than if the ureteral orifice is dilated or if an adjacent paraureteral diverticulum predisposes the child to reflux. We follow reflux nonoperatively if the upper tracts are normal, there is no infection, and the ureteral orifices look normal. We correct reflux if there is infection, the reflux is great in amount, the orifices are abnormal, and the problem persists on the follow-up examination.

Case 2 (Fig. 56-6): Valve Ablation and Further Reconstruction

This patient was referred at age 1 week with gram-negative septicemia and palpable bladder and kidneys. He was treated immediately with catheter drainage, using a 5-French feeding catheter, antibiotics, and intravenous therapy. Cystogram showed severe urethral valves with dilation and elongation of the prostatic urethra and a thick-walled bladder

with many cellules. Intravenous pyelography showed severe bilateral hydronephrosis with poor visualization of the upper tracts. One week later, when the infant was afebrile and metabolically stable, the valves were resected endoscopically. Retrograde ureterograms were performed at that time to visualize the upper tracts. Although the child thrived, studies 1 year later showed obstruction at both ends of the right ureter and left vesicoureteral reflux. Serum blood urea nitrogen (BUN) value was 28 mg/dl, creatinine level was 0.5 mg/dl, and creatinine clearance was 44 l/m² BSA/day. The refluxing left ureter was reimplanted to stop reflux, and the obstructive megaureter on the right was repaired. At age 1½ years, both ureteropelvic junctions were explored. A simple dismembered pyeloplasty was performed on both sides for mild obstruction, and the right upper ureter was tapered as well. When last seen at age 12 years, the patient was well and had a stable intravenous pyelography (IVP).

COMMENT. This patient clearly had associated ureteral disease that was not secondary to urethral valve obstruction. Therefore, this disorder was corrected when it did not improve after valve ablation. YV-plasty of the bladder neck was also performed.

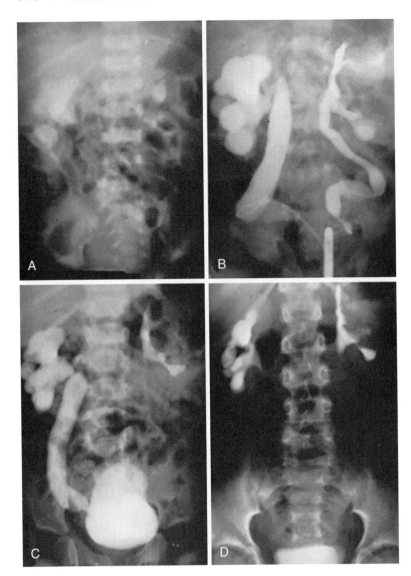

Figure 56–6. Case 2. Representative radiographs. *A*, Intravenous pyelogram (IVP) on admission at age 1 week, with poor bilateral function and hydronephrosis. *B*, Retrograde pyelogram at time of endoscopic valve resection showing bilaterally dilated, tortuous ureters—the right more than the left. *C*, Subsequent IVP at age 5 months. On the right side, there was partial obstruction at both ends of the ureters. On the left side, there was reflux and delayed emptying of the upper tract, with tortuosity at the ureteropelvic junction. *D*, Later IVP at age 6 years.

At age 7 years, a bladder neck narrowing procedure was done to correct the stress incontinence that resulted. This case serves to emphasize that the hypertrophied bladder neck that appears to be obstructive should be left alone in most cases. Furthermore, urodynamic evaluation should be performed to test bladder compliance in boys who have had urethral valves and continue to have dysfunctional voiding. Some can be helped with drugs, and others need bladder augmentation.

Case 3 (Fig. 56-7): Valve Ablation and Immediate Reconstruction of the Urinary Tract

When first referred, this infant was acutely ill with severe urinary infection. Blood chemical values showed BUN 70 mg/dl, and creatinine was 3.6 mg/dl. An IVP before admission provided poor bilateral visualization. Cystogram showed typical urethral valves and massive vesicoureteral reflux.

Four days of catheter drainage and supportive therapy with fluids and antibiotics dramatically improved his condition. Then, the valves were resected transurethrally. The ureteral orifices were widely dilated, allowing a view up into the ureters. It was thought, therefore, that the massive reflux would persist. The lower ureters were therefore shortened, tapered, and reimplanted. Six weeks later, the still tortuous and dilated upper ureters were repaired, resecting each ureteropelvic junction and tapering the upper ureters. Subsequent growth and development were normal. The patient is now age 30 years, is 6 ft, 3 inches tall, weighs more than 200 lb, and excelled in college basketball. BUN is 27 mg/dl, serum creatinine is 1.6 mg/dl, and creatinine clearance is 41 l/m² BSA/day.

COMMENT. Direct reconstruction was performed because massive reflux was likely to persist, causing urosepsis and further damage to the very hydronephrotic upper tracts. The patient developed temporary partial obstruction of the left lower ureter and

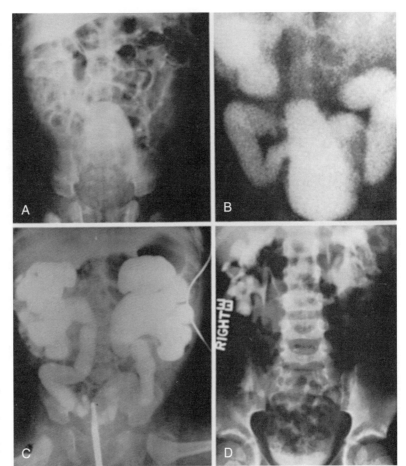

Figure 56-7. Case 3. *A,* Preoperative intravenous pyelogram (IVP) showing large bladder and poor visualization of upper urinary tracts. *B,* Preoperative cystogram showing massive reflux, tortuous ureters, and hydronephrosis. Urethra showed typical valves. If the cystogram is done first and there is no reflux, no need exists to obtain an IVP to visualize the upper tracts. *C,* Retrograde study at the time of valve resection and lower ureter repair, which is seldom done immediately and only in very severe cases. *D,* IVP at age 8 years. Appearance is the same on the study at 21 years.

also a small leak from the left upper ureteral repair. Both problems resolved with short-term nephrostomy drainage. This case emphasizes that complications can occur after ureteral repair in a small infant, but they do not preclude an excellent long-term result.

In our early experience with megaureter surgery, we tended to repair dilated upper ureters more often than we do today.[38, 41] However, if the upper ureters remain dilated, have ineffective peristalsis, and show persistent tortuosity of the ureteropelvic junction, we do not hesitate to undertake repair to optimize upper tract drainage. The upper ureter is never operated on first, for two reasons. First, correcting the lower ureter will often obviate the need for upper ureter surgery. Second, shortening and tapering the upper ureter can temporarily reduce the collateral blood supply of the lower ureter, which can cause ischemic necrosis of the lower ureter, if it should be operated on a short time later.

The initial radiographs of this critically ill 3-month-old infant were ominous. I believe that early complete repair salvaged the urinary tract because it stopped obstruction and reflux immediately. This maneuver prevented infection and deterioration of the hydronephrotic upper tracts. I do not think he

would have otherwise become a robust adult whose creatinine clearance value is 41 l/m² BSA.

Case 4 (Fig. 56-8): Valve Ablation and Surgery for Megaureter

This 3-month-old infant was referred with a weak urinary stream. The IVP showed remarkable ureteral tortuosity. Presenting in 1964, before modern endoscopes were available, valves were resected by open technique (long outmoded) and YV-plasty was performed to the bladder neck (not done today). The remarkable tortuosity and dilation of the ureters did not improve. Cinefluorography demonstrated bilateral ureterovesical junction obstruction. Although ureteral peristalsis was active, the contrast medium churned back and forth in the ureters, emptying poorly into the bladder. Therefore, 3 months later, the upper ureters were repaired. The lower ureters were repaired 2 months after the upper ureters. At age 11 years, the bladder neck and prostatic urethra were narrowed via a symphysis-splitting exposure to correct stress incontinence. The patient was a normal young adult until 19 years of age, when he died in an automobile accident.

COMMENT. This was the first patient upon whom I

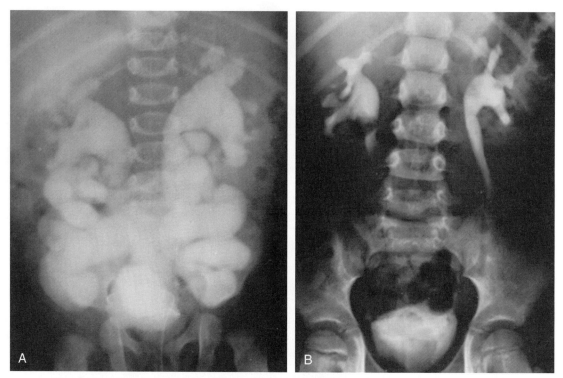

Figure 56–8. Case 4. A 3-month-old infant with weak urinary stream. *A,* Intravenous pyelogram (IVP) at age 3 months with good function by massively tortuous, dilated ureters. There was no reflux. Upper tracts did not change or empty better after valves were resected. *B,* Later IVP at age 12 years after staged reconstruction of ureters. Prior studies for a decade looked the same.

performed total revamping of the urinary tract in an era when ureterostomy and other types of urinary diversion were commonly done. In the past 25 years, lower ureter repair has been done *first,* not the reverse, as we did in this early case. The results served to convince me that reconstruction should be considered in cases in which valve resection alone does not clearly improve the appearance of the upper tracts. The patient should be followed closely after valve ablation to assess the upper tract drainage. We have not found radionuclide study with furosemide washout very helpful in assessing drainage, when the upper tracts are quite dilated. Furthermore, in my experience, the Whitaker antegrade pressure perfusion study[42] has not proven reliable in deciding whether a ureter is obstructed. This case also poignantly illustrates the loss of young men from preventable trauma.

Case 5 (Figs. 56–9 to 56–11): Obstruction of Anterior Urethra by Diverticulum and Massive Reflux

This patient was referred at age 9 weeks with acute urinary infection and an IVP showing massive bilateral hydronephrosis caused by an anterior urethral valve or diverticulum (see Fig. 56–9). Cystogram showed obstruction of the anterior urethra and massive reflux, as illustrated in Figures 56–10 and 56–11. To obtain the cystogram, a suprapubic needle was inserted into the bladder, because a small plastic feeding catheter merely curled up in the urethral diverticulum.

The urethral obstruction was relieved by incising the distal rim of the diverticulum by the same technique used for typical urethral valves. The ureteral orifices were so dilated that the endoscope could be passed into the lower ureters. It was elected, therefore, to perform bilateral shortening, tapering, and reimplantation. Radiographic follow-up showed improvement. At age 13 years, the patient's BUN level was 15 mg/dl and creatinine level was 0.7 mg/dl. The creatinine clearance measured 100 l/m² BSA/day. At age 27 years, the patient is well.

COMMENT. This type of urethral obstruction can occur in all degrees of severity, just like true urethral

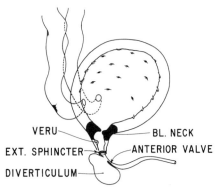

Figure 56–9. Case 5. Anatomy of a urethral diverticulum—the anterior rim creating a valve.

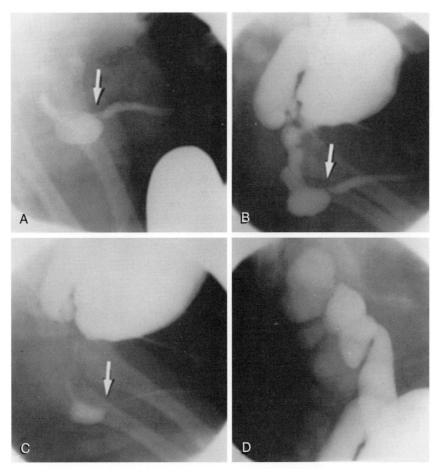

Figure 56–10. Case 5. Preoperative cystogram studies. *A,* A 5-French plastic feeding catheter is curled up in the diverticulum *(arrow)*. *B,* Voiding study obtained by suprapubic needle inserted in bladder to infuse contrast medium. Note valve-like obstruction from distal rim of diverticulum *(arrow)*. *C,* Contrast material retained in diverticulum *(arrow)*. *D,* Massive bilateral reflux.

valves. The obstructing rim of the diverticulum can be resected by an open operation on the urethra, or it can be done endoscopically. In one of our cases, there was a large stone in the diverticulum, which was best treated by an open operation.

Case 6 (Fig. 56-12): Secondary Valve Case with Previous Urinary Diversion

This 19-year-old man was referred for urinary reconstruction. Many previous operations had been performed. At age 2 years, operations included resection of valves, loop ureterostomies, ureteral reimplantations, and nephrostomies. At age 5 years, the ureterostomies were closed and an ileal loop conduit was performed. At age 7, cystostomy was performed for pyocystis. At age 13 years, a scrotal flap was used to repair a urethral stricture that had been caused by valve resection. There was an open perineal urethrostomy. The bladder held only 60 ml. The first operation consisted of removing the hairy scrotal flap, substituting a patch of penile skin, and closing the perineal urethrostomy. Cycling the bladder by filling through the suprapubic cystostomy increased its size to 200 ml. Five months later, undi-

version was performed. The bladder was augmented using cecum with an intussuscepted nipple for prevention of reflux. The left ureter was drained into the right renal pelvis, and the upper ureter on the right was drained into the terminal ileum. The operation lasted 13 hours.

His postoperative course was complicated by gastrointestinal bleeding from *Clostridium difficile,* which responded to appropriate treatment.

One year later, because there was stress incontinence, an operation was done to narrow the bladder neck from a suprapubic approach and taper the distal prostatic urethra through a perineal approach. The cecal nipple made to prevent reflux was partially prolapsed, although it was not refluxing. Therefore, it was replaced into the cecum and sewn to the adjacent cecal wall.

Five years after he was first treated, at age 24 years, the patient still had some stress incontinence. Therefore, a more radical narrowing of the bladder neck and prostatic urethra was performed via a symphysis splitting approach. This procedure made the patient entirely continent. However, he must empty by intermittent self-catheterization. He is now age 36 years, is in good general health, and has three

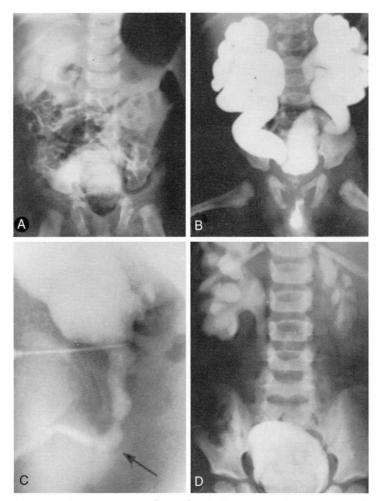

Figure 56–11. Case 5. Representative radiographs. *A*, Preoperative intravenous pyelogram (IVP) at age 9 weeks. Massive bilateral hydronephrosis with poor visualization of the left side. *B*, Preoperative cystogram showing massive reflux and hydronephrosis. This pediatric patient was managed by immediate reconstruction, because the lower ureters were widely dilated, leaving little chance that this reflux would subside. *C*, Voiding study via suprapubic needle, 6 months after reconstructive procedure. *Arrow* points to prior site of diverticulum—now almost normal in appearance after endoscopic resection. There was no urethral reflux. *D*, Later IVP at age 3½ years.

healthy children, despite the previous extensive surgery to his prostatic urethra.

COMMENT. This case illustrates the host of complications that can follow inexpert initial treatment of a boy with urethral valves. His treatment began with valve ablation via a perineal urethrostomy. A urethral stricture resulted. Ureterostomy, ureteral reimplantation, nephrostomy, and ileal loop urinary diversion followed. Among 186 urinary undiversion operations that I described, 66 were in male patients who had severe urethral valves and were referred for reconstruction after prior urinary diversions.[43]

Bladder augmentation was necessary because the bladder remained small, despite cycling with saline. If an ileocecal augmentation is used, the nipple must be sewn to the cecal wall to prevent its breakdown.[8] Bladder neck surgery was needed again to finally achieve continence, and this was accomplished through splitting the pubic symphysis.

I have used that approach with increasing frequency in the past several years, because it affords unparalleled access to the entire urethra from the bulb up through the newly created bladder neck.[44] A fundamental principle in surgery for incontinence is to be willing to reoperate if additional resistance is needed, stressing to the patient that intermittent catheterization may be required to empty when adequate outlet resistance is attained. Continence requires having a compliant bladder with adequate volume and a low enough pressure to not exceed outlet resistance. In this patient's mind, the ultimate outcome justified the series of operations required to achieve his present status.

☐ Conclusions

Urethral valves vary in severity and are more common than is generally appreciated. Endoscopic ablation should be possible without damaging the urethra, external urinary sphincter, or bladder neck. Some patients need nothing more. Others require

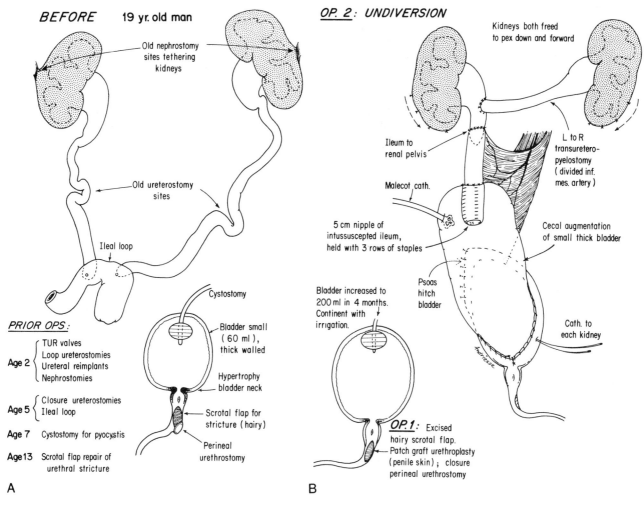

Figure 56–12. Case 6. *A*, Preoperative anatomy. *B*, Postoperative anatomy.

extensive reconstructive surgery for ureteral obstruction or reflux. Bladder augmentation is necessary, in some, to improve compliance and capacity. Many patients live with urinary diversions whose original pathology was urethral valves. They can undergo undiversions with present techniques.

REFERENCES

1. Young HH, Frontz WA, Baldwin JC: Congenital obstruction of the posterior urethra. J Urol 3:289–292, 1919.
2. Hendren WH: Posterior urethral valves in boys: A broad clinical spectrum. J Urol 106:298–307, 1971.
3. Nieh PT, Hendren WH: Obstructing posterior urethral valves in octogenarian. Urology 13:412–413, 1979.
4. Mueller SC, Marshall FF: Spectrum of recognized posterior urethral valves in the adult. Urology 22:139–142, 1983.
5. Bauer SB, Dieppa RA, Labib KK, Retik AB: The bladder in boys with posterior urethral valves: A urodynamic assessment. J Urol 121:769–773, 1979.
6. Campaiola JM, Perlmutter AD, Steinhardt GF: Noncompliant bladder resulting from posterior urethral valves. J Urol 134:708–710, 1985.
7. Gearhart JP, Albertsen PC, Marshall FF, Jeffs RD: Pediatric applications of augmentation cystoplasty: The Johns Hopkins experience. J Urol 136:430–432, 1986.
8. Hendren WH, Hendren RB: Bladder augmentation: Experience with 129 children and young adults. J Urol 144:445–453, 1990.
9. Tank ES, Carey TC, Seifert AL: Management of neonatal urinary ascites. Urology 16:270–273, 1980.
10. Brown T, Mandell J, Lebowitz RL: Neonatal hydronephrosis in the era of sonography. AJR 148:959–963, 1987.
11. Cremin BJ, Aaron IA: Ultrasonic diagnosis of posterior urethral valve in neonates. Br J Radiol 6:435–438, 1983.
12. Thomas DF, Irving HC, Arthur RJ: Pre-natal diagnosis: How useful is it? Br J Urol 57:784–787, 1985.
13. Hutton KA, Thomas DF, Davies BW: Prenatally detected posterior urethral valves: Qualitative assessment of second trimester scans and prediction of outcome. J Urol 158:1022–1025, 1997.
14. Freedman AL, Bukowski TP, Smith CA, et al: Fetal therapy for obstructive uropathy: Diagnosis specific outcomes. J Urol 156:720–723, 1996.
15. Sholder AJ, Maizels M, Depp R, et al: Caution in antenatal intervention. J Urol 139:1026–1029, 1988.
16. Bruce J, Stannard V, Small PG, et al: The operative management of posterior urethral valves. J Pediatr Surg 22:1081–1086, 1987.
17. Whitaker RH, Sherwood T: An improved hook for destroying posterior urethral valves. J Urol 135:531–532, 1986.
18. Zaontz MR, Firlit CF: Percutaneous antegrade ablation of posterior urethral valves in infants with small caliber urethras: An alternative to urinary diversion. J Urol 36:247–248, 1986.
19. Lal R, Bhatnagar V, Mitra DK: Urethral structures after fulgu-

ration of posterior urethral valves. J Pediatr Surg 33:518–519, 1998.

20. Hendren WH: "Urethral Valves: Diagnosis and Endoscopic Resection." Film available from Eaton Film Library, Norwich, CT, and the Film Library of the American College of Surgeons, Chicago, 1974.

21. Johnston JH: Temporary cutaneous ureterosomy in the management of advanced congenital urinary obstruction. Arch Dis Child 38:161–167, 1963.

22. Leape LL, Holder TM: Temporary tubeless urinary diversion in children. J Pediatr Surg 5:288–291, 1970.

23. Dwoskin JY: Management of the massively dilated urinary tract in infants by temporary diversion and single-stage reconstruction. Urol Clin North Am 1:515–525, 1974.

24. Arap S, Monti P, Nahas WC, et al: Vesicostomy: A temporary urinary diversion. J Urol 91:429–433, 1985.

25. Perlmutter AD, Patil J: Loop cutaneous ureterostomy in infants and young children: Late results in 32 cases. J Urol 107:655–659, 1972.

26. Rushton HG, Parrott TS, Woodard JR, Walther M: The role of vesicostomy in the management of anterior valves in neonates and infants. J Urol 138:107–109, 1987.

27. Sober I: Pelvioureterostomy-en-Y. J Urol 107:473–476, 1972.

28. Williams DI, Cromie WH: Ring ureterostomy. Br J Urol 47:789–792, 1975.

29. Rosen MA, Roth DR, Gonzales ET Jr: Current indications for cutaneous ureterostomy. Urology 43:92–96, 1994.

30. Close CE, Carr MC, Burns ME, et al: Lower urinary tract changes after early valve ablation in neonates and infants: Is early diversion warranted? J Urol 157:984–988, 1997.

31. Tietjen DN, Gloor JM, Husmann DA: Proximal urinary diversion in the management of posterior urethral valves: Is it necessary? J Urol 158:1008–1010, 1997.

32. Duckett JW Jr: Current management of posterior urethral valves. Urol Clin North Am 1:471–483, 1974.

33. Aaronson IA: Posterior urethral valve: A review of 120 cases. S Afr Med J 17:418–422, 1984.

34. Glassberg KI: Current issues regarding posterior urethral valves. Urol Clin North Am 12:175–185, 1985.

35. Mitchell ME, Close CE: Early primary valve ablation for posterior urethral valves. Semin Pediatr Surg 5:66–71, 1996.

36. Smith GH, Canning DA, Schulman SL, et al: The long-term outcome of posterior urethral valves treated with primary valve ablation and observation. J Urol 155:1730–1734, 1996.

37. Hendren WH: Complications of ureterostomy. J Urol 120:269–281, 1978.

38. Hendren WH: Operative repair of megaureter in children. J Urol 101:491–507, 1969.

39. Hendren WH: A new approach to infants with severe obstruction: early complete reconstruction. J Pediatr Surg 5:184–199, 1970.

40. Warshaw BL, Hynes LC, Trulock TS, Woodard JR: Prognostic features in infants with obstructive uropathy due to posterior urethral valves. J Urol 133:240–243, 1985.

41. Hendren WH: Complications of megaureter repair in children. J Urol 113:238–254, 1975.

42. Whitaker RH: Methods of assessing obstruction in dilated ureters. Br J Urol 45:15–20, 1973.

43. Hendren WH: Urinary tract refunctionalization after long-term diversion: A 20 year experience with 177 patients. Ann Surg 212:478–495, 1990.

44. Peters CA, Hendren WH: Splitting the pubis for exposure in difficult reconstructions for incontinence. J Urol 142:527–531, 1989.

57

EXSTROPHY OF THE BLADDER

J. Patrick Murphy, MD

Exstrophy of the bladder is made up of a spectrum of conditions ranging from glanular epispadias to complete exposure of bladder and urethra on the abdominal wall. The condition is rare, and early surgical intervention at a center experienced with the care of these patients is crucial to optimize the chances of good functional results.

□ Historical Perspectives

The first description of exstrophy was written in 1597 by VonGrafenberg.[1] In the 1850s, several unsuccessful attempts at primary closure were reported, and over the subsequent 80 to 90 years, urinary diversion, primarily by ureterosigmoidostomy,[2, 3] was the mainstay of treatment.

A successful primary bladder closure in a female patient was reported by Young in 1942,[4] and in 1948, Michon reported successful closure in a male patient.[5] Over the following 30 years, bladder closure became more common, but success, as measured by continence, was poor.

Subsequently, the concept of staged bladder reconstruction was initiated, with early primary bladder closure, later penile and urethral reconstruction, and, ultimately, bladder neck reconstruction to enhance continence.[6, 7] In the past three decades, various refinements in this staged reconstruction technique have led to continence rates of as high as 80%. Further refinements continue to occur, with the idea of complete one-stage newborn repair emerging.[8] The history of bladder exstrophy continues to evolve.

□ Clinical Aspects

The incidence of classic bladder exstrophy is estimated to be 1 in 30,000 to 40,000 live births, with a male-to-female predominance of about 3 to 5:1.[9] The risk of exstrophy increases dramatically in children of patients with exstrophy, with a reported incidence of one in 70 live births.[10]

The exstrophy anomaly occurs some time between the 4th and 10th weeks of gestation. The most popular theory suggests that the defect is the result of an "overdevelopment" of the cloacal membrane, which prevents the medial ingrowth of mesenchyme that is necessary for normal lower abdominal wall formation. The cloacal membrane then ruptures, and the abdominal wall defect leaves the urethra and bladder to be exposed on the abdominal wall. If rupture of the membrane occurs before the cloaca divides into the urogenital sinus and rectum, cloacal exstrophy results.[11] Another theory based on studies of rat embryos postulates that it is the abnormal, more caudal insertion of the body stalk that prevents mesenchymal migration to the midline. The bladder and urethra or the cloaca, lacking the support of the normal abdominal wall, ruptures to form the exstrophy.[12]

The classic bladder exstrophy (exposed bladder plate, open urethra, wide pubic diastasis, low umbilicus, and wide rectus) is the most common presentation of the anomaly. The penis in the male patient characteristically is wide and short because of the attachment of the corporal bodies to the pubic rami that have not come together to form a symphysis (Fig. 57–1). The urethral plate is exposed on the dorsum of the penis and the cleft glans penis. The preputium is ventrally placed from the shaft of the penis.[13] The periprostatic nerves and the penile neurovascular bundles, which normally are paired dorsally on the fused corporal bodies, are displaced to lie lateral to the urethral plate.[14] The testicles are usually descended, and the vas deferens and ejaculatory ducts are normal. In most cases of bladder exstrophy, functional phallic reconstruction is possible.

The female exstrophic genitalia demonstrate a bifid clitoris and separation of the labia. The vagina is shortened and anteriorly displaced, and the uterus, ovaries, and tubes are generally normal. Duplication of uterus and vagina may occur (Fig. 57–2).

There are some unusual variants of exstrophy. Side-by-side duplication of the baldder may occur, with each bladder receiving one ureter, in which

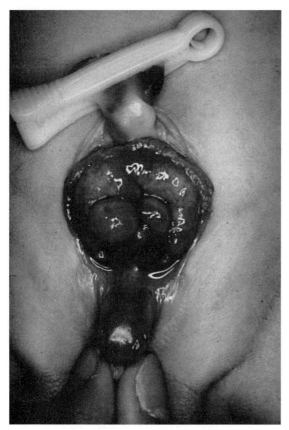

Figure 57–1. Classic bladder exstrophy in a male patient. Note the exposed bladder plate, low set umbilicus, and wide, shortened phallus.

characteristic pubic and rectus diastasis usually is present.

☐ Associated Anomalies

Musculoskeletal anomalies are related mostly to the diastasis of the symphisis pubis. The widened innominate bones account for the external rotation of the lower limbs and waddling gait seen in children with this disorder. Over time, this external rotation tends to correct itself, and few or no long-term defects in mobility occur.[15] The incidence of vertebral anomalies is slightly increased in exstrophy, and spinal dysraphism is more common in cloacal exstrophy.[15, 16] Inguinal hernias are common in the exstrophy complex and can generally be repaired at the time of initial bladder closure.

Anorectal anomalies are usually limited to anterior displacement of the rectum. Rectal prolapse can occur in exstrophy prior to bladder closure. Imperforate anus is uncommon, except in the cloacal exstrophy patient. Renal anomalies are uncommon; however, hydroureteronephrosis can occur, particularly if the bladder remains exposed for an extended period. Because the bladder is small and thick walled, hydronephrosis can occur following closure. Most surgeons recommend ureteral stents in the immediate postoperative period. Vesicoureteric reflux is common and is usually corrected at the time of bladder neck reconstruction.

☐ Treatment

Treatment of exstrophy begins immediately at birth. The bladder plate should be protected with a moist nonadherent covering. The umbilical clamp is removed and the umbilicus ligated to prevent trauma to the bladder plate. Physical examination determines bladder plate size, sexual identity, and

case one bladder may be closed and the other exstrophic. There may be a vertical duplication of the bladder, where the bladder in proximity with the umbilicus is exstrophic and the inferior bladder and urethra are normally formed. Superior vesical fissure is an exstrophy variant in which the dome of the bladder is open just below the umbilicus. The

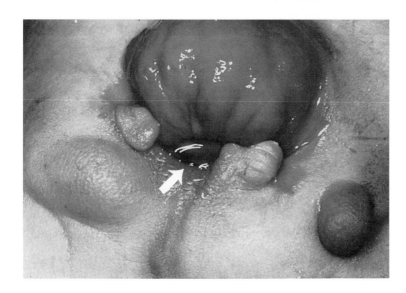

Figure 57–2. Female exstrophy with bifid clitoris, anterior vagina *(arrow)*, and separation of the labia.

genital size. Renal ultrasonography is done to evaluate for possible hydronephrosis.

Staged reconstruction of bladdder exstrophy is the time-proven and most common approach to surgical treatment.[15, 16] The first step consists of primary bladder and bladder neck closure in the first 48 to 72 hours of life to create an epispadias. Epispadias repair is the second stage, which in boys is performed at about 1 year of age. The third stage consists of bladder neck reconstruction, undertaken when the bladder capacity is greater than 60 ml and the child has social interest in urinary continence, usually at 3 to 5 years of age.

Simultaneous repair of exstrophy and epispadias in the neonate has been advocated by some[8, 19] with the hope of improving the long-term cosmetic and functional results, which at times can be less than ideal following staged reconstruction.[20] Early results are encouraging from some centers.[8, 19, 21] Others, however, are concerned that early complete closure may increase bladder outlet resistance, leading to severe reflux and upper tract deterioration. Critics of the neonatal one-stage repair believe there may be deleterious effects to bladder development and stability. They recommend the combined closure only in older infants or in those who have failed neonatal primary bladder closure.[22]

Certainly, the combined, single-stage newborn repair is appealing and would seem ideal if it led to improved functional and cosmetic results when compared with the time-honored functional staged reconstruction. Data from patients treated with combined closure represent follow-up of less than 8 years, with relatively low numbers of patients.[18, 20, 23, 24] Therefore, only time will dictate the best approach to the newborn with exstrophy. At this point, staged reconstruction is the most widely accepted technique.

BLADDER CLOSURE

Primary bladder closure is best accomplished in the first 72 hours of life. This timing takes advantage of the pliability of the newborn pelvis and may obviate the need for pelvic osteotomy. It also decreases the amount of edema and thickening of the bladder plate and makes the bladder closure easier. The technique of bladder closure is illustrated in Figure 57–3. The use of paraexstrophy skin flaps[25] demonstrated in the figure are rarely needed, and it is preferable to keep the urethral plate intact if at all possible.[24, 26] Placing the bladder deep in the pelvis, positioning the prostatic and membranous urethra as far posterior as possible (with approximation of the urogenital diaphragm soft tissue around the prostatic urethra and approximation of the pubic symphis) all enhance the success of closure and subsequent development of bladder capacity and continence.[24, 26]

Ureteral stenting and suprapubic drainage are advisable until edema of the bladder has subsided and adequate urinary drainage can be demonstrated, from both the ureters and the bladder neck. Maintenance of internal rotation of the legs with Buck's traction and leg wrapping is used for several weeks postoperatively or, if osteotomies are performed, external fixation is accomplished for 6 weeks.[27] Suppressive antibiotic therapy is continued until bladder neck reconstruction and correction of vesicoureteric reflux is done at the third stage. Ultrasonography, nuclear renal scan, intravenous pyelography, and contrast cystography all may be used to evaluate renal drainage and function as well as bladder capacity and reflux during the period leading up to bladder neck reconstruction.

EPISPADIAS REPAIR

Epispadias repair is usually performed at approximately 12 months of age. Straightening and lengthening of the penis with creation of a ventrally placed urethra is the goal of the repair. The commonly used technique[28] is illustrated in Figure 57–4 and accomplishes these goals in most cases. A reported modification of the repair that uses complete disassembly of the corporal bodies and ventral placement of the urethra is an alternative.[29] This repair provides excellent ventral placement of the urethra and good cosmetic results and has gained wide acceptance.[30] Techniques used commonly to repair hypospadias, such as preputial flaps or free skin or mucosal grafts, may be used occasionally to enhance the repair of the more difficult epispadias. Dressing and urinary diversion are similar to those used in hypospadias repairs.

BLADDER NECK RECONSTRUCTION

Bladder neck reconstruction to enhance continence is undertaken when the child is old enough to desire being continent and able to cooperate with the sometimes long and frustrating process of bladder training. Bladder capacity should be at least 60 ml, as measured with cystogram and/or cystoscopy under anesthesia.[26, 31, 32] Approximation of the pubis is thought by some surgeons to be important for successful urinary continence.[31–33] Therefore, osteotomy or repeat osteotomy may be considered at the time of the bladder neck procedure.

The technique of bladder neck reconstruction, as modified from Young-Dees-Leadbetter[34–36] is illustrated in Figure 57–5. The bladder is opened, and a cross-trigonal ureteral reimplantation is performed to correct reflux and move the ureters away from the bladder neck to provide adequate length for approximately 3 cm of bladder to be tubularized as a new bladder neck. The reconstruction is performed as illustrated, with tubularization of the mucosa and detrusor over an 8 French catheter. Suprapubic drainage is maintained over a period of 3 weeks prior to initiating voiding trials.[26] Close observation is important postoperatively to ensure

Text continued on page 760

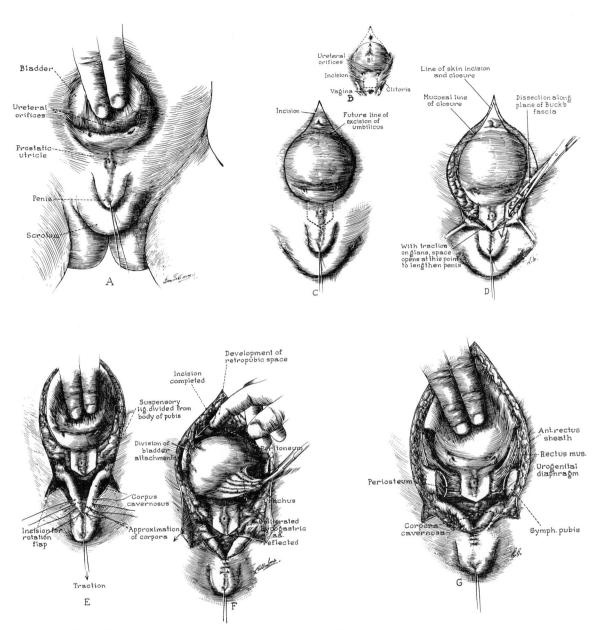

Figure 57–3. *A* to *O*, Steps in primary bladder closure following osteotomy or without osteotomy in the newborn less than 72 hours of age. *A, B, C,* and *D* depict the incision line around the umbilicus and bladder down to the urethral plate. If the male urethral groove is adequate, no transverse incision is made in the urethral plate for initial urethral lengthening.

E, Lateral skin incisions allow rotation of paraexstrophy skin to cover the elongated penis if the urethral groove has been transected.

F, Development of the retropubic space from below the area of umbilical dissection to facilitate separation of the bladder from the rectus sheath and muscle.

G, Medial fan of rectus muscle attaching behind the prostate to urogenital diaphragm. The urogenital diaphragm and anterior corpus are freed from the pubis in a subperiosteal plan.

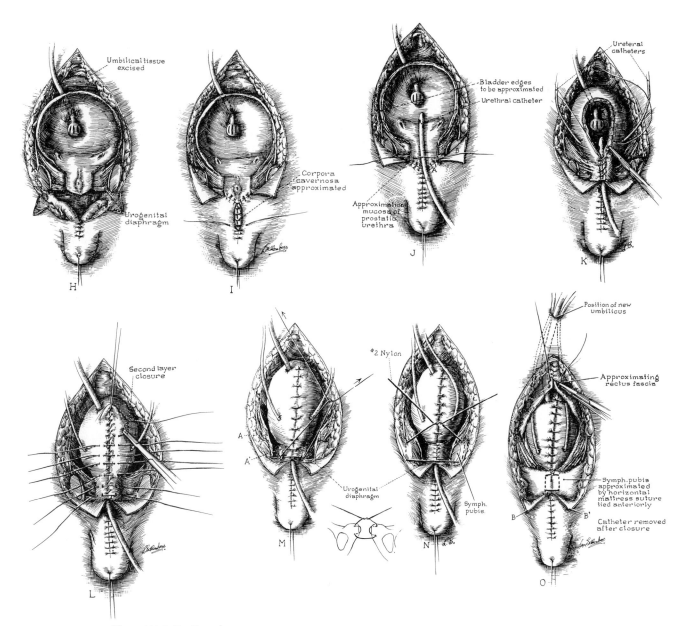

Figure 57–3 *Continued*

H to *L* depict the anastomosis of the paraexstrophy skin to the prostatic plate.

M, The urogenital diaphragm is closed with a separate layer of sutures if possible. Often, this maneuver is not possible.

N, Horizontal mattress sutures are tied on the external surface of symphysis while the assistant applies medial rotation of greater trocanters.

O, The catheter is removed from the closed bladder neck and urethra. Approximation of skin point B to B1 provides an anterior step from penile closure to abdominal wall closure. (Drawings by Leon Schlossberg.) (From Gearhart JP, Jeffs RD: Management of the exstrophy-epispadias complex and urachal anomalies. In Walsh PC, Campbell MF [eds]: Campbell's Urology [6th ed]. Philadelphia, WB Saunders, 1992, pp 1791–1794.)

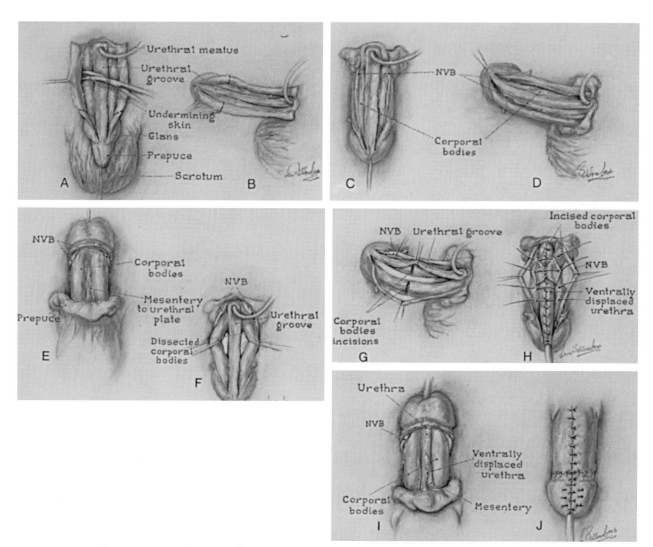

Figure 57–4. *A*, and *B*, Epispadias repair. Marking an incision of the urethral groove and mobilization of the penile skin.

C and *D*, Incision of the glans and exposure of the neurovascular bundles (NVB).

E and *F*, Separation of the urethral groove from the corporal bodies with dissection initially started from below.

G and *H*, Mobilization of neurovascular bundles from corporal bodies and incision in corporal bodies. Closure of urethral groove to tip of penis, closure of corporal incision displacing urethra ventrally. Further sutures placed distally to further bury urethra under corporal bodies.

I and *J*, Completed repair with urethra below corporal bodies and skin closure of penis. (Drawings by Leon Schlossberg.) (From Gearhart JP, Jeffs RD: Management of the exstrophy-epispadias complex and urachal anomalies. In Walsh PC, Campbell MF [eds]: Campbell's Urology [6th ed]. Philadelphia, WB Saunders, 1992, p 1798.)

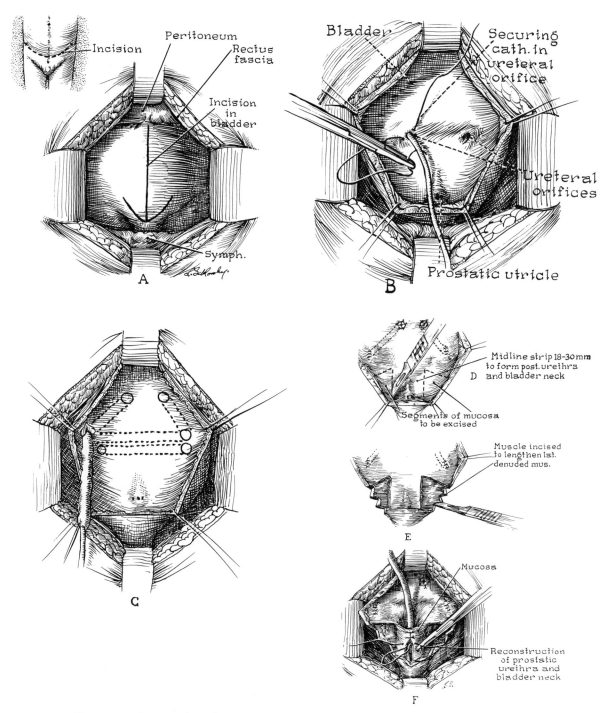

Figure 57–5. Steps in the Cohen transtrigonal or cephalotrigonal reimplantation of ureters and bladder neck reconstruction for continence.

A, Transverse bladder incision with vertical extension subsequently closed in midline to narrow bladder near bladder neck.

B to *F*, Ureteral mobilization with either transtrigonal or cephalotrigonal course for reimplantation. Mucosal strip of trigone to form bladder neck and prostatic urethra. Lateral denuded muscle triangles are lengthened by several small incisions to allow tailoring of the bladder neck reconstruction.

Illustration continued on following page

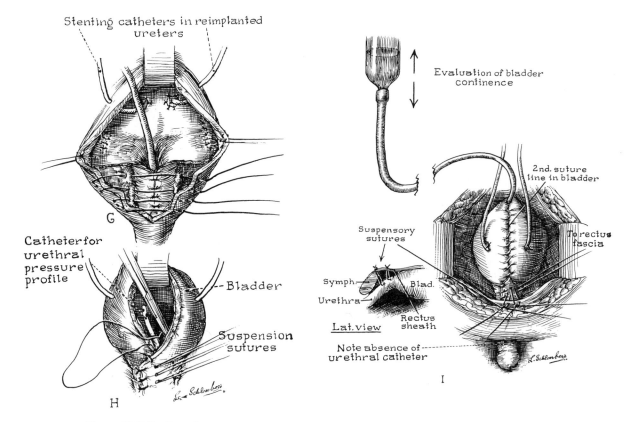

Figure 57–5 *Continued*

F to *H*, The double-breasted nature and exact suture placement of the bladder neck and reconstruction. A pressure profile catheter can be left and urethral pressure profile obtained prior to closure of the bladder dome. Suspension sutures are elevated manually to estimate the final urethral pressure profile.

I, Bladder neck and urethra are unstented. Drainage is by urethral catheters and suprapubic tube. Bladder outlet resistance is estimated by water manometer. (Drawings by Leon Schlossberg.) (From Gearhart JP, Jeffs RD: Management of the exstrophy-epispadias complex and urachal anomalies. In Walsh PC, Campbell MF (eds): Campbell's Urology [6th ed]. Philadelphia, WB Saunders, 1992, p 1800.)

adequate bladder emptying and avoid hydronephrosis. Prior to removing the suprapubic tube, urethra must be able to be catheterized. Some patients may require a temporary or long-term period of clean intermittent catheterization, which should be discussed with the parents preoperatively. Adequate bladder volume may take months to develop, and close observation is critical to prevent the development of progressive hydronephrosis and/or urinary infection.

Patients who do not develop adequate capacity for bladder neck reconstruction or who fail to gain adequate continence after a bladder neck procedure may require some form of urinary diversion. Bladder augmentation, combined with clean intermittent catheterization, either via the urethra or through a continent catheterizable stoma,[37] is the preferred diversion if an adequate bladder exists and urethral leakage is not a problem. For those who cannot have bladder augmentation, either because of inadequate capacity or urethral resistance, a continent catheterizable urinary reservoir made of bowel is the next choice. There may be rare instances in which non-continent diversion or ureterosigmoid anastomosis is the best option.

☐ Results

Complications of initial bladder closure include dehiscence of the closure, prolapse of bladder, or bladder outlet obstruction with hydronephrosis. Dehiscence is a relatively uncommon occurrence with the current surgical techniques and care. Experienced centers should expect an incidence of 5% or less. Bladder prolapse is more common, with an incidence of 10 to 15%, and outlet obstruction occurs in about 5% of cases.[26]

The most common complication of epispadias repair is urethrocutaneous fistula, the incidence of which is between 30 and 50%. The newer techniques of repair, with a more ventral placement of the urethra, have reduced the incidence of this complication.[28, 30] Residual dorsal chordee typically has been a long-term problem,[38] and secondary procedures for correction are common. Again, the newer techniques may reduce this problem.

Continence rates following bladder neck reconstruction range from 40 to 80%.[20, 24, 39–43] Achieving these rates of social continence requires careful follow-up, patience, and, often, multiple procedures. Certainly, the medical and surgical techniques needed to achieve long-term continence in these patients continue to evolve.

Bladder malignancy is significantly more common in patients who have had exstrophy. Adenocarcinoma, which is the most common malignancy in these cases is probably related to chronic inflammatory changes from exposure of the exteriorized bladder.[44] Squamous cell and rhabdomyosarcoma have also occurred.

Sexual function is possible in reconstructed exstrophy patients.[13, 45] There are numerous reports of pregnancies in female exstrophy patients and also of males who have fathered children.[46] Fertility in male patients is diminished, however. This fact is most likely a result of reconstruction of the urethra and bladder neck, which may result in injury to the ejaculatory system.

With experienced surgical care, there is potential for the exstrophy patient to become a well-adjusted individual with adequate sexual and bladder function. This potential is obviously influenced by the careful attention to the technical aspects of repair, but social and psychological care and follow-up have an equally important role.

REFERENCES

1. Murphy LJT: The History of Urology. Springfield, IL, Charles C. Thomas, 1972.
2. Syme J: Ectopia vesicase. Lancet 2:568, 1852.
3. Coffey RC: Transplantation of the ureter into the large intestine in the absence of a functioning bladder. Surg Gynecol Obstet 32:383–385, 1921.
4. Young HH: Exstrophy of the bladder: The first case in which a normal bladder and urinary control have been obtained by plastic operation. Surg Gynecol Obstet 74:729–731, 1942.
5. Michon L: Conservative operations for exstrophy of the bladder with particular reference to urinary incontinence. Br J Urol 20:167–169, 1948.
6. Leadbetter GW: Surgical correction of total urinary incontinence. J Urol 91:261–266, 1964.
7. Dewan PA: Historical trends in the management of bladder exstrophy. Pediatr Surg Int 10:289–297, 1995.
8. Ngan JH, Grady RW, Carr MC, Mitchell ME: An argument for complete one-stage anatomic repair of exstrophy in the newborn [abstract 970]. J Urol 157:248, 1997.
9. Lancaster PAL: Epidemiology of bladder exstrophy: A communication from the International Clearinghouse for Birth Defects monitoring systems. Teratology 36:221–227, 1987.
10. Shapiro E, Lepor H, Jeffs RD: The inheritance of the exstrophy–epispadias complex. J Urol 132:308–310, 1984.
11. Muecke EC: The role of the cloacal membrane in exstrophy: The first successful experimental study. J Urol 92:659, 1964.
12. Mildenberger H, Kluth D, Dzuiba M: Embryology of bladder exstrophy. J Pediatr Surg 23:166–170, 1988.
13. Woodhouse CRJ, Kellett MJ: Anatomy of the penis and its deformities in exstrophy and epispadias. J Urol 132:1122–1124, 1984.
14. Schlegel PN, Gearhart JP: Neuroanatomy of the pelvis in an infant with cloacal exstrophy: A detailed microdissection with histology. J Urol 141:583–585, 1989.
15. Kelly JH: Vesical exstrophy: Repair using radical mobilisation of soft tissues. Pediatr Surg Int 10:298–304, 1995.
16. Loder RT, Dayioglu MM: Association of congenital vertebral malformations with bladder and cloacal exstrophy. J Pediatr Orthoped 10:389–393, 1990.
17. Diamond DA, Jeffs RD: Cloacal exstrophy: A 22-year experience. J Urol 133:779–782, 1985.
18. Yeggappan L, Peppas DS, Gearhart JP, Jeffs RD: Bladder exstrophy: A twenty-one year experience with functional reconstruction in 87 consecutive patients followed from birth [abstract 973]. J Urol 157:249, 1997.
19. McLorie GA, Salle JP, Merguerian PA, et al: Simultaneous repair of bladder exstrophy and epispadias in male infants [abstract 157]. J Urol 159:43, 1998.
20. Schanne FJ, Lanchoney TF, McKitty S, et al: Long-Term follow-up for continence in patients with classic bladder exstrophy [abstract 159]. J Urol 159:43, 1998.
21. Grady RW, Carr MC, Lipski B, Mitchell ME: Complete primary repair of exstrophy [abstract 98]. Presented at the American Academy of Pediatrics Section on Urology Annual Meeting, San Francisco; October 19, 1998.
22. Gearhart JP, Mathews R, Taylor S, Jeffs RD: Combined bladder closure and epispadias repair in the reconstruction of bladder exstrophy. J Urol 160:1182–1185, 1998.
23. Dinlec CZ, Bauer SB, Hendren WH, et al: Response of the exstrophy bladder to staged reconstruction [abstract 158]. J Urol 159:44, 1998.
24. Kelly JH: Exstrophy and epispadias: Kelly's method of repair. In O'Neill JA, Rowe MI, Grosfeld JL, et al (eds): Pediatric Surgery (5th ed). St. Louis, Mosby-Year Book, 1998, pp 1732–1759.
25. Duckett JW: Use of paraexstrophy skin pedicle grafts for correction of exstrophy and epispadias repair. Birth Defects 13:175–179, 1977.
26. Gearhart JP: Bladder and urachal abnormalities: The exstrophy–epispadias complex. In Kelalis PP, King LR, Belman AB (eds): Clinical Pediatric Urology (3rd ed). Philadelphia, W.B. Saunders Company, 1992, pp 579–619.
27. Sponseller PD, Gearhart JP, Jeffs RD: lliac osteotomies for revision of bladder exstrophy failures. J Urol 146:137–140, 1991.
28. Gearhart JP, Sciortino C, Ben-Chaim J, et al: The Cantwell-Ransley epispadias repair in exstrophy and epispadias: Lessons learned. Urology 46:92–96, 1995.
29. Mitchell ME, Bagli DJ: Complete penile disassembly for epispadias repair: The Mitchell technique. J Urol 155:300–304, 1996.
30. Zaontz MR, Steckler RE, Dairiki Shortliffe LM, et al: Multicenter experience with the Mitchell technique for epispadias repair. J Urol 160:172–176, 1998.
31. Kramer SA, Kelalis PP: Assessment of urinary continence in epispadias: Review of 94 patients. J Urol 128:290–293, 1982.
32. Lepor H, Jeffs RD: Primary bladder closure and bladder neck reconstruction in classical bladder exstrophy. J Urol 130:1142–1145, 1983.
33. Gearhart JP, Jeffs RD: State of the art reconstructive surgery for bladder exstrophy at the Johns Hopkins Hospital. Am J Dis Child 143:1475–1478, 1989.
34. Young HH: An operation for the cure of incontinence associated with epispadias. J Urol 7:1–32, 1922.
35. Dees JE: Epispadias with incontinence in the male. Surgery 12:621–630, 1942.
36. Leadbetter GW Jr: Surgical correction of total urinary incontinence. J Urol 91:261–266, 1964.
37. Mitrofanoff P: Cystomie continente trans-appendiculaire dans le traitement des vessies neurologues. Chir Ped 21:297–305, 1980.
38. Kramer SA, Mesrobian HJ, Kelalis PP: Long term follow up of cosmetic appearance and genital function in male epispadias: Review of 70 cases, J Urol 135:543–547, 1986.
39. Canning DA, Gearhart JP, Oesterling JE, Jeffs RD: A computerized review of exstrophy patients managed during the past thirteen years [abstract 219]. J Urol 141(4–2):224A, 1990.
40. Chisholm TC: Exstrophy of the urinary bladder. In Kiesewetter WB (ed): Long-Term Follow Up in Congenital Anomalies.

Pediatric Surgical Symposium, Vol. 6. Pittsburgh, Pittsburgh Children's Hospital, 1979, p 31.

41. Conner JP, Lattimer JK, Hensle TW, Burbige KA: Primary bladder closure of bladder exstrophy: Long-term functional results in 137 patients. J Pediatr Surg 23:1102–1106, 1988.

42. Husmann DA, McLorie GA, Churchill BM: Closure of the exstrophic bladder: An evaluation of the factors leading to its success and its importance on urinary continence. J Urol 142:522–524, 1989.

43. Jeffs RD, Guice SL, Oesch I: The factors in successful exstrophy closure. J Urol 127:974–976, 1982.

44. Woodhouse CRJ, Strachan JR: Malignancy in exstrophy patients [abstract]. Presented at the British Association of Urological Surgeons, Scarborough, England; July 11, 1990.

45. Woodhouse CRJ, Ransley PC, Williams DI: The exstrophy patient in adult life. Br J Urol 55:632–635, 1983.

46. Burbige KA, Hensle TW, Chambers WL, et al: Pregnancy and sexual function in women with bladder exstrophy. Urology 28:12–14, 1986.

47. Shapiro E, Lepor H, Jeffs RD: The inheritance of the exstrophy–epispadias complex. J Urology 132:308–310, 1984.

58

HYPOSPADIAS

J. Patrick Murphy, MD

Hypospadias is a developmental anomaly characterized by a urethral meatus that opens onto the ventral surface of the penis, proximal to the end of the glans. The meatus may be located anywhere along the shaft of the penis, from the glans to the scrotum, or even in the perineum.

Chordee, which is ventral curvature of the penis, has an inconsistent association with hypospadias. The degree of chordee is ultimately more significant in the surgical treatment of hypospadias than in the initial location of the meatus. A subcoronal hypospadias with little or no chordee is much less complicated to repair than one with significant chordee and insufficient ventral skin. For this reason, when discussing the degrees of hypospadias, it is clinically more appropriate to use a classification system that refers to the meatal location after chordee has been released. Therefore, the system proposed by Barcat is the most clinically relevant and commonly used classification (Table 58–1).[1]

Normal phallic development occurs in the 7th to 14th week of gestation. By 6 weeks of gestation, the genital tubercle is formed anterior to the urogenital sinus. In the next week, two genital folds form caudal to the tubercle and a urethral plate forms between them. Under the influence of testosterone

TABLE 58–1. Hypospadias Classification According to Meatal Location After Release of Chordee

---

Anterior (65–70% of cases)

Glanular
Coronal
Distal penile shaft

Middle (10–15% of cases)

Middle penile shaft

Posterior (20% of cases)

Proximal penile shaft
Penoscrotal
Scrotal
Perineal

---

from the fetal testes, which begins to be produced at about 8 weeks of gestation, the inner genital folds fuse medially to form a tube that communicates with the urogenital sinus and runs distally to end at the base of the glans. The formation of the penile urethra is thus generally completed by the end of the first trimester.[2]

The glanular urethra forms as an ectodermal ingrowth on the glans, which deepens to meet the distal urethra that has formed from the closure of the endodermal genital folds. The capacious anastomosis of these two structures is the fossa navicularis.[3, 4] The formation of the glanular urethra occurs separately and is the last step in the formation of the completed urethra. This sequence probably accounts for the predominance of glanular and coronal hypospadias.

Dorsal to the developing urethra, mesenchymal tissue forms the paired corporal bodies. These are the major components of the erectile tissue and are invested by the tunica albuginea. Mesenchyme also forms Buck's fascia, dartos fascia, and corpus spongiosum.

The corpus spongiosum is the supportive erectile tissue that normally surrounds the urethra and communicates with the erectile tissue of the glans. Buck's fascia is the deep layer of fascia that surrounds the corporal bodies and invests the spongiosum. The dorsal neurovascular bundles are deep to this layer. Superficial to this layer is the dartos fascia, which is the loose subcutaneous layer that contains the superficial veins and lymphatics. These structures form subsequent to completion of the urethra by medial fusion of the outer genital folds, proceeding from the proximal to the distal aspect of the penis. This development accounts for how a fully formed urethra can have a poorly formed spongiosum and thin overlying skin with ventral tethering, despite the meatus being located at the tip of the glans.

Finally, the prepuce is formed, originating at the coronal sulcus. It gradually encloses the glans circumferentially.

Arrested development of the urethra may leave the meatus located anywhere along the ventral surface of the penis. Typically, this would lead to foreshortening of the ventral aspect of the penis distal to the meatus and to failure of the prepuce to form circumferentially.

□ Historical Perspectives

The first description of hypospadias and its surgical correction was reported in the 1st and 2nd centuries AD by the Alexandrian surgeons Heliodorus and Antyllus. They described the defect of hypospadias and its relationship to problems with urination and ineffective coitus. They further described a surgical treatment consisting of amputation of the glans distal to the hypospadiac meatus.[5, 6]

Little progress was made in the surgical treatment of hypospadias until the 19th century when two Americans, Mettauer and Bushe, described techniques using a trocar to establish a channel from the meatus to the glans. Dieffenbach also described a similar technique in the 1830s. None of these methods were very successful.[5]

In 1874, Theophile Anger reported the successful repair of a penoscrotal hypospadias, using the technique described in 1869 by Thiersch for the repair of epispadias, in which lateral skin flaps were tubularized to form the neourethra. Anger's report initiated the modern era of hypospadias surgery characterized by the use of local skin flaps.[7, 8] Duplay soon described his two-stage technique. In the first stage, the chordee was released; in the second stage, a ventral midline strip of skin was tubularized from the meatus out to the end of the glans. The tube was covered by undermining lateral skin flaps that were closed in the midline. Duplay did not believe that it was necessary to completely form the tube because he thought that epithelialization would occur even if an incomplete tube were buried under the lateral skin flaps.[6] Browne used this concept in his well-known "buried strip" technique, which was widely used in the early 1950s.[9] In the late 1800s, various other surgeons reported on penile, scrotal, and preputial flap techniques for multistage procedures. Several of them used the technique of burying the penis in the scrotum to obtain skin coverage, similar to the technique described by Cecil and Culp in the 1950s.[10]

Edmonds, in 1913, was the first to describe the transfer of preputial skin to the ventrum of the penis at the time of release of chordee. At a second stage, the Duplay tube was created to complete the urethral closure. Byars popularized this two-stage technique in the early 1950s.[11] Smith further improved on the procedure by denuding the epithelium of one of the lateral skin flaps to give a "pants-over-vest" closure and, thus reduce the risk of fistula formation.[12] Belt devised another preputial transfer two-stage procedure, which was popularized by Fuqua in the 1960s.[13]

Nove-Josserand, in 1897, was the first to report the use of a free, split-thickness skin graft in an attempt to repair hypospadias. Over the next 20 years, various other tissues were used as free grafts, including saphenous vein, ureter, and appendix. None of these procedures had any consistent success.[14] McCormack used a free, full-thickness skin graft in a two-stage repair.[15] Humby, in 1941, described a one-stage technique using the full thickness of the foreskin.[16] Devine and Horton later popularized this free preputial graft technique with very good results.[17]

In 1947, Memmelaar reported the use of bladder mucosa as a free graft technique in a one-stage repair.[18] Marshall, in 1955, selected bladder mucosa in a two-stage technique.[19] Urologists in China also experienced success with a primary repair using bladder mucosa. This technique was developed independently during a period in China of scientific and cultural isolation.[20] Buccal mucosa from the lip was used for urethral reconstruction in 1941 by Humby[16] and has recently gained renewed attention as a free graft technique.[21]

Improved techniques in preputial and meatal-based vascularized flaps since the 1970s to 1980s have greatly advanced the technique of hypospadias repair. Through the contributions of surgeons such as Mathieu, Barcat,[1] Mustardé,[22] Broadbent and associates,[23] Hodgson,[24] Horton, Devine, Standoli,[25] and Duckett,[26] the single-stage repair of even the most severe forms of hypospadias has become commonplace.

□ Clinical Aspects

INCIDENCE

The incidence of hypospadias has been estimated to be between 0.8 and 8.2 per 1000 live male births.[27] The variation probably represents some geographic and racial differences, but more significant is the exclusion of the more minor degrees of hypospadias in some reports. If all degrees of hypospadias, even the most minor, are included, then the incidence is probably 1 in 125 live male births.[28] Using the most quoted figure of 1 per 300 live male births, it can be assumed that more than 6000 males are born with hypospadias each year in the United States.[29]

ETIOLOGY

A defect in the androgen stimulation of the developing penis, which precludes complete formation of the urethra and its surrounding structures, is the ultimate cause of hypospadias. This defect can occur from deficient androgen production by the testes and placenta, from failure of testosterone to convert to dihydrotestosterone by the 5α-reductase enzyme, or from deficient androgen receptors in the penis. Various intersex conditions can cause deficiencies at any point along the androgen stimulation axis. These are discussed in Chapter 61.

The origin of routine hypospadias not associated with intersex conditions is unclear. An endocrine cause has been implicated by some reports that show a diminished response to human chorionic gonadotropin in some patients with hypospadias, suggesting delayed maturation of the hypothalamic-pituitary axis.[30, 31] Other reports have shown an increased incidence of hypospadias in monozygotic twins, suggesting an insufficient amount of human chorionic gonadotropin production by the single placenta to accommodate the two male fetuses.[32]

Environmental causes have also been implicated. A higher incidence of hypospadias in winter conceptions has been noted.[32] The maternal ingestion of progestin-like agents has been associated with hypospadias. However, this association is a weak one.[33, 34]

Genetic factors in the etiology of hypospadias are indicated by the higher incidence of the anomaly in first-degree relatives of hypospadic patients.[27, 34, 36] In one study that evaluated 307 families, the risk of occurrence of hypospadias in a second male sibling was 12%. If the index child and his father were affected, the risk for a second sibling increased to 26%. If the index child and a second-degree relative were affected, rather than the father, the risk of the sibling being affected was only 19%.[36] This pattern suggests a multifactorial mode of inheritance, with these families having a higher than average number of influential genes for creation of the anomaly.[36] A combination of the endocrine, environmental, and genetic factors ultimately determines the potential for developing the hypospadias complex in any one individual.

ANATOMY OF THE DEFECT

The clinical significance of the hypospadias anomaly is related to several factors. The abnormal location of the meatus and the tendency toward meatal stenosis result in a ventrally deflected and splayed stream. This fact makes the stream difficult to control and often makes it difficult for the patient to void while standing. The ventral curvature associated with chordee can lead to painful erections, especially with severe chordee. Impaired copulation and, thus, inadequate insemination is a further consequence of significant chordee. In addition, the unusual cosmetic appearance associated with the hooded foreskin, flattened glans, and ventral skin deficiency may have an adverse effect on the psychosexual development of the adolescent with hypospadias.[37–41] All of these factors are evidence that early surgical correction should be offered to all boys with hypospadias, regardless of the severity of the defect.

The distal form of hypospadias is the most common (see Table 58–1); frequently, there is little or no associated chordee (Fig. 58–1). The size of the meatus and the quality of the surrounding suppor-

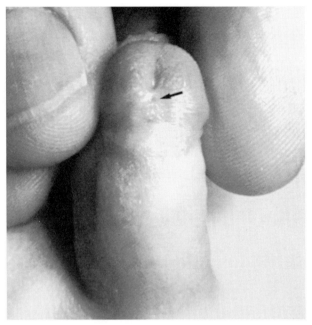

Figure 58–1. Distal hypospadias with stenotic meatus *(arrow)* located on glans with no chordee. The patient is a good candidate for meatal advancement and glanuloplasty (MAGPI).

tive tissue as well as the configuration of the glans are variable and ultimately determine the surgical procedure. Well-formed perimeatal skin, which is mobile, and a deep ventral glans groove may allow local perimeatal flaps to form the urethra (Fig. 58–2). In contrast, atrophic and immobile skin around the

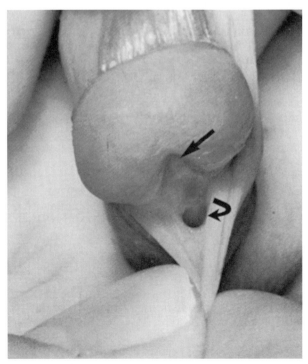

Figure 58–2. Patulous, subcoronal meatus *(curved arrow)* with mobile perimeatal skin and deep ventral glans groove *(straight arrow).* This is a good variant for meatal-based flap procedure.

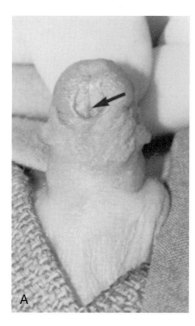
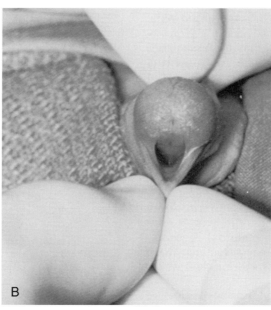

Figure 58-3. *A*, Previously circumcised penis with megameatus *(arrow)* intact circumferential prepuce. *B*, Large wide-mouthed meatus in the same penis as shown in *A*.

meatus may require tissue transfer from the preputium to form the neourethra.

An unusual variant of the distal hypospadias is the large wide-mouth meatus with a circumferential foreskin or megameatus intact prepuce variant (Fig. 58–3).[42] Owing to the intact prepuce, this variant is often not identified until a circumcision has been done. If clinicians discover hypospadias during circumcision, they should stop and preserve the foreskin, even if a dorsal slit has been done.

At times, the distally located meatus may be associated with significant chordee, sometimes of a severe degree (Fig. 58–4). The release of the chordee places the meatus in a much more proximal location, requiring more complicated transfers of skin to bridge the gap between the proximal meatus and the end of the glans.

When the meatus is located on the penile shaft, the character of the urethral plate (midline ventral shaft skin distal to the meatus) is important in determining what type of repair is possible. A well-developed and elastic urethral plate suggests minimal if any distal ventral curvature (Fig. 58–5). However, a thin atrophic urethral plate heralds a significant chordee. The proximal supportive tissue of the urethra is also important. If lack of spongiosum exists proximal to the hypospadic meatus, this portion of the native urethra is not substantial enough to incorporate in the repair (Fig. 58–6). Therefore, the urethra needs to be discarded back to the point of adequate spongiosum.

The position of the meatus at the penoscrotal, scrotal, or perineal location is usually associated with severe chordee, which requires release with a subsequent extensive urethroplasty (Fig. 58–7). This type is usually more predictable in the preoperative period as to the choice of repair than are some of the more distal types previously discussed.

Other anatomic elements of the anomaly that are important to consider include penile torsion, glans tilt, penoscrotal transposition, and chordee without hypospadias. These are discussed more completely in the section, Surgical Procedures.

ASSOCIATED ANOMALIES

Inguinal hernia and undescended testes are the most common anomalies associated with hypospadias. They occur from 7 to 13% of the time, with a

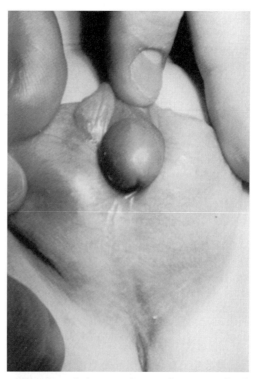

Figure 58–4. Scrotal hypospadias with severe chordee and marked penoscrotal transposition.

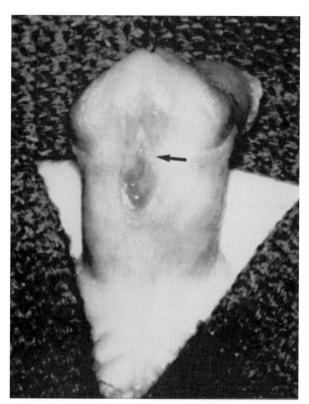

Figure 58–5. Midshaft hypospadias with elastic, well-developed urethral plate distal to the meatus *(arrow).* No significant chordee is present. This is a good variant for onlay island flap procedure.

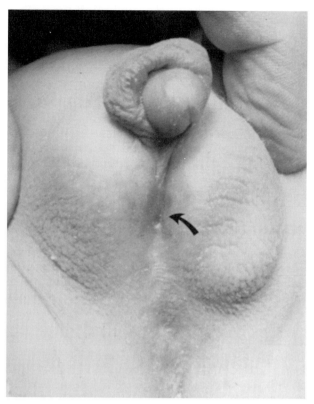

Figure 58–7. Perineal-scrotal hypospadias *(arrow)* with severe chordee and bifid scrotum.

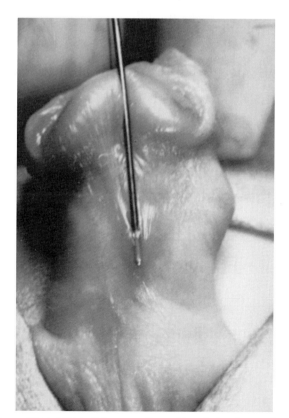

Figure 58–6. Midshaft hypospadias with a lack of spongiosum support proximal to meatus. Urethra needs to be opened back to an area of good spongiosum support at the penoscrotal position.

greater incidence when the meatus is more proximal.[43–45] An enlarged prostatic utricle is also more common in posterior hypospadias, with an incidence of about 11%.[44] Infection is the most common complication of a utricle, but surgical excision is rarely necessary.[46]

Several reports have been made of significantly high numbers of upper urinary tract anomalies associated with hypospadias,[47–50] suggesting that routine upper tract screening is necessary. However, when the association is studied selectively, it can be shown that the types of hypospadias that are at risk for surgically significant upper tract anomalies are the penoscrotal and perineal forms and those associated with other organ system abnormalities.[43, 45] When one, two, or three other organ system anomalies occur, the incidence of significant upper tract anomalies is 7%, 13%, and 37%, respectively. Associated myelomeningocele and imperforate anus carry a 33% and 46% incidence, respectively. In isolated posterior hypospadias, the incidence of associated upper tract anomalies is 5%.[45]

In middle and distal hypospadias, when not associated with other organ system anomalies, the incidence is similar to that of the general population.[43, 45, 51] Therefore, it is recommended that screening for upper urinary tract anomalies by voiding cystourethrogram and renal ultrasonography or intravenous pyelogram be done in patients with penoscrotal and perineal forms of hypospadias and in those with anomalies of at least one additional organ system. Screening should be done in patients with other known indications, such as a history of urinary tract infection, upper or lower tract obstructive symptoms, and hematuria, and a strong family history of urinary tract abnormalities.[52]

The intersex state is another potential disorder associated with hypospadias. This association is rare in the routine forms of hypospadias. Failure of testicular descent, micropenis, penoscrotal transposition (see Fig. 58–4), or bifid scrotum (see Fig. 58–7), when associated with hypospadias, are all signs of potential intersex problems and warrant evaluation with karyotype screening.[27, 53, 54]

TREATMENT

The advent of safe anesthesia, fine suture material, delicate instruments, and good optical magnification have allowed virtually all types of hypospadias to be repaired in younger pediatric patients. Generally, the repair is done on an outpatient basis. To deny a child the benefit of repair because the defect is "too mild" or the risk of complication is "too high" is inappropriate. The chance to make the phallus as normal as possible should be offered to all children, regardless of the severity of the defects.

Age at Repair

The technical advances over the past few decades have made it possible to repair hypospadias, in most cases, in the 1st year of life.[55–57] Controversy still exists with regard to the ideal age for repair. Some surgeons have suggested delaying repair until after the child is 2 to 3 years of age.[52, 58–60] However, most surgeons who deal routinely with the defect prefer to do the repair when the patient is 6 to 18 months old.[53, 54, 56, 57, 61, 62] One study compared the emotional, psychosexual, cognitive, and surgical risks for hypospadias. The "optimal window" recommended for repair was about 6 to 15 months of age (Fig. 58–8).[63] Unless other health or social problems require delay, the ideal time to complete penile reconstruction in the pediatric patient is between 6 and 12 months of age.[64] Anesthetic risk is low (see Chapter 3) and, at this age, postoperative care is much easier for the parents than it is when the child is a toddler.

Objectives of Repair

The objectives of hypospadias correction are divided into the following categories:
1. Complete straightening of the penis
2. Placing the meatus at the tip of the glans
3. Forming a symmetric, conically shaped glans
4. Constructing a neourethra uniform in caliber
5. Completing a satisfactory cosmetic skin coverage

If these objectives can all be attained, the ultimate goal of forming a "normal" penis for the child with hypospadias can be accomplished.

Straightening

Curvature of the penis is difficult to judge, at times, in the preoperative period. Artificial erection, by injecting physiologic saline in the corpora at the time of operation, allows for determination of the exact degree of curvature.[65] This curvature may be caused only by ventral skin or subcutaneous tissue tethering, which is corrected with the release of the skin and dartos layer.[66, 67] About 25% of the time, the curvature is secondary to true fibrous chordee,

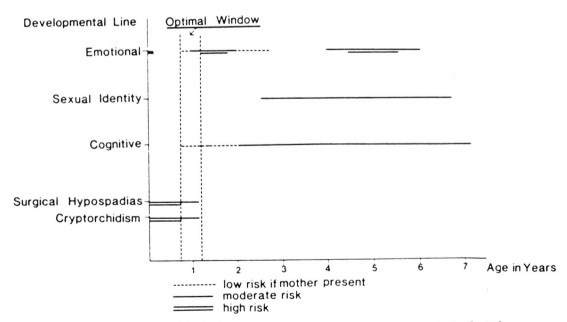

Figure 58–8. Evaluation of risk for hypospadias repair from birth to age 7 years. Optimal window is 6 months to 15 months of age. (From Schultz JR, Klykylo WM, Wacksman J: Timing of elective hypospadias repair in children. Pediatrics 71:342–351, 1983.)

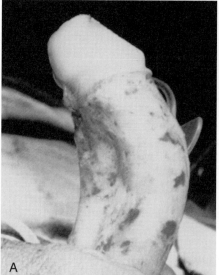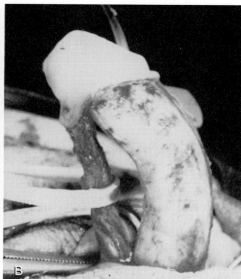

Figure 58–9. *A,* Chordee without hypospadias. The meatus is located at the tip of the glans with marked ventral curvature. *B,* Fibrous ventral tissue is all released. Urethra is mobilized, but curvature persists, indicating corporal body disproportion. This requires ventral patch or dorsal plication (see text).

A

B

which requires division of the urethral plate and excision of the fibrous tissue down to the tunica albuginea.[68]

Sometimes, even after extensive ventral dissection of chordee tissue, a repeat artificial erection still reveals the presence of significant ventral curvature. This finding is usually secondary to the uncommon problem of corporal body disproportion, which is caused by true deficiency of ventral corporal development. This problem can be treated by making a releasing incision in the ventral tunica albuginea and inserting either a dermal or tunica vaginalis patch to expand the deficient ventral surface.[69, 70] Another technique is to excise wedges of tunica albuginea dorsally with transverse closure to shorten this dorsal surface and straighten the penis.[71, 72] Other surgeons have had success with dorsal plication without excision of tunica albuginea.[73–75]

Ventral glans tilt is another problem, particularly in the distal variants. This problem is often corrected when the glansplasty is done. If the tilt persists, plication of the glans tissue to the dorsal corporal bodies can correct ventral tilt.[76, 77]

Axial rotation of the penis, or penile torsion, is another aspect of penile straightening that must be managed. This problem can generally be corrected by releasing the dartos layer as far proximal as possible on the penile shaft. This allows the ventral shaft to rotate back to the midline and corrects the torsion. Chordee or torsion can also occur without hypospadias. Management encompasses the entire spectrum of techniques when hypospadias is involved (Fig. 58–9).[78]

Placing the Meatus

Placing the meatus at the tip of the glans has not always been standard in hypospadias repair. The risk of complications was thought to be too great to routinely recommend procedures that would place the meatus beyond the subcoronal area.[79] Multistage repairs popular in the 1950s and 1960s were designed to attain only a subcoronal location of the meatus. Surgical techniques since then have improved sufficiently so that glans channeling and glans splitting techniques are used with minimal complications, making the distal tip meatus possible.

In glanular and subcoronal variants, the configuration of the meatus is the determining factor in what techniques move the meatus distally on the glans. Meatoplasty with or without dorsal advancement, distal urethral mobilization and tubularization, or meatal-based flaps are the methods selected in most cases of distal hypospadias.[80, 81] In the more proximal forms, creating the neourethra with local vascularized skin flaps or free grafts allows placement of the urethra at the end of the penis while glans channeling or glans splitting accomplishes placement of the meatus at the tip of the glans.[1, 17, 22, 26, 82–84]

Glans Shape

Creation of a symmetric, conically shaped glans is the objective of the glansplasty component of the repair. Approximating the lateral glanular tissue in the midline ventrally over a meatoplasty or meatal advancement corrects the flattened glans appearance to the more anatomically normal, conically shaped glans. Similarly, approximation of well-developed glans wings to the midline over a neourethra in a split glans restores the glans to its normal conical shape.

Urethral Construction

Formation of the neourethra can be accomplished by local skin flaps, various types of free grafts, or vascularized pedicle flaps. Local skin flaps may be formed from in situ skin or dorsal skin transferred to the ventrum in a previous stage. In either case, it is important to avoid making these flaps too narrow or thin at the risk of compromising their vascular supply. Free grafts depend on an adequately vascularized bed for survival; therefore, they should not be placed in a scarred channel. Well-vascularized subcutaneous tissue and skin must cover them to allow adequate neovascularization and survival of the graft.[17]

Mobilized vascularized flaps of preputium have a more reliable blood supply than free grafts. Therefore, if they are available, these flaps are the choice of most surgeons.[24, 26, 84, 85] They may be used as patches onto a strip of native urethral plate to complete the urethra, or they may be tubularized and used as bridges over the gap between a proximal native urethra and the end of the glans.[26, 86] A watertight closure of the well-vascularized neourethra is formed, with care being taken to make it uniform in caliber and of appropriate size for the age of the child. This closure helps avoid stricturing and forming of saccules, diverticula, and fistulas.

Cosmesis

Creating cosmetically appealing, well-vascularized skin coverage of the penile shaft after urethroplasty can sometimes be challenging. Transfer of vascularized dorsal preputial skin to the ventrum can be accomplished in several ways.

Buttonholes of the dorsal skin allow the penis to come through this defect, draping the distal preputium over the ventral surface of the penis.[19] This maneuver has the advantage of transferring well-vascularized skin over the repair, but it is not appealing cosmetically.

A more satisfactory method of transferring skin to the ventrum is by splitting the dorsal skin in the midline longitudinally and advancing the flaps around on either side to meet in the midline. This technique allows for a midline ventral closure, which simulates the median raphe, and allows for a subcoronal closure to the preputial skin circumferentially, which simulates the suture lines of a standard circumcision.[87, 88] Another adjunct in this closure is to advance lateral flaps of inner preputial skin from each side to the ventral midline of the penis at the time of glansplasty or closure of glans wings.[89] Approximating these flaps in the midline gives the appearance of an intact circumferential preputial collar, further enhancing the potential for an anatomically normal skin closure (see Fig. 58–14).

Some people, particularly those in European countries, prefer the appearance of a noncircumcised penis. In distal repairs, reconstruction of the preputium for a noncircumcised appearance can be accomplished in certain cases.[90] Correction of the more significant degrees of penoscrotal transposition is often necessary to avoid the feminizing appearance it causes. This step may be done at the time of the original repair, in some cases. However, when using vascularized pedicle flaps for the repair, it is usually safer to correct significant penoscrotal transposition with rotational flaps at a later time.[91–94]

□ Surgical Procedures

Due to the wide variation in the anatomic presentation of hypospadias, no single urethroplasty is applicable to every case. At times, a final decision regarding the degree of curvature and the ultimate location of the meatus cannot be made until the

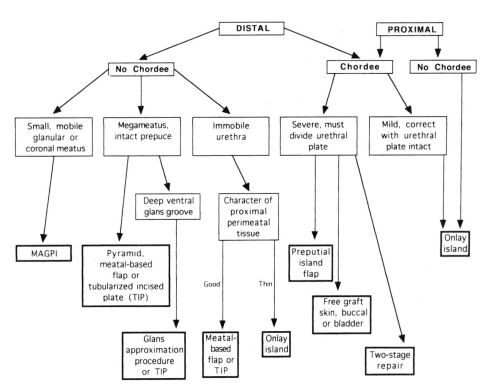

Figure 58–10. Flow diagram for types of repair in variants of hypospadias.

operation has started and an artificial erection is done. The surgeon who repairs hypospadias must be adaptable and experienced to deal with all variants of the defect. Versatility and experience with all options of surgical treatment are the keys to successful management of hypospadias. By recognizing the sometimes subtle nuances of meatal variation, glans configuration, and curvature character, the experienced surgeon can make the best choices as to the type of repair to use (Fig. 58–10).

☐ Specific Techniques

ANTERIOR VARIANTS

Many of the glanular and subcoronal types are amenable to the meatal advancement and glansplasty (MAGPI) type of repair (Fig. 58–11).[95] A stenotic meatus with good mobility of the urethra and a fairly shallow ventral glanular groove are the anatomic characteristics best suited for the MAGPI. A modification has been described that allows for this procedure in the more immobile urethra or the more proximal meatus. The technique involves advancing distally two flaps of the perimeatal cuff and approximating their medial borders to form the ventral floor of the neourethra. The glans is then approximated in the midline over the neourethra.[96]

A wide-mouth meatus is not amenable to the MAGPI repair. The meatal-based flap repair is often

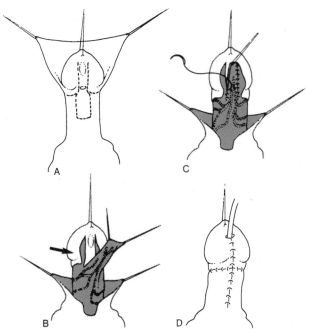

Figure 58–12. Meatal-based flap repair. *A,* Parallel incisions along ventral groove distal to meatus and formation of meatal-based flap proximal to meatus. *B,* Glans wings developed on either side of the urethral plate *(arrow)* to close over the neourethra later. Meatal-based flap is mobilized distally maintaining good, vascular soft tissue support. *C,* Flap is anastomosed to bilateral edges of urethral plate to form neourethra. *D,* Glans wings are closed over the neourethra in the midline giving conical glans configuration. Penile shaft is covered with dorsal foreskin advanced ventrally.

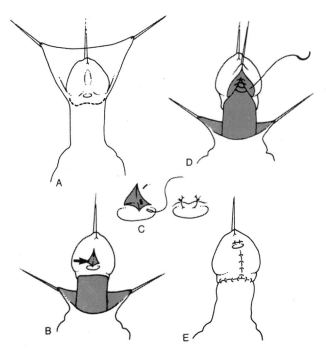

Figure 58–11. Meatal advancement and glanuloplasty repair. *A,* Circumferential subcoronal incision to deglove penile shaft skin. *B,* Longitudinal incision through ventral groove of glans *(arrow).* *C,* Transverse closure of glans groove incision to advance dorsal urethral plate and to open stenotic meatus. *D,* Glans tissue approximated ventrally in midline to restore conical configuration to glans. *E,* Completion of skin closure.

used effectively in this situation, if there is no chordee and if mobile, well-vascularized skin exists proximal to the meatus (Fig. 58–12).[97, 98] This repair works well when a moderately deep ventral groove exists, allowing the urethra to be placed deep in the glans to form a conically shaped glans after closure of the glans wings.

In rare instances, chordee may exist distal to the anterior meatus. In this case, a flip-flap repair may be applicable.[99] This repair divides the urethra distal to the meatus releasing any chordee. A proximal meatal-based flap is rotated distally and fits into a triangulated flap of the glans to reconstruct the urethra. The glans wing closure completes the repair. If the glans has a normal conical shape and a distal chordee exists, the proximal meatal-based flap is tubularized and rotated distally, tunneling it through a glans channel to locate the meatus at the tip of the glans.[23] I have used these two procedures only rarely. Transfer of a dorsal, preputial pedicle flap is more effective in my experience when distal chordee is present.

The glans approximation procedure is sometimes useful when a wide-mouth proximal glanular meatus exists with a very deep ventral groove (Figs. 58–13 and 58–14).[100] This repair can give a very good cosmetic result when done in the proper situation.

The pyramid procedure is well suited for the fish

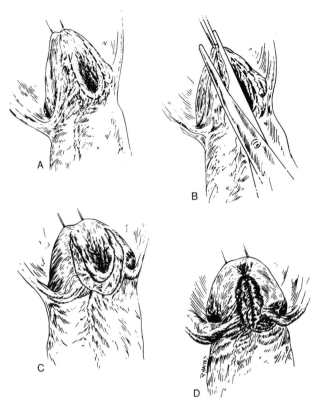

Figure 58–13. Glans approximation procedure (GAP). *A*, Deep ventral groove and patulous, coronal meatus with outline of proposed incision. *B*, Skin is excised along previously marked U-shaped line. *C*, De-epithelialized glans with urethral plate intact. *D*, Two-layer closure of glanular urethra with glans skin still open. (From Zaontz MR: The GAP (glans approximation procedure) for glanular/coronal hypospadias. J Urol 141:359–361, 1989.)

mouth type of meatus seen in the megameatus intact prepuce variant (Fig. 58–15).[42] This procedure is an extension of a previously described distal urethral tubularization technique.[77, 101] The meatal-based flap repair is also appropriate in this megameatus intact prepuce variant.

The tubularized incised plate urethroplasty is a modification of the Thiersch-Duplay tubularization, which involves a deep longitudinal incision of the urethral plate in the midline. This allows the lateral skin flaps to be mobilized and closed in the midline without tension. This procedure allows the wide-mouth meatus variant with a flat, shallow ventral groove to be repaired without the need for additional flaps.[102]

MIDDLE VARIANTS

The amount of ventral curvature generally dictates the type of repair in the middle and distal shaft hypospadias. When no significant chordee is present, the meatal-based flap repair can sometimes be done. A better technique is the onlay island flap repair (Fig. 58–16).[86] This procedure involves mobilizing an inner preputial flap on its pedicle and rotating it ventrally to lay it on the well-developed

dorsal urethral plate and to complete the tubularization of the neourethra. This technique is applicable to many forms of penile shaft hypospadias.

In milder degrees of chordee, the curvature can be corrected without dividing the urethral plate by taking down tethering bands lateral to the urethral plate or by dorsal plication techniques.[74, 75] This allows the onlay island flap repair technique to be used instead of the tubularized pedicle flap, which has a higher incidence of complications.[54] If significant chordee does exist, division of the urethral plate is necessary. This moves the meatus more proximal and requires treatment as described later.

PROXIMAL VARIANTS

Most of the proximal forms of hypospadias are associated with significant chordee, which requires division of the urethral plate, leaving a gap to be bridged between the proximal native urethra and the tip of the glans. This can be done with staged

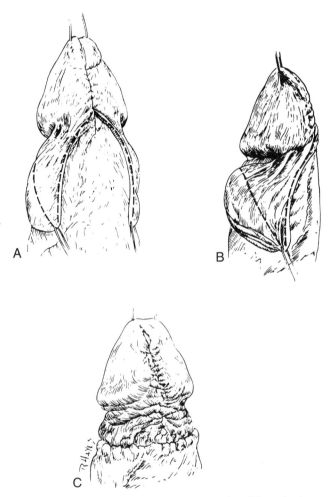

Figure 58–14. *A*, Glanular skin approximated and lateral wings of inner preputial skin outlined. *B*, Lateral view of outline for preputial collar. *C*, Lateral preputial wings closed in midline to give circumferential preputial collar. (From Zaontz MR: The GAP (glans approximation procedure) for glanular/coronal hypospadias. J Urol 141:359–361, 1989).

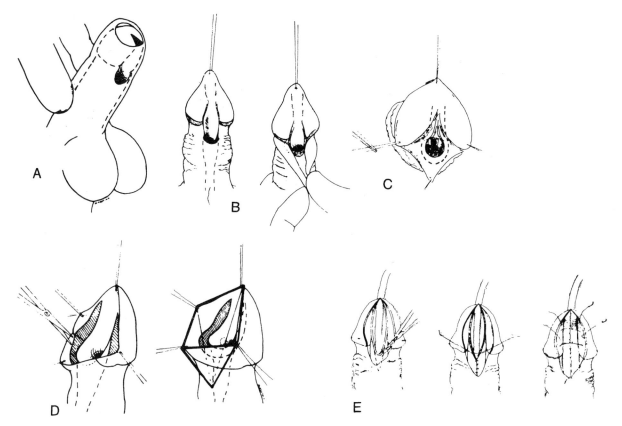

Figure 58–15. Pyramid technique. *A*, MIP variant, circumferential foreskin and hidden, coronal megameatus. *B*, Foreskin retracted showing megameatus. *C*, Tennis-racquet incision marked around meatus and along glans groove. *D*, Dissection around urethra to apex of inverted pyramid. *E*, Wedge reduction of urethra with closure of neourethra and glans in two layers. (From Duckett JW, Keating MA: Technical challenge of the megameatus intact prepuce hypospadias variant: The pyramid procedure. J Urol 141:1407–1409, 1989.)

Figure 58–16. Onlay island flap repair. *A*, Outline of incisions along well-developed urethral plate with no chordee. *B*, Mobilization of glans wings and shaft skin with urethral plate intact distal to meatus. Outline of inner preputial island flap that will be transposed ventrally for onlay completion of neourethra. *C*, Island flap transposed ventrally on pedicle. The first part of the anastomosis is completed. *D*, Remainder of anastomosis to complete neourethra to tip of glans. *E*, Glans wings are approximated over the neourethra in the ventral midline. The penile shaft is covered with the ventral advancement of dorsal foreskin.

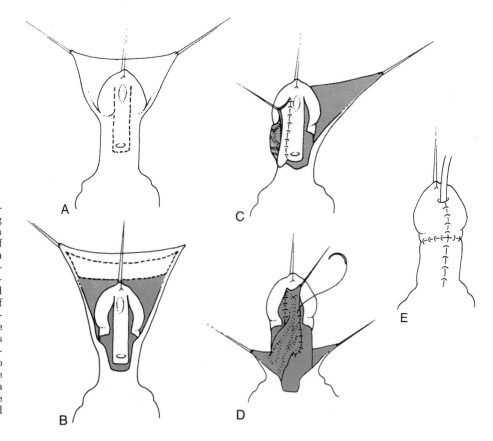

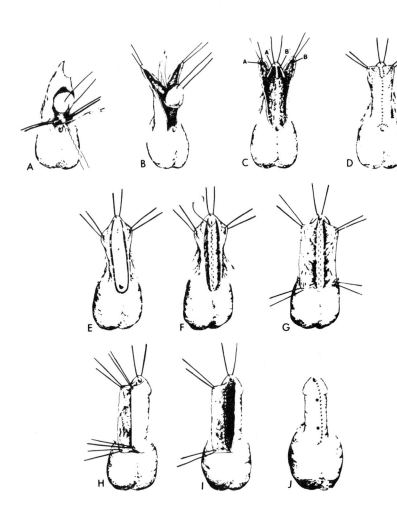

Figure 58–17. Two-stage Durham Smith repair. *A,* Release of chordee. *B,* Splitting of dorsal preputium. *C,* Denuded ventral glans before transposing preputial skin to ventrum. *D,* Transposition of dorsal foreskin to ventrum completes the first stage. *E,* U-shaped incision around the meatus and out onto glans. *F,* Tubularization of Duplay-type tube to form the neourethra. *G,* Second layer of soft tissue to reinforce suture line. *H to J,* Overlapping skin closure with de-epithelialization of inner flap gives a "double-breasted" closure of the skin. (From Belman AB: Urethra. In Kelalis PP, King LR, Belman AB [eds]: Clinical Pediatric Urology [2nd ed]. Philadelphia, WB Saunders, Philadelphia, 1985.)

Figure 58–18. Transverse preputial island flap tube repair. *A* and *B,* Release of chordee and degloving of penile shaft skin. *B,* Outline of inner preputial island flap. *C,* Tubularization of inner preputial island flap. *D,* Transposition of the tubularized island flap to the ventrum maintaining pedicle blood supply. *E,* Creation of a channel through glans tissue with sharp incisional and excisional technique. *F,* Island tube anastomosed to proximal native urethra, brought through glans channel and anastomosed to epithelium at tip of glans. *G,* Penile shaft covered with dorsal foreskin advanced ventrally. Skin closure completed.

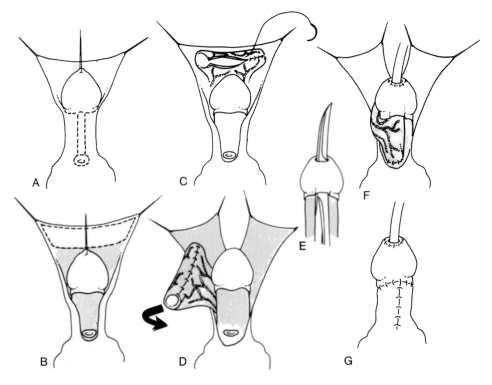

procedures in which coverage of the ventral penile shaft is attained by rotation of dorsal flaps to the ventrum with lateral tubularization to form the neourethra (Fig. 58–17).

Another method is the tubularized free graft anastomosed to the native urethra proximally and extended to the end of the glans by a tunneling or splitting technique. The most commonly used free grafts are full-thickness skin, bladder mucosa, or buccal mucosa. Preputial skin is much preferred to extragenital skin.[17, 103] If genital skin is not available, bladder or buccal mucosa may be the next best tissue.[21, 104, 105]

Vascularized flaps are a more physiologically sound alternative to free grafts. The transverse inner preputial island flap that is tubularized and transposed ventrally to form the neourethra is the preferred type of vascularized flap (Fig. 58–18).[26, 106] It provides good preputial skin with a reliable blood supply that does not rely on neovascularization for healing of the neourethra, as do free flaps. Occasionally, the length of the prepuce alone may not be adequate to bridge the defect to a very proximal meatus. In this case, the shiny non–hair-bearing skin around the meatus can be tubularized (Fig. 58–19), moving the proximal urethra to the penoscrotal junction. The preputial flap can then be used to reach the remainder of the distance to the end of the penis.[53]

In some cases, the penile shaft skin may be deficient enough to cause concern about ventral coverage after completion of the neourethra. The double-face island flap can solve this problem.[24] This technique leaves some of the outer preputial skin attached to the pedicle after tubularizing the inner preputial layer. This outer preputium is transferred to the ventrum with the pedicle and supplies the skin coverage of the ventral penile shaft. One study suggests that this double-face pedicle better preserves the blood supply to the flap.[107] However, the number of complications associated with the double-face island flap have not supported that theory.[55]

I prefer the transverse island flap in a one-stage procedure in most cases of proximal hypospadias with chordee. In the rare case in which the skin deficiency is so severe that a vascularized pedicle cannot be used or in which the chordee is so severe that a dermal or tunica vaginalis graft is required to correct corporal disproportion, I, as well as others, perform a two-stage repair.[108, 109] However, there are only a few cases in which the repair cannot be accomplished in one stage.

□ Technical Perspectives

OPTICAL MAGNIFICATION

Most surgeons agree that optical magnification is indispensable in hypospadias surgery. Standard operating loupes, ranging from 2.5-power to 4.5-power, are generally thought to be ideal for the magnifica-

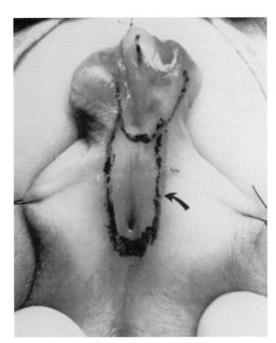

Figure 58–19. Outline of non–hair-bearing skin distal to scrotal meatus *(arrow)* that will be tubularized to move meatus to penoscrotal junction. Island flap tube will complete repair to end of glans.

tion needed for this type of surgery. Some workers advocate the use of the operating microscope and suggest an improved result with this technique.[110] Most surgeons have not believed that this degree of magnification is necessary for obtaining excellent results. In fact, the microscope may be overly cumbersome for any improvement in visualization that it may provide.[111]

SUTURES AND INSTRUMENTS

Fine absorbable suture is chosen by most surgeons to close the neourethra. Polyglycolic or polyglactin material is probably the most common choice of suture. However, some surgeons prefer the longer lasting polydiaxanone suture.[110] Permanent sutures of nylon or polypropylene, in a continuous stitch that is pulled out 10 to 14 days postoperatively, are recommended by some.[12, 56]

The type of optical magnification also determines the size of the suture. Generally, 6-0 or 7-0 suture is preferred. With the microscope, 8-0 or 9-0 may be used. Skin closure is best accomplished with either fine chromic (6-0 or 7-0) or plain catgut suture. Occasionally, small suture sinus tracts may occur along these stitches as they dissolve. These are less likely to occur with the plain gut sutures than with chromic sutures. I use only a few anchoring sutures of chromic and close the remaining skin with fast absorbing plain gut to avoid these suture sinuses.

The delicate instruments of ophthalmologic surgery are well designed for the precise tissue handling required in hypospadias repair. Small, single-toothed forceps or fine skin hooks allow tissue handling with minimal trauma. Standard microscopic tools are necessary for those who prefer the microscope over loupe magnification.

URINARY DIVERSION

The goal of the surgeon in any urinary diversion procedure in hypospadias repair is to protect the neourethra from the urinary stream for the initial healing phase. In theory, this diversion should decrease the complication rate, particularly fistula formation. The more traditional perineal urethrostomy and suprapubic cystostomy are uncomfortable and cumbersome to manage in the postoperative period. Small indwelling No. 6 or 8 French Silastic tubes left through the repair and just into the bladder allow drainage of the urine into the diaper in infants (Figs. 58–20 and 58–21).[111] This technique greatly facilitates the outpatient care of these pediatric patients. These stents are well tolerated by the patients. Problems with the stents becoming plugged or dislodged are uncommon.

Some surgeons favor a splint that traverses the repair but is not indwelling in the bladder.[110] The patient is allowed to void, but the stent protects the repair. I prefer the indwelling stent and leave it for 5 to 14 days, depending on the complexity of the repair. In older children who would not tolerate wearing a diaper, a No. 6 or 8 French Foley catheter may be used in the simpler distal repairs and a suprapubic cystostomy in the more complex repairs. Suprapubic drainage should be used in complex reoperations or in any repairs requiring a free graft. No diversion is necessary for simple distal procedures, such as meatoplasty or MAGPI. Simple small fistula repairs can be done without diversion.

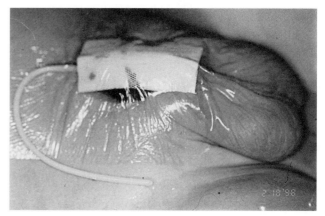

Figure 58–21. Occlusive dressing of transparent adhesive material in sandwich fashion on abdominal wall, with No. 6 French soft Silastic indwelling tube for urinary diversion.

DRESSINGS

Hypospadias dressings should apply enough gentle pressure on the penis to help with hemostasis and to decrease edema formation, without compromising the vascularity of the repair. They should also be waterproof, if possible, for at least the first 24 hours in those patients who have undergone urinary diversions that allow drainage into diapers. Various dressings accomplish this purpose. A silicon-foam dressing, which can be placed round the penis in a liquid state to later solidify, leaves a soft, mildly compressive dressing that is waterproof (see Fig. 58–20).[112] This dressing can be removed without difficulty several days postoperatively. Other dressings include transparent adhesive dressings wrapped around the penis or fixed to the abdominal wall in a sandwich-like fashion (see Fig. 58–21).[68] A DuoDerm dressing can be applied around the penis as an alternative, before using a transparent adhesive dressing.[110] In patients who undergo suprapubic diversion, a mildly compressive dressing of gauze and soft tape is ideal.

ANALGESIA

Postoperative pain is generally controlled with oral analgesics. Bladder spasms caused by indwelling catheters can be dealt with by methantheline bromide (Banthīne) and opium suppositories or by oral oxybutynin. A dorsal penile nerve block done intraoperatively with bupivacaine can help control postoperative pain.[113]

A caudal block is my preferred method for postoperative pain control.[114] In most cases, the patients are comfortable for the entire day and evening of surgery and are easily cared for at home with only oral analgesia.

☐ Complications

The type and incidence of complications vary with the particular form of repair. Attention to detail

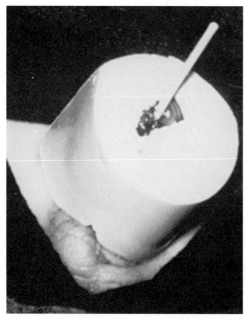

Figure 58–20. Foam dressing around the penis after hypospadias repair with No. 6 French Silastic tube left as an indwelling urethral catheter.

and meticulous technique are imperative to keep the incidence of all complications to a minimum. The following is a discussion of some of the general complications that can occur with all repairs.

BLEEDING

Intraoperative bleeding can, at times, be troublesome, but with careful attention to the control of bleeding by judicious use of point tip cautery, it can generally be kept to a minimum. Tourniquets or cutaneous infiltrations with dilute concentrations of epinephrine can be helpful, but they should not replace careful technique.[115] Postoperative bleeding is generally prevented by mildly compressive dressings. Subcutaneous hematomas may occur but generally do not need to be drained.

INFECTION

Wound infection is a rare problem in hypospadias repair, especially in the prepubertal patient. As long as good viability of tissue is maintained, infection should be a minor problem. Perioperative antibiotic prophylaxis is favored by some surgeons.[115] This is probably a reasonable precaution in an extensive repair, especially in the postpubertal patient. Urinary suppression with oral antibiotics is recommended with indwelling catheters that are open to drainage in the diaper.[68, 116, 117]

DEVITALIZED SKIN FLAPS

If the sloughing of skin coverage occurs, it is usually on the ventral surface of the penis where dorsal skin has been transposed. When the devascularized skin is over a well-vascularized bed of tissue, such as with a pedicle flap, primary healing generally occurs without sequelae. If the slough is over poorly vascularized tissue, such as a free graft, the result can be the breakdown of the repair. Careful attention to the transposing of well-vascularized tissue for coverage of the neourethra in all repairs is critical to avoid this problem.

FISTULAS

Urethrocutaneous fistulas are the most commonly reported complications of hypospadias surgery. They result from failure of healing at some point along the neourethral suture line and can range in size from pinpoint to large enough for all voided urine to exit at this point. Fistulas may also be associated with stenosis or distal stricture. Occasionally, small fistulas seen early postoperatively may close spontaneously. Surgical closure should be postponed until complete tissue healing has occurred, which requires at least 6 months.[118, 119] A small fistula may be closed by local excision of the fistula tract followed by closure of the urethral epithelium with fine absorbable suture. Approximating several layers of well-vascularized subcuta-

neous tissue over this closure is important to prevent recurrence. Urinary diversion is usually not necessary in small fistula repairs. Larger fistulas may require more complicated closures, with mobilization of tissue flaps or advancement of skin flaps to ensure an adequate amount of well-vascularized tissue for a multilayered closure.[118–121] Urinary diversion is often necessary with more complicated closures.

STRICTURES

Narrowing of the neourethra may occur anywhere along its course. However, the most common sites of stricture formation are at the meatus and at the proximal anastomosis. Most cases of meatal narrowing can be managed as an office procedure by gentle dilation in the first few weeks postoperatively. Occasionally, meatotomy or meatoplasty is needed, especially when associated with a proximal fistula or neourethral diverticulum. More proximal strictures can generally be treated by dilation or visual internal urethrotomy. However, open urethroplasty may sometimes be required with excision of the stricture and primary urethral anastomosis or patch graft urethroplasty.[118, 119, 122]

DIVERTICULUM

Saccular dilation of the neourethra may result from distal stenosis causing progressive dilation, contained urinary extravasation from the breakdown of the repair, or initial creation of an oversized segment of the neourethra. Classic bulging of the urethra ventrally with voiding is evident with significant diverticulum formation (Fig. 58–22). Urinary stasis with chronic inflammation is common. Obstruction can result from kinking of the urethra when the diverticulum distends with voiding. Repair requires excision of the redundant urethra with primary closure to restore a uniform caliber to the urethra.[123] Special attention should be paid to any narrowing of the neourethra distally, just as in fistula repair.

RETRUSIVE MEATUS

Retraction of the meatus from its original position at the tip of the glans to a proximal glanular or subcoronal position can occur with any repair. Retrusive meatus is caused by the failure of the glansplasty closure or the breakdown of devascularized distal neourethra. Retraction is a common problem when the MAGPI procedure is used in patients whose meatus is too proximal or when there is too much tension on the glansplasty closure.[124] Correction can usually be accomplished by a repeat glansplasty or a meatal-based flap procedure.[118, 124]

PERSISTENT CHORDEE

Residual ventral curvature following hypospadias repair can be a troublesome problem. It is usually

TABLE 58–2. Complications of Various Type of Repairs

	Number of Cases	Meatal Stenosis (%)	Retrusive Meatus (%)	Stricture (%)	Fistula (%)	Diverticulum (%)	Total (%)
MAGPI							
Hensle[128]	25	—	—	—	1 (4.0)	—	1 (4.0)
Issa[124]	142	—	5 (3.5)	—	—	—	5 (3.5)
Shapiro[129]	55	1 (1.8)	—	—	2 (3.6)	—	3 (5.4)
Livne[130]	63	—	2 (3.2)	—	—	—	2 (3.2)
Kass[131]	25	—	—	—	—	—	0 (0)
Keating[54]	225						(<1)
Duckett[132]	1100	—	7 (0.6)	—	5 (0.4)	—	12 (1.1)
Personal series	225	—	2 (0.8)	—	—	—	2 (0.8)
Meatal-Based Flap							
Rabinowitz[133]	59	—	1 (1.7)	—	—	—	1 (1.7)
Gonzales[134]	63	1 (1.6)	—	—	5 (7.9)	—	6 (9.5)
Retik[135]	294	1 (0.5)	—	—	1 (0.5)	—	2 (1.0)
Wacksman[98]	125	—	—	—	1 (0.8)	—	1 (0.8)
Belman[56]	30	—	—	—	3 (10.0)	—	3 (10.0)
Kass[131]	84	1 (1.2)	—	—	—	—	1 (1.2)
Elder[86]	34	1 (2.9)	—	—	—	—	1 (2.9)
Bellinger[136]	51	—	—	—	1 (2.0)	—	1 (2.0)
Personal series	241	4 (1.7)	—	—	2 (0.8)	—	6 (2.5)
Onlay Island Flap							
Elder[86]	50	—	—	—	1 (2.0)	—	1 (2.0)
Hollowell[74]	66						(8.0)
Keating[54]	43						(9.0)
Gearhart[137]	61	—	1 (1.6)	—	3 (5.0)	—	4 (6.6)
Personal series	158	—	—	—	4 (2.5)	1 (0.6)	5 (3.2)
Tube Island Flap							
Duckett[26]	100						(10.0)
Wacksman[98]	94						7 (7.4)
Keating[54]	34						(18.0)
Hollowell[74]	85						(15.0)
Kass[131]	77	—	—	—	1 (1.3)	—	1 (1.3)
Personal series	50	4* (8.0)	—	—	2 (4.0)	4* (8.0)	6 (12.0)
Free Graft (Preputium)							
Devine[17]	20	—	—	—	6 (30.0)	—	6 (30.0)
Hanna[138]	27	—	—	1 (3.7)	4 (14.8)	1 (3.7)	6 (22.2)
Hendren[139]	103	3 (2.9)	—	—	6 (5.8)	—	9 (8.7)
Rober[140]	81	—	—	7 (8.6)	28 (34.6)	—	35 (43.2)
Stock[141]	77	2 (2.5)	—	3 (3.8)	10 (12.9)	—	15 (19.5)
Bladder Mucosa							
Koyle[104]	16	1 (6.2)	—	—	1 (6.2)	—	2 (12.5)
Ransley[142]	47	9 (19.1)	—	1 (2.1)	10 (21.3)	—	20 (42.5)
Ehrlich[143]	79	—	—	8 (10.1)	2 (2.5)	4 (5.0)	14 (17.7)
Mollard[144]	76	14 (17.4)	—	15† (19.7)	—	—	29 (38.1)
Li[145]	113	6 (5.3)	—	8 (7.0)	—	—	14 (12.4)
Buccal Mucosa							
Burger[146]	6	1 (16.6)	—	—	3 (50.0)	—	3 (50.0)
Duckett[147]	18	5 (27.8)	—	1 (5.5)	1 (5.5)	—	7 (38.9)

*Same patients with meatal stenosis and diverticulum.
†Three of these 15 were failed grafts.
MAGPI, meatal advancement and glansplasty.

related to inadequate release of chordee at the original procedure. Increased ventral curvature occurring as the penis grows is at least a theoretical possibility. The artificial erection has made this complication much less common. Treatment of the problem is similar to the treatment of chordee without hypospadias. Degloving of the penis and takedown of any ventral tethering tissue is done, using the artificial erection technique to guide dissection.

Dorsal plication, ventral excision with patching, and division of the urethra may all be necessary.[119]

RECURRENT MULTIPLE COMPLICATIONS

Patients with recurrent multiple complications generally have experienced multiple failed repairs that have resulted in a combination of severe complications. Extensive fibrosis of the urethra with fis-

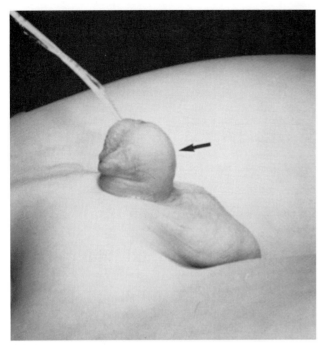

Figure 58–22. Neourethral diverticulum with bulging ventrally with voiding *(arrow).*

tulas, strictures, diverticula, and residual chordee may be present. The successful outcome of further repair depends on thorough evaluation of each complication and the use of all the techniques available to the surgeon experienced in hypospadias repair. Vascularized flaps or staging procedures are preferable to free grafts in a scarred phallus if tissue is available.[125] If a free graft must be used, it is important to obtain the most vascularized bed possible in which to place the graft. Bladder or buccal mucosa is probably the best tissue for a free graft in this type of situation.[21, 54, 119] In patients with severe scarring and ventral skin loss, a split thickness skin graft may be used for ventral coverage. This tissue may then be tubularized at a second stage.[126]

SEXUAL FUNCTION

Long-term results of hypospadias repairs with regard to erectile function, ejaculation, and fertility are not available for the children who have undergone repairs at a younger age over the past decade. Historically, sexual difficulties after hypospadias repair have been reported. These were thought to be related to psychosexual factors related to surgery later in childhood rather than to anatomic problems.[36, 41] Fertility has been assessed by semen analysis in patients after hypospadias repair.[38, 127] Higher rates of oligospermia are reported. These lower sperm counts generally occur in patients with associated anomalies, such as cryptorchidism, chromosome abnormalities, varicoceles, or torsion. In a patient with an anatomically successful hypospadias repair and no associated anomalies that might affect fertility, a high potential for fertility and an adequate

sexual function are expected. Only close observation of pediatric patients into their adulthood following hypospadias repair early in life will reveal the true incidence of sexual dysfunction and fertility problems.

RESULTS

A summary of the incidence of certain complications for commonly used procedures is given in Table 58–2. A personal series is included and represents those patients I have seen over a 10-year period (from 1987 to 1997). A follow-up of at least 6 months postoperatively is available for the patients included in this series.

REFERENCES

1. Barcat J: Current concepts of treatment. In Horton CE (ed): Plastic and Reconstructive Surgery of the Genital Area. Boston, Little, Brown & Co, 1973, pp 249–263.
2. Bellinger MF: Embryology of the male external genitalia. Urol Clin North Am 8:375–382, 1981.
3. Sommer JJ, Stephens FD: Dorsal urethral diverticulum of the fossa navicularis: Symptoms, diagnosis and treatment. J Urol 124:94–97, 1980.
4. Glenister TW: The origin and fate of the urethral plate in man. J Anat 88:413, 1954.
5. Rogers DO: History of external genital surgery. In Horton CE (ed): Plastic and Reconstructive Surgery of the Genital Area. Boston, Little, Brown & Co, 1973, pp 3–47.
6. Horton CE, Devine CJ, Baran N: Pictorial history of hypospadias repair techniques. In Horton CE (ed): Plastic and Reconstructive Surgery of the Genital Area. Boston, Little, Brown & Co, 1973, pp 237–243.
7. Bachus LH, de Felice CA: Hypospadias, then and now. Plast Reconstr Surg 25:146–160, 1960.
8. Creevy CD: The correction of hypospadias: A review. Urol Surv 8:2–47, 1958.
9. Browne D: An operation for hypospadias. Proc R Soc Med 41:466–468, 1949.
10. Culp OS: Hypospadias with and without chordee. In Horton CE (ed): Plastic and Reconstructive Surgery of the Genital Area. Boston, Little, Brown & Co, 1973, pp 315–320.
11. Byars LT: A technique for consistently satisfactory repair of hypospadias. Surg Gynecol Obstet 100:184–190, 1955.
12. Smith ED: Durham Smith repair of hypospadias. Urol Clin North Am 8:451–455, 1981.
13. Fuqua F: Renaissance of urethroplasty: The Belt technique of hypospadias repair. J Urol 106:782–785, 1971.
14. Coleman JW, McGovern JH, Marshall VF: The bladder mucosal graft technique for hypospadias repair. Urol Clin North Am 8:457–462, 1981.
15. McCormack RM: Simultaneous chordee repair and urethral reconstruction for hypospadias: Experimental and clinical studies. Plast Reconstr Surg 13:257, 1954.
16. Humby G: A one-stage operation for hypospadias. Br J Surg 29:84–92, 1941.
17. Devine CJ Jr, Horton DE: Hypospadias repair. J Urol 85:166–172, 1972.
18. Memmelaar J: Use of bladder mucosa in a one-stage repair of hypospadias. J Urol 58:68–73, 1947.
19. Marshall VF, Spellman RM: Construction of a urethra in hypospadias using vesical mucosal grafts. J Urol 73:335–342, 1955.
20. LiZhong-Chu, Zheng Yu-Hen, Sheh Ya-Xiong, et al: One-stage urethroplasty for hypospadias using a tube constructed with bladder mucosa—a new procedure. Urol Clin North Am 8:463–470, 1981.
21. Duckett JW, Coplen D, Ewalt D, et al: Buccal mucosal urethral replacement. J Urol 153:1660–1663, 1995.

22. Mustardé JC: One-stage correction of distal hypospadias and other people's fistulae. Br J Plast Surg 18:413–422, 1965.
23. Broadbent, TR, Woolf RM, Tosku E: Hypospadias: One-stage repair. Plast Reconstr Surg 27:154–159, 1961.
24. Hodgson NB: Use of vascularized flaps in hypospadias repair. Urol Clin North Am 8:471–481, 1981.
25. Standoli L: One-stage repair of hypospadias: Preputial island flap technique. Ann Plast Surg 9:81–88, 1982.
26. Duckett JW: The island flap technique for hypospadias repair. Urol Clini North Am 8:513–519, 1981.
27. Sweet RA, Schrott HG, Kurland R, Culp OS: Study of the incidence of hypospadias in Rochester, Minnesota, 1940–1970, and a case control comparison of possible etiologic factors. Mayo Clin Proc 49:52–58, 1974.
28. Duckett JW: Hypospadias. Pediatr Rev 11:37–442, 1989.
29. Duckett JW: Hypospadias. In Gillenwater Y, Frayhack JT, Howards SS, et al (eds): Adult and Pediatric Urology. Chicago, Year Book Medical, 1987, pp 1880–1915.
30. Allen TD, Griffin JE: Endocrine studies in patients with advanced hypospadias. J Urol 131:310–314, 1984.
31. Shima H, Ikoma F, Yabumoto H, et al: Gonadotropin and testosterone response in prepubertal boys with hypospadias. J Urol 135:539–542, 1986.
32. Roberts CJ, Lloyd S: Observations on epidemiology of simple hypospadias. BMJ 1:768–770, 1973.
33. Mau G: Progestins during pregnancy and hypospadias. Teratology 24:285–287, 1981.
34. Avellan L: The incidence of hypospadias in Sweden. Scand J Plast Reconstr Surg 9:129–139, 1975.
35. Avellan L: On etiological factors in hypospadias. Scand J Plast Reconstr Surg 11:115–123, 1977.
36. Bauer SB, Retik AB, Colodny AH: Genetic aspects of hypospadias. Urol Clin North Am 8:559–564, 1981.
37. Maier WA, Tewes G: Sexual function after operations for hypospadias according to Ombredanne. Progr Pediatr Surg 17:79–82, 1984.
38. Glassman CN, Machlus BJ, Kelalis PP: Urethroplasty for hypospadias: Long-term results. Urol Clin North Am 7:437–441, 1980.
39. Bracka A: A long-term view of hypospadias. Br J Plast Surg 42:251–255, 1984.
40. Svensson J, Berg R, Berg G: Operated hypospadias: Late follow-up. Social, sexual and psychological adaptation. J Pediatr Surg 16:134–135, 1981.
41. Berg R, Berg G: Penile malformation, gender identity and sexual orientation. Acta Psychiatr Scand 68:154–166, 1983.
42. Duckett JW, Keating MA: Technical challenge of the megameatus intact prepuce hypospadias variant: The pyramid procedure. J Urol 141:1407–1409, 1989.
43. Cerasaro TS, Brock WA, Kaplan GW: Upper urinary tract anomalies associated with congenital hypospadias: Is screening necessary? J Urol 135:537–538, 1986.
44. Shima H, Ikoma F, Terakowa T, et al: Developmental anomalies associated with hypospadias. J Urol 122:619–621, 1970.
45. Khuri FJ, Hardy BE, Churchill BM: Urologic anomalies associated with hypospadias. Urol Clin North Am 8:565–571, 1981.
46. Ritchey ML, Benson RC Jr, Kramer SA, et al: Management of müllerian duct remnants in the male patient. J Urol 140:795–799, 1988.
47. Fallon B, Devine CJ Jr, Horton CE: Congenital anomalies associated with hypospadias. J Urol 116:585–586, 1976.
48. Lutzker LG, Kogan SJ, Levitt SB: Is routine IV urography indicated in patients with hypospadias? Pediatrics 59:630–633, 1977.
49. Kennedy PA: Hypospadias: A twenty-year review of 489 cases. J Urol 85:814–817, 1961.
50. Neyman MA, Schirmer HKA: Urinary tract evaluation in hypospadias. J Urol 94:439, 1965.
51. McArdle R, Lebowitz R: Uncomplicated hypospadias and anomalies of the upper urinary tract. Need for screening? Urology 5:712–716, 1975.
52. Smith DS: Hypospadias. In Ashcraft KW (ed): Pediatric Urology. Philadelphia, WB Saunders, 1990, pp 353–395.
53. Sheldon CA, Duckett JW: Hypospadias. Pediatr Clin North Am 34:1259–1272, 1987.
54. Keating MA, Duckett JW: Recent advances in the repair of hypospadias. Surg Ann 22:405–425, 1990.
55. Wacksman J: Results of early hypospadias surgery using optical magnification. J Urol 131:516–517, 1984.
56. Belman AB, Kass EJ: Hypospadias repair in children less than 1 year old. J Urol 128:1273–1274, 1982.
57. Manley CB, Epstein ES: Early hypospadias repair. J Urol 125:698–700, 1981.
58. Kelalis PP, Bunge R, Barkin M, Perlmutter AD: The timing of elective surgery on the genitalia of male children with particular reference to undescended testes and hypospadias. Pediatrics 56:479–483, 1975.
59. Smith DS: Timing of surgery in hypospadias repair. Aust N Z J Surg 53:396–397, 1983.
60. Winslow BH, Horton CE: Hypospadias. Semin Urol 5:236–242, 1987.
61. Mackay A: Hypospadias repair under the age of 1 year. Aust N Z J Surg 53:449–452, 1983.
62. Duckett JW: Advances in hypospadias repair. Postgrad Med J 66(suppl 1):562–571, 1990.
63. Schultz JR, Klykylo WM, Wacksman J: Timing of elective hypospadias repair in children. Pediatrics 71:342–351, 1983.
64. Kass EJ, Jogan SJ, Manley CB, et al: Timing of elective surgery on the genitalia of male children with particular reference to the risks, benefits and psychological effects of surgery and anesthesia. Pediatrics 97:590–594, 1996.
65. Gittes RF, McClaughlin AP: Injection technique to induce penile erection. Urology 4:473–475, 1974.
66. Allen TD, Spence HM: The surgical treatment of coronal hypospadias and related problems. J Urol 100:504–508, 1968.
67. Devine CJ, Horton CE: Chordee without hypospadias. J Urol 110:264–271, 1973.
68. Duckett JW: Hypospadias. In Gillenwater JY, Grayhack JT, Howards SS, et al (eds): Adult and Pediatric Urology. St Louis, Mosby–Year Book, 1991, pp 2103–2140.
69. Horton CE, Devine CJ: Peyronie's disease. Plast Reconstr Surg 52:503, 1973.
70. Das S: Peyronie's disease: Excision and autografting with tunica vaginalis. J Urol 124:818, 1980.
71. Nesbit RM: Congenital curvature of the phallus. Report of three cases with description of corrective operation. J Urol 93:230–234, 1965.
72. Livne PM, Gibbons MD, Gonzales ET: Correction of disproportion of corpora cavernosa as cause of chordee in hypospadias. Urology 22:608–610, 1983.
73. Cendron J, Melin Y: Congenital curvature of the penis without hypospadias. Urol Clin North Am 8:389–395, 1981.
74. Hollowell JG, Keating MA, Snyder HM, et al: Preservation of the urethral plate in hypospadias repair: Extended applications and further experience with the onlay island flap urethroplasty. J Urol 143:98–101, 1990.
75. Baskin L, Duckett JW: Dorsal tunica albuginea plication (TAP) for hypospadias curvature. J Urol 151:1668–1671, 1994.
76. Lattimer JK, Vakili B, Smith AM: The dorsal tilt: An embellishment to any operation for hypospadias. J Urol 109:1035–1036, 1973.
77. King LR: Cutaneous chordee and its implications in hypospadias repair. Urol Clin North Am 8:397–402, 1981.
78. Hurwitz RS, Devine CJ, Horton CE, et al: Chordee without hypospadias. Dialogues in Pediatric Urology 9:1–8, 1986.
79. Mills C, McGovern J, Mininberg D, et al: An analysis of different techniques for distal hypospadias repair: The price of perfection. J Urol 125:701–702, 1981.
80. Gibbons MD, Gonzales ET: The subcoronal meatus. J Urol 130:739–742, 1983.
81. Gibbons MD: Nuances of distal hypospadias. Urol Clin North Am 12:169–174, 1985.

82. Hendren WH: The Belt-Fuqua technique for repair of hypospadias. Urol Clin North Am 8:431–450, 1981.

83. Belman AB: The Broadbent hypospadias repair. Urol Clin North Am 8:483–490, 1981.

84. Standoli L: Vascularized urethroplasty flaps: The use of vascularized flaps of preputial and penopreputial skin for urethral reconstruction in hypospadias. Clin Plast Surg 15:355–370, 1980.

85. Shapiro SR, Zaontz MR, Scherz HC: Hypospadias repair: Update and controversies, part 1. Dialogues in Pediatric Urology 13:1–8, 1990.

86. Elder JS, Duckett JW, Snyder HM: Onlay island flap in the repair of mid and distal penile hypospadias without chordee. J Urol 138:376–379, 1987.

87. Sadove RC, Horton CE, McRoberts JW: The new era of hypospadias surgery. Clin Plast Surg 15:341–354, 1988.

88. Snodgrass W, Decter RM, Roth DR, et al: Management of the penile shaft skin in hypospadias repair: Alternative to Byar's flaps. J Pediatr Surg 23:181–182, 1988.

89. Firlit CF: The mucosal collar in hypospadias surgery. J Urol 137:80–82, 1987.

90. VanDorpe EJ: Correction of distal hypospadias with reconstruction of the preputium. Plast Reconstr Surg 80:290–293, 1987.

91. Nonomura K, Koyanagi T, Imanaka K, et al: One-stage total repair of severe hypospadias with scrotal transposition: Experience in 18 cases. J Pediatr Surg 23:177–180, 1988.

92. Glenn JF, Anderson EE: Surgical correction of incomplete penoscrotal transposition. J Urol 110:603–605, 1973.

93. Ehrlich RM, Scardino PT: Simultaneous surgical correction of scrotal transposition and perineal hypospadias. Urol Clin North Am 8:531–537, 1981.

94. Ehrlich RM, Scardino PT: Surgical corrections of scrotal transposition and perineal hypospadias. J Pediatr Surg 17:175–177, 1982.

95. Duckett JW: MAGPI (meatoplasty and glanuloplasty). Urol Clin North Am 8:513–519, 1981.

96. Arap S, Mitre AI, De Goes GM: Modified meatal advancement glanuloplasty repair of distal hypospadias. J Urol 131:1140–1141, 1984.

97. Mathieu P: Traitement en un temps de l'hypospadias balanique et juxtabalanique. J Chir 39:481, 1932.

98. Wacksman J: Modification of the one-stage flip flap procedure to repair distal penile hypospadias. Urol Clin North Am 8:527–530, 1981.

99. Devine CJ Jr, Horton CE: Hypospadias repair. J Urol 118:188–193, 1977.

100. Zaontz MR: The GAP (glans approximation procedure) for glanular/coronal hypospadias. J Urol 141:359–361, 1989.

101. King LR: Hypospadias: A one-stage repair without skin graft based on a new principle: Chordee is sometimes produced by the skin alone. J Urol 103:660–662, 1970.

102. Snodgrass W: Tubularized incised plate urethroplasty for distal hypospadias. J Urol 151:464–465, 1994.

103. Hendren HW, Horton CE Jr: Experience with one-stage repair of hypospadias and chordee using free graft of prepuce. J Urol 140:1250–1264, 1988.

104. Koyle MA, Ehrlich RM: The bladder mucosa graft for urethral reconstruction. J Urol 138:1093–1095, 1987.

105. Decter RM, Roth DR, Gonzales ET: Hypospadias repair by bladder mucosal graft: An initial report. J Urol 140:1256–1258, 1988.

106. Duckett JW: Transverse preputial island flap technique for repair of severe hypospadias. Urol Clin North Am 7:423, 1980.

107. Hinman F: Blood supply to island flaps [abstract 254]. American Urological Association Annual Meeting. J Urol 143(suppl):252A, 1990.

108. Greenfield SP, Sadler BT, Wan J: Two stage repair for severe hypospadias. J Urol 152:498–501, 1994.

109. Retik AB, Bauer SB, Mandell J, et al: Management of severe hypospadias with two-stage repair. J Urol 152:749–751, 1994.

110. Shapiro SR, Wacksman J, Koyle MA, et al: Hypospadias repair: Update and controversies, part 2. Dialogues in Pediatric Urology 13:1–8, 1990.

111. Duckett JW: Hypospadias [discussion]. J Urol 136:272, 1986.

112. Gaylis FD, Zaontz MR, Dalton D, et al: Silicone foam dressing for penis after reconstructive pediatric surgery. Urology 33:296–299, 1989.

113. Goulding FJ: Penile block for postoperative pain relief in penile surgery. J Urol 126:337, 1981.

114. Reynolds PI, Rosen DA: Caudal analgesia for pediatric urologic procedures. Dialogues in Pediatric Urology 13:6–7, 1990.

115. Duckett JW, Kaplan GW, Woodard JR: Panel: Complications of hypospadias repair. Urol Clin North Am 7:443–454, 1980.

116. Sugar EC, Firlit CF: Urinary prophylaxis and postoperative care of children at home with an indwelling catheter after hypospadias repair. Urology 32:418–420, 1988.

117. Shohet I, Alagam M, Shafir R, et al: Postoperative catheterization and prophylactic antimicrobials in children with hypospadias. Urology 22:391–391, 1983.

118. Horton CE Jr, Horton CE: Complications of hypospadias surgery. Clin Plast Surg 15:371–379, 1988.

119. Retik AB, Keating MA, Mandell J: Complications of hypospadias surgery. Urol Clin North Am 15:223–236, 1988.

120. Walker RD: Outpatient repair of urethral fistula. Urol Clin North Am 8:582–582, 1981.

121. Zagula EM, Braren V: Management of urethrocutaneous fistulas following hypospadias repair. J Urol 130:743–745, 1983.

122. Scherz HC, Kaplan GW, Packer MG, et al: Post-hypospadias repair urethral strictures: A review of 30 cases. J Urol 140:1253–1255, 1988.

123. Zaontz MR, Kaplan WE, Maizels M: Surgical correction of anterior urethral diverticula after hypospadias repair in children. Urology 33:40–42, 1989.

124. Issa MM, Gearhart JP: The failed MAGPI: Management and prevention. Br J Urol 64:169–171, 1989.

125. Sheldon CA, Essig KA: Surgical strategies in the reconstruction of the failed hypospadias: Advantages and versatility of vascular based graft/flap techniques [abstract 250]. American Urological Association Annual Meeting. J Urol 143(suppl):251A, 1990.

126. Ehrlich RM, Alter G: Split-thickness skin graft urethroplasty and tunica vaginalis flaps for failed hypospadias repairs. J Urol 155:131–134, 1996.

127. Marberger H, Pauer W: Experience in hypospadias repair. Urol Clin North Am 8:403–419, 1981.

128. Hensle TW, Bedillo F, Burbige KA: Experience with the MAGPI hypospadias repair. J Pediatr Surg 18:692–694, 1983.

129. Shapiro SR: Complications of hypospadias repair. J Urol 131:518–522, 1984.

130. Livne PM, Gibbons MD, Gonzales ET Jr: Meatal advancement and glanulopasty: An operation for distal hypospadias. J Urol 131:95–98, 1984.

131. Kass EJ, Bolong D: Single stage hypospadias reconstruction without fistula. J Urol 144:520–522, 1990.

132. Duckett JW, Snyder HM: Meatal advancement and glanuloplasty hypospadias repair after 1000 cases: Avoidance of meatal stenosis and regression. J Urol 147:665–669, 1992.

133. Rabinowitz R: Outpatient catheterless modified Mathieu hypospadias repair. J Urol 138:1074–1076, 1987.

134. Gonzales ET Jr, Veeraghavan KA, Delaune J: The management of distal hypospadias with meatal-based vascularized flaps. J Urol 129:119–120, 1983.

135. Retik AB, Mandell J, Bauer SB, et al: Meatal based hypospadias repair with the use of a dorsal subcutaneous flap to prevent urethrocutaneous fistula. J Urol 152:1229–1231, 1994.

136. Bellinger MF: Technical modifications of the Mathieu urethroplasty [abstract 256]. American Urological Association Annual Meeting. J Urol 143(suppl):252A, 1990.

137. Gearhart JP, Borland RN: Onlay island flap urethroplasty: Variation on a theme. J Urol 148:1507–1507, 1992.

138. Hanna MK: Single-stage hypospadias repair: Techniques and results. Urology 21:30–35, 1983.

139. Hendren WH, Horton CE: Experience with one-stage repair of hypospadias and chordee using free graft of prepuce. J Urol 140:1259–1264, 1988.

140. Rober PE, Perlmutter AD, Reitelman C: Experience with 81, one-stage hypospadias/chordee repairs with free graft urethroplasties. J Urol 144:526–529, 1990.

141. Stock JA, Cortez J, Scherz HC, et al: The management of proximal hypospadias using a one-stage hypospadias repair with a preputial free graft for neourethral construction and a preputial pedicle flap for ventral skin coverage. J Urol 152:2335–2337, 1994.

142. Ransley PG, Duffy PG, Oesch IL, et al: The use of bladder mucosa and combined bladder mucosa/preputial skin grafts for urethral reconstruction. J Urol 138:1096–1098, 1987.

143. Ehrlich RM, Reda EF, Koyle MA, et al: Complications of bladder mucosa graft. J Urol 142:626–627, 1989.

144. Mollard P, Mouriguand P, Bringeon G, et al: Repair of hypospadias using a bladder mucosal graft in 76 cases. J Urol 142:1548–1550, 1989.

145. Li LC, Zhang X, Zhou SW, et al: Experience with repair of hypospadias using bladder mucosa in adolescents and adults. J Urol 153:1117–1119, 1995.

146. Burger RA, Muller SC, el-Damanhoury H, et al: The buccal mucosa graft for urethral reconstruction: A preliminary report. J Urol 147:662–664, 1992.

147. Duckett JW, Coplen D, Walt D, et al: Buccal mucosal urethral replacement. J Urol 153:1660–1663, 1995.

59

CIRCUMCISION

Stephen C. Raynor, MD

Circumcision, which is one of the most frequently performed surgical procedures, is done for therapeutic reasons, for perceived prophylactic benefits, or as a religious ritual. Rates of circumcision vary widely in different regions of the world, and this has led to much debate regarding its merits and indications.

□ Embryology

The development of the prepuce begins during the 3rd month of gestation as a fold of skin at the base of the glans. With growth, this skin extends distally, with the dorsal portion growing at a more rapid rate than the ventral component. Its proper development depends on the presence of androgens and androgen receptors. After closure of the glanular urethra, the growth of the ventral portion of the prepuce completes by the 5th month of gestation. Keratinization of the glans and inner epithelial surface of the prepuce then begins. Initially, the inner surface of the prepuce and the epithelium of the glans are fused. Lacunae then begin to form between the two surfaces, and an eventual separation of these two surfaces results. However, this separation remains incomplete at birth.[1]

As a result of this incomplete keratinization, the foreskin can be completely retracted in only about 5% of newborns. In 46% of newborns, the foreskin adhesions do not allow the meatus to be seen. The natural process of separation between the glans and the prepuce is a gradual one. Separation sufficient to allow complete retraction of the foreskin can be expected in 20% of boys by 6 months, 50% by 1 year, 80% by 2 years, and 90% by 3 years.[2] By age 17, all foreskins should be retractable.[3] Until this natural process of separation is complete, there is usually no need for forceful retraction of the foreskin and cleaning of the glans.

□ History and Incidence

There is evidence that circumcision has been practiced since ancient times; circumcision is de-

picted in bas relief on a tomb of ancient Egypt.[1] The Bible declares circumcision to be the sign of the covenant between God and the people of Israel.[4] It was reported that Columbus found circumcised natives on his arrival to the New World.[1] Today, there are wide variations in the rate of circumcision throughout the world. It has been estimated that one of six males in the world is circumcised.[5] There is a high rate of ritual circumcision in Jewish and Muslim populations, and circumcision is quite common in the United States. Black Africans, Australian aborigines, and people of the Near East also practice ritual circumcision.[5, 6] In contrast, ritual circumcision is rarely performed in Europe, China, and the Far East, and Central and South America.[5] Whereas there is general agreement on therapeutic indications for circumcision, there is much disagreement regarding the value of routine prophylactic newborn circumcision.

□ Indications

Phimosis is the inability to retract the foreskin. True phimosis, as opposed to the natural, delayed separation of the prepuce from the glans, is an uncommon event in infancy and is indicated by ballooning of the foreskin with urination. Paraphimosis occurs when the foreskin has been retracted behind the corona but is able to be brought back over the glans with difficulty or not at all. Both are considered indications for circumcision, though ardent opponents of circumcision would offer preputial stretching or preputial plasty as alternatives.[7–9] In one study, 10% of phimosis in older boys was due to lichen sclerosis et atrophicus and was seen as an indication for circumcision.[7] Balanitis is an infection of the glans, and posthitis is an infection of the prepuce. Recurrent infection with clinical scarring of the prepuce is an accepted indication for circumcision.[6, 11]

□ Routine Newborn Circumcision

Much has been written regarding routine newborn circumcision, and it has become a contentious and emotional issue. Confounding the argument is the lack of a clear understanding as to the precise function of the foreskin.[12] Consequently, circumcision has been presented as a symbol of the "therapeutic state,"[13] as a mutilating procedure,[14] as a religious ritual, and as prophylaxis against a variety of diseases. Circumcision is performed on the 8th day in the Jewish faith, traditionally being done by a mohel, a member of the Jewish faith trained in ritual circumcision. In Islamic countries, circumcision is considered traditional but not obligatory, with a wide variability in age at the time of circumcision.[15]

Many arguments have been put forth to justify routine newborn circumcision. As rates of circumcision have fallen in the United States, reports have appeared suggesting an increased rate of urinary tract infections in uncircumcised male infants. An initial report of infant urinary tract infections showed that in infants younger than 3 months of age, males predominated, with a disproportionately large number of these boys being uncircumcised.[16] Subsequent retrospective analysis of infants of families in the armed services suggested that uncircumcised infants have a 12-fold increased risk for urinary tract infection as compared with circumcised infants.[17–19] This increased incidence of infection is believed to be secondary to adherence of pathogenic bacteria to the prepuce.[20] It has also been suggested that there is an increased risk of urinary tract infections in uncircumcised young adults.[21] Critics have been quick to note that these studies all have been retrospective analyses and therefore are subject to significant bias.[22, 23] Others have suggested that colonization of the prepuce by nonmaternal uropathic bacteria could be prevented by strict rooming-in with the mother. Infection may result from colonization of the baby with maternal anaerobic gut flora.[24]

Another proposed benefit of circumcision is in the reduction of sexually transmitted diseases (STDs). There have been multiple studies examining the relationship between circumcision status and STDs. Studies have shown an increased risk of chancroid, syphilis, gonorrhea, candidiasis, and genital herpes,[25, 26] whereas others have found little support for or have refuted these findings altogether.[27, 28] It may be that the protective effect of circumcision against STDs may differ among developed and developing nations with poorer hygiene.[28] With the multiple confounding variables and lack of agreement between studies, there is not enough evidence to make a definitive recommendation for routine circumcision as a preventive measure against STDs.

Epidemiologic studies of HIV and AIDS have raised another argument for prophylactic circumcision. In Africa, there are regional differences in the rate of routine or ritual circumcision. As the HIV/AIDS epidemic has emerged on the continent, the patterns of disease have been correlated with circumcision status, with increased rates of HIV/AIDS in areas with low circumcision rates.[29] An analysis of 30 epidemiologic studies from Africa concluded that there was enough evidence that circumcision was associated with reduced HIV infection rates to consider male circumcision as a viable strategy to reduce HIV transmission.[30] A similar association between circumcision status and HIV has been noted in the United States, with uncircumcised homosexual men having a twofold increase in the risk of HIV infection.[31] Noncircumcision in the male partner also seems to be associated with an increased risk of transmission of HIV in heterosexual contacts.[32]

Perhaps the strongest argument for routine circumcision is as a protective measure against cancer of the penis. The etiology of penile cancer is unknown, but there appears to be an association with human papillomaviruses (HPV).[33] The incidence of penile cancer in the United States is approximately 1 case per 100,000, with nearly all cases occurring in uncircumcised men.[23, 34] This protective effect against penile cancer is diminished or lost when circumcision is done after the newborn period.[6, 34, 35] Other factors associated with cancer of the penis include smoking, a history of genital warts, penile rash or tear, and multiple sexual partners.[35] Critics of circumcision cite equally low rates of penile cancer in countries with low circumcision rates. This epidemiologic data combined with the extremely low incidence of penile cancer and the probable viral etiology has led some authors to conclude that the impact of routine newborn circumcision against penile cancer does not justify its widespread practice.[22, 33]

Taken together, the studies to date do not provide conclusive evidence regarding the practice of routine neonatal circumcision. Perhaps 10% of males not circumcised at birth will eventually require circumcision.[14] A longitudinal study comparing circumcised with uncircumcised males showed a higher risk of penile problems in infancy in the circumcised group, with a higher rate of problems in the uncircumcised group after infancy. By 8 years of age, the uncircumcised group had experienced 1.5 times the rate of penile problems.[36] After review of the data, the American Academy of Pediatrics in 1989 softened earlier recommendations against newborn circumcision, concluding that there may be potential benefits to newborn circumcision and the risks and benefits should be discussed with parents.[23] On their review of the data, the Canadian Pediatric Society felt that the risks and benefits of routine newborn circumcision were evenly balanced and concluded that routine newborn circumcision was not recommended.[32] Interestingly, in the United States, the decision regarding circumcision seems to be based more on social as opposed to medical concerns.[37]

□ Surgical Technique

Circumcision has been practiced for centuries and there have been numerous techniques developed. Common to all methods, the goal is removal of enough of the prepuce to uncover the glans, treat or prevent phimosis, and eliminate the possibility of paraphimosis. Whatever method is chosen, the surgeon must be familiar with and adept at the procedure with a resultant low complication rate. Informed consent should always be obtained prior to any circumcision.

□ Newborn Circumcision

Circumcision represents the most frequently performed male operation in the United States, with 61% of the newborn males born in 1987 being circumcised.[6] Newborn circumcision is most frequently performed with a circumcision device. These various devices may be a shield, used in the traditional Jewish circumcision; Mogen clamp; Gomco clamp; or Plastibell.[5] Prior to the procedure, the penis should be inspected for any congenital abnormality, such as a hypospadias or the presence of chordee, that might be a contraindication to circumcision.

Although the pain of newborn circumcision has been thought to be short-lived, studies have shown that circumcised infants have a stronger pain response to vaccination at 4 and 6 months of age.[38] This underscores the importance of providing adequate analgesia for this procedure. Effective relief of circumcision pain has been shown to be obtained by acetaminophen, topical lidocaine-procaine cream, as well as local nerve blocks.[39–42]

Even though most procedures are done outside the operating room, antisepsis is critical, because infection is a serious potential complication. In performing a Gomco circumcision, after prepping the field, the adhesions between the glans and the inner surface of the prepuce are bluntly separated. The extent of foreskin to be excised is then marked, either with a marking pen or with a crush of the dorsal prepuce done with a straight hemostatic forceps. A dorsal slit allows the appropriate-sized bell to be placed over the glans, inside the prepuce. The bell and foreskin are then brought through the opening in the base of the clamp, placed in the yoke which is tightened, followed by excision of the foreskin distal to the base of the clamp. Elecrocautery must never be used to excise the foreskin, because transmission of the electrical current to the shaft of the penis will take place. The bell is then released and removed, taking care not to disrupt the weld between the shaft skin and the remnant of the inner surface of the prepuce.

A Plastibell differs from the Gomco clamp in that the distal foreskin is strangulated, with a resulting slough of that tissue. After sterile prep and dorsal slit, the appropriate-sized Plastibell is placed over the glans and inside the prepuce and positioned. A string is then tied around the glans, being positioned in a groove in the bell. The excess foreskin is trimmed and the handle is broken off the bell. The foreskin remnant and bell are expected to slough off in 7 to 12 days.

□ Operative Circumcision

In older patients, circumcision is usually done in the operating room. Circumcision devices seem to be less adequate for the older patient, and sleeve resection of the foreskin is preferable. As shown in Figure 59–1, after prepping the operative field, any

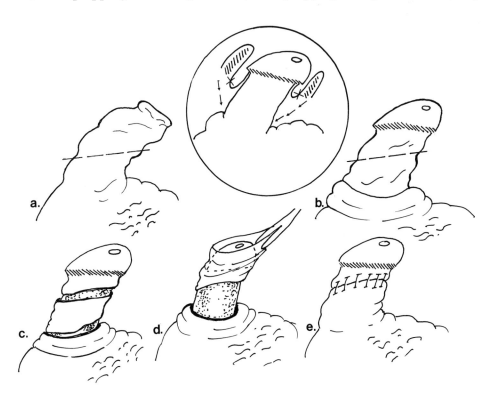

Figure 59–1. When performing a freehand circumcision, the initial incision is made in the shaft skin, leaving more skin ventrally (a). A second incision is then made in the subcoronal sulcus, leaving a generous cuff (b). The inset shows the amount of foreskin to be excised. The isolated foreskin (c) is then excised (d), and the shaft skin is sutured to the subcoronal skin (e).

remaining adhesions between the glans and foreskin are bluntly taken down.

After marking the subcoronal sulcus, the foreskin is incised along the base of the glans with the foreskin in its normal position. Less skin is to be excised from the ventral surface. Dissection is carried down to Buck's fascia. The prepuce is then retracted and an incision made in the subcoronal sulcus, leaving a generous cuff of subcoronal skin. Injury to the urethra must be avoided. The collar of foreskin that has been isolated is then excised and electrocautery is used to obtain meticulous hemostasis. The shaft skin is then approximated to the subcoronal skin using interrupted absorbable sutures.

□ Complications

When done by experienced hands, circumcision has a low complication rate of between 2 and 10%.[33] Bleeding is the most frequent complication and is generally minor. Infection is the second most common complication and generally is a minor problem. However, serious problems can result, including necrotizing fasciitis, sepsis, Fournier's gangrene, and meningitis.[6] Complications related to the excision of too little or too much foreskin include insufficient circumcision with postoperative phimosis or concealed penis. Other complications include skin bridges, inclusion cysts, iatrogenic hypospadias or epispadias, partial amputation of the glans, and the catastrophic loss of the penis when electrocautery was used with a metal circumcision device.

REFERENCES

1. Kaplan GW: Circumcision: An overview. Curr Probl Pediatr 7:1–33, 1977.
2. Gardner D: The fate of the foreskin. BMJ 2:1433–1437, 1949.
3. Oster J: Further fate of the foreskin. Arch Dis Child 43:200–203, 1968.
4. The Holy Bible.
5. Holman J, Lewis E, Ringler R: Neonatal circumcision techniques. Am Fam Physician 52:511–518, 1995.
6. Niku S, Stock J, Kaplan G: Neonatal circumcision. Urol Clin North Am 22:57–65, 1995.
7. Cuckow P, Rix G, Mouriquand P: Preputial plasty: A good alternative to circumcision. J Pediatr Surg 29:561–563, 1994.
8. Holmlund D: Dorsal incision of the prepuce and skin closure with dexon in patients with phimosis. Scand J Urol Nephrol 7:97–99, 1973.
9. Cooper C, Thomson G, Raine P: Therapeutic retraction of the foreskin in childhood. BMJ 286:186–187, 1983.
10. Meuli M, Briner J, Hanimann B, et al: Lichen sclerosus et atrophicus causing phimosis in boys: A prospective study with 5-year follow-up after complete circumcision. J Urol 152:987–989, 1994.
11. Escala J, Rickwood A: Balanitis. Br J Urol 63:196–197, 1989.
12. Taylor J, Lockwood A, Taylor A: The prepuce: Specialized mucosa of the penis and its loss to circumcision. Br J Urol 77:291, 1996.
13. Szasz T: Routine neonatal circumcision: Symbol of the birth of the therapeutic state. J Med Philos 21:137–148, 1996.
14. Weiss G, Weiss E: A perspective on controversies over neonatal circumcision. Clin Pediatr 33:726–730, 1994.
15. Sari N, Buyukunal S, Zulfikar B: Circumcision ceremonies at the Ottoman palace. J Pediatr Surg 31:920–924, 1996.
16. Ginsburg C, McCracken G: Urinary tract infections in young infants. Pediatrics 69:409–412, 1982.
17. Wiswell T, Enzenauer R, Cornish D, et al: Declining frequency of circumcision: Implications for changes in the absolute incidence and male-to-female sex ratio of urinary tract infections in early infancy. Pediatrics 79:338–342, 1987.
18. Wiswell T, Geschke W: Risks from circumcision during the first month of life compared with those for uncircumcised boys. Pediatrics 83:1011–1015, 1989.
19. Wiswell T, Hachey W: Urinary tract infection and the uncircumcised state: An update. Clin Pediatr 82:130–134, 1993.
20. Roberts J: Pathogenesis of non-obstructive urinary tract infections in children. J Urol 144(part 2):475–479, 1990.
21. Spach D, Stapleton A, Stamm W: Lack of circumcision increases the risk of urinary tract infection in young men. JAMA 267:679–681, 1992.
22. Poland R: The question of routine neonatal circumcision. N Engl J Med 822:1312–1315, 1990.
23. Schoen E, Anderson G, Bohon C, et al: Report of the task force on circumcision. Pediatrics 84:388–391, 1989.
24. Winberg J, Gothefors L, Bollgren I, et al: The prepuce: A mistake of nature? Lancet 1(8638):598–599, 1989.
25. Parker S, Stewart A, Wren M, et al: Circumcision and sexually transmitted disease. Med J Aust 2:288–290, 1983.
26. Cook L, Koutsky L, Holmes K: Circumcision and sexually transmitted diseases. Am J Public Health 84:197–201, 1994.
27. Laumann E, Masi C, Zuckerman E: Circumcision in the United States. Prevalence, prophylactic effects and sexual practice. JAMA 277:1052–1057, 1997.
28. Donovan B, Bassett I, Bodsworth N: Male circumcision and common sexually transmissible diseases in a developed nation setting. Genitourin Med 70:317–320, 1994.
29. Moses S: Geographical patterns of male circumcision practices in Africa: Association with HIV seroprevalence. Int J Epidemiol 19:693–697, 1990.
30. Moses S, Plummer F, Bradley J, et al: The association between lack of male circumcision and risk for HIV infection: A review of the epidemiological data. Sex Transm Dis 21:201–210, 1994.
31. Kreiss J, Hopkins S: The association between circumcision status and human immunodeficiency virus infection among homosexual men. J Infect Dis 168:1404–1408, 1993.
32. McCarthy K, Studd J, Johnson M: Heterosexual transmission of human immunodeficiency virus. Br J Hosp Med 48:404–408, 1992.
33. Fetus and Newborn Committee Canadian Pediatric Society: Neonatal circumcision revisited. CMAJ 154:769–780, 1996.
34. Schoen E: The relationship between circumcision and cancer of the penis. CA Cancer J Clin 41:306–309, 1991.
35. Maden C, Sherman K, Beckmann A, et al: History of circumcision, medical conditions, and sexual activity and risk of penile cancer. J Natl Cancer Inst 85:19–24, 1993.
36. Fergussen D, Lawton J, Shannon F: Neonatal circumcision and penile problems: An 8-year longitudinal study. Pediatrics 81:537–541, 1988.
37. Brown M, Brown C: Circumcision decision: The prominence of social concerns. Pediatrics 80:215–219, 1987.
38. Taddio A, Katz J, Iiersich A, et al: Effect of neonatal circumcision on pain response during subsequent routine vaccination. Lancet 849:599–603, 1997.
39. Howard C, Howard F, Weitzman M: Acetaminophen analgesia in neonatal circumcision: The effect on pain. Pediatrics 93:641–646, 1994.
40. Taddio A, Stevens B, Craig K, et al: Efficacy and safety of lidocaine-prilocaine cream for pain during circumcision. N Engl J Med 336:1197–1201, 1997.
41. Serour F, Cohen A, Mandelberg A, et al: Dorsal penile nerve block in children undergoing circumcision in a day-care surgery. Can J Anaesth 43:954–958, 1996.
42. Lenhart J, Lenhart N, Reid A, et al: Local anesthesia for circumcision: Which technique is most effective? J Am Board Fam Pract 10:13–19, 1997.

60

PRUNE-BELLY SYNDROME

Michael A. Keating, MD • Mark A. Rich, MD

Shortly after an initial description of its urologic findings by Parker[1] in 1895, Osler[2] assigned the graphic term of *prune-belly syndrome* (PBS) to a triad of findings that include the following:

1. Congenital absence, deficiency, or hypoplasia of the abdominal wall musculature
2. Urinary tract abnormalities characterized by a large hypotonic bladder (megacystis), dilated ureters, and dilated prostatic urethra
3. Bilateral cryptorchidism

As in most syndromes, the effects are not confined solely to classic manifestations, and other organs, including the kidneys, lungs, heart, extremities, and gastrointestinal (GI) tract, are frequently affected (Table 60–1).[3]

A variety of labels have been applied to this constellation of findings, including Eagle-Barrett syndrome, mesenchymal dysplasia, and abdominal musculature deficiency (AMD) syndrome.[4–6] The moniker of "prune" is bluntly descriptive but presents a negative connotation of the affected child. Nunn and Stephens coined the term *triad syndrome* to minimize emotional repercussions.[7] Nevertheless, the designation prune-belly remains the most widely accepted.

Owing to its inclusion of cryptorchidism, by definition, fully developed PBS occurs exclusively in male patients. Occasionally, a female patient exhibits abdominal walls that are phenotypically and histologically indistinguishable from those in males with PBS. Even more rarely, severe degrees of urinary tract ectasia occur.[8, 9] Female or male patients who manifest one or two components of PBS are probably best identified as having *pseudoprune disorder*. It is rare to have a normal urinary tract with the characteristic abdominal wall, although the converse is not true.[10]

☐ Incidence and Genetics

The incidence of PBS is probably similar to that of bladder exstrophy (1 per 35,000 to 50,000 live births).[11, 12] Despite this relative paucity, several cen-

ters have amassed considerable experience with PBS and its variants.[8, 13, 14]

Extensive testing has failed to implicate a genetic basis for the syndrome. No evidence has been found of autosomal recessive or single-gene inheritance, although PBS has been documented in siblings.[5, 15, 16] Sex-linked inheritance could explain the inordinate male predominance in the disorder but has never been shown. Instead, a complex polygenic transmission of autosomal dominant mutation having sex-limited expression that mimics X-linkage has been proposed.[17] Mosaicism has been reported in two siblings with PBS.[18] Cases associated with individ-

TABLE 60–1. Extragenitourinary Abnormalities

Pulmonary

Pulmonary hypoplasia
Pneumothorax
Pneumomediastinum
Lobar atelectasis

Cardiac

Tetralogy of Fallot
Ventricular septal defect
Atrial septal defect
Patent ductus arteriosus

Orthopedic

Pectus excavatum and carinatum
Varus deformity of feet
Dimpling of elbow or knee
Congenital hip dislocation
Severe leg maldevelopment

Gastrointestinal

Intestinal malrotation
Intestinal atresias
Gastroschisis
Omphalocele
Imperforate anus
Hepatobiliary anomalies
Hirschsprung's disease

Miscellaneous

Adrenal cystic dysplasia
Splenic torsion

ual chromosomal anomalies (trisomy 13 and 18, and Turner's syndrome) have also been reported and may suggest the involvement of multiple loci.[19–22] However, these types of chromosomal abnormalities are the exception and the karyotypic analysis is nearly always normal. The 100% discordance among twins strongly suggests another cause in most cases.[5, 11]

□ Etiology

EMBRYOLOGY

The lateral plate mesoderm of the embryo splits into a visceral layer (muscular coat of the gut) and a parietal or somatic layer (body wall). The coelom progressively enlarges between the two. In the caudal region, coelomic extension and lateral plate division do not occur. Here, the undivided mesoderm extends around the allantois and cloaca where its deeper layers form bladder wall musculature, ureters, and prostate. The superficial layers of the lateral plate mesoderm are necessary for closure of the anterior abdominal wall. Omphalocele and exstrophy result when midline approximation of mesoderm does not occur. Differentiation of the abdominal wall musculature is derived from the *lower thoracic somites*, which migrate into the plate.

A variety of theories have been proposed regarding the origin of PBS, although its precise cause remains unclear.[23] The *theory of yolk sac hindrance* implicates an error in the interplay of maturing abdominal wall and the yolk sac.[24] Normally, the yolk sac constricts as the mesoderm infolds and differentiates into the anterior abdominal wall. Its persistence could block this sequence, leaving abdominal wall redundancy as its aftermath. This could conceivably account for the anomalies of the urachus, bladder, and prostatic urethra found with PBS but does not explain its cryptorchidism and ureteral abnormalities.

The *mesodermal defect theory* speculates that a defect of the lateral plate mesenchyme disrupts the migration or differentiation of the thoracic somites, affecting myoblast development.[25] Histologic demonstrations of dystrophic abdominal musculature replaced by fibrous tissue surrounded by fascia perhaps support this theory.[26] Electron microscopy showing poorly organized muscle and Z-band fragmentation in the sarcomeres is thought to be more indicative of a developmental disturbance than an insult from lengthening or atrophy, as might be expected from bladder obstruction and abdominal distention.[27]

The mesodermal defect theory is clinically supported by the fourfold incidence of twinning seen with PBS (1:23 vs. 1:80 in the general population).[5] Every case in twins has been discordant for PBS. Theoretically, only one fetus receives adequate mesenchyme with initial divisions of the embryo's primitive streak. To its detriment, this theory does not account for the urinary tract abnormalities, cryptorchidism, or male predominance. However, it is plausible that a similar mesodermal error could affect the adjacent paraxial, intermediate, and lateral plate mesoderm essential to normal genitourinary development.[28] A lack of hormonal responsiveness by the primordial gubernaculum and prostate has also been implicated in the etiology of cryptorchidism and prostatic hypoplasia.[29] This type of defect would link the theories of mesodermal defect and bladder outlet obstruction.

The *theory of bladder obstruction and distention* has become the most widely accepted.[30] According to this explanation, urethral obstruction occurs during a critical "window" in development, which results in massive distention of the bladder and ureters. This, in turn, causes degeneration of the abdominal wall. Histologic studies demonstrating atrophic abdominal musculature rather than primitive muscle support the hypothesis.[31–33] Obstruction could explain the changes seen in bladder walls as well as the ureteral dilation and urachal patency that commonly occur. Early outlet obstruction also has obvious implications for the developing kidneys where dysplasia, oligohydramnios, and subsequent pulmonary hypoplasia often result. In this theory, the testes are also blocked by the distended bladder or fail to descend due to abdominal wall laxity and decreased intraabdominal pressures within, which normally act as an impetus to descend.

The exact mechanism of obstruction remains to be defined. Critics note that the majority of PBS infants are born without demonstrable urethral obstruction. In addition, the severity of the abdominal wall laxity does not correlate well with the degree of urinary tract dilation in many cases. Perhaps most perplexing is that PBS or cryptorchidism do not develop in the majority of babies with urethral valves or other bladder outlet obstructions. Nevertheless, it appears that transient obstruction is present at some point during fetal development and that *timing* is actually the factor most crucial to the appearance of PBS.[30, 34] Transient urethral valves or the hypoplastic prostate uniformly found in these boys are possible causal factors. With the latter, the weakened walls of the dysgenetic gland, lacking smooth muscle support, bulge dorsally and caudally. As a consequence, the unsupported membranous urethra twists anteriorly at its junction with the prostatic urethra. A flap-valve obstruction to flow results.[31] Posterior urethral obstruction would explain the male predominance.

Intraabdominal distentions unrelated to urinary tract obstruction have also been implicated. Fetal ascites, megacystis microcolon syndrome, and intestinal duplication cysts have all been observed with the bladder obstruction syndrome.[35–37] Such associations may play a role in cases of pseudoprune disorder, but they do not explain the urologic findings of PBS. In addition, these types of distentions do not usually cause abdominal wall laxity in most of the children in whom they occur.

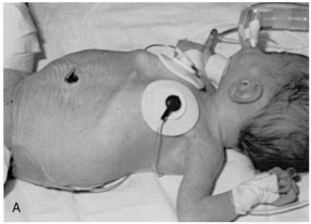

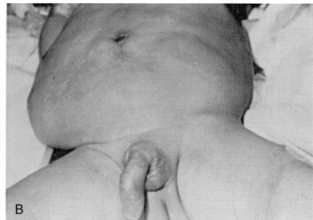

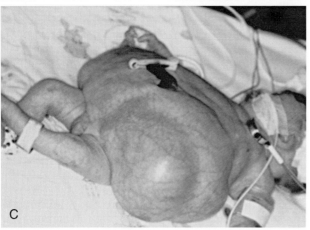

Figure 60–1. Variable degrees of abdominal wall laxity with prune-belly syndrome. *A*, Subtle wrinkling in less severely affected infant. *B*, Typical appearance. *C*, Severely affected newborn. (Part *C* courtesy of D.M. Joseph, MD.)

☐ Genitourinary Manifestations

ABDOMINAL WALL

Pathophysiology

A large degree of variability in the involvement of the abdominal wall musculature is seen (Fig. 60–1). Typically, the upper abdominal oblique and rectus muscles are well developed, whereas the lateral and ventral abdominal muscles are diffusely deficient, irregular, and often asymmetric.[38] Affected muscles (in decreasing order of frequency) include the transversus, rectus abdominis below the umbilicus, internal oblique, external oblique, and rectus above the umbilicus.[39] The abdominal wall periphery usually shows normal or near-normal muscle. In contrast, studies of affected areas show poorly organized muscle interspersed with dense collagenous tissue.[7, 27] At times, the lower medial aspect of the abdomen consists merely of skin, fat, and fibrous tissue condensed onto the peritoneum, making differentiation of the muscle layers difficult.[40] The innervation of the abdominal musculature and skin is normal.[7] However, electromyography shows little or no functional muscle in the lower central abdomen.[38] Nonspecific ultrastructural disorganization is seen at the cellular level.[27]

Clinical Correlates

The lax abdominal musculature fails to support the viscera within. The overlying skin is stretched in utero and results in a typically wrinkled appearance in the newborn. The thin and pliable abdominal wall allows easy palpation of the organs. Peristalsis of the intestine and ureter can often be observed immediately beneath its surface. A potbellied appearance typically evolves with continued development as the cutaneous wrinkling resolves with the accumulation of subcutaneous fat. Some abdominal tone is also gained in most children.[41]

The severity of the abdominal defect has no prognostic significance, although urinary tract involvement often correlates with ipsilateral abdominal wall involvement in cases of asymmetry.[10] The lack of abdominal wall support can pose a problem. For all practical purposes, rectus muscle continuity is lost. Infants with severe defects are typically unable to sit from the supine position; instead, they roll prone and raise themselves by pushing up. Developmental delay in motor skills that require balance and coordination (e.g., walking) is common.

Problems with respiratory toilet result from an impaired cough. Pulmonary secretions are difficult to expectorate without the assistance of the abdominal musculature. Respiratory infections are common. This deficit also increases the risk of pulmonary complications after general anesthesia.[42]

TESTICLES

Pathophysiology

The undescended testicles in PBS are usually located at the level of the iliac vessels, but more proximal positions have been described.[7, 43] Histologically, such testes are indistinguishable from normal age-matched gonads early in development.[44, 45] Biopsies in adults, however, have shown little or no germ cell maturation, even after the gonads have been repositioned into the upper scrotum or canal.[46] Whether these changes represent the natural progression of PBS cryptorchidism or are in some way influenced by the timing or technique of surgery is unclear.

Adnexal abnormalities have also been described. Epididymal detachment and atresia have been noted.[7] Vas deferens detachment has also been described. The architecture of the vas deferens is variable. Collagen replaces muscle in some cases. Others are thin-walled, tortuous, and segmentally atretic.[47] The gubernaculum is usually normal, and its course through the inguinal canal is direct, although malformations have been described that may contribute to cryptorchidism.[3, 45]

Clinical Correlates

Fertility has not been recorded with PBS, regardless of the age of orchiopexy.[46, 48] A variety of factors could contribute to infertility, including decreased germ cell potential, prostatic maldevelopment causing deficient seminal fluid, and retrograde ejaculation resulting from the wide open bladder neck that occurs. Absent ejaculation is a common finding in adulthood.[49] However, one study failed to demonstrate sperm in pre-ejaculate and postejaculate urine in five adults with PBS, further emphasizing impaired spermatogenesis.[46] Normal secondary sexual characteristics, erections, and orgasm usually occur in the adult with PBS. Testosterone production is usually good, although luteinizing hormone levels are elevated, an indication of Leydig cell damage. Several malignancies have been reported in PBS, yet the risk of malignancy appears to be no greater than that with other disorders involving intraabdominal testes.[50, 51]

KIDNEYS

Pathophysiology

Although the kidneys in patients with PBS can be normal, some degree of renal dysplasia (Potter's type II dysplasia) occurs in about 50%. Signs of disordered nephron development—embryonic tubules, cysts, cartilage, and mesenchyme—are thought to be indicative of a developmental insult rather than obstruction. Ureteral ectopy or some other abnormal interplay between the ureteral bud and renal blastema is implicated.[24, 52] Variable degrees of dysplasia occur within individual kidneys, sometimes interspersed between normal parenchyma. Wide ranges in involvement also occur between the kidneys of an affected patient, and functional asymmetry is common. One study found dysplasia in 25% of the parenchyma in 10 nephrectomy specimens; another found bilateral dysplasia affecting 30 to 70% of the kidneys in seven of nine autopsies.[53]

Variable degrees of hydronephrosis are also common. However, the parenchymal changes are not usually typical of other obstructive processes, such as ureteropelvic junction obstruction (e.g., Potter's type IV changes, pelvic thinning). In fact, the quality of the renal parenchyma is routinely much better than expected, given the degree of collecting system dilation. This suggests that the mechanism of dilation in PBS differs from that in other obstructive uropathies. It may be that hydronephrosis of the syndrome represents a low-pressure reflection of the same mesenchymal defect that has affected the lower urinary tract. True ureteropelvic junction obstruction or ureteral stenosis was found in only 6 of 80 patients in two reports.[54]

Radiographic Findings

Signs of renal dysmorphism are easily appreciated on excretory urography (Fig. 60–2). Rotational abnormalities are common and the kidneys have a lobulated outline. Calyceal clubbing and infundibular narrowing are also common. These changes have random distribution, however, and may be interspersed between normal calyces. The severity of pelvic dilation is variable, but disproportion usually occurs between generous distal ureters and less voluminous renal pelves. When changes appear, they are typically asymmetric.

Ultrasonography (US) provides useful information about renal size, the degree of pelvic and calyceal dilation, and differentiation of the parenchyma. The most severely dysplastic kidneys are small and hyperechoic, and have absent corticomedullary junctions. Radioisotope (technetium[99m] diethylenetriaminepentaacetic acid or glucoheptonate) scans help assess function and obstruction.

Clinical Correlates

The degree of dysplasia dictates the prognosis in the infant who survives the pulmonary sequelae of oligohydramnios. Dysplasia is typically more severe in children born with urethral stenosis or agenesis, megalourethra, or imperforate anus.[55, 56] The function of many of these kidneys is surprisingly good. Subsequent growth and development depends on the balance between viable renal tissue that remains and the demands required of it. Urologic management is directed at preserving this tissue by avoiding infections, the main risk to deterioration.

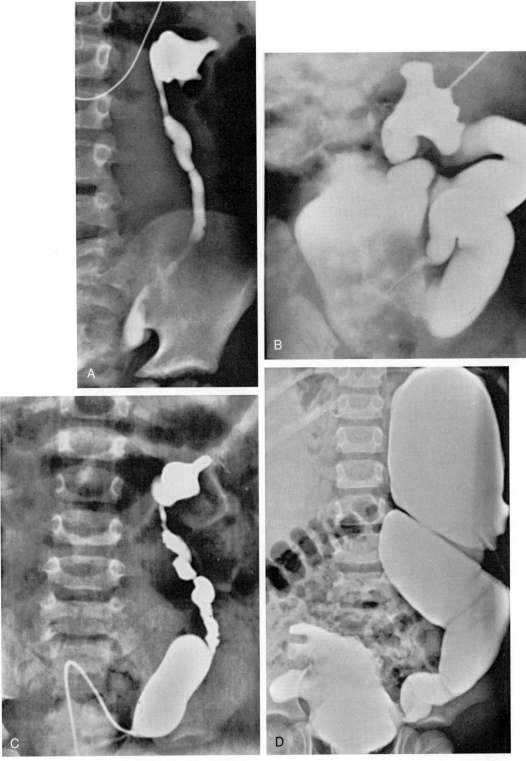

Figure 60–2. Variable degrees of dilation and dysmorphism of the upper urinary tract. *A*, Dysmorphic renal pelvis with mild ureteral dilation. *B*, Calyceal clubbing and tortuous "wandering" ureter. *C*, Dysmorphic pelvis with exaggerated dilation of distal ureteral spindle. *D*, Bizarre appearance of collecting system as well as bladder.

URETERS

Pathophysiology

Elongated, dilated, and tortuous ureters are the most common urinary tract abnormality in patients with PBS.[7] Like the other organs involved, the degree of impairment is variable. Studies show that affected ureters have a patchy distribution of smooth muscle interspersed with fibrocytes and collagen.[24] In some cases, the entire wall is composed of acellular hyaline ground substance, and differentiation into normal muscular layers is absent.[57] These changes can be segmental, but classically the lower ureter is involved preferentially to the upper, where greater densities of normal smooth muscle is found.[58, 59]

Ineffective peristalsis, the functional sequelae of these abnormalities, results from disruption of the neuromyogenic cohesiveness of ureteral smooth muscle by collagen.[60] Nerve plexus decrease and irregular nonmyelinated Schwann fibers have also been described.[59] Periureteral ganglion and other adjacent nerves are normal.[6] Vesicoureteral reflux is present in more than 75% of patients.[10] The orifices are often gaping and laterally displaced. Obstructions are rare.

Radiographic Findings

The diagnosis of PBS is frequently made by the appearance of the ureters on excretory urography or voiding cystourethrography (with reflux) (see Fig. 60–2). Exaggerated distal ureteral ectasia is a hallmark of the syndrome. The proximal ureter typically has a more normal caliber.[61] Varying degrees of almost bizarre dilation, sometimes interspersed with segments of narrowing, result in tortuous ureters that "wander" across the newborn abdomen. Fluoroscopy may show ineffective peristalsis. With continued growth, the ureters often straighten and peristalsis improves.

Clinical Correlates

The degree of ureteral dilation does not correlate with the status of the kidneys or the patient's prognosis (Fig. 60–3). However, these types of nonobstructive megaureters leave the system at risk for infection owing to urinary stasis. Pyelonephritis is common, especially when reflux is present. Preventing infection, eliminating reflux, and improving peristalsis become the goals of ureteral reconstruction when medical management is ineffective.

The proximal ureter is usually the better functioning and most normal portion. Abnormal ureter should be discarded. Operations that preserve the distal ureter (end ureterostomies or reimplantation with minimal resection) should usually be avoided.

BLADDER AND URACHUS

Pathophysiology

The bladder is typically enlarged and distorted. Like the ureter, its walls are thickened with connective tissue interspersed between sparse muscle layers.[61] At times, the muscular deficiency is so severe that portions of the bladder bulge under pressure and act like diverticula. Trabeculations are unusual, and muscular hypertrophy is absent even in rare cases in which outlet obstruction is also present.[62] The trigone is usually large and asymmetric, with ureteral orifices laterally positioned at its distal extent. Ureteral ectopia accounts for the high incidence of reflux.[63]

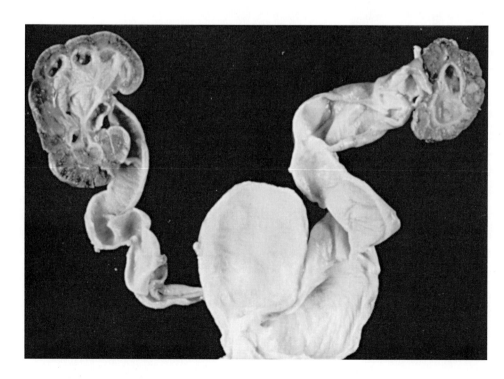

Figure 60–3. Postmortem specimen of a newborn with prune-belly syndrome and severe pulmonary hypoplasia shows dilated ureters having thickened walls. Both kidneys demonstrated renal dysplasia. (Courtesy of C. Galiani, MD.)

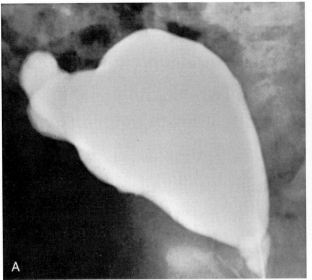

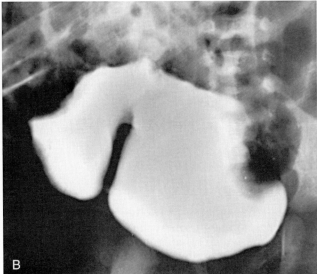

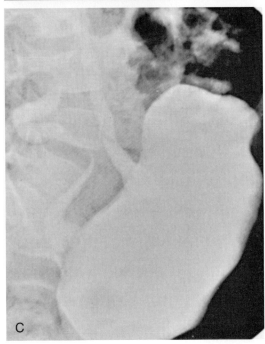

Figure 60–4. Radiographic examples of a typically large, misshapen prune-belly syndrome bladder. *A*, Fixation to the umbilicus by urachal remnants is evident. *B*, "Waisting" of the bladder dome during voiding results in pseudodiverticulum. *C*, Vesicoureteral reflux is present in most cases.

Radiographic Findings

Voiding cystourethrography usually shows a large misshapen bladder (Fig. 60–4). A patent urachus is sometimes present at the dome and commonly occurs in cases of urethral atresia, providing a "pop-off" for the obstructed bladder.[56] Fixation of the bladder to the umbilicus via urachal remnants creates an hourglass shape as detrusor contractions produce a waist-like effect during voiding. This muscular action can exclude the dome from the emptying process, causing it to act like a pseudodiverticulum. The bladder neck is usually wide open during voiding, and its junction with the dilated and triangular prostatic urethra is poorly defined. This configuration contrasts sharply with the findings of urethral valves and other outlet obstructions, in which the bladder neck is narrowed from muscular hypertrophy above the dilated prostatic urethra.

Clinical Correlates

A few patients with PBS have relatively normal urodynamics, with normal flow rates, voiding pressures, and complete bladder emptying. A larger group exhibits abnormal voiding dynamics with delayed sensation to void and increased volumes caused by reflux and reduced contractility. Despite this, nearly half can spontaneously void to completion. The remainder are found with an imbalance between intravesical voiding pressures and outflow resistance.[64] Significant postvoid residuals result. In some cases, voiding patterns improve with age. In others, an increase in residual urine or decompensation with an inability to void occurs.[65, 66] Upper urinary tract deterioration is more likely with significantly abnormal bladder dynamics. Elevated resting pressures and residual urine impair the emptying of already compromised ureters. Intermittent catheterization is a simple and effective means of facilitating bladder emptying. Surgery to improve bladder mechanics is less successful. Partial cystectomy only transiently lessens volume in most cases.

PROSTATE AND PROSTATIC URETHRA

Pathophysiology

Generalized hypoplasia of the prostatic epithelium occurs, although some scantily distributed acinar tissue remains. Tubules may be present in the posterior portion of the gland, but fibrous tissue replaces its anterior portion, where smooth muscle normally predominates.[67, 68] This loss of muscular support causes the dilated configuration of the gland and is implicated in the "functional obstruction" theory proposed for PBS.[69] The verumontanum can be completely absent or sometimes takes on a dimpled configuration.

Radiographic Findings

The prostatic urethra is classically wide and elongated at the bladder neck and tapers at the level of the urogenital diaphragm (Fig. 60–5).[10, 67] Prominent posterior bulging is seen, and utricular diverticula are common. The triangular appearance of the gland can mimic that of posterior urethral valves. Valves have been described with PBS, but their presence represents a coincidence rather than an association.[70]

Clinical Correlates

The discrepancy between the caliber of the prostatic and membranous urethras gives the erroneous impression of mechanical obstruction. Urethral obstructions (atresia, stenosis, diverticulum, diaphragm, and valves) were found in one third of cases in one series. However, an origin entirely different from that of classic posterior urethral valves could usually be implicated.[26] Urodynamics have consistently failed to document functional outlet obstruction in most patients, although in utero obstructions remain a possibility.[7, 32, 71] Cystoscopy occasionally reveals redundant folds of mucosa that can occlude the anterior membranous urethra as the prostatic urethra distends. These are labeled "type IV valves" or "pseudovalves" and should be resected at the 12-o'clock position. Improved bladder emptying does not uniformly occur, however, depending on the quality of detrusor contractions.

ANTERIOR URETHRA

The anterior and penile urethra are usually normal, but atresia or significant hypoplasia occasionally occurs in the membranous or bulbar positions (18% in one series).[72] Urachal patency is required for survival. Extreme degrees of urethral ectasia are also seen, some of which may be progressively dilated with indwelling catheters.[73]

An association with both types of congenital *megalourethra* has also been documented (Fig. 60–6).[74]

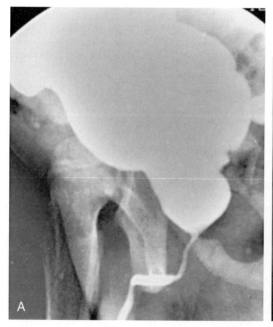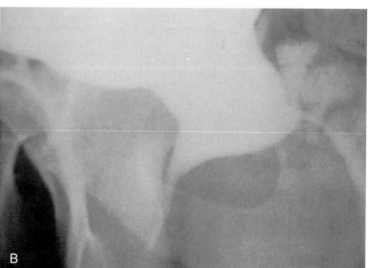

Figure 60–5. Voiding cystourethrography is instrumental to the diagnosis of prune-belly syndrome. *A,* Note wide open bladder neck and beak-like narrowing at the membranous urethra. *B,* Utricular diverticulum and posterior bulging are common. A smooth-walled bladder is present in each case.

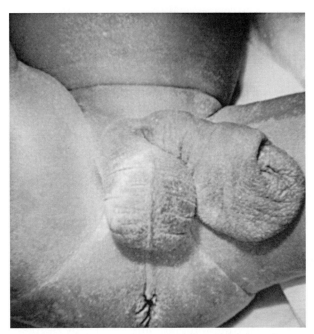

Figure 60–6. Gross appearance of scaphoid megalourethra in a child with prune-belly syndrome.

Scaphoid megalourethra, the less severe and more common variety, is found with an absent corpus spongiosum. *Fusiform* megalourethra is associated with absent corpora cavernosa.[75] Mild urethral dilations are frequent (as many as 70%), but clinically significant megalourethra is rare.[67] The converse is not true, however, with PBS being common in patients with megalourethra. In one review, nearly half of 26 patients with scaphoid megalourethra and all 5 with fusiform variants had PBS.[76] When necessary, the principles of hypospadias repair are used to excise redundant urethra and reconstruct its lumen to normal caliber. In rare instances, a vesicostomy is necessary to vent the bladder until the urethra can be corrected.

☐ Associated Nonurologic Anomalies

Nonurologic problems are found in as many as three fourths of patients with PBS.[77] The deformities of the extremities and pulmonary hypoplasia are directly related to the problems noted with the urinary tract and the insult of oligohydramnios. PBS continues to be reported with other malformations in smaller series or case reports in which coincidental associations probably exist or some etiologic significance has been postulated.[78–81]

GASTROINTESTINAL

The GI malformation most commonly seen with PBS is *malrotation* secondary to universal mesentery and unattached cecum.[82] In theory, decreased intraabdominal pressures fail to seat the colon against the posterior abdominal wall, thus delaying or preventing the fusion of its dorsal mesentery. An incidence of 40% has been cited.[83] Clinically significant malrotation with its sequelae of obstruction and volvulus is less common. Some clinicians have recommended routine radiographic evaluations of the GI tract to assess the relative risks.[84]

Other GI anomalies reported with PBS include atresia of the colon and small intestine, gastroschisis, splenic torsion, persistent cloaca, omphalocele, and paucity of intralobar bile ducts.[79, 84–88] Hirschsprung's disease has also been described.[89] Historically, aganglionosis was considered a factor in the urinary dilation of PBS.[90] The theory was later disproved when studies showed normal distribution of ureteral ganglion cells.[7, 91]

Functional "megacolon" does occur, however, and chronic constipation from the lack of abdominal wall musculature poses a formidable problem. Imperforate anus and rectal atresia also occur, usually in more severely affected patients who have urethral atresia.[92] Diverting colostomy is required in the case of high imperforate anus, rectourinary fistula, or pelvic hypoplasia. Abdominal wall laxity can challenge the placement of an ostomy and fitting of an appliance.[41]

CARDIAC

Any child born with PBS requires a thorough assessment of cardiovascular status. Cardiovascular anomalies occur in approximately 10% of PBS cases, in which such anomalies may represent the manifestation of a common embryogenetic insult.[93] Patent ductus arteriosus and atrial and ventricular septal defects are the most common. Tetralogy of Fallot also occurs.

MUSCULOSKELETAL

Musculoskeletal abnormalities of the lower extremities have been reported in one third to one half of patients with PBS.[26, 77, 94] The majority of these abnormalities are the aftermath of in utero compression. Talipes, scoliosis, and congenitally dislocated hips are the most common, requiring orthopedic management. Milder manifestations include dimples of the elbows and knees. Other malformations include polydactylism and arthrogryposis.[10, 83, 95] Compression of the iliac vessels by a distended bladder are implicated in patients with hypoplasia of a limb.

PULMONARY

The importance of the kidneys to pulmonary development is underscored by the respiratory findings with PBS. In one series of neonatal autopsies, pulmonary hypoplasia was the cause of death in 30% of cases.[26] Newborns with pulmonary hypoplasia who survive and those with milder forms of the syndrome remain susceptible to episodes of recurrent pneumonia and lobar atelectasis. The latter is secondary to the musculoskeletal disorder rather than parenchymal disease. Elements of gas trapping and restrictive lung disease have been shown.[96] Exercise limitation also occurs, and pulmonary function testing has demonstrated decreased expiratory pressure, low work rates, and decreased V_{O_2} in most cases.[97] The defect in pulmonary toilet undoubtedly increases the risk of postoperative pulmonary complications.[42, 98]

Flaring of the costal margins and other chest wall deformities routinely accompany PBS. Pectus carinatum is also common, and kyphoscoliosis results from the lack of a counterbalance to the paraspinous muscles. Chest radiographs routinely show flattening of the diaphragms, flaring of the rib cage, and drawing in of the lower sternum. Other findings might include rare congenital cystic adenomatoid malformation or pneumomediastinum and pneumothorax as harbingers of hypoplastic lungs.[99]

☐ Clinical Presentations and Evaluation

ANTENATAL DIAGNOSIS

The use of antenatal US has obvious implications for the fetus with PBS. The bladder and kidneys can be appreciated by 14 to 16 weeks of gestation. The findings of dilated ureters, enlarged bladder, and flaccid abdominal wall may denote the presence of PBS.[100] Although in utero intervention has been used, the enthusiasm for these types of efforts has since waned for the following reasons[37, 101]:

1. The diagnostic validity of prenatal US is suboptimal. False-positive and false-negative assessments of obstructive uropathy are common.[102-104] Disorders that can mimic PBS include urethral valves, megacystis-microcolon-hypoperistalsis syndrome, high-grade reflux, hydrocolpos, gastroschisis, and omphalocele.
2. The presence of urinary tract dilation may not imply significant obstruction. This concept is probably more true of the low-pressure collecting systems of PBS than those of any other urinary tract abnormality.[105]
3. Ectatic changes in the urinary tract are usually not detectable until after significant embryologic insult has occurred. This would negate the benefit of later decompression.[106, 107]

Serial assessment of the fetus with presumed PBS should be done on a regular basis. In rare instances, dystocia presents an indication for urinary tract decompression, or the interval development of oligohydramnios warrants early delivery or antenatal intervention.[101] Termination of pregnancy can be considered in cases with severe renal dysplasia. The testing of urinary electrolytes and enzymatic assays of tubular damage can also be done.

POSTNATAL DIAGNOSIS
Initial Assessment

The diagnosis of PBS is suspected in any newborn with abdominal wall laxity and nonpalpable testes. The presence of oligohydramnios is also suggestive. Examination reveals many of the stigmata of the syndrome, including the thin, wrinkled abdominal wall that allows easy palpation of the viscera. Urologic involvement rarely represents an emergency, but surveys of the *nonurologic systems* affected by PBS are necessary. Radiographs of the chest are obtained to assess pulmonary development and to rule out pneumothorax or pneumomediastinum. The anus, rectum, and heart are also examined.

Early Observation

The newborn with PBS is closely monitored during the first few days of life, with particular attention being paid to respiratory function. Serial analyses of renal function gradually reflect the degree of renal dysplasia and functional capacity after a few days. Frequent urine cultures are also obtained. The urinary stream should be normal, but suprapubic bladder massage can be used to facilitate bladder drainage. Prophylactic antibiotics are given before radiologic instrumentation and are continued when significant degrees of hydroureteronephrosis or reflux are present.

Radiographic Studies

Urinary US is recommended as an initial study to provide information about renal differentiation, the severity of hydroureteronephrosis, and the quality of the bladder. *Voiding cystourethrography* remains instrumental to the diagnosis and helps identify reflux and bladder outlet obstruction while giving some idea of bladder dynamics. Both studies are done during the first few days of life.

Functional imaging with nuclear scintigraphy is typically deferred for several weeks, allowing for the changes of transitional renal physiology to improve the quality of the study. Scans in newborns have less validity in quantifying obstruction, especially when renal dysplasia or significant hydronephrosis is present. Premature evaluations of the kidneys tend to confuse the picture in systems that are almost always nonobstructive.

☐ Management

The clinical implications of PBS occur as a spectrum, like most other syndromes. Variability between the degrees of abdominal wall laxity, hydroureteronephrosis, and renal dysplasia are expected. Attempts to classify children with these conditions to perhaps standardize their management have been of equivocal value owing to this variability (Table

TABLE 60–2. Classification Scheme for
Prune-Belly Syndrome*

Category 1

Pulmonary hypoplasia or pneumothorax
Oligohydramnios
Renal dysplasia
Possible urethral obstruction or patent urachus
Club feet
Stillborn or limited survival

Category 2

Typical prune-belly syndrome external features, such as lax
    abdominal muscles
Uropathy of full-blown syndrome with diffuse
    hydroureteronephrosis
Renal dysplasia common but less severe than in Category 1
Urosepsis or gradual azotemia may or may not develop

Category 3

External prune-belly syndrome features mild or incomplete
Less severe uropathy
Normal renal function
Little or no urologic reconstructive surgery needed

*Classification scheme proposed for prune-belly syndrome demonstrates
the difficulty categorizing patients, especially when the category relates to
treatment, which must be individualized.

60–2).[6, 14] Instead, the urologic management of PBS
must be individualized.

After delivery, the affected infant's immediate
prognosis is dictated by his or her pulmonary status.
Newborns with significant renal impairment are
born with pulmonary hypoplasia. Stillborn delivery
or death soon after delivery can be expected of
most.[61, 77] For others, adequate amounts of amniotic
fluid have been present in utero, and pulmonary
development is acceptable. Instead, the infant's
long-term prognosis depends on his or her renal
status. Two factors must be considered: the first is
the magnitude of irreversible renal dysplasia, and
the second is the degree of damage that the kidneys
incur from recurrent infections or, less commonly,
unrecognized obstruction. These are generally
avoidable and become the focus of radiologic surveillance and any therapy, medical or surgical, that
might be recommended.

CONTROVERSIES IN MANAGEMENT

How to best preserve renal function in children
with PBS remains the subject of debate. Some clinicians advocate an aggressive surgical approach, believing that the benefits of complete urinary reconstruction outweigh its technical and anesthetic
risks.[108–111] In theory, eliminating reflux and urinary
stasis should decrease the incidence of infection
and progressive renal parenchymal damage. But, although radiographic appearance is often improved,
it remains unclear as to whether the operative effort
makes a significant difference. In one series, for
example, serum creatinine and ureteral configuration remained stable, but only 33% of the patients
were rendered free of recurrent urinary tract infec-

tion (UTI).[112] In addition, despite these efforts,
chronic renal failure develops in a significant number of children, especially those with impaired function at presentation.[77] These types of findings have
led proponents of a minimally invasive approach to
contend that the management of the hydronephrosis
and reflux of PBS is different from that in other
disorders.[10, 43, 113, 114]

We recommend surgical intervention when management with prophylactic antibiotics and observation is unsuccessful in preserving renal function
and preventing bacteriuria. Other clinicians, using
a similar approach and having more than 30 years'
follow-up in some cases, reported stable serum creatinine in 75% of patients who had normal renal
function as newborns (Fig. 60–7).[43] Ureteral function
and flow improves in many patients who receive
nonoperative treatment.[115] Some proponents of conservative treatment contend that tapering the PBS
ureter decreases caliber but does not improve peristalsis and drainage owing to intrinsic muscular deficiencies.[58, 116] In any case, unless functional deterioration results from refractory infection, little
evidence exists to suggest that surgical intervention
improves renal function in patients with PBS (Fig.
60–8). These concepts in management are no different than those used with primary vesicoureteral reflux.

It requires patience to refrain from addressing
some of these impressively distorted urinary tracts,
especially during the neonatal period. At times, the
results of extensive reconstruction, which include
tapered reimplantation of megaureters combined
with reduction cystoplasty as well as orchiopexy,
can be impressive.[111] However, the following should
be remembered:

1. A surgical procedure cannot reverse renal dysplasia
2. These low-pressure systems result from ureteral smooth muscle deficiency rather than obstruction
3. The technical and anesthetic challenges presented by PBS urinary tract are not without
risk[117]

☐ Infection

The aim of any form of therapy, medical or surgical, is directed toward keeping the child infection-
free. The importance of UTIs to the prognosis is
underscored by the description of renal insufficiency in 8 of 19 children with PBS who survived
the perinatal period. Nephrectomy specimens
showed dysplastic changes in only 25% of the renal
parenchyma. Instead, reflux nephropathy and
chronic pyelonephritis were largely involved in
most cases.[53] Antibiotics are required in neonates
and on a long-term basis to prevent damage. UTIs
disrupt a delicate balance that exists in many of
these urinary tracts. Endotoxins from gram-negative
organisms can impair ureteral peristalsis and blad-

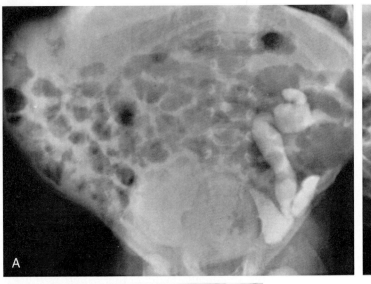

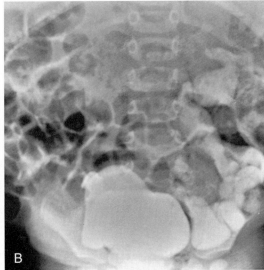

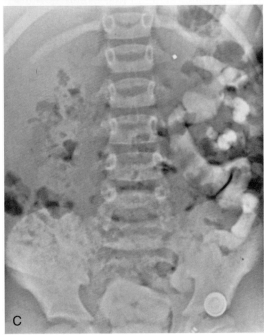

Figure 60–7. Child with prune-belly syndrome having large bladder, solitary left kidney, and no reflux managed with observation alone. *A,* Excretory urogram of the newborn. *B,* Radiographic appearance at 2 years of age. *C,* Appearance at 7 years of age. Renal function remained normal (creatinine level of 1.1). Note the lessening ureteral tortuosity with continued development.

der emptying, causing further dilation and stasis. Once begun, UTIs in PBS can be difficult to eradicate without facilitating drainage and, even then, can be difficult to treat.

DIVERSION AND DRAINAGE

The status of the kidneys and the dynamics of the urinary tract become readily apparent during the first months of life. Deteriorating renal function is usually caused by dysplasia, a finding that can be confirmed by renal biopsy, if necessary. Adequate drainage becomes the critical factor for a small subset of newborns with urethral obstruction or for patients of any age with recalcitrant infections. A number of techniques can be used to vent the urinary tract, each with its own drawbacks. Application is selective. Otherwise, urinary dynamics can

be disrupted so that obligate surgical reconstruction is required of a system that might not need it.

Percutaneous Nephrostomy

Tubes occasionally provide temporary drainage or are used to assess nadir renal function.[118] If improvement in renal function occurs with proximal decompression, a case can be made for more permanently diverting or reconstructing the collecting system. Otherwise, surgical drainage does not make a difference.

Pyelostomy

Pyelostomy is reserved for the renal pelvis that is so redundant that a more distal diversion might not provide adequate drainage.[119] This diversion pro-

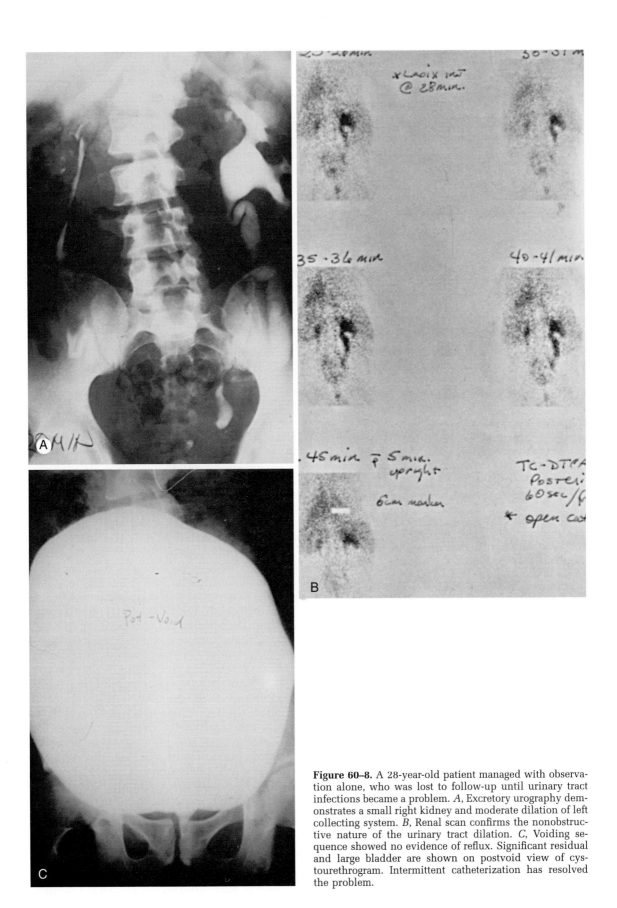

Figure 60–8. A 28-year-old patient managed with observation alone, who was lost to follow-up until urinary tract infections became a problem. *A*, Excretory urography demonstrates a small right kidney and moderate dilation of left collecting system. *B*, Renal scan confirms the nonobstructive nature of the urinary tract dilation. *C*, Voiding sequence showed no evidence of reflux. Significant residual and large bladder are shown on postvoid view of cystourethrogram. Intermittent catheterization has resolved the problem.

vides optimal drainage and preserves the ureteral blood supply crucial to the success of later undiversion.[120]

Cutaneous Ureterostomy

Ureterostomy is useful only when proximal diversion is preferred but the renal pelvis is too small to create a pyelostomy. The technique can jeopardize ureteral vascularity and compromise the more anatomically normal proximal ureter. Proximal stomas are difficult to fit with an appliance after open drainage to diapers is no longer tolerated.

Vesicostomy

Vesicostomy usually provides adequate drainage. Concerns that upper tract drainage is ineffective are unfounded.[115] We have noted that the ureteral decompression in PBS does not occur to the same degree as that with vesicostomy for truly obstructive uropathy, probably owing to intrinsic myopathy and secondary dilation. The Blocksom technique is simple and effective, but a more generous stoma is made in PBS to help the bladder empty.[121] Stomal stenosis seems to be more of a problem and revisions are occasionally necessary. No collection devices are worn, and closure is simply done around the age of toilet training. Concerns that creation of a vesicostomy adversely alters bladder dynamics are unfounded.

DETRUSOR DYNAMICS

As an alternative to diversion, some procedures are directed at improving the dynamics of bladder emptying. Two such techniques, reduction cystoplasty and urethrotomy, have been met with mixed enthusiasm.

Reduction Cystoplasty

Laplace's law supports the belief that decreasing the size of a misshapen, enlarged bladder might improve its emptying.[122] This seems truer of bladders distorted by urachal pseudodiverticula that are excluded from the emptying process. Fluoroscopy helps assess this possibility. Reduction cystoplasty is rarely, if ever, indicated as a primary procedure but is often routinely done with ureteral reconstruction.[111] When reduction cystoplasty seems appropriate, a variety of different techniques can be used, including domectomy with midline bladder reapproximation, detrusor plication, and mucosal excision with pants-over-vest approximation of the underlying detrusor.[57, 113] Paired pedicle flaps of rectus muscle to augment emptying have also been tried.[123] The gradual reappearance of bladder ectasia is common, however, despite a reduction that seems successful early after surgery.

Urethrotomy (Sphincterotomy)

Incising the urethra can decrease outlet resistance in some children, despite the fact that the external sphincter and urethra are usually normal. In theory, weakened detrusor contractions are unable to overcome membranous and bulbous urethral elasticity. Unbalanced voiding results.[64] Urodynamic improvement and reduction in residual urine after urethrotomy have been reported, but the technique carries the risk of sphincter damage and, with it, urinary incontinence.[66, 124]

Medical Management

Intermittent catheterization has assumed a primary role in the management of PBS when bladder emptying is a problem. In most children, significant UTIs are not increased by such manipulation. Some boys have trouble with the technique owing to discomfort. When this is the case, a continent vesicostomy should be considered.

MEGAURETER REVISION

The decision to correct the megaureters found with PBS is based either on recurrent UTIs resulting from reflux or on obstruction. The severity of reflux alone does not serve as a criterion for its correction, unlike reflux in normal subjects. Successful revision of a megaureter depends on achieving a balance between inadequate reduction, which leads to recurrent reflux, and excessive tailoring, which potentially leads to stenosis and obstruction. The challenge of working with the dysgenetic ureter and recipient bladder of PBS is not taken lightly. One report describes ureterovesical junction obstruction in 6 of 15 patients who required megaureter revision and persistent reflux in 4 others.[110]

When correction is required, meticulous technique, minimal handling, and preservation of periureteral vascularity are crucial. Poorly functioning, ectatic distal ureter should be discarded. Healthy proximal ureter is used in reconstruction. Mobilization of the kidneys is sometimes necessary to eliminate unsuitable ureter and enable a tension-free anastomosis to the bladder. Imbrication can be used to tailor the less dilated megaureter with little risk to the vascularity. However, the more dilated megaureter requires the traditional excisional method to eliminate the bulk that results with plication. *Transureteroureterostomy* is an ideal option when both ureters require revision. Reimplantation is done by relying on the best ureter being repositioned into the abnormal bladder.[108]

ABDOMINOPLASTY

The management of the abdominal wall abnormality varies according to its severity. Solutions range from braces and corsets to a variety of surgical procedures aimed at improving cosmesis and optimiz-

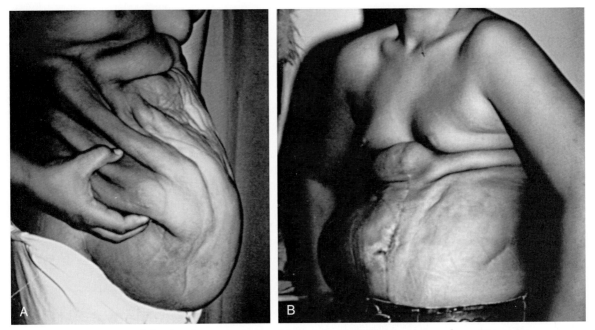

Figure 60–9. Abdominoplasty—vertical revision. *A,* Preoperative appearance shows impressive distortion of abdominal wall in a teenager. *B,* Postoperative appearance, although not perfect, shows significant improvement.

ing function of whatever normal musculature remains. Vertical abdominal wall revisions can be successful, although some patients see their laxity return after seemingly successful early results.[10, 125] A midline incision with skin revision that allows a double-breasted plication of the fascia may improve outcomes (Fig. 60–9).[126] Another novel modification includes resection of the poorly developed lateral musculofascial segments adjacent to the umbilicus and midline rectus muscles, which are preserved as an island (Fig. 60–10).[127] Loss of the umbilicus has occurred in our hands and tailoring of the redundant skin still presents a problem.

The results with smile-like incisions that extend from one costovertebral area to the other have been encouraging.[38] This approach permits excision of the most severely affected musculature and creates a waist for the patient that allows for more normal-fitting of clothes. The cosmetic result is good but not perfect (Fig. 60–11) with this technique as with the others. Nevertheless, the psychological and cosmetic benefits of abdominoplasty outweigh its risks in children with PBS and is usually recommended. Excellent exposure is provided if other urinary reconstruction is planned. In addition, improved voiding efficiency with decreased postvoid residuals has been shown after successful abdominoplasty.[128] Wound healing is not compromised by the abnormal composition of the abdominal wall.

ORCHIOPEXY

The role and timing of orchiopexy remain somewhat controversial. Regardless of the normal histology of the gonads early in development, correcting gonadal position has not been shown to make a difference in sperm-forming potential. Despite this bleak outlook for fertility, we advocate orchiopexy at an early age to maximize gonadal development, enable surveillance of malignancy, and provide psychological benefit.

There are technical advantages to performing orchiopexy during the neonatal period, often in concert with abdominoplasty, vesicostomy, or urinary tract reconstructions.[112] The flaccid abdomen offers excellent exposure of the retroperitoneum and easy mobilization of the testes, whose vascular and vasal mesentery are typically long and lax. Dependent scrotal position can be achieved without ligating the testicular vessels. Success rates of nearly 90% have been described in children younger than 2 years of age.[110] However, a group of high intraabdominal testes remain, especially in older boys, which have insufficient cord length to reach the scrotum. In this case, the Fowler-Stephens method is used by dividing the spermatic vessels and mobilizing the testicle on peritoneum containing the vessels of the vas deferens.[129] Success rates with the Fowler-Stevens maneuver of nearly 80% have been reported.[130]

☐ Future Trends

Historically, the mortality rates of infants born with PBS have been as high as 20% during early infancy and 50% during the first 2 years of life. Pulmonary complications accounted for many of the early deaths. Renal failure or sepsis was responsible for most later deaths.[91, 131–133] Some clinicians had attributed this grave outlook in part to conservative

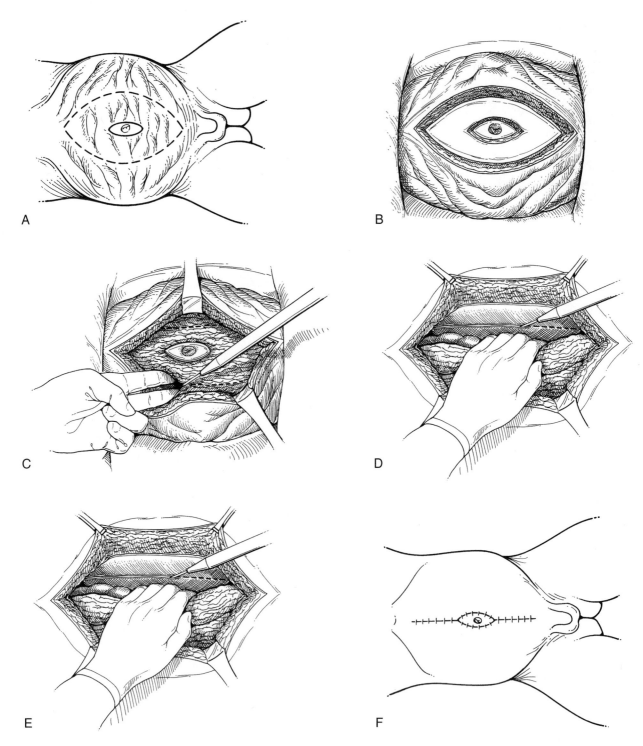

Figure 60–10. Monfort abdominoplasty. *A,* Skin incisions circumscribe umbilicus and define areas of adjacent abdominal wall redundancy to be removed. *B,* Excision of skin (epidermis and dermis alone) using electrocautery. *C,* Abdominal wall central plate incised at lateral borders of the rectus muscle on either side, creating a central musculofascial plate. *D,* The parietal peritoneum overlying the lateral abdominal wall musculature is scored with electrocautery. *E,* Edges of the central plate are sutured along the scored line. *F,* Excess skin removed and midline approximation envelops previously isolated umbilicus. (From Woodward JR, Perez LM: Prune-belly syndrome. In Marshall FF [ed]: Operative Urology. Philadelphia, WB Saunders, 1996.)

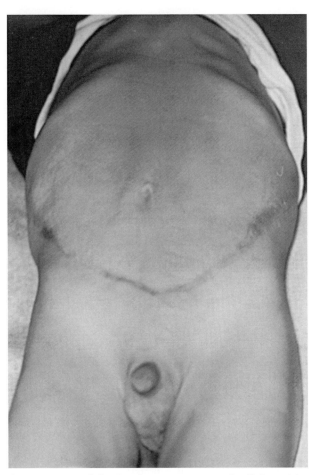

Figure 60–11. Abdominoplasty—transverse "smile" revision. Postoperative appearance in older child.

medical treatment.[134] Others implicated excessive surgical intervention.[6]

Increased survival rate and longevity appear to be the trend, regardless of whether the treating physician takes a conservative or aggressive approach with the syndrome. This undoubtedly stems from a better understanding of the natural history of PBS, earlier identification of its accompanying problems, and improved medical and surgical methods for its treatment. The management controversy will continue and new techniques could swing the therapeutic pendulum. Managing renal dysplasia in infants using peritoneal dialysis as a preempt to transplantation is a typical example. If affected children are nurtured to a suitable age, organ transplantation is not adversely affected by the syndrome.[135] Earlier identification, in utero management, and futuristic medicine raise new ethical and socioeconomic issues that are yet to be resolved. In any event, the outlook for the child born with PBS is much brighter than it has been in the past.

ACKNOWLEDGMENT

We would like to acknowledge the many contributions of the late John Duckett to our understanding of the pathogenesis and treatment of prune-belly syndrome. Many of the ideas presented herein are John's.

REFERENCES

1. Parker RW: Case of an infant in whom some of the abdominal muscles were absent. Trans Clin Soc London 28:201, 1895.
2. Osler W: Congenital absence of the abdominal muscle, with distended and hypertrophied urinary bladder. Bull Johns Hopkins Hospital 12:331–333, 1901.
3. Williams DI, Burkholder GV: The prune belly syndrome. J Urol 98:244–251, 1967.
4. Eagle JF, Barrett GS: Congenital deficiency of abdominal musculature with associated genitourinary abnormalities: A syndrome–reports of 9 cases. Pediatrics 6:721–736, 1950.
5. Ives EJ: The abdominal muscle deficiency triad syndrome—experience with ten cases. In Bergsma D (ed): Birth Defects: Original Series. Baltimore, Williams & Wilkins, 1974, pp 127–137.
6. Welch KJ, Kearney GP: Abdominal musculature deficiency syndrome: Prune-belly. J Urol 11:693–700, 1974.
7. Nunn IN, Stephens FD: The triad syndrome: A composite anomaly of the abdominal wall, urinary system, and testes. J Urol 86:782–794, 1961.
8. Rabinowitz R, Schillinger JF: Prune belly syndrome in the female subject. J Urol 118:454–456, 1977.
9. Aaronson IA, Cremin BJ: Prune belly syndrome in young females. Urol Radiol 1:151, 1980.
10. Bellah RD, States LJ, Duckett JW: Pseudoprune-belly syndrome: Imaging findings and clinical outcome. AJR Am J Roentgenol 167:1389–1393, 1996.
11. Garlinger P, Ott J: Prune belly syndrome—possible genetic implications. Birth Defects 10:173–180, 1974.
12. Baird PA, MacDonald EC: An epidemiologic study of congenital malformations of the anterior abdominal wall in more than half a million consecutive live births. Am J Hum Genet 33:470–478, 1981.
13. Goulding FG, Garrett RA: Twenty-five year experience with prune belly syndrome. Urology 12:329–332, 1978.
14. Woodard JR: The prune belly syndrome. Urol Clin North Am 5:75–93, 1978.
15. Adeyokunnu AA, Familusi JB: Prune belly syndrome in two siblings and a first cousin. Am J Dis Child 136:23–25, 1982.
16. Gaboardi F, Sterpa A, Thiebat E, et al: Prune-belly syndrome: Report of three siblings. Helv Paediatr Acta 37:283–288, 1982.
17. Riccardi VM, Grum CM: The prune-belly syndrome: Heterogeneity and superficial X-linkage mimicry. J Med Genet 14:266, 1977.
18. Harley LM, Chen Y, Rattner WH: Prune belly syndrome. J Urol 108:174–176, 1972.
19. Beckman H, Rehder H, Rauskolb R: Prune belly sequence associated with trisomy 13 [letter to the editor]. Am J Med Genet 19:603–604, 1984.
20. Frydman M, Magenis RE, Mohandas TK, et al: Chromosome abnormalities in infants with prune belly anomaly: Association with trisomy 18. Am J Med Genet 15:145–148, 1983.
21. Lubinsky M, Doyle K, Trunca C: The association of "prune-belly" with Turner's syndrome. Am J Dis Child 134:1171–1172, 1980.
22. Halbrecht I, Komlos L, Shabtai F: Prune belly syndrome with chromosomal fragment. Am J Dis Child 123:518, 1972.
23. Greskovich FJ III, Nyberg Jr LM: The prune-belly syndrome: A review of its etiology, defects, treatment, and prognosis. J Urol 140:707–712, 1988.
24. Stephens FD: Morphology and embryogenesis of the triad. In Stephens FD (ed): Congenital Malformations of the Urinary Tract. New York, Praeger, 1983, pp 485–511.
25. Bruton OC: Agenesis of abdominal musculature with genitourinary and gastrointestinal tract anomalies. J Urol 66:607–611, 1951.
26. Wigger HJ, Blanc WA: The prune belly syndrome. Pathol Ann 12:17–39, 1977.

27. Minninberg DT, Mantoya F, Okada, K, et al: Subcellular muscle studies in the prune belly syndrome. J Urol 109:524–526, 1973.

28. Smith DW: Recognizable Patterns of Human Malformations. Philadelphia, WB Saunders, 1970, p 5.

29. Fallon B, Welton M, Hawtry C: Congenital anomalies associated with cryptorchidism. J Urol 127:91–93, 1982.

30. Gonzalez R, Reinberg Y, Burke B, et al: Early bladder outlet obstruction in fetal lambs induces renal dysplasia and the prune-belly syndrome. J Pediatr Surg 25:342–345, 1990.

31. Moerman P, Fryns J, Goddeeris P, et al: Pathogenesis of the prune-belly syndrome: A functional urethral obstruction caused by prostatic hypoplasia. Pediatrics 73:470–475, 1984.

32. Pagon RA, Smith DW, Shepard TH: Urethral obstruction malformation complex: A cause of abdominal muscle deficiency and the "prune belly." J Pediatr 94:900–906, 1979.

33. Burton BK, Dillard RG: Brief clinical report: Prune belly syndrome: Observations supporting the hypothesis of abdominal overdistension. Am J Med Genet 17:669–672, 1984.

34. Fitzsimons RB, Keohane C, Galvin J: Prune-belly syndrome with ultrasound demonstration of reduction of megacystis in utero. Br J Radiol 58:374–376, 1985.

35. Monie IW, Monie BJ: Prune belly syndrome and fetal ascites. Teratolgy 19:111–113, 1979.

36. Shapiro I, Sharf M: Spontaneous intrauterine remission of hydrops fetalis in one identical twin: Sonographic diagnosis. J Clin Ultrasound 13:427–430, 1985.

37. Nakayama KD, Harrison MR, Chinn DH, et al: The pathogenesis of prune belly. Am J Dis Child 138:834–836, 1984.

38. Randolph J, Cavett C, Eng G: Surgical correction and rehabilitation for children with "prune-belly" syndrome. Ann Surg 193:757–762, 1981.

39. Housden LG: Congenital absence of the abdominal muscles. Arch Dis Child 9:219–232, 1934.

40. Affi AK, Rebiez JM, Andonian SJ, et al: The myopathology of the prune belly syndrome. J Neurol Sci 15:153–165, 1972.

41. Aschraft KW: Prune belly syndrome. In Ashcraft KE (ed): Pediatric Urology. Philadelphia, WB Saunders, 1990, pp 257–267.

42. Karamanian A, Kravath R, Nagashima H, Gentsch HH: Anaesthetic management of "prune belly" syndrome. Br J Anaesthesiol 46:897–899, 1974.

43. Woodhouse CRJ, Ransley PG, Williams DI: Prune belly syndrome—report of 47 cases. Arch Dis Child 57:856–859, 1982.

44. Orvis BR, Bottles K, Kogan BA: Testicular histology in fetuses with the prune belly syndrome and posterior urethral valves. J Urol 139:335, 1988.

45. Massad CA, Cohen MB, Kogan BA, et al: Morphology and histochemistry of infant testes in the prune belly syndrome. J Urol 146:1598, 1991.

46. Woodhouse CRJ, Snyder HM: Testicular and sexual function in adults with prune belly syndrome. J Urol 133:607–609, 1985.

47. Tayakkanonta K: The gubernaculum testis and its nerve supply. Aust N Z J Surg 33:61–68, 1963.

48. Woodard JR, Parrott TS: Orchiopexy in the prune belly syndrome. Br J Urol 50:348–351, 1978.

49. Asplund J, Laska J: Prune belly syndrome at the age of 37. Scand J Urol Nephrol 9:297–300, 1975.

50. Woodhouse CRJ, Ransley PG: Teratoma of the testis in the prune belly syndrome. Br J Urol 55:580–581, 1983.

51. Sayre R, Stephens R, Chonko AM: Prune belly syndrome and retroperitoneal germ cell tumor. Am J Med 81:895–897, 1986.

52. Schwarz RD, Stephens FD, Cussen LJ: The pathogenesis of renal dysplasia, II: The significance of lateral and medial ectopy of the ureteric orifice. Invest Urol 19:97–100, 1981.

53. Manivel JC, Pettinata G, Reinberg Y, et al: Prune belly syndrome: Clinicopathologic study of 29 cases. Pediatr Pathol 9:691–711, 1989.

54. Snow BW, Duckett JW: The prune belly syndrome. In Retik AB, Cukier J (eds): Pediatric Urology. Baltimore, Williams & Wilkins, 1987, pp 253–270.

55. Potter EL: Abnormal development of the kidney. In Potter EL (ed): Normal and Abnormal Development of the Kidney. Chicago, Year Book Medical, 1972, pp 154–220.

56. Rogers LW, Ostrow PT: The prune belly syndrome. Report of 20 cases and description of a lethal variant. J Pediatr 83:786–793, 1973.

57. Hanna MK, Jeffs RD, Sturgess JM, et al: Ureteral structure and ultrastructure. Part III. The congenitally dilated ureter (megaureter). J Urol 117:24–27, 1977.

58. Palmer JM, Tesluk H: Ureteral pathology in the prune belly syndrome. J Urol 111:701–707, 1974.

59. Ehrlich RM, Brown WJ: Ultrastructural anatomic observations of the ureter in the prune-belly syndrome. Birth Defects 13:101–103, 1977.

60. Gearhart JP, Lee Br, Partin AW, et al: A quantitative histological evaluation of the dilated ureter of childhood, II: Ectopia, posterior urethral valves and the prune belly syndrome. J Urol 153:172–176, 1995.

61. Berdon WE, Baker DH, Wigger HJ, et al: The radiologic and pathologic spectrum of the prune belly syndrome. Radiol Clin North Am 15:83–92, 1977.

62. Stephens FD: Idiopathic dilatations of the urinary tract. J Urol 112:819–822, 1974.

63. Mackie GG, Stephens FD: A correlation of renal dysplasia with position of the ureteral orifice. J Urol 114:274–280, 1975.

64. Snyder HM, Harrison NW, Whitfield HN, et al: Urodynamics in the prune-belly syndrome. Br J Urol 48:663–670, 1976.

65. Lee ML: Prune-belly syndrome in a 54-year-old man. JAMA 237:2216–2217, 1977.

66. Kinahan TJ, Kravath R, Nagashima H, et al: The efficacy of bladder emptying in the prune belly syndrome. J Urol 148:600, 1992.

67. Kroovand RL, Al-Ansari RM, Perlmutter AD: Urethral and genital malformations in prune-belly syndrome. J Urol 127:94–96, 1982.

68. Deklerk DP, Scott WW: Prostatic maldevelopment in prune-belly syndrome: A defect in prostatic stromal-epithelial interaction. J Urol 120:341–344, 1978.

69. Popek EJ, Tyson RW, Miller GJ, et al: Prostate development in prune belly syndrome (PBS)—lower tract obstruction or primary mesenchymal defect? Pediatr Pathol 11:1, 1991.

70. Aaronson IA: Posterior urethral valve masquerading as the prune belly syndrome. Br J Urol 55:508–512, 1983.

71. Stephens FD, Gupta D: Pathogenesis of the prune belly syndrome. J Urol 152:2328, 1994.

72. Reinber Y, Chelimsky G, Gonzalez R: Urethral atresia and the prune belly syndrome: Report of 6 cases. Br J Urol 72:112–114, 1993.

73. Passerini-Glazel G, Araguna F, Chiozza L, et al: The PADUA (progressive augmentation by dilating the urethra anterior) procedure for the treatment of severe urethral hypoplasia. J Urol 140:1247–1250, 1988.

74. Sellers BB: Congenital megalourethra associated with prune belly syndrome. J Urol 116:814–815, 1976.

75. Stephens FD: Congenital Malformations of the Rectum, Anus, and Genitourinary Tracts. Edinburgh, Livingstone, 1963.

76. Shrom SH, Cromie WJ, Duckett JW: Megalourethra. Urology 17:152–156, 1981.

77. Geary DF, MacLusky IB, Churchill BM, et al: A broader spectrum of abnormalities in the prune belly syndrome. J Urol 135:324–326, 1986.

78. Lockhart JL, Reeve HR, Bredael JJ, et al: Siblings with prune belly syndrome and associated pulmonic stenosis, mental retardation, and deafness. Urology 14:140–142, 1978.

79. Short KL, Groff DB, Cook L: The concomitant presence of gastroschisis and prune belly syndrome in a twin. J Pediatr Surg 20:186–187, 1985.

80. Wilson SK, Moore GW, Hutchins GM: Congenital cystic adenomatoid malformation of the lung associated with abdominal musculature deficiency (prune belly). Pediatrics 62:421–424, 1978.

81. Shorey P, Lobo G: Ocular anomalies in abdominal deficiency syndrome. Am J Ophthalmol 108:193–194, 1989.

82. Silverman FM, Huang N: Congenital absence of the abdominal muscle associated with malformation of the genitourinary and alimentary tracts: Report of cases and review of literature. Am J Dis Child 80:91–124, 1950.
83. Metrick S, Brown RH, Rosenblum A: Congenital absence of the abdominal musculature and associated anomalies. Pediatrics 19:1043–1052, 1957.
84. Wright JR, Barth RF, Neff JC, et al: Gastrointestinal malformations associated with prune belly syndrome: Three cases and a review of the literature. Pediatr Pathol 5:421–448, 1986.
85. Potter EL, Craig JM: Pathology of the Fetus and the Infant (3rd ed). Chicago, Year Book Medical, 1975.
86. Teramoto R, Opas LM, Andrassy R: Splenic torsion with prune belly syndrome. J Pediatr 98:91–92, 1981.
87. Petersen DS, Fish L, Cass AS: Twins with congenital deficiency of abdominal musculature. J Urol 107:670–672, 1972.
88. Aanpreung P: Beckwith B, Gelansky SH, et al: Association of paucity of interlobular bile ducts with prune belly syndrome. J Pediatr Gastroenterol Nutr 16:81, 1993.
89. Cawthern TH, Bottene CA, Grant D: Prune-belly syndrome associated with Hirschsprung's disease. Am J Dis Child 133:652–653, 1979.
90. Henley WL, Hyman A: Absent abdominal musculature, genitourinary anomalies and deficiency in pelvic autonomic nervous system. Am J Dis Child 86:795–798, 1953.
91. McGovern JS, Marshall VF: Congenital deficiency of the abdominal musculature and obstructive uropathy. Surg Gynecol Obstet 108:289–305, 1959.
92. Morgan CL Jr, Grossman H, Novak R: Imperforate anus and colon calcification in association with prune belly syndrome. Pediatr Radiol 7:19–21, 1978.
93. Adebonojo FO: Dysplasia of the abdominal musculature with multiple congenital anomalies: Prune belly or triad syndrome. J Natl Med Assoc 65:327–333, 1973.
94. Loder RT, Guiboux J, Bloom DA, et al: Musculoskeletal aspects of prune-belly syndrome. Am J Dis Child 146:1224–1229, 1992.
95. Brinker MR, Palutsis RS, Sarwark JF: The orthopaedic manifestations of prune-belly (Eagle-Barrett) syndrome. J Bone Joint Surg Am 77:251–257, 1995.
96. Crompton CH, MacLusky IB, Geary DF: Respiratory function in the prune-belly syndrome. Arch Dis Child 68:505–506, 1993.
97. Ewig JM, Griscom NT, Wohl ME: The effect of the absence of abdominal muscles on pulmonary function and exercise. Am J Respir Crit Care Med 153:1314–1321, 1996.
98. HanningtonKiff JG: Prune-belly syndrome and general anesthesia. Br J Anaesthesiol 42:649–652, 1970.
99. Weber KJ, Rivard G, Perreault G: Prune belly syndrome associated with congenital cystic adenomatoid malformation of the lung. Am J Dis Child 132:316–317, 1978.
100. Shih W, Greenbaum LD, Baro C: In utero sonogram in prune belly syndrome. Urology 20:102–105, 1982.
101. Gadziala NA, Kavada CY, Doherty FJ, et al: Intrauterine decompression of megalocystis during the second trimester of pregnancy. Am J Obstet Gynecol 144:355–356, 1982.
102. Glazer GM, Filly RA, Callen PW: The varied sonographic appearance of the urinary tract in the fetus and newborn with urethral obstruction. Radiology 144:563–568, 1982.
103. Elder JS, Duckett JW, Snyder HM: Intervention for fetal obstructive uropathy. Has it been effective? Lancet 10:1007, 1987.
104. Clarke NW, Gough DCS, Cohen SJ: Neonatal urological ultrasound: Diagnostic inaccuracies and pitfalls. Arch Dis Child 64:578–580, 1989.
105. Keating MA: A different perspective of the perinatal primary megaureter. In Kramer SA (ed): Problems in Urology—Recent Advances in Pediatric Urology. Vol. 3. (No. 4). Philadelphia, JB Lippincott, 1990, pp 583–595.
106. Sholder AJ, Maizels M, Depp R, et al: Caution in antenatal intervention. J Urol 139:1026, 1988.
107. Freedman AL, Bukowski TP, Smith CA, et al: Fetal therapy for obstructive uropathy: Diagnosis specific outcomes. J Urol 156:720–723, 1996.
108. Hendren WH: Restoration of function in the severely decompensated ureter. In Johnson JH, Scholtmeijer RJ (eds): Problems in Paediatric Urology. Amsterdam, Excerpta Medica, 1972, pp 1–56.
109. Jeffs RD, Comisarow RH, Hanna MK: The early assessment for individualized treatment in the prune-belly syndrome. Birth Defects 13:97–99, 1977.
110. Fallat ME, Skoog SJ, Belman BA, et al: The prune belly syndrome: A comprehensive approach to management. J Urol 142:802–805, 1989.
111. Woodard JR, Zucker I: Current management of the dilated urinary tract in prune belly syndrome. Urol Clin North Am 17:407–418, 1990.
112. Woodard JR, Parrott TS: Reconstruction of the urinary tract in prune-belly uropathy. J Urol 119:824–828, 1978.
113. Williams DI, Parker RM: The role of surgery in the prune-belly syndrome. In Johnston JH, Goodwin WF (eds): Reviews of Pediatric Urology. Amsterdam, Excerpta Medica, 1974, pp 315–331.
114. Tank ED, McCoy G: Limited surgical intervention in the prune belly syndrome. J Pediatr Surg 18:688–691, 1983.
115. Duckett JW, Knutrud O, Hohenfellner R, et al: Prune belly syndrome. Dialogues Pediatr Urol 3, 1980.
116. Woodhouse CRJ, Kellett MJ, Williams DI: Minimal surgical interference in prune-belly syndrome. Br J Urol 51:475–480, 1979.
117. Driekorn K, Palmtag W, Robal L: The prune belly syndrome: Treatment of terminal renal failure by hemodialysis and renal transplantation. Eur Urol 3:245–247, 1977.
118. LiPuma JP, Haaga JR, Bryan PJ, et al: Percutaneous nephrostomy in neonates and infants. J Urol 132:722–724, 1984.
119. Schmidt JD, Hawtrey CE, Culp DA, et al: Experience with cutaneous pyelostomy diversion. J Urol 109:990–992, 1973.
120. Randolph JG: Total surgical reconstruction for patients with abdominal muscular deficiency (prune belly) syndrome. J Pediatr Surg 12:1033–1043, 1977.
121. Duckett JW: Cutaneous vesicostomy in children: The Blocksom technique. Urol Clin North Am 1:485–495, 1974.
122. Perlmutter AD: Reduction cystoplasty in prune belly syndrome. J Urol 116:356–362, 1976.
123. Messing EM, Dibbell DG, Belzer FO: Bilateral rectus femoris pedicle flaps for detrusor augmentation in the prune belly syndrome. J Urol 134:1202, 1985.
124. Cukier J: Resection of the urethra in the prune belly syndrome. Birth Defects 13:95–96, 1977.
125. Stephenson KL: A new approach to the treatment of abdominal musculature agenesis and plastic reconstruction. Surgery 2:413, 1953.
126. Erlich RM, Lesavoy MA, Fine RN: Total abdominal wall reconstruction in the prune belly syndrome. J Urol 136:282–285, 1986.
127. Monfort G, Guys JM, Bocciardi A, et al: A novel technique for reconstruction of the abdominal wall in the prune belly syndrome. J Urol 146:639–640, 1991.
128. Smith CA, Smith EA, Parrott TS, et al: Voiding function in patients with the prune-belly syndrome after Monfort abdominoplasty. J Urol 159:1657–1679, 1998.
129. Fowler R, Stephens FD: The role of testicular vascular anatomy in the salvage of the high undescended testis. Aust N Z J Surg 29:92–106, 1959.
130. Gibbons MD, Cromie WJ, Duckett JW Jr: Management of the abdominal undescended testicle. J Urol 122:76–79, 1979.
131. Barnhouse DH: Prune belly syndrome. Br J Urol 44:356–360, 1972.
132. Burke EC, Shin MH, Kelalis PP: Prune-belly syndrome: Clinical findings and survival. Am J Dis Child 117:668–671, 1969.
133. Lattimer JK: Congenital deficiency of the abdominal musculature and associated genitourinary abnormalities: A report of 22 cases. J Urol 79:343–352, 1958.
134. Walbaum RS, Marshall VF: The prune belly syndrome: A diagnostic therapeutic plan. J Urol 103:668–674, 1970.
135. Reinberg Y, Manivel JC, Fryd D, et al: The outcome of renal transplantation in children with the prune belly syndrome. J Urol 142:1541–1542, 1989.

61

INTERSEX

Ronald J. Sharp, MD

☐ History

Hermaphroditism has been described since antiquity. Rabbinical commentaries on Adam and Eve describe Adam as androgenous. The creation of Eve signifies the separation of the two sexes. Mosaic law recounted detailed descriptions of behavioral norms, which were a mixture of male and female privileges and restrictions for the hermaphroditic individual. The origin of the word *hermaphrodite* is uncertain. In ancient Greece, Hermaphrodito was a minor deity whose parents were Hermes and Aphrodite.[1] The Roman poet Ovid created a myth surrounding the nymph Salmacis many years later, which said that Salmacis' advances were rebuffed by Hermaphrodito. She pleaded with the gods to unite her with him in one body. The gods complied, and from that time on, Hermaphrodito had the sex organs of both. Another theory on the origins of the word comes from ancient Greece. Stone columns served as property markers. They often bore the head, bust and genitalia of a god. Their purpose was to impart fertility to the crops. The columns were referred to as Hermes. Later, the head and busts of female goddesses were placed on the columns; hence, the word *hermaphrodite*.[1] Oriental and Greek civilizations thought of hermaphrodites as superhuman and included them in much of their art (Figs. 61–1 and 61–2). Plato, Aristotle, Galen, and Hippocrates were among many early physicians and philosophers whose hypotheses on the origin of the intersex child were based on natural phenomena. This is in marked contrast to the Romans, who saw the birth of such children as an evil omen and promptly destroyed them by drowning or abandoning them in an open field to die of exposure.[1, 2] This fear and loathing of the intersex child persisted throughout the Dark Ages. Antide Colles of Dole (1599) was accused of having intercourse with the devil, as "evidenced" by her ambiguous genitalia. She was tortured until she confessed to the act and then burned at the stake for her "sin." Ambrose Pare published a paper called "Monsters and Marvels" in 1573, which was the beginning of the naturaliza-

tion and medicalization of intersex and other congenital disorders.[3, 4–7]

☐ Epidemiology

In the United States, South America, and most of Western Europe, female pseudohermaphroditism secondary to congenital adrenal hyperplasia (CAH) is the most common intersex disorder. In a large Brazilian study of almost a million live births, 89 were found to have intersex disorders, 50% of which were CAH. This translates into 1 in 10,000 live births. The researchers found intersex disorders in 1 of 350 stillborn infants.[8, 9] In the United States, 1 of 128 in the population are heterozygous for CAH. One in 82 and 1 of 11 of the population are heterozygous for the same gene in Canada and Upic Eskimos, respectively.[10, 11]

In South Africa, true hermaphroditism is the most common disorder. Karyotypes in true hermaphro-

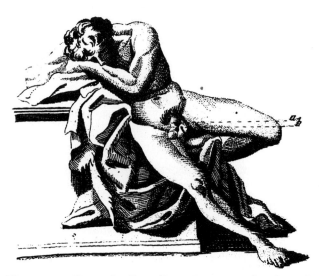

Figure 61–1. Hermaphrodites. (From Epstein J: Altered Conditions: Disease, Medicine, and Storytelling. New York, Routledge, 1995.)

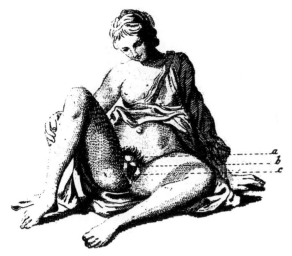

Figure 61–2. Hermaphrodites. (From Epstein J: Altered Conditions: Disease, Medicine, and Storytelling. New York, Routledge, 1995.)

dites vary geographically. 46 XX predominates in South Africa and the United States. More than 50% are mosaics in Europe, and virtually all are 46XY in Japan. There have been 449 cases of true hermaphroditism recorded in the world literature since 1899. Twenty-five percent were diagnosed after the age of 20.[12–18]

One type of male pseudohermaphroditism, 5-alpha reductase deficiency, is an autosomal recessive trait. It has been discovered in very diverse cultures, ranging from New Guinea, Turkey, and the Dominican Republic to the United States.[10, 11, 19, 20] Testicular feminization syndrome occurs in 1 in 20,000 to 64,000 male births.[21]

□ Embryology

In 1947, some ingenious experiments were designed that demonstrated that two discrete substances, produced by the fetal testes, mediated male sexual differentiation. If these substances were absent, female development would ensue. The stated conclusion was that, "In man, female sex differentiation is the innate tendency of the gonadal and genital primordia, against which maleness must be actively imposed."[15] The fetus is completely dimorphic during the first 4 to 6 weeks of development. Normal male development depends on a number of complex timed steps. Normal female development can occur even in the absence of an ovary.[22] Primitive germ cells, originating in the yolk sac, migrate to the urogenital ridge, where they receive instruction from Y chromosome–produced testis-determining factor (TDF), which directs development of a testis. From this point, the remainder of male development is orchestrated by the testes. Once stimulated by TDF, the germ cells are surrounded by seminephrous tubules, which contain the sertoli cells. These cells produce two very important hor-

mones, müllerian-inhibiting substance (MIS) and androgen-binding protein. MIS inhibits the development of the ipsilateral müllerian structures. Androgen-binding protein seems to a play a role in enhancing the action ipsilaterally of testosterone on the development of wolffian ducts. Leydig's cells are next to arrive and form up just outside of the sertoli cells. The Leydig's cells produce testosterone that acts locally and possibly ipsilaterally to advance the development of the wolffian ducts. Systemic testosterone is converted to dihydrotesterone by the action of 5-alpha reductase, which is located more abundantly in the external genital area. Both testosterone and dihydrotestosterone act on the androgen receptor. Dihydrotestosterone elicits a much stronger response and is responsible for the development of the external genitalia. Androgen receptors have been demonstrated in almost every tissue of the body except for the spleen.[19, 23–25]

□ Classification

The classification system currently used to describe the various intersex disorders has its origins in the Greek mythologic word *hermaphrodite*. In 1876,[26] the prefixes *true* and *false* (pseudo) were added to *hermaphrodite* to clarify the anatomic differences within the overall spectrum of possibilities. This distinction was based on the gonadal morphology. Thus, a male pseudohermaphrodite is one with the external appearance of a female but the gonads of a male, where as a female pseudohermaphrodite demonstrates male external genitalia and female internal genitalia. The true hermaphrodite is one that conforms to the original description of having the characteristics and gonads of both sexes. This classification system requires that the gonad can be reasonably classified. Those with dysgenetic or streak gonads do not fit well into this gonadal-based classification; therefore, a fourth category, mixed gonadal dysgenesis, was added. Another classification system based on chromosomal morphology is more precise and avoids the emotionally charged words used to describe the various disorders.[27]

Because the original system is so entrenched, we use it in this chapter to avoid confusion.

□ Pathophysiology

Normal male sexual differentiation can be roughly broken down into three phases. The first is the establishment of chromosomal sex, which directs the second phase, gonadal sex. In the third phase, the testes are responsible for the hormones that orchestrate male phenotypic development.[19] Normal female differentiation occurs, even in the absence of a gonad.[28] TDF is produced by genes on the short arm of the Y chromosome. Much evidence points to the SRY gene in this region as the most likely candidate. Mutations in this gene result in a wide range of abnormalities, from dysgenesis to cryptorchidism to XY females.[27, 29–31] Mutations affecting normal testicular development range from point mutations of a single amino acid to large deletions. Polymerase chain reaction (PCR) analysis allows researchers to pinpoint abnormalities in this and many other genes responsible for normal sexual development.[32] The appearance of the sertoli cells heralds the onset of testicular differentiation. MIS produced by the sertoli cells is one of the first products of the developing testes. MIS is produced in postnatal girls by the granulosa cells. The chromosome for MIS is located on gene 19, and its receptor, on gene 12. Expression of MIS seems to be affected only by mutations of the MIS gene and not by gonadal dysgenesis. It functions to block the differentiation of the müllerian ducts in the fetus, inhibits aromatase in granulosa cells of the ovary in preadolescent girls, and possibly inhibits steroidogenesis in the prepubertal boy. This is supported by the fact that MIS levels remain elevated in boys until puberty and suppressed in girls until puberty, at which point the opposite occurs. MIS levels are useful in the evaluation of intersex states and cryptorchidism. Normal levels vary widely, necessitating testosterone levels and possibly human chorionic gonado-

tropin (hCG) stimulation tests to make a final determination in some cases.[25, 33–36] See Table 61–1. Testosterone, the next hormone to be produced, acts locally and systemically. It is converted to dihydrotestosterone by 5-alpha reductase peripherally, which potentiates its action on certain tissues, particularly the genital ridge area, where the bipotential genital premordia differentiate into normal male genitalia. The action of testosterone, both locally and peripherally, is dependent on its molecular configuration and the androgen receptor. Complete absence of the androgen receptor, which has been discovered, defines the null phenotype. Individuals with this condition are anatomically perfect females who lack body hair. PCR analysis has demonstrated a huge range of abnormalities of the AR gene. In some cases, a point mutation with a single amino acid substitution has been shown to result in complete testicular feminization. Phenotypic aberrations range from cryptorchidism and hypospadias to complete testicular feminization. The degree of aberration does not seem to correlate with the location or the extent of abnormality of the AR gene. With continued PCR analysis of individuals with androgen insensitivity, a predictable pattern may emerge.[37–44]

Androgen receptors have been demonstrated in

TABLE 61–1. Serum Müllerian-Inhibiting Substance and Testosterone Levels for 18 Patients with Intersex Abnormalities

Case No.	Diagnosis	Karyotype	Age	Serum MIS (ng/ml)	Serum Testosterone (ng/dl)	Anatomy
1	M pseud	46,XY	1 wk	20	35*	Ambiguous genitalia
2	M pseud	46,XY	3 days	5	34*	Ambiguous genitalia
			6 mo	10	—	
3	M pseud	46,XY	3 days	52	116	Ambiguous genitalia
			6 mo	25	—	
4	M pseud	46,XY	6 mo	16	10*	Ambiguous genitalia
			10 mo	7	—	
5	M pseud	46,XY	4.5 yr	49	4*	Bilateral labial testes
				0		(after bilateral gonadectomy)
6	T fem	46,XY	5 yr	73†	4*	Bilateral inguinal testes
7	T fem	46,XY	4.5 yr	68	<3*	Bilateral labial testes
8	T fem	46,XY	18 yr	37	1050	Bilateral intraabdominal testes
9	True herm	45,X/46,XY	3 wk	5.5	260	Bilateral ovotestes; normal uterus
10	True herm	46,XX/46,XY	2 wk	7	230	Bilateral ovotestes; normal uterus
			2.5 mo	10	—	(after partial gonadectomy)
			2.7 mo	0	—	(after complete gonadectomy)
11	True herm	46,XX	4 yr	8†	<20*	Surgical exploration pending
12	MGD	45,X/46,XY/47,XYY	1 wk	12	65*	Streak gonads; normal uterus
13	MGD	46,XY	5 wk	3	349	Dysgenetic gonads; normal uterus
			5 mo	0	—	(after bilateral gonadectomy)
14	CAH	46,XX	8 mo	0	—	High vaginal atresia
15	CAH	46,XX	2 yr	0	—	High vaginal atresia
16	Cloacal exstrophy	—	2 days	10	—	Bilateral immature testes
			2 wk	0	—	(after bilateral gonadectomy)
17	? Anorchia	—	20 mo	9.5	—	Negative examination, US
18	? Anorchia	—	3.5 yr	41†	<10*†	Negative examination, US, hCG stimulation

*Serum testosterone level within the expected range for "normal" females of that age.
†Serum MIS/testosterone levels measured at the end of an hCG stimulation test.
CAH, congenital adrenal hyperplasia; hCG, human chorionic gonadotropin; MGD, mixed gonadal dysgenesis; MIS, müllerian-inhibiting substance; M pseud, male pseudohermaphroditism; T fem, testicular feminization; True herm, true hermaphroditism; US, ultrasound. (From Gustafson ML, Lee MM, Asmundson L, et al: Müllerian-inhibiting substance in the diagnosis and management of intersex and gonadal abnormalities. J Pediatr Surg 28:439–444, 1993.)

every tissue with the exception of the spleen.[23] There is convincing evidence that the external genitalia and the internal sexual ducts are not the only areas masculinized by the effects of androgenic hormones. The brain may very well be "masculinized" by the effects of androgen in the fetus and possibly in the very early neonatal period. Brain masculinization is suggested by animal studies, natural experiments, and human "social engineering." Studies have been done in sheep in which the female fetuses were treated with male hormone after phenotypic development was complete. These ewes demonstrated male social behavior after birth. This was manifested by mounting other ewes and aggressive behavior toward rams. These same experiments and results have been verified in other species.[45] The natural experiments are several. The most striking is that of a Dominican kindred of 34 subjects with 5-alpha reductase deficiency. Nineteen of these children were raised unambiguously as females, and only one of the original 19 has maintained the female gender role assignment beyond puberty. The same result was found in an isolated tribe in New Guinea, especially remarkable in this culture where strict gender segregation is practiced. There are several case reports of undiagnosed genotypic female children with CAH raised as male (Fig. 61–3). Most are married and lead normal lives in that role.[4, 6, 7] In CAH children diagnosed early, there is a 50% incidence of homosexual orientation.[46] A study in CAH patients showed a direct correlation between salt wasting (severity) and percent homosexual preference. The examples of "social engineering" are case reports and by themselves prove nothing but seem to support this thesis. The most remarkable is the story of Joan/John, who was born a normal male twin (originally named John) and suffered a penile amputation during a newborn circumcision gone awry. John was renamed Joan, and a genitoplasty was carried out in infancy. The family did everything to raise Joan as a girl and maintained very close contact and follow-up with the institution that was managing her case. "Joan," when interviewed

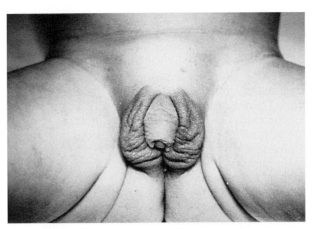

Figure 61–4. Newborn adrenogenital syndrome.

as an adult, now says he felt from an early age that he was male and that the efforts of his physicians and parents to make him female left him confused. When his father finally told him the true story of his infancy, he was relieved and changed his role to that of male. He underwent genital reconstruction and is now happily married.[47] There is a remarkably similar story of a Laotian child with mixed gonadal dysgenesis who was raised unambiguously from infancy as female. He changed gender role during his teenage years.[48] The story of John is especially important, as it appears that his case was the basis for much of the reasoning that went into arbitrary neonatal sex assignment. Sex assignment is currently based on the surgeon's ability to construct adequate genitalia rather than the potential hormonal imprinting that likely occurs before birth. It appears that cultural and social influences alone may not be sufficient to define gender role.[19, 49–59]

FEMALE PSEUDOHERMAPHRODITISM

In North America and Europe, female pseudohermaphroditism appears to be the most common intersex disorder (Figs 61–4 and 61–5). It occurs as a result of various enzymatic deficiencies in the

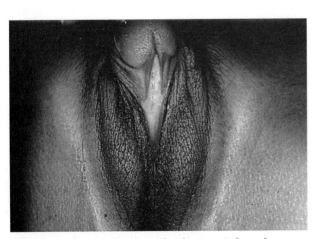

Figure 61–3. Genetic female with adrenogenital syndrome presented as a teenager for his ureteroplasty.

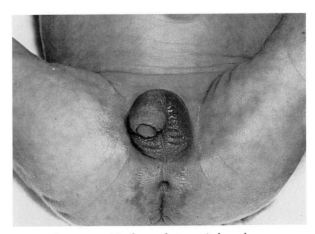

Figure 61–5. Newborn adrenogenital syndrome.

steroidogenic pathway leading to the synthesis of cortisol; i.e., CAH. CAH becomes manifest in the autosomal recessive state. Of the general population, it is estimated that 1 in 128 in the United States, 1 in 82 in Canada and 1 in 11 among Yupic Eskimos are heterozygous for this gene.[10] Incidence in the general population is 1 in 10,000 live births. In the Yupic Eskimo population, the incidence is 1 in 684 live births.[27, 60] Maternal drug ingestion and tumors of pregnancy are less common causes.[27] The biosynthetic pathways leading to the synthesis of cortisol and testosterone are illustrated (Fig. 61–6). A deficiency of 21-hydroxylase accounts for more than 90% of cases of CAH. The effects of three of the enzyme deficiencies involved in corticosteroid synthesis are listed (see Table 61–1). The severity of a particular enzymatic deficiency is variable and likely depends on the nature of the mutation in the gene for that particular enzyme. This variation in severity accounts for the marked ambiguity and severe salt wasting found in some children with 21-hydroxylase deficiency, whereas others have the nonclassic form of CAH manifested by subfertility, precocious puberty, hirsutism, and slight clitoromegaly. CAH is just as common in male patients.[27, 12]

MALE PSEUDOHERMAPHRODITISM

Male pseudohermaphroditism can be defined as the condition of an XY individual having incomplete masculinization or complete feminization of the external genitalia (Fig. 61–6). Clinically, these children range from having severe hypospadias and cryptorchidism to complete testicular feminization.[61] The etiologic possibilities in male pseudohermaphroditism are numerous, and the various points at which abnormal development may occur are listed (Table 61–2). Aberrations can occur at the chromosomal, gonadal, hormonal, and receptor levels.

An XY female could be explained by translocation of the TDF region of the Y chromosome to the X chromosome. It is known that the pseudoautosomal regions of the short arms of the X and Y chromosome recombine during male meiosis. Because the

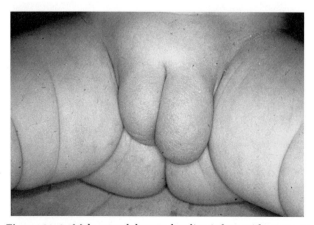

Figure 61-6. Male pseudohermaphrodite infant with testes in labioscrotal fold.

TABLE 61-2 Etiological Possibilities in Male Pseudohermaphroditism

Chromosomal Level

XY female (TDF locus translocated to X chromosome)
Abnormal TDF

Gonadal Level

Abnormal TDF receptor
Testicular dysgenesis
Leydig's cell abnormality
Qualitative or quantitative abnormality of testosterone
Sertoli cell abnormality
Qualitative or quantitative defect MIF
Gonadotropin deficiency

Hormonal Level

Enzymatic deficiency testosterone biosynthetic pathway
   20,22-desmolase
   20α-hydroxylase
   3β-hydroxysteroid dehydrogenase
   17α-hydroxylase
   17,20-desmolase
   17β-ketosteroid reductase

Dihydrotestosterone Deficiency

5a-reductase abnormality

Androgen Response

Receptor abnormality
   Quantitative
   Qualitative
Congenital anomalies involving the gastrointestinal and
   genitourinary systems

MIF, müllerian-inhibiting factor; TDF, testis-determining factor.

TDF region is very close to this area, translocation of this segment could occur.[61] This may account for the facts that 1 in 20,000 phenotypic male patients is 46XX and that there is a smaller number of XY female patients.[62] There is also the possibility that TDF or its receptor may be abnormal.

Testicular dysgenesis in male pseudohermaphroditism is distinguished from mixed gonadal dysgenesis by the fact that two testes are present in testicular dysgenesis and both are dysgenetic. In mixed gonadal dysgenesis, one gonad is classically streak and the other is a dysgenetic testis. The timing of testicular dysgenesis is critical. If it occurs before 8 weeks, the child may have a normal female phenotype. If it occurs after 20 weeks, the child will have a normal male phenotype because the differentiation of the external genitalia is completed by this time. If the dysgenesis occurs between 8 and 20 weeks, a spectrum of genital ambiguity may result. An abnormality of Leydig's cell function or blunted response to hCG could result in low levels of testosterone production. Leydig's cell hypoplasia and agenesis have been reported.[42, 63, 64] Sertoli cell abnormalities or absence may result in decreased levels or absence of müllerian-inhibiting factor. The absence of the sertoli cells, which are necessary for nurturing and preserving the germ cells, may also result in infertility. The various enzyme deficiencies that result in decreased or defective testosterone production are autosomal recessive traits (Table 61–3).[65, 66]

TABLE 61-3. Diminished Androgen
Production: Enzymatic Deficiencies
(All Autosomal Recessive)

20,22-desmolase
20α-hydroxylase
3β-hydroxysteroid dehydrogenase
17α-hydroxylase
17,20-desmolase
17β-ketosteroid reductase

Failure of conversion of testosterone to dihydrotestosterone results from a 5-alpha reductase deficiency, which is an autosomal recessive trait. Children with this disorder often virilize markedly at puberty if the gonads are intact. The severity of the enzymatic defect is dependent on the nature of the chromosomal defect.[66] Androgen receptor abnormalities account for a sizable portion of male pseudohermaphrodites. Receptor abnormalities are X-linked recessive traits. There is a tremendous spectrum of phenotypes, ranging from simple hypospadias to complete testicular feminization. Recent work with PCR analysis has demonstrated a wide variety of abnormalities at the chromosomal level, ranging from single amino acid substitutions to large deletions. The fact that normal levels of cytoplasmic receptor are found should not be confounding, as the receptor may not bind to the DNA molecule or, if bound, cannot transcribe. The extent of the chromosomal abnormality does not seem to correlate with the degree of ambiguity. This may account for the proliferation of syndromes described (e.g., Reifenstein's, Gilbert-Dreyfuss, Lubbs). In time, as more androgen-resistant children are examined by PCR analysis, some predictive patterns may arise that can be useful for sex assignment and treatment.

TRUE HERMAPHRODITISM

True hermaphroditism exists when both testicular and ovarian tissue is present (Fig. 61–7). A lateral true hermaphrodite has a testis on one side and an ovary on the opposite side. In such a case, the internal ducts are congruent with the ipsilateral gonad.[67] The majority of true hermaphrodites, however, have an ovotestis.[60]

Various hypotheses have been advanced to account for true hermaphroditism. The 46XX/XY individual usually has unilateral ovary and contralateral testes, as opposed to an ovotestis combination. The 46XY true hermaphrodite may be a chimera with an undetected 46XX cell line. Postzygotic mutation of the SRY gene has recently been reported to occur in part of the gonadal tissue. This mutation was found only in the gonadal tissue and indicates that each cell in the primordial gonad needs to have the SRY gene present for a normal testis to develop.[32] This finding could explain the presence of an ovotestis. Many 46XX true hermaphrodites are HY antigen positive or have Y-specific DNA sequences, indicating a translocation of the Y segment.[27, 68, 69] Histologically normal ovarian tissue with numerous follicles is usually present.[12, 27, 60] Pregnancy and live births have been reported at least 14 times in true hermaphrodites.[27, 70] The testicular component of either a unilateral testis or ovotestis is often dysgenetic. This histologic finding may explain the infertility and poor virilization seen at puberty in children raised as male.[71–73] However, there have been two reports of male true hermaphrodites who have fathered children.[18] At puberty, those with a male assignment may need hormonal replacement, as the dysgenetic testis may not be responsive enough for normal development.[12, 72, 74]

MIXED GONADAL DYSGENESIS

Children with mixed gonadal dysgenesis do not fit well into the gonad-based intersex classification. They classically have a testis on one side, a streak ovary on the opposite, and sex chromosomal mosaicism.[24, 75] Variations include unilateral gonadal agenesis and tumor, bilateral streak gonads, or a gonad on one side and a tumor on the opposite. One suggested classification system is based on the belief that these disorders are variations of Turner's syndrome, with mosaicism for several different cell lines—the most common of which is 46X46XY. The absence of the second X chromosome is thought to lead to an incomplete formation of the follicular mantle around the oocyte, which may lead to degeneration of the oocytes and formation of a streak ovary. Meiotic nondisjunction is a likely etiology in the majority of these single cell line depletion syndromes.[27] Included in this classification are some pure XY patients with gonadal dysgenesis (Swyer's syndrome), sometimes associated with the absence of gonads or, more commonly, with bilateral streak gonads. This may occur because of failure of germ cell migration, teratogenic destruction of early testis, repressor gene action on the testicular determinant locus, or abnormal gonadal receptors for these gene products.[27] These children are especially prone to developing tumors. In children with gonadal dys-

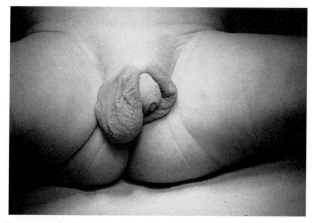

Figure 61–7. True hermaphrodite infant. Note gonadal asymmetry.

genesis, the presence of a Y chromosome or even indirect evidence of a Y chromosome is associated with increased risk of tumor formation.

This classification, however, does not explain the five patients in one series who were 46XY but had testes and contralateral streak gonad and, in one case, dysgerminoma. The authors of this study were not able to prove the presence of mosaicism. A postzygotic mutation of the primordial gonad could account for this finding.[76]

☐ Clinical Presentation

Sex assignment is usually made in the first seconds of life by the obstetrician or midwife. This assignment is based solely on the appearance of the external genitalia. When there is uncertainty, a chain of events of great import to the child and his or her family is initiated. How these events are handled by medical practitioners will determine in great part the future happiness of this child and the family. Many cases of intersex, however, go undiagnosed until puberty or later.[14] In a report of 17 patients who presented at age 11 years or older, 41% presented with sexual dysfunction, 6% with infertility, 24% with amenorrhea, 6% with gynecomastia, 6% with cryptorchidism, and 12% with abdominal pain.[14, 17, 18] In a study of 20 patients with severe hypospadias and undescended testes, all 20 were proven to have an intersex disorder. Ten were male pseudohermaphrodites, four had mixed gonadal dysgenesis, one was a true hermaphrodite, one was a XX male, and one had Klinefelter's syndrome.[77] Other reports indicate a 25 to 50% incidence of intersex when hypospadias and cryptorchidism are found.[61, 75, 77, 78, 79] Twenty-five percent of true hermaphrodites present at 20 years or older. Gynecomastia and periodic hematuria are the most common presenting complaints.[67] Drash syndrome is characterized by ambiguous genitalia and nephropathy, which rapidly progresses to renal failure. Those with this syndrome are at very high risk of developing Wilms's tumors and gonadal tumors. It is recommended that they undergo prophylactic nephrectomy and gonadectomy early in their course.[80] CAH, the most common intersex disorder in the United States, may first present with life-threatening adrenal crisis. This may occur anywhere from the 4th day of life to the 4th year. The prelude consists of poor feeding, vomiting, diarrhea, and significant weight loss over a very short period. Untreated, this complication is rapidly fatal in both female and male patients with CAH.[81]

PATIENT HISTORY

Once an intersex anomaly is discovered, a careful history should be obtained. A pedigree is constructed, with attention to relatives with genital abnormalities, infertility, hernias, and unexplained early deaths. Drug usage of any type, especially seizure medications, during pregnancy should be determined. Maternal virilization may result from tumors of the ovary or adrenal gland. Maternal blood for testosterone and dehydroepiandrosterone should be drawn if maternal virilization is noted.[24, 82]

PHYSICAL EXAMINATION

Blood pressure and pulse should be accurately measured. A detailed general and genital examination should be carried out. Subtle findings suggestive of an intersex disorder, such as heterochromia of the iris or skin mottling, may be indicative of chimerism found in true hermaphroditism. Areolar and/or scrotal hyperpigmentation may indicate high melanocyte-stimulating hormone levels, which result from maximum stimulation of adrenocorticotropic hormone. This is often seen in more severe forms of CAH. The phallus should be carefully examined to see if there is a midline frenulum, which is more often seen in normal males, whereas a hypertrophied clitoris will often have only lateral folds. The location of the opening of the urogenital sinus/urethra should be noted and documented. The phallus should be measured from symphysis to the stretched tip, and the girth noted. The labial scrotal folds should be examined for the presence of gonads. This examination is facilitated by applying lotion to the groin and the examiner's hand. Gentle sweeping motions from the area of the internal ring to the labioscrotal fold will pick up even the smallest remnant of a gonad. The gonadal examination can give one a general idea of the diagnosis. Bilateral symmetry is indicative of female or male pseudohermaphroditism, whereas asymmetry is indicative of true hermaphroditism or mixed gonadal dysgenesis. A bimanual rectopelvic examination often can reveal the presence of müllerian structures.

LABORATORY AND RADIOLOGIC EVALUATION

Buccal smears are of historical interest only and need not be obtained.[20, 83] A rapid analysis for chromosomes, which can be obtained within 12 hours, is much more precise. At the same time that blood for the karyotype is drawn, serum 17-hydroxyprogesterone, dehydroepiandrosterone (DHEA), cortisone, electrolytes, blood urea nitrogen, and glucose should be determined. Serum electrolytes should be closely monitored until a firm diagnosis is made. 17-Hydroxyprogesterone will be elevated in the cord blood of all infants, but it drops precipitously in the first 24 hours of life. Children with CAH have persistent elevation of their 17-hydroxyprogesterone and/or DHEA. Serum MIS levels may be obtained. Absent or very low levels indicate the absence of testes, the presence of ovaries, severe testicular dysgenesis, or a defect in the MIS gene.[84] Plasma renin levels may be elevated in the face of mineralocorticoid deficiency.[30] While awaiting the serum studies, a genitogram should be performed to determine the anatomy of the internal genital ducts. The tip of an 8-French Foley catheter inflated with 5 cc of air is inserted into the urogenital sinus, and the balloon is held firmly against the perineum. Contrast material is gently injected by syringe under fluoroscopy. By this method, one can fill the urethra, bladder, and vagina, if present, and possibly demonstrate a cervical dimple at the apex of the vagina (Fig. 61–8).

A gonadal biopsy is necessary in all children, with the exception of those with CAH whose diagnosis can be established by karyotyping and serum steroid precursor assay. The biopsy is necessary to determine the gonadal sex of the child and should be pole to pole if an ovotestis is suspected.[14] Laparoscopy gives a much more detailed view of the pelvis.[40] Gonadal biopsy could then be done through a much smaller incision. Cysto-vaginoscopy during this procedure is useful to further define the internal anatomy. The results of the gonadal biopsy and karyotyping serve to classify children into the other three major categories: male pseudohermaphroditism, true hermaphroditism, and mixed gonadal dysgenesis. Male pseudohermaphrodites will require further study to define the etiology of their ambiguity and their subsequent treatment.[66] A biopsy of the genital skin for culture should be obtained. The biopsy is used to assay for 5-alpha reductase and also to determine androgen receptor binding. Serum levels of testosterone, dihydrotestosterone, luteinizing hormone (LH), follicle-stimulating hormone (FSH), DHEA, and androstenedione should be drawn. An hCG stimulation test is next done to help distinguish between hypogonadism and end-organ unresponsiveness. It also allows for the evaluation of the pituitary gonadal axis. A total of 5000 units/m² of hCG is given subcutaneously. Testosterone, FSH, LH, and β-hCG levels are draw at 48 and 120 hours. An elevated β-hCG level indi-

cates that the drug was given. Depressed levels of FSH and LH indicate that the pituitary is normally responsive. If the 48-hour testosterone level is twice basal or greater, one can assume that a normally responsive testis is present. If no rise in testosterone is noted, the child is anorchic or has dysgenetic testes. If the 120-hour testosterone level is less than twice basal, then one must assume that an enzyme deficiency is present, causing a decrease in testosterone production.[19] PCR analysis should be carried out for androgen receptor, 5-alpha reductase, and 21-hydroxylase.

□ Treatment

Intersex disorders should be considered a psychosocial emergency.[9, 51] They should be cared for at centers with a well-organized management team. Early expeditious care of these infants will alleviate parental fear and anxiety and afford the child the best chance for a happy life.[6, 7, 85] Great care must be taken not to give an arbitrary sex assignment. There should be one spokesman for the team to avoid confusion.

GENDER ASSIGNMENT

Once the diagnostic evaluation has been completed, determination of sex assignment and appropriate surgical reconstruction should be carried out in the neonatal period. Factors considered in sex assignment may include
- Anatomy
- Diagnosis
- Age at diagnosis
- Potential fertility
- Gonadal sex
- Parental desires
- Socioethnic background
- Genetic sex
- Androgen imprinting

The standard teaching is that anatomy, except in CAH patients, dictates sex assignment in the newborn. That arbitrary sex assignment made in the newborn period is undoubtedly best for the patient is refuted by the high transition rates from female to male assignment in long-term studies and several key case reports.[14, 46, 86, 87] The idea that anatomy was key in making early decisions was based on the fact that it is easier to make a functional vagina than a functional penis. This is no longer the case. There are several centers around the world that report excellent results with penile construction. A recent report of 11 boys, seven of whom were prepubertal, described a one-stage penile construction (Figs. 61–8 and 61–9). The surgery included urethral reconstruction, coaptation of erogenous nerves, and aesthetic refinements. All of the postpubertal patients report erogenous sensibility in the reconstructed phallus.[88] This same group reported eight patients who had a prosthesis placed, six of which

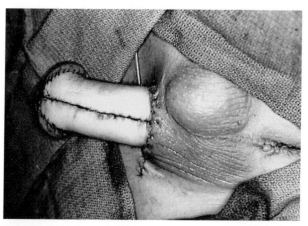

Figure 61–8. Modern phallic construction techniques aim to produce a phallus that will allow the patient to void while standing, will experience return of tactile and erogenous sensibility, will contain enough bulk to retain a penile stiffener, will be aesthetically acceptable to the patient, will grow through childhood, and will have a low incidence of donor site morbidity. (From Gilbert DA, Winslow BH: Penis construction. Semin Urol 5:262–269, 1987.)

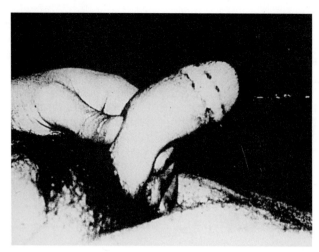

Figure 61–9. Constructed phallus. (Courtesy of David A. Gilbert, MD, Norfolk, Virginia.)

remain functional.[89] Penile construction is now a viable option. It should be limited, however, to centers where surgeons have the requisite skills.[88–99]

Diagnosis dictates female assignment in XX neonates with CAH because all of these patients are potentially fertile and have normal internal anatomy. Attempts to change gender after a certain period should be very carefully considered. Children older than 1 year should have their current sex assignment supported and enhanced surgically, where appropriate. Potential fertility, gonadal sex, parental desires, and socioethnic background are factors that must be taken into consideration in those cases where proper assignment is not clear. Genetic sex is important only in the sense that it may raise the question of prenatal androgen imprinting of the brain in those children who have functioning androgen receptors. If one is not necessarily limited by anatomy, androgen imprinting becomes a very important consideration.

Female Pseudohermaphroditism

All CAH children diagnosed in the neonatal period should be given a female sex assignment. Medical management can be very difficult but must be instituted very soon after diagnosis. Cortisol therapy to overcome the deleterious effects of the enzymatic block that has produced the genital ambiguity must be carefully monitored, because both overtreatment and undertreatment with cortisol result in growth retardation, whereas undertreatment leads to further virilization. The fact that excess androgen is converted to estrogen, limiting bone growth, was discovered by an experiment of nature. A 28-year-old man, who was 203 cm tall and still growing, was found to totally lack estrogen receptors.[100] A new medical treatment for CAH has been suggested based on this observation. The treatment protocol includes flutamide (an antiandrogen) and testolactone, which inhibits the conversion of androgen to estrogen.[100] Adrenalectomy for treatment of CAH has

been proposed but is certainly not universally advocated.[101]

Maternal treatment with prenatal dexamethasone is currently being studied. This would theoretically obviate the genital deformity due to CAH and would be beneficial to the affected fetus, but it may be harmful to a fetus who does not have this metabolic disorder.[102]

True Hermaphroditism

Tradition suggests that if a true hermaphrodite presents in the neonatal period, he or she should be assigned female sex.[103–105] Questionable fertility potential as a male and the risk of testicular tumor are the stated reasons. There have been some reports of paternity in true hermaphrodites, and the risk of tumor is real but small.[103] If the external genitalia are well masculinized, there is a good possibility that androgen imprinting has occurred. Hypospadias repair and a testicular prosthesis would afford a good cosmetic and functional result in this setting. Socioethnic background and parental desires may play a prominent role in sex determination in the case of true hermaphrodites. If true hermaphroditism is discovered later, the assigned sex of rearing should be supported.

Once assignment has been made, appropriate genital reconstruction should be carried out. All discordant gonadal and internal ductal tissue should be removed.[67] The determination of MIS levels is useful to assess the completeness of testicular tissue removal. If a male assignment is made, the child should be monitored for development of a testicular tumor. Male children should probably undergo an hCG stimulation test just prior to puberty to assess the functional capability of the native testicular tissue. If it is inadequate, they may require steroid supplementation during puberty.[12]

Mixed Gonadal Dysgenesis

The dysgenetic gonads in these children are very tumor prone. Tumors have been reported in the newborn period. Early bilateral gonadectomy and later appropriate hormonal replacement should be considered.[12, 106] Female sex assignment in the newborn has been the rule, but there is no compelling reason for this recommendation.[48] If the external genitalia are sufficiently masculinized for hypospadias repair, male assignment can be considered. These children should demonstrate a good response to testosterone treatment prior to hypospadias repair. Once a sex assignment has been made, appropriate genital reconstruction is carried out in the newborn period for girls and at around 6 months of age in boys. Discordant internal ducts and dysgenetic gonads should be removed.[78]

Male Pseudohermaphroditism

Proper sex assignment in this group of patients is very challenging. One might consider those with

5-alpha reductase deficiency and those with testicular feminization syndrome to be at opposite extremes. All patients with testicular feminization syndrome (complete lack or nonfunction of the androgen receptor) should be given a female sex assignment, and all patients with 5-alpha reductase deficiency should be given a male assignment if the condition is discovered in infancy.[19, 107] The condition of most children in each of these groups is not discovered until much later.[51] Gonadectomy after puberty is recommended in children with testicular feminization syndrome because of the high tumor potential.[21, 83] The children who fall in between these two extremes pose a difficult problem.[108] The high transition rates from female to male later in life suggest that the decision of female sex assignment in the neonatal period may be wrong 50% of the time.[14, 109] This is one area where PCR analysis of the androgen receptors in all of these children may be of great benefit. At present, it is best to do a testosterone trial prior to definitive assignment. If there is a good response, then male assignment can be considered. This will delay assignment beyond the neonatal period, which is not optimal but is exceedingly important. The decision should be reached well before 1 year of age.

FEMINIZING GENITOPLASTY

Feminizing genitoplasty should be carried out in the neonatal period.[20, 110, 111] The goal of genitoplasty is to create external genitalia that are as normal as

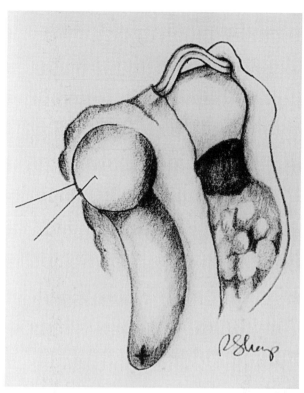

Figure 61–11. Clitoroplasty—mobilization of neurovascular bundle.

possible in both form and function. Genitoplasty usually involves two phases—clitorolabioplasty and vaginoplasty. We prefer to do the clitorolabioplasty in the neonatal period and the vaginoplasty at the time of puberty. Others prefer to do both at the same time.[103] Clitoroplasty is preferable to clitoridectomy, which often results in poor cosmetic appearance and decreased or absent sensation. Clitoral recession results in poor cosmetic results and painful erections in more than 50% of patients, but sensation was well preserved. The currently recommended technique of clitoral reduction with preservation of the neurovascular supply results in a good cosmetic result and normal sensation.[26, 112–116] Several techniques have been advocated (Figs. 61–10 to 61–17).

The technique we use is a modification of that recommended by Mollard.[117] We do not remove the wedge of skin. We make a single incision, which, when retracted, gives good access to the corpora. Anastomosis of the corpora recesses the glans. The prepuce folds over and makes a very adequate labia minora. At the same time, we do a cutback of the urogenital sinus, which helps define the labia majora. If the labia majora are redundant, we do not attempt to reduce them at this time, as they often shrink with time. If the labia majora remain redundant, a portion can be used for a subsequent vaginoplasty.

Vaginoplasty in the newborn period has been advocated and made easier because there remains some neonatal estrogen effect on the vagina.[103, 110, 118] Where there has been minimal masculinization, a

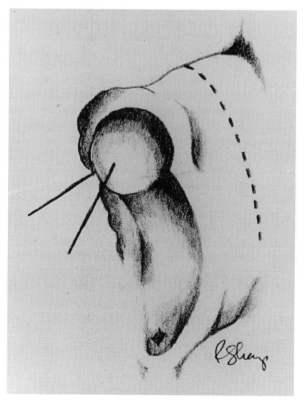

Figure 61–10. Clitoroplasty.

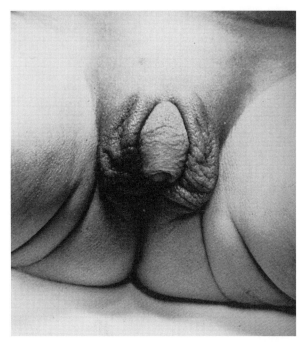

Figure 61–12. Patient A—preoperative view of adrenogenital syndrome.

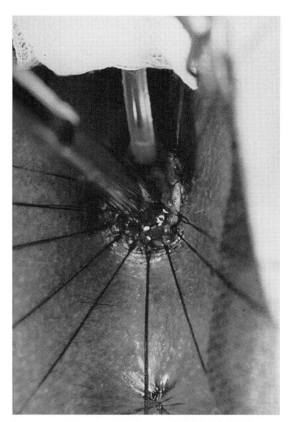

Figure 61–14. Patient A—postvaginoplasty, age 12 years.

simple cutback vaginoplasty is all that is necessary. It is important to ascertain the point at which the vagina arises from the urogenital sinus. If the vagina arises proximal to the external sphincter, a cutback vaginoplasty may injure the external sphincter and render the patient incontinent.[13, 103] Incontinence has not been a problem in patients who underwent repair with a posterior sagittal approach in one expert's hands.[119] We have used a similar approach with some minor modifications in three postpubertal girls without any evidence of incontinence (see Figs. 61–14 and 61–17). Early vaginoplasty is often associated with stenosis.[120, 121] If the vaginoplasty is delayed until puberty, the patient will usually be

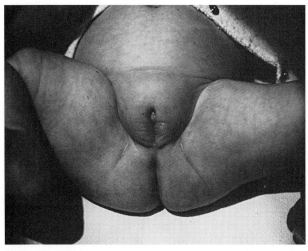

Figure 61–13. Patient A—postoperative view of clitoral reduction.

motivated to help with her dilation to prevent introital stenosis.

In male pseudohermaphrodites, where a neovagina must be created, several techniques have been advocated. A technique using split-thickness skin grafts has been popular for many years.[122] This technique, as modified, was used for 92 vaginal reconstructions with excellent results.[123] This operation should be reserved for the older patient, as it requires cooperation and motivation. The squamous epithelium most closely simulates the normal vaginal epithelium. The functional results have been excellent in long-term studies.[124]

Colon or ileal segments can be used for vaginal construction. These segments are less likely to stricture than split-thickness skin grafts. The downside is the appearance and excessive mucus production.[125, 126] Patients with a shortened vagina, as in those with testicular feminization, can be treated with progressive dilation when they reach puberty.[30]

Hypospadias repair can be safely carried out at any age. We prefer to proceed at about 6 months. Treatment with intramuscular testosterone prior to repair often doubles the size of the penis and often results in more redundant, better vascularized skin for the repair.[20, 127, 128] For the details of hypospadias repair see Chapter 58.

"Sex is what you see, gender is what you feel: Comfort with each is necessary for happiness."[129] Hopefully, if these children are managed with com-

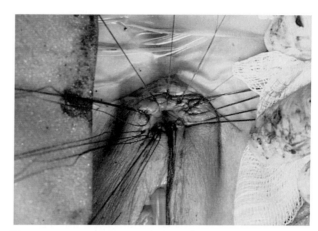

Figure 61–17. Patient B—postvaginoplasty, posterior sagittal approach.

passion and skill, we will afford them the best chance for a happy and full life.

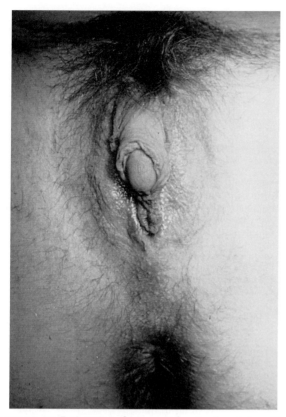

Figure 61–15. Patient B—adrenogenital not referred for clitoroplasty until age 18. Preoperative.

REFERENCES

1. Kiefer J: The hermaphrodite as depicted in art and medical illustration. Trans Am Assoc Genito Urinary Surg 58:121–172, 1966.
2. Bartsocas C, Bartsocas CS: Goiters, dwarfs, giants and hermaphrodites. Prog Clin Biol Res 200:1–18, 1985.
3. Julia Epstein (ed): Altered Conditions: Disease, Medicine and Storytelling. New York, Routledge, 1995.
4. New MI, Kitzinger ES: President's address: Pope Joan: A recognizable syndrome. J Clin Endocrinol Metab 76:3–13, 1993.
5. Bakan R: Queen Elizabeth I: A case of testicular feminization? Med Hypotheses 17:277–284, 1985.
6. Capizzi PJ, Horton CE: A case of colonial gender conflict: Thomas (Thomasine) Hall. Ann Plastic Surg 23:320–322, 1989.
7. Jones HW Jr: A long look at the adrenogenital syndrome. Johns Hopkins Med J 145:143–149, 1979.
8. Castilla EE, Orioli IM, Lugarinho R, Dutra G: Epidemiology of ambiguous genitalia in South America. Am J Med Genet 27:337–343, 1987.
9. Ladee-Levy JV: Ambiguous genitalia as a psychosocial emergency. Z Kinderchir 39:178–181, 1984.
10. Muram D, Dewhurst J: Inheritance of intersex disorders. Can Med Assoc J 130:121–125, 1984.
11. Kasik JW, Woods R, Nelson RM: Antenatal prediction of sex. Acta Obstet Gynecol Scand 65:659–660, 1986.
12. Aaronson A: True hermaphroditism. A review of 41 cases with observations on testicular histology and function. Br J Urol 57:775–779, 1985.
13. Donahoe PK, Hendren WH: Perineal reconstruction in ambiguous genitalia: Infants raised as females. Ann Surg 200:363–371, 1984.
14. Roslyn JJ, Fonkalsrud EW, Lippe B: Intersex disorders in adolescents and adults. Am J Surg 146:138–144, 1983.
15. Jost A, Vigier B, Perchellet JP: Studies on sex differentiation in mammals. Rec Progr Horm Res 29:1–6, 1973.
16. Hanna, MK: Vaginal construction. Urology 29:272–275, 1987.
17. Nichter LS, Freislag JA: Emergency operation in the true hermaphrodite. Surg Gynecol Obstet 156:493–496, 1983.
18. Raspa RW, Subramaniam AP, Romas NA: Intermittent hematuria and groin pain. Urology 28:133–136, 1986.
19. Wilson JD, Griffin JE, Russell DW: Steroid 5α-reductase 2 deficiency. Endocr Rev 14:577–593, 1993.
20. Rajendran R, Hariharan S: Profile of intersex children in South India. Ind Pediatr 32:666–671, 1995.

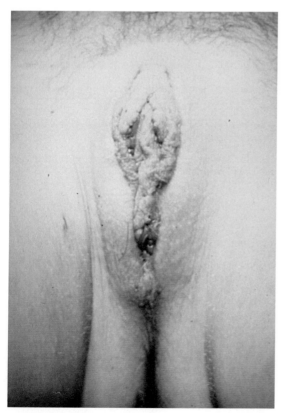

Figure 61–16. Patient B—1 month postclitoroplasty.

21. Hussain AP, Hussain M: Testicular feminisation syndrome. J Ind Med Assoc 82:334–335, 1984.

22. Biglieri EG: A prismatic case. 17α-Hydroxylase deficiency: 1963–1966. J Clin Endocrinol Metab 82:48–50, 1997.

23. Takeda H, Chodak G, Mutchnik S, et al: Immunohistochemical localization of androgen receptors with mono- and polyclonal antibodies to androgen receptor. J Endocrinol 126:17–25, 1990.

24. McGillivray BC: Genetic aspects of ambiguous genitalia. Pediatr Clin North Am 39:307–317, 1992.

25. Forest MG: Serum müllerian inhibiting substance assay—a new diagnostic test for disorders of gonadal development. N Engl J Med 336:1480–1486, 1997.

26. Klebs E: In Herschwald A (ed): Handbuch der pathologischen Anatomie. Berlin, Zweit Abtheilung, 1876, p 718.

27. Reindollar RH, Tho SPT, McDonough PG: Abnormalities of sexual differentiation: Evaluation and management. Clin Obstet Gynecol 30:697–713, 1987.

28. Jost A: Récherches sur la differenciacion sexuelle de l'embryon de lapin. III Role des gonades foetales dans la differentiation sexuelle somatigue. *Arch Anat Micr Morphol Exp* 36:271–315, 1947.

29. Ferguson-Smith MA, Goodfellow PN: SRY and primary sex-reversal syndromes. In Scriver CR (ed): Metabolic and Molecular Bases of Inherited Disease (7th ed). New York: McGraw-Hill, 1995.

30. Rosenfield RL, Lucky AW, Allen TD (eds): The Diagnosis and Management of Intersex. Chicago, Year Book, pp 1–156, 1980.

31. Scully RE: Gonadoblastoma. Cancer 25:1340–1356, 1970.

32. Braun A, Kammerer S, Cleve H, et al: True hermaphroditism in a 46, XY individual, caused by a postzygotic somatic point mutation in the male gonadal sex-determining locus (SRY): Molecular genetics and histological findings in a sporadic case. Am J Hum Genet 52:578–585, 1993.

33. Lee MM, Donahoe PK, Silverman BL, et al: Measurements of serum müllerian-inhibiting substance in the evaluation of children with nonpalpable gonads. N Engl J Med 336:1480–1486, 1997.

34. Lee MM, Donahoe PK, Hasegawa T: Müllerian inhibiting substance in humans: Normal levels from infancy to adulthood. J Clin Endocrinol Metab 81:571–576, 1996.

35. Cass DT, Hutson J: Association of Hirschsprung's disease and müllerian inhibiting substance deficiency. J Pediatr Surg 27:1596–1599, 1992.

36. Rey R, Al-Attar L, Louis F, et al: Testicular dysgenesis does not affect expression of anti-müllerian hormone by sertoli cells in premeiotic seminiferous tubules. Am J Pathol 148:1689–1698, 1996.

37. La Spada AR, Wilson EM, Lubahn DB, et al: Androgen receptor gene mutations in X-linked spinal and bulbar muscular atrophy. Nature 352:77–79, 1991.

38. Quigley CA, Friedman KJ, Johnson A, et al: Complete deletion of the androgen receptor gene: Definition of the null phenotype of the androgen insensitivity syndrome and determination of carrier status. J Clin Endocrinol Metab 74:927–933, 1992.

39. Edelstein RA, Carr MC, Caesar R, et al: Detection of human androgen receptor mRNA expression abnormalities by competitive PCR. DNA Cell Biol 13:265–273, 1994.

40. McDougall EM, Clayman RV, Anderson K: Laparoscopic gonadectomy in a case of testicular feminization. Urology 42:201–204, 1993.

41. Quigley CA, Evans BAJ, Simental JA, et al: Complete androgen insensitivity due to deletion of exon C of the androgen receptor gene highlights the functional importance of the second zinc finger of the androgen receptor in vivo. Mol Endocrinol 6:1103–1112, 1992.

42. Eil C, Austin RM, Sesterhenn I, et al: Leydig cell hypoplasia causing male pseudohermaphroditism: Diagnosis 13 years after prepubertal castration. J Clin Endocrinol Metab 58:441–448, 1984.

43. Saito S, Kumamoto Y: The number of spermatogonia in various congenital testicular disorders. J Urol 141:1166–1168, 1989.

44. Brown TR, Migeon CJ: Androgen receptors in normal and abnormal sexual differentiation. Adv Exp Med Biol 196:227–255, 1986.

45. Chalmers C, Book B, Foxcroft GR, Hunter RHF: Luteinizing hormone response to an oestradiol challenge in 5 intersex pigs possessing ovotestes. J Reprod Fert 87:455–461, 1989.

46. Money, J: The concept of gender identity disorder in childhood and adolescence after 39 years. J Sex Marital Ther 20:163–177, 1994.

47. Diamond M, Sigmundson HK: Sex reassignment at birth. Long-term review and clinical implications. Arch Pediatr Adolesc Med 151:298–304, 1997.

48. Reiner WG: Case study: Sex reassignment in a teenage girl. J Am Acad Child Adolesc Psychiatry 35:799–803, 1996.

49. Stoller RJ: The "bedrock" of masculinity and femininity: Bisexuality. Arch Gen Psychiat 26:207–212, 1972.

50. Imperato-McGinley J, Gautier T, Pichardo M, Shackleton C: The diagnosis of 5α-reductase deficiency in infancy. J Clin Endocrin Metabol 63:1313–1318, 1986.

51. Canty TG: The child with ambiguous genitalia. A neonatal surgical emergency. Ann Surg 186:272–281, 1977.

52. Imperato-McGinley J, Miller M, Wilson JD, et al: A cluster of male pseudohermaphrodites with 5α-reductase deficiency in Papua New Guinea. Clin Endocrinol 34:293–298, 1991.

53. Imperato-McGinley J, Peterson RE, Gautier T, Sturla E: Male pseudohermaphroditism secondary to 5α-reductase deficiency—a model for the role of androgens in both the development of the male phenotype and the evolution of a male gender identity. J Steroid Biochem 11:637–645, 1979.

54. Herdt GH, Davidson J: The Sambia "Turnim-Man": Sociocultural and clinical aspects of gender formation in male pseudohermaphrodites with 5-alpha-reductase deficiency in Papua New Guinea. Arch Sex Behav 17:33–56, 1988.

55. Imperato-McGinley J, Peterson RE, Gautier T, Sturla E: Androgens and the evolution of male-gender identity among male pseudohermaphrodites with 5α-reductase deficiency. N Engl J Med 300:1233–1237, 1979.

56. Diffmann RW, Kappes ME, Kappes MH: Sexual behavior in adolescent and adult females with congenital adrenal hyperplasia. Psychoneuroendocrinology 17:153–170, 1992.

57. Dorner G: Sex-specific gonadotropin secretion, sexual orientation and gender role behaviour. Exp Clin Endocrinol 86:1–6, 1985.

58. Dorner G, Docke F, Gotz F, et al: Sexual differentiation of gonadotrophin secretion, sexual orientation and gender role behaviour. J Steroid Biochem 27:1081–1087, 1987.

59. Gladue BA, Green R, Hellman RE: Neuroendocrine response to estrogen and sexual orientation. Science 225:1496–1499, 1984.

60. New MI, Josso N: Disorders of gonadal differentiation and congenital adrenal hyperplasia. Endocrinol Metab North Am 17:339–366, 1988.

61. Iyengar JK, Rohatgi M, Menon PSN, et al: Clinical, cytogenetic and hormonal profile in extreme hypospadias with bilaterally descended testes. Ind J Med Res 83:604–609, 1986.

62. Hodgkin J: Everything you always wanted to know about sex. Nature 331:300–301, 1988.

63. Lee PA, Rock JA, Brown TR, et al: Leydig cell hypofunction resulting in male pseudohermaphroditism. Fertil Steril 37:675, 1982.

64. Schwartz M, Imperato-McGinley J, Peterson RE, et al: Male pseudohermaphroditism secondary to an abnormality in Leydig cell differentiation. J Clin Endocrinol Metab 53:123, 1981.

65. Pagnon RA: Diagnostic approach to the newborn with ambiguous genitalia. Pediatr Adolesc Endocrinol 34:1019–1031, 1987.

66. Berkovitz GD, Lee PA, Brown TR, et al: Etiologic evaluation of male pseudohermaphroditism in infancy and childhood. Am J Dis Child 138:755–759, 1984.

67. Kropp BP, Keating MA, Moshang T, Duckett JW: True hermaphroditism and normal male genitalia: An unusual presentation. Urology 46:736–739, 1995.

68. Skordis NA, Stetka DG, MacGillivray MH, Greenfield SP: Familial 46,XX males coexisting with familial 46,XX true hermaphrodites in same pedigree. J Pediatr Surg 110:244–248, 1986.
69. Hadjiathanasiou CG, Brauner R, Lortat-Jacob S, et al: True hermaphroditism: Genetic variants and clinical management. J Pediatrics 125:738–744, 1994.
70. Gooren LJG: Reversal of the LH response to oestrogen administration after orchidectomy in a male subject with the androgen insensitivity syndrome. Horm Metabol Res 19:138, 1987.
71. Grace HJ: Intersexuality: Definitions, diagnosis and dilemmas. Arch Androl 17:129–131, 1986.
72. McDaniel EC, Nadel M, Woolverton WC: True hermaphrodite with bilaterally descended ovotestes. J Urol 100:77–81, 1968.
73. Van Niekerk WA: True hermaphroditism: An analytic review with a report of 3 new cases. Am J Obstet Gynecol 126:890–907, 1976.
74. Salvatierra O, Skaist LB, Morrow JW: True hermaphroditism discovered 10 years after hypospadias repair: Report of 2 cases. J Urol 98:111–115, 1967.
75. Salle B, Hedinger C: Gonadal histology in children with male pseudohermaphroditism and mixed gonadal dysgenesis. Acta Endocrinol 64:211–227, 1970.
76. Donahoe PK, Hendren WH: Intersex abnormalities in the newborn infant. In Holder TH, Ashcraft KW (eds): Pediatric Surgery. Philadelphia, W.B. Saunders, pp 858–890, 1980.
77. Rohatgi M, Menon PSN, Verma IC, Iyengar JK: The presence of intersexuality in patients with advanced hypospadias and undescended gonads. J Urol 137:263–267, 1987.
78. Ritcey ML, Benson RC Jr, Kramer SA, Kelalis PP: Management of müllerian duct remnants in the male patient. J Urol 140:795–799, 1988.
79. O'Brien WM, Gibbons MD: Hypospadias. Am Fam Physician 39:183–191, 1989.
80. Jensen JC, Ehrlich RM, Hanna MK, et al: A report of 4 patients with the Drash syndrome and a review of the literature. J Urol 141:1174–1176, 1989.
81. Donohoue PA, Parker K, Migeon CJ: Congenital adrenal hyperplasia. In Scriver CR (ed): Metabolic and Molecular Bases of Inherited Disease (7th ed). New York: McGraw-Hill, 1995.
82. Haymond MW, Weldon VV: Female pseudohermaphroditism secondary to a maternal virilizing tumor. J Pediatr 82:682–686, 1973.
83. Schneider KM, Becker JM, Krasna IH: Surgical management of intersexuality in infancy and childhood: Ann Surg 168:255–261, 1968.
84. Gustafson ML, Lee MM, Asmundson L, et al: Müllerian inhibiting substance in the diagnosis and management of intersex and gonadal abnormalities. J Pediatr Surg 28:439–444, 1993.
85. Oppenheimer A: Consideration on anatomical, and psychic reality in relation to an intersexual patient. Int J Psycho Anal 76:1191–1204, 1995.
86. De Jong TPVM, Boemers TML: Neonatal management of female intersex by clitoro-vaginoplasty. J Urol 154:830–832, 1995.
87. Money J: Pediatric sexology and hermaphroditism. J Sex Marital Ther 11:139–156, 1985.
88. Gilbert DA, Jordan GH, Devine CJ Jr, et al: Phallic construction in prepubertal and adolescent boys. J Urol 149:1521–1526, 1993.
89. Jordan GH, Alter GJ, Gilbert DA, et al: Penile prosthesis implantation in total phalloplasty. J Urol 152:410–414, 1994.
90. Gilbert DA, Horton CE, Terzis JK, et al: New concepts in phallic reconstruction. Ann Plast Surg 18:128–136, 1987.
91. Vorstman B, Horton CE, Winslow BH: Repair of secondary genital deformities of epispadias/exstrophy. Clin Plast Surg 15:381–391, 1988.
92. Perovic S: Phalloplasty in children and adolescents using the extended pedicle island groin flap. J Urol 154:848–853, 1995.
93. Husmann DA, McLorie GA, Churchill BM: Phallic reconstruction in cloacal exstrophy. J Urol 142:563–564, 1989.
94. Sadove RC, Sengezer M, McRoberts JW, Wells MD: One-stage total penile reconstruction with a free sensate osteocutaneous fibula flap. Plast Reconstr Surg 92:1314–1325, 993.
95. Gilbert DA, Jordan GH, Devine CJ Jr, Winslow BH: Microsurgical forearm "cricket bat-transformer" phalloplasty. Plast Reconstr Surg 90:711–716, 1992.
96. Gilbert DA, Williams MW, Horton CE, et al: Phallic reinnervation via the pudendal nerve. J Urol 140:295–299, 1988.
97. Kai-Xiang C, Ru-Hong Z, Su Z: Cheng's method for reconstruction of a functionally sensitive penis. Plast Reconstr Surg 99;87–92, 1997.
98. Gilbert DA, Winslow BH: Penis construction. Semin Urol 5:262–269, 1987.
99. Stolar CJH, Wiener ES, Hensle TW, et al; Reconstruction of penile agenesis by a posterior sagittal approach. 22:1076–1080, 1987.
100. Merke DP, Cutler GB Jr: New approches to the treatment of congenital adrenal hyperplasia. JAMA 277:1073–1076, 1997.
101. Van Wyk JJ, Gunther DF, Ritzen EM, et al: The use of adrenalectomy as a treatment for congenital hyperplasia. J Clin Endocrinol Metab 81:3180–3190, 1996
102. Mercado AB, Wilson RC, Cheng KC, et al: Prenatal treatment and diagnosis of congenital adrenal hyperplasia owing to steroid 21-hydroxylase deficiency. J Clin Endocrinol Metab 80:2014–2020, 1995.
103. Donahoe PK, Powell DM, Lee MM: Clinical management of intersex abnormalities. Curr Probl Surg 28:513–579, 1991.
104. Simpson JL: Diagnosis and management of genital ambiguity. Am J Obstet Gynecol 128:137–145, 1977.
105. Luks FI, Hansbrough F, Klotz DH Jr, et al: Early gender assignment in true hermaphroditism. J Pediatr Surg 23:1122–1126, 1988.
106. Petersen L, Kock K, Jacobsen BB: Germ cell neoplasms in three intersex patients with 46, XY karyotype. Int Urol Nephrol 24:633–639, 1992.
107. Hammar B, Michowitz M, Solowiejczyk M: Testicular feminization syndrome. Am Surg 46:457–460, 1980.
108. Boczkowski K: Franciszek Neugebauer (1856–1914)—Pioneer in the study of hermaphroditism. Bull Pol Med Sci Hist 9:155–157, 1966.
109. Money J, Lobato C: Matched pair of siblings concordant for 46, XY hermaphroditism with female sex assignment and discordant for erotosexual outcome. Psychiatry 51:65–79, 1988.
110. De Jong T, Boemers TML: Neonatal management of female intersex by clitorovaginoplasty. J Urol 154:830–832, 1995.
111. Shaw RW, Farquhar JW: Female pseudohermaphroditism associated with danazol exposure in utero. Case report. Br J Obstet Gynecol 91:386–389, 1984.
112. Allen LE, Hardy BF, Churchill BM: The surgical management of the enlarged clitoris. J Urol 128:351–354, 1982.
113. Caufriez A: Male pseudohermaphroditism due to 17-ketoreductase deficiency: Report of a case without gynecomastia and without vaginal pouch. Am J Obstet Gynecol 154:148–149, 1986.
114. Barrett TM, Gonzales ET: Reconstruction of the female external genitalia. Urol Clin North Am 7:455–463, 1980.
115. Randolph JG, Hung W: Reduction clitoroplasty in females with hypertrophied clitoris. J Pediatr Surg 5:224–231, 1970.
116. Spence HM, Allen TD: Genital reconstruction in the female with the adrenogenital syndrome. Br J Urol 45:126–130, 1973.
117. Mollard P, Juskiewenski S, Sarkissian J: Clitoroplasty in intersex: A new technique. Br J Urol 53: 363–371, 1981.
118. Gonzalez R, Fernandes ET: Single-stage feminization genitoplasty. J Urol 143:776–778, 1990.
119. Pena A, Filmer B, Bonilla E, et al: Transanorectal approach for the treatment of urogenital sinus: Preliminary report. J Pediatr Surg 27:681–685, 1992.
120. Jones HW, Verkauf BS: Surgical treatment in congenital

adrenal hyperplasia: Age at operation and other prognostic factors. Obstet Gynecol 36:1–10, 1970.

121. Lobe TE, Woodall DL, Richards GE, et al: The complications of surgery for intersex: Changing patterns over two decades. J Pediatr Surg 22:651–652, 1987.

122. McIndoe AH, et al: An operation for the cure of congenital absence of the vagina. J Obstet Gynecol 45:490–494, 1938.

123. Wiser WL, Bates GW: Management of agenesis of the vagina. Surg Gynecol Obstet 159:108–112, 1984.

124. Masters WH, Johnson VE: Human Sexual Inadequacy. Boston, Little, Brown, pp 214–250, 1970.

125. Goligher JC: The use of pedicled transplants of sigmoid or other parts of the intestinal tract for vaginal construction. Ann R Coll Surg Engl 65:353–355, 1983.

126. Laub DR, Laub DR II, Biber S: Vaginoplasty for gender confirmation. Clin Plast Surg 15:463–470, 1988.

127. Gearhart JP, Jeffs RD: The use of parenteral testosterone therapy in genital reconstructive surgery. J Urol 138:1077–1078, 1987.

128. Lee PA: Micropenis. Pediatr Adolesc Endocrinol 19:149–154, 1989.

129. Benjamin H: Sex is what you see, gender is what you feel; comfort with each is necessary for happiness. Presented at International Gender Symposium; Norfolk, VA; 1972.

62

RENOVASCULAR HYPERTENSION

James C. Stanley, MD

Renal artery occlusive disease is an uncommon but exceedingly important form of surgically correctable hypertension in children. The underlying renal artery stenoses represent a heterogeneic group of complex lesions that must be carefully defined before undertaking operative therapy. Although pediatric renovascular hypertension has been the subject of many reports, few centers have reported more than an anecdotal experience with the surgical treatment of this disease.[1–9]

☐ Clinical Presentation

The precise frequency of pediatric renovascular hypertension is unknown, yet its clinical relevance has been firmly established. Manifestations of this disease are variable. Older children may have silent elevations of their blood pressure, but many have a history of cephalalgia and fatigability. Younger children and infants with severe hypertension often exhibit failure to thrive. Seizures affect occasional patients, and some children present with fixed neurologic deficits due to cerebral hemorrhage. Increased awareness of the serious consequences of untreated hypertension in children has resulted in renovascular disease being recognized in many children whose blood pressure elevations were noted during routine physical examination.

Children with renovascular hypertension in the largest reported series had a mean age of 10.6 years, with no gender predilection noted.[7] In this series, the mean duration of preoperative hypertension was 14.2 months. Preoperative blood pressures decreased significantly from an average of 181/117 mm Hg without medication to an average of 158/104 mm Hg with drug therapy. Blood pressure after surgical therapy averaged 117/73 mm Hg. These data are similar to those of other large clinical experiences.

High blood pressure in children usually represents a secondary form of hypertension. This is because essential hypertension is rarely, if ever, encountered in infants and children. Thus, the mere presence of modest or severe blood pressure eleva-

tions in a child should generate a suspicion of renovascular etiology. Children with this disease, like their adult counterparts, are often resistant to drug therapy.[7] Although it has been suggested that medical therapy is appropriate in certain younger patients,[10, 11] uncontrolled hypertension and its clinical sequelae usually preclude nonoperative management of this illness. Severe deterioration of renal function has been an infrequent finding among children with nonmalignant renovascular hypertension, even when the entire renal mass appears to be at risk from bilateral disease or when unilateral disease affects a solitary kidney.

☐ Pathology of Renal Artery Stenotic Disease

Intimal fibroplasia and atypical medial-perimedial fibrodysplasia are the most common histologic types of renal artery disease affecting children.[7] Such dysplastic lesions account for 90% of cases of pediatric renovascular hypertension. Nearly all of the remaining 10% of children exhibit inflammatory renal artery occlusive disease of varying etiologies. Trauma and emboli are rare causes of sustained hypertension in children, although both may cause renal infarction and acute transient blood pressure elevations.

Ostial lesions account for nearly 70% of pediatric renovascular stenoses (Fig. 62–1). In most cases, the primary vessel defect is considered to be developmental. These proximal stenoses often are encountered in patients who have neurofibromatosis or abdominal aortic narrowing. The renal artery lesions usually represent hypoplastic vessels, having an external hourglass appearance. Dysplastic intimal and medial changes invariably contribute to the stenosis, characterized by loss of smooth muscle, increases in ground substances, and fragmentation and excessive accumulations of elastic tissue (Fig. 62–2). Intimal fibroplasia in these lesions is considered a secondary phenomenon, occurring as a consequence of turbulent flow through the narrowed vessel.

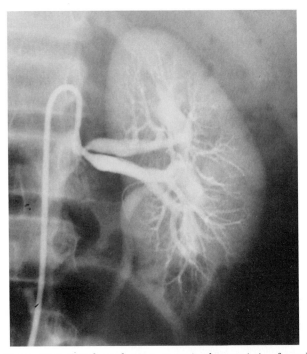

Figure 62–1. Ostial renal artery stenosis characteristic of renal artery occlusive disease associated with neurofibromatosis or developmental abdominal aortic narrowing. (From Stanley JC, Fry WJ: Pediatric renal artery occlusive disease and renovascular hypertension: Etiology, diagnosis, and operative treatment. Arch Surg 116:669–676, 1981. Copyright 1981, American Medical Association.)

Mid-renal artery lesions, appearing as either focal or long tubular stenoses, account for about 20% of pediatric renovascular stenoses (Fig. 62–3). Focal lesions usually represent eccentric dysplastic mesenchymal tissue projecting into the arterial lumen. Tubular lesions are characterized by circumferential medial fibroplasia with secondary intimal proliferation. Certain of these lesions may be the sequela of trauma or intraluminal thrombotic events incurred early in life.

Isolated segmental lesions, appearing almost web-like, affect 5% of these children (Fig. 62–4). Umbilical catheter-related embolism may be a cause of these lesions in some children. Coexistent segmental and middle main renal artery stenoses affect an additional 5% of these patients. The latter lesions, unlike ostial disease, occur most often in patients not manifesting stigmata of neurofibromatosis or aortic narrowing.

Developmental events responsible for the various stenoses encountered in children with renovascular hypertension are poorly defined.[12–14] Failure of the normal transition of fetal mesenchymal tissue to vascular smooth muscle or altered organization and growth of this smooth muscle may cause arrested development of the two dorsal aortas in utero or the fused aortas during early infancy. This may lead to aortic narrowing and subsequent renal artery stenoses. In fact, patients with abdominal aortic coarctation or hypoplasia often exhibit coexisting renal ar-

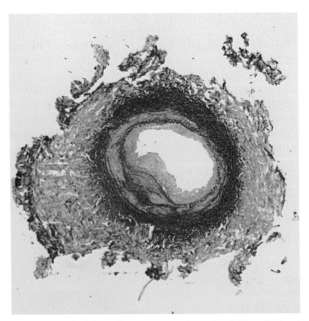

Figure 62–2. Ostial renal artery stenosis. Intimal fibroplasia, duplication of the internal elastic lamina, medial thinning, and excessive adventitial elastic tissue characterize this developmentally narrowed renal artery with a luminal diameter of less than 0.5 mm. Cross-section. (Reprinted from Am J Surg, 142, Stanley JC, Graham LM, Whitehouse WM Jr, et al, Developmental occlusive disease of the abdominal aorta, splanchnic and renal arteries, pp 190–196, 1981, with permission from Excerpta Medica Inc.)

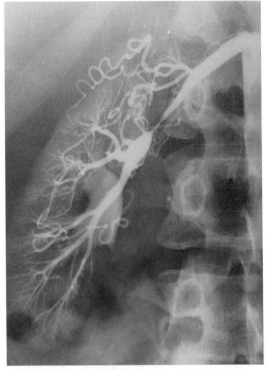

Figure 62–3. Midrenal artery smooth focal stenosis characteristic of intimal fibroplasia. (From Stanley JC, Fry WJ: Renovascular hypertension secondary to arterial fibrodysplasia in adults. Arch Surg 110:922–928, 1975. Copyright 1975, American Medical Association.)

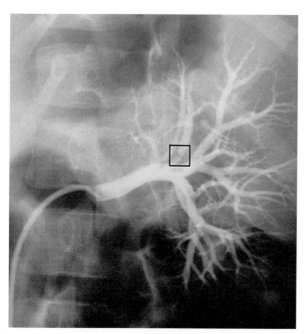

Figure 62–4. Segmental renal artery stenosis affecting a second-order intraparenchymal vessel. The focal, web-like lesion is associated by minimal poststenotic arterial dilation. (From Stanley JC, Fry WJ: Pediatric renal artery occlusive disease and renovascular hypertension: Etiology, diagnosis, and operative treatment. Arch Surg 116:669–676, 1981. Copyright 1981, American Medical Association.)

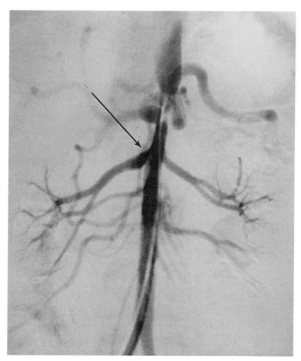

Figure 62–5. Suprarenal abdominal aortic coarctation with two arteries to each kidney and an ostial stenosis of the right superior pole vessel *(arrow)*. (Reprinted from Am J Surg, 142, Stanley JC, Graham LM, Whitehouse WM Jr, et al, Developmental occlusive disease of the abdominal aorta, splanchnic and renal arteries. Am J Surg 142:190–196, 1981, with permission from Excerpta Medica Inc.)

tery stenoses and renovascular hypertension (Figs. 62–5 and 62–6). Viruses such as rubella that are cytocidal or those that inhibit cell replication may contribute to impaired aortic growth in some children. In other cases, these lesions may reflect the aftermath of an earlier inflammatory disease, such as Takayasu's aortoarteritis.[15] Finally, neurofibromatosis, a disorder commonly coexisting with aortic hypoplasia, may include mesenchymal tissue abnormalities that directly interfere with development of normal smooth muscle and result in renal artery narrowing.[16–18]

Detection of multiple renal arteries to one or both kidneys in nearly 80% of patients with abdominal aortic narrowing lends support to the developmental etiology of many renovascular lesions.[7, 19] Under usual circumstances, the two dorsal aortas fuse at about the same embryonic time that the multiple metanephric branches disappear, leaving a single renal artery in 65 to 75% of the population. Persistence of a single renal artery is alleged to result from its obligate hemodynamic advantage over adjacent metanephric vessels. Aortic abnormalities that cause flow disturbances in the vicinity of the origin of a principal renal artery may diminish its hemodynamic advantage, thus permitting persistence of adjacent metanephric channels.

Ostial narrowing of the celiac and superior mesenteric arteries affects 22% of patients with abdominal aortic coarctation or hypoplasia.[19] These stenoses may be hemodynamically insignificant in young patients but may become functionally important as

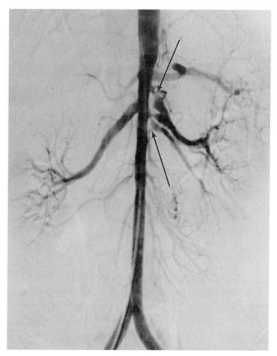

Figure 62–6. Diffuse abdominal aortic narrowing from the level of the celiac artery to the aortic bifurcation. Severe ostial stenoses affecting multiple left renal arteries *(arrows)*. (From Graham LM, Zelenock GB, Erlandson EE, et al: Abdominal aortic coarctation and segmental hypoplasia. Surgery 86:519–529, 1979.)

the patient becomes older, owing to a failure of these vessels to grow. In fact, evolving stenoses of the celiac artery have been associated with late recurrences of hypertension, following what initially were considered successful splenorenal revascularization operations.

The developmental aortic narrowings, like the renal artery stenoses, appear to represent diminutive vessels, often having an hourglass shape. The locations of the abdominal aortic narrowings are at renal level in 52% of patients, suprarenal in 11%, and infrarenal in 25%.[19] The remaining 12% of children exhibit diffuse aortic hypoplasia, usually limited to the abdominal aorta. Aortic tissues in the coarcted or hypoplastic vessel invariably exhibit intimal fibroplasia with increased basophilic medial ground substances without evidence of active inflammation.

□ Diagnostic Studies

The role of laboratory tests in establishing the presence of renovascular hypertension in children deserves specific comment.

HYPERTENSIVE UROGRAPHY

Hypertensive urograms are of limited usefulness. Nevertheless, urographic findings supporting existence of unilateral renovascular disease include the following: (1) delay in contrast appearance within the ischemic kidney's collecting system; (2) renal length discrepancies, the ischemic kidney being shorter than the normal kidney; (3) hyperconcentration of contrast within the ischemic kidney's collecting system on later films; and (4) ureteral or renal pelvic collecting system notching caused by collateral vessels.

Size differences become relevant when length discrepancies are greater than 0.5 cm in children younger than 15 years of age or greater than 1.0 cm in older children. Unfortunately, abnormal hypertensive urograms have been documented in only 27% of children with proved renovascular hypertension who were subsequently cured of their disease by operation.[6] This is likely a result of the existence of bilateral renal artery stenoses or unilateral segmental disease, which are not detected by hypertensive urography.

ARTERIOGRAPHIC STUDIES

Arteriographic studies are essential to confirm the presence and define the extent of renovascular disease in children. Collateral vessels circumventing a stenosis confirm the lesion's hemodynamic and functional importance. A pressure gradient of 10 to 15 mm Hg across a stenosis causes development of such collateral vessels, and this pressure change is a clear cause of excess release of renin from the kidney. Collateral vessels have been observed in 88% of children with renovascular hypertension.[6]

DUPLEX ULTRASONOGRAPHY

Deep abdominal duplex ultrasonography of the renal arteries in children has had limited clinical application. Because of the two-dimensional aspects of ultrasonography, direct imaging may not always reveal the degree of a stenosis. Velocity studies are more reliable for identification of hemodynamically important renal artery stenoses. Peak velocity in the range of 180 to 200 cm/sec and a renal artery–to–aortic velocity ratio approaching 3.5 are diagnostic. Because it is impossible to discriminate among lesions exceeding a 60% cross-sectional narrowing, as well as to recognize small accessory or segmental vessel disease, this technology must be used cautiously in children as a means of excluding a diagnosis of renovascular hypertension.

ANGIOTENSIN-CONVERTING ENZYME INHIBITORS

Administration of angiotensin-converting enzyme (ACE) inhibitors in children may provide for better blood pressure control, but impaired renal function may follow use of such agents, and this, in fact, may be a marker of the existence of renovascular hypertension. ACE inhibitor renal nuclide scans have been suggested to be useful in detecting reduced renal blood flow in children, but validation of these studies has not been forthcoming.[20, 21]

RENAL VEIN:RENIN RATIOS

Elevated plasma renin activity occurs in about 85% of children with renovascular hypertension. It is generally accepted that renal vein:renin ratios, comparing renin activity in venous blood samples from each kidney, suggest functionally important renal artery stenotic disease when greater than 1.48. In one large series, the mean renal vein:renin ratio among those benefiting from operation was 2.07.[6] However, 20% of these children had a renal vein:renin ratio of less than 1.48, of whom most had either distal segmental branch disease or severe bilateral main renal artery stenoses. Clearly, renal vein:renin ratios lose their diagnostic value in cases of bilateral disease with similarly elevated renin secretion from both kidneys. Owing to such false-negative study results, these ratios are of limited usefulness in children with renovascular hypertension.

RENAL-TO-SYSTEMIC RENIN INDEX

Individual kidney renin activity, expressed as a renal-to-systemic renin index, allows for a more accurate identification of patients who have functionally important renal artery stenosis, regardless of the bilaterality of the disease. The renal-to-systemic renin index is calculated by subtracting systemic renin activity from renal vein renin activity and dividing the remainder by the systemic renin activity. Systemic renin activity is usually assayed from infrarenal vena caval blood samples. Although renin kinetics in hypertensive children have not been as thoroughly studied as in adults, a beneficial response after unilateral surgical therapy is likely to occur when the involved ipsilateral kidney has a renal-to-systemic renin index of greater than 0.48 (representing renin hypersecretion) and when the index from the contralateral kidney approaches 0 (representing renin suppression).[6] Among children cured by unilateral operations in one large experience, the mean ischemic kidney renal-to-systemic renin index was 1.04 and the contralateral index was 0.01. Among children cured by bilateral interventions, the mean renal-to-systemic renin index for the most ischemic kidney was 3.14, and the contralateral index was 2.33. Thus, renin index data, documenting renin hypersecretion and suppression, provide useful preoperative prognostic information. This becomes particularly important when determining the appropriateness of unilateral versus bilateral renal revascularization.

□ Treatment

Surgical intervention for pediatric renovascular hypertension must be individualized. Certain operations have become relatively well standardized.[7, 22, 23] Exposure is critical to successful renal revascularization in children. A supraumbilical transverse incision is preferred, carried from the opposite midclavicular line to the posterior axillary line on the side of the affected renal artery. The incision is extended into both flanks for bilateral reconstruction. Transverse abdominal incisions offer distinct technical advantages over vertical midline abdominal incisions. The renal vessels and abdominal aorta are exposed by incising the lateral parietes and reflecting the colon, duodenum, and pancreas medially. This extraperitoneal exposure provides better visualization of the renal arteries than is possible through an anterior approach at the base of the mesocolon and small bowel mesentery.

Before clamping the aorta or renal arteries, the patient is systemically anticoagulated with intravenous heparin, 150 U/kg. Similarly, before clamping the renal artery, a diuresis is established, facilitated by intravenous administration of mannitol, 0.17 g/kg. The heparin anticoagulation is reversed at the conclusion of the arterial reconstruction with intravenous administration of protamine sulfate, 1.5 mg/ 100 units of previously administered heparin.

REIMPLANTATION OF A RENAL ARTERY

Reimplantation of a renal artery into the aorta or an adjacent renal artery, after its transection beyond the stenosis, has become a preferred manner of treating children whose stenotic disease is limited to the origin of the main renal artery or a segmental artery (Figs. 62–7 to 62–9).[7] In these circumstances, the transected renal artery to be implanted is spatulated anteriorly and posteriorly so as to create a generous anastomotic orificial patch. An aortotomy or an arteriotomy on an adjacent artery is made of a length that usually is a little over twice the diameter of the renal artery, to permit creation of a generous anastomosis. These anastomoses usually are created using interrupted monofilament sutures. A continuous suture is appropriate for creation of larger aortic anastomoses in older adolescents.

AORTORENAL BYPASS

Aortorenal bypass with an internal iliac artery graft has been used most often when a bypass is required in children (Fig. 62–10).[7] The internal iliac artery should be excised to include a bifurcation branch at its distal end. Incising the crotch between the branch and trunk of the artery allows for creation of a wide orificial opening for the aortic anas-

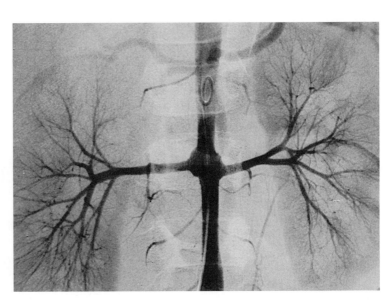

Figure 62–7. Aortic reimplantation of main renal arteries, beyond orificial stenoses.

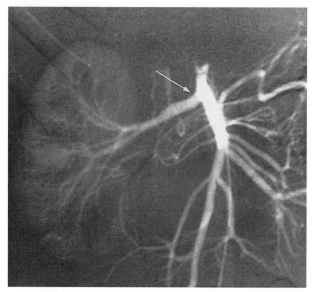

Figure 62–8. Reimplantation of right renal artery to superior mesenteric artery, in end-to-side fashion. (From Stanley JC, Zelenock GB, Messina LM, et al: Pediatric renovascular hypertension: A thirty-year experience of operative treatment. J Vasc Surg 21:212–227, 1995.)

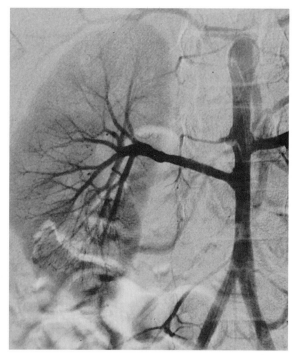

Figure 62–10. Aortorenal bypass with internal iliac artery graft. (From Stanley JC, Zelenock GB, Messina LM, et al: Pediatric renovascular hypertension: A thirty-year experience of operative treatment. J Vasc Surg 21:212–227, 1995.)

tomosis. The aortic anastomosis is completed in most children using a continuous monofilament suture interrupted in three or four places. The anastomosis of the graft to the distal renal artery is fashioned in an end-to-end manner. Spatulation of both vessel ends creates an ovoid anastomosis that is less apt to develop a late stricture than is a nonspatulated anastomosis (Fig. 62–11). Individual interrupted sutures are used to anastomose vessels 2 mm or less in diameter, with continuous sutures used for adult-sized vessel anastomoses. Multiple stenoses of small renal arteries are best managed by joining the transected vessels so that they form a larger common orifice to which the graft can be anastomosed.

Prosthetic grafts are inappropriate for most pediatric renal artery reconstructive procedures owing to technical limitations and the possibility of infection. Autogenous saphenous vein grafts are not recom-

mended because 60% degenerate and dilate, including 20% that exhibit severe aneurysmal changes.[7, 24] Continued expansion or embolization of mural thrombus has necessitated removing aneurysmal vein grafts. Placement of an external Dacron mesh around aortorenal vein grafts in children has been advocated as a means of preventing aneurysmal dilation.[2] Internal iliac artery grafts do not often undergo aneurysmal change. Late stenosis occurs in 5% of aortorenal vein grafts placed in children but is rarely seen with hypogastric artery grafts.

SPLENORENAL BYPASS

Splenorenal bypass with direct anastomosis of the splenic artery to the end of the left renal artery is

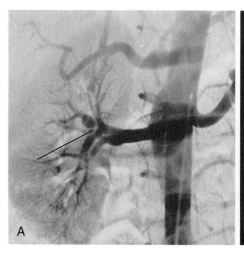
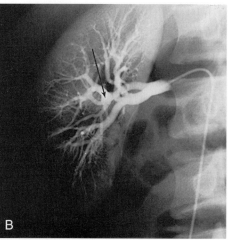

Figure 62–9. Reimplantation of segmental renal artery, beyond its stenosis, into adjacent segmental renal artery. *A,* Preoperative arteriogram documenting stenosis and poststenotic dilation (*arrow*). *B,* Postoperative arteriogram demonstrating widely patent anastomosis (*arrow*). (From Stanley JC, Zelenock GB, Messina LM, et al: Pediatric renovascular hypertension: A thirty-year experience of operative treatment. J Vasc Surg 21:212–227, 1995.)

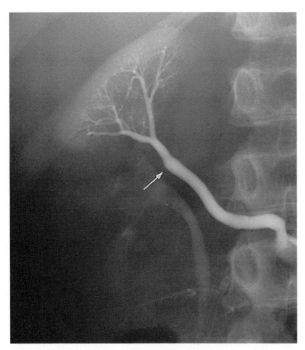

Figure 62–11. Ovoid appearance of a spatulated autogenous saphenous vein-segmental renal artery anastomosis *(arrow)* during immediate postoperative period. (From Fry WJ, Ernst CB, Stanley JC, et al: Renovascular hypertension in the pediatric patient. Arch Surg 107:692–698, 1973. Copyright 1973, American Medical Association.)

complicated by an unacceptable incidence of early thrombotic problems.[5, 25] Furthermore, many children with renovascular hypertension have normal-appearing celiac arteries at the time of their initial reconstructive procedure, only to manifest failure of the celiac artery to grow as the child becomes older. The latter may lead to recurrent hypertension. Unfortunately, there is no means of predicting whether a given celiac artery will subsequently become stenotic in a child being treated for renovascular hypertension.

EX VIVO REVASCULARIZATIONS

Renal autotransplantation as a routine treatment for pediatric renovascular hypertension is controversial. Although most surgeons favor in situ reconstructions, members of active kidney transplantation programs often perform this type of renal revascularization.[26, 27] The ability to perform a bench reconstruction for extensive renal artery stenotic disease should be in the armamentarium of all surgeons who undertake operative treatment of renovascular hypertension in children.

OPERATIVE DILATION

Operative dilation of segmental renal artery stenosis carries a relatively high incidence of thrombotic complications. Most pediatric renal artery narrowing represents true vessel hypoplasia. Vascular disruption is required for effective operative dila-

tion, or for percutaneous transluminal angioplasty (PTA), to relieve most stenotic lesions. Furthermore, PTA of first- or second-order segmental branch disease is often complicated by intimal fractures and irreparable intraparenchymal renal artery thromboses. Owing to these issues, PTA in children has not provided predictably good results.[28–30] Thus, unlike in adults, PTA has a limited role in the treatment of renovascular hypertension in children. In contrast, percutaneous transcatheter ablation of renal segments responsible for excess renin production by injection of alcohol may prove useful in select cases.[7, 31]

THORACOABDOMINAL AORTOAORTIC BYPASS

Thoracoabdominal aortoaortic bypass using expanded polytetrafluoroethylene (PTFE) or fabricated Dacron prostheses in conjunction with renal artery reconstructions has been a common operation performed for the management of abdominal aortic narrowing and concomitant renal artery disease[32–34] (Fig. 62–12). Extraperitoneal reflection of the abdominal viscera provides generous access to the proximal abdominal aorta and its renal branches in these cases. Renal artery autograft with the proximal end anastomosed to the aorta below the aortic bypass graft is less likely to occlude than one that is anastomosed to the thoracoabdominal prosthesis.

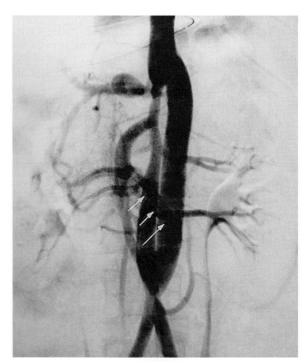

Figure 62–12. Thoracoabdominal bypass (Dacron venous graft) and aortorenal bypass to right renal artery *(arrows)* in a patient who had a suprarenal abdominal aortic coarctation and ostial stenosis of the right renal artery. (From Graham LM, Zelenock GB, Erlandson EE, et al: Abdominal aortic coarctation and segmental hypoplasia. Surgery 86:519–529, 1979.)

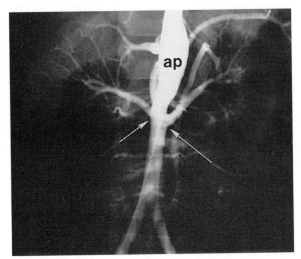

Figure 62–13. Aortoplasty (ap) of midabdominal aortic coarctation (PTFE patch) with bilateral reimplantation of renal arteries *(arrows)* in a patient who had a suprarenal abdominal aortic coarctation and bilateral renal artery ostial stenotic disease. (From Stanley JC, Brothers TE: Surgical treatment of renovascular hypertension in children. In Ernst CB, Stanley JC [eds]: Current Therapy in Vascular Surgery [2nd ed]. Philadelphia, BC Decker, 1991, pp 856–860.

PRIMARY PATCH AORTOPLASTY

Primary patch aortoplasty with prosthetic graft material for treatment of aortic narrowing, combined with reimplantation of the renal arteries into the normal aorta, is currently the preferred treatment for most combined pediatric renal artery and abdominal aortic lesions[7, 34] (Fig. 62–13). The patch, usually of expanded PTFE, should be wide enough that it does not become constrictive as the patient grows into adulthood. Avoidance of competitive parallel flow in the native aorta and a thoracoab-dominal bypass, absence of individual aortorenal bypass grafts, and a reduction in the number of anastomoses performed represent important advantages of such a single-stage patch aortoplasty and renal artery implantation technique.

□ Results of Operative Therapy

Outcomes from operations for pediatric renovascular hypertension should be judged by specifically defined criteria for age and gender,[35] as follows:

Cure, if no antihypertensive medications were administered for the preceding 6 months and blood pressure is below the 95th percentile expected for the child

Improved, if pressures are within normotensive ranges on drug therapy (excluding ACE inhibitors), or if diastolic pressures are greater than normal but at least 15% lower than preoperative levels

Failure, if diastolic pressures remain greater than established normal levels but are not 15% lower than preoperative values, or if ACE inhibitors are required to control the blood pressure

Cumulative experiences with the operative treatment of children with renovascular hypertension reveal excellent results (Table 62–1). A beneficial outcome should be anticipated in almost all patients. Although certain discrepancies exist from one center to the next regarding the number of primary arterial reconstructions versus primary nephrectomies, improved vascular surgical techniques have increased the likelihood of successful revascularization with preservation of renal parenchyma.

TABLE 62–1. Pediatric Renovascular Hypertension: Comparative Results of Surgical Treatment

Medical Center	No. of Patients	Primary Procedure		Secondary Procedures	Postoperative Status (%)*			Operative Mortality (%)
		Arterial Reconstruction	Nephrectomy		Cure	Improved	Failure	
University of Michigan[7] 1963–1993	57	67	7	20	79	19	2	0
Cleveland Clinic[5, 25] 1955–1977	27	22	11	5	59	18.5	18.5	4
University of California, Los Angeles[8] 1967–1977	26	19	11	7	84.5	7.5	4	4
Vanderbilt University[4]† 1962–1977	21	15	8	4	68	24	8	0
University of Pennsylvania[2] 1974–1987	17	30	0	1‡	76.5	23.5	0	0
University of California, San Francisco[9] 1960–1974	14	10	4	2	86	7	0	7

*Criteria for blood pressure response defined in cited publications. Operative mortality not included in failure category. Data expressed to nearest 0.5%.
†Results included data from four patients with parenchymal disease treated by nephrectomy.
‡Two revascularized kidneys considered to have become infarcted postoperatively were not removed in this series, but they would have represented a secondary procedure had they been removed.

REFERENCES

1. Benjamin SP, Dustan HP, Gifford RW Jr: Stenosing renal artery disease in children: Clinicopathological correlation in 20 surgically treated cases. Clev Clin Q 43:197–206, 1976.
2. Berkowitz HD, O'Neill JA Jr: Renovascular hypertension in children: Surgical repair with special reference to the use of reinforced vein grafts. J Vasc Surg 9:46–55, 1989.
3. Fry WJ, Ernst CB, Stanley JC, et al: Renovascular hypertension in the pediatric patient. Arch Surg 107:692–698, 1973.
4. Lawson JD, Boerth R, Foster JH, et al: Diagnosis and management of renovascular hypertension in children. Arch Surg 122:1307–1316, 1977.
5. Novick AC, Straffon RA, Stewart BH, et al: Surgical treatment of renovascular hypertension in the pediatric patient. J Urol 119:794–805, 1978.
6. Stanley JC, Fry WJ: Pediatric renal artery occlusive disease and renovascular hypertension: Etiology, diagnosis and operative treatment. Arch Surg 116:669–676, 1981.
7. Stanley JC, Zelenock GB, Messina LM, et al: Pediatric renovascular hypertension: A thirty-year experience of operative treatment. J Vasc Surg 21:212–227, 1995.
8. Stanley P, Gyepes MT, Olson DL, et al: Renovascular hypertension in children and adolescents. Radiology 129:123–131, 1978.
9. Stoney RJ, Cooke PA, Strong ST: Surgical treatment of renovascular hypertension in children. J Pediatr Surg 10:631–639, 1975.
10. Daniels SR, Loggie JMH, McEnery PT, et al: Clinical spectrum of intrinsic renovascular hypertension in children. Pediatrics 80:698–704, 1987.
11. Mirkin BL, Newman TJ: Efficacy and safety of captopril in the treatment of severe childhood hypertension: Report of the International Collaborative Study Group. Pediatrics 75:1091–1100, 1985.
12. Arnot RS, Louw HJ: The anatomy of the posterior wall of the abdominal aorta: Its significance with regard to hypoplasia of the distal aorta. S Afr Med J 47:899–902, 1973.
13. Maycok WD'A: Congenital stenosis of the abdominal aorta. Am Heart J 13:633–646, 1937.
14. Stanley JC, Graham LM, Whitehouse WM Jr, et al: Developmental occlusive disease of the abdominal aorta, splanchnic and renal arteries. Am J Surg 142:190–196, 1981.
15. Wada J, Kazui T: Long-term results of thoracoabdominal bypass graft for atypical coarctation of the aorta. World J Surg 2:891–896, 1978.
16. Greene JF, Fitzwater JE, Burgess J: Arterial lesions associated with neurofibromatosis. Am J Clin Pathol 62:481–487, 1974.
17. Mena E, Bookstein JJ, Holt JF, et al: Neurofibromatosis and renovascular hypertension in children. AJR Am J Roentgenol 118:39–45, 1973.
18. Roy P, Cartier P, Rojo-Ortega JM: Arterial hypertension and neurofibromatosis: Renal artery stenosis and coarctation of abdominal aorta. Can Med Assoc J 113:879–885, 1975.
19. Graham LM, Zelenock GB, Erlandson EE, et al: Abdominal aortic coarctation and segmental hypoplasia. Surgery 86:519–529, 1979.
20. Gauthier B, Trachtman H, Frank R, et al: Inadequacy of captopril challenge test for diagnosing renovascular hypertension in children and adolescents. Pediatr Nephrol 5:42–44, 1991.
21. Hamed RMA, Balfe JW, Ellis G: Use of the captopril test to assess renin responsiveness in children with hypertension and renal disease. Child Nephrol Urol 10:181–185, 1990.
22. Stanley JC: Surgical intervention in pediatric renovascular hypertension. Child Nephrol Urol 12:167–174, 1992.
23. Stanley JC, Whitehouse WM, Zelenock GB, et al: Reoperation for complications of renal artery reconstructive surgery undertaken for treatment of renovascular hypertension. J Vasc Surg 2:133–144, 1985.
24. Stanley JC, Ernst CB, Fry WJ: Fate of 100 aortorenal vein grafts: Characteristics of late graft expansion, aneurysmal dilatation, and stenosis. Surgery 74:931–944, 1973.
25. Martinez A, Novick AC, Cunningham R, et al: Improved results of vascular reconstruction in pediatric and young adult patients with renovascular hypertension. J Urol 144:717–720, 1990.
26. Jordan ML, Novick AC, Cunningham RL: The role of renal autotransplantation in pediatric and young adult patients with renal artery disease. J Vasc Surg 2:385–392, 1985.
27. Kent KC, Salvatierra O, Reilly LM, et al: Evolving strategies for the repair of complex renovascular lesions. Ann Surg 206:272–278, 1987.
28. Guzzetta PC, Potter BM, Ruley EJ, et al: Renovascular hypertension in children: Current concepts in evaluation and treatment. J Pediatr Surg 24:1236–1240, 1989.
29. Stanley P, Hieshima G, Mehringer M: Percutaneous transluminal angioplasty for pediatric renovascular hypertension. Radiology 153:101–104, 1984.
30. Watson AR, Balfe JW, Hardy BE: Renovascular hypertension in childhood: A changing perspective in management. J Pediatr 106:366–372, 1985.
31. Teigen CL, Mitchell SE, Venbrux AC, et al: Segmental renal artery embolization for treatment of pediatric renovascular hypertension. J Vasc Interv Radiol 3:111–117, 1992.
32. Lewis VD 3d, Meranze SG, McLean GK, et al: The midaortic syndrome: Diagnosis and treatment. Radiology 167:111–113, 1988.
33. Messina LM, Goldstone J, Farrell LD, et al: Middle aortic syndrome: Effectiveness and durability of complex arterial revascularization techniques. Ann Surg 204:331–339, 1986.
34. Stanley JC, Brothers TE: Midabdominal aortic coarctation and hypoplasia associated with renal artery stenosis. In Ernst CB, Stanley JC (eds): Current Therapy in Vascular Surgery (2nd ed). Philadelphia, BC Decker, 1991, pp 856–860.
35. National Heart, Lung and Blood Institute's Task Force on Blood Pressure Control in Children: Report of the second task force on blood pressure control in children. Pediatrics 79:1–25, 1987.

63

ADJUVANT THERAPY IN CHILDHOOD CANCER

Gerald M. Haase, MD •
Susan G. Kriessman, MD

☐ Overview of Chemotherapy Treatment for Childhood Cancer

The impressive improvement in cure rates for pediatric malignancies over the past 30 years could not have occurred without the development of multimodality therapy and the cooperative efforts of surgeons, pediatric oncologists, and radiation therapists from across the country. In the 1940s, with the use of wide surgical excision, about 20% of children with localized solid tumors could be cured of their malignancies. However, with the discovery of effective chemotherapeutic agents, pediatric oncologists joined together with surgeons and radiation therapists in cooperative groups and developed a scientific approach to the study of these agents, rapidly improving upon these statistics. Even in the earliest days of cancer therapy, it was the rare child who was not treated with the optimal standardized therapy, from which information was obtained and applied to the next generation of protocols. It was this carefully developed multimodality approach to the total care of the child with cancer that led to the implementation of similar systems in the treatment of adult malignancies and has led to the fact that almost 85% of children with cancer will outlive their malignancy.[1]

HISTORY OF PEDIATRIC ONCOLOGY

The first demonstration that chemotherapy could be effective therapy for childhood malignancies occurred in 1948, when Sidney Farber reported temporary remissions in children with acute lymphoblastic leukemia when the folic acid antagonist aminopterin was given.[2] Several years later, another folic acid antagonist, methotrexate, produced cures in choriocarcinoma.[3] As additional chemotherapeu-

tic agents were developed, these were combined in multidrug regimens that demonstrated significantly improved response rates and response duration compared with single agents. This was first demonstrated in children with acute lymphoblastic leukemia (ALL) and soon confirmed in Wilms' tumor.[4, 5]

The treatment of Wilms' tumor also served as a model for the successful use of multimodality therapy.[6] The adjuvant use of vincristine, actinomycin, and regional radiation therapy following surgical resection produced substantial improvements in cure rates. Similar approaches were adopted for the treatment of rhabdomyosarcoma, Ewing's sarcoma, lymphoma, and other solid tumors. The efficacy of chemotherapy in improving survival in nonmetastatic osteosarcoma patients following surgery was demonstrated in a randomized cooperative group trial. Patients who received adjuvant chemotherapy had a 66% disease-free survival, as compared with a 17% disease-free survival in the patients who received surgery alone.[7] This use of "adjuvant" chemotherapy to control micrometastases has now become standard practice for most solid tumors in children.

There have been many advances in pediatric oncology since these early discoveries, most of them attributable to continued collaboration of pediatric oncologists, surgeons, and radiation therapists within cooperative groups. With the development of improved supportive care measures, dose-intensive chemotherapy programs have been successful in improving outcome for patients with Burkitt's lymphoma, neuroblastoma, and other advanced-stage solid tumors.[8–10] Further improvements in outcome have been made by altering the schedule of chemotherapy administration, either by alternating effective groups of chemotherapeutic agents to overcome or prevent resistance[11] or administering agents by continuous infusion rather than bolus.[12] Improvements in radiation therapy have led to the development of intraoperative radiation therapy and radio-surgery techniques. Sharing of scientific knowledge and tumor samples within the cooperative groups has led to tremendous advances in the understanding of cell growth and regulation, the identification of cytogenetic abnormalities characteristic for specific malignancies, and the identification of oncogenes and tumor suppressor genes. All these taken together have led to profound improvements in the quality of life and survival of children with solid tumors.

EPIDEMIOLOGY AND SURVIVAL STATISTICS FOR CHILDHOOD CANCER

When compared with the adult incidence rate of cancer, the incidence of cancer in children is very small. However, while childhood cancer accounts for only 2% of all reported cancer cases, it accounts for 10% of all deaths among children and is the leading cause of death from disease among children.[13]

The distribution of types of cancer in childhood is very different from that in adults. Whereas the majority of all cancers in adults are of epithelial cell origin, less than 10% of childhood cancers fall into this category. Table 63–1 displays the distribution of cancer in children younger than 15 years.[14]

The incidence rates for specific cancers vary by age, sex, and race. Overall, the annual incidence rate for all types of childhood cancer is 133.3 per million children younger than 15 years. The peak incidence for childhood cancer is before the age of 2 years, with an incidence rate of more than 200 cases per million. The incidence then falls to a low of 82.5 cases per million at age 9 years, at which point it begins to climb again through the adolescent years. Prior to 2 years of age, central nervous system malignancies, neuroblastoma, acute myeloid leukemia, Wilm's tumor, and retinoblastoma account for the majority of diagnoses. Between ages 2 and 4, acute lymphoblastic leukemia is the most common childhood cancer. After age 9, the incidence of Hodgkin's disease, osteosarcoma, and Ewing's sarcoma begins to rise sharply.[13]

TABLE 63–1. Distribution of Cancer in Children Younger Than 15 Years

Type of Cancer	Distribution (%)
Acute lymphoblastic leukemia	23.2
Central nervous system tumors	20.7
Neuroblastoma	7.3
Non-Hodgkin's lymphoma	6.3
Wilms' tumor	6.1
Hodgkin's disease	5.0
Acute myeloid leukemia	4.2
Rhabdomyosarcoma	3.4
Retinoblastoma	2.9
Osteosarcoma	2.6
Ewing's sarcoma	2.1
All other cancers	16.4

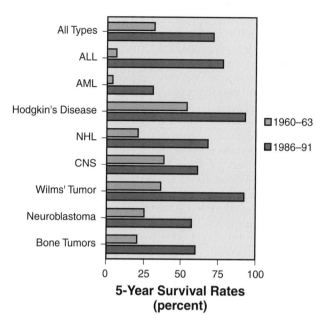

Figure 63–1. Comparison of patient survival during the period 1960–1963 versus 1986–1991 for the common childhood malignancies. (From Parker SL, Tong T, Bolden S, et al: Cancer statistics 1996. CA Cancer J Clin 65:5–27, 1996.)

According to the Surveillance, Epidemiology, and End Results program, the average annual incidence of childhood cancer has increased 10.8% between reporting year 1973 through 1974 and 1989 through 1990.[15] The percent change has been the greatest in ALL, non-Hodgkin's lymphoma, and central nervous system tumors. The change in reported incidence may be accounted for by improved reporting of cancer cases, improved identification and diagnosis of cancer, or a random fluctuation in the number of cases for the years studied. Concern has been raised as to the impact of environmental exposures resulting in increased cancer cases, but studies to date have not provided conclusive evidence for this assumption.

Survival from childhood cancer has improved dramatically over the past 30 years, so much so that the overall cure rate for childhood cancer is approaching 85%[16] and one of every 900 people between the ages of 16 and 44 years is a survivor of childhood cancer.[1] Figure 63–1 compares the survival statistics for specific cancers from 1960 through 1990.[17]

IMPORTANCE OF PATHOLOGY OF CHILDHOOD TUMORS IN SELECTING CHEMOTHERAPY

Unlike adult malignancies, which are primarily carcinomas, less than 10% of solid tumors of childhood are epithelial malignancies.[15] Although the spectrum of malignancies in childhood is more limited than in adults, exact diagnosis is often more difficult because of the prevalence of "small round blue-cell" tumors in childhood. These very primitive or embryonal malignancies often lack morphologically distinguishing characteristics. As a result, Ewing's sarcoma, neuroblastoma, lymphoma, small-cell osteosarcoma, and primitive neuroectodermal tumors, to name a few, may appear quite similar by simple light microscopy. An error in diagnosis of Ewing's sarcoma in a patient who actually has a lymphoma of bone would lead to vastly different therapy and poor outcome.

Exact diagnosis in pediatric oncology is crucial, as chemotherapy for childhood malignancies is carefully tailored to each specific tumor type. This has become even more important over the past two decades as pediatric oncologists have continued to better define prognostic subgroups for many tumors that help dictate the best therapy and the dose intensity of the therapy required for cure. Whereas the survival rate for patients with stages I to III Wilms' tumor with favorable histology is more than 90%[18] with standard therapy consisting of vincristine and actinomycin, with or without doxorubicin, a diagnosis of a Wilms' tumor with diffuse anaplasia carries a far worse prognosis and requires more intensive therapy for cure.

The initial step in the accurate diagnosis of a tumor is availability of adequate material on which to make the diagnosis. Therefore, it is crucial that during the initial surgical procedure, whether it be a biopsy or a resection, that tissue of adequate quantity and quality be obtained. The amount of tissue required for diagnostic purposes can be discussed with the pathologist and pediatric oncologist prior to the procedure to ensure the proper handling of the specimen (e.g., the need for fresh tissue, frozen samples, and fixed specimens for histologic and biologic diagnostic use).

While light microscopy remains the primary tool of pathologists they can now also rely on immunohistology, electron microscopy, DNA content of tumor, cytogenetic abnormalities, and specific tumor gene expression to establish a diagnosis. Consent is frequently obtained from families to allow any additional tumor tissue available after a diagnosis is established to be used for research to continue to advance understanding of tumor biology.

☐ Tumor Biology: Understanding Childhood Cancer and Treatment Principles

Cancer is a genetic event. Genetic alterations within a single cell, those that can be identified as a cytogenetic abnormality, the activation of an oncogene, or the loss of a tumor suppressor gene can all lead to the accumulation of cells lacking the ability to respond to growth-regulating signals and the subsequent development of a cancer. The study of malignant cell transformation has significantly contributed to the understanding of normal cell growth as well as the molecular origins of cancer; the ability to define tumors by their cytogenetic and molecular characteristics; and the future use of this information to fashion improved therapies for cancer.

CELL GROWTH AND REGULATION

Understanding normal cell growth and regulation is a prerequisite to understanding both the genetic basis for the development of childhood cancer and the mechanisms of action of chemotherapeutic agents designed to kill rapidly proliferating cancer cells. Normal cell growth occurs by the regulated progression of the cell through the cell cycle of DNA replication and mitosis, separated by two intervening growth phases called G_1 and G_2. Cells can temporarily leave the cell cycle and enter a resting state called G_0 (Fig. 63–2). Cells are instructed to proceed through the cell cycle by a series of external and internal stimuli. Binding of proteins (growth factors) to cell surface receptors stimulates a cascade of cytoplasmic signaling proteins (membrane kinases and signal transducers) that carries the stimuli to the nucleus, where other proteins (transcription factors) bind to the DNA, resulting in the expression of growth-regulating genes. When functioning normally, these genes promote or prevent cell division, direct the cell to differentiate, or initiate apoptosis, the process of programmed cell death.

Alterations in one or several of these signaling proteins can lead to the unregulated cell growth characteristics of cancer cells. Oncogenes result from mutation or overexpression of the normal growth-promoting proto-oncogenes. Tumor suppressor genes are normally present in cells and function as negative regulators to slow the process of proliferation and allow time for cellular repair. When oncogenes become activated or tumor suppressor gene function is lost, cells lose their ability to respond to the usual regulatory protein stimuli and proliferate rapidly. Rapid cell proliferation leads to accumulation of more genetic defects, activation of additional oncogenes, and loss of more negative regulators as the cells become increasingly more malignant. Through the study of chromosomal aberrations, more than 100 oncogenes and 12 tumor suppressor genes have now been identified.

CANCER CYTOGENETICS: A DIAGNOSTIC TOOL

The association of a consistent chromosomal aberration with a specific cancer was first made in 1960 with the discovery of the minute "Philadelphia chromosome" (9;22)(q34;q11) in chronic myeloid leukemia.[19] With the discovery of chromosomal

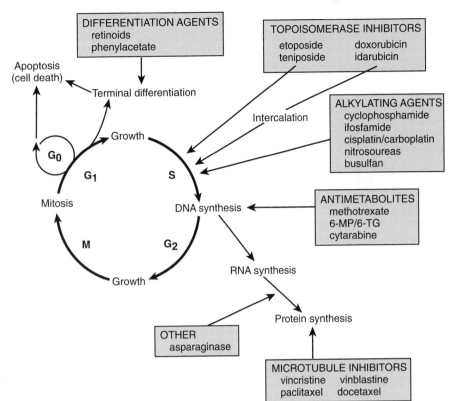

Figure 63–2. The cell cycle. Normal cell growth proceeds through DNA replication (S) and mitosis (M) separated by two growth phases (G₁ and G₂). Cells leave the cell cycle to enter a resting phase (G₀) to differentiate or to die. Chemotherapy agents act at specific sites along the cell cycle as indicated. (Adapted from Balis FM, Holcenberg JS, Poplack DG: General principles of chemotherapy. In Pizzo P, Poplack D (eds): Principles and Practice of Pediatric Oncology (3rd ed). Philadelphia, Lippincott-Raven, 1997, p 219.)

banding techniques in the 1970s, cancer cytogeneticists were first able to identify subchromosomal deletions, inversions, and translocations occurring in cancer cells. Study of these aberrant regions led to the identification of oncogenes and tumor suppressor genes, a process that is continuing today.

The presence of consistent cytogenetic abnormalities associated with a specific childhood leukemia or solid tumor helps in both cancer diagnosis and assignment of prognosis. Specific cytogenetic aberrations have been identified in rhabdomyosarcoma, Ewing's sarcoma, synovial sarcoma, germ cell tumors, medulloblastomas, neuroblastomas, retinoblastomas, and Wilms' tumors.[20] Finding one of these distinct translocations, deletions, or inversions can often aid the pathologist in making the correct diagnosis when faced with a histologically indistinct small round blue-cell tumor. Chromosomal aberrations can also help assign prognosis. The finding of a chromosome 1q deletion, the presence of double minute chromatin bodies, or the presence of homogeneous staining regions in neuroblastoma confers a poor prognosis.[21]

The process of using specific translocations for diagnostic purposes is now enhanced by the use of the techniques of fluorescent in situ hybridization, which allows for the localization and visualization of a single gene on a chromosome using fluorescent DNA probes. Unlike standard cytogenetic analysis, which requires 5 to 14 days for the cancer cells to proliferate in culture before a karyotype can be obtained, this technique can be performed directly on tumor cells.[22]

☐ Chemotherapy Principles in Pediatric Oncology

The goal of chemotherapy treatment for childhood malignancy is to maximize tumor kill while maintaining acceptable side effects. Clinical trials have led to the development of standard combination chemotherapy regimens for most childhood cancers. Increased understanding of tumor biology and improved supportive care have allowed for the administration of increased doses of chemotherapy (increased dose intensity) and changes in chemotherapy administration schedules to maximize tumoricidal effects. Adjuvant therapy (following local control measures) has remained the mainstay of cancer therapy, but neoadjuvant chemotherapy (prior to definitive local control measures) has proved to be effective in patients with metastatic disease and in localized tumors to begin to control microscopic metastatic disease immediately.

IDENTIFYING ACTIVE CHEMOTHERAPEUTIC AGENTS: PHASES I THROUGH III CLINICAL TRIALS

Chemotherapy drugs go through a long series of basic laboratory studies prior to being tested for activity in humans. Drugs are tested in cell culture for ability to inhibit or destroy cancer cells; then, promising agents are extensively tested in laboratory animals before the most active enter clinical trials in humans.

In the clinical development of promising anticancer agents, the first step is to define a tolerable dose. Phase I clinical trials are designed as dose escalation studies to determine the maximally tolerated dose of a new drug given as a single agent. The dose of the agent is slowly increased in successive cohorts of patients until dose-limiting toxicity is consistently observed. The dose level immediately lower than the dose resulting in consistent toxicity is then selected to begin phase II trials. In a phase II trial, a consistent dose of the agent is tested for efficacy in a variety of tumor types to establish the spectrum of activity of the agent. Once an agent has demonstrated activity in a specific cancer, this agent is tested for efficacy when combined with other known active agents in that tumor system.

"Standard" therapy for a specific tumor type is established through phase III clinical trials. Classically, phase III trials utilize a prospective randomized design to compare two previously established effective chemotherapy combinations. By randomly assigning new patients to treatment on one or the other chemotherapy "arm" of the study, the most effective chemotherapy combination can be established and the toxicities of the two regimens compared. At the conclusion of the trial, the chemotherapy regimen with the greatest efficacy and the least toxicity is selected as the standard regimen for that tumor system. Subsequent phase III trials then compare new regimens to this established standard therapy. It is through the development of phase I through III clinical trials within national cooperative groups that advances in cancer cures have been made. Individual patients benefit from clinical trials by having the most effective combination chemotherapy programs available to them, and cancer patients in general benefit from the continued advances and new information generated by these trials.

COMBINATION CHEMOTHERAPY

Combination chemotherapy remains the mainstay of treatment of childhood cancer. In the 1960s, the benefits of combining several drugs together was demonstrated first for ALL. Complete remission using single agents could only be expected in about half of the patients, whereas the combination of four or five drugs produced remission rates of more than 95%.[23] In the patients achieving remission with a single agent, resistance developed within 6 to 9 months, and relapse occurred. Long-term remission rates were higher with combination chemotherapy, demonstrating the ability to overcome or prevent chemotherapy resistance.

Several biologic models have been devised to attempt to explain this observation. The most well known is the Goldie–Coldman hypothesis, which proposes that the response of any individual tumor to a chemotherapeutic agent is dependent on both the sensitivity of that tumor to the agent and the inherent tendency of that tumor to accumulate mutations that will make it chemotherapy resistant. The chance of developing resistance is related to the mutation rate and the size of the tumor. This hypothesis predicts that once a single tumor cell develops resistance to a chemotherapeutic agent, the tumor cannot be cured using that agent alone. Therefore, the best chance to cure a tumor is to give all available active agents simultaneously, following local control measures, when the tumor burden is as low as possible and the chance of any tumor cells having acquired resistance is minimal.[24]

The agents used for combination chemotherapy must be carefully selected. Agents are selected for use in a combination chemotherapy regimen based on (1) demonstrated activity as a single agent in relapsed or refractory solid tumors, (2) differing mechanisms of action for cell killing, (3) non–cross resistance to prevent selection of a resistant clone, and (4) nonoverlapping toxicities to allow the drug to be given at the maximally effective dose and schedule.

This principle of designing combination chemotherapy regimens using non-cross resistant agents with non-overlapping toxicities has been successfully used for childhood solid tumor treatment for the past 25 years. The improvement in survival rates over this time period for neuroblastoma, Ewing's sarcoma, anaplastic Wilms' tumor, and osteosarcoma can be directly linked to effective combination chemotherapy treatment. For example, in Ewing's sarcoma, it was demonstrated that ifosfamide could induce responses in patients with recurrent disease who were previously treated with cyclophosphamide.[25] Shortly thereafter, it was discovered that response rates in recurrent Ewing's sarcoma could be significantly improved by the addition of etoposide to ifosfamide therapy.[26] Recently, the addition of ifosfamide and etoposide courses alternating with the previously standard Ewing's therapy of cyclophosphamide, doxorubicin, and vincristine produced a significant improvement in disease-free survival in patients with newly diagnosed Ewing's sarcoma.[11]

ADJUVANT AND NEOADJUVANT CHEMOTHERAPY

Adjuvant chemotherapy refers to the administration of chemotherapy to a patient with nonmetastatic disease following local therapy with surgery or radiation to eliminate micrometastases that may have already occurred before the appearance of clinically detectable disease. The use of adjuvant chemotherapy is supported by the finding that less than 20% of sarcoma and lymphoma patients with initially nonmetastatic solid tumors can be cured by surgery and/or radiation therapy alone.[27] In the majority of these patients, recurrence is at a distant site, lending strong support to the hypothesis that micrometastatic disease exists at the time of presentation for the majority of patients with clinical nonmetastatic disease. In Wilms' tumor, as many as

40% of patients can be cured with surgery and radiation therapy alone; however, survival can be increased to 90% with the addition of adjuvant combination chemotherapy.[28]

Because the goal of adjuvant chemotherapy is to prevent to appearance of metastatic disease, it is vital that chemotherapy begin as soon as possible after local control measures are completed. Major delays to allow recovery from surgery or radiation allow for growth of microscopic metastatic disease, increasing the chance for resistance to develop and decreasing overall response rates and survival. It is for this reason that most current chemotherapy regimens for childhood solid tumors recommend chemotherapy be given within 2 weeks of initial surgery. In Wilms' tumor, the National Wilms' Tumor Study Group recommends that the initial dose of actinomycin D begin within 5 days of nephrectomy.[29]

One approach to prevent delays in instituting chemotherapy in patients with nonmetastatic disease is to delay surgical resection until after several courses of chemotherapy can be administered. This is referred to as neoadjuvant chemotherapy, in which only a biopsy of the tumor is performed at diagnosis, and therefore chemotherapy can begin as soon as the diagnosis is established at a time when the distant tumor burden is at its lowest. This approach has become standard in the treatment of Ewing's sarcoma and osteosarcoma.[11, 30, 31] In these tumors, surgery and radiation are delayed for up to 3 to 4 months while alternating combinations of effective chemotherapy agents are administered. This approach has the theoretical advantage of minimizing the appearance of chemotherapy resistance; furthermore, delayed surgery may allow for a more complete or less morbid surgical resection and for pathologic assessment of tumor responsiveness to the chemotherapy agents on an individual patient basis. It should be kept in mind, however, that neoadjuvant chemotherapy is only of benefit for tumors for which a known highly effective combination chemotherapy program is available that limits the risk of tumor progression at the primary site.

SCHEDULE OF ADMINISTRATION

Children often tolerate chemotherapy better than adults because they have a superior and more rapid recovery from the toxic effects of treatment. Standard pediatric solid tumor chemotherapy protocols call for the administration of chemotherapy courses every 21 days to allow time for hematologic and organ recovery. Most combination chemotherapy programs are given over the first 1 to 5 days of the 21-day cycle. Historically, the next course of chemotherapy was withheld until the absolute neutrophil count was greater than $1000/mm^3$ and the platelet count was greater than $100,000/mm^3$. Over the past 5 years, the trend has been to maximize dose intensity and begin the next course when the absolute neutrophil count is greater than $750/mm^3$

and the platelet count greater than $75,000/mm^3$, as long as mucositis and/or diarrhea induced by chemotherapy has resolved. Proceeding with the next course of chemotherapy prior to organ recovery would result in cumulative tissue damage and increases the chance of death from infection, bleeding, or irreversible organ damage. When these criteria are adhered to the toxic death rate for standard combination chemotherapy programs is less than 5%.

Recently, changes in schedule of chemotherapy administration have led to improved efficacy of some agents. Etoposide is an epipodophyllotoxin that has been extremely effective in most pediatric solid tumors and in some epithelial cancers in adults. The mechanism of action is inhibition of topoisomerase II. Classically, etoposide has been given with an alkylator and infused over one hour. It has been demonstrated that continuous intravenous exposure to etoposide over 3 to 21 days is superior to a 1 to 24-hour infusion.[32, 33] In pediatric brain tumor patients, daily oral etoposide for 21 days was well tolerated and produced significant responses in patients with recurrent tumors.[34] This same schedule of continuous oral exposure to etoposide is currently being evaluated within the pediatric cooperative group setting in a variety of tumor systems. Continuous exposure to etoposide has the theoretical advantage of maintaining a continuous blockage of topoisomerase II and thus preventing tumor cell repair, ultimately leading to more effective tumor kill.

Prolonged exposure to combination chemotherapy agents in neuroblastoma and acute myeloid leukemia has led to improved responses.[35, 36] In neuroblastoma, patients with advanced-stage disease refractory to standard induction therapy had a 40% response rate when cisplatin, etoposide, and doxorubicin were given as a 96-hour continuous infusion along with daily bolus ifosfamide.[36]

Duration of chemotherapy programs for most pediatric solid tumors has classically been 1 year. As the dose intensity of chemotherapy programs has increased, the duration of therapy has decreased. The current intergroup osteosarcoma protocol consists of only 30 weeks of treatment. The National Wilms' Tumor Study III demonstrated that 11 weeks of therapy was as effective as 6 months for patients with low-stage disease.[18] In neuroblastoma, when intensive induction therapy is followed by consolidation with autologous stem cell transplant, the total duration of treatment is now 6 months.[37] As dose intensity of therapy increases, duration of chemotherapy may continue to decrease. In the future, biologic response modifiers and immunotherapies may be standardly used following completion of chemotherapy.

CHEMOTHERAPY DOSE INTENSITY

To develop an effective combination chemotherapy program, it is important to select not only the correct combination of agents but also the correct dose of each agent. The trend for the past 10 years in pediatric oncology has been to increase chemotherapy dose intensity, with the goal of maximizing efficacy. In designing dose-intensive programs, the individual toxicities of the agents to be intensified must be considered. The best agents to use in high doses are those with limited organ toxicity whose toxicity profile is mainly hematologic.

Most chemotherapeutic agents have a sigmoidal dose-response curve with a steep linear phase, followed by a plateau phase. The principle of chemotherapy dose intensity is to administer the maximum tolerated dose of the agent that falls within the linear phase of the dose-response curve in the shortest possible interval while maintaining tolerable toxicity. Dose intensity is defined as the amount of drug delivered per unit time, expressed as mg/m^2/week.[38] Therefore, dose intensity can be increased by giving higher doses of a chemotherapeutic agent, giving an agent more frequently, or both.

It has been demonstrated in animal systems that a twofold increase in administered cyclophosphamide dose can lead to a 10-fold increase in tumor cell kill,[39] whereas a decrease in dose intensity of as little as 20% in an osteosarcoma animal model can decrease the cure rate by 50%.[40]

Similar clinical observations have been made in childhood leukemia and osteosarcoma. A prospective clinical trial of high-risk ALL patients revealed that patients receiving less than 94% of the planned dose of chemotherapy during the intensive portion of therapy had a 5.5-fold increased risk of relapse.[41] In osteosarcoma, patients receiving less than 80% of the proposed chemotherapy doses had a threefold increased risk of relapse.[42]

The *positive impact* of increasing the dose intensity of therapy on improving response rate and survival duration has been demonstrated for Burkitt's lymphoma, osteosarcoma, Ewing's sarcoma, testicular cancer, breast cancer, and advanced ovarian cancer.[8-10, 38, 43-45] This finding has had a significant impact on the design of clinical trials for childhood solid tumors, with efforts focused on identifying the most effective agents to intensify and then maximizing supportive care to allow dose escalation.

In a retrospective meta-analysis of induction therapy used in 44 clinical trials for patients older than one year of age with disseminated neuroblastoma; the dose intensity of the most active agents had a significant impact on response, median survival, and median progression-free survival.[9] Cisplatin, teniposide, cyclophosphamide, and doxorubicin were identified as the most important agents to intensify to improve response in neuroblastoma. For Ewing's sarcoma and osteosarcoma, the dose intensity of doxorubicin has been identified as having the greatest impact on response and survival.[44] Improved response rates with high-dose cyclophosphamide (> 3 g/m^2) have been demonstrated in recurrent or refractory sarcomas.[46] With the concomitant use of hematopoietic growth factors to speed granulocyte recovery, chemotherapy doses of myelosuppressive agents often can be increased. For example, the standard dose of cyclophosphamide was 900 mg/m^2 in the Intergroup Rhabdomyosarcoma Study-I,[47] whereas the current Intergroup Rhabdomyosarcoma Study-V protocol uses cyclophosphamide at 2.2 g/m^2/dose, with granulocyte colony-stimulating factor (G-CSF) support as standard therapy—a 2.4-fold dose increase.

Increasing the dose intensity of active chemotherapy agents in pediatric clinical trials has been possible because of recent advances in supportive care to decrease or minimize the toxic effects on normal tissues that occur from higher-dose chemotherapy. The use of cytokines to speed recovery of white blood cells and platelets (G-CSF and interleukin-11)[48, 49] and the use of cardioprotectant agents to allow higher cumulative dose of doxorubicin to be used have helped in the development of new dose-intensive therapy for solid tumors.[50]

The most recent advance, the infusion of previously collected peripheral blood progenitor cells (PBPCs) to support repeated courses of dose-intensive submyeloablative chemotherapy, has allowed dose intensity in multiple chemotherapy cycles to be increased further than was previously possible.

Several pediatric studies have demonstrated that collection of PBPCs from children as small as 10 kg is feasible.[51] PBPCs have been effective in engrafting pediatric patients following myeloablative chemoradiotherapy.[52, 53] In myeloablative therapy, "supralethal" doses of chemotherapy are given, and hematopoietic recovery will only occur if a stem cell source (either PBPCs or bone marrow) is infused into the patient following completion of the myeloablative regimen. PBPCs are also effective in enhancing recovery following submyeloablative chemotherapy.[54] In submyeloablative regimens, hematopoietic recovery usually occurs in 3 to 4 weeks when combined with growth factor or PBPC support but would ultimately occur without these methods of support in 6 to 10 weeks.

A study performed at James Whitcomb Riley Hospital for Children has successfully utilized repetitive PBPC collections to support newly diagnosed neuroblastoma patients through four courses of submyeloablative dose-intensive chemotherapy prior to consolidation with a myeloablative PBPC transplant.[54] Another trial in high-risk brain tumor patients also demonstrated the feasibility of sequential high-dose chemotherapy with PBPC support to successfully mitigate hematopoietic toxicity. In this study, as chemotherapy doses were escalated, nonhematologic toxicities became dose-limiting.[55]

The Children's Cancer Group (CCG) is currently conducting a clinical pilot study to further investigate the feasibility of repetitive collection, storage, and infusion of PBPCs for use with multicycle dose-intensive chemotherapy in newly diagnosed neuroblastoma patients. Patients receive two induction courses of high-dose cyclophosphamide with continuous-infusion doxorubicin and vincristine. At the time of hematopoietic recovery from the second course, patients have PBPC collected using a specialized apheresis machine, and then cells are cryopreserved and stored. These cells are reinfused following the first consolidation chemotherapy course, which consists of high-dose cyclophosphamide, etoposide, and carboplatin. Collection and infusion of PBPCs is repeated a total of three times during the three consolidation chemotherapy courses. GCSF is given daily following the infusion of PBPCs to further speed hematopoietic recovery. For this pilot study, the toxicity of the chemotherapy agents used is primarily hematopoieitic, with minimal organ toxicity. The goal of this protocol is to both time-compress chemotherapy courses and administer higher doses of chemotherapy, leading to significant increases in dose intensity.

☐ Chemotherapeutic Agents

CLASSES OF AGENTS AND THEIR MECHANISMS OF ACTION

The rational design of combination chemotherapy programs requires an understanding of the mechanism of action, the site of metabolism, the rate of drug clearance, and the toxicity profile for each drug. Most chemotherapy agents work by interfering with DNA or RNA synthesis, transcription, or repair. Unfortunately, these agents are not selective for cancer cells, and the same metabolic pathways are disrupted in normal cells, leading to the toxic effects observed with chemotherapy treatment.

It is important to understand the nomal cell cycle to understand how each chemotherapy agent interferes with the normal cell growth and repair processes of the cell. A normal cell proceeds through the four phases of the cell cycle in an orderly fashion. Checkpoints are in place to slow growth and allow for needed repairs to prevent the accumulation of DNA or RNA errors. Malignant cells are usually lacking in some or most of these checkpoints and as a result may be more susceptible to the toxic effects of chemotherapeutic agents. Figure 63–2 illustrates the normal cell cycle and indicates the site of action of the major chemotherapeutic agents.

Chemotherapy agents can be divided into classes by their mechanism of action. The classes of agents include alkylating agents including cisplatin and its analogues, antimetabolites, topoisomerase inhibitors, antimicrotubule agents, differentiation agents, and miscellaneous nonclassified agents. Understanding the individual mechanisms of action helps in the design of drug combinations with additive or synergistic antitumor effects. The most common agents from each class, their mechanism of action, common side effects, and tumors in which they are active are listed in Table 63–2.

ACUTE CHEMOTHERAPY TOXICITY AND SUPPORTIVE CARE

Most acute toxicities in childhood solid tumor therapy are reversible. Toxicity is greatest in the normal cells with the highest rate of turnover. Therefore, normal bone marrow cells, mucosal lining cells, liver cells, and hair cells are frequently affected. The most common side effects from combination chemotherapy include nausea and vomiting, myelosuppression, hair loss, mucositis, diarrhea, liver function test abnormalities, and allergic reactions.

Myelosuppression is an expected side effect of almost every treatment program for childhood solid tumors. Transfusions of packed cells and platelets are frequent. Of greatest concern is the risk of severe life-threatening bacterial or fungal infections that occur during episodes of neutropenia. In dose-intensive regimens, more than 75% of chemotherapy courses result in hospitalization for fever, with the incidence of bacteremia ranging from 10 to 20% per course.[56]

Several chemotherapeutic agents have very specific toxicities. For example, vincristine and doxorubicin are vesicants and can cause severe skin and tissue necrosis if the drug extravasates into the subcutaneous tissue. Doxorubicin and related anthracyclines have cumulative cardiotoxic effects, and the total lifetime anthracycline dose must be limited for each patient to minimize the risk of developing congestive heart failure. Cisplatin has toxic renal effects and is often combined with another nephrotoxic agent, ifosfamide, in treatment of osteosarcoma and neuroblastoma. Vincristine and vinblastine can cause cumulative peripheral neuropathies, and drug doses frequently need to be altered to prevent significant morbidity. These toxicities must be considered when designing therapeutic programs; aggressive supportive care and close patient monitoring are mandatory.

Some of the success in improving outcome for children with cancer is attributable to advances made in supportive care. Routine use of hematopoeitic growth factors, specifically G-CSF, results in more rapid granulocyte recovery and shorter hospitalizations for fever and neutropenia.[48] Recently, interleukin-11 (rhIL-11) has demonstrated efficacy in enhancing platelet recovery, decreasing the depth of the platelet nadir, and decreasing platelet transfusions requirements.[49, 57, 58] It has been well tolerated in children and will be extremely beneficial in combination regimens that induce severe thrombocytopenia.[58]

The gastrointestinal tract is injured by certain chemotherapy agents, specifically cytarabine, anthracyclines, and high-dose methotrexate. Leukovorin, a folate derivative, can be given to "rescue" normal mucosal and bone marrow cells from the effects of high-dose methotrexate. As of yet, there is no rescue known for the mucositis and diarrhea that occur from other agents. Use of rhIL-11, in addition to

TABLE 63-2. Common Chemotherapy Agents

Class of Agent	Mechanism of Action	Antitumor Activity	Acute Toxicities
Alkylating Agents			
Mustards			
Nitrogen mustard	Alkylation, DNA cross-linking	Hodgkin's disease	Myelo, N/V, alopecia, mucositis, phlebitis vesicant
Melphalan	Alkylation, DNA cross-linking	Rhabdo, for BMT. Ewing's sarcoma, NB	Myelo, mucositis, N/V, alopecia, VOD (HD)
Cyclophosphamide	(Prodrug) alkylation, DNA cross-linking	Rhabdo, Wilms', NB, Ewing's sarcoma	Myelo, immuno, N/V, alopecia, cystitis, SIADH, cardiac (HD), lung (HD), VOD (HD)
Ifosfamide	Alkylation, DNA cross-linking	Ewing's sarcoma, rhabdo, osteosarcoma, NB	Myelo, N/V, alopecia, hepatic, renal, cystitis, neuro
Busulfan	Alkylation, DNA cross-linking	Leukemia	Myelo, skin, lung, alopecia
Nitrosoureas			
BCNU	DNA cross-linking	CNS tumors, lymphoma	Myelo, N/V, alopecia, lung, renal
CCNU	DNA cross-linking	CNS tumors, lymphoma	Myelo, N/V, alopecia, lung, renal
Tetrazines			
Dacarbazine (DTIC)	DNA methylation	Hodgkin's disease, sarcomas, NB	Myelo, hepatic, flu-like illness, N/V, alopecia
Other alkylators			
Thiotepa	Alkylation, DNA cross-linking	CNS tumors, for BMT, sarcomas, NB	Myelo, N/V, alopecia, diarrhea, mucositis, skin, VOD (HD)
Procarbazine	(Prodrug) methylation; free radical formation	Hodgkin's disease, CNS tumors	Myelo, N/V, rash, allergy, mucositis
Platinum agents			
Cisplatin	DNA/platinum adduct formation; DNA cross-linking	Osteosarcoma, NB, hepatoblastoma, germ cell tumors, CNS tumors	N/V (severe), alopecia, myelo, renal, neuro mucositis, neuro, ototoxicity
Carboplatin	DNA/platinum adduct formation; DNA cross-linking	NB, CNS tumors, retinoblastoma, sarcomas in HD	Myelo (severe plts), N/V (mild), renal and ototoxicity rare
Antimetabolites			
Methotrexate	Inhibitor dihydrofolate reductase; interferes with folate metabolism	Leukemia, lymphoma, osteosarcoma in HD	Myelo, rash, mucositis, hepatic, renal (HD)
5-Fluorouracil	(Prodrug) inhibits thymidine synthesis	Hepatoblastoma, carcinomas	Myelo, N/V, mucositis, diarrhea, hyperpigmentation, neuro
Cytarabine	(Prodrug) incorporated into DNA; inhibits DNA replication	Leukemia, lymphoma	Myelo, malaise, N/V, mucositis, diarrhea, neuro (HD), eye (HD), skin (HD)
6-Mercaptopurine 6-Thioguanine	(Prodrug) inhibits purine synthesis	Leukemia	Myelo, N/V, hepatic, mucositis
Topoisomerase Inhibitors			
Epipodophyllotoxins			
Etoposide	Non-DNA–binding topoisomerase II inhibitor; stabilizes DNA double-strand breaks	NB; Ewing's sarcoma, rhabdo, germ cell tumors, leukemia, CNS tumors, lymphoma	Myelo, N/V, rash, allergy, low BP, alopecia, mucositis, hepatic (HD)
Teniposide	Same as etoposide	NB; leukemia	Myelo, N/V, rash, allergy, low BP, alopecia, mucositis, hepatic (HD)
Anthracyclines			
Doxorubicin	DNA intercalation, free radical formation, topoisomerase II inhibitor	Wilms' tumor, Ewing's sarcoma, NB, lymphoma, leukemia	Myelo, N/V, alopecia, mucositis, diarrhea, phlebitis, vesicant, hepatic, cardiac
Daunorubicin	Same as doxorubicin	Leukemia, lymphoma	Myelo, N/V, alopecia, mucositis, diarrhea, phlebitis, vesicant, hepatic, cardiac
Actinomycin D	Same as doxorubicin	Wilms' tumor, rhabdo, Ewing's sarcoma	Myelo, N/V, alopecia, mucositis, hepatic, vesicant
Bleomycin	DNA intercalation, free radical formation	Germ cell tumors, Hodgkin's disease, lymphoma	Myelo, skin, allergy, mucositis, lung
Camptothecin analogue			
Topotecan	Topoisomerase I inhibitor	In phase II testing in osteosarcoma and NB	Myelo, N/V, alopecia, mucositis, diarrhea, hepatic

TABLE 63–2. Common Chemotherapy Agents *Continued*

Class of Agent	Mechanism of Action	Antitumor Activity	Acute Toxicities
Antimicrotubule Agents			
Vinca alkyloids			
Vincristine	Binds tubulin, prevents microtubule formation, blocks mitosis	Sarcomas, leukemia, Hodgkin's disease, Wilms' tumor, lymphoma	Constipation, neuro, vesicant, SIADH
Vinblastine	Same as vincristine	Hodgkin's disease, germ cell tumors	Myelo, mucositis, vesicant
Taxanes			
Paclitaxel (Taxol)	Binds microtubules, blocks microtubule depolymerization, blocks mitosis	Ovarian carcinoma	Myelo, alopecia, mucositis, paresthesias, hypersensitivity
Docetaxel (Taxotere)	Same as paclitaxel	In phase II testing in sarcomas and other solid tumors	Myelo, alopecia, skin, hypersensitivity, flu, retention, paresthesias, mucositis
Differentiation Agents			
Retinoids			
Cis-retinoic acid	Binds to retinoic acid receptor; induces differentiation	NB	Skin, mucositis, eye, pseudotumor, hepatic, electrolyte
All trans retinoic acid	Same as cis-retinoic acid	APML; in phase II testing in Wilms' tumor, NB	Skin, mucositis, eye, pseudotumor, hepatic, electrolyte
Fenretinide	Same as cis-retinoic acid	To begin testing in NB	To be tested
Miscellaneous Nonclassified			
Corticosteroids	Lympholysis, multiple other effects not well classified	Leukemia (ALL), lymphoma	Weight gain, high BP, high glucose, mood change, many others
L-Asparaginase, PEG-asparaginase	Asparagine depletion, inhibition of protein synthesis	Leukemia (ALL), lymphoma	Anorexia, hepatic, pancreatitis, coagulopathy, neuro

BCNU, lomustine; BMT, bone marrow transplant; BP, blood pressure; CCNU, carmustine; CNS tumors, central nervous system tumors; HD, high dose; myelo, myelosuppression; NB, neuroblastoma; neuro, neurologic toxicity; N/V, nausea and vomiting; rhabdo, rhabdomyosarcoma; SIADH, syndrome of inappropriate antidiuretic hormone; VOD, veno-occlusive disease.

Data from Balis FM, Holcenberg JS, Poplack DG: General principles of chemotherapy. In Pizzo P, Poplack D (eds): Principles and Practice of Pediatric Oncology (3rd ed). Philadelphia, Lippincott-Raven, 1997, pp 215–272; Ratain M, Teicher B, O'Dwyer P, et al: Pharmacology of cancer chemotherapy. In DeVita V, Hellman S, Rosenberg S (eds): Cancer: Principles and Practice of Oncology. Philadelphia: Lippincott-Raven, 1997, pp 375–385; Dorr R, Von Hoff D: Drug monographs. In Dorr R, Von Hoff D (eds): Cancer Chemotherapy Handbook. Norwalk, CT, Appleton and Lange, 1994, p 129.

enhancing platelet production, may help speed recovery from gastrointestinal injury following chemotherapy. Early studies demonstrate rapid reversal of gut toxicity with the use of rhIL-11 following radiation.[59]

Renal toxicity can occur from the use of cisplatin, ifosfamide, and high-dose methotrexate. Cisplatin causes renal tubular damage, leading to elevation of blood urea nitrogen and creatinine. Often this is reversible. Both ifosfamide and cisplatin cause renal electrolyte wasting, called Fanconi's syndrome, in which hypokalemia, hypocalcemia, hypophosphatemia, and hypomagnesemia can occur. Renal injury from these agents can be decreased by hyperhydration and forced diuresis. Ongoing studies with the organic thiophosphate compound amifostine show promise in preventing cisplatin-induced renal injury. Amifostine may also have protective effects against neurologic and cumulative bone marrow toxicities.[60] Mesna can prevent hemorrhagic cystitis resulting from cyclophosphamide and ifosfamide by binding to the bladder toxic acrolein metabolites.[61]

It is anticipated that supportive care measures will continue to improve. In the future, some of the toxic effects of chemotherapy on bone marrow may be ameliorated by the use of gene therapy to transfer chemotherapy resistance genes into normal hematopoieitic progenitor cells. This would allow higher doses of chemotherapy to be given without myelosuppression. Preliminary in vitro and animal studies have shown that hematopoietic progenitor cells can be made more resistant to nitrosoureas.[62]

LONG-TERM SIDE EFFECTS OF CANCER THERAPY IN CHILDREN

In light of the fact that 1 of every 900 adults will soon be a survivor of childhood cancer,[1] emphasis on diagnosis, treatment, and prevention of late effects of childhood cancer therapy has become essential.

In general, tissues with the highest cell turnover rate are the most susceptible to acute toxicities of chemotherapy. Usually, acute toxicities are reversible but may be persistent and lead to late effects. Tissues that replicate slowly or that can no longer regenerate may be susceptible to long-term or late effects of therapy. Children are more susceptible to certain late effects of therapy than adults by virtue of the fact that their tissues are still growing, and damage to these tissue may affect growth, fertility, and neuropsychologic development.

All aspects of combined-modality treatment can contribute to late effects of childhood cancer therapy. Chemotherapy agents have been associated with specific late toxicities (see Table 63–2). Radiation therapy can significantly inhibit further growth of bone, muscle, heart, and kidney within the radiation field, as well as affecting fertility. Certain surgical procedures can be associated with late sequelae, as with scoliosis following thoracotomy, impotence after retroperitoneal lymph node dissection, and limited mobility after amputation.

Growth retardation is the late effect unique to children. The degree of impairment depends on the dose of chemotherapy or radiation and the age of the child at time of therapy. The younger the child at the time of the insult, the more severe the sequelae. More than 50% of childhood brain tumor patients treated with 3000 cGy or more to the whole brain will have severe growth retardation, with adult height being less than the fifth percentile.[63] Cranial irradiation can lead to growth hormone deficiency, which will result in poor linear growth unless growth hormone replacement is given. Patients who have received total body radiation or spinal radiation may not be able to achieve their full height potential because the irradiated bones have limited growth potential, even with growth hormone stimulation.[64]

In addition to poor overall growth, therapy can cause other musculoskeletal problems including scoliosis, avascular necrosis, osteoporosis, and atrophy or hypoplasia of tissues. Radiation therapy to the head and neck results in hypoplasia of the jaw, orbit, or neck, with associated atrophy of the soft tissues. Associated endocrine, dental, and psychological consequences may also occur.[65] Aseptic necrosis of bone may affect as many as 10% of high-risk ALL patients as a result of chronic steroid use. Osteoporosis occurs as a result of steroid treatment and from high-dose radiation, as used for sarcoma therapy.

Most children who receive chemotherapy for solid tumors do not experience neuropsychologic dysfunction. Patients treated for brain tumors and those receiving cranial radiation for ALL are the exception and can experience severe decline in IQ. Compared with their siblings, patients treated with cranial irradiation for ALL were significantly more likely to enter a special education or learning disabled program.[66]

Specific organs are often affected by chemotherapy. Heart, liver, lung, thyroid, and gonadal function can be impaired. Gonadal dysfunction (azospermia, amenorrhea) frequently results from alkylator treatment. Therapy with mechloethamine, vincristine, prednisone, and procarbazine resulted in azospermia in 80 to 100% of all males.[67] Combination chemotherapy programs for childhood Hodgkin's disease have been adjusted to replace mechlorethamine with cyclophosphamide and eliminate dacarbazine from standard treatments to attempt to decrease the infertility risk. It should be noted that the children of childhood cancer survivors are not at an increased risk for congenital anomalies.[68]

Cardiotoxicity from anthracycline antibiotics has been a problem in the treatment of Ewing's sarcoma, osteosarcoma, and lymphomas. Use of continuous-infusion anthracycline can decrease the risk of cardiac muscle damage, and subsequent congestive heart failure.[69] Another new strategy has been the use of the cardioprotectant dexrazoxone to prevent anthracycline-induced cardiotoxicity.[50] Until a safe dose of anthracycline given with dexrazoxone can be defined, the cumulative lifetime dose of anthracycline continues to be limited to 450 mg/m², a level at which less than 5% of patients experience clinical congestive heart failure.[70]

Pulmonary toxicity is a source of significant late toxicity of cancer therapy. Many alkylating agents and radiation therapy contribute to pulmonary fibrosis, resulting in decreased lung volume, lung compliance, and diffusing capacity. The nitrosoureas and bleomycin are the most common agents to cause pulmonary fibrosis. In Hodgkin's disease, when bleomycin is given followed by mantle irradiation, the risk of pulmonary toxicity is increased.[71] Whole-lung irradiation, as given for pulmonary metastasis in Wilms' tumor and Ewing's sarcoma, also can result in pulmonary impairment.

Other significant organ-related late effects include hypothyroidism following radiation in Hodgkin's disease, chronic renal insufficiency from cisplatin therapy, chronic cystitis from cyclophosphamide or ifosfamide treatment, and prolonged hypogammaglobulinemia and T lymphocyte dysfunction following multiple high-dose alkylators for bone marrow transplant.[72]

One of the more significant late effects of cancer therapy is the risk of secondary malignancy. As the number of childhood cancer survivors increases, this has become a major concern. In a retrospective review of 1406 childhood cancer patients, the actuarial risk of a second malignant neoplasm was 5.6% at 25 years after diagnosis.[73] The risk of second malignancy is highest in the patients who received both chemotherapy and radiation therapy. Hodgkin's disease survivors have the highest secondary malignancy rates. The estimated actuarial incidence of any second cancer was 7% at 15 years after diagnosis. Breast cancer was the most common solid tumor, with an estimated actuarial incidence in women of 35% by age 40. These patients are also at risk to develop leukemia, non-Hodgkin's lymphoma, and thyroid carcinoma.[74] In some series of survivors of childhood Hodgkin's disease, the cumulative estimated incidence of second malignancies at 30 years has ranged from 18 to 31%[75, 76] Patients who have received additional multimodality therapy for recurrent Hodgkin's disease have the highest risk of second tumors. Patients with soft-tissue sarcomas, retinoblastoma, and Ewing's sarcoma who receive high-dose radiation to the primary lesion are at increased risk for secondary osteosarcoma within the radiation field.[77] In the past 10 years, etoposide has been recognized as causing secondary acute myeloid leukemia, usually of the M4 or M5 subtype, with a short latency period (1 to 3 years from exposure) and a characteristic chromosomal translocation involving chromosome 11q23.[78]

As new advances in combination chemotherapy treatment result in an increase in childhood cancer survival of as much as 1% per year, the challenge for the future is to maintain the excellent survival rates while altering therapy to prevent late toxicity.

□ Principles of Immunotherapy

The human immune system is designed to identify and destroy foreign cells. One of the great mysteries of oncology is why a patient's immune system is unable to eliminate malignant cells. Studies in the mid-1990s indicate that some tumor cells may express a protein, Fas ligand, that conveys a "death signal" to T lymphocytes, causing them to undergo apoptosis and therefore be useless in fighting the cancer.[79] Immunotherapy is a new branch of cancer therapy being developed to enhance or stimulate the natural products of the immune system (lymphocytes, antibodies, and cytokines) to better recognize and destroy cancer cells.

The immune system is composed of many cell types, but the lymphocyte has the primary role in controlling immune function. B lymphocytes function by secreting antibodies that mediate cell destruction by binding compliment or causing opsinization, resulting in phagocytosis by macrophages. T lymphocytes can directly interact with specific cell-surface antigens on a target cell and cause cell lysis through cytotoxic granule release or programmed cell death. These cytotoxic T lymphocytes are involved with tumor cell killing. To initiate this response, antigens must be presented to the T cell by antigen presenting cells (APCs) that express the antigens bound to major histocompatibility complex (MHC) proteins in the presence of stimulatory cytokines. Cytokines or interleukins (e.g., interleukin-2, interferon alpha, tumor necrosis factor) are proteins produced by helper T lymphocytes and monocytes that help recruit other effector cells, including APCs, as well as regulate antibody production. The effector cells of the immune system (e.g., granulocytes, monocytes, macrophages, eosinophils, dendritic cells) can become tumor selective when activated by a specific antibody, a process called antibody-dependent cell-mediated cytotoxicity (ADCC).

Immunotherapy takes advantage of all these immune functions. The goal of immunotherapy is to improve the immunogenicity of a tumor and allow it to be recognized and targeted for destruction by the immune system. Immunotherapy can be divided into two major categories: active immunity and passive immunity.

ACTIVE IMMUNITY AND CANCER VACCINES

Active immunity involves the use of tumor vaccines made from autologous or allogeneic tumor-associated antigens. Vaccines have been made using whole tumor cells and partially purified or highly purified tumor antigens. Specific purified tumor antigens have been identified that can be made more immunogeneic by attachment to carrier proteins (adjuvants). The majority of all clinical trials using this type of tumor vaccine have been performed in melanoma patients. In a phase III study using purified GM2 ganglioside combined with bacille Calmette-Guérin (BCG) there was a trend toward improved survival for patients receiving vaccine versus low-dose cyclophosphamide and BCG. Among vaccine-treated patients, 86% produced an immunoglobulin M response.[80] A recent pilot study using GM2 ganglioside conjugated to keyhole limpet hemocyanin (KLH) and mixed with the adjuvant QS-21 produced high-titer immunoglobulin M antibodies in all patients.[81] Tumor vaccines using ganglioside for neuroblastoma are currently under development.

Another type of tumor vaccine in development is one designed to stimulate tumor-specific T cell immunity to tumor peptides, resulting in the generation of cytotoxic T lymphocytes. For this type of vaccine to be successful, it is necessary to modify the tumor peptide to stimulate antigen presentation to the T cell. The presentation of the antigen is often restricted to specific MHC alleles. Tumor cells themselves are poor APCs because they often lack expression of MHC class I and II proteins. Neuroblastoma murine tumor cells have been modified to express exogenous MHC class II genes. In a murine model, this resulted in enhanced presentation of tumor antigens directly to T cells, producing a potent in vivo tumor response.[82] Tumor cells can also be genetically engineered to overexpress cytokines (interleukin-2 [IL-2], granulocyte-macrophage colony stimulating factor [GM-CSF]) that activate APCs and other immune cells.[83, 84] Modified tumor vaccine studies designed to stimulate cytotoxic T lymphocytes are currently underway in melanoma patients.[80]

PASSIVE IMMUNITY

Passive immunity involves the use of monoclonal antibodies or cytotoxic effector cells produced in vitro and infused into the patient. Monoclonal antibodies have been tested in patients with neuroblastoma. Initially, monoclonal antibodies were developed and used for in vitro purging of autologous bone marrow prior to myeloablative transplant. Murine monoclonal antibodies have been raised to a glycolipid antigen, surface glycoproteins, and specific disialogangliosides GD2 and GD3 in neuroblastoma cells. The murine anti-GD2 antibody was the first to be used in clinical trials. Antibody to GD2 mediates antibody-dependent or complement-dependent cellular cytotoxicity, which can be enhanced by the addition of cytokines.[85] A phase II clinical trial of mouse monoclonal antibody to GD2 (called 3F8) in advanced neuroblastoma patients resulted in an immune response in 40% of patients.[86]

A more recent trial used a murine anti-GD2 antibody, 14.G2a, infused with IL-2, designed with the goal of enhancing ADCC. In this CCG trial, 33 patients with neuroblastoma or osteosarcoma were treated with a combination of IL-2 and escalating doses of 14.G2a antibody to determine 14.G2a's toxicity and efficacy. Toxicity included transient neurogenic pain, allergic reactions, and rash. One neuroblastoma patient had a partial response, three patients had decrease in bone marrow infiltrates, and one osteosarcoma patient had a complete response.[87] One drawback of murine monoclonal antibody therapy is that when these antibodies are repeatly infused into humans, most patients will ultimately produce a human-anti-mouse antibody, which renders further antibody treatment useless.

Recently, chimeric human-mouse antibodies have been produced that may decrease the risk of human-anti-mouse antibody generation.[87] This antibody was formed by fusing the Fab portion of the murine 14.G2a antibody to the human Fc constant regions of an IgG1 immunoglobulin to form the chimeric antibody ch14.18. This antibody has been tested in phase I trials[88] and is currently being used along with GM-CSF in neuroblastoma patients following bone marrow transplant. It is anticipated that the antibody will be most efficacious in the setting of minimal residual disease.

Another form of passive immunity is the generation of lymphocyte-activated killer cells and tumor-infiltrating lymphocytes. Other forms of immunotherapy involve the use of cytokine infusions such as interferon alpha, IL-2, and tumor necrosis factor to stimulate immune reaction against tumor cells. Adoptive immunotherapy with interferon alpha has produced significant responses in chronic myeloid leukemia (CML). In renal cell carcinoma and metastatic melanoma, continuous infusion of IL-2 produced a 20% remission rate.[89] IL-2 is being studied in the CCG to treat the minimal residual disease state in childhood acute myeloid leukemia following completion of chemotherapy. Interferon alpha 2a combined with all trans retinoic acid is currently being studied as salvage therapy for patients with Wilms' tumor and neuroblastoma by the CCG.

IMMUNOTOXINS

Immunotoxins are a new class of immunopharmacologic agents that combine monoclonal antibodies conjugated to toxins derived from plants or bacteria to specifically target tumor cell antigens. Some of these agents have demonstrated promising results in patients with lymphoid malignancies.[90] To be effective, an immunotoxin must recognize a specific antigen on the surface of the cell. The target antigen should not be present on peripheral blood cells. Once bound to the target antigen, the immunotoxin complex must be internalized for the toxin to kill the cell.

The immunotoxin, B43-PAP, which is currently being studied in the treatment of B lineage ALL, meets all these criteria. This immunotoxin is composed of the antibody B43 specific for the CD19 antigen on B lineage ALL blasts conjugated to the plant toxin pokeweed antiviral protein (PAP). Currently, B43-PAP is in phase II testing within the CCG in newly diagnosed high-risk ALL patients who show a slow early response to induction chemotherapy.

The field of immunotherapy is still in the early stages of development, but improved understanding of immune mechanisms and ability to genetically alter tumor cells may lead to advances in the near future.

☐ Local Tumor Control

In addition to systemic treatment, local tumor control is important in pediatric oncology. Metastatic disease is more readily eradicated in young patients compared with in adults when the primary lesion has been adequately treated. A number of modalities may be employed to control local disease.[91]

RADIATION ONCOLOGY

An understanding of the biologic principles of radiation therapy in childhood cancer is important. Radiation may directly affect cellular DNA or produce reactive free radicals that indirectly damage genetic material and interfere with the reproductive capacity of normal or malignant tissues. The effect of ionizing radiation on tumors depends on the number of actively reproducing cells at the time of exposure and the length of the cellular regeneration cycle. Because most of the damage is indirect and focused on reproduction, malignant lesions usually show a delayed effect to radiation therapy. The tumor may begin to shrink or eventually disappear weeks to months after treatment. At some dose of therapy, the response of the malignant tissues becomes exponential, but further damage to normal adjacent cells may also occur.

Acute reactions to ionizing radiation depend on this balance between replication and cell death and seem to be affected by increased time intervals between dose fractions that allow enhanced cellular repopulation. The radiation fraction size has a small impact on what volume of cells are acutely destroyed. Conversely, the chronic effects of therapy primarily depend on the total exposure dose and the size of each treatment fraction. The therapeutic ratio may be enhanced by exploiting the difference between the early and late radiation effects. Techniques may be utilized that reduce the late effects by lowering the dose per fraction and increasing the number of fractions delivered over the conventional treatment time. A further strategy would be to accelerate this dose fractionation by reducing the overall radiation time and thereby providing rapidly proliferating tumors less opportunity for repopulation.

Radiation therapy may be combined with surgery in a strategic manner to deliver the highest effective dose to a well-defined site yet minimize the dose to surrounding normal structures.[92] By combining these two modalities, maximal advantage can be taken from their basic differential effects. Large, resectable tumors may be grossly removed, but the peripheral tissues may contain microscopic disease. Radiation is most effective for this peripheral burden of micrometastases and yet would be less effective for the central bulk of the tumor. Although each approach has advantages, it is logical to combine these two modalities sequentially to maximize local tumor control. Preoperative radiation therapy may permit a smaller treatment area because the operative bed has not been manipulated. In larger tumors, its use may reduce the lesion volume sufficiently to allow a subsequent resection. Also, potential tumor seeding during operative removal may be reduced because the cells that may be surgically disseminated have been rendered incapable of reproducing. Conversely, preoperative radiation may delay the surgical procedure to allow tissue recovery. Also, the extent of disease, which is usually defined and staged at operation, is less certain, and the radiation therapy plan may be adversely affected by inappropriate downstaging of the tumor. Finally, dose limitations may preclude retreatment if the surgical margin remains histologically positive for tumor cells.

For these reasons, many combined strategies employ postoperative radiation such that the treatment fields and doses are determined after surgical resection and histologic assessment.[92] Higher doses generally can be delivered postoperatively because the target sites and volumes have been more accurately defined. Specifically, doses to the periphery of the tumor can be fine-tuned, depending on the presence of gross, microscopic, or no residual disease. However, postoperative delivery may require a wider treatment area after extensive surgical manipulation. Also, adhesions or scarring over vascular or other vital structures may increase the risk of radiation toxicity.

The management of soft-tissue sarcoma provides a model for the adjunctive role of radiation therapy because neither surgery nor radiation alone usually completely controls local disease in the head and neck, extremity, trunk or retroperitoneum.[93] In extremity lesions, radiation also allows more conservative resection with limb sparing. Whereas preopera-

tive therapy can decrease tumor cell implantation and spread at surgery, it may compromise wound healing and histologic evaluation of the primary tumor. Nevertheless, local tumor control rates of 75 to 98% have been achieved, with limb salvage rates greater than 80%. Unfortunately, wound complications occur in as many as 40% of patients. Recent use of neoadjuvant radiation at more modest doses (30 Gy total) has decreased the complication rate while maintaining excellent (>95%) 5-year local control and ultimate limb salvage.[94] Postoperative radiotherapy also may be advantageous. In a large adult sarcoma series, doses between 60 and 70 Gy provided 80% local tumor control and functional limb salvage.[95] The wound complication rate was less than 10%.

Finally, there are several aspects of radiation treatment in pediatric patients that deserve special consideration. Attention must be paid to the issues of immobilizing or sedating children so ionizing doses can be targeted to the desired area without inappropriate exposure of surrounding tissues. It can be difficult to balance the doses required for antitumor efficacy with the risks of adverse reactions in young patients. Pediatric radiation oncologists may use lower treatment doses and accept a higher recurrence rate to ensure lower toxicity, especially in critical developing organs such as the brain. Also, the normal "tolerance" of organs or tissues may be adversely affected when chemotherapeutic agents are utilized. The long-term effects of combined modality therapy must be considered in regard to musculoskeletal and dental tissues, CNS and neuropsychological sequelae, and endocrine and gonadal dysfunction, as well as direct effects on the heart, lungs, or kidneys.[96] The following sections describe techniques that allow safe, efficacious doses of radiation to be delivered, often in combination with surgical excision, to produce the maximal therapeutic benefit.

BRACHYTHERAPY

Brachytherapy is radiation treatment in which the ionizing source is in contact with the lesion, usually within the initial tumor volume. The dose distribution generally depends on the inverse square law, and the most commonly employed isotopes have short half-lives and may be shielded readily. Catheters are placed in the tumor during surgery and may be loaded with temporary or permanent implant sources. Remote afterloading may decrease radiation exposure to personnel and family members and can be performed in the patient's room or on an outpatient basis. Low-dose rate sources such as cesium provide about 1 cGy per minute, whereas high-dose rate sources such as iridium provide about 100 cGy per minute.

Intraoperative brachytherapy with iridium-192 (^{192}Ir) implants delivering 45 Gy has been effective in sarcomas.[97] In this series, the 5-year local control rate with the brachytherapy boost was 82%, compared with 67% with external beam radiation alone. The greatest benefit (90 vs. 65%) was in patients with histologic high-grade tumors. Because interstitial implants allow continuous-dose delivery over a much shorter time, they offer a radiobiologic advantage in high-grade tumors with rapid cell growth kinetics. Close cooperation between surgeon and radiation oncologist during the procedure is critical to ensure the most effective mapping of the tumor bed target.

Pediatric patients with soft-tissue sarcomas can also benefit from specialized radiation treatment strategies. If children have microscopic residual disease after surgery and chemotherapy, radiation produces excellent local tumor control.[98] Hyperfractionated radiotherapy is tolerated just as well as single-fraction treatments. This technique employs smaller doses given as several fractions per day over the same overall treatment time, so that a higher total dose is delivered with similar tissue toxicity. Boosts with interstitial implantation may be particularly well suited for extremity lesions in children that present areas of limited radiation volume because of considerations for future growth and development.

High-precision interstitial radiotherapy techniques have also been beneficial in CNS tumors. The addition of 60-Gy brachytherapy to patients with high-grade gliomas significantly enhanced median survival time compared with patients who received chemotherapy and external beam radiotherapy alone.[99] Interstitial thermoradiotherapy combined with brachytherapy employing ^{192}Ir further increased survival when compared with brachytherapy boost alone in this high-risk group of patients.[100] Younger patients with brain tumors seem to benefit most from therapy boosts after external beam radiation. Among 159 adults with primary glioblastoma, iodine-125 (^{125}I) implants at a median dose of 55 Gy were employed after surgery (75% incomplete resections).[101] The best outcome was achieved in the 18 to 29-year-old group, with a 78% median survival at 3 years.

Unfortunately, radiation therapy to the CNS may cause necrosis, arteritis, leukoencephalopathy, or radiation-induced tumors. Benign meningiomas have developed in children who received initial high-dose cranial radiation for malignant brain tumors, and some patients experienced a short latency period between treatment and tumor development.[102] The carcinogenic effect of radiation therapy on brain tumors also has been theorized in more than 100 cases of malignant intracranial tumors.[103] These patients could be clinically differentiated from those with spontaneous brain tumors, and their outcome was particularly unfavorable.

Recent experience with complex soft-tissue sarcomas and dermoid tumors continues to be favorable. An institutional review of 12 patients who underwent interstitial implantation at surgery followed by manual afterloading with ^{192}Ir has been retrospectively analyzed.[104] The low dose rate technique provided a boost of as much as 20 Gy to external beam radiation, so that a total dose of at least 60 Gy was delivered. The 3-year survival rate was 83%, with only two locoregional failures. There was an overall 32% complication rate, which was considered acceptable because excellent local control was achieved while radical surgical procedures were avoided. Similar encouraging results with brachytherapy have been reported in a variety of adult malignancies, including breast, prostate, and biliary tract cancer.[105–107] Wound complications were related to the time interval between the operation and brachytherapy. If the "boost" dose was 10 to 20 Gy, only 38% of patients experienced early wound complications, and all were minor, requiring no surgical intervention or delay in adjuvant therapy.[108]

The brachytherapy experience in children is more limited and has been employed in a heterogeneous variety of tumors. Implants of ^{125}I or ^{192}Ir were placed in the tumor bed of 18 patients at the time of primary resection of brain tumors, sarcoma, neuroblastoma, rhabdomyosarcoma, hepatoblastoma, and pancreatic cancer.[109] Two implants were afterloaded. Because of advanced disease, only three patients are long-term survivors. However, local tumor control was achieved in 13 instances, with only two patients experiencing treatment-related morbidity. Further evaluation of external beam or interstitial irradiation in 37 children with synovial sarcoma has been completed.[110] Ionizing radiation was delivered to 16 primary lesions, and durable local control was achieved in 14 patients, 10 of whom are long-term survivors. Although there was no benefit to adjuvant radiation after a complete surgical resection, there was significant local control benefit in lesions with incomplete resection or partial chemotherapy response.

High dose rate brachytherapy has been successfully utilized in pediatric patients (Fig. 63–3). Low dose rate techniques require sedation, immobilization, long exposure times, and hospitalization, even with low-energy sources. High dose rate therapy is delivered in a few minutes, which is particularly helpful in young children. The short therapy duration also allows rapid reinstitution of systemic chemotherapy. The morbidity is usually related to skin or mucosal reactions, which may progress as a "recall" phenomenon in patients treated with radiosensitizing agents such as anthracyclines.[111] Recent experience demonstrated effective local control in a variety of childhood sarcomas.[112] Eleven of 13 patients received 36 Gy as a fractionated dose, and 2 children received a similar dose with combined brachytherapy and external beam treatment. Three tumors recurred, but 11 patients were surviving disease-free 41 months after therapy. Half the patients demonstrated mild to moderate skin and mucosal reactions, but only one had grade 3 toxicity. Bone and organ growth were maintained, and the long-term cosmetic appearance was good.

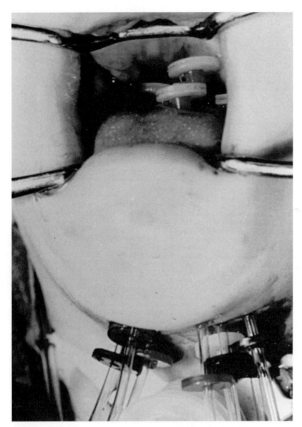

Figure 63–3. A 3-month-old infant with rhabdomyosarcoma in the base of the tongue. Eight high-dose rate brachytherapy catheters were placed delivering 36 Gy in 12 fractions over 8 days. The child is alive and disease-free and has a good cosmetic result 7 years after treatment. (Courtesy of Subir Nag, MD, Chief of Brachytherapy, Ohio State University, Columbus, Ohio.)

INTRAOPERATIVE RADIATION

Intraoperative radiation therapy (IORT) can be an important adjunctive measure to external beam radiation for local tumor control of advanced adult cancer.[113] IORT allows the radiation dose to be directly applied to the target area while shielding adjacent structures. Whenever disease remains in surgically inaccessible areas, IORT may be an effective adjunct. Most applications of IORT in children would include for unresectable disease at diagnosis, delayed primary or second-look procedures, residual lesions, or local tumor recurrence.

Preliminary outcomes suggest that this modality may be beneficial. A report of 59 pediatric patients with various tumor diagnoses showed the value of doses in the 10 to 17 Gy range, delivered with 5 to 11 MEV electrons to a tissue depth of up to 3 cm.[114] Ten of 11 patients with histologically benign but locally aggressive tumors achieved local control. There was a 75% local tumor control rate among the 48 patients with malignant lesions. The largest patient group included 25 children with neuroblastoma, of whom 15 survived a mean of 51 months after IORT. Although half of the stage IV patients were surviving at the time of the initial report, fol-

low-up 3 years later detected only a 38% survival in these children with metastatic disease.[115]

Other series have reported similar results with minor technique variations. In a series of eight children with advanced tumors, a dose of 3 to 15 Gy was delivered with 6 to 13 MEV electrons.[116] Five patients received additional external beam radiation, and local tumor control was achieved in 63% of the cases. There was minimal increase in the operative time and no increase in the complication rate. A subsequent experience with 11 locally advanced or recurrent abdominal tumors in children was also encouraging.[117] In this series, 10 to 25 Gy were administered with 6 to 15 MEV electrons over one to five treatment fields per patient. Again, neuroblastoma was an important target, with three of the four children alive for a mean of 117 months.

Although the operation is ideally undertaken in suites containing linear accelerators, most centers require interdepartmental transfer, and the guidelines for this maneuver have been described.[118] IORT requires more generous incisions and greater degree of tissue mobilization than standard tumor resections. Intracavitary exposure must provide adequate space to place the electron beam accelerator cones and exclude normal organs from the radiation field (Fig. 63–4). IORT should be employed whenever there is concern regarding the original tumor bed or the resection margin adjacent to normal organs or vascular adventitia. In older adolescents or adults, multiple-field matching of IORT applicators and frequent use of customized lead shields can be employed to protect uninvolved tissues.[119] In most infants and children, uninvolved structures can be adequately mobilized so that treatment cones can be placed without cumbersome shielding. For extensive areas of treatment, multiple nonoverlapping fields may be utilized. All surgical dissection must be performed prior to leaving the operating room, as further exploration is potentially dangerous while the patient is in the radiation therapy suite. Proper anesthetic management is critical for these complex procedures, and the techniques have been well established.[120] After radiation therapy, the patient is transported back to the surgical suite for completion of the operation, which generally consists only of ascertaining hemostasis and wound closure.

Earlier experience with IORT demonstrated some treatment-related complications.[121] Three patients required surgical intervention for fibrotic ureteral strictures or renal artery stenosis. In two cases, the injured structures were within a supplemental external beam treatment field. Two children developed neuropathies, one transiently after IORT alone and one permanently after combined therapy with external beam radiation. Nevertheless, all patients were survivors for up to 42 months' follow-up. Currently, more extensive dissection of normal structures and avoidance of overlapping radiation fields have decreased the complication rate.[114] In this series, there was no acute intestinal injury or neuropathy. One superficial wound infection occurred, but there

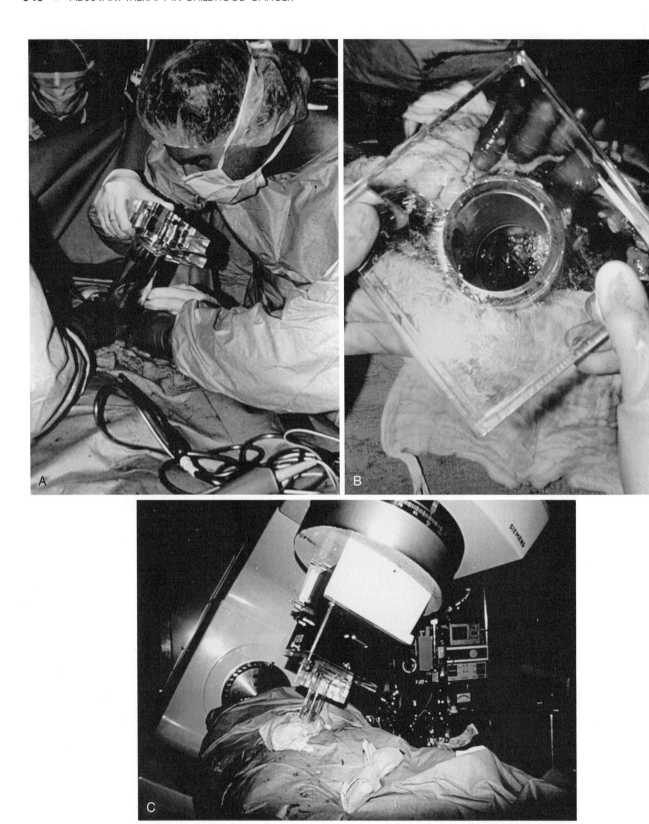

Figure 63–4. *A,* The surgeon places a lucite treatment cone for intraoperative radiation therapy in the abdomen of a child with a recurrent celiac axis neuroblastoma after maximum gross tumor resection has been achieved. *B,* The treatment field inside the cone encompasses the residual tumor bed and excludes normal organs from the radiation field. *C,* Electron beam therapy is accomplished with a linear accelerator, which delivers a single dose of 15 Gy with 11 MEV electrons to a tissue depth of 3 cm. There were no posttreatment complications and the child is surviving with no evidence of disease more than 4 years after therapy.

were no deep intracavitary infections. One child had an episode of self-limited pancreatitis, and two children suffered postoperative intussusception. One patient had undergone a laminectomy and radiation for a paraspinous tumor and developed scoliosis during long-term follow-up. The overall complication rate was similar to that in a matched group of patients who underwent tumor resection alone without IORT.

STEREOTACTIC RADIOTHERAPY

There are now sophisticated sterotactic radiotherapy techniques for the treatment of intracranial neoplasms, which require precise radiation volume definition, localization of normal structures, acurate determination of tumor and adjacent tissue dosage, and careful patient immobilization. Intracranial targets are usually irregular in shape, and treatment planning requires matching the treatment volume to the target in three dimensions with avoidance of adjacent critical normal structures.[122]

Radiation produces acute degenerative necrosis with inflammation, phagocytosis of necrotic debris with peripheral vascular proliferation, and eventual prominent glial scarring.[123] Benign tumors are more slowly proliferating and would be good targets for a single large radiation dose. Conversely, malignant tumors that are rapidly proliferating would respond better to fractionated doses, which would be less damaging to the surrounding normal slow growing brain cells. The concept of stereotactic radiotherapy combines the target and dose localization of single-dose "radiosurgery" with the biologic advantage of dose fractionation. This treatment modality has been made possible by the development of relocatable stereotactic frames and dedicated linear accelerators.[124]

Field shaping is critical to optimize dose delivery in stereotactic radiosurgery. Conformed therapy utilizes a digitally reconstructed computed tomographic image. The use of multiple static beams at different gantry positions and table angles is appropriate for large targets. Most recently, dynamic collimation with simultaneous rotation of treatment couch and gantry allows more sophisticated field shaping and precise treatment of deep-seated irregular lesions.

Evidence suggests that dose-response relationships exist, with improved survival over a range from 45 to 60 Gy.[125] There may be a response ceiling at 60 Gy without further benefit up to 80 Gy. However, radiation therapy for highly malignant disease processes may require total cumulative doses exceeding 100 Gy. The maximum tolerated dose for treatment of patients with recurrent, previously irradiated primary and metastatic brain lesions based on tumor diameter, has recently been established.[126] These doses ranged from 15 Gy to 27 Gy for lesions that ranged from 20 mm to 40 mm in diameter.

Among 61 patients treated for low-grade gilomas using stereotactic radiotherapy, at a dose of 50 to 60 Gy, there were no field recurrences or marginal failures at a median follow-up time of 18 months.[127] In eight children between the ages of 9 and 18 years with benign arteriovenous malformations, the radiosurgery technique was completely successful, and the neurocognitive evaluation 6 years after treatment demonstrated good performance.[128] It was felt that the minimally invasive nature of the procedure contributed to the successful physical and psychological recovery. In high-grade astrocytomas, stereotactic techniques have controlled disease with substantially decreased toxicity from symptomatic radiation necrosis.[129] Radiosurgical techniques can be used to treat metastatic lesions in the brain with response rates greater than 80%, low morbidity, and local failure rates less than 20%. The modality may be more cost-effective than surgery and reduce hospitalization time. While fractionated stereotactic radiotherapy achieves precise target treatment in pediatric brain tumors and has minimal acute effects, longer-term follow-up is still necessary to evaluate the therapeutic efficacy.[130]

Intracranial tumor therapy is also enhanced by the recent availability of surgical navigation technology, which gathers, stores, and reformats three-dimensional images of an intracranial lesion within the surgical field.[131] This intraoperative guidance system allows the surgeon to define the tumor borders for a safer and more complete resection. Complete surgical resections can be achieved in 90% of patients, with less than 10% morbidity and less than 1% mortality. Interactive systems are being devised that integrate radiologic data with the actual patient anatomy at surgery.[132] These newer systems are functionally superior to previously used stereotatic devices. A recently developed "viewing wand" has demonstrated excellent anatomic detail, identified critical structures, and adjusted surgical trajectories in a series of 250 patients undergoing various neurosurgical procedures.[133] The use of computed tomography or magnetic resonance imaging is superior to intraoperative ultrasound (US) in characterizing deep lesions. Intraoperative navigation also provides real-time video processing with computer-generated virtual images of anatomic structures and has been successfully applied to the difficult skull-based lesions and complex craniofacial tumor operations.[134–136]

☐ Innovative Adjunctive Techniques

CRYOSURGERY

The basic principle involved in cryosurgery is the in situ destruction of tissue by the freeze-thaw process. As the frozen tissue thaws, the circulation returns, and for a brief period the tissue may appear almost normal. However, as endothelial cell damage, thrombosis, edema, and vascular stasis develop, the microcirculation progressively fails and cell death ensues.[137] The mechanism of tissue response is multifactorial and highly dependent on the rate of cooling. When this technique is applied to cancer, the goal is to devitalize the same volume of neoplastic tissue by freezing as would have been excised with a local resection. The most important tumoricidal mechanism appears to be the rapid freezing, slow thawing, and immediate repetition of this cycle.[138]

Presently, intraoperative ultrasound allows precise placement into the center of tumors of vacuum-insulated cryoprobes that can monitor the progression of the freeze margin in real time.[139] Liquid nitrogen is circulated through the tip of the probes, achieving temperatures in the range of -160 to $-180°C$. Central placement of the probe is critical because the freeze ball extends symmetrically in all directions. This technique has been successfully utilized with lesions in the breast, liver, bladder, and prostate, as well as with intraocular tumors and benign and malignant skin lesions.

Cryosurgery was employed in 60 patients with primary liver tumors, with a 5-year survival of 12%.[140] However, if the tumor was less than 6 cm in diameter, the local control was improved and the survival rate was 38% at 5 years. In a series of 18 patients with unresectable liver metastases from colon cancer, 4 (22%) were alive without evidence of disease at a median follow-up of 29 months.[141] In a larger series of both primary and metastatic liver lesions, 110 patients were treated with cryosurgery, resulting in a local tumor control rate of 24% at a median 14-month follow-up.[142] Recent reports have described a disease-free survival of as much as 23% at 18 months mean follow-up.[143] Overall survival was achieved in 60% of patients with primary tumors. The incidence of major complications in most series is less than 5%. Leukocytosis and low-grade fevers are common. Local hemorrhage from the probe tract is easily controlled by pressure or packing with hemostatic agents. Hepatic enzyme elevation to about twice normal usually occurs and spontaneously resolves within the first postoperative week. Pleural effusion, myoglobinuria, hemorrhage, biliary leak, or abscess formation is rare.

Cryosurgery has been successfully employed for aneurysmal bone cysts,[144] aggressive benign bone tumors, or low-grade malignancies.[145] Although cryosurgery offers the advantage of preserving supportive function of bone in these skeletal tumors, complications do occur. Most importantly, intraoperative venous gas embolism may rarely produce hemodynamically significant events.[146] It has been suggested that end-tidal nitrogen tension may be monitored intraoperatively to analyze the clinical incidence of this complication.

INTRACAVITARY HYPERTHERMIA AND CHEMOTHERAPY

Hyperthermia has a selective, often lethal, effect on neoplastic cells in vitro and in vivo. High temperatures may sensitize malignant tissues to the cytotoxic effects of ionizing radiation and chemotherapy by inhibiting DNA repair and increasing cellular membrane permeability to chemotherapeutic and other agents. Thermoradiotherapy combines interstitial hyperthermia with brachytherapy and has been utilized to increase median survival time to 23.5 months in malignant gliomas.[100] Multivariant analysis suggested that the hyperthermia had increased the survival. A similar approach was used for recurrent malignant astrocytomas.[147] Three symptomatic patients underwent ^{192}Ir brachytherapy at a 50 Gy dose accompanied by 915-MHz microwave antenna heating for 1 hour. Two patients were symptomatically improved, and the overall survival was 7, 12, and 15 months.

Hyperthermia has also been synergistically combined with a number of chemotherapeutic agents, including doxorubicin, melphalan, cisplatin, bleomycin, and mitomycin-C.[148] The maximal cytotoxic effects are seen after a brief exposure to chemotherapy in the presence of hyperthermia. There appears to be a differential response experimentally between malignant microvasculature and normal blood vessels.[149] Regional hyperthermia also prolongs the half-life of cisplatin after intraperitoneal administration, thereby enhancing its antitumor effects without increasing systemic toxicity. A similar strategy has also been employed with intrathoracic administration of cisplatin.[150]

Intracavitary installation of chemotherapeutic agents without hyperthermia has been used with a variety of pediatric solid tumors.[151] Intracavitary cisplatin at doses between 50 and 210 mg/m² was instilled in the chest or abdomen, with thiosulfate protection in 11 children with rhabdomyosarcoma or pulmonary tumors, including lung metastases from sarcomas. Serum levels were at least comparable to those obtained by intravenous drug administration, and resolution or improvement of effusions or ascites occurred in four patients. There were no intracavitary local recurrences, and two patients were surviving for more than 3 years while two other children were alive more than 8 years after diagnosis. Because most of the patients had also received systemic therapy, the exact contribution of intracavitary cisplatin to outcome could not be assessed. However, the safety of this approach was ascertained, and the low incidence of local recurrence in a group of high-risk relapsed patients suggests that direct installation of these agents may be effective in children with malignant tumors, especially in situations in which high local concentrations of chemotherapeutics would be beneficial.

CHEMOEMBOLIZATION

The regional delivery of chemotherapy for hepatic tumors is possible because the liver has a dual blood supply, with the hepatic artery contributing approximately 25% of the parenchymal flow to normal cells, whereas malignant hepatic lesions derive nearly all of their blood supply from this source. This allows a selective delivery of cytotoxic agents to tumor. In addition, the liver can withstand regional dose escalation because of its ability to detoxify via "first-pass" kinetics. Whereas foreign body embolization produced temporary arterial occlusion and transient palliative effects, the most durable responses were achieved when chemotherapeutic agents were infused distal to the ligated hepatic artery.[152] The therapeutic strategy involves infusing high concentrations of chemotherapy and prolonging the dwell time with a variety of embolic materials (Fig. 63–5). A series of adult patients with unresectable hepatocellular carcinoma demonstrated responses when chemotherapy was suspended in embolic agents.[153] When doxorubicin, mitomycin-C, and cisplatin were combined with gelfoam, 11 of 26 patients showed a tumor reduction of greater than 50% by imaging studies without toxic mortality. If cisplatin was suspended in lipiodal, partial tumor responses could be detected in 33 of 71 patients.[154] The same technique was employed in a variety of liver tumors, including metastatic colon cancer and ocular melanoma.[155] A 23% partial response rate was noted, and the patients had a 7-month mean survival. In a large review of 800 patients from several series treated palliatively for hepatocellular carcinoma, partial response rates of 60 to 83% were noted.[156] Overall patient survival at 3 years ranges from 18 to 51%. Among 90 patients with metastatic colorectal carcinoma, some decrease in tumor size was observed in 78 to 100% of patients, whereas the 1-year survival rate was 67%.

The number of prospective randomized trials in unresectable hepatocellular carcinoma is small. A recent study compared chemoembolization with conservative therapy.[157] The 96 patients received ei-

ther cisplatin suspended in lipiodal and gelatin sponge or supportive care only. Most patients receiving chemoembolization showed a significant decrease in tumor size by imaging study, lower alpha-fetoprotein levels, and even relief of portal obstruction compared with the conservatively treated group. Although there was a trend that favored survival with chemoembolization, the difference was not statistically significant. Of note, 60% of the patients in the treatment arm developed liver failure, which parallels previous experience. Most patients treated with this method have elevation in liver function tests, abdominal pain, nausea, vomiting, fever, ascites, suppressed hematopoiesis, and thrombocytopenia. Some patients have developed diabetes, and occasional patients have developed renal failure.

The pediatric experience with chemoembolization is quite small, although isolated cases of limited success have been reported.[158, 159] This technique has also been extended to hepatic malignancies in infancy.[160] The largest experience in childhood liver tumors has been recently reported.[161] A suspension of cisplatin, doxorubicin, and mitomycin-C mixed with bovine collagen and radiopaque contrast material was utilized in 11 children with unresectable or recurrent lesions. Six patients had progressive hepatoblastoma, two had unresectable hepatocellular carcinoma, two had undifferentiated hepatic sarcomas, and one had chronic cirrhosis and a newly diagnosed unresectable hepatocellular carcinoma. All children except the one with cirrhosis had received previous systemic chemotherapy. The six hepatoblastoma patients had initial partial response, as measured by imaging and alphafetoprotein levels. Three patients underwent subsequent surgical resection, but one progressed and died whereas two

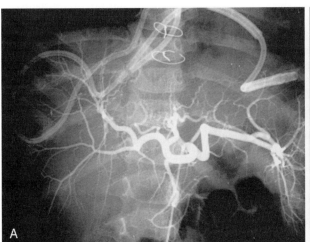 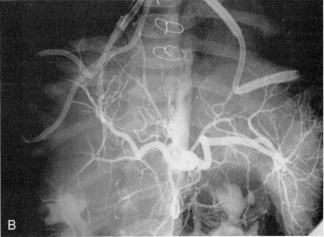

Figure 63–5. *A*, Celiac axis injection before embolization showing slight tortuosity of distal branches of the anterior superior segment of the right lobe, the middle hepatic artery, and the medial segment of the left lobe. (Courtesy of Philip Stanley, MD, Pediatric Hematology-Oncology, UCLA School of Medicine, Los Angeles, California.) *B*, Post-embolization injection of celiac axis showing marked peripheral attenuation of branches of the right and left lobes secondary to deposition of collagen laden with chemotherapy agent. (Courtesy of Philip Stanley, MD, Pediatric Hematology-Oncology, UCLA School of Medicine, Los Angeles, California.)

survived more than 15 months. The other three also eventually died from known progressive disease. Of the three children with hepatocellular carcinoma, one underwent surgical resection and was a long-term survivor for more than 65 months, one was alive with disease for more than 36 months, and one (with cirrhosis) died of progressive liver failure with no evidence of malignancy. One of the two patients with hepatic sarcoma was still alive, but he had progressive disease. Most of the patients experienced fever, nausea, vomiting, transient coagulopathy, and pain during chemoembolization. Only the patient with cirrhosis developed significant toxicity, with a severe tumor lysis syndrome, coagulopathy, and central nervous system hemorrhage. Overall, hepatic chemoembolization is feasible in young patients, with tolerable toxicity, and represents a reasonable therapeutic alternative in persistent, unresectable or recurrent hepatoblastoma or in nonmetastatic hepatocellular carcinoma.

LYMPHATIC MAPPING

Accurate staging of regional disease continues to be important in pediatric and adult tumors. The initial draining lymph node, the so-called sentinel node, is reportedly predictive of regional nodal metastases in a variety of tumors.[162] Intraoperative lymphatic mapping using vital dye injections reliably localizes this node, draining the site of a primary tumor. If the sentinel node has no histologic evidence of metastases, the related regional lymphatic bed is highly likely to be tumor free and the morbidity of lymphadenectomy could be avoided. However, substantial experience is required to undertake the tedious process of dissecting along the dye-stained lymphatic ducts and still avoid the common local wound complications, including seroma, infection, and necrosis.

Subsequent reports describe a less-invasive yet equally accurate method of localizing the sentinel node utilizing radionuclide labeling with technetium-99 (^{99}Tc) sulphur colloid.[163] Gamma probe localization provides many advantages, including a broad time interval during which detection of the initial draining node is possible. Gamma camera images detected nodal uptake as early as 10 minutes following injection, and the uptake persisted for at least 5 hours. This technique allows sentinel node localization prior to making the skin incision and yet permits accurate intraoperative verification of nodal position and completeness of excisional biopsy. The adjacent lymphatic bed can also be scanned to verify that the count does not exceed background levels.

Lymphoscintigraphy is also a reliable indicator of lymphatic drainage from cutaneous melanoma of the head, neck, and trunk.[164] A radiolabeled tracer of ^{99}Tc sulphur colloid or human serum albumin was injected prior to wide local excision of the primary lesion. Of 297 patients reviewed, 181 underwent elective dissection of the lymph node basins identified by the lymphoscintigraphy, and 27% had melanoma detected within the dissected basin. Of these, seven developed nodal metastases as their site of first recurrence, and all were within the area predicted by the original scan. The other 116 patients were observed, and 14% developed lymph node metastases as their first sign of recurrence. Only one of these patients, who developed rapidly progressive disease, had lymph node metastases in an area not predicted by the scan. Overall, 70 of 71 patients had documented lymphatic metastases occur in a predicted lymph node bed, confirming that cutaneous lymphoscintigraphy can be reliably used to guide therapy in high-risk melanoma.

Lymph node localization by gamma probe scanning has also been extended to breast cancer management.[165] In addition, the techniques of vital dye mapping and lymphoscintigraphy have been combined to maximize the accuracy in both melanoma and breast cancer.[166] Sentinel lymph nodes were identified in 92% of patients, and there were no false-negative scans. When blue dye and radiolocalization were combined in 110 patients with melanoma, the sentinel lymph node was identified in 99.5% of patients.[167] In this study, the method was highly accurate in detecting lymph node involvement, with a 3% false-negative rate and no false-positive results.

The implications of sentinel lymph node mapping are important in pediatric tumors such as rhabdomyosarcoma. In the Intergroup Rhabdomyosarcoma Studies I and II, the positive regional lymph node incidence was 12 to 17%. However, most of these patients did not undergo lymph node sampling. More recently, when the majority of patients actually did have a lymph node biopsy, the incidence of detecting disease rose to 40%.[168] These findings were also confirmed subsequently in the Intergroup Rhabdomyosarcoma Study III, which demonstrated that when regional lymph nodes were biopsied, 39% contained metastatic disease.[169] In this study, patient survival improved because those with positive regional lymph nodes underwent radiation therapy to the involved lymphatic bed. Currently, the following technique is being used in children with extremity rhabdomyosarcoma. On the day before operation, the patient is injected around the palpable lesion or the previous incision site with 0.2 to 0.5 ml of ^{99}Tc sulphur colloid. Immediately preoperatively, the same area is injected with 0.5 to 1.0 ml of vital blue dye. When a hand-held gamma probe is used, signal localization parallels the presence of the blue dye in the lymphatic channels leading to the sentinel lymph node. This tissue is stained blue and scans positive, and excisional biopsy is performed for histologic assessment, which should predict involvement of the remaining lymphatic bed. No therapy is necessary for negative biopsies. Histologically positive tissue leads to lymph node dissection and regional lymphatic radiation.

RADIO RECEPTOR GUIDED SURGERY

The concept of radioimmune guided surgery (RIGS) incorporates the use of monoclonal antibodies (MoAbs) to tumor-associated antigens labeled with gamma-emitting isotopes.[170] The antibody is usually administered 3 to 4 weeks prior to the anticipated surgical procedure, such that at the time of operation, background counts are low and tissue is considered positive when the ratio of activity to background is greater than 1.5:1. The tumor is excised, and resection margins, regional lymph node sites, and remote intracavitary areas are scanned. Positive regions undergo biopsy or are removed as appropriate. When this technique was employed in primary colorectal cancer, 30 of 36 patients had positive study results, and they were in unexpected areas in 80% of cases. In 34% of the cases, patients were upstaged, and the operating room strategy was changed 25% of the time.[171]

More recent studies were undertaken with a second-generation MoAb CC49, which is specific for tumor-associated glycoprotein 72, a pancarcinoma antigen found in colorectal, breast, prostate, and ovarian cancer.[172, 173] In 22 patients with recurrent colorectal carcinoma, 51 sites were detected by RIGS, and 44 showed histologically positive tumor.[174] Occult disease was detected in 10 patients, which resulted in a major change in the surgical procedure. Further studies with recurrent colorectal carcinoma confirmed the value of this technology. Indium-111 (^{111}In)-labeled anti-carcinoembryonic antigen MoAbs were employed, and occult disease in the cecum and retroperitoneum was detected. The gamma probe detected 86% of all grossly obvious tumors, and for histologically confirmed tumors, the probe detected 100%.[175] In this setting, RIGS verified that complete surgical resection had been attained. In addition, RIGS using the newest MoAb labeled with ^{125}I identified different patterns of tumor dissemination from those noted by standard operative staging techniques.[176] It is suggested that removal of all "positive" tissue, even in remote areas, may improve survival.

However, antibody tumor targeting can be associated with problems. If the tumor is heterogenous, much of the TAG MoAb will not localize on the tumor and may have toxic systemic effects.[177] These concerns may be exacerbated by variable antibody distribution and binding affinity. Furthermore, the murine origin of the MoAb with the potential for anaphylaxis and the slow circulation clearance time of whole antibodies would require a long interval between injection and surgery.

A wide variety of endocrine and nonendocrine tumors contain high-affinity receptors for somatostatin.[178] Thus, radiolabeled somatostatin could be expected to be useful for tumor localization and staging. Neuroendocrine tumors such as carcinoid, insulinoma, pheochromocytoma, medullary carcinoma of the thyroid, small-cell carcinoma of the lung, neuroblastoma, and medulloblastoma express high densities of somatostatin receptors. Octreotide, an octapeptide analogue, has a more clinically useful half-life of 90 to 120 minutes than the native compound and provides superior receptor binding affinity and more favorable clearance characteristics to enhance the ratio of tumor to background distribution.[179] Iodine-123 (^{123}I)-labeled analogues are poorly visualized in the upper abdomen because of hepatobiliary excretion. Therefore, techniques using an ^{111}In label have been developed.[180]

Several tumors that affect children, including lymphomas and Hodgkin's disease, also express somatostatin receptors.[181] Of particular importance in pediatric tumors is the elevated expression of neuropeptide receptor genes in neuroblastoma, such that 90% of patients with this tumor have visualization by ^{111}In-labeled octreotide scintigraphy.[182] The level of uptake matches that seen with iodine-131 (^{131}I)-labeled metaiodobenzylguanidine radionuclide scanning. The prognostic significance of somatostatin binding also has become apparent, in that receptor expression may be downregulated in more aggressive tumors.[183] All patients who demonstrated high-affinity receptors on their tumors survive, whereas 60% of those who were receptor negative died.[184] In confirmatory studies, receptor-positive patients had a median relapse-free survival of 23 months compared with receptor-negative patients, who all rapidly progressed and died.[185]

An approach to take advantage of these characteristics would be to combine the diagnostic imaging provided by somatostatin receptor expression with the radioimmune-guided surgical methods of intraoperative detection of occult tumor. Because high-affinity receptors have been identified on both primary and metastatic neuroblastoma, radiolabeled analogues could improve anatomic staging of disease, define surgical margins of resection, and ensure that occult tumor sites are detected and removed. To test this hypothesis, six children with Evans stage III or IV neuroblastoma underwent operation after receiving systemic administration of ^{125}I-tyr^3-octreotide.[186] Tissue that was grossly suspicious for tumor or was gamma probe scanning positive was excised. Binding of octreotide to the malignant tissue was detected in the five children with known neuroblastoma and documented by histopathology, immunohistochemistry, and microautoradiography. Intraabdominal uptake occurred within 15 minutes, was greatest in the hepatobiliary system, and decreased over 24 hours. Viable neuroblastoma was detected in 15 of 17 sites with radioreceptor binding. Four of these specimens in three children were from unexpected occult sites of malignancy. Seven other specimens demonstrated no binding, and five of these were negative by histopathology. RIGS was 100% sensitive and 71% specific in neuroblastoma and may provide more accurate disease staging and assessment of surgical excision.

A standard procedure has evolved for RIGS (Fig. 63–6). An intravenous injection of 2 to 15 microcuries per milliliter of radioligand is performed imme-

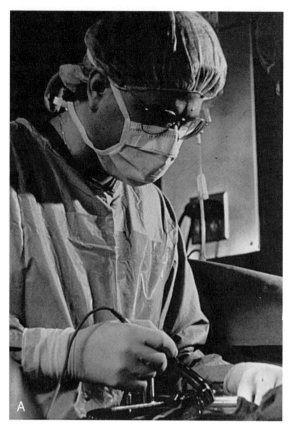

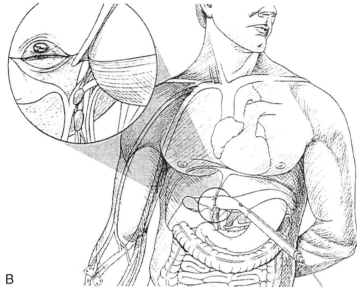

Figure 63–6. *A,* The surgeon uses the handheld gamma detecting probe intraoperatively to determine the background counts and to seek tissue with increased radioactive signal. (Courtesy of Frederick Cope, PhD, Director, Discovery Research, Neoprobe Corporation, Dublin, Ohio.) *B,* This diagrammatic sketch depicts the findings from a typical adult case whereby an occult metastatic site in the liver from a colonic primary lesion was detected by increased audible signal and numerical radioactivity level. (Courtesy of Frederick Cope, PhD, Director, Discovery Research, Neoprobe Corporation, Dublin, Ohio.)

diately before the surgery. Intraoperatively, the hand-held gamma-detecting probe determines the background count from a remote site, and this level is squelched. The radioactivity above background is perceived as an audible signal with intensity and frequency directly proportional to the binding level. Probes are now available that provide a visual signal and a voice prompt that state the numerical radioactivity level. A ratio of at least 2:1 tissue to normal background is considered positive. Routine formal exploration is undertaken. All gross tumor and tissue with increased radioactive signal is removed or biopsied.

In addition to intracavitary application, radiolabeled scanning can also guide detection and biopsy of skeletal and extremity lesions. [99]Tc methylene diphosphonate is employed to localize a wide spectrum of lesions in bone. External scanning techniques identify a bony lesion that may be difficult to detect using surface skin markers. Inaccurate placement of the skin incision may also occur after patient movement and complicates the localization process. Intraoperative gamma probe detection was used successfully in five patients with bony lesions.[187] The radionuclide was injected 4 to 12 hours preoperatively, and the underlying bone lesion was precisely localized so that a more limited procedure for biopsy or excision could be undertaken. This technique can be successfully applied to the broad spectrum of neoplastic or benign processes that accumulate technetium.

MINIMALLY INVASIVE IMAGING

Appropriate management of liver neoplasms requires the accurate detection of all intrahepatic masses. Despite an array of noninvasive external imaging techniques, 20 to 40% of all such lesions are missed.[188] Intraoperative ultrasound is considered an accurate modality for detection of these occult tumors. Sonography was employed at operation in 45 patients with liver neoplasms, 80% of which were metastatic disease.[189] This intraoperative method identified 97% of the lesions that were ultimately diagnosed, whereas routine inspection and palpation found 78% and preoperative imaging detected 67% of the tumors. The planned operative strategy was changed in half of the patients, and in 19 of these, the change was based primarily on the intraoperative ultrasonographic findings.

Because the use of intraoperative imaging has had an impact on the management of hepatic, biliary, and pancreatic surgery, applications have been developed to provide US for minimally invasive surgical procedures. This strategy is important because thoracoscopy and laparoscopy are increasingly performed, and accurate imaging could shorten operative time, reduce tissue manipulation and damage, facilitate surgical decisions and perhaps reduce the operative complication rate. In fact, very recent reports have examined the feasibility of US-guided laparoscopic cryosurgery for hepatic tumors.[190] Laparoscopic intraoperative US has been primarily restricted by the location and size of the access ports through which the transducer is placed. The configuration and depth of the field of view is critical, and a square view field is optimal.[191] Addition of a Doppler signal would provide audio information and spectral analysis display regarding flow and velocity characteristics of vascular structures. The color Doppler provides directional flow information and allows differentiation of vascular structures from those that are ductal or cystic.

Experience with a rigid transducer probe during minimal access surgery in 176 patients demonstrated successful target organ visualization in more than 80% of cases.[192] Scanning at a frequency of 5 to 7.5 MHz allows a 10 to 12 cm depth of penetration for viewing. The development of angulating ultrasonic probes provides greater flexibility for surgical manipulation. A new convex scanner can be placed through a 10-mm trocar site and has the capability to be angled 90 degrees upward and 45 degrees downward.[193] The inclusion of real-time sonography and color flow Doppler facilitates imaging examination of the liver, biliary tree, pancreas, spleen, and virtually all other intraabdominal organs. Most recently, technical innovations have allowed development of a three-dimensional imaging modality that can be utilized during laparoscopy. For example, simultaneous real-time magnetic resonance imaging can now be undertaken through the laparoscope.[194] Dynamic gadolinium-enhanced viewing also can be provided. This imaging guidance would allow interstitial laser therapy of lesions in solid organs to be undertaken. Because this has now been successfully performed in animal models, the methodology can be introduced into clinical practice in an appropriate investigational setting.

This chapter has emphasized the adjunctive treatment strategies that may accompany surgery in the management of neoplastic disease. Systemic, cytotoxic, and immune therapies may provide response, long-term survival, or cure by eradicating micrometastases. In addition, a variety of ionizing radiation techniques and other innovations may provide local tumor control as a part of the overall treatment plan.

REFERENCES

1. Bleyer WA: The impact of childhood cancer on the United States and the world. CA Cancer J Clin 40:355, 1990.
2. Farber S, et al: Temporary remissions in acute leukemia in children produced by folic acid antagonist, 4-aminopteroylglutamic acid (aminopterin). N Engl J Med 238:787, 1948.
3. Li MC, Hertz R, Spencer D, et al: Effect of methotrexate upon choriocarcinoma and chorioadenoma. Proc Soc Exptl Bio Med 93:361, 1956.
4. Frei E III, Freireich EJ, Gehan E, et al: Studies of sequential and combination antimetabolite therapy in acute leukemia: 6-Mercaptopurine and methotrexate. Blood 18:431, 1961.
5. Green DM, Jaffe N: Wilms' tumor—model of a curable pediatric malignant solid tumor. Cancer Treat Rev 5:143, 1978.
6. D'Angio GJ, Evans AE, Breslow N, et al: The treatment of Wilms' tumor: Results of the National Wilms Tumor Study. Cancer 38:647, 1976.
7. Link MP, et al: The effect of adjuvant chemotherapy on relapse-free survival in patients with osteosarcoma of the extremity. N Engl J Med 314:1600, 1986.
8. Schwenn MR, Blattner SR, et al: HiC-COM: A 2 month intensive chemotherapy regimen for children with stage III and IV Burkitt's lymphoma and B-cell acute lymphoblastic leukemia. J Clin Oncol 9:133–138, 1991.
9. Cheung NK, Heller G: Chemotherapy dose intensity correlates strongly with response, median survival and median progression-free survival in metastatic neuroblastoma. J Clin Oncol 9:1050–1058, 1991.
10. Antman K, Ayash L, Elias A, et al: A phase II study of high dose cyclophosphamide, thiotepa, and carboplatin with autologous marrow support in women with measurable advanced breast cancer responding to standard therapy. J Clin Oncol 10:102–110, 1992.
11. Grier H, Krailo M, Link M, et al: Improved outcome in nonmetastatic Ewing's sarcoma and PNET of bone with the addition of ifosfamide and etoposide to vincristine, adriamycin, cyclophosphamide, and actinomycin: A Children's Cancer Group and Pediatric Oncology Group report. J Clin Oncol 13(suppl):421, 1994.
12. Clark PI, Slevin ML, Joel SP, et al: A randomized trial of two etoposide schedules in small-cell lung cancer: The influence of pharmacokinetics on efficacy and toxicity. J Clin Oncol 12:1427–1435, 1994.
13. Parker SL, Tong T, Bolden S, et al: Cancer Statistics, 1997. CA Cancer J Clin 47:5–27, 1997.
14. Gurney JG, Severson RK, Davis S, Robinson LL: Incidence of cancer in children in the United States. Cancer 75:2186–2195, 1995.
15. Miller BA, Ries LA, Hankey BF, et al (eds): SEER Cancer Statistics Review 1973–1990. NCI Publ No. (NIH) 93-2789. Bethesda, MD: NCI, 1993.
16. Bleyer WA: The U.S. Pediatric Cancer Clinical Trials Programmes: International implications and the way forward. Eur J Cancer 33:1439, 1997.
17. Parker SL, Tong T, Bolden S, Wingo PA: Cancer statistics 1996. Ca Cancer J Clin 65:5–27, 1996.
18. D'Angio GJ, Breslow N, Beckwith JB, et al: Treatment of Wilms' tumor: Results of the Third National Wilms' Tumor Study. Cancer 64:349, 1989.
19. Nowell P, Hungerford D: A minute chromosome in human chronic granulocytic leukemia. Science 132:1497, 1960.
20. Kreissman SG: Molecular genetics: Toward an understanding of childhood cancer. Semin Pediatr Surg 2:2–10, 1993.
21. Brodeur GM: Neuroblastoma: Clinical applications of molecular parameters. Brain Pathol 1:45, 1990.
22. Pinkel D, Gray JW, Trask B, et al: Cytogenetic analysis by invitro hybridization with flourescently labeled nucleic acid probes. Cold Spring Harbor Symp Quant Biol 51:151–157, 1986.
23. Henderson EH, Samaha RJ: Evidence that drugs in multiple combinations have materially advanced the treatment of human malignancies. Cancer Res 29:2272, 1969.
24. Goldie JH, Coldman AJ: A mathematic model for relating the drug sensitivity of tumors to the spontaneous mutation rate. Cancer Treat Rep 63:1727, 1979.
25. Pratt CB, Horowitz ME, Meyer WH, et al: A phase II trial of ifosfamide in the children with malignant solid tumors. Cancer Treat Rep 71:131–135, 1987.
26. Miser JS, Kinsella TJ, Triche TJ, et al: Ifosfamide with Mesna uroprotection and etoposide: An effective regimen in the treatment of recurrent sarcomas and other tumors of children and young adults. J Clin Oncol 5:1191–1198, 1987.
27. Balis FM, Holcenberg JS, Poplack DG: General principles of chemotherapy. In Pizzo P, Poplack D (eds): Principles and Practice of Pediatric Oncology. (3rd ed). Philadelphia, Lippincott-Raven, 1997, pp 216.
28. D'Angio GJ, Evans AE, Breslow N, et al: The treatment of Wilms' tumor: Results of the National Wilms Tumor Study. Cancer 38:633, 1976.
29. Green DM, Breslow NE, Evans I, et al: The effect of chemotherapy dose intensity on the hematological toxicity of treatment for Wilms' tumor: A report from the National Wilms' Tumor Study. Am J Pediatr Hematol Oncol 16:207–212, 1994.
30. Picci P, Rougraff BT, Bacci G, et al: Prognostic significance

of histopathologic response to chemotherapy in nonmetastatic Ewing's sarcoma of the extremities. J Clin Oncol 11:1763, 1993.

31. Provisor AJ, Ettinger LJ, Nachman JB, et al: Treatment of nonmetastatic osteosarcoma of the extremity with preoperative and postoperative chemotherapy: A report from the Children's Cancer Group. J Clin Oncol 15:76, 1997.

32. Slevin ML, Clark PI, Joel SP, et al: A randomized trial to evaluate the effect of schedule on the activity of etoposide in small-cell lung cancer. J Clin Oncol 7:1333–1340, 1989.

33. Thompson DS, Hainsworth JD, Hande KR, et al: Prolonged administration of low-dose infusional etoposide in patients with etoposide-sensitive neoplasms: A phase I/II study. J Clin Oncol 11:1322–1328, 1993.

34. Chamberlain MC, Grafe MR: Recurrent chiasmatic-hypothalamic glioma treated with oral etoposide. J Clin Oncol 13:2072–2076, 1995.

35. Woods WG, Kobrinsky N, Buckley JD, et al: Timed-sequential induction therapy improves postremission outcome in acute meyloid leukemia: A report from the Children's Cancer Group. Blood 87:4979, 1996.

36. Campbell LA, Seeger RC, Harris RE, et al: Escalating doses of continuous infusion combination chemotherapy for refractory neuroblastoma. J Clin Oncol 11:623, 1993.

37. Stram DO, Matthay KK, O'Leary M, et al: Consolidation chemoradiotherapy and autologous bone marrow transplant versus continued chemotherapy for metastatic neuroblastoma: A report of two concurrent Children's Cancer Group Studies. J Clin Oncol 14:2417, 1996.

38. Hryniuk W, Levine MN: Analysis of dose intensity for adjuvant chemotherapy trials in stage II breast cancer. J Clin Oncol 4:1162, 1986.

39. Frei E, Canellos GP: Dose: A critical factor in cancer chemotherapy. Am J Med 69:585, 1980.

40. Skipper H: Data and analysis having to do with the influence of dose intensity and duration of treatment (single drugs and combinations) on lethal toxicity and the therapeutic response of experimental neoplasms. Booklets 13 and 2–13. Birmingham, AL: Southern Research Institute, 1986, 1987.

41. Gaynon P, Steinherz P, Bleyer WA, et al: Association of delivered drug dose and outcome for children with acute lymphoblastic leukemia and unfavorable presenting features. Med Pediatr Oncol 19:221, 1991.

42. Bacci G, Picci P, Avella M, et al: The importance of dose-intensity in neoadjuvant chemotherapy of osteosarcoma: A restrospective analysis of high-dose methotrexate, cisplatinum and Adriamycin used preoperatively. J Chemother 2:127, 1990.

43. Broun R, Nichols CR, Kneebone P, et al: Long-term outcome of patients with relapsed and refractory germ cell tumors treated with high-dose chemotherapy and autologous bone marrow rescue. Ann Intern Med 117:124–128, 1992.

44. Smith MA, Ungerleider RS, Horowitz ME, Simon R: Influence of doxorubicin dose intensity on response and outcome for patients with osteogenic sarcoma and Ewing's sarcoma. J Natl Cancer Inst 83:1460–1470, 1991.

45. Kaye SB, Lewis CR, Dave J, et al: A randomized study of two doses of cisplatin and cyclophosphamide in epithelial ovarian cancer. Lancet 340:678, 1992.

46. Collins C, Mortimer J, Livingston RB, et al: High dose cyclophosphamide in the treatment of refractory lymphomas and solid tumor malignancies. Cancer 63:228–232, 1989.

47. Crist WM, Garnsey L, Beltangody MS, et al: Prognosis in children with rhabdomyosarcoma: A report of the Intergroup Rhabdomyosarcoma Studies I and II. J Clin Oncol 8:443–452, 1990.

48. Householder SE, Rackoff W, Goldman J, et al: A case-control retrospective study of the efficacy of granulocyte colony stimulating factor in children with neuroblastoma. Am J Pediatr Hematol Oncol 16:132, 1994.

49. Tepler I, Elias L, Smith JW II, et al: A randomized placebo-controlled trial of recombinant human interleukin-11 in cancer patients with severe thrombocytopenia due to chemotherapy. Blood 87:3607, 1996.

50. Lipshultz SE: Dexrazoxane for protection against cardiotoxic effects of anthracyclines in children. J Clin Oncol 14:328, 1996.

51. Lasky L, Fox S, Smith J, et al: Collection and use of peripheral blood stem cells in very small children. Bone Marrow Transplant 7:281–284, 1991.

52. Takaue Y, Watanabe T, Kawano Y, et al: Isolation and storage of peripheral blood hematopoietic stem cells for autotransplantation into children with cancer. Blood 74:1245–1251, 1989.

53. Fukuda M, Kojima S, Matsumoto K, et al: Autotransplantation of peripheral blood stem cells mobilized by chemotherapy and recombinant human granulocyte colony-stimulating factor in childhood neuroblastoma and non-Hodgkin's lymphoma. Br J Haematol 80:327–331, 1992.

54. Kreissman S, Moss T, Breitfeld P, et al: Repeated peripheral blood stem cell collection and infusion is feasible in pediatric neuroblastoma as support for rapidly administered cycles of dose intensive chemotherapy. J Clin Oncol 15(suppl):460, 1996.

55. Jakacki R, Jamison C, Heifetz S, et al: Feasibility of sequential high-dose chemotherapy and peripheral blood stem cell support for pediatric central nervous system malignancies. Med Pediatr Oncol 29:553–559, 1997.

56. Kreissman SG, Rackoff W, Lee M, et al: High dose cyclophosphamide with carboplatin: A tolerable regimen suitable for dose intensification in children with solid tumors. J Pediatr Hematol Oncol 19:309, 1997.

57. Gordon MS, McCaskill-Stevens WJ, Battiato LA, et al: A phase I trial of recombinant human interleukin 11 (Neumega rgIL-11 growth factor) in women with breast cancer receiving chemotherapy. Blood 87:3615, 1996.

58. Ali-Nazir A, Davenport G, Reaman G, et al: A phase I/II trial of rhIL-11 following ifosfamide, carboplatin, and etoposide (ICE) chemotherapy in pediatric patients with solid tumors or lymphoma. J Clin Oncol 15(suppl):274, 1996.

59. Sonis S, Muska A, O'Brien J, et al: Alterations in the frequency, severity, and duration of chemotherapy induced mucositis in hamsters by interleukin-11. Eur J Cancer 31:261, 1995.

60. Kemp G, Rose P, Lurain J, et al: Amifostine pretreatment for protection against cyclophosphamide-induced and cis-platin-induced toxicities: Results of a randomized control trial in patients with advanced ovarian cancer. J Clin Oncol 14:2101, 1996.

61. Shaw IC, Graham MI: Mesna—a short review. Cancer Treat Rev 14:67, 1987.

62. Moritz T, MacKay W, Glassner B, et al: Retrovirus-mediated expression of DNA repair protein in bone marrow protects hematopoietic cells from nitrosourea-induced toxicity in vitro and in vivo. Cancer Res 55:2608, 1995.

63. Oberfield SE, Allen JC, Pollack J, et al: A Long-term endrocrine sequalae after treatment of medulloblastoma: Prospective study of growth and thyroid function. J Pediatr 108:219, 1986.

64. Huma Z, Boulad F, Black P, et al: Growth in children after bone marrow transplantation for acute leukemia. Blood 86:819, 1995.

65. Larson DL, Kroll S, Jaffe N, et al: Long-term effects of radiotherapy in childhood and adolescence. Am J Surg 160:348, 1990.

66. Haupt R, Fears T, Robison L, et al: Educational attainment in long-term survivors of childhood acute lymphoblastic leukemia. JAMA 272:1427, 1994.

67. Whitehead E, Shalet SM, Morris-Jones PH, et al: Gonadal function after combination chemotherapy for Hodgkin's disease in childhood. Arch Dis Child 57:287, 1982.

68. Green DM, Zevon MA, Lowrie G, et al: Congenital anomalies in children of patients who received chemotherapy for cancer in childhood or adolescence. N Engl J Med 325:141, 1991.

69. Legha SS, Benjamin RS, Mackay B, et al: Reduction of doxorubicin cardiotoxicity by prolonged continuous infusion. Ann Intern Med 96:133, 1982.

70. Nicholson HS, Mulvihill JJ: Late effects of therapy in survivors of childhood and adolescent osteosarcoma. Cancer Treat Res 62:45, 1993.

71. Ginsberg SJ, Comis RL: The pulmonary toxicity of antineoplastic agents. Semin Oncol 9:34, 1982.

72. Blatt J, Copeland DR, Bleyer WA: Late effects of childhood cancer and its treatment. In Pizzo PA, Poplack DG (eds): Principles and Practice of Pediatric Oncology (3rd ed.) Philadelphia, Lippincott-Raven Publishers, 1997, p 1303.

73. Green DM, Zevon MA, Reese PA, et al: Second malignant tumors following treatment during childhood and adolescence. Med Pediatr Oncol 22:1, 1994.

74. Bhatia S, Robison LL, Oberlin O, et al: Breast cancer and other second neoplasm after childhood Hodgkin's disease. N Engl J Med 334:745, 1996.

75. Jenkin D, Greenberg M, Fitzgerald A: Second malignant tumours in childhood Hodgkin's disease. Med Pediatr Oncol 26:373, 1996.

76. Sankila R, Garwicz S, Olsen JH, et al: Risk of subsequent malignant neoplasms among 1,641 Hodgkin's disease patients diagnosed in childhood and adolescence: A population-based cohort study in the five Nordic countries. J Clin Oncol 14:1442, 1996.

77. Smith MB, Xue H, Strong L, et al: Forty year experience with second malignancies after treatment of childhood cancer: Analysis of outcome following the development of the second malignancy. J Pediatr Surg 28:1342, 1993.

78. Smith MA, Rubinstein L, Ungerleider RS: Therapy-related acute myeloid leukemia following treatment with epipodophyllotoxins: Estimating the risks. Med Pediatr Oncol 23:86, 1994.

79. Hahne M, Rimoldi D, Schroter M, et al: Melanoma cell expression of Fas (Apo-1/CD95) ligand: Implications for tumor immune escape. Science 274:1363, 1996.

80. Restifo NP, Snzol M: Cancer vaccines. In DeVita VT, Hellman S, Rosenberg SA (eds): Cancer: Principles and Practice of Oncology (5th ed.) Philadelphia, Lippencott-Raven Publishers, 1997, p 3033.

81. Helling F, Zhang S, Shang A, et al: GM2-KLH conjugate vaccine: Increased immunogenicity in melanoma patients after administration with immunological adjuvant QS-21. Cancer Res 55:2783, 1995.

82. Hock RA, Reynolds BD, Tucker-McClung CL, et al: Murine neuroblastoma vaccines produced by retroviral transfer of MHC class II genes. Cancer Gene Ther 3:314, 1996.

83. Dranoff G, Jaffee E, Lazenby A, et al: Vaccination with irradiated tumor cells engineered to secrete murine granulocyte-macrophage colony stimulating factor stimulates potent, specific, and long-lasting anti-tumor immunity. Proc Natl Acad Sci U S A 90:3539, 1993.

84. Uchiyama A, Hoon DSB, Morisaki T, et al: Transfection of interleukin-2 gene into human melanoma cells augments cellular immune response. Cancer Res 53:949, 1991.

85. Ziegler MM, Ishizu H, Nagabuchi E, et al: A comparative review of the immunobiology of murine neuroblastoma and human neuroblastoma. Cancer 79:1757, 1997.

86. Cheung NK, Burch L, Kushner BH, et al: Monoclonal antibody 3F8 can effect durable remissions in neuroblastoma patients refractory to chemotherapy: A phase II trial. In Evans AE, D'Angio GJ, Knudson AG, Seeger RC (eds): Advances in Neuroblastoma Research. New York, Wiley-Liss, 1991, p 395.

87. Frost JD, Hank JA, Reahman GH, et al: A phase I/IB trial of murine monoclonal anti-GD2 antibody 14.G2a plus interleukin-2 in children with refractory neuroblastoma. A report of the Children's Cancer Group. Cancer 80:317, 1997.

88. Handgretinger R, Anderson K, Lang P, et al: A phase I study of human mouse chimeric antiganglioside GD2 antibody ch14.18 in patients with neuroblastoma. Eur J Cancer 31A:261–267, 1995.

89. Rosenberg SA: Principles of cancer management: Biologic therapy. In DeVita VT, Hellman S, Rosenberg SA (eds): Cancer: Principles and Practice of Oncology (5th ed.) Philadelphia, Lippincott-Raven Publishers, 1997, p 364.

90. Grossbard ML, Press OW, Appelbaum FR, et al: Monoclonal antibody-based therapies of leukemia and lymphoma. Blood 80:863–878, 1992.

91. Bertsch H, Rudoler S, Needle MN, et al: Emergent/urgent irradiation in pediatric oncology: Patterns of presentation, treatment, and outcome. Med Pediatr Oncol 30:101, 1998.

92. Eisbruch A, Lichter AS: What a surgeon needs to know about radiation. Ann Surg Oncol 4:516, 1997.

93. Liu L, Glicksman AS: The role of radiation in the management of soft tissue sarcoma. Med Health RI 80:32, 1997.

94. Temple WJ, Temple CLF, Arthur K, et al: Prospective cohort study of neoadjuvant treatment in conservative surgery of soft tissue sarcomas. Ann Surg Oncol 4:586, 1997.

95. Lindberg RD, Martin RG, Romsdahl MM, et al: Conservative surgery and postoperative radiotherapy in 300 adults with soft-tissue sarcomas. Cancer 47:2391, 1981.

96. Fryer CJH: Principles of pediatric radiatioin oncology. In Holland JF, Frei E, Bast RC, et al (eds): Cancer Medicine, Baltimore, Williams & Wilkens, 1996, pp 2899–2905.

97. Harrison LB, Franzese F, Gaynor JJ, et al: Long-term results of a prospective randomized trial of adjuvant brachytherapy in the management of completely resected soft tissue sarcomas of the extremity and superficial trunk. Int J Radiat Oncol Biol Phys 27:259, 1993.

98. Donaldson S, Breneman J, Asmar L, et al: Hyperfractionated radiation in children with rhabdomyosarcoma—results of an intergroup rhabdomyosarcoma pilot study. Int J Radiat Oncol Biol Phys 32:903, 1995.

99. Green SB, Shapiro WR, Burger PC, et al: A randomized trial of interstitial radiotherapy (RT) boost for newly diagnosed malignant glioma: Brain Tumor Cooperative Group (BTCG) trial 8701. Proc Am Soc Clin Oncol 13:174, 1994.

100. Stea B, Rossman K, Kittelson J, et al: Interstitial irradiation versus interstitial thermoradiotherapy for supratentorial malignant gliomas: A comparative survival analysis. Int J Radiat Oncol Biol Phys 30:591, 1994.

101. Sneed PK, Prados MD, McDermott MW, et al: Large effect of age on the survival of patients with glioblastoma treated with radiotherapy and brachytherapy boost. Neurosurgery 36:898, 1995.

102. Starshak RJ: Radiation-induced meningioma in children: Report of two cases and review of the literature. Pediatr Radiol 26:537, 1996.

103. Kaschten B, Flandroy P, Reznik M, et al: Radiation-induced gliosarcoma: Case report and review of the literature. J Neurosurg 83:154, 1995.

104. Burmeister BH, Dickinson I, Bryant G, et al: Intra-operative implant brachytherapy in the management of soft-tissue sarcomas. Aust NZ J Surg 67:5, 1997.

105. Pieters BR, Maher M, Gerbaulet AL, et al: Brachytherapy in the management of breast cancer: A review. Cancer Treat Rev 21:527, 1995.

106. D'Amico AV, Coleman CN: Role of interstitial radiotherapy in the management of clinically organ-confined prostate cancer: The jury is still out. J Clin Oncol 14:304, 1996.

107. Leung J, Guiney M, Das R: Intraluminal brachytherapy in bile duct carcinomas. Aust NZ J Surg 66:74, 1996.

108. Dalton RR, Lanciano RM, Hoffman JP, et al: Wound complications after resection and immediate postoperative brachytherapy in the management of soft-tissue sarcomas. Ann Surg Oncol 3:51, 1996.

109. Healey EA, Shamberger RC, Grier HE, et al: A 10-year experience of pediatric brachytherapy. Int J Radiat Oncol Biol Phys 32:451, 1995.

110. Fontanesi J, Pappo AS, Parham DM, et al: Role of irradiation in management of synovial sarcoma: St. Jude Children's Research Hospital experience. Med Pediatr Oncol 26:264, 1996.

111. Nag S, Grecula J, Ruymann FB: Aggressive chemotherapy, organ-preserving surgery, and high-dose-rate remote brachytherapy in the treatment of rhabdomyosarcoma in infants and young children. Cancer 72:2769, 1993.

112. Nag S, Olson T, Ruymann F, et al: High-dose-rate brachytherapy in childhood sarcomas: A local control strategy preserving bone growth and function. Med Pediatr Oncol 25:463, 1995.

113. Merrick HW, Dobelbower RR, Konski AA: Intraoperative radiation therapy for pancreatic, biliary and gastric carcinoma: The U.S. experience. Front Radiat Ther Oncol 25:246, 1991.

114. Haase GM, Meagher DP Jr, McNeely LK, et al: Electron beam intraoperative radiation therapy for pediatric neoplasms. Cancer 74:740, 1994.

115. Leavey PJ, Odom LF, Poole M, et al: Intra-operative radiation therapy in pediatric neuroblastoma. Med Pediatr Oncol 28:424, 1997.

116. Aitken D, Hopkins G, Archambeau J, et al: Intraoperative radiotherapy in the treatment of neuroblastoma: Report of a pilot study. Ann Surg Oncol 2:343, 1994.

117. Schomberg PJ, Gunderson LL, Moir CR, et al: Intraoperative electron irradiation in the management of pediatric malignancies. Cancer 79:2251, 1997.

118. Archambeau JO, Aitkin D, Potts TM, et al: Cost-effective, available-on-demand intraoperative radiation therapy. Int J Radiat Oncol Biol Phys 15:775, 1988.

119. Sindelar WF, Hoekstra HJ, Kinsella TJ: Surgical approaches and techniques in intraoperative radiotherapy for intra-abdominal, retroperitoneal, and pelvic neoplasms. Surgery 103:247, 1988.

120. Friesen RH, Morrison JE Jr, Verbrugge JJ, et al: Anesthesia for intraoperative radiation therapy in children. J Surg Oncol 35:96, 1987.

121. Ritchey ML, Gunderson LL, Smithson WA, et al: Pediatric urologic complications with intraoperative radiation therapy. J Urol 143:89, 1990.

122. Shrieve DC, Kooy HM, Tarbell NJ, et al: Fractionated stereotactic radiotherapy. In DeVita VT, Hellman S, Rosenberg SA (eds): Important Advances in Oncology. Philadelphia, Lippincott-Raven Publishers, 1996, pp 205–224.

123. Mehta MP: The physical, biologic, and clinical basis of radiosurgery. Curr Probl Cancer 19:265, 1995.

124. Gill SS, Thomas DG, Warrington AP, et al: Relocatable frame for stereotactic external beam radiotherapy. Int J Radiat Oncol Biol Phys 20:599, 1991.

125. Bleehan NM, Stenning SP: A Medical Research Council trial of two radiotherapy doses in the treatment of grades 3 and 4 astrocytoma. Br J Cancer 64:769, 1991.

126. Shaw E, Scott C, Souhami L, et al: Radiosurgery for the treatment of previously irradiated recurrent primary brain tumors and brain metastases: Initial analysis of Radiation Therapy Oncology Group protocol (RTOG) 9005. Int J Radiat Oncol Biol Phys 30:166, 1994.

127. Shaw EG, Scheithauer BW, O'Fallon JR. Management of supratentorial low-grade gliomas. Semin Radiat Oncol 1:23, 1991.

128. Riva D, Pantaleoni C, Devoti M, et al: Radiosurgery for cerebral AVMs in children and adolescents: The neurobehavioral outcome. J Neurosurg 86:207, 1997.

129. Shrieve DC, Alexander E III, Wen PY, et al: Comparison of stereotactic radiosurgery and brachytherapy in the treatment of recurrent glioblastoma multiforme. Neurosurgery 36:275, 1995.

130. Dunbar SF, Tarbell NJ, Kooy HM, et al: Sterotactic radiotherapy for pediatric and adult brain tumors: Preliminary report. Int J Radiat Oncol Biol Phys 30:531, 1994.

131. Kelly PJ: Volumetric stereotactic surgical resection of intraaxial brain mass lesions. Mayo Clin Proc 63:1186, 1988.

132. Barnett GH, Steiner CP, Weisenberger J: Target and trajectory guidance for interactive surgical navigation systems. Stereotact Funct Neurosurg 66:91, 1996.

133. Sipos EP, Tebo SA, Zinreich SJ, et al: In vivo accuracy testing and clinical experience with the ISG viewing wand. Neurosurgery 39:194, 1996.

134. Wagner A, Ploder O, Enislidis G, et al: Virtual image guided navigation in tumor surgery—technical innovation. J Craniomaxillofac Surg 23:271, 1995.

135. Robinson JR, Golfinos JG, Spetzler RF: Skull base tumors: A critical appraisal and clinical series employing image guidance. Neurosurg Clin North Am 7:297, 1996.

136. League D: Interactive, image-guided, stereotactic neurosurgery systems. AORN J 61:360, 1995.

137. Rubinsky B, Lee CY, Bastacky J, et al: The process of freezing and the mechanism of damage during hepatic cryosurgery. Cryobiology 27:85, 1990.

138. Gage AA: Cryosurgery in the treatment of cancer. Surg Gynecal Obstet 174:73, 1992.

139. Ravikumar TS, Steele GD: Hepatic cryosurgery. Surg Clin North Am 69:433, 1989.

140. Zhou XD, Tang ZY, Yu YQ, et al: Clinical evaluation of cryosurgery in the treatment of primary liver cancer. Report of 60 cases. Cancer 61:1889, 1988.

141. Onik G, Rubinsky B, Zemel R, et al: Ultrasound-guided hepatic cryosurgery in the treatment of metastatic colon carcinoma. Cancer 67:901, 1991.

142. Ravikumar TS, Buenaventura S, Salem RR, et al: Intraoperative ultrasonography of liver: Detection of occult liver tumors and treatment by cryosurgery. Cancer Detect Prevent 18:131, 1994.

143. Crews KA, Kuhn JA, McCarty TM, et al: Cryosurgical ablation of hepatic tumors. Am J Surg 174:614, 1997.

144. Marcove RC, Sheth DS, Takemoto S, et al: The treatment of aneurysmal bone cyst. Clin Orthop 311:157, 1995.

145. Devitt A, O'Sullivan T, Kavanagh M, et al: Surgery for locally aggressive bone tumors. Irish J Med Sci 165:278, 1996.

146. Schreuder HWB, VanBeem HBH, Veth RPH: Venous gas emoblism during cryosurgery for bone tumors. J Surg Oncol 60:196, 1995.

147. Seegenschmiedt MH, Karlsson UL, Black P, et al: Thermoradiotherapy for brain tumors. Am J Clin Oncol 18:510, 1995.

148. Miller RC, Richards M, Baird C, et al: Interaction of hyperthermia and chemotherapy agents: Cell lethality and oncogenic potential. Int J Hypertherm 10:89, 1994.

149. Perez CA, Patterson JH, Emami B: Evaluation of 45°C hyperthermia and irradiation. Am J Clin Oncol 16:469, 1993.

150. Doi O, Kodama K, Tatsuta M, et al: Effectiveness of intrathoracic chemotherapy for malignant pleurisy due to Ewing's sarcoma: A case report. Int J Hyperthermia 6:963, 1990.

151. Boyer MW, Moertel CL, Priest JR, et al: Use of intracavitary cisplatin for the treatment of childhood solid tumors in the chest or abdominal cavity. J Clin Oncol 13:631, 1995.

152. Coldwell DM, Stokes KR, Yakes WF: Embolotherapy: Agents, clinical applications, and techniques. Radiographics 14:623, 1994.

153. Venook AP, Stagg RJ, Lewis BJ, et al: Chemoembolization for hepatocellular carcinoma. J Clin Oncol 8:1108, 1990.

154. Shibata J, Fujiyama S, Sato T, et al: Hepatic arterial injection chemotherapy with cisplatin suspended in an oily lymphographic agent for hepatocellular carcinoma. Cancer 64:1586, 1989.

155. Feun LG, Reddy KR, Yrizzarry JM, et al: A phase I study of chemoembolization with cisplatin and Lipiodol for primary and metastatic liver cancer. Am J Clin Oncol 17:405, 1994.

156. Soulen MC: Chemoembolization of hepatic malignancies. Oncology 8:77, 1994.

157. Trinchet JC, Rached AA, Beaugrand M: A comparison of Lipiodol chemoembolization and conservative treatment for unresectable hepatocellular carcinoma. N Engl J Med 332:1256, 1995.

158. Sue K, Ikeda K, Nakagawara A, et al: Intrahepatic arterial injections of cisplatin-phosphatidylcoline-lipiodol suspension in two unresectable hepatoblastoma cases. Med Pediatr Oncol 17:496, 1989.

159. Nakagawa N, Cornelius A, Kao SC, et al: Transcatheter oily chemoembolization for unresectable malignant liver tumors in children. J Vasc Interv Radiol 4:353, 1993.

160. Ogita S, Tokiwa K, Taniguchi H, et al: Intraarterial chemotherapy with lipid contrast medium for hepatic malignancies in infants. Cancer 60:2886, 1987.

161. Malogolowkin MH, Stanley P, Steele DA, et al: Feasibility and toxicity of chemoembolization for children with liver tumors. J Clin Oncol, in press.

162. Morton DL, Wend D, Wong JH, et al: Technical details of intraoperative lymphatic mapping for early stage melanoma. Arch Surg 127:392, 1992.

163. Alex JC, Weaver DL, Fairbank JT, et al: Gamma-probe-

guided lymph node localization in malignant melanoma. Surg Oncol 2:303, 1993.

164. Berger DH, Feig BW, Podoloff D, et al: Lymphoscintigraphy as a predictor of lymphatic drainage from cutaneous melanoma. Ann Surg Oncol 4:247, 1997.

165. Krag DN, Weaver DL, Alex JC, et al: Surgical resection and radiolocalization of the sentinel lymph node in breast cancer using a gamma probe. Surg Oncol 2:335, 1993.

166. Guiliano AE, Leirgan DM, Guenther JM, et al: Lymphatic mapping and sentinel lymphadenectomy for breast cancer. Ann Surg 220:391, 1994.

167. Kapteijn BA, Nieweg EO, Liem I, et al: Localizing the sentinel node in cutaneous melanoma: Gamma probe detection versus blue dye. Ann Surg Oncol 4:156, 1997.

168. LaQuaglia MP, Ghavimi F, Peneberg D, et al: Factors predictive of mortality in pediatric extremity rhabdomyosarcoma. J Pediatr Surg 25:238, 1990.

169. Andrassy RJ, Corpron CA, Hays DM, et al: Extremity sarcomas: An analysis of prognostic factors from the Intergroup Rhabdomyosarcoma Study III. J Pediatr Surg 31:191, 1997.

170. LaValle GJ, Chevinsky A, Martin EW: Impact of radioimmunoguided surgery. Semin Surg Oncol 7:167, 1991.

171. Arnold MW, Schneebaum S, Berens A, et al: Radioimmunoguided surgery challenges traditional decision making in patients with primary colorectal cancer. Surgery 112:624, 1992.

172. Thor A, Ohuchi N, Szpak CA, et al: Distribution of oncofetal antigen tumor associated glycoprotein-72 defined by monoclonal antibody B72.3. Cancer Res 46:3118, 1986.

173. Arnold MW, Schneebaum S, Berens A, et al: Intraoperative detection of colorectal cancer with radioimmunoguided surgery and CC49, a second-generation monoclonal antibody. Ann Surg 216:627, 1992.

174. Schneebaum S, Papo J, Graif M, et al: Radioimmunoguided surgery benefits for recurrent colorectal cancer. Ann Surg Oncol 4:371, 1997.

175. Kuhn JA, Corbisiero RM, Buras RR, et al: Intraoperative gamma detection probe with presurgical antibody imaging in colon cancer. Arch Surg 126:1398, 1991.

176. Bertsch DJ, Burak WE, Young DC, et al: Radioimmunoguided Surgery for colorectal cancer. Ann Surg Oncol 3:310, 1996.

177. Aftab F, Stoldt HS, Testori A, et al: Radioimmunoguided surgery and colorectal cancer. Eur J Surg Oncol 22:381, 1996.

178. Reubi JC, Krenning EP, Lamberts SWJ, et al: Somatostatin receptors in malignant tissues. J Steroid Biochem Mol Biol 37:1073, 1990.

179. Lamberts SWJ, Krenning EP, Reubi J-C: The role of somatostatin and its analogs in the diagnosis and treatment of tumors. Endo Rev 12:450, 1991.

180. Bakker WH, Albert R, Bruns C, et al: [¹¹¹In-DTPA-D-Phe¹]-octreotide, a potential radiopharmaceutical for imaging of

somatostatin receptor-positive tumors: Synthesis, radiolabeling, and in vitro validation. Life Sci 49:1583, 1991.

181. Reubi JC, Waser B, van Hagen M, et al: In vitro and in vivo detection of somatostatin receptors in human malignant lymphomas. Int J Cancer 50:895, 1992.

182. Krenning EP, Kwekkeboom DJ, Bakker WH, et al: Somatostatin receptor scintigraphy with [¹¹¹In-DTPA-D-Phe¹]- and [¹²³I-Tyr³]-octreotide: The Rotterdam experience with more than 1000 patients. Eur J Nucl Med 20:716, 1993.

183. Maggi M, Baldi E, Finetti G, et al: Identification, characterization, and biological activity of somatostatin receptors in human neuroblastoma cell lines. Cancer Res 54:124, 1994.

184. O'Dorisio MS, Chen F, O'Dorisio TM, et al: Characterization of somatostatin receptors on human neuroblastoma tumors. Cell Growth Diff 5:1, 1994.

185. Moertel CL, Reubi JC, Scheithauer BS, et al: Somatostatin receptors (SS-R) are expressed and correlate with prognosis in childhood neuroblastoma. Proc Am Soc Pediatr Res 27:146A, 1990.

186. Martinez DA, O'Dorisio MS, O'Dorisio TM, et al: Intraoperative detection and resection of occult neuroblastoma: A technique exploiting somatostatin receptor expression. J Pediatr Surg 30:1580, 1995.

187. Krag DN, Ford PV, Patel M, et al: A simplified technique to resect abnormal bony radiolocalizations using a gamma counter. Surg Oncol 1:371, 1992.

188. Wernecke K, Rummeny E, Bongartz G, et al: Detection of hepatic masses in patients with carcinoma: Comparative sensitivities of sonography, CT, and MR imaging. AJR Am J Roentgenol 157:731, 1991.

189. Kane RA, Hughes LA, Cua EJ, et al: The impact of intraoperative ultrasonography on surgery for liver neoplasms. J Ultrasound Med 13:1, 1994.

190. Tandan VR, Litwin D, Asch M, et al: Laparoscopic cryosurgery for hepatic tumors. Experimental observations and a case report. Surg Endosc 11:1115, 1997.

191. Jakimowicz JJ: Laparoscopic intraoperative ultrasonography, equipment, and technique. Semin Laparosc Surg 1:52, 1994.

192. Jakimowicz JJ: Review: Intraoperative ultrasonography during minimal access surgery. J R Coll Surg Edinb 38:231, 1993.

193. Röthlin M, Largiadèr F: New, mobile-tip ultrasound probe for laparoscopic sonography. Surg Endosc 8:805, 1994.

194. Klotz HP, Flury R, Erhart P, et al: Magnetic resonance-guided laparoscopic interstitial laser therapy of the liver. Am J Surg 174:448, 1997.

195. Ratain M, Teicher B, O'Dwyer P, et al: Pharmacology of cancer chemotherapy. In DeVita V, Hellman S, Rosenberg S (eds): Cancer: Principles and Practice of Oncology. Philadelphia: Lippincott-Raven, 1997, pp 375–385.

196. Dorr R, Von Hoff D: Drug monographs. In Dorr R, Von Hoff D (eds): Cancer Chemotherapy Handbook. Norwalk, CT, Appleton and Lange, 1994, p 129.

64

RENAL NEOPLASMS

Denis R. King, MD • Jonathan I. Groner, MD

☐ Wilms' Tumor

HISTORY

Although Max Wilms cannot be credited with the initial description of nephroblastoma, his 1899 monograph entitled *Mixed Tissue Tumors of the Kidney* established the term *Wilms' tumor* as part of the standard nomenclature.[1] Effective treatment of children with nephroblastoma was not possible during Wilms' lifetime. At that time, surgical management was the only therapeutic modality available, and nephrectomy in children with Wilms' tumor was attended by an unacceptable operative mortality rate, frequent recurrence, and an overall survival rate of perhaps 5%. Because surgical management provided such a consistently poor outcome, in 1916 Friedlander recommended radiation as an appropriate therapeutic alternative.[2]

In 1938, Ladd reviewed the available literature on Wilms' tumor and described a standardized perioperative management plan and surgical technique, which in his experience decreased the operative mortality rate from 23 to 7%.[3] Ladd emphasized the importance of optimal preoperative preparation with blood transfusion and fluid administration, transperitoneal exposure, and initial control of the renal vascular pedicle. Strict adherence to these principles not only decreased the perioperative morbidity and mortality rates but also resulted in a cure rate of 20% for those patients undergoing treatment at the Boston Children's Hospital during the 1930s.

Gross and Neuhauser built on this firm foundation of meticulous care with the addition of routine postoperative abdominal radiation therapy.[4] In 1950, these pioneers of multimodal management were able to report a consecutive series of 38 patients with no postoperative deaths and an estimated cure rate of 47%. At that time, the authors summarized the status of chemotherapy as ". . . nothing will be mentioned here since there is little of value which can be offered . . . , however, rapid strides are being made in this field . . . ."[4]

In 1954, Farber introduced actinomycin D as an effective adjuvant chemotherapeutic agent and, during the next 10 years, a dramatic improvement in the survival rate was observed.[5, 6] By the mid-1960s, both actinomycin D and vincristine had been demonstrated to be useful in managing children with Wilms' tumor, and in some medical centers, survival rates were approaching 80%.[7] Since the late 1970s, most of the advances in the clinical management of children with Wilms' tumor have been based on clinical trials performed by the National Wilms' Tumor Study Group (NWTS) in the United States and the Nephroblastoma Study Group of the International Society of Paediatric Oncology (SIOP) in Europe.

EPIDEMIOLOGY

Wilms' tumor is the most common renal malignancy observed in childhood, with an incidence of 8 in 1 million children younger than 15 years of age. In the United States, these tumors develop in approximately 450 children each year. The occurrence rate has been reported to be relatively constant in most Caucasian populations (6 to 9 cases per million person-years), which has prompted the use of Wilms' tumor as the index cancer against which the incidence rates of other childhood malignancies can be compared.[8] A recent review of data from the International Agency for Research on Cancer demonstrated that children from the East Asian countries have a much lower risk of developing nephroblastoma (3 to 4 cases per million person-years), whereas children in African countries and African Americans have a higher incidence (>10 cases per million person-years).[9] Aniridia, hemihypertrophy, cryptorchidism, hypospadias, Wiedemann-Beckwith syndrome (WBS), Drash's syndrome, Klippel-Trenaunay syndrome, Perlmann's syndrome, and specific cytogenetic abnormalities have all been reported to confer an increased risk for developing Wilms' tumor.

In 1972, Knudson and Strong proposed a two-stage mutational model that attempted to explain the clustering of some of the epidemiologic characteristics observed in children with Wilms' tumor.[10] According to their hypothesis, nephroblastoma could occur in either hereditary or sporadic forms. Two mutations were required to allow a tumor to develop. In some children, the first mutation was thought to occur prezygotically (hereditary type, e.g., aniridia and hypospadias), whereas in others, both mutations were thought to occur postzygotically (sporadic type, e.g., hemihypertrophy). Many of the demographic features of patients with Wilms' tumor are consistent with this hypothesis. On the basis of this epidemiologic data, a number of recommendations of practical significance to the clinician have been formulated.

Age, Gender, and Bilaterality

Of the 5085 patients registered on the various NWTS protocols between 1969 and 1990, a small but statistically significant preponderance of females (male-to-female ratio: 1:1.1) was observed.[11] The age at diagnosis was somewhat younger for the boys (median 41.5 mo vs. 46.9 mo for the girls). Similar observations have been made in the clinical trials performed under the auspices of SIOP.[12] Bilateral Wilms' tumors were observed in 358 of the NWTS patients (7%). Eighty-five percent of the bilateral tumors were synchronous in nature. Patients with bilateral Wilms' tumors were much younger at diagnosis (mean = 31.9 mo). In children with unilateral disease, 516 had multicentric tumors (12%). The relative preponderance of females was substantially higher in patients with multicentric (57%) and bilateral (58.3%) tumors.[11, 12]

Aniridia

The association between sporadic aniridia and Wilms' tumor was reported in 1964.[13] Twenty-six patients in the NWTS were reported to have aniridia (0.75%), which represents a risk approximately 600 times higher than normal.[14] In one report of 20 children with sporadic aniridia, Wilms' developed in 7 (35%) before age 4 years.[15] Patients with aniridia are known to have a deletion on the short arm of chromosome 11.[16] All children with aniridia should have a physical examination and abdominal ultrasound (US) every 3 months for the first 2 years of life and every 6 months thereafter until 4 years of age.[17-19]

Hemihypertrophy

Hemihypertrophy was recognized in 112 children in the NWTS experience (2.2%), which represents a thousand-fold increase in risk.[14] Sixty percent of these patients are female and 16% have bilateral tumors. Age at diagnosis is similar to that of children with unilateral tumors. Careful follow-up of all children with hemihypertrophy is suggested. Wilms' tumors have been reported in the offspring of a woman with hemihypertrophy.[20]

Genitourinary Anomalies

Cryptorchidism and hypospadias have population incidences of 0.7% and 1.0%, respectively, but these anomalies have been described in 5.2% of the boys enrolled in NWTS studies.[14] Bilateral tumors are much more common in patients with these genitourinary abnormalities (23%). Mean age at diagnosis was 31 months, which suggests the possibility that a prezygotic mutation occurred as described in children with aniridia. The incidence of both cryptorchidism and hypospadias is substantially lower in the SIOP studies (35 to 50% of NWTS rates), which may reflect significant population differences between the United States and Europe.[12]

Familial Wilms' Tumor

A family history of Wilms' tumor is present in 1.4% of patients.[21] The relationship involved a parent or sibling in half of the cases and a more distant relative (e.g., cousin or uncle) in the others. Parent-to-child transmission occurred in less than 10% of the cases. The inheritance likely is consistent with an autosomal dominant trait with variable penetrance. Bilateral tumors were more frequent (16%) and early age of presentation was common.

Other Considerations

Children with WBS have a 6 to 10% risk of developing hepatoblastoma, adrenal cortical carcinoma, and Wilms' tumor during childhood. Frequent US examinations have been recommended for patients with WBS.[22] Drash's syndrome affects male infants with pseudohermaphroditism, Wilms' tumor, and degenerative renal disease, which often progresses to end-stage renal disease during the 1st year of life.[23] The risk of malignancy may warrant prophylactic nephrectomies soon after developing end-stage renal disease.[24] Although several epidemiologic studies have suggested it, paternal occupation has not been found to be a major risk factor.[25, 26]

MOLECULAR GENETICS

Many studies have confirmed the heterogeneity of the Wilms' tumor gene, and several chromosomal loci have been implicated in the development of nephroblastoma.[27-30] WT-1 is a tumor suppressor gene that maps to the p13 region on chromosome 11 (11p13). This gene is constitutionally deleted in all children with WAGR syndrome (Wilms' tumor, aniridia, genitourinary abnormalities, and mental retardation) and in 5 to 10% of sporadic Wilms' tumors.[27] A second Wilms' tumor suppressor gene has been demonstrated at the 11p15 locus, which is also the site of the chromosomal abnormality associated with the familial form of WBS. At least one other gene must be involved because many patients with familial Wilms' tumor do not have any abnormalities at either the 11p13 or 11p15 locus.

In addition to the WT-1 and WT-2 tumor suppressor genes, which appear to be important in the development of nephroblastoma, genetic abnormalities in chromosomes 16q and 1p have been demonstrated to be associated with an aggressive form of the disease. A study that evaluated 232 Wilms' tumors from the NWTS identified a higher than normal loss of heterozygosity (LOH) on chromosomes 11p (33%), 16q (17%), and 1p (12%).[31] Despite the fact that there was no association between LOH and either stage or histology, the patients with LOH on chromosome 16q had a statistically significant increase in the incidence of tumor recurrence (three times normal) and a 12-fold higher mortality rate. LOH on 1p was also associated with a higher risk of recurrence and death, whereas abnormalities on 11p had no effect on outcome. The tumor suppressor gene p53 also has a role in the aggressive form of Wilms' tumor. There is a high incidence of p53 mutations in anaplastic Wilms' tumors, suggesting that genetic alterations at this locus are required for the development of anaplastic histology.

CLINICAL PRESENTATION

The typical patient with Wilms' tumor is a healthy thriving preschooler who has an asymptomatic abdominal mass that is discovered either by the parents during bath time or the physician during a routine office examination. Other clinical manifestations that may prompt a diagnostic evaluation include hypertension and hematuria. On physical examination, a large, smooth, firm mass is palpable, arising beneath the costal margin. The lesion is nontender and relatively immobile and usually does not cross the midline. Occasionally, a child may have abdominal pain, fever, and anemia as a result of tumor necrosis with intraparenchymal or subcapsular bleeding. Pediatric patients with this constellation of symptoms are difficult to distinguish from those with neuroblastoma. Infrequently, a Wilms' tumor ruptures freely into the peritoneal cavity and the child has signs and symptoms of an acute abdomen.

The extraabdominal portion of the physical examination is normal in most patients with Wilms' tumor. Control of hypertension may be required preoperatively. Intravenous extension of the tumor may be manifest as a cardiac murmur, hepatosplenomegaly, ascites, prominent abdominal wall veins, varicocele, or gonadal metastases.

DIAGNOSTIC IMAGING

The imaging studies for a suspected Wilms' tumor are designed to establish the following:
    Nature of the mass
    Organ of origin
    Presence of functioning contralateral renal tissue
    Presence of bilateral disease
    Patency of the inferior vena cava and renal vein
    Presence of distant metastases

Accordingly, the initial studies usually consist of standard chest and abdominal radiographs. The chest film is scrutinized for evidence of parenchymal metastases. Linear calcifications may be observed on the abdominal radiographs of patients with Wilms' tumor, whereas fine-stippled calcium deposits are typical of neuroblastoma. Sonographic demonstration of a solid tumor necessitates a detailed US examination of the renal vein, inferior vena cava, and right atrium to evaluate intravascular involvement. Some experts believe that most children with nephroblastoma do not require sophisticated imaging studies, but others believe that computed tomographic (CT) scans should be obtained routinely.[32–34]

CT of the abdomen using both intravenous and oral contrast helps delineate the extent of the tumor, the presence of a functioning contralateral kidney, and the possibility of bilateral disease (Fig. 64–1). A chest CT is usually obtained, but this examination should not be used as the sole criterion of pulmonary metastases. Although the sensitivity of a chest CT is high, the specificity is low. If the thoracic CT scan is positive and the chest radiograph is normal, the NWTS-5 protocol recommends either that treatment be based on the pathologic stage of the abdominal tumor or that a biopsy of the lung lesion be obtained to confirm the presence of pulmonary metastases.[35, 36] A percutaneous needle biopsy of the abdominal mass should not be performed. This procedure provides no significant information for the surgeon and tumor seeding in the needle tract has been reported.[37]

SURGICAL MANAGEMENT

The surgeon has two basic responsibilities: to accomplish a complete resection of all viable tumor

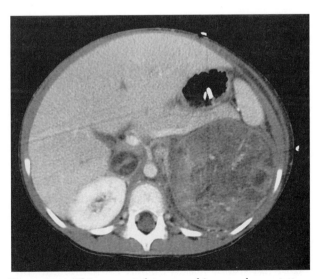

Figure 64–1. This computed tomographic scan demonstrates a left-sided Wilms' tumor and an anatomically normal contralateral kidney. In addition, the lack of contrast material in the inferior vena cava indicates the presence of tumor extension with obstruction of the vessel.

TABLE 64-1. Wilms' Tumor—NWTS-5
Staging System

Stage I

The tumor is limited to the kidney and was completely
  resected.
The renal capsule has an intact outer surface.
The tumor was not ruptured or biopsied before removal.
The vessels of the renal sinus are not involved.
There is no evidence of tumor at or beyond the margins of
  resection.

Stage II

The tumor extends beyond the kidney, but was completely
  resected.
There is regional extension of tumor (i.e., penetration of the
  renal capsule or extensive invasion of the renal sinus).
The blood vessels outside the renal parenchyma, including
  those of the renal sinus, contain tumor.
The tumor was biopsied (except for fine needle aspiration), or
  there was spillage of tumor before or during surgery that is
  confined to the flank and does not involve the peritoneal
  surface.
There is no evidence of tumor at or beyond the margins of
  resection.

Stage III

Residual nonhematogenous tumor is present and confined to
  the abdomen. Any one of the following may occur:
    Lymph nodes within the abdomen or pelvis are found to be
      involved by tumor (renal hilar, paraaortic, or beyond).
    The tumor has penetrated through the peritoneal surface.
    Tumor implants are found on the peritoneal surface.
    Gross or microscopic tumor remains postoperatively.
    The tumor is not completely resectable because of local
      infiltration into vital structures.
    Tumor spill not confined to the flank occurred either before
      or during surgery.

Stage IV

Hematogenous metastases or lymph node metastases outside the
  abdominopelvic region are present.

Stage V

Bilateral renal involvement is present at diagnosis.

---

tissue and to provide accurate staging information, so that appropriate adjuvant therapy can be prescribed (Table 64–1). A unilateral radical nephroureterectomy is performed, in most cases.

The operative procedure is performed through a generous transverse supraumbilical incision. Thoracic extension is rarely necessary. A midline incision is preferred if intravascular involvement has been identified preoperatively. The abdominal cavity is explored for evidence of peritoneal implants and lymphatic or hematogenous metastases. The tumor is inspected for areas of subcapsular hemorrhage, cystic degeneration, or dense soft tissue attachment, which might be susceptible to rupture and result in diffuse peritoneal contamination. A tumor biopsy should not be performed. The retroperitoneal vessels and veins coursing over the surface of the tumor are evaluated critically, and the infrahepatic vena cava is visualized and palpated. If venous engorgement is observed, intravascular extension should be suspected. In this situation, proximal control of the involved vessels becomes a prior-

ity to prevent tumor embolization. The contralateral kidney is examined both visually and by palpation. Suspicious-looking areas should be biopsied or excised.

The nephrectomy is initiated by incising the peritoneum at the base of the small bowel mesentery to expose the retroperitoneal structures. The ureter is isolated as it crosses the pelvic brim. The anterior surface of the aorta or vena cava is cleared of overlying lymphatic and adventitial tissue up to the level of the left renal vein. The involved renal artery and vein are ligated in sequential fashion, and the surrounding soft tissue attachments of the kidney are divided. A formal lymphadenectomy is not required, but care should be taken to ensure that all enlarged periaortic lymph nodes are included with the specimen and that an adequate sampling of hilar nodes is obtained.[38]

The adrenal gland may be left in situ if the tumor involves the lower pole of the kidney; however, it is usually included with the surgical specimen for upper pole lesions. If the tumor is densely adherent to or has invaded adjacent organs, such as diaphragm, pancreas, or colon, portions of these structures may be removed in continuity as long as total gross resection can be achieved safely. If, in the opinion of the surgeon, a complete resection cannot be accomplished safely, a tumor biopsy should be performed and the nephrectomy delayed until after chemotherapy has been initiated.[39] On occasion, transdiaphragmatic biopsy of basilar pulmonary nodules may be obtained to provide complete clinicopathologic staging. The margins of resection are marked with a few titanium clips. Large numbers of clips should not be used for intraoperative hemostasis because the quality of follow-up diagnostic imaging studies would be compromised. The specimen is marked on the superior and anterior surfaces so that the pathologist can provide an appropriate orientation and accurate report on margins. Ideally, the tumor should be examined by the pathologist before formalin fixation.

Partial nephrectomy, which has been recommended by some authors, is discussed here only to be condemned.[40–44] This procedure has no role in managing a unicentric, unilateral Wilms' tumor in a child with an anatomically normal contralateral kidney. The cure rate for localized tumors is so high (95%) and the incidence of renal failure is so low (0.25%) that no compelling argument for nephron-sparing surgery can be made.[45] Partial nephrectomy should be reserved for patients with preexisting abnormalities in the contralateral kidney, bilateral Wilms' tumors, Wilms' tumor and a single kidney, and possibly Wilms' tumor and nephroblastomatosis because these patients are at risk for developing metachronous bilateral lesions.

Venous Extension

The propensity for extension of tumor into adjacent venous tributaries is a well-known characteristic of Wilms' tumor and fatal tumor emboli have been reported both at presentation and during surgery.[46, 47] The ability to recognize venous involvement preoperatively may be of major therapeutic significance. Decisions must be made regarding the primary therapeutic modality (surgery or chemotherapy), the anticipated need for cardiopulmonary bypass, the selection of the most appropriate incision, and the conduct of the operative procedure with reference to early control of major vascular structures and minimal tumor manipulation. The outcome for patients with venous extension should not be different from those with simple intrarenal tumors as long as a careful preoperative evaluation is provided and appropriate intraoperative technique is used. The clinical manifestations of intravascular extension have been well described.[48]

Two hundred and eleven of the 1865 patients enrolled in NWTS-3 had extension of tumor into the renal vein (11.3%).[49] Physical findings of venous tumor were documented in only 1 child who had a varicocele, but hematuria was observed in 38%. A correct preoperative diagnosis was established in only 5 children (0.2%), and the accuracy of the various imaging studies was disappointing. Unilateral nonfunction was apparent on intravenous pyelography in 21 of 153 (14%) patients. Of the 115 US studies obtained, intravascular tumor was confirmed on a single occasion (0.9%). CT demonstrated intravascular extension in 1 of the 78 studies reviewed (1.3%). Inferior vena cavography was the most accurate modality used, identifying tumor thrombus in 4 of the 23 patients evaluated (17%).

Renal vein extension was apparent at the time of nephrectomy in 61 patients (32%), but in most instances, the intravascular tumor was not appreciated until the pathologist examined the surgical specimen. En bloc removal of the kidney and the tumor thrombus was possible in 198 patients, but gross residual intravascular disease was left behind in 4 others. Intraoperative tumor spill was a common problem (local in 45 and diffuse in 37), but no tumor emboli were reported. The outcome for children with renal vein extension was identical to that with intrarenal tumors of similar stage and histologic type. The 2-year relapse-free survival rates were 90% for stage II lesions, 79% for stage III, and 74% for stage IV. Despite the inaccuracy of preoperative assessment, renal vein extension did not represent a critical factor in the surgical management of most of these children.

Extension of tumor thrombus into the vena cava or atrium represents a much more significant technical challenge for the surgeon.[50] This phenomenon was observed in only 4% of the patients enrolled in NWTS-3.[51] Physical findings that suggested intravascular involvement were documented in only 5 of the 77 patients: varicocele (2), hepatomegaly (2), and congestive heart failure (1). Gross hematuria was noted in 30%. An accurate preoperative diagnosis was achieved in 48 children (62%). Unilateral nonfunction was apparent on 28% of the intrave-

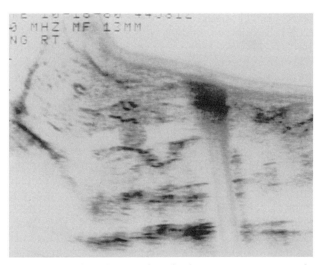

Figure 64–2. This ultrasound study demonstrates tumor in the inferior vena cava. The vessel is patent above and below the intravascular mass.

nous pyelograms. US was diagnostic in 33 of 56 patients overall (59%) and in 14 of 15 patients with atrial involvement (Fig. 64–2). CT demonstrated caval extension on 16 occasions (42%), and contrast studies of the inferior vena cava demonstrated intravascular tumor in 20 of the 23 patients studied (87%) (Fig. 64–3).

The extent of involvement was infrahepatic in 47

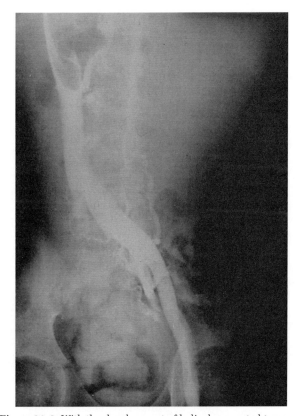

Figure 64–3. With the development of helical computed tomography, venography is infrequently necessary. This study shows an obstructing lesion in the inferior vena cava.

(61%), intrahepatic in 14 (18%), and atrial in 16 (21%). En bloc excision of the renal tumor and the intravascular extension was achieved in 31 patients. Separate removal was performed on 40 occasions. Cardiopulmonary bypass was used in 8 of the patients who had atrial extension. Six children required partial resection of the inferior vena cava. The remaining 57 underwent extraction of the intravascular tumor thrombus through a separate incision in the vena cava or the renal vein orifice. A total of 14 patients were left with gross residual disease within the cava. No operative deaths occurred, but complications were common. Massive hemorrhage (>50 ml/kg) occurred in 33% of these patients. Occlusion of the inferior vena cava was documented postoperatively in 5 patients. The outcome for children with caval and atrial extension in NWTS-3 was not related to the level of vena caval involvement, the extent of tumor spillage, or the presence of residual disease following surgery. Stage and histology of the primary tumor were the only factors of prognostic significance. Overall survival of children with caval and atrial extension was not different from that of children with intrarenal lesions of similar stage and histology.

Complete excision of the caval tumor extension en bloc with the primary nephrectomy specimen is the preferred approach when appropriate, and a carefully considered strategy for resection of Wilms' tumors with intravascular extension has been published.[52] Preoperative radiation and chemotherapy offer the potential benefit of decreasing the morbidity of surgical management, however. A recent retrospective review of 30 NWTS patients confirmed the wisdom of this approach.[53] Fifteen of the children had caval involvement and 15 had atrial extension. With initial chemotherapy, the intravascular mass decreased in size in 23 patients (77%) and resolved

completely in 7 (23%). Only 4 of the 15 children with atrial extension required a median sternotomy and/or cardiopulmonary bypass, and only 3 had residual intravascular tumor. No tumor emboli were reported. Two children died before surgery: in 1 with anaplastic histology, progressive disease developed, and the 2nd died of toxicity from the chemotherapy. The 2-year survival rate of 70% was reasonable, considering that 23% of the patients had anaplastic histology and 77% had either stage IV or V disease. On the basis of this information, it seems most appropriate to treat all cases of intrahepatic or suprahepatic tumor extension with preoperative chemotherapy. This strategy may also be useful for the occasional patient who represents a particularly high risk for surgical intervention owing to a very large locally invasive primary tumor, extensive metastatic disease, massive ascites, or unstable metabolic status.[39, 54, 55]

Bilateral Wilms' Tumor

In contrast to the relatively standardized care available for children with unilateral Wilms' tumor, children with bilateral disease pose a variety of difficult problems (Fig. 64–4).[56–59] There were 204 of 3300 NWTS-1, 2, and 3 patients who had synchronous bilateral tumors.[14] Females predominated in a ratio of 2:1. The patients were first seen at an average age of 25 months versus 44 months for patients with unilateral tumors. Hemihypertrophy (5.4%) and genitourinary anomalies (16%) are two to four times more common in patients with bilateral tumors.

Recent advances in imaging capabilities have led some authors to suggest that contralateral renal exploration is no longer necessary.[60, 61] The experience of patients with synchronous bilateral Wilms' tu-

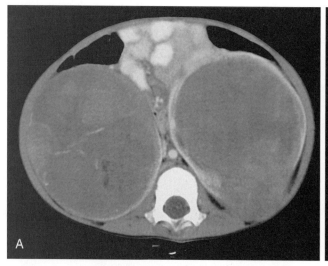
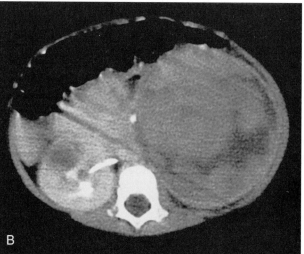

Figure 64–4. *A,* This computed tomographic scan demonstrates huge bilateral Wilms' tumors, which fill virtually the entire abdominal cavity. There is no obvious segment of normal renal tissue available to salvage by partial nephrectomy. *B,* Although the tumor in the right kidney is small in comparison to the mass on the left side, it is in close proximity to the hilar vessels, and achieving a clean resection would be difficult.

mors in NWTS-4 has been compiled.[62] Of the 122 patients reported, 95 had US and 119 underwent either CT or magnetic resonance imaging studies. In nine children (7%), the presence of bilateral disease was missed. Lesions 3 cm or smaller were missed by both US (47%) and CT (16%). It is the NWTS recommendation that contralateral exploration continue to be performed routinely.

In children with bilateral Wilms' tumor, multicentric involvement in one or both kidneys is common (61%). The incidence of unfavorable histology (UH) is 10%, which is similar to that in patients with unilateral tumors. Discordant pathology (favorable on one side and unfavorable on the other) was observed in 40% of the cases with anaplasia, which emphasizes the need to obtain biopsy samples of all discrete lesions in both kidneys. Lymph node involvement was documented in 18%, and this was associated with a poorer prognosis (56 vs. 85% survival at 3 years). Nodal tissue should be obtained at the initial abdominal exploration so that chemotherapy appropriate for the stage of disease can be provided.

A review of patients enrolled in NWTS-2 and 3 confirmed the efficacy of delaying definitive surgery until after chemotherapy had been administered. The overall survival rate of the 145 children studied was 76% at 3 years.[57] Comparable results have been reported by SIOP investigators who achieved a cumulative survival of 64% at 10 years for bilateral Wilms' tumor.[63] A recent evaluation of the renal salvage procedures performed in 98 children with bilateral Wilms' tumor enrolled in NWTS-4 indicated that 72% of the kidneys at risk were able to be preserved and total gross removal of viable tumor was achieved in 88% of the patients.[64] Survival at 4 years was 82%. The current results of multimodal therapy for bilateral Wilms' tumor appear to validate the conservative philosophy of surgical management recommended in the NWTS protocol.

In patients with bilateral disease, the objective is to preserve as much renal tissue as possible. Current recommendations include the following:

Nephrectomy is avoided at the initial laparotomy
Excisional biopsy or partial nephrectomy is appropriate if two thirds of the renal parenchyma can be preserved
Biopsy specimens are obtained from all discrete lesions in both kidneys
Lymph node sampling is accomplished (both hilar and paraaortic) to facilitate accurate staging
Chemotherapy is given appropriate for the stage of the most advanced unilateral lesion

A second-look operative procedure is performed 6 weeks later to attempt removal of all viable tumor. Partial nephrectomy and excisional biopsy are the recommended procedures. If complete removal of tumor tissue is not accomplished during the second-look procedure, chemotherapy is resumed and a third laparotomy is planned within 6 months. At the third operation, a definitive resection should be completed. Options include the entire range of procedures from local enucleation of small residual tumors to bilateral nephrectomy with plans for dialysis and eventual transplantation, if necessary.[65]

Bench surgery with autotransplantation and intraoperative radiotherapy (both in situ and ex vivo) have been successfully used and should be considered before proceeding to bilateral nephrectomy.[66–68] If UH is identified, renal preservation becomes a secondary therapeutic goal. In this situation, aggressive surgical management and chemotherapy must be pursued. In the NWTS studies, the survival of children with bilateral tumors with UH characteristics was 16% compared with 84% of those with favorable histopathologic features.

Metachronous bilateral tumors have been observed in 1.5% of the patients enrolled in the NWTS studies.[69, 70] The incidence of metachronous lesions has decreased significantly from 3.1% in NWTS-1 to 1.3% in a later 5-year cohort, which suggests that current chemotherapy regimens suppress premalignant tumor foci. Girls again were affected twice as often as boys. The interval between initial diagnosis and the appearance of the second tumor ranged from 68 to 2810 days (median 541 days). In the SIOP experience, 96% of the metachronous tumors were diagnosed within 42 months.[63]

The original tumors of all patients with metachronous lesions had favorable histologic characteristics. One third of the primary lesions were described as multicentric and some form of nephroblastomatosis was recognized in 72% of patients. Some of the metachronous lesions may have been overlooked at the initial operation owing to an inadequate examination of the contralateral kidney. Children with evidence of multicentricity or nephroblastomatosis should undergo quarterly US examinations of the contralateral kidney. The overall prognosis for patients with metachronous bilateral tumors was less favorable than those with synchronous lesions. NWTS has reported a 39% disease-free survival rate, whereas SIOP has achieved a favorable outcome in 56%.[63, 69]

PATHOLOGY

Favorable and Unfavorable Histology

Wilms' tumors are composed of blastemal, stromal, or epithelial elements. Any one cell type may predominate, or a mixed tissue pattern may be observed.[71]

In the NWTS-1 experience, 25 patients had anaplastic and 24 patients had sarcomatous histology.[72] Although these "unfavorable" variants were observed in only 11.5% of the patients enrolled in NWTS-1, they accounted for 52% of the deaths. The mortality rate for children with UH was 57%, in sharp contrast to the 7% incidence of tumor-related deaths in the 378 patients with favorable histologic (FH) features. On the basis of this report, histopathology was defined as the single most important prognostic factor for children with Wilms' tumor.[73]

TABLE 64-2. NWTS-3: Outcome
by Histologic Subtype

Histology	Patients	Relapse-Free at 2 y (%)	Survival at 3 y (%)
Favorable	1031	88	93
Anaplastic	52	58	62
Sarcomatous	52	75	80
Rhabdoid	29	19	19

Subsequent studies have further refined understanding of these lesions.[74, 75]

The sarcomatous subtypes (clear cell sarcoma and rhabdoid tumors) are no longer considered to be variants of Wilms' tumor. These lesions are classified as distinct malignant tumors of the kidney (Table 64-2).

Anaplastic tumors continue to be considered an unfavorable histopathologic variant of nephroblastoma.[76] The overall incidence of anaplastic Wilms' tumor, combining data from both NWTS-2 and NWTS-3, is 5.6%.[77] A report from the NWTS of 58 patients with unilateral anaplastic tumors established the following:

The prognosis of stage I anaplastic Wilms' tumors is similar to that of stage I FH. In NWTS-3, only one of the 17 stage I patients with anaplasia developed recurrence (6%).

Children with anaplastic tumors are typically older than those with FH (mean age at diagnosis = 62 mo vs. 47 mo).

Overall survival rate for children with UH (anaplastic only) was 62%, which included the 27 stage I patients with good prognosis. Only 16 of the 41 stage II, III, and IV patients were alive at 2 years without evidence of recurrence (39%).

The prognosis for children who experience relapse is poor. Of the 17 children with anaplasia in whom recurrence developed, 15 died (88%), despite initiation of aggressive retrieval chemotherapy.

Recurrent tumor was most frequently observed in the lung (10) and tumor bed (8).

Pathologic characteristics that were associated with a particularly adverse outcome included the observation of anaplastic tissue in extrarenal tumor sites (e.g., lymph nodes and renal sinus) and a predominantly blastemal pattern in the primary tumor.

A retrospective analysis of the 47 anaplastic Wilms' tumor patients in NWTS-2 revealed no difference in survival rate between children with diffuse and focal anaplasia. This change has been attributed to the addition of doxorubicin to therapy. Additionally, it was found that anaplastic tumors were present in 11% of patients older than 36 months but only in 3% in younger patients. Anaplastic features were observed in 4% of Caucasian patients in contrast to 13% of African American or Hispanic children. Anaplastic tumors metastasized to lymph nodes much more commonly than did FH tumors (30 vs. 16%).

Cassady—Stage I Lesions

In NWTS-5, a subset of stage I tumors has been defined which is not treated with adjuvant chemotherapy. The "surgery only" trial includes stage I FH lesions weighing less than 550 g in children up to 24 months of age. These criteria were initially proposed by Cassady in 1973, and recent follow-up studies and a review of the NWTS 1, 2, and 3 experience confirms that these children have an excellent prognosis.[78–80] The tumors in this group of patients do not usually demonstrate the adverse microsubstaging variables that are associated with relapse in stage I FH tumors, which include (1) the presence of an inflammatory pseudocapsule, (2) renal sinus invasion, (3) tumor in intrarenal vessels, and (4) capsular invasion.[81, 82]

Nephroblastomatosis

A clear association exists between nephroblastomatosis and Wilms' tumor. Most investigators consider this lesion to be premalignant.[83] Nephroblastomatosis is associated with an increased risk of asynchronous tumor development in the contralateral kidney.[74] Nephroblastomatosis is defined histologically by the presence of persistent metanephric tissue in the kidney after the 36th week of gestation. Microscopic foci of perilobar nephroblastomatosis have been documented in 1% of infant kidneys at post-mortem examination but exist in 25 to 40% of children with Wilms' tumor. In NWTS-2, metachronous bilateral tumors developed in 5% of pediatric patients with *perilobar* nephroblastomatosis and in 16% of those with *intralobar* lesions.

Recommendations for the clinical management of children with histologic evidence of nephroblastomatosis must be based on an analysis of relative risk. If nephroblastomatosis is discovered incidentally in a child without Wilms' tumor, the risk of subsequent development of a nephroblastoma has been estimated at 1%. Under this circumstance, no therapeutic intervention or intensive diagnostic follow-up program is recommended. If multiple foci of ipsilateral nephroblastomatosis are observed in a patient with a unilateral Wilms' tumor, however, routine follow-up with quarterly US examinations of the remaining kidney appears to be prudent because the risk of metachronous tumor is between 5 and 16%. When resecting a suspected unilateral Wilms' tumor, if small nodules of nephroblastomatosis are observed in the contralateral kidney, a biopsy or conservative excision that does not place the remaining renal tissue in jeopardy is advised. The overall favorable experience with bilateral Wilms' tumor recorded during the past two decades in the various NWTS studies should temper the surgeon's enthusiasm for removing all abnormal-appearing tissue.

RADIATION AND CHEMOTHERAPY

Clinical management of children with Wilms' tumor is continuously evolving. The NWTS-1 was initiated in 1969 as a cooperative venture by Acute Leukemia Group-B, Children's Cancer Study Group, and Southwest Oncology Group. Since 1969, four major clinical trials have been completed under the aegis of the NWTS, and a fifth study has been initiated.[84–88]

National Wilms' Tumor Study-1

The initial NWTS clinical trial (October 1969 to December 1973) enrolled 606 patients and allowed a number of important observations.[84] Postoperative radiation therapy offered no benefit for children with stage I tumors. A combination of actinomycin D and vincristine provided a better outcome for patients with stage II and III tumors. UH, regional lymph node metastases, tumor weight greater than 250 g, age older than 2 years, and single-agent chemotherapy were identified as factors associated with an increased risk of relapse and death.[73, 85] Parameters that had little or no correlation with survival included tumor laterality, capsular penetration, vascular invasion, direct regional tumor extension, and intraoperative tumor spill. Without doubt, the recognition of a subset of tumors with UH represented a landmark in the understanding of the biology of Wilms' tumor.[72]

National Wilms' Tumor Study-2

The objectives of NWTS-2 (October 1974 to July 1978) were to establish the ideal duration of chemotherapy for children with group I disease and to study the efficacy and toxicity of doxorubicin as a third chemotherapeutic agent in children with group II, III, and IV tumors.[86]

Six months of actinomycin D and vincristine were as good as 15 months for stage I patients. The addition of doxorubicin for stage II and III FH patients improved the relapse-free survival rate from 75 to 90% but with no improvement in the 2-year survival rate. Three drugs were no better than two in the stage IV patients. The outcome of children with UH was much worse than that of those with FH (54 vs. 90% survival rate at 2 years). Patients with regional lymph node involvement also fared poorly (54 vs. 82% 2-year survival rate). The risk of death as a result of therapy (e.g., drug toxicity and infection) remained acceptably low (2%).[87] The incidence of preoperative diagnostic error was reduced from 5% in NWTS-1 to 1.6%.

National Wilms' Tumor Study-3

The third NWTS (May 1979 to November 1985) involved 1439 children.[88, 89] The incidence of UH (10.4%), bilateral tumors (6.5%), and erroneous preoperative diagnoses (2.3%) was similar to that of the previous clinical trials.

In children with stage I-FH tumors, no differences in relapse or survival rate was seen by giving actinomycin D and vincristine for 10 weeks or 6 months. The outcome for patients with stage I tumors was not dependent on histology. The outcome for stage II FH patients was not improved by the addition of doxorubicin, whereas children with stage III FH tumors did slightly better on triple-agent therapy. Children with stage IV FH tumors were not improved by the addition of cyclophosphamide to the standard triple-agent chemotherapy protocol. Radiation therapy (2000 cGy) failed to improve the outcome of children with stage II FH lesions. In the stage III patients randomized to receive either 1000 or 2000 cGy, no differences in relapse or survival rate were attributable to radiation dose.

National Wilms' Tumor Study-4

The stated aims of the NWTS-4 (1986 to 1994) were to simplify, shorten, and refine the various treatment protocols.[90] Pulse intensive (PI) and standard chemotherapy were compared on protocols of either 6 or 15 months' duration. A total of 3107 patients were registered on NWTS-4, and although the final report is not yet published, some preliminary findings are available.[91]

PI chemotherapy regimens were less toxic

PI chemotherapy is more economical than standard chemotherapy

There was no difference in the 2-year relapse-free survival between the PI and standard chemotherapy protocols

There was no difference in the 2-year relapse-free survival between 6 and 15 months of therapy

Minimal treatment for children with diffuse anaplasia should consist of vincristine, actinomycin D, doxorubicin, and cyclophosphamide

Relapse-free and overall survival rates for all NWTS-4 patients at 4 years are 88% and 95%, respectively

National Wilms' Tumor Study-5

The objectives of the NWTS-5 are to study the biology of Wilms' tumor by determining whether LOH on chromosomes 16q and 1p and increased tumor cell DNA are associated with a poorer prognosis. In addition, new chemotherapy protocols are being evaluated for high-risk patients with diffuse anaplasia, clear cell sarcoma, and rhabdoid tumors, and a surgery-only strategy will be used for Cassady stage I FH tumors.[35]

LATE EFFECTS

One measure of success in managing children with cancer is the increasing concern about the possible late effects of therapy. It has been estimated that the survival rate for children currently being enrolled on the various NWTS protocols exceeds 85%.[92] One of the primary goals of the NWTS-4 and -5 studies has been to minimize the intensity and duration of therapy for patients in the good prognostic categories.

Second Malignant Neoplasms

The records of 487 children with Wilms' tumor who had been treated at the Dana-Farber Cancer Institute between 1927 and 1981 were reviewed.[93] In 11 patients (2%), second primary malignancies developed 7 to 34 years after treatment (median 17 years). Ten of the 11 lesions were cancers of soft tissue origin that arose in the radiation field. Analysis of these data indicated that the cumulative probability of developing a second cancer was 6% at 20 years and 18% at 34 years. Similar results have been reported by the late effects study group, NWTS, and SIOP.[94–96]

Of the 2438 patients enrolled on NWTS protocols between 1969 and 1982, second malignant neoplasms (SMNs) developed in 15.[92] This observed incidence of second tumors was eight times higher than expected. At 10 years, SMNs had developed in approximately 1% of the survivors. The spectrum of tumors included 6 with leukemia or lymphoma, 3 with hepatocellular carcinoma, and 3 with soft tissue sarcomas. Children with Wilms' tumor who achieve late survival status require ongoing medical surveillance for the development of SMNs during their adult life.

Reproductive Problems

Other areas of late effects that represent well-documented problems for Wilms' tumor survivors are fertility, pregnancy, and premature or low birth weight infants. In 1982, a review of the reproductive histories of 36 Wilms' tumor survivors (27 women and 9 men) revealed a significant increase in perinatal mortality rate (6.7%), primarily as a result of prematurity and low birth weight.[97] The majority of problem pregnancies were observed in women who had undergone abdominal radiotherapy. The risk of low birth weight babies in this subset of patients was 30%. The offspring of male survivors were not at increased risk. The incidence of major congenital anomalies was not higher than normal. In none of the children did Wilms' tumors or other malignancies develop during the follow-up period.

Another study reported 17 perinatal deaths and 17 low birth weight babies of 114 pregnancies in radiated female Wilms' tumor survivors.[98] In contrast, only 2 of the 77 pregnancies (3%) in nonirradiated women or the wives of male survivors produced an adverse result. It has been suggested that all female survivors of therapy for Wilms' tumor undergo prenatal counseling and that all who become pregnant be referred to a high-risk pregnancy program.[99]

In a review of 787 NWTS-1 and NWTS-2 patients, other problems were documented to occur with increased frequency with longer follow-up.[95] Scoliosis

and musculoskeletal abnormalities were seven times more common in children given radiation therapy. Benign tumors developed in 10.5% of the radiated patients. Cardiovascular problems were infrequent even in the children who had been given doxorubicin (Adriamycin). The cumulative frequency of doxorubicin cardiomyopathy was only 1.7% at 15 years after diagnosis, but in children who were treated with doxorubicin and whole lung irradiation, the incidence increased to 5.4%. There was no apparent increase in the incidence of neuropsychiatric problems in patients who had been given vincristine.[95]

☐ Clear Cell Sarcoma

Clear cell sarcoma of the kidney (CCSK) was initially included as one of the UH variants of Wilms' tumor.[72] When the histologic, ultrastructural, and clinical characteristics of this tumor were reviewed, an unusual propensity for osseous metastases was recognized and the term *bone metastasizing renal tumor of childhood* was suggested.[100] Subsequent studies have confirmed the characteristic morphologic and clinical features of CCSK, which is no longer considered a variant of nephroblastoma but rather a distinct malignant tumor of renal origin that occurs in about 20 patients per year in the United States.[71]

Of the 2841 patients reviewed in the NWTS between 1969 and 1986, 120 were diagnosed as CCSK (4.2%).[101] The mean age at presentation was 36.7 months. Boys were more commonly affected (male-to-female ratio 1.7:1). No physical characteristics distinguish this lesion from a Wilms' tumor at the time of laparotomy. On cut surface, the tumor is tan. Cystic spaces are often present, but hemorrhage and necrosis are infrequent. Most CCSKs have a recognizable histologic pattern, which consists of "sharply defined polygonal cells with water-clear cytoplasm and ovoid-to-rounded vesicular nuclei, in which nucleoli are inconspicuous."[71] One important histologic feature is the presence of "spaced fibrovascular septa coursing throughout the tumor, often forming vascular arcades that divide the tumor cells into cords or columns." The ultrastructural features of this tumor have been defined.[101]

As far as clinical management is concerned, a number of important observations have been made. No cases of multicentric or bilateral CCSK have been reported. The incidence of bone metastases in children with CCSK is 23%.[102, 103] In comparison, osseous metastases developed in only 0.3% of all children entered in the NWTS-3. Standard radiographic techniques were more accurate than radionuclide scans in identifying the osseous lesions, but both imaging techniques should be used because the studies are frequently complementary. CCSK patients have a significantly increased risk of development of cerebral metastases (17%), which dictates the need to obtain brain scans in addition to the osseous imaging studies.[102] The prognosis of the children in whom bone metastasis developed was poor, with 3 of 19 reported long-term survivors (16%).[103]

The treatment of children with CCSK differs somewhat from that of children with Wilms' tumor. Current recommendations indicate that all patients with CCSK (stages I through IV) undergo nephrectomy, receive abdominal radiation therapy to the tumor bed (1080 cGy), and receive a four-drug, 6-month, chemotherapy regimen, which includes vincristine, doxorubicin, etoposide, cyclophosphamide, and mesna.[35] The prognosis for children with CCSK has improved dramatically since the addition of doxorubicin to the chemotherapy protocol (Table 64–3). In NWTS-1 and NWTS-2, in 31 cases of CCSK, 20 patients experienced relapse (65%) and 15 died (48%). In contrast, the 58 children with CCSK on in NWTS-3 who received actinomycin D, vincristine, and doxorubicin had a 6-year relapse-free survival rate of 64% and an overall survival rate of 72%.[104] Late recurrence continues to be a significant problem, with 30% of the relapses occurring more than 2 years after diagnosis.[105]

☐ Rhabdoid Tumors

Rhabdoid tumors of the kidney (RTK) are the least common (10 cases per year in the United States) but most lethal renal malignancies of childhood (see Table 64–2). This lesion was also included in the original description of unfavorable Wilms' tumor variants but is now recognized as a distinct lesion that probably arises from cells of neural crest origin in the renal medulla.[106]

The 79 confirmed cases of RTK entered on NWTS protocols since 1969 represent 1.8% of the renal neoplasms registered.[107] The rhabdoid tumor is an aggressive lesion that appears early in childhood. The mean age at diagnosis was 16.8 months. Boys were more commonly affected (male-to-female ratio, 1.5:1). In contrast to Wilms' tumor, few RTKs are confined to the kidney at the time of diagnosis. Hypercalcemia is a relatively common manifestation. Some authors have proposed that the diagnosis of rhabdoid tumor may be suggested by characteristic features on CT. The lobular appearance of the tumor, a crescent-shaped subcapsular fluid collection, and low-attenuation areas of hemorrhage and necrosis circumscribing tumor nodules are diagnostic imaging findings present in 71% of patients with rhabdoid tumors.[108, 109] At laparotomy, rhabdoid tumors typically appear as bulky lesions that consistently involve the medial portion of the kidney and distort the hilar structures. Intravascular extension is common, but surface lobulation is not. All patients with RTK had unilateral lesions. On cut section, the tumor is gray-pink and friable. Satellite lesions are frequently visible. Nine major morpho-

TABLE 64–3. Wilms' Tumor—NWTS-5 Treatment Recommendations

Stage	Histology	Features	Surgery	Radiation	Chemotherapy	
I	FH	Age <24 mo Tumor weight <550 g	Nephrectomy	None	None	Abdominal US and chest radiograph q 3 mo × 2 y
I	FH	Age >24 mo Tumor weight >550 g	Nephrectomy	None	A	
	UH	Focal or diffuse anaplasia			V	18wk
II	FH		Nephrectomy	None	A V	18 wk
II	UH	Focal anaplasia	Nephrectomy	1080 cGy to abdomen	A V	24 wk 24 wk
III	FH UH	Focal anaplasia			D	
IV	FH UH	Focal anaplasia	Nephrectomy	1080 cGy to abdomen (if UH or primary tumor stage III) 1200 cGy to thorax	A V D	24 wk
V	FH		Initial biopsy Delayed resection	As needed	A V	Second-look laparotomy at 6 wk
II–IV	UH	Diffuse anaplasia	Nephrectomy	1080 cGy to abdomen 1200 cGy to thorax if IV	V D E C M	24 wk

A, actinomycin D; C, cyclophosphamide; D, doxorubicin; E, etoposide; FH, favorable histology; M, mesna; UH, unfavorable histology; US, ultrasonography; V, vincristine.

TABLE 64–4. Staging of Renal Adenocarcinoma

Stage	Definition
I	Tumor contained within renal capsule
II	Tumor spread to perinephric fat but within Gerota's fascia
III-A	Venous tumor thrombus
III-B	Regional lymph node metastasis
III-C	Venous tumor thrombus and regional lymph node metastasis
IV-A	Direct invasion of adjacent organs outside Gerota's fascia
IV-B	Distant metastasis

logic patterns have been described on light microscopy, and the ultrastructural features have been defined.[107] Virtually all rhabdoid tumors stain positive for vimentin, whereas the affinity for other antibodies including cell adhesion molecules (CAM) 5.2, epithelial membrane antigen, neuron-specific enolase (NSE), and S-100 protein is quite variable.[110]

In contrast to the children with CCSK, clinical management of RTK has not proven successful. Despite triple-agent chemotherapy (actinomycin D, vincristine, and doxorubicin), no improvement in outcome has occurred. Survival rate at 3 years is less than 20%.[110] Of the 57 RTK patients registered on NWTS protocols with developed relapse, 55 died as a result of tumor progression (96%). Metastases arose in multiple sites, but pulmonary lesions were most frequent (70%). Children with RTK also have a propensity for developing primary brain tumors.[111] In one report, intracranial tumors that were histologically distinct from the primary renal lesions developed in 14% of the patients, and brain scans are recommended as part of the initial evaluation of all children with rhabdoid tumors of the kidney.[111]

Current treatment recommendations include a 6-month, three-drug chemotherapy protocol using carboplatin, etoposide, cyclophosphamide, and mesna.[35] Abdominal radiation (1080 cGy) should be provided for patients with stage III lesions. The role of autologous bone marrow transplantation in this disease process has not been defined.

☐ Renal Adenocarcinoma

Adenocarcinoma of the kidney is distinctly uncommon in the pediatric age group, representing less than 1% of all the renal cancers diagnosed in children and adolescents.[71] Although the majority of the reports on pediatric patients are retrospective reviews of institutional experiences dating back 20 or 30 years, an analysis of these papers provides some consistent information for the clinician.[112–116]

Most renal cell carcinomas occur in older children and adolescents. The classic triad of abdominal pain, hematuria, and flank mass described in adults is less frequent in childhood. Many of the patients

have malaise, lethargy, weight loss, and fever. Renal cell carcinoma staging is presented in Table 64–4.[117] Approximately 50% of the pediatric patients reported in the literature had localized tumors (stages I and II) and the remainder were seen first with advanced stage disease (stages III and IV). The most common metastatic sites are lung, liver, and bone. Patient outcome is directly related to the clinicopathologic stage at presentation (Table 64–5). The recommended surgical management for patients with renal cell adenocarcinoma is radical nephroureterectomy with regional lymphadenectomy, and an overall survival rate of 50% should be anticipated. As far as adjuvant treatment is concerned, radiation therapy has no role in managing patients with localized renal cell carcinoma, but radiation has been used successfully to control symptomatic metastatic lesions.[118] Renal cell carcinoma is acknowledged to be resistant to virtually all chemotherapeutic agents.[118] The best treatment approach currently available for patients with metastatic disease is immunomodulation using recombinant interleukin-2 and interferon-α. Unfortunately, the use of immunotherapeutic agents produces response rates of only 15 to 20% and durable responses and cures are an unattainable goal.

☐ Congenital Mesoblastic Nephroma

Congenital mesoblastic nephroma (CMN) was established as a distinct renal tumor in 1967 when the characteristic clinicopathologic features of the lesion were described.[119] Before this report, CMN had been considered a variant of Wilms' tumor and many infants had been subjected to potentially morbid treatment with both radiation and chemotherapy. In 1973, a review of 48 cases reaffirmed the benign nature of CMN and established nephrectomy as the treatment of choice, without the need for adjuvant radiation or chemotherapy.[120]

CMN accounts for approximately 5% of pediatric renal tumors or approximately 20 cases per year in the United States. More than 90% of these tumors are discovered during the 1st year of life. Mesoblas-

TABLE 64–5. Clinicopathologic Stage at Presentation

Author	Year	No.	Stage I	II	III	IV
Raney et al[116]	1983	20	5	7	3	5
Lack et al[112]	1985	17	6	4	4	3
Bruce and Gough[114]	1990	6	3	1	1	1
Broeckner[113]	1991	6	1	1	2	2
Aronson et al[115]	1996	22	7	1	—	14
Survival			21:22	9:14	4:10	1:25
			95%	64%	40%	4%

tic nephroma is the most common renal tumor *only in the first 3 months of life.* Beginning at 4 months of age, Wilms' tumor is diagnosed more frequently. There are no cases of bilateral mesoblastic nephroma. Prenatal detection has been described in a dozen cases. In most instances, polyhydramnios preceded discovery of the tumor. Preterm labor, low birth weight, and hydrops fetalis have been reported.[121, 122]

In 1982, the patients with CMN who had been registered with the NWTS protocols were reviewed.[123] The 51 cases represented 2.8% of the NWTS study population. The mean age at diagnosis was 3.4 months. Male infants were more frequently affected (male-to-female, 1.8:1). A palpable abdominal mass was the most common presenting feature (94%). Hematuria was observed in 9 patients (18%). Although complete excision was achieved in 43 patients, local extension of tumor into the perirenal soft tissues prevented the surgeon from achieving clear surgical margins in 8 others and intraoperative tumor rupture was a common problem (20%). Despite the difficulties with surgical management, patient outcome was extremely favorable; 50 children were described as survivors. Only 1 patient had recurrent intraabdominal tumor. The single death recorded in this series occurred in a neonate in whom neutropenia and sepsis developed following chemotherapy. This study affirmed the role of surgical excision as the sole therapeutic modality for most children with CMN.

Ninety-five percent of congenital mesoblastic nephromas are cured by appropriate surgical therapy alone. A radical nephrectomy with generous margins around all gross tumor is critical to prevent recurrence. Particular attention must be paid to the hilum and great vessels owing to the tendency of this tumor to send finger-like projections into the perirenal soft tissues in this area. The surgical specimen should include the entire kidney, the ureter, the renal vessels, the perihilar soft tissue, and the perivascular soft tissue around the great vessels.

The recurrence risk for mesoblastic nephroma is about 5% and postoperative diagnostic imaging surveillance is suggested. Monthly abdominal US examinations combined with chest radiographs every 2 or 3 months should be performed for at least 12 months and then at less frequent intervals. Despite the relatively benign appearance of these tumors, reports continue to be published detailing aggressive behavior in mesoblastic nephromas.[124–128] It has been proposed that mesoblastic nephroma is part of a spectrum of mesenchymal renal tumors of varying malignant potential. In this classification, mesoblastic nephroma represents the benign variant and spindle cell sarcoma the malignant extreme, and there is a "gray zone" with lesions of intermediate aggressiveness that histologically have either focal or diffuse increased cellularity and mitotic rates.[129]

For more than two decades, the gray zone lesions have been the focus of controversy and confusion.[130, 131] The terms *cellular, atypical,* and *rarely metastatic mesoblastic nephroma* have all been used to describe tumors with histologic characteristics suggestive of aggressive behavior. The term *cellular* is preferred over *atypical* because 66% of CMN have come to be recognized as predominantly cellular. Twenty-four percent have *classic* histology, and the remaining 10% are mixed tumors.[71]

In 1986, a review of 18 cases of cellular mesoblastic nephroma found that 7 (39%) had recurred.[132] No specific histopathologic features were predictive of recurrence. Although older infants had an increased risk of recurrent disease, adjuvant therapy could not be advised on the basis of age alone. The only factor that predicted recurrence was a positive surgical margin, which was usually noted at the medial edge of the resected specimen. On the basis of these data, it was suggested that cellular CMNs that were completely excised did not require adjuvant chemotherapy. Patients with residual disease, positive margins, or tumor rupture should be considered appropriate candidates for chemotherapy. Vincristine, doxorubicin, and cyclophosphamide have been recommended. However, only one third of recurrent mesoblastic nephromas respond to chemotherapy or radiation. These tend to be rapidly growing lesions that are controlled only by aggressive surgical resection. In a collected series of 28 cases of recurrent mesoblastic nephromas, the majority presented in the retroperitoneal area; however, there were 7 pulmonary and 3 brain metastases, and 11 deaths occurred among the 28 patients.

REFERENCES

1. Daun R, Leier W, Roth H, et al: Wilms—a man, a syndrome. Kinderchir 44:327–329, 1989.
2. Friedlander A: Sarcoma of the kidney treated by the roentgen ray. Am J Dis Child 12:238, 1916.
3. Ladd WE: Embryoma of the kidney (Wilms' tumor). Ann Surg 108:885–902, 1938.
4. Gross RE, Neuhauser EBD: Treatment of mixed tumors of the kidney in childhood. Pediatrics 6:843–852, 1950.
5. Farber S, Toch R, Sears EM, et al: Advances in chemotherapy of cancer in man. In Greestein JP, Haddow A (eds): Advances in Cancer Research. Vol. 4. New York, Academic Press, 1956, pp 1–71.
6. Farber S, D'Angio G, Evans A, et al: Clinical studies of actinomycin-D with special reference to Wilms' tumor in children. Ann N Y Acad Sci 89:421–425, 1960.
7. Sutow WW, Thurman WG, Windmiller J: Vincristine (leurocristine) in the treatment of children with metastatic Wilms' tumor. Pediatrics 32:880–887, 1963.
8. Breslow N, Beckwith JB: Epidemiological features of Wilms' tumor: Results of the National Wilms' Tumor Study. J Natl Cancer Inst 68:429–436, 1982.
9. Stiller CA, Parkin DM: International variations in the incidence of childhood renal tumors. Br J Cancer 62:1026–1030, 1990.
10. Knudson AG, Strong LC: Mutation and cancer: A model for Wilms' tumor of the kidney. J Natl Cancer Inst 48:313–324, 1972.
11. Breslow N, Olshan A, Beckwith JB, et al: Epidemiology of Wilms' tumor. Med Pediatr Oncol 21:172–181, 1993.
12. Pastore G, Carli M, Lemerle J, et al: Epidemiological features of Wilms' tumor: Results of studies by the International Society of Paediatric Oncology (SIOP). Med Pediatr Oncol 16:7–11, 1988.
13. Miller RW, Frammeni JF, Manning MD: Association of

Wilms' tumor with aniridia, hemihypertrophy and other congenital malformations. N Engl J Med 270:922–927, 1964.

14. Breslow N, Beckwith JB, Ciol M, et al: Age distribution of Wilms' tumor: Report from the National Wilms' Tumor Study. Cancer Res 48:1653–1657, 1988.

15. Pilling GP IV: Wilms' tumor in seven children with congenital aniridia. J Pediatr Surg 10:87–96, 1975.

16. Framcke U, Holmes LB, Atkins L, et al: Aniridia—Wilms' tumor association: Evidence for specific relation of 11q 13. Cytogenet Cell Genet 24:185–192, 1979.

17. Craft AW, Parker L, Stiller C, et al: Screening for Wilms' tumour in patients with aniridia, Beckwith syndrome, or hemihypertrophy. Med Pediatr Oncol 24:231–234, 1995.

18. DeBaun MR, Brown M, Kessler L: Screening for Wilms' tumor in children with high-risk congenital syndromes: Considerations for an intervention trial. Med Pediatr Oncol 27:415–421, 1996.

19. Palmer N, Evans AE: The association of aniridia and Wilms' tumor: Methods of surveillance and diagnosis. Med Pediatr Oncol 11:73–75, 1983.

20. Meadows AT, Lichtenfeld JL, Koop CE: Wilms' tumor in three children of a woman with congenital hemihypertrophy. N Engl J Med 291:23–24, 1974.

21. Breslow N, Olson J, Moksness J, et al: Familial Wilms' tumor: A descriptive study. Med Pediatr Oncol 27:398–403, 1996.

22. Shah KJ: Beckwith-Weidemann syndrome: Role of ultrasound in its management. Clin Radiol 34:313–319, 1983.

23. Drash A, Sherman F, Hartmann WH, et al: A syndrome of pseudohermaphroditism, Wilms' tumor, hypertension, and degenerative renal disease. J Pediatr 76:585–593, 1970.

24. Jensen JC, Ehrlich RM, Hanna MK, et al: A report of 4 patients with the Drash syndrome and a review of the literature. J Urol 141:1174–1176, 1989.

25. Bunin GR, Nass CC, Kramer S, et al: Parenteral occupation and Wilms' tumor: Results of a case-control study. Cancer Res 49:725–729, 1989.

26. Olshan AF, Breslow NE, Daling JR, et al: Wilms' tumor and paternal occupation. Cancer Res 50:3212–3217, 1990.

27. Grundy P, Coppes M: An overview of the clinical and molecular genetics of Wilms' tumor. Med Pediatr Oncol 27:394–397, 1996.

28. Grundy P, Koufos A, Morgan K, et al: Familial predisposition to Wilms' tumour does not map to the short arm of chromosome 11. Nature 336:374, 1988.

29. Koufos A, Grundy P, Morgan K, et al: Familial Wiedemann-Beckwith syndrome and a second Wilms' tumor locus both map to 11p 15.5. Am J Hum Genet 44:711–719, 1989.

30. Huff V, Amos CI, Douglass EC, et al: Evidence for genetic heterogeneity in familial Wilms' tumor. Cancer Res 57:1859–1862, 1977.

31. Grundy PE, Telzerow PE, Breslow N, et al: Loss of heterozygosity for chromosomes 16q and 1p in Wilms' tumors. Cancer Res 54:2331–2333, 1988.

32. D'Angio GJ, Rosenberg H, Sharples K, et al: Position paper: Imaging methods for primary renal tumors of childhood: Costs versus benefits. Med Pediatr Oncol 21:205–212, 1993.

33. Ditchfield MR, De Camp JF, Waters KD, et al: Wilms' tumor: A rational use of preoperative imaging. Med Pediatr Oncol 24:93–96, 1995.

34. Cohen MD: Commentary: Imaging and staging of Wilms' tumors: Problems and controversies. Pediatr Radiol 26:307–311, 1996.

35. National Wilms' Tumor Study Group: NWTS-5 Protocol. Children's Cancer Group, Arcadia, CA, 1995.

36. Green DM, Fernbach DJ, Norkool P, et al: The treatment of Wilms' tumor patients with pulmonary metastases detected only with computed tomography: A report from the National Wilms' Tumor Study. J Clin Oncol 9:1776–1781, 1991.

37. Lee IS, Nguyen SI, Shanberg AM: Needle tract seeding after percutaneous biopsy of Wilms' tumor. J Urol 153:1074–1076, 1995.

38. Othersen HB, deLorimier A, Hrabovsky E, et al: Surgical evaluation of lymph node metastases in Wilms' tumor. J Pediatr Surg 25:330–331, 1990.

39. Ritchey ML, Pringle KC, Breslow NE, et al: Management and outcome of inoperative Wilms' tumor: A report of National Wilms' Tumor Study-3. Ann Surg 220:683–690, 1994.

40. Polascik TJ, Pound CR, Meng MV, et al: Partial nephrectomy: Technique, complications, and pathological findings. J Urol 154:1312–1318, 1995.

41. Sagalowsky AL: Indications and techniques for nephron sparing surgery. J Urol 154:1319–1320, 1995.

42. McLorie GA, McKenna PH, Greenberg M, et al: Reduction in tumor burden allowing partial nephrectomy following preoperative chemotherapy in biopsy proven Wilms' tumor. J Urology 146:509–513, 1991.

43. Moorman-Voestermans CGM, Starlman CR, Delemarre JFM: Partial nephrectomy in unilateral Wilms' tumor is feasible without local recurrence [abstr]. Med Pediatr Oncol 23:218, 1994.

44. Wilinas JA, MaGill L, Parham DM, et al: The potential for renal salvage in nonmetastatic unilateral Wilms' tumor. Am J Pediatr Hematol Oncol 13:342–344, 1991.

45. Ritchey ML, Green DM, Patrick RM, et al: Renal failure in Wilms' tumor patients: A report from the National Wilms' Tumor Study Group. Med Pediatr Oncol 26:75–80, 1996.

46. Shurin SB, Gauderer MWL, Dahms BB, et al: Fatal intraoperative pulmonary embolization of Wilms' tumor. J Pediatr 101:559–562, 1982.

47. Zakowski M, Edwards RH, McDonough ET: Wilms' tumor presenting as sudden death due to tumor embolism. Arch Pathol Lab Med 114:605–608, 1990.

48. Grosfeld JL, Weber TR: Surgical considerations in the treatment of Wilms' tumor. In Gonzales-Crussi F (ed): Wilms' Tumor (Nephroblastoma) and Related Neoplasms of Childhood. Boca Raton, FL, CRC Press, 1984, pp 263–283.

49. Ritchey ML, Othersen HB Jr, de Lorimier AA, et al: Renal vein involvement with nephroblastoma: A report of the National Wilms' Tumor Study-3. Eur Urol 17:139–144, 1990.

50. Nakayama VK, de Lorimier AA, O'Neill JA, et al: Intracardiac extension of Wilms' tumor: A report of the National Wilms' Tumor Study. Ann Surg 304:693–697, 1986.

51. Ritchey ML, Kelalis PP, Breslow N, et al: Intracaval and atrial involvement with nephroblastoma: Review of National Wilms' Tumor Study-3. J Urol 140:1113–1118, 1988.

52. Thompson WR, Newman K, Seibel N, et al: A strategy for resection of Wilms' tumor with vena cava or atrial extension. J Pediatr Surg 27:912–915, 1992.

53. Ritchey ML, Kelalis PP, Haase GM, et al: Preoperative therapy for intracaval and atrial extension of Wilms' tumor. Cancer 71:4104–4110, 1993.

54. Kogan SJ, Marans H, Santorineau M, et al: Successful treatment of renal vein and vena caval extension of nephroblastoma by preoperative chemotherapy. J Urol 13:312–317, 1986.

55. Bray GL, Pendergrass TW, Schaller RT, et al: Preoperative chemotherapy in the treatment of Wilms' tumor diagnosed with the aid of fine needle aspiration biopsy. Am J Pediatr Hematol Oncol 8:75–78, 1986.

56. Bishop HC, Tefft M, Evans AE, et al: Survival in bilateral Wilms' tumor—review of 30 National Wilms' Tumor Study cases. J Pediatr Surg 12:631–638, 1977.

57. Blute ML, Kelalis PP, Offord KP, et al: Bilateral Wilms' tumor. J Urol 138:968–973, 1987.

58. Asch MJ, Siegel S, White L, et al: Prognostic factors and outcome in bilateral Wilms' tumor. Cancer 56:2524–2529, 1985.

59. Laberge J, Nguyen LT, Homsey YL, et al: Bilateral Wilms' tumors: Changing concepts in management. J Pediatr Surg 22:730–735, 1987.

60. Koo AS, Koyle M, Hurwitz RS, et al: The necessity of contralateral surgical exploration in Wilms' tumor with modern noninvasive imaging technique: A reassessment. J Urol 144:416–417, 1990.

61. Kessler O, Franco I, Jayabose S, et al: Is contralateral exploration of the kidney necessary in patients with Wilms' tumor? J Urol 156:693–695, 1996.

62. Ritchey ML, Green DM, Brewlos NB, et al: Accuracy of

current imaging modalities in the diagnosis of synchronous bilateral Wilms' tumor—a report from the National Wilms' Tumor Study Group. Cancer 75:600–604, 1995.
63. Coppes MJ, de Kraker J, van Dijken PJ, et al: Bilateral Wilms' tumor: Long-term survival and some epidemiologic features. J Clin Oncol 7:310–315, 1989.
64. Horwitz JR, Ritchey ML, Moksness J, et al: Renal salvage procedures in patients with synchronous bilateral Wilms' tumors: A report from the National Wilms' Tumor Study Group. J Pediatr Surg 31:1020–1025, 1996.
65. Ehrlich RM, Shanberg AM, Asch MJ, et al: Bilateral nephrectomy for Wilms tumor. J Urol 136:308–311, 1986.
66. Anderson KD, Altman RP: Selective resection of malignant tumors using bench surgical techniques. J Pediatr Surg 11:881–882, 1976.
67. Longaker MT, Harrison MR, Adzick NS, et al: Nephron-sparing approach to bilateral Wilms' tumor: In situ or ex vivo surgery and radiation therapy. J Pediatr Surg 25:411–414, 1990.
68. Debaker A, Lamote J, Keuppens F, et al: In situ cooling of the kidney facilitates curative excision of tumors with preservation of renal function. J Pediatr Surg 30:1338–1340, 1995.
69. Jones B, Hrabovsky E, Kiviat N, et al: Metachronous bilateral Wilms' tumor: National Wilms' Tumor Study. Am J Clin Oncol 5:545–550, 1982.
70. Kim TH, Norkool P, Beckwith JB, et al: Metachronous bilateral Wilms' tumor—a follow up report of the National Wilms' Tumor Study. Med Pediatr Oncol 17:313–314, 1989.
71. Beckwith JB: Renal Tumors. In Askin FB, Stocker JT (eds): Pathology of Solid Tumors in Children. New York, Chapman & Hall Medical, 1998, pp 1–23.
72. Beckwith JB, Palmer NF: Histopathology and prognosis of Wilms tumor: Results from the first National Wilms' Tumor Study. Cancer 41:1937–1948, 1978.
73. Breslow NE, Palmer NF, Hill LR, et al: Wilms' tumor: Prognostic factors for patients without metastases at diagnosis. Cancer 41:1577–1589, 1978.
74. Beckwith JB: Wilms' tumor and other renal tumors of childhood: A selective review from the National Wilms' Tumor Study Pathology Center. Hum Pathol 14:481–492, 1983.
75. Beckwith JB: Wilms' tumor and other renal tumors of childhood: An update. J Urol 136:320–324, 1986.
76. Bonadio JF, Storer B, Norkool P, et al: Anaplastic Wilms' tumor: Clinical and pathologic studies. J Clin Oncol 3:513–520, 1985.
77. Zuppan CW, Beckwith JB, Luckey DW: Anaplasia in unilateral Wilms' tumor: A report from the National Wilms' Tumor Study Pathology Center. Hum Pathol 19:1199–1209, 1988.
78. Cassady JR, Tefft M, Filler RM, et al: Considerations in the radiation therapy of Wilms' tumor. Cancer 32:598–608, 1973.
79. Larsen E, Perez-Atayde A, Green DM, et al: Surgery only for the treatment of patients with Stage I (Cassady) Wilms' tumor. Cancer 66:264–266, 1990.
80. Green DM, Breslow NE, Beckwith JB, et al: Treatment outcomes in patients less than 2 years of age with small, Stage I, favorable-histology Wilms' tumors: A report from the National Wilms' tumor study. J Clin Oncol 11:91–95, 1993.
81. Green DM, Beckwith JB, Weeks DA, et al: The relationship between microsubstaging variables, age at diagnosis, and tumor weight of children with stage I/favorable histology Wilms' tumor: A report from the National Wilms' Tumor Study. Cancer 74:1817–1820, 1994.
82. Weeks DA, Beckwith JB, Luckey DW: Relapse-associated variables in stage I favorable histology Wilms' tumor: A report of the National Wilms' Tumor Study. Cancer 60:1204–1212, 1987.
83. Hennigar RA, Othersen HB Jr, Garvin AJ: Clinicopathologic features of nephroblastomatosis. Urology 33:259–269, 1989.
84. D'Angio GJ, Evans AE, Breslow N, et al: The treatment of Wilms' tumor: Results of the National Wilms' Tumor Study. Cancer 38:633–646, 1976.
85. Leape L, Breslow NE, Bishop HC: The surgical treatment of Wilms' tumor: Results of the National Wilms' Tumor Study. Ann Surg 187:351–356, 1978.
86. D'Angio GJ, Evans A, Breslow N, et al: The treatment of Wilms' tumor: Results of the second National Wilms' Tumor Study. Cancer 47:2301–2311, 1981.
87. Jones B, Breslow NE, Takashima J: Toxic deaths in the second National Wilms' Tumor Study. J Clin Oncol 2:1028–1033, 1984.
88. D'Angio GJ, Breslow NE, Beckwith JB, et al: Treatment of Wilms' tumor: Results of the third National Wilms' Tumor Study. Cancer 64:349–360, 1989.
89. Breslow NE, Sharples K, Beckwith JB, et al: Prognostic factors in nonmetastatic, favorable histology Wilms' tumor: Results of the third National Wilms' Tumor Study. 68:2345–2353, 1991.
90. National Wilms' Tumor Study Group: NWTS-4 Protocol. Children's Cancer Group, Arcadia, CA, 1986.
91. Green DM: Paediatric oncology update: Wilms' tumour. Eur J Cancer 33:409–418, 1997.
92. Breslow NE, Norkook PA, Olshan A, et al: Second malignant neoplasms in survivors of Wilms' tumor: A report from the National Wilms' Tumor Study. J Natl Cancer Inst 80:592–595, 1988.
93. Frederick PL, Yan JC, Sallan S, et al: Second neoplasms after Wilms' tumor in childhood. J Natl Cancer Inst 71:1205–1209, 1983.
94. Meadows AT, Baum E, Fossati-Bellani F, et al: Second malignant neoplasms in children: An update from the Late Effects Study Group. J Clin Oncol 3:532–538, 1985.
95. Evans AE, Norkool P, Evans I, et al: Late effects of treatment for Wilms' tumor: A report from the National Wilms' Tumor Study Group. Cancer 67:331–336, 1991.
96. Carli M, Frascella E, Tournade MF, et al: Second malignant neoplasms in patients treated on SIOP Wilms' tumour studies and trials 1, 2, 5, and 6. Med Pediatr Oncol 29:239–244, 1997.
97. Green DM, Fine WE, Li Frederick: Offspring of patients treated for unilateral Wilms' tumor in childhood. Cancer 49:2285–2288, 1982.
98. Li FB, Gimbrere K, Gelber RD, et al: Outcome of pregnancy in survivors of Wilms' tumor. JAMA 257:216–219, 1987.
99. Byrne J, Mulvihill JJ, Connelly RR, et al: Reproductive problems and birth defects in survivors of Wilms' tumor and their relatives. Med Pediatr Oncol 16:233–240, 1988.
100. Marsden HB, Lawler W, Kumar PM: Bone metastasizing renal tumor of childhood: Morphological and clinical features, and differences from Wilms' tumor. Cancer 42:1922–1928, 1978.
101. Haas JE, Bonadio JF, Beckwith JB: Clear cell sarcoma of the kidney with emphasis on ultrastructural studies. Cancer 54:2978–2987, 1984.
102. Beckwith JB, Norkool P, Breslow N, et al: Clinical observations in children with clear-cell sarcoma of the kidney [abstr]. Proc Am Assoc Cancer Res 27:200, 1986.
103. Feusner JH, Beckwith JB, D'Angio GJ: Clear cell sarcoma of the kidney: Accuracy of imaging methods for detecting bone metastases. Report from the National Wilms' Tumor Study. Med Pediatr Oncol 18:225–227, 1990.
104. Green DM, Breslow NE, Beckwith JB, et al: Treatment of children with clear-cell sarcoma of the kidney: A report from the National Wilms' Tumor Study Group. J Clin Oncol 12:2132–2137, 1994.
105. Kusumakumary P, Chellam VG, Rojymon J, et al: Late recurrence of clear cell sarcoma of the kidney. Med Pediatr Oncol 28:355–357, 1997.
106. Haas JE, Palmer NF, Weinberg AG, et al: Ultrastructure of malignant rhabdoid tumor of the kidney: A distinctive renal tumor of children. Hum Pathol 12:646–657, 1981.
107. Weeks DA, Beckwith JB, Mierau GW, et al: Rhabdoid tumor of kidney: A report of 111 cases from the National Wilms' Tumor Study Pathology Center. Am J Surg Pathol 13:439–458, 1989.
108. Sisler CL, Siegel MJ: Malignant rhabdoid tumor of the kidney: Radiologic features. Radiology 172:211–212, 1989.
109. Agrons GA, Kingsman KD, Wagner BJ, et al: Rhabdoid tu-

mor of the kidney in children: A comparative study of 21 cases. AJR Am J Roentgenol 168:447–451, 1997.

110. Vujanic GM, Sandstedt B, Harms D, et al: Rhabdoid tumor of the kidney: A clinicopathological study of 22 patients from the International Society of Paediatric Oncology (SIOP) nephroblastoma file. Histopathology 28:333–340, 1996.

111. Bonnin JM, Rubinstein LJ, Palmer NG, et al: The association of embryonal tumors originating in the kidney and in the brain. Cancer 54:2137–2146, 1984.

112. Lack EE, Cassady JR, Sallan SE: Renal cell carcinoma in childhood and adolescence: A clinical and pathological study of 17 cases. J Urol 133:822–828, 1985.

113. Broeckner B: Renal cell carcinoma in children. Urology 38:54–56, 1991.

114. Bruce J, Gough DCS: Long-term follow-up of children with renal carcinoma. Br J Urol 65:446–448, 1990.

115. Aronson DC, Medary I, Finlay JL, et al: Renal cell carcinoma in childhood and adolescence: A retrospective survey for prognostic factors in 22 cases. J Pediatr Surg 31:183–186, 1996.

116. Raney RB, Palmer N, Sutow WW, et al: Renal cell carcinoma in children. Med Pediatr Oncol 11:91–98, 1983.

117. Robson CJ: Staging of renal cell carcinoma. In Renal Tumors: Proceedings of the First International Symposium on Kidney Tumors. New York, Alan R Liss, 1982.

118. Bukowski RM: Natural history and therapy of metastatic renal cell carcinoma. The role of interleukin-2. Cancer 80:1198–1220, 1997.

119. Bolande RP, Brough AJ, Izant RJ Jr: Congenital mesoblastic nephroma of infancy. A report of eight cases and the relationship to Wilms' tumor. Pediatrics 40:272–278, 1967.

120. Bolande RP: Congenital mesoblastic nephroma of infancy. In Rosenberg HS, Bolande RP (eds): Perspectives in Pediatric Pathology. Chicago, Year Book Medical, 1973, pp 227–250.

121. Haddad B, Haziza J, Touboul C, et al: The congenital mesoblastic nephroma: A case report of prenatal diagnosis. Fetal Diagn Ther 11:61–66, 1996.

122. Liu Y, Mai Y, Chang CC, et al: The presence of hydrops fetalis in a fetus with congenital mesoblastic nephroma. Prenat Diagn 16:363–365, 1996.

123. Howell CG, Othersen HB, Kiviat NE, et al: Therapy and outcome in 51 children with mesoblastic nephroma: A report of the National Wilms' Tumor Study. J Pediatr Surg 17:826–831, 1982.

124. Fu YS, Kay S: Congenital mesoblastic nephroma and its recurrence: An ultrastructural observation. Arch Pathol 96:66–70, 1973.

125. Joshi VV, Kay S, Milsten R, et al: Congenital mesoblastic nephroma of infancy: Report of a case with unusual clinical behavior. Am J Clin Pathol 60:811–816, 1973.

126. Walker D, Richard GA: Fetal hamartoma of the kidney: Recurrence and death of patients. J Urol 119:352–353, 1973.

127. Heidelberger KP, Ritchey ML, Dauser RC, et al: Congenital mesoblastic nephroma metastatic to the brain. Cancer 72:2499–2502, 1993.

128. Ali AA, Finlay JL, Gerald WL, et al: Congenital mesoblastic nephroma with metastasis to the brain: A case report. Am J Pediatr Hematol Oncol 16:361–364, 1994.

129. Beckwith JB: Mesenchymal renal neoplasms of infancy revisited. J Pediatr Surg 9:803–805, 1974.

130. Joshi VV, Kasznica J, Walters TR: Atypical mesoblastic nephroma. Pathologic characterization of a potentially aggressive variant of conventional congenital mesoblastic nephroma. Arch Pathol Lab Med 110:100–106, 1986.

131. Beckwith JB, Weeks DA: Congenital mesoblastic nephroma. When should we worry? Arch Pathol Lab Med 110:98–99, 1986.

132. Gormley TS, Skoog SJ, Jones RV, et al: Cellular congenital mesoblastic nephroma: What are the options? J Urol 142:479–483, 1989.

65

NEUROBLASTOMA

Edward M. Kiely, FRCSI, FRCS, FRCPCH •
Gillian Barker, FRCS

Although neuroblastoma has probably affected children since antiquity, recognition of its separate identity is recent. Deaths caused by infectious conditions were common and greatly overshadowed the smaller number of deaths resulting from malignancy. The neural origin of neuroblastoma was first proposed by Virchow in 1864, and succeeding years brought a slow acquisition of understanding of the condition.[1] Marchand is credited with recognizing the similarity of neuroblastoma cells to the cells of the sympathetic nervous system in 1891.[2] Several reports dealt with stage 4S disease and, by the early years of the 20th century, pathologic features of the condition had been defined.[3-6] The name *neuroblastoma* was devised by James Homer Wright in 1910 and rapidly supplanted previous names.[5] Hutchison, in 1907, wrote a clear description of metastatic neuroblastoma although he considered it a sarcoma.[7]

The first recorded successful resection was undertaken by Willard Bartlett of St. Louis, Missouri, in 1914; he removed a 470-g tumor from an 11-month-old boy.[8] This patient was alive and well 15 years later.[9] An intimation of the enigmatic behavior of this tumor was provided by Cushing and Wolbach in 1927.[10] They described maturation of a neuroblastoma into a ganglioneuroma over a 10-year period.

By 1934, Blacklock in Glasgow wrote that neuroblastoma was the fourth most common type of malignancy in children.[11] In 1938, Redman noted 275 reported cases in the literature.[12] Radiotherapy was first used in three patients in 1928, none of whom survived.[13] A report from Boston in 1940 suggested that radiotherapy improved survival.[14]

In 1953, Phillips evaluated the results of a substantial series from the Memorial Hospital in New York and described the use of nitrogen mustard derivatives.[15] Survival rates of those with advanced disease were dismal. In 1955, Koop recommended "a major surgical insult" to the tumor because, in his hands, this resulted in a better outcome.[16] The experience at St. Jude Hospital with combination chemotherapy was published in 1965, but overall results remained poor.[17]

□ Incidence and Natural History

The incidence of neuroblastoma varies somewhat between different racial groups.[18] In predominantly Caucasian populations, the age-standardized rate is 7 to 12 per 1 million and accounts for 6 to 10% of all childhood cancers. Thirty percent of neuroblastomas occur in the 1st year of life, 50% occur between 1 and 4 years of age, and only 5% occur after age 10 years. The reason for the 1.3:1 male predominance is not clear.

In 1963, Beckwith and Perrin described the presence of incidental neuroblastoma nodules in the adrenals of infants younger than 3 months of age who were dying of unrelated conditions.[19] These nodules varied in size from 0.4 to 9.5 mm and were found in 0.3 to 1.0% of their two series of autopsies.[19] Whether these nodules would have regressed or might have developed into future neuroblastoma is not clear. Subsequent data from the Japanese screening program suggest that even larger neuroblastoma masses may regress.[20]

The etiology of neuroblastoma is unknown. Rare familial cases are described, often with multiple primary tumors, but most cases are sporadic.[21] The tumor arises from sympathetic neuroblast cells derived from the neural crest. Neuroblast migration occurs from paravertebral ganglia into the adrenal medulla, mainly during early fetal life.[22] Once a neoplasm develops, local extension occurs with vascular encasement and invasion of adjacent structures. Metastases occur to lymph nodes, bone, bone marrow, liver, and skin. Apart from infants with stage 4S disease, secondary spread is usually associated with large primary tumors and may occur late in the natural history of the disease.

□ Pathology

On macroscopic inspection, neuroblastomas are frequently soft with areas of necrosis and hemorrhage. More mature areas of tumor are firm and grayish white in color.

Histologically, the immature neuroblasts are seen as sheets of dark blue cells with scanty cytoplasm set in a delicate vascular stroma. Rosette formation, consisting of a ring of neuroblasts around a neurofibrillary core, is a characteristic feature but is often absent. With differentiation toward mature ganglion cells, the eosinophilic cytoplasm becomes more abundant and the nuclei show well-defined nucleoli.[23] The combination of immature neuroblasts in a predominantly mature tumor is considered to be a ganglioneuroblastoma.

Attempts have been made to use the histologic appearance of these tumors to predict the clinical outcome. In the era of molecular biology, the use of histologic reading systems may seem an anachronism. However, the appearance under the microscope is presumably a reflection of the biologic properties of the tumor and pathologic grading remains useful.

Of the many systems that have evolved, the Shimada classification is perhaps the most widely applied.[24] This system was devised after evaluation of the microscopic appearances of 295 untreated neuroblastoma specimens stained with hematoxylin and eosin. The microscopic features assessed included the stroma, the degree of differentiation of neuroblastoma cells, and the nuclear morphology (mitosis and karyorrhexis). From the nuclear morphology, a mitosis-karyorrhexis index (MKI) was calculated by counting the number of mitotic or karyorrhectic cells per 5000 cells. A low index was less than 100 cells per 5000, intermediate was 100 to 200, and high was more than 200. Based on these assessments, two prognostic groups were distinguished: good prognosis and poor prognosis.

The good prognosis group met the following criteria:

Age younger than 1½ years with any degree of differentiation and a low MKI

Children with stroma-rich tumors and well-differentiated or intermixed degrees of differentiation

Age 1½ to 5 years with more mature histology and a low MKI

The poor prognosis group met the following criteria:

Children with all other tumors that had undifferentiated histology and a high MKI

Age 1½ to 5 years with undifferentiated histology and a high or an intermediate MKI

Age 5 years and older

Children with tumors with a nodular pattern

In the original publication, 87% of those in the good prognosis group survived; only 7% of children in the poor prognosis group survived.

☐ Sites of Disease

Because neuroblastomas arise from neuroblasts of the sympathetic nervous system, they may be found anywhere that sympathetic cells are found, predominantly in the ganglia of the sympathetic chains from neck to pelvis, in other preaortic and pelvic ganglia, and in the adrenal medulla. The adrenal medulla is the most common site of origin (40 to 60% of the total), followed by other retroperitoneal sites (20%), mediastinum (10%), pelvis (2 to 6%), and neck (about 2%).[25, 26] Most children have metastatic disease at the time of presentation (62 to 70%).[25, 26] Localized disease is present in about 25% and stage 4S disease in 10%.[26] Antenatal diagnosis has been described, but it is too early to know whether this will have an impact on the total number of patients with neuroblastoma or on the subsequent survival rate. Prenatally diagnosed tumors are mainly adrenal (93%) with favorable biologic features, and 67% have localized (stage 1) disease.[27]

☐ Markers of Disease Activity

A series of biochemical and molecular markers of disease activity and behavior is available. Some of these measurements are within the range of all hospital laboratories, and some are available only to more specialized centers.

BIOCHEMICAL MARKERS

Several biochemical markers of disease are found in patients' blood serum. These include neuron specific enolase (NSE), lactate dehydrogenase (LDH), and ferritin.

NSE is a glycolytic enzyme expressed by cells of the central and peripheral nervous system and by neuroblastoma cells. Levels of NSE higher than 15 ng/ml are considered abnormal. High levels of NSE (>100 ng/ml) correlate with advanced stages of disease and reduced survival rates.[28–30]

Serum LDH levels may also be an independent prognostic variable. Patients with measurements of less than 1500 IU/ml have improved survival rates. In general, low levels are associated with a more favorable biologic profile.[31–33]

Ferritin is the major tissue iron-binding protein. The circulating level is related to tissue iron stores. Neuroblastoma cells produce ferritin, which may be detected in serum.[34] Although ferritin may be found in the cells of the primary tumor, high serum levels are unusual in patients with low stage disease.[35] High serum ferritin (>142 ng/ml) is a feature of those with stage 3 and stage 4 disease and is associated with a worse outcome. Furthermore, in patients with advanced disease, low (<75 ng/ml), intermediate (75 to 142 ng/ml), and high (>142 ng/ml) levels are associated with different outcomes.[35] Increasing serum ferritin levels at diagnosis were associated with diminishing progression-free survival (PFS).

MOLECULAR MARKERS

The explosion of knowledge about cellular genetics has been followed by a slower accrual of understanding of the factors involved in tumor genesis and tumor behavior. This increased knowledge has not, so far, led to improved treatment or to significant changes in outcome. A wide variety of molecular abnormalities have been detected in neuroblastoma cells including N-*myc* amplification, chromosome 1p deletion, DNA ploidy and DNA index, CD44 expression, TRKA expression, and multidrug resistance–associated protein (MRP).

The normal locus for the N-*myc* proto-oncogene is on the short arm of chromosome 2. Amplification of this sequence in neuroblastoma was first described in 1983.[36] N-*myc* amplification has been shown repeatedly to correlate with advanced stage and with disease progression.[32, 37–40] Overall, about 25% of patients with neuroblastoma show N-*myc* amplification.[39] Those with stages 1, 2, and 4S disease do not usually show amplification; about 50% of those with stage 3 and 4 disease do. About 10% of infants with neuroblastomas show N-*myc* amplification.[41] In general, N-*myc* amplification correlates with disease progression independent of age and stage.[32, 39, 42]

The significance of amplified N-*myc* in those with low-stage disease is somewhat uncertain. The numbers involved are usually small. Review of a Pediatric Oncology Group (POG) study suggested that fewer than 5% of those with localized disease showed amplification.[43] N-*myc* amplification is also associated with unfavorable histologic features.[39] This combination was associated with a 13% PFS in a Children's Cancer Study Group (CCSG) report. Diploid DNA content is more frequently found in tumors with N-*myc* amplification and is associated with a poor outcome.[32, 38, 42] There is a correlation between N-*myc* amplification and chromosome 1p deletion. Both are associated with an aggressive clinical course.[44, 45]

Unlike the situation in other tumors, the presence of hyperdiploid DNA content is associated with a lower stage and an improved prognosis.[46] Hyperdiploid tumors are more commonly found in infants than in older children and constitute the majority of low-stage tumors in all age groups.[42, 46] Tumors with diploid or near-diploid DNA content are found in about two thirds of children with stage 3 and 4 disease. When associated with N-*myc* amplification, the prognosis is even worse.[38] Chemosensitivity may also be related to ploidy, with diploid tumors responding poorly.[42] Finally, thoracic tumors, which carry a better prognosis, are more likely than nonthoracic tumors to be hyperdiploid.[31]

A number of chromosomal deletions and translocations have been described in neuroblastomas. Deletion of the short arm of chromosome 1 appears to be the most useful prognostically. It seems likely that a tumor suppressor gene or genes reside in the deleted region. Deletion of this gene then allows tumor development and progression. 1p loss of heterozygosity (LOH) is strongly associated with N-*myc* amplification.[44, 47] 1p LOH is found in 19 to 33% of all neuroblastomas and correlates with elevated ferritin and LDH levels.[45, 48] Patients who might oth-

erwise be thought to be at low risk owing to low tumor stage and who do not have N-*myc* amplification may be identified by deleted 1p chromosome to be at high risk.[48]

CD44 is a cell surface glycoprotein involved in cell-to-cell and cell-to-matrix interactions. Unusually, CD44 expression is correlated with improved survival in neuroblastoma and with absence of N-*myc* amplification.[41, 49, 50] CD44 was expressed in 84% of patients in a prospective study.[41] All those with stages 1, 2, and 4S expressed CD44. In those with stage 4 disease, seven of eight infants showed expression of CD44 and 15 of 32 older patients did also. In this study, there was a strong inverse relationship between CD44 expression and N-*myc* copy numbers. Normal N-*myc* and CD44 expression were the strongest predictors of survival.

The proto-oncogene TRKA encodes a tyrosine kinase nerve growth factor receptor. TRKA expression was found in 91% of 77 neuroblastomas, with a high level of expression being found in 82%.[51] There was a strong correlation between low stage, age younger than 1 year, and normal N-*myc* copy number and TRKA expression.[51, 52] High levels of expression predicted a favorable outcome. Low levels of TRKA expression were associated with advanced stage, older age, and N-*myc* amplification. TRKA expression has prognostic value even in those tumors with normal N-*myc* copy number.

Treatment failure in patients with advanced disease is manifest by resistance of the tumor to a wide variety of chemotherapeutic agents. Recently, a gene on chromosome 16 has been found to mediate resistance to vinca alkaloids, anthracyclines, and epipodophyllotoxins. This gene encodes a membrane-bound glycoprotein termed the *multidrug-resistance-associated protein (MRP)*. MRP is probably expressed in all neuroblastomas, with higher levels recorded in those with advanced clinical stages. High levels correlated with N-*myc* amplification and with lower survival. The effect of high levels of MRP expression is independent of N-*myc* expression and TRKA expression.[52]

☐ Screening

More than 85% of neuroblastomas excrete elevated levels of catecholamine metabolites.[53, 54] These are readily detectable by standard laboratory techniques. The most common metabolites measured are vanillylmandelic acid (VMA) and homovanillic acid (HVA). VMA is the main breakdown product of adrenaline and noradrenalin. HVA is the main breakdown product of dopa and dopamine.[53]

The ability to detect elevated levels has led to several attempts at screening in the infant population to detect neuroblastomas before the development of metastases. Initially, there was considerable enthusiasm for neuroblastoma screening.[55, 56] Subsequently, however, it has become apparent that screening had detected an increased number of tu-

TABLE 65-1. International Neuroblastoma Staging System Criteria

Stage	Definition
1	Localized tumor with complete gross excision, with or without microscopic residual disease; representative ipsilateral lymph nodes negative for tumor microscopically (nodes attached to and removed with the primary tumor may be positive).
2A	Localized tumor with incomplete gross excision; representative ipsilateral nonadherent lymph nodes negative for tumor microscopically.
2B	Localized tumor with or without complete gross excision, with ipsilateral nonadherent lymph nodes positive for tumor. Enlarged contralateral lymph nodes must be negative microscopically.
3	Unresectable unilateral tumor infiltrating across the midline,* with or without regional lymph node involvement *or* Localized unilateral tumor with contralateral regional lymph node involvement *or* Midline tumor with bilateral extension by infiltration (unresectable) or by lymph node involvement.
4	Any primary tumor with dissemination to distant lymph nodes, bone, bone marrow, liver, skin, or other organs (except as defined for stage 4S).
4S	Localized primary tumor (as defined for stage 1, 2A, or 2B), with dissemination limited to skin, liver, and bone marrow† (limited to infants <1 year of age).

*The midline is defined as the vertebral column. Tumors originating on one side and crossing the midline must infiltrate to or beyond the opposite side of the vertebral column.

†Marrow involvement in stage 4S should be minimal (i.e., <10% of total nucleated cells identified as malignant on bone marrow biopsy or on marrow aspirate). More extensive marrow involvement would be considered to be stage 4. The metaiodobenzylguanidine scan (if performed) should be negative in the marrow.

mors that have an inherently good prognosis without detecting the poor prognosis tumors that become manifest later in older children.[57] The Quebec screening program screened infants at 3 weeks and 6 months of age over a 5-year period. Roughly twice as many neuroblastomas were found as would have been expected, but there was no decrease in cases presenting later with advanced disease. In general, neuroblastoma detected by screening is characterized by low stage and favorable biologic features.[58] Therefore, evidence suggests that there is a group of infants with neuroblastoma who have a good prognosis and whose disease is detectable by screening. Most of these tumors regress.[20] Furthermore, disease in patients older than 1 year of age, who have a much less favorable prognosis by other measures, is not detectable by screening in infancy.

☐ Staging

Staging systems are used to document disease extent at diagnosis and to stratify and modify treatment in response to outcome. A plethora of staging systems have been used in children with neuro-

blastoma, a reflection on the difficulties encountered in trying to achieve a cure in these patients. This has made comparisons among different therapies difficult to evaluate. In 1986, an international conference representing most of the larger oncology groups recommended criteria for diagnosis, staging, and response in patients with neuroblastoma.[59] These criteria have subsequently been revised and appear to have considerable support across national boundaries.[60] The International Neuroblastoma Staging System (INSS) is shown in Table 65-1. This is based on clinical and surgical criteria and carries features of the older Evans and POG systems.[23, 61] The POG system is shown in Table 65-2. Doubtless, the revised INSS will be superseded in turn by a system incorporating biologic features.

About 25% of patients have localized stage 1 and 2 disease. Stage 4S disease is present in 10%. Those with locally advanced and metastatic disease constitute the remainder, 62 to 70%.[26, 31]

☐ Presentation

Neuroblastoma commonly presents insidiously with vague symptoms. Presenting symptoms may be due to the mass or to the presence of metastases. Malaise, weight loss, fever, and sweating are common symptoms. Bone and joint pain, the result of metastatic disease, may initially be diagnosed as juvenile arthritis. Periorbital ecchymosis or proptosis, the result of skull secondaries, may initially be attributed to nonaccidental injury but should draw attention to the possibility of a neuroblastoma.

Tumors in the neck are usually found due to a visible mass. Those in the chest may be unexpected findings on a chest radiograph obtained for persisting or recurrent mild respiratory symptoms. Oc-

TABLE 65-2. Pediatric Oncology Group Staging Criteria

Stage	Definition
A	Complete gross resection of primary tumor, with or without microscopic residual. Intracavitary lymph nodes, not adhered to and removed with primary (nodes adhered to or without tumor resection may be positive for tumor without upstaging patient to stage C), histologically free of tumor. If primary is in abdomen or pelvis, liver is histologically free of tumor.
B	Grossly unresected primary tumor. Nodes and liver same as stage A.
C	Complete or incomplete resection of primary tumor. Intracavitary nodes not adhered to primary histologically positive for tumor. Liver as in stage A.
D	Any dissemination of disease beyond intracavitary nodes (i.e., extracavitary nodes, liver, skin, bone marrow, bone).
D(S)	Evans IVS. Evans stage I or II except for metastatic tumor in liver, bone marrow, or skin.

TABLE 65–3. International Neuroblastoma Staging System Criteria for Diagnosis of Neuroblastoma

---

Unequivocal pathologic diagnosis* is made from tumor tissue by light microscopy (with or without immunohistology, electron microscopy, and increased urine or serum catecholamines or metabolites†)

or

Bone marrow aspirate or trephine biopsy contains unequivocal tumor cells* (e.g., syncytial or immunocytologically positive clumps of cells) and increased urine or serum catecholamines or metabolites†

---

*If histology is equivocal, karyotypic abnormalities in tumor cells characteristic of other tumors, such as t(11-22), then exclude a diagnosis of neuroblastoma, whereas genetic features characteristic of neuroblastoma (1p deletion, N-*myc* amplification) would support this diagnosis.
†Catecholamines and metabolites include dopamine, homovanillic acid, and vanillylmandelic acid; levels must be >3.0 SD above the mean per milligram creatinine for age to be considered increased, and at least two of these must be measured.

casionally, Horner's syndrome is noted with apical thoracic tumors.

Pelvic tumors may interfere with bowel and bladder function and come to light during investigations for sphincter disturbances.

The majority of abdominal tumors are found due to symptomatic metastatic disease. Finally, a number of neuroblastomas present with locomotor disturbance and progressive paraplegia, the result of extradural cord compression.

On examination, abdominal neuroblastomas are usually hard, irregular, and fixed. Less commonly, tumors in infancy are smooth and ballotable. Pelvic tumors may be palpable on abdominal examination or rectal examination. An enlarged bladder from urine retention or palpable feces from constipation are features of pelvic lesions.

Infants with stage 4S disease may show multiple skin nodules. Frequently, however, these children have increasing abdominal distention from enlarging hepatomegaly. This may progress to the point at which breathing is impaired and ventilator support is required.

Hypertension is not unusual and may be due to catecholamine secretion or renal artery compression. Hypertension was documented in 19% of 59 children with newly diagnosed neurogenic tumors. The blood pressure did not correlate with urinary catecholamine secretion. The hypertension resolved following tumor resection or chemotherapy.[62]

□ Paraneoplastic Syndromes

Rare forms of presentation include the dancing eye (opsomyoclonus) syndrome and intractable diarrhea. Opsomyoclonus syndrome is characterized by progressive cerebellar ataxia with frequent jerking movements of the muscles of the limbs and trunk. In addition, opsoclonus is manifest by rapid, chaotic, conjugate eye movements. More than half of these patients have a thoracic primary tumor.[63] Developmental delay is common in these children, although the prognosis in terms of survival is favorable.

Intractable diarrhea as a presenting symptom is uncommon and is due to vasoactive intestinal polypeptide (VIP) secretion by the tumor. It is more common in those with ganglioneuromas and ganglioneuroblastomas than in those with neuroblastomas.[64] Diarrhea commencing after initiation of treatment of a stage 4 neuroblastoma has been recorded.[65]

□ Diagnosis

The diagnosis is suspected on clinical grounds from the history and physical findings. Confirmation of the diagnosis is by a combination of laboratory and radiologic investigation and by tissue examination. Staging investigations are then completed. Table 65–3 shows the INSS criteria for the diagnosis of neuroblastoma. Using these criteria, a positive tissue diagnosis is considered essential. Table 65–4 shows the INSS recommendations for assessing extent of disease.

TABLE 65–4. International Neuroblastoma Staging System Staging Investigations

Tumor Site	Recommended Tests
Primary tumor	CT or MRI scan with three-dimensional measurements; MIBG scan, if available.
Metastatic Sites	*Recommended Tests*
Bone marrow	Bilateral posterior iliac crest marrow aspirates and trephine (core) bone marrow biopsies required to exclude marrow involvement. A single positive site documents marrow involvement. Core biopsies must contain at least 1 cm of marrow (excluding cartilage) to be considered adequate.
Bone	MIBG scan; ^{99m}Tc scan required if MIBG scan is negative or unavailable, and plain radiographs of positive lesions are recommended.
Lymph nodes	Clinical examination (palpable nodes), confirmed histologically. CT scan for nonpalpable nodes (three-dimensional measurements).
Abdomen and Liver	CT or MRI scan with three-dimensional measurements.
Chest	Anteroposterior and lateral chest radiographs. CT and MRI necessary if chest radiograph is positive or if abdominal mass/nodes extend into chest.

CT, computed tomography; MIBG, metaiodobenzylguanidine; MRI, magnetic resonance imaging.

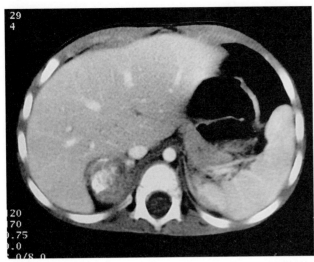

Figure 65–1. Computed tomography scan of stage 1, right adrenal neuroblastoma.

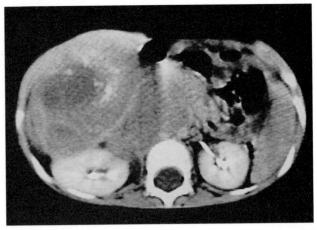

Figure 65–3. Computed tomography scan of stage 3, right-sided neuroblastoma. At operation, this tumor had invaded beyond the left side of the spine.

☐ Laboratory Investigations

Estimation of urinary catecholamine metabolites is the initial diagnostic screen. Urinary VMA and HVA are elevated in the majority of children with neuroblastoma.

The evaluation must include full blood count, serum biochemistry, and liver and renal function tests. Serum ferritin, LDH, and NSE should also be measured.

☐ Imaging

The sequence of imaging investigations performed depends on the clinical presentation and local facilities. Most children obtain plain radiographs and ultrasonography (US). Dystrophic calcification is seen on more than 50% of plain radiographs.[26] In addition to radiologic examination of the anatomic site in question, children must have a chest radiograph. Lateral views are often helpful in the presence of mediastinal tumors.

US is helpful as a screening test to establish whether a mass is solid or cystic. Neuroblastoma does not have a diagnostic US appearance. It generally shows a mixed echo pattern with areas of calcification and necrosis. Frequently, however, an experienced ultrasonographer recognizes the heterogeneous echo pattern and this, combined with the anatomic location and pattern of growth, allows a fairly confident diagnosis. US is of limited use in the chest and in the pelvis.

For accurate anatomic detail, contrast-enhanced computed tomography or magnetic resonance imaging (MRI) is necessary. The two are complementary rather than interchangeable. For most purposes, computed tomography with contrast provides the

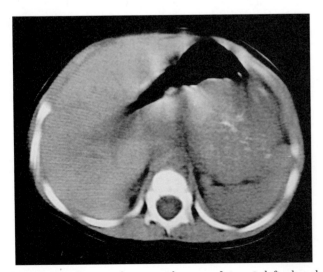

Figure 65–2. Computed tomography scan of stage 2, left adrenal neuroblastoma.

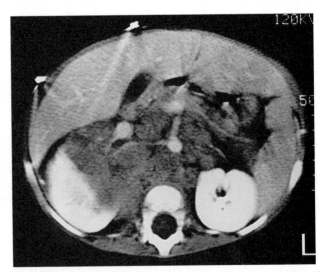

Figure 65–4. Computed tomography scan of stage 4, right adrenal neuroblastoma, displacing and encasing the great vessels at the level of the superior mesenteric artery.

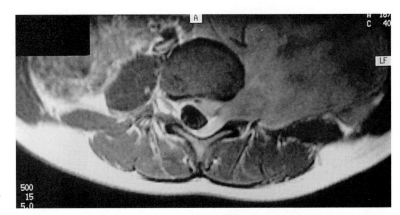

Figure 65–5. Magnetic resonance imaging scan showing left-sided dumbbell tumor.

necessary detail regarding site, consistency, and relation to vital structures; MRI gives detailed information regarding soft tissue changes, liver involvement, and, most valuably, the anatomy of intraspinal extension. Because multiplanar images are possible, full information is available on tumor extent. It is the investigation of choice in dumbbell tumors and gives superior images to myelography. Bone involvement is also readily seen on MRI scanning. Representative scans are shown in Figures 65–1 to 65–6.

Skeletal metastases may be seen on plain radiography with periosteal erosion, radiolucencies, and pathologic fractures. Routine identification of metastatic skeletal disease is best performed by isotope scanning. Radiolabeled metaiodobenzylguanidine (MIBG) is regarded as a sensitive method of detecting bone and bone marrow disease.[66] MIBG is labeled with ^{123}I or [131]I. Figure 65–7 shows extensive neuroblastoma demonstrated on an MIBG scan. MIBG scans have a false-negative rate and are best complemented by ^{99m}Tc methylene diphosphonate (MDP) bone scanning.[67] The present INSS criteria suggest using MIBG scanning when available and ^{99m}Tc scanning only if the MIBG is negative. Widespread skeletal involvement, demonstrated on a technetium scan, is shown in Figure 65–8.

☐ Tissue Biopsy

Tissue diagnosis is regarded as essential. The tissue may be obtained by aspiration or trephine of bone marrow or by biopsy of primary or accessible secondary disease. Sufficient tissue should be obtained both for diagnosis and for the completion of cytogenetic studies.

☐ Treatment

The management of a patient with neuroblastoma involves a multidisciplinary team. The composition

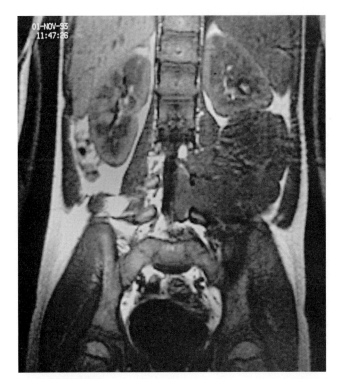

Figure 65–6. Magnetic resonance imaging scan of left-sided dumbbell tumor (coronal view).

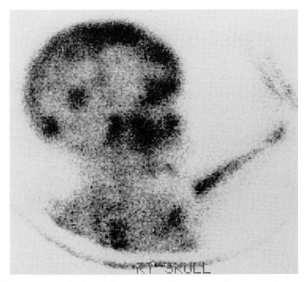

Figure 65–7. Metaiodobenzylguanidine scan showing extensive metastatic neuroblastoma.

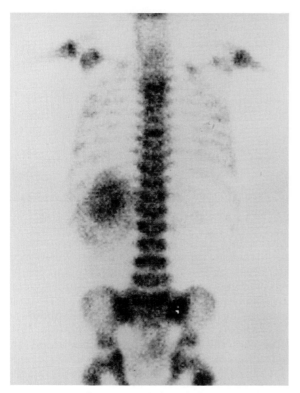

Figure 65–8. ^{99m}Technetium methylene diphosphonate bone scan showing widespread vertebrae and skeletal metastatic disease.

of the team varies among institutions. Treatment modalities include chemotherapy, surgery, and radiotherapy. These are provided, in turn, by pediatric oncologists, pediatric surgeons, and pediatric radiotherapists. Indispensable contributions are made by pediatric radiologists and pathologists.

The surgeon's role is to excise tumors where possible, to perform biopsies when necessary, and to provide vascular access.

The management of those with stage 1 disease is by operation. These relatively uncommon tumors are usually amenable to complete resection. Ideally, those with stage 2 disease should also undergo complete excision. This may not be feasible or even advisable when injudicious attempts to clear all tumor may be hazardous. Examples include tumors extending into intervertebral foramina and apical thoracic tumors close to the stellate ganglion. There are also instances in which a course of chemotherapy might be advisable to facilitate surgery.

The management of dumbbell tumors with spinal cord compression is controversial. Opinion fluctuates between the use of chemotherapy and urgent laminectomy. A recent report from France supports the use of primary chemotherapy, with surgery being reserved for those who have rapidly deteriorating neurologic status.[68] This article confirms the high incidence of thoracic tumors in this group of patients and the excellent outcome. Either way, surgery is often advised for residual extradural tumor followed concurrently or later by excision of the extraspinal component.

The trend in managing those with stage 3 and 4 disease is toward delayed surgery after chemotherapy. Posttreatment tumors are less vascular and are more amenable to complete resection.[69, 70]

For those with stage 4S disease, management is tailored to the patient. Neonates with hepatomegaly are at greater risk and may require intensive treatment.[26, 71] The use of ventral hernias to enlarge the abdomen has been associated with a high mortality rate.[72] Older infants with stage 4S disease frequently show maturation and regression of disease in the absence of any treatment.[73] Resection of the primary tumor confers no benefit in terms of survival rate.[74] Some centers remove the primary tumor if it persists and other evidence of disease has regressed.

CHEMOTHERAPY

Chemotherapy protocols undergo constant modification and refinement. The aim is to limit therapy to those with a good prognosis and to intensify treatment for those with a poor prognosis. At the present time, combination chemotherapy is the mainstay of treatment for those with advanced disease.

A considerable number of chemotherapy protocols are in use worldwide. For those with advanced disease, chemotherapy is often followed by delayed surgical excision. In many protocols, myeloablative therapy using total body irradiation (TBI) or melphalan is used, followed by bone marrow transplantation (BMT).[75, 76] Agents used in combination include cyclophosphamide, ifosfamide, vincristine, cisplatin, carboplatin, doxorubicin, etoposide, and melphalan. BMT is mostly performed with autologous purged bone marrow.

Such toxic treatment carries its own risks. Death resulting from treatment has been reported in up to 20% of cases. Lesser complications from the treatment include sepsis, hemorrhage, and veno-occlusive disease.[75]

The INSS response criteria are listed in Table 65–5. The response to chemotherapy is usually assessed after 3 to 4 months of induction chemotherapy.

SURGICAL THERAPY

The aim of surgery is to remove all tumor. In lower stages, resection is usually possible. In advanced cases, resection may present some difficulty.

Standard techniques suffice for the rare cervical tumors. Thoracic tumors similarly do not usually present serious surgical obstacles. The majority arise from the sympathetic chain and lie in the costovertebral angle. Encasement of major vessels is not common. Tumors arising in the upper thoracic ganglia may encroach on the stellate ganglion. Excision may then result in a Horner's syndrome. Although standard thoracotomy incisions are satisfactory for most thoracic tumors, apical tumors and those extending into the neck may present problems with

TABLE 65-5. International Neuroblastoma Staging System Response Criteria

Response	Primary Tumor	Metastatic Sites*
CR	No tumor	No tumor; catecholamines normal
VGPR	Decreased by 90–99%	No tumor; catecholamines normal; residual ^{99m}Tc bone changes allowed
PR	Decreased by >50%	All measurable sites decreased by >50%
		Bones and bone marrow: number of positive bone sites decreased by >50%. No more than 1 positive bone marrow site allowed
MR	No new lesions; >50% reduction of any measurable lesion (primary or metastases) with <50% reduction in any other; <25% increase in any existing lesion	
NR	No new lesions; <50% reduction but <25% increase in any existing lesion	
PD	Any new lesion; increase of any measurable lesion by >25%; previous negative marrow positive for tumor	

*One positive marrow aspirate or biopsy allowed for PR if this represents a decrease from the number of positive sites at diagnosis.
CR, complete response; MR, minimal response; NR, no response; PD, progressive disease; PR, partial response; VGPR, very good partial response.

access. The trap door incision extends along the upper border of the clavicle, vertically through the manubrium as far as the third interspace, and then laterally through the third intercostal space. Once the sternomastoid muscle is transected, the whole flap can be reflected laterally.[77, 78]

Dumbbell thoracic tumors connected to an intraspinal component may be difficult to remove completely. There is no consensus as to whether intraspinal disease should be removed before or after the thoracic component or even during the same surgery. The authors' practice is to request initial removal of the intraspinal tumor. Postoperative swelling of a spinal extension after thoracic operation might otherwise jeopardize the cord.

Excision of abdominal tumors presents some difficulties. With stage 3 and 4 tumors, it is usual to encounter encasement of both the great vessels and main visceral vessels. Whatever technique is used, the aim is to preserve the vessels while clearing the tumor. Again, with locally advanced tumors, excision is impossible without incising the tumor.

Detailed accounts of the surgical technique used to excise advanced neuroblastoma are uncommon.[79, 80] Because the main problems are encountered with major blood vessels, the logical approach is to display all the vascular anatomy before tumor excision. Neuroblastoma does not usually invade the tunica media of major blood vessels, whether they are arteries or veins. Consequently, a subadventitial plane exists around all the major vascular structures. This plane may be entered and maintained with a knife. Knife dissection is not commonly used in pediatric surgery, but for this operation it is nearly essential. Optical magnification, bipolar diathermy, and a table-mounted retractor complete the list of essentials.

The majority of abdominal tumors arise in the upper abdomen. Surgical approaches vary between thoracoabdominal and upper transverse abdominal incisions. The colon is reflected medially on its mesentery to expose the retroperitoneum. On the left side, the spleen, pancreas, and stomach are also

mobilized and all viscera placed in an intestinal bag to reduce desiccation and serosal trauma.

Once the colon is reflected, the full extent of the tumor is apparent. There are three phases to the operation: vessel display, vessel clearance, and tumor removal. The first is the most difficult and the most important.

Dissection may commence proximally or distally. In either case, control of the thoracic aorta gives added security. The diaphragm may be incised above the proximal limit of the tumor to enter the chest and display the lower thoracic aorta. Once this vessel has been identified and a sling placed, the decision is made whether to proceed from above or from below. In general, it is easier to commence distally and proceed proximally.

The first phase of the procedure begins below where the vessels emerge from the tumor. On the left side, this normally means the external iliac or common iliac artery. On the right side, the corresponding vein is usually first encountered.

The tunica adventitia is picked up by the surgeon and by the assistant and incised along the middle of the vessel. The subadventitial layer is then entered. By applying traction and countertraction, the surgeon and assistant ensure that the correct plane opens once the overlying tissue and tumor are incised. Once the subadventitial plane is displayed, the dissection moves proximally to encounter and incise the tumor down into the same plane. The lengths of the incision usually vary from 2 to 5 cm at a time. Hemostasis is secured with bipolar diathermy. As long as the vessel is kept in sight and the incision is in the 12-o'clock position relative to the vessel, then this maneuver is safe.

At the level of the bifurcation, the direction of the incision changes and continues along the middle of the great vessel proximally. On the left side, the inferior mesenteric artery is the first of the visceral vessels to be encountered. Its presence is noted by the position of the vessel in the mesentery before it is found on the aorta. Cautious dissection along the aorta usually brings the root of the vessel into view before any damage is done.

The next vessel to be found is the left renal vein crossing the aorta above the gonadal arteries. The tumor is often adherent to the aorta at this level, but persistence is usually rewarded. The vein is commonly surrounded by tumor and lies a variable distance from the aorta. Surprisingly, careful incision of the tumor down toward the aorta often reveals the bluish color of the vein before it is in any danger. Once part of the vein wall has been exposed, a 5-cm to 7-cm length should be mobilized circumferentially to facilitate dissection of the underlying aorta. Once again, the axis of dissection is longitudinal along the middle of the vein, establishing the subadventitial plane and then maintaining this plane around the circumference of the vein.

The left gonadal vein is usually encountered as it enters the renal vein and may be divided if necessary. The left adrenal vein is often seen at this stage as well and is best left intact during this portion of the procedure. The inferior vena cava is usually well to the right. Infrequently, a large posterior tributary from the hemiazygous system enters the renal vein just to the left of the aorta. Division of this tributary is often necessary. On occasion, division of the left renal vein may be necessary and is usually well tolerated as long as the hilum of the kidney is not dissected and the kidney is not mobilized from its bed.

Once the vein can be moved, the left renal artery must be found. The anterior aortic wall is exposed posterior to the vein and cautious dissection on the left side of the aorta brings the origin of the left renal artery into view. Dense adherence of tumor to aorta is unusual at this level or indeed from here proximally to the diaphragm.

The superior mesenteric artery (SMA) lies just proximal to the level of the renal artery; therefore, the direction of the blade changes from the 12-o'clock position to the 1-o'clock to 2-o'clock position on the aortic wall. The knife should still come down in perpendicular fashion onto the aorta. The pace of the operation often slows at this time, although this phase of the operation is generally straightforward. Incision of the tumor continues as before until the proximal edge of the tumor has been incised. The median arcuate ligament and part of the diaphragm are usually incised as well.

The roots of the celiac and SMA are then exposed by clearing the anterior wall of the aorta. Each is then dissected in turn by incision in the longitudinal axis of the vessel in the subadventitial plane. The SMA is dealt with first because it appears more robust and has a straight, predictable, course. The celiac looks more fragile. The trunk of the celiac is longer than expected. The phrenic arteries may come off the aorta separate from the celiac but more commonly arise from the celiac trunk. More distally on the celiac is found the trifurcation into left gastric, splenic, and hepatic arteries. As before, all of these vessels are exposed by incision in their long

axes as far as is necessary. Dense adherence of tumor to celiac and SMA is exceptional.

The only remaining visceral artery of note is the right renal artery, which lies deep to the SMA. Exposure of this vessel usually awaits tumor clearance. It must, however, be in view before a decision on left nephrectomy is made.

Vessel exposure is then complete and vessel clearance begins. The SMA and celiac arteries are cleared circumferentially, and once these arteries are mobile, the surrounding tumor is removed piecemeal. The area between celiac artery and diaphragm presents no problems. Tissue to the right of the celiac and along the hepatic artery is less accessible, particularly when the right crus of the diaphragm is involved. For this reason, it may be necessary to incise the lesser omentum and open the lesser sac. If there is considerable bulk of tumor in this area, it can be approached later from the right side.

Tumor between celiac and SMA obscures the splenic vein and its junction with the superior mesenteric vein. The safest course is to expose the splenic vein down to its termination. If there is a substantial mass of tumor around the portal vein, it should be left until a later phase of the operation.

The main bulk of tumor may then be excised. This is done by first completing the clearance of the left renal artery. It is better to expose the origin of the right renal artery before dissecting the left renal artery. The first branch from the left renal artery is the adrenal artery and this is sacrificed. The branch to the apical segment of the kidney often arises quite proximally and division of this vessel may be unavoidable. This results in a small apical infarct. The renal artery is followed as far as is necessary and occasionally into the hilum. Each branch of the artery is followed and cleared in turn.

The proximal aorta is cleared of tumor to the left and posteriorly. The lumbar arteries are preserved where possible. All that remains is to dissect the tumor from the diaphragm, posterior abdominal wall, and upper pole of left kidney.

Subsequently, tumor below the left renal hilum and around the inferior mesenteric artery is resected. Dissection of the ureter is often bloody but tumor is rarely attached to it. Lumbar arteries are preserved if possible. It is not clear how many of these may be sacrificed before spinal cord damage occurs. On occasion, five lumbar arteries have been divided without sequelae. The safest course is to preserve as many as possible.

By clearing and mobilizing the lower abdominal aorta, the surgeon may encounter substantial prevertebral tumor. This is easily overlooked. Incision down onto vertebral bodies reveals the extent of disease in this location.

Right-sided tumors are managed in similar fashion: the colon is reflected, the duodenum mobilized, and the cava dissected in similar fashion. If any tumor remains from a left-sided dissection, the right paraaortic region is also approached in this manner.

Mobilization of the liver from its bed often facilitates dissection of a large right adrenal mass and eases the search for the right adrenal vein.

Access to pelvic tumors may be difficult because the majority occur presacrally or just lateral to this area below the brim of the pelvis. Lower midline, transverse, or Pfannenstiel incisions are frequently used. For improved access, a modified Pfannenstiel incision, extended to the anterior superior spines on either side, is useful. The rectus sheath is developed proximally in the usual manner. The rectus bellies are then detached from the pubis by dividing the tendons on the anterior aspect of the bone. Laterally, the muscles are divided, staying well above the inguinal canals. This incision gives unrivaled access to the pelvis.

It is well to dissect and control part of the internal iliac vessels unless the tumor lies in the hollow of the sacrum. Review of the anatomy of the internal iliac vessels and the sciatic nerve aid in this dissection. Most of these tumors may be dissected without difficulty unless they are very large. As in any cancer operation, the priority is tumor excision but at a reasonable price. The pelvic autonomic nerves are at risk, potentially affecting continence and potency. It is usually feasible to preserve at least one of the hypogastric nerves to preserve ejaculation.[81]

SURGICAL COMPLICATIONS

Complications of surgery do not feature prominently in the literature. One report of five operative mishaps found that four of the surgical injuries occurred in infants.[82] Two of these children later died. The authors noted a paucity of surgical complications reported in the literature, but uncontrollable hemorrhage was the predominant cause of operative or early postoperative deaths.

In our own series of more than 170 neurogenic tumors, there were two perioperative deaths. The first was a 4-year-old in whom severe hypoglycemia developed after a 4:1 blood transfusion during the course of a stage 3 neuroblastoma resection. In the second child, the abdominal aorta and splenic artery ruptured on the 8th postoperative day. In addition to these fatalities, we are aware of one child who lost the left kidney after left renal vein thrombosis as a postoperative event.

A more notable problem has been postoperative diarrhea, which has developed in about one third of the patients undergoing extensive retroperitoneal dissection. Clearance of the SMA and celiac arteries appears to be causative.[83] In most of those who survived, the diarrhea was permanent, despite the use of loperamide.

RADIOTHERAPY

Radiotherapy has been used for many years in children with neuroblastoma. Currently, it is mainly used to treat residual disease, progressive hepatomegaly in patients with stage 4S disease, or TBI

before BMT and, more recently, as targeted radiotherapy.

The use of radiotherapy to residual tumor has been the subject of conflicting reports. In the late 1950s, Gross and colleagues were encouraged by a 2-year survival rate of 64% achieved after radiotherapy to residual tumor.[25] More recently, radiotherapy combined with chemotherapy has been used to enhance resectability.[84] It seems clear that those with stage 1 and 2 disease do not benefit from radiotherapy even if macroscopic disease remains after surgery.[85, 86] The place of radiotherapy in managing stage 3 and 4 patients is unclear.

Infants with rapidly growing hepatomegaly with stage 4S disease are vulnerable. Radiotherapy is frequently used in these circumstances, but the results, especially in neonates, are poor. There is a 46% mortality rate in neonates who have hepatomegaly at birth.[71] Death results from the complications of an enlarged liver, despite radiotherapy. In older infants, response to radiotherapy has been more encouraging, although it is slow and unpredictable.[72, 87]

As part of megatherapy, TBI is used to achieve marrow ablation before BMT.[76] Finally, the benefits of targeted radiotherapy using ^{131}I-MIBG are awaited. Targeted MIBG treatment used as initial therapy in 33 patients with advanced disease found a complete response in one patient and partial response (>50% reduction) in 18 patients.[88] The application of this type of therapy may expand in the future.

☐ Outlook

The outlook for children with neuroblastoma has improved considerably since the 1970s. The failure to influence the course of those with advanced unfavorable disease has engendered pessimism, but, overall, the outlook has improved. Survival figures from the POG investigators record an overall survival rate of 58% in 1335 patients enrolled between 1980 and 1990.[31] Data from the United Kingdom National Registry of Childhood Tumors suggests that the 5-year actuarial survival rate was 15% of those born between 1971 and 1973 and 43% for those born in the years 1983 to 1985. The survival rate was unchanged 3 years later.[89]

MATURATION TO GANGLIONEUROMA

Since the report of spontaneous maturation of a neuroblastoma, the possibility of spontaneous cure has received much attention.[10] The incidence of this occurrence is unknown. In 1968, a report recorded only one spontaneous cure in 133 patients with neuroblastoma.[90] The patient was a neonate with skin and lymph node metastases. Two such patients in a series of 217 neuroblastoma patients were reported in 1959.[25] Both were infants, one aged 6 weeks and one 11 months, with unresectable pelvic and mediastinal neuroblastoma. In both, the tumors were undetectable 25 and 20 years later. More recently, spontaneous regression has been reported in untreated tumors found on screening.[20] Twelve of 25 patients with tumors less than 5 cm in diameter were followed up for periods ranging from 4 to 27 months. Tumor size diminished in 11 of the 12 on repeated US examination. The ultimate fate of these patients is not yet known.

The natural history of neuroblastoma also includes patients with an indolent course. Late progression and death has been described 17 years after diagnosis, with the clinical course being marked by periods of tumor activity and inactivity.[91]

EARLY DETECTION AND SCREENING

Tumor detected antenatally exhibits a favorable biologic profile.[27] N-*myc* amplification has not been described to date and the DNA index is usually greater than 1. In addition, only 5% have metastatic stage 4 disease. Interestingly, 44% were cystic at the time of diagnosis. Unusually, 2 of the 55 reviewed patients had lung metastases. Overall survival rate was 90% in this group of patients.

The outlook for tumors found on screening is favorable, with 92% survival rate being reported in an early study.[55] Spontaneous regression is common in this group.

BIOCHEMICAL MARKERS

The absolute levels of *catecholamine metabolite* excretion do not have prognostic values. However, the VMA-to-HVA ratio is related to survival, with lower survival rate being recorded when the ratio was less than 1.5.[53, 54]

In a CCSG report dealing with patients with locally advanced or metastatic disease, the probability of PFS at 2 years was 76% for those with low levels of serum ferritin and 23% for those with high levels.[35] Children older than 12 months with stage 4 disease and high serum ferritin levels had a 3% 2-year PFS versus 21% for those with low levels.

In this study, the lowest survival rate was associated with the highest levels of serum ferritin. A POG study showed survival rates of 45% and 17% for those with low and high levels of serum ferritin, respectively. In the same POG review, LDH values of greater or less than 1500 IU/ml were associated with survival rates of 24% and 77%, respectively. The prognostic value of high levels of LDH is maintained even in infants.[32]

In patients with stage 3 disease, survival rate was 20% in those with NSE levels of greater than 100 ng/ml, compared with a 57% survival rate in those with lower levels.[29] Corresponding figures for infants with stage 4S disease were 25% survival rate with the higher levels of NSE and 100% survival rate in patients whose NSE levels were less than 100 ng/ml.

MOLECULAR MARKERS

The presence of N-*myc* amplification is associated with a worse outcome. Only 6 of 181 patients with localized tumors had N-*myc* amplification in a recent study.[43] Two of these six patients died: both had unfavorable histology. By contrast, patients with N-*myc* amplification and advanced disease had survival rates varying from less than 10% to about 40% depending on age, ploidy, histology, and other features.[31, 38, 39] One study showed a 16% 3-year survival rate in those with N-*myc* amplified tumors.[41] Another study recorded an overall 24% survival rate for those with N-*myc* amplified tumors compared with a 77% survival rate in those without amplification.[31]

In patients with stage 4S disease, tumor regression may occur in early life despite N-*myc* amplification. N-*myc* amplification was noted in 5 of 10 patients with stage 4S disease.[92] At the time of the report, 3 of the 5 patients were dead and the 4th was alive with disease. Two of the patients who died had shown initial regression with later relapse. In most studies, multivariate analysis confirms the predictive power of N-*myc* amplification independent of age and stage.

Most evidence suggests that chromosome 1p deletion is a reliable predictor of a poor outcome. 1p deletion in those with stages 1, 2, and 4S was associated with a 12% mean 3-year event-free survival rate.[48] For those without 1p deletion, the corresponding figure was 75%. In those with stages 3 and 4 disease and 1p deletion, none survived 3 years without adverse events. The corresponding figure was 53% for those without 1p deletion. Infants with 1p LOH showed a 3-year event-free survival rate of 32%. All the other infants survived in the absence of 1p LOH. A POG study showed that, in all patients, 1p deletion was associated with a 32% 4-year survival rate compared to 76% for those without the abnormality.[45] When 1p deletion is associated with N-*myc* amplification, 4-year survival was 7%.

Diploid DNA content worsens the prognosis overall, 58% versus 28% mortality rate for those with aneuploid DNA content.[31] Analysis showed 94% 2-year disease-free survival rate in those with near triploid neuroblastoma compared to 45% for those with diploid or near diploid DNA content.[38] This figure decreased to 11% in those with N-*myc* amplification in addition. Finally, a recent POG study of neuroblastoma in infancy showed a 94% 3-year survival rate in those with hyperdiploid tumors versus 55% in those with diploid tumors.[32]

CD44 expression is associated with improved survival rate. One study reported 81% 3-year survival rates in CD44-positive tumors against 7% in those with CD-negative tumors.[41] Absence of CD44 expression combined with N-*myc* amplification was a particularly bad combination, 9% 3-year survival rate. In those with stage 4 disease, event-free survival rate was 35% in CD44-positive tumors and 7% in those lacking CD44 expression.

The prognostic benefit of high levels of TRKA expression was demonstrated by an 86% survival rate in patients whose TRKA was high versus 14% in those with low levels in one study and 91% survival rate versus 46% in another.[51, 52] In addition, the association of low TRKA expression and high N-*myc* copy number was uniformly fatal.

Histopathologic classification and MKI demonstrate excellent correlation between the good prognosis group (87% survival rate) and the poor prognosis group (7% survival rate).[24] Unfavorable histology coupled with N-*myc* amplification carries the worst prognosis.[39]

AGE AT PRESENTATION

Children younger than 12 months of age at diagnosis have an 84% survival rate compared to 42% for older children.[31] Infants with advanced disease also have an improved outlook. Biopsies of infants' tumors rarely show N-*myc* amplification and usually demonstrate favorable histology. When survival was correlated with ploidy, infants with hyperdiploid tumors showed a 95% 3-year estimated survival rate compared to 55% in those with diploid tumors.[32] At the other extreme, neuroblastoma in older children, adolescents, and adults is marked by an indolent but inexorably downhill course. Two recent studies record only a 17% event-free survival rate in one and 6% in the other.[93, 94]

SYNDROMES

Patients being seen with paraneoplastic syndromes have a surprisingly low mortality rate. In a literature review of 28 cases, 2-year survival rate of 89% was noted in those with opsomyoclonus, although, in another study, 64% had persisting cerebellar signs and 36% had developmental delay.[63, 95] Those with vasoactive intestinal polypeptide secreting tumors are much less common and the tumors are often more mature. We have dealt with only two such patients, and both tumors were ganglioneuromas. In addition to the risk from the tumor, there is a substantial risk from the secretory diarrhea.[65]

SITE OF ORIGIN

In the late 1950s, there was roughly a 50% cure for cervical, thoracic, and pelvic tumors compared to 25% for those with adrenal primaries.[25] Twenty years later, 100% survival rate was reported for those with cervical and pelvic primaries, 75% for those with thoracic primaries, and 28% for those with abdominal tumors.[26] In the mid-1990s, there was a reported 83% survival rate for those with thoracic primary tumors contrasted with 53% for other locations.[31] Hyperdiploid DNA content is seen in the majority of infants with cervical and thoracic primaries.[32]

SPINAL CANAL EXTENSION

Dumbbell tumors are also associated with high survival rates: 97% in a recent study of 42 patients.[68] In this study, 26 (62%) of the patients had neurologic impairment. Complete neurologic recovery was recorded in two thirds of these patients. By contrast, an earlier study from Great Ormond Street recorded 13 (61%) survivors of 21 patients with spinal cord compression.[96] Ten of the 13 survivors had residual neurologic impairment, however, with neonatal patients having the worst outcome.

STAGING

Using the POG staging system, there is a recorded 89% survival rate in patients with stage A tumors.[61] A CCSG study confirmed the excellent prognosis (90% PFS) in those with stage II disease.[97] This study also showed that survival was not dependent on achieving complete surgical resection. Data from Memorial Sloan-Kettering Hospital confirmed the good prognosis for those with INSS stage 1 disease—10 of 10 patients treated with surgery alone were disease-free at 5-year follow-up.[98] Survival figures by INSS staging showed stage 1, 95%, stage 2A, 88%, and stage 2B, 100%.[86] Only 13 of 93 patients were given any treatment other than surgical.

ADJUVANT THERAPY

For those with locally advanced or metastatic disease, multiagent chemotherapy combined with myeloablative treatment has resulted in improved survival rates. Most of the follow-up periods are short. Recent CCSG data show a 3-year progression-free survival rate of 25% for these groups.[76] The Japanese Study Group showed 70% 3-year survival rates for stage 3 and 45% for stage 4 disease.[99] For the whole group, 5-year survival rate was 44% for those with N-*myc* amplification and 54% for those without. The POG study reports a survival rate of 39% for stage D disease.[31]

COMPLETENESS OF EXCISION

The exact contribution of surgery to these survival figures is uncertain. We and others have been unable to confirm the beneficial effect of complete versus incomplete resection.[79, 100] Other groups have shown improved survival rates in children undergoing complete versus incomplete resection (59% vs. 47%).[101] Data after 20 months of follow-up from the CCSG showed 59% survival rate for children with poor risk neuroblastoma after complete resection versus 26% survival rate after partial resection.[102] Finally, a retrospective review of 28 patients suggested improved survival and progression-free survival for those who had undergone complete surgical resection. Three-year survival rates were 40% as opposed to 15% for those who had an incomplete resection.[103]

STAGE 4S

Earlier reports of 84% survival rates in infants with stage 4S disease are not supported by more recent data in which a survival rate of only 50% was seen.[72, 104] Multiorgan impairment—respiratory compromise, oliguria, thrombocytopenia, leg edema—especially when severe, is associated with a poor outcome. Neonates with multiorgan impairment rarely survive.[71]

REFERENCES

1. Virchow R: Die Krankenhafte Geschwulste. Vol. 2. Berlin, Germany, Hirschwald, 1864, p 149.
2. Marchand F. Beitr z Kenntnis der Glandula Carotica und der Nebennieren. Festschr. f R Virchow Intern Beitr z Wissesch. Med Berlin I:535, 1891.
3. Parker RW: Diffuse (?) sarcoma of liver, probably congenital. Trans Path Soc Lond 31:290–293, 1880.
4. Dalton N: Infiltrating growth in liver and suprarenal capsule. Trans Path Soc Lond 36:247–251, 1885.
5. Wright JH: Neurocytoma or neuroblastoma: A kind of tumor not generally recognised. J Exp Med 12:556–561, 1910.
6. Dunn JS: Neuroblastoma and ganglio-neuroma of the suprarenal body. J Path Bact 19:456–476, 1915.
7. Hutchison R: On suprarenal sarcoma in children with metastases in the skull. Q J Med 1:33–38, 1907.
8. Lehman EP: Neuroblastoma: With report of a case. J Med Res 36:309–326, 1917.
9. Lehman EP: Adrenal neuroblastoma in infancy—15 year survival. Ann Surg 95:473, 1932.
10. Cushing H, Wolbach SB: The transformation of a malignant paravertebral sympathicoblastoma into a benign ganglioneuroma. Am J Pathol 3:203–216, 1927.
11. Blacklock JWS. Neurogenic tumors of the sympathetic system in children. J Path Bact 39:27–48, 1934.
12. Redman JL, Agerty HA, Barthmaier OF, et al: Adrenal neuroblastoma. Report of a case and review of the literature. Am J Dis Child 56:1097–1112, 1938.
13. Holmes GW, Dresser R: Roentgenologic observations in neuroblastoma. JAMA 91:1246–1248, 1928.
14. Farber S: Neuroblastoma. Am J Dis Child 60:749–750, 1940.
15. Phillips R: Neuroblastoma. Ann R Coll Surg Engl 12:29–47, 1953.
16. Koop CE, Kiesewetter WB, Horn RC: Neuroblastoma in childhood. An evaluation of surgical management. Pediatrics 16:652–657, 1957.
17. James DH, Hustu O, Wrenn EL, et al: Combination chemotherapy of childhood neuroblastoma. JAMA 194:123–126, 1965.
18. Stiller CA, Parkin DM: International variations in the incidence of neuroblastoma. Int J Cancer 52:538–543, 1992.
19. Beckwith JB, Perrin EV: In situ neuroblastomas: A contribution to the natural history of neural crest tumors. Am J Pathol 45:1089–1104, 1963.
20. Yamamoto K, Hanada R, Tanimura M, et al: Natural history of neuroblastoma found by mass screening. Lancet 349:1102, 1997.
21. Kushner BH, Gilbert F, Helson L. Familial neuroblastoma: Case reports, literature review, and etiologic considerations. Cancer 57:1887–1893, 1986.
22. Berry CL, Keeling JW: Neuroblastoma. In Berry CL (ed): Pediatric Pathology (3rd ed). London, Springer-Verlag, 1996, p 869.
23. Evans AE, D'Angio GJ, Randolph J: A proposed staging for children with neuroblastoma. Cancer 27:374–378, 1971.
24. Shimada H, Chatten J, Newton WA, et al: Histopathologic prognostic factors in neuroblastic tumors: Definition of subtypes of ganglioneuroblastoma and an age-linked classification of neuroblastomas. J Natl Cancer Inst 73:405–416, 1984.
25. Gross RE, Farber S, Martin LW: Neuroblastoma sympatheticum: A study and report of 217 cases. Pediatrics 23:1179–1191, 1959.
26. Grosfeld JL, Baehner RL: Neuroblastoma: An analysis of 160 cases. World J Surg 4:29–38, 1980.
27. Acharya S, Jayabose S, Kogan SJ, et al: Prenatally diagnosed neuroblastoma. Cancer 80:304–310, 1997.
28. Zeltzer PM, Marangos PJ, Parma AM, et al: Raised neuron-specific enolase in serum of children with metastatic neuroblastoma: A report from the Children's Cancer Study Group. Lancet 2:361–363, 1983.
29. Zeltzer P, Marangos PJ, Sather H, et al: Prognostic importance of neuron specific enolase levels in widespread and localized neuroblastoma. Proc Am Soc Clin Oncol 3:13, 1984.
30. Wong KY, Hann HL, Marangos P, et al: Prognostic factors in patients with stage III neuroblastoma. Proc Am Soc Clin Oncol 3:85, 1984.
31. Morris JA, Shochat S, Smith EI, et al: Biological variables in thoracic neuroblastoma: A Pediatric Oncology Group Study. J Pediatr Surg 30:296–303, 1995.
32. Bowman LC, Castleberry RP, Cantor A, et al: Genetic staging of unresectable or metastatic neuroblastoma in infants: A Pediatric Oncology Group Study. J Natl Cancer Inst 89:373–380, 1997.
33. Shuster JJ, McWilliams NB, Castleberry R, et al: Serum lactate dehydrogenase in childhood neuroblastoma. Am J Clin Oncol 15:295–303, 1992.
34. Hann HL, Levy HM, Evans AE: Serum ferritin as a guide to therapy in neuroblastoma. Cancer Res 40:1411–1413, 1980.
35. Hann HL, Evans AE, Siegel SE, et al: Prognostic importance of serum ferritin in patients with stages III and IV neuroblastoma: The Children's Cancer Study Group experience. Cancer Res 45:2843–2848, 1985.
36. Schwab M, Alitalo K, Klempnauer K-H, et al: Amplified DNA with limited homology to myc cellular oncogene is shared by human neuroblastoma cell lines and a neuroblastoma tumor. Nature 305:245–248, 1983.
37. Brodeur GM, Seeger RC: Amplification of N-myc in untreated human neuroblastoma correlates with advanced disease stage. Science 220:1121–1124, 1984.
38. Bourhis J, DeVathaire F, Wilson GD, et al: Combined analysis of DNA ploidy index and N-myc genomic content in neuroblastoma. Cancer Res 51:33–36, 1991.
39. Shimada H, Stram DO, Chatten J, et al: Identification of subsets of neuroblastomas by combined histopathologic and N-myc analysis. J Natl Cancer Inst 87:1470–1476, 1995.
40. Brodeur GM: Molecular basis for heterogeneity in human neuroblastomas. Eur J Cancer 31A:505–510, 1995.
41. Combaret V, Gross N, Lasset C, et al: Clinical relevance of CD44 cell-surface expression and N-myc gene amplification in a multicentric analysis of 121 pediatric neuroblastomas. J Clin Oncol 14:25–34, 1996.
42. Look AT, Hayes FA, Shuster JJ, et al: Clinical relevance of tumor cell ploidy and N-myc gene amplification in childhood neuroblastoma: A Pediatric Oncology Group Study. J Clin Oncol 9:581–591, 1991.
43. Cohn SL, Look AT, Joshi VV, et al: Lack of correlation of N-myc gene amplification with prognosis in localized neuroblastoma: A Pediatric Oncology Group Study. Cancer Res 55:721–726, 1995.
44. Fong C-T, Dracopoli NC, White PS, et al: Loss of heterozygosity for the short arm of chromosome 1 in human neuroblastomas: Correlation with N-myc amplification. Proc Natl Acad Sci U S A 86:3753–3757, 1989.
45. Maris JM, White PS, Beltinger CP, et al: Significance of chromosome 1p loss of heterozygosity in neuroblastoma. Cancer Res 55:4664–4669, 1995.
46. Look AT, Hayes FA, Nitschke R, et al: Cellular DNA content as a predictor of response to chemotherapy in infants with unresectable neuroblastoma. N Engl J Med 311:231–235, 1984.
47. Brodeur GM, Green AA, Hayes A, et al: Cytogenetic features of human neuroblastomas and cell lines. Cancer Res 41:4678–4686, 1981.
48. Caron H, van Sluis P, de Kraker J, et al: Allelic loss of chromosome 1p as a predictor of unfavorable outcome in patients with neuroblastoma. N Engl J Med 334:225–230, 1996.

49. Favrot MC, Combaret V, Lasset C: CD44—a new prognostic marker for neuroblastoma [letter]. N Engl J Med 329:1965, 1993.

50. Combaret V, Lasset C, Frappaz D, et al: Evaluation of CD44 prognostic value in neuroblastoma: Comparison with the other prognostic factors. Eur J Cancer 31A:545–549, 1995.

51. Nakagawara A, Arima-Nakagawara M, Scavarda NJ, et al: Association between high levels of expression of the TRK gene and favorable outcome in human neuroblastoma. N Engl J Med 328:847–854, 1993.

52. Norris MD, Bordow SB, Marshall GM, et al: Expression of the gene for multidrug-resistance-associated protein and outcome in patients with neuroblastoma. N Engl J Med 334:231–238, 1996.

53. Laug WE, Siegel SE, Shaw KNF, et al: Initial urinary catecholamine metabolite concentrations and prognosis in neuroblastoma. Pediatrics 62:77–83, 1978.

54. LaBrosse EH, Com-Nougué C, Zucker J-M, et al: Urinary excretion of 3-methoxy-4-hyhroxymandelic acid and 3-methoxy-4-hydroxyphenylacetic acid by 288 patients with neuroblastoma and related neural crest tumors. Cancer Res 40:1995–2001, 1980.

55. Sawada T: Outcome of 25 neuroblastomas revealed by mass screening in Japan [letter]. Lancet 1:377, 1986.

56. Woods WG, Tuchman M: Neuroblastoma: The case for screening infants in North America. Pediatrics 79:869–873, 1987.

57. Woods WG, Tuchman M, Robison LL, et al: A population-based study of the usefulness of screening for neuroblastoma. Lancet 348:1682–1687, 1996.

58. Kaneko Y, Kanda N, Maseki N, et al: Current urinary mass screening for catecholamine metabolites at 6 months of age may be detecting only a small portion of high-risk neuroblastomas: A chromosome and N-*myc* amplification study. J Clin Oncol 8:2005–2013, 1990.

59. Brodeur GM, Seeger RC, Barrett A, et al: International criteria for diagnosis, staging and response to treatment in patients with neuroblastoma. J Clin Oncol 6:1874–1881, 1988.

60. Brodeur GM, Pritchard J, Berthold F, et al: Revisions of the international criteria for neuroblastoma diagnosis, staging and response to treatment. J Clin Oncol 11:1466–1477, 1993.

61. Nitschke R, Smith EI, Schochat S, et al: Localized neuroblastoma treated by surgery: A Pediatric Oncology Group Study. J Clin Oncol 6:1271–1279, 1988.

62. Weinblatt ME, Heisel MA, Siegel SE: Hypertension in children with neurogenic tumors. Pediatrics 71:947–951, 1983.

63. Altman AJ, Baehner RL: Favorable prognosis for survival in children with coincident opso-myoclonus and neuroblastoma. Cancer 37:846–852, 1976.

64. Swift PGF, Bloom SR, Harris F: Watery diarrhea and ganglioneuroma with secretion of vasoactive intestinal peptide. Arch Dis Child 50:896–899, 1975.

65. Tiedemann K, Pritchard J, Long R, et al: Intractable diarrhea in a patient with vasoactive intestinal peptide-secreting neuroblastoma. Eur J Pediatr 137:217–219, 1981.

66. Nadel HR: Nuclear oncology in children. In Nuclear Medicine Annual. Philadelphia, Lippincott-Raven, 1996, pp 143–193.

67. Gordon I, Peters AM, Gutman A, et al: Skeletal assessment in neuroblastoma—the pitfalls of iodine-123-MIBG scans. J Nucl Med 31:129–134, 1990.

68. Plantaz D, Rubie H, Michon J, et al: The treatment of neuroblastoma with intraspinal extension with chemotherapy followed by surgical removal of residual disease. Cancer 78:311–319, 1996.

69. Moss TJ, Fonkalsrud EW, Feig SA, et al: Delayed surgery and bone marrow transplantation for widespread neuroblastoma. Ann Surg 206:514–520, 1987.

70. Shamberger RC, Allarde-Segundo A, Kozakewich HPW, et al: Surgical management of stage III and IV neuroblastoma: Resection before or after chemotherapy? J Pediatr Surg 26:1113–1117, 1991.

71. Hsu LL, Evans AE, D'Angio GJ: Hepatomegaly in neuroblastoma stage 4S: Criteria for treatment of the vulnerable neonate. Med Pediatr Oncol 27:521–528, 1996.

72. Wilson PCG, Coppes MJ, Solh H, et al: Neuroblastoma stage IV-S: A heterogeneous disease. Med Pediatr Oncol 19:467–472, 1991.

73. Haas D, Ablin AR, Miller C, et al: Complete pathologic maturation and regression of stage IVS neuroblastoma without treatment. Cancer 62:818–825, 1988.

74. Guglielmi M, de Bernardi B, Rizzo A, et al: Resection of primary tumor at diagnosis in stage IV-S neuroblastoma: Does it affect the clinical course? J Clin Oncol 14:1537–1544, 1996.

75. Ladenstein R, Favrot M, Lasset C, et al: Indication and limits of megatherapy and bone marrow transplantation in high-risk neuroblastoma: A single centre analysis of prognostic factors. Eur J Cancer 29A:947–956, 1993.

76. Matthay KK, O'Leary MC, Ramsay NK, et al: Role of myeloablative therapy in improved outcome for high risk neuroblastoma: Review of recent Children's Cancer Group results. Eur J Cancer 31A:572–575, 1995.

77. Steenburg RW, Ravitch MM: Cervico-thoracic approach for subclavian vessel injury from compound fracture of the clavicle: Considerations of subclavian-axillary exposures. Ann Surg 157:839–846, 1963.

78. Pranikoff T, Hirschl RB, Schnaufer L: Approach to cervicothoracic neuroblastomas via a trap door incision. J Pediatr Surg 30:546–548, 1995.

79. Kiely EM: The surgical challenge of neuroblastoma. J Pediatr Surg 29:128–133, 1994.

80. Tsuchida Y, Honna T, Kamii Y, et al: Radical excision of primary tumor and lymph nodes in advanced neuroblastoma: Combination with intensive induction chemotherapy. Pediatr Surg Int 6:22–27, 1991.

81. Kedia KR, Markland C, Fraley EE: Sexual function following high retroperitoneal lymphadenectomy. J Urol 114:237–239, 1975.

82. Azizkhan RG, Shaw A, Chandler JG: Surgical complications of neuroblastoma resection. Surgery 97:514–517, 1985.

83. Rees H, Markley MA, Kiely EM, et al: Diarrhea after resection of advanced abdominal neuroblastoma: A common management problem. Surgery: 123:568–572.

84. Smith EI, Krous HF, Tunell WP, et al: The impact of chemotherapy and radiation therapy on secondary operations for neuroblastoma. Ann Surg 191:561–568, 1980.

85. Ninane J, Pritchard J, Morris Jones PH, et al: Stage II neuroblastoma: Adverse prognostic significance of lymph node involvement. Arch Dis Child 57:438–442, 1982.

86. Evans AE, Silber JH, Shpilsky A, et al: Successful management of low-stage neuroblastoma without adjuvant therapies: A comparison of two decades, 1972 through 1981 and 1982 through 1992, in a single institution. J Clin Oncol 14:2504–2510, 1996.

87. Suarez A, Hartmann O, Vassal G, et al: Treatment of stage IV-S neuroblastoma: A study of 34 cases treated between 1982 and 1987. Med Pediatr Oncol 19:473–477, 1991.

88. De Kraker J, Hoefnagel CA, Caron H, et al: First line targeted radiotherapy, a new concept in the treatment of advanced stage neuroblastoma. Eur J Oncol 31A:600–602, 1995.

89. Stiller CA: Trends in neuroblastoma in Great Britain: Incidence and mortality, 1971–1990. Eur J Cancer 29A:1008–1012, 1993.

90. Fortner J, Nicastri A, Murphy ML: Neuroblastoma: Natural history and results of treating 133 cases. Ann Surg 167:132–142, 1968.

91. Vogel JM, Coddon DR, Simon N, et al: Osseous metastases in neuroblastoma. A 17-year survival. Cancer 26:1354–1360, 1970.

92. Nakagawara A, Sasazuki T, Akiyama H, et al: N-*myc* oncogene and stage IV-S neuroblastoma. Cancer 65:1960–1967, 1990.

93. Franks LM, Bollen A, Seeger RC, et al: Neuroblastoma in adults and adolescents: An indolent course with poor survival. Cancer 79:2028–2035, 1997.

94. Blatt J, Gula MJ, Orlando SJ, et al: Indolent course of advanced neuroblastoma in children older than 6 years at diagnosis. Cancer 76:890–894, 1995.

95. Senelick RC, Bray PF, Lahey ME, et al: Neuroblastoma and

myoclonic encephalopathy: Two cases and a review of the literature. J Pediatr Surg 8:623–631, 1973.

96. Punt J, Pritchard J, Pincott JR, et al: Neuroblastoma: A review of 21 cases presenting with spinal cord compression. Cancer 45:3095–3101, 1980.

97. Matthay KK, Sather HN, Seeger RC, et al: Excellent outcome of stage II neuroblastoma is independent of residual disease and radiation therapy. J Clin Oncol 7:236–244, 1989.

98. Kushner BH, Cheung N-KV, LaQuaglia MP, et al: International neuroblastoma staging system stage 1 neuroblastoma: A prospective study and literature review. J Clin Oncol 14:2174–2180, 1996.

99. Suita S, Zaizen Y, Kaneko M, et al: What is the benefit of aggressive chemotherapy for advanced neuroblastoma with N-*myc* amplification: A report from the Japanese Study Group for the treatment of advanced neuroblastoma. J Pediatr Surg 29:746–750, 1994.

100. Shorter NA, Davidoff AM, Evans AE, et al: The role of surgery in the management of stage IV neuroblastoma: A single institution study. Med Pediatr Oncol 24:287–291, 1995.

101. Tsuchida Y, Yokoyama J, Kaneko M, et al: Therapeutic significance of surgery in advanced neuroblastoma: A report from the Study Group of Japan. J Pediatr Surg 27:616–622, 1992.

102. Haase GM, O'Leary MC, Ramsay NKC, et al: Aggressive surgery combined with intensive chemotherapy improves survival in poor-risk neuroblastoma. J Pediatr Surg 26:1119–1124, 1991.

103. Chamberlain RS, Quinones R, Dinndorf P, et al: Complete surgical resection combined with aggressive adjuvant chemotherapy and bone marrow transplantation prolongs survival in children with advanced neuroblastoma. Ann Surg Oncol 2:93–100, 1995.

104. D'Angio GJ, Evans AE, Koop CE: Special pattern of widespread neuroblastoma with a favourable prognosis. Lancet 1:1046–1049, 1971.

66

LESIONS OF THE LIVER

Michael P. La Quaglia, MD, FRCS

Advances in the treatment of hepatic tumors have been based on an appreciation of the surgical anatomy (Fig. 66–1).[1–3] Hepatic lobectomy for childhood hepatoblastoma was suggested in 1969, and the use of adjuvant chemotherapy and radiation soon followed.[4–8] In 1975, a survey by the members of the Surgical Section of the American Academy of Pediatrics emphasized the difference in biologic virulence between hepatocellular carcinoma and hepatoblastoma and the importance of complete surgical resection of the primary tumor for ultimate cure.[9] Successful hepatectomy and liver transplantation for hepatoblastoma was reported in 1987.[10] A series of 15 patients who underwent transplantation for hepatic malignancies was reported in 1992.[11]

☐ Benign Hepatic Tumors

One third of childhood liver tumors are benign.[12] Benign tumors include vascular malformations, adenomas, focal nodular hyperplasia, mesenchymal hamartomas, and various types of cysts.

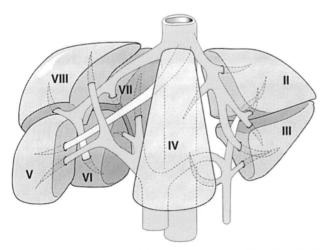

Figure 66–1. The segmental hepatic anatomy as defined by Couinaud.[2, 3] A comprehensive understanding of the hepatic segmental divisions is necessary for successful hepatic resection.

HEMANGIOMAS AND VASCULAR MALFORMATIONS

Hemangiomas have endothelial-lined vascular spaces that can vary in size and extent.[13–15] Venous malformations and cavernous hemangiomas are distinguished by a lack of cellularity and large vascular spaces. Hemangioendotheliomas are highly proliferative cellular lesions of variable malignant potential. Arteriovenous malformations are the rarest pathologic subtype and have naturally occurring anastomoses between arteries and veins. All of these vascular tumors may be associated with significant shunting that results in congestive heart failure (CHF).

Incidence

The overall incidence of endothelial-lined vascular tumors of the liver in childhood is unknown because many cases are asymptomatic. Vascular lesions make up 13 to 18% of symptomatic hepatic tumors in childhood.[9, 12, 16] Hepatic hemangiomas are twice as common in female patients.[13]

Presentation and Diagnosis

An abdominal mass is probably the most frequent sign of a vascular tumor of the liver. Cutaneous hemangiomas suggest possible visceral lesions. A systolic bruit can sometimes be heard over the liver. Large lesions may produce CHF. Rarely, jaundice, disseminated intravascular coagulation, or hemorrhagic shock from intraperitoneal bleeding may be observed.[17] The diagnosis is confirmed by magnetic resonance imaging (MRI) rather than arteriography.[18] The extent and nature of the vascular lesion are often accurately defined by this study. Biopsy may result in massive hemorrhage.

Treatment

Many hepatic hemangiomas regress after the 1st year of life. CHF requires digoxin and diuretic therapy. If the heart failure does not resolve, hepatic artery embolization or ligation may be necessary.[19, 20] Hepatic arterial embolization may control symptoms, but collateral vessels may make subsequent resection or embolization difficult. Hepatic resection may be required in refractory cases of CHF. Blood loss in these complicated procedures may be reduced using hemodilution techniques.[21–23] Transfusion of blood and platelets may be required for disseminated intravascular coagulation.

Rupture of a vascular tumor usually requires hepatic resection. Arterial embolization may temporarily control bleeding, allow stabilization, and result in a more controlled operative procedure.[20]

Outcome

The overall prognosis for benign hepatic vascular lesions is good. Most patients do not require operative intervention, and most cellular lesions regress after the 1st year of life. Angiosarcomatous degeneration of benign hemangioendotheliomas has been reported, often following radiotherapy of a benign hemangioendothelioma.[16, 24]

FOCAL NODULAR HYPERPLASIA AND HEPATOCELLULAR ADENOMA

Focal nodular hyperplasia (FNH) and hepatocytic adenomas are more common in adults than in children. Both lesions occur with type I glycogen storage disease.[25, 26] Both tumors have been correlated with a high-estrogen environment.[26] Hepatic adenomas are seen in patients undergoing androgen therapy for hematologic disorders, in patients undergoing danazol therapy, and in women taking oral contraceptives.[27–29] In one report, 5 of 39 unresected hepatic adenomas developed hepatocellular carcinoma.[30]

Epidemiology

These lesions make up less than 2% of hepatic tumors in childhood.[16] Most patients are younger than 5 years of age at presentation. There is a female predominance.[31] Focal nodular hyperplasia has been reported in an infant exposed antenatally to corticosteroids.[32]

Presentation and Diagnosis

Patients usually have an asymptomatic mass. Adenomas are more likely to be symptomatic and may rupture, producing shock and acute abdominal pain.

Both lesions are encapsulated on imaging studies. Because FNH is associated with fibrous septa, abdominal ultrasonography (US) and computed tomography (CT) may show a distinctive central "scar" by which it is distinguished from adenoma (Fig. 66–2). Adenomas are seen as encapsulated by US or CT, but histologically they may resemble hepatocellular carcinoma.

Treatment

Adenomatous lesions should be removed because they may be or may become hepatocellular carcinomas. They may rupture and bleed.[33] Removal usually requires a segmental resection. Embolization is an option if the adenoma is not resectable. Some unresectable and all asymptomatic cases of FNH may simply be observed.

Outcome

Most patients do well after resection for adenoma or FNH. In one study of eight patients with FNH and two with an adenoma, six were long-term survivors.[34] Three patients with FNH survived resection and two survived nonoperative management. One patient who died of leukemia had an FNH lesion found at autopsy. One of the two patients with an adenoma survived hepatic lobectomy and the second died of postoperative hemorrhage.

MESENCHYMAL HAMARTOMA

Mesenchymal hamartomas are usually solitary hepatic masses presenting in infants. They often have

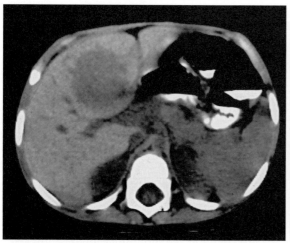
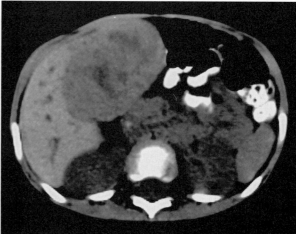

Figure 66–2. Computed tomography scan of a patient with focal nodular hyperplasia.

multiple cysts lined with biliary epithelium surrounded by distended lymphatics and actively growing mesenchyme. It is postulated that mesenchymal hamartomas arise in areas of focal intrahepatic biliary atresia.[35, 36] Another hypothesis is that these lesions arise in conjunction with vascular anomalies, which would explain the occurrence of small hemangiomas observed in close proximity.[37]

Epidemiology

Mesenchymal hamartomas make up 6% of primary liver tumors in childhood. There is a male predominance. Two thirds of these tumors are diagnosed in children younger than 1 year of age, although presentation in teenagers has been described. The mean age at diagnosis is 16 months.[38]

Presentation and Diagnosis

The majority of mesenchymal hamartomas present as an asymptomatic, enlarging abdominal mass.[37] Their size may produce respiratory distress or vena caval obstruction. The most useful diagnostic modalities are US, CT, and MRI. Often, an open biopsy is required to confirm the diagnosis.

Treatment

Anatomic resection is preferred. Hamartomas have a capsule that facilitates enucleation of large, centrally located lesions that are not amenable to lobectomy. Marsupialization of a large hamartoma may be done if enucleation is not possible.

Outcome

Patients do well with all forms of therapy. In one study of 18 patients, the 13 available for follow-up were all well 1 month to 24 years after treatment (mean, 5 years).[38]

SOLITARY CYSTS

Solitary, congenital, nonparasitic liver cysts in childhood are extremely rare and are frequently discovered as incidental findings on US or CT performed for other reasons.[39–41] The wall of these simple cysts usually has three layers. The lining is cuboidal, columnar, or squamous epithelium. Vascular elements make up the middle layer, and the outer layer is made up of compressed hepatocytes, collagen, muscle fibers, and bile ducts.[42] They contain straw-colored, clear fluid. They are predominantly found in the right, anteroinferior hepatic lobe (segment V). Occasionally, they are pedunculated.

The diagnosis is usually by US, although MRI or Doppler US is necessary to determine proximity to the portal and hepatic vessels. Nine percent of solitary cysts produce jaundice by compression of the extrahepatic biliary ducts. Cysts discovered incidentally at laparotomy should be left alone if they are less than 5 cm in diameter. Aspiration of cysts that are between 5 and 10 cm in diameter should be performed to confirm the diagnosis.

Asymptomatic solitary cysts do not require therapy. Pain, rupture, or torsion require surgical treatment. Percutaneous aspiration as therapy is usually followed by recurrence unless ethanol is injected. More commonly, operative intervention is required. Cysts that are not adherent to essential structures are excised. Occasionally, marsupialization is a viable alternative. The rare communication between cyst and biliary ducts may be identified by the injection of contrast media into the cyst or by aspiration of bile from it. This is followed by excision of the cyst wall. Hepatic lobectomy may be necessary for symptomatic cysts that adhere to major vessels or if there has been previous inflammation.[43]

MULTICYSTIC DISEASE

Adult type polycystic disease involving the liver has been effectively treated by right hepatic lobectomy, sparing the left hepatic lobe.[44]

ECHINOCOCCAL CYSTS

Echinococcus granulosus (cystic hydatid) and *Echinococcus multilocularis* (alveolar hydatid) produce the most serious human cestode infection in the world.[45, 46] The liver is the most common site of echinococcal cyst formation. The right hepatic lobe is the more frequently involved and the growth rate of the cysts is approximately 1 cm per year.[47] *E. granulosus* forms a cyst, containing its own daughter cysts, that is surrounded by a tough fibrous capsule. These cysts can attain a size of 20 cm that compresses but does not invade adjacent hepatic tissue. *E. multilocularis* daughter cysts infiltrate into adjacent tissues, simulating a malignancy. Early cysts are usually asymptomatic, and small ones can resolve spontaneously or after treatment with albendazole. Larger cysts may cause abdominal enlargement, hepatomegaly, pain, pressure, and vomiting. Rupture of the cysts spreads scolices throughout the peritoneal cavity.

Solitary *E. granulosus* cysts can be treated at laparotomy by cyst aspiration followed by injection of a scolicidal agent such as 3% saline or cetrimide. The cyst must be carefully walled off from the peritoneal cavity. The cyst lining is then removed (pericystectomy).[48] Spillage of protoscolices can result in dissemination or anaphylaxis. A 1997 randomized trial compared albendazole given in a dose of 10 mg/kg/day for 8 weeks followed by percutaneous drainage with operative pericystectomy. The albendazole/drainage regimen was associated with fewer complications and a shorter hospitalization when used to treat simple hydatid cysts (*E. granulosus*).[49] Alveolar hydatid disease (*E. multilocularis*) must be treated by complete resection with a margin of normal hepatic tissue as if one were treating a malignancy.

□ Malignant Hepatic Tumors

In developed nations, primary liver tumors constitute approximately 1.1% of childhood malignancies. There are about 1.4 cases per million children in the United States.[50, 51]

HEPATOBLASTOMA

Epidemiology

Hepatoblastoma is the most common primary hepatic tumor of childhood, making up 43% of cases in one large series. The male-to-female ratio is 1.7:1.[52, 53] Although there are sporadic reports of hepatoblastoma in adults, the median age at presentation is about 18 months and most cases occur before age 3 years.[9] There are several reports of hepatoblastoma occurring in siblings.[54-57] Hepatoblastoma is known to occur with familial polyposis, Gardner's syndrome, and Beckwith-Wiedemann syndrome.[58-68] There is also a correlation between low birth weight and the development of hepatoblastoma.[69] Hepatoblastoma has also been reported along with other congenital anomalies such as cleft palate, cardiovascular and renal anomalies including multicystic kidney, and absence of the right adrenal gland.[68, 70]

PATHOLOGY

Hepatoblastomas are divided into five subtypes that are separable based on light microscopy criteria: fetal, embryonal, mixed mesenchymal, macrotrabecular, and anaplastic or small cell. The importance of subtyping in hepatoblastoma is the association between prognostic risk and subtype that is illustrated in Table 66–1.[71, 72] Multiple studies have concluded that the fetal histologic subtype is associated with an improved prognosis. In contrast, patients with the rare anaplastic variant usually do poorly. Extramedullary hematopoiesis is characteristically present and may be related to constitutive cytokine production by the tumor cells.[73] Calcification is sometimes noted in these tumors, and there is one report of a patient with osteosarcomatous elements in the hepatoblastoma and associated pulmonary metastases.[74]

Biology and Molecular Biology

There are few cellular models of hepatoblastoma. One cell line clearly expressed the oncogenes c-*myc* and Ha-*ras* as well as the epidermal growth factor receptor. Growth factors that were required for maximal growth included 10% fetal bovine serum, insulin, transferrin, hydrocortisone, and epidermal growth factor.[75] Antibodies that blocked the epidermal growth factor receptor inhibited cell growth. The significance of oncogene expression is undetermined.

In another study, elevated hepatocyte growth factor (HGF) levels were found in the serum of 10 of 22 (45%) patients with hepatoblastoma. The hepatocyte growth factor receptor, c-*met*, was identified on the surface of the epithelial component of these tumors.[76] Addition of hepatocyte growth factor causes proliferation in hepatoblastoma-derived cell lines.

The well-known thrombocytosis associated with untreated hepatoblastoma as well as the presence of extramedullary hematopoiesis in these tumors is intriguing. The platelet count is markedly elevated in most patients at diagnosis with platelet counts ranging into the millions. Hepatoblastoma cells have been shown to secrete interleukin-1, erythropoietin, and stem cell factor, which may account for the thrombocytosis.[77]

Cytogenetics

Losses of heterozygosity on chromosome 11p15.5 and 1p36 have both been described in hepatoblastoma.[78, 79] Investigations into both these regions suggest that each may contain a tumor suppressor gene. There is also a high incidence of trisomy 20 and trisomy of all or part of chromosome 2.[80, 81]

Presentation

The hepatoblastoma patient is most commonly first seen with an asymptomatic abdominal mass discovered by the parent or the pediatrician.[82] Failure to thrive is more common than significant weight loss. Some patients are seen acutely with tumor rupture.[83, 84] Hepatoblastoma may rarely produce sexual precocity.[85-87] Imaging studies often show a large tumor with evidence of central necrosis (Fig. 66–3). Hepatoblastomas are uncommonly multifocal or show extrahepatic dissemination.

Alphafetoprotein

Serum alphafetoprotein (AFP) is a well-established tumor marker used in the diagnosis of hepatoblastoma and for monitoring therapeutic response.[88-91] The normal AFP level is less than 20 ng/ml, but levels up to 7.7×10^6 ng/ml have been

TABLE 66-1. Relative Risk and Histopathologic Subtype for Hepatoblastoma

Histopathologic Subtype	Relative Risk of Death from Disease
Fetal	1.07*
Embryonal	1.74
Mixed epithelial-mesenchymal	0.53
Macrotrabecular pattern	1.20
Small cell undifferentiated (anaplastic)	3.71

*Risk of death adjusted for age, sex, and stage compared to other histologic subtypes.

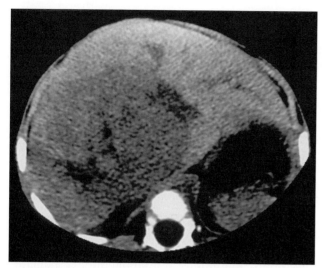

Figure 66–3. Computed tomography scan of a patient with hepatoblastoma.

seen with hepatoblastoma. A mean AFP level for hepatoblastoma patients of almost 3×10^6 ng/ml was compared with the mean of almost 200,000 ng/ml measured in children with hepatocellular carcinoma.[92] Subfractionation of AFP may help differentiate hepatoblastoma, hepatocellular carcinoma, endodermal sinus tumor, and benign liver disease.[93, 94] A return to normal AFP levels has been demonstrated with clinical or radiographic disappearance of hepatoblastoma.[95, 96] A large, early decrease in AFP levels may be a predictor of survival. It has been postulated but not proved that a low initial AFP level is associated with a decreased survival rate.[97, 98] Anaplastic hepatoblastomas may be associated with lower AFP levels.[99]

Staging

Most studies have used the clinical grouping defined by the Children's Cancer Group and the Pedi-

TABLE 66–2. Clinical Groups for Pediatric Epithelial Hepatic Malignancies

Intergroup Liver Tumor Clinical Group	Criteria	Relative Risk of Death from Disease
I	Complete resection as initial treatment	0.16
IIA	Complete resection after chemotherapy or irradiation	0.57
IIB	Residual disease confined to one lobe	
III	Disease involving both lobes	2.87*
IIIB	Regional nodes involved	
IV	Distant parenchymal metastases (extent of primary tumor is irrelevant)	3.51

*Relative risk was assessed for stages II and III patients collectively. The relative risk is compared to other stages. Relative risk refers to hepatoblastoma patients.

atric Oncology Group (Table 66–2). There is a trend, however, to use the TNM classification (Table 66–3).[100]

Treatment

Survival, in most subtypes, is dependent on removal of the primary liver tumor and adjuvant chemotherapy.[98, 101–107] Doxorubicin, vincristine, 5-fluorouracil, cisplatin, and ifosfamide have been reported to be effective in various combinations.[108, 109] There have been more complications with combinations that include doxorubicin. The recommendation for initial treatment of hepatoblastomas is with cisplatin, 5-fluorouracil, and vincristine. Young infants who undergo complete resection may receive a shortened course of adjuvant single-agent doxorubicin, which is well tolerated. Completely resected hepatoblastomas with fetal histology may not require adjuvant chemotherapy.

About 46% of hepatic malignancies are resectable at diagnosis.[110] Often, tumors are not resectable if they are large and involve both lobes. Preoperative (neoadjuvant) chemotherapy typically reduces the tumor mass and allows resection.[111] An initial biopsy is required to confirm the diagnosis. For unresectable tumors, the biopsy procedure should include placement of long-term vascular access for chemotherapy. A second laparotomy is performed if imaging studies show a good response to the neoadjuvant chemotherapy and the tumor appears resectable. *Complete resection of the primary tumor is necessary for survival* and may require extended hepatic resection and complex biliary reconstructions. The patient continues with chemotherapy after definitive resection.

Outcome

In one study, the 1-year survival rate for patients with metastases was no different from those with localized tumors.[95] Patients with metastatic disease may have survival rates approaching 50%. If the

TABLE 66–3. TNM Staging for Hepatic Malignancies

Stage Grouping	TNM Status
Stage I	T1, N0, M0
Stage II	T2, N0, M0
Stage III	T1, N1, M0
	T2, N1, M0
	T3, N0, M0
Stage IVA	T4, any N, M0
Stage IVB	Any T, any N, M1

T0, N0, and M0 mean no evidence of the primary tumor, regional nodes, and distant metastases respectively. T1, solitary tumor <2 cm; T2, solitary tumor <2 cm with vascular invasion or multiple tumors limited to one lobe without vascular invasion, or >2 cm but with no vascular invasion; T3, solitary tumor >2 cm with vascular invasion, multiple tumors limited to a lobe with vascular invasion; T4, multiple tumors in more than one lobe or involvement of a major branch of the portal or hepatic vein.

primary lesion is resected, pulmonary metastases resolve with chemotherapy. Resection is sometimes required for larger or persistent metastatic lesions.[112–114] Some radiation oncologists have treated pulmonary metastases with 18 to 20 Gy administered by external beam radiotherapy similar to that used for Wilms' tumors.[115]

An overall survival rate of 60 to 70% is achievable with stages I to III hepatoblastoma, except in the very aggressive small cell (anaplastic) variant. If there is residual gross disease in the liver, survival rate declines to zero. Microscopic residual disease may be eradicated with continued chemotherapy or external beam radiotherapy to the liver. Factors determined by multivariate analysis to be independent predictors of a bad prognosis include a high TNM stage, unresectable gross tumor, bilobar involvement and multifocality, an AFP level of less than 100 or greater than 10^5 ng/ml, distant metastases, embryonal histology, and vascular invasion.[116]

Future Directions

Hepatic transplantation for unresectable primary lesions can be effective for tumors that are confined to the liver.[11, 117–120] Chemoembolization using thrombogenic materials that also contain cisplatin or doxorubicin delivers 50 to 100 times the dose to the embolized segment of tumor.[121] Early results indicate that some unresectable hepatoblastomas may become resectable using this technique.[122–125] Other approaches include treatment with anti-AFP antibodies and viral transfection vectors to attack malignant hepatic cells.

HEPATOCELLULAR CARCINOMA (HEPATOMA)

Epidemiology

Hepatocellular carcinoma accounts for 23% of pediatric liver tumors but is rare in infants and young children.[12, 126] Some reported cases in children younger than 5 years may have been hepatoblastomas.[9] The incidence of hepatoma is bimodal with an early peak at 5 years and a second peak between 13 and 15 years of age. The fibrolamellar variant of hepatocellular carcinoma presents at a median age of 20 years and it is rarely seen before age 10. Hepatoma occurs from 1.3 to 3.2 times more commonly in male patients except in areas endemic for hepatitis B where the ratio is reversed (0.2:1). In the United States, approximately 35 to 40 new pediatric cases of hepatocellular carcinomas are diagnosed per year.

Hepatitis B and C are risk factors for hepatocellular carcinoma. Hepatitis B surface antigens are found in 85% of cases in the Far East but in only 10 to 25% of cases in the United States. The highest risk is in those patients with chronic active hepatitis.[100] An intense program of vaccination against hepatitis B has reduced the incidence of hepatocel-

lular carcinoma in Taiwan.[127] Hepatitis C antibodies are found in 20% of patients with hepatocellular carcinoma. There is a report of a hepatocellular carcinoma developing in an infant with a history of neonatal hepatitis.[128]

Other conditions associated with the development of hepatocellular carcinoma include cirrhosis, α_1-antitrypsin deficiency, tyrosinemia, aflatoxin ingestion, hemochromatosis, hepatic venous obstruction, androgen and estrogen exposure, and the Alagille syndrome (arteriohepatic dysplasia).[129]

Pathology

Hepatocellular carcinomas are highly invasive and often multicentric at diagnosis. Tumor cells are larger than normal hepatocytes and pleomorphic with prominent nucleoli. Extramedullary hematopoiesis is not seen. Invasiveness is a hallmark of these tumors. Extrahepatic dissemination to portal lymph nodes, lungs, and bones is frequent at diagnosis and strongly affects the survival rate. The natural progression of hepatocellular carcinoma is capsular invasion followed by extracapsular extension, then vascular invasion, and, finally, intrahepatic metastases.[130] There is a strong correlation between intrahepatic metastases and portal vein thrombosis. This suggests that efferent tumor vessels anastomose to the portal rather than the hepatic veins, allowing intrahepatic spread and explaining the multicentricity that is such a hallmark of hepatocellular carcinoma.

The fibrolamellar variant hepatoma seen in older children and young adults was thought to have a better prognosis, but studies indicate that, in comparable stages, survival is similar.[131]

Biology and Molecular Biology

Cytogenetic data indicate that chromosomal abnormalities are complex, but no consistent patterns have been established.[132, 133]

Presentation

Children and adolescents with hepatocellular carcinoma frequently have anorexia, malaise, nausea and vomiting, and significant weight loss. About 40% have a palpable abdominal mass, and about the same number have pain with or without a mass.[50] Jaundice is an uncommon feature. The AFP level is elevated in approximately 85% of patients, with most levels being more than 1000 ng/ml.[100] Although elevated, these levels are usually lower than those measured in hepatoblastoma patients. Up to 10% of patients may first be seen with tumor rupture and a hemoperitoneum.[100]

Staging

The staging schemes listed for hepatoblastoma are also used for hepatocellular carcinoma (see Tables

66–2 and 66–3). A CT scan of a 5-year-old patient with hepatocellular carcinoma and bony metastases at diagnosis is shown in Figure 66–4.

Treatment

The primary treatment of hepatocellular carcinoma is complete surgical resection, without which long-term survival is not possible. This is often impossible, however, owing to multicentric tumor, extrahepatic extension, vascular invasion, and distant metastases. The same chemotherapy protocols used for hepatoblastoma are also applied to hepatocellular carcinomas in childhood. Cisplatin, in particular, has had activity against hepatocellular carcinoma.[134] Owing to the poor survival rate, new and innovative approaches are under investigation.

Unresectable hepatocellular carcinomas can be palliated with chemoembolization, percutaneous intralesional injection of ethanol, and cryotherapy.[125, 135–138] All of these techniques are of limited efficacy owing to tumor size and spread.

Outcome

The overall survival rate from hepatocellular carcinoma in childhood approaches zero and it remains a therapeutic dilemma. Resection of localized lesions occasionally results in long-term survival.[139–143]

Future Directions

Gene therapy with viral vectors that attack dividing cells is being investigated. Hepatocytes rarely divide unless stimulated by liver resection. Viruses (e.g., herpesvirus) attack dividing cells and can be molecularly manipulated to contain cytokine genes or other molecules that can attack cells.[144]

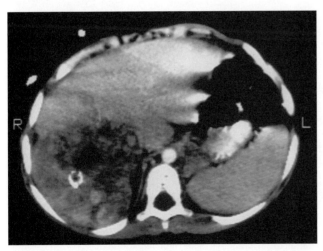

Figure 66–4. Computed tomography scan of a patient with hepatocellular carcinoma. The patient has multifocal disease within the liver and metastases to hilar nodes and bone at diagnosis.

RHABDOMYOSARCOMA OF THE EXTRAHEPATIC BILE DUCTS

Only 10 cases of embryonal rhabdomyosarcoma of the extrahepatic bile ducts were reported in the Intergroup Rhabdomyosarcoma Studies I and II constituting 0.8% of tumors in those studies.[145] The patients range in age from 1 to 9 years at diagnosis. The typical presentation includes intermittent jaundice, loss of appetite, and episodes of cholangitis (Charcot's triad). Hepatomegaly or a palpable abdominal mass are frequent.[146, 147] The diagnosis may be confused with hepatitis with resultant delay in specific therapy.

US demonstrates a hilar or intrahepatic mass that may be confused with a choledochal cyst.[148, 149] CT or MRI may provide information about extension and metastases but do not establish the diagnosis. Open biopsy of a hilar lymph node or the primary tumor should be done carefully so as not to enter the bile ducts. Histologically, the tumors are of the embryonal subtype and often demonstrate botryoid characteristics similar to other rhabdomyosarcomas that arise in a hollow viscus. Distant metastases develop in approximately 40%, but death is most often due to the effects of local invasion.[146]

It is probably better to establish the diagnosis with a biopsy, institute chemotherapy, and resect the tumor at a second-look procedure. At the initial biopsy, hilar and left gastric lymph nodes are removed to determine whether radiotherapy will be added. Six of the 10 Intergroup Rhabdomyosarcoma Studies patients who underwent initial resection had microscopic or minimal gross disease left behind. However, the 4 survivors were in this group. There were no survivors in 4 patients in whom resection was not attempted. Roux-en-Y jejunostomy is the favored bile duct reconstruction. Intraoperative cholangiography is recommended to ensure adequate bile drainage.

Three consecutive patients reported from a single institution all presented with jaundice, cachexia, and a mass.[150] The tumor arose in the common hepatic duct in two children and the left hepatic duct in the third. Intrahepatic extension made initial resection impossible. Two of these patients are alive and disease-free at 9 months and 14 years, whereas the third died of progressive disease at 33 months. All received adjuvant radiotherapy and multiagent chemotherapy. Jaundice was not a late problem.

MALIGNANT MESENCHYMOMA OF THE LIVER

Malignant mesenchymoma is a rare primary hepatic neoplasm that occurs in children aged 5 to 16 years.[151–153] A painful right upper quadrant abdominal mass is the usual presenting symptom. These tumors often appear hypodense (dark) on CT and have a bright peripheral fibrous pseudocapsule (Fig. 66–5).[154] They can be confused with cystic liver disease.[155, 156] They are composed of primitive mes-

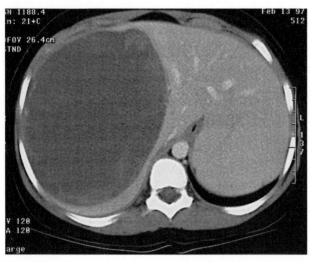

Figure 66–5. Computed tomography scan of a patient with malignant mesenchymoma. The tumor appears dark or cystic with an enhancing periphery.

enchymal cells with occasional small cysts and ducts lined with benign appearing epithelium.[157] Malignant mesenchymomas are treated with surgical resection, adjuvant chemotherapy, and radiotherapy, but most patients relapse and die of progressive disease.[152, 153, 158]

LEIOMYOSARCOMA

There is an increasing incidence of smooth muscle tumors in patients with HIV infection.[159, 160] Leiomyosarcoma of the liver has been reported in more than 20 patients, the youngest of whom was 9 years old. Adjuvant therapy is ineffective, and these tumors must be resected for control. They tend to be of low grade or even have an indeterminate malignant

potential. Supportive and antiretroviral therapy should be maintained through the perioperative period.

HEPATIC METASTASES

The liver is a relatively frequent site of metastatic disease in childhood. Non-Hodgkin's lymphoma, neuroblastoma, rhabdomyosarcoma, rhabdoid tumors, Wilms' tumor, the desmoplastic small round cell tumor, adrenal cortical carcinoma, osteogenic sarcomas, and a host of other malignancies may metastasize to the liver. There are few data to determine the correct surgical approach to these lesions. Criteria for surgical removal of hepatic metastases include control of the primary site, a solitary or limited number of metastases, good performance status, and a reasonable expectation of prolonged survival or cure.

HEPATIC RESECTION

Imaging

At present, Doppler US combined with MRI of the liver gives adequate information concerning the vascular and biliary anatomy. In Figure 66–6A, the origin of the right portal vein and the anterior and posterior sectorial branches to the right lobe are visualized (*arrows*). Between these branches is the right hepatic vein. Figure 66–6B is a magnetic resonance cholangiogram that illustrates the biliary anatomy. The hepatic ducts, common bile duct, and gallbladder are easily seen. Combinations of MRI techniques with and without the use of contrast agents usually gives all the information necessary to assess resectability, and arteriography is rarely indicated.

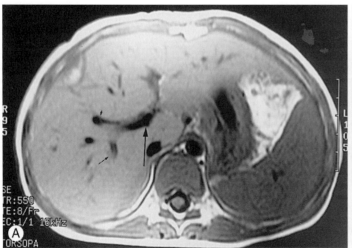
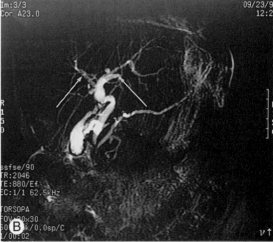

Figure 66–6. *A,* Magnetic resonance imaging scan of the liver illustrating the vascular detail obtained with this technique. The *long arrow* points to the origin of the right hepatic vein and the *shorter arrows* indicate the anterior and posterior sectorial branches. The right hepatic vein can be seen between these branches. The left portal vein is also visible. *B,* Magnetic resonance cholangiogram. The *arrows* indicate the right and left hepatic ducts. The common bile duct and gallbladder can be easily seen.

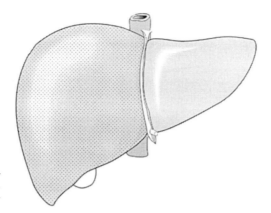

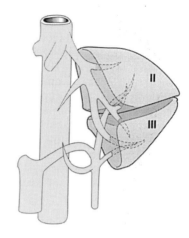

Figure 66–7. Margins of an extended right hepatic lobectomy. Only segments I, II, and III remain.

Surgical Anatomy

The schema of hepatic anatomy most useful for the surgeon is based on the work of Coineaud (see Fig. 66–1). The portal and hepatic veins subdivide the liver into eight segments. Segment I, the caudate lobe, is considered separate from the others owing to its unique vascular supply. It is essentially a third hepatic lobe.

Incisions

Hepatic resection is usually performed through a bilateral subcostal incision. Frequently, this must be extended vertically in the midline to allow visualization of the inferior vena cava at the confluence of the hepatic veins. Raising a small skin flap in the midline and incising just the midline fascia can sometimes be done. This avoids the upper skin extension and allows a more cosmetic closure. A right thoracoabdominal incision is sometimes required in patients with large lesions that arise high in the right lobe with or without diaphragmatic invasion. This is a good approach as well if caval resection is planned because it facilitates control of the supradiaphragmatic vena cava and access to the right atrium. A left thoracoabdominal incision is rarely required.

Right and Extended Right Hepatic Lobectomy

Right hepatic resections are the most frequently performed (60%). After division of the suspensory ligaments, dissection is directed to the hilus where the hilar plate extending from the gallbladder is divided to expose the bifurcation of the hepatic artery and portal vein. The hepatic veins and the vascular structures at the hilum are examined, and a decision to go ahead with resection is made. If the tumor is resectable, it is best to ligate the right hepatic artery and the right portal vein at this point. This reduces flow through the right hepatic vein and facilitates its dissection. Attempts at early control of the hepatic vein before hilar vascular control can result in hepatic vein injury and hemorrhage. Placing the patient in the Trendelenburg position reduces pressure in the inferior vena cava and hepatic veins and minimizes the risk of air embolus. Figure 66–7 illustrates the margins of an extended right hepatic lobectomy. Only segments II and III and the caudate lobe (not shown) remain.

Next, unnamed hepatic veins that extend from the retrohepatic vena cava to the right hepatic lobe are ligated and divided. For large right-sided tumors, a large unnamed hepatic vein is found before the main right hepatic vein. Just below the right hepatic

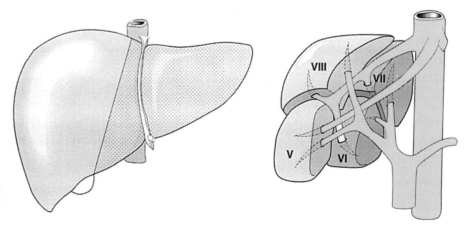

Figure 66–8. The margins of a left hepatic lobectomy. Segments V, VI, VII, and VIII remain.

vein, a ligamentous structure is encountered on the right side of the vena cava. After this is divided, the right hepatic vein is ligated. Essentially, a vascular isolation of the right lobe is carried out before division of the hepatic substance. The liver is divided with the hepatoduodenal ligament clamped (Pringle's maneuver). In an extended right hepatic lobectomy, the middle hepatic vein is ligated and all or a major part of segment IV is removed. Usually, the middle hepatic vein is suture ligated within the hepatic substance during transection. Elective hepatic resections do not usually need drainage.[161]

Left and Extended Left Hepatic Lobectomy

A left hepatic resection begins with ligamentous division as on the right. If the tumor is resectable, the first step is hilar ligation of the left hepatic artery and left branch of the portal vein. The left lobe is separated from the caudate by dissection through the sinus venosus. This facilitates identification of the left and middle hepatic veins, which usually form a common trunk. The liver is transected after extrahepatic vascular isolation of the resected segment and performance of a Pringle maneuver. In an extended left hepatectomy, all or most of segments V and VIII are removed. Figure 66–8 depicts the margins of a left hepatic lobectomy.

Hepatic Regeneration

In most patients, there is a rapid recovery to the normal volume for age.[162, 163] This occurs despite administration of postoperative chemotherapy.

REFERENCES

1. Bismuth H: Surgical anatomy of the liver. Recent Results Cancer Res 100:179–184, 1986.
2. Couinaud C: [Surgical anatomy of the liver. Several new aspects]. Chirurgie 112:337–342, 1986.
3. Couinaud C: [The anatomy of the liver]. Ann Ital Chir 63:693–697, 1992.
4. Martin LW, Woodman KS: Hepatic lobectomy for hepatoblastoma in infants and children. Arch Surg 98:1–7, 1969.
5. Holton CP, Burrington JD, Hatch EI: A multiple chemotherapeutic approach to the management of hepatoblastoma: A preliminary report. Cancer 35:1083–1087, 1975.
6. Ito J, Johnson WW: Hepatoblastoma and hepatoma in infancy and childhood: Light and electron microscopic studies. Arch Pathol 87:259–266, 1969.
7. Shafer AD, Selinkoff PM: Preoperative irradiation and chemotherapy for initially unresectable hepatoblastoma. J Pediatr Surg 12:1001–1007, 1977.
8. Fegiz G, Rosati D, Tonelli F, et al: A case report of hepatoblastoma treated by chemotherapy and hepatic lobectomy. World J Surg 1:407–414, 1977.
9. Exelby PR, Filler RM, Grosfeld JL: Liver tumors in children in the particular reference to hepatoblastoma and hepatocellular carcinoma: American Academy of Pediatrics Surgical Section Survey—1974. J Pediatr Surg 10:329–337, 1975.
10. Heimann A, White PF, Riely CA, et al: Hepatoblastoma presenting as isosexual precocity. The clinical importance of histologic and serologic parameters. J Clin Gastroenterol 9:105–110, 1987.
11. Tagge EP, Tagge DU, Reyes J, et al: Resection, including

12. transplantation, for hepatoblastoma and hepatocellular carcinoma: Impact on survival. J Pediatr Surg 27:292–296, 1992.
12. Finegold MJ: Tumors of the liver. Semin Liver Dis 14:270–281, 1994.
13. Mulliken JB: Diagnosis and natural history of hemangiomas. In Mulliken JB, Young AE (eds): Vascular Birthmarks: Hemangiomas and Malformations. Philadelphia, WB Saunders, 1988, pp 41–62.
14. Ehren H, Mahour GH, Isaacs H Jr: Benign liver tumors in infancy and childhood: Report of 48 cases. Am J Surg 145:325–329, 1983.
15. Ishak KG: Primary hepatic tumors in childhood. Prog Liver Dis 5:636–667, 1976.
16. Weinberg AG, Finegold MJ: Primary hepatic tumors of childhood. Hum Pathol 14:512–537, 1983.
17. Hobbs KE: Hepatic hemangiomas. World J Surg 14:468–471, 1990.
18. Powers C, Ros PR, Stoupis C, et al: Primary liver neoplasms: MR imaging with pathologic correlation. Radiographics 14:459–482, 1994.
19. de Lorimier AA, Simpson EB, Baum RS, et al: Hepatic-artery ligation for hepatic hemangiomatosis. N Engl J Med 277:333–337, 1967.
20. Takvorian P, Floret D, Valette PJ, et al: [Hepatic rupture after puncture biopsy: Value of embolization. Apropos of a case with hepatoblastoma]. Pediatrie (Bucur) 43:531–533, 1988.
21. Kitahara S, Makuuchi M, Ishizone S, et al: Successful left trisegmentectomy for ruptured hepatoblastoma using intraoperative transarterial embolization. J Pediatr Surg 30:1709–1712, 1995.
22. Schaller RT Jr, Schaller J, Morgan A, et al: Hemodilution anesthesia: A valuable aid to major cancer surgery in children. Am J Surg 146:79–84, 1983.
23. Schaller RT Jr, Schaller J, Furman EB: The advantages of hemodilution anesthesia for major liver resection in children. J Pediatr Surg 19:705–710, 1984.
24. Costello SA, Seywright M: Postirradiation malignant transformation in benign haemangioma. Eur J Surg Oncol 16:517–519, 1990.
25. Saito Y, Karasawa F, Kohno M, et al: [Anesthetic management and metabolic control of a patient with von Gierke's disease (glycogen storage disease type I) associated with hepatic adenoma. Masui 33:1395–1399, 1984.
26. Sakatoku H, Hirokawa Y, Inoue M, et al: Focal nodular hyperplasia in an adolescent with glycogen storage disease type I with mesocaval shunt operation in childhood: A case report and review of the literature. Acta Paediatr Jpn 38:172–175, 1996.
27. Scott LD, Katz AR, Duke JH, et al: Oral contraceptives, pregnancy, and focal nodular hyperplasia of the liver. JAMA 251:1461–1463, 1984.
28. Graf KJ, Meyer zum Buschenfelde KH: [Liver cell tumor induction by oral contraceptives]. Dtsch Med Wochenschr 105:61–65, 1980.
29. Fermand JP, Levy Y, Bouscary D, et al: Danazol-induced hepatocellular adenoma. Am J Med 88:529–530, 1990.
30. Foster JH, Berman MM: The malignant transformation of liver cell adenomas. Arch Surg 129:712–717, 1994.
31. Nagorney DM: Benign hepatic tumors: Focal nodular hyperplasia and hepatocellular adenoma. World J Surg 19:13–18, 1995.
32. Prasad VK, Aronson DC, Gerald WL, et al: Hepatic focal nodular hyperplasia in an infant antenatally exposed to steroids [letter]. Lancet 346:371, 1995.
33. Westaby D, Portmann B, Williams R: Androgen related primary hepatic tumors in non-Fanconi patients. Cancer 51:1947–1952, 1983.
34. Lack EE, Ornvold K: Focal nodular hyperplasia and hepatic adenoma: A review of eight cases in the pediatric age group. J Surg Oncol 33:129–135, 1986.
35. Dehner LP, Ewing SL, Sumner HW: Infantile mesenchymal hamartoma of the liver. Histologic and ultrastructural observations. Arch Pathol 99:379–382, 1975.
36. Okeda R: Mesenchymal hamartoma of the liver—an autopsy

case with serial sections and some comments on its pathogenesis. Acta Pathol Jpn 26:229–236, 1976.

37. Srouji MN, Chatten J, Schulman WM, et al: Mesenchymal hamartoma of the liver in infants. Cancer 42:2483–2489, 1978.

38. DeMaioribus CA, Lally KP, Sim K, et al: Mesenchymal hamartoma of the liver: A 35-year review. Arch Surg 125:598–600, 1990.

39. Hernandez-Siverio N, Gomez Culebras MA, Garcia Santos J, et al: [Solitary, non-parasitic hepatic cyst in childhood]. An Esp Pediatr 28:269–270, 1988.

40. Pul N, Pul M: Congenital solitary nonparasitic cyst of the liver in infancy and childhood. J Pediatr Gastroenterol Nutr 21:461–462, 1995.

41. Romer KH, Motsch H, Freitag J, et al: [Solitary non-parasitic liver cyst in childhood]. Zentralbl Chir 109:270–272, 1984.

42. Jones RS: Surgical management of non-parasitic liver cysts. In Blumgart LH (ed): Surgery of the Liver and Biliary Tract. London, Churchill Livingstone, 1994, pp 1211–1218.

43. Iwatsuki S, Todo S, Starzl TE: Excisional therapy for benign hepatic lesions. Surg Gynecol Obstet 171:240–246, 1990.

44. Marcellini M, Palumbo M, Caterino S, et al: Adult polycystic liver disease in childhood. A case report. Ital J Surg Sci 16:217–221, 1986.

45. De Rosa F, Teggi A: Treatment of *Echinococcus granulosus* hydatid disease with albendazole. Ann Trop Med Parasitol 84:467–472, 1990.

46. Sailer M, Soelder B, Allerberger F, et al: Alveolar echinococcosis of the liver in a six-year-old girl with acquired immunodeficiency syndrome. J Pediatr 130:320–323, 1997.

47. Suwan Z: Sonographic findings in hydatid disease of the liver: Comparison with other imaging methods. Ann Trop Med Parasitol 89:261–269, 1995.

48. Vara-Thorbeck R, Morales OI, Vara-Thorbeck C: [Echinococcosis of the liver: Its surgical treatment based on 178 personal cases]. Zentralbl Chir 111:188–195, 1986.

49. Khuroo MS, Wani NA, Javid G, et al: Percutaneous drainage compared with surgery for hepatic hydatid cysts. N Engl J Med 337:881–887, 1997.

50. Ni YH, Chang MH, Hsu HY, et al: Hepatocellular carcinoma in childhood. Clinical manifestations and prognosis. Cancer 68:1737–1741, 1997.

51. SEER Cancer Statistics Review, 1973–1992: Tables and Graphs. Bethesda, National Cancer Institute, 1995. NIH Publication Number 96-2789.

52. Lampkin BC, Wong KY, Kalinyak KA, et al: Solid malignancies in children and adolescents. Surg Clin North Am 65:1351–1386, 1985.

53. Leonard AS, Alyono D, Fischel RJ, et al: Role of the surgeon in the treatment of children's cancer. Surg Clin North Am 65:1387–422, 1985.

54. Fraumeni JF Jr, Rosen PJ, Hull EW, et al: Hepatoblastoma in infant sisters. Cancer 24:1086–1090, 1969.

55. Napoli VM, Campbell WG Jr: Hepatoblastoma in infant sister and brother. Cancer 39:2647–2650, 1977.

56. Ito E, Sato Y, Kawauchi K, et al: Type 1a glycogen storage disease with hepatoblastoma in siblings [published erratum appears in Cancer 60:723, 1987]. Cancer 59:1776–1780, 1987.

57. Surendran N, Radhakrishna K, Chellam VG: Hepatoblastoma in siblings. J Pediatr Surg 24:1169–1171, 1989.

58. Phillips M, Dicks-Mireaux C, Kingston J, et al: Hepatoblastoma and polyposis coli (familial adenomatous polyposis) [clinical conference]. Med Pediatr Oncol 17:441–447, 1989.

59. LeSher AR, Castronuovo JJ Jr, Filippone AL Jr: Hepatoblastoma in a patient with familial polyposis coli [see comments]. Surgery 105:668–670, 1989.

60. Giardiello FM, Petersen GM, Brensinger JD, et al: Hepatoblastoma and APC gene mutation in familial adenomatous polyposis. Gut 39:867–869, 1996.

61. Iwama T, Mishima Y: Mortality in young first-degree relatives of patients with familial adenomatous polyposis. Cancer 73:2065–2068, 1994.

62. Li FP, Thurber WA, Seddon J, et al: Hepatoblastoma in families with polyposis coli. JAMA 257:2475–2477, 1987.

63. Hartley AL, Birch JM, Kelsey AM, et al: Epidemiological and familial aspects of hepatoblastoma. Med Pediatr Oncol 18:103–109, 1990.

64. Krush AJ, Traboulsi EI, Offerhaus JA, et al: Hepatoblastoma, pigmented ocular fundus lesions and jaw lesions in Gardner syndrome. Am J Med Genet 29:323–332, 1988.

65. Tsai SY, Jeng YM, Hwu WL, et al: Hepatoblastoma in an infant with Beckwith-Wiedemann syndrome. J Formos Med Assoc 95:180–183, 1996.

66. Koishi S, Kubota M, Taniguchi Y, et al: Myelodysplasia in a child with Beckwith-Wiedemann syndrome previously treated for hepatoblastoma with multi-agent chemotherapy [letter]. J Pediatr Hematol Oncol 18:419–420, 1996.

67. Vaughan WG, Sanders DW, Grosfeld JL, et al: Favorable outcome in children with Beckwith-Wiedemann syndrome and intraabdominal malignant tumors. J Pediatr Surg 30:1042–1045, 1995.

68. Kosseff AL, Herrmann J, Gilbert EF, et al: Studies of malformation syndromes of man XXIX: The Wiedemann-Beckwith syndrome. Clinical, genetic and pathogenetic studies of 12 cases. Eur J Pediatr 123:139–166, 1976.

69. Ikeda H, Matsuyama S, Tanimura M: Association between hepatoblastoma and very low birth weight: A trend or a chance? [see comments]. J Pediatr 130:557–560, 1997.

70. Rao PS, Krishna A, Rohatgi M: Multicystic kidney in association with hepatoblastoma—a case report. Jpn J Surg 19:583–585, 1989.

71. Gonzalez-Crussi F, Upton MP, Maurer HS: Hepatoblastoma: Attempt at characterization of histologic subtypes. Am J Surg Pathol 6:599–612, 1982.

72. Lack EE, Neave C, Vawter GF: Hepatoblastoma: A clinical and pathologic study of 54 cases. Am J Surg Pathol 6:693–705, 1982.

73. von Schweinitz D, Schmidt D, Fuchs J, et al: Extramedullary hematopoiesis and intratumoral production of cytokines in childhood hepatoblastoma. Pediatr Res 38:555–563, 1995.

74. Alcantar VC: [Hepatoblastoma associated with osteosarcoma]. Rev Mex Pediatr 52:389–392, 1985.

75. Manchester KM, Warren DJ, Erlandson RA, et al: Establishment and characterization of a novel hepatoblastoma-derived cell line. J Pediatr Surg 30:553–558, 1995.

76. von Schweinitz D, Gluer S, Fuchs J, et al: [Hepatocyte growth factor in pediatric hepatoblastoma]. Langenbecks Arch Chir Suppl Kongressbd 114:37–40, 1997.

77. von Schweinitz D, Hadam MR, Welte K, et al: Production of interleukin-1 beta and interleukin-6 in hepatoblastoma. Int J Cancer 53:728–734, 1993.

78. Kraus JA, Albrecht S, Wiestler OD, et al: Loss of heterozygosity on chromosome 1 in human hepatoblastoma. Int J Cancer 67:467–471, 1996.

79. Albrecht S, von Schweinitz D, Waha A, et al: Loss of maternal alleles on chromosome arm 11p in hepatoblastoma. Cancer Res 54:5041–5044, 1994.

80. Stocker JT: Hepatoblastoma. Semin Diagn Pathol 11:136–143, 1994.

81. Swarts S, Wisecarver J, Bridge JA: Significance of extra copies of chromosome 20 and the long arm of chromosome 2 in hepatoblastoma. Cancer Genet Cytogenet 91:65–67, 1996.

82. Chen WJ, Lee JC, Hung WT: Primary malignant tumor of liver in infants and children in Taiwan. J Pediatr Surg 23:457–461, 1988.

83. Kuo CY, Liu HC, Chang MH, et al: Hepatoblastoma in infancy and childhood: A clinical and pathological study of 32 cases. Acta Paediatr Sin 32:79–87, 1991.

84. Brown BF, Drehner DM, Saldivar VA: Hepatoblastoma: A rare pediatric neoplasm. Mil Med 158:51–55, 1993.

85. Arshad RR, Woo SY, Abbassi V, et al: Virilizing hepatoblastoma: Precocious sexual development and partial response of pulmonary metastases to cis-platinum. CA Cancer J Clin 32:293–300, 1982.

86. Galifer RB, Sultan C, Margueritte G, et al: Testosterone-producing hepatoblastoma in a 3-year-old boy with precocious puberty. J Pediatr Surg 20:713–714, 1985.

87. McArthur JW, Toll GD, Russfield AB, et al: Sexual precocity

attributable to ectopic gonadotropin secretion by hepatoblastoma. Am J Med 54:390–403, 1973.

88. Van Tornout JM, Buckley JD, Quinn J, et al: Rate and magnitude of decline in alphafetoprotein (AFP) levels in treated children with unresectable or metastatic hepatoblastoma (HB) are indicators of outcome: A report from the Children's Cancer Group [abstract]. Proceedings of the Annual Meeting of the American Society of Clinical Oncology 12:A1408, 1993.

89. Alpert ME, Seeler RA: Alpha fetoprotein in embryonal hepatoblastoma. J Pediatr 77:1058–1060, 1970.

90. Pritchard J, Da Cunha A, Cornbleet MA, et al: Alpha feta (alpha FP) monitoring of response to Adriamycin in hepatoblastoma. J Pediatr Surg 17:429–430, 1982.

91. Heinrich UE, Bolkenius M, Daum R, et al: Virilizing hepatoblastoma—significance of alpha-1-fetoprotein and human chorionic gonadotropin as tumor markers in diagnosis and follow-up. Eur J Pediatr 135:313–317, 1981.

92. Ortega JA, Krailo MD, Haas JE, et al: Effective treatment of unresectable or metastatic hepatoblastoma with cisplatin and continuous infusion doxorubicin chemotherapy: A report from the Children's Cancer Study Group. J Clin Oncol 9:2167–2176, 1991.

93. Tsuchida Y, Terada M, Honna T, et al: The role of subfractionation of alpha-fetoprotein in the treatment of pediatric surgical patients. J Pediatr Surg 32:514–517, 1997.

94. Saraswathi A, Malati T: Clinical relevance of alphafetoprotein microheterogeneity in alphafetoprotein-secreting tumors. Cancer Detect Prev 18:447–454, 1994.

95. Van Tornout JM, Buckley JD, Quinn JJ, et al: Timing and magnitude of decline in alpha-fetoprotein levels in treated children with unresectable or metastatic hepatoblastoma are predictors of outcome: A report from the Children's Cancer Group. J Clin Oncol 15:1190–1197, 1997.

96. Walhof CM, Van Sonderen L, Voute PA, et al: Half-life of alpha-fetoprotein in patients with a teratoma, endodermal sinus tumor, or hepatoblastoma. Pediatr Hematol Oncol 5:217–227, 1988.

97. von Schweinitz D, Hecker H, Harms D, et al: Complete resection before development of drug resistance is essential for survival from advanced hepatoblastoma—a report from the German cooperative pediatric liver tumor study hb-89. J Pediatr Surg 30:845–852, 1995.

98. von Schweinitz D, Wischmeyer P, Leuschner I, et al: Clinico-pathological criteria with prognostic relevance in hepatoblastoma. Eur J Cancer 30A:1052–1058, 1994.

99. Tsunoda Y, Okamatsu T, Iijima T, et al: Non-alpha-fetoprotein-producing anaplastic hepatoblastoma cell line [letter]. In Vitro Cell Dev Biol Anim 32:194–196, 1996.

100. Brower ST, Hoff PM, Jones DV, et al: Pancreatic cancer, hepatobiliary cancer, and neuroendocrine cancers of the GI tract. In Pazdur R, Coia LR, Hoskins WJ, Wagman LD (eds): Cancer Management: A Multidisciplinary Approach. Huntington, NY, PRR, 1998, pp 113–148.

101. Douglass EC, Reynolds M, Finegold M, et al: Cisplatin (DDP)/vincristine (VCR)/5-fluorouracil (5FU) therapy for hepatoblastoma: A Pediatric Oncology Group (POG) study [meeting abstract]. Proceedings of the Annual Meeting of the American Society of Clinical Oncology 10:A1075, 1991.

102. Staines A, Cullen S, Guiney EJ, et al: Combination chemotherapy in the treatment of hepatoblastoma. Pediatr Hematol Oncol 7:205–207, 1990.

103. Langevin AM, Pierro A, Liu P, et al: Adriamycin and cisplatinum administered by continuous infusion preoperatively in hepatoblastoma unresectable at presentation. Med Pediatr Oncol 18:181–184, 1990.

104. Gauthier F, Valayer J, Thai BL, et al: Hepatoblastoma and hepatocarcinoma in children: Analysis of a series of 29 cases. J Pediatr Surg 21:424–429, 1986.

105. Quinn JJ, Altman AJ, Robinson HT, et al: Adriamycin and cisplatin for hepatoblastoma. Cancer 56:1926–1929, 1985.

106. von Schweinitz D, Hecker H, Harms D, et al: Complete resection before development of drug resistance is essential for survival from advanced hepatoblastoma—a report from the German Cooperative Pediatric Liver Tumor Study HB-89. J Pediatr Surg 30:845–852, 1995.

107. von Schweinitz D, Burger D, Bode U, et al: [Results of the HB-89 Study in treatment of malignant epithelial liver tumors in childhood and concept of a new HB-94 protocol]. Klin Padiatr 206:282–288, 1994.

108. Douglass EC, Reynolds M, Finegold M, et al: Cisplatin, vincristine, and fluorouracil therapy for hepatoblastoma: A Pediatric Oncology Group study. J Clin Oncol 11:96–99, 1993.

109. von Schweinitz D, Byrd DJ, Hecker H, et al: Efficiency and toxicity of ifosfamide, cisplatin and doxorubicin in the treatment of childhood hepatoblastoma. Study Committee of the Cooperative Paediatric Liver Tumour Study HB89 of the German Society for Paediatric Oncology and Haematology. Eur J Cancer 33:1243–1249, 1997.

110. Ortega JA, Krailo MD, Haase GE, et al: Effective treatment of unresectable or metastatic hepatoblastoma with cisplatin and continuous infusion doxorubicin chemotherapy: A report from the Children's Cancer Study Group. J Clin Oncol 9:2167–2176, 1991.

111. Reynolds M: Conversion of unresectable to resectable hepatoblastoma and long-term follow-up study. World J Surg 19:814–816, 1995.

112. Rivilla Parra F, Gamez Arance M, Fernandez Sanchez A, et al: [Surgery of lung metastasis in childhood]. Cir Pediatr 2:58–60, 1989.

113. Black CT, Luck SR, Musemeche CA, et al: Aggressive excision of pulmonary metastases is warranted in the management of childhood hepatic tumors. J Pediatr Surg 26:1082–1086, 1991.

114. Passmore SJ, Noblett HR, Wisheart JD, et al: Prolonged survival following multiple thoracotomies for metastatic hepatoblastoma. Med Pediatr Oncol 24:58–60, 1995.

115. Habrand JL, Nehme D, Kalifa C, et al: Is there a place for radiation therapy in the management of hepatoblastomas and hepatocellular carcinomas in children? [see comments]. Int J Radiat Oncol Biol Phys 23:525–531, 1992.

116. von Schweinitz D, Hecker H, Schmidt-von-Arndt G, et al: Prognostic factors and staging systems in childhood hepatoblastoma. Int J Cancer 74:593–599, 1997.

117. Koneru B, Flye MW, Busuttil RW, et al: Liver transplantation for hepatoblastoma. The American experience. Ann Surg 213:118–121, 1991.

118. Barton JW, Keller MS: Liver transplantation for hepatoblastoma in a child with congenital absence of the portal vein. Pediatr Radiol 20:113–114, 1989.

119. Achilleos OA, Buist LJ, Kelly DA, et al: Unresectable hepatic tumors in childhood and the role of liver transplantation. J Pediatr Surg 31:1563–1567, 1996.

120. Superina R, Bilik R: Results of liver transplantation in children with unresectable liver tumors. J Pediatr Surg 31:835–839, 1996.

121. Malogolowkin MH, Stanley P, Daniels J, Ortega JA: Chemoembolization (CE) for progressive hepatoblastoma (HB) in children [meeting abstract]. Proc Annu Meet Am Soc Clin Oncol 12:A1450, 1993.

122. Berthold F, Schultheis KH, Aigner K, et al: [Combination chemotherapy and chemoembolization in the treatment of primary inoperable hepatoblastoma]. Klin Padiatr 198:257–261, 1986.

123. Clouse ME, Perry L, Stuart K, et al: Hepatic arterial chemoembolization for metastatic neuroendocrine tumors. Digestion 55(suppl 3):92–97, 1994.

124. Order SE, Siegel JA, Principato R, et al: Preliminary experience of infusional brachytherapy using colloidal 32P. Ann Acad Med Singapore 25:347–351, 1996.

125. Maini CL, Scelsa MG, Fiumara C, et al: Superselective intra-arterial radiometabolic therapy with I-131 Lipiodol in hepatocellular carcinoma. Clin Nucl Med 21:221–226, 1996.

126. Primary liver cancer in Japan: Sixth report. The Liver Cancer Study Group of Japan. Cancer 60:1400–1411, 1987.

127. Chang MH, Chen CJ, Lai MS, et al: Universal hepatitis B vaccination in Taiwan and the incidence of hepatocellular carcinoma in children. Taiwan Childhood Hepatoma Study Group [see comments]. N Engl J Med 336:1855–1859, 1997.

128. Moore L, Bourne AJ, Moore DJ, et al: Hepatocellular carci-

noma following neonatal hepatitis. Pediatr Pathol Lab Med 17:601–610, 1997.

129. Wegmann W, Evison J, Schaub N, et al: [Liver cell carcinoma as a late complication of Alagille syndrome (arteriohepatic dysplasia)]. Leber Magen Darm 26:157–158, 161–163, 1996.

130. Toyosaka A, Okamoto E, Mitsunobu M, et al: Pathologic and radiographic studies of intrahepatic metastasis in hepatocellular carcinoma; the role of efferent vessels. HPB Surg 10:97–103, 1996.

131. Greenberg M, Filler RM: Hepatic tumors. In Pizzo PA, Poplack DG (eds): Principles and Practice of Pediatric Oncology. Philadelphia, JB Lippincott, 1989, pp 697–711.

132. Terris B, Ingster O, Rubbia L, et al: Interphase cytogenetic analysis reveals numerical chromosome aberrations in large liver cell dysplasia. J Hepatol 27:313–319, 1997.

133. Lowichik A, Schneider NR, Tonk V, et al: Report of a complex karyotype in recurrent metastatic fibrolamellar hepatocellular carcinoma and a review of hepatocellular carcinoma cytogenetics. Cancer Genet Cytogenet 88:170–174, 1996.

134. Bower M, Newlands ES, Habib N: Fibrolamellar hepatocellular carcinoma responsive to platinum-based combination chemotherapy. Clin Oncol (R Coll Radiol) 8:331–333, 1996.

135. Takayasu K, Moriyama N, Muramatsu Y, et al: Hepatic arterial embolization for hepatocellular carcinoma. Comparison of CT scans and resected specimens. Radiology 150:661–665, 1984.

136. Ryu M, Shimamura Y, Kinoshita T, et al: Therapeutic results of resection, transcatheter arterial embolization and percutaneous transhepatic ethanol injection in 3225 patients with hepatocellular carcinoma: A retrospective multicenter study. Jpn J Clin Oncol 27:251–257, 1997.

137. Crews KA, Kuhn JA, McCarty TM, et al: Cryosurgical ablation of hepatic tumors. Am J Surg 174:614–618, 1997.

138. Ravikumar TS: The role of cryotherapy in the management of patients with liver tumors. Adv Surg 30:281–291, 1996.

139. Ehrlich PF, Greenberg ML, Filler RM: Improved long-term survival with preoperative chemotherapy for hepatoblastoma. J Pediatr Surg 32:999–1002, 1997.

140. Stringer MD, Hennayake S, Howard ER, et al: Improved outcome for children with hepatoblastoma. Br J Surg 82:386–391, 1995.

141. Hata Y: The clinical features and prognosis of hepatoblastoma: Follow-up studies done on pediatric tumors enrolled in the Japanese pediatric tumor registry between 1971 and 1980, part I: Committee of Malignant Tumors, Japanese Society of Pediatric Surgeons. Jpn J Surg 20:498–502, 1990.

142. Moore SW, Hesseling PB, Wessels G, et al: Hepatocellular carcinoma in children. Pediatr Surg Int 12:266–270, 1997.

143. Weitman S, Ochoa S, Sullivan J, et al: Pediatric phase II cancer chemotherapy trials: A Pediatric Oncology Group study. J Pediatr Hematol Oncol 19:187–191, 1997.

144. Karpoff HM, D'Angelica M, Blair S, et al: Prevention of hepatic tumor metastases in rats with herpes viral vaccines and gamma-interferon. J Clin Invest 99:799–804, 1997.

145. Ruymann FB, Raney RB Jr, Crist WM, et al: Rhabdomyosarcoma of the biliary tree in childhood. A report from the Intergroup Rhabdomyosarcoma Study. Cancer 56:575–581, 1985.

146. Lack EE, Perez-Atayde AR, Schuster SR: Botryoid rhabdomyosarcoma of the biliary tract. Am J Surg Pathol 5:643–652, 1981.

147. Nagaraj HS, Kmetz DR, Leitner C: Rhabdomyosarcoma of the bile ducts. J Pediatr Surg 12:1071–1074, 1977.

148. Friedburg H, Kauffmann GW, Bohm N, et al: Sonographic and computed tomographic features of embryonal rhabdomyosarcoma of the biliary tract. Pediatr Radiol 14:436–438, 1984.

149. Geoffray A, Couanet D, Montagne JP, et al: Ultrasonography and computed tomography for diagnosis and follow-up of biliary duct rhabdomyosarcomas in children. Pediatr Radiol 17:127–131, 1987.

150. Martinez-F LA, Haase GM, Koep LJ, et al: Rhabdomyosarcoma of the biliary tree: The case for aggressive surgery. J Pediatr Surg 17:508–511, 1982.

151. Flemming P, Lang H, Georgii A: [Mesenchymal tumors of the liver: Their frequency and histopathological diagnostic problems in surgical investigations]. Verh Dtsch Ges Pathol 79:116–119, 1995.

152. Newman KD, Schisgall R, Reaman G, et al: Malignant mesenchymoma of the liver in children [see comments]. J Pediatr Surg 24:781–783, 1989.

153. Vetter D, Bellocq JP, Amaral D, et al: [Hepatic undifferentiated (or embryonal) sarcoma. Diagnostic and therapeutic problems apropos of botryoid rhabdomyosarcoma]. Gastroenterol Clin Biol 13:98–103, 1989.

154. Ros PR, Olmsted WW, Dachman AH, et al: Undifferentiated (embryonal) sarcoma of the liver: Radiologic-pathologic correlation. Radiology 161:141–145, 1986.

155. Orozco H, Mercado MA, Takahashi T, et al: [Undifferentiated (embryonal) sarcoma of the liver: Report of a case]. Rev Invest Clin 43:255–258, 1991.

156. Tozzi MC, Tarani L, Di Nardo R, et al: The hepatic malignant mesenchymoma: A case report. Eur J Pediatr 151:488–491, 1992.

157. Gallivan MV, Lack EE, Chun B, et al: Undifferentiated ("embryonal") sarcoma of the liver: Ultrastructure of a case presenting as a primary intracardiac tumor. Pediatr Pathol 1:291–300, 1983.

158. Kadomatsu K, Nakagawara A, Zaizen Y, et al: Undifferentiated (embryonal) sarcoma of the liver: Report of three cases. Surg Today 22:451–455, 1992.

159. Ross JS, Del Rosario A, Bui HX, et al: Primary hepatic leiomyosarcoma in a child with the acquired immunodeficiency syndrome. Hum Pathol 23:69–72, 1992.

160. Norton KI, Godine LB, Lempert C: Leiomyosarcoma of the kidney in an HIV-infected child. Pediatr Radiol 27:557–558, 1997.

161. Fong Y, Brennan MF, Brown K, et al: Drainage is unnecessary after elective liver resection. Am J Surg 171:158–162, 1997.

162. Wheatley JM, Rosenfield NS, Berger L, LaQuaglia MP: Liver regeneration in children after major hepatectomy for malignancy—evaluation using a computer-aided technique of volume measurement. J Surg Res 61:183–189, 1996.

163. Shamberger RC, Leichtner AM, Jonas MM, et al: Long-term hepatic regeneration and function in infants and children following liver resection. J Am Coll Surg 182:515–519, 1996.

67

TERATOMAS, DERMOIDS, AND OTHER SOFT TISSUE TUMORS

Jean-Martin Laberge, MD, FRCSC •
Luong T. Nguyen, MD, FRCSC •
Kenneth S. Shaw, MD, FRCSC

☐ Teratomas

Teratomas are generally divided into gonadal and extragonadal. This chapter focuses on extragonadal locations, the most common being sacrococcygeal.

EMBRYOLOGY AND PATHOLOGY

Teratoma, from the Greek *teratos* ("monster") and *onkoma* ("swelling"), is a term first applied by Virchow in 1869 to "sacrococcygeal growths."[1] Teratomas are composed of multiple tissues foreign to the organ or site in which they arise.[2] Although teratomas are sometimes defined as having the three embryonic layers (endoderm, mesoderm, and ectoderm), recent classifications include monodermal types.[2, 3]

Teratomas are thought by some to arise from totipotent primordial germ cells.[3, 4] These cells develop among the endodermal cells of the yolk sac near the origin of the allantois and migrate to the gonadal ridges during the 4th and 5th weeks of gestation (Fig. 67–1).[5] Some cells may miss their target destination and give rise to a teratoma anywhere from the brain to the coccygeal area, usually on the midline. Another theory has teratomas arising from remnants of the primitive streak or primitive node.[5–7] During the 3rd week of development, midline cells at the caudal end of the embryo divide rapidly and, in a process called *gastrulation,* give rise to all three germ layers of the embryo (Fig. 67–2).[5] By the end of the 3rd week, the primitive streak shortens and disappears. This theory would explain the more common occurrence of teratomas in the sacrococcygeal region. By either theory, the totipotent cells could give rise to monoclonal neoplasms. Recent evidence shows that whereas immature teratomas may be monoclonal, mature teratomas can be polyclonal, hence more like a hamartoma than a neoplasm.[8] This finding is compatible with a third theory, that teratomas are a form of incomplete twinning.[2, 3]

The primordial germ cell is the principal but possibly not the exclusive progenitor of a teratoma.[2] The recent trend is to include teratomas under the classification of germ cell tumors.[2–4] This histologic classification also includes germinomas (alias dysgerminomas), embryonal carcinomas, yolk sac tumors, choriocarcinomas, gonadoblastomas, and mixed germ cell tumors. Gonadal and extragonadal teratomas may have a different origin, explaining the different behavior according to tumor site.

Teratomas are fascinating tumors owing to the diversity of tissues they may contain and the varying degree of organization of these tissues. Many tumors contain skin elements, neural tissue, teeth, fat, cartilage, and intestinal mucosa, often with normal ganglion cells. These tissues are usually present as disorganized islands of cells with cystic spaces. Tumor sometimes consists of more organized tissue, such as small bowel, limbs, and even a beating heart; these have been called *fetiform teratomas* (Fig. 67–3).[2, 3, 6, 9, 10] When the mass includes vertebrae or notochord and a high degree of structural organization, the term *fetus in fetu* is used; this is viewed by some as a variant of conjoint twinning but is classified as a teratoma by others owing to the absence of a recognizable umbilical cord in its vascular pedicle.[3, 11] Whether teratomas are at one end of a spectrum that includes fetus in fetu, parasitic twins, conjoined twins, and normal twins is the subject of controversy.[3] One certainly cannot dismiss the many reports of teratomas associated with fetus in fetu in the same patient and with a twin pregnancy.[2, 3, 12–14]

Not only is the overall tissue architecture variable in teratomas but also there is a spectrum of cellular differentiation. Most benign teratomas are composed of mature cells, but 20 to 25% also contain

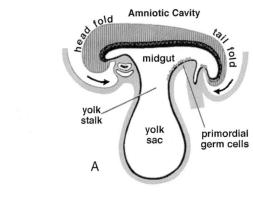

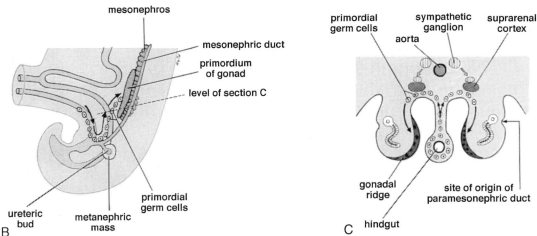

Figure 67–1. Commonly cited theory on the origin of teratomas. *A,* Drawing of embryo during the 4th week (longitudinal section), showing primordial germ cells at the base of the yolk sac. *B* and *C,* During the 5th week, these cells migrate toward the gonadal ridges. According to this theory, some cells could miss their intended destination. (Modified from Moore KL, Persaud TVN: The Developing Human. Philadelphia, WB Saunders, 1993, pp 71, 181.)

immature elements, most often neuroepithelium.[2–4] The degree of histologic immaturity is of proven prognostic significance only in ovarian teratomas.[3, 15] Immature tissue is considered normal and without any influence on prognosis in neonatal teratoma.[2, 6] In fact, spontaneous maturation of malignant tumors has been reported after partial excision of giant sacrococcygeal teratomas in two fetuses at 23 and 27 weeks' gestation.[16]

Teratomas may also contain or develop foci of malignancy, or a pure malignant germ cell tumor may be found in sites typical for teratomas, such as the mediastinum or sacrococcygeal area. Whether the lesion was malignant from the onset or the malignant cells destroyed and replaced the benign teratoma component is difficult to ascertain. The most common malignant component of a teratoma is the yolk sac tumor, also called *endodermal sinus tumor.* Other malignant germ cell tumors can occur, and, rarely, malignancy of other tissues composing the teratoma, such as neuroblastoma,[17] squamous cell carcinoma,[18] carcinoid,[19] and others, occurs. Malignancy at birth is uncommon but increases with age and with incomplete resection. An apparently mature teratoma may recur several months or years after resection as a malignant yolk sac tumor, illus-

trating the difficulties in histologic sampling of large tumors and the need for close follow-up.[2, 3]

Most yolk sac tumors and some embryonal carcinomas secrete alphafetoprotein (AFP), which can be measured in the serum and demonstrated in the cells by immunohistochemistry.[20] This marker is particularly useful to assess the presence of residual or recurrent disease. Levels are normally very high in neonates and decrease with time.[20, 21] The postoperative half-life is about 6 days. Persistently high levels may be an indication for further surgery or chemotherapy. Other markers that may be elevated are β-human chorionic gonadotropin (β-hCG), produced by choriocarcinomas, and rarely, carcinoembryonic antigen. Secretion of β-hCG by the tumor may be sufficient to cause precocious puberty.[22]

The genetic basis of teratomas is not yet understood. Most germ cell tumors appear to have an amplification, or isochromosome, in a region of the short arm of chromosome 12, designated i (12p).[3, 4, 23] This has been well described in adults but was not confirmed in one pediatric series, in which deletions on chromosomes 1 and 6 were found instead.[24] Oncogenes and tumor-suppressor genes did not appear to correlate with prognosis in one study,[25] whereas N-myc gene amplification was present in

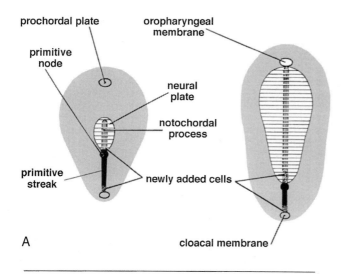

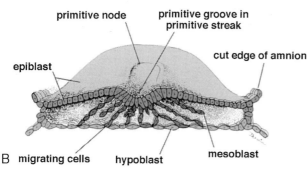

A

B migrating cells   hypoblast   mesoblast

Figure 67–2. Alternate theory on embryogenesis of teratomas. *A*, Sketches of dorsal views of the embryonic disk on days 17 and 18 showing the primitive streak and primitive node. *B*, Drawing of a transverse cut of the embryonic disk during the 3rd week. This shows that cells from the primitive streak migrate to form mesoblast (the origin of all mesenchymal tissues) and also displace the hypoblast to form the endoderm. Hence, remnants of these pluripotent primitive streak cells could give rise to teratomas and could account for the more frequent sacrococcygeal location. (From Moore KL, Persaud TVN: The Developing Human. Philadelphia, WB Saunders, 1993, pp 55–56.)

immature teratomas but absent in mature teratomas in another report.[26] The clinical usefulness of these findings remains to be determined.

ASSOCIATED ANOMALIES

Teratomas are usually isolated lesions. A well-recognized association is the triad of anorectal malformation, sacral anomaly, and a presacral mass.[27, 28] The presacral mass is usually a teratoma or an anterior meningocele, but duplication cysts and dermoid cysts have been described, as have combinations of these lesions.

An extensive review of the English and German literature published in 1989[29] found 51 cases and highlighted important facts. Twenty percent of patients are older than 12 years at the time of diagnosis, yet there are no reports of malignancy, in contrast with a 75% malignancy rate in patients older than 1 year who have the usual sacrococcygeal teratomas.[30] The female preponderance is only 1.5:1,

less than the 3:1 ratio noted in isolated sacrococcygeal teratomas. The familial predisposition, first recognized in 1974,[31] is noted in 57% of the cases; the inheritance is autosomal dominant. Although all variants of anorectal malformations have been described, by far the most common is anal or anorectal stenosis. In a recent report, this triad was present in 38% of all patients with anorectal stenosis and in 1.6% of patients with low imperforate anus.[32] Anal anomalies have also been reported in the absence of sacral defects. Hirschsprung's disease has been wrongly diagnosed in some cases,[4, 33, 34] indicating the need to eliminate the presence of a presacral mass by digital rectal examination, by a metal sound when the anus is too tight, or by imaging techniques.

Urogenital anomalies, such as hypospadias, vesicoureteral reflux, and vaginal or uterine duplications are other anomalies associated with teratomas.[29, 30, 35] Congenital dislocation of the hip was seen in 7% of patients with sacrococcygeal teratomas in one report, which also drew attention to vertebral anomalies and late orthopedic sequelae (see Fig. 67–3).[36] Central nervous system lesions, such as anencephaly, trigonocephaly, Dandy-Walker malformations, spina bifida, and myelomeningocele, may occur.[2, 3, 37–39] Another peculiar association with sacrococcygeal teratomas is a family history of twins in as many as 10% of the patients.[31, 40, 41] Although not confirmed in all series, this finding, combined with reports of simultaneous twin pregnancy or sequential familial occurrences of fetus in fetu and teratoma, supports the theory that teratomas are just one end of the spectrum of conjoint twinning.[2, 3, 10, 12, 14]

Klinefelter's syndrome is strongly associated with mediastinal teratoma[42] and has been reported in patients with intracranial[43] or retroperitoneal tumors.[44] It is estimated that 8% of male patients with primary mediastinal germ cell tumors have Klinefelter's syndrome, 50 times the expected frequency.[42] These tumors are often malignant, are the choriocarcinoma type, secrete β-hCG, and produce precocious puberty. Histiocytosis is also associated with mediastinal teratoma, both with[45, 46] and without Klinefelter's syndrome.[47] Other hematologic malignancies, such as acute leukemias[48, 49] and Hodgkin's disease,[50] occur rarely.

The following rare associations were reported, most often with nonsacrococcygeal lesions: trisomy 13,[51] trisomy 21, Morgagni's hernia,[52] congenital heart defects,[37, 39] Beckwith-Wiedemann syndrome,[53] pterygium,[54] cleft lip and palate,[37] and rare syndromes, such as Proteus[55] and Schinzel-Giedion syndromes.[56] The malformations listed do not include those caused by a mass effect from the teratoma itself.

DIAGNOSIS AND MANAGEMENT BY TUMOR SITE

Sacrococcygeal Teratoma

Sacrococcygeal tumors account for 35 to 60% of teratomas (gonadal included) in large series (Table

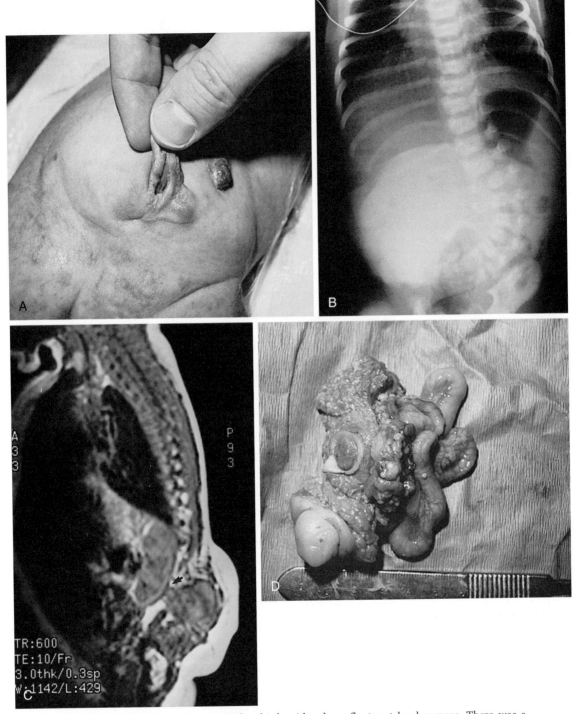

Figure 67–3. *A,* This child presented at birth with a large fluctuant lumbar mass. There was a family history of myelomeningocele in a great aunt. She also had an atrophic right leg with neurologic impairment below the L3 root and clubbing of the right foot. Note the ulcerated, arachnoid-looking area cranially and the pedunculated skin caudally, which had the appearance of a vulva and was oozing serous fluid. *B,* Plain radiographs showed a severe lumbosacral scoliosis with vertebral anomalies. Computed tomography confirmed the vertebral anomalies with spina bifida and demonstrated a pattern of intestine with inspissated or calcified meconium in the teratoma. *C,* Magnetic resonance imaging revealed that the mass extended into the retroperitoneum, where it was contiguous with the lower pole of the right kidney *(arrow). D,* At operation, normal-looking blind bowel loops were found deep to the vulva-like structure. Part of the mass extended along the spinal cord, which required dissection and untethering by the neurosurgeon. The pathologic diagnosis was a mature fetiform teratoma that contained, among many other things, two adrenals, two ovaries, renal tissue with some glomeruli and tubules, bone with bone marrow, and portions of stomach and small and large bowel. The child recovered well neurologically but required spinal instrumentation owing to progressive scoliosis at 2 years of age.

TABLE 67-1. Relative Frequency
of Teratomas by Site*

Site	No. of Cases (%)
Sacrococcygeal	290 (45)
Gonadal Ovary	176 (27)
Testis	31 (5)
Mediastinal	41 (6)
Central nervous system	30 (5)
Retroperitoneal	28 (4)
Cervical	20 (3)
Head	20 (3)
Gastric	3 (<1)
Hepatic	2 (<1)
Pericardial	1 (<1)
Umbilical cord	1 (<1)
Total	**643 (100)**

*Data are from five series of teratomas in children.
Modified from Dehner LP: Gonadal and extragonadal germ cell neoplasms: Teratomas in childhood. In Finegold M (ed): Pathology of Neoplasia in Children and Adolescents. Philadelphia, WB Saunders, 1986.

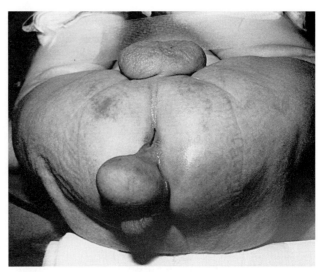

Figure 67–5. This patient presented at birth with a scrotum-like perianal mass with anal stenosis. An anoplasty was done with removal of the mass, which was not attached to the coccyx. Pathology showed only fibro-adipose tissue with smooth muscle, vascular structures, and cartilage, consistent with a hamartomatous process or caudal vestige (also called *tail remnant*).

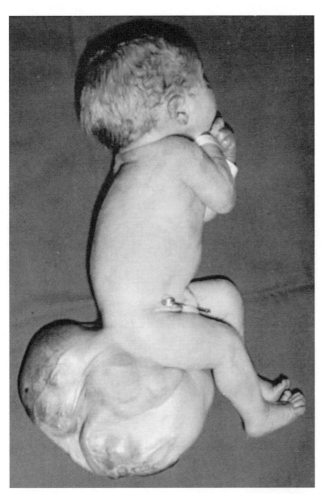

Figure 67–4. Infant with large sacrococcygeal teratoma. The infant and attached teratoma weighed 2363 g. The teratoma weighed 675 g. After surgical excision of the tumor, the infant weighed 1688 g. The external size of such a teratoma is not a deterrent to surgical excision because the attachment in large and small teratomas is similar.

67–1).[57–59] This is the most common tumor in the newborn, even when stillbirths are considered.[37] The estimated incidence is 1 per 35,000 to 40,000 live births.[3, 4]

Diagnosis

Most sacrococcygeal teratomas present a visible mass at birth, making the diagnosis obvious (Fig. 67–4). There is an unexplained female preponderance of 3:1.[30, 57] The main differential diagnosis is meningocele. Typically, meningoceles occur proximal to the sacrum and are covered by dura, but sometimes they are covered by skin. Examination of the child reveals bulging of the fontanelle on gentle pressure of a sacral meningocele, helping to establish the diagnosis before plain radiographs, ultrasonography (US), and magnetic resonance imaging (MRI) confirm it. The coexistence of meningocele with teratoma is well recognized in the familial form, but these are usually presacral. Rarely, a typical exophytic teratoma may have an intradural extension.[60] Other lesions in the differential diagnosis of neonatal sacrococcygeal masses include lymphangiomas, lipomas, tail-like remnants (Fig. 67–5), meconium pseudocysts, and several other rare conditions.[30, 61]

Although many neonates with sacrococcygeal teratomas do not have symptoms, some require intensive care due to prematurity, high-output cardiac failure, disseminated intravascular coagulation,[62] and bleeding within the tumor. Lesions with a large intrapelvic component may cause urinary obstruction. Besides looking for signs of a myelomeningocele, the physical examination always includes a rectal examination to evaluate any intrapelvic component. Imaging studies consist of plain anteroposterior and lateral radiographs of the pelvis and spine, looking for calcifications in the tumor and for spinal defects, and US of the abdomen, pelvis, and spine. Further preoperative studies are unnecessary in most newborns.

Diagnosis of purely intrapelvic teratomas is often delayed.[30] Children may present with constipation, urinary retention, an abdominal mass, or symptoms of malignancy, such as failure to thrive. Age is not a predictor of malignancy in teratomas at sites other than testicular, mediastinal, and sacrococcygeal.[2] The risk of malignancy is less than 10% at birth but more than 75% after 1 year of age for sacrococcygeal tumors, with the exception of familial presacral teratomas. The risk of malignancy is also high for incompletely excised lesions. Complete excision of the tumor should be carried out as soon as the neonate is stable enough to undergo the procedure. Serum markers should be drawn preoperatively for later comparison.

The diagnosis is often made on prenatal US, especially when this examination is routinely performed in the second trimester. The site of the lesion, its complex appearance, and intrapelvic extension with or without urinary tract obstruction are easily recognized. Most teratomas do not adversely affect the fetus or fetal life.

Repeated US assessment of tumor size is important because the fetus should be delivered by cesarean section if the tumor is larger than 5 cm or larger than the fetal diameter (Fig. 67–6).[63] Dystocia during vaginal delivery is associated with tumor rupture and hemorrhage and is an avoidable obstetric nightmare. The options in managing unexpected cases with dystocia include emergency cesarean completion of the partially delivered fetus, which has been intubated and ventilated after vaginal presentation of the head.[63]

Polyhydramnios with larger tumors may lead to premature labor. Tumors that are larger than the fetal biparietal diameter at diagnosis or that grow faster than the fetus are associated with a poor prognosis.[64] As the tumor gets extremely large, the fetus may develop placentomegaly or hydrops. This is a harbinger of impending fetal demise and should lead to urgent cesarean delivery. Open fetal surgery has been performed in three cases considered too premature to deliver,[63, 65] although others have reported survival after emergency delivery as early as 26 weeks' gestation.[66] Successful intrauterine endoscopic laser ablation was reported in one case.[67]

Operative Procedure

Adequate intravenous access and availability of blood products should be ascertained before starting the operation, especially with large tumors.

For most tumors, the major component of which is extrapelvic, the patient is placed in the prone position. If there is a significant intrapelvic or intraabdominal component, it may be wise to begin with a laparotomy. In our experience, most resections can be achieved completely in the prone position, especially if the internal portion is cystic. A safe approach when in doubt is to prepare the skin from the lower chest down to the toes, allowing the infant to be turned to the supine position without having to redrape. Vaseline packing in the rectum

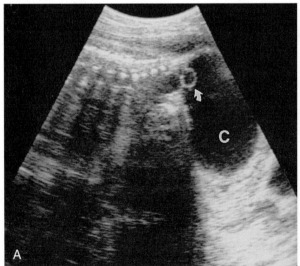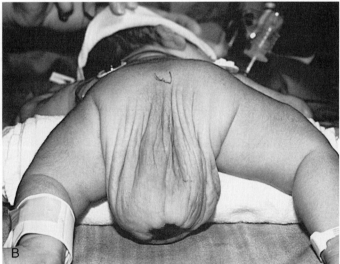

Figure 67–6. *A,* Ultrasound of a female fetus at 38 weeks' gestation, showing a large cystic mass (C) attached to the coccyx with tiny cysts anterior to the sacrum *(arrow).* An ultrasound at 18 weeks was normal. The cyst was gradually enlarging from an initial diameter of 9.5 cm at 31 weeks' gestation. The cyst was aspirated for 650 ml of fluid, permitting external version from breech to vertex. Two days later, when labor was induced, another 200 ml of fluid was removed to permit an uncomplicated vaginal delivery. *B,* Twenty-four hours postnatally, the lesion remained floppy with an area of skin ulceration, likely a consequence of excessive in utero distention. A mature cystic teratoma tissue confirmed histologically.

facilitates its identification throughout the procedure (Fig. 67–7). En bloc excision, including the coccyx, is preferable. Failure to remove the coccyx is associated with a high recurrence rate.[2–4] An acceptable gluteal crease and perineum is formed by the appropriate positioning of the perianal musculature.

Although the chevron incision has been used by most surgeons, a vertical incision leaves a nearly normal-looking median raphe (Fig. 67–8). Resection of the excess skin at the closure gives the best cosmetic result.

Several techniques have been described to help in the management of giant teratomas. These include intraoperative snaring of the aorta,[68] the use of extracorporeal membrane oxygenation and hypothermic perfusion,[69] and devascularization and staged resection.[66]

Prognosis

Fetuses with tumors diagnosed in utero have a survival rate in excess of 90% if the tumors are small and discovered by routine US. If a complicated pregnancy is the indication for US, the mortality rises to 60%. Nearly 100% of patients die when hydrops or placentomegaly occurs.[63] Dystocia or tumor rupture during delivery are probably underreported as a cause of mortality. In one series, 10% of patients died during transfer, all before the widespread use of antenatal US.[70]

In the absence of severe prematurity and intrapartum complications, the prognosis is dependent on the presence of malignancy and is therefore related to age at operation and completeness of resection. When the tumor is benign and completely excised, recurrence is less common than when the tumor is large and mostly solid.[71] The recurrent tumor may be benign or malignant, and benign metastatic tissue may become evident in lymph nodes.[72] Immature or fetal elements in gonadal teratomas are associated with a higher risk of aggressive behavior,[73] but this is not necessarily true for sacrococcygeal tumors.[2, 6] Whereas malignant recurrence of a "benign" teratoma may be as high as 15%,[7] the original benign diagnosis may have been due to sampling error or to an undetected residual microscopic focus of malignant tumor.[74] Patients whose tumors are resected after the newborn period have a higher risk of malignant recurrence, especially when there is an elevated AFP at diagnosis. The elevated AFP likely signifies the presence of malignancy in the original tumor.[75] It is important to follow all patients with physical examination, including rectal examination and serum markers, every 2 or 3 months for at least 3 years because most recurrences occur within 3 years of operation.[76]

Recurrent disease is usually local, but metastases to inguinal nodes, lung, liver, brain, and peritoneum can occur. The prognosis of a malignant tumor or a malignant recurrence was dismal until the advent of platinum-based chemotherapy.[74] Survival rates higher than 80% are now achieved, but the risk of late recurrences or second malignancies persist.[75, 77, 78]

A Children's Cancer Group (CCG) review illustrates the revised prognosis.[79] The mortality was 10% in 126 patients treated in 15 institutions from 1972 to 1994; 3 patients died of severe associated anomalies, 2 of hemorrhagic shock postoperatively, and 6 of combinations of severe prematurity, birth asphyxia due to failed vaginal delivery, and preoperative tumor rupture. Death from metastatic yolk sac tumor occurred in 1 patient, and a second patient with metastatic disease was lost to follow-up and is presumed dead. Thus, there were only 2 deaths from malignancy, despite a total of 20 yolk sac tumors (13 malignant at initial operation, 7 malignant recurrences after resection of "benign" teratomas). Owing to the effectiveness of current chemotherapy in treating recurrent disease and its toxicity in young infants, it appears that a completely excised malignant yolk sac tumor does not require adjuvant therapy. The patient should be closely monitored clinically and by serial AFP measurements.

In older patients, treatment of malignant tumors involves excision, chemotherapy, and monitoring by imaging studies and serum markers. For unresectable tumors, biopsy and chemotherapy are followed by excision of the primary tumor after adequate reduction has been obtained. Radiation therapy is usually reserved for local recurrence of malignant tumors. Patients with malignant tumors should be enrolled in a pediatric cooperative study or treated by their guidelines.

The prognosis for patients with a sacrococcygeal teratoma, in the current era of fetal diagnosis, is not dependent on classification[30] but rather on tumor size, physiologic consequences, histology, and associated anomalies. The prognosis of malignant tumors depends on tumor type, stage,[79] and location and patient age. Functional results in survivors have been reported as excellent in most series,[57, 59, 71] but recent reports draw attention to fecal and urinary continence problems as well as lower limb weakness.[80–82] Some of these problems are clearly related to associated anomalies[70] or to the presence of large presacral or intraabdominal tumors,[80] but they can occur after excision of purely extrapelvic benign tumors. A good outcome requires meticulous dissection along the tumor capsule, preservation and reconstruction of muscular structures, and long-term follow-up.

Thoracic Teratomas

The anterior mediastinum is the common site of thoracic teratomas, which account for 7 to 10% of all teratomas (see Table 67–1).[2, 3]

Mediastinal Teratomas

Mediastinal teratomas are diagnosed from the newborn period to adolescence or even adulthood.[2, 83] Most are located in the anterior mediastinum.[84] In

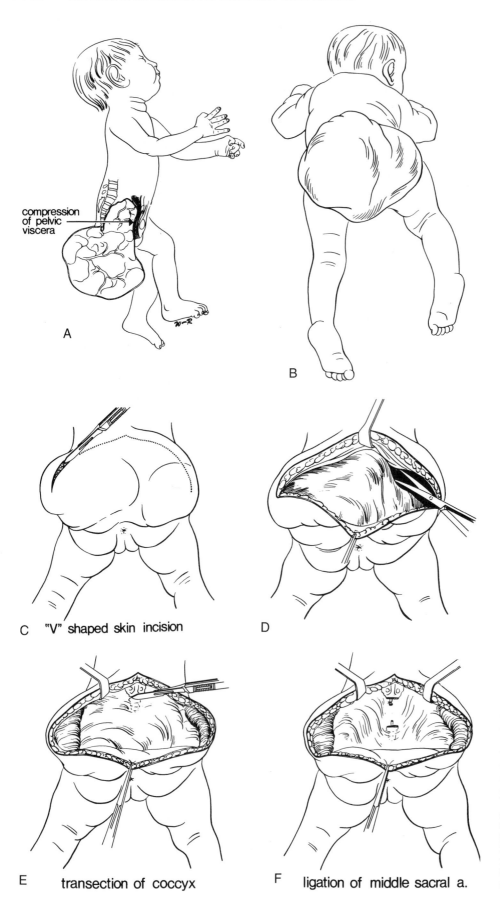

C "V" shaped skin incision

D

E transection of coccyx

F ligation of middle sacral a.

Figure 67–7. *A,* The teratomatous attachment may compress the rectum, vagina, and bladder anteriorly. *B,* The patient is placed on the operating table in a prone jackknife position, using general endotracheal anesthesia. An appropriate intravenous cannula should be placed in an arm vein. *C,* The incision is an inverted V shape to allow for excision of the tumor and to facilitate an eventually satisfactory cosmetic closure. The amount of skin excised is dependent on the size and shape of the tumor. *D,* The tumor is dissected from the gluteus maximus muscle. *E,* The coccyx is transected and removed in continuity with the tumor. *F,* The middle sacral artery is the major blood supply to the tumor and is ligated after transection of the coccyx.

compression of pelvic viscera

A

B

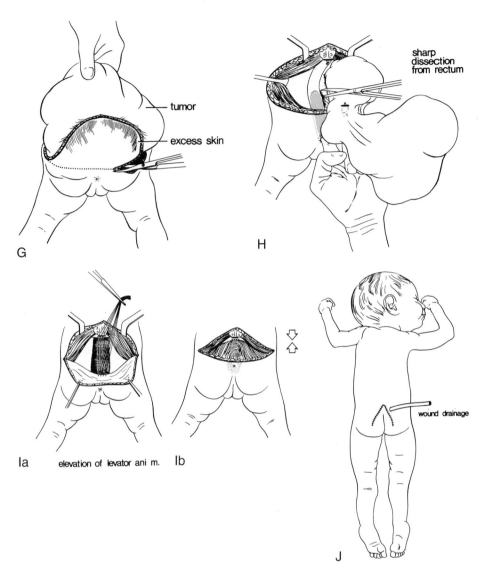

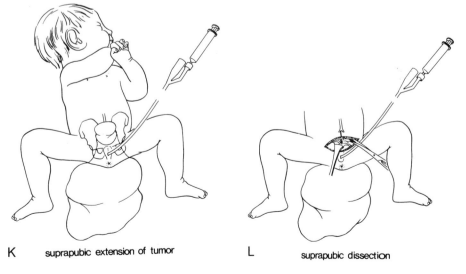

Figure 67–7 *Continued. G,* Excess skin is excised to facilitate closure. *H,* Because the tumor is adherent to the rectum, sharp dissection can be directed by placing a finger in the rectum. *I,* Placement of sutures between the anal sphincter and the presacral fascia (a). When the sutures are tied, the anal sphincter is pulled upward to the sacrum to form a gluteal crease (b). *J,* Drain is left in the surgical site for serosanguineous fluid discharge postoperatively. *K,* If tumor extends through the bony pelvis into the retroperitoneum, a urinary bladder catheter is inserted to facilitate suprapubic dissection. *L,* Lower abdominal transverse incision allows interruption of the middle sacral artery and dissection of the tumor from the sacrum and pelvis, which is eventually removed from the perineum.

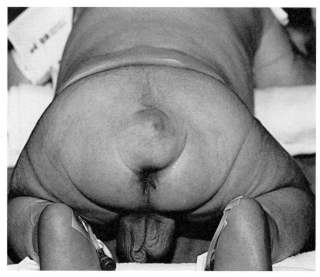

Figure 67–8. Smaller cystic teratoma at 1 month of age, initially mistaken for a hemangioma owing to its soft compressible nature and bluish skin discoloration. This tumor lends itself well to a longitudinal elliptical excision with midline closure, as in a posterior sagittal anorectoplasty.

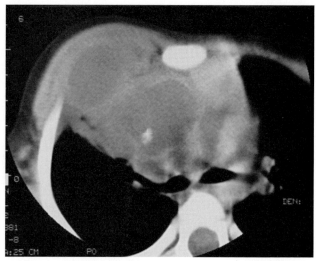

Figure 67–10. This 2-year-old was referred for a 5-cm by 5-cm hard fixed right chest wall mass that appeared suddenly during an upper respiratory infection. The computed tomography scan shows a bilobed lesion that extends through the chest wall and contains a small area of calcification. An incisional biopsy revealed pus-like material, containing ghost cells and calcified debris. Serum markers were normal. Complete excision of the mass required a right anterior thoracotomy and partial resection of an adherent right middle lobe. Pathologic examination revealed a ruptured mature teratoma with marked inflammatory reaction, containing foci of enteric, respiratory, and squamous mucosa; smooth muscle; salivary glands; pancreas; neuroglial tissue; and bone.

infants, respiratory distress is a common presenting manifestation, but in older children, the teratoma is often an incidental finding on chest radiograph (Fig. 67–9).[2] Mediastinal teratomas may present as a chest wall tumor and may even erode through the skin (Fig. 67–10). They can also erode into a bronchus, with hemoptysis as the initial manifestation. There is a strong association with Klinefelter's syndrome, and in these cases, choriocarcinoma in the teratoma often leads to precocious puberty.[2, 22, 85] Histiocytosis has

also been reported with mediastinal teratoma, both with and without Klinefelter's syndrome.[40, 46, 47, 85]

Histologically, the presence of immature tissue does not affect the prognosis in children younger

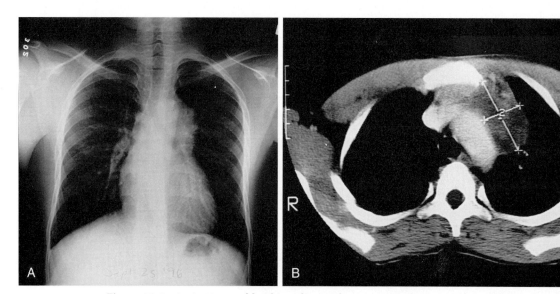

Figure 67–9. *A,* A 13-year-old African boy with an asymptomatic anterior mediastinal mass discovered on routine immigration chest radiograph. *B,* The computed tomography scan shows a heterogeneous mass adjacent to the aorta, suggestive of a neoplasm (thymoma or lymphoma). While considering a fine-needle aspiration biopsy, ultrasonography was done and suggested the presence of cysts with debris (not shown). Magnetic resonance imaging (not shown) confirmed the presence of cystic components as well as fat. A mature teratoma was excised through a small left anterior mediastinotomy, removing the left second costal cartilage.

than 15 years.[2] After 15 years of age, mediastinal teratomas have a high incidence of malignant behavior.[2] The tumor should be excised either through a median sternotomy or a thoracotomy.[2, 85] Smaller tumors may be approached through an anterior mediastinotomy (see Fig. 67–9) or by thoracoscopy, although tumor seeding is a concern with the latter. Chemotherapy is required for malignant lesions as adjuvant therapy or preoperatively for unresectable tumors.

Intrapericardial Teratomas

Intrapericardial teratomas are most commonly seen in the newborn period or in utero, with evidence of cardiorespiratory distress or nonimmune fetal hydrops.[2, 3, 86] They are a leading cause of massive pericardial effusion in the neonate.[3] Delay in diagnosis could be fatal.

On US, a cystic or solid teratoma is located anterior to the right atrium and ventricle with attachments to the great vessels.[86] In older infants, it may present with respiratory distress or poor feeding. It is not rare that the tumor may be found incidentally on chest radiograph. The only treatment is surgical excision. On histologic examination, these teratomas are usually composed of mature tissue with or without neuroglial components.[2, 3]

Intracardiac Teratomas

Intracardiac teratomas are rare and arise from the atrium or ventricle. Many can be cured by surgical resection.[2]

Abdominal Teratomas

The most frequent abdominal teratomas are the gonadal teratomas which are discussed in other chapters.

Retroperitoneal Teratomas

Retroperitoneal teratomas occur outside the pelvis, often in a suprarenal location. They represent about 5% of all childhood teratomas, and 75% occur in children younger than 5 years.[2, 3] Usually, the tumor is discovered as an abdominal mass that can compress the gastrointestinal tract, causing symptoms such as vomiting and constipation.[87]

Abdominal radiographs may show calcifications or bony structures within the tumor (Fig. 67–11). US, computed tomography (CT), and assessment of serum markers are the investigations used. Surgical excision is often easily performed. Malignancy is uncommon.[2, 87] Occasionally, differentiation from a teratoid Wilms' tumor may be difficult. The retroperitoneal site is the most common for the fetus in

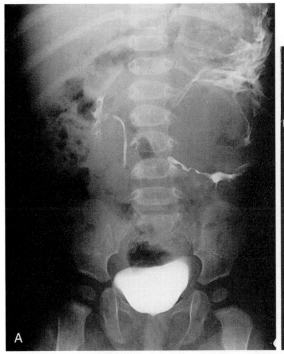
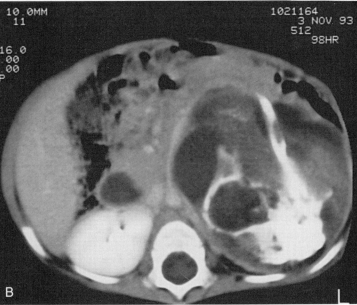

Figure 67–11. This 7-month-old girl was found to have an abdominal mass on routine examination. *A,* Plain films showed a large calcified left upper quadrant mass, which can be seen to displace the kidney inferiorly after injection of intravenous contrast. Ultrasonography (not shown) revealed multiple cystic areas. *B,* This was confirmed by computed tomography scan, which also revealed areas of fat density, making teratoma much more likely than neuroblastoma. The mature teratoma contained all types of cerebral and cerebellar tissues; respiratory, transitional, and squamous epithelium; sebaceous and salivary glands; smooth muscle; cartilage; and fat. Serum markers were normal.

fetu malformations and intermediate fetiform teratomas.[2, 3]

Gastric Teratomas

Gastric teratomas are rare lesions seen most commonly in infant boys.[2, 40, 88] They account for 1% of all teratomas. Clinically, the tumors present with hematemesis or vomiting due to gastric outlet obstruction.[2, 3, 40, 88, 89] A palpable mass is common. The tumor is an exophytic mass in the lesser curvature or posterior wall of the stomach, and the whole stomach may be involved.

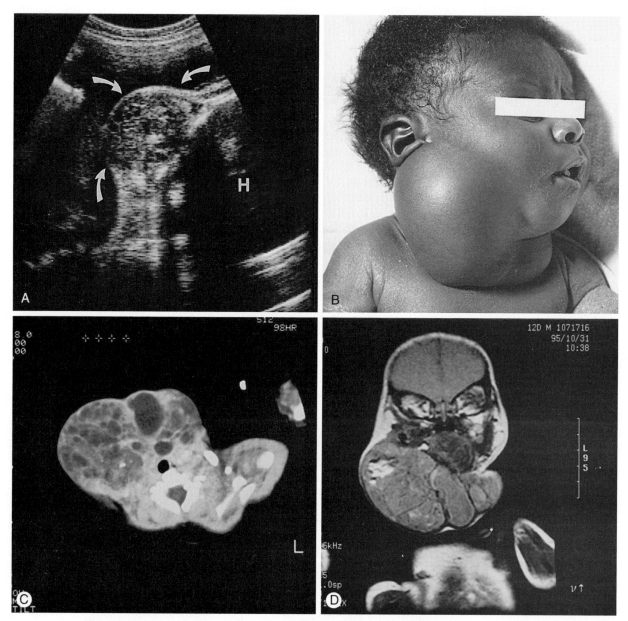

Figure 67–12. *A,* Fetal ultrasound at 34 weeks' gestation showing a 7-cm cervical mass of mixed echogenicity, containing blood flow by Doppler (arrows point to the mass, head is marked H). *B,* After birth by cesarean section, the child presented with only mild tachypnea despite the large right cervical mass extending to the left. Parts of the mass transilluminated, suggesting the diagnosis of hygroma. *C,* Computed tomography scan of the lower cervical area shows intact trachea and multiple cysts. This was initially interpreted as compatible with a hygroma, although an area of calcification was identified retrospectively. *D,* Magnetic resonance imaging confirmed the presence of fat, which appears bright on T1-weighted images as well as on the proton density–weighted imaging sequence shown here. At operation, the mass appeared to originate from the right lobe of the thyroid gland. It contained epithelium-lined cysts, cartilage, bone, glandular tissue, and complex papillary structures; there was a predominance of neuroepithelial tissue with a few small areas of immature, neuroblastoma-like tissue. Preoperative vanillylmandelic acid levels were normal. Postoperatively, the patient required thyroid hormone supplementation due to subclinical hypothyroidism (elevated thyroid-stimulating hormone with normal thyroxine and triiodothyronine levels).

Most gastric teratomas are benign with mature and immature tissue, mostly neuroglial tissue. Benign peritoneal gliomatosis has been found incidentally in hernia sacs 10 months after resection of a gastric teratoma in the newborn period, illustrating the unusual behavior of some of these tumors.[90] Surgical excision is curative. Recurrence and malignancy are rare.[91]

Others

Other rare sites of abdominal teratomas include liver, kidney, intestine, bladder, prostate, uterus, mesentery, and abdominal wall.[2, 3, 92–94]

Head and Neck Teratomas

More than 10% of teratomas in children originate from the neck, head, and central nervous system.[2, 3, 95, 96] The neck, nasopharynx, oral cavity, and orbit are the most common extracranial sites. Most of these tumors are recognized at or shortly after birth and are associated with an increased incidence of stillbirth. They can also be diagnosed by prenatal US (Fig. 67–12).[97, 98]

Cervical Teratomas

Cervical teratomas represent up to 8% of all teratomas.[17, 98] Large tumors can be seen in utero by US.[97] These tumors present as a cervical cystic mass, which may compromise the airway and require immediate intubation or tracheostomy.[99] Death may result from tracheal compression or deviation.[17, 100, 101] Prenatal diagnosis permits cesarean section and establishment of an airway by the surgical team before the cord is clamped.[101] Extension of tumor to the mediastinum may cause pulmonary hypoplasia, which increases respiratory morbidity and mortality.[2, 3] The tumor is usually well defined and may contain calcifications. The differential diagnosis includes cystic hygroma, congenital goiter, and branchial cleft cyst (see Fig. 67–12).[100] Investigation should include plain radiographs, US, and measurement of AFP and β-hCG as well as urinary catecholamine metabolites. CT and MRI may be useful to establish the diagnosis and to define the anatomic relationships.

Complete excision is performed through a wide collar incision. The tumor is usually not difficult to separate from the strap muscles and the fascial planes, but the pretracheal fascia is sometimes very adherent. Often, the site of origin cannot be identified, but in many instances, the tumor is firmly attached to and appears to originate from the thyroid gland; a thyroid lobectomy should be performed in these cases. The terms *thyrocervical* and *cervicothyroidal* are often used to describe cervical teratomas.[2, 3] Generally, the tumor is composed of both mature and immature neuroglial tissue, but cartilage and bronchial epithelium are not uncommon.[17, 100, 102] In 35% of cases, the tumor contains thyroid tissue. Cervical teratomas are usually benign, but malignancy has been reported, even in infants. A report

from the CCG showed that 20% of tumors clearly contained malignant elements—most often neuroblastoma, but also teratocarcinoma, neuroblastoma-like tumor, and neuroectodermal tumor.[17] Complete excision in the newborn period results in a survival rate of 80 to 90%. A prognostic classification for cervical teratomas takes into account birth status, age at diagnosis, and presence of respiratory distress.[102] In neonates without respiratory distress, the mortality rate was 2.7%, compared with 43.4% in those with respiratory compromise.

Craniofacial Teratomas

Craniofacial teratomas include a spectrum of lesions which may be life-threatening.

EPIGNATHUS. Epignathus is a term used to describe teratomas protruding from the mouth (Fig. 67–13). These tumors arise from the soft or hard palate in the region of Rathke's pouch.[103, 104] They generally fill the oral cavity and extend out through the mouth. They can prevent fetal swallowing, which leads to polyhydramnios. Surgical excision is mandatory. They are usually benign, and recurrence is rare. A high degree of organization often gives them the appearance of a parasitic fetus.

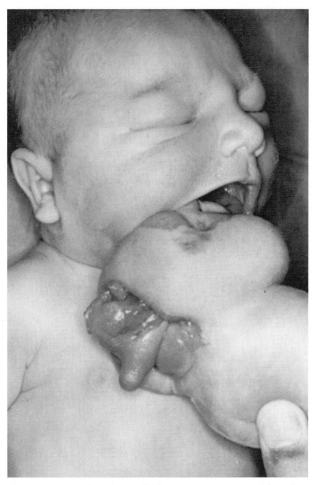

Figure 67–13. Epignathus, which is a teratoma protruding from the mouth.

PHARYNGEAL TERATOMAS. Pharyngeal teratomas arise from the posterior aspect of the nasopharynx. Large tumors can interfere with fetal swallowing to produce polyhydramnios, cause severe respiratory distress at birth, and lead to stillbirth.[2] Most pharyngeal teratomas are benign, and the treatment is surgical excision.[99]

OROPHARYNGEAL TERATOMAS. Oropharyngeal teratomas represent 2% of all teratomas.[105] These tumors can originate from the tongue, sinuses, mandible, and tonsils. Airway compromise requires immediate care at the time of delivery. Most tumors are benign, and recurrence is uncommon after complete resection.[105]

ORBITAL TERATOMAS. Orbital teratomas usually present at birth with unilateral proptosis in a normal, full-term neonate.[106] They grow rapidly, but the eye is intact. Occasionally, the tumor extends intracranially. The proptotic eye may rupture due to prolonged exposure. Histologically, these tumors are benign and contain mature tissue and immature neuroglial elements. Surgery is the treatment of choice, and the eye can usually be preserved.[2, 106]

MIDDLE EAR TERATOMAS. Middle ear teratomas may be difficult to differentiate from hereditary cholesteatoma. They are benign tumors, but surgery is difficult owing to the location of the tumor and the deformation of the middle ear. Ossiculoplasty is sometimes necessary.[107, 108]

Intracranial Teratomas

Intracranial teratomas generally present with symptoms of space-occupying lesions. These lesions account for only 2 to 4% of all teratomas, but they represent nearly 50% of brain tumors in the first 2 months of life.[2, 3, 40, 109] Most are benign in neonates but malignant in older children and young adults.[40, 109–112] These teratomas can appear in utero and cause massive hydrocephalus. Massive teratoma, causing skull rupture at delivery, has been reported.[110] The pineal gland is the most common site of origin, but intracranial teratomas may be seen in different areas, such as the hypothalamus, ventricles, cerebellum, and suprasellar region.[40, 111]

Pineal gland teratomas can secrete chorionic gonadotropin hormone, causing precocious puberty. In infants younger than 2 years, obstructive hydrocephalus is the most common clinical finding. In older children, symptoms of an increase of intracranial pressure are most common. The diagnosis can be made by using skull radiographs, US, CT, or MRI.

Treatment of intracranial teratomas is difficult and many are unresectable. The only long-term survivors are the ones who have the mass completely resected. Palliative shunting to reduce intracranial pressure is of little long-term benefit.[40] Perinatal mortality is high, with only a 6% survival when diagnosed in the fetus or newborn.[3]

Miscellaneous Sites

Teratomas have been reported in other sites, such as skin, perianal region well away from the coccyx,

umbilical cord (possibly associated with omphalocele), and placenta.[2, 3, 113, 114]

☐ Dermoid, Epidermoid, and Related Cysts

DERMOID CYSTS

Dermoid cysts are congenital cysts that are lined by skin with fully mature pilosebaceous structures.[115, 116] They are the result of sequestration of skin along lines of embryonic closure. The head and neck are the sites of predilection, but they have been described on other midline sites, including the sacral area, perineal raphe, scrotum, and presternal area.[116] The so-called *dermoids of the ovary* are in fact cystic teratomas and are discussed in Chapter 73.

Typical locations on the head are under the lateral part of the eyebrow (Fig. 67–14), the scalp, the glabella, the tip of the nose, the orbit, and the palate, where they are associated with a cleft.[117] They also occur intracranially and in the spinal canal.[118]

Dermoids are usually rounded, soft, and often fixed to deep tissues or to bone. They usually present as a painless mass of 1 or 2 cm in diameter but can grow up to 4 cm or more if untreated. Some are associated with a sinus tract, especially those on the nose. This site is also typical for intracranial extension and a familial occurrence.[118] Dermoids in the head area are usually deep to muscles and often cause an indentation in the outer table of the skull. They can even erode through both bony tables and extend intracranially. A skull radiograph may show the defect, but it may be normal if the cyst is situated over a fontanelle or an unfused suture. CT is essential in those cases, and neurosurgical consultation is advisable.[118]

Dermoids deep to the lateral part of the eyebrow are usually approached through an incision just above the eyebrow because an incision within the eyebrow leaves a more visible scar. We have been impressed with an alternative incision, through the palpebral crease. This requires a slightly longer incision and more retraction but leaves an invisible scar (see Fig. 67–14). This approach also has the advantage of allowing access to the orbit for the rare cases in which the cyst penetrates through the orbital bone in a dumbbell fashion.

Dermoids in the cervical area are usually midline, mostly suprahyoid or submental. Because they are deep within muscles, they tend to move with swallowing just as thyroglossal duct cysts do. On US, they usually appear echogenic and are often misinterpreted as being solid rather than cystic. They can be differentiated intraoperatively by their yellowish appearance and their soft, buttery content with sebaceous material and hair; this appearance alleviates the need for a hyoidectomy.

Dermoid cysts should be excised because they tend to grow and may rupture or become infected,

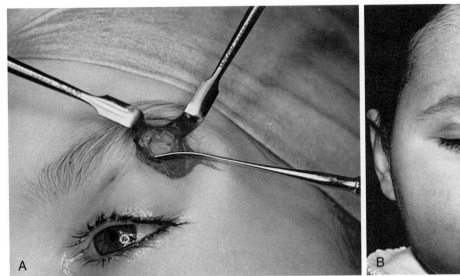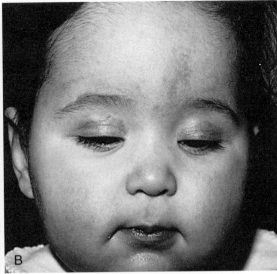

Figure 67–14. *A*, Dermoid cyst deep to the lateral part of the left eyebrow is approached through an incision made in the palpebral crease, taken through the muscle, which is then retracted upward, exposing the cyst lying on the periosteum. *B*, A different patient shown 1 month after excision of a right eyebrow dermoid through a palpebral skin incision. (*A* courtesy of Patricia Bortoluzzi, MD, FRCSC.)

resulting in a more difficult excision and a higher risk of recurrence.

EPIDERMAL CYSTS

Epidermal or epidermoid cysts have a wall composed of true epidermis, as seen on the skin surface and in the infundibulum of hair follicles (hence, they are also called *infundibular cysts*).[115] They do not contain pilosebaceous units or hair. Some have a congenital origin like that of dermoid cysts, whereas others are acquired, either spontaneously arising from hair follicles or secondary to trauma with implantation of epidermis into the dermis or subcutaneous tissue.

Epidermal cysts are slowly growing, formed by desquamation of epithelial cells. They are round, intradermal or subcutaneous lesions that stop growing after having reached 1 to 5 cm in diameter. They occur most commonly on the face, scalp, neck, and trunk (i.e., hair-bearing areas). They may be associated with a small sinus tract or dimpling of the skin. In the neck and infraclavicular area, they may be confused with branchial cleft remnants. Preauricular sinuses and cysts are often considered epidermal cysts. Epidermoid cysts of the spleen are discussed in Chapter 46.

Some patients may have more than one cyst, but the presence of multiple cysts, especially on the scalp and face, should raise the possibility of Gardner's syndrome.[115, 116] The cysts contain dry cheesy or horny material and lack skin appendages on histology. Treatment is excision, which often can be achieved under local anesthesia, even in young children. The use of a topical anesthetic cream (EMLA) before excision, a 30-gauge needle for infiltration of the local anesthetic, and occasionally sedation with

oral chloral hydrate or midazolam makes it possible to avoid a general anesthetic for superficial lesions.

Preauricular cysts are better excised under general anesthesia owing to their deep attachment to the helix cartilage.[117] Spontaneous rupture of any epidermal cyst leads to an intense foreign-body reaction, and the child presents with an abscess-like mass. This may require incision and drainage but often can be "cooled" with antibiotics and local warm compresses. This mode of presentation increases the risk of cyst recurrence after excision and often results in a wider scar than would have occurred with earlier excision. Infection of the cyst may also be caused by bacteria tracking along the small sinus tract that is sometimes present. These lesions rarely degenerate to epidermoid or basal cell carcinomas.[118] The treatment of asymptomatic preauricular sinuses is controversial, but certainly excision should be carried out in the presence of a palpable cyst or discharge of material from the sinus tract.

Epidermoid cysts of the skull and central nervous system share some similarities with dermoids, but they usually become symptomatic at an older age, between 20 and 40 years.[119] Most are thought to have a congenital origin, although iatrogenic and inflammatory mechanisms are likely for intraspinal epidermoids (caused by multiple lumbar punctures, especially when using a needle without stylet) and middle ear epidermoids (cholesteatomas), respectively.

TRICHILEMMAL CYSTS

Trichilemmal cysts, also called *pilar* or *sebaceous cysts*, are thought to arise from hair follicles.[115] Most are acquired and appear in adulthood. They often show an autosomal dominant inheritance pattern and are solitary in only 30% of the cases.[115] Some authors classify these as epidermoid or epidermal cysts.[118]

☐ Soft Tissue Tumors

Numerous soft tissue tumors have been described and are of mainly ectodermal and mesodermal origin. Some of these pediatric neoplasms are classified in Table 67–2. Tumors covered in other chapters are indicated. Only those soft tissue tumors likely to be encountered by pediatric surgeons are discussed here. More extensive discussions of soft tissue tumors are available.[120, 121] Many soft tissue tumors are cutaneous or subcutaneous and are amenable to excision under local anesthesia.

Epidermis

Pyogenic Granulomas

Pyogenic granulomas are solitary polypoid capillary hemangiomas often associated with trauma or local irritation. They are commonly found on the skin as red, raised, occasionally bleeding lesions or in the mouth in association with pregnancy.[122] They are easily treated with topical silver nitrate or liquid nitrogen or ligature of the polyp neck. Excision or electrocautery are rarely needed.

TABLE 67–2. Classification of Soft Tissue Tumors That Occur in Children

Tissue	Benign	Malignant
Ectoderm		
Epidermis	Dermoid cyst, calcifying epithelioma (pilomatrixoma)	Epidermoid cancer
Sweat gland	Hidradenoma	Adenocarcinoma
Sebaceous gland	Sebaceous cyst	Epidermoid cancer
Melanocytes (see Chap. 70)	Nevus	Malignant melanoma
Nerve tissue	Neurofibroma	Neurofibrosarcoma
Mesoderm		
Undifferentiated	Mesenchymoma, myxoma	Malignant mesenchymoma
Fibrous tissue	Fibroma, fibromatosis, keloid	Fibrosarcoma
Vascular tissue (see Chap. 71)	Hemangioma, lymphangioma, glomus	Hemangioendothelioma
Adipose tissue	Lipoma, lipoblastoma	Liposarcoma
Muscle (see Chap. 69)	Rhabdomyoma	Rhabdomyosarcoma
Synovial tissue	Giant cell synovioma, ganglion cyst, synovial cyst	Malignant synovioma

Skin Papillomas

Skin papillomas resemble skin tags of mucous membrane and occur at birth or in childhood.[123] Sessile variants may be called *verrucae*, whereas the projections are termed *acrochordon*. Treatment is by simple excision.

Warts

Warts are uncommon before 4 years of age but are a common pediatric complaint.[123] Various subtypes of human papillomavirus affect different body areas.[122] Verrucae spread through families, sports teams, and schoolmates and are most common on the hands and feet.[123] Topical treatment includes salicylic or trichloroacetic acid, liquid nitrogen, or fine-tip electrocautery. Excision is occasionally required.

Condylomata acuminata occur in the perineal skin and suggest but do not prove child sexual abuse. The virus may be transmitted by hand contact during diaper changes in infants or acquired at birth during vaginal delivery, but the lesions may take months to develop. One study suggested that sexual abuse was an unlikely source of transmission in children under 3 years of age if there were no other signs of abuse.[124] These lesions have a core of connective tissue covered in epithelium occurring as solitary or cauliflower-like lesions. Spontaneous regression is known, but topical podophyllin may be required. Some cases may necessitate electrocautery under general anesthesia to enable a thorough rectoscopic and vaginoscopic assessment and treatment.

Aberrant Skin Glands

Aberrant skin glands appear as rough, yellow-brownish skin resembling nevi or xanthoma. Histologic examination reveals adenoid hyperplasia, but a potential for later malignant change is reported, and therefore excision of these lesions is recommended.[123]

Calcifying Epithelioma of Malherbe

The calcifying epithelioma of Malherbe or *pilomatrixoma* is a solitary benign calcifying tumor of hair follicles. This is one of the most common acquired soft tissue lesions in children. Clinically, a circumscribed, firm, mobile, intracutaneous or subcutaneous nodule is palpable, with occasional yellowish or bluish coloration. These lesions are most common before the age of 20 years, and 60 to 70% are found in the head and neck region.[122] Only 2 to 3% are multiple, and most are less than 1 cm, although lesions up to 4 cm have been reported.[122, 125] They are more common than sebaceous cysts in younger patients. Local excision is indicated.[125]

Sweat Gland Lesions

Sweat gland pathology results from disorders of the sebaceous, apocrine, or eccrine adnexal structures of the skin. One series reported that only 1.7%

of pediatric skin biopsies showed these lesions.[122] *Hidradenoma* originates from the ductal portion of the sweat gland and produces multiple small flesh-colored papules on the face, neck, and upper chest during puberty and adolescence. Two subtypes are of interest: the eruptive form results in many lesions in a short period, whereas the clear cell variant causes solitary and occasionally painful lesions.[122] Sweat gland carcinomas are rare and are rarely differentiated enough to subtype confidently.[122] They may be locally aggressive and metastasize to the local lymph nodes. Treatment primarily involves resection with individualized adjuvant therapy.

Malignant Epithelial Tumors

Malignant epithelial tumors are rare in children.[123] General treatment principles include wide local excision and radiotherapy for prevention of recurrence.[123] Only 1% of all basal cell carcinomas occur in children. The basal cell nevus syndrome[126] is an autosomal dominant disease with basal cell lesions of the eyes, nose, and cheeks in association with anomalies of the mouth, skin, skeleton, central nervous system, eyes, and genitals. These patients may have concomitant xeroderma pigmentosum. Epidermoid or squamous cell carcinoma is also found in xeroderma pigmentosum patients.[122] Epidermoid cancers in pediatric transplant recipients have also been reported.[122]

Nerve Tissue

Neurofibromas

A neurofibroma is a benign neoplasm of abnormal proliferation of Schwann cells usually of peripheral nerves. When multiple or associated with multiple café-au-lait spots, neurofibromatosis type 1 (NF-1), or Recklinghausen's disease, an autosomal dominant disorder, may be diagnosed. The NF-1 gene appears to produce a tumor-suppression product, and neurofibromatosis may be a disease to which the two-hit genetic hypothesis applies.[127] The diagnosis may be delayed, but children in affected probands are usually diagnosed earlier, even by antenatal US.[128, 129] Neurofibromas of the mucosa are associated with multiple endocrine neoplasia type 2B and can present in childhood before medullary thyroid carcinoma or pheochromocytoma.[130] The NF-2 gene has been associated with acoustic neuromas.

NF-1 has several clinical forms, which are summarized in Table 67–3.[131] Because operative management is not curative of a genetic disorder, a multidisciplinary team supports patients and parents through decision making, treatment, rehabilitation, and developmental challenges (Fig. 67–15). Malignant degeneration to neurofibrosarcoma and associated malignancies[132] may necessitate US, CT, or MRI studies of new complaints. These imaging modalities are useful in following larger or deeper neurofibromas as well. Rapid growth is an ominous sign

TABLE 67–3. Clinical Patterns in Neurofibromatosis

Clinical	Description
Fibroma molluscum	Hundreds or thousands of pedunculated nodules; number makes resection impractical
Plexiform neurofibroma	Occur usually in the face and scalp, causing bony deformity by pressure erosion; resections for cosmesis may be repeated because curative resection is rare
Elephantiasis nervorum	With neurofibromas of the extremities, these cause greatly thickened skin simulating limb hypertrophy; resection is done to manage disfigurement
Thoracic neurofibroma	May have intraspinal extension (dumbbell tumor); have a high incidence of malignancy
Visceral neurofibroma	May affect intestine, kidney, and bladder because of the presence of associated nerves; when large, neurofibrosarcoma incidence increases
Skeletal syndromes	Include kyphoscoliosis, pseudarthrosis of tibia and ulna
Cranial syndromes	Meningiomas, gliomas, and optic gliomas have been reported
Endocrine syndromes	Sexual precocity, medullary thyroid carcinoma, and pheochromocytoma have been reported
Cardiovascular syndromes	Heart is rarely involved, but coarctation of the aorta and renal artery lesions have been reported

of neurofibrosarcoma. Excision or debulking may be combined with chemotherapy and radiotherapy.[133] Radiotherapy does not appear to be useful in slowing down progression of benign disease but has been documented to cause neurofibrosarcoma.[134] Treatment with chemotherapy and interferon-α has not been proved to be of benefit.

Xanthomas

Xanthoma is a tumor of lipid-laden histiocytes or foam cells forming yellowish skin nodules. It may be due to uncontrolled diabetes mellitus or biliary tract obstruction, which unbalances triglyceride and cholesterol metabolism leading to accumulation in histiocytes. Xanthomas are typical features of Alagille's syndrome (syndromic paucity of bile ducts) and familial hypercholesterolemia (Fig. 67–16). Correcting the underlying disorder reverses these cases, but excisional biopsy may be indicated for bothersome lesions or diagnostic purposes.

MESODERM

Undifferentiated Mesenchyme

Mesenchymomas

Mesenchymoma is a mixed mesenchymal tumor of two or more cellular elements not commonly

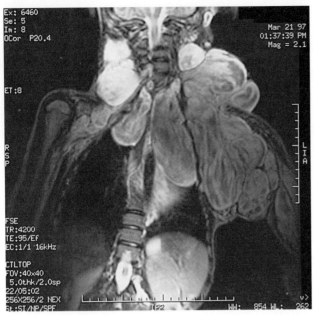

Figure 67–15. Magnetic resonance imaging study of a young boy with extensive neurofibromatosis type I who had undergone two previous cervical laminectomies to remove plexiform neurofibromas that were causing symptomatic cord compression. The left neck mass was enlarging, causing tracheal deviation and growing along the cervical nerve roots. This boy also had increasing left arm weakness and pain. A trial of chemotherapy with vincristine and actinomycin D did not stop progression of the disease.

associated (not including fibrous tissue). It can occur after radiotherapy or chemotherapy.[135] These lesions are usually benign in children and occur primarily in the head, neck, and extremities. Rib lesions in neonates and liver lesions are also described.[136] Malignant mesenchymoma is the corresponding sarcoma and is rare.

Myxomas

A myxoma is a benign primitive connective tissue cell and stroma tumor resembling mesenchyme. It occurs mainly in the heart, producing symptoms by obstruction of normal blood flow, and is removed using cardiopulmonary bypass.

Fibrous Tissue

Fibromas

A fibroma is a lesion composed of fibrous or fully developed connective tissue occurring as lytic bone lesions, breast lumps, finger swelling, and other forms.[136] *Fibromatosis* presents usually in infancy with multiple firm rubbery masses in the soft tissues, mostly in the lower extremities and head and neck. When congenital and generalized, death may occur in the first weeks of life, due mainly to pulmonary lesions.[136]

NODULAR FASCIITIS. Nodular fasciitis is the most common fibrous tissue tumor or self-limiting reactive process.[137] These tumors may be subcutaneous, intramuscular, or fascial in location and are commonly found in the head and neck of children.[137] Half of cases are associated with discomfort, and one fourth of lesions occur in patients younger than 20 years. Excisional biopsy is necessary to differentiate these rapidly growing lesions from a malignancy.

FIBROSARCOMAS. Fibrosarcoma is a neoplasm producing collagen that otherwise lacks cellular differentiation. It is the most common sarcoma of children younger than 1 year.[138] Treatment is complete excision coupled with systemic adjuvant chemotherapy. Preoperative chemotherapy may be of benefit. Radiotherapy for local recurrence may be required.

Congenital Epulis

Congenital epulis is a benign granular cell tumor occurring almost exclusively in girls at or immediately after birth. It originates from the maxillary dental mucosa and averages 1 to 2 cm in diameter.[139] Its exact nature is not clear. Some classify it under

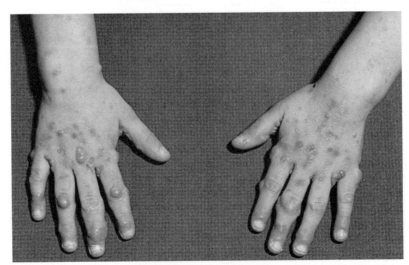

Figure 67–16. Multiple xanthomas in a child with Alagille's syndrome.

tumors of peripheral nerves, whereas others consider it a fibrous tumor, hence the synonym *granular cell fibroblastoma*. Spontaneous regression is unusual, and simple excision is curative.[139]

Keloid

A keloid is a sharply elevated, irregularly shaped, progressively enlarging scar caused by excessive collagen in the dermis during connective tissue repair. Unlike the hypertrophic scar (which does not progress), a keloid may recur after excision. Treatment by intradermal injection of steroids, pressure garments (as in some burn patients), and cryosurgery may be attempted. Rarely, judicious excision with radiotherapy may be employed.[140] Keloids developing after minor procedures are common. Their incidence is higher in black patients.

Desmoid Tumors

Desmoid tumors are fibrous tumors that usually arise from musculoaponeurotic tissue of the skull or abdominal cavity—hence, the modern name *musculoaponeurotic fibromatosis*.[141] They are not encapsulated and are locally invasive, although they do not metastasize. They are associated with Gardner's syndrome.

When they arise from the retroperitoneum, complete resection may be impossible without risking damage to splanchnic vessels. High-dose radiotherapy or interstitial brachytherapy may be considered for residual tumor.[138] Steroid therapy (tamoxifen, prednisone) and nonsteroidal therapy (indomethacin and sulindac) have been used in recurrent and inoperable tumors.[142]

Vascular Glomus

A glomus tumor is an uncommon pediatric lesion consisting of a meshwork of fine arterioles connected to veins and intertwined with nerve tissue. Children have a greater tendency to develop multiple tumors than do adults, possibly representing autosomal dominant inheritance.[136] The lesions on the skin are discrete blue-black spots and may be extremely painful if present under nails. Excision is the preferred treatment.

Adipose Tissue

A lipoma is a benign, soft, rubbery, encapsulated tumor of adipose tissue composed of mature fat cells occurring on the trunk, neck, and forearms. Lipomas represented 94%, lipoblastoma 4.7%, and liposarcoma 1.3% of adipose tumors in one series.[143] All are slow-growing tumors. Diagnosed often before 3 years of age, lipoblastoma may be superficial and well encapsulated or deep and infiltrative. Definitive treatment of adipose tumors is complete resection. Chemotherapy may play a role in treating residual liposarcoma. Local recurrence rates for lipoblastoma and liposarcoma are about 10 to 20%.[143] Characterized by a myxoid stroma, em-bryonal lipoblasts, and mature fat cells, the myxoid variant of liposarcoma is similar histologically to lipoblastoma. Tumor karyotyping may be useful in differentiating these adipose tumors.[143]

Liposarcoma arises from the intermuscular fascia, where embryonal lipoblasts exhibit variable differentiation with occasional nuclear atypia. The myxoid variant is the most common and metastasizes late if at all. The dedifferentiated subtype is highly malignant and may coexist with spindle cell sarcoma.

Synovial Tissue

Synovial Cysts

Synovial cysts or *ganglion cysts* arise from joints or tendon sheaths, resulting in firm 0.5- to 2-cm, mucin-filled lesions with a fibrous capsule. They are most common on the hand, especially on the dorsum of the wrist, but also occur on the ankle, foot, and popliteal fossa (where they are called Baker's cysts). One fourth of the latter occur in children younger than 6 years.[144]

Pathology texts separate synovial cysts that have a true synovial lining (such as Baker's cysts) from ganglia, which are thought to be degenerative and are without a synovial lining.[145, 146] Clinicians, however, usually use both terms interchangeably.[147] Symptoms of pain and weakness occur, but most children present with an asymptomatic mass. Spontaneous resolution of all types of synovial cysts is common in children. Surgery is reserved for patients with persistently symptomatic lesions.[147] Classic treatment includes traumatic disruption ("strike it with the family Bible") or steroid injection. Both should be discouraged due to high recurrence risk and associated pain. Use of nonsteroidal antiinflammatory agents, coupled with rest or wrist splinting, is usually sufficient if the cyst causes transient discomfort.

Giant Cell Synoviomas

The giant cell synovioma is a benign tumor of the tendon sheath, generally occurring before 10 years of age.[136] It occurs in the fingers (75 to 80% of cases) on the volar aspect. Treatment by resection results in a 10 to 15% recurrence rate.[136] Malignant synovioma or synoviosarcoma represents 5 to 10% of soft tissue malignancies in patients younger than 20 years.[148] Most occur near the knee, but they are also found in the head and neck, anterior abdominal wall, and inguinal area. The mass may be palpable or reveal itself as calcification on radiograph. Cure by wide excision without chemotherapy can often be achieved, but neurovascular anatomy related to the tumor may necessitate microsurgical reconstruction if not amputation. The calcifying subtype has a better 5-year survival rate (83%) than the noncalcifying subtypes (25 to 50%).[149]

REFERENCES

1. Virchow R: Ueber Die Sakralgeschwulst Des Schliewener Kindes. Klin Wschr 46:132, 1869.

2. Dehner LP: Gonadal and extragonadal germ cell neoplasms: Teratomas in childhood. In Finegold M (ed): Pathology of Neoplasia in Children and Adolescents. Philadelphia, WB Saunders, 1986, pp 282–312.
3. Isaacs H: Germ cell tumors. In Isaacs H (ed): Tumors of the Fetus and Newborn. Philadelphia, WB Saunders, 1997, pp 15–38.
4. Skinner MA: Germ cell tumors. In Oldham KT, Colombani PM, Foglia RP (eds): Surgery of Infants and Children: Scientific Principles and Practice. Philadelphia, Lippincott-Raven, 1997, pp 653–662.
5. Moore KL, Persaud TVN: The Developing Human. Philadelphia, WB Saunders, 1993.
6. Isaacs H: Tumors. In Gilbert-Barness E (ed): Potter's Pathology of the Fetus and Infant. St Louis, CV Mosby, 1997, pp 1242–1331.
7. Bale PM: Sacrococcygeal developmental abnormalities and tumors in children. Perspect Pediatr Pathol 1:56, 1984.
8. Sinnock KL, Perez-Atayde AR, Boynton KA, et al: Clonal analysis of sacrococcygeal "teratomas." Pediatr Pathol Lab Med 16:865–875, 1996.
9. Chadha R, Bagga D, Malhortra CJ, et al: Accessory limb attached to the back. J Pediatr Surg 28:1615–1617, 1993.
10. de Lagausie P, de Napoli Cocci S, Stempfle N, et al: Highly differentiated teratoma and fetus-in-fetu: A single pathology? J Pediatr Surg 32:115–116, 1997.
11. Heifetz SA, Alrabeeah A, Brown BS, et al: Fetus in fetu: A fetiform teratoma. Pediatr Pathol 8:215–226, 1988.
12. Hanquinet S, Damry N, Heimann P, et al: Association of a fetus in fetu and two teratomas: US and MRI. Pediatr Radiol 27:336–338, 1997.
13. Drut RM, Drut R, Fontana A, et al: Mature presacral sacrococcygeal teratoma associated with a sacral "epignathus." Pediatr Pathol 12:99–103, 1992.
14. Parizek J, Nemecek S, Pospisilova B, et al: Mature sacrococcygeal teratoma containing the lower half of a human body. Childs Nerv Syst 8:108–110, 1992.
15. Kooijman CD: Immature teratomas in children. Histopathology 12:491–502, 1988.
16. Graf JL, Housely HT, Albanese CT, et al: A surprising histological evolution of preterm sacrococcygeal teratomas. J Pediatr Surg 33:177–179, 1998.
17. Azizkhan RG, Haase GM, Applebaum H, et al: Diagnosis, management, and outcome of cervicofacial teratomas in neonates: A Children's Cancer Group Study. J Pediatr Surg 30:312–316, 1995.
18. Hijiya N, Horikawa R, Matsushita T, et al: Malignant mediastinal germ-cell tumors in childhood: A report of two cases achieving long-term disease-free survival. Am J Pediatr Hematol-Oncol 11:437–440, 1989.
19. Stringer DA, Sprigg A, Kerrigan D: Malignant carcinoid within a recurrent sacrococcygeal teratoma in childhood. Can Assoc Radiol J 41:105–107, 1990.
20. Tsuchida Y, Endo Y, Saito S, et al: Evaluation of alpha fetoprotein in early infancy. J Pediatr Surg 13:155–162, 1978.
21. Wu JT, Book L, Sudar K: Serum alpha fetoprotein (AFP) levels in normal infants. Pediatr Res 15:50–52, 1981.
22. Derenoncourt AN, Castro-Magana M, Jones KL: Mediastinal teratoma and precocious puberty in a boy with mosaic Klinefelter syndrome. Am J Med Genet 55:38–42, 1995.
23. Rodriguez E, Reuter VE, Mies C, et al: Abnormalities of 2q: A common genetic link between rhabdomyosarcoma and hepatoblastoma? Genes Chromosom Cancer 3:122–127, 1991.
24. Perlman EJ, Cushing B, Hawkins E, et al: Cytogenetic analysis of childhood endodermal sinus tumors: A Pediatric Oncology Group Study. Pediatr Pathol 14:695–708, 1994.
25. Kruslin B, Hrascan R, Manojlovic S, et al: Oncoproteins and tumor suppressor proteins in congenital sacrococcygeal teratomas. Pediatr Pathol Lab Med 17:43–52, 1997.
26. Ishiwata I, Ishiwata C, Soma M, et al: N-myc gene amplification and neuron specific enolase production in immature teratomas. Virchows Arch A Pathol Anat Histopathol 418:333–338, 1991.
27. Currarino G, Coln D, Votteler T: Triad of anorectal, sacral, and presacral anomalies. AJR Am J Roentgenol 137:395–398, 1981.
28. Ng WT, Ng TK, Cheng PW: Sacrococcygeal teratoma and anorectal malformation: Case reports. Aust N Z J Surg 67:218–220, 1997.
29. Tsuchida Y, Watanasupt W, Nakajo T: Anorectal malformations associated with a presacral tumor and sacral defect. Pediatr Surg Int 4:398–402, 1989.
30. Altman RP, Randolph JG, Lilly JR: Sacrococcygeal teratoma: American Academy of Pediatrics Surgical Section Survey—1973. J Pediatr Surg 9:389–398, 1974.
31. Ashcraft KW, Holder TM: Hereditary presacral teratoma. J Pediatr Surg 9:691–697, 1974.
32. Lee S-C, Chun Y-S, Jung S-E, et al: Currarino triad: Anorectal malformations, sacral bony abnormality, and presacral mass—a review of 11 cases. J Pediatr Surg 32:58–61, 1997.
33. Shaija JK: Anorectal malformation presenting as Hirschsprung's disease: A case report. East Afr Med J 72:130–131, 1995.
34. Sonnino RE, Chou S, Guttman FM: Hereditary sacrococcygeal teratoma. J Pediatr Surg 24:1074–1075, 1989.
35. Subbarao P, Bhatnagar V, Mitra DK: The association of sacrococcygeal teratoma with high anorectal and genital malformations. Aust N Z J Surg 64:214–215, 1994.
36. Lahdenne P, Heikinheimo M, Jaaskelainen J, et al: Vertebral abnormalities associated with congenital sacrococcygeal teratomas. J Pediatr Orthop 11:603–607, 1991.
37. Werb P, Scurry J, Ostor A, et al: Survey of congenital tumors in perinatal necropsies. Pathology 24:247–253, 1992.
38. Sadove AM, Kalsbec JE, Ellis FD, et al: Orbital teratoma associated with trigonocephaly. Plast Reconstr Surg 88:1059–1063, 1991.
39. Aughton DJ, Sloan CT, Milad MP, et al: Nasopharyngeal teratoma ("hairy polyp"), Dandy-Walker malformation, diaphragmatic hernia, and other anomalies in a female infant. J Med Genet 27:788–790, 1990.
40. Rowe MI, O'Neill JA, Grosfeld JL, et al: Teratomas and germ cell tumors. In Rowe MI, O'Neill JA, Grosfeld JL, et al (eds): Essentials of Pediatric Surgery. St Louis, CV Mosby, 1995, pp 296–305.
41. Gross RE, Clatworthy HW Jr, Meeker IA Jr: Sacrococcygeal teratomas in infants and children: A report of 40 cases. Surg Gynecol Obstet 92:341–354, 1951.
42. Hasle H, Jacobsen BB, Aschenfeldt P, et al: Mediastinal germ cell tumour associated with Klinefelter syndrome: A report of case and review of the literature. Eur J Pediatr 151:735–739, 1992.
43. Casalone R, Righi R, Granata P, et al: Cerebral germ cell tumor and XXY karyotype. Cancer Genet Cytogenet 74:25–29, 1994.
44. Hachimi-Idrissi S, Desmytere S, Goossens A, et al: Retroperitoneal teratoma as first sign of Klinefelter's syndrome. Arch Dis Child 72:163–164, 1995.
45. Zon R, Orazi A, Neiman RS, et al: Benign hematologic neoplasm associated with mediastinal mature teratoma in a patient with Klinefelter's syndrome: A case report. Med Pediatr Oncol 23:376–379, 1994.
46. Beasley SW, Tiedemann K, Howat A, et al: Precocious puberty associated with malignant thoracic teratoma and malignant histiocytosis in a child with Klinefelter's syndrome. Med Pediatr Oncol 15:277–280, 1987.
47. Sasou S, Nakamura SI, Habano W, et al: True malignant histiocytosis developed during chemotherapy for mediastinal immature teratoma. Human Pathol 27:1099–1103, 1996.
48. Aurer I, Nemet D, Uzarevic B, et al: Mediastinal malignant teratoma and acute myeloid leukemia in a patient with Klinefelter's syndrome: Comparison of DNA content in the two malignancies. Acta Oncol 33:705–706, 1994.
49. Koo CH, Reifel J, Kogut N, et al: True histiocytic malignancy associated with a malignant teratoma in a patient with 46XY gonadal dysgenesis. Am J Surg Pathol 16:175–183, 1992.
50. Goetsch SJ, Hadley GP: Hodgkin's disease following successful treatment of gastric teratoma in a neonatal female. Pediatr Pathol Lab Med 15:455–461, 1995.

51. Dische MR, Gardner HA: Mixed teratoid tumors of the liver and neck in trisomy 13. Am J Clin Pathol 69:631–637, 1978.
52. Quah BS, Menon BS: Down syndrome associated with a retroperitoneal teratoma and Morgagni hernia. Clin Genet 50:232–234, 1996.
53. Falik-Borenstein TC, Korenberg JR, Davos I, et al: Congenital gastric teratoma in Wiedemann-Beckwith syndrome. Am J Med Genet 38:52–57, 1991.
54. Akguner M, Karaca C, Karatas O, et al: Mentosternal pterygium with teratoma. Ann Plast Surg 37:201–203, 1996.
55. Zachariou Z, Krug M, Benz G, et al: Proteus syndrome associated with a sacrococcygeal teratoma: A rare combination. Eur J Pediatr Surg 6:249–251, 1996.
56. Robin NH, Grace K, DeSouza TG, et al: New finding of Schinzel-Giedion syndrome: A case with a malignant sacrococcygeal teratoma. Am J Med Genet 47:852–856, 1993.
57. Billmire DF, Grosfeld JL: Teratomas in childhood: Analysis of 142 cases. J Pediatr Surg 21:548–551, 1985.
58. Schropp KP, Lobe TE, Rao B, et al: Sacrococcygeal teratoma: The experience of four decades. J Pediatr Surg 27:1075–1079, 1992.
59. Tapper D, Lack EE: Teratomas in infancy and childhood: A 54-year experience at the Children's Hospital Medical Center. Ann Surg 198:398–410, 1983.
60. Powell RW, Weber ED, Manci EA: Intradural extension of a sacrococcygeal teratoma. J Pediatr Surg 28:770–772, 1993.
61. West K, Touloukian RJ: Meconium pseudocyst presenting as a buttock mass. J Pediatr Surg 23:864–865, 1988.
62. Murphy JJ, Blair GK, Fraser GC: Coagulopathy associated with large sacrococcygeal teratomas. J Pediatr Surg 27:1308–1310, 1992.
63. Flake AW: Fetal sacrococcygeal teratoma. Semin Pediatr Surg 2:113–120, 1993.
64. Veschambre R, Wartanian B, Lebouvier L, et al: Facteurs pronostiques anténatals des tératomes sacro-coccygiens. Rev Fr Gynecol Obstét 88:325–330, 1993.
65. Adzick NS, Crombleholme TM, Morgan MA, et al: A rapidly growing fetal teratoma. Lancet 349:538, 1997.
66. Robertson FM, Crombleholme TM, Frantz ID, et al: Devascularization and staged resection of giant sacrococcygeal teratoma in the premature infant. J Pediatr Surg 30:309–311, 1995.
67. Hecher K, Hackeloer B-J: Intrauterine endoscopic laser surgery for fetal sacrococcygeal teratoma. Lancet 347:470, 1996.
68. Lindahl H: Giant sacrococcygeal teratoma: A method of simple intraoperative control of hemorrhage. J Pediatr Surg 23:1068–1069, 1988.
69. Lund DP, Soriano DG, Fauza D, et al: Resection of a massive sacrococcygeal teratoma using hypothermic hypoperfusion: A novel use of extracorporeal membrane oxygenation. J Pediatr Surg 30:157–159, 1995.
70. Shanbhogue LKR, Bianchi A, Doig CM, et al: Management of benign sacrococcygeal teratoma: Reducing mortality and morbidity. Pediatr Surg Int 5:41–44, 1990.
71. Bilik R, Shandling B, Pope M, et al: Malignant benign neonatal sacrococcygeal teratoma. J Pediatr Surg 28:1158–1160, 1993.
72. Ouimet A, Russo P: Fetus in fetu or not? J Pediatr Surg 24:926–927, 1989.
73. Norris HJ, Zirkin HJ, Benson WL: Immature (malignant) teratoma of the ovary: A clinical and pathologic study of 58 cases. Cancer 37:2359–2372, 1976.
74. Gilcrease MZ, Brandt ML, Hawkins EP: Yolk sac tumor identified at autopsy after surgical excision of immature sacrococcygeal teratoma. J Pediatr Surg 30:875–877, 1995.
75. Malogolowkin MH, Ortega JA, Kraila M, et al: Immature teratomas: Identification of patients at risk of malignant recurrence. J Natl Cancer Instit 81:870–874, 1989.
76. Hawkins EP, Isaacs H, Cushing B: Occult malignancy in neonatal sacrococcygeal teratomas: A report from a combined Pediatric Oncology Group and Children's Cancer Group Study. Am J Pediatr Hematol Oncol 15:406–409, 1993.
77. Shanbhogue LKR, Gough DCS, Jones PM: Malignant sacro-coccygeal teratoma: Improved survival with chemotherapy. Pediatr Surg Int 4:202–204, 1989.
78. Dewan PA, Davidson PM, Campbell PE, et al: Sacrococcygeal teratoma: Has chemotherapy improved survival? J Pediatr Surg 22:274–277, 1987.
79. Rescorla FJ, Sawin RS, Coran AG, et al: Long-term outcome of infants and children with sacrococcygeal teratomas: A report from the Children's Cancer Group. J Pediatr Surg 33:171–176, 1998.
80. Malone PS, Spitz L, Kiely EM, et al: The functional sequelae of sacrococcygeal teratoma. J Pediatr Surg 25:679–680, 1990.
81. Havranek P, Hedlund H, Rubenson A, et al: Sacrococcygeal teratoma in Sweden between 1978 and 1989: Long-term functional results. J Pediatr Surg 27:916–918, 1992.
82. Boemers TML, van Gool JD, de Jong TPVM, et al: Lower urinary tract dysfunction in children with benign sacrococcygeal teratoma. J Urol 151:174–176, 1994.
83. Lewis BD, Hurt RD, Payne WS, et al: Benign teratomas of the mediastinum. J Thorac Cardiovasc Surg 86:727–731, 1983.
84. Sidani AH, Oberson R, Deleze G, et al: Infected teratoma of lower posterior mediastinum in a six-year-old boy. Pediatr Radiol 21:438–439, 1991.
85. Chaussain JL, Lemerle J, Roger M, et al: Klinefelter syndrome, tumor, and sexual precocity. J Pediatr 97:607–609, 1980.
86. Sumner TE, Crowe JE, Klein A, et al: Intrapericardial teratoma in infancy. Pediatr Radiol 10:51–53, 1980.
87. Augé D, Satgé D, Sauvage P, et al: Les tératomes rétropéritonéaux de la période néonatale. Ann Pediatr (Paris) 40:613–621, 1993.
88. Senocak ME, Kale G, Buyukpamukcu N, et al: Gastric teratoma in children including the third reported female case. J Pediatr Surg 25:681–684, 1990.
89. Haley T, Dimler M, Hollier P: Gastric teratoma with gastrointestinal bleeding. J Pediatr Surg 21:949–950, 1986.
90. Coulson WF: Peritoneal gliomatosis from a gastric teratoma. Am J Clin Pathol 94:87–89, 1990.
91. Bourque CJ, Mackay AJ, Payton D: Malignant gastric teratoma: Case report. Pediatr Surg Int 12:192–193, 1997.
92. Shah RS, Kaddu SJ, Kirtane JM: Benign mature teratoma of the large bowel: A case report. J Pediatr Surg 31:701–702, 1996.
93. Misugi K, Reiner CB: A malignant true teratoma of liver in childhood. Arch Pathol 80:409–412, 1965.
94. Chiba T, Iwami D, Kikuchi Y: Mesenteric teratoma in an 8-month-old girl. J Pediatr Surg 30:120, 1995.
95. Filston HC: Hemangiomas, cystic hygromas, and teratomas of the head and neck. Semin Pediatr Surg 3:147–159, 1994.
96. Kountakis SE, Minotti AM, Maillard A, et al: Teratomas of the head and neck. Am J Otolaryngol 15:292–296, 1994.
97. Schoenfeld A, Edelstein T, Joel-Cohen SJ: Prenatal ultrasonic diagnosis of the fetal teratoma of the neck. Br J Radiol 51:742–744, 1978.
98. Garmel SH, Crombleholme TM, Semple JP, et al: Prenatal diagnosis and management of fetal tumors. Semin Perinatal 18:350–365, 1994.
99. Byard RW, Jimenez CL, Caroebter BF, et al: Congenital teratomas of the neck and nasopharynx: A clinical and pathological study of 18 cases. J Pediatr Child Health 26:12–16, 1990.
100. Ward RF, April M: Teratomas of the head and neck. Otolaryngol Clin North Am 22:621–629, 1989.
101. Langer JC, Tabb T, Thompson P, et al: Management of prenatally diagnosed tracheal obstruction: Access to the airway in utero prior to delivery. Fetal Diagn Ther 7:12–16, 1992.
102. Jordan RB, Gauderer MW: Cervical teratomas: An analysis. Literature review and proposed classification. J Pediatr Surg 23:583–591, 1988.
103. Hatzihaberis F, Stamatis D, Staurinos D: Giant epignathus. J Pediatr Surg 13:517–518, 1978.
104. Wilson JW, Gehweiler JA: Teratoma of the face associated with a patent canal extending into the cranial cavity (Rathke's pouch) in a three-week-old child. J Pediatr Surg 5:349–359, 1970.

105. Sauter ER, Diaz JH, Arensman RM, et al: The perioperative management of neonates with congenital oropharyngeal teratomas. J Pediatr Surg 25:925–928, 1990.
106. Lee GA, Sullivan TJ, Tsikleas GP, et al: Congenital orbital teratoma. Aust N Z J Ophthalmol 25:63–66, 1997.
107. Navarro Cunchillos M, Bonachera MD, Navarro Cunchillos M, et al: Middle ear teratoma in a newborn. J Laryngol Otol 110:875–877, 1996.
108. Parnes LS, Sun AH: Teratoma of the middle ear. J Otolaryngol 24:165–167, 1995.
109. Odell JM, Allen JK, Badura RJ, et al: Massive congenital intracranial teratoma: A report of two cases. Pediatr Pathol 7:333–340, 1987.
110. Washburne JF, Magann EF, Chauhan SP, et al: Massive congenital intracranial teratoma with skull rupture at delivery. Am J Obstet Gynecol 173:226–228, 1995.
111. Hunt SJ, Johnson PC, Coons SW, et al: Neonatal intracranial teratomas. Surg Neurol 34:336–342, 1990.
112. Greenhouse AH, Neubürger KT: Intracranial teratoma of the newborn. AMA Arch Neurol 3:718–724, 1960.
113. Jona JZ: Congenital anorectal teratoma: Report of a case. J Pediatr Surg 31:709–710, 1996.
114. Kreczy A, Alge A, Menardi G, et al: Teratoma of the umbilical cord: Case report with review of the literature. Arch Pathol Lab Med 118:934–937, 1994.
115. Lever WF, Schaumburg-Lever G: Tumors and cysts of the epidermis. In Lever WF, Schaumburg-Lever G (eds): Histopathology of the Skin (7th ed). Philadelphia, JB Lippincott, 1990, pp 523–571.
116. Mascaro JM, Torras H, Iranzo P: Cutaneous tumors in childhood. In Ruiz-Maldonado R, Parish LC, Beare JM (eds): Textbook of Pediatric Dermatology. Philadelphia, Grune & Stratton, 1989, pp 715–726.
117. Rowe MI, O'Neill JA, Grosfeld JL, et al: Miscellaneous skin lesions. In Rowe MI, O'Neill JA, Grosfeld JL, et al (eds): Essentials of Pediatric Surgery. St Louis, CV Mosby, 1995, pp 819–828.
118. Hurwitz S: Cutaneous tumors in childhood. In Hurwitz S (ed): Clinical Pediatric Dermatology (2nd ed). Philadelphia, WB Saunders, 1993, pp 198–241.
119. Baxter JW, Netsky MG: Epidermoid and dermoid tumors: Pathology. In Wilkins RH, Rengachary SS (eds): Neurosurgery. New York, McGraw-Hill, 1985, pp 655–661.
120. Enzinger FM, Weiss SW: Soft Tissue Tumors (3rd ed). St Louis, CV Mosby, 1995.
121. Webber BL, Parham DM: Soft tissue tumors other than rhabdomyosarcoma and peripheral neuroepithelioma. In Parham DM (ed): Pediatric Neoplasia: Morphology and Biology. Philadelphia, Lippincott-Raven, 1996, pp 205–218.
122. Dehner LP: Skin and supporting adnexae. In Dehner LP (ed): Pediatric Surgical Pathology (2nd ed). Baltimore, Williams & Wilkins, 1987, pp 1–103.
123. Lindsay WK: Congenital defects of the skin, muscles, connective tissues, tendons, and hands. In Welch KJ, Randolph JG, Ravitch MM, et al (eds): Pediatric Surgery. Vol. 2 (4th ed). Chicago, Year Book Medical, 1986, pp 1479–1499.
124. Cohen BA, Honig P, Androphy E: Anogenital warts in children. Arch Dermatol 126:1575–1580, 1990.
125. Schlecter R, Hartsough NA, Guttman FM: Multiple pilomatricomas (calcifying epitheliomas of Malherbe). Pediatr Dermatol 2:23–25, 1984.
126. Graham JK, McJimsey BA, Hardin JC: Nevoid basal cell carcinoma syndrome. Arch Otolaryngol Head Neck Surg 87:72–77, 1968.
127. Serra E, Purg S, Otero D, et al: Confirmation of a double-hit model for the NF-1 gene in benign neurofibromas. Am J Hum Genet 61:512–519, 1997.
128. Friedman JM, Birch PH: Type 1 neurofibromatosis: A descriptive analysis of the disorder in 1,728 patients. Am J Med Genet 70:138–143, 1997.
129. Drouin V, Marret S, Petitcolas J, et al: Prenatal US abnormalities in a patient with generalized neurofibromatosis type 1. Neuropediatrics 28:120–121, 1997.
130. Pujol RM, Matias-Buiu X, Miralles J, et al: Multiple idiopathic mucosal neuromas: A minor form of multiple endocrine neoplasia type 2B or a new entity? J Am Acad Dermatol 37:349–352, 1997.
131. Adkins JC, Ravitch MM: Neurofibromatosis-Von Recklinghausen's disease. In Welch KJ, Randolph JG, Ravitch MM, et al (eds): Pediatric Surgery. Vol. 2 (4th ed). Chicago, Year Book Medical, 1986, pp 1500–1504.
132. Hamanaka S, Hamanaka Y, Yamashita Y, et al: Leiomyoblastoma and leiomyomatosis of the small intestine in a case of Von Recklinghausen's disease. J Dermatol 24:117–119, 1997.
133. Raney RB, Littman P, Jarrett P, et al: Results of multimodal therapy for children with neurogenic sarcoma. Med Pediatr Oncol 7:229, 1979.
134. Chu JY, O'Connor DM, Danis RK: Neurofibrosarcoma at irradiation site in a patient with neurofibromatosis and Wilms' tumor. Cancer 31:333–335, 1981.
135. Mulvihill JJ: Childhood cancer, the environment and heredity. In Pizzo PA, Poplack DG (eds): Principles and Practice of Pediatric Oncology (2nd ed). Philadelphia, JB Lippincott, 1993, pp 11–29.
136. Dehner LP: Soft tissue, peritoneum, and retroperitoneum. In Dehner LP (ed): Pediatric Surgical Pathology (2nd ed). Baltimore, Williams & Wilkins, 1987, pp 869–938.
137. Enzinger FM, Weiss SW: Benign fibrous tissue tumors. In Enzinger FM, Weiss SW (eds): Soft Tissue Tumors (3rd ed). St Louis, CV Mosby, 1995, pp 165–199.
138. Miser JS, Pritchard DJ, Triche TJ, et al: The other soft tissue sarcomas of childhood. In Pizzo PA, Poplack DG (eds): Principles and Practice of Pediatric Oncology (2nd ed). Philadelphia, JB Lippincott, 1993, pp 823–840.
139. Enzinger FM, Weiss SW: Benign tumors of peripheral nerves. In Enzinger FM, Weiss SW (eds): Soft Tissue Tumors (3rd ed). St Louis, CV Mosby, 1995, pp 871–872.
140. Hurwitz S: Tumors of fat, muscles, and bone. In Hurwitz S (ed): Clinical Pediatric Dermatology (2nd ed). Philadelphia, WB Saunders, 1993, p 233.
141. Rosai J: Soft tissues. In Rosai J (ed): Ackerman's Surgical Pathology (8th ed). St Louis, CV Mosby, 1996, pp 2021–2135.
142. Enzinger FM, Weiss SW: Fibromatoses. In Enzinger FM, Weiss SW (eds): Soft Tissue Tumors (3rd ed). St Louis, CV Mosby, 1995, pp 201–229.
143. Miller GG, Yanchar NL, Magee JF, et al: Lipoblastoma and liposarcoma in children: An analysis of 9 cases and review of the literature. Can J Surg 41:455–458, 1998.
144. Dehner LP: Bone and joints. In Dehner LP (ed): Pediatric Surgical Pathology (2nd ed). Baltimore, Williams & Wilkins, 1987, pp 939–1025.
145. Enzinger FM, Weiss SW: Benign soft tissue tumors of uncertain type. In Enzinger FM, Weiss SW (eds): Soft Tissue Tumors (3rd ed). St Louis, CV Mosby, 1995, pp 1039–1066.
146. Rosai J: Bones and joints. In Rosai J (ed): Ackerman's Surgical Pathology (8th ed). St Louis, CV Mosby, 1996, pp 1917–2020.
147. Angelides AC: Ganglions of the hand and wrist. In Green DP (ed): Operative Hand Surgery (3rd ed). New York, Churchill Livingstone, 1993, pp 2157–2172.
148. Buck P, Mickelson MR, Bonfiglo M: Synovial sarcoma: Review of 33 cases. Clin Orthop 156:211–215, 1981.
149. Varela-Duran J, Enzinger FM: Calcifying synovial sarcoma. Cancer 50:345–352, 1982.

68

LYMPHOMAS

Alan S. Gamis, MD, MPH

Lymphomas are a result of chromosomal alterations permitting uncontrolled growth of cells of lymphoid origin. Lymphomas are the second most common solid tumors that occur in childhood (behind brain tumors and ahead of neuroblastoma) and make up 15% of all childhood solid tumors diagnosed annually in children. Almost 1200 new childhood cases are diagnosed each year.

Lymphomas have classically been divided into two distinct groups: Hodgkin's disease (HD) and non-Hodgkin's lymphoma (NHL). Both *typically* present with enlarged lymph nodes and may have systemic symptoms of fever and fatigue, extra lymphatic spread, or both. However, these two types of lymphoma also have clear differences. HD typically presents as an indolent process, whereas NHL most often presents with symptoms of rapid onset. Due to rapid tumor growth, children with NHL often have associated anatomic and metabolic comorbidities of such a degree that diagnosis and treatment constitutes a medical emergency.

These two lymphomas are truly a study of contrasts, exemplified in the evolution of their therapy. HD has for years been one of the most curable cancers. Now, with markedly improved treatment protocols, NHL has nearly equivalent cure rates.[1] Owing to the historically high survival rates of HD, its therapy has focused on the reduction of intensity. NHL therapy, owing to its previously poor prognosis, has focused on intensification of treatment. The role of surgery in lymphoma is aimed at the rapid attainment of adequate and properly preserved biopsy material to permit the pathologist to make the diagnosis of the *specific type and subtype* of lymphoma. Except for certain situations, attempts to resect lymphomas at the time of presentation have no role in the modern management of lymphomas.

☐ Hodgkin's Disease

Thomas Hodgkin, in 1832, reported on the gross necropsy examination of seven patients who had generalized lymphadenopathy and splenomegaly without evidence of infection or inflammation.[2] Histologic description of the Reed-Sternberg (RS) cell, the pathognomonic multinucleated giant cell, came later.[3, 4] Even though the etiology of HD remains unclear, therapeutic intervention began soon after the discovery of x-rays.

With the understanding of contiguous spread of HD, the application of radiation to adjacent nodal areas resulted in improvement in survival.[5] Limitations of diagnostic radiologic techniques led to the practice of laparotomy with splenectomy and celiac node and liver biopsy for the purpose of staging and targeting therapy.[6] This has properly been described as the *model for the careful staging of cancer as a required prerequisite to the design of therapy*, which is a hallmark of oncologic practice today.[7, 8]

Chemotherapy combinations have made HD one of the most curable cancers, with rates of cure typically exceeding 90% for patients presenting with nondisseminated disease. With this high expectation for cure, attention since the late 1980s in pediatric oncology has focused on the reduction of long-term sequelae of treatment. Chemotherapy has evolved from an adjunctive role to a primary one, with the hope of eliminating the need for radiation altogether. When radiation therapy is needed, the focus has been to reduce both the size of the fields and the doses used. The chemotherapy agents used, of which there have been two classic combinations (MOPP—nitrogen *m*ustard, vincristine (*O*ncovin), *p*rocarbazine, *p*rednisone; and ABVD—*A*driamycin, *b*leomycin, *v*inblastine, *d*acarbazine), have also evolved to reduce long-term sequelae. Hybrids of these combinations have reduced the doses delivered to the patient with equivalent results and less toxicity.

INCIDENCE AND EPIDEMIOLOGY

HD is the sixth most common type of childhood cancer, with about 500 children diagnosed annually; it constitutes 44% of all childhood cases of lymphoma. There is a gradual trend of increasing incidence with increasing age (Fig. 68–1). Beyond the

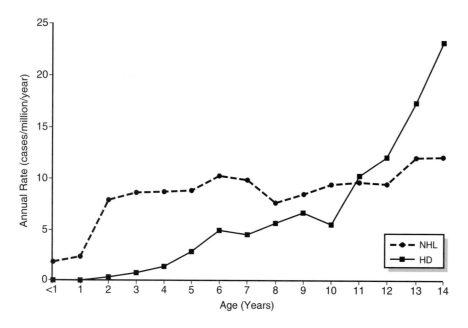

Figure 68–1. Incidence rates for lymphomas in children younger than 15 years. HD, Hodgkin's disease; NHL, non-Hodgkin's lymphoma. Adapted from Gurney JG, Severson RK, Davis S, Robison LL: Incidence of cancer in children in the United States. Cancer 75:2186–2195, 1995.

age of 11 years, it is the most common of the two types of lymphoma. There is a slight male predominance (1.32:1), most pronounced in the youngest children.[9] HD occurs more often in Caucasians than African Americans (1.55:1). Familial clusters of HD have been reported. Whether this represents risk due to environmental exposure (infectious) or genetics is uncertain. Monozygotic twins of HD patients are at greater risk of developing HD than dizygotic twins,[10] strongly implicating genetics as a principle risk factor. Among young adults, there is an increased risk of HD with higher socioeconomic status,[11] smaller families, fewer infectious exposures as young children, and later exposure to infections.[11, 12] These risks implicate a delayed infectious exposure as a principal factor.

Most likely, it is a combination of genetic risk and infectious exposure that predisposes a young adult to HD. Immunodeficiency may be the link between these two risk factors; HD is more prevalent in HIV–infected patients,[13, 14] and patients with HD have a higher incidence of cellular immunodeficiency at the time of diagnosis.[15] Etiologic theories focus primarily on the Epstein-Barr virus (EBV). Genomic material from EBV has been found in RS cells in up to 79% of patients with HD.[16–19] There is a higher risk of HD in patients with a history of infectious mononucleosis[20] and with previously high titers to EBV.[21]

One hypothesis that incorporates these factors suggests the following sequence:

1. Either a genetic, iatrogenic, or viral immunosuppression
2. Subsequent or coincidental EBV infection or oncogenetic rearrangement in a lymphoid precursor cell
3. Further genetic alterations, followed by
4. Clonal expansion of lymphoid cells with morphologic features of RS cells, finally resulting in

5. The clinical syndrome known as HD, diagnosed by the presence of RS cells[22]

CELL BIOLOGY

Diagnosis of HD requires the dual finding of the diagnostic RS cell and a reactive cellular background.[23] The RS cell is a large cell (15 to 45 μm) with an "owl's eye" appearance, owing to a bilobed nucleus. The RS cell often makes up no more than 2% of the involved tissues. The cellular background is a reactive, pleomorphic mixture of inflammatory cells, including reactive lymphocytes, histiocytes, plasma cells, eosinophils, neutrophils, and fibroblasts with varying degrees of fibrosis and sclerosis. The RS cell is thought to be the neoplastic cell in HD that creates this reactive background through the abundant release of various cytokines.[24] Evidence suggests the RS cell has a B-lymphocytic origin.[25]

The Rye classification divides HD into the following four primary morphologic classifications:

1. Nodular sclerosing (the most common)
2. Mixed cellularity
3. Lymphocyte predominant
4. Lymphocyte depleted[26]

The nodular sclerosing subtype is seen in 40% of younger patients and in 70% of adolescents with HD.[27] It is characterized by tumor nodules surrounded by broad sclerotic bands arising from a thickened fibrotic capsule.[23] This subtype has a strong predilection for involvement of the lower cervical, supraclavicular, and mediastinal lymph nodes.

The mixed cellular subtype is found in 30% of cases and has an increased incidence in younger children.[9] RS cells are typically increased in number. The lymph node architecture is often completely effaced by the RS cells and their surrounding reactive cells. This subtype often presents with advanced, widely disseminated disease in extranodal sites.

The lymphocyte-predominant subtype is seen in 10% to 15% of children, typically younger patients with localized disease. Histology shows benign-appearing lymphocytes with an occasional RS cell. This subtype can be misdiagnosed as reactive hyperplasia.

The lymphocyte-depleted subtype is rare in children but is common in HIV patients.[28] Histologically, there are rare lymphocytes with many RS cells and numerous, bizarre, malignant reticular cells. This type often presents with widespread disease involving the bone and bone marrow.

Reported 5-year survival rates by histologic subtype were as follows: lymphoctye predominant, 83.9%, nodular sclerosing, 82.2%, mixed cellularity, 68.1%; and lymphocyte depleted, 36.4%.[29] All types are currently treated similarly; the poorer outcome of the latter two types may reflect their typically higher stage at diagnosis.

CLINICAL PRESENTATION

Children present with painless enlarged lymph nodes typically in the cervical or supraclavicular nodal groups. These nodes are usually rubbery and fixed and can be either single or matted. Occasionally, owing to rapid growth, tenderness may be present. Tumor lysis syndrome is rarely seen in children with HD.

More than 90% of patients with HD present with involvement of the cervical or mediastinal nodal groups.[30] HD tends to spread from the cervical nodes of one side of the neck to the mediastinum before it spreads to the contralateral cervical nodes. The mixed cellularity and lymphocyte-depleted subtypes have more widespread involvement than the nodular sclerosing or lymphocyte-predominant subtypes.

Mediastinal disease is most common in female patients older than 12 years and in those with constitutional symptoms.[31] Mediastinal disease may present with significant respiratory compromise due to compression of the airway.[28] These patients may present with dyspnea on exertion, shortness of breath at rest, persistent cough, or stridor. They may have recently been treated for presumed asthma or bronchiolitis without radiographic examination. Patients with a mediastinal lymphoma may have orthopnea and are most comfortable in an upright, forward-leaning position. The physician must be vigilant for mediastinal disease because it may be silent until a patient is sedated for radiologic or surgical procedures. These patients may prove impossible to aerate even with intubation owing to distal major airway obstruction. It is imperative that all patients with suspected lymphoma (HD *or* NHL) have a chest radiograph before *any* sedation or procedure. These patients may also have signs of superior vena caval obstruction.[32]

Three fourths of patients have no systemic symp-

toms at the time of initial diagnosis. The other one fourth have one or more constitutional symptoms (also known as *B symptoms*), including weight loss of more than 10% in the previous 6 months, unexplained fever with temperatures higher than 38°C, or night sweats.[30] Pruritus, fatigue, and anorexia are other nonspecific symptoms seen in HD patients. Anemia and thrombocytopenia, both infrequent, may be due either to marrow involvement with HD or to immune cytopenias.[33, 34]

DIAGNOSIS

The diagnostic evaluation should include physical, laboratory, and radiologic examination (Table 68–1). Physical examination should pay close attention not only to the obviously involved nodal groups but also to adjacent groups, keeping in mind the propensity for contiguous spread. The number of involved nodal groups in stage II patients (more than four) has been associated with a worse prognosis and should be carefully determined.[35] The size of the palpated nodal masses should be determined and recorded. Bulky disease (nodes or nodal aggregates larger than 10 cm or mediastinal tumor width more than one third of intrathoracic width on a posteroanterior chest radiograph or computed tomography [CT] scan) is associated with worse outcome in patients with early-stage disease and necessitates additional therapy to achieve equivalent outcomes.[36–38] Auscultation of the airway, palpation of the abdomen, and examination of distant nodal groups are also critical.

Laboratory examination should include full blood counts and chemistries, including hepatic function tests, lactate dehydrogenase (LDH) levels, and erythrocyte sedimentation rate (ESR). Serum copper and ferritin levels may also be obtained. However, there are no clinical findings pathognomonic for HD.

Ultimately, the diagnosis awaits the biopsy of in-

TABLE 68-1. Diagnostic and Staging Evaluation of Hodgkin's Disease at Presentation

Complete physical examination with documentation of involved nodal groups (including measurements of nodes) and involved extralymphatic organs
Complete blood count, chemistry panel including hepatic function tests, erythrocyte sedimentation rate, copper, ferritin, lactate dehydrogenase level
Chest radiograph to evaluate for possible mediastinal disease and airway compression
Computed tomography scans of areas identified on physical examination (also include chest, neck, and abdomen)
Gallium scan
Bone scan
Excisional biopsy of node
Bone marrow biopsies and aspirates (bilateral)
Lymphangiogram (optional)
Staging laparotomy (mandatory if considering radiation therapy alone) with splenectomy, nodal sampling, and wedge biopsies of hepatic lobes

volved sites, most commonly an excised lymph node. Fresh specimens should be placed in a sterile container and delivered quickly to the pathologist for processing. Formalin should never be used. For patients critically ill at diagnosis, such as those with severe airway obstruction, diagnosis by alternative methods should be strongly considered. Alternative methods may include nodal biopsy with local anesthetic alone, CT-guided percutaneous needle biopsy of a mass, aspiration of pleural effusion, or bone marrow biopsy and aspirate.

STAGING

Further evaluation of a patient with HD is required to determine accurately the extent of disease at diagnosis and thus the stage of disease (Table 68–2).[38] HD is further subdivided into asymptomatic (A) and symptomatic (B) subcategories. Patients with symptomatic HD have a worse prognosis and require chemotherapy in addition to radiation therapy. Patients with symptoms are more apt to have distant, widespread disease.[39]

Therapy for HD rests on the staging results. Until recently, all patients underwent both clinical and pathologic staging. Clinical staging includes physical, laboratory, and radiologic evaluations. Pathologic staging requires laparotomy with splenectomy, nodal sampling, and wedge biopsies of hepatic lobes. Lymphangiography has been reported to be more sensitive than CT in the assessment of possible abdominal nodal disease in cases in which there was a subsequent staging laparotomy.[40, 41] Other investigators reported no difference[42] and also that the expertise required to perform lymphangiography is not widespread. CT examination is used most frequently.[43]

Staging laparotomy has been shown to "up-stage" disease in up to 35% of patients as compared with CT staging.[44, 45] However, with the use of systemic chemotherapy and the de-emphasis on radiation therapy, this no longer appears to have a significant impact on treatment or outcome.[46, 47] Staging laparotomy should continue to be used in patients destined to be treated with radiation therapy alone because the presence of abdominal disease has a significant impact on therapy.[48–51] Gallium scans are useful in identifying unrecognized sites of disease at presentation and for following disease regression with and after therapy.

Patients with nodular sclerosing mediastinal disease often have persistently enlarged cervical and mediastinal nodes after therapy. If these sites were gallium avid at presentation, a negative gallium scan indicates a nonneoplastic cause of persistent nodal enlargement.[52–55] It is also important to be aware of the phenomenon of thymic rebound after therapy, which may result in both an enlarging mediastinal mass on CT and a positive gallium scan. The experienced radiologist recognizes this phenomenon by its timing (within the first 6 months after therapy has been completed) and by the normal (though enlarged) homogeneous appearance of the thymic tissue. However, false-negative interpretations can occur, and close follow-up of these patients is critical. A positive bone marrow examination upgrades the patient to a stage IV status, which necessitates much more intensive chemotherapy.

TREATMENT

Treatment of HD has been by radiation therapy alone, combinations of radiation and chemotherapy, and most recently, chemotherapy without radiation therapy. Three themes guide modern pediatric HD therapy. First, for patients with early-stage or low-stage HD (stage I–III), reduction of therapy duration and intensity reduces long-term sequelae while maintaining high cure rates. The second theme is the elimination of radiation therapy in patients with early- or low-stage HD. The third theme is the intensification of therapy in patients with advanced-stage HD (stage IV) and identification of new and more effective regimens to increase their relapse-free survival. Most children with HD are enrolled or registered with the National Cancer Institute–sponsored cooperative groups—Children's Cancer Group and Pediatric Oncology Group. Treatment should be coordinated through one of the centers associated with these two groups.

Principles of Radiation Therapy

HD is a radiosensitive neoplasm. Radiation therapy given to the sites of disease and contiguous

TABLE 68-2. Ann Arbor Staging Classification for Hodgkin's Disease

Stage	Definition
I	Involvement of a single lymph node region (I) or of a single extralymphatic organ or site (I_E)
II	Involvement of two or more lymph node regions on the same side of the diaphragm (II) or localized involvement of an extralymphatic organ or site and its regional lymph node(s) with involvement of one or more lymph node regions on the same side of the diaphragm (II_E)
III	Involvement of lymph node regions on both sides of the diaphragm (III), which may be accompanied by involvement of the spleen (III_S) or by localized involvement of an extralymphatic organ or site (III_E) or both (III_{SE})
IV	Disseminated (multifocal) involvement of one or more extralymphatic organs or tissues with or without associated lymph node involvement or isolated extralymphatic organ involvement with distant (nonregional) nodal involvement

Adapted from Carbone PP, Kaplan HS, Husshoff K, et al: Report of the Committee on Hodgkin's Disease Staging Classification. Cancer Res 31:1860–1861, 1971.

clinically uninvolved areas is known as *extended-field irradiation*. More recently, *involved-field irradiation* coupled with chemotherapy has been shown to provide excellent local control (97%).[56] Finally, a *shrinking-field* technique is used when possible. This requires repeated measurements to reduce the radiation field continually as the primary tumor shrinks.

Megavoltage therapy reduces the scatter seen with cobalt-60 and is given preferentially with a 4- to 8-MeV linear accelerator. Recent evidence suggests doses of 4000–4400 cGy to diseased areas and 3000–4000 cGy to contiguous areas. Further reduction in radiation dosage to less than 2500 cGy is possible when used in conjunction with systemic chemotherapy.[56]

The side effects of radiation therapy, which include cosmetic defects, growth retardation, endocrinologic sequelae, and secondary malignancy, are compelling reasons to eliminate radiation therapy completely in the treatment of children with HD. Chemotherapy combinations are the principal therapy for HD in children, and radiation, if used, is given in low doses and to limited areas. The small subgroup of children in whom radiation may still be considered front-line therapy are the fully grown adolescent boys with localized disease (stages I and IIA). The use of alkylating agents in this particular group results in reduced fertility. Because growth is complete, radiation does not result in cosmetic deformities owing to arrest of bone growth. Conversely, radiation therapy for adolescent girls should be given only after strong consideration of the increased risk of breast cancer known to result from irradiation of breast tissue at this critical age.[57–61]

Principles of Chemotherapy

Chemotherapy is the mainstay of treatment of growing children with HD. For patients with early-stage HD, the MOPP or ABVD regimen is administered over 12 months; both have resulted in excellent outcomes.[62, 63] Recognition of the sequelae of this "full-dose" regimen has led to newer combinations of therapy. Hybrid protocols have either replaced the agents with the worst sequelae (e.g., cyclophosphamide replacing nitrogen mustard) or have used them at much lower doses. In addition, the number of chemotherapy cycles or overall duration has been significantly decreased.[37, 64] Full treatment is now given monthly for four to six cycles.

Stage-Related Therapy

Therapy for HD is dictated almost exclusively by the stage in which the child presents. An exception to this is that stage II and III patients with symptoms typically receive six courses of therapy instead of four. Current recommendations are for patients with stage I or II disease to receive four cycles of chemotherapy with an additional two cycles dependent on the presence of bulky disease, number of involved

nodal sites, and demonstrated incomplete remission after four cycles. Patients with stage III disease and those with adverse risk factors should receive six cycles of therapy. Patients with bulky mediastinal disease should probably receive radiation therapy in addition to systemic chemotherapy. Stage IV patients should receive more intensive regimens of systemic chemotherapy and involved-field radiation. Blood or marrow stem cell transplantation is reserved for patients who are refractory to systemic chemotherapy or whose disease has relapsed less than 1 year after achieving complete remission. Those whose disease relapses later than 1 year after achieving remission can often be salvaged with additional conventional chemotherapy.

RESULTS

More than 90% of patients treated with combinations of chemotherapy and radiation therapy enter into complete remission.[65, 66] Many patients, especially those with the nodular sclerosing subtype, may have persistent adenopathy or mediastinal enlargement for months or years after therapy. Although most are cured, close monitoring of these patients is critical. For those who do not enter remission with today's front-line chemotherapy and radiation therapy combinations, the prognosis is poor, and intensification with the use of stem cell transplantation should be considered.[67]

For patients with stage I or II disease, combined therapy typically results in higher than 90% 5-year disease-free survival (DFS) rates; for stage III patients, higher than 80% 5-year DFS; and for stage IV patients, higher than 60% DFS.

Acute Complications

Acute complications of therapy in children with HD are due either to the tumor itself or to the therapy administered. Overwhelming sepsis is the acute complication of splenectomy for staging. This risk is increased by the effects of chemotherapy. Fever in the neutropenic patient necessitates hospitalization and intravenous antibiotic therapy. Bone marrow suppression may necessitate transfusions of either red blood cells or platelets. Specific chemotherapy agents used may have acute complications, such as nausea and vomiting, restrictive pulmonary disease (bleomycin, irradiation), extravasation burns (nitrogen mustard, vincristine, vinblastine, doxorubicin), and chemical phlebitis (nitrogen mustard, vinblastine, dacarbazine). To alleviate these risks, central venous catheters are often placed.

Long-Term Complications

Radiation to bone often results in growth arrest, causing cosmetic deformities years later. This may result in shortening of the clavicles in patients receiving mantle irradiation or shortened height in those receiving radiation to the spine.[68] Radiation to the neck often results in permanent hypothyroidism[69] and increases the risk of developing thyroid cancer.[70, 71] If radiation is to be given to the pelvis of a female patient, gonadopexy should be considered to remove the ovaries from the field of radiation.[72]

Second malignancies are a major concern.[73] The relative risk of a second malignancy in HD patients carries a 15-year actuarial risk of 7 to 23%.[74–76] These second cancers include leukemia and solid tumors. One study recently found a decrease in secondary leukemia among patients treated with the newer hybrid regimens,[76] likely a result of reduction in nitrogen mustard and procarbazine in MOPP therapy.[77, 78] Patients treated with ABVD do not have an increased risk of developing leukemia. Splenectomy has repeatedly been shown to increase the risk of leukemia in HD patients treated with chemotherapy.[49–51] Solid tumors, including lung, stomach, melanoma, bone, and soft tissue, have accounted for most of the second malignancies, with a cumulative incidence of about 13% at 15 to 19 years of follow-up.[79] This increased risk of solid tumors is primarily related to radiation,[80, 81] possibly with an additive risk when subsequent chemotherapy is administered in relapse patients.[82] Radiation exposure to the adolescent breast has been shown to increase the risk of secondary breast cancer to as high as 35% by 40 years of age.[57–59, 61, 73] For all types of secondary cancer, adolescents appear to be at greater risk than younger children.[71, 83]

Other long-term sequelae include pericarditis or myocardiopathy secondary to mantle irradiation, and the use of doxorubicin (in ABVD regimens), which effects up to 13% of patients.[83, 84] Pulmonary toxicity caused by bleomycin or irradiation affected up to 9% of children, but this high incidence appears to be decreasing with the use of hybrid regimens and low-dose involved-field irradiation. Female infertility and early menopause are primarily a result of exposure of the ovaries to radiation,[85, 86] which is less likely to occur if the ovaries are surgically moved out of the field of radiation.[72] Male patients have a significant rate (30 to 40%) of gonadal dysfunction at the time of diagnosis.[87] After six courses of MOPP therapy, most male patients are sterile.[88] There is no similar effect when ABVD is used.[89] Spermatogenesis is only transiently affected by pelvic irradiation for HD. Although spermatogenesis is significantly affected by MOPP therapy, testosterone production appears unimpaired.

☐ Non-Hodgkin's Lymphoma

In contrast to Hodgkin's disease, the presentation, treatment, and outcome of NHL are dramatically different in children and adults. Most adults with NHL have low-grade or intermediate-grade lymphomas, whereas virtually all children present with advanced or disseminated disease (stages III to IV). These lymphomas typically present with a rapidly expanding mass over a short time. It is this propensity for rapid growth that makes the diagnostic evaluation in a child with suspected NHL urgent, approaching a medical emergency. Of all the childhood tumors, NHL has the greatest chance of acute complications preceding therapy. Anatomic impingement of mediastinal tumors on the airway, nasopharyngeal tumors on the orbits, bowel obstruction with or without intussusception, and metabolic derangements due to spontaneous tumor lysis are common. Understanding the initial anatomic and metabolic complications, improved methods of determining the subtypes of NHL, and better chemotherapy combinations have led to the achievement of the most dramatic improvements in survival of all childhood tumors during the past several decades.[90] The other major change in NHL therapy for children has been the virtual elimination of radiation from treatment regimens.

INCIDENCE AND EPIDEMIOLOGY

The 666 annual pediatric NHL cases diagnosed account for 6.3% of all childhood cancers, 8.7% of solid tumors, and 57% of lymphomas. Before the age of 11 years, NHL is the most common of the two types of lymphoma. There is a high male-to-female ratio of 2.6:1. This large difference is present throughout childhood. The risk in Caucasian children is 1.7 times that in African American children.

There are two small peaks in occurrence of NHL at 6 to 7 years of age and again at 12 to 14 years (see Fig. 68–1). These peaks coincide with the two most common histologic types of NHL: the 6- to 7-year-olds overwhelmingly have small noncleaved cell lymphoma (SNCCL) of B-cell origin, and the teenagers typically have lymphoblastic lymphoma (LBL) of T-cell origin.

NHL of B-cell origin, either SNCCL or large cell lymphoma (LCL), occurs more often in patients with prior EBV exposure, in patients with a history of immune suppression, and in equatorial Africa.[91–93] EBV infection in the immune-compromised child probably has a role either in the development of or the predisposition to B-cell NHL.[94, 95] For T-cell NHL (LBL) or anaplastic LCL, no such etiologic correlations have been made.

CLASSIFICATION

The Revised European-American Classification of Lymphoid Neoplasms (REAL)[96] has been developed in an effort to eliminate the confusion surrounding the lymphoma subtypes caused by the prior classification schemes. This is a consensus classification based on morphologic, immunologic, and cytogenetic characteristics that also describes the typical clinical presentation, the course, and the putative cell of origin. The reader is referred to this summary for further detailed information.[96]

Unlike the myriad subtypes of NHL seen in adults, childhood NHL primarily consists of just three subtypes: SNCCL, 39%; LBL, 28%; and LCL, which may have B-cell or T-cell origin and is usually anaplastic, 26%. The first two are "small, round, blue cell tumors," which are differentiated from neuroblastoma, rhabdomyosarcoma, and Ewing's sarcoma by the presence of an immunocytochemical marker called the *leukocyte common antigen* (LCA) CD45, present in the NHL cell.

SNCCL has classically been divided into Burkitt's and non-Burkitt's (Burkitt-like in the REAL classification) subtypes. These tumors are of a mature B-cell origin, with flow cytometric immunophenotyping revealing the presence of surface immunoglobulin M, several B-cell markers, and HLA-DR antigen. These two types of SNCCL differ histologically in their degree of pleomorphism, but they appear to have no clinical differences.[97] Burkitt's cells are medium-sized cells with round nuclei containing multiple (2 to 5) nucleoli, abundant basophilic cytoplasm, and cytoplasmic lipid vacuoles. Owing to the extreme rates of proliferation and spontaneous cell death seen in Burkitt's lymphoma, the macrophages that consume the dying Burkitt's cells give rise to the classic "starry-sky" appearance.[96]

LBLs are distinguished by round or convoluted nuclei, fine dispersed chromatin, inconspicuous nucleoli, and scant cytoplasm. In most of these tumors, flow cytometry reveals the presence of the T-cell markers, CD3 and CD7, with variable positivity of CD2 and CD5. This subtype is classified as a precursor T-cell neoplasm in the REAL classification.[96]

LCLs are a heterogeneous group of neoplasms. Histologically, about half are immunoblastic, 40% are large noncleaved cell, and 5% are large cleaved cell.[98] Flow cytometry shows relatively equal frequencies of B-cell and T-cell origin, 36% and 33%, respectively, with 30% of indeterminate origin.[99, 100] A unique subset, identified by the immunophenotype, CD30+ (the antigen identified by the Ki-1 monoclonal antibody[101]), is recognized morphologically by its anaplastic characteristics, including very large cells with abundant cytoplasm, atypical lobulated nuclei, and prominent nucleoli. These cells exhibit a cohesive pattern with a typical lymph node sinusoidal invasion. In the REAL classification, this is referred to as *anaplastic large cell lymphoma*.[96] This subtype has in the past also been referred to as *malignant histiocytosis*. Most of these children (60%) have a T-cell immunophenotype.[99, 102] Originally thought to be uncommon in children, recent studies reveal that it accounts for 40 to 50% of LCL cases.[99, 100, 103, 104] These cells are also immunophenotypically positive for CD25, CD71, and CD1a. CD30 is also found on the RS cells in HD, but these two entities are clearly different on a clinical level, with anaplastic LCL more similar to other NHLs than to HD.[102]

CELL BIOLOGY

Cancer is a result of (1) the inappropriate or unregulated expression of a gene, at either the wrong time in a cell's cycle or in the wrong cell, (2) abnormal combinations of genes producing proteins not normally present in cells, or (3) the loss of gene expression and their products required for cellular control. These first two categories encompass the protooncogenes and oncogenes, and the last comprises the tumor-suppressor genes.

Lymphomas arise from precursors of lymphocytes at various stages of maturation, primarily caused by errors in transcriptional factor control and production, as a result of protooncogenes and oncogenes. Early B and T cells normally splice together different segments of their immunoglobulin and T-cell–receptor genes to generate the diverse proteins capable of binding foreign antigens.[105] In lymphoid cancers, this system goes awry as a result of the inadvertent splicing (juxtaposition) of transcription factor genes (protooncogenes) to one of these regions. This leads to the abnormal and unregulated expression of this gene (now an oncogene) and the production of its oncoprotein. It is this oncoprotein that eventually leads to the cell's malignant transformation (by a variety of mechanisms) and hence its uncontrolled growth. The reader is referred elsewhere for more detailed descriptions of normal and oncologic gene regulation and expression (transcription).[105–108] This neoplastic process typically occurs as a result of nonrandom chromosomal translocations or inversions, although deletions and insertions of DNA sequences likely also contribute to the malignant transformation.

Burkitt's lymphoma is the tumor in which this phenomena was originally described.[109] The translocation involving chromosomes 8 and 14 was first identified in Burkitt's cells in 1976.[110] As a result of this translocation, t(8; 14), the *c-myc* oncogene located on chromosome 8q24, is juxtaposed to the immunoglobulin receptor subunit gene on chromosome 14q32 (immunoglobulin heavy-chain gene). This translocation is found in both African (endemic) and American (sporadic) patients with Burkitt's lymphoma, although the exact breakpoints on chromosome 8 differ.[111] In a smaller percentage of patients with Burkitt's lymphoma, *c-myc* is juxtaposed to chromosome 2p11 (κ immunoglobulin light-chain gene), t(2;8), or 22q11 (λ light-chain gene), t(8;22).[112] It is thought that an increased pool of B cells, either through chronic stimulation, as in the case of malaria, or through inhibition of cell death, as in the case of EBV, increases the chance occurrence of these translocations.[113, 114] The oncoprotein, *MYC*, normally controls progression through G1 into the S phase of the cell cycle, but as a result of these translocations, its expression is dysregulated, leading to uncontrolled lymphoproliferation.[115]

For T-cell lymphomas or LBLs, translocations are found less often. The translocations known to date result in the juxtaposition of several different oncogenes to T-cell–receptor (TCR) genes located on chromosomes 14q11 (TCR α/δ) and 7 (TCR β).[105, 115] Nonrandom translocations found in LBLs of T-cell origin include t(11;14), t(1;14), t(10;14), t(7;19), t(8;14), and t(1;7) and involve the oncogenes *RHOMB1 & 2* (11p13 and 15), *TAL1* (1p32), *HOX11* (10q24), *LYL1* (19p13), *MYC* (8q24), and *LCK* (1p34). The cytogenetic translocation most often found in LCL patients is that associated with the Ki-1, CD30[+] anaplastic LCLs. In this tumor, t(2;5),[116] when present, results in the juxtapositioning of the *ALK* tyrosine kinase gene on chromosome 5q35 to a ribosomal assembly gene, *NPM*, on chromosome 2p23.[117] This produces an abnormal oncoprotein, NPM-ALK (p80), normally absent in cells.

CLINICAL PRESENTATION

By Initial Site of Disease

Children with NHL present with extranodal disease and typically have disease that spreads by routes other than contiguous nodal pathways. The abdomen is the site of disease in 31% of children, the mediastinum in 27%, and the head and neck in 29%.[1] Other sites include peripheral nodes, bone, and skin. Most abdominal disease primary tumors are due to SNCCL, whereas most mediastinal and intrathoracic primary tumors are due to LBL. Disease that presents primarily in the peripheral nodes and bones is often due to LCL, and skin involvement is primarily associated with the Ki-1[+] LCL subtype.[100, 118, 119] Correlating with this distribution and the known age peaks of the two types of small cell lymphomas, abdominal primary tumors occur more often in children younger than 10 years, whereas mediastinal primary tumors are more likely to occur in adolescents.

Children with abdominal primary tumors may present with nausea, vomiting, abdominal pain, and changes in bowel habits; on physical examination, they are found to have an abdominal mass in any of the quadrants. They may present with an acute abdomen due either to intussusception (typically a result of NHL in Peyer's patches) or small bowel obstruction, perforation of an involved bowel wall, or presence as an ileocecal mass mimicking acute appendicitis.[120] A child with intussusception who is older than 5 years must be considered to have NHL until proved otherwise. NHL must always be in the differential diagnosis of a 5- to 10-year-old child presenting with an abdominal mass. Radiographic evaluation with either CT or ultrasound typically reveals a homogeneous mass with or without evidence of central necrosis arising either from the retroperitoneum or the bowel walls. Accompanying adenopathy and metastatic dissemination to the liver and spleen are often seen. The bowel loops may simply be shifted away from the mass or may show evidence of intussusception or obstruction.

Children with mediastinal primary tumors may present with minimal symptomatology, such as a mild cough or audible wheeze suggestive of asthma, or may present with obstruction of the airway. These patients may also have the superior vena caval syndrome. They may assume a forward-leaning position and have orthopnea, shortness of breath, and dyspnea on exertion. A chest radiograph is an essential component of the patient's initial evaluation before any sedation or procedure. A chest radiograph and CT scan of the chest reveal the widened mediastinum with often dramatic narrowing of the trachea and bronchi. Pleural or pericardial effusions may be revealed by CT, magnetic resonance imaging (MRI), or echocardiography.[121]

Patients with head and neck lymphomas may present with a history of rapidly progressive adenopathy, recent onset of snoring at night, mouth breathing, bad breath, epistaxis, proptosis or periorbital edema, diplopia, extraocular muscle paralysis (entrapment in this case), cranial nerve paralysis, and sudden blindness. Physical examination of the nares, oral cavity, and extraocular movements is critical and may reveal signs not appreciated as abnormal by the child. The presence of asymmetric and painless tonsillar hypertrophy should also alert the clinician to the possibility of NHL.[122] Radiographic evaluation with CT reveals a homogeneous mass, often with destruction of the adjacent bony structures.

Bone primary tumors produce localized tenderness seen as lytic lesions on the radiograph.[123–125] NHL may present as a skin ulcer that does not heal or as a subcutaneous nodule. Patients with central nervous system (CNS) disease may have no symptoms, seizures, or signs and symptoms related to the location of tumor infiltration.

Laboratory findings at the time of diagnosis are dependent on the amount of tumor present (regardless of the histologic subtype). Most patients have an elevated ESR. Patients with large tumor burdens typically have high LDH values, which can be followed as a tumor marker. The degree of LDH elevation has been used as an adverse prognostic factor.[1, 126, 127] Laboratory signs of tumor lysis include elevated uric acid, phosphorus, and potassium levels, often with a low calcium level. Some patients may already be in renal failure at the time of presentation, with elevated creatinine levels. Hematologic values are nonspecific. Cytopenias should raise the suspicion of marrow involvement. Cerebrospinal fluid pleocytosis may or may not be present in patients with CNS involvement.

Sixty-one percent of affected children have advanced or disseminated (stage III to IV) disease at diagnosis.[1, 128] Fourteen percent of patients present with some bone marrow involvement. Patients with less than 25% lymphoblasts in the bone marrow are classified as having lymphoma, whereas those with more than 25% lymphoblasts are diagnosed as having leukemia. CNS involvement is seen in 3%.[1]

By Histologic Subtype

Denis Burkitt, in Uganda, described a rapidly growing tumor involving the nodes around the jaw.[129] Later, it was determined that although this is a common presentation of patients with endemic Burkitt's lymphoma (African), patients with sporadic Burkitt's (American) more typically had presentation of disease either in the abdomen or the nasopharynx.[130] Endemic Burkitt's patients have accompanying abdominal disease in roughly half of cases, and sporadic Burkitt's patients have jaw involvement about 15 to 20% of the time.[131] Sporadic Burkitt's patients also have a higher incidence of marrow involvement (21% compared with rates of 7%) but lower CNS dissemination (11% compared with 17%).

About two thirds of SNCCL patients have disseminated or advanced disease (defined as stage III to IV) at diagnosis.[132] LBL patients most often are adolescents presenting with supradiaphragmatic disease, either intrathoracic or head and neck. Disseminated disease is present in nearly 90% of LBL patients at diagnosis.[132] In LBL patients, involvement of the marrow has been seen in about one fourth of children and CNS disease in 10%.[132] LCL patients may have presentations in all sites but have a higher prevalence than the other two subtypes in skin, bone, and peripheral nodes.[118, 125] Disseminated disease in LCL patients is also present at diagnosis in up to 65% of patients[132] (Table 68–3). Involvement of the marrow (2%) or CNS (0%) in LCL patients is rare.[132]

In Immunodeficient Patients

In patients with congenital or acquired immunodeficiency, presentation varies from polyclonal plasmacytic hyperplasia, most often in nasopharyngeal nodes or tonsils, to a clonal polymorphic lymphoma slowly arising in the lymph nodes or extranodal sites, to widely disseminated rapidly progressive immunoblastic lymphoma.[133, 134] This entity has become more common with the use of more potent antirejection drugs after solid organ or bone marrow transplantation.[135]

TABLE 68–3. Prevalence of Primary Sites Among the Three Primary Types of Childhood Non-Hodgkin's Lymphoma

Primary Site	SNCCL	LBL	LCL
Abdomen	56%	3%	25%
Intrathoracic	2%	65%	21%
Head and neck	34%	23%	29%
Peripheral nodes	2%	7%	11%
Other	5%	3%	14%
Total	**100%**	**100%**	**100%**

LBL, lymphoblastic lymphoma; LCL, large cell lymphoma; SNCCL, small noncleaved cell lymphoma.
Adapted from Murphy SB, Fairclough DL, Hutchison RE, Beard CW: Non-Hodgkin's lymphomas of childhood: An analysis of the histology, staging, and response to treatment of 338 cases at a single institution. J Clin Oncol 7:186–193, 1989.

DIAGNOSIS

Children initially suspected to have NHL should be evaluated urgently; the rapidity of tumor growth may create, overnight, a life-threatening complication. Once suspected, a concerted and well thought-out plan of evaluation is important to achieve diagnosis as quickly as possible (see Table 68–1).

The diagnosis awaits the biopsy of involved sites, most commonly an excised lymph node or percutaneous core-sample needle biopsy. It is critical that the excised tissue is quickly delivered fresh and sterile to the pathologist for processing. There must be enough tissue for cytogenetic and molecular genetic evaluations. Formalin should never be used. NHL patients often have severe airway obstruction, and diagnosis by alternative methods should be considered. NHL patients explored for acute abdominal illness should have ample tissue for the pathologist. If resection of bowel is required owing to perforation or obstruction from intussusception, total resection of the lymphoma should be considered. *This is the one instance in which resection of a lymphoma may be beneficial.* Resection definitely reduces the stage of the patient's disease, improves survival, and reduces the amount of therapy required.[136] For all other patients, resection of the mass provides no improvement in staging or long-term cure and delays the time to initiation of chemotherapy. With chemotherapy alone, more than 90% of patients enter complete remission.

Pathologic evaluation of the excised material should include general histochemical techniques used to distinguish a lymphoma from other tumors and to subtype the lymphoma. Flow cytometry analysis of cell-surface markers determines the immunophenotype of the lymphoma. Cytogenetic evaluation for diagnostic translocations and DNA analysis using either Southern blot or the polymerase chain reaction allows for detection of the pathognomonic oncogenes (gene rearrangements) even in the absence of identifiable cytogenetic translocations.[137] These are all essential components of the initial diagnosis and should be performed at an institution capable of performing *all* of them. Therapy differences between the subtypes of lymphoma are such that assignment to the wrong subtype due to a lack of adequate diagnostic material greatly impacts the chance of cure. These evaluations may be performed with biopsy material from any involved site, including the primary mass, enlarged lymph nodes, effusions, and bone marrow.

NHL patients should have a lumbar puncture for cytocentrifuged cerebrospinal fluid analysis, although those with localized abdominal SNCCL and those with LCL are unlikely to have CNS disease. Bilateral iliac crest biopsies and aspirates allow for the marrow examination necessary to distinguish NHL from leukemia.

STAGING

Staging is important in the determination of therapeutic planning. The most widely used staging schema is the St. Jude's, or Murphy, staging system[138] (Table 68–4). This system divides cases into localized (stage I or II) and disseminated or advanced (stage III or IV) disease. Involvement of the CNS or marrow immediately places the patient in the stage IV category. Patients with more than 25% bone marrow involvement are by definition diagnosed with leukemia rather than lymphoma. This includes patients with B-cell or Burkitt's leukemia (L3 leukemia morphologic classification) and T-cell leukemia. The former patients are treated on B-cell NHL protocols with much better results than previously obtained on acute lymphoblastic leukemia (ALL) regimens. Many of the B-cell NHL protocol results reported in the literature include these patients in their stage IV populations. The T-cell leukemia patients remain on ALL protocols, but there are many similarities between these protocols and those used in LBL therapy.

PROGNOSTIC RISK FACTORS

The stage of the lymphoma at diagnosis is a strong predictor of outcome.[1] Prediction of a patient's eventual outcome with stratification of high-risk (for relapse) patients to more intensive or novel therapies and low-risk patients to shorter, more moderate therapies is the goal of prognostic factor development. The therapy given must be considered whenever reviewing prognostic factors reported in NHL. It has been shown definitively that therapy based on histology is of critical importance in the successful outcome of patients.[128]

For SNCCL patients, marrow involvement has

TABLE 68–4. St. Jude's (Murphy) Stages for Childhood Non-Hodgkin's Lymphoma

Stage	Definition
I	Single tumor (extranodal) or single anatomic area (nodal), excluding mediastinum or abdomen
II	Single tumor (extranodal) with regional node involvement On same side of diaphragm: a) Two or more nodal areas b) Two single (extranodal) tumors with or without regional node involvement Primary gastrointestinal tract tumor (usually ileocecal) with or without associated mesenteric node involvement, grossly completely resected
III	On both sides of diaphragm: a) Two single tumors (extranodal) b) Two or more nodal areas All primary intrathoracic tumors (mediastinal, pleural, thymic) All extensive primary intraabdominal disease; unresectable All primary paraspinal or epidural tumors regardless of other sites
IV	Any of the above with initial central nervous system or bone marrow involvement (<25%)

From Murphy SB: Classification, staging and end results of treatment of childhood non-Hodgkin's lymphomas: Dissimilarities from lymphomas in adults. Semin Oncol 7:332–339, 1980.

been an adverse factor for DFS and overall survival (OS).[128] Patients with CNS involvement in both SNCCL and LBL have predictably worse outcomes,[128] although in SNCCL patients, this is probably attributable more to tumor burden than to the presence of CNS disease alone.[139]

LCL patients have their own unique prognostic characteristics, and these are likely to change in the future as this entity is better described and therapy is more appropriately administered according to subtype. Skin involvement at presentation in LCL patients has been shown to be a poor prognostic indicator.[136] In patients with advanced LCL disease, the presence of CD30+ cells has indicated a better OS,[140] although in other studies, there has been no effect on prognosis.[99] B-cell immunophenotype has been shown to improve prognosis.[99] Current staging methods do not appear to carry the same prognostic significance in LCL patients,[99, 103] although in some studies, there are survival differences between stages.[100] Patients with intrathoracic primary tumors have a better prognosis than those with primary tumors elsewhere.[140]

TREATMENT

Therapy for childhood NHL is based on the knowledge that this tumor is extremely chemosensitive. The duration of therapy for SNCCL and LCL has been shortened to 6 months or less because it became apparent that most if not all patients were relapsing within the first 6 to 8 months of therapy. Despite reductions of therapy, no increases in relapse have been seen. Virtually all relapses occur within the first 2 years.[126–128, 141, 142] SNCCL (B-cell) therapy has shown clear improvements when escalated methotrexate and ara-C doses are added to cyclophosphamide and prednisone.[136, 142, 143]

The duration of therapy for LBL remains 33 weeks to 32 months depending on the extent of disease and the particular protocol. Attempts to shorten therapy have led to increased relapses. The most effective regimens for LBL have been similar to the intensive T-cell ALL protocols in current use.

For SNCCL and LCL, there is no increase in DFS or OS with radiation therapy[103, 118, 143]; CNS relapse is effectively prevented with intrathecal chemotherapy.[139] Some type of CNS prophylaxis is thought to be required for all patients with NHL, except those with localized, resected SNCCL or LCL gastrointestinal primary tumors.[141]

Although radiation has been administered to areas of LBL bulk disease, its need is uncertain.[145] Radiation therapy has been used for CNS prophylaxis, but the substitution of intrathecal chemoprophylaxis has not led to increased CNS relapses. Radiation therapy for LBL patients with CNS or testicular disease remains an important part of their treatment.

Several additional therapeutic points deserve mention. Steroids should not be given before a diagnosis has been established because the rapid necrosis induced in the lymphoma makes subtype determination difficult if not impossible. Once adequate tissue is available for the pathologist, chemotherapy, including steroids, is an excellent method for rapid reduction of life-threatening masses. Because of the extreme sensitivity of NHL, it is not unusual to have symptoms resolve completely within 24 hours and to have patients be in complete radiographic remission within 7 days. Tumor destruction is so impressive that many protocols now call for a period of reduced dose chemotherapy for the first week of therapy to prevent the tumor lysis syndrome.

Immunodeficient patients most often have B-cell lymphoma, either small or large cell. For patients with ongoing iatrogenic immune suppression, reduction of the immunosuppressive agent with or without acyclovir may be adequate to induce remission in up to 75% of cases.[146] However, this may not be possible due to the risk of transplant rejection. Interferon alpha has been used with mixed success in these patients and may exacerbate rejection. A small proportion of patients with localized disease may be cured with surgical resection of the involved nodal tissue. When the lymphoma is resistant to these techniques, chemotherapy regimens are used, although mortality has been higher in these immunodeficient patients than in immunocompetent patients.

RESULTS

Today, typically 90 to 100% of patients with NHL achieve complete remission.[103, 141, 147] Patients with localized disease have an overall excellent prognosis regardless of histologic subtype, with DFS rates exceeding 90 to 95%. SNCCL patients with advanced disease are experiencing marked improvements in outcome, with DFS rates exceeding 80% in the most recent trials. LBL patients with disseminated disease have DFS rates exceeding 65 to 70% in most trials. Treatment failures occur typically within the first 2 years after diagnosis, although LCL patients more often have late relapses.

Acute Complications

Depending on the tumor burden present at diagnosis, patients may present with a constellation of significant metabolic derangements known as *tumor lysis syndrome*. This includes hyperuricemia, hyperphosphatemia, hyperkalemia, and hypocalcemia. Life-threatening acute renal failure may occur in as many as 30% of patients without proper treatment.[7] Spontaneous necrosis of the tumor or any manipulation, including transfusion or surgery, may induce a sudden worsening of this syndrome. Adequate hydration (>3000 ml/m^2/day) and prevention of acidosis are essential. Patients should be placed on either allopurinol to reduce the production of uric acid through inhibition of xanthine oxidase, or the experimental agent, urate oxidase, which cleaves uric acid into allantoin, a soluble byproduct. Despite these measures, about 5% of patients require

dialysis to treat either hyperuricemia, hyperphosphatemia, or hyperkalemia.[132, 149]

In addition to the acute airway and intestinal obstructions caused by NHL, blindness may result from a nasopharyngeal primary tumor, and seizures or increased intracranial pressure may result from a CNS primary tumor or metastases.

Because chemotherapy for NHL is myelosuppressive, infection is a significant risk for NHL patients.[128] In one recent study, 63% of the NHL deaths were due to infection. Most patients require transfusion support during treatment owing to myelosuppression. The chemotherapy itself may cause acute complications, including severe chemical burns caused by extravasation of certain vesicant agents (vincristine, anthracyclines). Because most children require the placement of central venous catheters to facilitate their therapy, thrombosis of these lines has become a common complication.[150]

Long-Term Complications

As long-term survival of NHL patients has improved, the concern about sequelae has increased. These sequelae include potential long-term cardiac dysfunction resulting from anthracycline exposures,[84] infertility as a result of the alkylating agents used,[151] and secondary leukemias caused by epipodophyllotoxins (VP16, VM 26) and alkylating agents used in the NHL regimens.[152] Patients must be followed closely so that early identification of adverse sequelae and proper intervention can be achieved and good quality of life maintained in these long-term survivors.

REFERENCES

1. Murphy SB, Fairclough DL, Hutchison RE, Berard CW: Non-Hodgkin's lymphomas of childhood: An analysis of the histology, staging, and response to treatment of 338 cases at a single institution. J Clin Oncol 7:186–193, 1989.
2. Hodgkin T: On some morbid appearances of the absorbent glands and spleen. Med Chirurg Trans 17:68–114, 1832.
3. Sternberg C: Uber eine eigenartige unter dem Bilde der Pseudoleukemaemie verlaufende Tuberculose des lymphatischen Apparetes. Ztschr Heilk 19:21–92, 1898.
4. Reed D: On the pathological changes in Hodgkin's disease: With especial reference to its relation to tuberculosis. Johns Hopkins Hosp Rep 10:133–196, 1902.
5. Gilbert R: Radiotherapy in Hodgkin's disease. AJR Am J Roentgenol 41:198–240, 1939.
6. Kaplan HS, Rosenberg SA: The management of Hodgkin's disease. Cancer 36:796–803, 1975.
7. Hellman S: Thomas Hodgkin and Hodgkin's disease: Two paradigms appropriate to medicine today. JAMA 265:1007–1010, 1991.
8. Zantinga AR, Coppes MJ: Thomas Hodgkin (1798–1866): Pathologist, social scientist, and philanthropist. Med Pediatr Oncol 27:122–127, 1996.
9. Kung FH: Hodgkin's disease in children 4 years of age or younger. Cancer 67:1428–1430, 1991.
10. Mack TM, Cozen W, Shibata DK, et al: Concordance for Hodgkin's disease in identical twins suggesting genetic susceptibility to the young-adult form of the disease. N Engl J Med 332:413–418, 1995.
11. Grufferman S, Delzell E: Epidemiology of Hodgkin's disease. Epidemiol Rev 6:76–106, 1984.

12. Gutensohn N, Cole P: Childhood social environment and Hodgkin's disease. N Engl J Med 304:135–140, 1981.

13. Reynolds P, Sunders LD, Layefsky ME, et al: The spectrum of acquired immunodeficiency syndrome (AIDS)–associated malignancies in San Francisco, 1980–1987. Am J Epidemiol 137:19–30, 1993.

14. Hessol NA, Katz MH, Liu JY, et al: Increased incidence of Hodgkin disease in homsexual men with HIV infection. Ann Intern Med 117:309–311, 1992.

15. Riggs S, Hagemeister FB: Immunodeficiency states: A predisposition to lymphoma. In Fuller LM, Hagemeister FB, Sullivan M, et al (eds): Hodgkin's Disease and Non-Hodgkin's Lymphomas in Adults and Children. New York, Raven, 1988, p 451.

16. Ambinder RF, Browning PJ, Lorenzana I, et al: Epstein-Barr virus and childhood Hodgkin's disease in Honduras and the United States. Blood 81:462–467, 1993.

17. Herbst H, Steinbrecher E, Niedobitek G, et al: Distribution and phenotype of Epstein-Barr virus–harboring cells in Hodgkin's disease. Blood 80:484–491, 1992.

18. Knecht H, Odermatt B, Bachmann E, et al: Frequent detection of Epstein-Barr virus DNA by the polymerase chain reaction in lymph node biopsies from patients with Hodgkin's disease without genomic evidence of B- or T-cell clonality. Blood 78:760–767, 1991.

19. Khan G, Norton AJ, Slavin G: Epstein-Barr virus in Hodgkin disease. Cancer 71:3124–3129, 1993.

20. Rosdahl N, Larsen SO, Clemmesen J: Hodgkin's disease in patients with previous infectious mononucleosis: 30 Years' experience. BMJ 2:253–256, 1974.

21. Evans AS, Gutensohn NM: A population-based case-control study of EBV and other viral antibodies among persons with Hodgkin's disease and their siblings. Int J Cancer 34:149–157, 1984.

22. Haluska FG, Brufsky AM, Canellos GP: The cellular biology of the Reed-Sternberg cell. Blood 84:1005–1019, 1994.

23. Lukes RJ, Butler JJ: The pathology and nomenclature of Hodgkin's disease. Cancer Res 26:1063–1083, 1966.

24. Gruss HJ, Pinto A, Duyster J, et al: Hodgkin's disease: A tumor with disturbed immunological pathways. Immunol Today 18:156–163, 1997.

25. Schwartz RS: Hodgkin's disease: Time for a change. N Engl J Med 337:495–496, 1997.

26. Lukes RJ, Craver LF, Hall TC, et al: Report of the nomenclature committee. Cancer Res 26:1311, 1966.

27. Donaldson SS, Link MP: Childhood lymphomas: Hodgkin's disease and non-Hodgkin's lymphoma. In Moosa AR, Robson MC, Schimpff SC (eds): Comprehensive Textbook of Oncology. Baltimore, Williams & Wilkins, 1986, p 1161.

28. Hudson MM, Donaldson SS: Hodgkin's disease. In Pizzo PA, Poplack DG (eds): Principles and Practice of Pediatric Oncology (3rd ed). Philadelphia, Lippincott-Raven, 1997, p 523.

29. Medeiros LJ, Greinor T: Hodgkin's disease: SEER population-based data 1973–1987. Cancer 75(suppl 1):357–369, 1995.

30. Mauch PM, Kalish LA, Kadin M, et al: Patterns of Hodgkin disease: Implications for etiology and pathogenesis. Cancer 71:2062–2071, 1993.

31. Maity A, Goldwein JW, Lange B, et al: Mediastinal masses in children with Hodgkin's disease. Cancer 69:2755–2760, 1992.

32. Jeffery GM, Mead GM, Whitehouse JM: Life-threatening airway obstruction at the presentation of Hodgkin's disease. Cancer 67:506–510, 1991.

33. Xiros N, Binder T, Anger B, et al: Idiopathic thrombocytopenic purpura and autoimmune hemolytic anemia in Hodgkin's disease. Eur J Hematol 40:437–441, 1988.

34. Levine AM, Thornton P, Forman SJ, et al: Positive Coombs test in Hodgkin's disease: Significance and implications. Blood 55:607–611, 1980.

35. Cosset J, Henry Amar M, Meerwadt J, et al: The EORTC trials for limited stage Hodgkin's disease. Eur J Cancer 28A:1847–1850, 1992.

36. Longo D, Russo A, Duffey P, et al: Treatment of advanced stage massive mediastinal Hodgkin's disease: The case for combined modality therapy. J Clin Oncol 9:227–235, 1991.

37. Vecchi V, Pileri S, Burnelli R, et al: Treatment of pediatric Hodgkin's disease tailored to stage, mediastinal mass, and age. Cancer 72:2049–2057, 1993.

38. Carbone PP, Kaplan HS, Husshoff K, et al: Report of the Committee on Hodgkin's Disease Staging Classification. Cancer Res 31:1860–1861, 1971.

39. Mauch P, Larson D, Osteen R, et al: Prognostic factors for positive surgical staging in patients with Hodgkin's disease. J Clin Oncol 8:257–265, 1990.

40. Castellino RA, Hoppe RT, Blank N, et al: Computed tomography, lymphography, and staging laporatomy: Correlations in initial staging of Hodgkin's disease. AJR Am J Roentgenol 143:37–41, 1984.

41. Mansfield CM, Fabian C, Jones S, et al: Comparison of lymphangiography and computed tomography scanning in evaluating abdominal disease in stages III and IV Hodgkin's disease. Cancer 66:2295–2299, 1990.

42. Dudgeon DL, Miller K, Ghory MJ, et al: The efficacy of lymphangiography in the staging of pediatric Hodgkin's disease. J Pediatr Surg 21:233–235, 1986.

43. Castellino RA: Diagnostic imaging evaluation of Hodgkin's disease and non-Hodgkin's lymphoma. Cancer 67:1177–1180, 1991.

44. Muraji T, Hays DM, Siegel SE, et al: Evaluation of the surgical aspects of staging laparotomy for Hodgkin's disease in children. J Pediatr Surg 17:843–848, 1982.

45. Mendenhall NP, Cantor AB, Williams JL, et al: With modern imaging techniques, is staging laparotomy necessary in pediatric Hodgkin's disease? A Pediatric Oncology Group Study. J Clin Oncol 11:2218–2225, 1993.

46. Gomez GA, Reese PA, Nava H, et al: Staging laparotomy and splenectomy in early Hodgkin's disease: No therapeutic benefit. Am J Med 77:205–210, 1984.

47. Jenkin D, Chan H, Freedman M, et al: Hodgkin's disease in children: Treatment results with MOPP and low-dose, extended field irradiation. CA Cancer Treat Rep 66:949–959, 1982.

48. Russel KJ, Donaldson SS, Cox RS, Kaplan HS: Childhood Hodgkin's disease: Patterns of relapse. J Clin Oncol 2:80–87, 1984.

49. Kaldor JM, Day NE, Clarke EA, et al: Leukemia following Hodgkin's disease. N Engl J Med 322:7–13, 1990.

50. Tura S, Fiacchini M, Zinzani PL, et al: Splenectomy and the increasing risk of secondary acute leukemia in Hodgkin's disease. J Clin Oncol 11:925–930, 1993.

51. Dietrich PY, Henry-Amar M, Cosset JM, et al: Second primary cancers in patients continuously disease-free from Hodgkin's disease: A protective role for the spleen? Blood 84:1209–1215, 1994.

52. Hagemeister FB, Fesus SM, Lamki LM, Haynie TP: Role of gallium scan in Hodgkin's disease. Cancer 65:1090–1096, 1990.

53. Cooper DL, Caride VJ, Zloty M, et al: Gallium scans in patients with mediastinal Hodgkin's disease treated with chemotherapy. J Clin Oncol 11:1092–1098, 1993.

54. Weiner M, Leventhal B, Cantor A, et al: Gallium-67 scans as an adjunct to computed tomography scans for the assessment of a residual mediastinal mass in pediatric patients with Hodgkin's disease. Cancer 68:2478–2480, 1991.

55. King SC, Reiman RJ, Prosnitz LR: Prognostic importance of restaging gallium scans following induction chemotherapy for advanced Hodgkin's disease. J Clin Oncol 12:306–311, 1994.

56. Donaldson SS, Link MP: Combined modality treatment with low-dose radiation and MOPP chemotherapy for children with Hodgkin's disease. J Clin Oncol 5:742–749, 1987.

57. Curtis RE, Boice JD Jr: Second cancers after radiotherapy for Hodgkin's disease. N Engl J Med 319:244–245, 1988.

58. Prior P, Pope DJ: Hodgkin's disease: Subsequent primary cancers in relation to treatment. Br J Cancer 58:512–517, 1988.

59. Kaldor JM, Day NE, Band P, et al: Second malignancies following testicular cancer, ovarian cancer, and Hodgkin's

disease: An international collaborative study among cancer registries. Int J Cancer 39:571–585, 1987.

60. Hancock SL, Horning SJ, Hoppe RT: Breast cancer after the treatment of Hodgkin's disease [abstract]. Int J Radiat Oncol Biol Phys 21:157, 1991.

61. Shapiro CL, Mauch PM: Radiation-associated breast cancer after Hodgkin's disease: Risks and screening in perspective. J Clin Oncol 10:1662–1665, 1992.

62. DeVita VT, Serpick A, Carbone PP: Combination chemotherapy in the treatment of advanced Hodgkin's disease. Ann Intern Med 73:881–895, 1970.

63. Bonnadonna G, Zucali R, Monfardini S, et al: Combination chemotherapy of Hodgkin's disease with Adriamycin, bleomycin, vinblastine, and imidazole carboximde versus MOPP. Cancer 36:252–259, 1975.

64. Hutchinson R, Fryer C, Krailo M, et al: Comparison of MOPP/ABVD with ABVD/XRT for treatment of advanced Hodgkin's disease in children (CCG-521). Proc ASCO 11:340, 1992.

65. Oberlin O, Leverger G, Pacquement H, et al: Low-dose radiation therapy and reduced chemotherapy in childhood Hodgkin's disease: The experience of the French Society of Pediatric Oncology. J Clin Oncol 10:1602–1608, 1992.

66. Hunger SP, Link MP, Donaldson SS: ABVD/MOPP and low-dose involved-field radiotherapy in pediatric Hodgkin's disease: The Stanford experience. J Clin Oncol 12:2160–2166, 1994.

67. Bonfante V, Santoro A, Viviani S, et al: Outcome of patients with Hodgkin's disease failing after primary MOPP-ABVD. J Clin Oncol 15:528–534, 1997.

68. Willman KY, Cox RS, Donaldson SS: Radiation-induced height impairment in pediatric Hodgkin's disease. Int J Radiat Oncol Biol Phys 28:85–92, 1994.

69. Constine LS, Donaldson SS, McDougall JR, et al: Thyroid dysfunction after radiotherapy in children with Hodgkin's disease. Cancer 53:878–883, 1984.

70. McHenry C, Jarosz H, Calandra D, et al: Thyroid neoplasia following radiation therapy for Hodgkin's lymphoma. Arch Surg 122:684–686, 1987.

71. Sankila R, Garwicz S, Olsen JH, et al: Risk of subsequent malignant neoplasms among 1641 Hodgkin's disease patients diagnosed in childhood and adolescence: A population-based cohort study in the five Nordic countries. J Clin Oncol 14:1442–1446, 1996.

72. Thibaud E, Ramirez M, Brauner R, et al: Preservation of ovarian function by ovarian transposition performed before pelvic irradiation during childhood. J Pediatr 121:880–884, 1992.

73. Bhatia S, Robison LL, Oberlin O, et al: Breast cancer and other second neoplasms after childhood Hodgkin's disease. N Engl J Med 334:745–751, 1996.

74. Tucker MA, Coleman CN, Cox RS, et al: Risk of second cancers after treatment for Hodgkin's disease. N Engl J Med 318:76–81, 1988.

75. Cimino G, Papa G, Tura S, et al: Second primary cancer following Hodgkin's disease: Updated results of an Italian multicentric study. J Clin Oncol 9:432–437, 1991.

76. van Leeuwen FE, Klokman WJ, Hagenbeek A, et al: Second cancer risk following Hodgkin's disease: A 20-year follow-up study. J Clin Oncol 12:312–325, 1994.

77. Tura S, Fiacchini M, Zinzani PL, et al: Splenectomy and the increasing risk of secondary acute leukemia in Hodgkin's disease. J Clin Oncol 11:925–930, 1993.

78. van Leeuwen FE, Chorus AM, van den Belt-Dusebout AW, et al: Leukemia risk following Hodgkin's disease: Relation to cumulative dose of alkylating agents, treatment with teniposide combinations, number of episodes of chemotherapy, and bone marrow damage. J Clin Oncol 12:1063–1073, 1994.

79. Dietrich PY, Henry-Amar M, Cosset JM, et al: Second primary cancers in patients continuously disease-free from Hodgkin's disease: A protective role for the spleen? Blood 84:1209–1215, 1994.

80. Biovin JF, O'Brien K: Solid cancer risk after treatment of Hodgkin's disease. Cancer 61:2541–2546, 1988.

81. Salloum E, Doria R, Shubert W, et al: Second solid tumors in patients with Hodgkin's disease cured after radiation or chemotherapy plus adjuvant low-dose radiation. J Clin Oncol 14:2435–2443, 1996.

82. Doria R, Holford T, Farber LR, et al: Second solid malignancies after combined modality therapy for Hodgkin's disease. J Clin Oncol 13:2016–2022, 1995.

83. Hancock SI, Tucker MA, Hoppe RT: Factors affecting late mortality from heart disease after treatment of Hodgkin's disease. JAMA 270:1949–1955, 1993.

84. Steinherz LJ, Steinherz PG, Tan CT, et al: Cardiac toxicity 4 to 20 years after completing anthracycline therapy. JAMA 266:1672–1677, 1991.

85. Damewood MD, Grochow LB: Prospects for fertility after chemotherapy or radiation for neoplastic disease. Fertil Steril 45:443–459, 1986.

86. Byrne J, Mulvihill JJ, Myers MH, et al: Effects of treatment on fertility in long-term survivors of childhood or adolescent cancer. N Engl J Med 317:1315–1321, 1987.

87. Chapman RM, Sutcliffe SB, Malpas JS: Male gonadal dysfunction in Hodgkin's disease: A prospective study. JAMA 243:1323–1328, 1981.

88. Aubier F, Flamant F, Brauner R, et al: Male gonadal function after chemotherapy for solid tumors in childhood. J Clin Oncol 7:304–309, 1989.

89. Santoro A, Bonadonna G, Valgussa P, et al: Long-term results of combined chemotherapy-radiotherapy approach in Hodgkin's disease: Superiority of ABVD plus radiotherapy versus MOPP plus radiotherapy. J Clin Oncol 5:27–37, 1987.

90. Novakovic B: U.S. childhood cancer survival, 1973–1987. Med Pediatr Oncol 23:480–486, 1994.

91. Magrath IT: The pathogenesis of Burkitt's lymphoma. Recent Adv Cancer Res 55:133–270, 1990.

92. Hanto DW, Frizzera G, Gajl-Peczalska KJ, et al: Epstein-Barr virus, immunodeficiency, and B cell lymphoproliferation. Transplantation 39:461–472, 1985.

93. Cohen JI: Epstein-Barr virus lymphoproliferative disease associated with acquired immune deficiency. Medicine 70:137–160, 1991.

94. Shibata D, Weiss LM, Nathwani BN, et al: Epstein-Barr virus in benign lymph node biopsies from individuals infected with the human immunodeficiency virus is associated with concurrent or subsequent development of non-Hodgkin's lymphoma. Blood 77:1527–1533, 1991.

95. Neri A, Barriga F, Inghirami G, et al: Epstein-Barr virus infection precedes clonal expansion in Burkitt's and acquired immunodeficiency syndrome–associated lymphomas. Blood 77:1092–1095, 1991.

96. Harris NL, Jaffe ES, Stein H, et al: A revised European-American classification of lymphoid neoplasms: A proposal from the International Lymphoma Study Group. Blood 84:1361–1392, 1994.

97. Hutchison RE, Murphy SB, Fairclough DL, et al: Diffuse small noncleaved cell lymphoma in children, Burkitt's versus non-Burkitt's types. Cancer 64:23–28, 1989.

98. Nathwani BN, Griffith RC, Kelly DR, et al: A morphologic study of childhood lymphoma of the diffuse "histiocytic" type. The Pediatric Oncology experience. Cancer 59:1138–1142, 1987.

99. Hutchison RE, Berard CW, Shuster JJ, et al: B-cell lineage confers favorable outcome among children and adolescents with large-cell lymphoma: A Pediatric Oncology Group study. J Clin Oncol 13:2023–2032, 1995.

100. Sandland JT, Pui CH, Santana VM, et al: Clinical features and treatment outcome for children with CD30+ large-cell non-Hodgkin's lymphoma. J Clin Oncol 12:895–898, 1994.

101. Falini B, Pileri S, Pizzolo G, et al: CD30 (Ki-1) molecule: A new cytokine receptor of the tumor necrosis factor receptor superfamily as a tool for diagnosis and immunotherapy. Blood 85:1–14, 1995.

102. Fillipa DA, Ladanyi M, Wollner N, et al: CD30 (Ki-1)–positive malignant lymphomas: Clinical, immunophenotypic, histologic, and genetic characteristics and differences with Hodgkin's disease. Blood 87:2905–2917, 1996.

103. Reiter A, Schrappe M, Tiemann M, et al: Successful treat-

ment strategy for Ki-1 anaplastic large-cell lymphoma of childhood: A prospective analysis of 62 patients enrolled in three consecutive Berlin-Frankfurt-Munster Group studies. J Clin Oncol 12:899–908, 1994.

104. Kaden ME: Ki-1/CD30⁺ (anaplastic) large-cell lymphoma: Maturation of a clinicopathologic entity with prospects of effective therapy. J Clin Oncol 12:884–887, 1994.

105. Cline MJ: The molecular basis of leukemia. N Engl J Med 330:328–336, 1994.

106. Rosenthal N: Regulation of gene expression. N Engl J Med 331:931–933, 1994.

107. Lebowitz RM, Albrecht S: Molecular biology in the diagnosis and prognosis of solid and lymphoid tumors. Cancer Invest 10:399–416, 1992.

108. Look AT, Kirsch IR: Molecular basis of childhood cancer. In Principles and Practice of Pediatric Oncology (3rd ed). Pizzo PA, Poplack DG (eds): Philadelphia, Lippincott-Raven, 1997, pp 37–74.

109. Dalla-Fevera R, Bregni M, Erikson J, et al: Human *c-myc* oncogene is located on region of chromosome 8 that is translocated in Burkitt lymphoma cells. Proc Natl Acad Sci U S A 79:7824–7827, 1982.

110. Zech L, Haglund U, Nilsson K, et al: Characteristic chromosomal abnormalities in biopsies and lympoid-cell lines from patients with Burkitt and non-Burkitt lymphomas. Int J Cancer 17:47–56, 1976.

111. Shiramizu B, Barriga F, Neequaye J, et al: Patterns of chromosomal breakpoint locations in Burkitt's lymphoma: Relevance to geography and Epstein-Barr virus association. Blood 77:1516–1526, 1991.

112. Bernheim A, Berger R, Lenoir G: Cytogenetic studies on African Burkitt's lymphoma cell lines: t(8;14), t(2;8), and t(8;22) translocations. Cancer Genet Cytogenet 3:307–315, 1981.

113. Lam KM, Syed N, Whittle H, Crawford DH: Circulating Epstein-Barr virus B cells in acute malaria. Lancet 337:876–878, 1991.

114. Henderson S, Rowe M, Gregory G, et al: Induction of bcl-2 expression by Epstein-Barr virus latent membrane protein 1 protects infected B cells from programmed cell death. Cell 65:1107–1115, 1991.

115. Sandlund JT, Downing JR, Crist WM: Non-Hodgkin's lymphoma in childhood. N Engl J Med 1238–1248.

116. Le Beau MM, Bitter MA, Franklin WA, et al: The t(2;5)(p23;q35): A recurring chromosomal abnormality in sinusoidal Ki-1+ non-Hodgkin's lymphoma (Ki-1+ NHL). Blood 72(suppl):247, 1988.

117. Shiota M, Fujimoto J, Takenaga M, et al: Diagnosis of t(2;5)(p23;q35)–associated K-1 lymphoma with immunohistochemistry. Blood 84:3648–3652, 1994.

118. Kadin ME, Sako D, Berliner N, et al: Childhood Ki-1 lymphoma presenting with skin lesions and peripheral lymphadenopathy. Blood 68:1042–1049, 1986.

119. Howat AJ, Thomas H, Waters KD, et al: Malignant lymphoma of bone in children. Cancer 59:335–339, 1987.

120. Meyers PA, Potter VP, Wolner N, et al: Bowel perforation during initial treatment of childhood non-Hodgkin's lymphoma. Cancer 56:259–261, 1985.

121. Tesoro-Tess JD, Biasi S, Balzarini L, et al: Heart involvement in lymphomas. Cancer 72:2484–2490, 1993.

122. Ridgway D, Wolff LJ, Neerhout RC, Tilford DL: Unsuspected non-Hodgkin's lymphoma of the tonsils and adenoids in children. Pediatrics 79:399–402, 1987.

123. Ghelman B: Radiology of bone tumors. Orthoped Clin North Am 20:287–312, 1989.

124. Clayton F, Butler JJ, Ayala AG, et al: Non-Hodgkin's lymphoma in bone. Cancer 60:2494–2501, 1987.

125. Wollner N, Lane JM, Marcove RC, et al: Primary skeletal non-Hodgkin's lymphoma in the pediatric age group. Med Pediatr Oncol 20:506–513, 1992.

126. Finlay JL, Anderson JR, Cecalupo AJ, et al: Disseminated nonlymphoblastic lymphoma of childhood: A Children's Cancer Group study, CCG-552. Med Pediatr Oncology 23:453–463, 1994.

127. Schwenn MR, Blattner SR, Lynch SR, et al: HiC-COM: A 2-month intensive chemotherapy regimen for children with stage III and IV Burkitt's lymphoma and B-cell acute lymphoblastic leukemia. J Clin Oncol 9:133–138, 1991.

128. Anderson JR, Jenkin RDT, Wilson JF, et al: Long-term follow-up of patients treated with COMP or LSA₂L₂ therapy for childhood non-Hodgkin's lymphoma: A report of CCG-551 from the Children's Cancer Group. J Clin Oncol 11:1024–1032, 1993.

129. Burkitt D: A sarcoma involving the jaws in African children. Br J Surg 46:218–223, 1958.

130. Shad A, Magrath I: Malignant Non-Hodgkin's lymphomas in children. In Principles and Practice of Pediatric Oncology (3rd ed). Pizzo PA, Poplack DG (eds): Philadelphia, Lippincott-Raven, 1997, pp 545–587.

131. Sariban E, Donahue A, Magrath IT: Jaw involvement in American Burkitt's lymphoma. Cancer 53:141–146, 1984.

132. Reiter A, Schrappe M, Parwaresch R, et al: Non-Hodgkin's lymphomas of childhood and adolescence: Results of a treatment stratified for biologic subtypes and stage. A report of the Berlin-Frankfurt-Munster Group. J Clin Oncol 13:359–372, 1995.

133. Levine AM: Acquired immunodeficiency syndrome–related lymphoma. Blood 80:8–20, 1992.

134. Knowles DM, Cesarman E, Chadburn A, et al: Correlative morphologic and molecular genetic analysis demonstrates three distinct categories of posttransplantation lymphoproliferative disorders. Blood 85:552–565, 1995.

135. Ho M: Risk factors and pathogenesis of posttransplant lymphoproliferative disorders. Transplant Proc 27:38–40, 1995.

136. Reiter A, Zimmerman W, Zimmerman M, et al: The role of initial laparotomy and second look surgery in the treatment of abdominal B-cell non-Hodgkin's lymphoma of childhood. A report of the BFM group. Eur J Pediatr Surg 4:74–81, 1994.

137. Downing JR, Shurtleff SA, Zielenska M, et al: Molecular detection of the (2;5) translocation of non-Hodgkin's lymphoma by reverse transcriptase-polymerase chain reaction. Blood 85:3416–3422, 1995.

138. Murphy SB: Classification, staging and end results of treatment of childhood non-Hodgkin's lymphomas: Dissimilarities from lymphomas in adults. Semin Oncol 7:332–339, 1980.

139. Haddy TB, Adde MA, Magrath IT: CNS involvement in small noncleaved cell lymphoma: Is CNS disease per se a poor prognostic sign? J Clin Oncol 9:1973–1982, 1991.

140. Sandlund JT, Santana V, Abromowitch M, et al: Large cell non-Hodgkin's lymphoma of childhood: Clinical characteristics and outcome. Leukemia (Engl) 8:30–34, 1994.

141. Meadows AT, Sposto R, Jenkin RD, et al: Similar efficacy of 6 and 18 months of therapy with four drugs (COMP) for localized non-Hodgkin's lymphoma of children: A report from the Children's Cancer Study Group. J Clin Oncol 7:92–99, 1989.

142. Patte C, Philip T, Rodary C, et al: High survival rate in advanced-stage B-cell lymphomas and leukemias without CNS involvement with a short intensive polychemotherapy: Results from the French Pediatric Oncology Society of a randomized trial of 216 children. J Clin Oncol 9:123–132, 1991.

143. Bowman WP, Shuster JJ, Cook B, et al: Improved survival for children with B-cell acute lymphoblastic leukemia and stage IV small noncleaved-cell lymphoma: A Pediatric Oncology Group study. J Clin Oncol 14:1252–1261, 1996.

144. Sullivan MP, Ramirez I: Curability of Burkitt's lymphoma with high-dose cyclophosphamide: High dose methotrexate therapy and intrathecal chemoprophylaxis. J Clin Oncol 3:627–636, 1985.

145. Tubergen DG, Krailo MD, Meadows AT, et al: Comparison of treatment regimens for pediatric lymphoblastic non-Hodgkin's lymphoma: A Children's Cancer Group Study. J Clin Oncol 13:1368–1376, 1995.

146. Swinnen LJ, Mullen GM, Carr TJ, et al: Aggressive treatment for postcardiac transplant lymphoproliferation. Blood 86:3333–3340, 1995.

147. Link MP, Donaldson SS, Berard CW, et al: Results of treatment of childhood localized non-Hodgkin's lymphoma with combination chemotherapy with or without radiotherapy. N Engl J Med 322:1169–1174, 1990.
148. Cohen LF, Balow JE, Magrath IT, et al: Acute tumor lysis syndrome: A review of 37 patients with Burkitt's lymphoma. Am J Med 68:486–491, 1980.
149. Allegretta GJ, Weisman SJ, Altman AJ: Oncologic emergencies I: Metabolic and space-occupying consequences of cancer and cancer treatment. Pediatr Clin North Am 32:601–611, 1985.
150. Korones DN, Buzzard CJ, Asselin BL, et al: Right atrial thrombi in children with cancer and indwelling catheters. J Pediatr 128:841–846, 1996.
151. Pryzant RM, Meistrich ML, Wilson G, et al: Long-term reduction I sperm count after chemotherapy with and without radiation therapy for non-Hodgkin's lymphomas. J Clin Oncol 11:239–247, 1993.
152. Sandoval C, Pui CH, Bowman LC, et al: Secondary acute myeloid leukemia in children previously treated with alkylating agents, intercalating topoisomerase II inhibitors, and irradiation. J Clin Oncol 11:1039–1045, 1993.

69

RHABDOMYOSARCOMA

Edward M. Barksdale, Jr., MD •
Eugene S. Wiener, MD

Rhabdomyosarcoma (RMS) is the most common soft tissue sarcoma of childhood. These tumors are a heterogeneous group of highly malignant cancers that are characterized by extensive local invasion and early hematologic and lymphatic dissemination. They belong to the class of "small round blue cell" tumors of childhood, a group that includes neuroblastoma, Ewing's sarcoma, peripheral neuroectodermal tumors, non-Hodgkin's lymphoma, and leukemia. Although these tumors have the histologic features of striated skeletal muscle, they may arise anywhere in the body, including sites where skeletal muscle is absent.

The clinical manifestations of this disease depend on the primary site at presentation. Therapeutic management of these tumors has been extensively refined since the 1960s and is dependent on three principal factors: primary tumor location, extent of disease, and tumor histology. This chapter gives an overview of the critical features in the evaluation and management of RMS.

□ History

Weber, a German pathologist, first described this tumor in the female genitourinary tract in 1854.[1] Subsequent reports appeared in the literature, but the first correlative description of the clinical course, histology, and prognosis was not reported until 1946.[2]

Horn and Enterline devised the prototype for the modern classification system of RMS in 1958. They identified four principal subtypes of RMS: embryonal, alveolar, botryoid, and pleomorphic (Table 69–1).[3] Recently, this system was further modified and consists of three major groups based on histology and prognosis: favorable (botryoid and spindle cell), intermediate (embryonal), and poor (alveolar and undifferentiated) (Table 69–2).[4, 5]

The prognosis for these tumors remained poor until approximately 30 years ago. This poor prognosis coupled with the sporadic numbers of patients in any single institution inspired the development of the Intergroup Rhabdomyosarcoma Study (IRS) in 1972 to standardize the diagnosis, classification, and prospective management of these patients.[6] Subsequently, the prognosis has improved from a dismal 15% to the present survival rate of greater than 70%.[7, 8] There have been four completed studies since the inception of the IRS. These include IRS-1 (1972–1978), IRS-II (1978–1984), IRS-III (1984–1989), and IRS-IV (1989–1996). Comprehensive reports of therapy and prognosis have been published from all except IRS-IV, which is currently being formulated. IRS-V is under development.[9, 10]

□ Epidemiology

RMS is the most common soft tissue sarcoma of childhood and accounts for about 250 new cases annually in the United States.[11–13] There is a bimodal distribution of presentation, with the initial peak occurring in children between 2 and 5 years of age

TABLE 69–1. Third Intergroup Rhabdomyosarcoma Study Patient Distribution by Histology

Histology	Total (%)†
Alveolar	19
Embryonal	54
Botryoid	4.5
Pleomorphic	<1
EOE*	3
Undifferentiated	6
Other	13

*Extraosseous Ewing's (no longer included as rhabdomyosarcoma variant).

†1062 total evaluable patients.

Data from Crist W, Gehan EA, Ragab AH, et al: The Third Intergroup Rhabdomyosarcoma Study. J Clin Oncol 13:610–630, 1995.

TABLE 69–2. International Classification of Rhabdomyosarcoma

Favorable Prognosis

Botryoid
Spindle cell

Intermediate Prognosis

Embryonal
Pleomorphic

Poor Prognosis

Alveolar
Undifferentiated

and a second peak occurring in children between 10 and 19 years (Fig. 69–1).[9, 14] Seventy percent of the patients are younger than 10 years of age. The annual incidence of RMS is about 8 per million children with a 1.4:1 male predominance. There is no significant racial predilection for this pediatric malignancy.[15, 16]

Several epidemiologic studies have been performed that suggest that maternal radiation exposure and recreational drug use (cocaine) may be important prenatal risk factors for the development of RMS.[17, 18] Other epidemiologic studies demonstrate that approximately one third of RMS cases are associated with at least one congenital anomaly. The principal organ systems involved include the genitourinary, nervous, gastrointestinal (GI), and cardiovascular systems.[19] A number of inherited syndromes demonstrate a predisposition for developing RMS. These include the Li-Fraumeni syndrome, Werner's syndrome, tuberous sclerosis, neurofibromatosis, and basal cell nevus syndrome.[20] There

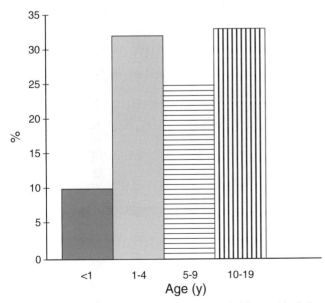

Figure 69–1. The bimodal age distribution of children with rhabdomyosarcoma in toddlers and teenagers is shown. (Data from Crist W, Gehan EA, Ragab AH, et al: The Third Intergroup Rhabdomyosarcoma Study. J Clin Oncol 13:610–630, 1995.)

seems to be a significant correlation between the incidence of breast cancer in the mothers of children with RMS; this increased risk is 3 to 13.5 times greater than control subjects.[21–23] These findings strongly implicate a genetic predisposition toward the development of RMS.

☐ Pathology

Although RMS belongs to the class of small round blue cell tumors of childhood, there are distinct light microscopic, ultrastructural, and molecular features that allow definitive diagnosis in most cases. The hallmark of diagnosis is based on the similar histologic appearance of these tumors with normal fetal skeletal muscle before innervation.[3, 24–26] The identification of rhabdomyoblasts or cells of myogenic lineage with cytoplasmic cross striations by light microscopy permits the classification of tumors as RMS, in most instances. The two principal histologic variants of RMS, embryonal and alveolar, each have distinguishing histopathologic and molecular features.[27–29]

The embryonal variant makes up about 60% of RMS cases. These tumors typically are composed of either round cells or spindle-shaped cells that are sparsely cellular with rich amounts of stroma. Individual rhabdomyoblasts are eosinophilic, with cross striations seen in the majority of tumors. The botryoid and spindle cell variants of these tumors are often discussed as distinct subtypes owing to their more favorable prognosis. The botryoid (Greek *botrys*, "grapes") tumors typically occur in cavitary structures within the GI tract, genitourinary tract, or head and neck nonparameningeal sites. Grossly, these tumors have a polypoid appearance with small, round cells and a distinct myxoid matrix of cells in the submucosa known as the cambium layer.[30, 31] The spindle cell or leiomyomatous variants are distinguished by a storiform growth pattern with low cellularity and few rhabdomyoblasts. These histiotypes primarily occur in the paratesticular region.[32]

The alveolar variant is characterized by fibrovascular septa that form pulmonary alveoli-like spaces that contain monomorphous round malignant cells. The rhabdomyoblasts aggregate in a syncytium of large multinucleated cells with scant cytoplasm. The solid alveolar subtype has features identical to the typical alveolar morphology but lacks any alveolar pattern. The tumor cells are packed closely together with dense collagen bands between individual tumor cells but scant stroma. Several tumor histologies may appear within a single specimen; however, the presence of any alveolar components constitutes an alveolar RMS. The alveolar RMS has a poorer prognosis. Undifferentiated RMS is a tumor that lacks any histologic features of myogenous differentiation. The prognosis is extremely poor.[31]

Most RMS cases are easily diagnosed via light microscopy. Undifferentiated or poorly differentiated tumors may share features with nonrhabomyosarcomatous tumors. A variety of immunohistochemical, ultrastructural, and molecular assays are available to facilitate the diagnosis. A panel of antibodies specific to skeletal muscle or muscle-specific proteins are useful. Desmin and muscle-specific actin (HHF-35) are the two most widely used of the many available.[33, 34] Often, the use of a combination of markers is advised to improve diagnostic accuracy. MyoD, a family of myogenic transcription regulatory proteins, which include MYF3, MYF4, MYF5, and MYF6, are specific lineage markers for RMS.[28, 35–37]

Electron microscopy can be a powerful adjunctive tool in making or refining the diagnosis. The ultrastructural features visualized by electron microscopy include well-defined sarcomeres with Z bands and variable orientation, Z bands with and without insertion of thick and thin elements (myosin and actin filaments), hexagonal array of thick and thin elements, and a single file alignment of ribosomes along the thick filaments.[31, 38–40] The molecular techniques are useful in detecting the characteristic translocation between the long arms of chromosomes 2 and 13 present in alveolar RMS or the loss of heterozygosity on chromosome 11, characteristic of embryonal tumors.[28]

☐ Molecular Biology

Recent research has delineated molecular biologic features that may distinguish alveolar and embryonal tumors. The alveolar histologic subtype is characterized by the reciprocal translocation between the long arms of chromosomes 2 and 13, t(2:13)q35;q14. This translocation positions 5′ sequences of PAX3, a transcriptional regulator to 3′ sequences of FKHR (a forkhead transcription factor). Subsequently, the PAX3-FKHR fusion product transcriptional activation domain differs from the usual domain for PAX3 and more potently activates transcription than does PAX3. This supersedes the transcriptional programs that normally control growth and differentiation of muscle. Hence, dysregulation of normal PAX3 activity may prevent terminal differentiation of myogenic precursors.[41, 42] Although embryonal tumors do not have a typical translocation, many of these tumors may be distinguished by the loss of heterozygosity of the short arm of chromosome 11 (11p). The molecular techniques of reverse transcriptase polymerase chain reaction and fluorescence in situ hybridization may therefore be useful in assisting and refining the histiotype diagnosis in RMS.[43]

☐ Clinical Presentation

RMS has protean clinical manifestations and its presentation is highly dependent on the age of the patient, location of the primary disease, and pres-

ence of metastatic disease. The major location of tumors by incidence are as follows: head and neck, 35%; genitourinary, 26%; extremities, 19%; other, 20% (Fig. 69–2).[10] Head and neck tumors are typically subdivided into three principal groups based on their behavior. The subgroups are orbital sites (10%); parameningeal sites (15%), which include the nasopharyngeal sites, nasal cavity, and paranasal sinuses, infratemporal fossa and middle ear; and nonparameningeal sites (10%) including scalp, face and oral cavity, oropharynx, hypopharynx, and neck. In general, these tumors are of embryonal histology and have an intermediate to excellent prognosis.[44] Many patients with these lesions of the head and neck are first seen with an asymptotically enlarging mass or visual disturbances, proptosis, or strabismus. Progressive enlargement of these nonparameningeal masses may manifest as bloody or mucous drainage from the nose, eye, or mouth. Parameningeal tumors tend to present late and may locally invade the central nervous system, manifesting with cranial nerve deficits, meningeal irritation, or brainstem symptoms.[45]

Genitourinary RMS accounts for 26% of all tumors. Two distinct subtypes of this group exist based on location. The bladder-prostate site accounts for 10% of all RMS cases and nonbladder-nonprostate sites (paratesticular sites, vulva, vagina, and uterus) account for 16% of all RMS.

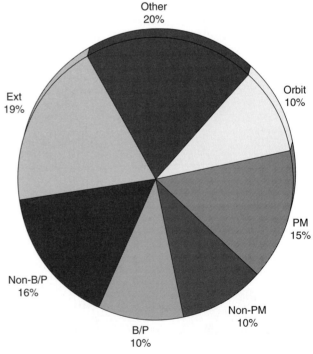

Figure 69–2. Site distribution rhabdomyosarcoma in Intergroup Rhabdomyosarcoma Study III. PM, parameningeal head/neck; non-PM, nonparameningeal head and neck; B/P, bladder-prostate; non-B/P, vagina, vulva, uterus, and paratestes; Ext, extremity; Other, trunk, perineum, paraspinal, retroperitoneum, and the like. (Data from Crist W, Gehan EA, Ragab AH, et al: The Third Intergroup Rhabdomyosarcoma Study. J Clin Oncol 13:610–630, 1995.)

The principal pattern of presentation for patients with bladder-prostate tumors includes symptoms of hematuria or bladder outlet obstruction. Prostatic RMS has a greater propensity relative to bladder for early hematologic dissemination to the bone marrow and lungs.[46, 47] Vaginal RMS appears primarily in prepubertal girls and usually presents with a polypoid mass extruding from the vaginal orifice or bloody mucoid vaginal discharge. Uterine RMS characteristically occurs in older children and teenagers and often presents as a painless pelvic mass.[48, 49] In boys, the soft tissue of areas around the testicle and spermatic cord, also known as the paratesticular region, are sites of RMS. These paratesticular sites account for 6% of all RMS cases. These tumors present as a painless scrotal or inguinal mass in prepubertal and postpubertal males. Early dissemination to regional lymph nodes is common.[47, 50] Morphologically, most genitourinary RMSs are of embryonal histology and have an intermediate prognosis. The botryoid tumors of the bladder and uterus and the paratesticular tumors with spindle cell morphology, however, have an excellent prognosis.[48, 51]

Extremity RMS occurs more commonly in the legs than in the arms and accounts for 9% of all RMS cases. The lesions may appear as symptomatic or asymptomatic masses in the involved extremity. These are aggressive tumors that may initially present with symptomatic disease in the sites of regional nodal involvement or disseminated metastases. They are of characteristic alveolar histology and have a poor to intermediate prognosis.[52]

RMS may arise in a variety of "other" sites that include the abdominal wall, retroperitoneum, biliary tract, thorax, diaphragm, and essentially any visceral organ in the abdomen or chest. These tumors often become large and bulky before they are detected. They may produce symptoms based on luminal obstruction of the GI or genitourinary tract, neural impingement, or obstructive jaundice. Their prognoses are typically guarded or poor owing to their late presentation and alveolar histology.[54, 55]

□ Diagnostic Evaluation

The goal of diagnostic evaluation of the child with a soft tissue sarcoma is to identify the extent of local disease and the presence of regional nodal or distant metastatic disease because the diagnostic approach critically guides therapy. A complete history and physical examination are the mainstays of the initial clinical evaluation. However, owing to the indolent course and protean manifestations of the soft tissue sarcomas, these alone are inadequate to make a complete diagnosis and fully evaluate the extent of disease. Definitive diagnosis requires pathologic evaluation of tumor tissue. The laboratory workup should include a complete blood count, urinalysis, electrolyte, blood urea nitrogen, and creatinine levels. Liver function tests are useful to assess for evidence

of metastatic disease or extrinsic compression of the biliary structures. Bone marrow aspiration and biopsy should be routinely used to assess for the evidence of skeletal metastases. A chest radiograph and a chest computed tomography (CT) scan are also important elements of the initial evaluation. In cases of head and neck parameningeal tumors or other tumors with meningeal involvement, a lumbar puncture is also a critical component of the evaluation.

The initial history, physical examination, and diagnostic studies direct further areas of investigation based on the site and extent of metastatic disease. CT scan with triple contrast (oral, intravenous, and rectal) is useful when evaluating sites of intraabdominal and pelvic disease. Magnetic resonance imaging evaluation is most useful in evaluating tumors in the extremities, chest wall (trunk), and parameningeal head and neck sites. In cases of vascular encasement or spinal canal extension, magnetic resonance imaging may be of great use in the surgical planning.

□ Therapy

The approach to therapy of RMS should incorporate the coordinated multidisciplinary efforts of medical, surgical, and radiation oncologists in conjunction with pathologists. Although the treatment for RMS is site specific, several universal principles of surgical management are important. These general principles should provide the foundation for the preoperative planning and intraoperative decision making. These principles include the following:

1. Initial complete primary resection with negative gross and microscopic margins is the ideal. There is no role for tumor debulking.
2. Plan primary excisions to be extensive enough to include any pseudocapsule.
3. Although the goal is initial complete excision, avoid extensive primary resections. Often, an initial incisional biopsy followed by neoadjuvant therapy and secondary excision has a better prognosis than an inadequate initial procedure.
4. Complete muscle compartment resection is not necessary in extremity tumors as long as there are negative tumor margins.
5. Biopsy clinically suspicious lymph nodes, as determined by physical examination and radiologic imaging, at the time of primary surgery. Alternatively, treat them as though they are positive and use regional nodal irradiation.[30]

This approach to therapy is based on the IRS clinical grouping system. These groups are determined by the completeness of resection at initial definitive surgery, node involvement, and presence of distant metastasis (Tables 69–3 and 69–4).

TABLE 69-3. Intergroup Rhabdomyosarcoma Study Clinical Groups

Group	Description
I	Completely resected
II	Total gross resection
	a. Microscopic residual (positive margins)
	or
	b. Positive regional nodes removed
	or
	c. a and b and/or microresidual tumor in nodes
III	Gross residual
	Local or regional
IV	Distant metastasis (at diagnosis)
	Lung, liver, brain, bone marrow, omentum
	Pleural or peritoneal implants
	Nonregional nodes
	Positive cytology:
	Cerebrospinal fluid
	Pleural
	Abdominal

TABLE 69-5. Primary Site Reexcision
of Rhabdomyosarcoma

	Primary Site Reexcision	Group IIa	Group I
3-y survival	91%	74%	73%
5-y survival	87%	67%	68%
P value	N/A	0.016	0.024
Total patients	**41**	**113**	**73**

Data from Hays DM, Lawrence W Jr, Wharam M, et al: Primary reexcision for patients with "microscopic residual" tumor following initial excision of sarcomas of trunk and extremity sites. J Pediatr Surg 24:5–10, 1989.

□ Primary Reexcision

The presence of microscopic residual disease after an apparently complete primary resection is not an unusual finding in RMS. Several retrospective reviews have shown that there is a clear survival advantage in patients following complete gross resection without microscopic residual disease (clinical group I) compared with those with microscopic residual disease after resection (clinical group II).

These reviews suggest that there is a distinct role for primary site reexcision or pretreatment reexcision of inadequately excised tumors, particularly in the extremity and trunk sites. Some evidence suggests that there also may be a role for the primary reexcision of all clinical group I tumors, but this remains an area of controversy. Clearly, evidence supports a role for primary reexcision in clinical group II patients following initial resection (Table 69–5).[55, 56]

□ Second-Look Operations

Most patients who are diagnosed with RMS have nonmetastatic extensive local disease that precludes primary resection (clinical group II).[30] As seen in other pediatric solid tumors such as neuroblastoma, Wilms' tumor, and hepatoblastoma, which, when at initial presentation are too extensive for a safe primary resection, there is a role for initial chemotherapy or radiation therapy.

Initially unresectable lesions may respond and be rendered resectable, resulting in the clinical downstaging of these patients into more favorable prognostic groups. Support for this approach has been demonstrated in a retrospective review of patients evaluated in IRS-III. The investigators evaluated 257 patients with clinical group III having RMS of all sites except the pelvis. "Second-look" surgery was performed in those patients with complete response (CR), partial response (PR), and nonresponse (NR) to presurgical neoadjuvant therapy. Nearly 75% of the PR and NR subjects were found on pathologic evaluation to be converted to the CR category. The 3-year survival rate of these regrouped PR and NR patients was found to closely parallel that of the patients found to be CR at the time of their secondary exploration (73% vs. 80%). Furthermore, this approach obviated the need for more aggressive che-

TABLE 69-4. Primary Tumor Site Stratified by Clinical Group

Site	Total (%)	Group I (%)	Group II (%)	Group III (%)	Group IV (%)
All sites		20	21	45	14
Head and neck	35	8	25	59	7
Orbit	10	3	42	53	2
Parameningeal	15	3	6	78	14
Nonparameningeal	10	22	35	39	4
Genitourinary	26	35	15	44	5
GU non-B/P*	16	53	22	20	5
GU B/P†	10	8	6	80	5
Extremity	19	32	26	19	23
Other‡	20	10	15	46	29

*Vulvar, vaginal, uterine, and paratesticular sites.
†Bladder and prostate sites.
‡Trunk, perineum, and retroperitoneum.
B/P, bladder-prostate; GU, genitourinary.

motherapy and radiation regimens associated with more acute and long-term toxicity. The goal of these second-look observations should always be to provide a complete resection of the tumor. Patients left with residual tumor have a meager survival rate of 28%. The orbital, head and neck, and genitourinary tumors are an exception because their outcome favors long-term survival in the absence of complete surgical resection.[57–61]

☐ Chemotherapy

Advances in systemic chemotherapy have been crucial in the markedly improved prognosis of patients diagnosed with RMS in the past 25 years. The increased understanding of the biology of this malignancy has allowed for more tailored therapeutic regimens. The principal goals of chemotherapy in RMS are to eradicate microscopic residual disease following surgical resection and to reduce tumor burden to levels that will allow for complete surgical resection. Although a number of agents, including vincristine, cyclophosphamide, actinomycin D, and doxorubicin, have individual antitumor activity against RMS, multiagent treatment regimens have been the mainstay of therapy since the initiation of the IRS protocols. Typically, these agents are given in an intense induction regimen and continued in a maintenance program for 12 to 18 months.[62, 63]

There has been some degree of variability in each of the IRS studies as to the chemotherapeutic drugs of choice. The multimodal therapies are currently in a state of dynamic evolution based on insights gained by the review of survival and toxicity data from previous protocols. In the earlier IRS protocols, drug choice was dependent on clinical stage and tumor histology.[9, 10] Current treatment of RMS is based on the clinical grouping system and the Lawrence Gehan pretreatment classification system.[11, 64] This pretreatment staging system is based on analysis of prognostic variables in IRS-II patients and is based more on tumor biology and natural history than on degree of surgical resection as in the IRS groupings. The pretreatment staging is based on clinical and imaging evaluation done before definitive therapy (including surgery) is instituted (Tables 69–6 and 69–7). This staging system is being tested in IRS-IV.

Consequently, therapy is a complex matrix of decisions determined by the extent of disease, prognostic factors, local-regional residual disease, and site of the primary tumor. The chemotherapeutic agents in IRS-IV include combinations of vincristine, actinomycin D, cyclophosphamide, doxorubicin (Adriamycin), etoposide, ifosfamide, and melphalan.[30]

LOCALIZED DISEASE

In IRS-IV, those patients with clinical group I tumors in favorable sites (paratesticular or orbital

TABLE 69-6. Prognostic Variables in Nonmetastatic Rhabdomyosarcoma

Variables	4-Year Survival (%)
Size	
≤5 cm	81
>5 cm	64
Nodes	
N_0	73
N_1	63
Primary Sites	
Orbit	91
Superficial head and neck	88
Paratesticles, vagina, uterus	94
Parameningeal head and neck	65
Bladder prostate	67
Extremities	68
Other	57

Data from Lawrence W Jr, Gehan EA, Hays DM, et al: Prognostic significance of staging factors of the UICC staging system in childhood rhabdomyosarcoma: A report from the Intergroup Rhabdomyosarcoma Study (IRS-11). J Clin Oncol 5:46–54, 1987.

sites), independent of histology, receive double-drug therapy consisting of vincristine and actinomycin D (VA), whereas the remaining clinical group I patients are randomized among three triple-drug regimens: VAC (vincristine, actinomycin D, cyclophosphamide), VAI (vincristine, actinomycin D, ifosfamide), and VIE (vincristine, ifosfamide, etoposide).

Patients in clinical group II with nonmetastatic

TABLE 69-7. Pretreatment Staging Classification

Stage	Site	T-Size	N	M
I	Orbit Head/neck* GU non-B/P†	a or b	N_0, N_1, or N_x	M_0
II	GU B/P‡ Extremity Parameningeal Other§	a	N_0 or N_x	M_0
III	GU B/P‡ Extremity Parameningeal Other	b	N_0, N_1, N_x	M_0
IV	All sites	a or b	N_0, N_1, N_x	M_1

*Nonparameningeal head and neck tumors.
†Paratestes, vagina, vulva.
‡Bladder and prostate tumors.
§Trunk, perineum, retroperitoneum.
T, tumor size.
  a, ≤5 cm.
  b, >5 cm.
N, regional nodes.
  N_0, not clinically involved uterine tumors.
  N_1, clinically involved.
  N_x, clinical nodal status unknown.
M, metastasis.
  M_0, no distant metastases.
  M_1, distant metastases.
B/P, bladder prostate; GU, genitourinary; non-B/P, vagina, vulva, uterus, and paratestes.

tumors (except orbital tumors) are randomized to one of the same three triple-drug regimens and receive conventional radiation therapy for microscopic residual disease. Clinical group II orbital tumors receive the double-drug therapy VA.[63]

LOCALLY INVASIVE NONMETASTATIC TUMORS

Clinical group III patients at all sites are randomized to one of the same three triple-drug regimens—VAC, VAI, and VIE—as in IRS-IV.

DISTANT METASTATIC DISEASE

Despite the advent of more complicated and aggressive treatment strategies, little progress has been made toward improving the dismal prognosis of metastatic RMS. Current therapy in IRS-IV uses an aggressive randomization of vincristine and melphalan versus etoposide (VP-16) and ifosfamide versus doxorubicin and ifosfamide given for 1 year, with VAC given as a rescue for treatment failures or relapse. Many patients have transient responses to initial chemotherapy, but, typically, metastatic disease recurs within 18 to 24 months of diagnosis and the patients die of their disease.

The most favorable prognosis for these patients is a 25% survival rate. New drugs are being developed and studied for their efficacy against metastatic disease. Novel treatment paradigms use dose intensification techniques either alone or in combination with total body irradiation and pretherapy autologous bone marrow (stem cell) harvesting followed by marrow purging techniques and autologous bone marrow transplantation. Hematopoietic growth factors such as granulocyte colony-stimulating factor and granulocyte-macrophage colony-stimulating factor may be used in conjunction with these methods to hasten marrow recovery. Although these techniques hold great theoretical promise, preliminary data are discouraging.[65]

☐ Radiation

The primary role of radiation therapy is as an adjunct to other therapies either to control local microscopic or macroscopic residual disease following resection or for therapy of involved regional lymph nodes. The efficacy of external beam radiation in RMS is well documented.[66–68] In early IRS-I studies, radiation doses of 6000R were found to be very effective at achieving local control but with significant long-term morbidity, including skeletal deformities ("micropelvis," scoliosis, and growth retardation), central nervous system impairments, and secondary malignancies (lymphoma).[30, 69] Subsequent IRS studies have shown that doses of 4000 to 5500 cGy are associated with less toxicity but higher rates of locoregional recurrence.

Several major concepts regarding XRT have

emerged from the IRS. Doses between 4000 and 4500 cGy are adequate to control microscopic residual disease in most patients. Higher doses between 4500 and 5000 cGy are indicated to achieve local control in large tumors (>5 cm) and gross residual disease.[9] There appears to be no role for XRT in treating uninvolved regional lymph nodes. There appears to be a higher risk of local failure in patients with tumors larger than 5 cm. IRS-IV guidelines for XRT are primarily based on the clinical group and are independent of age and histology.[30]

Current IRS protocols use external beam radiation therapy to the site of primary tumor in clinical groups II, III, and IV, regardless of the pretreatment stage. Radiation therapy is not indicated in patients with completely excised node negative tumors (clinical group), but it is given to patients with pretreatment stage III lesions who are in clinical group I. These protocols also indicate that metastatic foci of disease undergo radiation therapy, although many centers do not comply with this recommendation. Positive regional lymph nodes are treated with XRT to the full extent of the tissue tolerance.[10]

Using hyperfractionation techniques (twice daily therapy) to improve therapeutic response and reduce late complications, brachytherapy using newer interstitial isotopes, and radiomimetic chemotherapeutic agents all offer the potential for achieving greater local cure rates while minimizing local and systemic toxicities.[68, 71–73]

☐ Site-Specific Treatment Strategies

HEAD AND NECK

The head and neck regions are the most common sites for RMS, making up about 35% of such tumors. RMS is the most common nonlymphomatous tumor of the neck. These head and neck tumors are rapidly growing malignancies that often evade early detection owing to their protean manifestations. These are a heterogeneous group of tumors and may be subcategorized into three distinct regions: (1) orbit, (2) nonparameningeal tumors (e.g., cheek, neck, temporal, scalp, parotid, oropharynx, or larynx), and (3) cranial-parameningeal lesions (nasopharynx, middle ear, nasal cavity, paranasal sinuses, mastoid region, pterygopalatine, and infratemporal fossae).

The prognosis is best for those tumors arising in the orbital regions. Incisional biopsy alone followed by chemotherapy is usually sufficient. Seldom is radical enucleation needed.[59, 60] Nonparameningeal tumors should undergo wide local primary excision with negative margins, when possible, without creating significant cosmetic or functional deficits. Clinically positive lymph nodes should be biopsied at the time of primary surgery, but formal neck dissection is unnecessary.[59] Parameningeal tumors are treated with limited biopsy followed by chemotherapy and irradiation. Skull-based resection techniques are used in selected patients. Those patients with meningeal invasion should undergo intrathecal chemotherapy.[61]

GENITOURINARY TRACT

Genitourinary tract RMSs are common and can be subdivided into two principal categories based on location: bladder-prostate sites and vulvovaginal-uterine-paratesticular sites.

RMS of the bladder is bulky and most frequently arises at the trigone, markedly limiting successful attempts at bladder salvage. Major advances toward less aggressive and more functional approaches to managing these sites has evolved significantly with each subsequent IRS.[74, 75]

Previously, bladder and prostate RMS were treated with anterior or total pelvic exenteration with permanent urinary and GI diversion.[76] A significant reduction in the rate of radical cystectomy from greater than 50% in the previous series to 30% had been achieved without compromising survival. These efforts at bladder conservation have been promoted to maintain functional outcome without jeopardizing patient survival. A total of 171 patients with primary bladder tumors were enrolled in the IRS-I through IRS-III trials. Partial cystectomy was performed in 40 of these patients resulting in a 78% disease-free survival rate from 2 to 16 years. This compares favorably with the overall survival rate of 79% for the remaining patients with bladder RMS. Although lower tract dysfunction occurred in one fourth of these patients, renal failure developed in none of them, and the remainder had adequate function (Figs. 69–3 and 69–4).[77]

Trigonal RMS should be treated with adjuvant chemotherapy and radiation following diagnostic cystoscopy and biopsy. These tumors may respond slowly to therapy. Serial cystoscopy and biopsy are used to follow up patients receiving therapy to assess response. In the absence of clinical response or in the setting of progressive disease or early failure of therapy, radical extirpative procedures should be performed. Survival seems not to be adversely affected by delaying surgery during attempts at achieving local control.[78] Sometimes, less aggressive procedures may be performed such as partial cystectomy with ureteral reimplantation. Patients with prostate RMS who respond favorably to therapy may be candidates for bladder conservation and prostatectomy with urethral and/or bladder neck reconstruction. Patients who require more extensive procedures usually should be treated with rectal sparing anterior exenteration.[79]

RMS of the reproductive tract may involve the uterus, vagina, or vulva regions. Uterine and vaginal tumors are primarily of embryonal histology, whereas vulva RMS is usually alveolar.[51] Original therapeutic regimens used early radical extirpative surgery followed by chemotherapy and radiation.[76] Presently, presurgical adjuvant chemoradiation is used to reduce local tumor burden to facilitate less

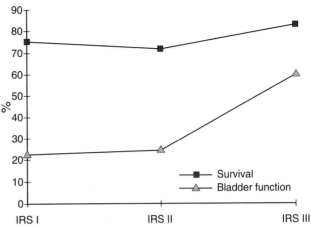

Figure 69–3. Preservation of bladder function along with patient survival in successive Intergroup Rhabdomyosarcoma Study (IRS) studies. In IRS-I, management was extensive surgery including exenteration followed by chemotherapy. In IRS-II, strategy was to preserve bladder function with primary chemotherapy and delayed radiation therapy. The outcome was slight decrease in patient survival rate with no improvement in bladder retention. In IRS-III with intensive chemotherapy and early radiation therapy, bladder salvage was 60% and patient survival rate increased to 83%. (Data from Crist W, Gehan EA, Ragab AH, et al: The Third Intergroup Rhabdomyosarcoma Study. J Clin Oncol 13:610–630, 1995; and Hays DM, Raney RB, Ragab A, et al: Retention of functional bladders among patients with vesicle/prostatic sarcomas in the intergroup rhabdomyosarcoma studies [IRS] [1978–1990] [abstract]. Med Pediatr Oncol 19:423, 1991.)

aggressive surgery or eliminate the need for resection at all.

Uterine tumors typically present in adolescent girls with a mean age of 14 years. IRS-III and IRS-IV reviews emphasize the functional benefits of less aggressive surgery following neoadjuvant chemotherapy without significant decremental changes in survival but innumerable long-term functional benefits.

Vaginal RMS usually occurs in girls younger than 2 years of age and it presents with either exophytic or intramural lesions. Their tumors are typically located in the anterior wall of the vagina and may involve the bladder or urethra. Total primary resection for many of these tumors would necessitate an anterior pelvic exenteration; however, neoadjuvant therapy has also been useful in facilitating less aggressive surgery. In the IRS-III and IRS-IV studies, there were 24 patients with vaginal RMSs, most of whom had clinical group III disease arising from the anterior wall of the vagina. Most of these patients received neoadjuvant therapy. Of the seven patients who eventually underwent tumor resection (radical anterior pelvic exenteration [1], hysterectomy and vaginectomy [1], hysterectomy [1], and subtotal vaginectomy [2]), all but one had no viable tumor in their specimen. The remaining patient had only mature rhabdomyoblasts. Hence, most patients with vaginal RMS have a favorable outcome with limited local resection or biopsy followed by adjuvant chemotherapy. Radical resections and radiation therapy are usually not required. Vulva lesions are relatively

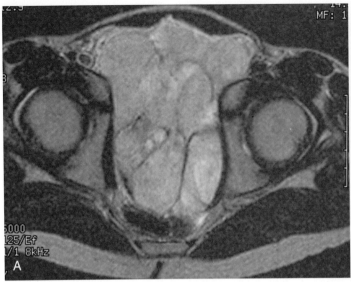
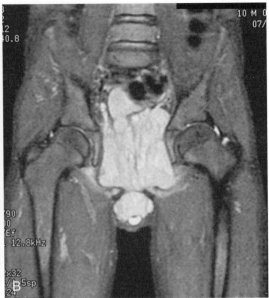

Figure 69–4. Magnetic resonance imaging sagittal and coronal views in a boy with prostate rhabdomyosarcoma. The large tumor originates from prostate and extends into the pelvis, almost to the umbilicus. This tumor responded to intensive chemotherapy and radiation. Bladder function has been preserved without local recurrence 3 years later.

rare, occurring in children with a mean age of 8 years. These tumors respond well to extensive local excision and adjuvant therapies. Ipsilateral inguinal node sampling often provides therapeutically relevant information.[80, 81]

Paratesticular RMS arises in the distal spermatic cord or tissues adjacent to the testicle. Tumors presenting in this manner should be managed as potential testicular cancers with a radical transinguinal orchidectomy. If previous transscrotal biopsy has been performed or there is invasion of the scrotal skin, then an ipsilateral hemiscrotectomy should be performed.[83] Retroperitoneal lymph node dissection is not necessary in patients with clinically negative lymph nodes by diagnostic imaging techniques and is requisite only in those patients with previously incompletely excised tumors or clinically positive nodes on preoperative evaluation.[84] The survival of patients with paratesticular RMS has improved dramatically with the advent of multimodal therapy.

EXTREMITY

Extremity RMS comprises approximately 20% of all sites and has the worst prognosis of tumors arising in the most common location with up to 25% of the patients having metastatic disease at the time of presentation.[11] Often, these tumors are amenable to complete primary tumor resection unless this would involve an amputation, debilitation, or disability. Otherwise, initial biopsy followed by chemotherapy with second-look resection should be widely used in the surgical therapy of patients with extremity RMS.[57, 85]

The principal prognostic factors for tumors in this location include size greater than 5 cm, nodal metas-

tases, distant metastases, and older age at the time of presentation. Owing to the strong tendency toward early nodal metastasis, nodal sampling techniques should be performed (Fig. 69–5).[86, 87]

TRUNK

Included in this category of RMS are tumors of the chest wall, paraspinal regions, lung or pleura, and heart. Most of these tumors arise from the chest wall and typically present with wide local infiltrative invasion of the adjacent tissues. Primary reexcision should be performed in the setting of those patients with residual microscopic disease following initial resections. In IRS-II and III, 76 patients diagnosed with trunk RMS were entered for study. The majority of the patients were clinical group II, with 25% of the patients in clinical group IV. Survival data for each clinical group was as follows: group I, 59%; group II, 75%; group III, 44%; and group IV, 0%. Paradoxically, the survival rate in group II was better than in group I patients.[88, 89] This is likely related to the presence of microscopic residual disease following an apparent total primary resection: all the group II patients received adjuvant radiation therapy to the resection bed and none of the group I patients did.

RMS may also occur in the lung, but it is rare, and it has been reported with increased frequency in patients with congenital lung lesions such as cystic adenomatoid malformations. Although these tumors are often resectable, they typically present with pleural, chest wall, and nodal metastases.[90, 91]

RETROPERITONEAL TUMORS

Retroperitoneal RMS usually presents as a large, ill-defined tumor that is unresectable at initial presentation. RMS typically has a radiographic appearance that resembles neuroblastoma. Diagnostic biopsy confirms the diagnosis. Intensive multimodal chemotherapy and radiotherapy are required to achieve some degree of tumor regression to allow resection. The role of second-look operations may be critical in achieving a favorable outcome in these patients. The overall prognosis in this group is poor, with best reports demonstrating less than a 30% survival rate.[92]

BILIARY TRACT TUMORS

RMS may appear at multiple sites within the biliary tract, including the ampulla of Vater, common bile duct, or common hepatic duct. These are typically bulky botryoid tumors that present with symptoms of abdominal pain, fever, and jaundice. Transient common bile duct obstruction may occur as the tumor embolizes distally and occludes the ampulla of Vater, leading to jaundice and cholangitis. This presentation mimics that of choledochal cysts but can be distinguished by a solid mass seen on diagnostic ultrasound or abdominal CT scan. The abdominal CT scan is useful in fully delineating the extent of local and metastatic disease for therapeutic planning.

Typically, widespread metastatic disease is present at diagnosis and the prognosis is generally poor, despite aggressive therapies. Nevertheless, diagnosis can be confirmed by endoscopic retrograde cholangiopancreatography, transhepatic cholangiography, or transabdominal biopsies. Radical surgical resection with biliary tract reconstruction followed by aggressive adjuvant chemoradiotherapy appears to offer the only chance for cure.[92–94]

OTHER SITES

RMS may appear in other sites such as the perianal and perineal regions, buttocks, and anterior abdominal wall. Perianal and perineal tumors tend to appear in the region of the anal sphincters and pelvic floor muscles.[96] These tumors may appear as painless subcutaneous nodules or as condylomatous-appearing lesions at the vaginal or anal orifices. Often, tumors in this location are present at birth. Alternatively, they may manifest as constipation or dysuria in children. Prognosis in these patients is variable. Tumor histology is predominantly alveolar but significant numbers of tumors have embryonal histology.

The goal of therapy in patients without metastatic disease at diagnosis is the complete removal of tumor with maximal functional preservation followed by adjuvant chemoradiotherapy.[96] In patients with metastatic disease at diagnosis, the goal is to control local and disseminated disease; often complete local resection is not possible.

☐ Metastatic Disease

Metastatic disease in RMS portends a poor prognosis. Despite the significant advances in survival rate since the initiation of the IRS studies, there has been incremental outcome improvement in patients with metastatic disease. The most common sites of metastasis are the lung (58%), bone (33%), regional lymph nodes (33%), liver (22%), and brain (20%).[10] Lung metastases are often multiple at presentation and not amenable to pulmonary metastatectomy. Nevertheless, histologic confirmation of suspicious lung lesions should be made in patients with RMS or in patients with RMS who are undergoing treatment.

Not all primary sites have the same propensity for metastasis. Extremity (23%), parameningeal (13%), retroperitoneum, and trunk sites have a tendency toward early metastasis. Orbital, nonparameningeal, head and neck, and genitourinary sites have the lowest rates of metastasis.[10, 29]

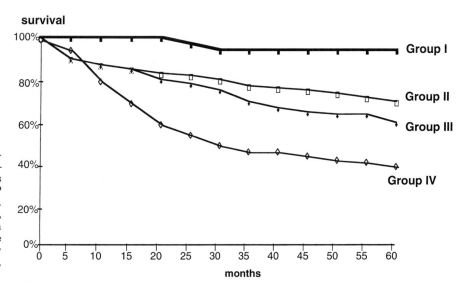

Figure 69–5. Survival curves in children with extremity rhabdomyosarcoma by clinical group. Group I versus all, P <.001; group I versus IIa, P <.002; group IV versus all, P <.05. (Data from Andrassy RJ, Corpron LA, Hays D, et al: Extremity sarcomas: An analysis of prognostic factors from the Intergroup Rhabdomyosarcoma Study [IRS] II. J Pediatr Surg 31:191–196, 1996.)

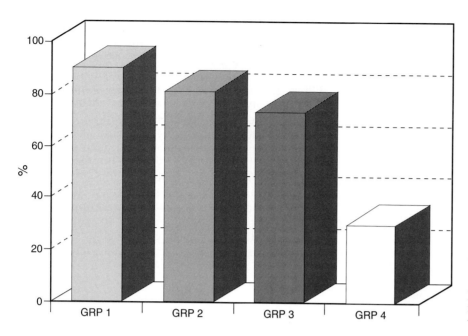

Figure 69–6. Five-year survival by clinical group in Intergroup Rhabdomyosarcoma Study III. (Data from Crist W, Gehan EA, Ragab AH, et al: The Third Intergroup Rhabdomyosarcoma Study. J Clin Oncol 13:610–630, 1995.)

□ Survival and Outcome

The overall survival rate for patients with RMS has improved remarkably since the initiation of the IRS. The incremental improvement in survival rate has occurred across almost all clinical groups. The overall survival rate has increased from less than 20% to approximately 70% in IRS-III (Fig. 69–6).[10] The survival rate and prognosis as previously outlined are dependent on multivariate factors.

Recently, additional emphasis has been placed on quality of life issues. Numerous long-term sequelae have been identified and prospective randomized trials within the context of the IRS have been designed to ameliorate or eliminate these. Examples of these adverse consequences to surgery, radiation, or chemotherapy include extremity amputation, pelvic exenteration, growth delay, gonadal dysfunction, hemorrhagic cystitis, and myocardial dysfunction.[97–101]

The focus on risk-based treatment regimens has resulted in fewer radical surgical resections without compromising outcome.[10] This becomes particularly important in the surgical management of those sites of RMS associated with greatest risk for high local recurrence and poor prognosis (e.g., extremity, trunk, retroperitoneum, and perineum). IRS-V will address this issue of local control in patients with extensive local disease (group III).

REFERENCES

1. Weber CO: Anatomische untersuchung einer hypertropische zunge nebst bemerkungen ueber neubildung guergestreifter muskelfasern. Virchow Arch Pathol Anat 7:115–121, 1894.
2. Stout AP: Rhabdomyosarcoma of the skeletal muscles. Ann Surg 123:442–447, 1946.
3. Horn RC, Enterline HT: Rhabdomyosarcoma: A clinicopathological study and classification of 39 cases. Cancer 58:181–199, 1958.
4. Newton WA Jr: Classification of rhabdomyosarcoma. In Harms D, Schmidt D (eds): Current Topics in Pathology. Berlin: Springer-Verlag, 1995, pp 241–258.
5. Newton WA, Soule EH, Hamoudi AB: Histopathology of childhood sarcomas, Intergroup Rhabdomyosarcoma Studies I and II: Clinicopathologic correlation. J Clin Oncol 6:67–75, 1988.
6. Malogolowkin MH, Ortega JA: Rhabdomyosarcoma of childhood. Pediatr Ann 17:251–268, 1988.
7. Sutow WW, Sullivan MP, Reid HL, et al: Prognosis in childhood rhabdomyosarcoma. Cancer 25:1384–1390, 1970.
8. Maurer HM, Beltangady M, Gehan EA, et al: The Intergroup Rhabdomyosarcoma Study I: A final report. Cancer 61:209–220, 1988.
9. Maurer HM, Gehan EA, Beltgandy M, et al: The Intergroup Rhabdomyosarcoma Study II. Cancer 71:1904–1922, 1993.
10. Crist W, Gehan EA, Ragab AH, et al: The Third Intergroup Rhabdomyosarcoma Study. J Clin Oncol 13:610–630, 1995.
11. Lawrence W Jr, Gehan EA, Hays DM, et al: Prognostic significance of staging factors of the UICC staging system in childhood rhabdomyosarcoma: A report from the Intergroup Rhabdomyosarcoma Study (IRS-II). J Clin Oncol 5:46–54, 1987.
12. Kramer S, Meadows AT, Jarrett P, et al: Incidence of childhood cancer: Experience of a decade in a population based registry. J Natl Cancer Inst 70:49–55, 1985.
13. Miller RW, Young JL, Novakovic B: Childhood Cancer. Cancer 75:395–405, 1995.
14. Grosfeld JL, Webber TR, Weetman RM, et al: Rhabdomyosarcoma in childhood: Analysis of survival in 98 cases. J Pediatr Surg 18:141–145, 1985.
15. Maurer HM, Moon T, Donaldson M, et al: The Intergroup Rhabdomyosarcoma Study: A Preliminary Report. Cancer 40:2015–2026, 1977.
16. Young JL, Ries LG, Silverberg E, et al: Cancer incidence, survival, and mortality for children younger than 15 years. Cancer 58:598–603, 1986.
17. Grufferman S, Schwartz AG, Ruymamm FB, et al: Parents' use of cocaine and marijuana and increased risk of RMS in their children. Cancer Causes and Control 4:217–224, 1993.
18. Grufferman S, Gula MJ, Olshan A, et al: In utero x-ray exposure and risk of childhood rhabdomyosarcoma. Paper presented at: Society for Epidemiologic Research 4th Annual Meeting; June 11, 1991; Buffalo, NY.
19. Ruymann FB, Maddux H, Ragab A, et al: Congenital anomalies associated with rhabdomyosarcoma: A report from the Intergroup Rhabdomyosarcoma Study. Med Pediatr Oncol 16:33–39, 1988.

20. Li FP, Fraumeni JF Jr, Mulviihill JJ, et al: A cancer family syndrome in 24 kindreds. Cancer Res 48:5358–5562, 1988.
21. Birch JM, Harley AK, Marsden HB, et al: Excess risk of breast cancer in the mothers of children with soft tissue sarcomas. Br J Cancer 49:325, 1984.
22. Li FP, Fraumeni JF Jr: Rhabdomyosarcoma in children: Epidemiologic study and identification of a familial cancer syndrome. J Natl Cancer Inst 43:1365–1373, 1969.
23. Lynch HT, Wush AJ, Halan WI, et al: Association of soft tissue sarcomas, leukemia, and brain tumors in families affected by breast cancer. Am Surg 39:199–206, 1973.
24. Stout AP: Tumors of the soft tissues. Atlas of Tumor Pathology, Section II, Fasicle 5. Washington, DC, Armed Forces Institute of Pathology, 1953.
25. Wolbach SB: A malignant rhabdomyoma of skeletal muscle. Arch Pathol 5:775–786, 1928.
26. Agamoulis DP, Dasu S, Krill CE Jr: Tumors of skeletal muscle. Human Pathol 17:778–795, 1986.
27. Strobbe AD, Dargeon HW: Embryonal rhabdomyosarcoma of the head and neck in children and adolescents. Cancer 3:826–836, 1950.
28. Scrable H, Witte D, Shimada H, et al: Molecular differential pathology in rhabdomyosarcoma. Genes Chromosom Cancer 1:23–35, 1989.
29. Riopelle JL, Teriault JP: Sur une forme meconnue de sarcome des parties moelles. Ann Anat Pathol (Pans) 1:88–111, 1956.
30. Wexler LH, Helman LJ: Pediatric soft tissue sarcomas. CA Cancer J Clin 44:211–247, 1994.
31. Tsokos M: The diagnosis and classification of childhood rhabdomyosarcoma. Semin Diagn Pathol 11:26–38, 1994.
32. Leuschner I, Newton WA Jr, Schmidt D, et al: Spindle cell variants of embryonal rhabdomyosarcoma in the paratesticular region: A report of Intergroup Rhabdomyosarcoma Study. Am J Surg Pathol 17:221–230, 1993.
33. DeJong AS, van Kessel-van Vark JA, Albus-Latter CE, et al: Skeletal muscle acting as a tumor marker in the diagnosis of rhabdomyosarcoma in childhood. Am J Surg Pathol 9:467–474, 1985.
34. Truong LD, Rangdaeny S, Cagle P, et al: The diagnostic utility of desmin. Am J Surg Pathol 10:680–686, 1986.
35. Li L, Olson EN: Regulation of muscle cell growth and differentiation by the MyoD family of helix-loop helix proteins. Adv Cancer Res 58:95–119, 1992.
36. Dias P, Parham DM, Shapiro DN, et al: Myogenic regulatory protein (MyoD1) expression in childhood solid tumors: Diagnostic utility in rhabdomyosarcoma. Am J Pathol 137:1283–1291, 1990.
37. Parham DM: The molecular biology of childhood rhabdomyosarcoma. Semin Diagn Pathol 11:39–46, 1994.
38. Morales AR, Fine G, Horn RC Jr: Rhabdomyosarcoma: An ultrastructural appraisal. Pathol Ann 7:81–106, 1972.
39. Mierau GW, Favara BE: Rhabdomyosarcoma in children. Cancer 46:2035–2040, 1980.
40. Ghadially FN: Myofilaments in rhabdomyoma and rhabdomyosarcoma. In Ultrastructural Pathology of the Cell and Matrix: A Test and Atlas of Physiological and Pathological Alterations in the Fine Structure of Cellular and Extracellular Components. London, Butterworths, 1988, pp 854–901.
41. Sublett JE, Jeon IS, Shapiro DN: The alveolar rhabdomyosarcoma PAX3/FKHR fusion protein is a transcriptional activator. Oncogene 11:545–552, 1995.
42. Fredericks WJ, Galili N, Mukhopadhyay S, et al: The PAX3-FKHR fusion protein created by the t(2;13) translocation in alveolar rhabdomyosarcomas is a more potent transcriptional activator than PAX3. Mol Cell Biol 15:1522–1535, 1995.
43. Barr FG, Chatten J, D'Cruz CM, et al: Molecular assays for chromosomal translocations in the diagnosis of pediatric soft tissue sarcomas. J Am Med Assoc 273:553–557, 1995.
44. Raney RB Jr: Rhabdomyosarcoma and related tumors of the head and neck in childhood. In Maurer HM, Ruymann FB, Pochedly C (eds): Rhabdomyosarcoma and Related Tumors in Children and Adolescents. Boca Raton, FL, CRC Press, 1991, pp 319–331.

45. Wiener ES: Head and neck rhabdomyosarcoma. Semin Pediatr Surg 3:203–206, 1994.
46. McLorie GA, Abara OE, Churchill M, et al: Rhabdomyosarcoma of the prostate in childhood: Current challenges. J Pediatr Surg 24:977–981, 1989.
47. Andrassy RJ, Wharman MD, Raney RB: Genitourinary rhabdomyosarcoma in childhood: Principles of treatment. In Raghavan D, Scher HL, Leibel SA, Lange PH (eds): Principles and Practice of Genitourinary Oncology. Philadelphia, Lippincott-Raven, 1997, pp 1039–1044.
48. Broecker BH, Plowman N, Pritchard J, et al: Pelvic rhabdomyosarcoma in children. Br J Urol 61:427–431, 1988.
49. Raney RB, Hays DM, Lawrence W Jr, et al: Paratesticular rhabdomyosarcoma in childhood. Cancer 42:729–736, 1978.
50. Copeland LJ, Gershenon DM, Saul PB, et al: Sarcoma botryoides of the female genital tract. Obstet Gynecol 66:262–266, 1985.
51. Hays DM, Shimada H, Raney RB Jr, et al: Sarcomas of the vagina and uterus: The Intergroup Rhabdomyosarcoma Study. J Pediatr Surg 20:718–724, 1985.
52. LaQuaglia MP: Extremity RMS: Biological principles, staging and treatment. Semin Surg Oncol 9:510–519, 1993.
53. Raney RB, Ragab AH, Ruymann FB, et al: Soft-tissue sarcomas of the trunk in childhood: Results of the Intergroup Rhabdomyosarcoma Study Committee. Cancer 49:2612–2616, 1982.
54. Crist WM, Raney, RB, Tefft M, et al: Soft-tissue sarcoma arising in the retroperitoneal space in children: A report from the Intergroup Rhabdomyosarcoma Study. Cancer 56:2125–2132, 1985.
55. Hays DM, Lawrence W Jr, Whavam M, et al: Primary reexcision for patients with "microscopic residual" tumor following initial excision of sarcomas of trunk and extremity sites. J Pediatr Surg 24:5–10, 1989.
56. Cofer BR, Wiener ES: Rhabdomyosarcoma. In Andrassy RJ (ed): Pediatric Surgical Oncology. Philadelphia, WB Saunders, 1998, pp 221–237.
57. Hays D, Raney RB, Crist WM, et al, for the IRS Committee: Secondary surgical procedures to evaluate primary tumor status in patients with chemotherapy responsive stage III and IV sarcomas: A report from the Intergroup Rhabdomyosarcoma Study. J Pediatr Surg 25:1100–1105, 1990.
58. Wiener E, Lawrence W, Hays D, et al: Survival is improved in clinical group III children with complete response established by second-look operations in the Intergroup Rhabdomyosarcoma Study (IRS II). Med Pediatr Oncol 19:399, 1991.
59. Wiener ES: Head and neck rhabdomyosarcoma. Semin Pediatr Surg 3:203–206, 1994.
60. Fiorillo A, Migliorati R, Grinaldi M, et al: Multidisciplinary treatment of primary orbital rhabdomyosarcoma: A single institution experience. Cancer 67:560–563, 1991.
61. Blatt J, Snyderman C, Wollman MR, et al: Delayed resection in the management of non-orbital rhabdomyosarcoma of the head and neck in Childhood. Med Pediatr Oncol 29:294–298, 1997.
62. Antwan KH: Adjuvant therapy of sarcomas of soft tissue. Semin Oncol 24:556–560, 1997.
63. Flamant F, Hill H: The improvement in survival associated with combined chemotherapy in childhood rhabdomyosarcoma: A historical comparison of 545 patients in the same center. Cancer 53:2417–2421, 1984.
64. Ortega J, Ragab AH, Gehan EA, et al: A feasibility, toxicity and efficacy study of ifosfamide, actinomycin D and vincristine for the treatment of childhood rhabdomyosarcoma. A report of the Intergroup Rhabdomyosarcoma Study-IV pilot study. Am J Pediatr Hematol Oncol 15:15–20, 1993.
65. Pappo AS, Shapiro DN, Crist WM, Maurer HM: Biology and Therapy of Pediatric Rhabdomyosarcoma. J Clin Oncol 13:2133–2139, 1995.
66. Dritschilo A, Weichselbaum R, Cassady JR, et al: The role of radiation therapy in the treatment of soft tissue sarcomas of childhood. Cancer 42:1192–1203, 1978.
67. Donaldson SS: Rhabdomyosarcoma: Contemporary status and future directions. Arch Surg 124:1015–1020, 1989.

68. Nag S, Grecula J, Ruymann FB: Aggressive chemotherapy, organ-preserving surgery, and high dose remote brachytherapy in the treatment of rhabdomyosarcoma in infants and young children. Cancer 72:2769–2776, 1993.
69. Tefft M, Lattin PB, Jereb B, et al: Acute and late effects on normal tissues following combined chemo- and radiotherapy for childhood rhabdomyosarcoma and Ewing's sarcoma. Cancer 37:1201–1214, 1976.
70. Donaldson S, Asmar L, Breneman J, et al: Hyperfractionated radiation in children with rhabdomyosarcoma—results of an intergroup rhabdomyosarcoma pilot study. Int J Radiat Oncol Biol Phys 32:903–911, 1995.
71. Mandell L, Ghavimi F, Peretz T, et al: Radiocurability of microscopic disease in childhood rhabdomyosarcoma with radiation doses less than 4000 cGy. J Clin Oncol 8:1536–1542, 1990.
72. Mandell L, Ghavimi E, Exelby P, et al: Preliminary results of alternating combination chemotherapy and hyperfractionated radiotherapy in advanced rhabdomyosarcoma. Int J Radiat Oncol Biol Phys 15:197, 1988.
73. Kinsella TJ, Glatstein E: Clinical experience with intravenous radiosensitizers in unresectable sarcomas. Cancer 59:908–915, 1987.
74. Hays DM: Bladder/prostate rhabdomyosarcoma: Results of the multi-institutional trials of the Intergroup Rhabdomyosarcoma Study. Semin Surg Oncol 9:520–523, 1993.
75. Hicks BA, Hensle T, Barlige KA, et al: Bladder management in children with genitourinary sarcoma. J Pediatr Surg 28:1019–1022, 1993.
76. Grosfeld JL, Smith JP, Clatwortay HW Jr: Pelvic rhabdomyosarcoma in infants and children. J Urol 107:673–675, 1972.
77. Hays DM, Raney RB, Ragab A, et al: Retention of functional bladders among patients with vesicle/prostatic sarcomas in the intergroup rhabdomyosarcoma studies (IRS) (1978–1990) [abstract]. Med Pediatr Oncol 19:423, 1991.
78. Hays DM, Raney RB, Wharam M, et al: Children with vesical rhabdomyosarcoma (RMS) treated with partial cystectomy with neoadjuvant or adjuvant chemotherapy with or without radiotherapy. J Pediatr Hematol Oncol 17:46–52, 1995.
79. LaQuaglia MP, Ghavimi F, Herr H, et al: Prognostic factors in bladder and bladder-prostate rhabdomyosarcoma. J Pediatr Surg 25:1066–1072, 1990.
80. Burger RA, Riedmiller H, Gutjahr P, et al: Extent of surgery in rhabdomyosarcoma of urogenital structures. Eur Urol 16:114–122, 1989.
81. Hays DM, Raney RB, Lawrence W, et al: Rhabdomyosarcoma of the female urogenital tract. J Pediatr Surg 16:828–834, 1981.
82. Andrassy R, Hays D, Raney RB, et al: Conservative surgical management of vaginal and vulvar pediatric rhabdomyosarcoma: Report from the Intergroup Rhabdomyosarcoma Study-III. J Pediatr Surg 30:1034–1037, 1995.
83. Corpron C, Andrassy R, Hays D, et al: Conservative management of uterine pediatric rhabdomyosarcoma: A report from the Intergroup Rhabdomyosarcoma Study II and IV pilot. J Pediatr Surg 30:942–944, 1995.
84. Wiener ES, Lawrence H, Hays D, et al: Retroperitoneal node biopsy in paratesticular rhabdomyosarcoma. J Pediatr Surg 29:171–177, 1994.
85. Lawrence W Jr, Hays DM, Heyn R, Beltangandy M: Surgical lessons from the Intergroup Rhabdomyosarcoma Study (IRS) pertaining to extremity tumors. World J Surg 12:676–684, 1988.
86. Andrassy RJ, Corpron LA, Hays D, et al: Extremity sarcomas: An analysis of prognostic factors from the Intergroup Rhabdomyosarcoma Study (IRS) II. J Pediatr Surg 31:191–196, 1996.
87. Mandell L, Ghavimi F, LaQuaglia M, et al: Prognostic significance of regional lymph node involvement in childhood extremity rhabdomyosarcoma. Med Pediatr Oncol 18:466–471, 1990.
88. Raney RB, Ragab AH, Ruymann FB, et al: Soft tissue sarcomas of the trunk in childhood: Results of the Intergroup Rhabdomyosarcoma Study. Cancer 49:2612–2616, 1982.
89. Wiener ES, Hays DM: Rhabdomyosarcoma in extremity and trunk sites. In Maurer HM, Ruymann FB, Pochedly C (eds): Rhabdomyosarcoma and related tumors in children and adolescents. Boca Raton, FL, CRC Press, 1991.
90. Murphy JJ, Blair GK, Fraser GC, et al: Rhabdomyosarcoma arising within congenital pulmonary cysts: Report of three cases. J Pediatr Surg 27:1364–1367, 1992.
91. Shariff S, Thomas JA, Shetty N, et al: Primary pulmonary rhabdomyosarcoma in children with a review of literature. J Surg Oncol 38:261–264, 1988.
92. Crist WM, Raney RB, Tefft M, et al: Soft tissue sarcoma arising in the retroperitoneal space in children: Results of the Intergroup Rhabdomyosarcoma Study Committee. Cancer 56:2125–2132, 1985.
93. Lack EE, Perez Atayde AR, Schuster SR: Botyroid rhabdomyosarcoma of the biliary tract: Report of five cases with ultrastructural observation and review. Am J Surg Pathol 5:643–652, 1981.
94. Akers RD, Mearle EN: Sarcoma botryoides of the bile ducts with survival. J Pediatr Surg 6:474–479, 1971.
95. Bar-Maor JA, Rudis E, Ben Arush M, et al: Rhabdomyosarcoma of the common bile duct imitating choledochal cyst. Pediatr Surg Intl 4:277–279, 1989.
96. Raney RB, Crist W, Hays D, et al: Soft tissue sarcoma of the perineal region in childhood: A report from the Intergroup Rhabdomyosarcoma Studies I and II, 1972 through 1984. Cancer 65:2787–2792, 1990.
97. Heyn RM: Late effects of therapy in rhabdomyosarcoma. J Clin Oncol 4:287–304, 1985.
98. Raney B, Tefft M, Heyn R, et al: Ascending myelitis after intensive chemotherapy and radiation therapy in children with cranial parameningeal sarcoma. Cancer 69:1498–1506, 1992.
99. Heyn R, Haeberlen V, Newton WA, et al: Second malignant neoplasms in children treated for rhabdomyosarcoma. J Clin Oncol 11:262–270, 1993.
100. Raney B Jr, Heyn R, Hays DM, et al: Sequelae of treatment in 109 patients followed for 5 to 15 years after diagnosis of sarcoma of the bladder and prostate: A report from the Intergroup Rhabdomyosarcoma Study Committee. Cancer 71:2387–2394, 1993.
101. Hughes LL, Baruzzi MJ, Ribeiro RC, et al: Paratesticular rhabdomyosarcoma: Delayed effects of multimodality therapy and implications for current management. Cancer 73:476–482, 1994.

70

NEVUS AND MELANOMA

Tom Jaksic, MD, PhD • James F. Nigro, MD •
M. John Hicks, MD, DDS, PhD

Nevus is a general term that refers to any skin lesion appearing at or after birth. Virtually all epidermal and dermal components have the potential to proliferate in an abnormal fashion to form nevi, and hence an extensive dermatologic nomenclature exists. Clinically and pathologically, however, nevi may be appropriately divided into two broad groups: nonmelanocytic (containing no melanocytes) and melanocytic (formed from the abnormal growth of melanocytes). Nonmelanocytic nevi, with the exception of sebaceous nevi, carry little risk for the evolution of malignancy and are commonly treated conservatively unless cosmetic concerns exist. Melanocytic nevi can evolve into malignant melanoma and in the instances of dysplastic (Clark's) nevus syndrome and congenital melanocytic nevi, this transformation occurs with some frequency. The pediatric surgeon must thus be knowledgeable about nonmelanocytic lesions primarily to avoid overtreatment and about melanocytic nevi to obviate undertreatment.

The incidence of malignant melanoma is increasing at a higher rate than any other cancer in the United States, and this neoplasm may arise de novo or from preexisting melanocytic nevi. Diagnostic delay often occurs in children, perhaps because there is a lack of awareness among physicians that melanoma does occur in this age group. As a consequence of the poor results of therapy for metastatic melanoma, effective intervention is based on prevention, early recognition, and adequate surgical excision.

☐ Nonmelanocytic Nevi

Nonmelanocytic nevi make up a heterogeneous group of skin abnormalities that may be of concern from a cosmetic standpoint, that occasionally are associated with congenital syndromes, but that usually do not carry a significant risk for malignant transformation. Nevus sebaceus is an exception in that it predisposes to the development of basal cell carcinoma.

EPIDERMAL NEVUS

Epidermal nevi are benign, well-circumscribed lesions characterized by a keratotic thickening of the uppermost layers of the skin. Although usually present at birth, epidermal nevi may not be clinically evident until early childhood. Solitary lesions are most common, but it is not unusual to observe individuals with more than one epidermal nevus. They may be located anywhere on the cutaneous surface including the trunk, extremities, face, scalp, and genitalia. The shape is usually linear, and the texture is typically verrucous or velvety. Other morphologic features such as size and color are highly variable. Most epidermal nevi measure several centimeters in length, or less, but extensive lesions can extend along an entire limb or traverse the chest, abdomen, or back. The color of an epidermal nevus can range from yellow to dark brown and, on occasion, the lesion may appear hypopigmented in comparison to the skin tone of the affected individual. Treatment of these lesions is unnecessary unless the nevus results in cosmetic disfigurement.

The epidermal nevus syndrome is a rare condition characterized by widespread epidermal nevi and associated cardiovascular and central nervous system abnormalities.

INFLAMMATORY LINEAR VERRUCOUS EPIDERMAL NEVUS

This variant of epidermal nevus presents as an erythematous, pruritic or painful, linear, warty eruption at birth or during childhood. The unpleasant symptoms of these persistent lesions warrant more aggressive therapy than that recommended for typical epidermal nevi. Application of topical or intralesional corticosteroids may be helpful, although resistant lesions often require surgical excision or dermabrasion.

NEVUS SEBACEUS

Nevus sebaceus (also known as nevus sebaceous of Jadassohn) usually presents at birth as a solitary, yellowish-orange plaque on the scalp.[1] The distinctive yellow-orange color is a result of immature sebaceous glands that are the major histologic feature of this lesion. Nevus sebaceus is well circumscribed, hairless, oval to round in shape, and usually less than 2 to 3 cm in diameter. Much larger or multiple lesions are rare.

Initially, the nevus is flat, but by adulthood the texture is roughened or papillomatous and has been likened to the peel of an orange. Nevus sebaceus occurs anywhere on the body, but the scalp and face are most commonly affected. Approximately 15% of nevus sebaceus cases undergo neoplastic transformation during adolescence or adulthood. The tumor most frequently associated with nevus sebaceus is basal cell carcinoma followed by syringocystadenoma papilliferum (a benign apocrine gland derived neoplasm). A variety of other tumors, including squamous cell carcinoma and malignant eccrine poroma, have also been described with nevus sebaceus. It is recommended that the nevus sebaceus be excised before puberty because neoplastic changes happen after adolescence.

NEVUS COMEDONICUS

Nevus comedonicus is a well-circumscribed plaque made up of grouped keratin-plugged hair follicles. It is usually present at birth but may be first noted in adolescence. Lesions consist of numerous pinpoints of firm, dark papules that resemble open comedones. They can occur anywhere over the hair-bearing surfaces of the skin. Treatment options include lactic acid–containing moisturizers or topical tretinoin to reduce the hyperkeratotic surface; more troublesome lesions can be surgically excised.[2] Nevus comedonicus does not have malignant potential.

CONNECTIVE TISSUE NEVUS

Connective tissue nevi are dermal malformations that are secondary to abnormalities in collagen or elastin fibers. They present as subtle, flesh-colored, small elevations in the skin, without marked epidermal change. Their texture may be smooth or pebbly and their diameter may range from several millimeters to several centimeters. Solitary or multiple lesions can be located anywhere on the body. Presentation occurs at birth, during infancy, or at any point throughout childhood.[3]

When connective tissue nevi are associated with tuberous sclerosis, they are termed *shagreen patches* and are considered one of the important cutaneous signs of the syndrome. Buschke-Ollendorf syndrome is characterized by connective tissue nevi (termed *dermatofibrosis lenticularis disseminata*) in association with osteopoikilosis that manifests radiologi-

cally as focal sclerotic areas of dysplasia in the long bones, pelvis, hands, and feet. Connective tissue nevi do not have a propensity for malignant degeneration and surgical treatment is not indicated.

NEVUS ANEMICUS

This unusual birthmark presents at birth or during early childhood as a well-circumscribed hypopigmented patch.[4] It is secondary to a localized abnormal constriction of the cutaneous vasculature.[5] These lesions have no malignant potential, and treatment is not necessary because the cosmetic abnormality is quite subtle in most cases.

NEVUS ACHROMICUS (NEVUS DEPIGMENTOSUS)

A decreased number of functional melanocytes in the affected skin account for this benign birthmark. Nevus achromicus can occur at birth or during early childhood and presents as a well-circumscribed hypopigmented patch that can have a variety of shapes including round, oval, linear, or whorled. The hypopigmentation may be enhanced with Wood's lamp illumination. Treatment is not indicated.

BECKER'S NEVUS

This irregular hyperpigmentation with overlying terminal hair growth is typically seen in male adolescents. The pigmentary change is due to increased melanin in the basal layer of the epidermis rather than a proliferation of melanocytes.[6] Therefore, Becker's nevus is not considered a risk for malignant transformation. These lesions are frequently noted over the back, shoulder, or upper arm. Becker's nevus is usually large, measuring 10 to 20 cm in diameter. Enhanced androgen sensitivity may explain why these lesions are more common in young men, although this condition may also develop in girls.[7] Treatment of the pigmentation, hypertrichosis, or both may be attempted with lasers. Shaving, depilatories, and electrolysis can also address the issue of hair overgrowth. Surgical excision is generally not attempted because of the large size and relatively inconspicuous location of these nevi.

☐ Melanocytic Nevi

Melanocytic nevi are benign collections of melanocytes in the skin that may be congenital or acquired, large or small, solitary or multiple, routine or problematic. Although all melanocytic nevi have a theoretical risk of malignant transformation to melanoma, this risk is small for individual lesions. Nevertheless, patients with melanocytic nevi should be observed with care. When individual nevi appear unusual or change over time, surgical intervention is required. Dysplastic (Clark's) nevus syndrome and large or giant congenital melanocytic nevi are particularly linked to the evolution of malignant melanoma.

HISTOLOGIC CHARACTERISTICS OF MELANOCYTES, NEVUS CELLS, AND MALIGNANT MELANOMA

Melanocytes provide a protective function from the harmful effects of sun exposure.[8–10] These cells are derived from the neural crest and during embryogenesis migrate to the skin, hair follicles, and the retina. Melanocytes produce a complex black-brown pigment polymer—melanin—whose functions include absorption of ultraviolet light, scavenging cytotoxic intermediates, and possibly aiding in the normal development of the nervous system. Melanocytes form melanin in membrane-bound vesicles called *melanosomes*. Melanocytes, nevus cells, and melanoma cells differ markedly in their cytologic appearance, organization, and biologic characteristics.[11–15]

Melanocytes are characterized by dendritic cytoplasm containing melanosomes, solitary cell arrangement without melanocyte-to-melanocyte contact, location along the basal cell layer of the epidermis, small regular nuclei, and rare mitotic activity. Nevus cells have similar nuclear morphology to that described for melanocytes; however, they lose contact inhibition, tend to cluster in close apposition, and may migrate from the basal layer of the epidermis to the papillary dermis. Nevus cells also retain melanosomes, have an absence of dendritic processes, and are round to ovoid in shape. Melanoma cells share some features of nevus cells, such as lack of dendritic processes, round to spindle shape, and loss of contact inhibition. They also demonstrate pleomorphism, irregular hyperchromatic nuclei, prominent nucleoli, and have readily detectable mitotic activity. Melanoma cells possess the ability to invade the superficial epidermis (Pagetoid spread), the underlying papillary and reticular dermis, and the subcutis, as well as to metastasize via lymphatic and vascular channels to the draining lymph node basin and to distant sites such as the lung.

JUNCTIONAL NEVUS

Junctional nevi are the most common type of acquired pigmented nevi in childhood. Nevus cells predominate at the epidermal-dermal junction, with some extension into the upper portions of the dermis. This results in relatively flat lesions that are usually oval or round with an even tan to brown pigmentation. However, some junctional nevi may be irregular in shape or color. Junctional nevi may occur anywhere on the body and are small in size with most ranging from several millimeters to 1 cm in diameter.

INTRADERMAL NEVUS

Although intradermal nevi can occur in pediatric patients, they are most commonly seen in adults. Clinically, they present as dome-shaped or pedunculated papules ranging in size from several millimeters to more than 1 cm. Pigmentation is usually uniform and varies from flesh toned to dark brown. The head and neck are the sites most frequently affected by intradermal nevi. Histologically, nests of nevus cells are limited to the dermis.

COMPOUND NEVUS

The term *compound nevus* refers to lesions that contain both junctional and intradermal proliferations of nevus cells. Clinically, it resembles a junctional nevus but may be more papular in texture. Although it can be seen in infancy, it is more common in older children and adults.

HALO NEVUS

Small pigmented lesions surrounded by a rim of hypopigmentation are termed *halo nevi*. They are typically seen in adolescents and are most commonly located over the trunk, especially the back. The rim of hypopigmentation measures several millimeters in diameter. The etiology is unclear, although it has been proposed that as yet undefined immune mechanisms destroy the pigment-containing melanocytes and nevus cells.[16] Ultimately, the entire lesion resolves with an eventual return of normal pigmentation in the affected area. Treatment is unnecessary unless the pigmented portion of the halo nevus appears atypical; then, excision of the entire lesion, including the halo, is recommended.

BLUE NEVUS

Blue nevi have a bluish-black appearance caused by the presence of spindle-shaped melanocytes in lower portions of the dermis. The distorted appearance of the deep pigmentation on the skin surface is referred to as the *Tyndall effect*. Blue nevi are typically small (2 to 3 mm), round, well-circumscribed, and located over the dorsum of the hands and feet. They may be present at birth but can occur at any age and seem to be more common in women.

Most blue nevi remain completely benign over time, although they are commonly excised because of their ominous dark pigmentation. Cellular blue nevi are a variant that tend to be greater than 1 cm in diameter and histologically are composed of aggregates of densely packed cells in the dermis. Cellular blue nevi have a low but definite risk of malignant transformation and should be excised with a narrow margin.[17]

NEVUS OF OTA AND ITO

These nevi are composed of large, irregular patches of bluish-gray pigmentation. Nevus of Ota is located in the periorbital region with a distribution related to the first and second branches of the trigeminal nerve. Nevus of Ito refers to the same type of lesion with a location over the supraclavicular and scapular skin.

These nevi are most common in female Asian patients but also occur in African Americans, Hispanics, and Native Americans. Histologically, these nevi are composed of dendritic melanocytes in the upper dermis. There is essentially no malignant potential, although rare cases of malignant melanoma have been associated with nevus of Ota. Treatment options for cosmetic purposes include laser ablation (Q-switched ruby) and cosmetic cover-up.[18]

SPITZ NEVUS

Spitz nevi are characterized by sudden onset and rapid growth during childhood or early adolescence. They are dome-shaped, reddish-tan, firm papules that commonly occur on the face and rarely exceed 1 cm in diameter (Fig. 70–1). Spitz nevi were originally termed *benign juvenile melanomas* because their histologic features can resemble those of malignant melanomas.[19] The presence of epithelioid and spindle cells may confuse pathologists who have limited pediatric experience (Fig. 70–2). Complete excisional biopsy of Spitz nevi is recommended because recurrent, partially removed lesions may be misinterpreted histologically as malignant.

SPECKLED LENTIGINOUS NEVUS

Also known as *nevus spilus*, this nevus is a tan patch of hyperpigmentation with dark brown freckling within the patch. Histologically, these nevi are similar to other acquired melanocytic nevi and theoretically have a small potential for malignant transformation.[20] They may be present at birth or appear by early childhood, and they can be located virtually anywhere on the skin surface. Sizes range up to

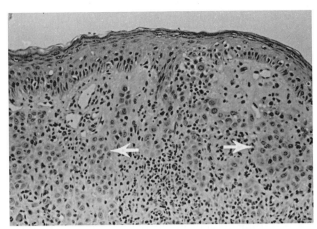

Figure 70–2. Spitz nevus histology with numerous intradermal cell nests *(arrows)* with an epithelioid character, abundant cytoplasm, and prominent nucleoli. This type of nevus may be confused with malignant melanoma on histopathologic examination.

several centimeters in diameter. Their extent generally makes surgical excision impractical. Observation of these nevi and biopsy of changes suspicious for malignancy is the management of choice.

CLARK'S NEVUS (DYSPLASTIC NEVUS)

Clark's nevi, also known as *atypical melanocytic moles* or *dysplastic nevi*, were first described in 1978.[21] They are common, with an incidence of about 5% in Caucasian populations. Clark's nevi may be familial or occur sporadically.[22] Lesions typically present in early adulthood; however, it is not uncommon to see Clark's nevi in young children. Clark's nevi are usually larger than common acquired melanocytic nevi with diameters ranging from 5 to 15 mm. Color is variable with multiple shades of brown, tan, and red often present within single lesions. The "fried egg" configuration of a lighter pigmented flat base with a central raised darkly pigmented center is the classic description of dysplastic nevi (Fig. 70–3). The borders tend to be poorly circumscribed with the appearance of pigment "bleeding into" the normal surrounding skin. The histologic characteristics of Clark's nevus are depicted in Figure 70–4. Although they can occur anywhere on the body, Clark's nevi seem to favor the trunk and scalp more than the extremities.

The relationship between Clark's nevi and malignant melanoma remains controversial with wide-ranging opinions regarding the role of these nevi as true markers for malignancy. Patients with sporadically occurring Clark's nevi are probably at greater risk for developing malignant melanoma over a lifetime when compared to those with common acquired melanocytic nevi or no nevi at all.[22]

This risk likely increases with increasing numbers of dysplastic nevi in a given individual. Nevertheless, the likelihood of a given dysplastic nevus transforming into malignant melanoma is small. True familial dysplastic nevi have a more significant

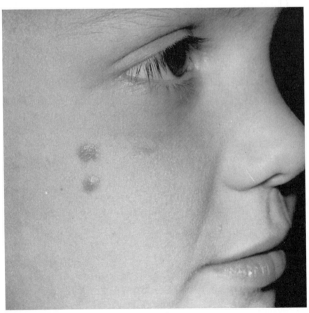

Figure 70–1. Two Spitz nevi of the face.

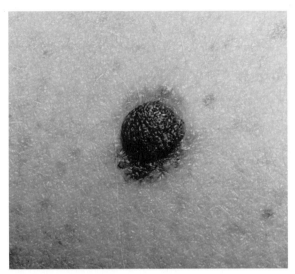

Figure 70–3. Clark's nevus (dysplastic nevus) with "fried egg" appearance.

relationship with malignant melanoma. Patients are considered to have the dysplastic nevus syndrome if they have dysplastic nevi and at least two family members have dysplastic nevi. The risk of malignancy increases further when there is a family history of melanoma. In those patients with two or more relatives with dysplastic nevi and melanoma, the lifetime risk for malignancy is greater than 50%.[23, 24]

Patients with Clark's nevi should be observed closely for new or changing lesions. Nevi that have an atypical appearance or have changed abruptly require total excision. First-degree relatives should have a complete skin examination and be monitored on a regular basis if noted to have dysplastic nevi. Routine excision of all dysplastic-appearing nevi is not recommended because the risk of melanoma developing in a given nevus is small and because malignant melanoma frequently develops de novo

without an associated preexisting nevus. Thus, a patient's risk for developing melanoma cannot be eliminated by prophylactic surgical removal of all dysplastic nevi and the resultant cost, trauma, and potentially disfiguring scar formation further mitigate against this approach.

CONGENITAL MELANOCYTIC NEVI

Congenital melanocytic nevi (CMN) are characterized qualitatively as small (<1.5 cm diameter), large, and giant (>9 cm diameter in the newborn or >20 cm diameter in the adult), although the distinction between large and giant nevi is often blurred in the literature. Small congenital melanocytic nevi occur in 1% of newborns and may be present anywhere on the body.

The pigmentation is typically uniform, with colors ranging from tan to dark brown, and the borders are well demarcated. Lesions may thicken and grow coarse terminal hairs over time. The lifetime risk for developing malignant melanoma in a small congenital nevus is unknown but is probably less than 5%.[25] There is no consensus regarding the specific treatment of small CMN. Evidence suggests that the risk for melanoma does not usually occur until after adolescence; therefore, it is reasonable to observe benign-appearing small CMN during childhood and recommend excision when patients can easily tolerate local anesthesia. It must be stressed, however, that any significant changes in lesion appearance should prompt immediate excision. Scalp lesions that are difficult to examine may warrant prophylactic excision (Fig. 70–5). In contrast, lesions such as those over the fingertips or eyelids may best be left intact and observed for change rather than risking functional impairment secondary to surgical excision.

Large or giant CMN typically affect the trunk and scalp but may involve any portion of the skin sur-

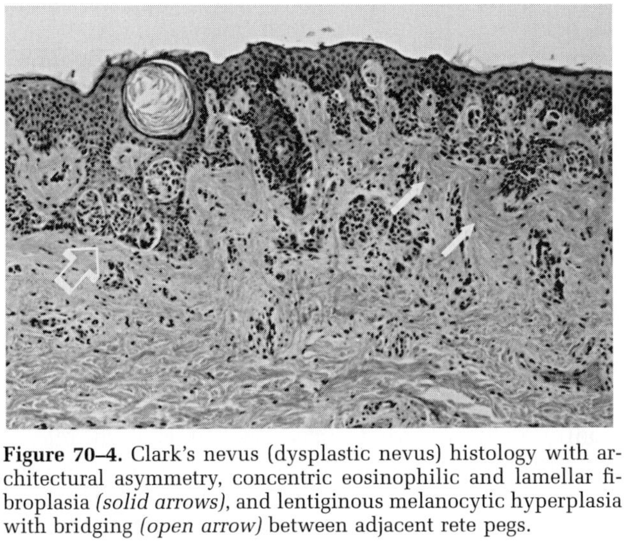

Figure 70–4. Clark's nevus (dysplastic nevus) histology with architectural asymmetry, concentric eosinophilic and lamellar fibroplasia *(solid arrows)*, and lentiginous melanocytic hyperplasia with bridging *(open arrow)* between adjacent rete pegs.

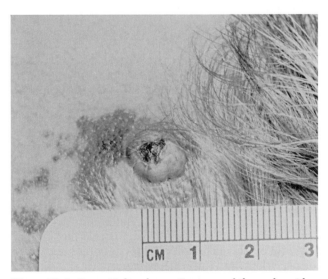

Figure 70–5. Congenital melanocytic nevus of the scalp with a melanoma arising from it (raised centrally pigmented lesion).

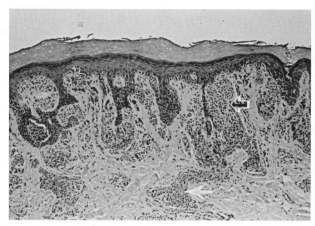

Figure 70–6. Congenital melanocytic nevus histology characterized by nevus cells extending from the dermal-epidermal junction *(open arrow)* along skin appendage structures into the deep dermis *(solid arrow).*

face. Color can range from tan to black and lesions usually contain a variety of hues. The surface may be flat, jagged, or nodular, with increased thickness usually occurring with advancing age. Extensive terminal hair growth is frequently present. Smaller, round satellite lesions often occur adjacent to the main nevus. The histologic characteristics of congenital melanocytic nevi are outlined in Figure 70–6. Unlike in small CMN, melanomas in large and giant congenital melanocytic nevi may develop early in infancy or childhood. Giant congenital melanocytic nevi can be associated with neurocutaneous melanosis, especially if the nevus is present over the scalp. Proliferation of melanocytes in the central nervous system can lead to increased intracranial pressure, seizure disorders, developmental delay, and malignant melanoma of the central nervous system.[26] The surgical treatment of large and giant congenital nevi is discussed in a later section, along with other prevention strategies for malignant melanoma.

☐ Pediatric Malignant Melanoma

The incidence of malignant melanoma is increasing at a higher rate than any other cancer in the United States, with the current lifetime risk being approximating 1 in 87 people.[27] Two percent of cases occur in patients younger than 20 years of age, and 0.3 to 0.4% of melanomas appear in prepubertal children.[28] A recent study in Sweden showed that the incidence of malignant melanoma during adolescence has doubled over the past 10 years.[29] Diagnostic delay is present in up to 60% of pediatric cases of malignant melanoma, perhaps owing to a lack of awareness among physicians that melanoma does occur in children.[30] Late diagnosis can adversely affect survival because metastatic childhood melanoma follows an aggressive course with a 5-year survival rate of only 34%, as compared to a 5-

year survival rate of 77% for localized disease.[31] Owing to the poor results of therapy for metastatic melanoma, effective intervention is based on prevention, early recognition, and adequate surgical excision.

PREVENTION

It has been estimated that 80% of melanoma is caused by repeated acute sun exposure, although the precise mechanism has not been determined.[32] Case-control studies indicate that a history of frequent sunburn accompanied with blistering during childhood and adolescence is associated with an elevated risk of developing malignant melanoma as an adult.[33] Furthermore, children living in the southern United States during adolescence appear to have an increased incidence of malignant melanoma.[34] In pediatric melanomas, boys have a predominance of head and trunk primary lesions, whereas girls have more arm and leg primary malignancies; however, the overall incidence is approximately the same in both genders. Australia, which is the country with the highest incidence of malignant melanoma, has embarked on a prevention campaign that educates children to (1) avoid direct sunlight during the middle of the day, (2) wear clothing and hats to limit sun exposure, and (3) as an adjunct, apply sunscreens. Twenty percent of the world's melanomas develop in black Africans and in Asians, hence darker skin pigmentation does not preclude the evolution of melanoma.[32]

Other risk factors for melanoma development in children include giant congenital melanocytic nevi, dysplastic (Clark's) nevus syndrome, xeroderma pigmentosa, and immunodeficiency states. Ten percent of melanomas are familial, and various mutations have been linked with the disease including an autosomal dominant gene with incomplete penetrance.[35] Melanoma is also the most common tumor that may be acquired transplacentally by the fetus from an affected mother. Multiorgan involvement is frequent in the transplacental cases, and the prognosis is usually poor, although spontaneous regression has been occasionally reported.[31]

Congenital melanoma may arise in giant or large congenital nevi, with the majority of malignant transformations occurring later in childhood. Large congenital nevi occur in 1 in 1000 to 1 in 20,000 newborns, and garment nevi, which involve a large surface area such as the back or a whole limb, occur in 1 in 500,000 newborns. The incidence of malignant transformation in large or giant congenital nevi is generally quoted as approximately 5%, with a range of 2 to 20% having been reported. The malignancies that evolve are predominantly melanomas, although other neuroectodermal tumors are sometimes present. Prophylactic removal in early life is usually recommended, because the risk of melanoma in the 1st year of life (8.6 per 10,000) is seven times greater than the risk of general anesthesia. Excision of giant congenital nevi should extend to the fascia, because the majority of melanomas arising in these lesions do not originate in the epidermis. Occasionally, even deeper excisions are required if nevic rests are present at the resection margins. Garment nevi often cannot be excised, and thus careful clinical examination throughout the patient's life is recommended, with prompt biopsy of all new or enlarging nodules (Fig. 70–7).[31]

DIAGNOSIS

Melanoma may be accurately diagnosed clinically and at an early stage in most cases. Generally, any change in size, shape, or color of a pigmented lesion over a period of weeks to months is suspicious. The following seven-point checklist has been validated as a sensitive screening method for the early detection of melanoma[36]:

Three Major Features

1. Change in size
2. Change in shape
3. Change in color

Four Minor Features

4. Inflammation
5. Bleeding or crusting
6. Sensory changes
7. Lesion diameter of greater than 7 mm

A pigmented lesion with a major feature demands detailed assessment with likely biopsy, whereas each of the minor features should engender careful follow-up. Other suggestive findings, sometimes referred to as the *"A, B, C, D" of melanoma* follow[37]:

*A*symmetry (one side of the lesion differs from the other)
*B*order irregularity
*C*olor variegation (usually different shades of brown)
*D*iameter (large)

The characteristic clinical and histologic features of malignant melanoma are demonstrated (Figs.

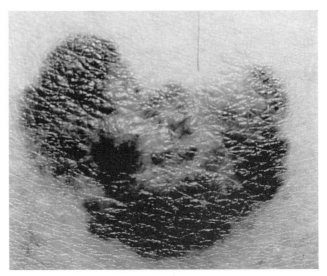

Figure 70–8. Malignant melanoma demonstrating asymmetry, border irregularity, and color variegation.

70–8 and 70–9). Because 50% of melanomas arise without a preexisting lesion, it is necessary to assess any new pigmented lesion carefully and to perform a complete skin examination, including the scalp. Inspection alone is up to 80% accurate in identifying malignant melanoma.[37] Other techniques, which have been used in an effort to enhance diagnostic sensitivity in high-risk patients, are full-body photographs, epiluminescence microscopy (magnification and oil immersion applied to a lesion to assess details below the lesion surface), and computer-based image analysis using digitized pictures.

Biopsy remains the unequivocal method to assess suspicious pigmented lesions. Tumor thickness and skin penetration are the most important prognostic factors; therefore, complete excision, including some adipose tissue, is the preferred method. If the lesion is large or the anatomic location requires tissue sparing, then a punch biopsy of the region

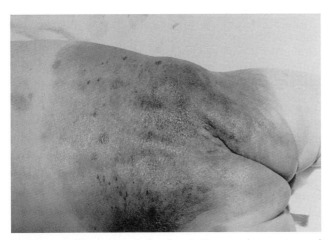

Figure 70–7. Giant congenital melanocytic nevus (garment nevus) of the back and buttock in a neonate.

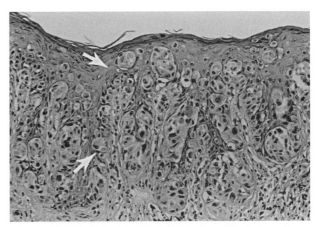

Figure 70–9. Superficial spreading melanoma histology with pagetoid invasion of the epidermis by malignant melanoma cells *(arrows)* and microinvasion of the underlying superficial papillary dermis. This is considered to be the radial growth phase of melanoma.

TABLE 70-1. Staging System
for Malignant Melanoma

Stage	Pathologic Findings
1	Tumor <1.5 mm thick
2	Tumor ≥1.5 mm thick and/or satellites present within 2 cm of primary tumor
3	Regional lymph nodes with tumor and/or in-transit disease
4	Distant metastatic disease

TABLE 70-3. Clark's Classification
for Malignant Melanoma

Level	Depth of Penetration
I	In situ
II	Extends into papillary dermis
III	Extends to the junction of the papillary and reticular dermis
IV	Extends into the reticular dermis
V	Invades the subcutaneous tissue

that clinically appears to be the thickest is acceptable. Transection of a melanoma at the time of biopsy does not adversely affect survival.[38]

For all new cases of melanoma, a thorough examination of the whole skin and regional lymph nodes is required. Any lymph node with an abnormally firm or rubbery consistency should be biopsied. For patients with primary melanomas 1 mm or greater in thickness, a baseline chest radiograph and liver function tests are indicated. Computed tomography of the head, chest, abdomen, and pelvis are necessary in all patients with nodal or distant metastatic disease. When leptomeningeal involvement is suspected, magnetic resonance imaging is useful. Positive emission tomography, after intravenous injection of ^{18}F-labeled glucose, may be the most sensitive method to detect distant melanoma metastases and is currently being evaluated for clinical application.[39]

STAGING AND PROGNOSIS

The staging system used by the American Joint Commission on Cancer for malignant melanoma is outlined in Table 70–1. Before the mid-1950s, pediatric melanoma was thought to be less aggressive than the adult disease owing to the erroneous classification of Spitz nevi as melanomas.

It is recognized that both pediatric and adult melanomas have a prognosis that is dependent on tumor thickness or level of invasion.[40] The 5-year survival rates of patients with primary malignant melanomas related to Breslow tumor thickness in millimeters are listed in Table 70–2. The level of invasion of malignant melanoma may also be determined according to the Clark classification (Table 70–3). Nodal metastases are rare in patients with lesions

TABLE 70-2. Breslow Tumor Thickness
Related to 5-Year Survival

Tumor Thickness (mm)	% 5-Year Survival
<0.75	95%
0.76–1.49	80%
1.50–4.00	60%
>4.00	<50%

less than 1.5 mm in thickness, whereas nodal metastases develop in two thirds of children with melanomas greater than 1.5 mm in thickness (or Clark's levels IV and V).[41, 42] As discussed previously, metastatic disease in childhood is associated with a 34% 5-year survival rate.[31]

TREATMENT

Successful treatment of malignant melanoma is based on the prompt and adequate excision of the primary lesion. The resection margins, which the surgeon selects, should be based on tumor thickness, although anatomic constraints may modulate decision making. The 1992 National Institutes of Health consensus conference on early melanoma recommended 0.5-cm margins for melanoma in situ.[43] Those lesions that invade the skin but do so at a depth of less than 1 mm are routinely removed with a resection margin of 1 cm.[44] A prospective randomized trial in tumors with a depth less than 2 mm showed a 3% local recurrence rate with a 1-cm resection margin, contrasted with a 0% local recurrence rate with 2-cm resection margin; however, this did not translate into any significant survival difference between the two groups after a mean follow-up of 55 months.[45]

A randomized trial of 2-cm resection margins compared to 4-cm resection margins for tumors between 1 and 4 mm thickness, with a mean follow-up of 6 years, also failed to show a survival benefit for the wider excision.[46] No randomized prospective trials are available to assess excision margins for melanomas greater than 4 mm in thickness, although a 3-cm resection margin is usually used in an effort to minimize local recurrence. Table 70–4 summarizes a set of reasonable guidelines for determining resection margins in malignant melanoma based on tumor thickness.[35]

The excision of regional lymph nodes on a prophylactic basis remains controversial. Three randomized, prospective clinical trials are available for review.[47–49] A study of more than 500 patients randomized between prophylactic excision of regional nodes and expectant management (with salvage nodal excision only if the nodes became clinically suspicious) demonstrated no difference in the survival rates between groups.[47] A smaller, single-center trial that compared immediate prophylactic

TABLE 70-4. Tumor Thickness and
Recommended Resection Margins

Tumor Thickness (mm)	Resection Margin (cm)
In situ	0.5
<1	1.0
1–4	2.0 (in anatomic regions where the function of a vital structure would be compromised, a 1.0-cm margin is acceptable)
>4	3.0 (no prospective trials available)

lymphadenectomy, delayed elective lymphadenectomy, and lymphadenectomy if nodes became clinically positive also did not show any survival differences between groups.[48] A more recent randomized trial that enrolled more than 700 patients with melanomas between 1 and 4 mm in thickness again did not prove any significant survival benefit for the prophylactic lymph node dissection group compared with the cohort managed expectantly.[49] A retrospective subgroup analysis of this study did, however, suggest that patients younger than 60 years of age with tumor thickness between 1 and 2 mm may have a significant survival benefit with prophylactic node dissection.[49]

Partially in response to the controversy regarding prophylactic lymph node dissection and its associated morbidity of lymphedema, the concept of sentinel node biopsy has evolved. This technique consists of the simultaneous injection of blue dye and subdermal radioactive tracer adjacent to the patient's melanoma. A gamma counter is used to isolate the first regional node, which is then locally excised and submitted for pathologic analysis, by frozen section. If the node is positive for melanoma, a formal lymph node dissection is started. The false-negative rate of this technique may be as low as 1%.[50] However, given the absence of any completed clinical trials to ascertain survival benefit, sentinel node biopsy remains an experimental modality.

The controversy regarding regional lymph node dissection does not extend to those melanoma patients with clinically apparent lymph node involvement. A therapeutic regional lymphadenectomy is usually performed as an attempt at salvage. The reported 5-year survival rates are all less than 50% and vary inversely with the number of lymph nodes involved; survival rates tend to be lower in truncal than in extremity tumors.[51] Melanomas may also spread hematogenously to any organ, and surgery for metastatic disease is rarely indicated except for palliation. Selected patients with isolated metastases and a long disease-free interval, such as those with secondary adrenal melanomas, may benefit from excision of the metastatic deposits; however, the number of subjects studied is limited and broad conclusions are impossible.[52]

Chemotherapy for metastatic disease is associated with a 20% response rate for the best single agent, dacarbazine, and up to 50% for combination chemotherapy.[35] Unfortunately, the response to systemic chemotherapy is short and the improvement in survival rate is low. Regional chemotherapy for limb melanoma with melphalan and recombinant tumor necrosis factor applied through a hyperthermic perfusion circuit does extend the disease-free interval but accomplishes little in terms of improving length of survival.[53] Adjuvant systemic chemotherapy protocols, administered in patients without known metastases, have also been ineffective in prolonging life.

Radiotherapy is rarely used in the primary treatment of cutaneous melanoma, and its use as an adjuvant therapy to improve regional control remains investigative.[54] The main indications for radiotherapy are for the palliative treatment of unresectable local disease, brain metastases, and bone metastases.[54] Some evidence exists that immunotherapy for malignant melanoma, including the use of interleukin-2, interferons, and monoclonal antibodies directed against cell surface antigens, may be useful in selected patients.[55] The use of melanoma vaccines, as an adjuvant treatment, is also currently being investigated in randomized trials and appears to have low toxicity and potential benefit.[56]

REFERENCES

1. Domingo J, Helwig E: Malignant neoplasms associated with nevus sebaceous of Jadassohn. J Am Acad Dermatol 1:545–556, 1979.
2. Richard JW, Mills O, Leyden JJ: Naevus comedonicus: Treatment with retinoic acid. Br J Dermatol 86:528–529, 1972.
3. Uitto J, Santa Cruz DJ, Eisen A: Connective tissue nevi of the skin: Clinical, genetic and histopathologic classification of hamartomas of the collagen, elastin, and proteoglycan type. J Am Acad Dermatol 3:441–461, 1980.
4. Happle R, Koopman R, Mier PD: Hypothesis: Vascular twin naevi and somatic recombination in man. Lancet 1:367–378, 1990.
5. Mountcastle EA, Diestlelmeier M, Lupton GP: Nevus anemicus. J Am Acad Dermatol 14:628–632, 1986.
6. Tate PR, Hodge SJ, Owen LG: A quantitative study of melanocytes in Becker's nevus. J Cutan Pathol 7:404–409, 1980.
7. Person JR, Longcope C: Becker's nevus: An androgen-mediated hyperplasia with increased androgen receptors. J Am Acad Dermatol 10:235–238, 1984.
8. Quevedo WC Jr, Fleischmann RD: Developmental biology of mammalian melanocytes. J Invest Dermatol 75:116–121, 1980.
9. Hearing VJ, Jimenez M: Mammalian tyrosinase: The critical regulatory control point in melanocytic pigmentation. Int J Biochem 19:1141–1147, 1987.
10. Prota G: Recent advances in the chemistry of melanogenesis in mammals. J Invest Dermatol 75:122–127, 1980.
11. Elder DE, Clark WH Jr, Elenitsas R, et al: The early and intermediate precursor lesions of tumor progression in the melanocytic system: Common acquired nevi and atypical (dysplastic) nevi. Semin Diagn Pathol 10:18–35, 1993.
12. Cochran AJ, Bailly C, Paul E, et al: Nevi, other than dysplastic and Spitz nevi. Semin Diagn Pathol 10:3–17, 1993.
13. Bhuta S: Electron microscopy in the evaluation of melanocytic tumors. Semin Diagn Pathol 10:92–101, 1993.
14. Gallagher RP, McLean DI: The epidemiology of acquired melanocytic nevi. Dermatol Clin 13:595–603, 1995.
15. Schleicher SM, Lim SJM: Congenital nevi. Int J Dermatol 34:825–829, 1994.

16. Berman B, Shaieb AM, France DS, et al: Halo congenital melanocytic nevus: In vitro immunologic studies. J Am Acad Dermatol 19:954–960, 1988.
17. Goldenhersch MA, Savin RC, Barnhill RL, et al: Malignant blue nevus: Case report and literature review. J Am Acad Dermatol 19:712–722, 1988.
18. Geronemus RG: Q-switched ruby laser therapy of nevus of Ota. Arch Dermatol 128:1618–1622, 1992.
19. Casso EM, Grin-Jorgensen CM, Grant-Kels JM: Spitz nevi. J Am Acad Dermatol 27:901–913, 1992.
20. Wagner RF, Cottel WI: In situ malignant melanoma arising in a speckled lentiginous nevus. J Am Acad Dermatol 20:125–126, 1989.
21. Clark WH Jr, Reimer RR, Greene MH, et al: Origin of familial malignant melanomas from heritable melanocytic lesions: The B-K mole syndrome. Arch Dermatol 114:732–738, 1978.
22. Greene MH, Clark WH Jr, Tucker MA, et al: Acquired precursors of cutaneous malignant melanoma: The familial dysplastic nevus syndrome. N Engl J Med 312:91–97, 1988.
23. Halpern AC, Guerry D IV, Elder DE, et al: Dysplastic nevi as risk markers of sporadic (non-familial) melanoma. Arch Dermatol 127:995–999, 1991.
24. Greene MH, Clark WH Jr, Tucker MA, et al: High risk of malignant melanoma in melanoma prone families with dysplastic nevi. Ann Intern Med 102:458–486, 1985.
25. Kraemer KH, Greene MH, Tarone R, et al: Dysplastic nevi and cutaneous melanoma risk. Lancet 2:1076–1077, 1983.
26. Mehregan AH, Mehregan DA: Malignant melanoma in childhood. Cancer 71:4096–4103, 1993.
27. Rigal DS, Friedman RJ, Kopf AW: The incidence of malignant melanoma in the United States: Issues as we approach the 21st century. J Am Acad Dermatol 34:839–847, 1996.
28. Boddie AW, Smith JL, McBride CM: Malignant melanomas in children and young adults: Effect of diagnostic criteria on staging and end results. South Med J 71:1074–1078, 1978.
29. Berg P, Lindelof B: Differences in malignant melanoma between children and adolescents. Arch Dermatol 133:295–297, 1997.
30. Melnik MK, Urdaneta LF, Al-Jurf AS, et al: Malignant melanoma in childhood and adolescence. Am Surg 52:142–147, 1986.
31. Ceballos PI, Ruiz-Maldonado R, Mihm MC: Current concepts: Melanoma in children. N Engl J Med 332:656–662, 1995.
32. Armstrong BK, Kricker A: How much melanoma is caused by sun exposure? Melanoma Res 3:395–401, 1993.
33. Holman CD, Armstrong BK: Pigmentary traits, ethnic origin, benign nevi, and family history as risk factors for cutaneous melanoma in children. J Natl Cancer Inst 72:257–266, 1984.
34. Weinstock MA, Golditz GA, Willet WC, et al: Nonfamilial cutaneous melanoma incidence in women associated with sun exposure before 20 years of age. Pediatrics 84:199–204, 1989.
35. Rivers JK: Melanoma. Lancet 347:803–807, 1996.
36. Healsmith MF, Bourke JF, Osbourne JE, Graham-Brown RAC: An evaluation of the revised seven-point checklist for the early diagnosis of cutaneous malignant melanoma. Br J Dermatol 130:48–50, 1994.
37. Rigel DS: Malignant melanoma: Incidence issues and their effect on diagnosis and treatment in the 1990s. Mayo Clin Proc 72:367–371, 1997.
38. Lederman JS, Sober AJ: Does wide excision as the initial diagnostic procedure improve prognosis in patients with cutaneous melanoma? J Dermatol Surg Oncol 12:697–699, 1986.
39. Gritters LS, Francis IR, Zayaduy KR: Initial assessment of positron emission tomography using 2-flourine-18-flouro-2-deoxy-D-glucose in the imaging of malignant melanoma. J Nucl Med 34:1420–1427, 1993.
40. Williams ML, Pennella R: Medical progress. Melanoma, melanocytic nevi, and other melanoma risk factors in children. J Pediatr 124:833–845, 1994.
41. Rao BN, Hayes FA, Pratt CB, et al: Malignant melanoma in children: Its management and prognosis. J Pediatr Surg 25:198–203, 1990.
42. Moss AL, Briggs JC: Cutaneous malignant melanoma in the young. Br J Plast Surg 39:537–541, 1986.
43. NIH Consensus Development Panel on Early Melanoma. Diagnosis and treatment of early melanoma. JAMA 268:1314–1319, 1992.
44. Veronesi U, Cascinelli N: Narrow excision (1-cm margin): A safe procedure for thin cutaneous melanoma. Arch Surg 126:438–441, 1991.
45. Veronesi U, Cascinelli N, Adamus J, et al: Thin stage I primary cutaneous malignant melanoma. N Engl J Med 318:1159–1162, 1988.
46. Balch CM, Urist MM, Karakousis CP, et al: Efficacy of 2-cm surgical margins for intermediate-thickness melanomas (1 to 4 mm): Results of a multi-institutional randomized surgical trial. Ann Surg 218:262–269, 1993.
47. Veronesi U, Adamus J, Bandiera BC, et al: Inefficacy of immediate node dissection in stage I malignant melanoma of the limbs. N Engl J Med 297:627–630, 1977.
48. Sim FH, Taylor WF, Pritchard DJ, Soule EH: Lymphadenectomy in the management of stage I malignant melanoma: A prospective randomized study. Mayo Clin Proc 61:697–705, 1986.
49. Balch CM, Soong SJ, Bartolucci AA, et al: Efficacy of an elective regional lymph node dissection of 1 to 4 mm thick melanoma for patients 60 years of age or younger. Ann Surg 224:255–266, 1996.
50. Morton DL, Wen DR, Wong JH, et al: Technical details of intraoperative mapping for early stage melanoma. Arch Surg 127:392–399, 1992.
51. Morton DL, Wanek L, Nizze A, et al: Improved long-term survival after lymphadenectomy of melanoma metastatic to regional nodes. Ann Surg 214:491–501, 1991.
52. Branum GD, Epstein RE, Leight GS, et al: The role of resection in the management of melanoma metastatic to the adrenal gland. Surgery 109:127–131, 1991.
53. Krementz ET, Carter RD, Sutherland CM, et al: Regional chemotherapy for melanoma: A 35-year experience. Ann Surg 220:520–535, 1994.
54. Geara FB, Ang KK: Radiation therapy for malignant melanoma. Surg Clin North Am 76:1383–1398, 1996.
55. Kirkwood JM: Systemic therapy of melanoma. Curr Opin Oncol 6:204–211, 1994.
56. Kuhn CA, Hanke CW: Current status of melanoma vaccines. Dermatol Surg 23:649–655, 1997.

71

HEMANGIOMAS AND LYMPHANGIOMAS

Gustavo Stringel, MD

☐ Hemangiomas and Arteriovenous Malformations

Hemangiomas are the most common tumors of infancy and the most common congenital anomalies in human beings.[1-3] *Hemangioma* is a nonspecific term that has been traditionally applied to benign tumors of vascular tissues, vascular birthmarks, and vascular malformations. Hemangiomas are present in about 1.1 to 2.6% of all newborns; this number increases to 10% by 1 year of age.[4]

The origin of hemangiomas and other congenital vascular lesions is not clear, but they appear to be the result of faulty embryogenesis. They can be arterial, venous, or combined.[5] Other theories abound.[6-11]

Some hemangiomas undergo spontaneous involution after a period of rapid growth.[12] This observation was a landmark in dictating treatment policy and in trying to recognize the lesions that are more likely to involute in order to avoid overtreatment. It is still not possible to predict with confidence which lesions will or will not regress spontaneously.

PATHOGENESIS

Studies report evidence that dermal vascularization begins at about the 35th day of gestation, continuing after birth for several months. The adult type of vascular pattern is established by about the 4th month of life.[13-15]

Angiogenic factors appear to play an important role in the growth and involution of hemangiomas. The high endothelial growth in proliferating hemangiomas is similar to the capillary proliferation in tumors. This rapid growth appears to be stimulated by angiogenesis.[16, 17] Angiogenic factors act in two ways: directly on the vascular endothelium to stimulate mitosis and indirectly through host helper cells, such as macrophages and mast cells.

Heparin released from mast cells stimulates migration of endothelial cells and capillary growth.[18] Heparin alone enhances angiogenesis, but heparin combined with cortisone inhibits the process of angiogenesis. This effect may be independent of glucocorticoid or mineralocorticoid activity.[15, 19] The angiogenic effect of heparin released by mast cells can be blocked by protamine. Other known inhibitors of angiogenesis are a constituent factor present in viable cartilage and some corticosteroids.[20] The concept of angiogenic inhibition has been supported by the effect of corticosteroids in the involution process of some hemangiomas. Angiostatin, an internal fragment of plasminogen, is a potent inhibitor of angiogenesis, which selectively inhibits endothelial cell proliferation. It has been postulated that this potent, specific, and nontoxic angiogenesis inhibitor will find wide clinical use to potentiate and improve the treatment of malignant tumors and other angiogenic diseases.[21]

The functional role of the macrophage is now recognized to extend far beyond its original role as a scavenger cell. Macrophages produce both stimulators and inhibitors of angiogenesis, in either a positive or negative fashion.[22] Rapidly growing hemangiomas are infiltrated by macrophages and mast cells, whereas involuting hemangiomas and vascular malformations have minimal monocytic infiltration. It has been postulated that macrophage infiltration of hemangiomas most likely results from a cell-derived chemotactic mediator. This substance could be the glycoprotein called *monocyte chemoattractant protein-1* (mcp-1), which is a specific chemoattractant for macrophages and monocytes in vitro. This chemoattractant protein is produced by perivascular smooth muscle cells in proliferative hemangiomas but not in stable, regressing hemangiomas or other lymphatic and venous malformations.

The expression of mcp-1 can be downregulated by physiologic doses of dexamethasone and interferon alpha. Additionally, interferon alpha has been shown to inhibit endothelial cell migration toward a chemotactic stimulus. Hence, the additional effect of interferon alpha may be to decrease macrophage recruitment and activation. This may in part explain the good results obtained with dexamethasone and interferon alpha in the treatment of proliferative hemangiomas.[23] E-selectin, an endothelial cell–specific leukocyte adhesion molecule, has been found to have a high expression in proliferative hemangiomas and to decline significantly in the involutive phase of hemangioma specimens. It is believed that E-selectin may be a marker for proliferating endothelium.[24] This important area of investigation is constantly developing and in the future may provide improvements in the treatment of patients with angiogenic diseases.

CLASSIFICATION

The most widely accepted classification divides hemangiomas into capillary, cavernous, and mixed lesions.[15] Another commonly used classification correlates the physical characteristics of the vascular lesions with future behavior.[1] There are five types of hemangiomas in this classification:

Type 1: Neonatal staining
Type 2: Intradermal capillary hemangiomas
    A. Salmon patch
    B. Port-wine stain
    B. Spider angioma
Type 3: Juvenile hemangiomas
    A. Strawberry mark
    B. Strawberry capillary hemangioma
    C. Capillary cavernous hemangioma
Type 4: Arteriovenous fistulas
    A. Arterial hemangioma
    B. Hemangiomatous giantism
Type 5: Cirsoid angioma (racemose aneurysm)[1]

Some clinical characteristics of commonly described hemangiomas[1] are as follows:

- Neonatal staining can affect the base of the neck, forehead, and sacrum. Fading usually occurs spontaneously.
- Salmon patch is a faint variety of intradermal hemangiomas that is light pink to rust. It usually does not change over a period of years.
- Port-wine stains are deep in color. They do not enlarge but, with time, often develop hyperkeratotic patches or knobs on their surfaces. These changes probably represent abnormalities of cutaneous nerve endings.
- Spider angiomas have a small, central, dermal arteriole with a network of radiating intradermal capillaries that spread out in stellar fashion. These lesions are small, and they can be multiple. They appear at 3 to 4 years of age. They can regress spontaneously over a period of years.
- Juvenile hemangiomas are congenital vascular malformations characterized by significant regression during childhood. They can be unpredictable. Some regress after a period of rapid growth, but others continue to proliferate and cause complications. About 73% of these lesions are present at birth and 85% are present by the

1st year of life. About 65% occur in girls and 35% in boys.
- The strawberry mark is characterized by a pale halo of skin that surrounds a radiating telangiectasia.
- The strawberry capillary hemangioma may appear at birth or shortly thereafter. It can appear with a period of frighteningly rapid growth, with an intense red color. The lesion may be circumscribed or elevated with lobulations. It is usually compressible. Before regression, significant complications can develop.
- Congenital arteriovenous fistulas differ significantly from acquired or traumatic fistulas. The congenital type has multiple and diffuse anastomoses with the surrounding vasculature. About 50% occur in the head and neck.
- Arterial hemangiomas are present as pulsatile masses with bruits, thrills, palpable hypertrophy of supplying arteries, hyperthermia, venous dilations, and occasional redness over the skin. They appear in early childhood and sometimes early adulthood. These masses respond to hormonal fluctuations. Cutaneous or superficial involvement can produce significant bleeding episodes. Hemangiomatous giantism can be an additional manifestation of congenital arteriovenous fistulas.

In a biologic classification of vascular birthmarks, lesions are divided into two major types: hemangiomas and vascular malformations.[25, 26] *Hemangiomas* are vascular tumors that enlarge by rapid cellular proliferation; 30% are present at birth as a red macule, and the female-to-male ratio is 3:1. These tumors develop a rapid postnatal proliferation and undergo slow involution. They may develop primary platelet trapping with thrombocytopenia (Kasabach-Merritt syndrome). Angiographic features consist of well-circumscribed, intense lobular or parenchymal staining with equatorial vessels. Bone changes and limb hypertrophy are rare.

Vascular malformations are all present at birth but may not be evident. They show commensurate growth. They may expand as a result of trauma, sepsis, or hormonal changes. The female-to-male ratio is 1:1. They can develop primary venous stasis with localized consumptive coagulopathy. Angiographically, they can have low flow with phleboliths and ectatic channels or high flow with enlarged tortuous arteries and arteriovenous shunting. Low-flow lesions can affect skeletal muscles by distortion or hypoplasia, and high-flow lesions can produce distortion, destruction, and limb hypertrophy.

Congenital hemangiomas can be detected as early as the second trimester of pregnancy by high-resolution prenatal ultrasonography (US). They present as full-blown hemangiomas at birth. These lesions do not grow any further after birth, possibly because they present during or after the proliferative phase. Shunting through a large intrauterine hemangioma can cause hydrops fetalis, a complication associated with high mortality. These hemangiomas are difficult to treat. Corticosteroids should not be given owing to the risk of premature closure of the ductus arteriosus, diminished glomerular filtration with salt retention, and gastrointestinal complications. Interferon alpha-2a is an effective antiangiogenic drug, but the interferon family also regulates growth and differentiation. On the basis of current knowledge, neither of these drugs should be given during pregnancy, unless there is a real threat to the life of an otherwise healthy fetus.[27]

In some lesions, overlapping of clinical characteristics is common, and future behavior is unpredictable. In some cases, the Doppler assessment of flow pattern[28] and the quantitation of biologic markers may help to identify the involuting type of hemangioma.

DIAGNOSIS

After a thorough physical examination, investigations may be indicated if complications are present or if surgical intervention is contemplated. Coagulation studies should be done if platelet trapping is suspected. On US, a hemangioma appears hypoechoic, well defined, of heterogenous texture, with cystic and sinusoidal spaces, and possibly containing phleboliths. US is enhanced by use of color Doppler imaging, especially if flow is demonstrated.[28-30]

Use of technetium 99m–labeled red blood cells is a quick and noninvasive diagnostic modality, but it does not define anatomic involvement.[31] This diagnostic modality may be useful in monitoring therapeutic effects and in detecting residual or recurrent vascular lesions.[32] Cavernous hemangiomas have been visualized by indium[111] octreotide scan. The visualization of hemangiomas by this technique would indicate a high density of somatostatin receptors within the hemangioma. At present, the clinical implications of this finding are unclear.[33]

Computed tomography (CT), especially with contrast-agent injection, can delineate the extent and involvement of the hemangioma and can help to differentiate hemangiomas from lymphatic anomalies.[34] Magnetic resonance imaging (MRI) is most useful in intramuscular hemangiomas, in which a high signal intensity with a characteristic serpiginous pattern is shown. Definition of muscle groups and muscle atrophy is good with MRI.[35] In small localized lesions, contrast-enhanced MRI may offer a significant advantage over other techniques.[36]

Conventional angiography should be reserved for cases in which embolization or surgical intervention is contemplated. Intravenous digital subtraction angiography is relatively noninvasive but does not have the resolution of conventional techniques.[37] Angiography can provide information about the size of the lesions and feeding vessels and can distinguish between hemangiomas and vascular malformations.

Biopsy of a hemangioma or a vascular malformation is rarely indicated. When the diagnosis is uncertain or when the threat of malignancy must be excluded, biopsy may be necessary.

COMPLICATIONS

Complications of hemangiomas are cosmetic and functional.[15] They can be secondary to hemorrhage (Fig. 71–1), ulceration (Fig. 71–2), infection, necrosis, airway obstruction, and cardiac failure. Platelet trapping can cause coagulopathy (Kasabach-Merritt syndrome) or disseminated intravascular coagulation (Fig. 71–3). Periorbital hemangiomas can cause astigmatism, ptosis, strabismus, amblyopia, and blindness (Fig. 71–4).[38] Hemangiomas in individual organs and systems can cause serious problems, depending on size and location. Some hemangiomas can compromise vital structures.[39, 40]

TREATMENT

The treatment of congenital vascular anomalies is based on an understanding of the clinical behavior and natural history of the individual lesions. True hemangiomas[25] grow rapidly for the first 12 months of life and involute by 5 to 7 years of age. Congenital vascular malformations[26] can involve blood vessels and lymphatics and have no potential for involu-

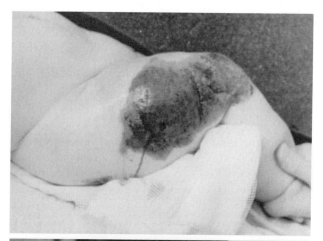

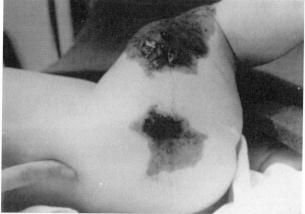

Figure 71–1. Large hemangioma of the lower extremity with hemorrhage.

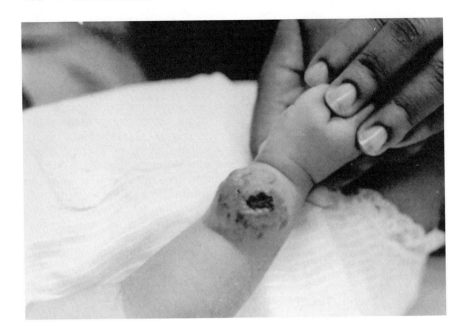

Figure 71–2. Hemangioma of the upper extremity with ulceration.

tion. Their clinical manifestation depends on hemodynamics, size, and anatomic location. It is sometimes difficult to distinguish between a hemangioma and a vascular malformation.

Many earlier methods of treatment, such as artificial ulceration with inoculation of infection, CO_2 snow-freezing, and thermocautery, are not now recommended.

Other therapeutic options include observation, compression, sclerosis, radiation therapy, chemotherapy, systemic steroids, interferon alpha, intralesional steroids, embolization, surgical excision, and laser ablation.

Observation

Uncomplicated hemangiomas and other vascular lesions are treated conservatively. Most hemangio-

mas involute spontaneously, whether they are capillary, cavernous, or mixed. These lesions leave little cosmetic or functional disability. In many cases, the cosmetic result is much better than that offered by surgical intervention (see Fig. 71–4).[12, 39] Educating parents about the hemangioma may reduce their distress.[41]

Compression Treatment

Two types of compression treatment are useful.[39] *Continuous compression*[42] is applied with bandages, garments, or splints. *Intermittent pneumatic compression*[43] is applied with a Jobst pump or Wright linear pump. The mechanism of action of this mode of treatment is unknown. Compression may promote vessel emptying with endothelial damage and proliferation with thrombosis, which causes early invo-

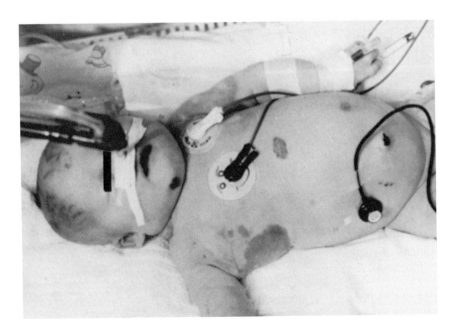

Figure 71–3. Large hemangioma of the chest with disseminated intravascular coagulation.

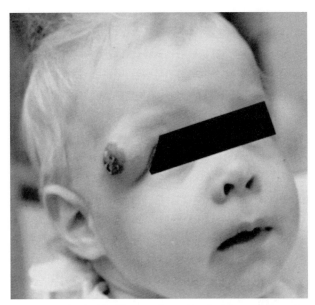

Figure 71–4. Periorbital hemangioma involuted spontaneously.

lution of the hemangioma. Hemangiomas of the extremities, abdomen, and parotid gland have been successfully treated with compression.[44] Compression treatment, which is safe and effective, should be attempted in accessible hemangiomas, including those with complications (Figs. 71–5 and 71–6).

The lesion must be accessible for intermittent pneumatic compression to be effective. Circumferential pressure is desirable. The pressure should be applied, preferably 24 hours a day, over the whole hemangioma. Compliance from parents is essential.[43]

Sclerotherapy

Sclerosing solutions are both tissue irritants and thrombogenic agents that provoke an inflammatory tissue reaction, which causes fibrosis and obliteration of vascular channels. Preparations used in the past, such as boiling water, sodium morrhuate, sodium psylliate, and quinine urethrone, have been abandoned due to pain and allergic reactions.[45, 46] Good results have been reported by some clinicians, using 1% and 3% sodium tetradecyl sulfate (Sotradecol), which we prefer, or 3% hydroxypolyethoxydodecan plus trichlorisobutyl alcohol plus spirit (Sclerovein).[46]

Treatment can be instituted as an outpatient procedure with no anesthesia. Each of the sclerosing agents is injected through a 25-gauge needle deeply into the lesion in various directions. About 0.1 to 0.2 ml of the solution is instilled with each thrust. The skin surface of the hemangioma is avoided to prevent necrosis. The total amount injected should not exceed 1 ml in children and 2 ml in adults. The maximum safe dose is unknown. Up to 10 treatments have been given with intervals of 3 to 4 weeks between treatments. Postinjection swelling and pain are expected.[45, 46]

Radiation

Radiation treatment of hemangiomas is controversial, although there are still some advocates.[15, 47] Complications of radiotherapy include damage to the bony epiphysis, breasts, gonads, skin, lens, and thyroid gland.[39] Carcinoma and sarcoma have also been reported after radiation treatment.[1, 48] Postirradiation complications increase when high total doses are delivered.

With modern radiation techniques, however, careful dosage delivered by an experienced radiotherapist makes the use of this modality justifiable in exceptional cases, such as the patient who has not responded to other forms of treatment and in whom surgical intervention is considered too hazardous.

Chemotherapy

Isolated reports of treatment of hemangiomas with chemotherapy have appeared in the literature. In one patient, a large facial hemangioma was successfully treated with intraarterial nitrogen mustard.[49] Four other children with life-threatening complications secondary to inoperable hemangiomas were successfully treated with cyclophosphamide. The

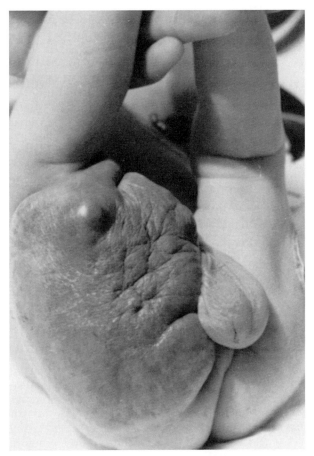

Figure 71–5. Giant hemangioma of the lower extremity with cardiac failure and platelet trapping in a newborn. This hemangioma resolved with intermittent pneumatic compression.

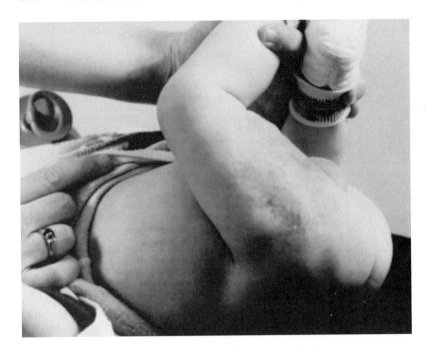

Figure 71–6. Giant hemangioma shown in Figure 71–5, after involution.

10 mg/kg/day dose was used intravenously for the short chemotherapy course.[50]

Systemic Steroid Treatment

The mechanism of action of systemic steroids in hemangiomas is unknown.[15, 39, 51] Steroids were first given for the treatment of thrombocytopenia associated with hemangiomas.[52] The size of the hemangioma was reduced under steroid treatment. Subsequently, many other reports have appeared confirming the beneficial effect of steroids on hemangiomas.[1, 53] Immature proliferating hemangiomas respond better to steroid treatment than do mature hemangiomas and vascular malformations (Figs. 71–7 and 71–8).[1, 53]

Recommended prednisone dosages include 10 to 40 mg/day for 9 weeks[1, 40, 41] and 2 to 3 mg/kg/day for 4 weeks, followed by alternate-day therapy for up to 6 weeks.[54] Other schedules recommend 2 to 4 mg/kg/day for 2 to 4 weeks after the hemangioma is stable or is beginning to regress. Treatment continues for 1 more month before the dose is tapered.[15] Some authors suggest that the response to steroids may be dose dependent and recommend initiating therapy with high-dose prednisone. This schedule recommends prednisone, 5 mg/kg/day, in four daily divided doses. This dosage should be used for no less than 6 weeks and for as long as 12 weeks.[55]

Megadose methylprednisolone has been used successfully in children with hemangiomas and Kasabach-Merritt syndrome. The treatment protocol consists of 30 mg/kg/day for 3 days, 20 mg/kg/day for 4 days, and subsequently 10, 5, 2, and 1 mg/kg/day for 1 week, with each dose given all at once before 8:00 AM. A potential complication may be anaphylaxis or severe asthmatic episodes; these adverse reactions have been observed in patients receiving parenteral prednisolone. In addition, injections of methylprednisolone containing alcohol as a preservative may have associated toxic effects in neonates.[56, 57] Steroid treatment always should be tapered gradually and never stopped abruptly.

Interferon Alpha

Interferon alpha was initially developed as an antiviral agent. It was noted to affect the growth of Kaposi's sarcoma and, in one patient, to treat

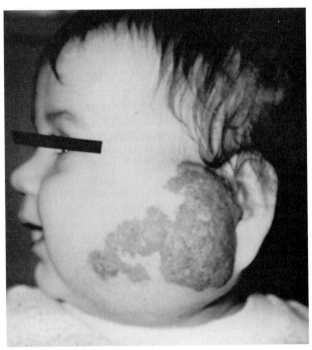

Figure 71–7. Large hemangioma of the parotid gland is treated with steroids and compression.

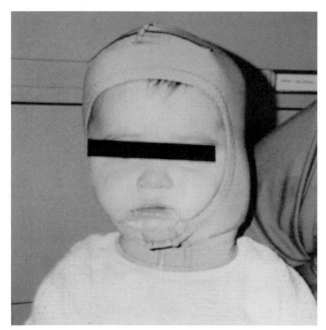

Figure 71–8. Patient in Figure 71–7 is treated with continuous compression garment.

pulmonary hemangiomatosis successfully.[58] It has been used with success to treat life-threatening hemangiomas and refractory hemangiomas not responsive to other modalities of treatment.[59] Immediate improvement of Kasabach-Merritt syndrome and associated coagulopathy has been reported. Interferon alpha-2a induces early involution of large hemangiomas. However, complete involution may take a long time.

The mechanism of action of interferon is not clearly understood. It appears to block migration and proliferation of endothelial cells, acting as an angiogenic inhibitor. It may also inhibit the effects of specific growth factors on the proliferation of endothelial cells, smooth muscle cells, or fibroblasts by decreasing the production of collagen or by enhancing the production and release of endothelial cell prostacyclin. It is also possible that interferon alpha-2a inhibits endothelial proliferation by blocking the action of basic fibroblast growth factor, which is known to be a potent angiogenic stimulant.

The recommended dosage of interferon alpha-2a is 3 million U/m²/day subcutaneously. Long-term therapy is recommended for an average of 12 to 18 months. It is usually well tolerated without any significant toxic effects, even in small children.

Potential short-term side effects of interferon alpha-2a (at 6 to 12 months) include mild fever, malaise, leukopenia, and abnormal liver transaminase levels. Long-term complications include interstitial nephritis, nephrotic syndrome, autoimmune diseases such as systemic lupus erythematosus, hemolytic anemia, thyroiditis, and thyrotoxicosis. Side effects are usually reversible by stopping the medication temporarily or permanently. In one reported case, therapy was discontinued due to irrita-

bility and poor oral intake.[58–61] In one report, interferon was unsuccessful in the treatment of large hemangiomas in four children; however, interferon alpha-2b was used.[62]

Other sporadic failure reports indicate that this drug may not always be effective and that more experience is needed to evaluate its applications further. At present, interferon alpha-2a is recommended in the treatment of complex hemangiomas, especially those with significant complications. Interferon is not a replacement for other traditional therapeutic modalities, which may be indicated in individual cases. Interferon is not effective in the treatment of vascular or lymphatic malformations.[58–61]

Intralesional Steroids

Most of the reports of successful treatment of hemangiomas with direct intralesional steroids have appeared in the ophthalmic literature.[14, 38, 63] Satisfactory results and few complications encourage the use of this technique in hemangiomas other than periorbital.[63] Intralesional injection of steroids in lesions situated around the eye and in the upper part of the face should be done with caution by experienced physicians. Reported complications include swelling, central retinal occlusion, eyelid necrosis, and sclerodermiform linear atrophy.[64, 65] Other potential complications include hirsutism, infection, adrenal suppression, cushingoid facies, ocular perforation, and the associated risk of a general anesthetic.[65]

Some surgeons recommend injection using general anesthesia. Others perform the procedure on an outpatient basis, without anesthesia. Generally, a 26- to 30-gauge needle is used. A mixture of triamcinolone acetonide (2 to 100 mg per injection) and betamethasone acetate (0.3 to 15 mg per injection) is recommended, in a total volume from 0.1 to 5 ml. The dose and volume are individualized for the size of the lesion. The most frequent dose used has been 20 mg of triamcinolone acetonide and 3 mg of betamethasone acetate, in a total volume of 1 ml.[63–65]

Injections are done directly into the hemangioma in different directions through the same needle hole. Direct pressure is applied for 2 to 10 minutes to prevent bleeding. Intralesional steroid injection appears to be effective in some hemangiomas, especially in the periorbital region, but this technique is certainly not free of complications.

Embolization

Embolization involves the deposition of thrombus-inducing material in the lumen of a blood vessel through an arterial catheter placed under fluoroscopic and contrast medium control. Embolization is attempted when the lesion is not amenable to other treatment or in preparation for surgical excision. Especially useful when the major complication is cardiac failure, the technique is also useful in

Kasabach-Merritt syndrome and hemorrhage. Occlusion of the blood vessel can be temporary, semipermanent, or permanent according to the material used. An experienced interventional radiologist is essential to success and to avoid embolization to normal tissues.

Many different embolizing materials have been employed. Some of the most popular include methacrylate spheres, balloon catheters, cyanoacrylate tissue adhesives, silicone rubber, wool and cotton, absorbable gelatin sponge, polyvinyl alcohol sponge, autologous blood clot, autologous muscle, and metallic coils.[66–68]

Surgical Excision

Surgical removal of a hemangioma is done only when complications occur and when the lesion has not responded to more conservative measures (Fig. 71–9). The surgical approach depends on the size and location of the hemangioma. As much information as possible is obtained from radiologic and other diagnostic studies.

The theory of removing a hemangioma during early infancy while it is still small and before it grows too large is not logical because it is impossible to predict the behavior of the hemangioma. The small lesion may never grow. If it does, it may also involute spontaneously. To undertake major surgical resection of the hemangioma is unwise and deforming during the period of rapid growth or when coagulation is not adequate. Preoperative embolization, which is valuable in decreasing the blood loss and the size of the hemangioma, is done when available.[66–68] Small hemangiomas that interfere with function, such as a periorbital or eyelid hemangioma, are removed when they are not amenable to other conservative treatment.

Vascular malformations may eventually require surgical excision because the potential for involution is minimal.[25, 26] If uncomplicated, the lesion should be treated conservatively for as long as possible. The task of removing this difficult and some-

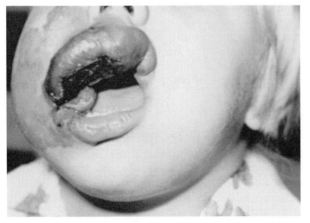

Figure 71–9. Large vascular malformation of the face was refractory to treatment.

times massive malformation is reserved for those who can deal with the inherent potential complications of such treatment.[1, 11, 67, 69] In some cases, excision is absolutely indicated, sometimes on an urgent basis, due to complications. The patient should understand that the cosmetic or functional result may sometimes be worse than the original disease.

Hypotensive anesthesia and total circulatory arrest with profound hypothermia have permitted excision of lesions that were previously inaccessible to surgical intervention.[70]

Laser Treatment

One of the most significant advances in cutaneous surgery and in the treatment of hemangiomas (especially port-wine stains) has been the advent of laser technology.[71] A laser beam may be aimed at a specific target or lesion where it produces its effect as it is absorbed.[72] More than a dozen different lasers have been used either clinically or experimentally.[73, 74] Lasers can be used to coagulate, cut, or ablate tissue.[71–73]

The CO_2 laser (10,600 nm) emits in the infrared light portion of the electromagnetic spectrum, acts by vaporization of water within cells, and offers no selectivity. The argon laser's two wavelengths (488 and 514 nm) are absorbed mainly by hemoglobin in dermal blood vessels. The Nd:YAG laser (1060 nm) is not readily absorbed by hemoglobin or water and penetrates deeper in the tissues. The main disadvantage of argon, CO_2, and Nd:YAG laser treatment of vascular skin lesions has been scarring.[72, 73] Scarring appears to be less when dye laser (577 nm) is used, but experience with this laser is still limited. Initial experience with treatment of port-wine stain in children showed that results were not as good as in adults because lesions were not as heavily pigmented with hemoglobin. Modification of dosages and postlaser care have improved these results.[71]

The flash lamp-pumped pulsed dye laser (585 nm) has been successfully used to treat superficial and deep proliferative hemangiomas, including ulcerated hemangiomas. It has been postulated that selective photothermolysis may arrest the development of the hemangioma and induce its remission.[74, 75]

Spider angiomas can be effectively treated with argon, CO_2, and dye lasers. Strawberry hemangiomas have been successfully treated with argon and Nd:YAG lasers. Port-wine stains in children appear to respond better to the tunable dye laser (577 nm) with less chance of scarring, but satisfactory results have also been obtained with argon and CO_2 lasers.

Laser treatment is not a panacea. It should be applied judiciously by a therapist experienced with treating children.

☐ Associated Syndromes

KASABACH-MERRITT SYNDROME

In 1940, Kasabach and Merritt reported a 2-month-old infant with a rapidly enlarging hemangioma of the thigh, thrombocytopenia, and hemorrhagic diathesis.[76] The thrombocytopenia responded to external irradiation and radium needle implants. Since this original report, more than 100 cases have appeared in the literature; the association of thrombocytopenia, consumption coagulopathy, and hemangioma is now recognized as the Kasabach-Merritt syndrome.[77]

The syndrome is usually associated with a large or "giant" hemangioma and has a high mortality rate (37%). The main cause of death is bleeding. The mechanism for the consumption of the clotting factors is unclear.[78, 79]

No one single mode of treatment is effective; many may be necessary. Some treatments include heparin, aspirin, dipyridamole, antifibrinolytics, aminocaproic acid, exchange transfusion, steroids, and interferon. Eradication of the hemangioma is the most definite form of therapy.

DIFFUSE NEONATAL HEMANGIOMATOSIS AND BENIGN NEONATAL HEMANGIOMATOSIS

Benign neonatal hemangiomatosis is a condition in which multiple small, bright red to purple capillary hemangiomas, ranging in size from pinhead to 20 mm, appear during the first few weeks of life. Only the skin is affected. This self-limited disease, with likely involution by the 4th month of life,[80] should be distinguished from diffuse neonatal hemangiomatosis,[81] which is often a fatal disorder characterized by widespread capillary hemangiomas that involve skin and visceral organs. Complications include high-output cardiac failure, gastrointestinal bleeding, hydrocephalus, and consumption coagulopathy.

MAFFUCCI'S SYNDROME

The association of hemangiomatosis and multiple enchondromatosis is known as Maffucci's syndrome. First described in 1881,[15, 82] this entity can be a cause of dwarfism, deformity, and malignancy. The most serious complication, the development of malignancy in about 23% of reported cases, is usually a transformation of one or more enchondromas to chondrosarcomas. Sarcomatous degeneration of hemangiomas or lymphangiomas can also occur.

KLIPPEL-TRENAUNAY SYNDROME

In 1900, Klippel and Trenaunay described a triad of port-wine stain, varicose veins, and hypertrophy of the involved extremity.[83] In 1907, Parkes-Weber described the same syndrome associated with arteriovenous fistulas.[84]

Klippel-Trenaunay syndrome can affect upper or lower extremities. It can be monomelic or multimelic. It can also involve the trunk and abdominal viscera.[82, 85] Careful clinical and radiologic assessment of the affected limb should be done at regular intervals to assess leg length discrepancy and to formulate an approach for prevention and treatment of overgrowth.

Intermittent pneumatic compression[85] can be useful, if started at an early age, but compliance is necessary. This compression is indicated when edema, lymphedema, and angiomatosis are present (Fig. 71–10). The size of the limb can be effectively

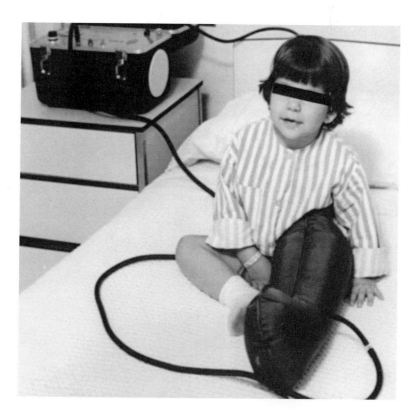

Figure 71–10. Patient is treated with intermittent pneumatic compression.

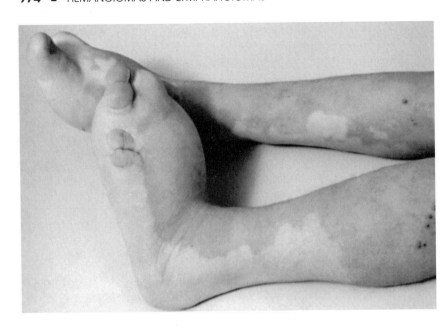

Figure 71–11. Severe case of Klippel-Trenaunay syndrome involves both lower extremities.

reduced, and varicose veins and arteriovenous fistulas can be controlled. Appropriate garments (Jobst) are required for continuous compression. Skin care is important to prevent ulcers and infections. Cellulitis, which is common, should be treated promptly with antibiotics, limb elevation, and bed rest.

Epiphysiodesis is reserved for major incapacitating leg length discrepancy, usually more than 3.8 cm.[86] Amputation and remodeling of limbs are sometimes necessary to improve function and cosmesis (Figs. 71–11 and 71–12). Excision of varicose

veins is contraindicated (Fig. 71–13).[85] Ligation of arteriovenous fistulas has been disappointing.

Percutaneous sclerotherapy can be performed in selected patients to treat symptomatic venous malformations. When this modality of treatment is contemplated, it is important to delineate the venous system by venography or MRI. These studies delineate the presence of arteriovenous fistulas and help prevent embolization of important structures. It is important to remember that the deep venous system is absent in 20% of patients with Klippel-Trenaunay syndrome. In these patients, embolization of super-

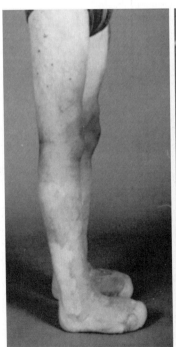
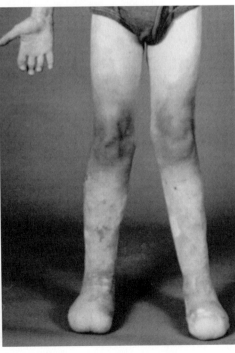

Figure 71–12. Patient in Figure 71–11 after compression treatment and surgical remodeling of limbs.

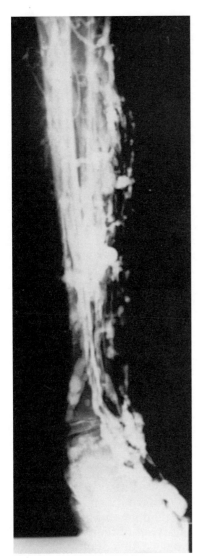

Figure 71–13. Venogram in a case of Klippel-Trenaunay syndrome demonstrates massive varicosities.

ficial veins can cause complications. Complications of sclerotherapy include skin necrosis, nerve palsy, hemoglobinuria, and allergic reactions with anaphylaxis.[87, 88] Emotional and supportive management is extremely important.

PROTEUS SYNDROME

The Proteus syndrome (named after the Greek god Proteus who could change his shape at will to prevent capture) is a congenital hamartomatous disorder described in 1983.[89] It has a wide range of clinical manifestations and can sometimes have overlapping clinical features with Klippel-Trenaunay syndrome. It is now believed that John Merrick ("the Elephant Man") had Proteus syndrome and not neurofibromatosis. This condition is sporadic, with equal gender incidence. Characteristic clinical features include asymmetric overgrowth, increased stature, macrodactyly, soft tissue hypertrophy, syndactyly of the toes, epidermal nevi, vascular nevi

(which may include port-wine stain, angiomatous lesions, and lymphangiomas), and soft subcutaneous masses representing complex hamartomatous malformations. Management of this condition is individualized, and treatment is directed to complications.[90, 91]

INTRAMUSCULAR HEMANGIOMA

Skeletal muscle hemangioma constitutes 0.8% of all hemangiomas. About 45% are in the lower extremity, with 18.9% in the quadriceps.[92] These tumors are usually discovered during childhood and adolescence. Occasionally, the malformation is palpable, but most become apparent due to recurrent pain and swelling.[92, 93] Functional impairment with deformity, motion limitation, and muscle weakness can be present.

Plain radiographs can sometimes show calcifications. CT and MRI accurately determine the extent of the involvement and sometimes resectability (Fig. 71–14).[34, 35] Arteriography helps to identify feeding vessels.

The first priority is to exclude malignancy.[94] Compressive stockings can sometimes be useful in preventing episodes of pain and thrombosis. Steroid treatment has limited value. Total or near-total removal of the lesion with ligation of all major feeding

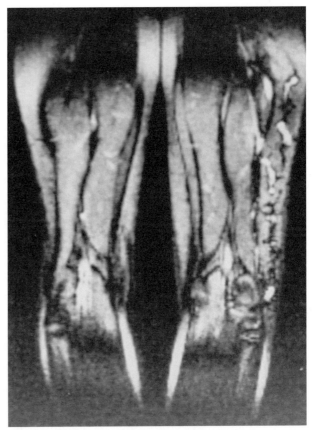

Figure 71–14. Subcutaneous and intramuscular hemangioma of the lower extremity is demonstrated by magnetic resonance imaging.

vessels is the treatment of choice. Embolization can be helpful to occlude major arteriovenous fistulas and may be beneficial before surgical intervention to decrease blood loss.

PYOGENIC GRANULOMA

Pyogenic granuloma is an acquired inflammatory proliferative lesion, which sometimes can resemble a capillary hemangioma. Although the term implies an infective origin, the cause of this lesion is unknown. Pyogenic granulomas have a predilection for the face and neck. They are more common in children and young adults. Sometimes, they can be associated with true hemangiomas. Histologically, the lesion is similar to ordinary granulation tissue, but it often shows proliferating endothelium.[95, 96] Recurrent bleeding is the main complication. Cosmesis can be a problem when the lesion is on the face.

Treatment by cauterization with silver nitrate applicators is usually successful, but recurrence is a problem. Electrocoagulation and laser treatment are both effective. When the lesion is pedunculated, a simple silk ligature can stop the bleeding and cure it, but the base of the friable granuloma should not be cut. Surgical removal is rarely indicated except in recurrent or difficult cases.

LYMPHATIC MALFORMATIONS

The spectrum of lymphatic anomalies can vary from the simple isolated lymphangioma that involves skin to the severe lymphatic malformation that involves different organs and anatomic regions. Their clinical manifestations differ from a simple swelling or a mass to ascites, chylothorax, lymphedema, respiratory problems, and many more.[97–99] Lymphatic malformations can be seen in any lymphatic-bearing anatomic region, but they are more common in rich lymphatic areas, such as the neck, axilla, mediastinum, groin, and retroperitoneum.[100, 101]

The basic function of the lymphatic vessels is to drain protein-rich fluid that has leaked from capillaries. They return the fluid to the blood and maintain equilibrium in the interstitial fluid.[97, 102] The lymphatic pressure is normally zero or negative. With a poorly developed or absent basement membrane, this pressure allows for intercellular diffusion of plasma proteins and lipids that are too large for reabsorption through the venous system.[103]

The four layers of lymphatics are as follows:
1. The superficial primary lymphatics are valveless; they form a capillary lymphatic network.
2. The subdermal or secondary lymphatics are larger; they have valves, and they drain the superficial lymphatics.
3. The third deep layer drains both systems; these lymphatics also have valves and a muscular wall.
4. The intramuscular lymphatic system exists

and functions independently of the superficial dermal systems.

The abdominal cisterna chyli and the thoracic duct complex collect the lymphatic drainage from the abdominal viscera and the extremities. The thoracic duct carries lymphatic drainage from all of the body except for the right side of the head and neck, right arm, and right side of the chest. Those areas are drained by the right lymphatic trunk. The thoracic duct drains into the left jugular–subclavian angle and the right lymphatic trunk into the right jugular–subclavian area.[104] Movement of lymphatic fluid depends on an intrinsic pump and valves and on extrinsic factors, such as muscle contraction, arterial pulses, respiratory movement, and massage.[105]

Lymphangiomas derive from a growth anomaly or arrest in the normal development of the lymphatic system. The embryologic development of the lymphatic system is not clearly understood. The discovery of jugular sacs by Saxer in 1876 was a landmark in the understanding of the evolution of the lymphatic system.[98]

Controversy exists about the development and connection between the sacs and the lymphatic system. Two theories try to explain this development: the *centrifugal theory*[106–108] and the *centripetal theory*.[109] According to the centrifugal theory, the lymphatics develop as mesenchymal spaces that grow centrifugally and continuously from the lymphatic sacs and eventually join the venous system. The centripetal theory proposes that lymphatic vessels develop in mesenchymal clefts and form continuous channels. They follow the centripetal flow of lymph and eventually join the venous system. These two theories do not completely explain the development of the different types of lymphatic anomalies. Some authorities suggest that lymphangioma and lymphedema are interrelated developmental anomalies.[97] Others propose that lymphatic proliferation or lymphangiogenesis plays an important role in the development and clinical behavior of lymphologic syndromes.[110]

Classification

The traditional classification divides lymphangioma into four groups[98, 101, 111, 112]: (1) capillary lymphangioma, (2) cavernous lymphangioma, (3) cystic lymphangioma (cystic hygroma), and (4) lymphangiohemangioma.

Capillary Lymphangioma

Lymphangioma simplex presents as superficial, slightly elevated, clear, smooth papules or wart-like vesicles. They can be single or multiple. They involve the oral region, especially the tongue. They can also involve other areas, particularly the genitals.

Lymphangioma circumscriptum is similar to simplex but has a deeper subcutaneous component of lymphatic cisterns. The circumscriptum type can involve the face, chest, and extremities. Lesions can be small or can involve large areas of the body. Histologically, the simplex type shows thin, dilated lymphatic channels in the dermis and epidermis. The circumscriptum type has a deep subcutaneous component. No communication of normal lymphatics and lymphangioma exists in the same anatomic area.

Complications include pain, recurrent infection, seepage of lymphatic fluid and blood, and cosmetic problems. Treatment consists of surgical excision, cryotherapy with liquid nitrogen, electrocoagulation, and laser treatment. Lymphangioma simplex responds well to treatment. In lymphangioma circumscriptum, the deeper component must be removed to avoid recurrence. Skin removal is often a limiting factor. Some clinicians advocate raising the skin flaps, removing the deeper component, and leaving enough skin for good cosmetic closure. The superficial component often disappears spontaneously.[113] CO_2 laser treatment has been reported to provide good results with few recurrences.[114]

Cavernous Lymphangioma

Cavernous lymphangiomas are characterized by superficial and deep small lymphatic spaces and dilated lymph channels, lined by endothelial cells. Smooth muscle may be present in the vessel wall.[111] Cavernous lymphangiomas can affect any area of the body and may extend deep into the muscles and surrounding tissue. Cavernous lymphangiomas are more commonly present in the tongue, cheek, thorax, extremities, and retroperitoneum. They usually occur at birth or during infancy, but they can occur later in life. Enlargement of lymphangioma can follow infection and trauma. Lymphedema may be associated with large lesions.

Complications are related to infection and functional interference, caused by pressure on adjacent tissues. Cosmesis and leaking of lymphatic fluid can also be a problem. Bleeding into a lymphangioma can cause confusion with a hemangioma. Complete removal of the lymphangioma is the treatment of choice, but often this is not possible.[98]

Spontaneous resolution of cavernous lymphangiomas has been documented[115, 116]; for this reason, some physicians recommend expectant treatment in asymptomatic cases.[111, 117] Children with macroglossia should be carefully observed for the development of complications. Tracheostomy may be needed when airway obstruction occurs. Partial glossectomy may be necessary in some cases.[101]

CO_2 laser has been successful in treating head and neck lymphangiomas and lesions that involve the airway passages.[118, 119] Supportive and prompt treatment of infection with antibiotics is extremely important.

Cystic Hygroma

Cystic hygroma has multiloculated cystic spaces lined by endothelial cells. They are separated by fine walls that contain numerous smooth muscle cells mixed with fibrous tissue.[111] Their incidence is about 1 in 12,000 births.[102] About 50 to 65% appear at birth, and 80 to 90% appear by the 2nd year of life.[120] Clinically, they occur as large, soft cystic masses with distortion of the associated anatomic area (Fig. 71–15). About 75% occur in the neck with predilection for the left side, mainly the posterior triangle, and 20% occur in the axillary region. The rest are usually distributed among the mediastinum, retroperitoneum, pelvis, and groin.[98, 103, 112]

Cystic hygromas are believed to be the result of maldevelopment of the lymphatic jugular sacs, with failure of these structures to connect or drain into the venous system. The diagnosis is usually made by physical examination. Transillumination can help to differentiate cystic hygromas from solid

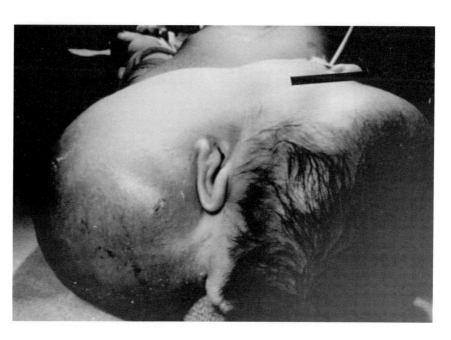

Figure 71–15. Large cystic hygroma of the neck in a newborn infant. (Courtesy of Sterling Blocker, MD.)

masses. US is helpful to confirm the diagnosis, especially in superficial lesions. US is less valuable for demonstrating extension into deep structures of the neck, thoracic cavity, and retroperitoneum.[121] MRI can clearly demonstrate the relationship of the lymphangioma to soft tissues, muscle, and vascular structures. MRI is especially useful in the diagnosis of orbital lymphangiomas.[122]

Complications

Most cystic hygromas show a growth proportional to that of the child. Often, however, they increase rapidly in size with no apparent precipitating cause. Cystic hygromas can also increase in size after trauma, infection, or bleeding into the cystic spaces.

Respiratory obstruction is the most significant complication (Fig. 71–16). Large hygromas can involve the oropharynx and trachea. About 3 to 5% extend into the mediastinum. *Dysphagia* is caused by the involvement of the hypopharynx and esophagus. Other complications are *inflammation* and *infection*. *Hemorrhage* into the cyst and nerve compression can cause paresthesias and pain. Erosions into a major vessel with exsanguinating hemorrhage is rare but has been reported. Dental *malocclusion* and mandibular abnormalities have been reported, secondary to large cervical cystic hygromas.[123]

The prenatal US diagnosis of nuchal or posterior cervical cystic hygroma has important implications because this lesion has been associated with other congenital anomalies, especially chromosomal abnormalities.[124, 125] It carries a high mortality rate, especially with *hydrops* and *lymphedema*. The prenatal, US-based diagnosis of fetal cystic hygroma requires a careful search to exclude other anomalies. Amniocentesis with chromosomal analysis should be done with subsequent genetic and family counseling.

Treatment

Surgical Excision

The treatment of cystic hygroma depends on the clinical presentation, the size of the lesion, the anatomic location, and the complications. The best treatment is meticulous, complete excision of the lesion, but this is often impossible. The removal of some cystic hygromas is a formidable task. Many complications can occur, including recurrence, fistula formation, infection, damage to vascular structures, damage to nerves, and cosmetic deformity. Nerve damage has been reported to the 7th, 9th, 10th, 11th, and 12th cranial nerves as well as to the sympathetic system and brachial plexus. The surgical mortality rate has varied from 2 to 6%.[98, 101, 112]

Most surgeons agree that removal of the cystic hygroma is the treatment of choice, but the question of timing of the intervention has not been answered. Some recommend immediate excision; others prefer to wait until the child is 2 to 6 months of age. When a hygromas shows progressive enlargement with associated symptoms, treatment should not be delayed.

Cystic hygromas are not neoplastic tumors. Radical resection with removal of major vessels and nerves is not indicated. Owing to the difficulty in removing some lesions, alternative modes of treatment have been tried with variable success. Aspiration is not effective owing to the multiloculated spaces and the rapid reaccumulation of fluid. Bleeding and infection can result. Incision and drainage are not indicated except in infected cases to drain purulent fluid collections and to relieve airway obstruction temporarily in emergency cases. As a general rule, radiation should not be used unless other modes of treatment have failed or are contraindicated.

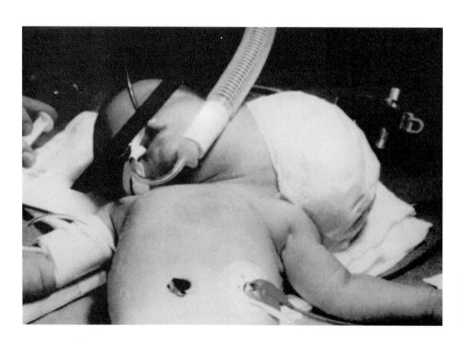

Figure 71–16. Large cervical cystic hygroma is complicated by respiratory obstruction. (Courtesy of Sterling Blocker, MD.)

Sclerotherapy

Sclerosing agents, as an alternative to surgical excision, have been met with some skepticism. Injection of boiling water and sodium morrhuate have shown disappointing results. The sclerosing agents currently in use are bleomycin, OK-432, and doxycycline. Fibrin glue (Tissucol) has been used with good results.

Bleomycin has been the recommended therapy in selected cases of lymphangiomas.[126, 127] Some advocate using bleomycin as a primary therapy, in preference to operative resection, but recommend excision as the best option for intraabdominal or life-threatening cases of cystic hygroma.[128, 129]

Microspheres in oil-bleomycin fat emulsions (BLM, 9 mg/ml) appear to be more effective than other preparations. Injection of 0.3 to 0.6 mg/kg is recommended through a 21-gauge needle into the cavity of the lymphangioma after aspiration of as much lymphatic fluid as possible. Bleomycin hydrochloride also has been used with good results.[129]

Owing to the side effects and complications, patients need to be admitted to the hospital for observation. These include fever, diarrhea, vomiting, infection, bleeding, respiratory distress, marked swelling, induration, erythema, vesiculation, and scarring. A second bleomycin treatment after 6 weeks has been recommended for patients whose initial response is not satisfactory.[128]

OK-432 is a sclerosant produced by incubating *Streptococcus pyogenes* of human origin with penicillin G potassium.[130] The recommended treatment is the intracystic injection of 0.1 mg in 10 ml of saline solution (0.9% wt/vol) immediately after the aspiration of as much lymphatic fluid as possible. If aspiration is difficult, OK-432 can be injected into the lesion at a few sites until the lesion becomes tense. The total volume injected should not exceed 20 ml.[131, 132] A second intralesional injection of OK-432 can be repeated in 3 to 6 weeks if the lesion has not resolved. Injections can be continued every 4 to 6 weeks.[131] Common side effects include fever for 2 to 4 days and local inflammatory reaction with tenderness, erythema, or swelling of the lesions, which lasts for 3 to 7 days.[131, 132]

Satisfactory results with percutaneous sclerotherapy using doxycycline have been reported.[133] The dose of injectable doxycycline ranges from 5 to 20 mg/ml. Percutaneous pigtail catheters are introduced under CT guidance to facilitate the drainage of lymphatic fluid and to deliver the sclerosing agent. The sclerosing agent is mixed with iohexol, diluted 1:4 to make it radiopaque. The volume injected is adjusted depending on the volume of the lymphangiomatous cavity and has ranged from 5 to 100 ml. Because the injection of doxycycline is extremely painful, it requires aggressive pain control. Other adverse reactions include fever and cellulitis.[133] The experience with this agent in the treatment of lymphangioma is limited at present.

Fibrin glue has been effective in treating cystic lymphangioma.[134] The cystic space is punctured with a catheter over the needle device; the needle is removed, and the catheter is left in place. The lymphatic fluid is aspirated until dry. Injection of fibrin glue in an amount equal to 10 to 15% of the volume aspirated is done through the same catheter. The procedure can be repeated several times, and several cystic spaces can be treated in the same session. No complications were noted.[134]

Swelling of the lymphangioma is the most dangerous side effect of injection of sclerosing agents. Swelling can cause airway compromise, especially when the lesion is located in the cervical area and mediastinum. It has been advocated that, for better control, injection should be done with the patient under general anesthesia and that the patient should be observed in the hospital for 24 hours after the injection.[133]

INTRAABDOMINAL LYMPHANGIOMA

Intraabdominal cystic and cavernous lymphangiomas are rare. They are usually found incidentally during abdominal surgery, through lymphangiography, or at postmortem examination. Retroperitoneal lesions are often difficult to differentiate from mesenteric lesions. They generally appear in early infancy; 90% are detected before the child is 2 years of age. Most of the time, the children do not have symptoms, but the lymphangiomas can be detected as palpable, soft, cystic masses in the abdomen.[135]

The enlarging mass can cause partial intestinal obstruction and displacement of kidneys, ureters, and other organs. It can occur as an acute abdominal emergency and can mimic appendicitis. Other reported complications include bleeding into the cyst after trauma, infection, perforation, volvulus, and rupture.[101, 135]

US and CT are the best diagnostic modalities.[136] The best treatment is complete surgical removal of the lymphangioma, if possible. If the lesion is not amenable to complete surgical excision, partial excision should be done—as much should be removed as possible without sacrificing vital structures. Unresectable cysts are unroofed or marsupialized to the peritoneal cavity. Use of argon-beam ablation was successful in treating one patient with life-threatening total abdominal lymphangiomatosis.[137] Another patient with severe nonresectable intraabdominal lymphangioma responded well to long-term total parenteral nutrition (TPN).[138] Patients are treated with antibiotics to prevent infection. If the lymphangioma is not completely removed, careful follow-up is indicated due to the possibility of recurrence.

LYMPHANGIECTASIA

Intestinal Lymphangiectasia

Intestinal lymphangiectasia is a rare disorder characterized by the presence of dilated lymphatic channels throughout all the intestinal layers and the mesentery. It can be congenital or secondary to other disorders.[139] This usually generalized lymphatic disorder can be associated with lymphedema of the extremities and chylous effusions in the peritoneum and pleura. Clinical manifestations are secondary to protein-losing enteropathy, hypoalbuminemia, and edema.[140] Other abnormalities include lymphopenia, impaired neutrophil function with impaired cell-mediated immunity, splenic atrophy, diarrhea, steatorrhea, failure to thrive, and growth retardation.[141] Intestinal lymphangiectasias can appear with abdominal pain, nausea, vomiting, and hypocalcemic seizures. The diagnosis can be suggested by radiologic studies, but it is confirmed by endoscopic intestinal biopsy findings. Lymphoma can be associated with intestinal lymphangiectasias; sometimes, it needs to be excluded from the differential diagnosis.

The primary treatment of intestinal lymphangiectasia is supportive, with correction of fluid and electrolyte imbalance and dietary manipulation. A low-fat, high-protein diet is recommended, supplemented with medium-chain triglycerides to bypass intestinal lymphatics. Surgical intervention is rarely indicated. Attempts at lymphovenous anastomoses have produced poor results. Improvement was reported in one patient treated with antiplasmin therapy.[142]

Congenital Pulmonary Lymphangiectasia

Congenital pulmonary lymphangiectasia is a rare anomaly that appears with intractable respiratory distress in the newborn. It may result from a diffuse dysplasia of the lymphatic network. This anomaly is characterized by generalized dilation of the pulmonary lymphatics.[143] Pulmonary lymphangiectasia has been classified into three different groups[144]: (1) as part of generalized lymphangiectasias, (2) as secondary to pulmonary venous hypertension or venous obstruction, and (3) as isolated lesions.

Pulmonary lymphangiectasias should always be considered in association with Noonan's syndrome (Turner's phenotype) and also in yellow-nail syndrome. A radiograph of the chest usually demonstrates reticulation, with a mottled linear pattern throughout the lung fields and occasional cystic areas.[145] Treatment is supportive, but localized lesions may be amenable to surgery.

Lymphangiectasia of the Bone

Lymphangiectasias of the bone are rare. They are also called "vanishing bone disease." More common in teenagers, they occur with severe osteolysis and deforming bone lesions. Treatment is usually unsuccessful. Progression of the disease has been arrested after radiotherapy.[146]

CHYLOUS ASCITES

Chylous ascites is secondary to accumulation of chyle in the peritoneal cavity. In adult patients,

chylous ascites is usually secondary to inflammatory conditions, intraabdominal malignancy, and lymphoma. It may also follow surgical procedures.[147] In children, the cause is often unknown, especially in infants and children younger than 2.5 years. In this pediatric group, no apparent cause was found in about 75% of the cases.[148] The term *congenital* has been applied to some cases that appear shortly after birth. Chylous ascites has been found in association with inguinal hernias, umbilical hernias, scrotal edema, Nissen fundoplication, intestinal malrotation, and child abuse.[104, 149, 150]

The main clinical finding is abdominal distention, caused by the accumulation of chyle. Other signs and symptoms are usually related to the increasing intraabdominal pressure with impairment of the venous return and respiratory embarrassment.

The diagnosis is confirmed by aspiration and laboratory analysis of the ascitic fluid.

The initial treatment of chylous ascites is conservative. Nutrition should be improved and intestinal lymphatic flow of chyle decreased. A diet high in protein and containing medium-chain triglycerides is started as soon as possible. Medium-chain triglycerides are absorbed directly into the portal circulation, bypassing the lymphatics and decreasing the lymphatic flow. Repeated paracentesis may be necessary to relieve symptoms. If diet fails, feeding should be completely stopped and TPN started. Even if prompt response to TPN is obtained, this treatment should be continued for 3 to 4 weeks to avoid recurrence. Resolution of persistent chylous ascites with use of somatostatin analogue (octreotide) and TPN has been reported in one case.[151]

Surgical exploration is reserved for patients who fail to improve on TPN or who have an identified surgically correctable lesion.[152] Leaking lymphatics can be found and repaired in some patients. An effort is made to expose the root of the mesentery, especially around the origin of the superior mesenteric artery. Some children completely recover after exploration and external drainage. In intractable cases, peritoneovenous shunts have been placed with some success.[104, 147, 148] In one reported case, control of chylous ascites was achieved with use of a circuit for extracorporeal recirculation of the ascites fluid from the peritoneal cavity into the superior vena cava; a hemofilter was incorporated into the circuit to remove excess water and electrolytes while retaining proteins, fat, and white cells.[153]

CHYLOTHORAX

Chylothorax is the accumulation of chyle in the pleural space. In the neonate, it represents the most common cause of pleural effusion in the first few days of life. The cause in this group of pediatric patients is probably a malformation of the thoracic duct. Chylothorax can also follow birth trauma. When the cause is not clear, the term *spontaneous chylothorax* is applied. Congenital chylothorax has been defined as an accumulation of pleural chylous effusion, without obvious cause, in infants 3 months of age or younger.[154]

Chylothorax has occurred after peritonitis, after blunt thoracic trauma, and with spinal cord injuries. It can also occur in association with neoplasms, mediastinal infections (e.g., tuberculosis, filariasis), and aortic aneurysms.[155]

Postoperative chylothorax has been reported after almost every known thoracic procedure, including insertion of central venous lines by subclavian puncture and translumbar aortography. In children, postoperative chylothorax occurs in 0.25 to 0.5% of thoracic cases, most commonly after cardiovascular operations.[151] The chylothorax can be caused by direct injury to the thoracic duct or by lymphatic injury during thymic dissection, especially when electrocautery is applied. If a chylous leak is identified during a thoracic procedure, it should be surgically repaired.

The clinical picture and the severity of the condition are determined by the volume and rate of chyle lost. Chronic and profuse losses are followed by malnutrition, fluid and electrolyte imbalance, and acid-base problems. Prolonged loss of T cells in chyle can decrease the patient's immunologic response to infection. Rapid accumulation of chyle can lead to severe respiratory problems.

The diagnosis is based on the identification of chyle in the pleural fluid. The presence of chylomicrons is pathognomonic of chylothorax.[156]

After the diagnosis is established, the pleural cavity is drained by repeated thoracentesis or chest tube. Thoracostomy tube drainage is preferred when persistent fluid accumulation is expected, when a pneumothorax is present, or when a recurrent large pleural effusion causes respiratory distress.

Supportive management and nutritional support are extremely important. Children with postoperative chylothorax are often debilitated, and they have compromised cardiovascular function. Most patients respond to nonsurgical treatment with a medium-chain triglyceride diet or fasting with TPN and pleural drainage. Thoracic duct ligation should be done in patients who do not respond to conservative management.[151–156] If no improvement is noted after 2 weeks of fasting and TPN, operative treatment should be undertaken. In adults, drainage of more than 1000 ml/day of chyle for more than 7 days is taken as an indication for surgery. In children, daily drainage of 100 ml/year-of-age/day or more than 15 ml/kg/day has been recommended as an indication for surgical intervention.[151, 157]

Operations for chylothorax include pleurodesis, pleuroperitoneal shunting, application of fibrin glue, ligation of leaking lymphatics, and ligation of the thoracic duct. Some of these procedures can be done by either thoracoscopy or thoracotomy. Commonly, thoracic duct ligation is done using the thoracic approach, but it can also be accomplished through the abdomen.[158, 159] We have successfully treated persistent chylothorax in a child using thoracoscopic thoracic duct ligation, TPN, and somatostatin analogue (octreotide).

LYMPHEDEMA

Lymphedema is the abnormal accumulation of lymphatic fluid in the interstitial tissue caused by maldevelopment of the lymphatic system or by lymphatic obstruction. Lymphedema can be primary (idiopathic) or secondary (Fig. 71–17).[160] The cause of primary lymphedema is not clear. Secondary lymphedema can be caused by trauma, neoplasia, infection, filariasis, radiotherapy, and surgical excision of lymph nodes (postmastectomy).

Primary lymphedema can be classified according to the age of onset: *congenital* (at birth and shortly after), *praecox* (before 35 years of age), and *tarda* (after 35 years of age). The most common type of primary lymphedema is lymphedema praecox; it is usually seen in women in the second and third decades of life.[160] Primary lymphedema has been subclassified according to the lymphangiographic pattern of the lymph vessels in (1) aplasia with no subcutaneous lymphatics; (2) hypoplasia with small lymph vessels and few lymph nodes; and (3) hyperplasia with large, tortuous, and varicose lymphatic channels.

Milroy's disease is lymphedema that is congenital and hereditary. Meige's disease is a familial form of lymphedema praecox with onset in the first or sec-

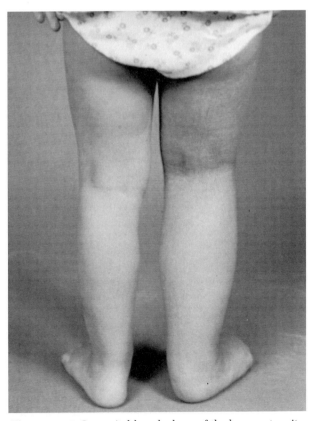

Figure 71–17. Congenital lymphedema of the lower extremity.

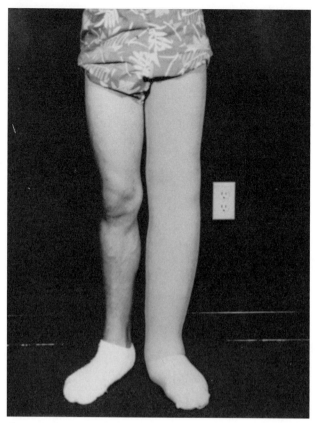

Figure 71–18. Lymphedema praecox is treated with Jobst garment.

potential complications than when done with oil-based dye, but experience with this technique is still limited.[160] Multiscintigraphic imaging is a relatively noninvasive method of investigating lymphedema and extremity enlargement and is useful in differentiating venous and lymphatic malformations in children. It involves the use of technetium[99m] antimony sulfide colloid for the lymphatics, technetium[99m] diethylenetriaminepentaacetic acid (DTPA) for capillary and interstitial areas, and technetium[99m]-labeled red blood cells for the venous system.[161]

Other diagnostic modalities include CT, venography, and biopsy. These studies are often unnecessary. They have limited value except in some cases in which primary lymphedema is difficult to distinguish from secondary lymphedema.[160–162]

The clinical course of primary lymphedema is unpredictable; some cases progress to a huge deforming extremity with functional impairment, whereas others remain the same. Complications of lymphedema include lymphangitis, cellulitis, functional disabilities, and cosmetic and psychological problems.

Lymphangiosarcoma, a rare and aggressive malignancy, most commonly occurs in secondary lym-

ond decade. Both Milroy's and Meige's diseases are autosomal dominant and relatively rare.

Primary lymphedema has been associated with other congenital anomalies, including intestinal and thoracic lymphangiectasias, chylous ascites, chylothorax, lymphangiomatosis, congenital heart disease, and Fabry's disease. Several genetic syndromes have also been associated with lymphedema, including Noonan's syndrome, yellow-nail syndrome, distichiasis (duplication of eyelashes), Turner's syndrome, and cerebrovascular malformations.

The increased incidence of lymphedema praecox in females has been attributed to a higher estrogen level and a lower subcutaneous tissue pressure in girls than in boys. Trauma and infection have also been reported to precipitate or aggravate lymphedema.

A combination of factors may act on a congenitally deficient lymphatic system to cause stasis of lymphatic fluid and to cause or aggravate lymphedema. Primary lymphedema is more common in the lower extremities but can also occur in the upper extremities and genitals. The main clinical presentation is that of a spontaneous, painless swelling of the lower extremities. The swelling is usually soft, smooth, and nonpitting.

The diagnosis of primary lymphedema is best established by a thorough clinical history and physical examination. Lymphangiography with water-soluble nonionic contrast material may have fewer

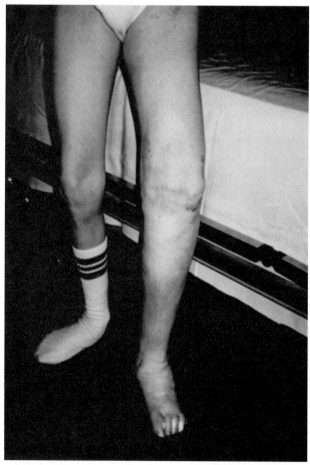

Figure 71–19. Patient with Klippel-Trenaunay syndrome with severe lymphedema.

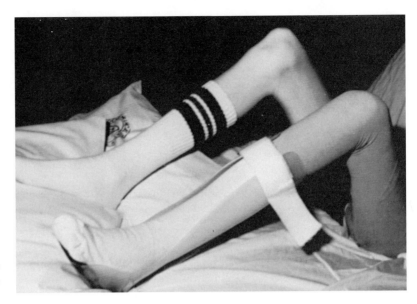

Figure 71–20. Patient in Figure 71–19 after treatment with intermittent pneumatic compression, Jobst garment, and splinting of the ankle.

phedema but can also occur in chronic primary lymphedema.

Treatment

Most patients with lymphedema respond to conservative treatment. Surgical intervention is seldom indicated except in difficult cases with extreme disabilities or recurrent complications.

Medical Management

Elevation of the extremity can be useful in some patients, but this form of therapy is difficult to enforce in an active child. Supportive stockings of the Jobst type are useful. These stockings are especially effective when combined with intermittent pneumatic compression (Fig. 71–18). The intermittent pneumatic compression is best used overnight and the elastic garments during the day. Rapid reduction of size is usually obtained, but the decrease is difficult to maintain due to lack of patient compliance. The elastic garment must be applied as soon as the patient wakes up in the morning and worn throughout the day (Figs. 71–19 and 71–20).

Skin care is extremely important to prevent breakdown and infection. Infection should be treated promptly with antibiotics and bed rest. Diuretics, anticoagulants, and other pharmacologic agents have limited value in the treatment of children with lymphedema.[102, 160] Two patients with idiopathic unilateral lymphedema improved with dietary restriction of long-chain triglycerides.[162]

Surgical Treatment

Many surgical techniques have been attempted in the treatment of lymphedema. The two basic goals have been to encourage lymph drainage and to remove lymphedematous tissue.[104] Ideally, appropriate lymphatic flow is reestablished. Implants of different material, such as silk, nylon, fascia, and rubber, have generally failed to provide long-term relief of the lymphedema. Omental flaps have not produced good results, despite early successful reports. Experimental data have shown that the absorptive capacity of mammalian omentum is limited. Pedicle flaps and myocutaneous flaps have failed to provide consistently good results.

A variety of lymphatic anastomoses have been tried, including lymph node-to-venous anastomosis, lymph vessel-to-vein anastomosis, and lymphatico-lymphatic anastomosis. Some of these techniques are theoretically attractive but require microsurgical expertise. They have not produced uniformly good results.

Excision techniques can produce good results in some patients. Split- and full-thickness skin grafts have some drawbacks, such as hypertrophic scarring, sensory loss in the skin, graft loss, scar contracture, keratoses, ulcerations, and aggravation of edema in the feet. Staged excision of subcutaneous tissue and skin may produce reasonably good results in selected patients. Staged excision has less risk of complications than does grafting, but necrosis of the flaps, sensory difficulty, and inadequate reduction in the size of the limb can occur. Surgery for cosmetic reasons alone is contraindicated because disproportion persists along with scars from the procedure. Function takes priority over cosmesis. Emotional support to patient and family is extremely important.

REFERENCES

1. Edgerton MT: The treatment of hemangiomas with special reference to the role of steroid therapy. Ann Surg 183:517–532, 1976.
2. MacCollum DW, Martin LW: Hemangiomas in infancy and childhood: A report based on 6479 cases. Surg Clin North Am 36:1647–1663, 1956.
3. Glowacki J, Mulliken JB: Mast cells in hemangiomas and vascular malformations. Pediatrics 70:48–51, 1982.
4. Amir J, Metzker A, Krikler MB, et al: Strawberry hemangioma in preterm infants. Pediatr Dermatol 3:331–332, 1986.
5. Watson WL, McCarthy WD: Blood and lymph vessel tu-

mors: A report of 1056 cases. Surg Gynecol Obstet 71:569–588, 1940.

6. Reinhoff WF Jr: Congenital arteriovenous fistula, an embryological study, with the report of a case. Bull Johns Hopkins Hosp 35:271, 1924.

7. Pack GT, Miller TR: Hemangiomas, classification, diagnosis, and treatment. Angiology 1:405–410, 1950.

8. Szilagyi DE, Smith RF, Elliot JP, et al: Congenital arteriovenous anomalies of the limbs. Arch Surg 111:423, 1976.

9. De Takats G: Vascular anomalies of the extremities. Surg Gynecol Obstet 55:227–237, 1932.

10. Gomes MM, Bernatz PE: Arteriovenous fistulas: A review and 10-year experience at the Mayo Clinic. Mayo Clin Proc 45:81–102, 1970.

11. Hurwitz DJ, Kerber CW: Hemodynamic considerations in the treatment of arteriovenous malformations of the face and scalp. Plast Reconstr Surg 67:421–432, 1981.

12. Lister WA: Natural history of strawberry nevi. Lancet 1:1429–1434, 1938.

13. Ryan TJ: Structure, pattern, and shape of the blood vessels of the skin. In Jarrett A (ed): The Physiology and Pathophysiology of the Skin: The Nerves and Blood Vessels. London, Academic Press, 1973, p 577.

14. Johnson CL, Holbrook KA: Development of human embryonic and fetal dermal vasculature. J Invest Dermatol 93(suppl 2):10S–17S, 1989.

15. Esterly NB: Cutaneous hemangiomas, vascular stains and malformations, and associated syndromes. Curr Probl Pediatr 26:3–39, 1996.

16. Folkman J: Tumor angiogenesis. Adv Cancer Res 43:175–201, 1985.

17. Folkman J, Klagsbrun M: Angiogenic factors. Science 235:442, 1987.

18. Azizkhan RG, Azizkhan JC, Zetter BR, et al: Mast cell heparin stimulates migration of capillary endothelial cells in vitro. J Exp Med 152:931–944, 1980.

19. Folkman J: Toward a new understanding of vascular proliferative disease in children. Pediatrics 74:850–856, 1984.

20. Roche WR: Mast cells and tumor angiogenesis: The tumor mediated release of endothelial growth factor from mast cells. Int J Cancer 36:721–728, 1985.

21. O'Reilly MS: Angiostatin: An endogenous inhibitor of angiogenesis and tumor growth. In Goldberg ID, Rosen EM (eds): Regulation of Angiogenesis. Basel, Birkhäuser, 1997, pp 273–292.

22. Polverini PJ: Role of the macrophage in angiogenesis-dependent diseases. In Goldberg ID, Rosen EM (eds): Regulation of Angiogenesis. Basel, Birkhäuser, 1997, pp 11–28.

23. Isik FF, Rand RP, Gruss JS, et al: Monocyte chemoattractant protein-1 mRNA expression in hemangiomas and vascular malformations. J Surg Res 61:71–76, 1996.

24. Kraling BM, Razon MJ, Boon LM, et al: E-selectin is present in proliferating endothelial cells in human hemangiomas. Am J Pathol 148:1181–1191, 1996.

25. Mulliken JB, Glowacki J: Hemangiomas and vascular malformations in infants and children: A classification based on endothelial characteristics. Plast Reconstr Surg 69:412–422, 1982.

26. Mulliken JB: Classification of vascular birthmarks. In Mulliken JB, Young AE (eds): Vascular Birthmarks: Hemangiomas and Malformations. Philadelphia, WB Saunders, 1988, pp 24–37.

27. Boon LM, Enjolras O, Mulliken JB: Congenital hemangioma: Evidence of accelerated involution. J Pediatr 128:329–335, 1996.

28. Salgarello G, Rosselli D, Salgarello M, et al: Immature angiomas: The importance of the Doppler exam in diagnosis and prognosis. Angiology 38:368–377, 1987.

29. Derchi LE, Balconi G, De Flaviis L, et al: Sonographic appearances of hemangiomas of skeletal muscle. J Ultrasound Med 8:263–267, 1989.

30. Yang WT, Ahuja A, Metreweli C, et al: Sonographic features of head and neck hemangiomas and vascular malformations: Review of 23 patients. J Ultrasound Med 16:39–44, 1997.

31. Sloan GM, Bolton LL, Miller JH, et al: Radionuclide-labeled red blood cell imaging of vascular malformation in children. Ann Plast Surg 21:236–241, 1988.

32. Inoue Y, Wakita S, Ohtake T, et al: Use of whole-body imaging using Tc-99m RBC in patients with soft-tissue vascular lesions. Clin Nucl Med 21:958–959, 1996.

33. Winter PF, Lapke J, Winek R: Subcutaneous cavernous hemangioma visualized on an indium-111–octreotide scan. J Nucl Med 37:1516–1517, 1996.

34. Christenson JT, Gunterberg B: Intramuscular hemangioma of the extremities: Is computerized tomography useful? Br J Surg 72:748–750, 1985.

35. Yuh WT, Kathol MH, Sein MA, et al: Hemangiomas of skeletal muscle: MR findings in five patients. AJR Am J Roentgenol 149:765–768, 1987.

36. Memis A, Arkun R, Ustun EE, et al: Magnetic resonance imaging of intramuscular hemangiomas with emphasis on contrast enhancement patterns. Clin Radiol 51:198–204, 1996.

37. Brunelle FO, Chaumont P, Teillac D, et al: Facial vascular malformations in children: Conventional and digital, diagnostic, and therapeutic angiography. Pediatr Radiol 18:377–382, 1988.

38. Reyes BA, Vazquez-Botet M, Capo H: Intralesional steroid in cutaneous hemangioma. J Dermatol Surg Oncol 15:828–832, 1989.

39. Stringel G, Mercer S: Giant hemangioma in the newborn and infants. Clin Pediatr 23:498–502, 1984.

40. Enjolras O, Riche MC, Merland JJ, et al: Management of alarming hemangiomas in infancy: A review of 25 cases. Pediatrics 85:491–498, 1990.

41. Shakin-Kunkel EJ, Zager RP, Hausman CL, et al: An interdisciplinary group for parents of children with hemangiomas. Psychosomatics 35:524–532, 1994.

42. Mangus DJ: Continuous compression treatment of hemangiomata. Plast Reconstr Surg 49:490–493, 1972.

43. Stringel G: Giant hemangioma: Treatment with intermittent pneumatic compression. J Pediatr Surg 22:7–10, 1987.

44. Totsuka Y, Fukuda H, Tomita K: Compression therapy for parotid hemangiomas in infants. J Craniomaxillofac Surg 16:366–370, 1988.

45. Woods JE: Extended use of sodium tetradecyl sulfate in treatment of hemangiomas and other related conditions. Plast Reconstr Surg 79:542–549, 1987.

46. Govrin-Yehudain J, Moscona AR, Calderon N, et al: Treatment of hemangiomas by sclerosing agents: An experimental and clinical study. Ann Plast Surg 18:465–469, 1987.

47. Furst CJ, Lundell M, Holm LE: Radiation therapy of hemangiomas, 1909–1959. Acta Oncol 26:33–36, 1987.

48. Mulliken JB: Treatment of hemangiomas. In Mulliken JB, Young AE (eds): Vascular Birthmarks: Hemangiomas and Malformations. Philadelphia, WB Saunders, 1988, pp 77–103.

49. Rush BF: Treatment of giant cutaneous hemangioma by intraarterial injection of nitrogen mustard. Ann Surg 164:921–923, 1966.

50. Hurvitz CH, Alkalay AL, Sloninsky L, et al: Cyclophosphamide therapy in life-threatening vascular tumors. J Pediatr 109:360–363, 1986.

51. Zwifach B, Shorr E, Black MM: The influence of the adrenal cortex on behavior of terminal vascular bed. Ann N Y Acad Sci 56:666, 1953.

52. Zarem HA, Edgerton MT: Induced resolution of cavernous hemangiomas following prednisone therapy. J Plast Reconstruct Surg 39:76–83, 1967.

53. Fost NC, Esterly NB: Successful treatment of juvenile hemangioma with prednisone. J Pediatr 72:351–357, 1968.

54. Hurwitz S: Vascular disorders of infancy and childhood. In Clinical Pediatric Dermatology. Philadelphia, WB Saunders, 1981, pp 190–196.

55. Sadan N, Wolach B: Treatment of hemangiomas of infants with high doses of prednisone. J Pediatr 128:141–146, 1996.

56. Ozsoylu S: Megadose methylprednisolone therapy for Kasabach-Merritt syndrome. J Pediatr 129:947, 1996.

57. Sadan N, Wolach B: Reply. J Pediatr 129:947–948, 1996.

58. White CW, Sondheimer HM, Crouch EC, et al: Treatment of pulmonary hemangiomatosis with recombinant interferon alpha-2a. N Engl J Med 320:1197–1200, 1989.
59. Ricketts RR, Hatley RM, Corden BJ, et al: Interferon alpha 2-a for the treatment of complex hemangiomas of infancy and childhood. Ann Surg 219:605–614, 1994.
60. Ohlms LA, Jones DT, McGill TJ, et al: Interferon alpha 2-a therapy for airway hemangiomas. Ann Otol Rhinol Laryngol 103:1–8, 1994.
61. MacArthur CJ, Senders CW, Katz J: The use of interferon alpha 2-a for life-threatening hemangiomas. Arch Otolaryngol Head Neck Surg 121:690–693, 1995.
62. Teillac-Hamel D, De Prost Y, Bodemer C, et al: Serious childhood angiomas: Unsuccessful alpha 2-b interferon treatment. A report of four cases. Br J Dermatol 129:473–476, 1993.
63. Sloan GM, Reinisch JF, Nichter LS, et al: Intralesional corticosteroid therapy for infantile hemangiomas. Plast Reconstr Surg 83:459–466, 1989.
64. Cogen MS, Elsas FJ: Eyelid depigmentation following corticosteroid injection for infantile adnexal hemangioma. J Pediatr Ophthalmol Strabismus 26:35–38, 1989.
65. Vazquez-Botet R, Reyes BA, Vasquez-Botet M: Sclerodermiform linear atrophy after the use of intralesional steroids for periorbital hemangioma: A review of complications. J Pediatr Ophthalmol Strabismus 26:124–127, 1989.
66. Olcott C, Newton TH, Stoney RJ, et al: Intraarterial embolization in the management of arteriovenous malformations. Surgery 79:3–12, 1976.
67. Schrudde J, Petrovici V: Surgical treatment of giant hemangioma of the facial region after arterial embolization. Plast Reconstr Surg 68:878–889, 1981.
68. Burrow PE, Lasjaunias PL, Ter Brugge KG, et al: Urgent and emergent embolization of lesions of the head and neck in children: Indications and results. Pediatrics 80:386–394, 1987.
69. Persky MS: Congenital vascular lesion of the head and neck. Laryngoscope 96:1002–1015, 1986.
70. Mulliken JB, Murray JE, Castaneda AR, et al: Management of a vascular malformation of the face using total circulatory arrest. Surg Gynecol Obstet 146:168–172, 1978.
71. Brauner GJ, Schliftman A: Laser surgery for children. J Dermatol Surg Oncol 13:178–186, 1987.
72. Tan OT, Gilchrest BA: Laser therapy for selected cutaneous vascular lesions in the pediatric population: A review. Pediatrics 82:652–662, 1988.
73. Wheeland RG, Walker NP: Lasers 25 years later. Int J Dermatol 25:209–216, 1986.
74. Barlow RJ, Walker NP, Markey AC: Treatment of proliferative hemangioma with the 585 nm pulsed dye laser. Br J Dermatol 134:700–704, 1996.
75. Lacour M, Syed S, Linward J, et al: Role of the pulsed dye laser in the management of ulcerated capillary hemangiomas. Arch Dis Child 74:161–163, 1996.
76. Kasabach HH, Merritt KK: Haemangioma with extensive purpura. Am J Dis Child 59:1063–1070, 1940.
77. Larsen EC, Zinkham WH, Eggleston JC, et al: Kasabach-Merritt syndrome: Therapeutic considerations. Pediatrics 79:971–980, 1987.
78. El-Dessouky M, Azmy AF, Raine PA, et al: Kasabach-Merritt syndrome. J Pediatr Surg 23:109–111, 1988.
79. Cohen BA: Hemangiomas in infancy and childhood. Pediatr Ann 16:17–26, 1987.
80. Messaritakis J, Anagnostakis D, Feingold M: Benign neonatal hemangiomatosis. Am J Dis Child 140:447–448, 1986.
81. Golitz LE, Rudihoff J, O'Meara OP: Diffuse neonatal hemangiomatosis. Pediatr Dermatol 3:145–152, 1986.
82. MacPherson RI, Letts RM: Skeletal diseases associated with angiomatosis. J Can Assoc Radiol 29:90–100, 1978.
83. Klippel M, Trenaunay P: Du naevus variqueux osteohypertrophique. Arch Gen Med (Paris) 185:641–672, 1900.
84. Parkes-Weber F: Angioma formation in connection with hypertrophy of limbs and hemihypertrophy. Br J Dermatol 19:231–235, 1907.
85. Stringel G, Dastous J: Klippel-Trenaunay syndrome and

other cases of lower limb hypertrophy: Pediatric surgical implications. J Pediatr Surg 22:645–650, 1987.
86. McCullough CJ, Kenwright J: The prognosis in congenital lower limb hypertrophy. Acta Orthop Scand 50:307–313, 1979.
87. De Lorimier AA: Sclerotherapy for venous malformations. J Pediatr Surg 30:188–194, 1995.
88. Kanterman RY, Witt PD, Hsieh PS, et al: Klippel-Trenaunay syndrome: Imaging findings and percutaneous intervention. AJR Am J Roentgenol 167:989–995, 1996.
89. Wiedemann HR, Burgio GR, Aldenhoff P, et al: The Proteus syndrome: Partial gigantism of the hands and/or feet, nevi, hemihypertrophy, subcutaneous tumors, macrocephaly or other skull anomalies, and possible accelerated growth and visceral affections. Eur J Pediatr 140:5–12, 1983.
90. Sansom JE, Jardine P, Lunt PW, et al: A case illustrating Proteus and Klippel-Trenaunay syndrome overlap. J R Soc Med 86:478–479, 1993.
91. Vaughn RY, Lesher JL Jr, Chandler FW, et al: Histogenesis of vascular tumors in the Proteus syndrome. South Med J 87:228–232, 1994.
92. Allen PW, Enzinger FM: Hemangioma of skeletal muscle. Cancer 29:8–22, 1972.
93. Cohen AJ, Youkey JR, Clagett CP: Intramuscular hemangioma. JAMA 249:2680–2682, 1983.
94. Agamanolis DP, Dasu S, Krill CE: Tumors of skeletal muscle. Hum Pathol 17:778–795, 1986.
95. Mills SE, Cooper PH, Fechner RE: Lobular capillary hemangioma: The underlying lesion of pyogenic granuloma. Am J Surg Pathol 4:471–480, 1980.
96. Dehner LP: Skin and supportive adnexae. In Dehner LP (ed): Pediatric Surgical Pathology. Baltimore, Williams & Wilkins, 1987, pp 1–103.
97. Levine C: Primary disorder of the lymphatic vessels: A unified concept. J Pediatr Surg 24:233–240, 1989.
98. Kennedy TL: Cystic hygroma-lymphangioma: A rare and still unclear entity. Laryngoscope 99:1–10, 1989.
99. Mulliken JB: Vascular malformations of the head and neck. In Mulliken JB, Young AE (eds): Vascular Birthmarks. Philadelphia, WB Saunders, 1988, pp 301–342.
100. Ninh TN, Ninh TX: Cystic hygroma in children: Report of 126 cases. J Pediatr Surg 9:191–195, 1974.
101. Fonkalsrud EW: Malformations of the lymphatic system and hemangioma. In Ashcraft KW, Holder TM (eds): Pediatric Surgery. Philadelphia, WB Saunders, 1980, pp 1042–1061.
102. Lewis JM, Wald ER: Lymphedema praecox. J Pediatr 104:641–648, 1984.
103. Savage RC: The surgical management of lymphedema. Surg Gynecol Obstet 160:283–290, 1985.
104. Ablan CJ, Littooy FN, Freeark RJ: Postoperative chylous ascites: Diagnosis and treatment. A series report and literature review. Arch Surg 125:270–273, 1990.
105. Foldi M: Anatomical and physiological basis for physical therapy of lymphedema. Experientia Suppl 33:15–18, 1978.
106. Sabin FR: On the origin of the lymphatic system from the veins, and the development of the lymph hearts and thoracic duct in the pig. Am J Anat 1:367–389, 1902.
107. Goetsch E: Hygroma colli cysticum and hygroma axillare: Pathological and clinical study and report of 12 cases. Arch Surg 36:394–479, 1938.
108. Lewis FT: The development of the lymphatic system in rabbits. Am J Anat 5:95–116, 1905.
109. Huntington GS, McClure CF: The anatomy and development of the jugular sac in the domestic cat. Am J Anat 10:177–183, 1910.
110. Witte MH, Witte CL: Lymphangiogenesis and lymphologic syndromes. Lymphology 19:21–28, 1986.
111. Williams HB: Hemangiomas and lymphangiomas. Adv Surg 15:317–349, 1981.
112. Stal S, Hamilton S, Spira M: Hemangiomas, lymphangiomas, and vascular malformations of the head and neck. Otolaryngol Clin North Am 19:769–797, 1986.
113. Browse NL, Whimster I, Stewart G, et al: Surgical management of lymphangioma circumscriptum. Br J Surg 73:585–588, 1986.

114. Eliezri D, Sklar JA: Lymphangioma circumscriptum: Review and evaluation of carbon dioxide laser vaporization. Dermatol Surg Oncol 14:357–364, 1988.

115. Grabb WC, Dingman RO, O'Neal RM, et al: Facial hamartomas in children: Neurofibroma, lymphangioma and hemangioma. Plast Reconstr Surg 66:509–527, 1980.

116. Broomhead IW: Cystic hygroma of the neck. Br J Plast Surg 17:225–231, 1964.

117. Wilson ME, Parker PL, Chavis RM: Conservative management of childhood orbital lymphangioma. Ophthalmology 96:484–490, 1989.

118. White B, Adkins WY: The use of carbon dioxide laser in hand and neck lymphangioma. Lasers Surg Med 6:293–295, 1986.

119. Kennerdell JS, Maroon JC, Garrity JA, et al: Surgical management of orbital lymphangioma with the carbon dioxide laser. Am J Ophthalmol 102:308–314, 1986.

120. Bill AH, Sumner DS: A unified concept of lymphangioma and cystic hygroma. Surg Gynecol Obstet 120:79–86, 1965.

121. Sheth S, Nussbaum AR, Hutchins GM, et al: Cystic hygromas in children: Sonographic pathologic correlation. Radiology 162:821–824, 1987.

122. Siegel MJ, Glazer HS, St Amour TE, et al: Lymphangiomas in children: MR imaging. Radiology 170:467–470, 1989.

123. Osborne TE, Levin LS, Tilghman DM, et al: Surgical correction of mandibulofacial deformities secondary to large cervical cystic hygromas. Oral Maxillofac Surg 45:1015–1021, 1987.

124. Pijpers L, Reuss A, Stewart PA, et al: Fetal cystic hygroma: Prenatal diagnosis and management. Obstet Gynecol 72:223–224, 1988.

125. Cohen MM, Schwartz S, Schwartz MF, et al: Antenatal detection of cystic hygroma. Obstet Gynecol Surv 44:481–490, 1989.

126. Tanigawa N, Shimomatsuya T, Takahashi K, et al: Treatment of cystic hygroma with the use of bleomycin fat emulsion. Cancer 60:741–749, 1987.

127. Tanaka K, Inomata Y, Utsonomiya H, et al: Sclerosing therapy with bleomycin emulsion for lymphangioma in children. Pediatr Surg Int 5:270–273, 1990.

128. Orford J, Barker A, Thonell S, et al: Bleomycin therapy for cystic hygroma. J Pediatr Surg 30:1282–1287, 1995.

129. Okada A, Kubota A, Fukuzawa M, et al: Injection of bleomycin as a primary therapy of cystic lymphangioma. J Pediatr Surg 27:440–443, 1992.

130. Ogita S, Tsuto T, Tokiwa K, et al: Intracystic injection of OK-432: A new sclerosing therapy for cystic hygroma in children. Br J Surg 74:690–691, 1987.

131. Ogita S, Tsuto T, Nakamura K, et al: OK-432 therapy in 64 patients with lymphangioma. J Pediatr Surg 29:784–785, 1994.

132. Schmidt B, Schimpl G, Hollwarth ME: OK-432 therapy of lymphangiomas in children. Eur J Pediatr 155:649–652, 1996.

133. Molitch HI, Unger EC, Witte CL, et al: Percutaneous sclerotherapy of lymphangiomas. Radiology 194:343–347, 1995.

134. Castañon Garcia-Alix M, Margarit Mallol J, Garcia Baglietto A, et al: Linfangioma quistico: Tratamiento con adhesivo de fibrina. Control evolutivo. Cir Pediatr 9:36–39, 1996.

135. Roisman I, Manny J, Fields S, et al: Intraabdominal lymphangioma. Br J Surg 76:485–489, 1989.

136. Blumhagen JD, Wood BJ, Rosenbaum DM: Sonographic evaluation of abdominal lymphangiomas in children. J Ultrasound Med 6:487–495, 1987.

137. Rothenberg SS, Pokorny WJ: Use of argon beam ablation and sclerotherapy in the treatment of a case of life-threatening total abdominal lymphangiomatosis. J Pediatr Surg 29:322–323, 1994.

138. Michaud L, Gottrand D, Turck D, et al: Recurrent gastrointestinal bleeding associated with an abdominal lymphangioma: Treatment by parenteral nutrition. J Pediatr Gastroenterol Nutr 17:449–450, 1993.

139. Bolton RP, Cotter KL, Losowsh MS: Impaired neutrophil function in intestinal lymphangiectasia. J Clin Pathol 39:876–880, 1986.

140. Gallo-Van Ess DM, Strasburger VC, Turetsky RA: Intestinal lymphangiectasia in an adolescent. J Adolesc Health Care 7:259–264, 1986.

141. Asakura H, Miura S, Morishita T, et al: Endoscopic and histopathological study on primary and secondary intestinal lymphangiectasia. Dig Dis Sci 26:312–320, 1981.

142. Mine K, Matsubayashi S, Nakai Y, Nakagawa T: Intestinal lymphangiectasia markedly improved with antiplasmin therapy. Gastroenterol 96:1596–1599, 1989.

143. Gardner TW, Domm AC, Brock CE, et al: Congenital pulmonary lymphangiectasis. Clin Pediatr 22:75–78, 1983.

144. Noonan JA, Walters LR, Reeves JT: Congenital pulmonary lymphangiectasia. Am J Dis Child 120:314–319, 1970.

145. Yiu WL, Snow J, Smith WL, et al: Localized pulmonary lymphangiectasia. AJR Am J Roentgenol 145:269–270, 1985.

146. Kurczynski E, Horwitz SJ: Response of lymphangiectasis to radiotherapy. Cancer 48:255–256, 1981.

147. Unger SW, Chandler JG: Chylous ascites in infants and children. Surgery 93:455–461, 1983.

148. Dillard RP, Stewart AG: Total parenteral nutrition in the management of traumatic chylous ascites in infancy. Clin Pediatr 24:290–292, 1985.

149. Parys SC, Hart MH: Chylous ascites following a Nissen fundoplication. J Pediatr Gastroenterol Nutr 15:181–183, 1992.

150. Benhaim P, Strear C, Knudson M, et al: Posttraumatic chylous ascites in a child: Recognition and management of an unusual condition. J Trauma 39:1175–1177, 1995.

151. Shapiro AM, Bain VG, Sigalet DL, et al: Rapid resolution of chylous ascites after liver transplantation using somatostatin analog and total parenteral nutrition. Transplantation 61:1410–1411, 1996.

152. Stringel G, Mercer S, Bass J: Surgical management of persistent postoperative chylothorax in children. Can J Surg 27:543–546, 1984.

153. Rector FE Jr, Whittlesey G: Effective control of chylous ascites: An alternative approach. J Pediatr Surg 28:76–77, 1993.

154. Jalili F: Medium chain triglycerides and total parenteral nutrition in the management of infants with congenital chylothorax. South Med J 80:1290–1293, 1987.

155. Jayabose S, Kogan S, Berezin S, et al: Combined occurrence of chyloperitoneum and chylothorax after surgery and chemotherapy for Wilms' tumor. Cancer 64:1790–1795, 1989.

156. Teba L, Dedhia HV, Bowern R, et al: Chylothorax review. Crit Care Med 13:49–52, 1985.

157. Bond SJ, Guzzetta PC, Snyder ML, et al: Management of pediatric postoperative chylothorax. Ann Thorac Surg 56:469–473, 1993.

158. Rheuban KS, Kron IL, Carpenter MA, et al: Pleuroperitoneal shunts for refractory chylothorax after operation for congenital heart disease. Ann Thorac Surg 53:85–87, 1992.

159. Merrigan BA, Winter DC, O'Sullivan GC: Chylothorax. Br J Surg 84:15–20, 1997.

160. Smeltzer DM, Stickler GB, Schirger M: Primary lymphedema in children and adolescents: A follow-up study and review. Pediatrics 76:206–218, 1985.

161. Mandell GA, Alexander MA, Harcke HT: A multiscintigraphic approach to imaging of lymphedema and other causes of congenitally enlarged extremity. Semin Nucl Med 23:334–346, 1993.

162. Soria P, Cuesta A, Romero H, et al: Dietary treatment of lymphedema by restriction of long-chain triglycerides. Angiology 45:703–707, 1994.

72

HEAD AND NECK SINUSES AND MASSES

John H. T. Waldhausen, MD •
David Tapper, MD

The wide variety of lesions involving the head and neck in children can be subdivided by etiology into those that result from infection, trauma, or neoplasm and those of congenital origin. The more common benign neoplasms are hemangiomas, lymphangiomas, and cystic hygromas. They are discussed in Chapter 71. Malignant neoplasms of childhood (e.g., neuroblastoma, lymphoma, and rhabdomyosarcoma), which occur as primary and metastatic masses in the head and neck, lesions of the thyroid and parathyroid, as well as traumatic injuries of the head and neck, are also discussed in other chapters.

In this chapter, common congenital head and neck malformations are discussed and inflammatory lesions are reviewed.

☐ Lesions of Embryonic Origin

Congenital cysts and sinuses that appear in the neck result from embryonic structures that have failed to mature or have persisted in an aberrant fashion.[1, 2] Successful treatment of a child with a mass or sinus in the head or neck requires accurate identification of the lesion as well as a planned course of therapy. Both diagnosis and therapy depend on a working knowledge of the embryologic origin and differentiation of the head and neck structures.[3, 4] This knowledge is particularly important because *complete* surgical resection of cartilaginous remnants, of remnants of the branchial arch and cleft structures, and of midline fusion abnormalities is imperative to avoid recurrence.

REMNANTS OF EMBRYONIC BRANCHIAL APPARATUS

Embryology

During the 4th to 8th week after fertilization, four pairs of well-developed ridges (branchial arches)

dominate the lateral cervicofacial area of the human embryo.[5] These four pairs are accompanied by two rudimentary pairs, which are analogous to the gill apparatus of lower forms.[2, 5] No true gill mechanisms are found in any stage of the human embryo. These pharyngeal arches and clefts are formed without a true connection between the outer ectodermal clefts and the inner endodermal pharyngeal pouches (Fig. 72-1).

The mature structures of the head and neck are derivatives of several branchial arches and their intervening clefts.[5, 6] The first branchial arch forms the mandible and contributes to the maxillary process of the upper jaw.[6-8] Abnormal development of the first branchial arch results in a host of facial deformities, including cleft lip and palate, abnormal shape or contour of the external ear, and malformed internal ossicles.[6, 8] The first branchial cleft contributes to the tympanic cavity and eustachian tube. Microtia and aural atresia occur with failure of the first branchial cleft to develop.[5, 6] The second arch forms the hyoid bone and the cleft of the tonsillar fossa.[1, 2] The third cleft migrates lower in the neck to form the inferior parathyroid glands and the thymus.[9, 10] The descent of the fourth cleft stops higher in the neck to form the superior parathyroid glands. The fourth pouch has added significance in that its ventral portion develops into the ultimobranchial body, which contributes thyrocalcitonin-producing parafollicular cells to the thyroid gland.[9]

Clinical Aspects

Complete fistulas are more common than external sinuses. Both are more common than branchial cysts, at least during childhood.[10, 11] In adults, cysts predominate.[10] By definition, all branchial remnants are truly congenital and are present at birth.[8, 11] Cysts developing from branchial structures usually appear later in childhood than do sinuses, fistulas, and

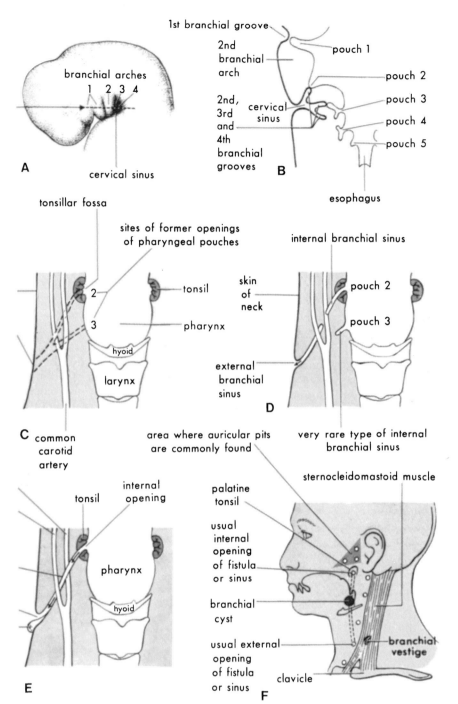

Figure 72–1. *A,* The head and neck region of a 5-week-old embryo. *B,* Horizontal section through the embryo illustrating the relationship of the cervical sinus to the branchial arches and pharyngeal pouches. *C,* The adult neck region indicating the former sites of openings of the cervical sinus and the pharyngeal pouches. The broken lines indicate possible courses of branchial fistulas. *D,* The embryologic basis of various types of branchial sinuses. *E,* A branchial fistula resulting from persistence of parts of the second branchial cleft and the second pharyngeal pouch. *F,* Possible sites of branchial cysts and openings of branchial sinuses and fistulas. A branchial vestige is also illustrated. (From Moore KL: The Developing Human: Clinically Oriented Embryology. Philadelphia, WB Saunders, 1977.)

cartilaginous remnants, which appear in infancy.[8] Commonly, the tiny external opening of the fistula and the external sinuses remain unnoticed for some time. Spontaneous mucoid drainage from the ostium usually heralds its presence and initiates the parent's concern and the reason for the child's referral.

The first clinical presentation may be an infected mass as a result of the inability of the thick mucoid material to spontaneously drain. Infection is, however, less common in fistulas and external sinuses than in cysts.[1] The cutaneous openings are occasionally marked by skin tags or cartilage remnants. The tract itself may be palpable. A cord-like structure

can be felt ascending in the neck by hyperextending the child's neck and making the skin taut. Compression along the tract may produce mucoid material exiting from the ostium.

First branchial anomalies are rare. Cysts present as swellings posterior or anterior to the ear or inferior to the earlobe in the submandibular region. External openings, if found, are located inferior to the mandible in a suprahyoid position. One third open into the external auditory canal.[12] The tract may be intimately associated with, or course through, the parotid gland. This and the proximity of the seventh nerve make resection difficult. Preauricular cysts, sinuses, and skin tags with or without cartilaginous remnants are not included in this group of anomalies.

The external ostium of the second branchial cleft is along the anterior border of the sternocleidomastoid muscle, generally at the junction of the lower and middle thirds.[10] Remnants of the second branchial cleft are more common than those of the first cleft.[10] Owing to its embryonic origin, the second cleft tract penetrates platysma and cervical fascia, to ascend along the carotid sheath to the level of the hyoid bone. Remnants may be found anywhere along this course. The residual tract turns medially between the branches of the carotid artery, behind the posterior belly of the digastric and stylohyoid muscles, and in front of the hypoglossal nerve to end in the tonsillar fossa (Fig. 72–2).[10] Although the internal opening can be anywhere in the nasopharynx or oropharynx, it is most commonly found in the tonsillar fossa. About 10% of second branchial remnants are bilateral.[10]

It is unusual to find cysts and sinuses from the third branchial cleft.[2, 6] When found, they are in the same area as those of the second cleft but ascend posterior to the carotid artery rather than through the bifurcation.[6] The fistula pierces the thyrohyoid membrane and enters the pyriform sinus.

Fourth branchial fistulas are exceedingly rare, and it may be difficult to differentiate these from other associated anomalies. Fourth pouch cysts are also highly unusual and need to be differentiated from laryngoceles. Fistula tracts originate at the apex of the pyriform sinus, descend beneath the aortic arch, and then ascend anterior to the carotid artery to end in the vestigial cervical sinus of His.[13]

Other anomalies arising from the third and fourth branchial pouches may present as cystic structures in the neck. Thymic cysts may occur as a result of incomplete degeneration of the thymal pharyngeal duct or of progressive cystic degeneration of epithelial remnants of Hassall corpuscles.[13] Most are found on the left side of the neck.

Parathyroid cysts may be located anywhere around the thyroid gland or in the mediastinum. These are usually not associated with biochemical abnormalities, although there are reports of hyperparathyroidism secondary to functioning cysts. The etiology of these cysts is not clear. They may be embryologic remnants of third and fourth branchial pouches or may represent cystic degeneration of adenomas or gradual enlargement of microcysts.[13]

Infection may develop at any time in these branchial remnants. From a technical standpoint, the surgical dissection is facilitated when the lesion is removed electively—before any infection. Scar formation and the risk of recurrence are also reduced. Persistent drainage and the possibility of infection remain the primary indications for surgical therapy. Squamous cell carcinoma has been reported in rare patients with branchial cleft cysts, but this complication does not appear until adulthood.[14]

Diagnosis

The presence of mucoid drainage from a small opening along the border of the sternocleidomastoid is indicative of a branchial cleft sinus. Palpating the tract and observing the mucoid discharge are confirmatory. Although colored dye or radiopaque material may be injected to delineate the tract, these manipulations generally are unnecessary. An accurate history from the parents is definitive. An understanding of the embryologic origin and proper surgical technique are necessary to ensure complete excision.

Cysts may be more difficult to diagnose. They lie deep to the skin along the anterior border of the sternocleidomastoid muscle.[1] They can usually be distinguished from cystic hygromas, which are subcutaneous and can be transilluminated. Ultrasonography (US) may be used to identify the cystic nature of a mass if it is not apparent by physical examination.[15, 16] In addition, real-time US with Doppler imaging can identify associated vascular structures. A skilled ultrasonographer can often help the pediatric surgeon identify important associated structures as well as characterize the type and location of the cystic structure located at the angle of the mandible. The differential diagnosis of a mass at the angle of the jaw is extensive and may include adenopathy, cystic hygromas, dermoids, and parotid lesions, as well as primary and metastatic neoplasms of lymphatic origin. The mass associated with torticollis is discussed later in this chapter. Definition of the exact etiology of the mass often requires surgical exploration.

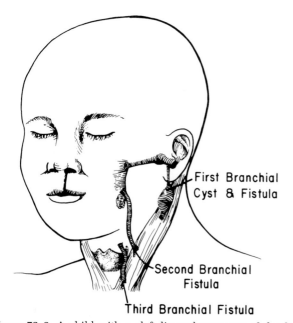

First Branchial Cyst & Fistula

Second Branchial Fistula

Third Branchial Fistula

Figure 72–2. A child with a cleft lip and remnants of the first three branchial systems. Note the important relationship to the sternocleidomastoid muscle and the fistula's origin. (From Welch KJ, Randolph JG, Ravitch MM, et al [eds]: Pediatric Surgery [4th ed]. Chicago, Year Book Medical, 1986, p 543.)

Treatment

The goal of treating all congenital neck sinuses, cysts, and fissures is complete excision, done electively, when no inflammation is present.[17] This procedure may be safely done at any age and, generally, the younger the better.[17] If the lesion is infected at clinical presentation, antibiotic therapy and warm soaks to encourage spontaneous drainage of mucoid plugs should precede definitive excision. Attempts at complete excision in an inflamed, infected field increase the risk of nerve injury, incomplete resection, and recurrence. A limited incision and drainage (I and D) procedure is sometimes necessary to resolve the infection. Although needle aspiration of branchial cysts is not recommended, it may be used in place of I and D to control infection. Repeated aspiration may be needed.

The outpatient operation to remove a branchial cleft sinus or cyst is performed using general anesthesia. The child is supine with slight hyperextension of the neck—maintained in position by a padded bean bag (Fig. 72–3). Generally, endotracheal intubation is required so that the anesthesiologist obtains a secure airway. A small transverse elliptical incision is made around the external opening and deepened beneath the cervical fascia. The initial dissection is along the inferior border of the incision, so that the ascending tract is identified from below and not injured. Although catheters and probes can be placed in the tract, use of a headlight and loupe magnification provide ample visualization to allow dissection of the tract from the investing muscle, fascia, and fat. Dissection proceeds cephalad, staying on the tract until visualization of the most superior portion of the tract becomes difficult. At this level, a second, more cephalad, parallel "stair-step" incision may be necessary for adequate exposure. The tract is pulled through the second incision, and the dissection is continued cephalad between the bifurcation of the carotid artery to the point where the tract inserts into the pharynx. The fistula is suture ligated with absorbable suture material. The wound is closed in layers with absorbable sutures. No drains are used.

Recurrences are rare and imply that a portion of the epithelium-lined tract was overlooked. The incidence of recurrence is higher in cases of previously infected lesions.

Branchial cysts free of infection are excised electively. Abscesses that are drained by incision or aspiration, or that drain spontaneously are treated with antibiotics to control secondary inflammation. Complete surgical excision is delayed until the inflammation subsides and the surrounding skin is supple. Recurrence is rare when the cyst is completely excised.

PREAURICULAR PITS, SINUSES, AND CYSTS

Embryology

Preauricular pits, cysts, and sinuses are not of true branchial cleft origin.[18] They represent ectodermal inclusions, which are related to embryonic ectodermal mounds that essentially form the auricles of the ear.[6] The sinuses are often short and end blindly. They never connect internally to the external auditory canal or eustachian tube.[18] They characteristically end in thin strands that blend with the periosteum of the external auditory canal. They tend to be familial and are often bilateral.[1] Preauricular cysts are located in the subcutaneous layer superficial to the parotid fascia. They seem deeper only if they become infected. The lining cells of these cysts and sinuses is stratified squamous epithelium. They do not contain hair-bearing follicles owing to their ori-

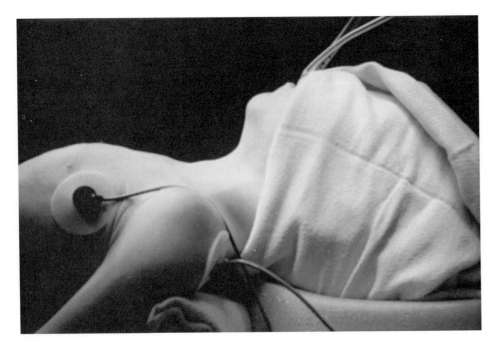

Figure 72–3. Positioning a child for neck surgery. Hyperextension of the head with support under the shoulders and stabilization with a bean bag keep the child in a stable position and facilitate exposure. Head of bed should be elevated 30 degrees to decrease venous pressure in the neck.

gin from the ectoderm associated with external ear formation.[17]

Clinical Aspects

Preauricular cysts and sinuses are commonly noted at birth. The parent may remark about the familial and bilateral nature of these lesions.[10] The sinuses do not commonly drain, and many pediatricians feel that excision is unnecessary. In those situations, no surgery is required. However, parents often report that sebaceous-like material drains from the sinus. The presence of drainage is an indication for surgical excision. Sinuses that drain are often connected to subcutaneous cysts that have an increased likelihood of staphylococcal infection. Ideally, these lesions should be completely excised before becoming infected (Fig. 72–4). Prior infection increases the difficulty of complete surgical excision, which increases the risk of recurrence.

Treatment

Complete surgical excision of the sinus tract and subcutaneous cyst to the level of the temporalis fascia is the treatment of choice in the uninfected draining sinus. It is important to avoid rupture of the sinus and to do a complete excision to decrease the risk of recurrence.[19] If infection supervenes, the lesion is treated with antibiotics and warm soaks to encourage drainage and control of the surrounding inflammation. Occasionally, as with infected

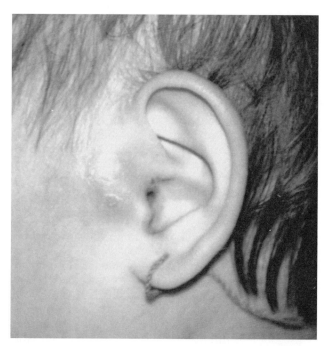

Figure 72–4. An infected preauricular cyst. The pit anterior to the helix is difficult to see. Note the swelling and skin changes anterior to the tragus. Preauricular sinuses that drain sebaceous material should be excised electively. Warm compresses and antibiotics allowed the inflammation to diminish. The cyst sinus was then completely excised.

branchial cysts, I and D or needle aspiration may be required to control the infection.

Surgical excision involves an elliptic incision with a small, chevron skin flap surrounding the sinus. The cyst is then dissected from the subcutaneous tissue and removed in its entirety.[18] The cyst or sinus may have multiple branches, making complete resection difficult. Removal of a small bit of adjacent cartilage reduces the risk of missing one of these branching tracts. The incidence of recurrence is as high as 42% owing to these multiple branches, and some clinicians have advocated an extended preauricular incision to enhance exposure.[19] Postoperative wound infection is also not uncommon.[19]

THYROGLOSSAL DUCT CYST

One of the most common lesions in the midline of the neck is the thyroglossal duct cyst.[4] Although it is embryonic in origin, it is rare for these lesions to occur in the newborn period.[1] More commonly, they are noted in preschool-age children.[1] Thyroglossal duct cysts are also common in young adults and, with the exception of thyroid goiter, are the most common midline neck masses.[12]

Embryology

Thyroglossal remnants produce midline masses from the base of the tongue to the pyramidal lobe of the thyroid gland. The embryogenesis of the thyroglossal duct is intimately involved with that of the thyroid gland, the hyoid bone, and the tongue.[9] The foramen cecum is the site of the development of the thyroid diverticulum.[9] In the embryo, this structure develops caudal to the central tuberculum impar, which is one of the pharyngeal buds that leads to the formation of the tongue.[9] As the tongue develops, the thyroid diverticulum descends in the neck, maintaining its connection to the foramen cecum.

The hyoid bone is developing from the second branchial arch at this time. The thyroid gland develops between the 4th and 7th week of gestation and descends into its pretracheal position in the neck.[20] As a result of these multiple events occurring simultaneously, the thyroglossal duct may pass in front of or behind the hyoid bone, but most commonly it passes through it. Normally, the duct disappears by the time the thyroid reaches its appropriate position. Thyroglossal duct cysts never have a primary external opening because the embryologic thyroglossal tract never reaches the surface of the neck.[20] A cyst can be located anywhere along the migratory course of the thyroglossal tract in the neck, if it fails to become obliterated (Fig. 72–5). Occasionally, the cysts attach to the pyramidal lobe or may be intrathyroidal.[21]

Complete failure of migration of the thyroid results in a lingual thyroid, which develops beneath the foramen cecum at the base of the tongue.[22] In this instance, there is no thyroid tissue in the neck.[22] The incidence of ectopic thyroid tissue in or near

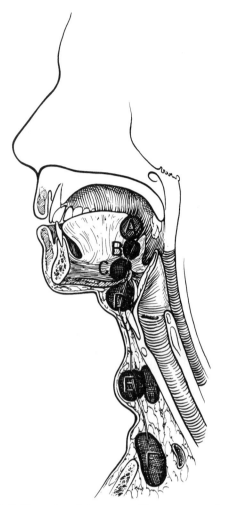

Figure 72–5. Thyroglossal duct cysts. These cysts can be located anywhere from the base of the tongue to behind the sternum. *A* and *B,* Lingual (rare). *C* and *D,* Adjacent to hyoid bone (common). *E* and *F,* Suprasternal fossa (rare). (From Welch KJ, Randolph JG, Ravitch MM, et al [eds]: Pediatric Surgery [4th ed]. Chicago, Year Book Medical, 1986, p 549.)

the duct is reported to be 10 to 45%, and some clinicians have advocated preoperative thyroid scanning to eliminate the possibility of an ectopic thyroid gland masquerading as a thyroglossal duct cyst.[23–25] Anatomic location may be useful in differentiating the two. Ninety percent of ectopic thyroid tissue lies at the base of the tongue, and thyroglossal duct cysts are rarely found there. A history should be obtained to elicit evidence of hypothyroidism, and consideration should be given to testing thyroid function. Abnormal thyroid function tests or a suspicious history should prompt a preoperative thyroid scan.[25] If ectopic thyroid tissue is found, the management becomes controversial, but some clinicians suggest a trial of medical suppression to decrease the size of the mass.

Clinical Aspects

Classically, the thyroglossal cysts are located in the midline at or just below the hyoid bone (Fig.

72–6). Suprahyoid thyroglossal cysts must be distinguished from submental dermoid cysts and from submental lymph nodes.[26] Rarely, the cysts are suprasternal in location.

The initial sign is usually a mass in the midline of the neck. Owing to the communication to the mouth via the foramen cecum, thyroglossal cysts can become infected with oral flora. Every effort should be made to excise these lesions before infection. Complete surgical excision of infected lesions is difficult and ill-advised. Risk of injury to the surrounding structures and incidence of recurrence are higher.

On physical examination, the thyroglossal duct cyst is smooth, soft, and nontender. To distinguish this lesion from the more superficial dermoid lesion, one should palpate the lesion while the child sticks out his or her tongue. Owing to its attachment to the foramen cecum, the thyroglossal duct cyst does not fully move when the tongue protrudes. This maneuver is more reliable than asking the child to swallow and determining whether the mass moves with swallowing.

The cyst is usually connected to the foramen cecum by single or multiple tracts, which pass through the hyoid. The duct lining is stratified squamous epithelium or ciliated pseudostratified columnar epithelium, with associated mucus-secreting glands.[9] The cyst contains a characteristic glairy mucus.

Treatment

Surgical excision is advised to avoid the complications of infection and due to the small risk (<1%) of cancer developing in the cyst.[25] Thyroglossal duct cyst is treated by complete excision of the cyst and its tract, upward to the base of the tongue (Fig. 72–7). Sistrunk, in 1920, described the excision of the central portion of the hyoid bone as necessary treatment to prevent recurrence.[27] Follow-up studies have confirmed these findings. The operation, as performed currently, must include the resection of the central portion of the hyoid bone.[28, 29] Several other studies have shown that there can be multiple smaller tracts connecting through the hyoid bone to the floor of the mouth, requiring wide resection of tracts above the hyoid.[28–30] If these suprahyoid tracts remain behind, the incidence of recurrence increases.[31] The best chance for successful resection is adequate wide resection at the initial procedure.[30]

The thyroglossal cyst is exposed through a transverse incision. The cyst has a characteristic appearance, distinctly different from thyroid tissue. The dissection should continue cephalad to the hyoid. Cutting the hyoid is simplified by using angled scissors, similar to Potts scissors. The base of the tract at the floor of the mouth is ligated with absorbable suture. The wings of the hyoid are not approximated. The wound is closed in layers. If the floor of the mouth is entered inadvertently, this can be repaired with absorbable suture. The wound is copiously irrigated. Occasionally, the dissection may be

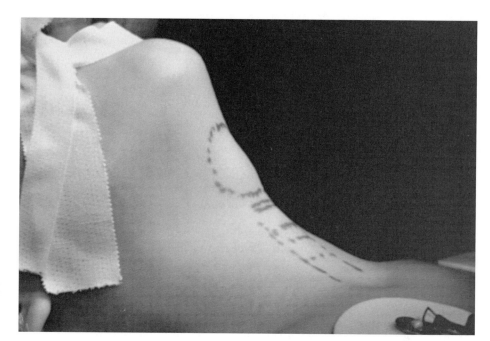

Figure 72–6. Classic thyroglossal duct cyst located in the midline just below the hyoid bone. Markings on the neck represent cricothyroid and tracheal rings.

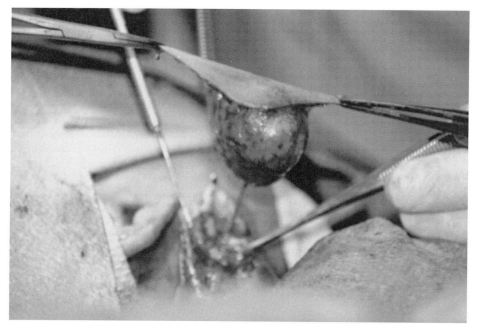

Figure 72–7. Complete excision of a previously infected thyroglossal duct cyst. Surrounding skin was removed due to changes related to previous infection. Note the well-defined tract leading toward the hyoid bone and the floor of the mouth. The operation was completed by excising the central portion of the hyoid and suture ligating the tract.

made simpler by having the anesthesiologist place his or her finger at the base of the child's tongue to identify the cephalad extent of the dissection.

With complete excision, including the central portion of the hyoid bone, the risk of recurrence is low.[31, 32]

DERMOID AND EPIDERMOID CYSTS

Dermoid cysts embryologically represent ectodermal elements, which were either trapped beneath the skin or failed to separate from the neural tube.[33, 34] Dermoids are differentiated from epidermoids histologically by the accessory glandular structures found in dermoids.[33] Dermoids contain sebaceous glands, hair follicles, connective tissues, and papillae.[33] Both contain sebaceous material within the cyst cavity.

The most common location for dermoids in children is along the supraorbital palpebral ridge. This lesion commonly appears as a characteristic swelling in the corner of the eyebrow. Although commonly attached to the underlying bony fascia, this lesion is movable and nontender. Occasionally, the mass may be dumbbell shaped and penetrate through the orbital bone. Midline dermoid cysts probably represent entrapment of epithelium of branchial arch origin at the time of embryologic midline fusion.[35] These cysts may be confused with midline thyroglossal duct cysts. Dermoids, however, are more superficial. As mentioned, they are movable when the tongue is forcibly protruded. Any midline scalp lesion suspected of being a dermoid should undergo preoperative evaluation with magnetic resonance imaging (MRI) to rule out intracranial extension. At operation, dermoid cysts lack a deep-seated tract connecting them to the hyoid bone or other neck structures.

Surgical excision is the treatment of choice for all dermoids and epidermoids. It is important to completely remove the capsule to decrease the risk of recurrence. Infection is possible secondary to repeated local trauma. Malignant degeneration of dermoids is also possible but rare.[35] Complete surgical excision is curative.

TORTICOLLIS

Etiology

Torticollis in childhood may be congenital or acquired. Congenital torticollis resulting from fibrosis and shortening in the sternocleidomastoid muscle is the most common type.[36–38] The shortening of the sternocleidomastoid muscle characteristically pulls the head and neck to the side of the lesion. The resulting "mass" represents the fibrous tissue palpable within the muscle. The etiology of this "fibrous tumor" is debatable.[39] The significant incidence of breech presentations and other abnormal obstetric positions has been used to support both the injury and the tumor etiology. Those who favor tumor see the abnormal presentation as the result of the fixed abnormal head position, whereas those who favor trauma see the difficult extraction as the cause of injury.[37, 40] No one theory completely explains this condition.

The etiology of acquired torticollis includes cervical hemivertebra and imbalance of the ocular muscles. In children in whom no identifiable muscular etiology is found, there is a high likelihood of Klippel-Feil anomalies or neurologic disorder as the cause.[41] Acquired torticollis should also raise the suspicion of otolaryngologic infection and the possibility of a neoplastic condition as the underlying cause.[42, 43]

Pathologically, the basic abnormality in congenital torticollis is endomysial fibrosis—the deposition of collagen and fibroblasts around individual muscle fibers that undergo atrophy.[39] The sarcoplasmic nuclei are compacted to form "muscle giant cells," which appear to be multinucleated.[39] The severity and distribution of fibrosis differ widely from patient to patient. Some cases of fibrosis occur bilaterally. The fact that mature fibrous tissue is present even in the neonate suggests that the disease begins well before birth and is probably not due to difficult delivery.

Diagnosis

In a series of 100 infants with torticollis, 66% had a "tumor" in the muscle and the other 34% had fibrosis but no tumor.[32, 44] A more recent series of 624 cases from China noted only 35.4% with a tumor.[45] In the typical case, the mass is not found in the newborn period but is noted at the first "well-baby" check-up, some 6 weeks after birth. The infant has the characteristic posture, with the face and chin rotated away from the affected side and the head tilted toward the ipsilateral shoulder.[40] Acquired torticollis may develop at any age, and it is important to keep in mind the various causes of the acquired lesion. Its appearance depends on the severity of the lesion, the distribution of the fibrosis, and the child's growth pattern. With time, facial and cranial asymmetry develop, which is likely to be irreversible by age 12 years.[46] A notable flattening of the facial structures on the side of the lesion occurs.

Treatment

Experience with this condition has shown that 80 to 97% of affected infants do not require operative treatment.[45, 47] The key to successful treatment is early recognition and prompt physical therapy.[38, 47] The longer the shortening of the muscle persists, the more facial and cranial asymmetry develops and the more the deeper cervical tissues become involved in the process.

In most instances, complete correction can be achieved by early range-of-motion and stretching exercises and positional changes with the baby in the crib. The parents should be taught to perform these exercises with the baby once or twice each day. One parent holds the child's shoulder down against a firm surface, and the other rotates the head toward the opposite shoulder. When the child's head is rotated toward the opposite shoulder, the muscle is gently kneaded along its entire course. Often, one parent can accomplish the stretching exercises by placing the baby on his or her lap, turning the baby's head, and gently extending the head and neck over the parent's knees. An additional maneuver is rearranging the baby's room, changing objects in the crib, and "forcing" the baby to look toward the side opposite the involved muscle. One study showed a mean duration of 4.7 months for successful nonoperative resolution.[48]

Some clinicians have suggested that the criterion for operation, regardless of age, is the development of facial hemihypoplasia.[38] In children with significant torticollis, facial hemihypoplasia is invariably present, and there is not always a linear relationship between the two conditions.[47] The muscle can be divided anywhere, but transection in the middle third, through lateral collar incision, is the simplest and provides the most aesthetically acceptable scar.[47, 49] Through this incision, one can divide the fascia colli of the neck, which is often tight and may need to be divided anteriorly as far as the midline and posteriorly to the anterior border of the trapezius. Intensive physiotherapy including full rotation of the neck in both directions and full extension of the cervical spine is instituted as soon as possible. Occasionally, in an older child, a splint is used to provide overcorrection and stretching of the muscle.[47, 49]

□ Inflammatory Lesions of Cervical Nodes

Enlarged cervical lymph nodes are by far the most common neck masses in childhood. In most instances, they are the result of nonspecific reactive hyperplasia.[1] The etiology is often viral or is related to an upper respiratory tract or skin infection. The adenitis resolves spontaneously. Most cases present with bilateral enlarged nodes. Because the anterior cervical nodes drain the mouth and pharynx, almost all upper respiratory and pharyngeal infections have some effect on the anterior cervical nodes. Enlarged cervical lymph nodes are frequently palpable in children between the ages of 2 and 10. Palpable nodes are uncommon in infants. A mass in a child younger than 2 years is more likely to be a cystic hygroma, thyroglossal duct cyst, dermoid cyst, or branchial cyst. The mass can often be diagnosed on clinical findings.[50]

Because the head contains so many structures through which bacteria or viruses may enter the body, the cervical lymph nodes frequently become involved in the infections and inflammatory diseases. Cervical nodes may also be the first clinical manifestations of various tumors, particularly those

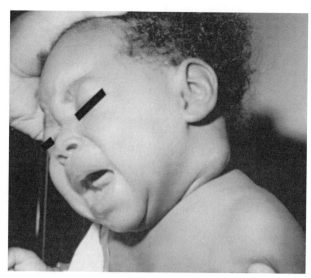

Figure 72–8. Acute suppurative cervical adenitis. Skin is shining and taut over the centralized abscess cavity.

of the lymphoma group.[1] The most frequent inflammatory lesion of the cervical lymph nodes is suppurative lymphadenitis (Figs. 72–8 and 72–9).[1] Others of importance are cat scratch disease, atypical mycobacterial lymphadenitis, and tuberculous lymphadenitis. Less common but important considerations in the differential diagnosis of cervical adenitis include Kawasaki's disease and AIDS.

ACUTE SUPPURATIVE CERVICAL LYMPHADENITIS

The most common cause of acute lymph node enlargement is a bacterial infection arising in the oropharynx or elsewhere in the drainage area.[51] The most common organisms are penicillin-resistant *Staphylococcus aureus* and *Streptococcus hemolyticus,* although cultures of the pus often yield a mixture of both or prove to be sterile.[51] *Staphylococcus*

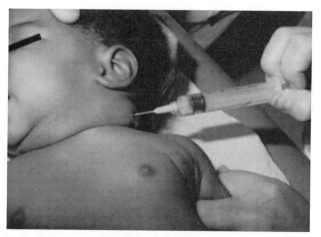

Figure 72–9. Aspiration of purulent material confirms the diagnosis of suppurative lymphadenitis. Frequently, repeated aspirations may be necessary to remove the majority of debris and can often obviate the need for formal incision and drainage.

may be more prevalent in infants.[52] Anaerobes, although common in the oropharynx, are not common pathogens in cervical adenitis. The diagnosis is usually apparent. Fever is variable and usually mild. Initial treatment with antibiotics is often followed by resolution without suppuration. Without treatment, the node often enlarges and becomes fluctuant, eventually leading to thinning of the overlying skin and abscess formation.

Needle aspiration can be both diagnostic and therapeutic. Aspiration of purulent material confirms the diagnosis. The material obtained can be cultured (see Fig. 72–9). Frequently, needle aspiration and drainage of the purulent material coupled with judicious antibiotic therapy may alleviate the necessity of formal I and D. Occasionally, repeated aspirations may be necessary.

If the child appears toxic or is quite young, hospitalization and intravenous antibiotics, including a β-lactamase–resistant antibiotic, may be helpful, but formal I and D is often required. The node can be incised and packed loosely with a Penrose drain. The parent can be taught to do irrigations through the Penrose drain, which encourages drainage of the residual debris. There is usually apparent improvement in 2 to 3 days, although antibiotic therapy should be continued for 10 days. Complete resolution of adenopathy may take weeks.

CHRONIC LYMPHADENITIS

Children occasionally have impressively enlarged nodes that do not seem to be acutely infected. The nodes are not as inflamed or as tender as in acute bacterial adenitis. Progression to fluctuation is unlikely. The child with this type of lymphadenopathy must be evaluated for tuberculosis, atypical mycobacterial infection, and cat scratch disease. Most children should receive a full 2-week course of an oral antistaphylococcal antibiotic. The same physician should examine the child on a number of occasions to assess the results of therapy. A single dominant lymph node present for longer than 6 to 8 weeks, which has not responded to appropriate antibiotic therapy, should be completely excised, fully cultured, and submitted for histologic examination to rule out the diagnosis of neoplasm. Nodes present in the supraclavicular space and posterior triangle tend to be more of a concern for malignancy than those found in the submandibular or anterior triangle.

MYCOBACTERIAL LYMPHADENITIS

Clinical Aspects

The prevalence and the relative incidence of infections caused by different mycobacteria vary with the success of preventive health measures in particular populations.[53] In developed countries, bovine mycobacteria have been eliminated from milk. Most mycobacterial lymphadenitis is caused by

the atypical mycobacteria of the *Mycobacterium avium-intracellulare-scrofulaceum* (MAIS) complex.[53] Internationally adopted terminology (MAIS) defines this group of 10 to 15 mycobacteria, which produce a specific and localized form of lymphadenitis.[28, 33, 53] The portal of entry is primarily through the mucous membranes of the pharynx. Lymphadenitis resulting from infection with *M. tuberculosis* is thought to be an extension of a primary pulmonary infection and usually involves the supraclavicular nodes.[54] Infection with the atypical strains usually involves higher cervical nodes, most commonly the submandibular or submaxillary.[54] This finding is consistent with the etiology being a primary infection and not pulmonary disease. Infection is most commonly seen between 1 and 5 years of age; occurrence before age 1 year is rare. The disease involves unilateral nodes, and dissemination is rare. Atypical mycobacteria enter from the environment and are not contagious, although the reservoir may be the mouth and oropharynx of apparently healthy children.[52] Person-to-person spread of disease has not been documented, and isolation is not necessary.

Infection with atypical mycobacteria is generally limited to the lymph nodes. Pediatric patients with atypical mycobacterial lymphadenitis are asymptomatic. The nodes are usually nontender. Spontaneous regression of atypical lymph node infection may occur but is likely to lead to breakdown of the nodes and sinus or fistula formation. The child with tuberculous scrofula usually is symptomatic. Most have pulmonary tuberculosis when the diagnosis is made.[55] It is rare for the infection to progress from cervical adenopathy to pulmonary disease if the initial chest roentgenograms are clear. Degeneration of nodes with abscess and fistula formation is unusual.

Diagnosis

In children, tuberculous or atypical mycobacterial lymphadenitis presents with a clinical picture of chronic lymph node hypertrophy.[56] Pulmonary tuberculosis on chest radiograph helps to identify the cause of the cervical swelling. Patients with MAIS usually have a normal chest roentgenogram. Skin testing helps differentiate these diseases. All children with tuberculosis should show positive test results to second-strength purified protein derivative (PPD). Children with atypical mycobacterial infection have either a negative or a doubtful skin test. If the initial PPD is inconclusive, second-strength PPD may help confirm the mycobacterial etiology. A history of familial exposure to tuberculosis should suggest tuberculosis as more likely than atypical mycobacteria. Although specific skin tests for atypical mycobacteria often provide positive results, it is difficult to obtain the appropriate antigen. Final diagnosis may depend on culture results or histopathology after excision of the involved nodes.[57]

Treatment

It is important to distinguish tuberculous from MAIS lymphadenitis because the treatment is significantly different. In human infections, antituberculous chemotherapy is required, usually resulting in marked resolution of the lymphadenopathy within a few months. Chemotherapy is continued for 2 years.[55] Surgical intervention in a human tuberculosis infection is confined to an excisional biopsy of a node, if the diagnosis cannot be made on other grounds. Most children with tuberculous lymphadenitis respond well to chemotherapy with standard drugs.

Treatment of MAIS infections is chiefly surgical.[58] Careful, thorough excision of the group of affected nodes (the one or two sentinel nodes) and adjacent smaller nodes is required. This procedure should ideally be performed before there is extensive ulceration of the overlying skin. Standard chemotherapy for tuberculosis is of no value in MAIS infections except in patients in whom a draining sinus develops after primary excision of infected nodes.[59] Children with atypical mycobacterial infection respond well to complete surgical excision without drug therapy.

CAT SCRATCH DISEASE

The incidence of cat scratch disease varies greatly in different parts of the world. In developed countries, cat scratch disease is the most common cause of nonbacterial chronic lymphadenopathy.[60, 61] It is most likely caused by a pleomorphic gram-negative bacillus, although recent attention has been turned to *Rochalimaea henselae*, an organism previously associated with disease in immunosuppressed hosts.[62, 63] The disease is usually transmitted via a superficial wound caused by a cat, dog, or monkey.[61] The healthy kitten is the most frequent vector.

The disease begins as a superficial infection or pustule forming in 3 to 5 days and is followed by regional adenopathy in 1 to 2 weeks. Generally, only one node is involved. Nodal involvement corresponds to inoculation site and the nodes that drain it. The axilla is the most commonly involved area.[1] The diagnosis can be confirmed by a skin test antigen prepared from the aspirate of an involved node.

Patients usually have tender lymphadenopathy and few systemic symptoms. On rare occasion, complications include encephalitis, retinitis, and osteomyelitis. The delay between wounding and subsequent lymphadenopathy can approach 30 days.[61] Careful history often elicits the cat contact.

No specific treatment exists for the disease. Antibiotics offer no help. Lymphadenopathy resolves spontaneously over a period of weeks to months with only occasional suppuration. Polymerase chain reaction studies for *R. henselae* on a fine needle aspirate may be useful when the diagnosis is in question, although this technique is not readily available in all hospitals.[63] Complete excision of the involved node is recommended to confirm the diagnosis, if necessary.

□ Salivary Glands

Surgical lesions of the salivary glands in children are unusual. This section addresses benign and inflammatory conditions of these glands.

RANULA

In children, a prominent, glistening, cystic mass occasionally develops below the tongue in the floor of the mouth. These cystic lesions generally arise from the sublingual glands and are known as *ranulae* (Fig. 72–10).[64] Most are simple cysts that result from the partial obstruction of the sublingual salivary duct.[64] The traditional ranula is a simple cyst lined with salivary ductal epithelium.

Occasionally, the sublingual duct can become completely occluded. The duct may rupture, which leads to the formation of a pseudocyst. The pseudocyst forms because amylase-containing secretions extravasate and erode or "plunge" into the neck muscles. This leads to the condition known as "plunging ranula."[65, 66] This lesion lacks a true epithelial lining.[65]

Many surgeons suggest marsupialization at the initial procedure for a simple ranula.[66] By incising the cyst and draining the contents, the mass rapidly decreases in size. Suturing the epithelium back on itself allows the partially occluded duct to drain. Marsupialization alone has a fairly high recurrence rate, and complete resection or marsupialization with packing may be preferable.[67, 68] Concurrent resection of the ipsilateral sublingual gland has been shown to decrease the rate of recurrence.[68]

The complex or plunging ranula requires a more extensive dissection into the neck to totally excise the pseudocyst and the atrophied sublingual gland.[66] This may be done by an intraoral approach

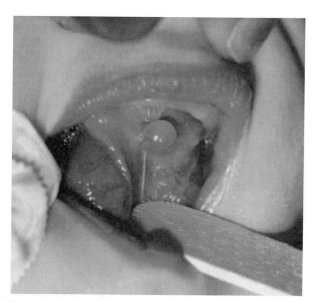

Figure 72–10. A simple cystic ranula located below the tongue, arising from the sublingual glands.

but may require a cervical incision. Dissection may be tedious in this inflamed area because the hypoglossal and lingual nerves run beneath the sublingual gland and become entrapped in the mass.

PAROTID HEMANGIOMA

This is the most common benign neoplasm affecting the major salivary glands commonly occurring in female infants at birth or within the first few months of life. They usually are confined to the intracapsular component of the gland and rarely involve the overlying subcutaneous tissues and skin. A surface sentinel lesion may be present. They appear as a spongy mass anterior to the ear. The diagnosis is usually evident on physical examination. Rarely is there a cutaneous component to the hemangioma. Growth may be rapid in the first few weeks of life. US is helpful, and MRI may also be useful in establishing the diagnosis. Most parotid hemangiomas involute by 4 to 6 years of age, and only 10% need surgical intervention. Surgical resection puts the seventh nerve at risk.

SIALADENITIS

Inflammation and swelling of the salivary glands are not common in children. Sialadenitis may present as an acute suppurative infection, a chronic infection, or a granulomatous replacement of the gland. *Acute suppurative sialadenitis* is most frequently seen in infants. The organism most often involved is *S. aureus*, followed by *Streptococcus* and group D *Pneumococcus*.[69]

The pathophysiology of *chronic sialadenitis* may involve duct-ectasia, stricture, and sialolithiasis. Sialectasis, a saccular dilation of the small, intercalated ducts that connect acini with striated ducts, is a common congenital abnormality of the gland. Sialolithiasis occurs much more commonly in the submandibular than in the parotid gland. Culture of material from the duct may not reveal pathogenic organisms. Recurrent bacterial infection without demonstrable obstruction is the primary problem in some cases.

Clinical Aspects

Sialadenitis is characterized by episodes of pain that may last from 1 to 7 days. Swelling and pain are isolated to the anatomic distribution of the gland and do not involve the overlying skin and subcutaneous tissue. Secretions are thick and flocculent. Bilateral involvement may occur over time, although each acute episode tends to be unilateral.

Diagnosis

Salivary gland abnormalities may follow diseases such as mumps. There may be tenderness, with cystic or solid swelling of the gland. The saliva coming from the duct of the involved gland is abnormal. Plain roentgenograms are useful in detecting radiopaque stones, which are seen four times more frequently in the submandibular than in the parotid gland.[70] Sialography remains the definitive study for ductal abnormalities, although it is associated with some discomfort and may require general anesthesia in younger children. High resolution US may demonstrate ductal ectasia.[70] Computed tomography has been used in children to evaluate vascularity and abscess formation. MRI may be useful in imaging the course of the facial nerve through the parotid gland.[71] Incisional biopsy is rarely indicated. The utility of fine needle aspiration is questionable.[72]

Treatment

Antibiotics may be useful in both acute and recurrent sialadenitis. Nonspecific therapy using sialagogues, with massage of the gland, may be helpful. Sialolithotomy or dilation with removal of demonstrated calculi is usually curative. Radical surgical treatment is rarely necessary in children.

REFERENCES

1. Filston HC: Head and neck—sinuses and masses. In Holder TM, Ashcraft KW (eds): Pediatric Surgery. Philadelphia, WB Saunders, 1980, pp 1062–1079.
2. Gray SW, Skandalakis JE: The pharynx and its derivatives. In Skandalakis JE, Gray SW: Embryology for Surgeons: The Embryological Basis for the Treatment of Congenital Defects. Philadelphia, WB Saunders, 1972, pp 15–62.
3. Guarisco JL: Congenital head and neck masses in infants and children. Part II. Ear Nose Throat J 70:75–82, 1991.
4. Telander RL, Deane SA: Thyroglossal and branchial cleft cysts and sinuses. Surg Clin North Am 57:779–796, 1977.
5. Moore GW, Hutchins GM, O'Rahilly R: The estimated age of staged human embryos and early fetuses. Obstetrics 139:500–506, 1982.
6. Burge D, Middleton A: Persistent pharyngeal pouch derivatives in the neonate. J Pediatr Surg 18:230–234, 1983.
7. Gaisford JC, Anderson VS: First branchial cleft cysts and sinuses. Plast Reconstr Surg 55:299–304, 1975.
8. Randall P, Royster HP: First branchial cleft anomalies. Plast Reconstr Surg 31:497–501, 1963.
9. Gray SW, Skandalakis JE, Akin JT Jr: Embryological considerations of thyroid surgery: Developmental anatomy of the thyroid, parathyroids, and the recurrent laryngeal nerve. Am Surg 42:621–628, 1976.
10. Soper RT, Pringle KC: Cysts and sinuses of the neck. In Welch K, et al (eds): Pediatric Surgery (4th ed). Chicago, Year Book Medical, 1986, pp 539–551.
11. Frazer JE, Bertwistle AP: The nomenclature of disease states caused by certain vestigial structures in the neck. Br J Surg 2:131–134, 1923.
12. Roback SA, Telander RL: Thyroglossal duct cysts and branchial cleft anomalies. Semin Pediatr Surg 3:142–146, 1994.
13. Benson MT, Dalen K, Mancuso AA, et al: Congenital anomalies of the branchial apparatus: Embryology and pathologic anatomy. Radiographics 12:943–960, 1992.
14. Khafif RA, Pricher R, Minkowitz S: Primary branchogenic carcinoma. Head Neck 11:153–163, 1989.
15. Reynolds JH, Wolinski AP: Sonographic appearance of branchial cysts. Clin Radiol 48:109–110, 1994.
16. Kraus R, Han BK, Babcock DS, et al: Sonography of neck masses in children. AJR Am J Roentgenol 146:609–613, 1986.
17. Lee K, Klein TR: Surgery of cysts and tumors of the neck. In Paparella MM, Shumrick DA (eds): Otolaryngology. Philadelphia, WB Saunders, 1973.

18. Singer R: A new technique for extirpation of preauricular cysts. Am J Surg 111:291–295, 1966.
19. Currie AR, King WW, Vlantis AC, et al: Pitfalls in the management of preauricular sinuses. Br J Surg 83:1722–1724, 1996.
20. Ward PA, Straham RW, Acquerelle M, et al: The many faces of cysts of the thyroglossal tract. Trans Am Acad Ophthalmol Otolaryngol 74:310–316, 1970.
21. Sonnino RE, Spigland N, Laberge JM, et al: Unusual patterns of congenital neck masses in children. J Pediatr Surg 24:966–969, 1989.
22. Katz AD, Zager WT: The lingual thyroid. Arch Surg 102:582–585, 1971.
23. Strickland AL, Macfee JA, VanWyk JJ, et al: Ectopic thyroid glands simulating thyroglossal duct cysts. JAMA 208:307–310, 1969.
24. Nanson EM: Salivary gland drainage into the thyroglossal duct. Surg Gynecol Obstet 149:203–205, 1979.
25. Radkowski D, Arnold J, Healy GB, et al: Thyroglossal duct remnants: Preoperative evaluation and management. Arch Otolaryngol Head Neck Surg 117:1378–1381, 1991.
26. Welch KJ, Tapper D, Vawter GP: Surgical treatment of thymic cysts and neoplasms in children. J Pediatr Surg 14:691–698, 1979.
27. Sistrunk WE: Technique of removal of cyst and sinuses of the thyroglossal duct. Surg Gynecol Obstet 46:109–112, 1928.
28. Bennett KG, Organ Jr CH, Williams GR: Is the treatment for thyroglossal duct cysts too extensive? Am J Surg 152:602–605, 1986.
29. Obiako MN: The Sistrunk operation for the treatment of thyroglossal cysts and sinuses. Ear Nose Throat J 64:196–201, 1985.
30. Hoffman MA, Schuster SR: Thyroglossal duct remnants in infants and children: Reevaluation of histopathology and methods for resection. Ann Otol Rhinol Laryngol 97:483–486, 1988.
31. Ein SH, Shandling B, Stephens CA, et al: Management of recurrent thyroglossal duct remnants. J Pediatr Surg 19:437–439, 1984.
32. Mukel RA, Calcaterra TC: Management of recurrent thyroglossal duct cyst. Arch Otolaryngol 109:34–36, 1983.
33. Gold BC, Skeinkopf DE, Levy B: Dermoid, epidermoid and teratomatous cysts of the tongue and the floor of the mouth. J Oral Surg 32:107–111, 1974.
34. Smirniotopoulos JG, Chiechi MV: Teratomas, dermoids, and epidermoids of the head and neck. Radiographics 15:1437–1455, 1995.
35. McAvoy JM, Zuckerbraun L: Dermoid cysts of the head and neck in children. Arch Otolaryngol 102:529–531, 1976.
36. Armstrong D, Pickerell K, Fetter B, et al: Torticollis: An analysis of 271 cases. Plast Reconstr Surg 35:14–19, 1965.
37. Dunn PM: Congenital sternomastoid torticollis: An intrauterine postural deformity. J Bone Joint Surg 55B:877–881, 1973.
38. Jones PG: Torticollis. In Welch KJ (ed): Pediatric Surgery (4th ed). Chicago, Year Book Medical, 1986, pp 552–556.
39. Mickelson MR, Cooper RR, Ponseti IV: Ultrastructure of the sternocleidomastoid muscle in muscular torticollis. Clin Orthop 110:11–18, 1975.
40. Dunn PM: Congenital postural deformities: Perinatal associations. Proc R Soc Med 65:735–739, 1972.
41. Ballock RT, Song KM: The prevalence of nonmuscular causes of torticollis in children. J Pediatr Orthop 16:500–504, 1996.
42. Kahn ML, Davidson R, Drummond DS: Acquired torticollis in children. Orthop Rev 20:667–674, 1991.
43. Bredenkamp JK, Maceri DR: Inflammatory torticollis in children. Arch Otolaryngol Head Neck Surg 116:310–313, 1990.
44. Ling CM, Low YS: Sternomastoid tumor and muscular torticollis. J Bone Joint Surg 41B:432–437, 1969.
45. Cheng JC, Au AW: Infantile torticollis: A review of 624 cases. J Pediatr Orthop 14:802–808, 1994.
46. Yu SW, Wand NH, Chin LS, et al: Surgical correction of muscular torticollis in older children. Chung Hua I Hsueh Tsa Chih Taipei 5:168–171, 1995.
47. Soeur R: Treatment of congenital torticollis. J Bone Joint Surg 38:35–40, 1940.
48. Emery C: The determinants of treatment duration for congenital muscular torticollis. Phys Ther 74:921–929, 1994.
49. Morrison DJ, McEwen GD: Congenital muscular torticollis: Observations regarding clinical findings, associated conditions, and results of treatment. J Pediatr Orthop 2:500–505, 1982.
50. Jones PG: Glands of the neck. In Welch K (ed): Pediatric Surgery (4th ed). Chicago, Year Book Medical, 1986, pp 517–520.
51. Hieber JP, Davis AT: Staphylococcal cervical adenitis in young infants. Pediatrics 57:424–426, 1976.
52. Bodenstein L, Altman RP: Cervical lymphadenitis in infants and children. Semin Pediatr Surg 3:134–141, 1994.
53. Altman RP, Margeleth AM: Cervical lymphadenopathy from atypical mycobacteria: Diagnosis and surgical treatment. J Pediatr Surg 10:419–422, 1975.
54. Belin RP, Richardson JD, Richardson DL, et al: Diagnosis and management of scrofula in children. J Pediatr Surg 9:103–107, 1974.
55. Kent PC: Tuberculous lymphadenitis: Not a localized disease process. Am J Med Sci 254:86–871, 1967.
56. Lincoln EM, Gilbert LA: Disease in children due to mycobacteria other than *Mycobacterium* tuberculosis. Am Rev Respir Dis 105:683–690, 1972.
57. Pinder SE, Colville A: Mycobacterial cervical lymphadenitis in children: Can histological assessment help differentiate infections caused by non-tuberculous mycobacteria from *Mycobacterium* tuberculosis? Histopathology 22:59–64, 1993.
58. MacKellar A: Diagnosis and management of atypical mycobacterial lymphadenitis in children. J Pediatr Surg 11:85–89, 1976.
59. Maridell F, Wright PF: Treatment of atypical *Mycobacteria* cervical adenitis with rifampin. Pediatrics 55:39–42, 1975.
60. Carithers HA: Cat scratch skin test antigen: Purification by heating. Pediatrics 60:928–929, 1977.
61. Carithers HA, Carithers CM, Edwards RO Jr: Cat scratch disease: Its natural history. JAMA 207:312–316, 1969.
62. Dolan MJ, Wong MT, Regnery RL, et al: Syndrome of *Rochalimaea henselae* adenitis suggesting cat scratch disease. Ann Intern Med 118:331–336, 1993.
63. Scott MA, McCurley TL, Vnencak-Jones CL, et al: Cat scratch disease: Detection of *Bartonella henselae* DNA in archival biopsies from patients with clinically, serologically, and histologically defined disease. Am J Pathol 149:2161–2167, 1996.
64. Quick CA, Lowell SH: Ranula and the sublingual salivary glands. Arch Orolaryngol 103:397–400, 1977.
65. Khafif RA, Schwartz A, Friedman E: The plunging ranula. J Oral Surg 33:537–541, 1975.
66. Roediger WE, Kay S: Pathogenesis and treatment of plunging ranulas. Surg Gynecol Obstet 144:862–864, 1977.
67. Yoshimura Y, Obara S, Kondoh T: A comparison of three methods used for treatment of ranula. J Oral Maxillofac Surg 53:280–282, 1995.
68. Baurmash HD: Marsupialization for treatment of oral ranula: A second look at the procedure. J Oral Maxillofac Surg 50:1274–1279, 1992.
69. Welch KJ: The salivary glands. In Welsh KJ, Randolph JG, O'Neill JA, et al (eds): Pediatric Surgery. Chicago, Year Book Medical, 1986, pp 487–502.
70. Seibert RW: Diseases of the salivary glands. In Bluestone CD, Stool SE, Kenna MA (eds): Pediatric Otolaryngology (3rd ed). Philadelphia, WB Saunders, pp 1093–1107, 1996.
71. Teresi LM, Kolin E, Lufkin RB, et al: MR imaging of the intraparotid facial nerve: Normal anatomy and pathology. AJR Am J Roentgenol 148:995–1000, 1987.
72. Batsakis JG, Sneige N, el-Naggar AK: Pathology consultation. Fine-needle aspiration of salivary glands: Its utility and tissue effects. Ann Otol Rhinol Laryngol 101:185–188, 1992.

73

PEDIATRIC GYNECOLOGY

Valerie K. Logsdon-Pokorny, MD • Susan Pokorny, MD

□ Gynecologic Conditions in the Fetus

With routine obstetric ultrasonography (US), gynecologic conditions can often be detected in the fetus. Current US technology is so refined that first trimester external genital ambiguities are detectable. The most commonly recognized fetal lesions are hypoechoic cystic structures in the lower abdomen, which are seen in the last trimester. This differential diagnosis should include ovarian cysts and hydromucocolpos as well as urachal cysts, bladder distention, enteric duplication, hydronephrosis, and mesenteric cysts.

OVARIAN CYST

In a normal pregnancy, the fetal ovarian cysts are stimulated by fetal gonadotropins before 28 weeks' gestation. By 28 weeks' gestation, the additive effects of fetal and maternal hormones contribute to a negative hypothalamic-pituitary feedback, which lowers fetal gonadotropins.[1] If a fetus with an ovarian cyst is delivered prematurely, before the mother contributes to the feedback, the fetal gonadotropin production maintains the cyst. The cyst eventually resolves. Certain other conditions contribute to the formation of fetal ovarian cysts even in the mature fetus, most commonly maternal diabetes, isoimmunization, nonimmune hydrops, and toxemia.

Fetal cysts may be classified as physiologic, functional, or neoplastic. The diagnostic workup and treatment of these cysts depend on their size and location.

Intrauterine decompression of a large fetal ovarian cyst is rarely reported, although such intervention is possible.[2] Cases of antenatal torsion have been reported in which the adnexa had autoamputated by the time the child was born. In utero decompression might have prevented the loss of the gonad (SF Pokorny and WJ Pokorny, unpublished data).[3–5]

HYDROMUCOCOLPOS

Hydromucocolpos results from obstruction of the lower genital tract. Usually, the fetus or neonate does not secrete enough mucus to produce a clinically detectable collection behind an obstruction; therefore, the exact origin of large fetal or neonatal hydromucocolpos cannot be easily explained. Obstruction is most commonly caused by an imperforate hymen, but it can be caused by vaginal agenesis or by a transverse vaginal septum. Cloacal anomalies may result in urinary hydrocolpos.

□ Gynecologic Conditions of the Neonate and Infant

Immediately following birth, the estrogen-primed endometrium and endocervix are shed. A small amount of bloody vaginal secretion is commonly noted. Withdrawal of maternal hormones also results in a rebound of the neonate's gonadotropin levels, which remain elevated throughout the first 1 to 2 years of life. Despite elevated gonadotropin levels, the neonatal ovaries respond only minimally, and circulating estradiol levels remain low. Furthermore, the hypothalamic-pituitary axis becomes sensitive to low estradiol levels, which results in a steady decrease of gonadotropins throughout the first few years of life.

OVARIAN CYST

Most antenatally detected ovarian cysts resolve over the first few months of postnatal life if they are simple, thin walled, and contain no debris. Historically, cysts larger than 4 cm were operated on to prevent torsion, rupture, or the possibility of malignancy. In one review of 170 patients with such cysts, 104 had oophorectomy (22 with simple cysts and 82 with complex cysts), 22 had cystectomy, and 1 had aspiration.[6] Cystectomy is a difficult procedure in the neonate even with microsurgical techniques, and sacrifice of the ovary frequently occurs. The natural history of untreated neonatal ovarian cysts is spontaneous resolution. Simple, asymptomatic cysts may safely be observed with US documentation of resolution. Simple cysts resolve in an average of 2.6 months (range 0.5 to 6 months).[6] Complex cysts or those that appear to produce discomfort may be surgically managed with the caveat of gonadal preservation kept in mind.

Because most cysts in the neonate are benign, another possibility for therapy is fine needle aspiration (FNA). However, FNA in women lacks diagnostic sensitivity and the recurrence rate in aspirated cysts is high; therefore, it should not be relied on for diagnosis. Aspiration of large, simple neonatal ovarian cysts has been reported in 11 patients with no complications and 1 recurrence.[6]

PERIURETHRAL CYST

Periurethral cysts may stretch the hymen. These cysts may be confused diagnostically with a small hydromucocolpos. If the suburethral area is carefully probed, an anteriorly placed vaginal introitus-hymenal perforation is found (Fig. 73–1). A probe or feeding tube can be guided posteriorly past the cyst into the vagina, proving hymenal patency. These cysts spontaneously resolve over the 1st month or so of neonatal life. They do not require excision or incision unless they become infected or cause symptoms.

□ Gynecologic Conditions of Childhood

After the impact of estrogen stimulation has waned at approximately 2 to 3 years of age, the girl

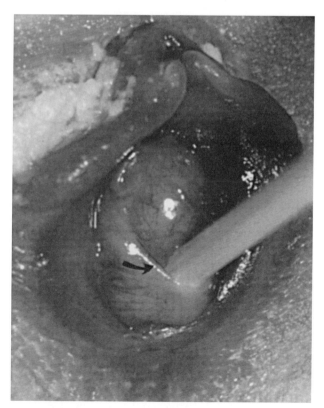

Figure 73–1. The hymen *(arrow)* was stretched thin over the yellowish periurethral cyst, which spontaneously resolved over several months.

enters a hypoestrogenic state.[7] During this period, which extends to the peripubertal period, the ovaries are quiescent. The vulva mucosa becomes thin and atrophic, similar to that of a postmenopausal female.

OVARIAN CYST

Between the 1st year of life and the onset of menses, the frequency of ovarian cysts is low. During these years, the pituitary gland secretes less gonadotropins than at any other time of the life cycle. This hormonal milieu makes the likelihood of a physiologic cyst small. Yet with the advent of US, cysts in girls have been more frequently discovered.

The majority of adnexal cysts found in girls are benign and may be either functional or neoplastic. Follicular cysts are the most common functional type, and teratoma is the most frequent neoplasm.[8] Adnexal masses are discovered when a girl has symptoms. Abdominal pain is the most common complaint, followed by the presence of a mass, constipation or diarrhea, urinary frequency or obstruction, vaginal bleeding, and weight gain. In younger girls with less space for masses, the symptoms may progress rapidly.

Enlarged ovaries in the pediatric population are susceptible to torsion. The infundibulopelvic pedicle is relatively longer in the child, facilitating torsion. Torsion produces a sudden onset of severe pain. Hemorrhage, rupture of a cyst, and infection of the adnexa also produce pain, but the onset is less dramatic. Irregular menstruation and precocious puberty may result from a functioning adnexal mass in a young girl. The diagnostic workup and treatment of these cysts depend on the child's symptoms, the size of the cyst, and the child's age. US with color flow Doppler has improved the diagnostic accuracy and helped differentiate ovarian pathology from acute appendicitis.

When an ovarian mass is associated with a rapid growth spurt, pubic or axillary hair, clitoromegaly, acne, primary thelarche, or thickening of the vulva mucosa, causes of precocious puberty should be investigated. If the bone age is advanced, and if signs of excess estrogen are present, a long bone survey is necessary to detect fibrous dysplasia characteristic of the Albright-McCune-Sternberg syndrome. Hormonal evaluation should include serum estradiol, androgen, luteinizing hormone, follicle-stimulating hormone, and thyroid-stimulating hormone. If these hormonal assays are all normal, the activity of the child's pituitary gland can be further investigated by a gonadotropin-releasing hormone stimulation test.

Although a simple autonomous ovarian cyst is the most common nonneoplastic cause of excess estrogen, ovarian neoplasms of the sex cord variety (e.g., granulosa and Sertoli-Leydig cell tumors) must be considered. These tumors are usually solid, but they can have cystic components. Secondary sexual characteristics related to estrogen secretion usually diminish or resolve once the tumor is removed. Except for acne, signs of androgen excess, including hirsutism and clitoromegaly, do not regress with tumor removal.

Enlarged ovaries in this age group have the same potential for torsion as in younger girls. The principles of management are the same as those discussed for the preceding group.

VULVOVAGINITIS

Pediatric vulvovaginitis is one of the most common pediatric entities seen in a gynecologist's office. The child has symptoms of vulvar pruritus, erythema, and dysuria or vaginal discharge. The differential diagnosis is important and includes single-organism vaginitis, vaginal foreign body, sarcoma botryoides, genital trauma, condyloma acuminata, urethral prolapse, dermatitis, *Enterobius vermicularis*, sexual abuse, and anaerobic vaginitis.

Multiple organisms have been cultured from the prepubertal vagina.[9] A single organism may dominate and be pathologic when the child has evidence of other infections such as upper respiratory infections (Fig. 73–2). The diagnosis is made by performing a vaginal culture. It is important that the laboratory be given specific directions to report all strains of organisms present in the culture. Unless

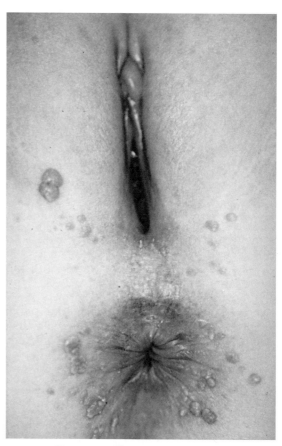

Figure 73–3. Human papillomavirus may have the same exophytic appearance in the child as in the adult. The perianal location of the lesions is common in children. Sexual abuse must be excluded.

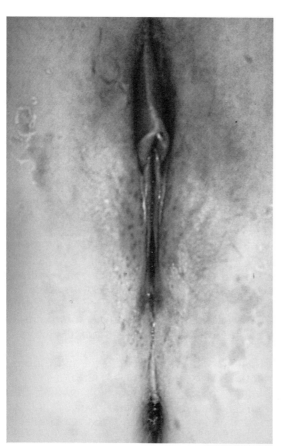

Figure 73–2. Vulvitis may be caused by a single organism. This 9-year-old diabetic girl had *Staphylococcus aureus* isolated from her vulva and vagina.

this is distinctly requested, the laboratory will report the culture as "normal vaginal flora," which is completely useless.

Most commonly, the bacteria cultured are enteric flora. The treatment for such a vaginitis should also be specific, using an antibiotic to which the bacteria are susceptible. Sexually transmitted disease must remain as a consideration. Vaginitis occurs in children with sexually transmitted diseases. If a child has been exposed to gonorrhea, vaginitis develops within a few days to a few weeks after exposure. This vaginitis is usually severe and consists of a profuse, purulent discharge. Salpingitis or pelvic inflammatory disease is rare in prepubertal children because the hormonally inactive endometrium does not allow bacterial ascent. Vaginal culture should be sent for documentation and appropriate antibiotic treatment instituted. Chlamydial infections are increasing in the pediatric population. Chlamydia causes a symptomatic vaginal infection but the organism is difficult to isolate. A culture should be performed from the vagina not the endocervix. Direct immunofluorescence tests should not be used.

Nonspecific vaginitis improves with local therapy. To keep the child's vulva cool, clean, and dry, the use of leotards or elastic pants should be avoided. The child should be bathed daily using a bland, nonmedicated and nonperfumed soap. The vulva should be patted dry and a blow dryer on a cool setting can be used to ensure dryness. When the child has a bowel movement, she should wipe from front to back using a soft white toilet paper without dye or perfumes. Hand washing should be stressed. If the vaginitis persists or recurs, or if blood is present, a vaginal foreign body must be suspected. Vaginoscopy, in that case, is the treatment of choice.

CONDYLOMA ACUMINATA (VENEREAL WARTS)

Venereal warts are being seen in epidemic proportions in children. When the lesions occur on the perineal skin and perianal areas, they are identified as warts (Fig. 73–3). When the lesions occur in the unestrogenized mucosa of the prepubertal child's vulva, they appear as necrotic, friable, exophytic lesions that are frequently flesh colored with small red punctations. These small punctations are the tips of capillaries that course through each papule (Fig. 73–4). Occasionally, the papilloma occurs as a large, nondescript, erythematous, friable, exophytic lesion—the origin of which remains unknown until excisional biopsy has been performed.

More than 50 strains of papillomavirus identified in condyloma exist, some of which are genital spe-

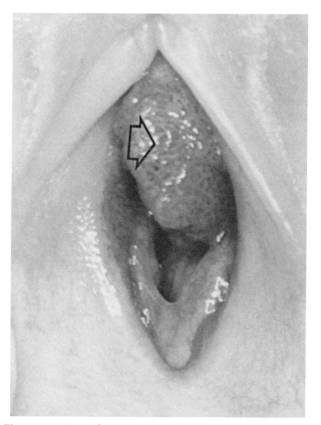

Figure 73–4. Typical appearance of a condyloma acuminatum on the unestrogenized periurethral mucosa of a 4-year-old child *(arrow)*. Note the small punctations, which represent capillaries that course through each papule of these very vascular lesions.

cific.[10] Typing of the specific strains is clinically available but impractical in most situations. Because certain strains are considered oncogenic, and because the presence of condyloma has both medicolegal and epidemiologic implications, a physician may be asked to obtain material to determine whether a child's condyloma are identical to those of a caretaker or molester. In these cases, typing of the papillomavirus associated with a given case can be very important.

Topical caustic agents or ablative procedures such as laser surgery or cryotherapy in an awake patient are not applicable to young children. Treatment consists of observation and excisional biopsy, with or without associated ablative procedures, which requires general anesthesia.

If a child has clinically evident condyloma acuminata before 2 years, the condyloma should be symptomatically managed because they may spontaneously resolve. In the older child, large condylomata may become inflamed. The constant discharge chaps the vulva as the child becomes more hypoestrogenic and she complains of pain and pruritus of the vulva. These symptoms dictate a more aggressive therapy.

The older child is more likely to have acquired the condyloma by sexual transmission. Excisional biopsy of the condyloma may be done for strain typing for epidemiologic and medicolegal reasons. While the child is anesthetized for the excisional biopsy, ablative procedures can be performed using a carbon dioxide laser. The appropriate children's protection agency should be consulted to investigate the child's environment for sexual abuse.

LABIAL-VULVAR AGGLUTINATION

Children with labial-vulvar agglutination are frequently brought to the attention of the pediatric surgeon by the gross anatomic distortion caused by this entity. Occasionally, the agglutination is so complete that it appears that no opening exists through which the child can urinate (Fig. 73–5).

Agglutination of the genital tissues typically does not occur until the child enters the hypoestrogenic state of childhood or has a florid vulvitis. Agglutination differs from the anatomy of an intersex disorder by appearance of the labia minora. In the child with congenital intersex disorder, because the androgen excess occurs early in embryonic life, the labia minora are incorporated into the clitoral hood or the anterior sheath of the penis-clitoris.

The etiology of labial-vulvar agglutination appears to be a combination of vulvitis and hypoestrogenic state. Many children with agglutination are totally asymptomatic; if followed up for a year, many experience spontaneous resolution.

If the child is symptomatic, treatment is aimed at removing the irritant that caused the vulvitis: caustic soap or shampoo, pinworms, Candida, or sexual abuse. If the child remains symptomatic with urethritis or vaginal pooling of urine, a 2- to 6-week course of topical estrogen cream resolves the aggluti-

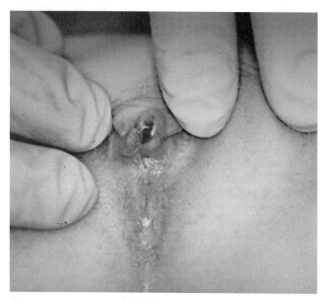

Figure 73–5. A 2-year-old child with almost complete agglutination of the labial and vulvar tissues. This child had no symptoms.

nation.[11] Manually forcing the agglutinated tissue apart is not appropriate. It causes unnecessary pain to the child and the resulting raw surfaces have a greater tendency to reagglutinate.

Rarely, a child has long-standing or severe agglutination in which the midline translucent anterior posterior membrane is not apparent. The agglutination has taken on the appearance of a skin bridge. In this case, the agglutinated tissue should be surgically separated using general anesthesia. The procedure is bloodless if laser or needle electrocautery is used. A short course of postoperative topical estrogen is appropriate.

GENITAL TRAUMA AND SEXUAL ABUSE

The management of most pediatric gynecologic conditions is distressing. Nowhere is this more apparent than with genital trauma. In the otherwise stable child, the goals are to determine the extent of the wound without additional trauma, to decide whether the wound can be managed by conservative nonsurgical means, and to discover whether the history of the injury is compatible with the findings.

Most falls onto objects result in wounds that are asymmetric or do not transect the hymen.[12] Midline wounds, particularly those that transect the hymen, have the greatest potential for penetrating into viscera above the vaginal apex because the vaginal canal is the weakest spot in the pelvic floor (Fig. 73–6). Midline, symmetric wounds that transect the hymen are likely associated with sexual assault. Although an occasional child may fall onto a broom handle, in all cases, the wound, the vagina, and the abdominal cavity (when the latter has been entered) should be irrigated and samples should be sent to a forensic laboratory to search for sperm.

If the patient is hemodynamically stable when

first seen, initial management should consist of placing a pressure bandage or ice pack against the perineum with the patient recumbent. The wound should be reevaluated frequently for hemostasis. Because the majority of these wounds are superficial, hemostasis is usually spontaneous. The next step is to generously lavage and clean the wound, clearing clots away so that the full extent of the wound can be visualized. The unestrogenized atrophic mucosa is vascular. Frequently, the amount of bleeding is excessive in relation to the severity of the wound. The child's caretakers and the nursing staff need to be forewarned that, with the child recumbent, blood pools in the vagina. When the child begins to ambulate or to void, a 4- to 5-ml clot will pass from the vagina.

If hemostasis cannot be achieved, the injury should be surgically repaired using general anesthesia. If any doubt exists about the extent of the wound or the integrity of the vaginal canal, an examination with anesthesia is warranted.

Deep perineal wounds must be débrided and drained using general anesthesia. Due to fecal contamination and associated bowel injury, a colostomy is occasionally necessary. Loose approximation of the wound margins to align the skin and to obtain hemostasis may be done with absorbable suture.

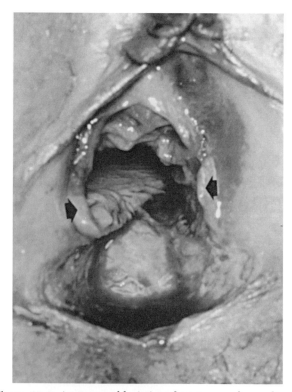

Figure 73–6. An 8-year-old victim of acute sexual assault who had small bowel herniating through the apex of the avulsed vagina. Note the abundant, although transected, amount of hymenal tissue *(arrows)* present, indicating that she had not had significant stretch trauma to her hymen before this episode of rape. (From Pokorny S, Pokorny W, Kramer W: Acute genital injury in the prepubertal girl. Am J Obstet Gynecol 166:1461–1466, 1992.)

Skin sutures not in the midline tend to tear out once the child resumes normal activity. Permanent sutures require a second anesthetic for removal.

Although perineal tissues have remarkable healing properties, the child and her caretakers must understand that she must remain inactive for a few days. If the child is allowed to be active, a small hematoma can expand into a hematoma of the labia majora and the ischiorectal fascia, which may require operative management.

A sexually abused child rarely has an acute injury. The majority of abusive activity does not involve attempts to penetrate the vagina. Nevertheless, it is important to recognize the hymenal changes that occur as a result of penetration.[13] Whether the sexually abused child is brought to the physician for repair of a remote genital injury or is seen for a regular checkup, the stretched hymen retracts into nubbins of tissue called *hymenal remnants* or *caruncles.*

VAGINAL FOREIGN OBJECTS

Although most girls deny any knowledge of the possibility of a foreign object in their vagina, this may be a cause of persistent vaginal drainage and bleeding.[14] Cultures of the drainage can be helpful because *Shigella, Streptococcus,* or any of the enteric organisms may produce a bloody discharge without the presence of a foreign object. If the culture findings do not identify a single pathogen or if the vaginal discharge persists after antibiotic therapy, vaginoscopy is necessary. Radiographic and US studies do not demonstrate many vaginal foreign objects. A preoperative rectal examination rarely aids in the detection of a small foreign object, but occasionally, with the child's cooperation and Valsalva maneuver, a larger foreign object can be milked out of the vagina.

The most common foreign objects recovered from the prepubertal vagina are wads of toilet paper, which appear occasionally just inside the vaginal orifice as a grayish mass. Removal by flushing may be possible. The vulva is anesthetized with viscous Xylocaine before inserting a lubricated 10 French catheter into the child's vagina. The vagina is flushed with a diluted povidone-iodine (Betadine) solution. If flushing is not successful or symptoms persist, vaginoscopy may be done using a cystoscope under anesthesia.

The irrigating capacity of this instrument allows expansion of the vagina so the entire canal and the cervix can be seen. A speculum cannot be opened sufficiently to see the entire vagina without damage to the hymen. An otoscope or the Cameron-Myers vaginoscope do not damage the hymen, but owing to their small portals, they are inefficient. Once identified, the foreign body can be removed.

Inflammation and trauma produce a characteristic papillary reaction of the unestrogenized vaginal mucosa. The mucosa appears roughened with small projections of approximately 1 to 2 mm in height.

The response to a chronic foreign body can be extensive with multiple polypoid projections that simulate a neoplastic process. Mucosal healing is facilitated by a 2-week course of estrogen cream applied to the vulva nightly.

LICHEN SCLEROSIS

Lichen sclerosis is a chronic condition of the epithelium and dermis characterized by thinning and atrophy of skin, which appears as small, white patches. The epidermis may be atrophic, acanthotic, or hyperkeratotic with elongated rete pegs and a homogeneous zone beneath the epidermis with inflammatory cells arranged in a band-like pattern.[15] These areas may cover the entire vulva but more characteristically form a "figure eight" pattern involving both the vulva and the perianal areas. This abnormal skin is sharply demarcated from the surrounding normal skin (Fig. 73–7). These lesions do not enter the vagina or spread laterally.

About 7% of all lichen sclerosis is seen in premenarchal girls. The peak age for diagnosis is between 6 and 8 years of age.[16] Most often, the patients complain of severe vulvar pruritus, soreness, bleeding, and discharge. The appearance is so typical that biopsy is rarely necessary. The etiology is unknown but local immunity factors may be involved.

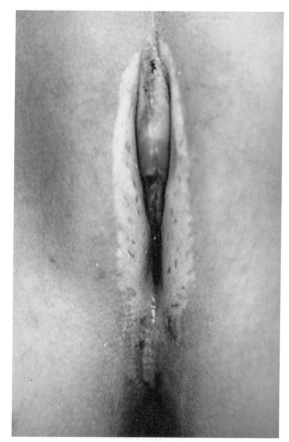

Figure 73–7. Lichen sclerosis diagnosed in a 5-year-old. There are frequently areas of hemorrhage that may mimic sexual abuse.

A variety of treatments to control symptoms have been tried, including vulvectomy, chloroquine, retinoids, antibiotic cream, topical estrogen, testosterone, and topical or systemic steroids; all have had only limited success. Topical steroids, including clobetasol propionate, beclomethasone dipropionate, and 1% hydrocortisone are currently recommended in addition to local vulvar care. The child should avoid straddle activities, tight clothing, and bathing with irritating soap. One study showed that lichen sclerosis in 11 of 22 girls diagnosed before age 7 years was cleared at puberty.[16]

□ Gynecologic Conditions of the Peripubertal Girl

The peripubertal girl is a child who has entered puberty but has not reached a stage of cyclic physiologic maturity. These girls have started breast development, but their first menstrual period may or may not have occurred. They do not ovulate regularly, but owing to follicle stimulation and ovarian activity, they experience lower abdominal pain. A variety of nonsurgical but painful situations result. On US evaluation, the ovaries may be enlarged with multiple follicles that give the appearance of polycystic ovaries. This is a normal progression of physiologic events.

OVARIAN CYST

The pathologically enlarged ovarian follicle is not painful unless it leads to torsion. Some peripubertal girls experience adnexal pain caused by intermittent torsion. Treatment with synthetic progesterone or with low-dose oral contraceptive pills reduces gonadotropin production and the size of the cyst. This hormonal approach for chronic pain is selected if the cyst is simple, 5 to 8 cm in size, and not torsed. Increased intensity or persistence of the pain are signs of torsion.

In addition to lower quadrant pain, torsion is suspected by US evidence of debris or hemorrhage within the cyst or by a thickening of the cyst wall. These sonographic findings can also be found with a hemorrhagic lutein cyst, dermoid cyst, or ectopic pregnancy. Therefore, the clinician must rely on other parameters when making the diagnosis.

In the peripubertal child, ectopic pregnancy must be considered in the differential diagnosis of adnexal cysts. The ability to diagnose this condition has improved dramatically over the years. Because the qualitative human chorionic gonadotropin (hCG) test is specific, a negative hCG excludes an ectopic pregnancy. A positive hCG requires further evaluation with US. Using traditional, transabdominal US, a normal intrauterine gestational sac should be reliably detected when the quantitative hCG reaches 6500 mIU/ml.[17] Transvaginal US allows reliable detection of intrauterine gestational sacs as early as the 1st week after the missed menstrual period. At this time, the hCG level with an intrauterine pregnancy ranges from 1000 to 2000 mIU/ml. If the quantitative hCG is 1500 mIU/ml or more and no intrauterine pregnancy is seen on transvaginal US, an ectopic pregnancy is likely.

Acute torsion of a right ovarian cyst frequently mimics appendicitis; both conditions require surgical intervention. Intermittent or partial torsion or leakage of caustic fluid or blood from a physiologic ovarian cyst is sometimes confused with the signs of early appendicitis.

INFECTED TUBE AND RUDIMENTARY UTERINE HORN

Pelvic inflammatory disease is a complex gynecologic entity in which etiology, complications, and treatment protocols are in a constant state of flux. The most serious complication is tuboovarian abscess (TOA), which, if not properly treated, has a high mortality rate. Although the treatment mainstay of TOA has been surgical drainage, a trend toward conservative management of bilateral TOA has come with the advent of newer antibiotics. No longer are bilateral salpingo-oophorectomy and hysterectomy warranted in most patients, particularly in young female patients who desire future fertility.

If abscessed pelvic viscera are not removed, proper drainage must be ensured. Long-term antibiotic therapy is necessary. Suppression of ovulation and the endometrium with low-dose oral contraceptive pills is advocated to diminish bacterial invasion.

The pediatric surgeon has a unique opportunity to manage a rare population of young women with TOA that results from menstrual accumulation in a rudimentary uterine horn. These müllerian anomalies often become evident only during the pubertal period. Many remain asymptomatic for several years following menarche. Some of these girls menstruate regularly from the more developed uterine horn, but ultimately poor drainage of the rudimentary horn leads to abscess formation. The surgical dilemma revolves around whether to remove or to drain the abscessed viscera. Drainage is probably the best initial course. After the inflammatory process is resolved, a more definitive study can be performed before surgical correction. The children most likely to have these anomalies are those with other urinary, cloacal, or rectal anomalies. Many of these children have had prior abdominal procedures during which the anomaly was overlooked.

□ Vaginal Anomalies

Developmental anomalies of the müllerian ducts include anomalies of the vagina, cervix, uterus, and fallopian tubes. Uterine and cervical anomalies are the most common. Vaginal anomalies are frequently accompanied by urinary tract anomalies.

An understanding of embryology is an absolute necessity to understanding vaginal anomalies. Three successive sets of excretory organs develop in human embryos: the pronephros, mesonephros, and metanephros. The mesodermal derivative pronephros is recognizable at week 3 of gestation. The pronephros give rise to the bilateral pronephric ducts, which migrate caudally toward the embryonic cloaca. The pronephric ducts, in turn, give rise to the mesonephric (wolffian) ducts. The metanephros become the true kidney.

During the 6th week, the paramesonephric (müllerian) ducts develop lateral to the mesonephric ducts. The müllerian ducts grow caudally where they fuse in the midline. The presence of the mesonephric duct is necessary for paramesonephric duct growth. The fused paramesonephric ducts invaginate the posterior wall of the urogenital sinus to form the müllerian tubercle. Unless inhibited, the müllerian system develops and the wolffian system regresses. Meanwhile, the cloaca is being divided by the urorectal septum into an anterior urogenital sinus and dorsal hindgut. The urogenital sinus becomes the bladder and the distal vagina, and the dorsal hindgut becomes the rectum and the anus. At the müllerian tubercle, endoderm proliferates to form the sinovaginal bulbs. These bulbs produce a solid vaginal plate that extends from the fused müllerian ducts downward. Lacunae form in the solid plate and eventually canalize to form the lumen of the vagina. This process occurs at about week 17 but is not complete until the late third trimester.

VAGINAL ATRESIA

Vaginal atresia is a failure of vaginal canalization. This failure of canalization may be complete, proximal, or distal. The vagina is malformed, but the uterus and the cervix are intact. Prepubertal children with vaginal atresia are asymptomatic; however, at the onset of puberty, they may be seen with hematocolpos or hematometra. The repair of vaginal atresia is complex and involves the creation of a neovagina using a variety of pull-through or graft techniques. Distal vaginal atresia can be treated with a perineal flap vaginoplasty, but proximal vaginal atresia may require abdominoperineal-vaginal pull-through.

VAGINAL AGENESIS

The typical form of vaginal agenesis is associated with uterine agenesis and is called the Mayer-Rokitansky-Küster-Hauser (MRKH) syndrome. This syndrome results from dysplasia of the müllerian ducts. It is second only to gonadal dysgenesis as a cause of primary amenorrhea and is estimated to occur in 1 in 4000 to 20,000 female births. Patients have a 46XX karyotype and normal endocrine and ovarian function.[18]

The diagnosis is usually made at menarche when amenorrhea is the presenting symptom. The exter-

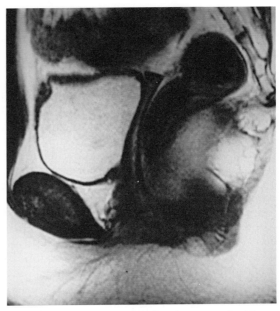

Figure 73–8. Magnetic resonance imaging scan of a 12-year-old with müllerian agenesis. There is complete lack of vagina or uterus in the space between the bowel and bladder. (Courtesy of Paula Woodard, MD, University of Utah School of Medicine.)

nal genitalia are normal but only a shallow vaginal pouch (1 to 6 cm long) is present. One must differentiate this condition from transverse vaginal septum and vaginal atresia. A physical examination alone most often does not lead to the diagnosis. US can be helpful, but with the advent of the pelvic coil, magnetic resonance imaging (MRI) has proved to be the most accurate (Fig 73–8).

Müllerian agenesis is often associated with renal anomalies. The reported incidence of renal anomalies is 34%, and the incidence of concomitant skeletal anomalies is 12 to 50%.

The nonsurgical approach to vaginal formation is a dilation involving graded Lucite dilators.[19] These dilators are used in conjunction with a bicycle seat apparatus.[20] The dilations are instituted after puberty when the introitus becomes toughened by endogenous estrogens. The girl must be able to rock her perineum on a firm surface that she can straddle. In essence, the girl is taught to identify the site of her neovagina, to place the smallest dilator against the spot, to hold the dilator in place by a light girdle or panties and sit on a narrow seat leaning slightly forward for 15 to 30 minutes at a time for at least 2 hours a day. The initial dilator is the smallest one available and extends 1 to 2 cm beyond the labia to ensure pressure. These dilators are capable of producing a vagina of adequate depth and width without additional intervention.

Surgical vaginal construction by the McIndoe technique involves creation of a neovagina using split thickness skin grafts implanted over a semirigid mold inserted into the potential vaginal space.[21] The mold is removed after 2 weeks and active vaginal dilation is continued. Neither of these techniques is applicable to the girl who has a uterus that will produce secretions.

VAGINAL DUPLICATION

Vaginal duplication may be the result of an isolated longitudinal vaginal septum or may be true vaginal duplication associated with a didelphic uterus. A longitudinal vaginal septum is a disorder of fusion. It is commonly seen in combination with urogenital sinus and cloacal anomalies. It may also occur as an isolated anomaly. The diagnosis is frequently delayed due to the complexity of anatomic abnormalities. The patient may experience cyclic abdominal pain, sciatic-like pain, or amenorrhea if both vaginal halves are occluded. Physical examination may reveal an abdominal or pelvic mass or sometimes purulent vaginal discharge caused by the infection of retained secretions. There is increased incidence of endometriosis among those with functional uterine tissue and vaginal obstruction. This isolated entity is repaired by vaginal septectomy or marsupialization of the obstructed side.

More often, vaginal duplication is seen in conjunction with a didelphic uterus. The didelphys occurs when there is complete failure of the paired müllerian ducts to fuse. This disorder is characterized by two hemiuteri and two cervices. A longitudinal vaginal septum is most often present. As long as both the vaginas are patent and drain to the exterior, there should be no signs or symptoms of this disorder. Although successful pregnancy in women with didelphic uteri is less likely than in the normal population, normal outcomes can be expected. Renal anomalies are also frequently seen in this disorder, including a double collecting system and renal agenesis. Very rarely is a uteroplasty indicated. Procedures to combine the uterine horns have been fraught with disaster and are not recommended.

IMPERFORATE HYMEN

The imperforate hymen and transverse vaginal septum are anomalies caused by failure of canalization. The hymen represents the junction of the sinovaginal bulb with the urogenital sinus. Imperforate hymen in an infant has been reported to spontaneously perforate by adolescence.

This diagnosis is usually made in the newborn period or at puberty. The newborn may be seen with mucocolpos, with the retained cervical mucus being stimulated by maternal estrogens (Fig. 73–9). The adolescent may be seen at puberty with hematocolpos or with urinary tract symptoms related to pelvic obstruction from a dilated uterus. The patient may complain of intermittent crampy abdominal pain, back pain, dysuria, and increased frequency of urination. Occasionally, a patient has urinary retention. Most patients have breast development yet are amenorrheic. The bulging hymenal membrane may appear bluish secondary to retained blood.

The diagnosis is made by physical examination or US. If there is any uncertainty regarding the anatomy, MRI demonstrates the uterus or cervix. The

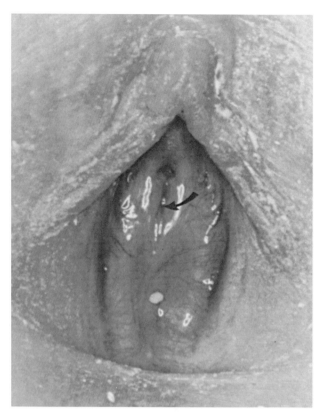

Figure 73–9. A seemingly imperforate hymen in a prepubertal female. A small probe could be passed into the vagina via a microperforate opening (*arrow*) in the suburethral area.

differential diagnosis includes ectopic ureter, hymenal cyst, hymenal skin tag, periurethral cyst, and vaginal cyst.

Unless mucocolpos is creating urinary symptoms, the hymen should be opened at puberty.

TRANSVERSE VAGINAL SEPTUM

The transverse vaginal septum results from an incomplete fusion between the müllerian duct and urogenital sinus. The septum is composed of fibrous tissue and of vascular and muscular elements covered by squamous epithelium. The septum is in the upper vagina in 46% of patients, in the midvagina in 40% of patients, and in the lower vagina in 14% of patients.[40] Its incidence varies from 1 in 2100 to 1 in 72,000. The presentation is similar to that of imperforate hymen with hydrocolpos, hematocolpos, and hematometra. There are few associated urologic anomalies.

It is imperative to know the level of obstruction and the thickness of the membrane before surgical excision. US and MRI establish whether the uterus and cervix are present. Transvaginal excision is possible if the septum is thin (1 to 2 cm). If it is thick, a combined abdominal-vaginal approach may be necessary. The mucosa of the lower and upper vaginal segment must be approximated in order to prevent stenosis. A very high septum or thick septum should be treated as an atretic vagina.

TABLE 73-1. Modified World Health Organization Comprehensive Classification of Ovarian Tumors

I. Common "epithelial" tumors
   A. Serous*
   B. Mucinous*
   C. Endometrioid*
   D. Clear cell*
   E. Brenner*
   F. Mixed epithelial
   G. Undifferentiated
   H. Mixed mesodermal tumors
   I. Unclassified
II. Sex cord-stromal tumors
   A. Granulosa stromal cell
      1. Granulosa cell
      2. Thecoma-fibroma
   B. Androblastomas; Sertoli-Leydig cell tumors
      1. Well-differentiated (Pick's adenoma, Sertoli cell tumor)
      2. Intermediate differentiation
      3. Poorly differentiated
      4. With heterologous elements
   C. Lipid cell tumors
   D. Gynandroblastoma
   E. Unclassified
III. Germ cell tumors
   A. Dysgerminoma
   B. Endodermal sinus tumor
   C. Embryonal carcinoma
   D. Polyembryoma
   E. Choriocarcinoma
   F. Teratomas
      1. Immature
      2. Mature (dermoid cyst)
      3. Monodermal (struma ovarii, carcinoid)
   G. Mixed forms
   H. Gonadoblastoma
IV. Soft tissue tumors not specific to the ovary
V. Unclassified tumors
VI. Secondary (metastatic) tumors
VII. Tumor-like conditions (e.g., pregnancy luteoma)

*Benign, borderline, or malignant.

☐ Ovarian Neoplasm

Ovarian neoplasms in the pediatric population present both a diagnostic and therapeutic dilemma. These tumors may be symptomatic or may be identified during an operation for some other problem. There are many different types of ovarian neoplasms. The surgeon need not have an encyclopedic knowledge of every type of tumor, but it is important to understand the surgical treatment of such disorders.

INCIDENCE

The true incidence of ovarian neoplasms is unknown. In a 20-year experience from a major children's hospital, only 63 patients with ovarian tumors were identified; 47 tumors were benign, 3 were embryonic teratoma, and 13 were malignant tumors.[8] The risk of malignancy is highest in younger children because they frequently have germ cell tumors. In girls younger than 18 years old, germ cell malignancies account for 60 to 74% of malignant

tumors, whereas stromal tumors represent 17 to 20% and epithelial cancers 4 to 12%.[22]

CLASSIFICATION

Ovarian neoplasms are classified according to their presumed cell of origin (Table 73–1) and are staged by multiple prognostic factors that are determined at operation, including nodal status, capsular rupture, peritoneal fluid cytology, peritoneal seeding, and site of metastasis (Table 73–2).

SYMPTOMS

The ovary does not become a pelvic organ until after puberty so abdominal pain is the most common

TABLE 73-2. Carcinoma of the Ovary: Staging Classification Using the FIGO Nomenclature

Stage	Description
I	Growth limited to the ovaries
IA	Growth limited to one ovary; no ascites present containing malignant cells; no tumor on the external surfaces; capsule intact
IB	Growth limited to both ovaries; no ascites present containing malignant cells; no tumor on the external surfaces; capsules intact
IC*	Tumor either stage IA or stage IB but with tumor on the surface of one or both ovaries; or with capsule ruptured; or with ascites present containing malignant cells or with positive peritoneal washings
II	Growth involving one or both ovaries with pelvic extension
IIA	Extension and/or metastases to the uterus and/or tubes
IIB	Extension to other pelvic tissues
IIC*	Tumor either stage IIA or stage IIB but with tumor on the surface of one or both ovaries; or with capsule(s) ruptured; or with ascites present containing malignant cells or with positive peritoneal washings
III	Tumor involving one or both ovaries with peritoneal implants outside the pelvis and/or positive retroperitoneal or inguinal nodes; superficial liver metastasis equals stage III; tumor is limited to the true pelvis but with histologically verified malignant extension to small bowel or omentum
IIIA	Tumor grossly limited to the true pelvis with negative nodes but with histologically confirmed microscopic seeding of abdominal peritoneal surfaces
IIIB	Tumor of one or both ovaries; histologically confirmed implants of abdominal peritoneal surfaces, none exceeding 2 cm in diameter; nodes negative
IIIC	Abdominal implants 2 cm in diameter and/or positive retroperitoneal or inguinal nodes
IV	Growth involving one or both ovaries with distant metastasis; if pleural effusion is present, there must be positive cytologic test results to allot a case to stage IV; parenchymal liver metastasis equal stage IV

*In order to evaluate the impact on prognosis of the different criteria for allotting cases to stage IC or IIC, it would be of value to know if rupture of the capsule was (1) spontaneous or (2) caused by the surgeon and if the source of the malignant cells detected was (1) peritoneal washings of (2) ascites.

Adapted from Changes in definitions of clinical staging for carcinoma of the cervix and ovary: International Federation of Gynecology and Obstetrics [Announcement]. Am J Obstet Gynecol 156:263, 1987.

symptom of an ovarian tumor in children. Other symptoms include a mass, constipation or diarrhea, vaginal bleeding, urinary obstruction or frequency, and weight gain. Vague gastrointestinal symptoms such as bloating, dyspepsia, and abdominal discomfort may be present. In a young girl, these symptoms may progress rapidly.

Ovarian tumors sometimes undergo torsion because the infundibulopelvic pedicle is long in the child. Torsion results in the sudden onset of pain. Other entities that may cause less acute pain include hemorrhage, rupture of a benign or malignant cyst, and infection. Unusual symptoms include fever, menstrual irregularities, and precocious puberty.

DIAGNOSIS

A palpable abdominal mass is the presenting symptom in more than 70% of girls. The nature of the mass may be determined by US, Doppler US, computed tomography, or MRI.

US differentiates solid, cystic, and complex tumors, but the correlation with the pathologic diagnosis is no better than 40%. The wall thickness and the presence or absence of internal debris, mural nodules, and fluid levels should be determined. The presence or absence of signs of metastatic disease such as ascites, lymphadenopathy, or peritoneal nodules should also be noted. No single US pattern for a particular lesion has been identified, and criteria suggested as indicative of a malignancy may often be misleading.[23] Malignant tumors are usually solid, although they may contain necrotic, cystic areas. Stippled calcification may be seen in dysgerminomas, whereas coarse calcification, teeth, bone, or calcified cartilage may be seen in benign or malignant teratomas.

Color Doppler US, assessing the blood flow to the ovary, may help to delineate the benign versus malignant nature of a mass. Transvaginal US probes are small yet are inappropriate for the neonate or prepubertal child.

In the evaluation of an ovarian mass, computed tomography and MRI better demonstrate the extent of tumor; these modalities are preferred over US for assessing malignant disease. They also allow a large, accurate view of the anatomy that is not operator dependent. MRI does not expose the child to ionizing radiation and more accurately identifies masses, showing an 87% correlation with the pathologic diagnosis.[24]

Ultimately, though, the correct diagnosis may not be established short of laparoscopy or laparotomy. The role of laparoscopy in the evaluation of pelvic masses in the young female patient is still being defined.

☐ Epithelial Tumor

Epithelial tumors are coelomic epithelial neoplasms that arise from the surface epithelium (mesothelium) of the ovary and its inclusion in the cortex. These tumors are seen much more frequently in adults and are rarely found in the prepubertal child. In a review of ovarian neoplasms in girls younger than 20 years of age, epithelial tumors were found in 19.3%, with a malignancy rate of 15.9%. Of these malignant tumors, 39.4% were of the serous type and 43.9% were of the mucinous type. Borderline malignant tumors were found in 30.4%, a much higher rate than in the adult.[25] There are no reports of clear cell or endometrioid tumors in premenarchal girls (Fig. 73–10).

Epithelial tumors are classified as benign, malignant, or borderline. *Benign* epithelial tumors can be managed conservatively by unilateral cystectomy or salpingo-oophorectomy (Fig. 73–11). Because preservation of ovarian function is important in these young patients, cystectomy should be the procedure of choice. The incidence of bilaterality warrants a biopsy of the contralateral ovary.

The epithelial lining in *borderline* tumors is stratified with atypia and pleomorphism but without stromal invasion. Borderline tumors have been traditionally treated with a unilateral salpingo-oophorectomy. More recently, cystectomy has been shown to have a similar outcome (Fig. 73–12). In one study, no recurrences were noted in ovaries from which a single borderline cyst with negative resectioned margins was removed.[26] Data on this tumor group in children are limited.

Malignant epithelial tumors in young patients are better differentiated, are lower stage, and have a

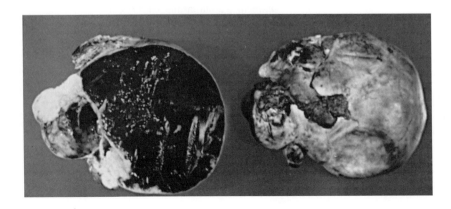

Figure 73–10. Serous cystadenocarcinoma presents as a solid irregular ovarian tumor. (Courtesy of Edward C. Klatt, MD, University of Utah School of Medicine.)

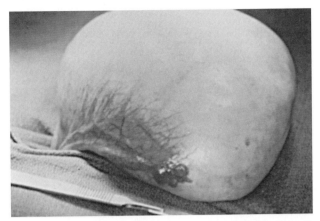

Figure 73–11. Large cystadenoma in an 11-year-old. Note the scalpel for relative size.

better 5-year survival rate.[22] Conservation of the contralateral ovary and the uterus may be contemplated for the purpose of preserving fertility, but the risk of a second ovarian malignancy may be unacceptable.[22] Occult malignancy in an otherwise normal appearing ovary has been reported in 12 to 24% of cases. The contralateral ovary must be biopsied before electing to preserve it and the uterus. Removal of the residual ovary is recommended when childbearing is over. Most oncologists, however, recommend total abdominal hysterectomy, bilateral salpingo-oophorectomy, omentectomy, and chemotherapy for disease in children.[27]

☐ Sex Cord Stromal Tumor

Sex cord stromal tumors (SCSTs) consist of granulosa cell tumors, Sertoli-Leydig cell tumors, and gonadoblastomas. They represent approximately 12%

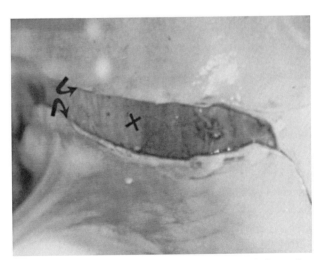

Figure 73–12. Cystectomy may be the procedure of choice for a benign or borderline ovarian mass. The cyst should be shelled out of the ovary. *Arrows* mark the ovarian tissue being peeled off the cyst *(X)*. The pedicle is in the lower left-hand corner. Many viable oocytes are in the thin ovarian tissue near the hilus.

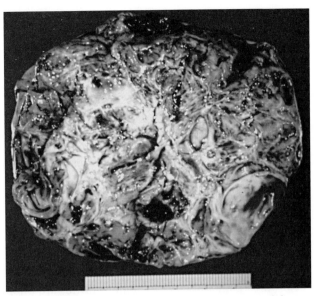

Figure 73–13. A granulosa-theca cell tumor of an adolescent ovary. (Courtesy of Edward C. Klatt, MD, University of Utah School of Medicine.)

of ovarian tumors in childhood and adolescence. They include most of the hormonally active tumors. Their incidence is related to age: 40% of ovarian neoplasms in girls younger than age 4 years were SCST, 30% in girls 5 to 9 years, 8% in girls 10 and 14 years, and 16% in those 15 to 17 years of age.[22]

GRANULOSA CELL TUMOR

The granulosa cell tumor may be comprised almost entirely of granulosa cells or contain variable numbers of theca cells and/or fibroblasts (Fig. 73–13). The combination tumor is much less likely to be malignant than the pure granulosa cell tumor. A pure thecoma is almost always benign. The juvenile granulosa cell tumor is histopathologically different than that of the adult granulosa cell tumor. It rarely has Call-Exner bodies and has a very high mitotic index.[28]

The most common symptoms of granulosa cell tumors are related to estrogen excess and consist of premature breast development (observed in 12 of 36 girls), vaginal bleeding (9 of 36), and development of mature female external genitalia (6 of 36).[28]

Most tumors present as stage I. These tumors are rarely bilateral and most children can be adequately treated with unilateral salpingo-oophorectomy. Bilateral oophorectomy, chemotherapy, and irradiation therapy in stage I disease do not improve outcome. However, this tumor frequently recurs later in life; therefore, long-term follow-up is needed. Chemotherapy is reserved for those with advanced or recurrent disease. Ten-year survival rate is nearly 80%.[29]

SERTOLI-LEYDIG CELL TUMOR

Sertoli-Leydig cell tumors are sex cord stromal tumors with evidence of maldifferentiation that were previously known as arrhenoblastoma or androblastoma. Androgen production is the hallmark of these tumors. In one series, one third of the patients presented with unequivocal evidence of androgen excess, and an additional 10% had a history suggesting androgen excess.[30]

This tumor is found only rarely in young girls. Most tumors are unilateral and rarely is there metastasis at the time of diagnosis. The treatment of these tumors includes unilateral salpingo-oophorectomy and procedures for staging. Chemotherapy and/or radiation seems beneficial in patients with poor differentiation or metastasis.

GONADOBLASTOMA

A gonadoblastoma is a tumor composed of a mixture of germ cells and cells resembling immature granulosa or Sertoli cells.

Chromosomal and gonadal abnormalities are often found in patients with this tumor. Most patients have 46XY or 45X/46XY karyotypes.[30] Eighty percent are phenotypically female. A pure gonadoblastoma is usually benign yet may be associated with dysgerminomas and other malignant germ cell tumors. There is a 33% incidence of bilateral involvement.[22] Due to the risk of malignancy, it is recommended that bilateral gonadectomy be performed when this tumor is encountered in phenotypic females with a Y chromosome in their karyotype.

□ Germ Cell Tumor

Germ cell tumors include endodermal sinus tumor, embryonal carcinoma, polyembryoma, choriocarcinoma, teratoma, immature teratoma, and dysgerminoma. They represent 15 to 20% of ovarian tumors. Sixty percent of ovarian tumors in female patients younger than age 20 years are germ cell neoplasms; 95% are benign cystic dermoid/teratomas. The younger the patient, the more likely the germ cell tumor is to be malignant.[31] Most often, these tumors are unilateral; therefore, a radical operation is not indicated. The opposite ovary should always be inspected. Before the advent of chemotherapy, many of these tumors were routinely fatal. Many chemotherapeutic regimens have been used to treat these tumors, but bleomycin, etoposide, cisplatin (BEP) and etoposide and cisplatin (EP) are the recommended combinations. VIP (VP-16, ifosfamide, cisplatin) has been used as a salvage regimen.[32] Recently, high-dose carboplatin, etoposide, and ifosfamide followed by autologous bone marrow transplantation have resulted in a 23 to 32% clinical response rate.[33] This may indeed be the treatment of the future.

BENIGN CYSTIC TERATOMA (MATURE TERATOMA, DERMOID)

Benign cystic teratomas arise from totipotential primordial germ cells and display ectodermal, me-

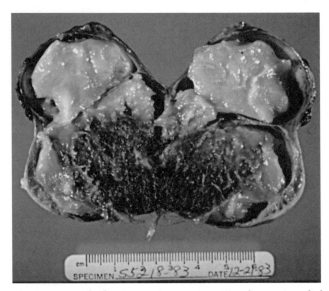

Figure 73–14. The benign cystic teratoma arises from primordial germ cells and displays endodermal, mesodermal, and ectodermal elements. Notice the hair present in this photo. (Courtesy of Edward C. Klatt, MD, University of Utah School of Medicine.)

sodermal, and endodermal elements microscopically.[29] Because these tumors contain adult-like tissues, they are considered mature. Dermoids have no significant malignant potential (Fig. 73–14).

Dermoids are the most common germ cell tumor found in the pediatric and adolescent population, making up 38.6% of ovarian neoplasms in girls and 57% of pediatric germ cell tumors. The occurrence of bilateral ovarian involvement is low (about 10%), yet high enough to warrant consideration.[27]

Teratomas usually present as do other ovarian mass lesions. US usually shows highly reflective cystic and solid echoes with areas of acoustic shadowing that obscure the back wall of the cyst, suggesting the "tip of the iceberg" sign.[34] Acoustic shadowing was seen in 70% of postpubertal girls and in 13% of prepubertal girls.[35] US fails to establish the exact diagnosis in 20% of patients.[34]

The ideal surgical treatment is to remove the teratoma, preserving some ovarian tissue. An incompletely resected dermoid may recur. Even if the tumor is large, with no ovarian tissue identified, enucleation of the tumor should be attempted. It has been shown that a preserved hilum that did not appear to contain recognizable ovarian tissue may provide ovarian function and return of normal menses. If the contralateral ovary is normal on intraoperative palpation or inspection, it is unlikely to be diseased and should not be bivalved or removed.

IMMATURE TERATOMA (IMMATURE GERM CELL TUMOR)

Immature teratomas are derived from three germ layers: ectoderm, mesoderm, and endoderm. They frequently contain immature or embryonic structures. These are most often completely solid and are highly malignant. Alphafetoprotein (AFP) is sometimes seen as a tumor marker and may be used to assess completeness of removal and recurrence. Bilateral involvement is rare, although the contralateral ovary may contain a mature teratoma in up to 5% of cases.[30]

If the tumor is limited to the ovary at the time of the initial operation, node sampling for staging and unilateral salpingo-oophorectomy should be performed. A more radical operation does not improve the prognosis. The prognosis directly correlates with the degree and extent of the immaturity of tissues.[36] This tumor is radioresistant. Except for those patients whose tumor is confined to the ovary (stage IA or IB), all patients should receive 6 to 12 months of postoperative chemotherapy. The prognosis has greatly improved since the mid-1980s with the advent of chemotherapy. In one report, 11 of 11 patients were alive without evidence of disease at 20 to 104 months of follow-up after surgery and multiagent chemotherapy.[37] Pregnancies, too, have been reported after this chemotherapy.

DYSGERMINOMA

Dysgerminoma is a malignant neoplasm of the primordial, sexually undifferentiated germ cells. Other aggressive germ cell elements may be found in these tumors. The histology of the tumor is classic: aggregates of large, uniform cells surrounded by varying amounts of connective tissue and stroma containing lymphocytes.

Dysgerminoma is the most common ovarian malignancy in the female adolescent. Fewer than 10% occur before menarche, yet 45% occur before age 20 years. Dysgerminoma makes up 16% of germ cell tumors and 11% of pediatric ovarian tumors. These tumors are bilateral in 10 to 20% of cases and are the most likely ovarian tumors to present in this manner.[22] The treatment of dysgerminoma depends on the stage at diagnosis.

Most patients are diagnosed at stage I. Dysgerminomas spread through the lymphatic system rather than by seeding over the peritoneal surface. Multiple node biopsies are essential to stage this tumor. When the tumor is grossly limited to the ovary and the nodes are negative, a conservative surgical approach is warranted. If the opposite ovary appears grossly normal, a wedge biopsy should be performed.[30] Dysgerminomas are radiosensitive. Radiation therapy, however, sacrifices the adolescent's endocrine and reproductive potential; an 80% or greater survival rate has been reported in these patients without adjuvant therapy. Two thirds of patients who have recurrence are salvaged with radiation.[30] With extensive spread of the tumor beyond the ovaries, as much gross tumor as possible should be removed. In patients with pure dysgerminoma, survival is related to stage, but 83% 5-year and 74% 10-year overall survival rates have been reported.[38]

ENDODERMAL SINUS TUMOR

Endodermal sinus tumor arises from undifferentiated and multipotential embryonal cells. This is the second most common malignant ovarian germ cell tumor seen in girls. The median age at diagnosis is 16 to 19 years. Sixty percent of patients are postmenarchal. Endodermal sinus tumor is also seen in very young patients. This tumor can be very aggressive.

AFP has been shown to be an excellent tumor marker both for diagnosis and monitoring of therapy. Surgery follows the same principles as for other ovarian tumors. Stages I and IA disease are treated with unilateral salpingo-oophorectomy.

Survival rate does not improve by removing the uninvolved uterus and contralateral ovary. No bilateral tumors were noted in 39 patients.[39] Stage II and higher tumors require total abdominal hysterectomy and bilateral salpingo-oophorectomy. The optimal treatment strategy appears to consist of appropriate removal of the primary tumor followed by intensive chemotherapy, including regimens of BVP (bleomycin, vinblastine, cisplatin) and BEP (bleomycin, VP-16 [etoposide], cisplatin) to achieve cure rates of 50 to 75%.[37] There have been reports of successful pregnancy after therapy for this tumor.

OVARIAN CHORIOCARCINOMA

Ovarian choriocarcinoma is a germ cell tumor differentiated toward trophoblastic structures (Fig. 73–15). It makes up 0.6% of all germ cell tumors, is most aggressive, and is frequently fatal.[27] hCG has proved to be a reliable tumor marker. Postoperative chemotherapy using a methotrexate-based regimen is frequently used.

EMBRYONAL CARCINOMA

Embryonal carcinoma is a distinct pathologic entity separate from the endodermal sinus tumor that resembles embryonal carcinoma of the adult testis. It is a rare malignant germ cell tumor seen as only 4 to 5% of all germ cell tumors. It makes up 6% of pediatric ovarian neoplasms and 8% of pediatric germ cell tumors.[27] The median age at diagnosis is 14 years.

Both hCG and AFP have been identified within these tumors. These are highly malignant tumors and require both surgery and postoperative chemotherapy. Most patients are first seen with stage I disease (60%), calling for unilateral salpingo-oophorectomy.[22] Postoperative chemotherapy should include one of the multiagent regimens. The survival rate is 40% at 5 years.

MIXED GERM CELL TUMOR

Mixed germ cell tumors are made up of more than one neoplastic germ cell element. Dysgerminoma is present in 80% of tumors, endodermal sinus tumor

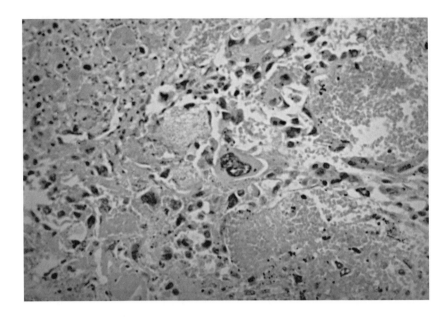

Figure 73–15. Ovarian choriocarcinoma. (Courtesy of Edward C. Klatt, MD, University of Utah School of Medicine.)

in 70%, immature teratoma in 53%, choriocarcinoma in 20%, and embryonal carcinoma in 16%.[22] Tumor markers are positive depending on the type and amount of elements contained in the tumor.

Mixed germ cell tumors represent 8% of all malignant germ cell tumors. More than 60% of cases present as stage I tumor and most have unilateral ovarian involvement.[22] Unilateral salpingo-oophorectomy is recommended because more extensive surgery does not improve prognosis. Surgical therapy alone is associated with approximately a 90% mortality rate. Chemotherapy is recommended, but the prognosis is poor.

ACKNOWLEDGMENT

This chapter is dedicated to the memory of the late William J. Pokorny, MD, who was a contributor to the first two editions of this text.—KWA

REFERENCES

1. Tapa Tapanainen J, Koivisto M, Vihko R, et al: Enhanced activity of the pituitary gonadal axis in premature human infants. J Clin Endocrinol Metab 52:235–238, 1981.
2. Landrum B, Ogburn PL, Feinberg S, et al: Intrauterine aspiration of a large fetal ovarian cyst. Obstet Gynecol 68:11S–14S, 1986.
3. Kennedy LA, Pinckney, LE, Currarino G, et al: Amputated calcified ovaries in children. Radiology 141:83–86, 1981.
4. Alrabeeah A, Galliani CA, Giacomantonio M, et al: Neonatal ovarian torsion: Report of three cases and review of the literature. Pediatr Pathol 8:143–149, 1988.
5. Avni EF, Godart S, Israel C, et al: Ovarian torsion cyst presenting as a wandering tumor in a newborn: Antenatal diagnosis and postnatal assessment. Pediatr Radiol 13:169–171, 1983.
6. Brandt ML, Luks, FI, Filiatrault D, et al: Surgical indications in antenatally diagnosed ovarian cysts. J Pediatr Surg 26:276–282, 1991.
7. Cowell CA: The gynecologic examination of infants, children, and young adolescents. Pediatr Clin North Am 28:247–266, 1981.
8. Ehren IM, Mahour GH, Isaacs H Jr: Benign and malignant ovarian tumors in children and adolescents: A review of 63 cases. Am J Surg 147:339, 1984.
9. Hammerschlag MR, Alpert S, Rosner I, et al: Microbiology of the vagina in children: Normal and potentially pathogenic organisms. Pediatrics 62:57–62, 1978.
10. Obalek S, Misiewicz J, Jablonska S, et al: Childhood condyloma acuminatum: Association with genital and cutaneous human papillomaviruses. Pediatr Dermatol 10:101–106, 1993.
11. Williams TS, Callen JP, Owen LG: Vulvar disorders in the prepubertal female. Pediatr Ann 15:588–605, 1986.
12. Pokorny SF, Pokorny WJ, Kramer W: Acute genital trauma in the prepubertal female. Am J Obstet Gynecol 166:1461–1466, 1992.
13. Pokorny SF, Kozinetz CA: Configuration and other anatomic details of the prepubertal hymen. Adolesc Pediatr Gynecol 1:97–103, 1988.
14. Paradise JE, English DW: Probability of vaginal foreign body in girls with genital complaints. Am J Dis Child 139:472–476, 1985.
15. Meffert JJ, Davis BM, Grimwood RE: Lichen sclerosis. J Am Acad Dermatol 32:393–416, 1995.
16. Flynt J, Gallup D: Childhood lichen sclerosus. Obstet Gynecol 53:79S–81S, 1979.
17. Barnhart K, Mennuti MT, Benjamin I, et al: Prompt diagnosis of ectopic pregnancy in an emergency department setting. Obstet Gynecol 84:1010, 1994.
18. Capraro VJ, Gallego MB: Vaginal agenesis. Am J Obstet Gynecol 124:98–107, 1976.
19. Frank R: The formation of an artificial vagina without operation. Am J Obstet Gynecol 35:1053, 1938.
20. Ingram JM: The bicycle seat stool in the treatment of vaginal agenesis and stenosis: A preliminary report. Am J Obstet Gynecol 140:867, 1981.
21. Hojsgaard A, Villadsen I: McIndoe procedure for congenital vaginal agenesis: Complications and results. Br J Plast Surg 48:97–102, 1995.
22. Huffman JW, Dewhurst DJ, Capraro VJ: Ovarian tumors in children and adolescents. In The Gynecology of Childhood and Adolescence (2nd ed). Philadelphia, WB Saunders, 1981, pp 277–349.
23. Surratt JT, Siegel MJ: Imaging of pediatric ovarian masses. Radiographics 11:533–548, 1991.
24. Aubel S, Wozney P, Edwards R: MRI of female uterine and juxta-uterine masses: Clinical application in 25 patients. Magnetic Resonance Imaging 9:485–491, 1991.
25. Deprest J, Moerman P, Corneillie P, et al: Ovarian borderline mucinous tumors in a premenarchal girl: Review on ovarian

epithelial cancer in young girls. Gynecol Oncol 45:219–224, 1992.

26. Lim-Tan SK, Dajigas HE, Scully RE: Ovarian cystectomy for serous borderline tumors: A follow-up study of 35 cases. Obstet Gynecol 72:775–780, 1988.

27. Breen JL, Bonamo JF, Maxson WS: Genital tract tumors in children. Pediatr Clin North Am 28:355–366, 1981.

28. Bjorkholm E, Silfversward C: Prognostic factors in granulosa-cell tumors. Gynecol Oncol 11:261–274, 1981.

29. Young RH, Scully RE: Ovarian Sertoli-Leydig cell tumors: A clinicopathological analysis of 207 cases. Am J Surg Pathol 9:543–569, 1985.

30. Kennedy AW: Ovarian neoplasms in childhood and adolescence. Semin Reprod Endocrinol 6:79–90, 1988.

31. Bulas DI, Ahlstrom PA, Sivit CJ: Pelvic inflammatory disease in the adolescent: Comparison of transabdominal and transvaginal sonographic evaluation. Radiology 183:435–439, 1992.

32. Chow SN, Yang JH, Lin YH, et al: Malignant ovarian germ cell tumors. Int J Gynecol Obstet 53:151–158, 1996.

33. Motzer RJ, Bajorin DF, Vlamis V, et al: Phase I trial with pharmacokinetic analysis of high-dose carboplatin, etoposide, and cyclophosphamide with autologous bone marrow transplantation in patients with refractory germ cell tumors. Cancer Res 53:3730–3735, 1993.

34. Lakkis WG, Martin MC, Gelfand MM: Benign cystic teratoma of the ovary: A 6-year review. Can J Surg 28:444–446, 1985.

35. Sisler CL, Siegel MJ: Ovarian teratomas: A comparison of the sonographic appearance in prepubertal and postpubertal girls. AJR Am J Roentgenol 154:139–141, 1990.

36. Bonazzi C, Peccatori F, Colombo N, et al: Pure ovarian immature teratoma, a unique and curable disease: 10 years' experience of 32 prospectively treated patients. Obstet Gynecol 84:598–604, 1994.

37. Chang FJ, Lai CH, Chu KK, et al: Treatment of malignant germ cell tumors of the ovary. J Formos Med Assoc 93:411–416, 1994.

38. LaPolla JP, Benda J, Vigliotti AP, et al: Dysgerminoma of the ovary. Obstet Gynecol 69:859–864, 1987.

39. Jimerson GK, Woodruff JD: Ovarian extraembryonal teratoma: Endodermal sinus tumor. Am J Obstet Gynecol 127:73–78, 1977.

40. Lodi A: Contributo clinico statistico sulle mal formazioni della vagina osservate nella: Clinica Obstetrica e Ginecologica di Milano dal 1906 al 1950. Ann Obstet Gine 73:1246, 1951.

74

BREAST DISEASES IN CHILDREN

Don K. Nakayama, MD

☐ Embryology

Formation of the breast occurs throughout embryonic and fetal life.[1] By the 4th week of embryonic development, the ectoderm thickens into a pair of longitudinal streaks in the ventral surface of the embryonic torso, the primitive mammary ridges. Breast tissue can develop anywhere along these "milk lines" that in the fully developed mammal extend from the axillae to the labia majora. The proximal and distal portions of each ridge atrophy by the 6th week. The ectoderm that remains in the pectoral area grows down into the underlying mesenchyme to form the primary mammary bud. From there, secondary buds begin to branch, forming early lactiferous ducts that are well established by 16 weeks. The buds respond to estrogenic hormonal stimulation by the maternal-placental-fetal unit during the last trimester, canalizing into ducts and enlarging en masse to form a true breast nodule during the final weeks of gestation.

The nipple and areola form during late fetal development. A mammary pit first appears at 12 weeks from down growth of the epidermis. A pigmented areola is first seen at 20 to 24 weeks, but a true nipple is not present until later in the perinatal period and is frequently inverted at birth.

☐ Anatomy and Physiology

The breast in the full-term newborn is a firm discrete nodule of white tissue up to 1 cm in diameter. The premature infant lacks a defined breast nodule and is particularly vulnerable to damage to the breast by an ill-placed surgical incision. The nodule may persist well into the 1st year of life, and may be more prominent at 6 months than earlier.[2] The nodule begins to involute in late infancy. Throughout prepuberty, small breasts are present in both boys and girls.

The ductal system of the infant breast ranges from rudimentary to one with well-developed terminal lobules but without an age-dependent progression of histology.[3] In contrast to the ductal anatomy, the ductal epithelium undergoes a progression of functional stages. A secretory epithelium in the first 3 days undergoes metaplasia into apocrine-type cells with cystic dilation of the ducts and alveoli over the 1st month. Over the next 2 years, the gland gradually involutes. The newborn breast is able to secrete milk, a response from elevated prolactin concentrations at birth.[4] Although, for the most part, secretory activity subsides within 3 to 4 weeks, immunohistochemical staining for casein remains strongly positive at 2 months and persists up to 7 months.[3] Two infants aged 9 and 18 months have been observed to secrete milk, long after prolactin concentrations have decreased and beyond any residual maternal hormonal effects, suggesting that endogenous hormones may actively affect breast function in early infancy.[4]

The onset of puberty is signaled by breast (thelarche; mean onset in North American females, 10.9 years) or pubic hair (pubarche; 11.2 years) development, although both are preceded by the onset of the adolescent growth spurt (9.2 years).[5, 6] Menarche follows an average of 2.3 years later.[7]

Thelarche is a response to the maturation of functional ovarian follicles.[7] Prolactin, glucocorticoids, and insulin have a permissive effect on breast development. With puberty, ovarian follicles begin estrogen synthesis. Estrogens circulate to the breast and stimulate ductal development and site-specific adipose deposition. Male adolescents fail to produce significant breast mass, primarily because they lack significant levels of circulating estrogen. Once started, the process usually progresses smoothly to maturity in about 3 years. The breast stages as defined by Marshall and Tanner are as follows[5]:

Stage 1: Preadolescent; elevation of papilla only

Stage 2: Breast bud stage; elevation of breast and areola as a small mound, enlargement of areola diameter

Stage 3: Further enlargement of breast and areola, with no separation of their contours

Stage 4: Projection of areola and papilla to form a secondary mound above the level of the breast

Stage 5: Mature stage; projection of papilla only, resulting from recession of the areola to the general contour of the breast.

☐ Pathophysiology

Female breast disease in pediatric age groups can be seen as an *a*berration of *n*ormal *d*evelopment and *i*nvolution (ANDI).[8] The breast undergoes a normal sequence of development, with each histologic and physiologic feature characteristic of each period: the breast first grows and develops into a functional breast, responds to cyclical changes of menstruation and pregnancy, then finally undergoes involution in late maturity. Disordered responses produce a corresponding sequence of breast conditions and disorders, with specific conditions being associated with each developmental state. The early reproductive period (menarche to 25 years) is the main period of lobular development in the breast. Under the ANDI concept, a fibroadenoma is not a typical benign tumor but a disorder of normal lobular development.[8] Stroma development during this period, if excessive, may result in juvenile hypertrophy. Exaggerated cyclic effects typical of a mature breast may result in cyclic mastalgia and nodularity. Table 74–1 summarizes the complete ANDI classification.

In early infancy, the breast foreshadows the histologic sequence of development and involution that will begin years later. As noted, the newborn breast develops lobules in response to maternal hormones. Over the next months of life it then undergoes invo-

lution. Although rare, benign conditions that result from breast involution may be encountered during infancy, such as periductal mastitis, nipple discharge, and nipple retraction.

Breast cancer represents the extreme end of the spectrum of developmental disorders. It is a disorder of the mature breast, apparently the cumulative product of genetic and hormonal influences over time.[9] It is extremely rare in pediatric age groups, almost exclusively seen in late adolescence when encountered. Although risk factors for breast cancer certainly involve events during childhood and adolescence (such as early menarche) and genetic influences (such as familial breast cancer), breast cancer is not a childhood disease.

☐ Disorders of Development and Growth

POLYTHELIA

Extra nipples and areolae may develop anywhere along the milk line from axilla to pubis. The most common location is on the chest below the actual breast. In a minority, a true accessory breast develops. Unsightly structures should be removed.

HYPOPLASIA AND APLASIA

True breast aplasia occurs in Poland syndrome.[10] Underlying chest wall structures, including pectoralis muscles and ribs, are absent or diminished in

TABLE 74-1. Aberrations of Normal Development and Involution of the Breast (ANDI)

| Stage (Peak Ages, y) | Normal Process | Aberration | | Disease State |
		Underlying Condition	Clinical Presentation	
Early reproductive period (15–25)	Lobule formation	Fibroadenoma	Discrete lump	Giant fibroadenoma, multiple fibroadenomas
	Stroma formation	Juvenile hypertrophy	Excessive breast development	
Mature reproductive period (25–40)	Cyclical hormonal effects on glandular tissue and stroma	Exaggerated cyclical effects	Cyclical mastalgia and nodularity (generalized or discrete)	
Involution (35–55)	Lobular involution (including microcysts, apocrine change, fibrosis, adenosis)	Macrocysts	Discrete lumps	
		Sclerosing lesions	Radiograph abnormalities (mastalgia lumps)	
	Ductal involution (including periductal round cell infiltrates)	Duct dilation	Nipple discharge	Periductal mastitis with bacterial infection and abscess formation
		Periductal fibrosis	Nipple retraction	
	Epithelial turnover	Mild epithelial hyperplasia		Epithelial hyperplasia with atypia

From Hughes LE: Aberrations of normal development and involution (ANDI)—an update. In Mansell RE (ed): Recent Developments in the Study of Benign Breast Disease. London, Parthenon Publishing, 1994, pp 65–73.

size. The ipsilateral upper extremity may also be affected. Reconstruction of the chest wall and placement of a mammary prosthesis or breast reconstruction by a variety of flap techniques are indicated.[11]

ATROPHY

Patients with atrophy of breasts that have undergone normal development should be evaluated for an underlying cause. Weight loss results in loss of fat from stroma and bilateral atrophy. Eating disorders may also be complicated by hypothalamic suppression and hypoestrogenism, further retarding breast growth.[12] In an otherwise well-nourished adolescent, endocrine disorders that result in low estrogen or increased androgens should be evaluated with appropriate hormone determinations.

Unilateral atrophy may occur in scleroderma.[12] It has been reported as a complication of infectious mononucleosis.[13]

VIRGINAL HYPERTROPHY

The cause of virginal hypertrophy is probably an end organ hypersensitivity to normal hormonal fluxes at the time of puberty.[14] Resected specimens may approach 8 to 10 kg. Histologically, breasts show proliferation of glandular tissue and resemble gynecomastia seen in boys.[12] A differential diagnosis must be considered in the evaluation of breast enlargement in adolescents and is summarized in Table 74–2.

The diagnosis is subjective and may depend in large part to the patient's own feelings. Tissue necrosis and rupture of the skin may result from sheer weight and justify reduction mammoplasty. There is little experience with medical therapy, although some improvement has been reported with danazol therapy.[15] Reduction mammoplasty is a safe and appropriate procedure for virginal hypertrophy.[16] Recurrence may occur due to continued growth of the residual tissue, requiring additional procedures.[17]

UNILATERAL HYPERTROPHY

Breast asymmetry may result from unilateral hypertrophy, a condition easily distinguished from hy-

TABLE 74–2. Differential Diagnosis of Breast Hypertrophy

Virginal hypertrophy
Inflammation
Giant fibroadenoma
Cystosarcoma phylloides
Hormone-secreting tumors of the ovary, adrenal gland, or pituitary gland
Lymphoma
Sarcoma
Adenocarcinoma

From Samuelov R, Siplovich L: Juvenile gigantomastia. J Pediatr Surg 23:1014–1015, 1988.

poplasia and aplasia. Some degree of asymmetry is normal and is detectable in many patients. Breast growth may magnify differences and may hamper the child psychologically, even though both breasts are completely clinically normal. Breast reduction of the enlarged breast is then indicated, once Tanner stage 5 breast maturity is reached.[18]

GYNECOMASTIA

Gynecomastia is the benign proliferation of glandular tissue of the male breast great enough to be felt or seen as an enlarged breast.[19] Male breast enlargement occurs physiologically in the newborn, adolescent, and older man. Breast development in the newborn is discussed previously. This discussion focuses on pubertal gynecomastia.

About 30 to 60% of boys exhibit gynecomastia. Prevalence first appears between 10 and 12 years of age. Highest prevalence is at 13 to 14 years, corresponding to Tanner stage 3 or 4. Involution is generally complete at 16 to 17 years. Imbalances between estrogen and androgen concentrations or effects may contribute to the development of gynecomastia during puberty. Testicular or adrenal neoplasms may overproduce estrogens. Peripheral conversion of androgens to estrogens may increase estrogen levels, as noted in pubic skin fibroblasts from patients with idiopathic gynecomastia, and if also present in the breast, may explain increased growth and development.[20] Decreased androgen levels or androgenic effects may result from primary defects of the testis, loss of tonic stimulation by pituitary gonadotrophins, or increased binding of androgens to sex-hormone-binding globulin. Displacement of androgens from their receptors by the many drugs associated with gynecomastia (e.g., spironolactone) may result in unopposed estrogen effects in sex-hormone-sensitive tissue, including the breast.

Histologic studies in the early stages of gynecomastia show marked duct epithelial cell proliferation, inflammatory cell infiltration, increased stromal fibroblasts, and enhanced vascularity. This proliferative stage, also known as the florid stage, may explain breast pain and tenderness that are typical of the clinical presentation. Epithelial proliferation and ductal dilation then both decrease, and the stroma begins to undergo fibrosis and hyalinization. Clinical resolution of breast enlargement and pain follow in 85% of cases, a fact that must be considered when contemplating treatment.

Painful, tender gynecomastia is a typical presentation in adolescent boys. The patient often recalls trauma to the breast; the injury more likely brought the lump to his attention than to have caused it. On palpation, true gynecomastia is a disk of rubbery tissue arising concentrically beneath and around the nipple and areola. This distinguishes it from pseudogynecomastia, increased amounts of adipose tissue beneath the breast causing prominence of the area. The differential diagnosis of gynecomastia is summarized in Table 74–3.

TABLE 74–3. Conditions Associated with Gynecomastia

Physiologic

Neonatal
Pubertal
Involutional

Pathologic

Neoplasms
  Testicular (germ cell, Leydig cell, Sertoli cell, sex cord)
  Adrenal (adenoma or carcinoma)
  Ectopic production of human chorionic gonadotropin
Primary gonadal failure
Secondary hypogonadism
Intersex
  Enzymatic defects of testosterone production
  Androgen insensitivity syndromes
  True hermaphrodism
Liver disease
Starvation, especially during the recovery phase
Renal disease and dialysis
Hyperthyroidism
Excessive extraglandular aromatase activity
Drugs
Idiopathic

From Braunstein GD: Gynecomastia. N Engl J Med 328:490–495, 1993. Copyright © 1993 Massachusetts Medical Society. All rights reserved.

Because pubertal gynecomastia is so prevalent, a thorough history and physical examination, especially of the testes, are sufficient in adolescent males. Reassurance and follow-up examinations at 6-month intervals are sufficient. Pubertal gynecomastia generally resolves within 1 year. Suggestive aspects of the personal medical history (especially drugs and medications), abnormal physical findings (particularly of the testes and genitalia), or pubertal gynecomastia that persists longer than 1 year should lead to a directed endocrinologic and oncologic workup. Drugs should be discontinued, if possible, and the patient reexamined in 1 month. Imaging studies of the testes and adrenal glands are necessary if a tumor is suspected.

The initial endocrinologic workup includes determinations of serum levels of human chorionic gonadotropin (hCG), luteinizing hormone (LH), testosterone, and estradiol (E2). Increased hCG suggests a testicular or extragonadal germ cell tumor and is evaluated with a testicular ultrasound (US). If the testes are normal, chest and abdominal computed tomography is indicated. The interpretation of decreased testosterone levels depends on LH: if elevated, primary hypogonadism is present; if normal or decreased, prolactin levels are checked for a possible prolactin-secreting tumor. If both testosterone and LH are elevated, thyroid hormone and thyroid-stimulating hormone levels are checked for the possibility of hyperthyroidism. Normal values suggest an androgen resistance syndrome. Elevated E2 with a normal or decreased LH suggests a Leydig or Sertoli cell tumor of the testis or an adrenal neoplasm.

The indications for therapy are severe pain, tenderness, or embarrassment sufficient to interfere with the patient's normal daily activities. Subcuta-

neous mastectomy through a periareolar incision is definitive treatment. Drugs have been used to treat gynecomastia, including testosterone, danazol, clomiphene, and tamoxifen. It is difficult to assess the efficacy of these various medical regimens because gynecomastia undergoes spontaneous regression in the vast majority of cases. Side effects from these medications do not justify drug therapy for pubertal gynecomastia.

☐ Inflammatory Lesions

BREAST TRAUMA AND FAT NECROSIS

Soft tissue injury to the breast may result from the familiar causes of blunt and penetrating mechanisms familiar to trauma surgeons. Shoulder harness restraints have been reported to cause subcutaneous rupture of the breast.[21] Most breast trauma is mild and self-limiting. Specific therapy is rarely required.

Fat necrosis is a benign condition that can mimic breast carcinoma. It is considered to result from breast trauma. A history of antecedent trauma is present in about 40% of cases. Areas of fat necrosis present as single or multiple firm, round, or irregular masses, often in the center of the breast near the areola. The masses may be painless, firm, immobile, and cause skin tethering and thickening, all features that suggest carcinoma. Speculated calcifications may be present on mammography, further suggesting the presence of a neoplasm.

Patients who are seen soon after breast injury with associated signs of trauma, such as ecchymosis and painful masses, may be observed for resolution. Patients who are seen later with painless masses require biopsy to rule out malignancy.

MASTITIS AND ABSCESS

Mastitis and breast abscess require appropriate antibiotic therapy against *Staphylococcus*, *Streptococcus*, and *Escherichia coli*. Areas of fluctuance or progression of inflammation while on antibiotics suggest the presence of an abscess that requires drainage. Mastitis in newborns responds in nearly all cases to intravenous antibiotics and warm packs to the affected breast. The decision to explore the infant breast for an abscess must be made with great care to avoid unnecessary damage that may result in breast deformity later in adolescence. An initial needle aspiration of suspicious areas is a prudent first step. If no pus is encountered, antibiotics are continued. Discovery of a true abscess requires incision and drainage.

Mastitis and abscess occur more commonly after thelarche. Causes include manipulation and breast-feeding, although in many cases the cause cannot be identified. Nursing may continue in cases that develop while breast-feeding. Adequate abscess drainage usually requires general anesthesia owing to loculations of pus and breast septations in the developing and mature breast.[1]

☐ Nipple Discharge

GALACTORRHEA

Galactorrhea is inappropriate lactation not related to pregnancy or that continues into postpartum in the absence of breast-feeding.[1] There are five pathophysiologic groups: neurogenic, hypothalamic, endocrine, drug-induced, and idiopathic. Neurogenic causes result from local breast and nipple irritation and stimulation. The most common hypothalamic cause of galactorrhea in adults is prolactinoma, a rare tumor in childhood and adolescence. Failure of sexual maturation often accompanies galactorrhea in children with these tumors.[22] Visual symptoms and headache were rare in children as compared to adults. Cessation of oral contraceptives, polycystic ovary, adrenal tumors, and gonadal tumors are rare causes of galactorrhea in adolescents.[1] Hypothyroidism in infants and children has been reported to be associated with galactorrhea and precocious puberty; nipple discharge ceases with correction of the underlying thyroid condition.[23, 24] Many drugs have been recognized as causes of adult galactorrhea, but seldom have been described in children.[1] Examples include neuroleptics, estrogens, and opiates.

Nipple discharge in boys is always abnormal and a cause must be sought. Prolactinoma is the most common cause in young boys.[25] If prolactin levels are high and evaluation of the sella turcica unrevealing, annual imaging of the sella is necessary until the end of puberty, even if galactorrhea resolves.

OTHER NIPPLE DISCHARGES

Nonmilky discharges include pus, cyst contents, and blood. Purulent discharges usually respond to antibiotics; chronic discharge may require drainage and duct excision. Serous drainage of brown to green fluid may indicate the presence of a communicating breast cyst and is usually self-limited. Bloody drainage is a sign of cancer in adults, but generally drainage is from an intraductal papilloma or duct ectasia in children and adolescents.[26] Excision of the abnormal duct is indicated.

☐ Mastalgia

Breast pain, or mastalgia, is a poorly characterized and underreported syndrome.[27] It accounts for about one fourth of visits to adult breast clinics and is the presenting symptom of breast cancer in 15% of cases. Its prevalence in young and adolescent girls is unknown.

Initial evaluation excludes localized lesions, benign and malignant, and inflammatory conditions. Pain is then characterized as cyclic or noncyclic. The distinction is important because the likelihood of response to drug treatment differs: cyclic pain is more likely to respond. Cyclic mastalgia usually occurs in the third decade of life. It is usually char-

TABLE 74–4. Breast Masses in Children

Physiologic
Normal breast bud
Premature thelarche
Pathologic
Inflammatory
Mastitis
Breast abscess
Fibrosis
Fat necrosis
Benign neoplasms
Hemangioma
Cyst
Lipoma
Papilloma
Malignant neoplasms
Metastatic (e.g., rhabdomyosarcoma, lymphoma)
Secretory carcinoma

acterized as bilateral, dull, burning, or aching. Pain starts 7 to 10 days before the onset of menses, building until menses, when the pain dissipates. Pain may persist throughout the cycle. Spontaneous resolution occurs in 22% of cases. Noncyclic mastalgia tends to occur a decade later and resolves in 50% of cases. Treatment includes removal of methylxanthines from the diet and reassurance. Evening primrose oil, danazol, and bromocriptine may be effective as adjunctive therapy.

☐ Breast Masses

EVALUATION OF BREAST MASSES

The age of the patient affects the differential diagnosis and hence the diagnostic approach (Tables 74–4 and 74–5). Patient age, history, and physical examination are sufficient to make the diagnosis in nearly all cases. Because primary breast cancer is so rare in pediatric age groups, observation has little risk and often is an appropriate step in determining the clinical diagnosis.[28] It is important, however, to follow up all lesions to resolution and to obtain further studies when lesions continue to grow or have features that are worrisome to the experienced clinician (e.g., hard consistency, irregular margins, fixation to chest wall or skin, regional lymphade-

TABLE 74–5. Breast Masses in Adolescents

Physiologic	Benign neoplasms
Thelarche	Fibroadenoma
Unilateral hypertrophy	Phyllodes tumor
	Cyst
Pathologic	Fibrocystic disease
	Neurofibroma
Inflammatory	Malignant neoplasms
Mastitis	Primary breast cancer
Breast abscess	Metastatic (e.g., lymphoma)
Fibrosis	
Fat necrosis	

nopathy). A directed workup in such cases may include fine needle aspiration for cytology, mammography, US examination, and ultimately biopsy.

PREPUBERTAL BREAST MASSES

Masses may occur in the prepubertal breast but are nearly always benign. The most important diagnosis to consider is asynchronous thelarche.[12] One breast bud may appear weeks to months ahead of the other. A breast bud is easily recognized as a disk of firm tissue beneath the areola. In such cases, biopsy is never indicated because it may lead to unilateral iatrogenic amastia.

CYSTS AND FIBROCYSTIC DISEASE

Benign simple cysts occur throughout childhood, but they are most common with the onset of breast development. They appear as soft, painless masses that are not fixed to surrounding breast tissue.[1] Needle aspiration of the cyst results in complete disappearance. Fluid may be serous or brown. Persistence of a mass after cyst aspiration is an indication for biopsy.

Fibrocystic disease is a disease of the mature breast, occurring most commonly in the fourth to fifth decades, and is generally not an issue in adolescents.[29] Masses that occur with fibrocystic disease may be asymptomatic or associated with mastalgia, worse in the perimenstrual period.[12] Resolution of the mass may occur over the course of one or two cycles. A persisting or dominant mass is aspirated for diagnostic and therapeutic reasons.

☐ Fibroadenomas

Fibroadenomas are the most common breast mass in pediatric age groups.[30] There are two variants that affect the pediatric age group: adult and juvenile. Adult fibroadenomas affect older adolescents and young women. They may be multiple in 10 to 15% of cases. The mass is small, measuring 1 to 2 cm in diameter. It is well circumscribed, rubbery in consistency, and mobile. Juvenile fibroadenomas affect younger adolescents around the time of puberty. In contrast to an adult fibroadenoma, the juvenile variant is much larger and may cause considerable breast asymmetry.

Fibroadenomas are considered to be benign, although adult fibroadenomas rarely harbor a carcinoma and juvenile variants may be related to phyllodes tumors.[1, 31] Clonal analysis shows that epithelial and stromal elements of the fibroadenoma are polyclonal, indicating a hyperplastic rather than a neoplastic process.[32] Adult fibroadenomas confer a small but definite increased risk (relative risk, 1.3 to 1.9) for breast cancer development.[30] Clonal analysis in three patients in whom phyllodes tumor of the breast developed after excision of a fibroade-

noma suggested that the former developed from the latter.[33]

Classic adult fibroadenomas can be safely followed up if the lesion exhibits the expected characteristic features: 1 to 2 cm, solitary, firm, rubbery, nontender, well circumscribed. Fine needle aspiration is useful in distinguishing fibroadenomas from carcinomas and phyllodes tumors, but differentiating fibroadenomas from other benign conditions is more difficult.[30] In one study of nonoperative management of adult fibroadenomas, 16% of clinically diagnosed adult fibroadenomas disappeared during 12 months.[34] Excision of those that persisted showed the clinical diagnosis to be accurate in 73% of cases, with the misdiagnoses being of other benign breast conditions. None was a malignancy. Because more than half (54%) of fibroadenomas in the study continued to grow during the period of observation, the authors concluded that the most expeditious course is to simply resect the mass.

Juvenile fibroadenomas should be excised soon after diagnosis to avoid further enlargement of the mass and preserve the architecture of the remaining normal breast tissue. The excision of either variant of fibroadenoma proceeds through an incision directly over the mass in following one of Langer's lines. The mass is held by a centrally placed suture or clamp and is removed with no more than a few millimeters of normal breast tissue. The same approach holds for larger juvenile fibroadenomas, sparing normal surrounding breast tissue. Further breast development is usually normal and symmetric as the tissue compressed by the tumor fills the defect over time.[12]

PHYLLODES TUMORS

Phyllodes tumors, formerly called cystosarcoma phyllodes, is a rare fibroepithelial tumor that ranges from benign (with significant risk for local recurrence) to malignant with rapidly growing metastases.[35] It ranges in size from 1 to 40 cm. Closely resembling a fibroadenoma, a phyllodes tumor appears well circumscribed grossly, but lacks a true capsule. Its surface has minute surface projections that can barely be seen. Owing to these features, complete surgical excision requires a 2-cm margin of normal breast parenchyma. Fibrous areas are interspersed by soft, fleshy areas, and cysts are filled with clear or semisolid bloody fluid, all features that distinguish it from a fibroadenoma. On microscopy, both epithelial and stromal elements show hyperplasia and may have areas of atypia, metaplasia, and malignancy. Characteristics of the stroma alone, however, determine whether a phyllodes tumor is malignant. The mean age of patients is in the fourth decade, about a decade older than for adult fibroadenoma. Phyllodes tumors have been recorded in both adolescent and prepubertal ages.[35]

Distinguishing phyllodes tumor from adenoma before operation is difficult, and a definitive diagnosis may require open excisional biopsy. Fine needle aspiration depends on the detection of a dimorphic pattern of stromal elements and benign epithelial tissue, although the technique may not yield a definitive diagnosis in all cases.[36] The mammographic appearance of phyllodes tumors resembles that of fibroadenomas, with smooth polylobulated margins.[35] US is useful if cysts are found within an otherwise solid mass, a characteristic of phyllodes tumor.

When the preoperative diagnosis is known, wide local excision with a 2-cm margin of normal breast tissue is recommended. Tumors that extend to the pectoralis fascia require removal of the muscle adjacent to the tumor. Owing to the similarity in appearance between a fibroadenoma and a phyllodes tumor, the latter is usually enucleated without a margin. About 20% of phyllodes tumors recur after resection with minimal or no margin. Most authorities recommend reexcision of normal breast tissue to obtain an adequate margin.[35]

Traditionally, malignant phyllodes tumors were treated with simple mastectomy. Recently, malignant tumors have been treated using wide local excision with 2-cm margins with acceptable results.[37] Lymph node metastases are not present, so lymph node dissection is not indicated.[36, 37]

Benign tumors more than 5 cm in diameter have a higher rate of recurrence (39%) than smaller ones (10%).[38] Both benign and malignant phyllodes tumors recur. Among recurrences in previously resected benign tumors, about 20% show malignant histologic transformation with a worse overall prognosis. Local recurrence of a benign tumor is reexcised, whereas most authorities recommend simple mastectomy for a recurrence of a malignant tumor.

☐ Breast Cancer

Although only 0.2% of primary breast cancers occur before age 25 years, they have been found in children younger than 5 years and in male as well as female adolescents.[39] More than 90% present as a breast mass. Nipple discharge is a presenting sign, on occasion.

Secretory carcinoma is a form that occurs relatively more frequently, but not exclusively, in children. It has a low-grade clinical behavior with a good prognosis for long-term survival after simple mastectomy.[40] Both boys and girls are affected; even though the sex ratio of girls to boys is 5:1, the youngest patient reported is a 3-year-old boy.[41] Even though most tumors measure 3 cm or less, lesions of 12 cm have been reported. Axillary lymph node involvement is present in about 20% of cases. Standard treatment is simple mastectomy, although some long-term survivors have been reported after excisional biopsy. Axillary node dissection is indicated if nodes are clinically involved. Recurrence after lumpectomy has been described in several reports. Long-term follow-up is imperative owing to the indolent nature of the disease and the risk for late recurrence.[39]

Nonsecretory breast cancers are less common than secretory breast cancers in pediatric age groups. Some large children's hospitals report no primary breast cancers in their series of pediatric breast masses.[28] They are reported exclusively in female adolescents and young adults and probably represent the leading edge of the prevalence distribution for adult primary breast cancer. They include histologic types seen in primary breast cancers in mature women: invasive intraductal (most common), invasive lobular, and signet ring.[42] Family history of breast cancer is a risk factor for early onset breast cancer and was present in one fourth of patients.[42] Treatment regimen is the same as for adult primary breast cancer, dictated by histology, stage, presence of hormone receptors, and patient menstrual status.

Metastatic carcinoma may involve the breast, with osteosarcoma, lymphoma, and rhabdomyosarcoma having been reported.[28, 42]

REFERENCES

1. Wiebke EA, Nieberhuber JE: Disorders of the breast. In Carpenter SE, Rock JA (eds): Pediatric and Adolescent Gynecology. New York, Raven Press, 1992, pp 417–431.
2. McKiernan J, Coyne J, Cahalane S: Histology of breast development in early life. Arch Dis Child 63:136–139, 1988.
3. Anbazhagan K, Bartek J, Monaghan P, et al: Growth and development of the human infant breast. Am J Anat 192:407–417, 1991.
4. McKiernan J, Hull D: Prolactin, maternal oestrogens and breast development in the newborn. Arch Dis Child 56:770–774, 1981.
5. Marshall WA, Tanner JM: Variations in pattern of pubertal changes in girls. Arch Dis Child 44:291–303, 1969.
6. Tanner JM, Davies PS: Clinical longitudinal standards for height and height velocity for North American children. J Pediatr 107:317–329, 1985.
7. Krasnow JS, Shapiro SS: Normal pubertal development. In Carpenter SE, Rock JA (eds): Pediatric and Adolescent Gynecology. New York, Raven Press, 1992, pp 49–64.
8. Hughes LE: Aberrations of normal development and involution (ANDI)—an update. In Mansell RE (ed): Recent Developments in the Study of Benign Breast Disease. London, Parthenon Publishing, 1994, pp 65–73.
9. Brinton LA, DeVesa SS, Weber BL, et al: Etiology and pathogenesis of breast cancer. In Harris JR, Lippman ME, Morrow M, et al (eds): Diseases of the Breast. Philadelphia, Lippincott–Raven, 1996, pp 159–306.
10. Ravitch MM: Poland's syndrome. In Ravitch MM: Congenital Deformities of the Chest Wall and Their Operative Correction. Philadelphia, WB Saunders, 1977, pp 233–271.
11. Shamberger RC, Welch KJ, Upton J III: Surgical treatment of thoracic deformity in Poland's syndrome. J Pediatr Surg 24:760–765, 1989.
12. Simmons PS: Diagnostic considerations in breast disorders of children and adolescents. Obstet Gynecol Clin North Am 19:91–102, 1992.
13. Haramis HT, Collins RE: Unilateral breast atrophy. Plast Reconstr Surg 95:916–919, 1995.
14. Samuelov R, Siplovich L: Juvenile gigantomastia. J Pediatr Surg 23:1014–1015, 1988.
15. Taylor PJ, Cumming DC, Corenblum B: Successful treatment of D-penicillamine-induced breast gigantism with danazol. BMJ [Clin Res] 282:362–363, 1981.
16. Evans GR, Ryan JJ: Reduction mammaplasty for the teenage patient: A critical analysis. Aesthetic Plast Surg 18:291–297, 1994.

17. Kupfer D, Dragman D, Broadbent R: Juvenile breast hypertrophy: Report of a familial pattern and review of the literature. Plast Reconstr Surg 90:303–309, 1992.
18. Fischl RA, Rosenberg I, Simon BE: Planning unilateral breast reduction for asymmetry. Br J Plast Surg 24:402–404, 1971.
19. Braunstein GD: Gynecomastia. N Engl J Med 328:490–495, 1993.
20. Bulard J, Mowszowicz I, Schaison G: Increased aromatase activity in pubic skin fibroblasts from patients with isolated gynecomastia. J Clin Endocrinol Metab 64:618–623, 1987.
21. Magnant CM: Fat necrosis, hematoma, and trauma. In Harris JR, Lippman ME, Morrow M, et al (eds): Diseases of the Breast. Philadelphia, Lippincott–Raven, 1996, pp 61–65.
22. Richmond IL, Wilson CB: Pituitary adenomas in childhood and adolescence. J Neurosurg 49:163–168, 1978.
23. Van Wyck JJ, Grumbach MM: Syndrome of precocious menstruation and galactorrhea in juvenile hypothyroidism: An example of hormonal overlap in pituitary feedback. J Pediatr 57:416–435, 1960.
24. Macaron C: Galactorrhea and neonatal hypothyroidism. J Pediatr 101:576–577, 1982.
25. Rohn RD: Galactorrhea in the adolescent. J Adolesc Health Care 5:37–49, 1984.
26. Turbey WJ, Buntain WL, Dudgeon DL: The surgical management of pediatric breast masses. Pediatrics 56:736–739, 1975.
27. Klimberg VS: Etiology and management of breast pain. In Harris JR, Lippman ME, Morrow M, et al (eds): Diseases of the Breast. Philadelphia, Lippincott–Raven, 1996, pp 99–106.
28. West KW, Rescorla FJ, Scherer LR III, et al: Diagnosis and treatment of symptomatic breast masses in the pediatric population. J Pediatr Surg 30:182–187, 1995.
29. Constantini M, Bucchi L, Dogliotti L, et al: Cohort study of women with aspirated gross cysts of the breast—an update. In Mansell RE (ed): Recent Developments in the Study of Benign Breast Disease. London, Parthenon Publishing, 1994, pp 227–239.
30. Houlihan MJ: Fibroadenoma and hamartoma. In Harris JR, Lippman ME, Morrow M, et al (eds): Diseases of the Breast. Philadelphia, Lippincott–Raven, 1996, pp 45–47.
31. Ozzello L, Gump FE: The management of patients with carcinomas in fibroadenomatous tumors of the breast. Surg Gynecol Obstet 160:99–104, 1985.
32. Noguchi S, Motomura K, Inaji H, et al: Clonal analysis of fibroadenoma and phylloides tumor of the breast. Cancer Res 53:4071–4074, 1993.
33. Noguchi S, Yokouchi H, Aihara T, et al: Progression of fibroadenoma to phylloides tumor demonstrated by clonal analysis. Cancer 76:1779–1785, 1995.
34. Wilkinson S, Anderson TJ, Rifkind E, et al: Fibroadenoma of the breast: A follow-up of conservative management. Br J Surg 76:390–391, 1989.
35. Petrek JA: Phyllodes tumors. In Harris JR, Lippman ME, Morrow M, et al (eds): Diseases of the Breast. Philadelphia, Lippincott–Raven, 1996, pp 863–869.
36. Stebbing JF, Nash AG: Diagnosis and management of phyllodes tumor of the breast: Experience of 33 cases at a specialist centre. Ann R Coll Surg Engl 77:181–184, 1995.
37. Palmer ML, De Risi DC, Pelikan A, et al: Treatment options and recurrence potential for cytosarcoma phyllodes. Surg Gynecol Obstet 170:193–196, 1990.
38. Chua CL, Thomas A: Cystosarcoma phyllodes tumors. Surg Gynecol Obstet 166:302–306, 1988.
39. Schydlower M: Breast masses in adolescents. Am Fam Phys 25:141–145, 1982.
40. Rosen PP: Invasive mammary carcinoma. In Harris JR, Lippman ME, Morrow M, et al (eds): Diseases of the Breast. Philadelphia, Lippincott–Raven, 1996, pp 393–444.
41. Karl SR, Ballantine TV, Zaino R: Juvenile secretory carcinoma of the breast. J Pediatr Surg 20:368–371, 1985.
42. Corpron CA, Black CT, Singletary SE, et al: Breast cancer in adolescent females. J Pediatr Surg 30:322–324, 1995.

75

ENDOCRINE DISORDERS AND TUMORS

Michael A. Skinner, MD •
Ruth D. Mayforth, MD, PhD

☐ Thyroid Gland

Diseases of the thyroid gland were demonstrated to occur in 36.7 of 1000 children in one population-based study of school-aged children in the United States.[1] About half of these are diffuse gland hypertrophy or simple goiter. Thyroiditis was the second most common abnormality, followed by thyroid nodules and functional disorders. Malignant neoplasms were exceedingly rare. Only two cases of papillary thyroid carcinoma were found in this population of nearly 5000 children followed for 3 years.

EMBRYOLOGY AND PHYSIOLOGY

The thyroid gland is the first endocrine organ to mature in fetal development, arising as an outpouching of the embryonic alimentary tract at about 24 days' gestation. The developing thyroid gland descends from the base of the tongue ventral to the hyoid bone and the larynx, to its final location by about 7 weeks' gestation. In about half of the population, a persistence of the thyroglossal diverticulum results in a pyramidal thyroid lobe. Accessory thyroid tissue may appear in the tongue or anywhere along the course of the duct. Rarely, nondescent results in a lingual thyroid.

Histologically, by the 11th week of gestation, colloid begins to form, and thyroxin (T_4) can then be demonstrated in the embryo. *Parafollicular cells,* or C cells, arise from the ultimobranchial bodies. These parafollicular cells then diffuse throughout the thyroid gland.

Thyroid hormones are synthesized at the interface between the follicular cell and the thyroglobulin. Thyroglobulin is recognized histologically as colloid. The first step in thyroid synthesis production is the iodination of tyrosine molecules, which are then coupled to form the definitive thyroid hormones T_4 and triiodothyronine (T_3). When free thyroid hormone reaches the nucleus of the target cell, the T_3 molecule interacts with the nuclear receptors, and the receptor–T_3 conjugate binds to DNA to regulate genetic transcription.[2] T_4 increases cellular oxygen consumption and the basal metabolic rate; stimulates protein synthesis; and influences carbohydrate, lipid, and vitamin metabolism.

The production and secretion of T_3 and T_4 are stimulated by thyroid-stimulating hormone (TSH) secreted by the pituitary, in response to thyrotropin-releasing hormone, which is, in turn, secreted by the hypothalamus. There are other peptides present within the thyroid gland, such as neuropeptide Y, substance P, cholecystokinin, and vasoactive intestinal peptide, which may assist in the production and secretion of thyroid hormones.[3]

DIAGNOSIS AND LABORATORY EVALUATION

The evaluation of a child whose history suggests thyroid disease should begin with a physical examination of the neck. The size and texture of the gland should be assessed. Diffuse enlargement in a euthyroid patient makes the diagnosis of simple colloid goiter more likely. Graves' disease should be suspected if there is diffuse enlargement and the child is hyperthyroid. Chronic lymphocytic (Hashimoto's) thyroiditis is classically associated with a gland whose texture is granular or pebbly. Firmness in the thyroid gland suggests an infiltrative process, whereas a very hard gland is more suspicious for neoplasia. Tenderness in the thyroid gland is most commonly associated with an acute inflammatory process. In addition to assessing the thyroid gland, the presence of enlarged neck lymph nodes should be specifically noted because thyroid carcinoma is often associated with local metastases before the primary tumor can be palpated.

Thyrotropin (TSH) is nearly always decreased in

the hyperthyroid state and elevated in hypothyroidism and is an extremely sensitive measure of this condition. The plasma free T_4 level is a measure of biologically active thyroid hormone, unaffected by protein binding. When total plasma T_3 and T_4 are measured, it is necessary to consider the level of thyroid-binding globulin to estimate the level of unbound biologically active hormone.

Several imaging modalities are available to assist in evaluating the thyroid gland. Radionuclide scintigraphy is probably the most commonly used test. The radioiodines ^{123}I and ^{131}I are most effective in detecting ectopic thyroid tissue or metastatic thyroid carcinoma, whereas technetium-99m pertechnetate produces superior imaging of thyroid gland nodules or tumors. Ultrasonography (US) is useful to delineate whether a neck mass actually arises from the thyroid and whether there are multiple nodules. US is currently used to screen for thyroid masses in children exposed to radiation following the Chernobyl disaster.[4]

NONNEOPLASTIC THYROID CONDITIONS

Goiter and Thyroiditis

The causes of thyromegaly in 152 affected children are listed in Table 75–1.[5] Most patients had simple adolescent colloid goiter. Physiologically, diffuse thyroid enlargement may be due to a defect in hormone production, related to autoimmune diseases, or a response to an inflammatory condition. Goiters are classified as diffusely enlarged or nodular and either toxic or euthyroid. Most children with goiters are euthyroid, and surgical resection is rarely indicated.

The differential diagnosis for diffuse thyroid enlargement is listed in Table 75–2. Laboratory evaluation should begin with a plasma free T_4 and TSH level. With a simple colloid goiter, the patient is euthyroid, US or scintigraphy reveals uniform enlargement, and serum thyroid antibody titers are normal. The etiology of this condition may be an autoimmune process.[6] The natural history of colloid goiter is not well known, but one study of adolescents found that, 20 years after diagnosis, nearly 60% of the glands were normal in size.[1] Exogenous thyroid hormone does not significantly enhance res-

TABLE 75–1. Etiology of Thyroid Gland Enlargement in 152 Children

Diagnosis	Frequency (%)
Simple goiter	83
Chronic lymphocytic thyroiditis	12.5
Graves' disease	2.5
Benign adenoma	1.5
Cyst	1
Total	**100**

Adapted from Jaksic J, Dumic M, Filipovic B, et al: Thyroid disease in a school population with thyromegaly. Arch Dis Child 70:103–106, 1994.

TABLE 75–2. Differential Diagnosis of Diffuse Thyroid Enlargement (Goiter) in Children

Autoimmune Mediated

Chronic lymphocytic (Hashimoto's) thyroiditis
Graves' disease
Simple colloid goiter

Compensatory

Iodine deficiency
Medications
Goitrogens
Hormone or receptor defect

Inflammatory Conditions

Acute suppurative thyroiditis
Subacute thyroiditis

olution of the goiter. In rare cases, resection may be indicated due to size or the suspicion of neoplasia.

Chronic lymphocytic (Hashimoto's) thyroiditis is another common cause of diffuse thyroid enlargement, occurring most frequently in female adolescents. This condition is part of the spectrum of autoimmune thyroid disorders. It is thought that CD4 T cells are activated against thyroid antigens and recruit cytotoxic CD8 T cells, which kill thyroid cells, to cause hypothyroidism.[7] Children are initially euthyroid and slowly progress to become hypothyroid. However, approximately 10% of children are hyperthyroid, a condition known as "Hashitoxicosis." The thyroid gland is usually pebbly or granular in texture and may be mildly tender.

Ninety-five percent of patients with chronic lymphocytic thyroiditis have elevated antithyroid microsomal antibodies or antithyroid peroxidase antibodies. Plasma thyroid hormone levels are normal or low, and TSH levels are elevated in 70% of patients. Thyroid imaging is usually not necessary if clinical and laboratory findings are strongly suggestive of the diagnosis. The radionuclide scan usually shows patchy uptake of the tracer and may mimic the findings in Graves' disease or multinodular goiter. The principal US finding is nonspecific, diffuse thyroid hypoechogenicity. Rarely, autoantibodies cannot be detected, and fine needle aspirate (FNA) may be needed to confirm the diagnosis. In as many as one third of adolescent patients, the thyroiditis resolves spontaneously, with the gland becoming normal and the antibodies disappearing. Thus, expectant management should be considered. Exogenous thyroid hormone should be administered in the hypothyroid patient, but in euthyroid children it is ineffective in reducing the size of the goiter.[8]

Subacute (de Quervain's) thyroiditis, a viral inflammation of the thyroid gland, is unusual in children. The thyroid is swollen, painful, and tender. Mild thyrotoxicosis results from injury to the thyroid follicles with release of thyroid hormone into the circulation. Serum T_3 and T_4 levels are elevated and TSH is decreased. Owing to thyroid follicular cell dysfunction, there is decreased radioactive iodine uptake, a finding that distinguishes subacute thyroiditis from Graves' disease. Histologically, granulomas and epithelioid cells may be seen. The treatment of subacute thyroiditis is symptomatic and generally consists of nonsteroidal antiinflammatory agents or steroids. The condition typically lasts 2 to 9 months, and complete recovery may be expected.

Acute suppurative thyroiditis is a bacterial infection of the gland. The gland is acutely inflamed, and the patient is septic. Patients are usually euthyroid. Staphylococci or mixed aerobic and anaerobic flora are common causal agents, and there may be a congenital pharyngeal sinus tract predisposing the patient to infection. Management consists of intravenous antibiotics. Abscess drainage may be necessary. The thyroid gland may be expected to recover completely.

Graves' Disease

Graves' disease, or diffuse toxic goiter, is the most common cause of hyperthyroidism in childhood. The condition is an autoimmune disease caused by the presence of immunoglobulins of the IgG class directed against components of the thyroid plasma membrane, possibly including the TSH receptor. These autoantibodies stimulate the thyroid follicles to increase iodide uptake and cyclic adenosine monophosphate production, leading to thyroid growth and inducing the production and secretion of increased thyroid hormone.

TSH-receptor antibodies are present in more than 95% of patients with active Graves' disease. The inciting event eliciting the antibody response against the TSH receptor is unknown. Reports have demonstrated that TSH-binding sites are present in a number of gram-positive and gram-negative bacteria, and it is possible that infection may elicit the production of antibodies that react with the TSH receptor.[9] An infectious etiology for Graves' disease is further supported by scattered epidemiologic reports of disease clustering.[10] Graves' disease is seen in girls about five times more commonly than in boys, and the incidence steadily increases throughout childhood, peaking in the adolescent years. Congenital Graves' disease, resulting from the transplacental passage of maternal antibodies, occurs in about 1% of babies born to women with active Graves' disease. The onset may be delayed until 2 to 3 weeks after birth.

In most children, the onset of Graves' disease develops over several months. Initial symptoms include nervousness, emotional lability, and declining school performance. Later, weight loss becomes evident, as does sweating, palpitations, heat intolerance, and general malaise. A smooth, firm, nontender goiter is present in more than 95% of cases. A bruit may be heard on auscultation. Exophthalmos is unusual in children, but a conspicuous stare may be evident. Laboratory evaluation generally reveals elevated free T_4 and decreased TSH level. In

10 to 20% of patients, there is only elevation of T_3, a condition known as *T_3 toxicosis.* The diagnosis of Graves' disease is definitively established by the presence of TSH-receptor antibodies.

Although the basic pathogenesis of Graves' disease is understood, no generally successful methods are available to correct the immunologic defect. The treatment of Graves' disease is palliative and is designed to decrease the production and secretion of thyroid hormone. The natural course of untreated Graves' disease is unpredictable. In some patients, the thyrotoxicosis may be persistent but variable in severity; in others, it may be cyclic with exacerbations of varying degree and duration.

Current treatment includes antithyroid medications, radioactive ^{131}I, and surgical resection.[11] In the United States, most pediatric endocrinologists initiate therapy with methimazole or propylthiouracil, which reduces thyroid hormone production by inhibiting follicle cell organification of iodide and the coupling of iodotyrosines. Propylthiouracil also inhibits peripheral conversion of T_4 to T_3 and may be the agent of choice if rapid alleviation of thyrotoxicosis is desired. Both agents may possess some immunosuppressive activity; this is suspected because there is usually a reduction in antithyroid antibodies. In most cases, methimazole is preferred due to its increased potency, longer half-life, and associated improved compliance. The initial adolescent dose is 30 mg once daily, which is reduced if the patient is younger. When the patient becomes euthyroid, as determined by normal T_3 and T_4 levels, the daily dose of methimazole should be reduced to 10 mg. T_3 and T_4 levels must be monitored. The thyroid gland decreases in size in about one half of patients. Thyroid enlargement with therapy signals either an intensification of the disease or hypothyroidism from overtreatment.

Side effects of methimazole include nausea, minor skin reactions, urticaria, arthralgias, arthritis, and fevers. The most serious reaction is an idiosyncratic agranulocytosis, occurring in fewer than 1% of patients. This may occur at any time during the course of treatment or even during a second course of the drug. The most common symptom of agranulocytosis is pharyngitis with fever, for which the patient should be warned to seek medical attention. In most cases, the granulocyte count increases 2 to 3 weeks after stopping the drug, but rare fatal opportunistic infections have been reported. Treatment with parenteral antibiotics during the recovery period has been recommended.

The goal when treating Graves' disease is to allow for natural resolution of the underlying autoimmune process. In general, the disease remission rate is approximately 25% after 2 years of treatment, with a further 25% remission every 2 years.[12] The resolution rate is decreased if TSH-receptor antibodies persist during and after treatment. The addition of T_4 to methimazole therapy resulted in a significantly lower incidence of disease recurrence in one study but not in another.[13, 14] The use of T_4 cannot be recommended in pediatric patients receiving antithyroid medications.

The thyroid gland must be ablated if there is resistance or severe reactions to the antithyroid medications. Both surgical resection and ablation with radioactive ^{131}I have complications. The advantages of ^{131}I therapy include its effectiveness, safety, ease of administration, and relatively low cost.[15] Even though the disease recurrence rate is low following radioiodine treatment, patients have a 50 to 80% incidence of long-term hypothyroidism.[16] Despite studies demonstrating no increased risk of cancer relative to the general population, there remain concerns over the possibility of teratogenic or carcinogenic effects of ^{131}I in children and adolescents.[15, 17] Reports have documented the safety and effectiveness of ^{131}I in treating hyperthyroidism in childhood, and the modality may be gaining favor among pediatric endocrinologists who manage Graves' disease.[18]

Either a subtotal or total thyroidectomy is indicated for patients who refuse radioiodine treatment or fail medical management, or for those children whose thyroid gland is so large that there are airway symptoms related to compression. An antithyroid medication should be administered to decrease T_3 and T_4 levels into the normal range before operation. Alternatively, β-blocking agents such as propranolol may be used to ameliorate the adrenergic symptoms of hyperthyroidism. In addition, Lugol's solution, 5 to 10 drops per day, should be administered for 4 to 7 days before thyroidectomy to reduce the vascularity of the gland.

The incidence of hypothyroidism following subtotal thyroidectomy is 12 to 54%, and the hypothyroidism may be subclinical in up to 45% of children.[15] When abnormal TSH levels are considered, the incidence of hyperthyroidism or hypothyroidism is even higher. The rate of recurrent hyperthyroidism is approximately 13%. It is likely that the relapse rate increases with time following surgery, and in the adult population, 30% of patients exhibit recurrent hyperthyroidism 25 years after their subtotal thyroidectomy.[11]

Hypothyroidism

Hypothyroidism may result from a defect anywhere in the hypothalamic-pituitary-thyroid axis and is rarely treated surgically. Approximately 90% of pediatric hypothyroidism is congenital, detected by neonatal screening programs, and results from dysgenesis of the thyroid gland. Two thirds of these babies have a rudimentary gland, and there is complete absence of thyroid tissue in the rest of the patients. The rudimentary gland may be ectopic (e.g., the base of the tongue). Maternal thyroid hormone may prevent symptoms even in children with complete thyroid agenesis. Ectopic thyroid tissue may supply a sufficient amount of T_4 for years or may prove to be insufficient later in childhood.

These unusual conditions may come to attention with the evaluation of a sublingual or midline neck mass. Surgeons must be mindful of the possibility of ectopic thyroid tissue when evaluating children with such masses. To ensure that all the functioning thyroid tissue is not inadvertently resected, radionuclide thyroid scanning should be considered before removing any unusual neck mass.

NEOPLASTIC THYROID CONDITIONS

Thyroid Nodules

Thyroid nodules are uncommon in children, but there is a relatively high likelihood of associated cancer. The incidence of malignancy in thyroid nodules has been about 20% in pediatric series.[19, 20] This cancer rate is lower than was reported in previous decades because there have been fewer children exposed to neck irradiation. Appropriate and prompt evaluation and management are important because the neoplasm may be at an early curable stage. A summary of pathologic results of several large series of children who underwent surgery for thyroid nodules is presented in Table 75-3. Other unlisted diagnostic possibilities for thyroid nodules include cystic hygroma, thyroglossal duct remnant, and germ cell tumor.

Girls have twice the incidence of thyroid nodules as boys.[21] In most patients, an asymptomatic mass in the lower anterior neck is the presenting symptom. It is impossible to differentiate benign from malignant lesions on clinical grounds, but a careful neck examination should be performed, especially to determine whether there are enlarged cervical lymph nodes. Unsuspected thyrotoxicosis resulting from an autonomously functioning nodule depresses the serum TSH. Thyroid imaging studies are unreliable in distinguishing benign from malignant

TABLE 75-3. Diagnoses in 251 Pediatric Patients Treated for Thyroid Nodules

No. Malignant	42 (17%)
Histologic subtype	
Papillary	29
Follicular	6
Mixed	2
Anaplastic	2
Medullary	2
Lymphoma	1
No. Benign	209 (83%)
Diagnosis	
Follicular adenoma	101
Thyroiditis	27
Thyroglossal cyst	5
Colloid nodule	59
Branchial cyst	5
Other	12

Data from Desjardins JG, Khan AH, Montupet P, et al: Management of thyroid nodules in children: a 20-year experience. J Pediatr Surg 22:736–739, 1987; Hung W, Anderson KD, Chandra RS, et al: Solitary thyroid nodules in 71 children and adolescents. J Pediatr Surg 27:1407–1409, 1992; and Yip FWK, Reeve TS, Poole AG, et al: Thyroid nodules in childhood and adolescence. Aust N Z J Surg 64:676–678, 1994.

nodules, but if US reveals multiple nodules, the diagnosis of thyroiditis becomes more likely. Because malignant nodules may be either solid or cystic, US does not differentiate them. Malignant nodules may be either functioning or nonfunctioning on thyroid scintiscan. A therapeutic trial of exogenous thyroid hormone to induce nodule regression is not recommended for children.

The usefulness of FNA cytology in pediatric patients has not been well defined. Pediatric surgeons have historically recommended the removal of thyroid nodules, and there have been few large studies defining the natural history of cytologically benign nodules in children. In one study of 57 children with thyroid nodules evaluated with aspiration, the incidence of malignancy was 18%.[22] One papillary carcinoma was initially misdiagnosed as benign but was recognized as a malignancy during follow-up. Approximately 80% of pediatric thyroid nodules are benign. If these could be accurately diagnosed without surgical removal, there may be significant potential savings in operative morbidity and cost.

In adolescent patients, FNA may be acceptable in evaluating thyroid nodules. The adolescent spectrum of thyroid disease is similar to that of adults. The incidence of malignancy in thyroid nodules in patients 13 to 18 years old was only 11% in one large series.[21] Benign nodules in adolescent patients can be followed up with serial physical examinations and US studies. Exogenous thyroid hormone to suppress benign thyroid nodules has not been shown to alter their natural history.

Surgical resection should be performed if the nodule is malignant or has indeterminate cytology, or if the size of a benign nodule increases. If a cystic thyroid lesion disappears after aspiration, surgery may be deferred. If the lesion recurs, it should be removed. Even though cyst fluid may be sent for cytologic analysis, the sensitivity of this test for determining the presence of cancer in children is unknown.[23]

There is a higher risk of malignancy in prepubertal children with thyroid nodules. The natural history of benign lesions in younger children is unknown, and the safety of nonoperative treatment has not been demonstrated. In children younger than 13 years, it is currently recommended that all thyroid nodules be removed. Preoperative US and thyroid scintigraphy aid in determining the anatomy.[19, 24]

Thyroid Carcinoma

Thyroid carcinoma represents about 3% of all pediatric malignancies in the United States. The peak incidence is between 10 and 18 years of age, and girls outnumber boys 2:1. Approximately 10% of all malignant thyroid tumors occur in children.

The incidence of childhood thyroid malignancy has decreased in most parts of the world since the mid-1970s owing to the reduced use of radiation to treat benign diseases. A marked increase of thyroid tumors has been noted in the Republics of Belarus and Ukraine following the 1986 Chernobyl nuclear power plant catastrophe.[25] The latency period for developing thyroid cancer following radiation exposure is about 4 to 6 years, and in the Belarus population, there has been a 62-fold increase in thyroid tumor incidence since the Chernobyl accident.

Treatment for a previous malignancy is another significant risk factor for thyroid carcinoma. Thyroid cancers constituted about 9% of second malignancies in one series.[26] Hodgkin's lymphoma is the most common malignancy associated with the subsequent thyroid cancer. Whereas most thyroid second neoplasms follow previous exposure of radiation to the neck, alkylating agents alone also predispose to thyroid cancer. The mean age at diagnosis of thyroid second neoplasms is 20 years, demonstrating the importance of careful surveillance for second tumors in children who have been successfully treated for cancer.

Various molecular biologic events may account for the disparity in behavior of the different histologic subtypes of thyroid cancer. RAS protooncogene mutations are found in about 20% of papillary tumors and 80% of follicular tumors.[27] Other studies have reported that RAS is frequently activated in benign follicular adenomas, suggesting that this genetic event occurs early in the transformation process.[28] An activating mutation of the RET protooncogene is found in about 35% of papillary thyroid cancers.[29] The RET protein is a receptor tyrosine-kinase molecule, which probably functions within the cell to regulate proliferation or differentiation.

In papillary thyroid tumors, the gene is activated by the fusion of the tyrosine kinase region of RET to another gene. This may occur through a chromosomal inversion, or a translocation event may fuse a gene from another chromosome into RET, forming the chimeric transforming gene.[30] Such a chimeric gene has been shown to cause transformation of cell lines in vitro, and this is probably one of the steps in transformation of thyroid cells to form papillary carcinomas. Finally, it is apparent that mutations in the TSH-receptor gene also may be responsible for some differentiated thyroid cancers.[31]

The RET protooncogene is also responsible for the development of medullary thyroid carcinoma. Various point mutations in RET are associated with the multiple endocrine neoplasia type 2 (MEN 2A, MEN 2B) syndromes and familial medullary thyroid carcinoma (FMTC). In addition, as many as 40% of sporadic nonfamilial medullary thyroid carcinomas possess RET mutations.[32] As a dominantly acting oncogene, it is likely that RET mutations perturb the intracellular signaling pathways to cause transformation of target thyroid cells.

Thyroid carcinoma generally presents clinically as a thyroid mass, sometimes with enlarged cervical lymph nodes. Regional lymph node metastases are present in three of four children when the disease is first detected (Table 75–4). The pathologic diagnosis can be established using either FNA cytology or frozen-section biopsy at operation. Papillary carci-

TABLE 75-4. Clinical Aspects of Differentiated Thyroid Cancer in Children from Six Large Pediatric Series

	Clinical Series					
	A	B	C	D	E	F
Total no. of patients	89	59	58	100	49	72
Mean age (y)	12.8	NA	11.9	13.3	14.0	11
Girls (%)	81	66	69	71	69	71
Histology (No.)						
Papillary	83	37	58	87	44	50
Follicular	6	19	0	7	4	21
Medullary	0	1	0	0	1	0
Other	0	2	0	6	0	0
Metastasis (%)	88	50	90	71	73	75
Median follow-up (y)	NA	11	28	20	7.7	13
Cancer mortality (%)	2.2	3.4	3.4	0	2.0	17

A, Harness JA, Thompson NW, McLeod MK, et al: Differentiated thyroid carcinoma in children and adolescents. World J Surg 16:547–554, 1992.

B, Samuel AM, Sharma SM: Differentiated thyroid carcinomas in children and adolescents. Cancer 67:2186–2190, 1991.

C, Zimmerman D, Hay ID, Gough IR, et al: Papillary thyroid carcinoma in children and adults: Long-term follow-up of 1039 patients conservatively treated at one institution during three decades. Surgery 104:1157–1163, 1988.

D, La Quaglia MP, Corbally MT, Heller G, et al: Recurrence and morbidity in differentiated thyroid carcinoma in children. Surgery 104:1149–1156, 1988.

E, Ceccarelli C, Pacini F, Lippi F, et al: Thyroid cancer in children and adolescents. Surgery 104:1143–1148, 1988.

F, Schlumberger M, De Vathaire F, Travagli JP, et al: Differentiated thyroid carcinoma in childhood: long term follow-up in 72 patients. J Clin Endocrinol Metab 65:1088–1094, 1987.

NA, data not available.

noma can usually be differentiated from benign conditions by either of these techniques. The functional status of the mass is determined by preoperative scintiscan. US may be helpful in planning the surgical procedure.[24] Because pulmonary metastases are frequent, a preoperative chest roentgenogram should be obtained.

There have been no clinical trials to determine whether total thyroidectomy, with lymph node dissection if the regional nodes are involved, is better than subtotal thyroidectomy.[33–35] Radioiodine ablative therapy is more effective after removal of the entire gland because there is less functioning endocrine tissue to take up the radionuclide. Surgeons preferring a lesser resection hold that differentiated thyroid carcinoma in children is an indolent disease and that survival is not clearly related to the extent of gland removal.[36, 37] The incidence of recurrent laryngeal nerve injury is 0 to 24%, and the reported frequency of permanent hypocalcemia is 6 to 27% in those patients having total thyroidectomy, although these complications occur less commonly in recent reports.[36, 38]

Multivariate analysis revealed that younger age at diagnosis and the histologic type of tumor were the only factors predictive of early disease recurrence in one retrospective review.[36] Children older than 12 years of age at diagnosis and with follicular histology were more likely to be cured at the initial procedure. Thus, tumor factors may be more important than treatment factors in determining the outcome. Major surgical complications occurred more frequently in younger children who had extensive resection of the gland.

Lobectomy with isthmus resection may be sufficient for tumors clearly isolated to one lobe, but thyroid cancer is bilateral in as many as 66% of cases, and about 80% of tumors exhibit multifocality.[35] Therefore, most pediatric surgeons believe that more aggressive thyroid gland resections are indicated and recommend that either a total or near-total thyroidectomy be performed for the management of differentiated thyroid cancer.

The recurrent laryngeal nerve should be identified and protected. A study has shown that, when tumor invades the recurrent laryngeal nerve, the nerve can be safely preserved without compromising survival; ^{131}I radiotherapy may successfully eradicate residual tumor.[39] Probably the most reliable way to preserve parathyroid gland function is to identify and autotransplant one or two of the glands into the sternocleidomastoid muscle or into the nondominant forearm.[40, 41] If regional nodes are suspicious for metastasis, a node dissection is recommended. In patients with locally advanced disease, it is especially important to remove as much of the thyroid gland as possible, to allow subsequent radioiodine scanning and treatment if the tumor recurs. Finally, after surgical resection, most investigators recommend that all patients with endocrine thyroid cancer be treated with exogenous thyroid hormone to suppress TSH-mediated stimulation of the gland.

The incidence of pulmonary metastasis at diagnosis of thyroid cancer in childhood is about 6%, but it almost never occurs in the absence of significant cervical lymph node metastasis.[37, 42] Pulmonary metastases require treatment with radioiodine. Plain chest roentgenograms may demonstrate the pulmonary disease in only about 60% of cases, so scanning with radioiodine is necessary. Pulmonary scintiscan may be falsely negative if there is significant residual thyroid gland remaining in the neck.[42]

The recurrence rate of thyroid cancer in children followed for 20 years is about 30%, and late deaths from persistent or recurrent disease are not uncommon.[35, 36] This underscores the importance of aggressive early treatment and relatively frequent long-term follow-up. An ^{131}I whole body scan should be performed approximately 6 weeks after the initial thyroid resection, followed by therapeutic doses of the radionuclide administered as necessary to treat residual metastatic disease.[33] A report of adult patients with differentiated thyroid cancer showed that routine ^{131}I treatment to ablate residual thyroid tissue resulted in fewer disease recurrences and improved survival rate among patients older than 40 years of age.[43] The implication of these results for pediatric patients is unclear.

After the initial treatment of differentiated thyroid cancer, diagnostic radioiodine scans should be repeated yearly to assess recurrence of the neoplasm. Thyroglobulin has been shown to be a useful marker of residual or metastatic thyroid cancer; the plasma level of this protein should be measured yearly, and an elevated value should raise the suspicion of recurrent disease.[44] It should be noted that the diagnostic accuracy of this test is significantly decreased in children who have residual thyroid tissue and in those who are taking thyroid hormone supplementation.

Medullary thyroid carcinoma (MTC) accounts for approximately 5% of thyroid neoplasms in children. Arising from the parafollicular C cells, MTC may occur either sporadically or in association with MEN 2A or MEN 2B, or the FMTC syndrome. MTC is usually the first tumor to develop in MEN patients and is the most common cause of death in this group. The neoplasm is particularly virulent in patients with MEN 2B and may occur in infancy.[45]

As with other pediatric thyroid neoplasms, the clinical diagnosis of MTC is usually made only after there is metastatic spread of the tumor to the adjacent cervical lymph nodes or to distant sites.[46] Surgical resection is the only effective treatment for MTC, underscoring the importance of early diagnosis and therapy before metastasis occurs. For this reason, current management of MTC in children from MEN 2 and FMTC kindreds relies on the presymptomatic detection of the RET protooncogene mutation responsible for the disease. Affected children with MEN 2A should undergo total thyroidectomy at approximately the age of 5 years, before the cancer spreads beyond the thyroid gland.[47, 48] Indeed, approximately 80% of children who have thyroidectomy based on the presence of the RET mutation already have foci of MTC within the thyroid gland.[48] Owing to the increased virulence of the MTC in children with MEN 2B, prophylactic thyroidectomy should be performed at approximately 1 year of age. Due to the high incidence of bilateral disease, complete removal of the thyroid gland is the recommended surgical management of MTC in children.[49] In addition, the lymph nodes in the central compartment of the neck, medial to the carotid sheaths and between the hyoid bone and the sternum, should be removed.

☐ Parathyroid Glands

EMBRYOLOGY AND PHYSIOLOGY

Parathyroid gland development begins about the 5th week of gestation, when the epithelium in the dorsal portions of the third and fourth pharyngeal pouches begins to proliferate, forming small nodules on the dorsal aspect of each pouch. During the 6th week of development, the parathyroid glands associated with the third pair of pharyngeal pouches migrate caudally with the thymic primordium, finally coming to rest on the dorsal surface of the thyroid gland low in the neck. The parathyroid glands arising from the fourth pharyngeal pouches also descend in the neck, ultimately resting superior to the other glands. Mobilization of calcium from the bones is directly stimulated by parathormone (PTH), a process that also requires vitamin D.

Hyperparathyroidism

PTH is secreted as an 84-amino acid protein, which is rapidly cleaved in the liver and kidney into the carboxyl-terminal, amino-terminal, and midregion fragments. The biologic activity of PTH resides in the amino-terminal segment, but the plasma level of this moiety is low, owing to its very short half-life in the circulation. The C-terminal fragment levels are 50- to 500-fold those of the N-terminal fragment, and most clinical assays of PTH measure C-terminal levels of the hormone. These assays are usually effective for the evaluation of hyperparathyroidism, but plasma levels of the C-terminal fragment may be selectively elevated if there is a component of renal failure. The laboratory hallmark of hyperparathyroidism is the finding of an inappropriately elevated plasma PTH level with hypercalcemia.

The differential diagnosis of hypercalcemia in childhood is presented in Table 75–5. Unlike hypercalcemia in adults, hypercalcemia in children is rarely related to a neoplasm. However, in rare cases, pediatric tumors may secrete a parathyroid-related polypeptide that elevates the calcium level. Neoplasms in which this has been reported include malignant rhabdoid tumor, mesoblastic nephroma, rhabdomyosarcoma, neuroblastoma, and lymphoma. In these patients, the PTH level is generally normal or decreased.

Primary Hyperparathyroidism

Primary hyperparathyroidism in childhood usually results from a solitary hyperfunctioning adenoma and more rarely from diffuse hyperplasia of all four glands.[50] Hyperparathyroidism resulting from hyperplasia in all four glands is a feature of MEN-I. Hyperparathyroidism develops in approximately 30% of patients having MEN 2A in their second or third decade of life.[51] At the time of prophylactic thyroidectomy for MEN 2, the parathyroid glands should be identified and autotransplanted

TABLE 75–5. Differential Diagnosis of Hypercalcemia in Childhood

Elevated parathyroid hormone level
  Primary hyperparathyroidism
  Secondary hyperparathyroidism
  Tertiary hyperparathyroidism
  Ectopic parathyroid hormone production
Hypervitaminosis D
Sarcoidosis
Subcutaneous fat necrosis
Familial hypocalcuric hypercalcemia
Idiopathic hypercalcemia of infancy
Thyrotoxicosis
Hypervitaminosis A
Hypophosphatasia
Prolonged immobilization
Thiazide diuretics

into the nondominant forearm.[40] If hyperparathyroidism develops, a portion of the heterotopic tissue may easily be removed from the forearm.

Surgical options for parathyroid gland hyperplasia involving all of the glands include either 3½ gland parathyroidectomy or total parathyroidectomy with heterotopic autotransplantation of some parathyroid tissue back into the nondominant forearm.[52] The latter approach has the advantage of avoiding repeated neck exploration if hyperparathyroidism should recur, and it has been shown to be safe in infants and children.[40, 48] Moreover, total parathyroidectomy with heterotopic autotransplantation has been shown to result in improved survival rate in infants with severe hypercalcemia.[52] Patients with total parathyroidectomy and autotransplantation require a short period of vitamin D and calcium supplementation until the heterotopic tissue begins to function.[40]

Primary hyperparathyroidism of infancy is a rare, often fatal, condition that usually develops within the first 3 months of life.[52, 53] Signs include hypotonicity, respiratory distress, failure to thrive, lethargy, and polyuria. The serum PTH is elevated. Pathologically, there is usually diffuse parathyroid gland hyperplasia. In about half of reported cases, there is a familial component to the disease. Early recognition and treatment are essential to allow normal growth and development of the baby.

The management of primary hyperparathyroidism in children is surgical. All four of the parathyroid glands should be identified and biopsied. An enlarged and adenomatous gland should be removed. If the other glands are normal, they should be marked with nonabsorbable sutures and left in place.

Familial Hypocalciuric Hypercalcemia

Familial hypocalciuric hypercalcemia differs from primary hypoparathyroidism in that PTH is normal but urinary excretion of calcium is low. Patients are usually asymptomatic with an elevated serum calcium level. Serum magnesium may also be elevated.

The disease is inherited as an autosomal dominant disorder caused by a heterozygous mutation in the Ca^{2+}-sensing receptor gene.[54] The parathyroid glands are normal, and there is usually no benefit to parathyroidectomy. If both parents are carriers, the neonate may have severe hypercalcemia. These infants have inherited mutations in both copies of the Ca^{2+}-sensing receptor gene and often have hyperplasia of all of their parathyroid glands, in which case they benefit from parathyroidectomy with transplantation of one gland.

Secondary Hypoparathyroidism

Secondary hypoparathyroidism occurs in children with renal insufficiency or malabsorption. PTH production is increased in response to decreased calcium levels. Affected patients typically respond to medical treatment designed to decrease intestinal phosphorus absorption, but in rare cases, severe renal osteodystrophy develops, manifested by skeletal fractures and metastatic calcifications. Especially severe cases of secondary hyperparathyroidism may be candidates for total parathyroidectomy with autotransplantation.[50]

Tertiary Hyperparathyroidism

Tertiary hyperparathyroidism occurs when there is persistent hyperfunction of the parathyroid glands even after the inciting stimulus has been removed. This is often seen in patients with chronic renal failure and secondary hyperparathyroidism who undergo renal transplantation. Tertiary hyperparathyroidism is commonly due to hyperplasia of all four glands, and children with this condition are candidates for total parathyroidectomy with autotransplantation.

□ Adrenal Glands

ANATOMY

The adrenal gland is made up of the cortex and the medulla. The adrenal cortex arises from embryonic mesoderm and is divided into three zones. The zona glomerulosa is the site of aldosterone production, and the zona fasciculata and the zona reticularis of the adrenal cortex produce cortisol, androgens, and small amounts of estrogens. The adrenal medulla is ectodermal in origin, arising from neural crest cells. It is innervated by preganglionic sympathetic nerves from the celiac plexus and synthesizes epinephrine, norepinephrine, and a small amount of dopamine.

Three arteries supply the adrenal gland. The superior adrenal artery is a branch of the inferior phrenic artery, the middle adrenal artery comes directly off the aorta, and the inferior adrenal artery arises from the renal artery. The right adrenal vein drains directly into the inferior vena cava, whereas the left adrenal vein enters the left renal vein.

ADRENAL MASSES

The differential diagnosis of adrenal lesions in childhood is listed in Table 75–6. Neuroblastoma accounts for greater than 90% of all childhood adrenal cancers. Computed tomography (CT) is about 80% sensitive for tumors 1 cm in size and almost 100% sensitive for 3- to 4-cm tumors. In most cases, CT cannot distinguish between functional and nonfunctional tumors or between malignant and benign disease.

Hypercortisolism, or Cushing's syndrome, is caused by the exogenous administration of corticosteroids, excessive endogenous production of corticosteroids, or uncontrolled pituitary production of adrenocorticotrophic hormone (ACTH). Patients exhibit hypertension, thin skin with easy bruising, acne, hirsutism, abdominal striae, muscle weakness, glucose intolerance, osteoporosis, menstrual irregu-

TABLE 75–6. Differential Diagnosis
of an Adrenal Mass

Functional Tumors

Adrenal adenoma
Adrenocortical carcinoma
Pheochromocytoma

Nonfunctional Tumors

Neuroblastoma
Adrenal cyst
Hemangioma
Leiomyoma
Leiomyosarcoma
Non-Hodgkin's lymphoma
Malignant melanoma

Metastatic Disease to the Adrenal Gland

Squamous cell carcinoma of the lung
Hepatocellular carcinoma
Breast cancer

Traumatic Adrenal Hemorrhage

Neonatal child abuse

larity, and psychiatric disturbances. Growth retardation and weight gain are common pediatric symptoms.[55] Infants tend to demonstrate generalized obesity, whereas older children may demonstrate the typical truncal obesity.[56]

Exogenous steroid administration is the most common cause of Cushing's syndrome in both children and adults. Endogenous causes of Cushing's syndrome can be broadly divided into ACTH-independent and ACTH-dependent causes (Table 75–7). Of the ACTH-independent causes, adrenal adenomas and adrenocortical carcinomas are more common in children younger than age 7 years, whereas hyperplasia predominates in older children and adults.[56, 57] ACTH-dependent Cushing's disease is caused by a pituitary microadenoma or more rarely by a macroadenoma, and it is the second most common cause of Cushing's syndrome in pediatric patients. The ACTH-dependent disease occurs in peripubertal patients who are first seen with weight

TABLE 75–7. Etiology of Cushing's Syndrome

Exogenous corticosteroid administration

ACTH-Dependent Causes

Cushing's disease (pituitary adenoma)
Ectopic ACTH production
Small cell bronchogenic carcinoma
Carcinoid tumors
Pancreatic islet cell carcinoma
Thymoma
Medullary thyroid carcinoma
Pheochromocytoma

ACTH-Independent Causes

Adrenal adenoma
Adrenocortical carcinoma
Adrenal hyperplasia

ACTH, adrenocorticotropic hormone.

gain and growth delay. Finally, hypercortisolism can rarely be caused by ectopic production of ACTH by tumors. In children, this is most frequently due to bronchial carcinoids. Other tumors that can produce ACTH are pulmonary neoplasms, neuroblastomas, pancreatic islet cell carcinomas, thymomas, carcinoids, medullary thyroid carcinomas, and pheochromocytomas.

The initial phase in the diagnosis of Cushing's syndrome is to screen for the syndrome; the second phase is to determine its etiology. Screening for Cushing's syndrome can be accomplished by measuring the plasma cortisol (normal levels are 15 to 20 µg/dl) at 8:00 AM and 6:00 PM to coincide with the diurnal variation in plasma cortisol, which is lost in Cushing's syndrome. The most sensitive screening test is the 24-hour urinary 17-hydroxycorticosteroid or free cortisol, which is greater than 150 µg/day in patients with Cushing's syndrome. The overnight dexamethasone suppression test is performed by administering 1 mg at 11:00 PM and measuring the plasma cortisol level the following morning at 8:00 AM. In normal individuals, ACTH is suppressed and the cortisol level is decreased by 50% or more of baseline (<5 µg/dl). This dose of dexamethasone is insufficient to cause suppression in patients with Cushing's syndrome.

Once established, further tests are used to determine the specific cause. The high-dose dexamethasone suppression test is used to distinguish pituitary causes from nonpituitary causes. An oral dose of 2 mg of dexamethasone is given every 6 hours for 48 hours (or 40 µg/kg/dose for infants). Urine is then collected for 24 hours to measure free cortisol and 17-hydroxysteroids. In patients with a pituitary neoplasm, the steroid excretion levels are suppressed to 50% of baseline. In patients with an adrenal adenoma or adrenocortical carcinoma and most patients with tumors that produce ACTH, the levels are not suppressed. Plasma ACTH levels are generally low or normal with adrenal causes of hypercortisolism, modestly elevated with pituitary neoplasms, and extremely elevated with tumors producing ectopic ACTH.

Magnetic resonance imaging (MRI) is the diagnostic study of choice for localizing pituitary lesions causing Cushing's disease. If the MRI of the pituitary gland is negative or equivocal, bilateral inferior petrosal sinus sampling can be performed to identify the source of ACTH.

Treatment of pituitary adenomas is transsphenoidal hypophysectomy, which leads to remission in about 85% of patients.[55] Treatment alternatives include mitotane (*o,p'*-DDD), pituitary radiation, and bilateral adrenalectomy, which should be performed as a last resort because this may actually stimulate pituitary tumor growth. Other symptoms and signs known as *Nelson's syndrome* are high ACTH levels and hyperpigmentation.

ADRENOCORTICAL CARCINOMA

Adrenocortical carcinomas have a bimodal age distribution, commonly presenting in the first and fifth decades of life. These tumors are rare in children, accounting for about 0.2% of all pediatric neoplasms.[58] Adrenocortical carcinoma has been associated with p53 mutations and the Li-Fraumeni and Beckwith-Wiedemann syndromes. Patients with adrenocortical cancer also have a higher incidence of other primary malignancies, especially medulloblastoma and astrocytoma.[59, 60] Adrenocortical carcinomas are aggressive tumors, with a mean survival of 2.9 months reported in patients with untreated tumors.[56] Patients are often seen late with stage III or IV disease.

About 95% of the adrenocortical carcinomas in children are functional, producing cortisol, aldosterone, androgens, or estrogens. Some tumors may synthesize more than one hormone, resulting in mixed syndromes. In children, 70 to 95% of adrenocortical carcinomas produce androgens that cause virilization rather than Cushing's syndrome. Boys with precocious puberty or girls with virilization should be evaluated for adrenocortical carcinoma. Rare reports of feminization by production of estrogens have been documented.

About 50% of patients with adrenocortical carcinoma have a palpable abdominal mass, although it is rarely a presenting complaint. In addition to having signs of virilization, children with adrenocortical carcinoma may have vague systemic symptoms including abdominal pain, weight loss, weakness, nausea, and anorexia. Adrenocortical carcinoma may metastasize to lungs, liver, and lymph nodes and rarely to brain, bone, or kidney. Nonfunctional tumors are rare and tend to have a more aggressive course.

Evaluation includes measurement of urinary 17-ketosteroids (androgen metabolites), 17-hydroxycorticosteroids (cortisol metabolites), urinary free cortisol, and serum testosterone and cortisol levels. The high-dose dexamethasone suppression test may be helpful in identifying Cushing's syndrome. Evaluation should also include CT scan of the chest, abdomen, and pelvis to determine the extent of the tumor and to evaluate for metastatic disease.

The only chance for cure is complete surgical resection of the tumor. However, debulking hormonally productive tumors may provide symptomatic relief to patients. Mitotane, or o,p'-DDD, is an adrenolytic agent that selectively causes adrenal gland necrosis and has been the most widely used chemotherapeutic agent. It is used for metastatic disease, for incompletely excised tumors, and for the hormonal effects of the tumors. Aminoglutethimide and metyrapone have also been used to ameliorate the symptoms related to hormone production. Mitotane has shown some limited benefit in the chemotherapeutic treatment of these tumors, eliciting a response in about one third of treated cases.[61]

The prognosis depends on the child's age and the resectability of the tumor. In one review of 55 children with adrenocortical carcinoma, the 2-year survival rates were 82% for children younger than 2 years old and 29% for children older than 2 years.

Survival rates were more than 67% if the tumors were completely excised, but there were no survivors after partial resection.[62] In another study, a mean survival of 5 years was reported for resectable tumors, with a mean 2.3-year survival for those with disease beyond the gland.[63]

Primary Hyperaldosteronism

Primary hyperaldosteronism is caused by the excessive production of aldosterone with consequent suppression of renin. In children, adrenocortical hyperplasia is the most common cause of primary hyperaldosteronism.[56] Rarely, primary hyperaldosteronism is caused by bilateral adrenal adenomas or adrenocortical carcinoma. Conn's syndrome, in which primary hyperaldosteronism is due to a unilateral adrenal adenoma, is rare but has been reported in children.[64] In adults, Conn's syndrome is the most common cause of primary hyperaldosteronism, occurring in 65 to 80% of cases, whereas bilateral adrenal hyperplasia of the zona glomerulosa causes primary hyperaldosteronism in 10 to 35% of cases.

Symptoms of primary hyperaldosteronism are generally vague. Patients have hypertension, muscle weakness, polydipsia, and polyuria. Hyperaldosteronism increases the total body sodium level and consequently increases the total body fluid volume. Renin and angiotensin formation is suppressed.

The diagnosis should be entertained in any child with hypertension and hypokalemia. Initial screening in children with hypertension involves checking a potassium level. Hypokalemia (<3.5 mEq/l) is consistent with primary hyperaldosteronism. The aldosterone level is elevated, the renin level is suppressed, and patients frequently also have a metabolic alkalosis. The diagnosis is confirmed by administering a saline load challenge; hypokalemia develops in patients with primary hyperaldosteronism, and they have high urinary potassium (>40 to 60 mEq/day) and aldosterone excretion. A high-sodium diet can be administered for 3 to 5 days, which fails to suppress aldosterone in patients with hyperaldosteronism. The serum aldosterone level must be drawn in the morning before the patient has arisen from the supine position.

Once established, it is important to distinguish between an aldosterone-secreting adenoma and bilateral adrenal hyperplasia. Aldosterone-secreting tumors generally produce much higher levels of aldosterone (>100 μg/dl) than are produced by adrenal hyperplasia. NP-59, or ^{131}I-6-β-iodomethyl-19-norcholesterol, is a cholesterol analogue that is taken up as cholesterol in the steroidogenic pathway. Dexamethasone suppression of ACTH-dependent adrenocortical tissue is followed by NP-59 administration. An adenoma is suggested if there is asymmetric adrenal uptake after 48 hours, whereas bilateral hyperplasia is suggested if the uptake is symmetric after 72 hours.

The treatment of a functional adrenal adenoma is

excision. The mortality rate from operative removal is generally less than 1%, with a cure rate of 75%. Treatment for patients with bilateral adrenal hyperplasia is with spironolactone.

Pheochromocytoma

A pheochromocytoma is a medullary adrenal tumor that produces an excess of catecholamines. About 90% of children demonstrate sustained catecholamine elevation, and 10% are episodically elevated. The catecholamines cause hypertension, tachycardia, sweating, headaches, and nervousness. Excessive catecholamines can produce a catecholamine-induced cardiomyopathy. Pheochromocytomas account for approximately 1% of hypertensive children, and they present at a mean age of 8 to 10 years.[65]

Only 10% of all pheochromocytomas are found in children.[66] Approximately 10% of pheochromocytomas are familial and may be associated with other syndromes such as the Hippel-Lindau syndrome, Recklinghausen's disease, tuberous sclerosis, Sturge-Weber syndrome, or MEN 2A or MEN 2B.[67] Familial pheochromocytomas independent of these syndromes have also been described.[68] In children, pheochromocytomas are more frequently associated with MEN 2 syndromes than in adults; pheochromocytomas associated with the MEN 2 syndrome are more likely to be bilateral and benign.

Pheochromocytomas are most common in the adrenal medulla, but they are found in extraadrenal locations in 30 to 40% of children.[69] Extraadrenal pheochromocytomas may be paravertebral, at the aortic bifurcation, and near the bladder. They have been reported in the neck and within the cranium.[70] Pheochromocytomas are bilateral in 25 to 30% of children, in contrast to only 10% of adults. About 3 to 6% of childhood pheochromocytomas are malignant.

A 24-hour urine sample for epinephrine and norepinephrine and their metabolites—metanephrine and vanillylmandelic acid—is needed to establish the diagnosis. CT and MRI can be useful in localizing the lesion. An isotope scan using ^{131}I-methaiodobenzylguanidine (MIBG), a norepinephrine analogue that accumulates in the storage vesicles in adrenal tumors, can be useful in locating extraadrenal tumors. Occasionally, selective adrenal venous sampling may be necessary to localize tumors that cannot be located by other means.

Preoperative preparation of the patient with a pheochromocytoma is crucial. These patients have an extracellular fluid volume deficit caused by chronic vasoconstriction, and a 2- to 3-week preoperative course using the α-blocking agent phenoxybenzamine makes up the volume deficit. If the patient is hypertensive or tachycardic, it may be necessary to add a β-blocker such as propranolol. Congestive heart failure may result if the α-blockade is not done before administering a β-blocker. This is especially important in patients with a catecholamine-induced cardiomyopathy.

A transabdominal surgical approach is generally used to allow evaluation of the contralateral adrenal gland and exploration for extraadrenal sites of tumor. It is important to isolate and ligate the adrenal vein early and to minimize manipulation of the tumor. Complete resection of a pheochromocytoma is considered curative, with an operative mortality rate of less than 3%. Metastatic disease should be removed, if possible. The contralateral adrenal gland should probably not be removed, especially if hyperplasia is identified in patients with MEN 2, because it may be many years before another pheochromocytoma develops.[71]

Chemotherapy should be considered preoperatively to shrink unresectable tumors and to treat residual and metastatic disease.[72] Radioactive MIBG has also been used to treat metastatic disease.[73] Following tumor resection, patients should be followed up throughout life for evidence of recurrence, which is highest in patients with MEN 2 in whom the most common site is the contralateral adrenal gland.[74–76]

CONGENITAL ADRENAL HYPERPLASIA

Congenital adrenal hyperplasia presents as a disorder of sexual ambiguity; it is discussed extensively in Chapter 61.

□ Precocious Puberty

In boys, precocious puberty is defined as the development of secondary sexual characteristics before the age of 9 years. In girls, the development of breasts (thelarche) before the age of 7.5 years, the development of pubic hair (pubarche) before the age of 8.5 years, or the onset of menses (menarche) before the age of 9.5 years is considered precocious. Precocious puberty can be complete or incomplete.

True or complete precocious puberty is due to the premature maturation of the hypothalamic-pituitary axis and results in gonadal enlargement as well as premature development of secondary sexual characteristics. The secondary sexual characteristics that develop in true precocious puberty are appropriate for the sex of the child and merely occur at a younger-than-appropriate age. In incomplete or pseudoprecocious puberty, only one secondary sexual characteristic develops prematurely, and it may or may not be appropriate for the patient's gender. Pseudoprecocious puberty is not due to pituitary gonadotropin secretion; rather, it is due to production of human chorionic gonadotropin (hCG), luteinizing hormone (LH), follicle-stimulating hormone (FSH), androgens, or estrogens, or it is due to stimulation of their receptors by the tumors.

PRECOCIOUS PUBERTY IN GIRLS

True precocious puberty, resulting from a premature activation of the hypothalamic-pituitary axis, is idiopathic in 75 to 95% of girls. The condition may be constitutional, that is, a normal variant that is simply at the younger age of a normal distribution curve. Neurogenic disturbances can cause true precocious puberty by interfering with inhibitory signals from the central nervous system (CNS) to the hypothalamus or by producing excitatory signals. Neurogenic disorders may include hydrocephalus, cerebral palsy, trauma, irradiation, chronic inflammatory disorder, or tumors, including hypothalamic hamartomas or pineal tumors.

McCune-Albright syndrome is an interesting disorder that can cause either true precocious puberty or pseudoprecocious puberty. Patients have a classic triad of precocious puberty, café-au-lait nevi with irregular "coast of Maine" borders, and polyostotic fibrous dysplasia. In these patients, autonomously functioning ovarian follicular cysts may develop, causing precocious puberty (see Chapter 73). Excess production of LH, FSH, or prolactin by pituitary adenomas has also been described. Other endocrine abnormalities, including acromegaly, Cushing's syndrome, and hyperthyroidism have been associated with this syndrome.[77]

Incomplete precocious puberty generally presents as isolated premature breast development (thelarche) or premature growth of pubic hair (pubarche). Premature pubarche is frequently caused by androgen excess. Isolated prepubertal menses is rare, and prepubertal vaginal bleeding is usually caused by a foreign body, sexual abuse, or tumors of the genital tract. Incomplete precocious puberty can be a normal variant or can be due to the production of hormones from neuroendocrine, adrenal, ovarian, or exogenous sources. In the Van Wyk-Grumbach syndrome, premature breast development is associated with hypothyroidism. Unlike most other causes of precocious puberty, growth is inhibited rather than stimulated. This syndrome may be due to the shared α-subunit of LH, FSH, and TSH. Tumors that produce excess quantities of LH or hCG can cause virilization.

PRECOCIOUS PUBERTY IN BOYS

As with girls, true precocious puberty in boys may be neurogenic, constitutional, or idiopathic. However, in boys, true precocious puberty is more often neurogenic than idiopathic.

The most common CNS tumor that causes precocious puberty is a hamartoma of the tuber cinereum. These hamartomas are ectopic hypothalamic tissue connected to the posterior hypothalamus. Because they are nonprogressive tumors and are in a surgically precarious location, they are generally treated with gonadotropin-releasing hormone (GnRH) agonists. Other disorders that can cause precocious puberty in boys are gliomas of the optic nerve or hypothalamus, astrocytomas, choriocarcinomas, meningiomas, rhabdomyosarcomas, neurofibrosarcomas, nonlymphocytic leukemia, ependymomas, neurofibromatosis type I, and germinomas. Other space-occupying lesions or causes of increased intracranial

pressure such as head trauma, suprasellar cysts, granulomas, brain irradiation, and hydrocephalus can also cause true precocious puberty. Some of these tumors or CNS conditions can cause both precocious puberty and growth hormone deficiency. In these patients, the growth rate may appear normal because the testosterone stimulates growth and compensates for the deficiency of growth hormone. However, the degree of growth is inadequate for the degree of pubertal development.

Incomplete precocious puberty can be caused by autonomous production of androgens or hCG. With many types of incomplete precocious puberty, the testes are not enlarged as they are with true precocious puberty. As with girls, the McCune-Albright syndrome can cause either true or pseudoprecocious puberty. Tumors producing hCG such as teratomas, chorioepitheliomas, hepatomas, hepatoblastomas, or germinomas of the pineal gland may lead to Leydig cell stimulation. Testotoxicosis is an autosomal recessive disorder in which premature Leydig cell maturation causes incomplete precocious puberty. The etiology in some families is due to the constitutive stimulation of the LH receptor and can cause the onset of precocious puberty at 1 to 4 years of age. Ketoconazole, spironolactone, and testolactone can be used to treat this disorder.

Excess androgen production causing virilization can be caused by congenital adrenal hyperplasia, specifically the 21-hydroxylase or the 11-hydroxylase enzymatic defects. During embryonic development, adrenal rests may be left in the testes. In untreated adrenal hyperplasia, ACTH stimulation may cause their enlargement and the secretion of androgens. These testes have an irregular appearance. Excess testosterone production can also be caused by interstitial cell tumors of the testes. Finally, exogenous administration of androgens or hCG (for undescended testes) can cause precocious puberty.

EVALUATION

For both boys and girls, evaluation of precocious puberty begins with a thorough history and physical examination. The Tanner stage should be carefully documented. In boys, the size and shape of the testes should be noted. In true precocious puberty, the testes generally enlarge symmetrically, whereas asymmetric or nodular enlargement is noted with Leydig cell tumors or adrenal rests. Feminization in boys may present as gynecomastia. The patient's height and weight should be measured and the growth curve should be examined. The bone age should also be determined. If the bone age and the height age closely correlate, it is likely that the presenting symptom is an extreme variant of normal. This simply requires close follow-up in 6 months to verify the diagnosis. However, if the bone age is abnormally accelerated relative to the height age, further investigation is warranted.

Serum estradiol, testosterone, and dehydroepiandrosterone sulfate (DHEAS) levels should be obtained. In girls, a vaginal smear for estrogen effect may be more sensitive than a serum estradiol level. Significantly elevated DHEAS levels are typically seen in adrenal tumors. Evidence of association with other syndromes may warrant measuring other hormone levels including prolactin, thyroid hormone, or cortisol. A GnRH test can be useful in determining whether the patient has complete or incomplete precocious puberty. Patients with true precocious puberty respond to GnRH with a typical pubertal pattern, whereas those with pseudoprecocious puberty have a minimal response to gonadotropin. Alternatively, a sleep-related increase in plasma LH levels can be diagnostic but is more cumbersome to obtain. In patients with feminizing or masculinizing features, US is useful to locate abdominal or pelvic masses. MRI should be used in patients with true precocious puberty to locate potential intracranial lesions.

TREATMENT

In general, tumors causing precocious puberty should be removed if they are surgically accessible. A number of agents have been used in the medical treatment of precocious puberty. True (gonadotropin-dependent) precocious puberty can be treated with GnRH agonists. Although initially these agents stimulate gonadotropin secretion, ultimately, GnRH receptors are down-regulated and LH and FSH secretion is subsequently decreased. Examples of GnRH agonists include deslorelin, buserelin, nafarelin, leuprolide, and triptorelin.

Other medications have been used in the medical treatment of incomplete precocious puberty. Medroxyprogesterone acetate, a progestational agent, can halt the progression of secondary sexual characteristic development and can prevent menstruation. It is not as effective, however, in slowing bone maturation. Ketoconazole is an antifungal agent that also inhibits the synthesis of testosterone by blocking the conversion of 17-hydroxyprogesterone to androstenedione. Testolactone competitively inhibits the aromatase enzyme that converts androgens to estrogens. Androgen antagonists include cyproterone acetate and spironolactone.

☐ Carcinoid Tumors

Carcinoid tumors arise from Kulchitsky cells, a type of enterochromaffin cell belonging to the APUD (amine precursor uptake and decarboxylation) family of cells. Carcinoid tumors can be broadly categorized according to their site of origin: the foregut, the midgut, and the hindgut. Foregut tumors account for approximately 5% of carcinoid tumors and can arise in the bronchus, stomach, or duodenum. Midgut tumors account for about 80 to 85% of carcinoid tumors. The majority of carcinoids arise from the appendix (46%), followed by the jejunum and ileum (28%), and the rectum (17%). Carcinoid tumors have also been found to arise from ovarian teratomas.

INTESTINAL CARCINOIDS

Intestinal carcinoids arise from Kulchitsky cells that normally reside in the crypts of Lieberkühn. Although most patients with carcinoid tumors are asymptomatic, those with symptoms may complain of obstruction, pain, or bleeding. Intestinal carcinoid tumors can cause an intense desmoplastic reaction in the mesentery, which shortens the mesentery and can narrow and kink the bowel.

Most appendiceal carcinoids are discovered incidentally when appendicitis develops. Carcinoid tumors in the midgut, and particularly those that have metastasized to the liver, may exhibit signs of the carcinoid syndrome, which include intermittent flushing, diarrhea, abdominal pain, and bronchoconstriction. These symptoms are likely related to serotonin, tachykinins, and other hormones secreted by the tumors that act on gastrointestinal and vascular smooth muscle. Serotonin is metabolized into 5-hydroxyindoleacetic acid (5-HIAA) in the liver and lungs and is subsequently excreted in the urine. Increased levels of vasoactive amines can eventually lead to the development of right-sided endocardial and valvular fibrosis.

Most appendiceal carcinoid tumors appear near the tip of the appendix and are benign. Even those that are malignant generally have a fairly indolent course. Tumors that are smaller than 2 cm rarely metastasize, whereas more than 80% of those greater than 2 cm have metastasized at the time of diagnosis.

Most pediatric patients are first seen with appendiceal carcinoids less than 2 cm, which can be treated with simple appendectomy. Right hemicolectomy is indicated for tumors greater than 2 cm, those close to the cecum, and those with mucin production.[78] Palliation for hepatic metastases can include hepatic arterial embolization or chemotherapy. For patients with symptoms of carcinoid syndrome, octreotide, a somatostatin analogue, frequently provides symptomatic relief.

Carcinoids are fairly indolent tumors. In one retrospective series of 40 children with appendiceal carcinoids, no recurrences or metastases were reported.[79] In adults, 5-year survival with complete resection is 75% and with hepatic metastases is 20%.[79-81]

BRONCHIAL CARCINOIDS

Bronchial carcinoids are the most common primary lung tumors in children. These tumors can secrete serotonin or 5-HIAA. They most frequently present with recurrent or persistent pneumonia secondary to obstruction of the bronchus by the tumor. Children commonly are seen with wheezing, atelectasis, and weight loss, in addition to the cough, pneumonitis, and hemoptysis that are frequently seen in adult patients.

Bronchial carcinoids can be diagnosed by bronchoscopy; they have a characteristic pink, friable mulberry appearance. In general, biopsy should not be attempted because the carcinoids have a propensity to hemorrhage, and usually these tumors have a classic gross appearance. If there is no evidence of lymph node involvement, segmental bronchial resection can be performed. However, lobectomy or pneumonectomy is usually required for treatment. These tumors are radiosensitive, and radiotherapy can be considered for unresectable disease. The prognosis following complete resection is excellent, with a 10-year survival rate of approximately 90%.[82, 83]

REFERENCES

1. Rallison ML, Dobyns BM, Meikle AW, et al: Natural history of thyroid abnormalities: Prevalence, incidence, and regression of thyroid diseases in adolescents and young adults. Am J Med 91:363–370, 1991.
2. Epstein FH: The molecular basis of thyroid hormone action. N Engl J Med 331:847–853, 1994.
3. Ahren B: Regulatory peptides in the thyroid gland—a review on their localization and function. Acta Endocrinologica 124:225–232, 1991.
4. Ito M, Yamashita S, Ashizawa K, et al: Childhood thyroid diseases around Chernobyl evaluated by ultrasound examination and fine needle aspiration cytology. Thyroid 5:365–368, 1995.
5. Jaksic J, Dumic M, Filipovic B, et al: Thyroid disease in a school population with thyromegaly. Arch Dis Child 70:103–106, 1994.
6. Fisher DA, Pandian MR, Carlton E: Autoimmune thyroid disease: An expanding spectrum. Pediatr Clin North Am 34:907–918, 1987.
7. Dayan CM, Daniels GH: Chronic autoimmune thyroiditis. N Engl J Med 335:99–107, 1996.
8. Rother KI, Zimmerman D, Schwenk WF: Effect of thyroid hormone treatment on thyromegaly in children and adolescents with Hashimoto disease. J Pediatr 124:599–601, 1994.
9. Tomer Y, Davies TF: Infection, thyroid disease, and autoimmunity. Endocrine Rev 14:107–120, 1993.
10. Phillips DI, Barker DJ, Rees Smith B, et al: The geographical distribution of thyrotoxicosis in England according to the presence or absence of TSH-receptor antibodies. Clin Endocrinol 23:283–287, 1985.
11. Franklyn JA: The management of hyperthyroidism. N Engl J Med 330:1731–1738, 1994.
12. Lippe BM, Landaw EM, Kaplan SA: Hyperthyroidism in children treated with long-term medical therapy: Twenty-five percent remission every two years. J Clin Endocrinol Metab 64:1241–1245, 1987.
13. Hashizume K, Ichikawa K, Sakurai A, et al: Administration of thyroxine in treated Graves' disease: Effects on the level of antibodies to thyroid-stimulating hormone receptors and on the risk of recurrence of hyperthyroidism. N Engl J Med 324:947–953, 1991.
14. McIver B, Rae P, Beckett G, et al: Lack of effect of thyroxin in patients with Graves' hyperthyroidism who are treated with an antithyroid drug. N Engl J Med 334:220–224, 1996.
15. Waldhausen JHT: Controversies related to the medical and surgical management of hyperthyroidism in children. Semin Pediatr Surg 6:121–127, 1997.
16. Berglund J, Christensen SB, Dymling JF, et al: The incidence of recurrence and hypothyroidism following treatment with antithyroid drugs, surgery, or radioiodine in all patients with thyrotoxicosis in Malmo during the period 1970–1974. J Intern Med 229:435–442, 1991.
17. Klein I, Becker DV, Levey GS: Treatment of hyperthyroid disease. Ann Intern Med 121:281–288, 1994.
18. Clark JD, Gelfand MJ, Elgazzar AH: Iodine-131 therapy of hyperthyroidism in pediatric patients. J Nucl Med 36:442–445, 1995.
19. Hung W, Anderson KD, Chandra RS, et al: Solitary thyroid nodules in 71 children and adolescents. J Pediatr Surg 27:1407–1409, 1992.
20. Desjardins JG, Khan AH, Montupet P, et al: Management of thyroid nodules in children: A 20-year experience. J Pediatr Surg 22:736–739, 1987.
21. Yip FWK, Reeve TS, Poole AG, et al: Thyroid nodules in childhood and adolescence. Aust N Z J Surg 64:676–678, 1994.
22. Raab SS, Silverman JF, Elsheikh TM, et al: Pediatric thyroid nodules: Disease demographics and clinical management by fine needle aspirajion biopsy. Pediatrics 95:46–49, 1995.
23. Mazzaferri EL: Management of a solitary thyroid nodule. N Engl J Med 328:553–559, 1993.
24. Newman KD: The current management of thyroid tumors in childhood. Semin Pediatr Surg 2:69–74, 1993.
25. Nikiforov Y, Gnepp DR: Pediatric thyroid cancer after the Chernobyl disaster: Pathomorphologic study of 84 cases (1991–1992) from the Republic of Belarus. Cancer 74:748–765, 1994.
26. Smith MB, Xue H, Strong L, et al: Forty-year experience with second malignancies after treatment of childhood cancer: Analysis of outcome following the development of the second malignancy. J Pediatr Surg 28:1342–1349, 1993.
27. Lemoine NR, Mayall ES, Wyllie FS, et al: Activated ras mutations in human thyroid cancers. Cancer Res 48:4459–4463, 1988.
28. Lemoine NR, Mayall ES, Wyllie FS, et al: High frequency of ras oncogene activation in all stages of thyroid tumorigenesis. Oncogene 4:159–164, 1989.
29. Bongarzone I, Butti MG, Coronelli S, et al: Frequent activation of ret protooncogene by fusion with a new activating gene in papillary thyroid carcinomas. Cancer Res 54:2979–2985, 1994.
30. Sozzi G, Bongarzone I, Miozzo M, et al: A t(10;17) translocation creates the RET/PTC2 chimeric transforming sequence in papillary thyroid carcinoma. Genes Chrom Cancer 9:244–250, 1994.
31. Paschke RP, Ludgate M: The thyrotropin receptor in thyroid diseases. N Engl J Med 337:1675–1681, 1997.
32. Eng C, Smith DP, Mulligan LM, et al: Point mutation within the tyrosine kinase domain of the RET proto-oncogene in multiple endocrine neoplasia type 2B and related sporadic tumours. Hum Mol Genet 3:237–241, 1994.
33. Harness JA, Thompson NW, McLeod MK, et al: Differentiated thyroid carcinoma in children and adolescents. World J Surg 16:547–554, 1992.
34. Ceccarelli C, Pacini F, Lippi F, et al: Thyroid cancer in children and adolescents. Surgery 104:1143–1148, 1988.
35. Schlumberger M, De Vathaire F, Travagli JP, et al: Differentiated thyroid carcinoma in childhood: Long term follow-up in 72 patients. J Clin Endocrinol Metab 65:1088–1094, 1987.
36. La Quaglia MP, Corbally MT, Heller G, et al: Recurrence and morbidity in differentiated thyroid carcinoma in children. Surgery 104:1149–1156, 1988.
37. Zimmerman D, Hay ID, Gough IR, et al: Papillary thyroid carcinoma in children and adults: Long-term follow-up of 1039 patients conservatively treated at one institution during three decades. Surgery 104:1157–1163, 1988.
38. de Roy van Zuidewijn DBW, Songun I, Kievit J, et al: Complications of thyroid surgery. Ann Surg Oncol 2:56–60, 1995.
39. Nishida T, Nakao K, Hamaji M, et al: Preservation of recurrent laryngeal nerve invaded by differentiated thyroid cancer. Ann Surg 226:85–91, 1997.
40. Wells SA Jr, Farndon JR, Dale JK, et al: Long term evaluation of patients with primary parathyroid hyperplasia managed by total parathyroidectomy and heterotopic autotransplantation. Ann Surg 192:451–458, 1980.
41. Skinner MA, Norton JA, Moley JF, et al: Heterotopic autotransplantation of parathyroid tissue in children undergoing total thyroidectomy. J Pediatr Surg 32:510–513, 1997.

42. Vassilopoulou-Sellin R, Klein MJ, Smith TH, et al: Pulmonary metastases in children and young adults with differentiated thyroid cancer. Cancer 71:1348–1352, 1993.
43. Mazzaferri EL: Thyroid remnant ^{131}I ablation for papillary and follicular thyroid carcinoma. Thyroid 7:265–271, 1997.
44. Kirk JM, Mort C, Grant DB, et al: The usefulness of serum thyroglobulin in the follow-up of differentiated thyroid carcinoma. Med Pediatr Oncol 20:201–208, 1992.
45. Samaan NA, Draznin MB, Halpin RE, et al: Multiple endocrine syndrome type IIb in early childhood. Cancer 68:1832–1834, 1991.
46. Gorlin JB, Sallan SE: Thyroid cancer in childhood. Endocrinol Metab Clin North Am 19:649–662, 1990.
47. Wells SA Jr, Chi DD, Toshima K, et al: Predictive DNA testing and prophylactic thyroidectomy in patients at risk for multiple endocrine neoplasia type 2A. Ann Surg 220:237–250, 1994.
48. Skinner MA, DeBenedetti MK, Moley JF, et al: Medullary thyroid carcinoma in children with multiple endocrine neoplasia types 2A and 2B. J Pediatr Surg 31:177–182, 1996.
49. Telander RL, Zimmerman D, van Heerden JA, et al: Results of early thyroidectomy for multiple endocrine neoplasia type 2. J Pediatr Surg 21:1190–1194, 1986.
50. Ross AJ, III: Parathyroid surgery in children. Prog Pediatr Surg 26:48–59, 1991.
51. Howe JR, Norton JA, Wells SA Jr: Prevalence of pheochromocytoma and hyperparathyroidism in multiple endocrine neoplasia type 2A: Results of long-term follow-up. Surgery 114:1070–1077, 1993.
52. Ross AJ, III, Cooper A, Attie MF, et al: Primary hyperparathyroidism in infancy. J Pediatr Surg 21:493–499, 1986.
53. Kulczycka H, Kaminski W, Wozniewicz B, et al: Primary hyperparathyroidism in infancy: Diagnostic and therapeutic difficulties. Klin Padiatr 203:116–118, 1991.
54. Pollak MR, Brown EM, Chou YH, et al: Mutations in the Ca(2+)-sensing receptor gene cause familial hypocalciuric hypercalcemia and neonatal severe hyperparathyroidism. Cell 75:1297–1330, 1993.
55. Magiakou MA, Mastorakos G, Oldfield EH, et al: Cushing's syndrome in children and adolescents. Presentation, diagnosis, and therapy. N Engl J Med 331:629–636, 1994.
56. Chudler RM, Kay R: Adrenocortical carcinoma in children. 16:469–479, 1989.
57. Grua JR, Nelson DH: ACTH-producing pituitary tumors. Endocrinol Metab Clin North Am 20:319–362, 1991.
58. Federici S, Galli G, Ceccarelli PL, et al: Adrenocortical tumors in children: A report of 12 cases. Eur J Pediatr Surg 4:21–25, 1994.
59. Wagner J, Portwine C, Rabin K, et al: High frequency of germline p53 mutations in childhood adrenocortical cancer. J Natl Cancer Inst 86:1707–1710, 1994.
60. Birch JM, Hartley AL, Tricker KJ, et al: Prevalence and diversity of constitutional mutations in the p53 gene among 21 Li-Fraumeni families. Cancer Res 54:1298–1304, 1994.
61. Teinturier C, Brugieres L, Lemerle J, et al: Adrenocortical carcinoma in children: Retrospective study of 54 cases. Arch Pediatr 3:235–240, 1996.
62. Sabbaga CC, Avilla SG, Schulz C, et al: Adrenocortical carcinoma in children: Clinical aspects and prognosis. J Pediatr Surg 28:841–843, 1993.
63. Cohn K, Gottesman L, Brennan M: Adrenocortical carcinoma. Surg 100:1170–1177, 1986.
64. Abasiyanik A, Oran B, Kaymakci A, et al: Conn syndrome in a child, caused by adrenal adenoma. J Pediatr Surg 31:430–432, 1996.
65. Januszewicz P, Wieteska-Klimczak A, Wyszynska T: Pheochromocytoma in children: Difficulties in diagnosis and localization. Clin Exp Hypertens 12:571–579, 1990.
66. Revillon Y, Daher P, Jan D, et al: Pheochromocytoma in children: 15 cases. J Pediatr Surg 27:910–911, 1992.
67. Gross DJ, Avishai N, Meiner V, et al: Familial pheochromocytoma associated with a novel mutation in the von Hippel-Lindau gene. J Clin Endocrinol Metab 81:147–149, 1996.
68. Albanese CT, Wiener ES: Routine total bilateral adrenalectomy is not warranted in childhood familial pheochromocytoma. J Pediatr Surg 28:1248–1251, 1993.
69. Atiyeh BA, Barakat AJ, Abumrad NN: Extra-adrenal pheochromocytoma. J Nephrol 10:25–29, 1997.
70. Kudoh Y, Kuroda S, Shimamoto K, et al: Intracranial pheochromocytoma—a case of noradrenaline-secreting glomus jugulare tumor. Jpn Circ J 59:365–371, 1995.
71. Lairmore TC, Ball DW, Baylin SB, et al: Management of pheochromocytomas in patients with the multiple endocrine neoplasia type 2 syndromes. Ann Surg 217:595–603, 1993.
72. Ein SH, Weitzman S, Thorner P, et al: Pediatric malignant pheochromocytoma. J Pediatr Surg 29:1197–1201, 1994.
73. Perel Y, Schlumberger M, Marguerite G, et al: Pheochromocytoma and paraganglioma in children: A report of 24 cases of the French Society of Pediatric Oncology. Pediatr Hematol Oncol 14:413–422, 1997.
74. Svab J, Navratil P: Experience with 33 operations for pheochromocytoma. Rozhl Chir 68:705–710, 1989.
75. Greene JP, Guay AT: New perspectives in pheochromocytoma [review]. Urol Clin North Am 16:487–503, 1989.
76. Caty MG, Coran AG, Geagen M, et al: Current diagnosis and treatment of pheochromocytoma in children. Experience with 22 consecutive tumors in 14 patients. Arch Surg 125:978–981, 1990.
77. Rosenfield RL: Puberty and its disorders in girls. Endocrinol Metab Clin North Am 20:15–42, 1991.
78. Deans GT, Spence RA: Neoplastic lesions of the appendix. Br J Surg 82:299–306, 1995.
79. Parkes SE, Muir KR, al Sheyyab M, et al: Carcinoid tumors of the appendix in children 1957–1986: Incidence, treatment and outcome. Br J Surg 80:502–504, 1993.
80. Corpron CA, Black CT, Herzog CE, et al: A half century of experience with carcinoid tumors in children. Am J Surg 170:606–608, 1995.
81. Deans GT, Spence RA: Neoplastic lesions of the appendix. Br J Surg 82:299–306, 1995.
82. Wang LT, Wilkins EWJ, Bode HH: Bronchial carcinoid tumors in pediatric patients. Chest 103:1426–1428, 1993.
83. Hancock BJ, Di Lorenzo M, Youssef S, et al: Childhood primary pulmonary neoplasms. J Pediatr Surg 28:1133–1136, 1993.

76

CONJOINED TWINS

Rowena Spencer, MD

The existence of cave drawings, carvings, and ceramic figurines of conjoined twins, as well as their occurrence in all kinds of animals, suggests that these malformations existed long before the human race finished descending from its ancestors. The fanciful and seemingly fictitious cases in early recorded history were probably based on distorted descriptions of actual examples: Janus, the two-faced Roman god of beginning and endings, was certainly a cephalopagus, and the multiheaded Hydra probably originated as dicephalus, perhaps as tricephalus.[1]

The first known attempt at surgical separation occurred during the 10th century in Byzantium in omphalopagus twins. They were cut apart when one died; the other died later.[2] In 1860, a physician reluctantly separated his own omphalopagus daughters, closing each 5.5-cm incision with three through-and-through sutures; one died but the other was well 5 years later.[3] An attempt to separate 7-year-old girls in 1899 was discontinued when a 3- to 4-cm by 10-cm union of the livers was found; however, a second physician determined (by experimental surgery in dogs) that the cut surface of the liver would heal, and the twins were successfully separated. One died of pneumothorax because the pleura was opened during surgery.[4] By the middle of the 20th century, conjoined twins were being separated with increasing frequency and success concomitant with the improvements being made in the care of pediatric surgical patients.

☐ Embryology

Because experimental human embryology is not ethical, the most logical means of answering the age-old question about whether fission or fusion is responsible for conjoined twins is to examine the end-product (the fetuses) and work back to the beginning (the early embryo).[5] One of the most important factors in this process is the umbilicus. The body of the very early embryo enlarges rapidly, bulging dorsally, and eventually overhanging the entire periphery of the disc, which becomes progressively smaller in proportion. The edges of the disc eventually "close down" around the umbilical cord, which is formed from the original body stalk and umbilical vessels and is surrounded by amnion. Thus the umbilicus comes to occupy the midventral aspect of the embryo, with possible duplication of the umbilicus giving a clue as to the number of embryonic discs involved in conjoined twins.

Late in the 3rd week after fertilization, the central nervous system is indicated on the dorsal aspect of the embryo by a deepening groove with an elevated ridge on each side. These ridges eventually fuse across the midline to convert the neural groove into the neural tube. The last portions to close are the cranial and caudal neuropores, which overhang the periphery of the embryonic disc. Craniopagus and pygopagus are thought to result from fusion of two embryos in the area of the neuropores and rachipagus from union in the midportion of the neural tube; they all have fusion of the skull or vertebral column, the meninges, and, often, the brain or spinal cord as well. These three types of twins always have entirely separate abdomens and umbilical cords, indicating that they did, indeed, arise from secondary fusion of two embryos on two separate embryonic discs.

The oropharyngeal and cloacal membranes occupy the rostral and caudal aspects of the embryonic disc. It is theorized that cephalopagus and ischiopagus, respectively, arise from union of two embryos in these areas, sharing all of the structures developing from and adjacent to these membranes. Also, the primordia of the diaphragm and the heart are actually outside the rostral edge of the embryonic disc, and if two embryos were to fuse in this primordial location, omphalopagus and thoracopagus, respectively, would result. In these four types of twins, the edges of the discs become united, usually resulting in a single shared umbilicus, umbilical cord, and abdomen. The 7% incidence of duplication of the placenta, the umbilicus, or some part of the umbilical cord in these four types of twins and the fact that some are actually diamniotic seem to support the theory that they, too, arise from secondary union of two separate embryonic discs.

On the other hand, it is possible that laterally

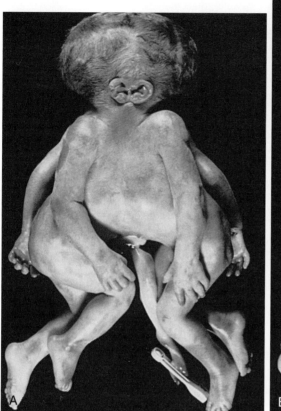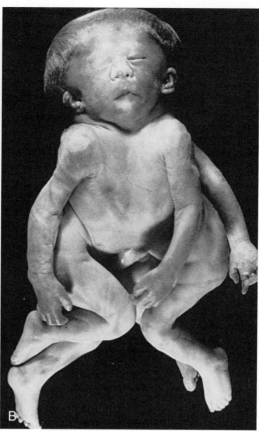

Figure 76–1. Cephalopagus. *A,* "Posterior" view. *B,* "Anterior" view. (Courtesy of Dr. M. C. Sault.)

united parapagus fetuses may result from two nearly parallel notochords developing on a single disc, but even here, 1% of these twins had duplication of the umbilicus, the umbilical cord, or the placenta.

Conjoined twins exhibit the effects of two embryologic derangements. The first, aplasia, occurs when the union is not directly symmetric and results in contiguous portions of two embryonic discs having insufficient space for complete development of all the structures destined to be formed there (Fig. 76–1A).

The second embryologic derangement affects midline structures at the site of union. These anatomic features are not simply buried but instead are divided vertically, diverted laterally, and reunited to form two new structures, which are often completely normal even though half of each is derived from a different embryo (see Fig. 76–1B).

All conjoined twins are united at homologous sites, but minimally united omphalopagus twins may be born "head to tail." Most twins consist of two complete fetuses, but infrequently, one fetus dies in early embryonic life, leaving parasitic structures always vascularized and occasionally even innervated by the autosite (the more normal twin).

☐ Identification and Classification

The incidence of conjoined twins is estimated to be 1 in 50,000 to 100,000 births. Approximately two thirds are female, and all pairs are of the same sex, including the several pseudohermaphrodites.

In conjoined twins, a distinction must be made between structures that are shared and those that belong only to one infant. As the twins are rarely united symmetrically, one conjoined aspect is broader than the other; this can be determined by measuring the distance between specific anatomic landmarks such as the nipples, acromion processes, or iliac spines (Fig. 76–2). When the twins lie in the position that exposes more of the abdomen(s), this broader aspect is referred to as the "secondary anterior" and the opposite surface as the "secondary posterior."[6] When necessary, laterality can be established by identifying the "anterior" surface of a conjoined heart or a single "anterior" falciform ligament or umbilicus. Only the craniopagus (and perhaps the rachipagus) cannot be identified in this way and must be labeled otherwise.

These "anterior" and "posterior" terms are always enclosed in quotation marks and never used in reference to an individual twin; those areas in each infant are referred to as dorsal and ventral. Using the "anterior" aspect as the point of reference, the twins now can be identified as twin-on-their-right and twin-on-their-left or simply right and left twins.

To avoid the confusion of Greek and Latin words and endings, the terms used to designate the different types of twins are used as singular and plural, noun and adjective.

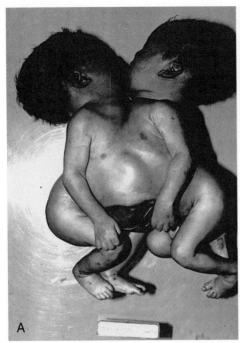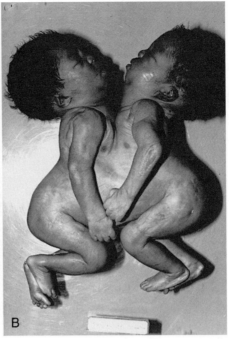

Figure 76–2. *A* and *B,* Thoracopagus showing the distance between the nipples on the "anterior" *(A)* and "posterior" *(B)* aspects of the union.

The most useful and logical classification of conjoined twins is based on the specific embryonic structure thought to be involved in the union (Table 76–1). There is one continuum from cephalopagus through thoracopagus to omphalopagus, with a graduated series of intermediate cases between them, a second from craniopagus through rachipagus to pygopagus, and a third between ischiopagus and parapagus.

The following information was garnered from the review of more than 1200 cases of conjoined twins (R. Spencer, unpublished data, 1998).

☐ Diagnosis and Treatment

GENERAL CONSIDERATIONS

The one third of conjoined twins that are possible candidates for separation include most omphalopagus, ischiopagus, and pygopagus; some craniopagus; and a very few thoracopagus and parapagus; but no cephalopagus (or probably rachipagus). In contrast, most parasites usually can be removed without difficulty.

A knowledge of the conjoined anatomy to be ex-

TABLE 76–1. Embryonic Classification of Conjoined Twins

Embryonic Aspect	Type	Incidence	Primordium	Union	Separability
Ventral (87%)					
Rostral (48%)	Cephalopagus	11%	Oropharyngeal membrane	Top of head to umbilicus	None
	Thoracopagus	19%	Heart	Thoracic, upper abdomen; conjoined heart	Rare
	Omphalopagus	18%	Diaphragm	Thoracic, upper abdomen; separate hearts	Likely 82% success
Caudal (11%)	Ischiopagus	11%	Cloacal membrane	Lower abdomen; genitourinary tract	Likely 63% success
Lateral (28%)	Parapagus	28%	Parallel notochords	Pelvis, variable trunk; diprosopus 2 faces; dicephalus 2 heads	Rare
Dorsal (13%)					
	Craniopagus	5%	Cranial neuropore	Cranial vault	Unlikely without sequelae
	Rachipagus	2%	Neural tube midportion	Vertebral column	None reported
	Pyopagus	6%	Caudal neuropore	Sacrum	Likely 68% success

pected in each type of union will indicate which areas require investigation and will protect the infants from unnecessary handling and exposure. Indications of potential complications include significantly asymmetric union, multiple malformations unrelated to the conjunction, an eccentric umbilicus, missing umbilical vessels, and severe lordosis or opisthotonus.

ANESTHETIC CONSIDERATIONS

The anesthesiologist must be aware of complications associated with the handling of two united patients; one potentially fatal problem is adrenal hypoplasia in one twin.[7] Also, in twins united in the thorax and abdomen, ventilation may have to be synchronized during anesthesia to ensure adequate respiratory exchange.[8]

As there are always some vascular anastomoses between the twins, holding one infant above the other to facilitate endotracheal intubation or placing them on different levels during surgery may result in the upper twin exsanguinating into the lower one. (In the original "Siamese" twins, exsanguination undoubtedly caused the death of Eng after his brother Chang died.) Unbalanced cross-circulation may also result in different transfusion requirements for the individual twins, particularly after some of the shared vessels have been divided; the twin with the stronger heart may become dangerously hypovolemic as a result of blood loss into the sibling, or the infant with a defective heart may collapse when suddenly deprived of the major source of circulating blood.

Both stabilization with rigid frames during operation and moving the twins to separate operating tables after separation are usually found to be unnecessary.

☐ Thoracopagus and Omphalopagus

Thoracopagus and omphalopagus (Figs. 76–2 and 76–3) are often indistinguishable externally, but the significant difference in survival indicates that they should be differentiated. Therefore, by definition, thoracopagus always have hearts that are united, if only by a single patent interatrial connection or by fusion of the muscular wall, whereas omphalopagus have two entirely separate hearts, rarely connected by a fibrous cord without a lumen.

The union in both thoracopagus and omphalopagus involves a variable amount of the lower thoracic wall, the supraumbilical abdominal wall, and the umbilicus, but does not extend to the pubis. Approximately one fourth have an omphalocele and almost all have some degree of lordosis, but the trachea and the lungs are not involved. The diaphragm, however, is almost invariably united. The fused upper small intestine, more common in thora-

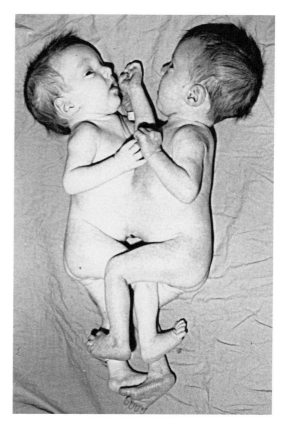

Figure 76–3. Omphalopagus.

copagus than in omphalopagus, has a mesentery from each twin and is a site of possible cross-circulation. Anomalies of the genitourinary (GU) tract are rare when the external genitalia are normal, and other malformations of any significance can be expected to show external evidence of their existence.

The hearts of thoracopagus are not only united but also quite anomalous, some retaining the primitive orientation of atria lying caudal to ventricles. The union usually involves the chambers, perhaps confined to the atria and/or coronary sinuses, but often including the ventricles as well. Only rarely is there simple fusion of the external surfaces of the muscular walls. The coronary arteries usually supply the ventricle from which the aorta arises, and the conducting system is assumed to be shared when the twins have identical heart rates and electrical activity.

The entire union in omphalopagus usually is less extensive than in thoracopagus, and when the bridge is small, the xiphoid will be conjoined, the hearts generally normal, the intestine separate, the liver minimally fused, and significant cross circulation rare. In one fifth of omphalopagus, however, one or both infants will have cardiac anomalies, many incompatible with independent existence. Also, extensive union of the sternum may presage a common pericardium with exocardia (ventral protrusion of the heart).

In view of the complexity of union of the mini-chambered and multichambered hearts with abnormal intercardiac and intracardiac septal defects, anomalous inflow and outflow tracts, and the possibility of shared coronary circulation and conducting systems, it may be necessary to accept the fact that the vast majority of thoracopagus are "accidents of nature" and the most compassionate decision is to "let nature take its course." Many physicians and theologians—and parents—believe that the treatment of these babies should consist of a warm blanket, a pacifier, and a bottle on demand while they are, literally, "loved to death." If it is believed that the twins can be separated, however, with the possibility that at least one infant can survive with an acceptable quality of life, suitable examination must be undertaken.

INVESTIGATION

Unless other indications exist, preoperative indagation in these twins can be confined to the cardiovascular and the gastrointestinal (GI) systems. Examination of the former should include not only the conjoined chambers and muscular walls but also the intrinsic circulation, the conducting system, and the possibility of cross-circulation through the internal mammary, intercostal, hepatic, and mesenteric vessels as well as abnormal channels.

Clinical symptoms indicate possible obstruction of the esophagus or small bowel. Possible fusion (without obstruction) of the upper small intestine is easily determined by administering a nonabsorbable colored material (i.e., charcoal) to one twin, and if the pigment subsequently appears only in one diaper, it can be assumed that the intestines and the biliary tracts are separate. When there is fusion of the duodenum, however, there may be serious problems in the liver or biliary tracts. Also, a huge saccular dilation of bowel (without distal obstruction) may be found in the lower portion of a fused segment of intestine. Union of the intestine rarely extends beyond the middle of the small bowel.

The livers are almost invariably fused, perhaps with intrahepatic or extrahepatic union of the biliary tracts. Conjoined bile ducts drain into a conjoined intestine, whereas separate common ducts may empty into either separate or united duodenums. Fusion of the pancreas is uncommon, but the anatomy of the pancreatic ducts usually is similar to that of the bile ducts. The arterial, portal, and venous circulation of the liver should be evaluated to determine that the entire circulation is adequate to ensure the viability of both livers and intestinal tracts. Occasionally, all hepatic veins drain into one heart and, rarely, the twins have two shared (not individual) livers; in this latter case, each liver occupies a conjoined epigastrium, placed symmetrically across the plane of junction.[9, 10] In these instances, the right twin usually supplies the hepatic artery and the common duct for the "anterior" liver and the left twin, for the "posterior" structures; the hepatic and portal venous systems are variable.

When surgery is postponed in these two types of twins, unbalanced cross-circulation may result in unequal weight gain or cardiac overload and subsequent failure in one twin. Asynchronous respiration can cause a problem until the twins learn to breathe simultaneously, and the lack of stability between the conjoined thoracic and abdominal cavities may result in an ineffective cough mechanism or serious respiratory problems when one twin cries vigorously and increases intraabdominal pressure of both. In addition, increasing lordosis may result in aspiration and/or accentuation of the ventral protrusion of the conjoined sternum.

OPERATIVE TREATMENT

The surgical approach is similar in thoracopagus and omphalopagus, except for the problems with cardiac union in the former. The twins should be placed on the operating table on their "posterior" aspect and the incision begun "anteriorly," as the heart and great vessels and the abdominal viscera are oriented toward this surface.

Omphalopagus with extensive union of the sternums may share a pericardium, but a small tunnel between two nearly separate pericardiums should be opened with care; it may contain a patent intercardiac vessel or a slender nonpatent cord connecting either the atria or the ventricles.

Approximately one tenth of thoracopagus are united only in the atria or the coronary sinus. In five of eight such cases, one infant died as soon as the connection was divided, some died because cardiac malformations rendered that twin nonviable, but others died perhaps because the sinoatrial node was ligated and/or divided.[11] The only thoracopagus known to have survived separation are 4 infants in 3 cases with uncomplicated atrial union, an 11% survival rate in 18 surgical cases.[12–14] In contrast, 82% of omphalopagus survived separation in 78 cases.

The handling of various sites of cross-circulation may pose serious problems during surgical separation, more often in thoracopagus. When there is inequality in the volume and direction of flow in the arterial and venous anastomoses, sequential interruption may result in one twin exsanguinating into the other. In some instances, it may be prudent to isolate all communicating vessels so that they can be occluded simultaneously and then divided individually.

The site of fusion may be the thickest part of conjoined livers. With asymmetric union, division into two approximately equal portions may cause a problem, and it may be impossible to divide one large liver. In several instances, hepatic necrosis, acute or chronic biliary obstruction, or nonviability of the intestine followed operation.[11, 14–18]

It is during the division of the livers that the twins should be monitored carefully because the abrupt disruption of significant cross-circulation may have a profound effect on one or both infants. Also, bradycardia and hypotension may result from obstruction of the hepatic veins and the inferior venae cavae during separation of the livers, particularly if the bodies of the infants are distracted to improve exposure of the surgical area.

The only problem usually associated with the division of the conjoined sternum is the possible opening of the closely adjacent pleura. Also, it may be difficult to reattach the diaphragm to a very short or bifurcated sternum without an intervening prosthesis.

Closure of the enormous surgical wound may be fraught with many difficulties. The first is covering the ventrally protruding sternum (similar to pectus carinatum) that results from long-standing lordosis and opisthotonus. A second, more serious problem involves the large space between the flared costal cartilages in extensively united sternums, as much as one fourth of the circumference of the thorax in each twin. The third difficulty, probably the most difficult to solve, is the exocardia in omphalopagus resulting from malposition of two hearts in a single pericardium; each heart may protrude as much as 2½ inches above the plane of the divided sternum and cannot be reduced into the thorax without obstructing the great vessels. A fourth problem may be replacing intestine that has forfeited the right of domicile after developing in a large omphalocele, possibly accentuated by severe lordosis and by the

diastasis recti associated with the conjunction of the upper abdominal wall.

Wound closure under tension must be avoided at all cost, as the resulting visceral and vascular compression or respiratory embarrassment may be fatal. In many instances, a prosthesis will be necessary unless part of the chest wall of a deceased twin can be used to close the defect in the surviving infant.

PARASITIC THORACOPAGUS AND OMPHALOPAGUS

The parasites of thoracopagus and omphalopagus (Fig. 76–4D), indistinguishable except for possible involvement of the heart, are affixed to the lower thorax and upper abdomen and often are completely separate from the umbilicus. They generally consist of rudimentary upper or lower extremities, genitalia, and abdominal viscera, and some are innervated. In the single thoracopagus parasite reported, the autosite died of failure of a shared multiventricular heart 3 weeks after surgery. Parasites were found in nearly one fourth of the omphalopagus; however, many of the autosites had an abnormal (but not conjoined) heart.

No blood vessels connecting the autosite and parasite need be preserved, but when the peritoneal cavities are shared, all parasitic viscera should be

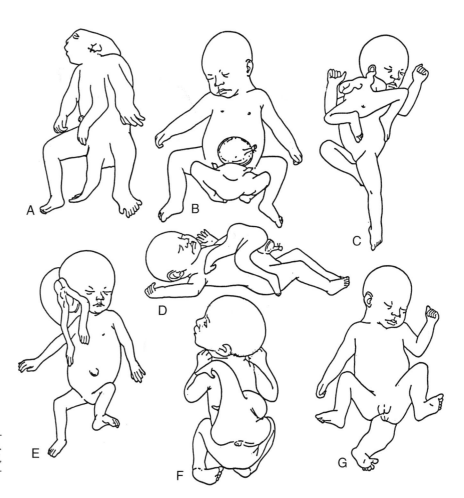

Figure 76–4. Parasitic twins. *A,* Parapagus. *B,* Ischiopagus. *C,* Cephalopagus. *D,* Thoracopagus or omphalopagus. *E,* Craniopagus. *F,* Rachipagus. *G,* Pygopagus.

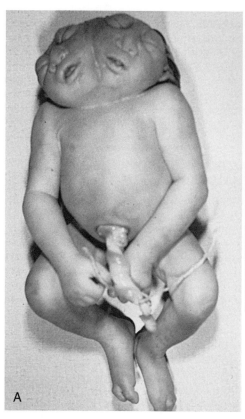

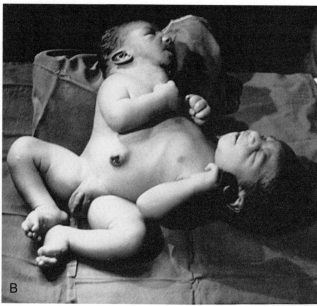

Figure 76–5. Parapagus. *A,* Diprosopus. *B,* Dicephalus.

removed (except perhaps a portion of a conjoined liver) to prevent subsequent gangrene of devascularized structures.

☐ Parapagus

The laterally united parapagus include a large range of cases that are always joined in the pelvis, with varying degrees of duplication in the cranial portion of the body and with four to seven extremities (Fig. 76–5). Surgical separation is feasible only when the upper portions of the trunks are sufficiently separate to provide a stable rib cage for each infant, usually when there are four arms, rarely when there are only three.

There is a continuum between parapagus and ischiopagus, both of which may have similar pelvic anatomy. All dibrachius, tribrachius, and dipus are classified as parapagus as they are rarely candidates for surgery, and all tetrabrachius tetrapus are included with ischiopagus as they usually can be separated. Distinction between the two types is made in the tetrabrachius tripus; if the heart is single or fused, the twins are included with parapagus, but if there are two separate hearts, they are classified as ischiopagus.

As the surgical problems are similar in both groups, the few surgically separated parapagus are discussed with ischiopagus.

PARASITIC PARAPAGUS

Parasitic parapagus are rare; only one case is known (see Fig. 76–4*A*).

☐ Ischiopagus

Ischiopagus are usually depicted lying flat on their backs, sharing the lower abdomen, pelvis, and perineum, with a pair of legs on each side and external genitalia between each pair of legs (Fig. 76–6). Classically, the two vertebral columns form a straight line, but the angle of ventral union can vary from 180 to 15 degrees; in the former, the twins are end to end, and in the latter, they are literally face to face. Also, the union may be somewhat lateral, this angle varying from 180 to approximately 90 degrees, resulting in fusion of contiguous "posterior" limb buds (ischiopagus tripus) and usually with some diminution of the genitalia on that aspect. About one half of ischiopagus have four legs, one third have only three, and the remaining one fifth are parasitic cases. The incidence of malformations is increased with any variation from the typical conjunction (extensive ventral, lateral, or caudal union) or other significant abnormalities (omphalocele in 20%, central nervous system in 10%, heart in 9%).

Even when the twins seem to be united symmetrically, an eccentric umbilicus will occupy the "anterior" aspect, and diminished external genitalia or legs closer together (or fused) will identify the "posterior."

In typical ischiopagus there are two sets of genitalia, each rotated 90 degrees from the normal orientation and both shared equally by both twins (Fig. 76–7*A*). Starting between the "anterior" pair of legs

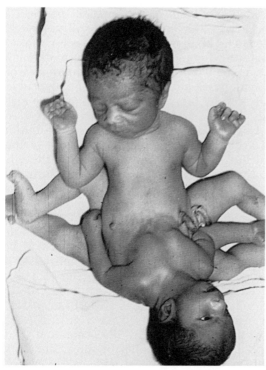

Figure 76–6. Ischiopagus. (From Spencer R: Surgical separation of Siamese twins. Surgery 39:827, 1956.)

on the female perineum, there are normal labia surrounding a clitoris, urethra, and vaginal orifice, then, in reverse order, another vaginal orifice, urethra, and clitoris surrounded by another set of labia

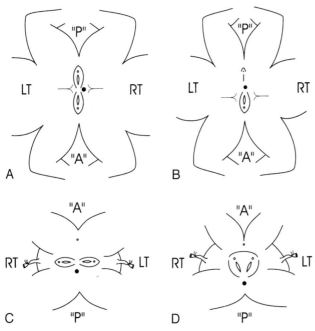

Figure 76–7. Perineum of ischiopagus and pygopagus. *A,* Symmetric ischiopagus. *B,* Asymmetric ischiopagus with diminution of "posterior" aspect. *C,* Symmetric pygopagus. *D,* Asymmetric pygopagus with diminution of "anterior" aspect. A, "anterior"; LT, left twin; P, "posterior"; RT, right twin.

between the "posterior" legs. Male genitalia are similarly oriented, with a penis and scrotum between each pair of legs.

One or both sets of genitalia may be united, rudimentary, or absent altogether (see Fig. 76–7*B*); single genitalia are almost invariably "anterior," while fused genitalia may occupy the center of the perineum or the dorsal aspect of the united buttocks. In male ischiopagus, two scrotums often surround a single penis with one or two urethras and/or multiple corpora cavernosa. In general, the more normal the genitalia, the more normal are the lower reproductive and urinary tracts.

In the pelvis of the classic female patient, behind the "anterior" symphysis pubis is a urinary bladder, then a uterus with attached fallopian tubes and ovaries, a rectum, another uterus, and finally another bladder behind the "posterior" symphysis. The ovaries and fallopian tubes are generally normal, but both uteri are frequently divided into two separate hemiuteri; the vagina may be double or septate, perhaps atretic, often ending in a persistent urogenital sinus. In male patients, the single rectum lies between the two bladders; the prostate and the vasa deferentia are usually normally related to the urethras, but occasionally the vasa deferentia empty into a ureter or directly into the bladder.

As a rule, each twin has two normal kidneys and ureters, the "anterior" ureters draining into the "anterior" bladder and the "posterior" ureters into the "posterior" bladder. A horseshoe kidney or crossed renal ectopia with double ureters usually contributes a ureter to each bladder. Anomalies interfering with renal function are infrequent, but anatomic malformations (solitary, ectopic, unrotated, fused kidneys) are relatively common.

In most patients, there are two normal (but shared) bladders and urethras, but rarely, the bladders are either septate or united, usually when there are other significant malformations. The dividing septum is not symphysis to symphysis, but oriented twin to twin, perhaps located under a conjoined mesorectum. The fusion is typically in the area of the bladder neck, with a rectovesical or rectourethral fistula entering and one or two urethras emerging from the bridge of union. Conjoined bladders are more common in males, the urethras often uniting in a single penis, but in females, the urethras usually end in a urogenital sinus or a cloaca. In two cases, the bladder emptied through a patent urachus.[19, 20]

The peritoneal cavities of ischiopagus are almost invariably united. The livers may be conjoined, but the bile ducts are separate. The distal half of the bowel usually is shared, but occasionally the GI tracts are entirely separate, the two rectums uniting in the pelvis, ending blindly, or emptying through one or two ani. Most often, the anal orifice is a rectoperineal fistula, stenotic, without proper sphincters, and unrelated to the one or two anal dimples that may be present. The orifice, normal or abnormal, is rarely in the midplane of junction between the two sets of external genitalia, but closer to one twin than the other.

Each twin has a wide diastasis pubis, the right pubis of one twin uniting with the left of the other to form one large pelvic girdle consisting of two symphyses pubis (at 90 and 270 degrees), two sacrums (at 0 and 180 degrees), and two pairs of innominate bones. Lateral union of the sacrums may result from reciprocal scoliosis of both lumbar areas; one vertebral column bends (not twists) toward the right and the other toward the left, thus bringing the lateral aspects of the sacrums together with the coccyges pointing "anteriorly." When the sacrums are shared or united, the contiguous ilia (one of each twin) will be distorted, and the dural sheaths or the spinal cords may be continuous from one twin to the other.

Minimally united ischiopagus (a fifth of the cases) are joined only in the umbilicus and the infraumbilical abdominal wall, some with union only in the umbilicus or in an omphalocele, some diamniotic, most with imperforate anus. Neither the bony pelvis nor the genitalia are involved, but there are always anomalies of the cloaca, with union of the urachus, bladder, or cloaca, along with the uterus. Of particular interest are three cases in which fetuses of 28-, 29-, and 40-weeks' gestation were found to have macerated or papyraceous parasitic twins of 13-, 9-, and 14-weeks' gestation, respectively, attached to the umbilical area of the autosite (M. Reynolds, oral communication, 1994).[21, 22]

INVESTIGATION

In symmetrically united ischiopagus tetrapus without other obvious malformations, the GU tracts are usually normal except for being shared. The entire anatomy must be studied thoroughly, however, particularly in the tripus, as very complicated intercommunications between the uterus, vagina, bladder, urethra, and/or rectum may result in complex variations of a partially or completely duplicated persistent urogenital sinus or cloaca. Possible vascular anastomoses (in the aortas or venae cavae, iliac, mesenteric, or hepatic vessels) should be visualized. The status of the lower intestine, especially the rectum(s), should be known, but unless other indications exist, no other indagation should be needed.

OPERATIVE TREATMENT

When possible, the initial portion of the incision should be planned so that the external genitalia can be assigned to either twin because intraoperative findings may negate a preoperative decision. The external and internal genitalia are vascularized by both twins; therefore, each infant can receive one set of genitalia and one bladder, with one ureter of each twin being removed from one bladder and reimplanted into the other. The ileum and the colon are generally long enough to be divided between the twins, but provision of a competent perineal anus for each twin may be impossible. All vascular connections can be divided, except possibly those supplying a third conjoined leg, which may be left for one twin or used to close the abdominal wound. Both symphyses pubis are divided, but the cut edges usually can be brought together to provide a stable pelvis.

In ischiopagus tripus, significant diminution of the "posterior" aspect of union results in the replacement of that symphysis by fused ilia and ischia, division of which may result in massive blood loss. A single bladder may be divided or given to one twin and the ureters rearranged as indicated, but a single urethra generally cannot be divided. When the "posterior" genitalia are defective or absent, however, intraoperative decisions will be affected by the configuration of the entire GU tract, perhaps also by the mental or physical potential of each twin. A single vulva may be divided and shared, but a single penis is given to one twin, the other perhaps to be raised as a girl. This raises ethical problems regarding the separation of these twins—the expected quality of life in intact twins compared to that of a child with half of a pelvis, a single leg, no genitalia, and preternatural openings for both the GI and the urinary tract.

The overall survival rate in the separation of ischiopagus tripus and tetrapus was 63% in 42 cases. The mortality rate was greatest in the newborn period when surgery was indicated by evisceration or death or nonviability of one twin.

As a rule, neither the tribrachius nor the tetrabrachius tripus classed as parapagus are suitable candidates for separation, but in rare cases, a viable infant may be salvaged by sacrificing a defective twin. Only six parapagus are known to have undergone surgery. Two-week-old tribrachius dipus girls had an interatrial connection between one normal and one abnormal heart; one infant was sacrificed and the other died 6 weeks later of multiple intraoperative and postoperative complications.[23] In two cases, tetrabrachius dipus were separated; one newborn lived after a defective twin was sacrificed (R. Spencer, unpublished data), and one of 3-year-old girls with subcutaneous union of the "posterior" arms survived.[24]

Three cases of parapagus tetrabrachius tripus had a single GU tract and, apparently, two normal hearts. One of two year-old girls died of a tight chest wall closure but two pairs of girls aged 5 and 12 months, respectively, survived.[18, 25, 26]

PARASITIC ISCHIOPAGUS

Parasitic ischiopagus account for a fifth of the cases, usually with one or two lower extremities on the ventral aspect of the pelvis, some occupying the diastasis pubis of the autosite and some being innervated by the autosite (see Fig. 76–4B). The genitalia, single or double, are in the location typical of ischiopagus—on the lateral aspects of the shared

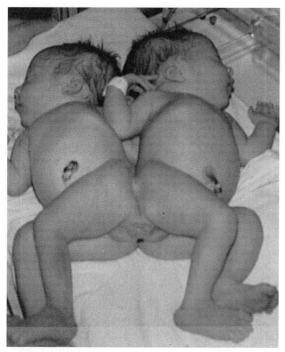

Figure 76–8. Pygopagus. (From Fournier L, Goulet C, Waugh R, et al: Anesthesia for separation of conjoined twins. Can Anaesth Soc J 23:427, 1976.)

perineum. Twelve of 16 autosites survived separation.

□ Pygopagus

Pygopagus are united dorsolaterally in the sacrum and the perineum, very rarely involving the "anterior" legs (Fig. 76–8). As the ventral portion of the trunk is free, the abdominal viscera are not involved and each twin has a separate umbilicus. Strangely, 60% of the cases are parasites, with male cases accounting for only 7% of the typical twins (2 of 27 cases) but 38% of the parasites.

Typically, there are two sets of normal genitalia, properly aligned to the symphysis of each twin and united "back to back" in the area of the fourchette (dorsally in relation to the individual twin) (see Fig. 76–7C). When the union is more extensive than usual, however, there may be one single shared "anterior" labium majus stretched across the plane of junction above the two relatively normal "posterior" labia (see Fig. 76–7D); only infrequently is the vagina or urethra Y-shaped or single. Usually, there is a single anus, not centered between the two sets of genitalia but on the "posterior" aspect; rarely, an "anterior" anus is represented by a sinus tract extending toward the conjoined rectum. Duplication of the anus is infrequent, and complete absence rare.

At first glance, the perineums of pygopagus and ischiopagus appear to be identical, each with two sets of genitalia properly oriented to an overlying symphysis pubis, united in the region of the four-

chette and with a single anus. However, the plane of junction extends *between* the genitalia in pygopagus, with each twin having an individual vulva and symphysis pubis (see Fig. 76–7C), but the plane of junction extends directly *through* the genitalia in ischiopagus, with both sets of genitalia and both symphyses pubis being shared equally by both twins (see Fig. 76–7A). The "anterior" aspect of the union is reduced in pygopagus, with the two sets of genitalia being brought together laterally (see Fig. 76–7D), but in ischiopagus, the "posterior" genitalia are reduced or absent whereas the "anterior" remain normal (see Fig. 76–7B).

Nearly half of pygopagus have significant anomalies of the central nervous system and/or vertebral column (hydrocephaly, myelomeningocele and meningocele, spina bifida, and rachischisis); the more lateral the union, the more frequent were these malformations.

Each twin has a complete, separate pelvic ring with an individual symphysis pubis and with the osseous fusion involving only the lateral portion of the sacrum and the coccyx. The dorsal aspect of the union is more extensive than the ventral and the caudal aspect is more extensive than the rostral; thus, there is aplasia of the dorsocaudolateral portion of each sacrum, the right of one twin and the left of the other. The contiguous "anterior" ilia (one of each twin) are usually separate but may be united by fibrous or fibrocartilaginous tissue. If the union involves the lumbar vertebrae, the twins are considered to be rachipagus.

In typical cases, 40% have a single dural tube extending from one twin to the other, several with fused or continuous spinal cords, thus supporting the theory that the primary union is in the caudal neuropore. The same proportion of parasites also have a neural connection with the autosite spinal cord.

Significant heart disease is rare in pygopagus and the upper GI tracts are entirely normal, but the two rectums generally unite a few centimeters above the anal canal. More than a fourth of cases have anatomic anomalies of the kidneys (agenesis, ectopia, and fusion) but normal renal function.

INVESTIGATION

The most important structures to be indagated before operation are the dura and the spinal cord, along with the site and extent of the sacral union. Also to be studied are the GU tract, the rectum, and the possible communication between major pelvic blood vessels: the aortas and venae cavae, the midsacrals, and the iliacs.

OPERATIVE TREATMENT

The union between the two sacrums may be fibrous or cartilaginous but is usually osseous, in which case surgical division may be accompanied by brisk hemorrhage. The spinal nerve roots may be united across the plane of union, so caution must be exercised, particularly on the ventral aspect where the sacral plexus will be located. If the spinal canals are united, the dura and/or the spinal cord may be continuous, and separation of the cords and/or cauda equina and closure of the dura must be meticulous to minimize neurologic damage and prevent cerebrospinal fluid fistula. Some degree of neurologic deficiency of the legs, as well as urinary and fecal incontinence, have been reported after operation.

Four surgical cases had fusion of the spinal cord, which was simply divided on the side of a severely defective twin or successfully separated (C. L. Fowler, oral communication).[27–29] In one case, both spinal cords bifurcated within the conjoined sacrum, where a spur of bone bridged the shared spinal canal (diastematomyelia); distal to this, the "anterior" branches of both cords fused together and could be separated only with magnification.[28] There is no contraindication to the division of any vascular connections; however, a severely defective twin may not survive ligation of major arterial and venous communication if the stronger heart of the normal twin has been providing circulation for both.

The external genitalia will not pose a problem if the twins are united dorsally ("back to back"), but with laterally united vulva, the "anterior" conjoined labium can be divided and half given to each twin. A septate vagina and a Y-shaped urethra will require reconstructive repair. The two rectums generally unite a few centimeters above the anus, but occasionally one rectum will end in a rectovaginal fistula. A sinus tract on the "anterior" aspect of the perineum (opposite the more normal "posterior" anus) will require careful dissection to determine whether it is actually a rectoperineal fistula.

The two pelvic peritoneal cavities generally are separated by a membranous septum, which need not be opened. As the lower portion of the pelvis is shared, reconstitution of the pelvic floor may be difficult or impossible.

Both twins survived in 8 of 11 surgical cases, and in each of the 3 others, a nonviable twin died during or shortly after operation.

PARASITIC PYGOPAGUS

Parasitic pygopagus are located on the dorsal aspect of the lower trunk, usually with a recognizable bony extremity, a direct neural connection to the autosite, and/or vestiges of other organ systems (see Fig. 76–4G). It may occupy the region between the coccyx and the anus, with the distinction between pygopagus parasite and sacrococcygeal tumor becoming difficult. Surgical removal of the parasite should pose no problems different from those of separation of two infants; 70% of the autosites survived.

☐ Craniopagus

The union in craniopagus twins involves only the head, including the cranial vault but not the fora-

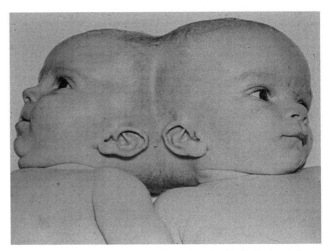

Figure 76–9. Craniopagus. (Courtesy Dr. D. E. Cameron.)

men magnum, the base of the skull, the vertebrae, the neck, or the trunk (Fig. 76–9). Craniopagus should not be confused with cephalopagus, the latter conjoined ventrally in the head and neck, the thorax, and the upper abdomen; craniopagus are not united in the face, but cephalopagus are. The rare rachipagus also may be conjoined in the head, but they are joined dorsally in the vertebral column as well.

The juncture in craniopagus, rarely symmetric, may involve the entire diameter of the head or only a portion thereof and may include the meninges, the venous sinuses, and even the brain itself. There is infinite variation in both axial and rotational orientation; the vertebral axes may form a straight line or any angle in any plane, and the twins may face either the same or exactly opposite directions or any point in between. All of these factors will affect the subsequent development, distortion, and displacement of the brain, its meninges, and its vascular system.

Other central nervous system malformations found in craniopagus are microcephaly, anencephaly, encephalocele, cysts and agenesis in various regions, and abnormalities of the ventricular system, as well as rachischisis and myelomeningocele.

The most useful classification of craniopagus simply describes the site of union (frontotemporal or frontoparietal in 25%, parietal in 45%, and occipital or occipitoparietal in 30%), even though this fails to include the dural venous sinuses, the most significant anatomic structures of all. It is the abnormalities of these vessels that doom the vast majority of these infants to living as intact conjoined twins or the significant risk of death or serious neurologic impairment following surgical separation.

If the conjunction is relatively small, only the scalp and the cranial vault are absent in the involved area, with simple osseous fusion, a thick bony ridge, or only a fibrous tissue symphysis at the site on union. When the union is extensive, particularly in the parietal region, the cranial bones may be displaced centrifugally, widely open, before they are united between the twins. Both brains are then contained in one large shared calvarium, which usually does not provide the same space as two normal skulls. In general, the more extensive the union, the greater the decrease in the relative volume of the conjoined crania and the greater the reciprocal pressure on the two developing brains.

The osseous junction of the cranium does not always coincide with the site of union of the underlying cerebra. The rapid growth of the brain may result in the herniation of the cerebral hemispheres of one twin into the cranial vault of the other, the resulting pressure resulting in distortion and displacement, atrophy, and even agenesis of affected areas. Even after birth, the growth of the brain is still disproportionately greater than that of the remainder of the body, increasing 135% in size during the 1st year.[30] This factor must be considered in the timing of surgical separation as neurologic impairment and developmental delay can be expected to increase postnatally.

Significant distortion of the brain will result in abnormality of the size, shape, and position of the ventricles; enlargement may indicate either deformity or obstruction in the ventricular system, but shared ventricles are invariably accompanied by fusion of the neural tissue itself. The dura in craniopagus may form a continuous single or double layer between the cerebra of the twins but will not form an intact layer if the cortex and/or leptomeninges are united. The dural defect may occupy virtually the entire area of union or occur only on one side, and, depending on the site and the angulation of union, the falx cerebri may be absent or defective in one or both twins.

The dura is divided into two layers, the meningeal and the endocranial periosteum, between which are the dural sinuses, which receive numerous tributaries from both the superficial and the deep venous systems. The sinuses are not true veins but simply spaces lined with a thin layer of endothelium; they have neither valves nor muscular or fibrous walls and consequently are very fragile. In addition, they are often triangular in cross section, fixed above to the overlying endosteum and on both sides where the two layers of dura are united. Unlike extracranial vessels, the sinuses are not movable within the surrounding tissue, and a circumferential ligature is likely to tear the sinus away from the points of fixation and result in severe hemorrhage.[31]

The factors that affect the configuration of the dural sinuses in craniopagus are the site and the size of the union as well as the rotational and axial alignment, all of which can be determined with various imaging techniques, using one twin (possibly the larger) as the fixed point. The location of the dural sinuses in the shared area and the direction of blood flow within them are not always predictable.

In the absence of the falx cerebri, the superior and inferior sagittal sinuses cannot develop; instead of a falx, many craniopagus have a short circumferential fold of dura around the periphery of the bridge between the two crania, resembling an abortive conjoined falx. This shared dural shelf, usually 1 cm or so wide, can be expected to contain a large venous sinus corresponding to the superior sagittal sinus. It may be completely circumferential, seen most often in symmetric parietal union of the entire vertex, or only semicircular, generally on the side where the dura is defective.

Abnormalities of the other large sinuses will depend on the location and the orientation of the union. With occipital or occipitoparietal union, the confluences and the transverse sinuses may be united, and in parietal union, twins facing in opposite directions may have contact between the frontal lobe of one and the tentorium of the other, so that the sinuses of the cerebral hemispheres of one twin drain into the transverse sinus or the confluence of the other.

Both twins will contribute multiple afferent veins to the shared sinuses, and division of these tributaries will result in venous congestion and necrosis of the underlying cortex. Also, the lack of a bony cranium across the site of union will preclude any communication between dural sinuses and the diploë of the skull, thus eliminating a possible source of collateral circulation when shared dural sinuses must be divided. In addition, the surgical removal of bone at the site of union may destroy anastomoses around the periphery of the bridge. Preexisting abnormalities and/or surgical disruption of the superior sagittal sinus and the venous lacunae may result in hydrocephaly after operation.

INVESTIGATION

The most important information to be obtained before surgery concerns the size of the bony defect and the location and interconnections of the dural venous sinuses.

OPERATIVE TREATMENT

The incision must be planned to provide adequate exposure, particularly when the junctions of the calvaria and the cerebra do not coincide, and to arrange for appropriate covering for the denuded cerebrum.

Other aspects that should be anticipated are:
1. Provision of adequate support of the brain to prevent gravitational deformation during surgical separation, especially when the union is extensive or asymmetric[32];
2. Prevention of air embolism from intentional or accidental openings in the dural sinuses; and
3. Control of the significant hemorrhage that may occur in dividing either the sinuses or the bony bridge, difficult because of inadequate exposure before the separation is complete.

The problems encountered with the shared sinuses may be insurmountable. Transverse division will destroy the venous drainage of some portion of the cortex of one or both twins, and simple longitudinal division will require intraluminal shunting, difficult because of the small size of the vessels. Theoretically, the superficial cerebral venous drainage might be diverted to the deep venous system by staged division of the tributaries, thereby encouraging the enlargement of collaterals with venous sinuses; in one case, this was followed by subsequent successful separation.[33] In several instances, all of the veins of one twin were divided, leaving the dural sinuses for the sibling, but this did not always result in saving either infant.

Arterial anastomoses signify union of the cortex, often in the depth of a fissure or a sulcus, thus indicating union before the development of the convolutions. They can be divided with impunity as there is adequate inflow from both directions; however, it may be difficult to determine where the united brains should be divided, particularly when complicated by inadequate exposure and lack of landmarks. There is apparently little or no neuronal connection between the twins even when cortex is united, but some parasites duplicate movements of the autosite.

Massive hemorrhage in at least 12 cases resulted in the death or neurologic damage of all except 2 of the infants involved. In 60 infants (30 pairs) whose surgical separation was attempted, only 7 emerged unscathed; 30 died, 17 were neurologically impaired, and 6 were reported before the ultimate outcome could be evaluated. Postoperative survival with normal neurologic status is most frequent with a small lateral union in the frontotemporal area with little or no axial rotation, and it is least often with a wide union in the midline parietal or occipital area with extensive rotation and acute dorsal angulation.

PARASITIC CRANIOPAGUS

Parasitic craniopagus in five cases consisted of extremities and genitalia attached to the temporal bone (see Fig. 76–4E), a parasitic head attached near the occiput, and rudiments of a head in the temporal region or in an occipital encephalocele.

☐ Rachipagus

Only a single typical rachipagus is known, twins joined dorsally from the top of the head down to the buttocks, each infant having four normal, properly oriented extremities (Fig. 76–10). The occipital bones were united but the foramina magna and the cervical vertebrae were free; then the vertebral arches were fused dorsally from the sixth thoracic to the third lumbar, where the vertebral columns were separate again. Only the skeleton was described in the original report.[34]

PARASITIC RACHIPAGUS

Parasitic rachipagus are united in the dorsal midline above the sacrum, involving the vertebrae and/

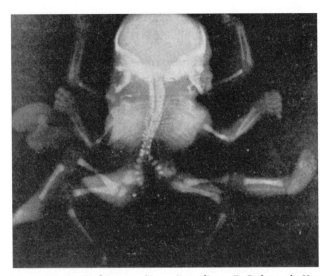

Figure 76–10. Rachipagus. (From Betoulieres P, Caderas de Kerleau J: Etude radiologique du squelette d'un monstre double janicephale-rachipage. Montpellier Med J 58:30, 1960.)

or a direct connection with the spinal cord, some capable of voluntary movement (see Fig. 76–4F). Of 20 cases, only 10 parasites were surgically removed; the autosite of 8 survived.

☐ Cephalopagus

Cephalopagus are united from the top of the head down to and including the umbilicus, with two faces on opposite sides of the single conjoined head (see Fig. 76–1). The structures shared by the twins include the forebrain and the optic chiasm; the entire face, pharynx, esophagus, and trachea; the stomach and upper small intestine; and two hearts, one on each aspect of the union. Most die before or during birth, and none live more than a few hours; under no circumstances can any of them be considered for surgical separation.

PARASITIC CEPHALOPAGUS

Parasitic cephalopagus in six cases consisted of vestigial remnants on the face and the ventral aspect of the trunk (see Fig. 76–4C); excision is usually possible.

REFERENCES

1. Reina E, Galvani G-A: Sopra un feto umano tricefalo. Atti dell'Accademi, Gioenia 8:203, 1834.
2. Pentogalos GE, Lascaratos JG: A surgical operation performed on Siamese twins during the 10th century in Byzantium. Bull Hist Med 58:99, 1984.
3. Bohm M: Ein Fall verwachsener Zwillingsfruchte (Xiphopage) gluchlich operative getrennt. Virchows Arch 36:152, 1866.
4. Chapot-Prevost E: Operabilidade de Rosalina e Maria. Rev Soc Med Cir do Rio de Jan 4:95, 1900.
5. Spencer R: Conjoined twins: Theoretical embryologic basis. Teratology 45:591, 1992.

6. Schwalbe E: Die Doppelbildungen. In Schwalbe E (ed): Die Morphologie der Missbildungen des Menschen und die Tiere. Teil II. Jena, Gustav Fischer, 1907.

7. Aird I: The conjoined twins of Kano. BMJ 1:831, 1954.

8. Kiesewetter WB: Surgery on conjoined (Siamese) twins. Surgery 59:860, 1966.

9. Marin-Padilla M, Chin AJ, Marin-Padilla TM: Cardiovascular abnormalities in thoracopagus twins. Teratology 23:101, 1981.

10. Spencer R, Robichaux WH, Seo J-W: Abnormal vasculature of the liver in thoracopagus twins: Case report. Pediatr Pathol Lab Med 17:315, 1997.

11. Patel B, Ho J, Sherry M, et al: Thoracoomphalopagus conjoined twins: Preoperative evaluation by scintigraphy. Am J Radiol 140:1113, 1983.

12. Messmer BJ, Hornchen H, Kosters C: Surgical separation of conjoined xiphopagus twins. Surgery 89:622, 1981.

13. Ramp JB, Baylor JR, Casamento VK, et al: Conjoined twins: A multidisciplinary approach. Neonatal Network 8:29, 1989.

14. Synhorst D, Matlak M, Roan Y, et al: Separation of conjoined thoracopagus twins joined at the right atria. Am J Cardiol 43:662, 1979.

15. Bloch EC, Karis JH: Cardiopagus in neonatal thoracopagus twins: Anesthetic management. Anesth Anal 59:304, 1980.

16. Micheli JL, Sadeghi J, Freeman C, et al: An attempt to separate xiphopagus twins sharing a common heart, liver, and duodenum. J Pediatr Surg 13:139, 1978.

17. Oberniedermayr A, Kriegel K, Westhues G: Der Munchner Siamesischen Zwillinge (zusammenfassender Bericht uber 2 Xiphopagen und 1 thorakopagen) Munch Med Wchnschr 25:1373, 1969.

18. O'Neill JA Jr, Holcomb GW 3rd, Schnaufer L, et al: Surgical experience with 13 conjoined twins. Ann Surg 208:299, 1988.

19. Root EH: Report of a case of composite monster: Monomphalic ischiopagus. JAMA 27:1238, 1896.

20. Lawson GW: Female pseudohermaphroditism in conjoined twin: Case report. Br J Obstet Gynaecol 87:1116, 1980.

21. Ornoy A, Navot D, Menashi M, et al: Asymmetry and discordance for congenital anomalies in conjoined twins: A report of six cases. Teratology 22:145, 1980.

22. Edmonds HW: Fetus omphalopagus parasiticus papyraceous, human: Report of a case with rare coincidental malformation of the autosite. Bull Int Assoc Med Mus 30:75, 1949.

23. Golladay ES, Williams GD, Seibert JJ, et al: Dicephalus dipus conjoined twins: A surgical separation and review of previously reported cases. J Pediatr Surg 17:259, 1982.

24. Spitz L, Stringer MD, Kiely EM, et al: Separation of brachio-thoraco-omphalo-ischiopagus bipus conjoined twins. J Pediatr Surg 29:477, 1994.

25. Chiu CT, Hou SH, Lai HS, et al: Separation of thoracopagus conjoined twins: A case report. J Cardiovasc Surg 35:459, 1994.

26. Cambio D: These twins survived separation. RN 57:54, 1994.

27. Gupta JM: Pygopagus conjoined twins. BMJ 2:868, 1966.

28. Gille P, Aubert D, Mourot M, et al: Separation de siamois pygopages. Chir Pediatr 24:100, 1983.

29. Votteler TP: Surgical separation of conjoined twins. AORN J 35:35, 1982.

30. O'Connell JEA: Craniopagus twins: Surgical anatomy and embryology and their implications. J Neurol Neurosurg Psychiatr 39:1, 1976.

31. Kapp JP, Schmidek HH: Surgery of the cerebral venous system. In Kapp JP, Schmidek HH (eds): Diseases of Cerebral Veins and Dural Sinuses. New York, Grune & Stratton, 1984, p 597.

32. Winston KR, Rockoff MA, Mulliken JB: Surgical division of craniopagi: Review article—57 references. Neurosurgery 21:782, 1987.

33. Roberts TS: Venous abnormalities in Siamese twins. In Kapp JP, Schmidek HH (eds): Diseases of Cerebral Veins and Dural Sinuses. New York, Grune & Stratton, 1984, p 355.

34. Betoulieres P, Caderas de Kerleau J: Etude radiologique du squelette d'un monstre double janicephale-rachipage. Montpellier Med J 58:30, 1960.

INDEX

■ ───

Note: Page numbers in *italics* refer to illustrations;
page numbers followed by the letter t refer to tables.

A,B,C,Ds, of malignant melanoma, 961
ABCDE mnemonic, definition of, 180–181
Abdomen, neuroblastoma in, 879. See
    also *Neuroblastoma.*
    surgical excision of, 883–885
    non-Hodgkin's lymphoma of, 934
    teratoma in, *915,* 915–917
    trauma to, 205–210
        assessment of, 187
        diagnosis of, 204–205
        diaphragmatic rupture in, 209–210
        duodenal injury in, 207, *208*
        hepatic injury in, 205–206, *206*
        hollow visceral injury in, 208–209,
            210
        pancreatic injury in, 207–208, *209*
        penetrating, 205
        retroperitoneal, 210
        splenic injury in, 206–207
Abdominal accessory lobe, in pulmonary
    sequestration, 282–283
Abdominal musculature deficiency (AMD)
    syndrome. See *Prune-belly syndrome.*
Abdominal wall, defects of, cesarean
    delivery of infant with, *642, 642*
    embryology of, 639–640, *639–640*
    epidemiology of, 640–641
    in gastroschisis, 642–645, *643–645*
    in omphalocele, 645–647, *645–647*
    prenatal screening for, *641,* 641–642
    Vanderbilt Children's Hospital experi-
        ence with, 647–648, 648t
    hernias of, 651–653. See also specific
        hernia, e.g., *Umbilical hernia.*
    in prune-belly syndrome, clinical corre-
        lates of, 789–790
        pathophysiology of, 789, *789*
Abdominoplasty, for prune-belly
    syndrome, 800–801, *801–803*
Abscess, anal, in Crohn's disease, 556,
    556
    breast, 1020
    cuff, as complication of surgery for
        Hirschsprung's disease, 465
    lung, 290–291, *291*
    pancreatic, 624–625
    pelvic, after appendectomy, 578, *578*
    perianal, 511
    perirectal, 511
    peritonsillar, 258
    retropharyngeal, 258
    soft tissue, 122
    splenic, 633
    tuboovarian, in peripubertal girl, 1006
Abuse, child, 226–227
        burn injury in, 159–160
        chronic subdural hematoma follow-
            ing, *224,* 227
        genital trauma in, 214–215, *1004,*
            1004–1005
Acalculous cholecystitis, 591

Accident(s), 188
    decannulation, as complication of extra-
        corporeal membrane oxygenation,
        102
    motor vehicle, prevention of, 188–189
ACE (angiotensin-converting enzyme)
    inhibitors, for renovascular
    hypertension, 824
Acetaminophen, postoperative pain relief
    with, 44
    after inguinal hernia repair, 660
N-Acetylcysteine irrigation, with
    enterotomy, for meconium ileus, 438
Achalasia, esophageal, 331–332, *332*
    surgical treatment for, 332
Achromicus nevus, 956
Acid(s), ingestion of, causing esophageal
        injury, 326
    causing gastric injury, 398
Acidosis, metabolic, as complication of
        total parenteral nutrition, 29
    in acute renal failure, 52
        management of, 55
    renal tubular, 50
        type IV, 50–51
Acquired immunodeficiency syndrome
    (AIDS). See *Human immuno-
    deficiency virus (HIV) infection.*
Actinomycin D, for Wilms' tumor, 859
    mechanism of action and toxicity of,
        838t
Actinomycosis, 295
Acupuncture, for burn patient, 166
Acute lymphoblastic leukemia, treatment
    of, B43-PAP immunotoxin in, 842
Acute relapsing pancreatitis, 622
Acute renal failure (ARF), in neonate,
        53–55
    clinical presentation of, 54
    diagnostic evaluation of, 54
    intrinsic, 53t, 53–54
    major causes of, 53t
    management of, 54–55
    postrenal, 53t, 54
    prerenal, 53, 53t
    postoperative, dialysis for, 52–53
        medical management of, 51–52, 52t
        pathophysiology of, 51
Acute splenic sequestration crisis (ASSC),
    634
Acute suppurative thyroiditis, 1027
Acyclovir, for infection, 120–121
Adenocarcinoma, of kidney, 870
    staging of, 870t
    of pancreas, 630
    of small intestine, associated with
        Crohn's disease, 554
Adenoma(s), aldosterone-secreting, 10–11
    hepatocellular, 892
Adenomatoid malformation, cystic,
    congenital. See *Congenital cystic
    adenomatoid malformation (CCAM).*

Adenomatous polyps, 562, 564
Adenosine diphosphate (ADP),
    endothelial inactivation of, 60
ADH (antidiuretic hormone), release of,
    circadian rhythm in, 727
Adhesion(s), platelet, 60–61
    postoperative, associated with appendi-
        citis, 578
Adhesive meconium peritonitis, 438, *439*
Adipose tissue, tumors of, 923
Adolescent(s), breast masses in, 1021t,
    1021–1022
    burns in, 159
ADP (adenosine diphosphate), endothelial
    inactivation of, 60
ADPKD (autosomal dominant polycystic
    kidney disease), 685–686
Adrenal glands, aldosterone-secreting
        adenoma of, 10–11
    anatomy of, 1032
    carcinoma of, 1033–1034
    congenital hyperplasia of, 11
    mass in, 1032–1033
        differential diagnosis of, 1033t
    pheochromocytoma of, 11
β₂-Adrenergic receptors, for hyperkalemia,
    52t
Adrenocortical carcinoma, 1033–1034
Advanced Trauma Life Support (ATLS)
        course, of American College of
        Surgeons, 179–181
Aerophagia, due to thoracic trauma, 191
Afibrinogenemia, 68
AFP. See *Alpha-fetoprotein (AFP).*
Aganglionosis, acquired, 456–457
    colonic, 453. See also *Hirschsprung's
        disease.*
    treatment of, 464
Age, gestational, as factor in extra-
        corporeal membrane oxygenation, 97
    malrotation related to, clinical presenta-
        tion of, 429t
    maternal, gastroschisis associated with,
        640
Agenesis, anorectal, without fistula, and
        imperforate anus, 475, 476
    repair of, 483
    pulmonary, bilateral, 284, *284*
        unilateral, 284
    renal, bilateral, 682
        unilateral, 681–682
Agglutination, of labial-vulvar tissue,
    1003–1004, *1004*
AIDS (acquired immunodeficiency
        syndrome). See *Human immuno-
        deficiency virus (HIV) infection.*
Air embolism, as complication of
        extracorporeal membrane
        oxygenation, 102–103
Airway(s), assessment and management
        of, in trauma patient, *182,* 182–183,
        193

ISBN 0-7216-7312-0

90038

9 780721 673127